ABRAMS'
Clinical Drug Therapy

Rationales for Nursing Practice

13th Edition

ABRAMS'
Clinical Drug Therapy

Rationales for Nursing Practice

Geralyn Frandsen, EdD, RN
Professor Emeritus
Maryville University
St. Louis, Missouri

Sandra Smith Pennington, PhD, RN
Administrator Emeritus
Rocky Mountain University of Health Professions
Provo, Utah
Professor Emeritus
Berea College
Berea, Kentucky

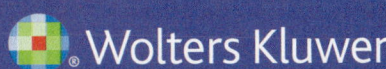 Wolters Kluwer

Philadelphia • Baltimore • New York • London
Buenos Aires • Hong Kong • Sydney • Tokyo

Not authorised for sale in United States, Canada, Australia, New Zealand, Puerto Rico, and U.S. Virgin Islands

Vice President and Publisher: Julie K. Stegman
Director, Nursing Education and Practice Content: Jamie Blum
Acquisitions Editor: Susan Hartman
Development Editors: Rose Foltz and Chelsea Neve
Editorial Coordinator: Sean Hanrahan
Editorial Assistant: Devika Kishore
Marketing Manager: Sarah Schuessler
Production Project Manager: Matthew West
Manager, Graphic Arts & Design: Stephen Druding
Art Director, Illustration: Jennifer Clements
Manufacturing Coordinator: Margie Orzech
Prepress Vendor: Straive

Thirteenth edition

Copyright © 2025 Wolters Kluwer

Copyright © 2021 Wolters Kluwer Copyright © 2018 Wolters Kluwer; Copyright © 2014, 2009 Wolters Kluwer Health | Lippincott Williams & Wilkins. Copyright © 2007, 2004, 2001 by Lippincott Williams & Wilkins. Copyright © 1998 by Lippincott-Raven Publishers. Copyright © 1995, 1991, 1987, 1983 by J. B. Lippincott Company. All rights reserved. This book is protected by copyright. No part of this book may be reproduced or transmitted in any form or by any means, including as photocopies or scanned-in or other electronic copies, or utilized by any information storage and retrieval system without written permission from the copyright owner, except for brief quotations embodied in critical articles and reviews. Materials appearing in this book prepared by individuals as part of their official duties as U.S. government employees are not covered by the above-mentioned copyright. To request permission, please contact Wolters Kluwer at Two Commerce Square, 2001 Market Street, Philadelphia, PA 19103, via email at permissions@lww.com, or via our website at shop.lww.com (products and services).

9 8 7 6 5 4 3 2 1

Printed in Mexico

Library of Congress Cataloging-in-Publication Data

ISBN: 978-1-9752-2232-1

This work is provided "as is," and the publisher disclaims any and all warranties, express or implied, including any warranties as to accuracy, comprehensiveness, or currency of the content of this work.

This work is no substitute for individual patient assessment based upon healthcare professionals' examination of each patient and consideration of, among other things, age, weight, gender, current or prior medical conditions, medication history, laboratory data and other factors unique to the patient. The publisher does not provide medical advice or guidance and this work is merely a reference tool. Healthcare professionals, and not the publisher, are solely responsible for the use of this work including all medical judgments and for any resulting diagnosis and treatments.

Given continuous, rapid advances in medical science and health information, independent professional verification of medical diagnoses, indications, appropriate pharmaceutical selections and dosages, and treatment options should be made and healthcare professionals should consult a variety of sources. When prescribing medication, healthcare professionals are advised to consult the product information sheet (the manufacturer's package insert) accompanying each drug to verify, among other things, conditions of use, warnings and side effects and identify any changes in dosage schedule or contraindications, particularly if the medication to be administered is new, infrequently used or has a narrow therapeutic range. To the maximum extent permitted under applicable law, no responsibility is assumed by the publisher for any injury and/or damage to persons or property, as a matter of products liability, negligence law or otherwise, or from any reference to or use by any person of this work.

shop.lww.com

I dedicate this edition to my family, my husband Gary, our daughter Claire, son-in-law John, son Joseph, daughter-in-law Allyson, and grandson Elliott.

Geralyn Frandsen

To my family, my daughter Jennifer, and granddaughter Liliana, my constant source of strength, inspiration, hope, and gratitude.

Sandra Smith Pennington

Contributors

CONTRIBUTORS TO THE 13TH EDITION

Lisa Albers, MSN, RN
Clinical Assistant Professor of Nursing
Catherine McAuley School of Nursing
Maryville University
St. Louis, Missouri
  Chapter 4: Pharmacology and the Care of Infants and Pediatric Patients

Jennifer Binggeli, PharmD, MBA, BCPS
Director of Remote Order Entry Operations
Largo, Florida
  Chapter 19: Drug Therapy With Aminoglycosides and Fluoroquinolones
  Chapter 20: Drug Therapy With Tetracyclines, Sulfonamides, and Urinary Antiseptics
  Chapter 21: Drug Therapy With Macrolides and Miscellaneous Anti-Infective Agents
  Chapter 31: Drug Therapy for Nasal Congestion and Cough
  Chapter 32: Drug Therapy to Decrease Histamine Effects and Allergic Response
  Chapter 33: Drug Therapy for Asthma, Airway Inflammation, and Bronchoconstriction

Vicki C. Callan, PhD, CRNA, CHSE
Associate Professor
Department of Nurse Anesthesia
Webster University
St. Louis, Missouri
  Chapter 50: Drug Therapy With Local Anesthetics
  Chapter 51: Drug Therapy With General Anesthetics

Ryan D. Dunn, PharmD
Division Infection Disease Pharmacist
Director of Pharmacy
HCA Florida Pasadena Hospital
St. Petersburg, Florida
  Chapter 18: Drug Therapy With Beta-Lactam Antibacterial Agents
  Chapter 24: Drug Therapy for Fungal Infections

Gary M. Frandsen, JD, MSN, RN
Associate Teaching Professor (Retired)
College of Nursing
University of Missouri–St. Louis
St. Louis, Missouri
  Chapter 22: Drug Therapy for Tuberculosis and *Mycobacterium avium* Complex Disease
  Chapter 35: Nutritional Support Products, Vitamins, and Mineral Supplements
  Chapter 44: Drug Therapy to Regulate Calcium and Bone Metabolism

Elizabeth Stuesse, MSN, RNC-OB, RNC-MNN, C-EFM, CLC, CCE, CHBE
Clinical Assistant Professor
Catherine McAuley School of Nursing
Maryville University
Women & Children Educator RN
Women's Education
Mercy Hospital
St. Louis, Missouri
  Chapter 6: Pharmacology and the Care of Pregnant or Lactating Females

Jennifer L. Taylor, PhD, RN, CNE
Associate Professor of Nursing
Catherine McAuley School of Nursing
Maryville University
St. Lois, Missouri
  Chapter 26: Drug Therapy for Hypertension
  Chapter 27: Drug Therapy for Dysrhythmias
  Chapter 30: Drug Therapy for Heart Failure

Dana Todd, PhD, APRN
Professor
BSN Program Director
Murray State University
Murray, Kentucky
  Chapter 7: Pharmacology and Female Health

CONTRIBUTORS TO THE 12TH EDITION

Lisa Albers, MSN, RN
Clinical Assistant Professor of Nursing
Catherine McAuley School of Nursing
Maryville University
Staff Nurse
SSM Health Cardinal Glennon Children's Hospital
St. Louis, Missouri
  Chapter 4: Pharmacology and the Care of Infants and Pediatric Patients

Vicki C. Coopmans, PhD, CRNA, CHSE
Associate Professor
Director of Clinical Education
Department of Nurse Anesthesia
Webster University
St. Louis, Missouri
  Chapter 50: Drug Therapy With Local Anesthetics
  Chapter 51: Drug Therapy With General Anesthetics

Ryan D. Dunn, PharmD
Division Infection Disease Pharmacist
HCA–West Florida Division
Largo, Florida
  Chapter 18: Drug Therapy With Beta-Lactam Antibacterial Agents
  Chapter 24: Drug Therapy for Fungal Infections

Gary M. Frandsen, JD, MSN, RN
Associate Teaching Professor
College of Nursing
University of Missouri–St. Louis
St. Louis, Missouri
   Chapter 22: Drug Therapy for Tuberculosis and *Mycobacterium avium* Complex Disease
   Chapter 35: Nutritional Support Products, Vitamins, and Mineral Supplements
   Chapter 44: Drug Therapy to Regulate Calcium and Bone Metabolism

Jennifer B. Miles, PharmD, MBA
Vice President of Pharmacy Services
HCA West Florida Division
HealthTrust
Largo, Florida
   Chapter 19: Drug Therapy With Aminoglycosides and Fluoroquinolones
   Chapter 20: Drug Therapy With Tetracyclines, Sulfonamides, and Urinary Antiseptics
   Chapter 21: Drug Therapy With Macrolides and Miscellaneous Anti-Infective Agents
   Chapter 31: Drug Therapy for Nasal Congestion and Cough
   Chapter 32: Drug Therapy to Decrease Histamine Effects and Allergic Response
   Chapter 33: Drug Therapy for Asthma, Airway Inflammation, and Bronchoconstriction

Vicki Moran, PhD, RN, MPH, CNE, CDE, PHNA-BC, TNS
Assistant Professor
Trudy Busch Valentine School of Nursing
Saint Louis University
St. Louis, Missouri
   Chapter 41: Drug Therapy for Diabetes Mellitus
   Chapter 42: Drug Therapy for Hyperthyroidism and Hypothyroidism

Sharon Souter, RN, PhD, CNE
Professor and Adjunct Faculty Member
University of Mary Hardin–Baylor
Belton, Texas
   Chapter 37: Drug Therapy for Peptic Ulcer Disease and Hyperacidity
   Chapter 52: Drug Therapy for Migraines and Other Headaches
   Chapter 54: Drug Therapy for Anxiety and Insomnia
   Chapter 57: Drug Therapy for Attention Deficit Hyperactivity Disorder and Narcolepsy

Elizabeth Stuesse, MSN, RNC-OB, RNC-MNN, C-EFM, CLC, CCE, CHBE
Clinical Assistant Professor
Catherine McAuley School of Nursing
Maryville University
Women & Children Educator RN
Women's Education
Mercy Hospital
St. Louis, Missouri
   Chapter 6: Pharmacology and the Care of Pregnant or Lactating Females

Jennifer L. Taylor, PhD, RN, CNE
Assistant Professor of Nursing
BSN Coordinator
Catherine McAuley School of Nursing
Maryville University
St. Lois, Missouri
   Chapter 26: Drug Therapy for Hypertension
   Chapter 27: Drug Therapy for Dysrhythmias
   Chapter 30: Drug Therapy for Heart Failure

Dana Todd, PhD, APRN
Professor
School of Nursing and Health Professions
Murray State University
Murray, Kentucky
   Chapter 7: Pharmacology and Female Health

Gladdi Tomlinson, RN, MSN
Professor of Nursing
Harrisburg Area Community College
Harrisburg, Pennsylvania
   Chapter 47: Drug Therapy for Myasthenia Gravis, Alzheimer Disease, and Other Conditions Treated With Cholinergic Agents
   Chapter 48: Drug Therapy for Parkinson Disease, Urinary Spasticity, and Disorders Requiring Anticholinergic Drug Therapy

Reviewers

Arlana Arsenault, RN
Instructor
Nursing School of Health and Natural Sciences
Fitchburg State University
Fitchburg, Massachusetts

Susan Beck, PhD, CNS, RN
Assistant Professor of Nursing
Bloomsburg University
Bloomsburg, Pennsylvania

Lynette DebellisMA, RN
Chair and Instructor
School of Nursing
Mount Saint Mary College
Newburgh, New York

Morgan L. Dutler, MSN
Faculty, Pharmacology
Purdue University Global
Des Moines, Iowa

Mary Francis, PhD Candidate, ACNP-BC
Assistant Professor, Nursing
Widener University
Chester, Pennsylvania

Jennifer Milligan, MS, RN, CCRN
Associate Clinical Professor, Nursing
Texas Woman's University
Denton, Texas

Katie Pawloski, MSN
Professor of Practice, Nursing
Utica University
Utica, New York

Sallyann Storer, DNP, CRNP
Clinical Assistant Professor
College of Nursing
University of Alabama in Huntsville
Huntsville, Alabama

Elizabeth Ann VandeWaa, PhD
Professor, Adult Health Nursing
University of South Alabama
Mobile, Alabama

Timothy J. Voytilla
Program Director
Associate of Science in Nursing
Keiser University
Gibsonton, Florida

Preface

Abrams' Clinical Drug Therapy: Rationales for Nursing Practice has a long tradition of guiding students and instructors through the practice of safe and effective medication administration. The 13th edition includes a Clinical Judgment case study for each section to assist in preparing you for the Next Generation NCLEX Examination. Quality and Safety Alerts for patient-centered care, patient safety, and evidence-based practice have been included in each chapter. To allow a quick review, significant information on the etiology and pathophysiology of disease has been placed on thePoint®. Drug therapy pertinent to the prevention and treatment of disease is provided in each chapter.

GOALS AND RESPONSIBILITIES OF NURSING CARE RELATED TO DRUG THERAPY

Varied goals and responsibilities inherent in safe medication administration are identified in each chapter. The following information will guide you in developing your own goals and responsibilities inherent to safe and effective nursing practice.

- Preventing the need for drug therapy, when possible, by promoting health and preventing conditions that require drug therapy.
- Using nonpharmacologic interventions alone or in conjunction with drug therapy. When used with drugs, such interventions may promote lower drug dosage, less frequent administration, and fewer adverse effects.
- Administering drugs accurately and taking into consideration patient characteristics such as age, weight, and hepatic and kidney function, which can influence drug response.
- Preventing or minimizing adverse effects by knowing the major adverse effects associated with particular drugs. It is important to assess patients with impaired hepatic and kidney function closely for adverse effects. The early recognition of adverse effects allows for the implementation of interventions to minimize their severity. All drugs cause adverse effects, and nurses must maintain a high index of suspicion that the development of new signs and symptoms may be drug induced.
- Understanding the effect produced if medications are combined with other medications, herbs, or foods.
- Teaching patients and families about the effects of medications. The nurse must instruct patients and families about the role and importance of their medications in treating particular illnesses, accurate administration of medications, nonpharmacologic treatments to use with or instead of pharmacologic treatments, and when to contact their healthcare provider.

ORGANIZATIONAL FRAMEWORK

The 10 sections of the textbook provide the reader with basic information about drug therapy as well as the administration of medications for the prevention and treatment of disease. The first section introduces the safeguards in place to promote drug safety, the Institute of Medicine Core Competencies, and medication administration. It also describes the nursing process and explains the application of the nursing process in the care of patients receiving drug therapy. The use of concept maps addresses priority considerations and nursing actions related to drug therapy. The second section addresses the effect medications have throughout the lifespan. The text introduces the effects of drugs on infants, children, older adults, pregnant and lactating patients, and drugs affecting male and female health. The remaining sections provide information on drug therapy related to systems, infections, and disease processes.

Each chapter opens with a case study, and its use throughout the chapter helps readers integrate information about a particular disease and its drug therapy so they can apply it. The chapters also have NCLEX-style questions distributed throughout to test knowledge of the content and its application to patient care. This approach will help the reader prepare for class examinations as well as the NCLEX itself.

At the end of each section, a clinical judgment case study is presented. The clinical reasoning case studies are on thePoint® to increase your knowledge of patient care and related drug therapy.

The chapters that focus on drug treatment for specific diseases use the prototype approach, allowing the reader to see the similarity in medications within each broad drug classification. Introduction and Overview sections provide the basis for understanding the drug therapy that prevents or treats the disease. Drug therapy sections summarize the medications, identifying the pharmacokinetics, action, use, adverse effects, contraindications, and nursing implications—including administration, assessment, and patient teaching. Many chapters address the effect of herbal supplements on prescribed medications. This information has become crucial for the maintenance of patient safety. Boxes containing patient teaching guidelines for a drug or class of drugs highlight crucial information the nurse should teach the patient and family.

RECURRING FEATURES

This updated edition includes new and revised features to enhance learning.

Chapter-Opening Features

- **Learning Objectives** summarize what the student should learn while reading the chapter and answering both the Clinical Application Case Study Questions and NCLEX Success questions, described below.
- A **Clinical Application Case Study** opens each chapter with a patient-focused clinical scenario. Throughout the chapter, the reader is asked **critical thinking questions** to apply chapter content, emphasizing a patient-centered and interdisciplinary approach to pharmacology.
- **Key Terms** with definitions help the reader understand the chapter's content.

Special Features

- **Quality and Safety Alerts**, presented in the context of the chapter discussion, alert the reader to important considerations regarding patient safety, patient-centered care, and evidence-based practice that are pertinent to drug therapy. These considerations emphasize safety as a primary objective in patient care.
- **Boxed Warnings** highlight serious or life-threatening adverse effects identified by the FDA as being associated with a drug.
- **Drugs at a Glance Tables**—which include **Canadian drug names**—summarize the routes and dosage ranges (for adults and for children) for each drug in the class. The prototype drug is indicated with an icon.
- **Drug Interactions** boxes highlight the risk of interactions as well as increased or decreased drug effects when drugs are combined with other medications.
- **Specific herbal and dietary interactions** with medications are included in the chapter sections that discuss preventing drug interactions.
- **Patient Teaching Guidelines** list specific information for the education of the patient and family.
- **NCLEX Success** sections interspersed throughout the chapter ask the student to answer NCLEX-style questions that pertain to the learning objectives and the information just presented. This feature helps students check and apply their knowledge as they read and assists them to prepare for patient care and for the NCLEX. The questions align to the terminology used on the NCLEX. The NCLEX Success questions exclusively use generic names for medications, which is consistent with the RN licensure examination.
- **Nursing Process Concept Maps** provide a succinct overview of drug therapy in terms of assessment, planning/goals, nursing interventions, and evaluation. Located at the end of each chapter, the nursing process concept maps provide the guidelines for drug therapy specifically related to nursing care. (Nursing diagnoses do not appear in these concept maps because nursing diagnoses are not tested on the NCLEX.)
- **Unfolding Patient Stories**, written by the National League for Nursing, are an engaging way to begin meaningful conversations in the classroom. These vignettes, which appear in relevant chapters, feature patients from Wolters Kluwer's *vSim for Nursing | Pharmacology* (codeveloped with Laerdal Medical) and DocuCare products; however, each Unfolding Patient Story in the book stands alone, not requiring purchase of these products.
- **Concept Mastery Alerts** clarify common misconceptions as identified by Lippincott's Adaptive Learning Powered by PrepU.

Chapter-Ending Features

- **References and Resources** provide sources on which content is based and direction for further reading.

Content on thePoint

- **Etiology and Pathophysiology** information for select diseases is available on thePoint. This allows students to make connections between the etiology and pathophysiology and pharmacologic management of a disease.
- **Clinical Reasoning Case Studies** focus on the action of the medication prescribed and the associated assessment of medication outcomes. These case studies are found on thePoint.
- **Key Concepts** available on thePoint summarize the most salient content that appears in each chapter.

A COMPREHENSIVE PACKAGE FOR TEACHING AND LEARNING

To further facilitate teaching and learning, a carefully designed ancillary package has been developed to assist faculty and students.

Resources for Instructors

Tools to assist with teaching this text are available upon its adoption on thePoint at http://thePoint.lww.com/Frandsen13e.

- The **Test Generator** lets you put together exclusive new tests from a bank containing more than 1,000 questions to help assess students' understanding of the material. Test questions are mapped to chapter learning objectives and page numbers.
- An extensive collection of materials is provided for each book chapter:
  - **PowerPoint Presentations** provide an easy way for you to integrate the textbook with your students' classroom experience, either via slide shows or handouts. Multiple-choice and true/false questions are integrated into the presentations to promote class participation and allow you to use i-clicker technology.
  - **Guided Lecture Notes** walk you through the chapters, objective by objective, and provide you with corresponding PowerPoint slide numbers.
  - **Discussion Topics** (and suggested answers) can be used as conversation starters or in online discussion boards.
  - **Assignments** (and suggested answers) include group, written, clinical, and Web assignments.
  - **Case Studies** with related questions (and suggested answers) give students an opportunity to apply their knowledge to a patient case similar to one they might encounter in practice.
  - **Learning Objectives** from the book.
- An **Image Bank** lets you use the photographs and illustrations from this textbook in your PowerPoint slides or as you see fit in your course.

Contact your sales representative or check out LWW.com/Nursing for more details and ordering information.

Resources for Students

An exciting set of free resources is available to help students review material and become even more familiar with vital concepts. Students can access all these resources on thePoint at http://thePoint.lww.com/Frandsen13e, using the codes printed in the front of their textbooks.

- **Concepts in Action Animations** bring physiologic and pathophysiologic concepts to life and enhance student comprehension.

- **Watch & Learn Video Clips** demonstrate nursing skills and appeal to visual and auditory learners.
- The following **online appendices**:
  - Appendix A: Answers for NCLEX Success
  - Appendix B: Answers for the Clinical Application Case Studies
  - Appendix C: Critical Thinking Questions and Answers
  - Appendix D: The International System of Units
  - Appendix E: Serum Drug Concentrations
- **Journal Articles** for each book chapter offer access to current research available in Wolters Kluwer journals.
- Plus **Etiology and Pathophysiology information for select diseases, Clinical Reasoning Case Studies, Key Concepts,** and **Heart and Breath Sounds**.

VSIM FOR NURSING

vSim for Nursing, jointly developed by Laerdal Medical and Wolters Kluwer Health, offers innovative scenario-based learning modules consisting of web-based virtual simulations, course learning materials, and curriculum tools designed to develop critical thinking skills and promote clinical confidence and competence. vSim for Nursing | Pharmacology includes 10 cases from the Simulation in Nursing Education—Pharmacology Scenarios. Students can progress through suggested readings, pre- and postsimulation assessments, documentation assignments, and guided reflection questions, and will receive an individualized feedback log immediately upon completion of the simulation. Throughout the student learning experience, the product offers remediation back to trusted Lippincott resources, including Lippincott Nursing Advisor and Lippincott Nursing Procedures—two online, evidence-based, clinical information solutions used in healthcare facilities throughout the United States. This innovative product provides a comprehensive patient-focused solution for learning and integrating simulation into the classroom.

Contact your Wolters Kluwer sales representative or visit http://thepoint.lww.com/vsim for options to enhance your pharmacology nursing course with vSim for Nursing.

LIPPINCOTT DOCUCARE

Lippincott DocuCare combines web-based academic electronic health record (EHR) simulation software with clinical case scenarios, allowing students to learn how to use an EHR in a safe, true-to-life setting, while enabling instructors to measure their progress. Lippincott DocuCare's nonlinear solution works well in the classroom, simulation lab, and clinical practice.

Contact your Wolters Kluwer sales representative or visit http://thepoint.lww.com/DocuCare for options to enhance your pharmacology nursing course with DocuCare.

A COMPREHENSIVE, DIGITAL, INTEGRATED COURSE SOLUTION: LIPPINCOTT® COURSEPOINT+

The same trusted solution, innovation, and unmatched support that you have come to expect from *Lippincott CoursePoint+* is now enhanced with more engaging learning tools and deeper analytics to help prepare students for practice. This powerfully integrated digital learning solution combines learning tools, case studies, virtual simulation, real-time data, and the most trusted nursing education content on the market to make curriculum-wide learning more efficient and to meet students where they are at in their learning. And now, it is easier than ever for instructors and students to use, giving them everything they need for course and curriculum success!

Lippincott CoursePoint+ includes the following:

- Engaging course content provides a variety of learning tools to engage students of all learning styles.
- A more personalized learning approach, including adaptive learning powered by PrepU, gives students the content and tools they need at the moment they need it, giving them data for more focused remediation and helping to boost their confidence.
- Varying levels of case studies, virtual simulation, and access to Lippincott Advisor help students learn the critical thinking and clinical judgment skills to help them become practice-ready nurses.
- Unparalleled reporting provides in-depth dashboards with several data points to track student progress and help identify strengths and weaknesses.
- Unmatched support includes training coaches, product trainers, and nursing education consultants to help educators and students implement CoursePoint+ with ease.

Acknowledgments

The expertise of our contributors and reviewers is a great example of how the power of collaboration improves outcomes, and we thank them. We also wish to thank the team at Wolters Kluwer who provided their expertise to this edition.

Contents

SECTION 1
THE CONCEPTUAL FRAMEWORK OF PHARMACOLOGY   1

1 The Foundation of Pharmacology: Quality and Safety   3
  Introduction   4
  Drug Sources   4
  Drug Classifications and Prototypes   4
  Drug Names   4
  Drug Marketing   5
  Pharmacoeconomics   5
  Pharmacogenomics   5
  Access to Drugs   5
  Drug Approval Processes: Food and Drug Administration   8
  Safety in Drug Administration   9
  Sources of Drug Information   12
  Strategies for Studying Pharmacology   13

2 Basic Concepts and Processes   14
  Introduction   15
  Drug Transport Through Cell Membranes   16
  Pharmacokinetics   16
  Pharmacodynamics   19
  Variables That Affect Drug Actions   21
  Adverse Effects of Drugs   25
  Toxicology: Drug Overdose   27

3 Medication Administration and the Nursing Process of Drug Therapy   32
  Introduction   33
  General Principles of Accurate Drug Administration   33
  Legal Responsibilities   34
  Medication Errors and Their Prevention   34
  Medication Orders   40
  Drug Preparations and Dosage Forms   41
  Calculating Drug Dosages   43
  Routes of Administration   45
  Nursing Process in Drug Therapy   50
  Integrating Evidence-Based Practice with the Nursing Process   58
  Herbal and Dietary Supplements   58
  Clinical Judgment in Practice   63

SECTION 2
DRUG THERAPY THROUGHOUT THE LIFESPAN   65

4 Pharmacology and the Care of Infants and Pediatric Patients   67
  Introduction   68
  Drug Safety in Pediatrics   68
  Pharmacotherapy in Pediatrics   68
  Medication Administration in Pediatrics   71

5 Pharmacology and the Care of Adults and Geriatric Patients   75
  Introduction   76
  Pharmacodynamics in Older Adults   76
  Pharmacokinetics in Older Adults   78
  Pharmacologic Care of Infections in Older Adults   79
  Medication Adherence and Aging   80

6 Pharmacology and the Care of Pregnant or Lactating Females   83
  Introduction   84
  Drug Therapy for Infertility   84
  Drugs Used in Pregnancy   86
  Fetal Therapeutics   89
  Maternal Therapeutics   89
  Drugs that Alter Uterine Motility: Tocolytics   92
  Drugs Used During Labor and Delivery at Term   93
  Lactation   95

7 Pharmacology and Female Health   99
  Introduction   100
  Overview of the Effects of Estrogens and Progestins   100
  Common Female Reproductive Health Conditions   100
  Estrogens   101
  Progestins   106
  Estrogen–Progestin Combinations   109

8 Pharmacology and Male Health   117
  Introduction   118
  Overview of Reproductive Health Problems in Males   118
  Androgens and Anabolic Steroids   119
  Phosphodiesterase Type 5 Inhibitors   123
  Adjuvant Medications Used to Treat Erectile Dysfunction   125
  5-Alpha Reductase Inhibitors   126
  Alpha$_1$-Adrenergic Blockers   128
  Clinical Judgment in Practice   132

SECTION 3
DRUGS AFFECTING THE HEMATOPOIETIC AND IMMUNE SYSTEMS   135

9 Drug Therapy for Coagulation Disorders   137
  Introduction   138
  Overview of Coagulation Disorders   138
  Anticoagulant Drugs   139
  Antiplatelet Drugs   150
  Thrombolytic Drugs   155
  Drugs Used to Control Bleeding   157

10 Drug Therapy for Dyslipidemia   161
  Introduction   162
  Overview of Dyslipidemia   162
  HMG-CoA Reductase Inhibitors   164
  Bile Acid Sequestrants   168

Fibrates 170
Cholesterol Absorption Inhibitor 171
PCSK9 Inhibitors 173
Miscellaneous Dyslipidemic Agent 174
Combination Therapy Used to Treat Dyslipidemia 174

11 Drug Therapy for Hematopoietic Disorders 178

Introduction 179
Overview of Hematopoiesis and Immune Function 179
Erythropoiesis-Stimulating Agents 180
Granulocyte Colony-Stimulating Factors 184
Interferons 186
Adjuvant Medications Used to Stimulate the Immune System: Interleukins 188

12 Drug Therapy: Immunizations 192

Introduction 193
Overview of Immunization 193
Individual Immunizing Agents 193
Keeping Up-to-Date with Immunization Recommendations 205

13 Drug Therapy to Decrease Immunity 208

Introduction 209
Overview of Altered Immune Function 209
Cytotoxic Immunosuppressive Agents 212
Conventional Antirejection Agents 216
Janus Kinase Inhibitor 219
Adjuvant Medications Used to Suppress Immune Function 221

14 Drug Therapy for the Treatment of Cancer 231

Introduction 232
Overview of Cancer 232
Cytotoxic Antineoplastic Drugs Used to Treat Cancer 234
Adjuvant Medications Used to Treat Cancer 252
Clinical Judgment in Practice 267

SECTION 4
DRUGS AFFECTING INFLAMMATION AND INFECTION 269

15 Inflammation, Infection, and the Use of Antimicrobial Agents 271

Introduction 272
Overview of Inflammation 272
Overview of Microorganisms 273

16 Drug Therapy to Decrease Pain, Fever, and Inflammation 285

Introduction 286
Overview of Pain, Fever, and Inflammation 288
Overview of Disorders that Produce Inflammation 288
Salicylates 291
Nonnarcotic Analgesic Antipyretic: Acetaminophen 294

Nonsteroidal Anti-Inflammatory Drugs 297
Propionic Acid Derivatives 297
Oxicam Derivatives 300
Acetic Acid Derivatives 302
Selective COX-2 Inhibitor: Celecoxib 305
Antigout Medication: the Mitotic Agent Colchicine 306
Uricosuric Agents 308

17 Drug Therapy With Corticosteroids 313

Introduction 314
Physiology of Endogenous Corticosteroids 314
Overview of Adrenal Cortex Disorders 315
Drug Therapy With Exogenous Corticosteroids 317

18 Drug Therapy With Beta-Lactam Antibacterial Agents 334

Introduction 335
Penicillins 336
Cephalosporins 340
Carbapenems 347

19 Drug Therapy With Aminoglycosides and Fluoroquinolones 352

Introduction 353
Aminoglycosides 353
Fluoroquinolones 357

20 Drug Therapy With Tetracyclines, Sulfonamides, and Urinary Antiseptics 364

Introduction 365
Tetracyclines 365
Sulfonamides 369
Adjuvant Medications Used to Treat Urinary Tract Infections: Urinary Antiseptics 372

21 Drug Therapy With Macrolides and Miscellaneous Anti-Infective Agents 376

Introduction 377
Macrolides 377
Miscellaneous Anti-Infective Agents 381

22 Drug Therapy for Tuberculosis and *Mycobacterium avium* Complex Disease 388

Introduction 389
Overview Of Tuberculosis and *Mycobacterium avium* Complex Disease 389
Isoniazid 392
Rifamycins 396
Adjuvant First-Line Antitubercular Drugs 399
First-Line Drug Combinations Used to Treat Tuberculosis 400
Second-Line Drugs Used to Treat Tuberculosis 400
Drugs Used to Treat *Mycobacterium avium* Complex Disease 400
Special Strategies to Increase Adherence to Antitubercular Drug Regimens 401

23 Drug Therapy for Viral Infections 404

Introduction 405
Overview of Viruses and Viral Infections 405
Drugs for COVID-19 410
Drugs for Herpesvirus Infections 415
Drugs for Respiratory Syncytial Virus 419
Monoclonal Antibody for Respiratory Syncytial Virus 421

Drugs for Influenza 422
Drugs for Hepatitis B: Nucleoside Analogs 425
Drugs for Hepatitis C 426
Drugs for Human Immunodeficiency Virus (Antiretroviral Drugs) 428
Cytochrome P450 Inhibitor 438
Combination Medication for HIV-1: Integrase Inhibitor, Reverse Transcriptase Inhibitor, Nucleoside, Reverse Transcriptase Inhibitor, Nucleotide 441

24 Drug Therapy for Fungal Infections 444
Introduction 445
Overview of Fungal Infections 445
Polyenes 446
Azoles 450
Echinocandins 454
Pyrimidine Analog 456
Miscellaneous Antifungal Agents for Superficial Mycoses 457

25 Drug Therapy for Parasitic Infections 462
Introduction 463
Overview of Parasitic Infections 463
Amebicides 463
Antimalarials 465
Anthelmintics 469
Scabicides and Pediculicides 471
Clinical Judgment in Practice 474

SECTION 5
DRUGS AFFECTING THE CARDIOVASCULAR SYSTEM 475

26 Drug Therapy for Hypertension 477
Introduction 478
Overview of Hypertension 478
Angiotensin-Converting Enzyme Inhibitors 484
Angiotensin II Receptor Blockers 488
Calcium Channel Blockers 491
Additional Medications Used to Treat Hypertension 494

27 Drug Therapy for Dysrhythmias 503
Introduction 504
Overview of Dysrhythmias 504
Class I Sodium Channel Blockers 506
Class IA 506
Class IB 510
Class IC 510
Class II Beta-Adrenergic Blockers 511
Class III Potassium Channel Blockers 513
Class IV Calcium Channel Blockers 516
Unclassified Antidysrhythmic Drugs 517
Drug Therapy in Emergency Resuscitation of Adults 518
Magnesium Sulfate 519

28 Drug Therapy for Coronary Heart Disease 521
Introduction 522
Overview of Coronary Artery Disease 522
Organic Nitrates 524
Beta-Adrenergic Blockers 529
Calcium Channel Blockers 531
Adjuvant Medications 534

29 Drug Therapy for Shock and Hypotension 539
Introduction 540
Overview of Acute Hypotension and Shock 540
Management of Hypotension and Shock 541
Adrenergic Drugs 541

30 Drug Therapy for Heart Failure 550
Introduction 551
Overview of Heart Failure 551
Drugs that Inhibit the Renin–Angiotensin System 555
Angiotensin Receptor–Neprilysin Inhibitors (ARNi) 555
Phosphodiesterase Inhibitors (Cardiotonic–Inotropic Agents) 557
Sinoatrial Node Modulators 559
Adjuvant Medications Used to Treat Heart Failure 560
Clinical Judgment in Practice 568

SECTION 6
DRUGS AFFECTING THE RESPIRATORY SYSTEM 571

31 Drug Therapy for Nasal Congestion and Cough 573
Introduction 574
Overview of Nasal Congestion and Other Respiratory Symptoms 574
Nasal Decongestants 575
Antitussives 578
Expectorants 580
Mucolytics 581
Herbal Remedies and Other Preparations 582
Combination Products 582

32 Drug Therapy to Decrease Histamine Effects and Allergic Response 586
Introduction 587
Overview of Hypersensitivity (Allergic) Reactions 587
First-Generation H_1 Receptor Antagonists 590
Second-Generation H_1 Receptor Antagonists 594
Third-Generation H_1 Receptor Antagonists 596

33 Drug Therapy for Asthma, Airway Inflammation, and Bronchoconstriction 601
Introduction 602
Overview of Asthma 602
Adrenergics 606
Anticholinergics 610
Xanthines 612
Corticosteroids 614
Leukotriene Modifiers 617
Immunosuppressant Monoclonal Antibodies 619
Adjuvant Medications Used to Treat Asthma 620
Clinical Judgment in Practice 624

SECTION 7
DRUGS AFFECTING THE KIDNEY AND DIGESTIVE SYSTEMS 627

34 Drug Therapy for Fluid Volume Excess 629
Introduction 630
Overview of Conditions Requiring Diuretic Agents 630
Loop Diuretics 631
Thiazide Diuretics 635
Potassium-Sparing Diuretics 637
Adjuvant Medications Used to Treat Fluid Volume Excess 640

35 Nutritional Support Products, Vitamins, and Mineral Supplements 644
Introduction 645
Overview of Altered Nutritional States 645
Fat-Soluble Vitamins 654
Water-Soluble Vitamins 658
Minerals 662
Nutritional Products 668

36 Drug Therapy for Weight Management 673
Introduction 674
Overview of Weight Management 674
Noradrenergic Sympathomimetic Anorexiants 679
Lipase Inhibitors 681
Glucagonlike Peptide-1 Receptor Agonists 683
Other Drugs Used for Weight Management 685
Herbal and Dietary Supplements Used for Weight Management 685

37 Drug Therapy for Peptic Ulcer Disease and Hyperacidity 689
Introduction 690
Overview of Peptic Ulcer Disease and GERD 690
Antacids 691
Histamine$_2$ Receptor Antagonists 693
Proton Pump Inhibitors 698
Adjuvant Medications Used to Treat PUD and GERD 701

38 Drug Therapy for Nausea and Vomiting 706
Introduction 707
Overview of Nausea and Vomiting 707
Phenothiazines 707
Antihistamines 710
5-Hydroxytryptamine$_3$ (5-HT$_3$) or Serotonin Receptor Antagonists 712
Substance P/Neurokinin 1 Antagonists 715
Miscellaneous Antiemetics 717
Nonpharmacologic Management 719

39 Drug Therapy for Constipation and Elimination Problems 722
Introduction 723
Overview of Constipation 723
Laxatives 724
Cathartics 728
Guanylate Cyclase-C Agonists 730
Miscellaneous Agents for Constipation 732

40 Drug Therapy for Diarrhea 736
Introduction 737
Overview of Diarrhea 737
Opiate-Related Antidiarrheal Agents 737
Adjuvant Medications Used to Treat Diarrhea 741
Clinical Judgment in Practice 746

SECTION 8
DRUGS AFFECTING THE ENDOCRINE SYSTEM 747

41 Drug Therapy for Diabetes Mellitus 749
Introduction 750
Overview of Diabetes 750
Insulins 753
Sulfonylureas 764
Biguanide 765
Alpha-Glucosidase Inhibitors 767
Thiazolidinediones 769
Meglitinides 769
Dipeptidyl Peptidase 4 Inhibitors 771
Amylin Analogs 773
Glucagonlike Peptide 1 Receptor Agonists (Incretin Mimetics) 774
Sodium–Glucose Cotransporter 2 (SGLT2) Inhibitors 776
Combination Drug Therapy for Type 2 Diabetes 777
Adjuvant Medications Used to Treat Diabetes 778

42 Drug Therapy for Hyperthyroidism and Hypothyroidism 782
Introduction 783
Overview of the Thyroid Gland 783
Antithyroid Drugs 786
Adjuvant Medication Used to Treat Hyperthyroidism 789
Thyroid Eye Disease Medications 790
Thyroid Drugs 790

43 Drug Therapy for Pituitary and Hypothalamic Dysfunction 796
Introduction 797
Overview of Pituitary and Hypothalamic Dysfunction 797
Anterior Pituitary Hormone Drugs for Growth Deficiency in Children 799
Posterior Pituitary Hormone Drugs for Diabetes Insipidus 803
Hypothalamic Hormone Drugs 805

44 Drug Therapy to Regulate Calcium and Bone Metabolism 811
Introduction 812
Overview of Calcium and Bone Metabolism 813
Calcium Preparations 815
Vitamin D 818
Bisphosphonates 820
Other Medications Used to Treat Bone Disorders and Hypercalcemia 823

45 Drug Therapy for Adrenal Cortex Disorders 827
Introduction 828
Overview of Addison Disease 828
Overview of Cushing Disease 829
Drugs Used to Treat Addison Disease 830

Drugs Used to Treat Cushing Disease 833
Glucocorticoid Receptor Antagonists 833
Clinical Judgment in Practice 839

SECTION 9
DRUGS AFFECTING THE AUTONOMIC AND CENTRAL NERVOUS SYSTEMS 841

46 Physiology of the Autonomic and Central Nervous Systems and Indications for the Use of Drug Therapy 843
Introduction 844
Structure and Function of the Autonomic Nervous System 844
Characteristics of Autonomic Drugs 850

47 Drug Therapy for Myasthenia Gravis, Alzheimer Disease, and Other Conditions Treated With Cholinergic Agents 852
Introduction 853
Overview of Myasthenia Gravis 853
Acetylcholinesterase Inhibitors (Indirect-Acting Cholinergics) 854
Immunosuppressive Therapy for Myasthenia Gravis 857
Overview of Alzheimer Disease 857
Cholinesterase Inhibitors: Reversible Indirect-Acting Cholinergics 858
N-Methyl-D-Aspartate Receptor Antagonist 860
Cholinesterase Inhibitor–N-Methyl-D-Aspartate Receptor Antagonist 861
Antiamyloid Monoclonal Antibody 861
Cholinergic Agonist 862
Irreversible Anticholinesterase Toxicity 863

48 Drug Therapy for Parkinson Disease, Urinary Spasticity, and Disorders Requiring Anticholinergic Drug Therapy 867
Introduction 868
Overview of Parkinson Disease 868
Dopamine Receptor Agonists 869
Catechol-O-Methyltransferase Inhibitors 875
Catechol-O-Methyltransferase Inhibitor and Decarboxylase Inhibitor/Dopamine Precursor 877
Overview of Anticholinergic Drugs 878
Belladonna Alkaloid and Derivatives 880
Centrally Acting Anticholinergics 883
Gastrointestinal Anticholinergics (Antisecretory/Antispasmodic) 885
Urinary Antispasmodics 886

49 Drug Therapy With Opioids 891
Introduction 892
Overview of Pain 892
Opioid Agonists 894
Opioid Agonists/Antagonists 903
Opioid Antagonists 906

50 Drug Therapy With Local Anesthetics 910
Introduction 911
Overview of Local Anesthesia 911
Amides 912
Esters 915

51 Drug Therapy With General Anesthetics 920
Introduction 921
Overview of General Anesthesia 921
Inhalation Anesthetics 922
Intravenous General Anesthetics 925
Neuromuscular Blocking Agents 928
Adjuvant Medications Used in General Anesthesia 931

52 Drug Therapy for Migraines and Other Headaches 935
Introduction 936
Overview of Headaches 936
Nonsteroidal Anti-Inflammatory Drugs (NSAIDs) 938
Acetaminophen, Aspirin, and Caffeine 940
Ergot Alkaloids 942
Triptans 944
Estrogen 947
Calcitonin Gene–Related Peptide Receptor Antagonist (Gepants) 948
Preventive Therapy for Migraine Headaches 949
Adjuvant Medications for Migraine Headaches 951

53 Drug Therapy for Seizure Disorders and Skeletal Muscle Disorders 953
Introduction 954
Overview of Epilepsy 954
Drugs Used to Treat Seizure Disorders 955
Other Antiepileptic Drugs 968
Miscellaneous Antiepileptic Drugs 982
Overview of Spinal Cord Injury 983
Drugs Used to Treat Muscle Spasms and Spasticity 984

54 Drug Therapy for Anxiety and Insomnia 992
Introduction 993
Overview of Anxiety 993
Overview of Sleep and Insomnia 993
Benzodiazepines 995
Nonbenzodiazepine Sedative–Hypnotic Agents 1001
Dual Receptor Antagonists 1003

55 Drug Therapy for Depression and Mood Disorders 1007
Introduction 1008
Overview of Depression 1008
Overview of Bipolar Disorder 1010
Tricyclic Antidepressants 1011
Selective Serotonin Reuptake Inhibitors 1013
Serotonin–Norepinephrine Reuptake Inhibitors 1017
Monoamine Oxidase Inhibitors 1019
Atypical Antidepressants 1021
Mood-Stabilizing Agents: Drugs Used to Treat Bipolar Disorder 1023
Other Medications Used to Treat Bipolar Disorder 1026
Ketamine Used to Treat Depression 1026

56 Drug Therapy for Psychotic Disorders 1029
Introduction 1030
Overview of Psychosis 1030
First-Generation Antipsychotics 1032
First-Generation Nonphenothiazines 1036
Second-Generation "Atypical" Antipsychotics 1038

57 Drug Therapy for Attention Deficit Hyperactivity Disorder and Narcolepsy 1046
Introduction 1047
Overview of Attention Deficit Hyperactivity Disorder 1047
Overview of Narcolepsy 1047
Stimulants 1048
Amphetamines 1049
Amphetamine-Related Drugs 1052
Other Medications Used to Treat Attention Deficit Hyperactivity Disorder and Narcolepsy 1055

58 Drug Therapy for Substance Use Disorders 1058
Introduction 1059
Overview of Substance Use 1059
Central Nervous System Depressant Use: Drug Therapy 1061
Benzodiazepines for Treatment of Alcohol Withdrawal 1061
Enzyme Inhibitors for Maintenance of Alcohol Sobriety 1064
Drugs Used to Reduce Cravings in Alcohol Use 1065
Opioid Agonists and Antagonists for Treatment of Opioid Use Disorder 1066
Central Nervous System Stimulant Abuse: Drug Therapy 1067
Psychoactive Substance Use: Drug Therapy 1067
Clinical Judgment in Practice 1070

SECTION 10
DRUGS AFFECTING THE EYE, EAR, AND SKIN 1073

59 Drug Therapy for Disorders of the Eye 1075
Introduction 1076
Basic Structure and Function of the Eye 1076
Overview of Disorders of the Eye 1076
Drug Therapy for the Diagnosis and Treatment of Ocular Disorders 1077
Drug Therapy for the Treatment of Glaucoma 1082
Combination Medications for Open-Angle Glaucoma 1089
Osmotic Drugs 1089
Drug Therapy for Ocular Infections and Inflammation 1090

60 Drug Therapy for Disorders of the Ear 1100
Introduction 1101
Overview of Disorders of the Ear 1101
Anti-Infective, Antiseptic, Glucocorticoid, and Acidifying Agents 1102
Fluoroquinolone: Ciprofloxacin 1104
Penicillin: Amoxicillin 1105
Adjuvant Medications to Treat Pain and Fever Related to Infections of the Ear 1107

61 Drug Therapy for Disorders of the Skin 1109
Introduction 1110
Overview of Drug Therapy for Skin Disorders 1110
Herbal Preparations for Skin Disorders 1117
Acne Vulgaris 1117
Retinoids 1119
Clinical Judgment in Practice 1124

Index 1127

AVAILABLE ON thePoint®

Appendix A: Answers for NCLEX Success
Appendix B: Answers for the Clinical Application Case Studies
Appendix C: Critical Thinking Questions and Answers
Appendix D: The International System of Units
Appendix E: Serum Drug Concentrations

Case Studies in This Book

CASES THAT UNFOLD ACROSS CHAPTERS

Unfolding Patient Stories: Junetta Cooper
Part 1: Chapter 1   11
Part 2: Chapter 26   494

Unfolding Patient Stories: Mary Richards
Part 1: Chapter 3   39
Part 2: Chapter 26   500

Unfolding Patient Stories: Danielle Young Bear
Part 1: Chapter 6   89
Part 2: Chapter 16   310

Unfolding Patient Stories: Rachel Heidebrink
Part 1: Chapter 7   113
Part 2: Chapter 9   146

Unfolding Patient Stories: Juan Carlos
Part 1: Chapter 12   205
Part 2: Chapter 41   764

Unfolding Patient Stories: Harry Hadley
Part 1: Chapter 19   360
Part 2: Chapter 61   1114

Unfolding Patient Stories: Yoa Li
Part 1: Chapter 32   599
Part 2: Chapter 49   900

Unfolding Patient Stories: Toua Xiong
Part 1: Chapter 33   623
Part 2: Chapter 60   1107

Unfolding Patient Stories: Jermaine Jones
Part 1: Chapter 35   670
Part 2: Chapter 55   1028

Unfolding Patient Stories: Suzanne Morris
Part 1: Chapter 37   705
Part 2: Chapter 44   826

CASES FEATURED IN INDIVIDUAL CHAPTERS

Chapter 1: The Foundation of Pharmacology: Quality and Safety
Clinical Application Case Study*   3

Chapter 2: Basic Concepts and Processes
Clinical Application Case Study*   14

Chapter 3: Medication Administration and the Nursing Process of Drug Therapy
Clinical Application Case Study*   32

Chapter 4: Pharmacology and the Care of Infants and Pediatric Patients
Clinical Application Case Study*   67
The Nursing Process   73

Chapter 5: Pharmacology and the Care of Adults and Geriatric Patients
Clinical Application Case Study*   75
The Nursing Process   81

Chapter 6: Pharmacology and the Care of Pregnant or Lactating Females
Clinical Application Case Study*   83
The Nursing Process   97

Chapter 7: Pharmacology and Female Health
Clinical Application Case Study*   99
The Nursing Process   115

Chapter 8: Pharmacology and Male Health
Clinical Application Case Study*   117
The Nursing Process   130

Chapter 9: Drug Therapy for Coagulation Disorders
Clinical Application Case Study*   137
The Nursing Process   159

Chapter 10: Drug Therapy for Dyslipidemia
Clinical Application Case Study*   161
The Nursing Process   176

Chapter 11: Drug Therapy for Hematopoietic Disorders
Clinical Application Case Study*   178
The Nursing Process   190

Chapter 12: Drug Therapy: Immunizations
Clinical Application Case Study*   192
The Nursing Process   206

Chapter 13: Drug Therapy to Decrease Immunity
Clinical Application Case Study*   208
The Nursing Process   229

Chapter 14: Drug Therapy for the Treatment of Cancer
Clinical Application Case Study*   231
The Nursing Process   265

Chapter 15: Inflammation, Infection, and the Use of Antimicrobial Agents
Clinical Application Case Study*   271
The Nursing Process   284

Chapter 16: Drug Therapy to Decrease Pain, Fever, and Inflammation
Clinical Application Case Study*   285
The Nursing Process   311

Chapter 17: Drug Therapy With Corticosteroids
Clinical Application Case Study*   313
The Nursing Process   332

Chapter 18: Drug Therapy With Beta-Lactam Antibacterial Agents
Clinical Application Case Study*   334
The Nursing Process   351

Chapter 19: Drug Therapy With Aminoglycosides and Fluoroquinolones
Clinical Application Case Study*   352
The Nursing Process   362

Chapter 20: Drug Therapy With Tetracyclines, Sulfonamides, and Urinary Antiseptics
Clinical Application Case Study*   364
The Nursing Process   374

Chapter 21: Drug Therapy With Macrolides and Miscellaneous Anti-Infective Agents
Clinical Application Case Study*   376
The Nursing Process   387

Chapter 22: Drug Therapy for Tuberculosis and *Mycobacterium avium* Complex Disease
Clinical Application Case Study*   388
The Nursing Process   402

Chapter 23: Drug Therapy for Viral Infections
Clinical Application Case Study*   404
The Nursing Process   442

Chapter 24: Drug Therapy for Fungal Infections
Clinical Application Case Study*   444
The Nursing Process   460

Chapter 25: Drug Therapy for Parasitic Infections
Clinical Application Case Study*   462
The Nursing Process   473

Chapter 26: Drug Therapy for Hypertension
Clinical Application Case Study*   477
The Nursing Process   501

Chapter 27: Drug Therapy for Dysrhythmias
Clinical Application Case Study*   503
The Nursing Process   519

Chapter 28: Drug Therapy for Coronary Heart Disease
Clinical Application Case Study*   521
The Nursing Process   537

Chapter 29: Drug Therapy for Shock and Hypotension
Clinical Application Case Study*   539
The Nursing Process   548

Chapter 30: Drug Therapy for Heart Failure
Clinical Application Case Study*   550
The Nursing Process   566

Chapter 31: Drug Therapy for Nasal Congestion and Cough
Clinical Application Case Study*   573
The Nursing Process   584

Chapter 32: Drug Therapy to Decrease Histamine Effects and Allergic Response
Clinical Application Case Study*   586
The Nursing Process   599

Chapter 33: Drug Therapy for Asthma, Airway Inflammation, and Bronchoconstriction
Clinical Application Case Study*   601
The Nursing Process   622

Chapter 34: Drug Therapy for Fluid Volume Excess
Clinical Application Case Study*   629
The Nursing Process   642

Chapter 35: Nutritional Support Products, Vitamins, and Mineral Supplements
Clinical Application Case Study*   644
The Nursing Process   671

Chapter 36: Drug Therapy for Weight Management
Clinical Application Case Study*   673
The Nursing Process   687

Chapter 37: Drug Therapy for Peptic Ulcer Disease and Hyperacidity
Clinical Application Case Study*   689
The Nursing Process   704

Chapter 38: Drug Therapy for Nausea and Vomiting
Clinical Application Case Study*   706
The Nursing Process   720

Chapter 39: Drug Therapy for Constipation and Elimination Problems
Clinical Application Case Study*   722
The Nursing Process   734

Chapter 40: Drug Therapy for Diarrhea
Clinical Application Case Study*   736
The Nursing Process   744

Chapter 41: Drug Therapy for Diabetes Mellitus
Clinical Application Case Study*   749
The Nursing Process   780

Chapter 42: Drug Therapy for Hyperthyroidism and Hypothyroidism
Clinical Application Case Study*   782
The Nursing Process   794

Chapter 43: Drug Therapy for Pituitary and Hypothalamic Dysfunction
Clinical Application Case Study*   796
The Nursing Process   810

Chapter 44: Drug Therapy to Regulate Calcium and Bone Metabolism
Clinical Application Case Study*   811
The Nursing Process   825

Chapter 45: Drug Therapy for Adrenal Cortex Disorders
Clinical Application Case Study*   827
The Nursing Process   838

Chapter 46: Physiology of the Autonomic and Central Nervous Systems and Indications for the Use of Drug Therapy
Clinical Application Case Study*   843
The Nursing Process   851

Chapter 47: Drug Therapy for Myasthenia Gravis, Alzheimer Disease, and Other Conditions Treated With Cholinergic Agents
Clinical Application Case Study*   852
The Nursing Process   865

Chapter 48: Drug Therapy for Parkinson Disease, Urinary Spasticity, and Disorders Requiring Anticholinergic Drug Therapy
Clinical Application Case Study* 867
The Nursing Process 889

Chapter 49: Drug Therapy With Opioids
Clinical Application Case Study* 891
The Nursing Process 908

Chapter 50: Drug Therapy With Local Anesthetics
Clinical Application Case Study* 910
The Nursing Process 918

Chapter 51: Drug Therapy With General Anesthetics
Clinical Application Case Study* 920
The Nursing Process 933

Chapter 52: Drug Therapy for Migraines and Other Headaches
Clinical Application Case Study* 935
The Nursing Process 952

Chapter 53: Drug Therapy for Seizure Disorders and Skeletal Muscle Disorders
Clinical Application Case Study* 953
The Nursing Process 990

Chapter 54: Drug Therapy for Anxiety and Insomnia
Clinical Application Case Study* 992
The Nursing Process 1005

Chapter 55: Drug Therapy for Depression and Mood Disorders
Clinical Application Case Study* 1007
The Nursing Process 1027

Chapter 56: Drug Therapy for Psychotic Disorders
Clinical Application Case Study* 1029
The Nursing Process 1044

Chapter 57: Drug Therapy for Attention Deficit Hyperactivity Disorder and Narcolepsy
Clinical Application Case Study* 1046
The Nursing Process 1057

Chapter 58: Drug Therapy for Substance Use Disorders
Clinical Application Case Study* 1058
The Nursing Process 1068

Chapter 59: Drug Therapy for Disorders of the Eye
Clinical Application Case Study* 1075
The Nursing Process 1098

Chapter 60: Drug Therapy for Disorders of the Ear
Clinical Application Case Study* 1100
The Nursing Process 1108

Chapter 61: Drug Therapy for Disorders of the Skin
Clinical Application Case Study* 1109
The Nursing Process 1122

*Note that each chapter has a Clinical Application Case Study that unfolds within that chapter. The page number for the introduction to the Clinical Application Case Study in each chapter is given here.

SECTION 1

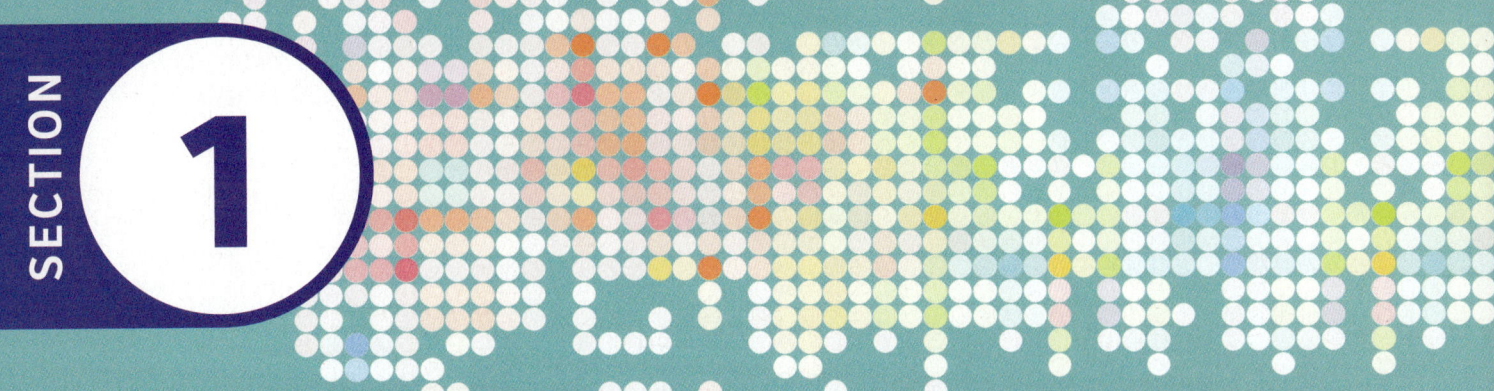

The Conceptual Framework of Pharmacology

Chapter 1 The Foundation of Pharmacology: Quality and Safety

Chapter 2 Basic Concepts and Processes

Chapter 3 Medication Administration and the Nursing Process of Drug Therapy

CHAPTER 1

The Foundation of Pharmacology: Quality and Safety

LEARNING OBJECTIVES

After studying this chapter, you should be able to:

1. Define a prototype drug.
2. Distinguish between generic and trade names of drugs.
3. Describe the five categories of controlled substances in relation to therapeutic use, potential for abuse, and regulatory requirements.
4. Identify the multiple safeguards and laws that are in place to promote drug safety in drug research, packaging, and approval processes.
5. Recognize initiatives designated to enhance safe drug administration.
6. Develop personal techniques for learning about drugs and using drug knowledge in patient care.
7. Identify authoritative sources of drug information.

CLINICAL APPLICATION CASE STUDY

Joan Clark, a senior nursing student, is preparing for the NCLEX-RN examination. As she reviews material, she examines safeguards in place to protect the public from injury due to medication administration.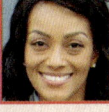

KEY TERMS

Biotechnology: process that may involve manipulating deoxyribonucleic acid (DNA) and ribonucleic acid (RNA) and recombining genes into hybrid molecules that can be inserted into living organisms (often *Escherichia coli* bacteria) and repeatedly reproduced

Brand (trade) name: manufacturer's chosen name for a drug, which is protected by a patent

Controlled substances: drugs, substances, and certain chemicals used to make drugs that are categorized by federal law according to therapeutic usefulness and potential for abuse; also known as scheduled drugs

Drug classifications: groups of medications that are classified according to their effects on particular body systems, their therapeutic uses, and their chemical characteristics

Generic name: chemical or official name of the drug that is independent of the manufacturer and often indicates the drug group

Over-the-counter (OTC) drugs: medications available for purchase without a prescription

Pharmacoeconomics: costs of drug therapy, including costs of purchasing, dispensing, storage, administration, and laboratory and other tests used to monitor patient responses; also considers losses due to expiration

Pharmacogenomics (also known as pharmacogenetics): study of how a person's genetic makeup, or genome, leads to variable responses to drugs; more generally refers to genetic polymorphisms that occur in a patient population, such as an ethnic group, as opposed to an individual person

Pharmacotherapy: use of drugs to prevent, diagnose, or treat signs, symptoms, and disease processes; also known as drug therapy

Placebo: inert substance containing no medication and given to reinforce a person's expectation to improve

Prescription drugs: medications that are ordered in writing by a licensed healthcare provider

Prototype: often the first drug of a particular drug class to be developed; usually the standard against which newer, similar drugs are compared

INTRODUCTION

Pharmacology is the study of drugs (chemicals) that alter the functions of living organisms. **Pharmacotherapy**, also known as drug therapy, is the use of drugs to prevent, diagnose, or treat signs, symptoms, and diseases. When prevention or cure is not a reasonable goal, relief of symptoms can greatly improve a patient's quality of life and ability to perform activities of daily living. Contemporary nursing guidelines require that nurses keep safety issues in mind when involved in the practice of pharmacotherapy.

Drugs given for therapeutic purposes are also called medications. These substances may be given for their local or systemic effects. Drugs with local effects, such as sunscreen lotions and local anesthetics, act mainly at the site of application. Those with systemic effects are taken into the body, circulated through the bloodstream to their sites of action in various body tissues, and eventually eliminated from the body. Most drugs are given for their systemic effects. Drugs are given for short-term acute disorders, such as pain or infection, or to relieve signs and symptoms of long-term disease processes, such as hypertension or diabetes.

DRUG SOURCES

Historically, drugs came from plants, animals, and minerals. Now, most drugs are synthetic compounds manufactured in laboratories. Chemists, for example, often create useful new drugs by altering the chemical structure of existing drugs. Such techniques and other technologic advances have enabled the production of new drugs as well as synthetic versions of many drugs originally derived from plants and animals. Synthetic drugs are more standardized in their chemical characteristics, more consistent in their effects, and less likely to produce allergic reactions. Semisynthetic drugs (e.g., many antibiotics) are naturally occurring substances that have been chemically modified.

Biotechnology is also an important source of drugs. This process may involve manipulating deoxyribonucleic acid (DNA) and ribonucleic acid (RNA) and recombining genes into hybrid molecules that can be inserted into living organisms (*Escherichia coli* bacteria are often used), which can be repeatedly reproduced. Each hybrid molecule produces a genetically identical molecule, called a clone. Cloning makes it possible to identify the DNA sequence in a gene and to produce the protein product encoded by a gene, such as insulin. Cloning also allows production of adequate amounts of the drug for therapeutic or research purposes. Biotechnology drugs constitute an increasing percentage of drugs now undergoing development, and this trend is expected to continue into the foreseeable future.

DRUG CLASSIFICATIONS AND PROTOTYPES

Drugs are classified according to their effects on particular body systems, their therapeutic uses, and their chemical characteristics. For example, morphine can be classified as a central nervous system depressant and a narcotic or opioid analgesic. The names of therapeutic classifications usually reflect the conditions for which the drugs are used (e.g., antidepressants, antihypertensives). However, the names of many drug groups reflect their chemical characteristics rather than their therapeutic uses (e.g., adrenergics, benzodiazepines). Many drugs fit into multiple groups because they have wide-ranging effects on the human body.

An individual drug that represents groups of drugs is called a **prototype**. The prototype, often the first drug of a particular drug class to be developed, is usually the standard with which newer drugs in the class are compared. For example, morphine is the prototype of the opioid analgesics, and penicillin is the prototype of the beta-lactam antibacterial drugs.

Drug classifications and prototypes are quite well established, and most new drugs can be assigned to a group and compared with a recognized prototype. However, some groups lack a universally accepted prototype, and some prototypes are replaced over time by newer, more commonly used drugs. In this text, information about the prototype is provided for each drug class.

DRUG NAMES

Individual drugs may have several different names, but the two that are most used are the generic (official) name and the brand (trade) name. The **generic name** (e.g., amoxicillin) is related to the chemical or official name and is independent of the manufacturer. The generic name often indicates the drug group (e.g., drugs with generic names ending in "cillin" are penicillins). In the United States, the United States Adopted Names Council assigns the generic name. The **brand (trade) name** is designated and patented by the manufacturer. For example, amoxicillin is manufactured by several pharmaceutical companies, some of which assign a specific trade name (e.g., Amoxil, Larotid) and several of which use only the generic name. In drug literature, trade names are capitalized, and generic names are presented in lowercase unless in a list or at the beginning of a sentence. Drugs may be prescribed and dispensed by generic or trade name. Generic equivalents are available for most drugs and can be substituted for trade-named drugs unless the prescriber requests the trade-named medication by writing "do not substitute" on the prescription. Generic drugs are required to be therapeutically equivalent and are less expensive than trade-named drugs.

> **Quality and Safety Alert: Safety**
>
> Using different drug names (i.e., generic or trade names) increases confusion and the risk of misuse. If the drug name on the package does not match the one on the prescription drug label, an individual may take too much medication or not take it at all.

NCLEX Success

1. The nurse is caring for a patient who has strong beliefs about not putting anything unnatural into their body. It is most accurate to say that most modern medications are
   A. natural products derived from plants
   B. natural products derived from minerals
   C. synthetic products manufactured in laboratories
   D. synthetic modifications of natural products

2. The nurse is taking care of a patient who is confused about the different medications they are prescribed. They note that some of the drug names have changed over the course of time they have been taking them. When counseling them, it is most important to keep the following statement in mind:
   A. A drug can belong to only one group or classification.
   B. A prototype drug is the standard by which similar drugs are compared.
   C. Drug groups and prototypes change frequently, and knowledge about a prototype cannot guide knowledge about other drugs in the same class.
   D. The generic name of a drug changes among manufacturers.

DRUG MARKETING

A patent protects a new drug for several years, during which time only the pharmaceutical manufacturer that developed it can market it. The company views this protection as a return on its investment in developing the drug, which might have required years of work and millions of dollars, and as an incentive to develop other drugs. Other pharmaceutical companies cannot manufacture and market the drug until the patent expires. However, for new drugs that are popular and widely used, other companies often produce similar drugs, with different generic and trade names.

PHARMACOECONOMICS

Pharmacoeconomics involves the costs of drug therapy, including costs of purchasing, dispensing (i.e., salaries of pharmacists, pharmacy technicians), storage, administration (i.e., salaries of nurses, costs of supplies), and laboratory and other tests used to monitor patient responses, as well as losses due to expiration. Length of illness or hospitalization is also a consideration. The goal of most pharmacoeconomic research is to identify drug therapy regimens that provide the desired benefits at the lowest cost.

PHARMACOGENOMICS

Pharmacogenomics is the study of how one's genetic makeup, or genome, affects the body's response to drugs. The term comes from the words *pharmacology* and *genomics* and is a combination of drugs and genetics. Information about a patient's pharmacogenomics helps providers choose the drugs and drug doses that are likely to work best for an individual. Because essentially all diseases and conditions have a genetic or genomic component, the use of this information in prevention, screening, diagnosis, and treatment and effectiveness enhances the likelihood of best practice in drug therapy. See Chapter 2 for additional information.

ACCESS TO DRUGS

Prescription and Nonprescription Drugs

Legally, American consumers have two ways to access therapeutic drugs. They can obtain them as **prescription drugs**, which require a written order. A licensed healthcare provider such as a physician, dentist, or nurse practitioner writes the prescription. Alternatively, they can purchase **over-the-counter (OTC) drugs**, which are medications that do not require a prescription. Various laws regulate these routes. Acquiring and using prescription drugs for nontherapeutic purposes by people who are not authorized to have the drugs or for whom they are not prescribed is illegal.

American Drug Laws and Standards

Current drug laws and standards have evolved over many years. Their main goal is to protect the public by ensuring that drugs marketed for therapeutic purposes are safe and effective. Table 1.1 further describes and summarizes the main provisions.

The Food, Drug, and Cosmetic Act of 1938 and its amendments regulate the manufacture, distribution, advertising, and labeling of drugs. The law also requires that official drugs (i.e., those listed in the United States Pharmacopeia and designated USP) must meet standards of purity and strength as determined by chemical analysis or by animal response to specified doses (bioassay). The Durham-Humphrey Amendment designates drugs that must be prescribed by a licensed physician or nurse practitioner and dispensed by a pharmacist. The U.S. Food and Drug Administration (FDA) is charged with enforcing the law.

TABLE 1.1
American Drug Laws and Amendments

Year	Name	Main Provision(s)
1906	Pure Food and Drug Act	Established official standards and requirements for accurate labeling of drug products Established the forerunner of FDA
1912	Shirley Amendment	Prohibited fraudulent claims of drug effectiveness
1914	Harrison Narcotic Act	Restricted the importation, manufacture, sale, and use of opium, cocaine, marijuana, and other drugs that the act defined as narcotics
1938	Food, Drug, and Cosmetic Act	Revised and broadened FDA powers and responsibilities; gave the FDA control over drug safety Required proof of safety from the manufacturer before a new drug could be marketed Authorized factory inspections Established penalties for fraudulent claims and misleading labels
1945	Amendment	Required governmental certification of biologic products, such as insulin and antibiotics
1951	Durham-Humphrey Amendment	Designated drugs that must be prescribed by a physician or nurse practitioner and dispensed by a pharmacist (e.g., controlled substances, drugs considered unsafe for use except under supervision by a healthcare provider, and drugs limited to prescription use under a manufacturer's new drug application)
1962	Kefauver-Harris Amendment	Required a manufacturer to provide evidence (from well-controlled research studies) that a drug was effective for claims and conditions identified in the product's labeling Gave the federal government the authority to standardize drug names
1970	Comprehensive Drug Abuse Prevention and Control Act; Controlled Substance Act	Regulated distribution of narcotics and other drugs of abuse Categorized these drugs according to therapeutic usefulness and potential for abuse Title II, Controlled Substances Act Updated or replaced all previous laws regarding narcotics and other dangerous drugs
1978	Drug Regulation Reform Act	Established guidelines for research studies and data to be submitted to the FDA by manufacturers Shortened the time required to develop and market new drugs
1983	Orphan Drug Act	Decreased taxes and competition for manufacturers who would produce drugs to treat selected serious rare diseases
1987		Established new regulations designed to speed up the approval process for high-priority medications
1992	Prescription Drug User Fee Act	Allowed the FDA to collect user fees from pharmaceutical companies, with each new drug application, to shorten the review time (e.g., by hiring more staff) Specified a review time of 12 mo for standard drugs and 6 mo for priority drugs
1993	NIH Revitalization Act	Requires inclusion of women and minorities in NIH-funded research studies, including phase III clinical drug trials
1997	FDA Modernization Act	Updated regulation of biologic products Increased patient access to experimental drugs and medical devices Accelerated review of important new drugs Allowed drug companies to disseminate information about off-label (non–FDA-approved) uses and costs of drugs Extended user fees
2002	Best Pharmaceuticals for Children Act	Encouraged pharmaceutical companies to conduct studies and label drugs for use in children Provided funds for 5 y for pediatric drug studies
2003	Medicare Prescription Drug Improvement and Modernization Act	Afforded the largest overhaul of Medicare in the 38-y history of the program Provided entitlement benefit for prescription drugs and other benefits for seniors and those with medical disabilities
2005	Combat Methamphetamine Epidemic Act	Established federal law that regulates retail over-the-counter sales of ephedrine, pseudoephedrine, and phenylpropanolamine products due to their use in the manufacturing of illegal drugs. Specifically, these drugs are: • Kept behind the counter or in a locked case • Limited in purchase to no more than 3.6 g a day and 9 g a month • Dispensed after purchasers produce identification and sign a sales log • Handled by employees who are properly trained Geared at curtailing clandestine production of methamphetamine

TABLE 1.1

American Drug Laws and Amendments (Continued)

Year	Name	Main Provision(s)
2008	Ryan Haight Online Pharmacy Consumer Protection Act	Applies to all controlled substances in all schedules Established federal law that it is illegal to deliver, distribute, or dispense a controlled substance by means of the internet unless the online pharmacy holds a modification of DEA registration authorizing it to operate as an online pharmacy
2018	Substance Use-Disorder Prevention that Promotes Opioid Recovery and Treatment (SUPPORT) for Patients and Communities Act	Dedicates more federal resources to combat the opioid crisis through alternate strategies for pain management, including increased focus on nonopioid pain relief, expanded treatment options for people with substance use disorders, greater access to APRN-delivered care and telehealth services Amends the Controlled Substances Act to permanently authorize Nurse Practitioners and provide a 5-y authorization for clinical nurse specialists, certified registered nurse anesthetists, and certified nurse-midwives to prescribe Medication-Assisted Treatments (MAT for opioid use disorders; expands Medicaid coverage for MAT)

APRN, Advanced Practice Registered Nurses; DEA, Drug Enforcement Administration; FDA, U.S. Food and Drug Administration; MAT, medication-assisted treatment; NIH, National Institutes of Health.

In addition, the Public Health Service regulates vaccines and other biologic products, and the Federal Trade Commission can suppress misleading advertisements of nonprescription drugs.

The Comprehensive Drug Abuse Prevention and Control Act was passed in 1970. Title II of this law, called the Controlled Substances Act, regulates the manufacture and distribution of narcotics, stimulants, depressants, hallucinogens, and anabolic steroids and requires the pharmaceutical industry to maintain physical security and strict record keeping for these drugs and substances. Drugs, substances, and certain chemicals used to make drugs are categorized into five distinct categories according to therapeutic usefulness and potential for abuse (Box 1.1) and are labeled as **controlled substances** (e.g., morphine is a C-II or Schedule II drug).

The Drug Enforcement Administration (DEA) enforces the Controlled Substances Act. Individual people and companies legally empowered to handle controlled substances must register with the DEA, keep accurate records of all transactions, and provide for secure storage. The DEA assigns prescribers a number, which they must include on all prescriptions they write for a controlled substance. Prescriptions for Schedule II drugs cannot be refilled; a new prescription is required. Nurses are responsible for storing controlled substances in locked containers, administering them only to people for whom they are prescribed, recording each dose given on agency narcotic sheets and on the patient's medication administration record, maintaining an accurate inventory, and reporting discrepancies to the proper authorities.

BOX 1.1 Categories of Controlled Substances

Schedule I

Drugs that have no accepted medical use, have lack of accepted safety, and have high abuse potentials: heroin, lysergic acid diethylamide (LSD), 3,4-methylenedioxy-methamphetamine (MDMA or ecstasy), mescaline, and peyote.

Schedule II

Drugs that are used medically and have high abuse potentials: opioid analgesics (e.g., codeine, hydromorphone, methadone, meperidine, morphine, oxycodone), central nervous system (CNS) stimulants (e.g., cocaine, methamphetamine), and barbiturate sedative–hypnotics (e.g., pentobarbital).

Schedule III

Drugs with less potential for abuse than those in Schedules I and II, but abuse of which may lead to psychological or physical dependence: androgens and anabolic steroids, some depressants (e.g., ketamine, pentobarbital), some CNS stimulants (e.g., methylphenidate), and mixtures containing small amounts of controlled substances (e.g., codeine, barbiturates not listed in other schedules). These drugs and substances have an accepted medical use in the United States.

Schedule IV

Drugs with an accepted medical use in the United States but with some potential for abuse: benzodiazepines (e.g., diazepam, lorazepam), other sedative–hypnotics (e.g., phenobarbital, chloral hydrate), and some prescription appetite suppressants (e.g., phentermine).

Schedule V

Products containing moderate amounts of controlled substances. They may be dispensed by the pharmacist without a physician's prescription but with some restrictions regarding amount, record keeping, and other safeguards. Included are cough suppressants containing small amounts of codeine and antidiarrheal drugs, such as diphenoxylate and atropine (Lomotil).

An approach known as medication-assisted treatment (MAT) may be used in the management of substance use disorders. MAT involves the use of FDA-approved medications in combination with counseling and behavioral therapies. The Substance Abuse and Mental Health Services Administration program provides a "whole-patient" approach to the treatment of substance use disorders that is consistent with the latest regulations that address the opioid crisis. The Substance Use-Disorder Prevention that Promotes Opioid Recovery and Treatment (SUPPORT) for Patients and Communities Act assists states in implementing updates to their plans of safe care and improving data sharing between states. It can help some people to sustain recovery.

> **Quality and Safety Alert: Patient-Centered Care**
>
> Although MAT provides an opportunity to address and treat opioid addiction, it is critical that people voluntarily consent to participation while in a criminal justice setting. The risk of undue influence from individuals in authority, particularly where sanctions are involved, requires protection of the decision-making rights and autonomy of individuals offered this treatment when facing legal sanctions.

In addition to federal laws, state laws also regulate the sale and distribution of controlled drugs. These laws may be more stringent than federal laws; if so, the stricter laws usually apply.

DRUG APPROVAL PROCESSES: FOOD AND DRUG ADMINISTRATION

The FDA is responsible for ensuring that new drugs are safe and effective before approving the drugs and allowing them to be marketed. The FDA reviews research studies (usually conducted or sponsored by pharmaceutical companies) about proposed new drugs; the organization does not test the drugs.

Testing Procedure

Since the 1962 Kefauver-Harris Amendment (see Table 1.1), newly developed drugs undergo extensive testing before being marketed for general use. A clinical trial proceeds through five phases if there is continuing evidence of drug safety and effectiveness. Initially, drug testing occurs in animals and small groups of humans (phase 0), and the FDA's Center for Drug Evaluation and Research (CDER) reviews the test results. Next, researchers perform clinical trials in more humans (phases 1–4), usually with a randomized, controlled experimental design that involves selection of subjects according to established criteria, random assignment of subjects to experimental groups, and administration of the test drug to one group and a control substance to another group.

In phase 1, a few doses are given to a certain number of healthy volunteers to determine safe dosages, routes of administration, absorption, metabolism, excretion, and toxicity. In phase 2, a few doses are given to a certain number of subjects with the disease or symptom for which the drug is being studied, and responses are compared with those of healthy subjects. In phase 3, the drug is given to different populations and different dosages and by using the drug in combination with other drugs. In double-blind, placebo-controlled designs, half of the subjects receive the new drug and half receive a **placebo** (an inactive substance similar in appearance to the actual drug, given to reinforce a person's expectation to improve), with neither subjects nor researchers knowing who receives which formulation. In crossover studies, subjects serve as their own control; each subject receives the experimental drug during half of the study and a placebo during the other half. Other research methods include control studies in which some patients receive a known drug rather than a placebo; in subject matching, patients are paired with other individuals of similar characteristics. Phase 3 studies help determine whether the potential benefits of the drug outweigh the risks. Testing may be stopped during any of the early phases if inadequate effectiveness or excessive toxicity becomes evident. In phase 4, the FDA allows the drug to be marketed and requires manufacturers to continue postmarketing monitoring and electronic report submission of the drug's safety and effectiveness.

Historically, drug research involved mainly young, white males. In 1993, Congress passed the National Institutes of Health (NIH) Revitalization Act, which formalized a policy of the NIH that women and racial and ethnic minorities be included in human subject research studies funded by the NIH and that they also be included in clinical drug trials. Now, major drug trials must recruit female subjects and include outcome data on females. In addition, all newly developed drugs must include sex-related effectiveness and safety information in the initial FDA application. Knowledge about the drug effects in females has increased but is still relatively limited because many commonly used drugs were developed before enactment of these regulations.

Subsequent withdrawal of approved and marketed drugs has occurred, usually because of serious adverse effects that become evident only when the drugs are used in a large, diverse population. In addition, over the past 25 years, the FDA has issued **BOXED WARNING ◆** about drugs that can cause serious adverse effects. The warning appears on the label, package insert, and any marketing literature; these boxed warnings are identified in this text (see Chapter 2 for additional information).

In response to growing public concern regarding health risks posed by approved drugs, the FDA requested that the Institute of Medicine (IOM) conduct an independent assessment of the FDA's drug safety system in the United States. Their report, released in 2006, recounted major deficiencies and made recommendations to improve risk assessment, surveillance, and the safe use of drugs. Ongoing assessment of deficiencies and identification of additional error reduction strategies persists.

Approval of Prescription and Nonprescription Drugs

The FDA's CDER approves many new prescription drugs annually, and it also approves drugs for OTC availability. With prescription drugs, a healthcare professional diagnoses the condition, often with the help of laboratory and other diagnostic tests and determines a need for the drug. With OTC drugs, the consumer must make these decisions, with or without consultation with a healthcare provider. The CDER handles the transfer of drugs from prescription to OTC status and may require additional clinical trials to determine the safety and effectiveness of

OTC use. For prescription drugs taken orally, the switch to OTC status may mean different indications for use and lower doses. FDA approval of a drug for OTC availability involves evaluation of evidence that the consumer can use the drug safely, using information on the product label, and shifts primary responsibility for safe and effective drug therapy from healthcare professionals to consumers.

Having drugs available OTC has potential advantages and disadvantages for consumers. Advantages include greater autonomy, faster and more convenient access to effective treatment, possibly earlier resumption of usual activities of daily living, fewer visits to healthcare providers, and possibly increased efforts by consumers to learn about their symptoms/conditions and recommended treatments. Disadvantages include inaccurate self-diagnoses and potential risks of choosing a wrong or contraindicated drug, delayed treatment by healthcare professionals, and development of adverse drug reactions and interactions. When a drug is switched from prescription to OTC status, sales and profits of pharmaceutical companies increase and costs of insurance companies decrease. Costs to consumers increase because health insurance companies do not cover most OTC drugs.

Clinical Application 1.1

Ms. Clark analyzes drug safety, including the national organizations charged with ensuring it.
- What is the role of the U.S. Food and Drug Administration (FDA) in the drug approval process?
- What is the role of the Drug Enforcement Administration (DEA) and the nurse with regard to controlled substances?

NCLEX Success

3. In understanding the use of controlled substances for patients, it is important that the nurse knows that controlled drugs are
   A. categorized according to prescription or nonprescription status
   B. regulated by state and local laws more than federal laws
   C. those that must demonstrate high standards of safety
   D. scheduled according to medical use and potential for abuse

4. A patient is asking what the difference is between a prescription for 800 mg of a medication that can be purchased on an OTC basis as a 200-mg tablet. To address this issue, it is important that the nurse knows that OTC drugs
   A. are considered safe for any consumer to use
   B. are not available for treatment of most commonly occurring symptoms
   C. often differ in indications for use and recommended dosages from their prescription versions
   D. are paid for by most insurance policies

SAFETY IN DRUG ADMINISTRATION

At least 4 million preventable adverse drug events costing more than 20 billion dollars occur in the healthcare system each year (Rodziewicz et al., 2022). As described previously, multiple safeguards to promote drug safety in packaging, drug laws, and approval processes are in place. Just as critical are safeguards to promote the safe administration of drugs at the point of care.

Rights of Medication Administration

Patient safety with medication administration begins by adhering to the rights of medication administration. The 11 rights of medication administration include the right drug, right dose, right patient, right assessment, right route, right time, right reason, right documentation, right patient education, right evaluation, and right to refuse the medication. These rights are goals of the medication administration process, and discussion of the effort to reduce medication errors and harm has expanded over the years. However, the focus on rights has been on the nurse and not the system in which medication administration takes place. Chapter 3 discusses the medication rights and their application to the nursing process.

Quality and Safety Alert: Quality Improvement

A qualitative study by Pfeiffer et al. (2020) examined double-checking in a drug administration process to detect the frequency and cause of potential medication errors by nurses prior to administering chemotherapy. Double checking by two nurses is intended to act as a safety barrier that reduces the likelihood of an error before the administration. The investigators compared the order against the prepared chemotherapy in 690 observed double-checks on an oncology floor and developed a category system for the inconsistencies that was applied independently by two researchers. In 22 observations (3.2%), 28 chemotherapy-related inconsistencies were detected; 11 observations were related to nonmatching information between order and drug label, while the other half were identified by nurses who recognized that further clarification of the information was required. In the researchers' analysis, 75% of the inconsistencies could be traced back to improper or wrong orders, which led to 33 subsequent or corrective actions.

Developing error-reduction strategies, such as double-checking in a medication process, can help ensure safe medication administrations, especially with high-risk drugs.

Prudent nursing actions support an organization's culture of safety by complying with processes (safety nets and fail-safe mechanisms) that are aimed at preventing and/or reducing environmental effects to prevent medication errors.

New technology in medication administration has expanded required competencies for safe medication administration. Electronic charting, automated drug-dispensing systems, and bar code medication administration have required enhanced nursing skills to manage these complex systems. The entire process of medication administration in a hospital is distracting, causing the nurse to lose focus on the task at hand; multiple interruptions and the extended hours that nurses work inevitably lead to the possibility of unintended consequences.

> **Quality and Safety Alert: Safety**
>
> Error-reduction strategies during medication administration include the following:
>
> - Having a "quiet zone" to prepare medications
> - Placing "quiet zone" signs at the entrance to the medication room or above the automated medication-dispensing system
> - Following protocols and checklists outlining medication administration
> - Wearing a sash or vest to signal others to avoid interrupting the nurse during medication administration
> - Educating staff to reduce interruptions of nurses administering medications
> - Having a drug guide available during drug administration
> - Verifying two patient identifiers to prevent instances of misidentification and near-miss error. The Joint Commission requires that two identifiers—such as a patient's full name, date of birth, and/or medical identification (ID) number—be used for every patient encounter.

Multiple national strategies have been implemented to reduce medication errors since the seminal work of the IOM (2000), which highlighted the breadth of preventable medical errors in the United States. Examining human factors and the response of nurses to workflow changes and technology have led to more successful system design, operation, and usability.

Quality and Safety Education for Nurses Initiative

Since 2005, the Quality and Safety Education for Nurses (QSEN) initiative has been committed to the continuous improvement in the quality and safety of healthcare systems by addressing the challenges of educating future nurses with the needed knowledge, skills, and attitudes in six areas: patient-centered care, teamwork and collaboration, evidence-based practice, quality improvement, safety, and informatics. Using the IOM competencies for nursing, QSEN faculty outlined prelicensure and graduate quality and safety competencies and associated performance targets for nursing. This initiative is the cornerstone of the 2021 American Association of Colleges of Nursing Essentials expectations that require nursing programs to transition to an outcomes-based competency framework designed to educate nurses for entry-level and advanced-level practice. Box 1.2 provides additional information.

National Patient Safety Goals

The Joint Commission is also concerned with implementing strategies to enhance safety and annually updates targeted patient safety goals related to medication safety. Outlined below are two areas of particular interest to medication administration safety.

"Do Not Use" List of Unacceptable Abbreviations

Over the last 20 years, the Joint Commission has played a key role in driving expectations around the standardization of terminology, definitions, abbreviations, acronyms, symbols, and dose designations related to medication ordering and administration.

> **BOX 1.2** *Drug Therapy Through a Lens of Quality and Safety*
>
> The Quality and Safety Education for Nurses (QSEN) Competencies (Cronenwett et al., 2007) have been valuable tools for curriculum development and student evaluation that support quality and safety in nursing practice. The QSEN domains (patient-centered care, teamwork and collaboration, safety, evidence-based practice, quality improvement, and informatics) remain a foundation on which the American Association of Colleges of Nursing (AACN) established a new paradigm to promote optimal patient care delivery.
>
> Through a lens of quality and safety, this text's Quality and Safety Alert feature supports nurses in fostering a spirit of inquiry on which to reflect before they act, reflect during action, and reflect on action. This approach during drug therapy leads to questions that help nurses determine best practices and promotes a practice attitude of continuous improvement.
>
> To intentionally apply a quality and safety framework for drug administration, nurses must consider a person-centered care focus, collaborate in interprofessional partnerships, apply evidence-based standards related to drug therapy, participate in continuous quality and safety improvement, and incorporate informatics and healthcare technologies in planning and managing the pharmacology needs of their patients.

> **Quality and Safety Alert: Quality Improvement**
>
> The Joint Commission has developed and updated a standardized list of abbreviations, acronyms, dose designations, and symbols that are not to be used in a healthcare organization, commonly called the "Do Not Use" list (Information Management standard IM.02.02.01) of prohibited definitions.

Table 1.2 lists these terms. Other organizations, such as the Institute for Safe Medication Practices (ISMP), have also identified and published additional error-prone abbreviations.

Targeted High-Risk Activities

The Joint Commission also requires performance measures related to safety in drug administration. Specifically, a healthcare facility must demonstrate safe medication management using risk-reduction activities with medication labeling and use of anticoagulant medications.

In the perioperative area and other procedural settings, all medications must be labeled in syringes and basins if transferred from the original packaging. This practice focuses on an identified risk point in medication administration.

TABLE 1.2

Official "Do Not Use" List*

Do Not Use	Potential Problem	Use Instead
U, u (unit)	Mistaken for "0" (zero), the number "4" (four), or "cc"	Write "unit"
IU (International Unit)	Mistaken for IV (intravenous) or the number 10 (ten)	Write "International Unit"
Q.D., QD, q.d., qd (daily)	Mistaken for each other	Write "daily"
Q.O.D., QOD, q.o.d., qod (every other day)	Period after the Q mistaken for "I" and the "O" mistaken for "I"	Write "every other day"
Trailing zero (X.0 mg)† Lack of leading zero (.X mg)	Decimal point is missed	Write X mg Write 0.X mg
MS	Can mean morphine sulfate or magnesium sulfate	Write "morphine sulfate"
MSO$_4$ and MgSO$_4$	Confused with one another	Write "magnesium sulfate"

*This list applies to all orders and all medication-related documentation that is handwritten (including free-text computer entry) or on preprinted forms.

†**Exception:** A "trailing zero" may be used only where required to demonstrate the level of precision of the value being reported, such as for laboratory results, imaging studies that report size of lesions, or catheter/tube sizes. It may not be used in medication orders or other medication-related documentation.

© The Joint Commission, 2021. Reprinted with permission.

Healthcare institutions that provide anticoagulant therapy must establish a defined process that has a positive impact on patient safety with this class of medications (see Chapter 9) and leads to better outcomes. It is necessary to develop a process for anticoagulant use related to education, standardized ordering, dispensing, administration, and monitoring. Routine short-term use of anticoagulants for prevention of venous thromboembolism is not included as an element of performance when it is expected that the patient's laboratory values will remain within or close to normal limits with the therapy.

High-Alert Medications

The ISMP identifies drugs that when used in error have a heightened risk of causing significant patient harm.

Unfolding Patient Stories: Junetta Cooper • Part 1

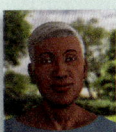

Junetta Cooper, a 75-year-old woman with chronic stable (exertional) angina pectoris secondary to coronary artery disease (CAD), is hospitalized. Junetta has had hypertension for 20 years that is well controlled with antihypertensives. Her morning medications include four oral medications, a transdermal patch, and an IV push medication. What measures can the nurse implement to prevent medication errors and ensure patient safety when preparing and administering these six medications? (Junetta Cooper's story continues in Chapter 26.)

Care for Junetta and other patients in a realistic virtual environment: *vSim for Nursing* (thepoint.lww.com/vSimPharm). Practice documenting these patients' care in DocuCare (thepoint.lww.com/DocuCareEHR).

Quality and Safety Alert: Technology

To reduce the chance of errors, strategies such as automatic alerts, automated dispensing devices, bar codes, computerized physician order entry, point of care drug resources, and standardizations of processes are important.

Box 1.3 lists drug classes and specific drugs that appear on the ISMP high-alert list.

Pregnancy Categories for Safety

As discussed in detail in Chapter 2, the Pregnancy and Lactation Labeling Rule in 2015 provided a new system that documents exposed known or potential maternal or fetal adverse reactions with individual drugs. This classification scheme replaced the A, B, C, D, and X pregnancy letter categories previously in use. The system has improved communication during counseling of people who are pregnant and lactating who need to take the medication. Providing the best available evidence on risks associated with drug exposure in pregnancy and lactation allows people to make better-informed and educated decisions for themselves and their children.

Beers Criteria for Potentially Inappropriate Medications Used in Older Adults

The American Geriatrics Society Beers Criteria, a list of medications that are generally considered best avoided generally in older adults and specifically in those with certain diseases, confirm that toxic medication effects and drug-related problems affect the safety of older adults. For a wide variety of reasons, the medications listed tend to cause adverse effects in this population and have been linked to poor health outcomes, including confusion, falls, and death. Further discussion of the Beers Criteria is found in Chapter 5.

BOX 1.3 — High-Alert Medications

Classes/Categories of Medications

Adrenergic agonists, IV (e.g., epinephrine, phenylephrine, norepinephrine)
Adrenergic antagonists, IV (e.g., propranolol, metoprolol, labetalol)
Anesthetic agents, general, inhaled, and IV (e.g., propofol, ketamine)
Antidysrhythmics, IV (e.g., lidocaine, amiodarone)
Antithrombotic agents (anticoagulants), including warfarin, low molecular weight heparin, IV unfractionated heparin, direct oral anticoagulants and factor Xa inhibitors (dabigatran rivaroxaban, apixaban, edoxaban, betrixaban, fondaparinux), direct thrombin inhibitors (e.g., argatroban, bivalirudin, dabigatran), thrombolytics (e.g., alteplase, reteplase, tenecteplase), and glycoprotein IIb/IIIa inhibitors (e.g., eptifibatide) cardioplegic solutions
Chemotherapeutic agents, parenteral and oral
Dextrose, hypertonic, 20% or greater
Dialysis solutions, peritoneal and hemodialysis
Epidural or intrathecal medications
Hypoglycemics, oral
Inotropic medications, IV (e.g., digoxin, milrinone)
Insulin, subcutaneous and IV
Liposomal forms of drugs (e.g., liposomal amphotericin B) and conventional counterparts (e.g., amphotericin B deoxycholate)
Moderate sedation agents, IV (e.g., dexmedetomidine, midazolam, lorazepam)
Moderate and minimal sedation agents, oral, for children (e.g., chloral hydrate, midazolam, ketamine [using the parenteral form])
Opiates, IV, transdermal, and oral (including liquid concentrates, immediate- and sustained-release formulations)
Neuromuscular blocking agents (e.g., succinylcholine, rocuronium, vecuronium)
Parenteral nutrition preparations
Sodium chloride for injection, hypertonic (greater than 0.9% concentration)
Sterile water for injection, inhalation, and irrigation (excluding pour bottles) in containers of 100 mL or more
Sulfonylurea hypoglycemics, oral (e.g., chloropropamide, glimepiride, glyburide, glipizide, tolbutamide)

Specific Medications

Epoprostenol (Flolan), IV
Insulin U-500 (special emphasis*)
Magnesium sulfate injection
Methotrexate, oral, nononcologic use
Opium tincture
Oxytocin, IV
Nitroprusside sodium for injection
Potassium chloride for injection concentrate
Potassium phosphate injection
Promethazine injection
Vasopressin, IV or intraosseous

*all forms of insulin, subQ, and IV are considered a class of high-alert medications. Insulin U-500 has been singled out for special emphasis to bring attention to the need for distinct strategies to prevent the types of errors that occur with this concentrated form of insulin

Reprinted with permission from the Institute for Safe Medication Practices (ISMP). (Copyright 2018). *ISMP's list of high-alert medications.* Retrieved November 7, 2021, from http://www.ismp.org/Tools/highalertmedications.pdf

NCLEX Success

5. Error-reduction strategies during medication administration include which of the following? (Select all that apply.)
   A. quiet zone signs at entrance to the medication room
   B. protocols and checklist outlining medication administration
   C. wearing a sash or vest to signal others to avoid interrupting the nurse during medication administration
   D. carrying several patients' prescanned medications on a tray
   E. educating staff to interrupt nurses administering medication only when they are in a patient's room

SOURCES OF DRUG INFORMATION

Sources of drug information include pharmacology and other textbooks, drug reference books, journal articles, point of care references, and internet websites. Textbooks provide information regarding groups of drugs in relation to therapeutic uses. Drug reference books and point of care referencing tools are most helpful concerning individual drugs. One authoritative source is Lippincott Advisor, which is a leading online evidence-based, nursing clinical decision support software at the point of care. The content in Lippincott Advisor supports compliance with current national guidelines, including those from the Agency for Healthcare Research and Quality and the American Association of Critical Care Nurses, and aligns with Joint Commission standards and components of the Magnet Recognition Program. A second authoritative source is *LexiComp Online*, reference handbooks, and desktop software by Wolters Kluwer, which are patient-centered drug references that provide drug content solutions to empower users to make the best possible evidence-based decision for each specific patient.

Numerous drug handbooks (e.g., *Nursing Drug Handbook*, published annually) and pharmacologic, medical, and nursing journals also contain information about drugs. Textbook chapters and journal articles often present information about drug therapy for patients with specific disease processes and may thereby facilitate application of drug knowledge in clinical practice.

Internet sites also contain drug information, but it is essential to assess their quality. A wide variety of information, ranging in accuracy, reliability, and value, is easily accessible.

Additionally, point of care clinical support references, such as UpToDate, provide quick access to drug information that supports evidence-based decision-making regarding drug therapy.

> Visit **thePoint** at http://thePoint.lww.com/Frandsen13e for answers to NCLEX Success questions (in Appendix A), answers to Clinical Application Case Studies (in Appendix B), and more!

Clinical Application 1.2

Ms. Clark also reviews additional strategies to promote the system safety in the administration of drugs at the point of care.
- What systemic issues in a hospital or nursing home have an impact on safe medication administration?
- What can the nurse do to avoid medication errors while dispensing medications?

STRATEGIES FOR STUDYING PHARMACOLOGY

- Concentrate on therapeutic classifications and their prototypes. For example, morphine is the prototype of opioid analgesics (see Chapter 49). Understanding morphine makes learning about other opioid analgesics easier because they are compared with morphine.
- Compare a newly encountered drug with a prototype or similar drug when possible. Relating the unknown to the known aids learning and retention of knowledge.
- Try to understand how the drug acts in the body. This understanding allows prediction of therapeutic effects and prediction, prevention, or minimization of adverse effects by early detection and treatment.
- Concentrate study efforts on major characteristics. Such characteristics include the main indications for use, common and potentially serious adverse effects, conditions in which the drug is contraindicated or must be used cautiously, and related nursing care needs.
- Keep an authoritative, up-to-date drug reference readily available. A drug reference is a more reliable source of drug information than memory, especially for dosage ranges. Use the reference freely when learning about an unfamiliar drug or when answering a question about a familiar one. Also, nurses have access to computerized databases of drug information through multiple electronic sources, and these can provide a ready source of up-to-date information.
- Use your own words when taking notes or writing drug information cards. Also, write notes, answers to review questions, definitions of new terms, and trade names of drugs encountered in clinical practice settings directly into your pharmacology textbook. The mental processing required for these activities helps in both initial learning and later retention and application of knowledge.
- Rehearse applying drug knowledge in nursing care by asking yourself, "What if I have a patient who is receiving this drug? What must I do to safely administer the drug? For what must I assess the patient before giving the drug, and for what must I observe in the patient after drug administration? What if my patient is an older adult or a child?"

REFERENCES AND RESOURCES

Ahmad, F. B., Rossen, L. M., & Sutton, P. (2021). *Provisional drug overdose death counts*. National Center for Health Statistics.

Alemar, D. (2021). *Utilizing the QSEN framework to redesign nursing orientation competencies*. Retrieved November 1, 2021, from https://qsen.org/utilizing-the-qsen-framework-to-redesign-nursing-orientation-competencies/

American Geriatrics Society. (2019). American Geriatrics Society 2019 updated AGS Beers criteria for potentially inappropriate medication use in older adults. *Journal of the American Geriatrics Society, 67*(4), 674–694. doi:10.1111/jgs.15767

Cronenwett, L., Sherwood, G., Barnsteiner, J., Disch, J., Johnson, J., Mitchell, P., Sullivan, D. T., & Warren, J. (2007). Quality and safety education for nurses. *Nursing Outlook, 55*(3), 122–131.

DiPiro, J., Yee, G. C., Posey, L. M., Haines, S. T., Nolin, T. D., & Ellingrod, V. (Eds.). (2020). *Pharmacotherapy: A pathophysiologic approach* (11th ed.). McGraw-Hill.

Hyatt, J. M., & Lobmaier, P. P. (2020). Medication assisted treatment (MAT) in criminal justice settings as a double-edged sword: Balancing novel addiction treatments and voluntary participation. *Health Justice, 8*, 7. https://doi.org/10.1186/s40352-020-0106-9

Institute for Safe Medication Practices. http://www.ismp.org

Institute of Medicine Committee on Quality of Health Care in America; Kohn, L. T., Corrigan, J. M., & Donaldson, M. S. (Eds.). (2000). *To err is human: Building a safer health system*. National Academies Press. doi:10.17226/9728

Institute of Medicine. (2003). *Health professions education: A bridge to quality*. National Academies Press.

Institute of Medicine. (2006). *Future of drug safety: Promoting and protecting the health of the public*. National Academies Press.

Institute of Medicine. (2007). *Preventing medication errors*. National Academies Press.

Larmené-Beld, K. H. M., Alting, E. K., & Taxis, K. (2018). A systematic literature review on strategies to avoid look-alike errors of labels. *European Journal of Clinical Pharmacology, 74*(8), 985–993. http://doi.org/10.1007/s00228-018-2471

Madden, E. F. (2019). Intervention stigma: How medication-assisted treatment marginalizes patients and providers. *Social Science & Medicine, 232*, 324–331. https://doi.org/10.1016/j.socscimed.2019.05.027

Pfeiffer, Y., Zimmermann C., & Schwappach, D.L.B. (2020). What are we doing when we double check? *BMJ Quality & Safety*. 29, 36-40. doi:10.1136/bmjqs-2019-009680.

Quality and Safety Education for Nurses (QSEN). http://www.qsen.org

QSEN Institute. (2013). *Competencies*. Retrieved November 8, 2021, from http://qsen.org/competencies/

Rodziewicz, T. L., Houseman, B., & Hipskind, J. E. (2022). Medical error reduction and prevention. In *StatPearls*. StatPearls Publishing

Scott, I. A., Pillans, P. I., Barras, M., & Morris, C. (2018). Using EMR-enabled computerized decision support systems to reduce prescribing of potentially inappropriate medications: A narrative review. *Therapeutic Advances in Drug Safety, 9*(9), 559–573. http://doi.org/10.1177/2042098618784809

The Joint Commission. (2022). *National patient safety goals*. Retrieved November 11, 2021, from https://www.jointcommission.org/-/media/tjc/documents/standards/national-patient-safety-goals/2022/npsg_chapter_hap_jan2022.pdf

U.S. Food and Drug Administration. *Frequently asked questions*. Retrieved November 5, 2021, from http://www.fda.gov/ForIndustry/FDABasicsforIndustry/ucm234634.htm

CHAPTER 2

Basic Concepts and Processes

LEARNING OBJECTIVES

After studying this chapter, you should be able to:

1. Describe the main pathways and mechanisms by which drugs cross biologic membranes and move through the body.
2. Explain each process of pharmacokinetics.
3. Recognize individual differences in patient drug responses related to genomic variations.
4. Discuss the clinical usefulness of measuring serum drug levels.
5. Describe major characteristics of the receptor theory of drug action.
6. Differentiate between agonist drugs and antagonist drugs.
7. Discuss mechanisms and potential effects of drug–drug interactions.
8. Explain drug-related and patient-related variables that affect drug actions.
9. Identify signs and symptoms that may occur with adverse drug effects on major body systems.
10. Discuss initial management considerations related to drug overdose and toxicity.
11. Discuss selected drug antidotes.

CLINICAL APPLICATION CASE STUDY

Doris Green, an 89-year-old widow with cardiovascular and kidney disease, takes a number of medications, including three medications to control her hypertension. She has recently switched to a new antihypertensive medication. She prides herself on being independent and able to manage on her own, despite failing memory and failing health.

You, as a home health nurse, visit Mrs. Green to assess the therapeutic and adverse effects of her antihypertensive medications and her adherence to the prescribed medical regimen. You plan to measure her blood pressure to check that it is within normal limits (for Mrs. Green), as well as assess her understanding of her antihypertensive medications and dosing regimen.

KEY TERMS

Absorption: process that occurs from the time a drug enters the body to the time it enters the bloodstream to be circulated

Agonist: drug that produces effects similar to those produced by naturally occurring hormones, neurotransmitters, and other substances

Antagonist: drug that inhibits cell function by occupying receptor sites

Antidote: substance that relieves, prevents, or counteracts the effect of a poison

Bioavailability: portion of a drug dose that reaches the systemic circulation and is available to act on body cells

Biotransformation: when drugs are altered from their original form into a new form by the body; also referred to as metabolism

Distribution: transport of drug molecules within the body; after a drug is injected or absorbed into the bloodstream, it is carried by the blood and tissue fluids to its sites of action, metabolism, and excretion

Enterohepatic recirculation: drugs or metabolites that are excreted in bile, reabsorbed from the small intestine, returned to the liver, metabolized, and eventually excreted in urine

Enzyme induction: production of larger amounts of drug-metabolizing enzymes by liver cells; process accelerates drug metabolism because larger amounts of the enzymes (and more binding sites) allow larger amounts of a drug to be metabolized during a given time

Enzyme inhibition: process in which a molecule binds to enzymes and inhibits their activity

Excretion: elimination of a drug from the body; effective excretion requires adequate functioning of the circulatory system and of the organs of excretion (kidneys, bowel, lungs, and skin)

First-pass effect: initial metabolism of some oral drugs as they are carried from the intestine to the liver by the portal circulatory system prior to reaching the systemic circulation for distribution to site of action

Hypersensitivity: immune-mediated reaction to a drug

Loading dose: dose larger than the regular prescribed daily dosage of a medication; used to attain a therapeutic blood level

Maintenance dose: quantity of drug that is needed to keep blood levels and/or tissue levels at a steady state or constant level

Nephrotoxicity: toxic or damaging effect of a substance on the kidney; potentially serious because kidney damage interferes with drug excretion, causing drug accumulation and increased adverse effects

Pharmacodynamics: reactions between living systems and drugs; drug actions on target cells and the resulting alterations in cellular biochemical reactions and functions

Pharmacogenomics (also known as pharmacogenetics): the study of how a person's genetic heritage leads to variable responses to drugs; more generally refers to genetic polymorphisms that occur in a patient population, such as an ethnic group, as opposed to an individual person

Pharmacokinetics: drug movement through the body to reach sites of action, metabolism, and excretion

Polymorphism: the occurrence of two or more clearly different forms (or phenotypes) in a species important in drug therapy because it explains the functionally different response to drugs in a general patient population or a specific individual or group

Prodrugs: initially inactive drugs that exert no pharmacologic effects until they are metabolized

Serum drug level: laboratory measurement of the amount of a drug in the blood at a particular time

Serum half-life: time required for the serum concentration of a drug to decrease by 50%; also called elimination half-life

INTRODUCTION

All body functions, all disease processes, and most drug actions occur at the cellular level. Drugs are chemicals that alter basic processes in body cells. They can stimulate or inhibit normal cellular functions; however, they cannot change the type of function that occurs normally. To act on body cells, drugs given for systemic effects must reach adequate concentrations in the blood and other tissue fluids surrounding the cells. Thus, they must enter the body and be circulated to their sites of action (target cells). After they act on cells, they must be eliminated from the body.

How do systemic drugs reach, interact with, and leave body cells? How do people respond to drugs? The answers to these questions are derived from cellular physiology, pathways, and mechanisms of drug transport, pharmacokinetics, pharmacodynamics, pharmacogenomics, and other basic concepts and processes that form the foundation of rational drug therapy and the content of this chapter.

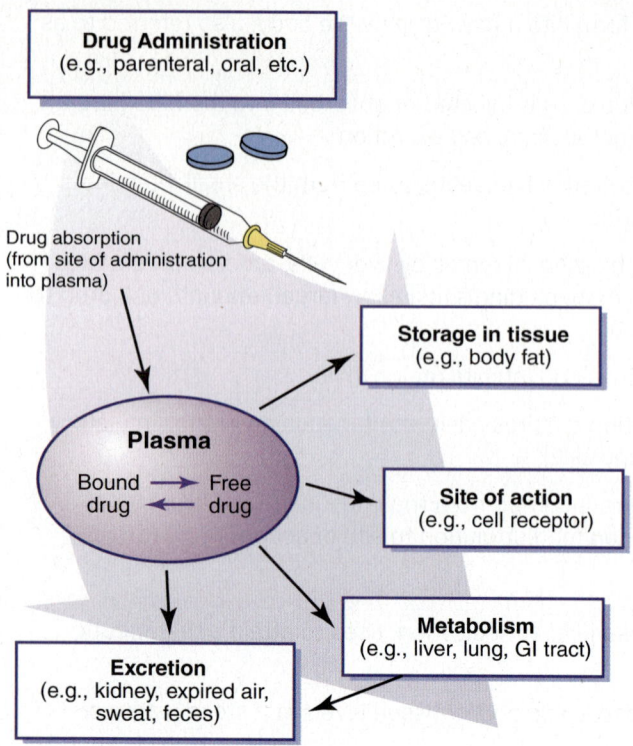

Figure 2.1. Entry and movement of drug molecules through the body to sites of action, metabolism, and excretion.

DRUG TRANSPORT THROUGH CELL MEMBRANES

Drugs must reach and interact with or cross the cell membrane to stimulate or inhibit cellular function. Unlike local effects of drugs that act at the site of contact, most drugs are given to affect body cells that are distant from sites of administration, causing systemic effects. To move through the body and reach their sites of action, metabolism, and excretion (Fig. 2.1), drug molecules must cross numerous cell membranes. For example, molecules of most oral drugs must cross the membranes of cells in the gastrointestinal (GI) tract, liver, and capillaries to reach the bloodstream, circulate to their target cells, leave the bloodstream and attach to receptors on cells, perform their action, return to the bloodstream, circulate to the liver, reach drug-metabolizing enzymes in liver cells, reenter the bloodstream (usually as metabolites), circulate to the kidneys, and be excreted in urine. Box 2.1 and Figure 2.2 describe the transport pathways and mechanisms used to move drug molecules through the body.

PHARMACOKINETICS

Pharmacokinetics involves drug movement through the body (i.e., "what the body does to the drug") to reach sites of action, metabolism, and excretion. Specific processes are absorption, distribution, metabolism, and excretion. Metabolism and excretion are often grouped together as drug elimination or clearance mechanisms. Overall, these processes largely determine serum drug levels; onset, peak, and duration of drug actions; therapeutic and adverse effects; and other important aspects of drug therapy.

Absorption

Absorption is the process that occurs from the time a drug enters the body to the time it enters the bloodstream to be circulated. Onset of drug action is largely determined by the rate of absorption; intensity is determined by the extent of absorption. Numerous factors affect the rate and extent of drug absorption, including dosage form, route of administration, blood flow to the site of administration, GI function, the presence of food or other drugs, and other variables. Dosage form is a major determinant of a drug's **bioavailability** (the portion of a dose

---

BOX 2.1 — Drug Transport Pathways and Mechanisms

Pathways

There are three main pathways of drug movement across cell membranes. The most common pathway is direct penetration of the membrane by lipid-soluble drugs, which are able to dissolve in the lipid layer of the cell membrane. Most systemic drugs are formulated to be lipid soluble, so they can move through cell membranes, even oral tablets and capsules that must be sufficiently water soluble to dissolve in the aqueous fluids of the stomach and small intestine.

A second pathway involves passage through protein channels that go all the way through the cell membrane. Only a few drugs are able to use this pathway because most drug molecules are too large to pass through the small channels. Small ions (e.g., sodium and potassium) use this pathway, but their movement is regulated by specific channels with a gating mechanism (a flap of protein that opens briefly to allow ion movement and then closes).

The third pathway involves carrier proteins that transport molecules from one side of the cell membrane to the other. All of the carrier proteins are selective in the substances they transport; a drug's chemical structure determines which carrier will transport it.

Mechanisms

Once absorbed into the body, drugs are transported to and from target cells by passive diffusion, facilitated diffusion, and active transport.

Passive diffusion, the most common mechanism, involves movement of a drug from an area of higher concentration to one of lower concentration. For example, after oral administration, the initial concentration of a drug is higher in the GI tract than in the blood. This promotes movement of the drug into the bloodstream. When the drug is circulated, the concentration is higher in the blood than in body cells, so that the drug moves (from capillaries) into the fluids surrounding the cells or into the cells themselves. Passive diffusion continues until a state of equilibrium is reached between the amount of drug in the tissues and the amount in the blood.

Facilitated diffusion is a similar process, except that drug molecules combine with a carrier substance, such as an enzyme or other protein.

In active transport, drug molecules are moved from an area of lower concentration to one of higher concentration. This process requires a carrier substance and the release of cellular energy.

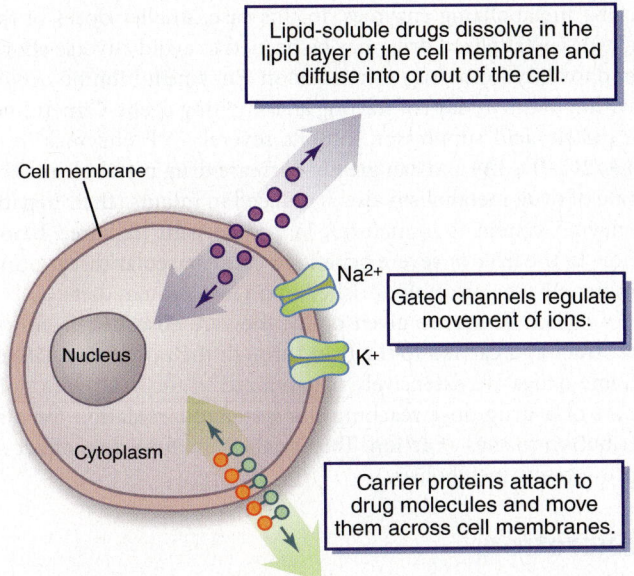

Figure 2.2. Drug transport pathways. Drug molecules cross cell membranes to move into and out of body cells by directly penetrating the lipid layer, diffusing through open or gated channels, or attaching to carrier proteins.

Distribution

Distribution involves the transport of drug molecules within the body. After a drug is injected or absorbed into the bloodstream, it is carried by the blood and tissue fluids to its sites of action, metabolism, and excretion. Most drug molecules enter and leave the bloodstream at the capillary level, through gaps between the cells that form capillary walls. Distribution depends largely on the adequacy of blood circulation. Drugs are distributed rapidly to organs receiving a large blood supply, such as the heart, liver, and kidneys. Distribution to other internal organs, muscle, fat, and skin is usually slower.

Protein binding is an important factor in drug distribution (Fig. 2.3). Most drugs form a compound with plasma proteins, mainly albumin, which act as carriers. Drug molecules bound to plasma proteins are pharmacologically inactive because the large size of the complex prevents their leaving the bloodstream through the small openings in capillary walls and reaching their sites of action, metabolism, and excretion. Only the free or unbound portion of a drug acts on body cells. As the free drug acts on cells, the decrease in plasma drug levels causes some of the bound drug to be released.

Protein binding allows part of a drug dose to be stored and released as needed. Some drugs also are stored in muscle, fat, or other body tissues and released gradually when plasma drug levels fall. These storage mechanisms maintain lower, more consistent blood levels and reduce the risk of toxicity. Drugs that are highly bound to plasma proteins or stored extensively in other tissues have a long duration of action.

Drug distribution into the central nervous system (CNS) is limited because the blood–brain barrier, which is composed of capillaries with tight walls, limits movement of drug molecules into brain tissue. This barrier usually acts as a selectively permeable membrane to protect the CNS. However, it also can make drug therapy for CNS disorders more difficult because drugs must pass through cells of the capillary wall rather than between cells. As a result, only drugs that are lipid soluble or have a transport system can cross the blood–brain barrier and reach therapeutic concentrations in brain tissue.

Drug distribution during pregnancy and lactation is also an important consideration (see Chapter 6). During pregnancy,

that reaches the systemic circulation and is available to act on body cells). An intravenous (IV) drug is virtually 100% bioavailable. In contrast, an oral drug is virtually always less than 100% bioavailable because some of it is not absorbed from the GI tract and some goes to the liver and is partially metabolized before reaching the systemic circulation.

Most oral drugs must be swallowed, dissolved in gastric fluid, and delivered to the small intestine (which has a large surface area for absorption of nutrients and drugs) before they are absorbed. Liquid medications are absorbed faster than are tablets or capsules because they need not be dissolved. Rapid movement through the stomach and small intestine may increase drug absorption by promoting contact with absorptive mucous membrane; it also may decrease absorption because some drugs may move through the small intestine too rapidly to be absorbed. For many drugs, the presence of food in the stomach slows the rate of absorption and may decrease the amount of drug absorbed.

Drugs injected into subcutaneous or intramuscular (IM) tissues are usually absorbed more rapidly than are oral drugs because they move directly from the injection site to the bloodstream. Absorption is rapid from IM sites because muscle tissue has an abundant blood supply. Drugs injected intravenously do not need to be absorbed because they are placed directly into the bloodstream.

Other absorptive sites include the skin, mucous membranes, and lungs. Most drugs applied to the skin are given for local effects (e.g., sunscreens). Systemic absorption is minimal from intact skin but may be considerable when the skin is inflamed or damaged. Also, some drugs are formulated in adhesive skin patches for absorption through the skin (e.g., clonidine, fentanyl, nitroglycerin). Some drugs applied to mucous membranes also are given for local effects. However, systemic absorption occurs from the mucosa of the oral cavity, nose, eye, vagina, and rectum. Drugs absorbed through mucous membranes pass directly into the bloodstream. The lungs have a large surface area for absorption of anesthetic gases and a few other drugs.

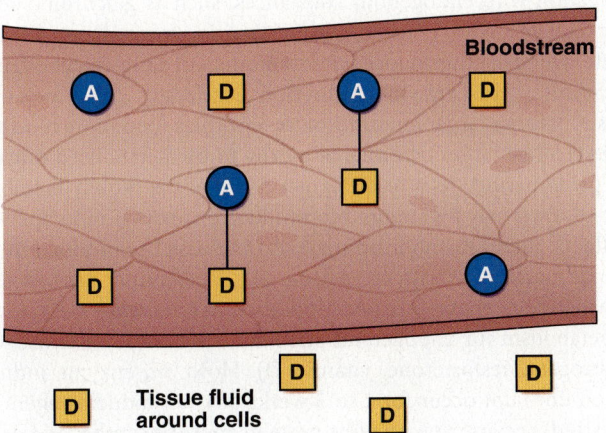

Figure 2.3. Plasma proteins, mainly albumin (A), act as carriers for drug molecules (D). Bound drug (A–D) stays in the bloodstream and is pharmacologically inactive. Free drug (D) can leave the bloodstream and act on body cells.

most drugs cross the placenta and may affect the fetus. During lactation, many drugs enter breast milk and may affect the nursing infant.

Metabolism

Metabolism, or **biotransformation**, is the method by which drugs are altered from their original form into a new form (biotransformed) by the body. Most often, an active drug is changed into inactive metabolites, which are then excreted. Some active drugs yield metabolites that are also active and that continue to exert their effects on body cells until they are metabolized further or excreted. Other drugs (called **prodrugs**) are initially inactive and exert no pharmacologic effects until they are metabolized. Most drugs are lipid soluble, a characteristic that aids their movement across cell membranes. However, the kidneys can excrete only water-soluble substances. Therefore, one function of metabolism is to convert fat-soluble drugs into water-soluble metabolites. Hepatic drug metabolism or clearance is a major mechanism for terminating drug action and eliminating drug molecules from the body. A genetic **polymorphism** is the occurrence of two or more clearly different forms (or phenotypes) in a species that influence metabolism by producing functionally different responses to drugs in ethnic groups or specific individuals compared to the general population.

Cytochrome P450 (CYP) enzymes in the liver metabolize most drugs. Red blood cells, plasma, kidneys, lungs, and GI mucosa also contain drug-metabolizing enzymes. The CYP system consists of several groups of enzymes, some of which metabolize endogenous substances and some of which metabolize drugs. The drug-metabolizing groups are labeled CYP1, CYP2, and CYP3. Individual members of the groups usually metabolize specific drugs; more than one enzyme participates in the metabolism of some drugs. In terms of importance in drug metabolism, the CYP3A4 enzymes are thought to metabolize about 50% of drugs; CYP2D6 enzymes about 25%; CYP2C8/9 about 15%; and CYP1A2, CYP2C19, CYP2A6, and CYP2E1 in decreasing order for the remaining 10%.

CYP enzymes are complex proteins with binding sites for drug molecules (and endogenous substances). They catalyze the chemical reactions of oxidation, reduction, hydrolysis, and conjugation with endogenous substances, such as glucuronic acid or sulfate. With chronic administration, some drugs stimulate liver cells to produce larger amounts of drug-metabolizing enzymes. This **enzyme induction** accelerates drug metabolism because larger amounts of the enzymes (and more binding sites) allow larger amounts of a drug to be metabolized during a given period. As a result, larger doses of the rapidly metabolized drug may be required to produce or maintain therapeutic effects. Rapid metabolism may also increase the production of toxic metabolites with some drugs (e.g., acetaminophen). Drugs that induce enzyme production also may increase the rate of metabolism for endogenous steroidal hormones (e.g., cortisol, estrogens, testosterone, vitamin D). However, enzyme induction does not occur for 1 to 3 weeks after an inducing agent is started, because new enzyme proteins must be synthesized.

Metabolism also can be decreased or delayed in a process called **enzyme inhibition**, in which a molecule binds to enzymes and inhibits their activity, which most often occurs with concurrent administration of two or more drugs that compete for the same metabolizing enzymes. In this case, smaller doses of the slowly metabolized drug may be needed to avoid adverse effects and toxicity from drug accumulation. Enzyme inhibition occurs within hours or days of starting an inhibiting agent. Cimetidine, a gastric acid suppressor, inhibits several CYP enzymes (e.g., 1A, 2C, 2D, 3A) and can greatly decrease drug metabolism. The rate of drug metabolism also is reduced in infants (their hepatic enzyme system is immature), in people with impaired blood flow to the liver or severe hepatic or cardiovascular disease, and in people who are malnourished or on low-protein diets.

When drugs are given orally, they are absorbed from the GI tract and carried to the liver through the portal circulation. Some drugs are extensively metabolized in the liver, with only part of a drug dose reaching the systemic circulation for distribution to sites of action. This is called the **first-pass effect** or presystemic metabolism.

Excretion

Excretion refers to elimination of a drug from the body. Effective excretion requires adequate functioning of the circulatory system and of the organs of excretion (kidneys, bowel, lungs, and skin). Most drugs are excreted by the kidneys and eliminated (unchanged or as metabolites) in the urine. Some drugs or metabolites are excreted in bile and then eliminated in feces; others are excreted in bile, reabsorbed from the small intestine, returned to the liver (called **enterohepatic recirculation**), metabolized, and eventually excreted in urine. Some oral drugs are not absorbed and are excreted in the feces. The lungs mainly remove volatile substances, such as anesthetic gases. The skin has minimal excretory function. Factors impairing excretion, especially severe kidney disease, lead to accumulation of numerous drugs and may cause severe adverse effects if dosage is not reduced.

NCLEX Success

1. A nurse practitioner (NP) has just changed a patient's medication from an oral form to a patch formulation to avoid the first-pass effect. The NP has explained it to the patient, but the patient still has questions and asks the nurse to explain again what is meant by the first-pass effect. The nurse would be most correct in explaining that this has to do with how
   A. drugs initially bind to plasma proteins
   B. initial kidney function is involved in drug excretion
   C. the drugs first reach their target cells
   D. initial metabolism of an oral drug occurs before it reaches the systemic circulation

2. A nurse is caring for a patient who has worsening liver disease. In monitoring their medication, it is important to know that a patient with liver disease may have impaired drug
   A. absorption
   B. distribution
   C. metabolism
   D. excretion

Serum Drug Levels

A **serum drug level** is a laboratory measurement of the amount of a drug in the blood at a particular time (Fig. 2.4). It reflects dosage, absorption, bioavailability, half-life, and the rates of metabolism and excretion. A minimum effective concentration (MEC) must be present before a drug exerts its pharmacologic action on body cells; this is largely determined by the drug dose and how well it is absorbed into the bloodstream. A toxic concentration is a level at which toxicity occurs; what is toxic for some patients is not toxic for others (see subsequent discussion). Toxic concentrations may stem from a single large dose, repeated small doses, or slow metabolism that allows the drug to accumulate in the body. Between these low and high concentrations is the therapeutic range, which is the goal of drug therapy—that is, enough drug to be beneficial but not enough to be toxic.

For most drugs, serum levels indicate the onset, peak, and duration of drug action. When a single dose of a drug is given, onset of action occurs when the drug level reaches the MEC. The drug level continues to climb as more of the drug is absorbed, until it reaches its highest concentration and peak drug action occurs. Then, drug levels decline as the drug is eliminated (i.e., metabolized and excreted) from the body. Although there may still be numerous drug molecules in the body, drug action stops when drug levels fall below the MEC. The duration of action is the time during which serum drug levels are at or above the MEC. When multiple doses of a drug are given (e.g., for chronic conditions), the goal is usually to give sufficient doses often enough to maintain serum drug levels in the therapeutic range and avoid the toxic range.

In clinical practice, measuring serum drug levels is useful in several circumstances:

- When drugs with a narrow margin of safety are given, because there is a small difference between their therapeutic and toxic doses (e.g., warfarin, gentamycin, lithium)
- To document the serum drug levels associated with particular drug dosages, therapeutic effects, or possible adverse effects
- To monitor unexpected responses to a drug dose such as decreased therapeutic effects or increased adverse effects
- When a drug overdose is suspected

Serum Half-Life

Serum half-life, also called elimination half-life, is the time required for the serum concentration of a drug to decrease by 50%. It is determined primarily by the drug's rates of metabolism and excretion. A drug with a short half-life requires more frequent administration than one with a long half-life.

When a drug is given at a stable dose, four or five half-lives are required to achieve steady-state concentrations and to develop equilibrium between tissue and serum concentrations. Because maximal therapeutic effects do not occur until equilibrium is established, some drugs are not fully effective for days or weeks. To maintain steady-state conditions, the amount of drug given must equal the amount eliminated from the body. When a drug dose is changed, an additional four to five half-lives are required to reestablish equilibrium; when a drug is discontinued, it is eliminated gradually over several half-lives.

PHARMACODYNAMICS

Pharmacodynamics involves drug actions on target cells and the resulting alterations in cellular biochemical reactions and functions (i.e., "what the drug does to the body").

Receptor Theory of Drug Action

Like the physiologic substances (e.g., hormones, neurotransmitters) that normally regulate cell functions, most drugs exert their effects by chemically binding with receptors at the cellular level (Fig. 2.5). Most receptors are proteins located on the surfaces of cell membranes or within cells. Specific receptors include enzymes involved in essential metabolic or regulatory processes (e.g., dihydrofolate reductase, acetylcholinesterase); proteins involved in transport (e.g., sodium–potassium adenosine triphosphatase) or structural processes (e.g., tubulin); and nucleic acids (e.g., DNA) involved in cellular protein synthesis, reproduction, and other metabolic activities.

When drug molecules bind with receptor molecules, the resulting drug–receptor complex initiates physiochemical reactions that stimulate or inhibit normal cellular functions. One type of reaction involves activation, inactivation, or other alterations of intracellular enzymes. Because enzymes catalyze almost all cellular functions, drug-induced changes can markedly increase or decrease the rate of cellular metabolism.

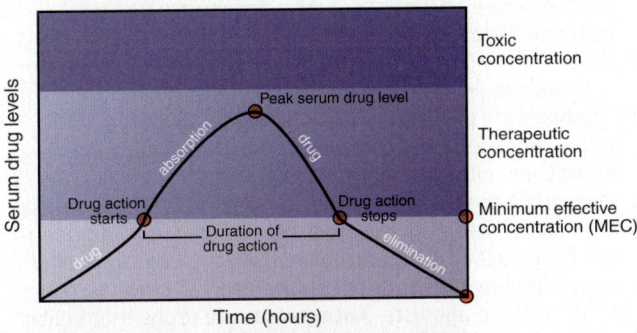

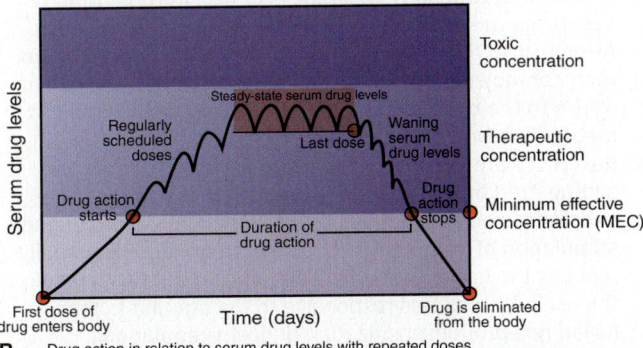

Figure 2.4. Serum drug levels with single **(A)** and multiple **(B)** oral drug doses. Drug action starts when enough drug is absorbed to reach the minimum effective concentration (MEC), continues as long as the serum level is above the MEC, wanes as drug molecules are metabolized and excreted (if no more doses are given), and stops when the serum level drops below the MEC. The goal of drug therapy is to maintain serum drug levels in the therapeutic range.

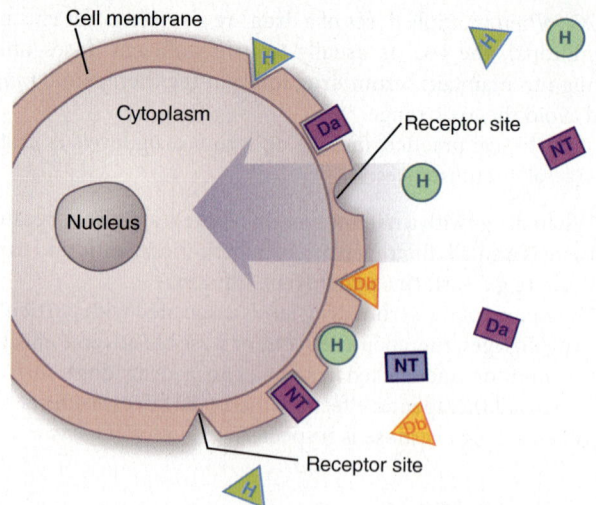

Figure 2.5. Cell membrane contains receptors for physiologic substances such as hormones (*H*) and neurotransmitters (*NT*). These substances stimulate or inhibit cellular function. Drug molecules (*Da* and *Db*) also interact with receptors to stimulate or inhibit cellular function.

For example, an epinephrine–receptor complex increases the activity of the intracellular enzyme adenylyl cyclase, which then causes the formation of cyclic adenosine monophosphate (cAMP). In turn, cAMP can initiate any one of many different intracellular actions, the exact effect depending on the type of cell.

A second type of reaction involves changes in the permeability of cell membranes to one or more ions. The receptor protein is a structural component of the cell membrane, and its binding to a drug molecule may open or close ion channels. In nerve cells, for example, sodium or calcium ion channels may open and allow movement of ions into the cell. This movement usually causes the cell membrane to depolarize and excite the cell. At other times, potassium channels may open and allow movement of potassium ions out of the cell. This action inhibits neuronal excitability and function. In muscle cells, movement of the ions into the cells may alter intracellular functions, such as the direct effect of calcium ions in stimulating muscle contraction.

A third reaction may modify the synthesis, release, or inactivation of the neurohormones (e.g., acetylcholine, norepinephrine, serotonin) that regulate many physiologic processes. Box 2.2 describes additional elements and characteristics of the receptor theory.

BOX 2.2 Additional Elements of the Receptor Theory of Drug Action

- The site and extent of drug action on body cells are determined primarily by specific characteristics of receptors and drugs. Receptors vary in type, location, number, and functional capacity.
- Most types of receptors occur in most body tissues, such as receptors for epinephrine and receptors for growth hormone, thyroid hormone, and insulin. Some occur in limited body tissues, such as receptors for opioids in the brain and subgroups of receptors for epinephrine in the heart (beta$_1$-adrenergic receptors) and lungs (beta$_2$-adrenergic receptors).
- Receptor type and location influence drug action. The receptor is often described as a lock into which the drug molecule fits as a key, and only those drugs able to bond chemically to the receptors in a particular body tissue can exert pharmacologic effects on that tissue. Thus, all body cells do not respond to all drugs.
- The number of receptor sites available to interact with drug molecules also affects the extent of drug action. Drug molecules must occupy a minimal number of receptors to produce pharmacologic effects. Thus, if many receptors are available but only a few are occupied by drug molecules, few drug effects occur. In this instance, increasing the drug dosage increases the pharmacologic effects. Conversely, if only a few receptors are available for many drug molecules, receptors may be saturated. In this instance, if most receptor sites are occupied, increasing the drug dosage produces no additional pharmacologic effect.
- Drugs vary even more widely than receptors. Because all drugs are chemical substances, chemical characteristics determine drug actions and pharmacologic effects. For example, a drug's chemical structure affects its ability to reach tissue fluids around a cell and bind with its cell receptors. Minor changes in drug structure may produce major changes in pharmacologic effects. Another major factor is the concentration of drug molecules that reach receptor sites in body tissues. Drug-related and patient-related variables that affect drug actions are further described later in this chapter.
- When drug molecules chemically bind with cell receptors, pharmacologic effects result from agonism or antagonism. **Agonists** are drugs that produce effects similar to those produced by naturally occurring hormones, neurotransmitters, and other substances. Agonists may accelerate or slow normal cellular processes, depending on the type of receptor activated. For example, epinephrine-like drugs act on the heart to increase the heart rate, and acetylcholine-like drugs act on the heart to slow the heart rate; both are agonists. **Antagonists** are drugs that inhibit cell function by occupying receptor sites. This strategy prevents natural body substances or other drugs from occupying the receptor sites and activating cell functions. After drug action occurs, drug molecules may detach from receptor molecules (i.e., the chemical binding is reversible), return to the bloodstream, and circulate to the liver for metabolism and the kidneys for excretion.
- Receptors are dynamic cellular components that can be synthesized by body cells and altered by endogenous substances and exogenous drugs. For example, prolonged stimulation of body cells with an excitatory agonist usually reduces the number or sensitivity of receptors. As a result, the cell becomes less responsive to the **agonist** (a process called receptor desensitization or down-regulation). Prolonged inhibition of normal cellular functions with an antagonist may increase receptor number or sensitivity. If the antagonist is suddenly reduced or stopped, the cell becomes excessively responsive to an agonist (a process called receptor up-regulation). These changes in receptors may explain why some drugs must be tapered in dosage and discontinued gradually if withdrawal symptoms are to be avoided.

Nonreceptor Drug Actions

Relatively few drugs act by mechanisms other than combination with receptor sites on cells. Drugs that do not act on receptor sites include the following:

- Antacids, which act chemically to neutralize the hydrochloric acid produced by gastric parietal cells and thereby raise the pH of gastric fluid.
- Osmotic diuretics (e.g., mannitol), which increase the osmolarity of plasma and pull water out of tissues into the bloodstream.
- Drugs that are structurally similar to nutrients required by body cells (e.g., purines, pyrimidines) and that can be incorporated into cellular constituents, such as nucleic acids, which interfere with normal cell functioning. Several anticancer drugs act by this mechanism.
- Metal chelating agents, which combine with toxic metals to form a complex that can be more readily excreted.

VARIABLES THAT AFFECT DRUG ACTIONS

Historically, expected responses to drugs were based on those occurring when a particular drug was given to healthy adult males (18 to 65 years of age) of average weight (150 lb [70 kg]). However, other groups (e.g., females, children, older adults, different ethnic or racial groups, patients with diseases or symptoms that the drugs are designed to treat) receive drugs and respond differently from healthy adult males. As a result, newer clinical trials include more representatives of these groups. In any patient, however, responses may be altered by both drug-related and patient-related variables.

Drug-Related Variables

Dosage

Dosage refers to the frequency, size, and number of doses; it is a major determinant of drug actions and responses, both therapeutic and adverse. If the amount is too small or administered infrequently, no pharmacologic action occurs because the drug does not reach an adequate concentration at target cells. If the amount is too large or administered too often, toxicity (poisoning) may occur. Overdosage may occur with a single large dose or with chronic ingestion of smaller doses.

Dosages recommended in drug literature are usually those that produce particular responses in 50% of the people tested. These dosages usually produce a mixture of therapeutic and adverse effects. The dosage of a particular drug depends on many characteristics of the drug (reason for use, potency, pharmacokinetics, route of administration, dosage form, and so on) and of the recipient (age; weight; state of health; and function of cardiovascular, kidney, and hepatic systems). Thus, recommended dosages are intended only as guidelines for individualizing dosages.

Even if the recommended dose controls a patient's symptoms, they may need a special **loading dose** at the beginning of drug therapy. This dose, which is larger than the regular prescribed daily dosage of a medication, is used to attain a more rapid therapeutic blood level of the drug. After the patient has been taking the drug for a few days, a **maintenance dose**, or quantity of drug that is needed to keep blood levels and/or tissue levels at a steady state, or constant level, is usually sufficient.

Route of Administration

Routes of administration affect drug actions and patient responses largely by influencing absorption and distribution. For rapid drug action and response, the IV route is most effective because the drug is injected directly into the bloodstream. For some drugs, the IM route also produces drug action within a few minutes because muscles have a large blood supply. The oral route usually produces slower drug action than parenteral routes. Absorption and action of topical drugs vary according to the drug formulation, whether the drug is applied to the skin or mucous membranes, and other factors.

Drug–Diet Interactions

A few drugs are used therapeutically to decrease food absorption in the intestinal tract. For example, orlistat (Xenical) decreases absorption of fats from food and is given to promote weight loss, and ezetimibe (Zetia) decreases absorption of cholesterol from food and is given to lower serum cholesterol levels. However, most drug–diet interactions are undesirable because food often slows absorption of oral drugs by slowing gastric emptying time and altering GI secretions and motility.

Quality and Safety Alert: Safety

Giving medications 1 hour before or 2 hours after a meal can minimize drug–diet interactions that decrease drug absorption.

In addition, some foods contain certain substances that react with certain drugs. One such interaction occurs between tyramine-containing foods and monoamine oxidase (MAO) inhibitor drugs. Tyramine causes the release of norepinephrine, a strong vasoconstrictive agent, from the adrenal medulla and sympathetic neurons. Normally, norepinephrine is quickly inactivated by MAO. However, because MAO inhibitor drugs prevent inactivation of norepinephrine, ingesting tyramine-containing foods with an MAO inhibitor may produce severe hypertension or intracranial hemorrhage. MAO inhibitors include the antidepressants isocarboxazid and phenelzine and the anti-Parkinson drugs rasagiline and selegiline.

Quality and Safety Alert: Safety

Tyramine-rich foods to be avoided by patients taking MAO inhibitors include aged cheeses, sauerkraut, soy sauce, tap or draft beers, and red wines.

Another type of interaction may occur between warfarin (Coumadin), an oral anticoagulant, and foods containing vitamin K. Because vitamin K antagonizes the action of warfarin, large amounts of spinach and other green leafy vegetables may offset the anticoagulant effects and predispose the person to thromboembolic disorders.

Another type of interaction occurs between the antibiotic tetracycline and dairy products, such as milk and cheese.

The drug combines with the calcium in milk products to form a nonabsorbable compound that is excreted in the feces.

Still, another interaction involves grapefruit. Grapefruit contains a substance that strongly inhibits the metabolism of drugs normally metabolized by the CYP3A4 enzyme. This effect greatly increases the blood levels of some drugs (e.g., the widely used "statin" group of cholesterol-lowering drugs), and the effect lasts for several days. Patients who take medications metabolized by the CYP3A4 enzyme should be advised against eating grapefruit or drinking grapefruit juice.

Drug–Drug Interactions

The action of a drug may be increased or decreased by its interaction with another drug in the body. Most interactions occur whenever the interacting drugs are present in the body; some, especially those affecting the absorption of oral drugs, occur when the interacting drugs are taken at or near the same time. The basic cause of many drug–drug interactions is altered drug metabolism. For example, drugs metabolized by the same enzymes compete for enzyme binding sites, and there may not be enough binding sites for two or more drugs. Also, some drugs induce or inhibit the metabolism of other drugs. Protein binding is also the basis for some important drug–drug interactions.

Interactions that can increase the therapeutic or adverse effects of drugs include the following:

- Additive effects, which occur when two drugs with similar pharmacologic actions are taken (e.g., ethanol + sedative drug increases sedative effects).
- Synergism, which occurs when two drugs with different sites or mechanisms of action produce greater effects when taken together (e.g., acetaminophen [nonopioid analgesic] + codeine [opioid analgesic] increases analgesic effects).
- Interference by one drug with the metabolism of a second drug, which may result in intensified effects of the second drug. For example, cimetidine inhibits CYP1A, CYP2C, and CYP3A drug-metabolizing enzymes in the liver and, therefore, interferes with the metabolism of many drugs (e.g., benzodiazepine antianxiety and hypnotic drugs, several cardiovascular drugs). When these drugs are given concurrently with cimetidine, they are likely to cause adverse and toxic effects because blood levels of the drugs are higher. The overall effect is the same as taking a larger dose of the drug whose metabolism is inhibited or slowed.
- Displacement (i.e., a drug with a strong attraction to protein-binding sites may displace a less tightly bound drug) of one drug from plasma protein–binding sites by a second drug, which increases the effects of the displaced drug. This increase occurs because the displaced drug, freed from its bound form, becomes pharmacologically active. The overall effect is the same as taking a larger dose of the displaced drug. For example, aspirin displaces warfarin and increases the drug's anticoagulant effects.

Interactions in which drug effects are decreased include the following:

- An **antidote** drug, which can be given to relieve, prevent, or counteract the toxic effects of another drug. For example, naloxone is commonly used to relieve respiratory depression caused by morphine and related drugs. Naloxone molecules displace morphine molecules from their receptor sites on nerve cells in the brain so that the morphine molecules cannot continue to exert their depressant effects.
- Decreased intestinal absorption of oral drugs, which occurs when drugs combine to produce nonabsorbable compounds. For example, drugs containing aluminum, calcium, or magnesium bind with oral tetracycline (if taken at the same time) to decrease its absorption and, therefore, its antibiotic effect.
- Activation of drug-metabolizing enzymes in the liver, which increases the metabolism rate of any drug metabolized mainly by that group of enzymes and therefore decreases the drug's effects. Several drugs (e.g., phenytoin, rifampin) and cigarette smoking are known enzyme inducers.

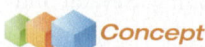 **Concept Mastery Alert**

Drug–drug interactions can either increase or decrease drug effects. A decrease in the therapeutic effect of a drug can be caused by the rate of absorption, distribution, metabolism, or excretion (pharmacokinetics) of the drug; therefore, the nurse should monitor for a delay in predicted therapeutic effects.

Patient-Related Variables

Age

The effects of age on drug action are especially important in neonates, infants, and older adults. In children, drug action depends largely on age and developmental stage. During pregnancy, drugs cross the placenta and may harm the fetus. Fetuses have no effective mechanisms for eliminating drugs because their liver and kidney functions are immature. Newborn infants (birth to 1 month) also handle drugs inefficiently. Drug distribution, metabolism, and excretion differ markedly in neonates, especially premature infants, because their organ systems are not fully developed. Older infants (1 month to 1 year) reach approximately adult levels of protein binding and kidney function, but liver function and the blood–brain barrier are still immature.

Children (1 to 12 years) have a period of increased activity of drug-metabolizing enzymes so that some drugs are rapidly metabolized and eliminated. Although the onset and duration of this period are unclear, a few studies have been done with particular drugs. Theophylline, for example, is eliminated much faster in a 7-year-old child than in a neonate or adult (18 to 65 years). After about 12 years of age, healthy children handle drugs similarly to healthy adults.

In older adults (65 years and older), physiologic changes may alter all pharmacokinetic processes. Changes in the GI tract include decreased gastric acidity, decreased blood flow, and decreased motility. Despite these changes, however, there is little difference in drug absorption. Changes in the cardiovascular system include decreased cardiac output and, therefore, slower distribution of drug molecules to their sites of action, metabolism, and excretion. In the liver, blood flow and metabolizing enzymes are decreased. Thus, many drugs are metabolized more slowly, have a longer action, and are more likely to accumulate with chronic administration. In the kidneys, there is decreased blood flow, decreased glomerular filtration rate, and decreased tubular secretion of drugs. All these changes tend to slow excretion and promote accumulation of drugs in the body. Impaired kidney and liver function greatly increase the risks of adverse drug effects. In addition, older adults are more likely to have acute and chronic illnesses that require the use of multiple drugs or long-term drug therapy. Thus, possibilities for interactions among drugs and between drugs and diseased organs are greatly multiplied.

Body Weight

Body weight affects drug action mainly in relation to dose. The ratio between the amount of drug given and body weight influences drug distribution and concentration at sites of action. In general, people who are heavier than average may need larger doses, provided that their kidney, hepatic, and cardiovascular functions are adequate. Recommended doses for many drugs are listed in terms of grams or milligrams per kilogram of body weight.

Pharmacogenomic Variations

Prescribers order drugs to cause particular effects in recipients. However, when some people receive the same drug in the same dose, by the same route, and in the same time interval, they may experience inadequate therapeutic effects or unusual or exaggerated effects, including increased toxicity. These interindividual variations in drug response are often attributed to genetic heritage, which produces differences in drug metabolism. The study of genetic variations in drug response is called **pharmacogenomics** (or pharmacogenetics).

Until recently, the emphasis of pharmacogenomics has been on forecasting adverse drug events in specific populations based on age, sex, or ethnicity. The focus has been on identifying inherited variability in metabolism among individuals that alters the uptake, effectiveness, and toxicity of drugs and makes some people react differently than anticipated.

Pharmacogenomic influences on drug response alter the pharmacologic effects of a drug. Specifically, the impact of genetic variability affects drug pharmacokinetics; pharmacodynamics; idiosyncratic reactions, such as hypersensitivity reactions; and/or the drug's effects on disease development, severity, or response to therapy.

Research has increased with awareness that genetic and ethnic characteristics are important factors and that diverse groups of people must be included in clinical trials. There is also increased awareness that each person is genetically unique and must be treated as an individual rather than as a member of a particular ethnic group.

Genetics

When most drugs enter the body, they interact with proteins (e.g., in plasma, tissues, cell membranes, drug receptor sites) to reach their sites of action, and they interact with other proteins (e.g., drug-metabolizing enzymes in the liver and other organs) to be biotransformed and eliminated from the body. Genetic characteristics that alter any of these proteins can alter drug responses. For example, metabolism of isoniazid, an antitubercular drug, requires the enzyme acetyltransferase. People may metabolize isoniazid rapidly or slowly, depending largely on genetic differences in acetyltransferase activity. Clinically, rapid metabolizers may need larger than usual doses to achieve therapeutic effects, and slow metabolizers may need smaller than usual doses to avoid toxic effects.

In addition, several genetic variations (called polymorphisms) of the CYP drug-metabolizing enzymes have been identified. Specific variations may influence any of the chemical processes by which drugs are metabolized. For example, CYP2D6 metabolizes several antidepressant, antipsychotic, and beta-adrenergic blocker drugs. About 7% of White people metabolize these drugs poorly and are at increased risk for drug accumulation and adverse effects. Conversely, codeine is also metabolized by CYP2D6 and, as a prodrug, is not active until it is converted into morphine in the liver. For ultrarapid metabolizers, the conversion of codeine to morphine occurs quickly and poses a risk for serious adverse effects, such as respiratory depression. CYP2C19 metabolizes diazepam, omeprazole, and some antidepressants. As many as 15% to 30% of individuals of Asian descent may metabolize these drugs poorly and develop adverse effects if dosage is not reduced.

Still another example of genetic variation in drug metabolism is that some people are deficient in glucose-6-phosphate dehydrogenase, an enzyme normally found in red blood cells and other body tissues. These people may have hemolytic anemia when given antimalarial drugs, sulfonamides, analgesics, antipyretics, and other drugs.

An increasing number of published pharmacogenomic studies and integration of next-generation sequencing technology for pharmacogenomic testing into patient care has shaped drug therapy regimens that maximize the therapeutic effects and minimize the adverse effects. The U.S. Food and Drug Administration (FDA) has updated drug labels with information that highlights the pharmacogenomic implications of specific drugs and has released a table of genomic biomarkers that have established roles in determining drug response. Many of the recommended tests for individual drugs are not routinely used for clinical decisions in part due to lack of education on potential benefit, limited guidelines for implementation of findings, and the potential delay of therapy when waiting for results.

> **Quality and Safety Alert: Safety**
>
> The FDA has included the effect of genomic variations in boxed warnings on drug labels highlighting known contraindications or precautions for individuals who require genotype-specific dosing. The nurse should recognize the role of pharmacogenomics in avoiding adverse drug reactions with an optimized drug dosage.

Ethnicity

Most drug information had been derived from clinical drug trials using White males. Interethnic variations became evident when drugs and dosages developed for White males produced unexpected responses, including toxicity, when given to people from other ethnic groups. One common variation is that African Americans respond differently to some cardiovascular drugs. For example, for African Americans with hypertension, angiotensin-converting enzyme (ACE) inhibitors and beta-adrenergic blocking drugs are less effective, and diuretics and calcium channel blockers are more effective. Also, African Americans with heart failure seem to respond better to a combination of hydralazine and isosorbide than do White American patients with heart failure.

Another variation is that people of Asian descent usually require much smaller doses of some commonly used drugs, including beta-adrenergic blockers and several psychotropic drugs (e.g., alprazolam, an antianxiety agent, and haloperidol, an antipsychotic). Some other documented interethnic variations are included in later chapters.

Sex

Most drug-related research has involved males, and the results have been extrapolated to females, sometimes with adjustment of dosage based on their usually smaller size and weight. Historically, sex was considered a minor influence on drug action except during pregnancy and lactation. Now, differences between males and females in responses to drug therapy are being increasingly identified, and since 1993, regulations require that major clinical drug trials include females. However, data on drug therapy in females are still limited. Some identified differences include the following:

- Females with depression are more likely to respond to the selective serotonin reuptake inhibitors (SSRIs), such as fluoxetine (Prozac), than to the tricyclic antidepressants (TCAs), such as amitriptyline (Elavil).
- Females with anxiety disorders may respond less well than males to some antianxiety medications.
- Females with schizophrenia seem to need smaller doses of antipsychotic medications than males. If given the higher doses required by males, females are likely to have adverse drug reactions.
- Females may obtain more pain relief from opioid analgesics (e.g., morphine) and less relief from nonopioid analgesics (e.g., acetaminophen, ibuprofen), compared with males.

Different responses in females are usually attributed to anatomic and physiologic differences. In addition to smaller size and weight, for example, females usually have a higher percentage of body fat, less muscle tissue, smaller blood volume, and other characteristics that may influence responses to drugs. In addition, females have hormonal fluctuations during the menstrual cycle. Altered responses have been demonstrated in some females taking clonidine, an antihypertensive; lithium, a mood-stabilizing agent; phenytoin, an anticonvulsant; propranolol, a beta-adrenergic blocking drug used in the management of hypertension, angina pectoris, and migraine; and antidepressants. In addition, a significant percentage of females with arthritis, asthma, depression, diabetes mellitus, epilepsy, and migraines experience increased symptoms premenstrually. The increased symptoms may indicate a need for adjustments in their drug therapy regimens. Females with clinical depression, for example, may need higher doses of antidepressant medications premenstrually, if symptoms exacerbate, and lower doses during the rest of the menstrual cycle.

There may also be differences in pharmacokinetic processes, although few studies have been done. With absorption, it has been noted that females absorb a larger percentage of an oral dose of two cardiovascular medications than males (25% more verapamil and 40% more aspirin). With distribution, females may have higher blood levels of medications that distribute into body fluids (because of the smaller amount of water in which the medication can disperse) and lower blood levels of medications that are deposited in fatty tissues (because of the generally higher percentage of body fat), compared with males. With metabolism, the CYP3A4 enzyme metabolizes more medications than other enzymes, and females are thought to metabolize the drugs processed by this enzyme 20% to 40% faster than males (and therefore may have lower blood levels than males of similar weight given the same doses). The CYP1A2 enzyme is less active in females so that those who take the cardiovascular drugs clopidogrel or propranolol may have higher blood levels than males (and possibly greater risks of adverse effects if given the same doses as males). With excretion, renally excreted medications may reach higher blood levels because a major mechanism of drug elimination, glomerular filtration, is approximately 20% lower in females.

In general, females given equal dosages or equal weight-based dosages are thought to be exposed to higher concentrations of medications compared to males. Although available data are limited, the main reasons postulated for the sex differences are that females have a lower volume of distribution, lower glomerular filtration, and lower hepatic enzyme activity (except for the medications metabolized by the CYP3A4 enzyme system, which is more active in females). As a result, all females should be monitored closely during drug therapy because they are more likely to experience adverse drug effects than are males.

Other Considerations
Preexisting Conditions

Various pathologic conditions may alter some or all pharmacokinetic processes and lead to decreased therapeutic effects or increased risks of adverse effects. Examples include the following:

- Cardiovascular disorders (e.g., myocardial infarction, heart failure, hypotension), which may interfere with all pharmacokinetic processes, mainly by decreasing blood flow to sites of drug administration, action, metabolism (liver), and excretion (kidneys).
- GI disorders (e.g., vomiting, diarrhea, inflammatory bowel disease, trauma or surgery of the GI tract), which may interfere with absorption of oral drugs.
- Hepatic disorders (e.g., hepatitis, cirrhosis, decreased liver function), which mainly interfere with metabolism. Severe liver disease or cirrhosis may interfere with all pharmacokinetic processes.
- Kidney disorders (e.g., acute or chronic kidney failure), which mainly interfere with excretion. Severe kidney disease may interfere with all pharmacokinetic processes.
- Thyroid disorders, which mainly affect metabolism. Hypothyroidism slows metabolism, prolonging drug action and slowing elimination. Hyperthyroidism accelerates metabolism, shortening drug action and hastening elimination.

Psychological Factors

Psychological considerations influence individual responses to drug administration, although specific mechanisms are unknown. An example is the placebo response. A placebo is a pharmacologically inactive substance. Placebos are used in clinical drug trials to compare the medication being tested with a "dummy" medication. Recipients often report both therapeutic and adverse effects from placebos.

Attitudes and expectations related to drugs in general, a particular drug, or a placebo influence patient response. They also influence compliance or the willingness to carry out the prescribed drug regimen, especially with long-term drug therapy.

Tolerance and Cross-Tolerance

Drug tolerance occurs when the body becomes accustomed to a particular drug over time so that larger doses must be given to produce the same effects. Tolerance may be acquired to the pharmacologic action of many drugs, especially opioid analgesics, alcohol, and other CNS depressants. Tolerance to pharmacologically related drugs is cross-tolerance. For example, a person who regularly drinks large amounts of alcohol becomes able to ingest even larger amounts before becoming intoxicated—this is tolerance to alcohol. If the person is then given sedative-type drugs or a general anesthetic, larger than usual doses are required to produce a pharmacologic effect—this is cross-tolerance.

Tolerance and cross-tolerance are usually attributed to activation of drug-metabolizing enzymes in the liver, which accelerates drug metabolism and excretion. They also are attributed to decreased sensitivity or numbers of receptor sites.

ADVERSE EFFECTS OF DRUGS

As used in this book, the term "adverse effects" refers to any undesired responses to drug administration, as opposed to therapeutic effects, which are desired responses. Most drugs produce a mixture of therapeutic and adverse effects; all drugs can produce adverse effects. Adverse effects may produce essentially any symptom or disease process and may involve any body system or tissue. They may be common or rare, mild or severe, and localized or widespread—depending on the drug and the recipient. Some adverse effects occur with usual therapeutic doses of drugs (often called side effects); most are more likely to occur and to be more severe with high doses. Box 2.3 describes common or serious adverse effects. Although adverse effects may occur in anyone who takes medications, they are especially likely to occur with some drugs (e.g., insulin, warfarin) and in older adults, who often take multiple drugs.

> **Quality and Safety Alert: Evidence-Based Practice**
>
> Although a list of drugs that should be avoided in older adults is available (Beers Criteria; see Chapter 5), older patients continue to experience significant use of potentially inappropriate medications (PIMs). In a cross-sectional study, Sharma et al. (2020) explored the prevalence of PIM prescriptions in 323 older adults as identified by Beers Criteria (2015 and 2019) at a tertiary care postgraduate teaching hospital. The study included 38.7% female patients and 61.3% male patients; 74% of patients were 65 to 70 years of age, and 78% of patients were illiterate. According to the Beers Criteria, the overall prevalence of PIMs prescribed in this older population was 60.1% in 2015 and 61.9% in 2019. Although diagnosis was not associated with the prescribing of PIMs, factors such as male gender, ages 76 to 80 years, and education at the 10th-12th grade level, were found to be significantly related to PIMs prescription. There is a need for increased awareness that the Beers Criteria present a list of medications where the risk of harm outweighs potential benefits. In nursing practice, it is vital to recognize risk associated with age-related changes and implement strategies to advocate for older adults and question the inappropriate use of drugs identified in the Beers Criteria when PIMs are ordered in the vulnerable older adult population.

Boxed Warnings

For some prescription drug groups and individual drugs that may cause serious or life-threatening adverse effects, the FDA requires drug manufacturers to place a warning formatted with a box or border around the text on the label of a prescription drug or in the literature describing it. The colloquial term  often describes these FDA-required warnings, and this term is used in this text. A boxed warning is the strongest warning that the FDA can give consumers and often includes prescribing or monitoring information intended to improve the safety of using the particular drug or drug group. In recent years, boxed warnings have been added to antidepressant drugs, nonopioid analgesics, and immediate-release opioid analgesics.

> *Concept Mastery Alert*
>
> When administering a drug with a boxed warning, the nurse should monitor the patient closely for adverse effects.

Pregnancy Categories

In 2015, the FDA implemented the Pregnancy and Lactation Labeling Rule and launched the phaseout of pregnancy categories on prescription drug labeling that stratified risk of fetal injury from drugs used as directed during pregnancy. The current system includes pregnancy exposure registries for individual drugs that document exposed known or potential maternal or fetal adverse reactions affecting pregnancy outcomes. The registries provide the best available evidence on risks associated with drug exposure in pregnancy and lactation that should lead to better-informed prescribing decisions. The data about individual prescription drugs during pregnancy and lactation help healthcare providers weigh the risks versus benefits when counseling pregnant and lactating patients to make data-informed decisions for themselves and their children. The pregnancy exposure registry collects health information from individuals who take prescription medicines or vaccines when pregnant as well as information on the newborn baby and compares it with those who have not taken the drug during pregnancy. Additional information about the need for pregnancy testing, contraception recommendations, and information about infertility as it relates to the drug is also reported. Labeling for over-the-counter (OTC) medications remains unchanged.

BOX 2.3 Common or Serious Adverse Drug Effects

Central Nervous System Effects

CNS effects may result from CNS stimulation (e.g., agitation, confusion, disorientation, hallucinations, psychosis, seizures) or CNS depression (e.g., impaired level of consciousness, sedation, coma, impaired respiration and circulation). CNS effects may occur with many drugs, including most therapeutic groups, substances of abuse, and over-the-counter preparations.

Gastrointestinal Effects

GI effects (e.g., nausea, vomiting, constipation, diarrhea) commonly occur. Nausea and vomiting occur with many drugs because of local irritation of the GI tract or stimulation of the vomiting center in the brain. Diarrhea occurs with drugs that cause local irritation or increase peristalsis. More serious effects include bleeding or ulceration (most often with nonsteroidal anti-inflammatory agents such as ibuprofen) and severe diarrhea/colitis (most often with antibiotics).

Hematologic Effects

Hematologic effects (excessive bleeding, clot formation [thrombosis], bone marrow depression, anemias, leukopenia, agranulocytosis, thrombocytopenia) are relatively common and potentially life threatening. Excessive bleeding is often associated with anticoagulants and thrombolytics; bone marrow depression is associated with anticancer drugs.

Hepatic Effects

Hepatic effects (hepatitis, liver dysfunction or failure, biliary tract disorders) are potentially life threatening. The liver is especially susceptible to drug-induced injury because most drugs are circulated to the liver for metabolism and some drugs are toxic to liver cells. Hepatotoxic drugs include acetaminophen (Tylenol), isoniazid (INH), methotrexate (Trexall), phenytoin (Dilantin), and aspirin and other salicylates. In the presence of drug- or disease-induced liver damage, the metabolism of many drugs is impaired. Besides hepatotoxicity, many drugs produce abnormal values in liver function tests without producing clinical signs of liver dysfunction.

Nephrotoxicity

Nephrotoxicity (nephritis, abnormal kidney function or failure) occurs with several antimicrobial agents (e.g., gentamicin and other aminoglycosides), nonsteroidal anti-inflammatory agents (e.g., ibuprofen and related drugs), and others. Nephrotoxicity is potentially serious because it may interfere with drug excretion, thereby causing drug accumulation and increased adverse effects.

Hypersensitivity

Hypersensitivity, which is an immune-mediated reaction to a drug, also called an allergy, may occur with almost any drug in susceptible patients. It is largely unpredictable and unrelated to dose. It occurs in those who have previously been exposed to the drug or a similar substance (antigen) and who have developed antibodies. When readministered, the drug reacts with the antibodies to cause cell damage and the release of histamine and other substances. These substances produce reactions ranging from mild skin rashes to anaphylactic shock. Anaphylactic shock is a life-threatening hypersensitivity reaction characterized by respiratory distress and cardiovascular collapse. It occurs within a few minutes after drug administration and requires emergency treatment with epinephrine. Some allergic reactions (e.g., serum sickness) occur 1 to 2 weeks after the drug is given.

Drug Fever

Drugs can cause fever by several mechanisms, including allergic reactions, damaging body tissues, interfering with dissipation of body heat, or acting on the temperature-regulating center in the brain. The most common mechanism is an allergic reaction. Fever may occur alone or with other allergic manifestations (e.g., skin rash, hives, joint and muscle pain, enlarged lymph glands, eosinophilia). It may begin within hours after the first dose if the patient has taken the drug before or within about 10 days of continued administration if the drug is new to the patient. If the causative drug is discontinued, fever usually subsides within 48 to 72 hours unless drug excretion is delayed or significant tissue damage has occurred (e.g., hepatitis). Many drugs have been implicated as causes of drug fever, including most antimicrobials.

Idiosyncrasy

Idiosyncrasy refers to an unexpected reaction to a drug that occurs the first time it is given. These reactions are usually attributed to genetic characteristics that alter the person's drug-metabolizing enzymes.

Drug Dependence

Drug dependence may occur with mind-altering drugs, such as opioid analgesics, sedative–hypnotic agents, antianxiety agents, and CNS stimulants. Dependence may be physiologic or psychological. Physiologic dependence produces unpleasant physical symptoms when the dose is reduced or the drug is withdrawn. Psychological dependence leads to excessive preoccupation with drugs and drug-seeking behavior.

Carcinogenicity

Carcinogenicity is the ability of a substance to cause cancer. Several drugs are carcinogens, including some hormones and anticancer drugs. Carcinogenicity apparently results from drug-induced alterations in cellular DNA.

Teratogenicity

Teratogenicity is the ability of a substance to cause abnormal fetal development when taken by patients who are pregnant. Drug groups considered teratogenic include antiepileptic drugs, "statin" cholesterol-lowering drugs, antidepressant drugs, nonopioid analgesics, and the antiflu drug oseltamivir (Tamiflu).

The labeling requirements for pregnancy and lactation for prescription drugs includes three subsections:

1. Pregnancy (includes labor and delivery):

The pregnancy subsection provides information about dosing and potential risks to the developing fetus and registry information that collects and maintains data on how pregnant women are affected when they use the drug or a vaccine. Contact information for the registries is included, and pregnant women are encouraged to enroll to help provide data on the effects of drug use or vaccines during pregnancy.

2. Lactation (includes nursing mothers)

Information in this subsection includes drugs that should not be used during breast-feeding, known human or animal data regarding active metabolites in milk, as well as clinical effects on the infant. Other information may include pharmacokinetic data like metabolism or excretion, a risk and benefit section, as well as considerations regarding timing of breast-feeding to minimize

3. Females and males of reproductive potential

In this newest subsection on females and males of reproductive potential, relevant information on pregnancy testing or birth control before, during, or after drug therapy and a medication's effect on fertility or pregnancy loss will be provided when available. When necessary, information about the need for pregnancy testing, contraception recommendations, and information about infertility as it relates to the drug will be included.

Clinical Application 2.1

- During your most recent visit (3 days ago), you instructed Mrs. Green to take her medication with a large glass of water and set up a daily pill calendar. You also checked her vital signs; her blood pressure was 148/70 mm Hg. Today, you recheck her vital signs, and her blood pressure is 96/60 mm Hg. You ask her about her medication, and she tells you she has been taking each medication according to the calendar three times a day. What future actions should the home health nurse take?

TOXICOLOGY: DRUG OVERDOSE

Drug toxicity (also called poisoning or overdose) results from excessive amounts of a drug and may damage body tissues. It is a common problem in both adult and pediatric populations. It may result from a single large dose or prolonged ingestion of smaller doses. Toxicity may involve alcohol or prescription, OTC, or illicit drugs. Clinical manifestations are often nonspecific and may indicate other disease processes. Because of the variable presentation of drug intoxication, healthcare providers must have a high index of suspicion so that toxicity can be rapidly recognized and treated.

When toxicity occurs in a home or outpatient setting and the victim is collapsed or not breathing, emergency aid can be obtained by dialing 911. If the victim is responsive, a poison specialist is available 24 hours a day, 7 days a week through the National Poison Control Center by phone at 1-800-222-1222. The caller is connected to a local Poison Control Center and, if possible, needs to tell the responding pharmacist or physician the name of the drug or substance that was taken as well as the amount and time of ingestion. The poison control consultant may recommend treatment measures over the phone or taking the victim to a hospital emergency department.

It is possible that the patient or someone else may know the toxic agent (e.g., accidental overdose of a therapeutic drug, use of an illicit drug, a drug taken in attempt of suicide). Often, however, multiple drugs have been ingested, the causative drugs are unknown, and the circumstances may involve traumatic injury or impaired mental status that make the patient unable to provide useful information. The main goals are starting treatment as soon as possible after drug ingestion, supporting and stabilizing vital functions, preventing further damage from the toxic agent by reducing absorption or increasing elimination, and administering antidotes when available and indicated. Box 2.4 describes general aspects of enteral management of toxicity, Table 2.1 lists selected antidotes, and relevant chapters noted discuss specific aspects of care.

Quality and Safety Alert: Safety

To reduce the risk of pulmonary aspiration, unconscious patients should not receive activated charcoal until the airway is secure. To decrease the risk of bowel obstruction, many patients are given a laxative (e.g., sorbitol) to aid removal of the charcoal–drug complex.

Most patients who overdose are treated in emergency departments and discharged to their homes. A few are admitted to intensive care units (ICUs), often because of unconsciousness and the need for endotracheal intubation and mechanical ventilation. Unconsciousness is a major toxic effect of several commonly ingested substances such as benzodiazepine antianxiety and sedative agents, TCAs, ethanol, and opioid analgesics. Serious cardiovascular effects (e.g., cardiac arrest, dysrhythmias, circulatory impairment) are also common and warrant admission to an ICU.

Clinical Application 2.2

- You see Mrs. Green again in a few days. She is taking three antihypertensive medications, and her blood pressure is 128/72 mm Hg. She tells you that she has been feeling better and that she is moving in with her daughter. What suggestions could you provide Mrs. Green's daughter regarding her mother's medication management?

NCLEX Success

3. A patient with an overdose of an oral drug usually receives which of the following?
   A. specific antidote
   B. activated charcoal
   C. syrup of ipecac
   D. strong laxative

4. The parent of a 14-month-old calls a nurse working in a pediatric clinic and reports that the child ingested an unknown number of sleeping pills about 4 hours ago and is now drowsy. The parent asks what they should do. The best response to give the parent is
   A. "Administer a dose of syrup of ipecac to ensure vomiting"
   B. "Call the Poison Control Center immediately"
   C. "Administer a strong laxative and observe for a response"
   D. "Call 911 to transport your child to the nearest emergency department"

5. Differences in CYP-450 drug-metabolizing enzymes are known to cause genetic variation in the drug metabolism of certain drugs that increase the risk of adverse effects. These include which of the following? (Select all that apply.)
   A. CYP2D6 metabolism of several antidepressant, antipsychotic, and beta-adrenergic blocker drugs increases the risk of drug accumulation and adverse effects.
   B. CYP2D6 metabolism of codeine in individuals who are ultrarapid metabolizers. The conversion of codeine to morphine occurs quickly and poses a risk of serious adverse effects, such as respiratory depression.
   C. CYP2C19 metabolism in some individuals of Asian descent. This may cause decreased drug metabolism of diazepam, omeprazole, and some antidepressants leading to adverse effects.
   D. Individuals with a deficiency of glucose-6-phosphate dehydrogenase may have hemolytic anemia when given antimalarial drugs, sulfonamides, analgesics, antipyretics, and other drugs.
   E. The CYP1A2 enzyme is less active in males, so males who take the cardiovascular drugs clopidogrel or propranolol may have higher blood levels than females (and possibly greater risks of adverse effects if given the same doses as females).

BOX 2.4 *Enteral Management of Toxicity*

Maintaining Airway, Breathing, and Circulation

The immediate priority is support of vital functions. Endotracheal intubation and mechanical ventilation may be required to maintain breathing (in unconscious patients), correct hypoxemia, and protect the airway to avoid brain injury, myocardial ischemia, and cardiac dysrhythmias. In serious poisonings, an electrocardiogram is indicated to assess for severe toxicity (e.g., dysrhythmias, ischemia). Cardiopulmonary resuscitation may be needed to maintain breathing and circulation. An intravenous (IV) line is usually needed to administer fluids and drugs, and invasive treatment or monitoring devices may be inserted. Endotracheal intubation and mechanical ventilation are often required to maintain breathing (in unconscious patients), correct hypoxemia, and protect the airway. Hypoxemia must be corrected quickly to avoid brain injury, myocardial ischemia, and cardiac dysrhythmias.

Drug Therapy

Serious cardiovascular and neurologic manifestations often require drug therapy.
- Hypotension and hypoperfusion may be treated with inotropic and vasopressor drugs to increase cardiac output and raise blood pressure. Dysrhythmias are treated according to advanced cardiac life support protocols.
- Recurring seizures or status epilepticus requires treatment with anticonvulsant drugs.
- For unconscious patients, as soon as an IV line is established, some authorities recommend a dose of naloxone (2 mg IV) for possible narcotic overdose and thiamine (100 mg IV) for possible brain dysfunction due to thiamine deficiency. A fingerstick blood glucose test should be done, and if hypoglycemia is indicated, a 50% dextrose solution (50 mL IV) should be given.

Ongoing Management

After the patient is out of immediate danger, a thorough physical examination and efforts to determine the drug(s), the amounts, and the time lapse since exposure are needed. If the patient is unable to supply needed information, anyone else who may be able to do so should be interviewed. It is necessary to ask about the use of prescription and over-the-counter drugs, alcohol, and illicit substances.
- There are no standard laboratory tests for poisoned patients, but baseline tests of liver and kidney function are usually indicated. Screening tests for toxic substances are not very helpful because test results may be delayed, many substances are not detected, and the results rarely affect initial treatment. Specimens of blood, urine, or gastric fluids may be obtained for laboratory analysis. Serum drug levels are needed when acetaminophen, alcohol, aspirin, digoxin, lithium, or theophylline is known to be an ingested drug, to assist with treatment.
- For most orally ingested drugs, the initial and major treatment is a single dose of activated charcoal. Sometimes called the "universal antidote," it is useful in many poisonings because it adsorbs many toxins and rarely causes complications. When given within 30 minutes

BOX 2.4 Enteral Management of Toxicity (Continued)

of drug ingestion, it decreases absorption of the toxic drug by about 90%; when given an hour after ingestion, it decreases absorption by about 37%. It is often given by nasogastric tube. The charcoal blackens subsequent bowel movements. If used with whole-bowel irrigation (WBI; see below), activated charcoal should be given before the WBI solution is started. If given during WBI, the binding capacity of the charcoal is decreased. Activated charcoal does not significantly decrease absorption of some drugs (e.g., ethanol, iron, lithium, metals).

- Multiple doses of activated charcoal may be given in some instances (e.g., ingestion of sustained-release drugs). Adverse effects of activated charcoal include pulmonary aspiration and bowel obstruction from impaction of the charcoal–drug complex.
- Ipecac-induced vomiting and gastric lavage are no longer routinely used because of minimal effectiveness and potential complications. Ipecac is no longer recommended to treat poisonings in children in home settings; parents should call a poison control center or a healthcare provider. Gastric lavage may be beneficial in serious overdoses if performed within an hour of drug ingestion. If the ingested agent delays gastric emptying (e.g., drugs with anticholinergic effects), the 1-hour time limit for gastric lavage may be extended. When used after ingestion of pills or capsules, the tube lumen should be of sufficient diameter to allow removal of pill fragments.
- WBI with a polyethylene glycol solution (e.g., Colyte) may be used to remove toxic ingestions of long-acting, sustained-release drugs (e.g., many beta-adrenergic blockers, calcium channel blockers, and theophylline preparations); enteric-coated drugs; and toxins that do not bind well with activated charcoal (e.g., iron, lithium). It may also be helpful in removing packets of illicit drugs, such as cocaine or heroin. When used, 500 to 2,000 mL per hour are given orally or by nasogastric tube until bowel contents are clear. Vomiting is the most common adverse effect. WBI is contraindicated in patients with serious bowel disorders (e.g., obstruction, perforation, ileus), hemodynamic instability, or respiratory impairment (unless intubated).
- Urinary elimination of some drugs and toxic metabolites can be accelerated by changing the pH of urine (e.g., alkalinizing with IV sodium bicarbonate for salicylate overdose), diuresis, or hemodialysis. Hemodialysis is the treatment of choice in severe lithium and aspirin (salicylate) poisoning.
- Specific antidotes can be administered when available and as indicated by the patient's clinical condition. Available antidotes vary widely in effectiveness. Some are very effective and rapidly reverse toxic manifestations (e.g., naloxone for opioids, specific Fab fragments for digoxin). When an antidote is used, its half-life relative to the toxin's half-life must be considered. For example, the half-life of naloxone, a narcotic antagonist, is relatively short compared with the half-life of the longer-acting opioids such as methadone, and repeated doses may be needed to prevent recurrence of the toxic state.
- Any patient in which intentional ingestion is suspected, should be evaluated by a mental health professional.

TABLE 2.1
Antidotes for Overdoses of Selected Therapeutic Drugs

Overdosed Drug (Poison)	Antidote	Route and Dosage Ranges	Comments
Acetaminophen (see Chapter 16)	Acetylcysteine (10% or 20% inhalation/oral solution, Acetadote 20% [200 mg/mL] injection solution)	PO 140 mg/kg initially, then 70 mg/kg every 4 h for 17 doses (72-h oral regimen) IV (Acetadote only): loading dose 150 mg/kg, diluted in 200 mL 5% dextrose, infused over 15 min Maintenance dose one: 50 mg/kg, diluted in 500 mL 5% dextrose, infused over 4 h Maintenance dose two: 100 mg/kg, diluted in 1,000 mL 5% dextrose, infused over 16 h (21-h IV regimen)	Dilute oral solution to a 5% solution with a cola or other soft drink for oral administration Follow instructions carefully and note that doses, amounts of diluent, and infusion times are different for the three total IV infusions Only the 72-h oral and 21-h IV regimens are FDA approved for acetaminophen overdose
Anticholinergics (atropine; see Chapter 48)	Physostigmine	IV, IM 2 mg; give IV slowly, over at least 2 min	Infrequently used because of its toxicity; consulting a regional poison center recommended. Should not be given to patients with a seizure disorder, overdose of unknown drugs, or overdose of drugs known to cause seizures in overdose (e.g., cocaine, lithium). In such circumstances, the risks of seizures outweigh drug benefits

(Continued on page 30)

TABLE 2.1

Antidotes for Overdoses of Selected Therapeutic Drugs (Continued)

Overdosed Drug (Poison)	Antidote	Route and Dosage Ranges	Comments
Benzodiazepines (see Chapter 54)	Flumazenil	IV 0.2 mg over 30 s; if no response, may give additional 0.3 mg over 30 s Additional doses of 0.5 mg may be given at 1-min intervals up to a total amount of 3 mg	Should not be given to patients with overdose of unknown drugs or drugs known to cause seizures in overdose (e.g., cocaine, lithium)
Beta-adrenergic blockers (see Chapter 27)	Glucagon	IV 50–150 mcg/kg (5–10 mg for adults) over 1 min initially, then 2–5 mg/h by continuous infusion as needed	Glucagon increases myocardial contractility and raises blood pressure. It does not act on beta-adrenergic receptors and is, therefore, not affected by beta-adrenergic blocking drugs
Calcium channel blockers (see Chapter 26)	Calcium gluconate 10%	IV 1 g over 5 min; may be repeated	Increases myocardial contractility
Cholinergics (see Chapter 47)	Atropine	Adults: IV 2 mg, repeated as needed Children: IV 0.05 mg/kg, up to 2 mg	If poisoning is due to organophosphates (e.g., insecticides), pralidoxime may be given with the atropine
Digoxin (see Chapter 30)	Digoxin immune Fab	IV 40 mg (one vial) for each 0.6 mg of digoxin ingested Reconstitute each vial with 4 mL water for injection, then dilute with sterile isotonic saline to convenient volume and give over 30 min, through 0.22-mcm filter. If cardiac arrest seems imminent, may give the dose as bolus injection	Recommended for severe toxicity; reverses cardiac and extracardiac symptoms in a few minutes Note: Serum digoxin levels increase after antidote administration, but the drug is bound and, therefore, inactive
Heparin (see Chapter 9)	Protamine sulfate	IV 1 mg/100 units of heparin, slowly, over at least 10 min; a single dose should not exceed 50 mg	
Iron (see Chapter 35)	Deferoxamine	IM 1 g every 8 h PRN IV 15 mg/kg/h if hypotensive	Indicated for serum iron levels >500 mg/dL or serum levels >350 mg/dL with GI or cardiovascular symptoms. Can bind and remove a portion of an ingested dose; urine becomes red as iron is excreted
Isoniazid (INH) (see Chapter 22)	Pyridoxine (vitamin B6)	IV 1 g per gram of INH ingested, at rate of 1 g every 2–3 min. If amount of INH unknown, give 5 g; may be repeated	Indicated for management of seizures and correction of acidosis
Lead	Dimercaptosuccinic acid (succimer; Chemet)	Children: PO 10 mg/kg every 8 h for 5 d followed by 10 mg/kg/dose every 12 h for 14 d; maximum: 500 mg/dose Adults: at same dosing parameters as children (off-label use)	Dimercaptosuccinic acid is dialyzable although the lead chelates are not
Opioid analgesics (see Chapter 49)	Naloxone (Narcan)	Adults: IM or intranasal (preferred) 0.4–2 mg PRN Children: IV (preferred) 0.1 mg/kg per dose; maximum dose 2 mg	Can be given by alternate routes as indicated

TABLE 2.1
Antidotes for Overdoses of Selected Therapeutic Drugs (Continued)

Overdosed Drug (Poison)	Antidote	Route and Dosage Ranges	Comments
Phenothiazine antipsychotic agents (see Chapter 56)	Diphenhydramine	Adults: IV 50 mg Children: IV 1–2 mg/kg, up to a total of 50 mg	Given to relieve extrapyramidal symptoms (movement disorders)
Thrombolytics (see Chapter 9)	Aminocaproic acid (Amicar)	PO, IV infusion, 5 g initially, then 1–1.25 g/h for 8 h or until bleeding is controlled; maximum dose, 30 g/24 h	
Tricyclic antidepressants (see Chapter 55)	Sodium bicarbonate	IV 1–2 mEq/kg initially, then continuous IV drip to maintain serum pH of 7.5	To treat cardiac dysrhythmias, conduction disturbances, and hypotension
Warfarin (see Chapter 9)	Vitamin K1	PO 5–10 mg daily IV (severe overdose) continuous infusion at rate no faster than 1 mg/min	

Visit thePoint® *at* http://thePoint.lww.com/Frandsen13e *for answers to NCLEX Success questions (in Appendix A), answers to Clinical Application Case Studies (in Appendix B), additional information on pathophysiology, and more!*

REFERENCES AND RESOURCES

Hinkle, J. L., Cheever, K. H., & Overbaugh, K. (2021). *Brunner & Suddarth's textbook of medical-surgical nursing* (15th ed.). Wolters Kluwer.

Krebs, K., & Milani, L. (2019). Translating pharmacogenomics into clinical decisions: Do not let the perfect be the enemy of the good. *Human Genomics, 13*(1), 39. https://doi.org/10.1186/s40246-019-0229-z

Olson, K. R. (2018). Poisoning. In M. Papadakis, S. J. McPhee, & M. W. Rabow (Eds.), *Current medical diagnosis & treatment 2019* (58th ed., pp. 1580–1610). McGraw-Hill.

Roden, D. M., Van Driest, S. L., Wells, Q. S., Mosley, J. D., Denny, J. C., & Peterson, J. F. (2018). Opportunities and challenges in cardiovascular pharmacogenomics: From discovery to implementation. *Circulation Research, 122*(9), 1176–1190. https://doi.org/10.1161/CIRCRESAHA.117.310965

Rodziewicz, T. L., & Hipskind, J. E. (Updated 2021 Aug 6). Medical error reduction and prevention. In *StatPearls [Internet]*. StatPearls Publishing. https://www.ncbi.nlm.nih.gov/books/NBK499956/

Rogers, M. A., Lizer, S., Doughty, A., Hayden, B., & Klein, C. J. (2017). Expanding RN scope of knowledge-Genetics/genomics: The new frontier. *Journal for Nurses in Professional Development, 33*, 56–63. https://doi.org/10.1097/NND.0000000000000340

Sayeed, S., Califf, R., Green, R., Wong, C., Mahaffey, K., Gambhir, S. S., Mega, J., Patrick-Lake, B., Frazier, K., Pignone, M., Hernandez, A., Shah, S. H., Fan, A. C., Krüg, S., Shaack, T., Shore, S., Spielman, S., Eckstrand, J., & Wong, C. A.; Project Baseline Health Study Research Group. (2021). Return of individual research results: What do participants prefer and expect? *PLoS One, 16*(7), e0254153. https://doi.org/10.1371/journal.pone.0254153

Sharma, R., Bansal, P., Garg, R., Ranjan, R., Kumar, R., & Arora, M. (2020). Prevalence of potentially inappropriate medication and its correlates in elderly hospitalized patients: A cross-sectional study based on Beers criteria. *Journal of Family & Community Medicine, 27*(3), 200–207. https://doi.org/10.4103/jfcm.JFCM_175_20

CHAPTER 3

Medication Administration and the Nursing Process of Drug Therapy

LEARNING OBJECTIVES

After studying this chapter, you should be able to:

1. Apply the rights of medication administration in the care of a patient.
2. Illustrate knowledge needed to administer medications to a patient.
3. Identify and interpret drug orders for medication administration.
4. Demonstrate the ability to calculate drug dosages accurately.
5. Apply the steps of the nursing process in the administration of medications.
6. Demonstrate safe and accurate administration of medications.
7. Apply evidence-based practice research in the administration of medications.
8. Identify alternative or complementary therapy that may potentiate, negate, or cause toxicity with prescribed medications.

CLINICAL APPLICATION CASE STUDY

Jacqueline Baranski has been admitted to the hospital for a total abdominal hysterectomy. This is the first postoperative day. She is currently taking lisinopril 10 mg PO daily and estradiol 1 mg PO. She is also receiving morphine sulfate by patient-controlled analgesia and heparin 5,000 units subcutaneously every 12 hours for 7 days.

KEY TERMS

Assessment: collection of patient data that affects drug therapy

Controlled-release: oral tablet or capsule formulations that maintain consistent serum drug levels; may also be referred to as extended release or sustained release

Dosage form: form in which drugs are manufactured; includes elixirs, tablets, capsules, suppositories, parenteral drugs, and transdermal systems

Enteric-coated: coating of a tablet or capsule that makes it insoluble in stomach acid

Evaluation: determining a patient's status in relation to stated goals and expected outcomes

Evidence-based practice: scientific evidence that yields the best practice in patient care

Interventions: planned nursing activities performed on a patient's behalf, including assessment, promotion of adherence to drug therapy, and solving problems related to drug therapy

Medication history: list of prescription medications, over-the-counter medications, herbal supplements, or illegal substances taken by the patient (both current and past)

Nursing diagnosis: description of patient problems or needs based on assessment data

Nursing process: systematic way of gathering and using information to plan and provide individualized patient care

Parenteral: injected administration; subcutaneous, intramuscular, or intravenous route

Planning/goals: expected outcomes of prescribed drug therapy

Rights of medication administration: assist to ensure accuracy in drug therapy; rights include right drug, right dose, right patient, right assessment, right route, right time, right reason, right documentation, right patient education, right evaluation, and right to refuse the medication

Topical: application of drugs (e.g., solutions, ointments, creams, or suppositories) to skin or mucous membranes

Transdermal: adsorption of drugs (e.g., skin patches) through the skin

INTRODUCTION

This chapter discusses the administration of medications and the implementation of the nursing process with medication administration. The purpose of administering medications is to evoke a therapeutic response. Giving medications to a patient is an important nursing responsibility in many healthcare settings, including ambulatory clinics, hospitals, long-term care facilities, schools, and homes. The basic requirements for accurate drug administration are the **rights of medication administration**, which are as follows:

- Right drug
- Right dose
- Right patient
- Right assessment
- Right route
- Right time
- Right reason
- Right to refuse the medication
- Right documentation
- Right patient education
- Right evaluation

These "rights" require knowledge of the drugs to be given and the patients who are to receive them as well as specific nursing skills and interventions. The implementation of the **nursing process** in the administration of medications provides a systematic way of gathering and using information to plan and provide individualized patient care as well as to evaluate the outcomes of that care. It involves both cognitive and psychomotor skills. Knowledge of, and skill in, the nursing process are required for drug therapy as in other aspects of patient care. The five steps of the nursing process are assessment, nursing diagnosis, planning and establishing goals for care, interventions, and evaluation as it is applied to medication administration. The nursing process is a way to assess a patient's needs, response to medications, and identification of adverse effects. In this textbook, the authors have chosen to eliminate the nursing diagnosis because it is not tested by the National Council of State Boards of Nursing. A concept map outlining the nursing process appears at the end of every chapter that discusses a specific group of drugs.

GENERAL PRINCIPLES OF ACCURATE DRUG ADMINISTRATION

The nurse adheres to the following principles:

- Follow the "rights" associated with medication administration consistently.
- Learn essential information about each drug to be given (e.g., indications for use, contraindications, therapeutic effects, adverse effects, any specific instructions about administration).
- Interpret the prescriber's order accurately (i.e., drug name, dose, frequency of administration). Question the prescriber if any information is unclear or if the drug seems inappropriate for the patient's condition.
- In the event a verbal or telephone order is given by a prescriber, write down the order or enter it in the computer, and then read the order back to the prescriber.
- Read labels of drug containers for the drug name and concentration (usually in milligrams per tablet, capsule, or milliliter of solution). Many medications are available in different dosage forms and concentrations, and it is extremely important to use the correct ones.
- Use only approved abbreviations for drug names, doses, routes of administration, and times of administration. For example, do not use U to refer to units. Instead, write out *units*. This promotes safer administration and reduces errors. Consult the "Do Not Use List," the safety guidelines published by The Joint Commission (see Table 1.2). Check the organization's website for details.
- Calculate doses accurately. Medical technology and infusion pumps have assisted in the accuracy of drug calculations, thus decreasing the nurse's responsibility for drug calculation. However, it is still important for the prescriber, pharmacist, and nurse to assess the dosage for accuracy.
- Measure doses accurately. Ask a colleague to double-check measurements of insulin and heparin, unusual doses (i.e., large or small), and any drugs to be given intravenously.
- Use the correct procedures and techniques for all routes of administration. For example, use appropriate anatomic landmarks to identify sites for intramuscular (IM) injections, follow the manufacturers' instructions for preparation and

administration of intravenous (IV) medications, and use sterile materials and techniques for injectable and eye medications.
- Seek information about the patient's medical diagnoses and condition in relation to drug administration (e.g., ability to swallow oral medications; allergies or contraindications to ordered drugs; new signs or symptoms that may indicate adverse effects of administered drugs; heart, liver, or kidney disorders that may interfere with the patient's ability to distribute, metabolize, or eliminate drugs).
- Verify the identity of all patients before administering medications; check identification bands on patients who have them (e.g., in hospitals or long-term care facilities).
- Omit or delay doses as indicated by the patient's condition, and report or record omissions appropriately.
- Be especially vigilant when giving medications to children, because there is a high risk of medication errors. Factors that place children at risk for medication errors and/or adverse effects include their wide ranges of age and weight, the issue of limited drug testing on children, and the challenge of limited sites for parenteral administration of medications. In addition, in many cases, the need for small volumes of fluid limits flushing between drugs (which may produce undesirable interactions with other drugs and IV solutions).
- According to The Joint Commission and the World Health Organization (WHO), patient safety is the prevention of errors and adverse effects. Each nurse and healthcare institution is responsible for internal and external reporting requirements for adverse drug events (ADEs), adverse drug reactions, and medication errors.
- Maintain up-to-date skills for medication administration and knowledge of theoretical drug information.

Clinical Application 3.1

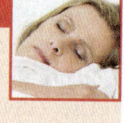

- Prior to administering the medications to Ms. Baranski, how does the nurse incorporate the rights of medication administration into the patient's care?
- Why is The Joint Commission's "Do Not Use" list so important in the prevention of medication administration errors?

NCLEX Success

1. A prescriber has written an order for an oral antihypertensive medication for a patient who is in rehabilitation following a stroke. Prior to administering the medication, which of the following nursing interventions is most important? (Select all that apply.)
   A. allowing the patient to take the medication with thickened liquids
   B. placing the patient in the sitting position
   C. assessing the patient's blood pressure
   D. assessing the patient's ability to swallow

LEGAL RESPONSIBILITIES

Registered and licensed practical nurses are legally empowered, under state nurse practice acts, to give medications ordered by licensed physicians, nurse practitioners, physician assistants, and dentists.

When giving medications, the nurse is legally responsible for safe and accurate administration. This means that the nurse may be held liable for not giving a drug or for giving a wrong drug or a wrong dose. In addition, the nurse is expected to have sufficient drug knowledge to recognize and question erroneous orders. If, after questioning the prescriber and seeking information from other authoritative sources, the nurse considers that giving a drug is unsafe, the nurse must refuse to give the drug. The fact that a physician wrote an erroneous order does not excuse the nurse from legal liability if they carry out that order.

The nurse also is legally responsible for actions delegated to people who are inadequately prepared for or legally barred from administering medications (e.g., nursing assistants). However, certified medical assistants (CMAs) may administer medications in physicians' offices, and certified medication aides (nursing assistants with a short course of training, also called CMAs) often administer medications in long-term care facilities.

The nurse who consistently follows safe practices in giving medications does not need to be excessively concerned about legal liability. The basic techniques and guidelines described in this chapter are aimed at safe and accurate preparation and administration. Most errors result when these practices are not followed.

Legal responsibilities in other aspects of drug therapy are less clear-cut. However, in general, nurses are expected to monitor patients' responses to drug therapy (e.g., therapeutic and adverse effects) and to teach patients safe and effective self-administration of drugs when indicated.

MEDICATION ERRORS AND THEIR PREVENTION

Medication errors continue to receive increasing attention from numerous healthcare organizations and agencies. Much of this interest stems from a 1999 report of the Institute of Medicine (IOM), which estimated that 44,000 to 98,000 deaths occur each year in the United States because of medical errors, including medication errors. The 2004 report of the IOM, *Keeping Patients Safe: Transforming the Work Environment of Nurses*, reported that the extended hours nurses work contribute to medication errors. Potential adverse patient outcomes of medication and other errors include serious illness, conditions that prolong hospitalization or require additional treatment, and death. Medication errors commonly reported include giving an incorrect dose, not giving an ordered drug, and giving an unordered drug. Specific drugs often associated with errors and ADEs include insulin, heparin, and warfarin. The risk of ADEs increases with the number of drugs a patient uses.

ADEs are injuries that result from the use of medications. Medication errors may or may not lead to injury, but the process or outcome of an error may provide the risk management team with strategies to improve patient care. Many years ago, the labels of heparin were very similar. This similarity resulted in an overdosage of heparin, leading to patient death. These drug errors led to changes in medication labeling. Potential adverse drug reactions pose a risk to the patient. A potential adverse drug reaction can also be termed a near miss. The nonpreventable adverse drug reaction is related to the chemical and pharmacologic properties that can result in an allergic or hypersensitivity reaction.

Medication errors may occur at any step in the drug distribution process, from the manufacturer to the patient, including prescribing, transcribing, dispensing, and administering. Many steps and numerous people are involved in giving the correct dose of a medication to the intended patient; each step or person has a potential for contributing to a medication error or preventing a medication error. All healthcare providers involved in drug therapy need to recognize risky situations, intervene to prevent errors when possible, and be extremely vigilant in all phases of drug administration. The most recent IOM publication, *The Future of Nursing 2020–2030: Charting a Path to Achieve Health Equity*, demonstrates that people of color, LGBTQI+ individuals, people with disabilities, people with lower incomes, and people living in rural communities have diminished access to quality healthcare. The social determinants of health and access to healthcare have an impact on individuals. For example, less education has been correlated with reduced patient understanding of medication adherence. In addition, lack of insurance or financial stability can impede a patient's ability to pay for healthcare and the medications required to treat comorbidities. Such factors result in inaccurate diagnoses and greater medication errors. Recommendations for prevention of medication errors have been developed by several organizations, including the IOM, the Agency for Healthcare Research and Quality (AHRQ), The Joint Commission, the Institute for Safe Medication Practices (ISMP), and the National Coordinating Council for Medication Error Reporting and Prevention (NCCMERP). Some sources of medication errors and recommendations to prevent them are summarized in Table 3.1.

TABLE 3.1
Medication Errors: Sources and Prevention Strategies

Sources of Errors	Recommendation to Prevent Errors
Drug Manufacturers • Drugs may have similar names that can lead to erroneous prescribing, dispensing, or administration. • For example, the antiseizure drug lamotrigine (Lamictal) has been confused with Lamisil, an antifungal drug; lamivudine, an antiviral drug; and others. • The FDA estimates that 10% of all reported medication errors result from drug name confusion. • In addition to similar names, many drugs, especially those produced by the same manufacturer, have similar packaging. This can lead to errors if container labels are not read carefully, especially if the products are shelved or stored next to each other. • Long-acting oral dosage forms with various, sometimes unclear indicators (e.g., LA, XL, XR), may be crushed, chewed, or otherwise broken so that the long-acting feature is destroyed. This can cause an overdose.	• FDA evaluation of proposed trade names in manufacturers' new drug applications in seeking FDA approval for marketing. • When choosing a trade name for a new drug, avoid names that are similar to drugs already on the market. • Design packaging so that all drugs from an individual manufacturer do not look alike in terms of color, appearance, etc. • Clearly designate long-acting drug formulations. • Use "Tall Man" lettering on drug labels to distinguish between generic drug with similar names (e.g., NICARdipine, NIFEdipine; vinBLAstine, VinCristine).
Healthcare Agencies • Prescribers, pharmacists, and nurses have a heavy workload, with resultant rushing of prescribing, dispensing, and administering medications. • They may also experience distractions by interruptions, noise, and other events in the work environment that make it difficult to pay needed attention to the medication-related task.	• Provide prescribers with CPOE technology and standardized drug order sheets; discourage handwritten drug orders; minimize verbal orders and state procedures to follow when verbal orders are necessary. Provide computerized technology (e.g., bar coding for patients; handheld scanning devices for nursing staff) to verify the drug, the dose, and the patient identity before administration of a dose and to record administration after a dose. Provide sufficient pharmacy staff to dispense medications. Provide sufficient nursing staff to administer medications. Try to provide a quiet and orderly work environment, with limited traffic, telephones, and other distractions. Provide adequate equipment for the required medication-related tasks. For pharmacies, this includes an adequate computer system for accessing databases of drug information and for detecting risks of adverse drug effects and drug–drug interactions. Standardize drug administration materials and equipment (e.g., infusion pumps) throughout the agency. Be sure that all professional staff members know and follow safety standards and medication reconciliation processes mandated by The Joint Commission.

(Continued on page 36)

TABLE 3.1

Medication Errors: Sources and Prevention Strategies (Continued)

Sources of Errors	Recommendation to Prevent Errors
Prescribers - May write orders illegibly - Order a drug that is not indicated by the patient's condition - Fail to order a drug that is indicated - Fail to consider the patient's age, size, kidney function, liver function, and disease process when selecting a drug or dosage - Fail to consider other medications the patient is taking, including prescription, over-the-counter, and herbal drugs - Lack sufficient knowledge about the drug - Fail to monitor for, or instruct others to monitor for, effects of administered drugs - Fail to discontinue drugs appropriately	- Use CPOE when available. - Be sure that any handwritten drug order is legible (e.g., printed in block letters if necessary), clear, and unambiguous. - Avoid or minimize the use of abbreviations. Consult The Joint Commission's "Do Not Use" List. - Use generic names of medications rather than brand names, and include the purpose of the drug. - Avoid verbal orders when possible. If a verbal order is necessary, have the person taking the order write the order and read it back, spelling drug names, dosages, routes, and so forth when indicated. - Review the patient's health status and other drugs being taken before ordering any new drug. Also, discontinue drugs appropriately when no longer needed. - Maintain a current knowledge base about new drugs and changes in uses of drugs for the relevant area of clinical practice.
Nurses - May have inadequate knowledge about a drug or about the patient receiving the drug - Not follow the rights to medication administration - Fail to question the medication order when indicated	- Be aware of agency policies and procedures about medication use, storage, administration, and recording. - Maintain an up-to-date knowledge base about drugs and their administration. - Make a diligent effort to learn about patients' health status and the drugs they are receiving. - Question or clarify any unclear drug orders. - Verify medication calculations with another nurse or a pharmacist, especially for children. - Recheck a single dose any time the amount seems unusually large or small. - Verify settings on drug infusion pumps with another nurse, when indicated. - Follow the rights of medication administration consistently. - Recheck the original drug order when a patient questions whether a particular drug dose should be taken. - Report errors, so that preventive efforts can be designed. - Discuss patients' medications during change-of-shift reports, including new and discontinued drugs, patients' responses to their medications, patient teaching about medications, and medications given 1–2 h before or after shift report.
Patients and Consumers - Outpatients may take drugs from several prescribers - Fail to inform one prescriber about drugs prescribed by another healthcare provider - Get prescriptions filled at more than one pharmacy - Fail to get prescriptions filled or refilled - Underuse or overuse an appropriately prescribed drug - Take drugs left over from a previous illness or prescribed for someone else - Fail to follow instructions for drug administration or storage - Fail to keep appointments for follow-up care - Fail to ask for information when needed	- Inform all healthcare providers about health status, any drug allergies, and all medications being taken (e.g., prescription, over-the-counter, herbal, and dietary supplements). - Ask prescribers to include the purpose of a drug on the label of all prescription medications. - If able, know names, strengths, doses, and the reason for use of all medications. - Follow instructions about when and how to take medications; do not increase amount or frequency of any medication without checking with a healthcare provider. Ask questions or request written instructions if needed. - If unable to take medications or if problems occur, discuss with a healthcare provider. Do not stop taking prescribed medications. - Maintain a current list of all medications being taken. Take the list or the medications to each visit to a healthcare provider. - Keep all medications in their original containers. - Read labels of medication containers every time a dose is taken. - Do not chew, crush, or break any tablets or capsules unless a healthcare provider says it is okay to do so.

CPOE, computerized provider order entry; FDA, Food and Drug Administration.

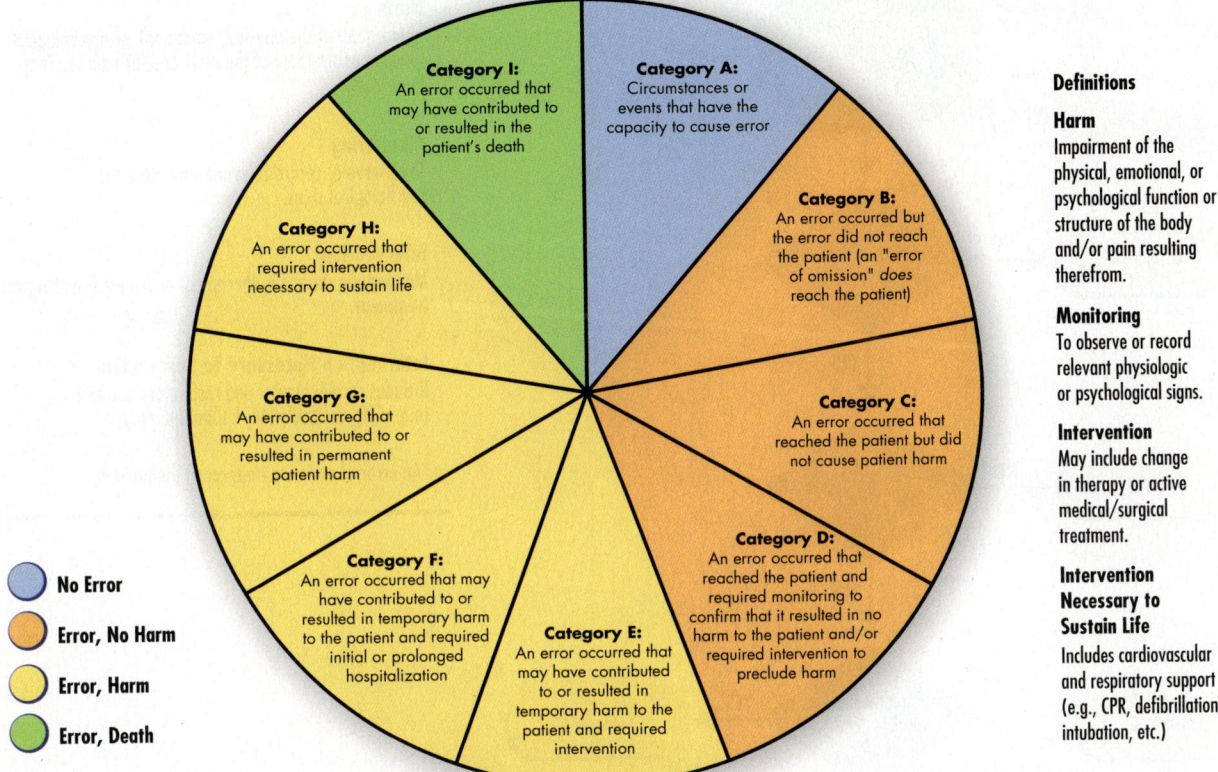

Figure 3.1. Index for categorizing medication errors, National Coordinating Council for Medication Error Reporting and Prevention. (NCC MERP Index for Categorizing Medication Errors. © 2023 National Coordinating Council for Medication Error Reporting and Prevention. All Rights Reserved. Retrieved from https://www.nccmerp.org/sites/default/files/indexColor2001-06-12.pdf)

The NCCMERP (2023), an independent council of 27 organizations, works to maximize the safe use of medications. It increases awareness of medication errors and promotes strategies to prevent further errors. It has developed an index (Fig. 3.1) and an algorithm (Fig. 3.2) for categorizing medication errors. This categorization of medication errors can be adopted by healthcare institutions. Using A through I, this system ranks medication errors according to the severity of their outcomes. Category A identifies circumstances that have the capacity to cause an error, and category I identifies an error that contributed to a patient's death. This system gives healthcare institutions the ability to track the rate of medication errors.

The WHO defines pharmacovigilance as "the science and activities related to the detection, assessment, understanding, and prevention of adverse drug effects or any possible drug-related problems." The domains of pharmacovigilance include adverse drug reactions or events, medication errors, counterfeit or substandard medications, lack of medication efficacy, misuse or abuse of medications, and medication interactions (World Health Organization, 2015). In 2020, the WHO identified that most adverse drug reactions are preventable. Some of the risks of adverse reactions include the following:

- Incorrect diagnoses
- Incorrect prescribed medications or incorrect dosages
- Undetected medical, genetic, or allergic reaction to medications
- Not following medication administration guidelines
- Drug to drug or drug to food/herbal interactions

The prevention of medication administration errors is key to safe patient care. A nurse must follow the guidelines to prevent errors in medication administration by using:

- Prefilled syringes, in which the syringes are prefilled when manufactured
- Bar codes, which contain information to maintain patient safety, such as the patient's allergies and contraindications related to the use of the medication (see Changes to Prevent Medication Errors)
- Tubing connectors for different routes of medications, which prevents the administration of a noncompatible medication
- Proper labeling, which is essential to prevent medication errors

The IOM report "*To Err is Human*" led to the development of "The Just Culture," with the goal to encourage healthcare providers to report mistakes. Jones et al. (2021) demonstrate that medication errors can be prevented with the establishment of "The Just Culture." The Just Culture aims to balance responsibility and accountability in nursing practice with the end goal of patient safety. The practice of threats and punishment does

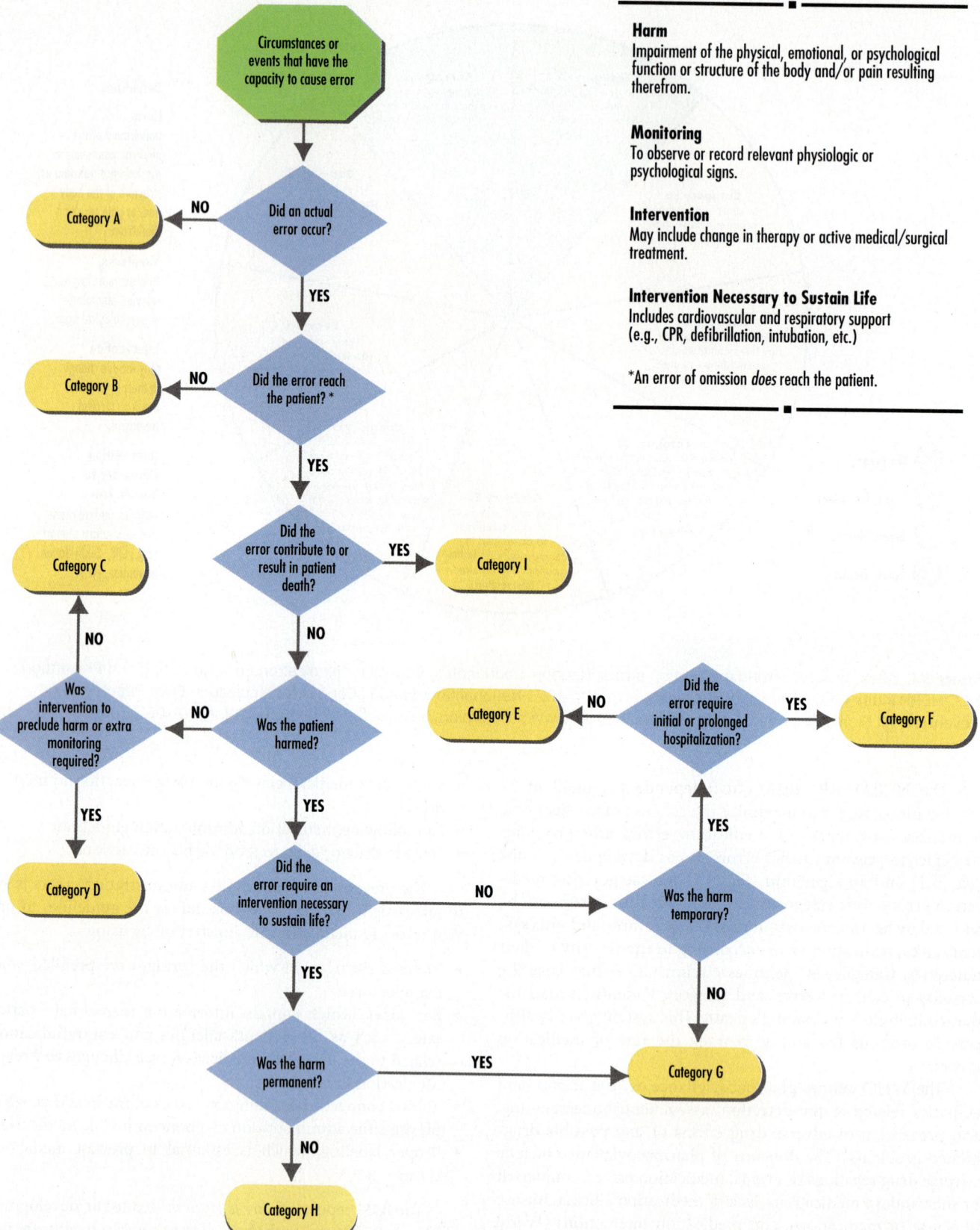

Figure 3.2. Algorithm for categorizing medication errors. (National Coordinating Council for Medication Error Reporting and Prevention. NCC MERP Index for Categorizing Medication Errors Algorithm. © 2023 National Coordinating Council for Medication Error Reporting and Prevention. All Rights Reserved. Retrieved from https://www.nccmerp.org/sites/default/files/algorColor2001-06-12.pdf)

not prevent medication errors, but nurses and nursing students must be held accountable for their actions. It is imperative that nurses and nursing students are knowledgeable about the medications to be administered. It has been reported that more than 35% of medication errors occur during the administration phase; every nurse must understand the cause of medication errors and how to reduce errors. In addition, the development of adverse drug events is commonly preventable. Nurses need to know drug–drug interactions, as well as interactions between drugs and food or herbal supplements.

Medication errors can occur despite a nurse's competence and vigilance. In the event of a medication error, the nursing profession and healthcare system must examine the root cause of the error and learn from it to develop strategies to prevent future errors. Prevention of errors must take an interdisciplinary approach involving all members of the healthcare team.

Unfolding Patient Stories: Mary Richards • Part 1

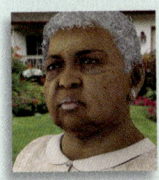

The nurse recommends docusate, a stool softener, for Mary Richards, an 82-year-old with heart failure, chronic atrial fibrillation, and hypertension. The provider informs the nurse that the order will be placed in the computer. When the nurse reviews the provider's orders, the only medication written is losartan 50 mg PO daily, which the nurse recognizes as an angiotensin receptor blocker used in the treatment of heart failure. Because losartan was not requested or discussed during patient rounds, how should the nurse proceed with this order? (Mary Richards' story continues in Chapter 26.)

Care for Mary and other patients in a realistic virtual environment: *vSim for Nursing* (thepoint.lww.com/vSimPharm). Practice documenting these patients' care in DocuCare (thepoint.lww.com/DocuCareEHR).

Medication Systems

Each healthcare facility has a system for distributing drugs. The unit dose system, in which most drugs are dispensed in single-dose containers for individual patients, is widely used. The pharmacist or pharmacy technician checks drug orders and stocks the medication in the patient's medication drawer. When a dose is due to be taken, the nurse removes the medication and gives it to the patient. Unit-dose wrappings of oral drugs should be left in place until the nurse is in the presence of the patient and ready to give the medication. It is essential that each dose of a drug be recorded on the patient's medication administration record (MAR) as soon as possible after administration.

Increasingly, institutions are using automated, computerized, locked cabinets for which each nurse on a unit has a password or code for accessing the cabinet and obtaining a drug dose. The pharmacy maintains the medications and replaces the drug when needed.

Controlled drugs, such as opioid analgesics, are usually kept as a stock supply in a locked drawer or automated cabinet and replaced as needed. The nurse must sign for each dose and record it on the patient's MAR. The nurse must comply with legal regulations and institutional policies for dispensing and recording controlled drugs.

Changes to Prevent Medication Errors

Changes in medication systems are being increasingly implemented, largely in efforts to decrease medication errors and improve patient safety. These changes include the following new processes and systems.

Computerized Provider Order Entry

In this system, a prescriber types a medication order directly into a computer. This decreases errors associated with illegible handwriting and erroneous transcription or dispensing. Computerized provider order entry (CPOE), which is already used in many healthcare facilities, is widely recommended as the preferred alternative to error-prone handwritten orders.

Bar Coding

In 2004, the Food and Drug Administration (FDA) passed a regulation requiring drug manufacturers to put bar codes on current prescription medications and nonprescription medications that are commonly used in hospitals. New drugs must have bar codes within 60 days of their approval. In hospitals, bar codes operate with other agency computer systems and databases that contain a patient's medication orders and MAR. The bar code on the drug label contains the identification number, strength, and dosage form of the drug, and the bar code on the patient's identification band contains the MAR, which can be displayed when a nurse uses a handheld scanning device. When administering medications, the nurse scans the bar code on the drug label, on the patient's identification band, and on the nurse's personal identification badge. A wireless computer network processes the scanned information; gives an error message on the scanner or sounds an alarm if the nurse is about to give the wrong drug or the right drug at the wrong time; and automatically records the time, drug, and dose given on the MAR. The FDA estimates that it will take about 20 years for all U.S. hospitals to implement this system of bar codes for medication administration.

For nurses, implementing the bar coding technology increases the time requirements and interferes with their ability to individualize patient care in relation to medications. Such a system works well with routine medications, but nonroutine situations (e.g., variable doses or times of administration) may pose problems. In addition, in long-term care facilities, it may be difficult to maintain legible bar codes on patient identification bands. Despite some drawbacks, bar coding increases patient safety, and therefore, nurses should support its development.

Point of Care

The medical centers of the U.S. Department of Veterans Affairs developed the point-of-care bar code–assisted software. Point of care is the time in which the nurse scans the bar-coded medication administered to the patient. This system uses bar code scanning that verifies the right drug, dose, patient, route, and time. The reason for the medication and subsequent documentation is the responsibility of the nurse administering the medication. This technology increases patient safety and accuracy of reporting. Using a handheld electronic device, the nurse scans the bar code and compares the medication being administered with what was ordered for the patient. Following receipt of the written order, the pharmacist enters, verifies, and profiles the order. Prior to administering the medication, the nurse confirms a match between the written and electronically profiled order. Before administering the medication, the nurse scans the patient's wrist band and medication. The device then verifies that it is the correct dose, correct time, and correct patient.

According to the FDA, hospitals have reduced medication administration errors since 2006 with the use of the bar coding technology at the point of care. Drawbacks to bar code technology have been identified. For example, bar codes on suppositories and IV solution bags can become unreadable. Also, as tubes of ointments are rolled from the bottom, the bar code may become difficult to decipher. Drug companies apply linear bar codes on pharmaceuticals. In 2011, President Barack Obama signed the executive order "Improving Regulation and Regulatory Review," requiring federal regulatory agencies to strengthen, complement, and modernize rules. The FDA chose to address the bar code rules.

Many countries use Bar Code Medication Administration (BCMA) to give medications. Workstations on wheels allow the nurse to bring the technology closer to the patient. The administration of medications with the BCMA technology has ensured that the medications available were only ordered for that patient.

Limiting Use of Abbreviations

The ISMP has long maintained a list of abbreviations that are often associated with medication errors, and The Joint Commission requires accredited organizations to maintain a "Do Not Use" list (e.g., write out unit of measurement, not "U"; write out international units, not "IU"; write out "daily," not qd) that applies to all prescribers and transcribers of medication orders. Other abbreviations are not recommended either. In general, it is safer to write out drug names and routes of administration and minimize the use of abbreviations, symbols, and numbers that are often misinterpreted, especially when handwritten.

Medication Reconciliation

This is a process designed to avoid medication errors such as omissions, duplications, dosing errors, or drug interactions that occur when a patient is admitted to a healthcare facility, transferred from one department or unit to another within the facility, or discharged home from the facility. It involves obtaining an accurate **medication history** about all drugs—a list of prescription medications, over-the-counter (OTC) medications, herbal supplements, or illegal substances taken by the patient (both current and past), including dose and frequency of administration—on entry into the healthcare facility (see later discussion on "Assessment"). The list of medications developed from the medication history is compared to newly ordered medications, and identified discrepancies are resolved. The list is placed in the medical record so that it is accessible to all healthcare providers, including the prescriber who writes the patient's admission drug orders. When the patient is transferred, the updated list must be communicated to the next healthcare provider. When a patient is discharged, an updated list should be given to the next provider and to the patient. The patient should be encouraged to keep the list up-to-date when changes are made in the medication regimen and to share the list with future healthcare providers.

> **Quality and Safety Alert: Evidence-Based Practice**
>
> Riordan et al. (2020) explored the pharmacovigilance and adverse drug reaction reporting knowledge, attitudes, and practices of healthcare professionals working in clinical trials. This was a mixed methods study with an online questionnaire and three semistructured interviews and focus groups. The online questionnaire revealed strong knowledge of pharmacovigilance. The participants were familiar with the practice of pharmacovigilance as evidenced by the monitoring and evaluation of adverse drug events, promotion of safe and effective use of medications, and knowledge of the benefit to risk assessment of medications and related risk management. The study participants valued pharmacovigilance training. In relation to reporting adverse drug reactions with clinical trials, the participants reported access to an adverse drug reaction portal was important. Knowledge of pharmacovigilance and the reporting of adverse drug reactions is important in maintenance of patient safety. The creation of a surveillance culture among nurses and healthcare team members administering medications ensures a culture that monitors and reports adverse drug reactions. The identification of the effects of new medications and reactions related to polypharmacy or comorbidities will be reported.

Clinical Application 3.2

- The nurse is checking Ms. Baranski's patient-controlled analgesia of morphine sulfate. The medication cartridge is empty and needs to be changed. What are the nurse's legal responsibilities when changing an opioid medication?
- What nursing interventions prevent medication errors?

NCLEX Success

2. The nurse is administering the first dose of an anti-infective agent. Which of the following assessments should the nurse make prior to administering the anti-infective agent?
   A. Assess the patient's temperature.
   B. Assess the patient's level of consciousness.
   C. Assess whether the patient is allergic to any anti-infective agent.
   D. Assess whether the patient has taken the medication previously.

MEDICATION ORDERS

Medication orders should include the full name of the patient; the name of the drug (preferably the generic name); the dose, route, and frequency of administration; and the date, time, and signature of the prescriber.

Orders in a healthcare facility may be typed into a computer (the preferred method) or handwritten on an order sheet in the patient's medical record. Occasionally, verbal or telephone

TABLE 3.2

Common Abbreviations

Routes of Drug Administration	
IM	intramuscular
IV	intravenous
PO	by mouth, oral
SL	sublingual
Sub-Q	subcutaneous
NAS	intranasal
Drug Dosages	
g	gram
IU	unit
mg	milligram
mcg	microgram
mL	milliliter
oz	ounce
tbsp	tablespoon
tsp	teaspoon
Times of Drug Administration	
ad lib	as desired
PRN	as needed
q4h	every 4 h
stat	immediately

> **NCLEX Success**
>
> 3. The nurse has administered lacosamide to the wrong patient. What is the first action the nurse should take?
>   A. Assess the patient's vital signs and level of consciousness.
>   B. Notify the physician.
>   C. Fill out an incident report.
>   D. Call the respiratory therapist for administration of oxygen.

orders are acceptable. When taken, they should be written on the patient's order sheet, signed by the person taking the order, and later countersigned by the prescriber. After the order is written, a copy is sent to the pharmacy, where the order is recorded, and the drug is dispensed to the appropriate patient care unit. In many facilities, pharmacy staff prepares a computer-generated MAR for each 24-hour period.

For patients in ambulatory care settings, the procedure is essentially the same for drugs to be given immediately. For drugs to be taken at home, written prescriptions are given. In addition to the previous information, a prescription should include instructions for taking the drug (e.g., dose, frequency) and whether the prescription can be refilled. Prescriptions for schedule II controlled drugs cannot be refilled.

To interpret medication orders accurately, the nurse must know commonly used abbreviations for routes, dosages, and times of drug administration (Table 3.2). As a result of medication errors that occurred because of incorrect or misinterpreted abbreviations, many abbreviations that were formerly used are now banned or are no longer recommended by The Joint Commission, the ISMP, and other organizations concerned with increasing patient safety. Thus, it is safer to write out such words as "daily" or "three times daily"; "at bedtime," "ounce," "teaspoon," or "tablespoon"; or "right," "left," or "both eyes" rather than using abbreviations, in both medication orders and in transcribing orders to the patient's MAR. If the nurse cannot read the physician's order or if the order seems erroneous, they question the order before giving the drug.

DRUG PREPARATIONS AND DOSAGE FORMS

Drug preparations and dosage forms vary according to the drug's chemical characteristics, reason for use, and route of administration. Some drugs are available in only one dosage form, and others are available in several forms. Table 3.3 and the following section describe characteristics of various dosage forms.

Dosage forms of systemic drugs include liquids, tablets, capsules, suppositories, and transdermal and pump delivery systems. Systemic liquids are given orally, or PO (Latin *per os*, "by mouth"), or by injection. Those given by injection must be sterile.

Administration of tablets and capsules is PO. Tablets contain active drug plus binders, colorants, preservatives, and other substances. Capsules contain active drug enclosed in a gelatin capsule. Most tablets and capsules dissolve in the acidic fluids of the stomach and are absorbed in the alkaline fluids of the upper small intestine. **Enteric-coated** tablets and capsules are coated with a substance that is insoluble in stomach acid. This substance delays dissolution until the medication reaches the intestine, usually to avoid gastric irritation or to keep the drug from being destroyed by gastric acid. Tablets for sublingual (under the tongue) or buccal (held in the cheek) administration must be specifically formulated for such use.

Several **controlled-release** dosage forms and drug delivery systems are available, and more continue to be developed. These formulations maintain more consistent serum drug levels and allow less frequent administration, which is more convenient for patients. Controlled-release oral tablets and capsules are called by a variety of names (e.g., timed release, sustained release, extended release), and their names usually include CR, SR, XL, or other indications that they are long-acting formulations. Most of these formulations are given once or twice daily. Some drugs (e.g., alendronate for osteoporosis, fluoxetine for major depression) are available in formulations that deliver a full week's dosage in one oral tablet. Because controlled-release tablets and capsules contain high amounts of drug intended to be absorbed slowly and act over a prolonged period of time, they should never be broken, opened, crushed, or chewed. Such an action allows the full dose to be absorbed immediately and constitutes an overdose, with potential organ damage or death. **Transdermal** (skin patch) formulations include systemically absorbed clonidine, estrogen, fentanyl, and nitroglycerin. These medications are slowly absorbed from the skin patches over varying periods of time (e.g., 1 week for clonidine and estrogen). Pump delivery

TABLE 3.3
Drug Dosage Forms

Dosage Forms and Their Routes of Administration	Characteristics	Considerations/Precautions
Tablets		
Regular: PO, gastrointestinal (GI) tube (crushed and mixed with water)	• Contain active drug plus binders, dyes, preservatives • Dissolve in gastric fluids	8 oz of water recommended, to promote dissolution and absorption
Chewable: PO	Colored and flavored, mainly for young children	Children may think tablets are candy; keep out of reach to avoid accidental overdose
Enteric coated: PO	Dissolve in the small intestine; mainly used for medications that cause gastric irritation	Do not crush; instruct patients not to chew or crush
Extended release (XL) (also called sustained release [SR], long acting [LA], and other names): PO	Slowly absorbed; effects prolonged, usually 12–24 h Contain relatively large amounts of active drug	**Warning:** Crushing to give orally or through a GI tube administers an overdose, with potentially serious adverse effects or death! *Never crush*; instruct patients not to chew or crush
Sublingual: Under the tongue	Dissolve quickly	
Buccal: Held in cheek	Medication absorbed directly into the bloodstream and exerts rapid systemic effects	Few medications formulated for administration by SL or buccal routes
Capsules		
Regular: PO	Contain active drug, fillers, and preservatives	8 oz of fluid recommended to promote dissolution and absorption
	Gelatin capsules dissolve in gastric fluid and release medication	
Extended release (XL); sustained release (SR); long-acting (LA): PO	Slowly absorbed; effects prolonged, usually 12–24 h Contain relatively large amounts of active drug	**Warning:** Emptying a capsule to give the medication orally or through a GI tube administers an overdose, with potentially serious adverse effects or death! Instruct patients not to bite, chew, or empty these capsules
Solutions		
Oral: PO, GI tube	Absorbed rapidly because they do not need to be dissolved	Use of appropriate measuring devices and accurate measurement is extremely important
Parenteral: IV, IM, Sub-Q, intradermal	Medications and all administration devices must be sterile IV produces rapid effects; Sub-Q is used mainly for insulin and heparin; IM is used for only a few drugs; intradermal is used mainly to inject skin-test material	Use of appropriate equipment and accurate measurement is extremely important. Insulin syringes should always be used for insulin, and tuberculin syringes are recommended for measuring small amounts of other drugs
Suspensions		
PO, Sub-Q (e.g., NPH, Lente insulins)	Particles of active drug are suspended in a liquid; the liquid must be rotated or shaken before measuring a dose	Drug particles settle to the bottom on standing. If not remixed, the liquid vehicle is given rather than the drug dose
Dermatologic Creams, Lotions, Ointments Topically to skin	Most are minimally absorbed through skin and exert local effects at the site of application; some (e.g., skin patches) are absorbed and exert systemic effects	*Formulations vary with intended uses and are not interchangeable.* When removed from the patient, skin patches must be disposed of properly to prevent someone else from being exposed to the active drug remaining in the patch

TABLE 3.3

Drug Dosage Forms (Continued)

Dosage Forms and Their Routes of Administration	Characteristics	Considerations/Precautions
Solutions and Powders for Oral or Nasal Inhalation, Including Metered Dose Inhalers (MDIs)	Oral inhalations are used mainly for asthma; nasal sprays for nasal allergies (allergic rhinitis). Effective with less systemic effect than oral drugs Deliver a specified dose per inhalation	Several research studies indicate that patients often do not use MDIs correctly; correct use is essential to obtaining therapeutic effects and avoiding adverse effects
Eye Solutions and Ointments	*Should be sterile* Packaged in small amounts for individual use	Can be systemically absorbed and cause systemic adverse effects
Throat Lozenges	Used for cough and sore throat	
Ear Solutions	Used mainly for ear infections	
Vaginal Creams and Suppositories	Used to treat vaginal infections	
Rectal Suppositories and Enemas	• Suppositories may be used to administer sedatives, analgesics, and laxatives • Medicated enemas may be used for constipation or inflammatory bowel diseases	Effects somewhat unpredictable because absorption is erratic

systems may be external or implanted under the skin and refillable or long acting without refills. Pumps are used to administer insulin, opioid analgesics, antineoplastics, and other drugs.

Solutions, ointments, creams, and suppositories are applied topically to the skin or mucous membranes. They are formulated for the intended route of administration. For example, several drugs are available in solutions for nasal or oral inhalation; they are usually self-administered as a spray into the nose or mouth.

Many combination products containing fixed doses of two or more drugs are also available. Commonly used combinations include analgesics, antihypertensive drugs, and cold remedies. Most are oral tablets, capsules, or solutions.

CALCULATING DRUG DOSAGES

When calculating drug dosages, the importance of accuracy cannot be overemphasized. Accuracy requires basic skills in mathematics, knowledge of common units of measurement, and methods of using data in performing calculations.

Systems of Measurement

The most commonly used system of measurement is the metric system, in which the meter is used for linear measure, the gram for weight, and the liter for volume. One milliliter (mL) equals 1 cubic centimeter (cc), and both equal 1 gram (g) of water. The household system, with units of drops, teaspoons, tablespoons, and cups, is infrequently used in healthcare agencies but may be used at home. Table 3.4 lists some commonly used equivalent measurements.

A few drugs are ordered and measured in terms of units or milliequivalents (mEq). Units express biologic activity in animal tests (i.e., the amount of drug required to produce a particular response). Units are unique for each drug. For example, concentrations of insulin and heparin are both expressed in units, but there is no relation between a unit of insulin and a unit of heparin. These drugs are usually ordered in the number of units per dose (e.g., NPH insulin 30 units subcutaneously every morning or heparin 5,000 units subcutaneously every 12 hours) and labeled in number of units per milliliter (U 100 insulin contains 100 units/mL; heparin may have 1,000, 5,000, or 10,000 units/mL). Milliequivalents express the ionic activity of a drug. Drugs such as potassium chloride are ordered and labeled in the number of milliequivalents per dose, tablet, or milliliter.

Mathematical Calculations

Most drug orders and labels are expressed in metric units of measurement. If the amount specified in the order is the same

TABLE 3.4

Selected Equivalent Measurements

Metric	Household
Weights	
1,000 mcg = 1 mg	
1,000 mg = 1 g	
30 g	1 oz
454 g	1 lb
1,000 g = 1 kg	2.2 lb
Liquids	
1 mL = 1 cc	
5 mL	1 tsp
30 mL	2 tbsp or 1 oz
250 mL	1 cup or 8 oz
500 mL	1 pint
1,000 mL = 1 L	1 quart

as that on the drug label, no calculations are required, and preparing the right dose is a simple matter. For example, if the order reads "ibuprofen 600 mg PO" and the drug label reads "ibuprofen 600 mg per tablet," it is clear that one tablet is to be given.

What happens if the order calls for a 600-mg dose and 200-mg tablets are available? The question is, "How many 200-mg tablets are needed to give a dose of 600 mg?" In this case, the answer can be readily calculated mentally to indicate three tablets. This is a simple example that also can be used to illustrate mathematical calculations. This problem can be solved by several acceptable methods; the following formula is relatively simple one:

$$\frac{D}{H} = \frac{X}{V}$$

D = desired dose (dose ordered, often in milligrams)
H = on-hand or available dose (dose on the drug label; often in mg per tablet, capsule, or milliliter)
X = unknown (number of tablets, in this example)
V = volume or unit (one tablet, in this example)

$$\frac{600 \text{ mg}}{200 \text{ mg}} = \frac{X \text{ tablet}}{1 \text{ tablet}}$$

Cross multiply:

$$200 X = 600$$

$$X = \frac{600}{200} = 3 \text{ tablets}$$

What happens if the order and the label are written in different units? For example, the order may read "amoxicillin 0.5 g" and the label may read "amoxicillin 500 mg/capsule." To calculate the number of capsules needed for the dose, the first step is to convert 0.5 g to the equivalent number of milligrams or convert 500 mg to the equivalent number of grams. *The desired or ordered dose and the available or label dose must be in the same units of measurement.* Using the equivalents (i.e., 1 g = 1,000 mg) listed in Table 3.4, an equation can be set up as follows:

$$\frac{1 \text{ g}}{1{,}000 \text{ mg}} = \frac{0.5 \text{ g}}{X \text{ mg}}$$

$$X = 0.5 \times 1{,}000 = 500 \text{ mg}$$

The next step is to use the new information in the formula, which then becomes

$$\frac{D}{H} = \frac{X}{V}$$

$$\frac{500 \text{ mg}}{500 \text{ mg}} = \frac{X \text{ capsules}}{1 \text{ capsule}}$$

$$500 X = 500$$

$$X = \frac{500}{500} = 1 \text{ capsule}$$

The same procedure and formula can be used to calculate portions of tablets or doses of liquids. These are illustrated in the following problems:

1. Order: 25 mg PO
   Label: 50-mg tablet

$$\frac{25 \text{ mg}}{50 \text{ mg}} = \frac{X \text{ tablet}}{1 \text{ tablet}}$$

$$50 X = 25$$

$$X = \frac{25}{50} = 0.5 \text{ tablet}$$

2. Order: 25 mg IM
   Label: 50 mg in 1 cc

$$\frac{25 \text{ mg}}{50 \text{ mg}} = \frac{X \text{ cc}}{1 \text{ cc}}$$

$$50 X = 25$$

$$X = \frac{25}{50} = 0.5 \text{ cc}$$

3. Order: 4 mg IV
   Label: 10 mg/mL

$$\frac{4 \text{ mg}}{10 \text{ mg}} = \frac{X \text{ mL}}{1 \text{ mL}}$$

$$10 X = 4$$

$$X = \frac{4}{10} = 0.4 \text{ mL}$$

Other Useful Formulas

Two other methods can be used to calculate the proper amount of medication to be administered to the patient. One is referred to as the two-ratio method. The other is referred to as the formula method.

Two-Ratio Method

The first ratio in this method is the known equivalent. The second ratio is the ordered dose.

Suppose a patient is having increasing pain at the end-of-life, the home care nurse notifies the physician of the patient's increased pain, and physician orders morphine sulfate to be increased from 5 to 10 mg. The home care nurse has a prescription for morphine sulfate, 5 mg per tablet. How many tablets of morphine sulfate should the home care nurse administer to the patient? The ratio is as follows (using the same mathematical symbols given earlier):

$$\frac{V}{H} = \frac{D}{X}$$

$$\frac{5 \text{ mg}}{1 \text{ tablet}} = \frac{10 \text{ mg}}{X \text{ mg}}$$

$$5X = 10$$

$$X = \frac{10}{5} = 2 \text{ tablets}$$

Formula Method

The easiest method to understand and use is the formula method. Supposing a nurse has acetaminophen 325 mg in 5 mL and needs to administer 650 mg orally. How many milliliters are administered? The drug formula is as follows (using the same mathematical symbols given earlier):

$$\frac{D}{H} \times V = X$$

$$\frac{650 \text{ mg}}{325 \text{ mg}} \times 5 \text{ mL} = X = 10 \text{ mL}$$

ROUTES OF ADMINISTRATION

Routes of administration depend on drug characteristics, patient characteristics, and desired responses. The major routes are oral (by mouth), **parenteral** (injected), and **topical** (applied to skin or mucous membrane). Each has advantages, disadvantages, indications for use, and specific techniques of administration (Table 3.5). Common parenteral routes are subcutaneous (Sub-Q), IM, and IV injections. Injections require special drug preparations, equipment, and techniques. The following section discusses general characteristics of the IV route, and Box 3.1 presents specific considerations.

Drugs for Injection

Injectable drugs must be prepared, packaged, and administered in ways to maintain sterility. Vials are closed containers with rubber stoppers through which a sterile needle can be inserted for withdrawing medication. Single-dose vials usually do not

TABLE 3.5

Routes of Drug Administration

Route and Description	Advantages	Disadvantages	Comments
Oral	Simple and can be used by most people Convenient; does not require complex equipment Relatively inexpensive	Dosage is unknown because some drug is not absorbed and some is metabolized in the liver before reaching the bloodstream Slow drug action Irritation of gastrointestinal (GI) mucosa by some drugs	The oral route should generally be used when possible, considering the patient's condition and ability to take or tolerate oral drugs
GI tubes (e.g., nasogastric, gastrostomy)	Allows use of GI tract in patients who cannot take oral drugs Can be used over long periods of time, if necessary May avoid or decrease injections	With nasogastric tubes, medications may be aspirated into the lungs Small-bore tubes often become clogged Requires special precautions to give correctly and avoid complications	Liquid preparations are preferred over crushed tablets and emptied capsules, when available Tube should be rinsed before and after instilling medication
Subcutaneous (Sub-Q) injection—injection of drugs under the skin, into the underlying fatty tissue	Relatively painless Very small needles can be used Insulin and heparin, commonly used medications, can be given Sub-Q	Only a small amount of drug (up to 1 mL) can be given Drug absorption is relatively slow Only a few drugs can be given Sub-Q	Sub-Q route is commonly used for only a few drugs because many drugs are irritating to Sub-Q tissues. Such drugs may cause pain, necrosis, and abscess formation if injected Sub-Q
Intramuscular (IM) injection—injection of drugs into selected muscles	May be used for several drugs Drug absorption is rapid because muscle tissue has an abundant blood supply	A relatively small amount of drug (up to 3 mL) can be given Risks of damage to blood vessels or nerves if needle is not positioned correctly	It is very important to use anatomic landmarks when selecting IM injection sites

(Continued on page 46)

TABLE 3.5

Routes of Drug Administration (Continued)

Route and Description	Advantages	Disadvantages	Comments
Intravenous (IV) injection—injection of a drug into the bloodstream	Allows medications to be given to a patient who cannot take fluids or drugs by GI tract. Bypasses barriers to drug absorption that occur with other routes. Rapid drug action. Larger amounts can be given than by Sub-Q and IM routes. Allows slow administration when indicated.	Time and skill required for venipuncture and maintaining an IV line. After it is injected, drug cannot be retrieved if adverse effects or overdoses occur. High potential for adverse reactions due to rapid drug action and possible complications of IV therapy (i.e., bleeding, infection, fluid overload, extravasation). Phlebitis and thrombosis may occur and cause discomfort or pain, take days or weeks to subside, and limit the veins available for future therapy.	The nurse should wear latex gloves to start IV infusions, for protection against exposure to bloodborne pathogens. Phlebitis and thrombosis result from injury to the endothelial cells that form the inner lining (intima) of veins and may be caused by repeated venipunctures, the IV catheter, hypertonic IV fluid, or irritating drugs.
Topical administration—application to skin or mucous membranes. Application to mucous membranes includes drugs given by nasal or oral inhalation; by instillation into the lungs, eyes, or nose; and by insertion under the tongue (sublingual), into the cheek (buccal), and into the vagina or rectum	With application to intact skin, most medications act at the site of application, with little systemic absorption or systemic adverse effects. Some drugs are given topically for systemic effects (e.g., medicated skin patches). Effects may last several days, and the patches are usually convenient for patients. With application to mucous membranes, most drugs are well and rapidly absorbed.	Some drugs irritate the skin or mucous membranes and cause itching, rash, or discomfort. With inflamed, abraded, or damaged skin, drug absorption is increased, and systemic adverse effects may occur. Application to mucous membranes may cause systemic adverse effects (e.g., beta-blocker eye drops, used to treat glaucoma, can cause bradycardia just as oral beta-adrenergic blockers can). Specific drug preparations must be used for application to skin, eyes, and sublingual, buccal, vaginal, and rectal sites.	When available and effective, topical drugs are often preferred over oral or injected drugs, because of fewer and/or less severe systemic adverse effects.

BOX 3.1 Principles and Techniques With Intravenous Drug Therapy

IV Administration Methods

- **Intravenous (IV) injection or IV push**: The direct injection of a medication into the vein.
  - The drug may be injected through an injection site on IV tubing or an intermittent infusion device.
  - Most IV push medications should be injected slowly. The time depends on the particular drug but is often 2 minutes or longer for a dose.
  - Rapid injection should generally be avoided because the drug produces high blood levels and is quickly circulated to the heart and brain, where it may cause adverse or toxic effects.
  - IV push may be useful with a few drugs or in emergency situations, slower infusion of more dilute drugs is usually preferred.
- **Intermittent IV infusion**: The administration of intermittent doses often diluted in 50 to 100 mL of fluid and infused over 30 to 60 minutes.
  - The drug dose is usually prepared in a pharmacy and connected to an IV administration set that controls the amount and flow rate.
  - Intermittent infusions are often connected to an injection port on a primary IV line, through which IV fluids are infusing continuously.
  - The purpose of the primary IV line may be to provide fluids to the patient or to keep the vein open for periodic administration of medications.
  - The IV fluids are usually stopped for the medication infusion and then restarted.
- **Intermittent Infusion Device**: Drug doses may also be infused through an intermittent infusion device (e.g., a saline lock) to conserve veins and allow freedom of motion between drug doses.
  - The devices decrease the amount of IV fluids given to patients who do not need them (i.e., those who are able to ingest adequate amounts of oral fluids) and those

BOX 3.1 Principles and Techniques With Intravenous Drug Therapy (Continued)

who are at risk of fluid overload, especially children and older adults. An intermittent infusion device may be part of an initial IV line or used to adapt a continuous IV for intermittent use.

- The devices include a saline lock or a resealable adapter added to a peripheral or central IV catheter. These devices must be flushed routinely to maintain patency.
- If the IV catheter has more than one lumen, all must be flushed, whether being used or not. Saline is probably the most commonly used flushing solution; heparin may also be used if recommended by the device's manufacturer or required by institutional policy.
- **Continuous IV Infusion:** Indicated for medications mixed in a large volume of IV fluid and infused continuously, over several hours. For example, vitamins and minerals (e.g., potassium chloride) are usually added to liters of IV fluids.
  - Greater dilution of the drug and administration over a longer time decrease risks of accumulation and toxicity, as well as venous irritation and thrombophlebitis.

Equipment

- **IV Supplies and Infusion Devices:** Equipment varies considerably from one healthcare agency to another. Nurses must become familiar with the equipment available in their work setting, including IV catheters, types of IV tubing, needles and needleless systems, types of volume-control devices, and electronic infusion devices (IV pumps).
- **Catheters** vary in size (both gauge and length), design, and composition (e.g., polyvinyl chloride, polyurethane, silicone).
  - The most common design type is over the needle; the needle is used to start the IV, and then, it is removed.
  - Choose a catheter to start an IV, one that is much smaller than the lumen of the vein is recommended.
    - This allows good blood flow and rapidly dilutes drug solutions as they enter the vein.
    - This, in turn, prevents high drug concentrations and risks of toxicity.
  - After a catheter is inserted, it is very important to tape it securely so that it does not move around; movement will increase the risk of venous irritation, thrombophlebitis, or infection. Apply a topical antibiotic or antiseptic ointment at the IV insertion site, followed by an occlusive dressing, and date and time the dressing. If irritation or occlusion develops, remove the catheter and insert a new catheter.
- **Peripheral Inserted Central Catheters:** Many medications are administered through peripherally inserted central catheters (PICC lines) or central venous catheters, in which the catheter tips are inserted into the superior vena cava, next to the right atrium of the heart. Central venous catheters may have single, double, or triple lumens. Other products, which are especially useful for long-term IV drug therapy, include a variety of implanted ports, pumps, and reservoirs.

Site Selection

IV needles are usually inserted into a vein on the hand or forearm; IV catheters may be inserted in a peripheral site or centrally. In general, recommendations are as follows:
- Start at the most distal location. This conserves more proximal veins for later use, if needed. Veins on the back of the hand and on the forearm are often used to provide more comfort and freedom of movement for patients.
- Use veins with a large blood volume flowing through them when possible. Many drugs cause irritation and phlebitis in small veins.
- When possible, avoid the antecubital vein on the inner surface of the elbow, veins over or close to joints, and veins on the inner aspect of the wrists. Reasons include the difficulty of stabilizing and maintaining an IV line at these sites and the fact that inner wrist venipunctures are very painful. *Do not perform venipuncture in foot or leg veins.* The risks of serious or fatal complications are too high.
- Rotate sites when long-term use (more than a few days) of IV fluid or drug therapy is required. Venous irritation occurs with longer duration of site use and with the administration of irritating drugs or fluids. When it is necessary to change an IV site, use the opposite arm if possible.
  - Most IV drugs are prepared for administration in pharmacies, and this is the safest practice. When a nurse must prepare a medication, considerations include the following points.
- Only drug formulations manufactured for IV use should be given IV. Other formulations contain various substances that are not sterile, pure enough, or soluble enough to be injected into the bloodstream. *In recent years, there have been numerous reports of medication errors resulting from IV administration of drug preparations intended for oral use!* Such errors can and should be prevented. For example, when liquid medications intended for oral use are measured or dispensed in a syringe (as they often are for children, for adults with difficulty in swallowing tablets and capsules, or for administration through a gastrointestinal [GI] tube), the syringe should have a blunt tip that will not connect to or penetrate IV tubing injection sites.
- Use sterile technique during all phases of IV drug preparation.
- Follow the manufacturer's instructions for mixing and diluting IV medications. Some liquid IV medications need to be diluted prior to IV administration, and powdered medications must be reconstituted with the recommended diluent. The diluent recommended by the drug's manufacturer should be used because different drugs require different diluents. In addition, be sure any reconstituted drug is completely dissolved to avoid particles that may be injected into the systemic circulation and lead to thrombus formation or embolism. A filtered aspiration needle should be used when withdrawing medication from a vial or ampule, to remove any particles in the solution. The filter needle should then be discarded, to prevent filtered particles from being injected when the medication is added to the IV fluid. Filters added to IV tubing also help to remove particles.
- Check the expiration date on all IV medications. Many drugs have a limited period of stability after they are reconstituted or diluted for IV administration.
- IV medications should be compatible with the infusing IV fluids. Most are compatible with 5% dextrose in water or saline solutions.
- If adding a medication to a container of IV fluid, invert the container to be sure the additive is well mixed with the solution.

(Continued on page 48)

BOX 3.1 Principles and Techniques With Intravenous Drug Therapy (Continued)

- For any IV medication that is prepared or added to an IV bag, label the medication vial or IV bag with the name of the patient, drug, dosage, date, time of mixing, expiration date, and the preparer's signature.
- Most IV medications are injected into a self-sealing site in any of several IV setups, including a scalp-vein needle and tubing; a plastic catheter connected to a heparin lock or other intermittent infusion device; or IV tubing and a plastic bag containing IV fluid.
- Before injecting any IV medication, be sure that the IV line is open and functioning properly (e.g., catheter not clotted, IV fluid not leaking into surrounding tissues, phlebitis not present). If leakage occurs, some drugs are very irritating to subcutaneous tissues and may cause tissue necrosis.
- Maintain sterility of all IV fluids, tubings, injection sites, drug solutions, and equipment coming into contact with the IV system. Because medications and fluids are injected directly into the bloodstream, breaks in sterile technique can lead to serious systemic infection (septicemia) and death.
- When two or more medications are to be given one after the other, flush the IV tubing and catheter (with the infusing IV fluid or with sterile 0.9% sodium chloride injection) so that the drugs do not come into contact with each other.
- In general, administer slowly to allow greater dilution of the drug in the bloodstream. Most drugs given by IV push (direct injection) can be given over 2 to 5 minutes, and most drugs diluted in 50 to 100 mL of IV fluid can be infused in 30 to 60 minutes.
- When injecting or infusing medications into IV solutions that contain other additives (e.g., vitamins, insulin, minerals such as potassium or magnesium), be sure that the medications are compatible with the other substances. Consult compatibility charts (usually available on nursing units) or pharmacists when indicated.
- IV flow rates are usually calculated in mL per hour and drops per minute.

contain a preservative and must be discarded after a dose is withdrawn. Multiple-dose vials contain a preservative and may be reused if aseptic technique is maintained.

Ampules are sealed glass containers, the tops of which must be broken off to allow insertion of a needle and withdrawal of the medication. Broken ampules and any remaining medication are discarded. When vials or ampules contain a powder form of the drug, a sterile solution of water or 0.9% sodium chloride must be added and the drug dissolved before withdrawal. When available, a filter needle is used to withdraw the medication from an ampule or vial because broken glass or rubber fragments may need to be removed from the drug solution. The filter needle is replaced with a regular needle before injecting the patient.

Many injectable drugs (e.g., morphine, heparin) are available in prefilled syringes with attached needles. These units are inserted into specially designed holders and used like other needle–syringe units.

Quality and Safety Alert: Safety

It is important to note that many such units, especially those from the same manufacturer, are similar, and their use may lead to medication errors if the label is not read carefully.

Equipment for Injections

Sterile needles and syringes are used to measure and administer parenteral medications; they may be packaged together or separately. Needles are available in various gauges and lengths. The term *gauge* refers to lumen size, with larger numbers indicating smaller lumen sizes. For example, a 25-gauge needle is smaller than an 18-gauge needle. Choice of needle gauge and length depends on the route of administration, the viscosity (thickness) of the solution to be given, and the size of the patient. Usually, a 25-gauge, 5/8-in needle is used for Sub-Q injections, and a 22- or 20-gauge, 1½-in needle is used for IM injections. Other needle sizes are available for special uses, such as for insulin or intradermal injections. When needles are used, avoid recapping them, and dispose of them in appropriate containers. Such containers are designed to prevent accidental needlestick injuries to healthcare and housekeeping personnel.

In many settings, needleless systems are used. These systems involve a plastic tip on the syringe that can be used to enter vials and injection sites on IV tubing. Openings created by the tip reseal themselves. Needleless systems were developed because of the risk of injury and spread of bloodborne pathogens, such as the viruses that cause acquired immunodeficiency syndrome and hepatitis B or C.

Syringes also are available in various sizes. The 3 mL size is often used. It is usually plastic and is available with or without an attached needle. Syringes are calibrated so that drug doses can be measured accurately. However, the calibrations vary according to the size and type of syringe.

Insulin and tuberculin syringes are used for specific purposes. Insulin syringes are calibrated to measure up to 100 units of insulin. Safe practice requires that *only* insulin syringes be used to measure insulin and that they be used for no other drugs. Tuberculin syringes have a capacity of 1 mL. They should be used for small doses of any drug because measurements are more accurate than with larger syringes.

Sites for Injections

Common sites for subcutaneous injections are the upper arms, abdomen, back, and thighs (Fig. 3.3). Sites for IM injections are the deltoid, ventrogluteal, and vastus lateralis muscles. It should be noted that most healthcare agencies no longer allow the administration of IM injections in the dorsogluteal site. It is important to review the policies and procedures of the institution before administering medications utilizing that site. To select the proper injection sites, the anatomical landmarks are identified (Fig. 3.4). Common sites for IV injections are the veins on the back of the hands and on the forearms (Fig. 3.5). Less common sites include intradermal (into layers of the skin), intra-arterial (into arteries), intra-articular (into joints), and intrathecal (into spinal fluid). Nurses may perform intradermal and intra-arterial injections (if an established arterial line is present); physicians perform intra-articular and intrathecal injections.

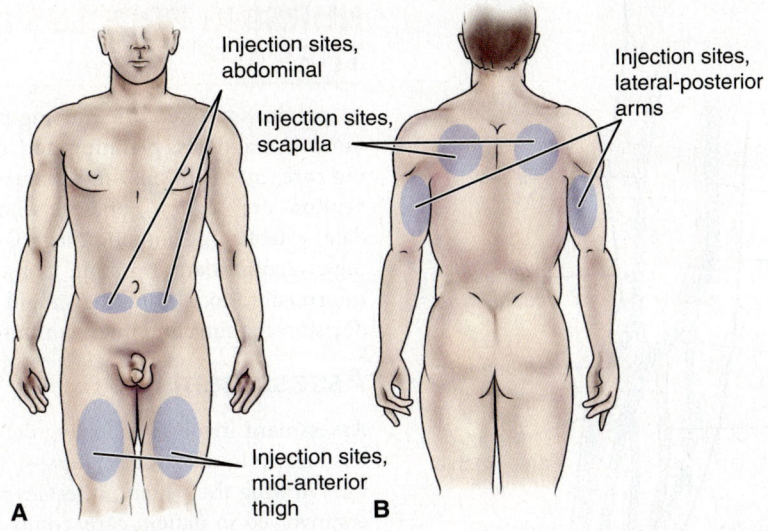

Figure 3.3. Subcutaneous injection sites.

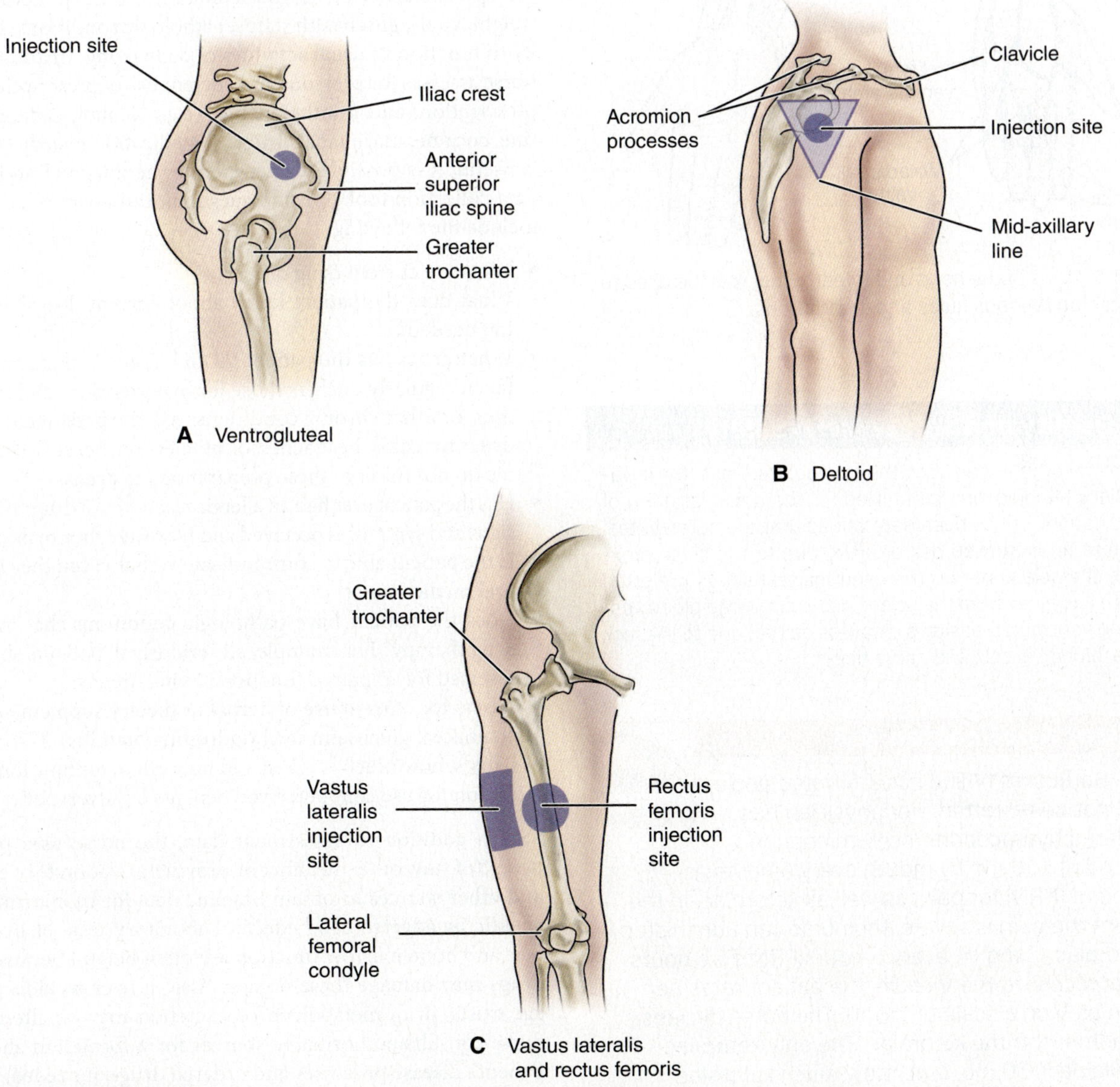

Figure 3.4. Anatomic landmarks and intramuscular (IM) injection sites. **A.** Ventrogluteal muscle. **B.** Deltoid muscle. **C.** Vastus lateralis and rectus femoris muscle.

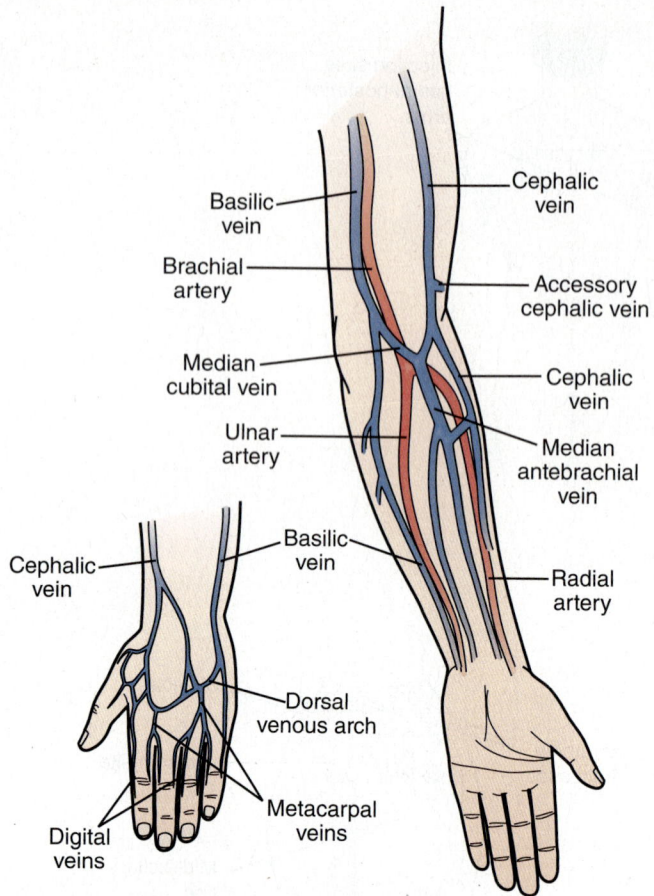

Figure 3.5. Veins of the hand and forearm that may be used to administer intravenous fluids and medications.

Quality and Safety Alert: Safety

It is not recommended that the dorsogluteal site for intramuscular (IM) injections be utilized for the administration of IM medications. It has been determined that the dorsogluteal site poses an increased risk of injury due to the close proximity to the sciatic nerve. The ventrogluteal site is preferred because it is away from the sciatic nerve and large blood vessels. The ventrogluteal site is also less painful due to the lack of large blood vessels and nerve fibers.

Clinical Application 3.3

- Ms. Baranski's IV line has infiltrated and will not be restarted. Her physician has ordered hydrocodone/acetaminophen (Vicodin) 500 mg by mouth every 6 hours as needed (PRN) for pain, as well as ketorolac. In the event the pain is severe, the nurse can administer ketorolac 15 mg IM every 6 hours PRN. Five hours after receiving the Vicodin, the patient rates her pain as 9 on a scale of 1 to 10. The nurse decides to administer the ketorolac. The only ketorolac available is 30 mg/1 mL. How much ketorolac should be administered?

NURSING PROCESS IN DRUG THERAPY

As previously stated, the nursing process involves assessment, nursing diagnosis, planning and establishing goals for nursing care, interventions, and evaluation. Assessment and intervention are "action" phases, whereas analyzing assessment data, establishing nursing diagnoses and goals, and performing evaluations are "thinking" phases. However, knowledge and informed, rational thinking should underlie all data collection, decision-making, and interventions.

Assessment

Assessment involves collecting data about patient characteristics known to affect drug therapy. This includes observing and interviewing the patient, interviewing family members or others involved in patient care, completing a physical assessment, reviewing medical records for pertinent laboratory and diagnostic test reports, and other methods. Initially (before drug therapy is started or on first contact), the nurse assesses age, weight, vital signs, health status, pathologic conditions, and ability to function in usual activities of daily living. In addition, the nurse assesses for previous and current use of prescription, nonprescription, and nontherapeutic (e.g., alcohol, caffeine, nicotine, cocaine, marijuana) drugs. A medication history (Box 3.2) is useful; it is possible to incorporate the information into any data collection tool. Specific questions and areas of assessment include the following:

- What are current drug orders?
- What does the patient know about current drugs? Is teaching needed?
- What drugs has the patient taken before? Include any drugs taken regularly, such as those for hypertension, diabetes mellitus, or other chronic conditions. Ask the patient about OTC drugs for colds, headaches, or indigestion, because some people do not think of these preparations as drugs.
- Has the patient ever had an allergic reaction to a drug? If so, what signs and symptoms occurred and how were they managed?
- Is the patient able to communicate verbally; can they swallow oral medications?
- Does the patient have pathologic conditions that influence drug therapy? For example, all seriously ill patients should be assessed for impaired function of vital organs.
- Assess for current use of herbal or dietary supplements (e.g., echinacea, glucosamine/chondroitin, vitamins). If so, ask for names, how much is taken and how often, for how long, their reason for use, and perceived benefits or adverse effects.

In addition to assessment data, the nurse uses progress notes (of any other healthcare providers), laboratory reports, and other sources to obtain baseline data for monitoring therapeutic or adverse drug effects. Laboratory tests of liver, kidney, and bone marrow function are often helpful because some drugs may damage these organs. Also, if liver or kidney damage exists, drug metabolism or excretion may be altered. The nurse consults authoritative sources for information about the patient's disease processes and ordered drugs, if needed.

After assessment data are obtained, they need to be analyzed to determine the patient's nursing care needs. Although

> **BOX 3.2 Medication History**
>
> Name _____ Age _____
> Health problems, acute and chronic
> Are you allergic to any medications?
> If yes, describe specific effects or symptoms.
>
> **Part 1: Prescription Medications**
>
> 1. Do you take any prescription medications on a regular basis?
> 2. If yes, ask the following about each medication.
>
> | Name | Dose |
> | Frequency | Specific times |
> | How long taken | Reason for use |
>
> 3. Do you have any difficulty in taking your medicines? If yes, ask to specify problem areas.
> 4. Have you had any symptoms or problems that you think are caused by your medicines? If yes, ask to specify.
> 5. Do you need help from another person to take your medicines?
> 6. Do you take any prescription medications on an irregular basis? If yes, ask the following about each medication.
>
> | Name | Dose |
> | Frequency | Reason for use |
> | How long taken | |
>
> **Part 2: Nonprescription Medications**
>
> Do you take over-the-counter medications?
>
> | | | Medication | | |
> |---|---|---|---|---|
> | Problem | Yes/No | Name | Amount | Frequency |
> | Pain | | | | |
> | Headache | | | | |
> | Sleep | | | | |
> | Cold | | | | |
> | Indigestion | | | | |
> | Heartburn | | | | |
> | Diarrhea | | | | |
> | Constipation | | | | |
> | Other | | | | |
>
> **Part 3: Social Drugs**
>
> | | Yes/No | Amount/day |
> |---|---|---|
> | Coffee | | |
> | Tea | | |
> | Cola drinks | | |
> | Alcohol | | |
> | Tobacco | | |
>
> **Part 4: Herbal or Dietary Supplements**
>
> Do you take any herbal or dietary supplements (e.g., ginkgo, glucosamine/chondroitin)? If so, ask for names, how much and how often taken, reason for use, perceived effectiveness, and any adverse effects.

listed as the first step in the nursing process for discussion purposes, assessment is a component of all steps and occurs with every contact with the patient. Ongoing assessment of a patient's health status and response to treatment is needed to determine whether nursing care requirements have changed. In general, nurses must provide care based on available information while knowing that assessment data are always relatively incomplete.

Nursing Diagnosis

A **nursing diagnosis**, as developed by the North American Nursing Diagnosis Association, describes patient problems or needs. It is based on assessment data and is individualized according to the patient's condition and the drugs prescribed. Thus, the number of nursing diagnoses needed to adequately reflect the patient's condition varies considerably. Because the NCLEX does not test nursing diagnoses, this textbook will focus on all aspects of the nursing process except nursing diagnoses.

Planning/Goals

The **planning/goals** phase describes the expected outcomes of prescribed drug therapy. As a general rule, goals are stated in terms of patient behavior, not nurse behavior. For example, the patient will

- Receive or take drugs as prescribed
- Experience relief of signs and symptoms
- Avoid preventable adverse drug effects
- Self-administer drugs safely and accurately
- Verbalize essential drug information
- Keep appointments for monitoring and follow-up
- Use any herbal and dietary supplements with caution and report such use to healthcare providers

Interventions

Interventions involve implementing planned activities and include any task performed directly with a patient or indirectly on a patient's behalf. Areas of intervention are broad and may include assessment, promoting adherence to prescribed drug therapy, and solving problems related to drug therapy, among others.

General interventions related to drug therapy include promoting health, preventing or decreasing the need for drug therapy, using nondrug measures to enhance therapeutic effects or decrease adverse effects, teaching, individualizing care, administering drugs, and observing patient responses. Some examples include the following:

- Promoting healthful lifestyles in terms of nutrition, fluids, exercise, rest, and sleep
- Performing hand hygiene and other measures to prevent infection
- Ambulating, positioning, and exercising
- Assisting to cough and deep breathe
- Applying heat or cold
- Increasing or decreasing sensory stimulation
- Scheduling activities to promote rest or sleep
- Recording vital signs, fluid intake, urine output, and other assessment data

The intervention of teaching patients and caregivers about drug therapy is essential because most medications are self-administered and patients need information and assistance to use therapeutic drugs safely and effectively. Adequate knowledge, skill, and preparation are required to fulfill teaching responsibilities. See Boxes 3.3, 3.4, and 3.5 for teaching aids to assist the nurse in this endeavor. Future chapters will address the patient teaching guidelines for medications discussed in each chapter.

Certain interventions exist with the administration of medications based on the route. No matter which route of medication administration is being implemented, it is important for the nurse to be uninterrupted during the time. The greatest number of failures within the medication administration

---

BOX 3.3 *Preparing to Teach a Patient or Caregiver*

- Assess learning needs, especially when new drugs are added or new conditions are being treated. This includes finding out what the person already knows about a particular drug. Do not assume that teaching is unneeded, even if the patient has been taking a drug for a while.
- Assess ability to manage a drug therapy regimen (i.e., read printed instructions and drug labels, remember dosage schedules, self-administer medications by ordered routes). A medication history (see Box 3.2) helps assess the patient's knowledge about drug therapy.
- From assessment data, develop an individualized teaching plan. This saves time for both nurse and patient by avoiding repetition of known material. It also promotes adherence to prescribed drug therapy.
- Try to decrease anxiety. Patients and caregivers may feel overwhelmed by complicated medication regimens. Provide positive reinforcement for effort.
- Choose an appropriate time (e.g., when the patient is mentally alert and not in acute distress from pain or other symptoms) and a place with minimal noise and distractions, when possible.
- Proceed slowly, in small steps; emphasize essential information; and provide opportunities to express concerns or ask questions.
- Provide a combination of verbal and written instructions, which is more effective than either alone. Minimize medical jargon, and be aware that patients may have difficulty understanding and retaining the material being taught because of the stress of the illness.
- When explaining a drug to a hospitalized patient, describe the name (preferably both the generic and a trade name), purpose, expected effects, and so on. The purpose can usually be stated in terms of symptoms to be relieved or other expected benefits. In many instances, the drug is familiar and can be described from personal knowledge. If the drug is unfamiliar, use available resources (e.g., drug reference books, computer drug databases, pharmacists) to learn about the drug and provide accurate information to the patient.
- When teaching a patient about medications to be taken at home, provide specific information and instructions about each drug, including how to take them and how to observe for beneficial and adverse effects. If adverse effects occur, teach them how to manage minor ones and which ones to report to a healthcare provider. In addition, discuss ways to develop a convenient routine for taking medications, so that usual activities of daily living are minimally disrupted. Allow time for questions, and try to ensure that the patient understands how, when, and why to take the medications.
- When teaching a patient about potential adverse drug effects, the goal is to provide needed information without causing unnecessary anxiety. Most drugs produce undesirable effects; some are minor, some are potentially serious. Many people stop taking a drug rather than report adverse reactions. If reactions are reported, it may be possible to continue the drug by reducing dosage, changing the time of administration, or other measures. If severe reactions occur, the drug should be stopped and the prescriber should be notified.
- Emphasize the importance of taking medications as prescribed throughout the teaching session and perhaps at times of other contacts. Common patient errors include taking incorrect doses, taking doses at the wrong times, omitting doses, and stopping a medication too soon. Treatment failure can often be directly traced to these errors.
- Reassess learning needs when medication orders are changed (e.g., when medications are added because of a new illness or stopped).

BOX 3.4 — Patient Teaching Guidelines for Safe and Effective Use of Prescription Medications

General Considerations

- Use drugs cautiously and only when necessary because all drugs affect body functions and may cause adverse effects.
- Use nondrug measures, when possible, to prevent the need for drug therapy or to enhance beneficial effects and decrease adverse effects of drugs.
- Do not take drugs left over from a previous illness or prescribed for someone else, and do not share prescription drugs with anyone else. The likelihood of having the right drug in the right dose is remote, and the risk of adverse effects is high in such circumstances.
- Keep all healthcare providers informed about all the drugs being taken, including over-the-counter (OTC) products and herbal or dietary supplements.
- Take drugs as prescribed and for the length of time prescribed; notify a healthcare provider if unable to take a medication. Therapeutic effects greatly depend on taking medications correctly. Altering the dose or time may cause underdosage or overdosage. Stopping a medication may cause a recurrence of the problem for which it was given or withdrawal symptoms. Some medications need to be tapered in dosage and gradually discontinued. If problems occur with taking a drug, report them to a healthcare provider. An adjustment in dosage or other aspect of administration may solve the problem.
- Follow instructions for follow-up care (e.g., office visits, laboratory or other diagnostic tests that monitor therapeutic or adverse effects of drugs). Some drugs require more frequent monitoring than do others. However, safety requires periodic checks with essentially all medications. With long-term use of a medication, responses may change over time with aging, changes in kidney function, and so on.
- Take drugs in current use (or an up-to-date list) to appointments with a healthcare provider.
- Get all prescriptions filled at the same pharmacy, when possible. This is an important safety factor in helping to avoid multiple prescriptions of the same or similar drugs and to minimize undesirable interactions of newly prescribed drugs with those already in use.
- Report any drug allergies to all healthcare providers, and wear a medical identification emblem that lists allergens.
- Ask questions (and write down the answers) about newly prescribed medications, such as the following:
  - What is the medicine's name?
  - What is it supposed to do (i.e., what symptoms or problems will it relieve)?
  - How and when do I take it, and for how long?
  - Should it be taken with food or on an empty stomach?
  - While taking this medicine, should I avoid certain foods, beverages, other medications, or certain activities (e.g., alcoholic beverages and driving a car should be avoided with medications that cause drowsiness or decrease alertness)?
  - What side effects are likely and what do I do if they occur?
  - Will the medication affect my ability to sleep or work?
  - What should I do if I miss a dose?
  - Is there a drug information sheet I can have?
- Store medications out of reach of children, and, to prevent accidental ingestion, never refer to medications as "candy."
- When taking prescription medications, talk to a doctor, pharmacist, or nurse before starting an OTC medication or herbal or dietary supplement. This is a safety factor to avoid undesirable drug interactions.
- Inform healthcare providers if you have diabetes or kidney or liver disease. These conditions require special precautions with drug therapy.
- If pregnant, consult your obstetrician before taking any medications prescribed by another physician.
- If breast-feeding, consult your obstetrician or pediatrician before taking any medications prescribed by another healthcare provider.

Self-Administration

- Develop a routine for taking medications (e.g., at the same time and place each day). A schedule that minimally disrupts usual activities is more convenient and more likely to be followed accurately.
- Take medications in a well-lighted area, and read labels of containers to ensure taking the intended drug. Do not take medications if you are not alert or cannot see clearly.
- Most tablets and capsules should be taken whole. If unable to take them whole, ask a healthcare provider before splitting, chewing, or crushing tablets or taking the medication out of capsules. Some long-acting preparations are dangerous if altered so that the entire dose is absorbed at the same time.
- As a general rule, take oral medications with 6 to 8 oz of water, in a sitting or standing position. The water helps tablets and capsules dissolve in the stomach, "dilutes" the drug so that it is less likely to upset the stomach, and promotes absorption of the drug into the bloodstream.
- Take most oral drugs at evenly spaced intervals around the clock. For example, if ordered once daily, take about the same time every day. If ordered twice daily or morning and evening, take about 12 hours apart.
- Follow instructions about taking a medication with food, on an empty stomach, or with other medications.
- If a dose is missed, most authorities recommend taking the dose if remembered soon after the scheduled time and omitting the dose if it is not remembered for several hours. If a dose is omitted, the next dose should be taken at the next scheduled time. Do not double the dose.
- If taking a liquid medication (or giving one to a child), measure with a calibrated medication cup or measuring spoon. A dose cannot be measured accurately with

(Continued on page 54)

BOX 3.4 Patient Teaching Guidelines for Safe and Effective Use of Prescription Medications (Continued)

household teaspoons or tablespoons because they are different sizes and deliver varying amounts of medication. If the liquid medication is packaged with a measuring cup that shows teaspoons or tablespoons, that should be used to measure doses, for adults or children.
- Use oral or nasal inhalers, eye drops, and skin medications according to instructions. If you are not clear how a medication is to be used, be sure to ask a healthcare provider. Correct use is essential for therapeutic effects.
- Report problems or new symptoms to a healthcare provider.
- Store medications safely, in a cool, dry place. Do not store them in a bathroom; heat, light, and moisture may cause them to decompose. Do not store them near a dangerous substance, which could be taken by mistake. Keep medications in the container in which they were dispensed by the pharmacy, where the label identifies it and gives directions. Do not mix different medications in a single container.
- Discard outdated medications; do not keep drugs for long periods. Drugs are chemicals that may deteriorate over time, especially if exposed to heat and moisture.

BOX 3.5 Patient Teaching Guidelines for Safe and Effective Use of Over-the-Counter Medications

- Read product labels carefully. The labels contain essential information about the name, ingredients, indications for use, usual dosage, when to stop using the medication or when to see a healthcare provider, possible adverse effects, and expiration dates.
- Use a magnifying glass, if necessary, to read the fine print. If you do not understand the information on labels, ask a physician, pharmacist, or nurse.
- Do not take over-the-counter (OTC) medications longer or in higher doses than recommended.
- Note that all OTC medications are not safe for everyone. Many OTC medications warn against use with certain illnesses (e.g., hypertension). Consult a healthcare provider before taking the product if you have a contraindicated condition. If taking any prescription medications, consult a healthcare provider before taking any OTC drugs to avoid undesirable drug interactions and adverse effects. Some specific precautions include the following:
  - Avoid alcohol if taking sedating antihistamines, cough or cold remedies containing dextromethorphan, or sleeping pills. Because all these drugs cause drowsiness alone, combining any of them with alcohol may result in excessive and potentially dangerous sedation.
  - Avoid OTC sleeping aids if you are taking a prescription sedative-type drug (e.g., for anxiety or nervousness).
  - Ask a healthcare provider before taking products containing aspirin if you are taking an anticoagulant (e.g., warfarin).
  - Ask a healthcare provider before taking other products containing aspirin if you are already taking a regular dose of aspirin to prevent blood clots, heart attack, or stroke. Aspirin is commonly used for this purpose, often in doses of 81 mg (a child's dose) or 325 mg.
- Do not take a laxative if you have stomach pain, nausea, or vomiting, to avoid worsening the problem.
- Do not take a nasal decongestant (e.g., pseudoephedrine [Sudafed], a multisymptom cold remedy containing phenylephrine products, that is, formulated to remove pseudoephedrine [e.g., Actifed], or an antihistamine–decongestant combination [e.g., Claritin D]) if you are taking a prescription medication for hypertension. Such products can raise blood pressure and decrease or cancel the blood pressure–lowering effect of the prescription drug. This could lead to severe hypertension and stroke. Loratadine (Claritin) is safe to take if you have hypertension.
- Store OTC drugs in a cool, dry place, in their original containers; check expiration dates periodically, and discard those that have expired.
- If pregnant, consult your obstetrician before taking any OTC medications.
- If breast-feeding, consult your pediatrician or family doctor before taking any OTC medications.
- For children, follow any age limits on the label.
- Measure liquid OTC medications with the measuring device that comes with the product (some have a dropper or plastic cup calibrated in milliliters, teaspoons, or tablespoons). If such a device is not available, use a measuring spoon. It is not safe to use household teaspoons or tablespoons because they are different sizes and deliver varying amounts of medication.
- Do not assume continued safety of an OTC medication you have taken for years. Older people are more likely to have adverse drug reactions and interactions because of changes in the heart, kidneys, and other organs that occur with aging and various disease processes.

system leading to medication errors occurs when the nurse is interrupted during administration of medications. Wang et al. (2021) observed the administration process of medications and determined that in 270 hours of observations, nurses were interrupted 3,424 times. In the acute care, extended care, and home care environments, the sources of the interruption events during the medication administration process included family members talking with the nurse, verbal interruptions by other healthcare team members, and cell phone calls related to patient care events. In the acute care environment, the use of cell phones has become common practice to communicate with the nurse. Currently, many call light systems have been enhanced by direct communication to the nurse's cell phone. The researchers concluded that nursing interruptions occur frequently, originate from many sources, have complex causes, and lead to negative outcomes. These interruptions can lead to medication errors. In other studies, the most common distractions reported by nurses were fatigue, unresolved patient issues, noise, and hunger. Nurses also reported greater frustration if they experienced distractions. The nursing unit manager and staff must develop strategies to minimize interruptions during the medication administration process.

> **Quality and Safety Alert: Safety**
>
> It is necessary to observe the following safety alerts relating to medication administration:
> - Do not interrupt a nurse who is administering medications.
> - Instruct staff members about the risk of medication administration error when a nurse is interrupted during medication administration.
> - Implement all rights of medication administration.
> - Do not use creative "work-arounds" with medication administration. Examples to be avoided include the following:
>   - Administering the medication without scanning the patient's wristband
>   - Administering the medication without scanning the medication bar code
>   - Scanning the medication package after the medication is administered
>   - Placing an identification (ID) band on another object and scanning it

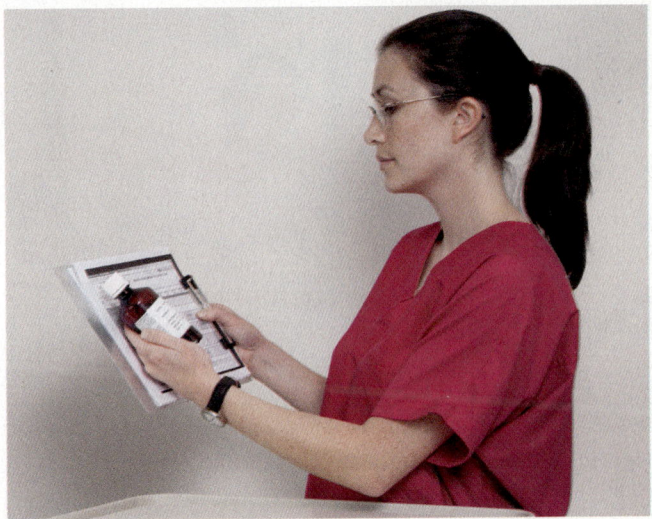

Figure 3.6. The nurse assesses the medication using the medication administration record.

The following sections present a list of guidelines for each route of medication administration. The process begins by checking the medication against the MAR (Fig. 3.6) and ends with the nurse documenting the medication administration (Fig. 3.7).

Oral Medication Administration

- Position the patient to prevent aspiration (Fig. 3.8).
- Open the unit-dose package at the patient's bedside, and place the capsule or tablet in a medicine cup.
- For liquid medications, place the cup at eye level and pour the desired amount of solution (Fig. 3.9). (Shake the elixir before measuring, if recommended by the manufacturer.)
- Administer medications with or without food as indicated to enhance absorption.
- For infants and children, administer liquid medications with a syringe or dropper.
- Hold liquid medications if the patient cannot take anything orally (Latin *nil per os*, or nothing by mouth [NPO]) or is vomiting, sedated, or unconscious.

Nasogastric or Gastrostomy Tube Medication Administration

- Administer liquid medications when available.
- Crush pills and dissolve in 30 mL of water. (Do not crush enteric-coated or extended-release medications, and do not empty the powdered medication in extended-release capsules.)
- Use a large catheter-tipped syringe to aspirate gastric fluid and assess pH.
- Rinse the tube and instill medication by gravity flow, and rinse the tube again with 50 mL of water. Do not allow the syringe to empty completely between additions of medication or water.
- Clamp off the tube from suction or drainage for at least 30 minutes.

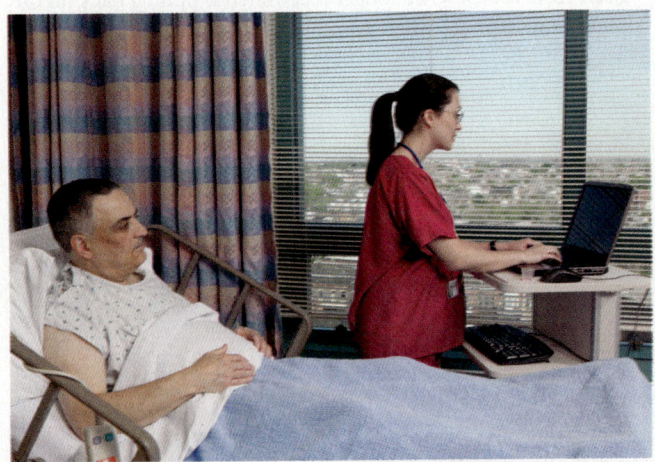

Figure 3.7. The nurse documents the administration of the medication in the electronic medical record.

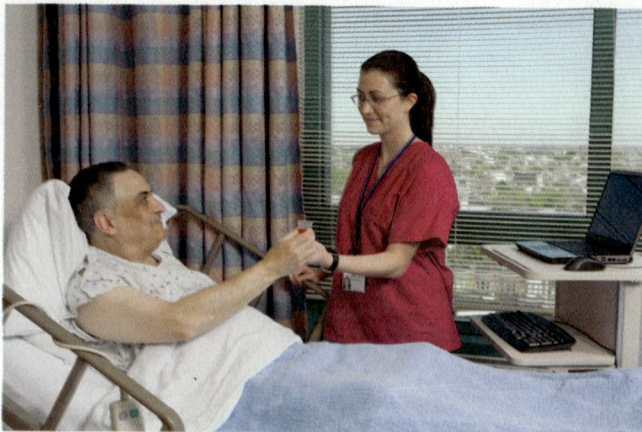

Figure 3.8. The nurse positions the patient to prevent aspiration.

Subcutaneous Medication Administration

- Use only sterile drug preparations labeled or commonly used for subcutaneous injections.
- Use a 25-gauge, 5/8-in needle for most subcutaneous injections.
- Select an appropriate injection site, based on patient preferences, drug characteristics, and visual inspection of possible sites. In long-term therapy, such as insulin, rotate injection sites. Avoid areas with lumps, bruises, or other lesions.
- Cleanse the site with an alcohol sponge.
- Tighten the skin or pinch a fold of skin and tissue between the thumb and fingers.
- Hold the syringe like a pencil and insert the needle quickly at a 45- or 90-degree angle. Use enough force to penetrate the skin and subcutaneous tissue in one smooth motion.
- Release the skin so that both hands are free to manipulate the syringe. *Never aspirate when giving heparin subcutaneously.* Wolicki and Miller (2021) provide detailed information on the administration of vaccines. *The Pink Book Home Page* can be accessed online by searching for "Vaccine Administration" at the Centers for Disease Control and Prevention (CDC). The vaccine should be inspected for damage, particulate matter, or contamination. The nurse should always check the beyond-use-date. No vaccines should be administered beyond the use date. Also, the CDC no longer recommends pulling back on the plunger to aspirate when administering a vaccine. It should be noted that the vaccine should be drawn up immediately prior to the vaccine administration. However, in the event of a large vaccination clinical, as seen with the distribution of the COVID-19 vaccines in 2021, predrawing vaccines is an option. In this case, it is imperative that strict quality control be instituted to ensure accuracy of administration.
- Remove the needle quickly and apply pressure for a few seconds.

Intramuscular Medication Administration

- Use only drug preparations labeled or commonly used for IM injections. Check label instructions for mixing drugs in powder form.
- Use a 1½-in needle for most adults and 5/8- to 1½-in needle for children, depending on the size of the patient.
- Use the smallest gauge needle that accommodates the medication. A 22-gauge is satisfactory for most drugs; a 20-gauge may be used for viscous medications.
- Select an appropriate injection site, based on the patient preferences, drug characteristics, anatomic landmarks, and visual inspection of possible sites. Rotate sites if frequent injections are being given, and avoid areas with lumps, bruises, or other lesions. *If the patient has had a mastectomy, do not administer any injection in the arm on the affected side.*
- Cleanse the site with an alcohol sponge.
- Tighten the skin, hold the syringe like a pencil, and insert the needle quickly at a 90-degree angle. Use enough force to penetrate the skin and subcutaneous tissue into the muscle in one smooth motion.
- Remove the needle quickly and apply pressure for several seconds.

> **Clinical Application 3.4**
> - Ms. Baranski's pain is not controlled with the Vicodin, and administration of ketorolac is necessary. What is the proper procedure for giving an IM injection?

Intravenous Medication Administration

- Use only drug preparations that are labeled for IV use.
- Check label instructions for the type and amount of fluid to use for dissolving or diluting the drug.
- Prepare drugs just before use, as a general rule. Also add drugs to IV fluids just before use.
- For venipuncture and direct injection into a vein, apply a tourniquet, select a site in the arm, cleanse the skin with an antiseptic (e.g., povidone–iodine or alcohol), insert the needle, and aspirate a small amount of blood into the syringe to be sure that the needle is in the vein. (*If the patient has had a mastectomy, do not administer any injection in the arm on the affected side.*) Remove the tourniquet and inject the drug slowly. Remove the needle and apply pressure until there is no evidence of bleeding.
- For administration by an established IV line:
  1. Check the infusion for patency and flow rate. Check the venipuncture site for signs of infiltration and phlebitis before each drug dose.
  2. For direct injection, cleanse an injection site on the IV tubing, insert the needle, and inject the drug slowly.

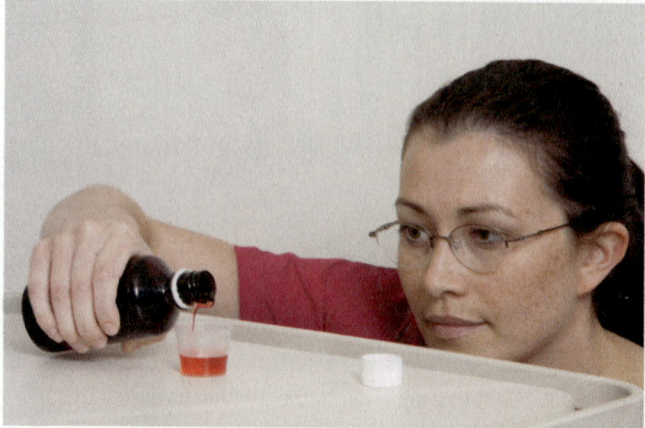

Figure 3.9. The nurse pours the liquid medication at eye level.

3. To use a volume-control set, fill it with 50 to 100 mL of IV fluid, and clamp it so that no further fluid enters the chamber and dilutes the drug. Inject the drug into the injection site after cleansing the site with an alcohol sponge and infuse, usually in 1 hour or less. After the drug is infused, add solution to maintain the infusion.
4. To use a "piggyback" method, add the drug to 50 to 100 mL of IV solution in a separate container. Attach the IV tubing and needle. Insert the needle in an injection site on the main IV tubing after cleansing the site. Infuse the drug over 15 to 60 minutes, depending on the drug.

- When more than one drug is to be given, flush the line between drugs. Do not mix drugs in syringes or in IV fluids unless the drug literature states that the drugs are compatible.
- When using an IV smart pump, be aware that it is a complex system that has a multistep process that can contribute to medication errors. In 2018, Giuliano identified six elements of the process to set up the smart pump; (1) select the drug, (2) select the dose, (3) select the infusion rate, (4) calculate and order the infusion, (5) program the infusion, and (6) deliver the infusion. The calculation, programming, and delivery of the infusion result in the greatest errors. In acute care settings and upon occasion in the home, secondary infusion by large volume IV smart pump is used. With the head-height differential method, the plastic hanger for lowering the primary bag must be extended completely. If the flow rate is ordered at 200 mL per hour or more, two plastic hangers fully extended may be needed to prevent primary fluid flow into the secondary infusion. When using the cassette method with the ICU Medical Plum, internal flow control valves actively direct flow from the primary or secondary bags. This system will not require the primary bag to be lowered (Giuliano et al., 2021).

> **Quality and Safety Alert: Patient Centered Care**
>
> If a catheter becomes clogged, do not irrigate it. Doing so may push a clot into the circulation and result in a pulmonary embolus, myocardial infarction, or stroke. It may also cause septicemia, if the clot is infected.

> **NCLEX Success**
>
> 4. The patient receives regular insulin 5 units subcutaneously. To what degree is the syringe held for the injection? (Select all that apply.)
>   A. 30 degrees
>   B. 45 degrees
>   C. 60 degrees
>   D. 90 degrees

Medication Administration to the Skin

- Use only drug preparations labeled for dermatologic use.
- Cleanse the skin, remove any previously applied medication, and apply the drug in a thin layer. For broken skin or open lesions, use sterile gloves, a tongue blade, or a cotton-tipped applicator to apply the drug.

Medication Administration to the Eye

- Use drug preparations labeled for ophthalmic use. Wash hands, open the eye to expose the conjunctival sac, and drop the medication into the sac, without touching the dropper tip to anything. Provide tissue for blotting any excess drug. If two or more eye drops are scheduled at the same time, wait 1 to 5 minutes before instillations.
- With children, prepare the medication, place the child in a head-lowered position, steady the hand holding the medication against the child's head, gently retract the lower lid, and instill the medication in the conjunctival sac.

Medication Administration to the Nose

- Have the patient hold their head back and drop the medication into the nostrils. Give the amount ordered.
- With children, place in a supine position with the head lowered, instill the medication, and maintain the position for 2 to 3 minutes. Then place the child in the prone position.

Medication Administration to the Ear

- Open the ear canal in adults by pulling the ear up and back for adults.
- Open the ear canal in children by pulling the ear down and back for children.
- Drop the medication on the side of the ear canal.

Medication Administration to the Rectum

- Lubricate the end with a water-soluble lubricant, wear a glove or finger cot, and insert into the rectum the length of the finger. Place the suppository next to the mucosal wall.
- If the patient prefers and is able, provide supplies for self-administration.

Medication Administration to the Vagina

- Use gloves or an applicator for insertion. If an applicator is used, wash thoroughly with soap and water after each use.
- If the patient prefers and is able, provide supplies for self-administration.

Evaluation

Evaluation involves determining the patient's response in relation to stated goals and expected outcomes. Some outcomes can be evaluated within a few minutes of drug administration (e.g., relief of acute pain after administration of an analgesic), but most require longer periods of time. Over time, the patient is likely to experience brief contacts with many healthcare providers, which increases the difficulty of evaluating outcomes of drug therapy. However, it is possible to manage difficulties by using appropriate techniques and criteria of evaluation.

General techniques include directly observing the patient's status; interviewing the patient or others about the patient's response to drug therapy; and checking appropriate medical records, including medication records and diagnostic test reports.

General criteria include progress toward stated outcomes, such as relief of symptoms, accurate administration, avoidance of preventable adverse effects, and compliance with instructions for follow-up monitoring by a healthcare provider. Specific criteria indicate the parameters that must be measured to evaluate responses to particular drugs (e.g., blood sugar with antidiabetic drugs, blood pressure with antihypertensive drugs).

INTEGRATING EVIDENCE-BASED PRACTICE WITH THE NURSING PROCESS

Evidence-based nursing practice requires a conscientious and continuing effort to provide high-quality care to patients by obtaining and analyzing the best available scientific evidence from research. Then, the scientific evidence is integrated with the nurse's clinical expertise and the patient's preferences and values to yield "best practices" for a patient with a particular disease process or health problem.

Evidence-based practice (EBP) may include any step of the nursing process, and it does not accept tradition or "that's the way we've always done it" as sufficient rationale for any aspect of nursing care. Requirements for implementing EBP include the following:

- Using research. Although professional nurses have always been encouraged to use research, EBP structures and formalizes the process. The nurse must use computer skills to search for the best evidence in making decisions about patient care. The search needs to be systematic; obtained data need to be critically analyzed for quality and relevance to the clinical situation.
- Keeping up-to-date in regard to research studies related to one's area of clinical practice. This includes reading research reports and analyzing them to determine their applicability.
- Considering levels of evidence to support clinical decision-making. Level A is the strongest level.
- Interpreting research evidence in relation to one's clinical expertise and patient choices to provide a scientific rationale for one's clinical decisions.
- Applying the available information to improve nursing care of an individual or group of patients.
- Evaluating the effectiveness of application. This means asking the question, Did the intervention improve the patient's condition?

HERBAL AND DIETARY SUPPLEMENTS

Complementary and alternative therapies, including herbal and dietary supplements, can be helpful in patient care. However, they can potentiate or negate the effects of prescribed medications, and it is important that the nurse evaluate the effects in a particular patient. Herbal and dietary supplements are commonly used, and patients who take them are likely to be encountered in any clinical practice setting. Herbal medicines, also called botanicals, phytochemicals, and nutraceuticals, are derived from plants. Other dietary supplements may be derived from a variety of sources. The 1994 Dietary Supplement Health and Education Act (DSHEA) defined a dietary supplement as "a vitamin, a mineral, an herb or other botanical used to supplement the diet." Under this law, herbs can be labeled according to their possible effects on the human body, but the products cannot claim to diagnose, prevent, relieve, or cure specific human diseases unless approved by the FDA.

To provide safe care, nurses need to know about their patient's use of herbal and dietary supplements. An additional impetus came from the IOM, which released a report on complementary and alternative conceptual medicine (CAM) in 2005 in which it recommended that "health profession schools incorporate sufficient information about…CAM into the standard curriculum at all levels to enable licensed professionals to competently advise their patients about CAM." The National Center for Complementary and Integrative Health, an agency of the U.S. Department of Health and Human Services and National Institutes of Health, funds and conducts research on CAM therapies. It seeks to answer questions on complementary health approaches. As Saper (2021) states, the increased usage of herbs and supplements is related to the belief that these substances will enhance health, diminish memory loss, and decrease arthritic pain and fatigue. Many individuals also believe that the use of naturally derived products is generally safe. However, the FDA has warned of the increased risk of drug interactions with the use of herbal supplements or complementary and alternative therapies. Dietary supplements can affect the absorption, metabolism, and distribution of prescribed or OTC medications. The most common drug-to-herb interactions occur with the administration of St. John's wort. For example, combining St. John's wort with a selective serotonin reuptake inhibitor will put the patient at risk for the development of serotonin syndrome.

More specifically, there are five major concerns associated with the nursing role in relation to herbal products and drug therapy, as follows:

1. Many of the products may not be safe because active ingredients and effects on humans are often unknown. Some contain heavy metals (e.g., lead) and other contaminants (e.g., pesticides); some contain prescription or nonprescription drugs. In addition, ingredients are not standardized and often differ from those listed on the product label.
2. Use of supplements may keep the patient from seeking treatment from a healthcare provider when indicated. This may allow disease processes to worsen and be more difficult to treat.
3. The products may interact with prescription drugs to decrease therapeutic effects or increase adverse effects. Dangerous interactions have been identified with St. John's wort and some herbs that affect blood clotting mechanisms.
4. Most products have not been studied sufficiently to evaluate their safety or effectiveness. In many studies, the products have not been standardized in terms of types or amounts of active ingredients. In addition, most reported studies have been short-term and with few subjects.
5. Many patients who use supplements do not tell their healthcare providers. This omission can lead to dangerous interactions when the supplements are combined with prescription or OTC drugs.

In general, nurses need to have an adequate knowledge base to assess patients who use herbal products and ensure that they do so safely. To develop and maintain a knowledge base, nurses (and patients) need to seek information from authoritative, objective sources rather than product labels, advertisements, or personal testimonials from family members, friends, or celebrities. Some resources are listed below:

- Commonly used supplements, some of which are described in Table 3.6. Later chapters describe selected supplements in more detail with some scientific support for their use. For example, Chapter 16 discusses some products reported to be useful in relieving pain, fever, inflammation, or migraines.
- Basic teaching guidelines about herbal and dietary supplements are presented in Box 3.6. This chapter provides general information. Later chapters have guidelines that may emphasize avoidance or caution in using supplements thought to interact adversely with prescribed drugs or particular patient conditions.

- Assessment guidelines. This chapter presents general information about the use or nonuse of supplements. Later chapters discuss specific supplements that may interact with particular drug group(s). For example, some supplements are known to increase blood pressure or risk of excessive bleeding.

Clinical Application 3.5

- Ms. Baranski says that a friend suggested that she take black cohosh for the hot flashes she is experiencing with menopause instead of the estrogen preparation her prescriber ordered. What information should the nurse teach Ms. Baranski regarding black cohosh in menopause?

NCLEX Success

5. During an initial nursing assessment, the patient reports that they are allergic to a particular medicine. What should the nurse ask the patient?
   A. What symptoms occurred when you had the allergic reaction?
   B. Did you need to take epinephrine (Adrenalin)?
   C. Did your physician think this information needed to be communicated?
   D. Have you ever overdosed on this medication?

TABLE 3.6

Herbal and Dietary Supplements

Name/Uses	Characteristics	Remarks
Black Cohosh		
Most often used to relieve symptoms of menopause (e.g., flushes, vaginal dryness, irritability) May also relieve premenstrual syndrome (PMS) and dysmenorrhea	Well tolerated; in overdose may cause nausea, vomiting, dizziness, visual disturbances, and reduced pulse rate Most clinical trials done with Remifemin, in small numbers of women; other trade names include Estroven and Femtrol	The World Health Organization identified the treatment of profuse sweating, irritability, and sleep disorders. Adverse effects have been associated with gastrointestinal upset and rashes. Not recommended for use longer than 6 mo (NIH, 2021)
Capsaicin		
Used to treat pain associated with neuralgia, neuropathy, and osteoarthritis Self-defense as the active ingredient in "pepper spray"	A topical analgesic that may inhibit the synthesis, transport, and release of substance P, a pain transmitter Derived from cayenne pepper Adverse effects include skin irritation, itching, redness, and stinging	Applied topically
Chamomile		
Used mainly for antispasmodic effects in the GI tract; may relieve abdominal cramping Decreases serum LDL cholesterol and triglycerides while raising HDL cholesterol	Usually ingested as a tea; may delay absorption of oral medications May cause contact dermatitis and severe hypersensitivity reactions, including anaphylaxis, in people allergic to ragweed, asters, and chrysanthemums May increase risks of bleeding	Few studies and few data to support use and effectiveness in GI disorders
Chondroitin		
Arthritis	Derived from the trachea cartilage of slaughtered cattle Usually taken with glucosamine Adverse effects may include GI upset, nausea, and headache	Several studies support use
Creatine		
Athletes take creatine supplements to gain extra energy, to train longer and harder, and to improve performance	An amino acid produced in the liver and kidneys and stored in muscles Causes weight gain, usually within 2 wk of starting use Legal and available in health food stores as a powder to be mixed with water or juice, as a liquid, and as tablets and capsules	Not recommended for use by children because studies have not been done and effects are unknown Nurses and parents need to actively discourage children and adolescents from using creatine supplements

(Continued on page 60)

TABLE 3.6

Herbal and Dietary Supplements (Continued)

Name/Uses	Characteristics	Remarks
Echinacea		
Most often used for the common cold but also advertised for many other uses (immune system stimulant, anti-infective)	Many species, but *E. purpurea* most often used medicinally Effects on immune system include stimulation of phagocytes and monocytes Contraindicated in persons with immune system disorders Hepatotoxic with long-term use	Hard to interpret validity of claims because various species and preparations used in reported studies Some evidence (level B) to support use in patients with the common cold, with possibly shorter durations and less severe symptoms
Feverfew		
Migraines, menstrual irregularities, arthritis	May increase risk of bleeding May cause hypersensitivity reactions in people allergic to ragweed, asters, daisies, or chrysanthemums May cause a withdrawal syndrome if use is stopped abruptly	Some studies support use in patients with migraine
Garlic		
Used to lower serum cholesterol and for other uses	Active ingredient thought to be allicin Has antiplatelet activity and may increase risk of bleeding Adverse effects include allergic reactions (asthma, dermatitis), dizziness, nausea, and vomiting	Some evidence that garlic has a small cholesterol-lowering effect; no reliable evidence to support other uses
Ginger		
Used mainly to treat nausea, including motion sickness and postoperative nausea	Inhibits platelet aggregation; may increase clotting time Gastroprotective effects in animal studies	Should not be used for morning sickness associated with pregnancy—may increase risk of miscarriage
Ginkgo Biloba		
Used mainly to improve memory and cognitive function in people with Alzheimer disease; may be useful in treating peripheral arterial disease	May increase blood flow to the brain and legs, improve memory, and decrease intermittent claudication (leg pain with walking) Inhibits platelet aggregation; may increase risks of bleeding with any drug that has antiplatelet effects (e.g., aspirin) Adverse effects include GI upset, headache, bleeding, and allergic skin reaction	Good evidence (level A) for small effects in treating dementia and claudication
Ginseng		
Used to increase stamina, strength, endurance, and mental acuity	Has various pharmacologic effects that vary with dose and duration of use Adverse effects include hypertension, nervousness, depression, insomnia, skin rashes, epistaxis, palpitations, and vomiting May increase risks of bleeding with any drug that has antiplatelet effects (e.g., aspirin) Increases risk of hypoglycemic reactions if taken with antidiabetic drugs Should not be taken with other herbs or drugs that inhibit monoamine oxidase (e.g., St. John's wort, selegiline); headache, mania, and tremors may occur	Insufficient evidence to support use for any indication A ginseng abuse syndrome, with insomnia, hypotonia, and edema, has been reported. Caution patients to avoid ingesting excessive amounts Instruct patients with cardiovascular disease, diabetes mellitus, or hypertension to check with their healthcare provider before taking ginseng Instruct any patient taking ginseng to avoid long-term use. Siberian ginseng should not be used longer than 3 wk
Glucosamine		
Osteoarthritis	Usually used with chondroitin Has beneficial effects on cartilage Adverse effects mild, may include GI upset, drowsiness	Several studies support use

TABLE 3.6

Herbal and Dietary Supplements (Continued)

Name/Uses	Characteristics	Remarks
Melatonin Used mainly for treatment of insomnia and prevention and treatment of jet lag	Several studies of effects on sleep, energy level, fatigue, mental alertness, and mood indicate some improvement, compared with placebo. Contraindicated in persons with hepatic insufficiency or a history of cerebrovascular disease, depression, or neurologic disorders. Adverse effects include altered sleep patterns, confusion, headache, sedation, and tachycardia	Patients with abnormal kidney function should use cautiously
St. John's Wort Used for treatment of depression, advertised as an "herbal Prozac"	Active component may be hypericin or hyperforin. Adverse effects include confusion, dizziness, GI upset, and photosensitivity. Interacts with many drugs; can decrease effectiveness of birth control pills, anticancer drugs, antivirals used to treat acquired immunodeficiency syndrome (AIDS), and organ transplant drugs (e.g., cyclosporine)	Good evidence (level A) for improvement in mild to moderate depression; not effective in major or serious depression. Should not be combined with monoamine oxidase inhibitors or selective serotonin reuptake inhibitor antidepressants. Use has declined since serious herb–drug interactions reported
Saw Palmetto Used to prevent and treat urinary symptoms in men with benign prostatic hyperplasia	May have antiandrogenic effects. Adverse effects may include GI upset and headache; diarrhea may occur with high doses	Some evidence (level B) of small beneficial effects with doses of 320 mg/d
Valerian Used mainly to promote sleep and allay anxiety and nervousness; also has muscle relaxant effects	Adverse effects with acute overdose or chronic use include blurred vision, drowsiness, dizziness, excitability, hypersensitivity reactions, and insomnia; also, risk of liver damage from combination products containing valerian and from overdoses averaging 2.5 g. Additive sedation if taken with other CNS depressants	Should not be combined with sedative drugs and should not be used regularly. Many extract products contain 40%–60% alcohol. Insufficient evidence to support use for treatment of insomnia

CNS, central nervous system; GI, gastrointestinal; HDL, high-density lipoprotein; LDL, low-density lipoprotein; NIH, National Institutes of Health.

BOX 3.6 — Patient Teaching Guidelines for General Information About Herbal and Dietary Supplements

- Herbal and dietary products are chemicals that have druglike effects in people. Unfortunately, their effects are largely unknown and may be dangerous for some people because there is little reliable information about them. For most products, little research has been done to determine either their benefits or adverse effects.
- The safety and effectiveness of these products are not regulated by laws designed to protect consumers, as are pharmaceutical drugs. As a result, the types and amounts of ingredients may not be identified on the product label. In fact, most products contain several active ingredients, and it is often not known which ingredient, if any, has the desired pharmacologic effect. In addition, components of plants can vary considerably, depending on the soil, water, and climate where the plants are grown. Quality is also a concern, as heavy metals (e.g., lead), pesticides, and other contaminants have been found in some products.
- These products can be used more safely if they are manufactured by a reputable company that states the ingredients are standardized (meaning that the dose of medicine in each tablet or capsule is the same).
- The product label should also state specific percentages, amounts, and strengths of active ingredients. With herbal medicines especially, different brands of the same herb vary in the amounts of active ingredients per recommended dose. Dosing is also difficult because a particular herb may be available in several different

(Continued on page 62)

> **BOX 3.6** **Patient Teaching Guidelines for General Information About Herbal and Dietary Supplements** (Continued)
>
> - dosage forms (e.g., tablet, capsule, tea, extract) with different amounts of active ingredients.
> - These products are often advertised as "natural." Many people interpret this to mean the products are safe and better than synthetic products. This is not true; "natural" does not mean safe, especially when taken concurrently with other herbals, dietary supplements, or drugs.
> - When taking herbal or dietary supplements, follow the instructions on the product label. Inappropriate use or taking excessive amounts may cause dangerous side effects.
> - Inform healthcare providers when taking any kind of herbal or dietary supplement to reduce risks of severe adverse effects or drug–supplement interactions.
> - Most herbal and dietary supplements should be avoided during pregnancy or lactation and in young children.
> - The American Society of Anesthesiologists recommends that all herbal products be discontinued 2 to 3 weeks before any surgical procedure. Some products (e.g., echinacea, feverfew, garlic, ginkgo, ginseng, valerian, and St. John's wort) can interfere with or increase the effects of some drugs, affect blood pressure or heart rhythm, or increase risks of bleeding; some have unknown effects when combined with anesthetics, other perioperative medications, and surgical procedures.
> - Store herbal and dietary supplements out of the reach of children.

Visit thePoint at http://thePoint.lww.com/Frandsen13e for answers to NCLEX Success questions (in Appendix A), answers to Clinical Application Case Studies (in Appendix B), and more!

REFERENCES AND RESOURCES

Giuliano, K. K. (2018). Intravenous smart pumps usability issues, intravenous medication administration error, and patient safety. *Critical Care Nurse Clinics of North America, 20*, 215–244.

Giuliano, K. K., Blake, J. W., & Butterfield, R. (2021). Secondary medication administration and IV smart pump setup: What every nurse needs to know. *American Journal of Nursing, 121*(8), 46–50.

Hinkle, J. H., Cheever, K. H., & Overbaugh, K. (2022). *Brunner & Suddarth's textbook of medical-surgical nursing* (15th ed.). Wolters Kluwer.

Institutes of Medicine Committee on the Use of Complementary and Alternative Medicine in the United States. (2005). *Complementary and alternative medicine in the United States*. National Academies Press. Retrieved September 25, 2021, from http://www.nap.edu/catalog/11182.html

Institutes of Medicine of the National Academies. (2004). *Keeping patients safe: Transforming the work environment of nurses*. National Academies Press.

Institute of Medicine of the National Academies. (2007). *Preventing medications errors*. National Academies Press.

Jones, J., Treiber, L., Shabo, R., et al. (2021). *Just culture, medication prevention, and second victim support: A better prescription for preparing nursing students for practice [White Paper]*. WellStar School of Nursing, WellStar College of Health and Human Services, Kennesaw State University.

National Academies of Sciences, Engineering, and Medicine. (2021). *The future of nursing 2020–2030: Charting a path to achieve health equity*. The National Academies Press. https://doi.org/10.17226/25982

National Center for Complementary and Integrative Health. (2021). *Dietary and herbal supplements*.

National Institutes of Health Office of Dietary Supplements. (2021). *Black Cohosh*. Retrieved September 25, 2021, from https://ods-od-nih-gov.proxy.library.maryville.edu/factsheets/BlackCohosh-HealthProfessional/

Riordan, D. O., Kinane, M., Walsh, K. A., Shiely, R., Eustace, J., & Bermingham, M. (2020). Stakeholders' knowledge, attitudes, and practices to pharmacovigilance and adverse drug reaction reporting in clinical trials: A mixed methods study. *European Journal of Clinical Pharmacology, 76*, 1363–1372. https://doi.org/10.1007/s00228-020-02921-0

Saper, R. B. (2021). Overview of herbal medicine and dietary supplements. *Up-To-Date*. Wolters Kluwer.

Taylor, C., Lynn, P., & Bartlett, J. L. (2019). *Fundamentals of nursing: The art and science of person-centered care* (9th ed.). Wolters Kluwer.

The Joint Commission National Patient Safety Guidelines Do Not Use List. (2020). Retrieved September 21, 2021, from https://www.jointcommission.org/standards/national-patient-safety-goals/-/media/36698dd44a574555a1f3103ed0ecfc74.ashx

Wang, W., Jin, L., Zhao, X., Li, Z., & Han, W. (2021). Current status and influencing factors of nursing interruption events. *The American Journal of Managed Care, 27*(6), e188–e196. doi:10.37765/ajmc.2021.88667. https://www.cdc.gov/vaccines/pubs/pinkbook/downloads/vac-admin.pdf

Wolicki, J., & Miller, E. (2021). *Vaccine administration, epidemiology, and prevention of vaccine-preventable diseases* (14th ed.). The Centers for Disease Control. Retrieved September 25, 2021.

World Health Organization. (2015). *WHO pharmacovigilance indicators: A practical manual for the assessment of pharmacovigilance systems*.

World Health Organization. (2020). *Ensuring medicines work safely for everyone*. Retrieved from https://www.who.int/news/item/02-11-2020-ensuring-medicines-work-safely-for-everyone

Zhu, J., & Weingart, S. N. (2021). Prevention of adverse drug events in hospitals. *Up-to-Date*. Wolters Kluwer.

Clinical Judgment in Practice: Section 1: The Conceptual Framework of Pharmacology

A 79-year-old female is admitted to the medical division of an acute care facility with a diagnosis of acute dehydration following a fall in her home. She was laying on the floor for 2 days after the fall, and as a result, she has not taken any medications for 2 days. Her blood pressure upon admission to the emergency department was 160/70. She takes enalapril 10 mg orally each morning for hypertension. Her other medications are ibuprofen 600 mg twice daily for arthritis, atorvastatin 20 mg for hyperlipidemia, and metformin 500 mg extended release for type 2 diabetes. Upon admission to the medical division, the patient is alert and oriented to person, place, and time. She is bruised on her left hip but does not have a fracture. The bruise is 10 cm × 7.5 cm. She complains of pain in her back and hip. She states her pain is 5 on a scale of 1 to 10. Her vital signs are 130/90, 72, 24, and 99.4. She has voided 30 mL of concentrated urine since admission. Her albumin level is 2.3 g/dL. The normal serum albumin is 3.4 to 5.4 g/dL. Her skin turgor tents when pinched. Her blood glucose is 130 mg/dL.

Step 1: Recognize Cues
Identify the relevant and important information from different sources, such as the medical history or subjective and objective data.

Answer: Temperature 99.4 orally, blood pressure 130/90, pulse 72 and regular, respirations 24. She has pain of 5 on scale of 1 to 10. She has a bruise on her left hip that measures 10 cm × 7.5 cm. Her skin turgor is poor with a serum albumin level of 2.3 g/dL. She has voided 30 mL of concentrated urine since admission to the hospital.

Step 2: Analyze Cues
Organize and link the recognized cues to the patient's clinical presentation.

Answer: You link her blood pressure of 160/70 and 130/90 to her missed enalapril doses for 2 days and the stress of her fall. In addition, her pain level of 5 will increase her blood pressure. Her albumin level is 2.3 g/dL due to dehydration. Her urine output is diminished and the urine is concentrated due to dehydration.

Step 3: Prioritize Hypotheses
Evaluate hypotheses and rank them according to priority, such as urgency, likelihood, risk, difficulty, and/or time. Cluster your findings to generate a list of problems (actual or potential) you believe the patient is experiencing or may experience and determine the level of urgency. Which problem is of the greatest concern?

Answer: The patient's altered fluid volume status is of greatest concern. If the patient is administered her medications, there will not be adequate distribution due to the diminished albumin levels. Protein binding is an important factor in drug distribution. Most drugs form a compound with plasma proteins, mainly albumin. Drug molecules bound to plasma proteins are pharmacologically inactive because the large size of the complex prevents their leaving the bloodstream through the small openings in capillary walls and reaching the sites of action, metabolism, and excretion. In addition, the patient's altered comfort related to pain in her left hip is of concern.

Step 4: Generate Solutions
Identify expected outcomes and use hypotheses to define a set of interventions for the expected outcomes.

Answer: The patient's dehydration has reduced her serum albumin level, and you recognize that the decrease in serum albumin level will prevent proper distribution of her medications. You anticipate the hospitalist's order of albumin solution of 12.5 g (250 mL) to be infused over 15 minutes. The serum albumin level will be reassessed in 2 hours, and if it is increased to 3.4 g/dL, you will administer acetaminophen 650 mg orally for pain. Following the infusion of albumin, you anticipate the patient is to receive D_5LR at 125 mL/hour.

Step 5: Take Actions
Implement the solutions that address the highest priorities.

Answer: You insert an IV in the patient's right hand and administer 250 mL albumin 12.5 g solution to be infused over 15 minutes.

Step 6: Evaluate Outcomes
Compare observed outcomes against expected outcomes.

Answer: The patient's albumin level was 3.6 g/dL 2 hours after the albumin infusion. She also continues to receive D_5LR at 125 mL/hour. Her urine output is 60 mL/hour. Her skin turgor has improved. Her pain is decreased to 2 on a scale of 1 to 10 one hour following acetaminophen 650 mg orally.

SECTION 2

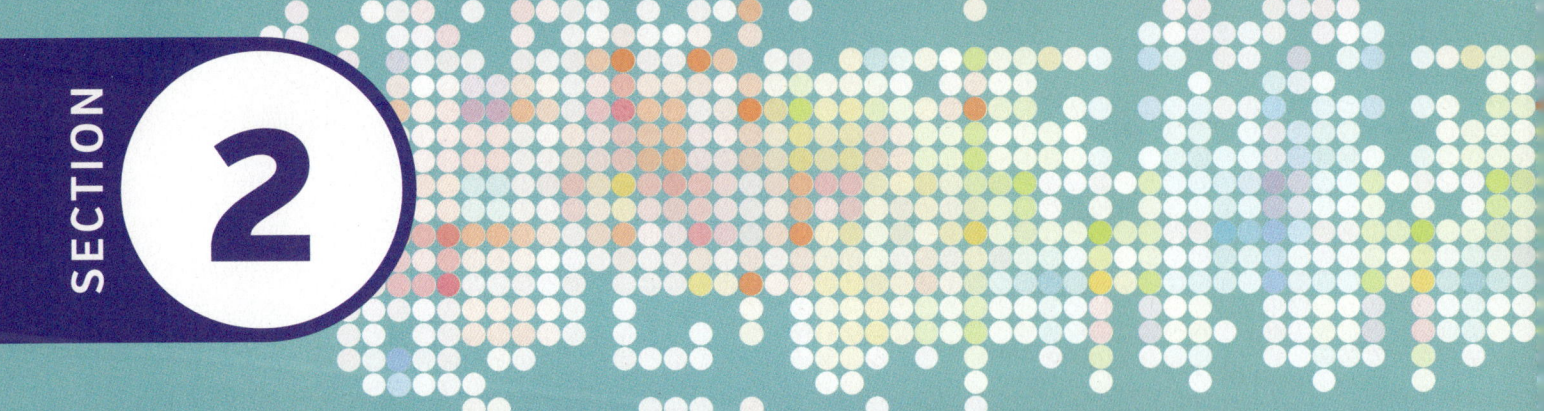

Drug Therapy Throughout the Lifespan

Chapter 4 Pharmacology and the Care of Infants and Pediatric Patients

Chapter 5 Pharmacology and the Care of Adults and Geriatric Patients

Chapter 6 Pharmacology and the Care of Pregnant or Lactating Females

Chapter 7 Pharmacology and Female Health

Chapter 8 Pharmacology and Male Health

CHAPTER 4

Pharmacology and the Care of Infants and Pediatric Patients

LEARNING OBJECTIVES

After studying this chapter, you should be able to:

1. Identify key characteristics of pediatric pharmacotherapy in children from birth to 18 years of age.
2. Describe the evolution of pediatric pharmacotherapy and the purpose of federal legislation in the development of current practice standards.
3. Describe methods for determining accurate pediatric dosing.
4. Explain differences in pharmacodynamic variables between children and adults.
5. Explain pharmacokinetic differences between children and adults.
6. Describe nursing interventions, based on child growth and development standards, to help ensure safe and effective medication administration to children.

CLINICAL APPLICATION CASE STUDY

Billy Lee, a 6-year-old boy, complains of shortness of breath. He is restless with expiratory wheezes. His parents report that Billy has a 2-day history of coldlike symptoms, with a productive cough and fever.

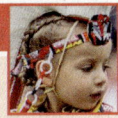

KEY TERMS

Blood–brain barrier: barrier in the central nervous system composed of capillaries with tight bonds, which acts to prevent the passage of most ions and large molecular weight compounds, including some drugs, from the blood to the brain

Body surface area: surface of a human body expressed in square meters

Child(ren): person(s) between birth and 18 years of age

Total body water: amount of water within the body (both intracellular and extracellular)

INTRODUCTION

Children naturally differ from adults. However, therapeutic indications and effects of drug therapy are similar in many ways. It is essential that nurses and other healthcare professionals understand the many ways children differ from adults because these differences present a challenge in medication dosing, administration, and management. For example, physiologic changes throughout development influence both the pharmacodynamic and pharmacokinetic actions of medications. A child's immature organ systems mean that molecular binding, receptor reactions, and intended actions of medications may not mimic those known for adults. Variables in absorption, distribution, metabolism, and excretion further complicate the medication process. Taken together, these differences indicate a need for vigilance in nursing management of pediatric pharmacotherapy.

Pediatrics includes the evaluation and management of all **children**—patients from birth to age 18. This group is further divided into five subgroups (Table 4.1), and each developmental group is characterized by a select set of physiologic changes that affect pharmacotherapy. The younger the patient, the greater the variation in medication action. Of course, many pediatric patients cannot verbalize adverse effects, and good assessment skills are crucial in evaluating all pediatric patients. It is also important to remember that as patients go through puberty, they begin to respond physiologically more like adults, but they are still immature psychologically and may lack the ability to dose, administer, or evaluate the effectiveness of their medications.

DRUG SAFETY IN PEDIATRICS

Legislation and Drug Testing

Many challenges in pediatric medication management involve the known physical differences in pediatric patients and the unknown action of drugs, often related to a lack of adequate information. Historically, researchers used only adults to test medications, and prescribers simply assumed that smaller doses would elicit the same results in smaller patients. However, pediatric pharmacotherapy began to change in 1994 when the U.S. Food and Drug Administration (FDA) enacted the Pediatric Rule, which compelled the pharmaceutical industry to submit all known data about the pharmacokinetics, safety, and efficacy of medications used for children (Connolly, 2018). The FDA continued the trend toward safer medication management for children when it passed the *U.S. Food and Drug Administration Modernization Act of 1997* (FDAMA), followed by the *2002 Best Pharmaceuticals for Children Act* (BPCA). These acts provide incentives to companies who perform research to determine the safety, efficacy, dosage, and unique risks associated with medications for children (AAP, 2020; Avant et al., 2018; Connolly, 2018).

The FDA continued to press for more research and better practice standards by issuing the *Pediatric Research Equity Act of 2003*, renewing the BPCA in 2007, and making the BPCA law in 2012. Since these measures were put in place, research has uncovered other gaps in pediatric studies, including a need for pediatric formulations, preclinical studies, and pediatric outcome measures. The *Food and Drug Administration Safety and Innovation Act (FDASIA)*, enacted in 2012, gives an overview of laws and regulations, an assessment of the pediatric program, and suggestions for improving pediatric research.

With the current emphasis on increased patient safety and decreased medication-related adverse events, it is especially important for pediatric practitioners to be at the forefront of current research and practice standards in pediatric pharmacotherapy. In recent years, focus has been on designing an e-prescribing system for pediatric patients and including parental health and English literacy in medication administration for children (AAP, 2020). Prescribers must still treat pediatric patients with drugs for which they lack information; therefore, they must always practice good assessment, dosing, and evaluation during the administration of any medication to a pediatric patient.

Clinical Application 4.1

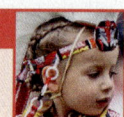

- Are Billy's medications chosen based on empiric evidence obtained from solid research performed on other 6-year-old boys?

Calculating Drug Dosages

The basis of pediatric drug dosing is weight, and determining drug dosages is highly dependent on the growth and development changes that occur across the lifespan. The prescriber uses weight alone to calculate pediatric dosages in an expression such as gentamicin 5 mg/kg/24 h or determines the **body surface area** (BSA), the surface of a human body expressed in square meters, using the child's weight (Table 4.2). Then the prescriber calculates the dose based on a known adult dose by using the following equation: pediatric dose = BSA/1.73 × adult dose.

According to Flint and Hall (2022), body surface area is used to ensure the therapeutic window for medication administration and the subsequent avoidance of adverse medication effects. However, significant variances in body surface area calculations may result in overdosing of some drugs or the inability to obtain a drug's targeted effects.

PHARMACOTHERAPY IN PEDIATRICS

Pharmacodynamics

Pharmacodynamics involves drug actions on target cells and the resulting alterations in cellular reactions and functions, which occur because of chemicals that bind with receptors at the cellular level. Most of these receptors are proteins on the

TABLE 4.1

Pediatric Age Groups

Premature infant	Less than 38 wk gestational age
Neonate	A full-term newborn 0–4 wk of age
Infant	Greater than 4 wk to 1 y of age
Child	Greater than 1–12 y of age
Adolescent	Greater than 12–18 y of age

TABLE 4.2

Body Surface Area[a]

Age	Average BSA (m²)
Neonate (newborn)	0.25
Child, 2 y	0.50
Child, 9 y	1.07
Child, 10 y	1.14
Child, 12–13 y	1.33
Man (older than 18 y)	1.90
Woman (older than 18 y)	1.60

[a]The following formula is used to calculate BSA:

$$BSA\ (m^2) = \sqrt{\frac{[height\ (cm) \times weight\ (lb)]}{3600}}$$

From Mosteller, R. D. (1987). Simplified calculation of body surface area. *The New England Journal of Medicine*, 317(17), 1098.

surface or within cells. Children's immature systems and changing body compositions mean that drugs affect them differently. Pharmacodynamic variables in pediatric patients are related to differences in target cell sites and changing numbers of protein receptors. Other causes of pharmacodynamic variability across the lifespan include differences in body composition, immature organ systems, and genetics. **Total body water** (the amount of water within the body, both intracellular and extracellular), fat stores, and protein levels change throughout childhood and greatly influence the effectiveness of drugs in the pediatric population (Kyle & Carman, 2020).

One example of a drug that has different pharmacodynamic actions in adults and children is thalidomide. In the 1960s, thalidomide was successful in decreasing morning sickness during pregnancy. However, it was soon apparent that it had severe teratogenic (adverse) effects on the fetus. This antiemetic drug resulted in severe limb abnormalities and often death for the fetus. Pharmacodynamic differences of positive drug action in pregnant adults and negative toxic effects to their unborn fetuses as seen in the use of thalidomide illustrate one of the many challenges of medication management of children versus adults.

Another example of pharmacodynamic issues in younger patients involves antidepressants. Initially, prescribers assumed that these drugs, widely used successfully in treating adults, could be safely used therapeutically in adolescents and children. However, by 2004, the FDA had found that these medications needed a **BOXED WARNING ◆** stating that antidepressants may play a causal role in inducing suicidality in pediatric patients. Years later, practitioners are still debating the use and risk of these drugs in children and adolescents because many feel the warning should be eliminated or amended based on recent research (Kelleher et al., 2020).

Clinical Application 4.2

- What nursing interventions would take priority in Billy's care?

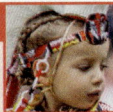

NCLEX Success

1. Medications should be individualized to ensure the best outcome. Individualizing drug therapy for a child involves which one of the following?
   - A. assessing the child's age and development level
   - B. administering an adult drug selection and dosage and observing for adverse reactions
   - C. deferring treatment until a better pediatric drug is developed
   - D. determining the child's diet and exercise needs

2. A pediatric patient is unable to tolerate montelukast (Singulair) for asthma and had a rash and abdominal pain. However, this drug works well for the child's parent, who experiences no adverse effects. The physician is aware that the child's reaction to the medication is most likely a reflection of their
   - A. inability to understand the purpose of the drug
   - B. hope that taking the drug will not be required
   - C. inability to swallow pills
   - D. genetic variability

Pharmacokinetics

Pharmacokinetics refers to the processes of drug absorption, distribution, metabolism, and elimination. The organ systems in pediatric patients vary widely in their growth and maturation compared with adult patients. This, in turn, greatly affects a prescriber's ability to dose pediatric drugs effectively. Newborn infants are a prime example because they process drugs very inefficiently. However, by age 12, children have grown and matured sufficiently to develop pharmacokinetic responses that resemble those of adults. To account for immature or impaired body systems in neonates and younger children, it is often necessary to dramatically change drug therapies. Drug effects are more varied in children and must be anticipated and carefully evaluated for after administration.

Absorption

Drug absorption in pediatrics is affected by the age of the child, gastric emptying, intestinal motility, routes of administration, and skin permeability. Careful thought to proper route, good monitoring, and anticipation of potential adverse effects can help ensure that intended outcomes are seen with administered drugs.

Age is one important factor in absorption of medications. During pregnancy, many drugs cross the placenta and may harm the fetus. During infancy, neonates have delayed, irregular gastric emptying and reduced gastric acidity. This delay potentially leads to greatly increased drug levels. The decreased acidity results in greater absorption of acid-labile medications or reduced absorption of weakly acidic medications.

In addition, the route of administration greatly affects absorption. Prescribers avoid the use of intramuscular (IM) injections in pediatric patients because of the associated pain and unpredictable absorption. Low blood flow to skeletal muscles and weak muscle contractions also contribute to the erratic absorption of IM injections. Thin and highly permeable skin increases the rate of absorption of topical drugs, and careful administration is important to avoid toxicity.

Distribution

Distribution of drugs in pediatric patients is dependent on percentage of body water, liver function, degree of protein binding, and the development of the blood–brain barrier.

Children differ from adults in the percentages of total body water. This includes the amount of water within the body, including the intracellular and extracellular compartments, plus the water in the gastrointestinal and urinary tracts (Fig. 4.1). In adults, total body water is approximately 60%, whereas in newborns, it is approximately 80%. This difference means that water-soluble drugs such as atenolol (Tenormin) and penicillin (Penicillin-G) are diluted easily and readily moved into intercellular tissue. As a result, serum drug concentrations are lower, and increased dosages of water-soluble drugs may be necessary to maintain therapeutic drug levels in neonates and premature infants.

In infants, immature liver function leads to very low plasma protein levels, which limits the amount of protein binding by drugs. Consequently, the serum concentrations of highly protein-bound drugs, including phenytoin (Dilantin), warfarin (Coumadin), ampicillin, and morphine (Duramorph), may be higher than expected, and toxicity may occur. By the end of the first year, protein-binding ability is at the adult level, and its effect on drug distribution is no longer a concern.

The **blood–brain barrier**, which is composed of capillaries with tight bonds in the central nervous system (CNS), prevents the passage of most ions and large molecular weight compounds—including certain drugs—from the blood to the brain. Although this barrier protects the CNS, it can make drug delivery to the neurons more difficult. In neonates, the blood–brain barrier is poorly developed; thus, drugs and other chemicals easily affect the CNS in young infants. The nurse must assess for increased drug effects or toxic results from drug administration and must be alert for other chemicals or drugs that may cause unwanted CNS effects such as vital sign irregularities, sedation, excitability, and seizures.

Metabolism

The enzyme cytochrome P450 (CYP450) in the liver metabolizes most drugs. In neonates, the ability to metabolize drugs is very low because of the immaturity of the liver and the resultant inability to break down drugs. To avoid toxicity, the prescriber needs to calculate drug doses carefully, and the nurse must monitor infants and young children closely until the liver is more mature—by the end of the second year.

Elimination

Excretion of most drugs occurs via the kidneys, and elimination in the urine follows. Young children have immature kidneys, a reduced glomerular filtration rate, and slower kidney clearance. Neonates are especially prone to increased levels of drugs that are eliminated primarily by the kidneys; the prescriber should dose appropriately, and the nurse should monitor carefully until kidney function reaches maturity—between 1 and 2 years of age.

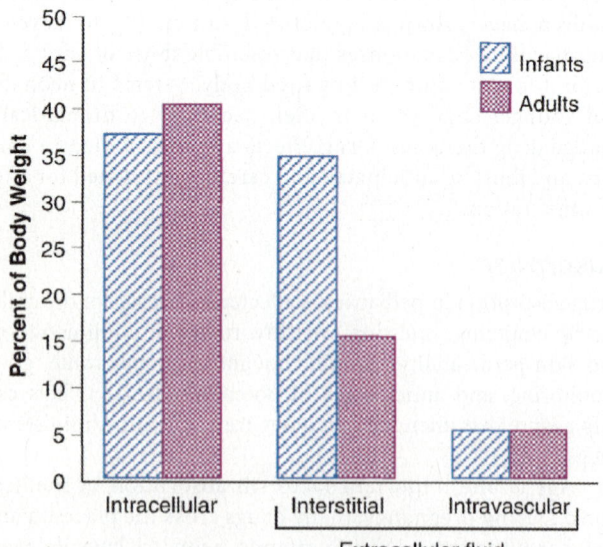

Figure 4.1. Graph indicating distribution on fluid in body compartments. Comparison between the infant and adult fluid distribution in body compartments shows that the adult total is about 60% of body weight, whereas the infant total is more than 70% of body weight. (Reprinted with permission from Hatfield, N. [2008]. *Broadribb's introductory pediatric nursing* [7th ed., Fig. 6-5]. Wolters Kluwer Health.)

Clinical Application 4.3

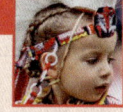

- How does the nurse know whether interventions designed to help Billy have been successful? What assessment data are warranted?

NCLEX Success

3. For a child with asthma, a prescriber has ordered albuterol (Proventil). Which one of the following important factors related to growth and development is most likely to affect absorption of this beta$_2$-adrenergic agonist?

    A. the ability of the child to cough up secretions
    B. the need to decrease the dose as the child's age increases
    C. the need to monitor the child for hypotension
    D. the ability of the child and caregivers to understand how to use the inhaler and spacer to administer the albuterol

4. A 3-month-old infant who receives fosphenytoin (Cerebyx) for a seizure disorder does not process this drug in the same way as an adult. Alterations in infant pharmacokinetics that influence drug action include which of the following concepts? (Select all that apply.)
   A. Drug response to oral medication in infants is slower than in adults.
   B. Neonates have a decreased response to drugs that affect the CNS.
   C. Infants have a decreased response to water-soluble drugs and an increased response to protein-bound drugs.
   D. By 3 months of age, drug response in infants is similar to that of adults.
   E. Characteristics of infant elimination may cause toxic drug effects.

MEDICATION ADMINISTRATION IN PEDIATRICS

Administering medications to infants and children presents its own set of challenges because of difficulties in communication, cooperation, and adherence. Trends in growth and development serve as the basis for care across different age groups, and the nurse must continue to focus on safety in all activities involving drug administration.

Infants

The focus in this age group is aimed at calculation of correct dosages, safety in administration, and teaching parents how to deliver medications correctly. Administering medication for infants includes a few key points related to infant growth and development.

- Oral medications are administered with a dropper or oral syringe into the inner aspect of the cheek, giving children time to swallow the medication as it is instilled.
- Some practitioners prefer giving oral medications through a nipple with a small amount of formula or breast milk, but this is controversial. Some authorities believe that infants may then refuse feedings if they associate food with the taste of the medication.
- Infants lack well-developed muscles. Thus, care is taken when medications or vaccinations can only be given by IM injections. Good practice involves using the smallest needle, preferably in the largest available muscle, the vastus lateralis.
- Many common medications come in suppository form, which makes administration easier in this age group.
- Comfort care is important with infants. They need holding and cuddling and are offered a pacifier with, or shortly after, medication administration.
- Intravenous (IV) sites for medication administration are often found in the scalp, hands, or feet, and a 22- to 24-gauge needle is frequently used.

Toddlers and Preschoolers

Toddlers are mobile and curious. Preschoolers are inquisitive and controlling. They generally love investigating but have short attention spans and want to exert their independence. The nurse involves toddlers and preschoolers in medication administration by having them hold items or choose the self-adhesive bandage or cup that will be used, but explanations should be short and simple, and adults need to control administration.

- To make oral medications more palatable, the nurse often mixes them with flavored syrups or fruit purees. Children may receive their favorite drink afterward.
- As toddlers develop bigger muscle mass, IM injections can move from the vastus lateralis to the ventrogluteal area.
- Reaction to suppositories is strong. Therefore, explanations should be short, and for successful administration, an assistant may be necessary.
- For toddlers, IV sites in the scalp are still occasionally appropriate, but for older toddlers and preschoolers, the feet, hands, or antecubital area are preferable.

 Quality and Safety Alert: Safety

The goal of the Pediatric Cough and Cold Safety Surveillance System, launched in 2008, was to understand the safety profile of cough and cold medications (CCMs). In 2018, this led to requiring prescription products that contain codeine to include "do not use in children less than 18 years old" on the label, a withdrawal of the concentrated infant formulations from manufacture, and reminders from the U.S. Food and Drug Administration to never use CCMs in children younger than 2 years of age.

School-Aged Children and Adolescents

School-aged children and adolescents are able to participate more in medication administration. They develop an ability to reason, and as they mature, the nurse can explain medication use in more detail. Often, these patients want to take medications independently, but they need supervision to make sure they take all of their medications at the correct times. Adolescents should be monitored, as they may try to self-medicate if prescription and over-the-counter (OTC) medications are available in the home. Careful tracking and good communication are essential to ensure safe medication practices for these patients.

- Some medications are available as chewable tablets or solutions. These work well for children who cannot swallow tablets or capsules.
- IM injections can be frightening for school-aged children and adolescents, and they need praise and encouragement. They often respond well to rewards after the injections have been completed.
- It is necessary to assess adolescents for risky behavior related to use of laxatives in eating disorders. The adolescent's use of prescription and OTC medication should also be assessed. It is important to assess the adolescent's use of alcohol or illegal drug use. Education on all of the effects of prescription, nonprescription, alcohol, and illegal drugs is imperative to promote patient safety.

- Important information about self-care related to medication administration provides good teaching points for this age group. Adolescents need explanations about the use of acne medications and antibiotics, including adverse effects. The nurse should tell adolescents who are taking birth control medications about possible decreased effectiveness with certain drugs and should also discuss the importance of preventive measures such as sun protection with many groups of medications.

Clinical Application 4.4

- What is the best way to teach Billy about his discharge plan, teach him how to use his inhaler, and review how to take his medications?

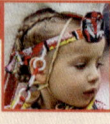

! Quality and Safety Alert: Safety

- Ensure that medications are dosed based on weight and calculated individually for each child.
- Ensure that electronic medical records are standardized to allow only kilograms and centimeters for pediatric weight and height entries.
- Use adequate measuring devices, graduated to tenths, for pediatric patients, and help make sure that these devices are available to caregivers.
- Administer oral medications only in oral syringes.
- Administer IV medications only in Luer lock syringes.
- Order, dispense, and administer medications based on individual dosages in milligrams, micrograms, units, and so on, not on variables such as tablets or milliliters, for which the concentration may vary.
- Administer IV medications using smart pump technology with safety systems enabled.
- Administer IV fluids and medications with syringe pump technology for smaller amounts over set times or at set rates, with safety systems enabled.
- Ensure a double-check system in prescribing, dispensing, and administering high-risk pediatric medications.
- Have access to current, pediatric-focused medication references.
- Collaborate with interdisciplinary team members on best practice solutions to pediatric medication management problems.
- Keep medications, including topicals and solutions, out of the reach of pediatric patients. Never store these in a crib or on a bedside table.
- Administer medications using a caring approach, involving knowledge of pediatric growth and development.
- Involve family or caregivers in the management of a child's medications, including teaching and demonstrating storage, safety, and proper administration of medications.

NCLEX Success

5. A 15-year old patient is prescribed an antibiotic to be administered IV. When starting the IV, the nurse notices many puncture marks in the patient's antecubital area. What question should the nurse ask following the IV insertion?
   A. "How often do you inject illegal drugs?"
   B. "Do you take other medications, or have you had tests done?"
   C. "Where do you get your drugs from?"
   D. "Do your parents know you use illegal drugs?"

6. A nurse is teaching a parent how to administer analgesic eardrops at home to a toddler with acute otitis media. Which statements by the parent indicate that teaching has been successful? (Select all that apply.)
   A. "I will let my child squirt in the eardrops so they won't fight me and he can feel independent."
   B. "I will use the holding technique you showed me to administer the medication once I have calmed my child."
   C. "I will give my child cold medication so they won't keep getting stuffy ears."
   D. "I will give the eardrops in my child's mouth if they won't let me put it in their ear because that will work for the pain, too."
   E. "If my child is also running a fever, I will give them an over-the-counter medication like acetaminophen (Tylenol) or ibuprofen (Motrin) according to the directions on the label."

THE NURSING PROCESS

A concept map outlines the nursing process related to drug therapy considerations in this chapter. Additional nursing implications related to the disease process should also be considered in care decisions.

Assessment
- Record the age, weight, and height of the child. Drug dosages are based on these values.
- Assess allergies and determine family allergy history.
- Assess growth and development related to age, cognitive, psychosocial, physiologic, and nutritional status.
- Assess medication history.
- Assess family understanding and cognitive level.
- Assess ability of patient and family to adhere to medication regimen.

Outcomes of Therapy
The patient will
- Receive the correct drug dose based on weight (recorded in kilograms).
- Receive a drug by the best route based on growth and development and therapeutic expectations.
- With the parents or caregiver, understand medication administration, action, use, and adverse effects. The child should be involved in all aspects of medication management as warranted by cognitive and growth and development levels.
- Maintain medication adherence.

Nursing Interventions
- Use appropriate pediatric drug references.
- Monitor closely for side effects related to immature liver and kidney function.
- Teach patients, especially nonverbal, young, or developmentally delayed children, and parents and/or caregivers about medication dosage, administration, therapeutic effects, adverse effects, and precautions.
- Communicate with patients, based on cognitive and growth and development levels, as well as parents and/or caregivers about all aspects of medication management and planning for care.
- Communicate with interdisciplinary team to advocate for the pediatric patient and ensure therapeutic medication management.
- Instruct parents and/or caregivers about the risk of using over-the-counter and alternative therapies without first consulting a health care practitioner.
- Advise parents and/or caregivers about safety practices related to medication storage, access, and administration.

Evaluation
- Evaluate the patient's response to the medication regimen.
- Evaluate the patient's and caregiver's understanding of the medication regimen.
- Evaluate the ability of the patient and caregiver to adhere to the medication regimen.

Visit thePoint at http://thePoint.lww.com/Frandsen13e for answers to NCLEX Success questions (in Appendix A), answers to Clinical Application Case Studies (in Appendix B), and more!

REFERENCES AND RESOURCES

American Academy of Pediatrics (AAP). (2020). *Medications in pediatrics: A compendium of AAP Clinical Practice Guidelines and Policies*. American Academy of Pediatrics.

Avant, D., Wharton, G., & Murphy, D. (2018). Characteristics and changes of pediatric therapeutic trials under the Best Pharmaceuticals for Children Act [BPCA]. *The Journal of Pediatrics, 192*, 8–12. doi:10.1016/j.jpeds.2017.08.048

Chike-Harris, K., & Kinyon-Munch, K. (2019). Asthma 101: Teaching children to use metered dose inhalers. *Nursing, 49*(3), 56–60. doi:10.1097/01.NURSE.0000552703.80996.43

Connolly, C. (2018). *Children and drug safety: Balancing risk and protection in Twentieth Century America*. Rutgers University Press.

Flint, B., & Hall, C. A. (2022). Body surface area. *National Library of Medicine National Center for Biotechnology Information*. March 26, 2022. StatPearls Publishing, LLC.

Food and Drug Administration (FDA). (2018). FDA drug safety communication: FDA requires labeling changes for prescription opioid cough and cold medicines to limit their use to adults 18 years and older. https://www.fda.gov/drugs/drug-safety-and-availability/fda-drug-safety-communication-fda-requires-labeling-changes-prescription-opioid-cough-and-cold

Hockenberry, M., Wilson, D., & Rodgers, C. (2019). *Wong's nursing care of infants and children* (11th ed.). Mosby Elsevier.

Institute for Safe Medication Practices (ISMP). (2015). *ISMP Part 1: Results of survey on pediatric medication safety, more is needed to protect hospitalized children from medication errors*. https://www.ismp.org/newsletters/acutecare/showarticle.aspx?id=110

Kelleher, K. J., Rubin, D., & Hoagwood, K. (2020). Policy and practice innovations to improve prescribing of psychoactive medications for children. *Psychiatric Services, 71*(7), 706–712. doi:10.1176/appi.ps.201900417

Kennedy, A. R., & Massey, L. R. (2019). Pediatric medication safety considerations for pharmacists in an adult hospital setting. *American Journal of Health-System Pharmacy, 76*(19), 1481–1491. https://doi-org.proxy.library.maryville.edu/10.1093/ajhp/zxz168

Kyle, T., & Carman, S. (2020). *Essentials of pediatric nursing* (3rd ed.). Wolters Kluwer Health.

Lim, S. Y., & Pettit, R. S. (2019). Pharmacokinetic considerations in pediatric pharmacotherapy. *American Journal of Health-System Pharmacy: AJHP: Journal of the American Society of Health-System Pharmacists, 76*(19), 1472–1480. doi:10.1093/ajhp/zxz161

Marufu, T., Takawira C., Bower, R., Hendron, E., & Manning, J. (2022). Nursing interventions to reduce medication errors in paediatrics and neonates: Systemic review and meta-analysis. *Journal of Pediatric Nursing, 62*, e139–e147. doi:10.1016/j.pedn.2021.08.024

Mosteller, R. D. (1987). Simplified calculation of body surface area. *The New England Journal of Medicine, 317*(17), 1098.

Schnur, M. B. (2017). Body mass index and body surface area: What's the difference between? *Lippincott Nursing Center*. https://www.nursingcenter.com/ncblog/august-2017/body-mass-index-and-body-surface-area-what-s-the-d

Tolley, C. L., Forde, N. E., Coffey, K. L., Sittig, D. F., Ash, J. S., Husband, A. K., Bates, D. W., & Slight, S. P. (2018). Factors contributing to medication errors made when using computerized order entry in pediatrics: A systematic review. *Journal of the American Medical Informatics Association: JAMIA, 25*(5), 575–584. doi:10.1093/jamia/ocx124

U.S. Food and Drug Administration (USFDA). (2015). *The Food and Drug Administration Safety and Innovation Act (FDASIA) Best Pharmaceuticals for Children Act and Pediatric Research Equity Act*. http://www.fda.gov/scienceresearch/specialtopics/pediatrictherapeuticsresearch/ucm509707.htm

CHAPTER 5

Pharmacology and the Care of Adults and Geriatric Patients

LEARNING OBJECTIVES

After studying this chapter, you should be able to:

1. Discuss pharmacodynamics and pharmacokinetic changes related to age in older adults.
2. Discuss the relevance of the Beers criteria to medication administration in the aging population.
3. Identify the physiologic changes associated with increased age related to pharmacokinetics (absorption, distribution, metabolism, and excretion) of medications.
4. Implement patient education about medications to prevent medication-related reactions and adverse effects.
5. Identify the pharmacologic care of the older adult diagnosed with infectious disease.
6. Discuss the effect of polypharmacy on the medication response of older adults.
7. Implement the nursing process in the care of the older adult with pharmacologic therapy.

CLINICAL APPLICATION CASE STUDY

Charles Franklin is a 75-year-old man with a diagnosis of an enlarged prostate. He has been experiencing insomnia for the past month and has begun taking acetaminophen in the form of Tylenol PM.

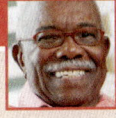

KEY TERMS

Adult: person who ranges in age from 19 to 64 years

Age-related changes: physiologic events due to increasing age, which affect drug responses

Older adult: person who is 65 years of age or older

Polypharmacy: use of several drugs during the same period

Risk to benefit ratio: poor outcome (adverse effects of medications) in relation to good outcome (desired medication effects); increases with increasing age

75

INTRODUCTION

Aging is a natural process that begins at birth. The most significant age-related changes begin in the **adult** years (19–64 years of age). **Age-related changes** are physiologic events, due to increasing age, which can affect drug responses. Most commonly, they occur in middle age and are related to heart disease, pulmonary insufficiency, cancer, arthritis, diabetes mellitus, obesity, substance use, and depression.

Older adults, people who are 65 years of age or older, are the largest consumers of healthcare. Chronic conditions have roots in the aging process. The most common health problems in older adults include arthritis, heart disease, decreased sensory perception, bone disorders, and diabetes mellitus. Older adults are also more prone to antibiotic-resistant infections. The treatment of chronic illnesses and associated comorbidities results in **polypharmacy**, the use of multiple medications. The interactions of medications can lead to greater complications and diminished mental status. In addition, the **risk to benefit ratio**, the relationship between the negative effects and the positive effects of a medication, increases as the patient ages. The nurse and the prescriber must consider the risk of associated adverse effects of those medications as well as possible benefits these medications might have in changing physiologic processes related to disease.

Rochon (2022) states that care must be taken in determining drug doses when prescribing to older patients. In premarketing drug trials, testing on older patients is extremely limited. From 2010 to 2019, Lau et al. sought to assess the representation of older adults in clinical trials for new drug applications (NDAs) and biologics license applications (BLAs). The study revealed data from 166 clinical trials with 229, 558 participants for 44 NDAs and BLAs that limited enrollment of the oldest adult groups aged 75 years and older with type 2 diabetes and non–small cell lung disease, along with adults 80 years or older with nonvalvular atrial fibrillation, insomnia, heart failure, or osteoporosis. The study also revealed that adults aged 60 to 74 years were enrolled in equal or greater proportion than that of the general population. The researchers found that the oldest adults were underrepresented in the evaluation of new drugs or biologics. Thus, it is important that future testing on new drugs and biologics be representative of the older and oldest adult populations.

Nurses must closely monitor and evaluate an older adult's reaction to any medication or combination of medications because many older adults have multiple comorbidities. On average, the older adult has at least five medical conditions for which they are prescribed medications at any given time.

PHARMACODYNAMICS IN OLDER ADULTS

Pharmacodynamics involves drug actions on target cells and the resulting alterations in cellular biochemical reactions and functions. In older adults, physiologic changes such as a reduced number of receptor sites for medications or reduced affinity to receptors alter the medication's ability to produce the desired effect. Older adults are prone to adverse drug reactions because of a decrease in the number of receptors needed for drug distribution. Beta-adrenergic agonists (Chapter 33) are less effective as a result of the decreased function of the beta-receptor system.

Nurses must be aware of other physiologic changes associated with increased age. For example, the volume of distribution of drugs may be increased based on the older adult's increase in body fat relative to the percentage of the skeletal muscle. The older adult's hepatic function declines leading to a significant amount of variability of drug metabolism. The decline in kidney function inhibits the adequate clearance of a drug. In addition, drug storage reservoirs increase with age. These physiologic changes interfere with drug distribution, limit effective drug metabolism, prolong half-life, and diminish drug excretion.

Cardiovascular disease is the number one cause of death in adults, including older adults. Hypertension affects 70% to 80% of older adults. In patients with hypertension, blood pressure control is key to preventing cardiovascular disease and stroke. Although a salt-reduction diet is often effective in the treatment of hypertension in younger adults, in older adults, lifestyle modifications alone may not be effective. Older adults who require antihypertensive medication should initially be prescribed a low-dose thiazide-type diuretic (Chapter 34), angiotensin-converting enzyme inhibitor, angiotensin II receptor blocker, or long-acting calcium channel blocker (Chapter 26). Beta-blockers should not be used as a primary treatment for systolic hypertension in the older adult population. Studies have shown that the use of beta-blockers may be worse than other agents in preventing stroke and may hasten death. This is particularly evident in older adults who have a history of smoking (Egan, 2021).

The use of digoxin (Lanoxin) (Chapter 30) in heart disease should not exceed 0.125 mg/day except when treating atrial fibrillation or supraventricular tachydysrhythmia. In atrial fibrillation, the maximum dose is 0.125 mg/day. For patients >70 years of age, low doses of 0.125 mg/day or every other day should be used. In supraventricular tachydysrhythmia, the digitalizing dose is 0.5 mg loading dose with an additional 0.125 to 25 mg every 6 to 8 hours. Do not exceed 0.75 to 1.5 mg (UpToDate, 2023). Digoxin has a low therapeutic index, placing patients at risk for adverse effects. Thus, administration of the medication with a reduced dose assists in maintaining safety.

Beers Criteria and Drug Burden Index

Dr. Mark Beers developed the Beers criteria list of potentially inappropriate medications used by the older adult population in 1997, and the American Geriatrics Society updated this list in 2023. The Beers Criteria for Potentially Inappropriate Medication Use in Older Adults is updated approximately every 3 to 4 years. It provides clinicians with the names of medications that are potentially inappropriate for use in older adults, listing drugs to be avoided and giving adjustments in dosages related to chronic kidney disease and diminished kidney function. An interdisciplinary panel of experts determines new criteria and updates existing criteria based on scientific evidence.

The 2019 update includes the two parts established in the 2015 review: (1) drugs for which dose adjustment is required based on kidney function and (2) drug–drug interactions (American Geriatrics Society, 2019 Beers Criteria Updated AGS Beers Criteria for Potentially Inappropriate Medication Use in Older Adults, 2019). The list does not include medications administered in the hospice and palliative care delivery systems. Many opioids are administered at the end of life. It is important to consider patients' needs for opioids in the treatment of chronic pain. The use of opioids in older adults requires patient assessment of response to treatment.

In nursing practice, it is vital to implement strategies to identify age-related changes associated with medication administration. According to Rochon (2022), 3% to 10% of all medical admissions are related to adverse drug events. Adverse drug events leading to overdose occur in two-thirds of the events. For the 2023 Beers criteria list of potentially inappropriate medication in older adults, visit thePoint http://thePoint.lww.com/Frandsen13e.

The Drug Burden Index is another approach to preventing adverse drug reactions in older adults. It identifies exposure to drugs with anticholinergic or sedative effects, the total number of medications, and the daily dosing. The increased drug burden for anticholinergic and sedative medications is associated with a community-based older adult's impaired performance related to mobility and cognitive testing. For example, zolpidem has been implicated in 21% of emergency department visits for adverse drug events related to this psychiatric medication taken among adults 65 years and older. A high Drug Burden Index is correlated with an increased risk for functional decline in community dwellers and increased risk of falls in residents of long-term care facilities (Rochon, 2021).

Anticholinergic medications are associated with multiple adverse drug effects. They result in memory impairment, confusion, hallucinations, dry mouth, blurred vision, constipation, nausea, urinary retention, impaired sweating, and tachycardia. Older adults diagnosed with benign prostatic hypertrophy are at greatest risk for the development of urinary retention related to the use of anticholinergic agents. In addition, patients diagnosed with narrow angle glaucoma have an increase in intraocular pressure related to the use of anticholinergics (Rochon, 2021).

> ### Quality and Safety Alert: Patient-Centered Care
>
> Drugs that contribute to or produce adverse effects in older adults include the following:
>
> - Amiodarone (Nexterone, Pacerone): potentially inappropriate as first-line therapy for atrial fibrillation, will cause acute hypotension
> - Amitriptyline hydrochloride: anticholinergic effects, sedation, and orthostatic hypotension
> - Cyclobenzaprine (Amrix, Fexmid): anticholinergic effects, weakness, serotonin syndrome
> - Dextromethorphan/quinidine: limited efficacy and increased risk of falls
> - Digoxin (Lanoxin): digoxin toxicity
> - Diphenhydramine hydrochloride: urinary retention
> - Flurazepam hydrochloride: sedation, hyperactivity, impaired mental alertness
> - Hydroxyzine hydrochloride: confusion and sedation
> - Ketorolac: gastrointestinal bleeding
> - Meperidine hydrochloride (Demerol): confusion
> - Methocarbamol (Robaxin): anticholinergic effects and weakness
> - Methyldopa: bradycardia and depression
> - Nitrofurantoin (Macrodantin): pulmonary and kidney toxicity, hepatotoxicity
> - Opioids with benzodiazepines and gabapentinoids: central nervous system (CNS) adverse effects and potential death
> - Rivaroxaban: caution required in patients older than age 75, increased risk of bleeding
> - Serotonin–norepinephrine reuptake inhibitors: avoid in patients who have experienced fractures or are prone to falls
> - Trimethoprim–sulfamethoxazole used with angiotensin-converting enzyme inhibitors or angiotensin receptor blockers: increased risk of hyperkalemia

Prevention of Adverse Effects

Strategies to prevent adverse drug reactions include the following:

- Assess a patient's health history and list of medications taken, including prescription medications, over-the-counter (OTC) medications, and herbal supplements.
- Assess blood urea nitrogen and creatinine clearance (CrCl) levels to determine the patient's ability to excrete the medications.
- Assess the ratio of alanine aminotransferase to aspartate aminotransferase to determine the patient's liver function and ability to metabolize drugs.
- Assess therapeutic drug levels as ordered by the prescriber to determine the medication effectiveness and prevention of toxicity.
- Educate the patient and family about all medications and possible drug–drug, drug–herb, and drug–diet interactions.
- Educate the patient and family about the generic and trade names of medications to prevent overmedication.
- Educate the patient and family to use one primary care provider who prescribes medications in consultation with other healthcare specialists.
- Educate the patient and family to have all prescriptions filled at one pharmacy.
- Assess the patient's adherence to the prescribed medications.
- Provide the patient with medication administration aids to increase adherence.

Clinical Application 5.1

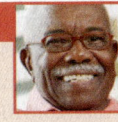

- What urinary effect is Mr. Franklin prone to developing since he began taking Tylenol PM?

NCLEX Success

1. A 75-year-old patient is having difficulty remembering to take all of their medications. Which of the following nursing interventions will assist the patient to improve adherence to the medication schedule?

   A. Have the patient's daughter administer the medications.
   B. Decrease the number of medications administered.
   C. Evaluate the patient's ability for self-care.
   D. Provide a medication administration aid.

PHARMACOKINETICS IN OLDER ADULTS

Aging results in physiologic changes that affect the absorption, distribution, metabolism, and excretion of medications. The most relevant physiologic change is the decreased function of vital organs needed for the pharmacokinetic processes. Frail, older adults are at greatest risk for altered drug responses. The more physically active older adults are, the less likely they will experience altered drug responses. Nurses can better plan for any potential adverse effects by assessing a patient's physical activity routine. Some medications place older adults at greater risk for adverse effects regardless of the physical activity level.

Healthcare providers prescribe many older adults anticholinergic agents, which are useful in the treatment of Parkinson disease, irritable bowel syndrome, and allergic reactions. The anticholinergic drug scale (ADS), which was developed and revised in 2006, measures anticholinergic effects on an ordinal scale of 0 to 3 (Carnahan et al., 2006). Patients with ADS scores of three or above have a higher risk of cognitive impairment. The study by Nissan et al. (2020) reveals that patients with high anticholinergic burden who were admitted for rehabilitation following hip fracture had lower functional abilities.

Indeed, many studies have reported that anticholinergic agents produce negative health outcomes in older adults. These outcomes increase the risk of falls, confusion, and diminished mental alertness. Attoh-Mensah et al. (2020) conducted a cross-sectional study in young–old (65 to 84 years) and old–old adults (85 years and older). The authors described background drugs as those possessing anticholinergic properties. There is growing evidence of adverse outcomes when both young–old and old–old adults are prescribed these medications or when they use the OTC versions of anticholinergic medications. Drugs with anticholinergic properties impair cognition in individuals as young as 55 years of age and should not be prescribed in patients aged 55 years and older. In addition, healthcare providers should educate young–old and old–old adults about the risk these medications pose, including OTC medications. Patients should avoid the use of such OTC drugs, which include first-generation histamine H_1 antagonists. The most common OTC medication is the prototype of this class, diphenhydramine, which was once available as Benadryl. Many preparations, such as Advil PM, Aleve PM, and Tylenol PM, contain this medication.

Absorption

In older adults, changes in the gastrointestinal (GI) tract include decreased gastric acidity, with an increase in the gastric pH, and delayed absorption or lack of absorption of medications that require this decreased pH. Other changes in the GI tract responsible for affecting drug absorption in older adults are decreased blood flow and decreased surface area to support absorption. Diminished gastric emptying also plays a role by causing the medication to remain in the stomach for a longer period. This factor increases the risk of developing nausea and vomiting, thus causing elimination of the medication in emesis and promoting fluid volume deficit.

In older patients, decreased circulation means that parenteral medications are also slowly absorbed. Decreased muscle mass and altered circulation can result in abnormal blood concentrations of medications administered intramuscularly.

In all cases, a slow rate of absorption can result in changes in peak serum drug levels. This factor may require greater dosages to be administered to produce therapeutic results.

Distribution

In older adults, physiologic factors that contribute to alterations in distribution of medications include diminished cardiac output, increased body fat, decreased body mass and body fluid, and decreased serum albumin. Aging results in body mass changes; the proportion of body fat increases while lean body mass decreases. These changes may have the following consequences:

- Lipid-soluble drugs such as the anesthetic agents stay in the fat tissue for a longer period of time. This places older adults at risk for respiratory depression following surgery.
- The amount of body fluid decreases in proportion to total body weight. Water-soluble drugs such as antibiotics are distributed in smaller volumes due to the decrease in total body fluid volume. This increases the risk of toxicity because drug concentrations are greater.
- Many medications require serum albumin to bind, transport, and distribute the medication to the target organ. If the amount of serum albumin is insufficient, the amount of free drug rises, and the effect of the drug is more intense.
- Medications are not distributed adequately due to the decreased circulation and diminished cardiac output.

Metabolism

Age-related physiologic changes of the liver affect the metabolism of medications. At approximately 60 years of age, the liver begins to decrease in size and mass. Hepatic circulation also decreases, lowering the rate of metabolism. The hepatic enzymes of the liver are decreased, altering the ability to remove metabolic by-products. It is important to understand that because older adults have a reduced metabolism, medications with a long half-life will remain in the body for a greater amount of time.

Pharmacogenomics is the science that uses information about the person's genetic make-up to select drug therapy. Genetic variations can alter drug metabolism and affect plasma concentrations. The potential benefit of genotyping provides more accurate information on drug metabolism to improve therapeutic outcomes. This is less biased than classifying drug response according to race. The FDA in 2020 established a Table of Pharmacogenetic Associations https://www.fda.gov/medical-devices/precision-medicine/table-pharmacogenetic-associations. This table provides sufficient evidence to suggest genetic variations and their effect on drug metabolism. For example, many older adults are prescribed statins to reduce cholesterol. The genetic variant SLCO1B1 may result in higher systemic concentrations of rosuvastatin or atorvastatin.

Excretion

The elimination of medications is vital in the prevention of adverse drug reactions. In older adults, physiologic changes associated with alterations in medication excretion include diminished kidney blood flow, number of functioning nephrons, glomerular filtration rate (GFR), and tubular secretion. The assessment of the patient's CrCl is an important indicator of the ability of the kidney system to eliminate the medication and prevent adverse drug effects. Dosages of medications should be lower in medications with an increased half-life. In most older adults, the serum creatinine remains within the normal range due to decreasing creatinine levels in association with a decrease in muscle mass. The GFR is the most reliable measure for evaluation of kidney function. Measuring the GFR is both complex and time consuming. The GFR is estimated by serum markers. Drug dosing guidelines have been developed using the Cockroft–Gault method.

The GFR is an overestimation of the CrCl, because creatinine is secreted by the proximal tubule and filtered by the kidneys. The GFR is the most accurate measure of the kidneys' ability to eliminate nitrogenous wastes, regulate the balance of electrolytes, fluids, acid–base, and mineral balance. It also assists in controlling blood pressure and synthesis along with secretion of erythropoietin and other hormones. The GFR is equal to the sum of the filtration rates or the functioning nephrons. The true GFR cannot be measured directly in humans; it is determined from serum levels of filtration markers. Creatinine is procured from the metabolism of creatinine in the skeletal muscle and dietary intake of cooked meat and released into the circulation at a proportionately constant rate. The differences in muscle masses between males and females contribute to the difference in mean serum creatinine levels. In addition, non-GFR determinants of serum creatinine include high or low muscle mass, patients with cirrhosis, serious chronic illness, chronic heart failure, amputations, neuromuscular disease, or individuals consuming a high protein or vegan diet. In the past, race was considered a non-GFR factor. As of 2021, race is no longer a factor in the creatinine value (Inker & Perrone, 2022).

Clinical Application 5.2

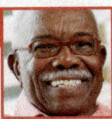

- Mr. Franklin asks the nurse in the emergency department why he could not urinate. What is the rationale for Mr. Franklin's urinary retention?

PHARMACOLOGIC CARE OF INFECTIONS IN OLDER ADULTS

In addition to changes in the absorption, metabolism, distribution, and excretion of medications, physiologic changes related to age also affect the response to infections in the older adult. Mody (2021) states that biologic and societal factors increase the older adult's susceptibility to infections, leading to poorer outcomes. Physiologic changes in the integumentary, pulmonary, and gastrointestinal system increase the risk of invasion by pathogenic organisms. In addition, changes in immunity and decreased production of cytokines increase the risk of infection. Chronic diseases impair immunity, thus increasing the susceptibility to infection.

Many older adults can experience serious infections without a fever. According to Mody (2021), frail older adults can also experience infections with a decline in temperature. When a change in mood or confusion develops in an older adult, the nurse must assess for the presence of infection.

The most common infection in adults aged 65 years and older is a urinary tract infection (UTI). Older adults should be treated for UTI in the presence of acute dysuria, increased frequency and urgency, hematuria, and costovertebral or suprapubic pain. Changes in cognition and vital sign abnormalities are indicative of acute UTI. Other common infections in older adults include pneumonia and infective endocarditis. When antibiotics are prescribed to treat an infection, the dosage should be determined based on the GFR, and the drug level must be monitored during therapy. For example, when administering vancomycin intravenously, the peak or trough levels and creatinine levels must be monitored closely to prevent impaired kidney function and hearing loss.

It is important to be aware that human immunodeficiency virus (HIV) in older adults can cause many drug interactions. Nurses must be cognizant of these interactions to maintain adequate hepatic and kidney function in older patients who have been diagnosed with HIV. Many older adults with HIV are experiencing the effects of long-term antiretroviral therapy, placing them at risk for kidney injury and bone loss.

Older adults also have diminished reactions to vaccine response. In recent years, communal living facilities have shown increased risk among older adults of developing viral, bacterial, and fungal infections, including SARS-CoV$_2$, which is noted with increased shortness of breath, cough, loss of taste and smell, headache, fever, and chills. COVID vaccines reduce the risk of morbidity and mortality in older adults. Vaccines are particularly important for older adults living in community-living, assisted living, and long-term care facilities.

NCLEX Success

2. A 68-year-old patient has been prescribed digoxin 0.125 mg. Based on the patient's age, what condition are they at risk for developing?
    A. diarrhea
    B. digoxin toxicity
    C. edema
    D. pulmonary embolism

3. An 85-year-old patient is administered a general anesthetic for repair of a hip fracture. Which of the following properties of the anesthetic place the patient at risk for respiratory depression?
    A. solubility in lipids
    B. solubility in water
    C. binding to cytochrome P450
    D. binding to muscle tissue

MEDICATION ADHERENCE AND AGING

As patients increase in age, they generally use a greater number of medications, both prescription and OTC, often with alternative therapies such as vitamins or herbal supplements. (As previously mentioned, the use of increased medications is known as polypharmacy.) Some older adults have difficulty remembering medications or maintaining appropriate administration schedules. Altered mental status and diminished visual acuity also contribute to improper medication use. Patients who have decreased vision may not be able to discriminate the dosing instructions or may not be able to see the amount of insulin drawn up in an insulin syringe.

Economic factors also contribute to nonadherence. Some older adults may have to choose between the cost of their medications and the ability to purchase food or pay for utilities. A multidisciplinary team approach is used to assist patients in obtaining medications. It is important for the prescriber to use generic medications and to order initially small quantities of medications so that an individual patient's reaction to the medication can be determined. In the event the medication needs to be changed, the financial burden on the patient will not be too great.

Starting slow and with low doses improves adherence to the medication regimen. Patients may describe not feeling well after using the prescribed medications, and starting with smaller doses minimizes these adverse effects. The administration of several medications concurrently can result in adverse effects. When adverse effects are experienced by older patients, they may not adhere to the recommended administration guidelines.

Being asymptomatic may contribute to nonadherence to a medication regimen. Many patients begin to feel better with the initiation of therapy and then discontinue medications altogether or miss individual doses. Patients and their families should be educated about adherence to medication regimens. This is particularly evident in patients being treated for hypertension. Patients who do not take antihypertensives as prescribed have an increased risk of a cardiovascular event. It is important that healthcare providers educate patients and families about medications and their use. To improve adherence, nurses and other healthcare providers should keep the care inexpensive, use generic preparations, provide easy to follow instructions, and use the fewest number of doses required. UpToDate recommends two types of patient education. "The Basics" recommends that patient education should be written in plain language at a fifth- to sixth-grade reading level. "Beyond the Basics" provides higher-level educational information that is at the 10th to 12th grade level (Egan, 2021).

Quality and Safety Alert: Evidence-Based Practice

Pariseault et al. (2021) identified a gap in research related to the management of polypharmacy and the value of nurse practitioners in providing care to older adults. The purpose of this study was to explore the experiences nurse practitioners have in caring for community-dwelling older adults experiencing polypharmacy. This qualitative study of 15 nurse practitioners revealed four themes: defining polypharmacy, communicating and collaborating, clinical judgment of nurse practitioners in relation to polypharmacy, and medication issues of older adults. Medication management in older adults is complex, and nurse practitioners have important roles in providing care. The authors identify the importance of improving communication and collaboration with other healthcare providers in medication prescribing and in managing polypharmacy for older adults.

NCLEX Success

4. A 68-year-old patient is receiving chemotherapy. What is the rationale for teaching the patient to drink eight glasses of water throughout the day following the administration of chemotherapy?
   A. Chemotherapy is toxic to the liver, and the water will reduce the adverse effects.
   B. The water will prevent the body from rejecting the medication.
   C. Chemotherapy is excreted in the kidneys and urine. The water will help eliminate it from the body.
   D. The water will prevent dehydration, an adverse effect of the medication.

5. A 78-year-old patient receiving treatment for hypertension has been having persistent headaches and difficulty with the prescribed medications. This is the third prescription the patient has received. The patient states, "I can't afford to get this filled and then stop it in a few days." Which statement is most appropriate for the nurse to communicate to the patient?
   A. Have the pharmacist give you a few pills to start.
   B. Take your other medication and then switch.
   C. Take the other medications back to the pharmacy for a refund.
   D. Save all your pills; you may need them again.

THE NURSING PROCESS

A concept map outlines the nursing process related to drug therapy considerations in this chapter. Additional nursing implications related to the disease process should also be considered in care decisions.

Assessment
- Assess the patient's knowledge of his or her medication regimen, including knowledge of the action and use of each medication administered.
- Assess the patient's ability to administer the medication correctly.
- Assess the patient for adverse effects of medications as well as drug–drug, drug–diet, and drug–herb interactions.
- Assess the patient's physiologic status with regard to the medication's pharmacokinetics (e.g., kidney function, liver function, cardiovascular function).
- Assess physiologic changes, such as the patient's ability to swallow.
- Assess body mass and its effect on medication absorption and distribution.
- Assess the patient's ability to maintain medication adherence based on memory, self-care, and caregiver's ability to assist in care.

Outcomes of Therapy
The patient will
- Take medications as prescribed.
- Tolerate medications based on kidney and liver function.
- Report adverse effects to primary care provider.
- Understand all aspects of medication administration, including action, use, and adverse effects.
- Maintain medication adherence.

Nursing Interventions
- Assess the patient's liver and kidney function as well as their circulation and changes in body mass affecting pharmacokinetics.
- Assess the patient's response to medication regimen.
- Assess the patient's ability to maintain medication administration.
- Assess for adverse effects of medications.
- Assess for the patient's adherence to medications.
- Instruct the patient and family about the use of medication administration aids.
- Instruct the patient and family about the administration of medications.
- Instruct the patient and family about the action, use, and adverse effects of medications.

Evaluation
- Evaluate the patient's response to the medication regimen.
- Evaluate the patient's and family's understanding of the medication regimen.
- Evaluate the patient's adherence to the medication regimen.

Visit thePoint® at http://thePoint.lww.com/Frandsen13e for answers to NCLEX Success questions (in Appendix A), answers to Clinical Application Case Studies (in Appendix B), and more!

REFERENCES AND RESOURCES

American Geriatrics Society. (2023). American Geriatrics Society 2023 updated AGS Beers criteria for potentially inappropriate medication use in older adults. Journal of the American Geriatrics Society. https://doi.org/10.1111/jgs.18372 https://agsjournals.onlinelibrary.wiley.com/doi/full/10.1111/jgs.18372

Attoh-Mensah, E., Loggia, G., Schumann-Bard, P., Morello, R., & Descatoire, P. (2020). Adverse effects of anticholinergic drugs on cognition and mobility: Cutoff for impairments in a cross-sectional study in young-old and old-old adults. Drugs & Aging, 37(4), 301–310. doi: 10.1007/s40266-019-00743-z

Carnahan, R. M., Lund, B. C., Perry, P. J., Pollack, B. G., & Culp, K. R. (2006). The anticholinergic drug scale as a measurement of drug-related anticholinergic burden: Associations with serum anticholinergic activity. Journal of Clinical Pharmacology, 46, 1481–1486. doi: 10.1177/0091270006292126

Egan, B. M. (2021). Treatment of hypertension in the elderly patient, particularly isolated systolic hypertension. UpToDate. Lexi-Comp, Inc.

Inker, L. A., & Perrone, R. D. (2022). Assessment of kidney function. UpToDate. Lexi-Comp, Inc.

Lau, S. W. J., Huang, Y., Hsieh, J., Wang, S., Liu, Q., Slattum, P. W., Schwartz, J. B., Huang, S., & Temple, R. (2022). Participation of older adults in clinical trials for new drug applications and biologics license application from 2010 through 2019. JAMA Network Open, 5(10), E2236149. doi: 10.1001/jamanetworkopen.2022.36149

Mody, L. (2021). Approach to infection in the older adult. UpToDate. Wolters Kluwer.

National Institute of Diabetes and Digestive and Kidney Diseases. (2021). Estimate glomerular filtration rate. Retrieved October 30, 2021, from https://www.niddk.nih.gov/health-information/professionals/clinical-tools-patient-management/kidney-disease/laboratory-evaluation/glomerular-filtration-rate/estimating

Nissan, R., Brill, S., & Hershkovitz, A. (2020). Association between anticholinergic drug prescription changes and rehabilitation outcome in post-acute hip fractured patients. Disability and Rehabilitation, 1–6. April 12, 2019. doi: 10.1080/09638288.2019.1576782

Norris, T. (2019). Porth's pathophysiology: Concepts of altered health states (10th ed.). Wolters Kluwer.

Olafuyi, O., Parekh, N., Wright, J., & Koenig, J. (2021). Inter-ethnic differences in pharmacokinetics—Is there more that unites than divides? Pharmacology Research & Perspectives doi: https://doi.org/10.1002/prp2.890

Pariseault, C. A., Sharts-Hopko, N., & Blunt, E. (2021). Nurse practitioners' experience of polypharmacy in community-dwelling older adults. Journal of the American Association of Nurse Practitioners, 33(10), 811–817. doi: 10.1097/JXX.0000000000000484

Rochon, P. (2022). Drug prescribing for older adults. UpToDate. Lexi-Comp, Inc.

Tantsiira, K., & Weiss, S. T. (2022). Overview of pharmacogenomics. UpToDate. Lexi-Comp, Inc.

UpToDate. (2023). Digoxin drug information. Lexi-Comp, Inc.

U.S. Food & Drug Administration. (2020). Table of pharmacogenetic associations. Retrieved March 11, 2023 from https://www.fda.gov/medical-devices/precision-medicine/table-pharmacogenetic-associations

Wang, J., Paul, S., Arbet, R. N., & Lin, A. C. (2023). Application of pharmacogenomics testing in a community-based facility. Hospital Pharmacy, 58(1), 98–105. doi: 10.1177/00185787221134693

CHAPTER 6

Pharmacology and the Care of Pregnant or Lactating Females

LEARNING OBJECTIVES

After studying this chapter, you should be able to:

1. Describe the etiology of infertility.
2. Describe the drugs used for infertility.
3. Identify the pregnancy-associated changes that affect drug pharmacokinetics.
4. Analyze the effect of teratogens on the fetus during development.
5. Identify the effects of herbal and dietary supplements on the patient and fetus during pregnancy.
6. Identify pharmacologic strategies to manage pregnancy-associated symptoms.
7. Identify the prototype drugs that alter uterine motility and describe these drugs.
8. Identify the prototype drugs used during labor and delivery and describe these drugs.
9. Discuss the use of drugs and herbs during lactation, including their effects on the infant.
10. Implement the nursing process in the care of patients who can become pregnant.

CLINICAL APPLICATION CASE STUDY

Lauren Ross is in the 36th week of pregnancy with her fourth child. During her weekly visit to the certified nurse midwife, her blood pressure is elevated, 164/112 mm Hg, on two consecutive readings taken 4 hours apart. The nurse midwife checks Lauren's urine for protein and determines that she is spilling protein in her urine. Ms. Ross has had mild epigastric pain and an unrelenting headache for the past 2 days. Also, her vaginal culture is positive for perinatal group B *Streptococcus*. In addition, during her pregnancy, she has been taking the antidepressant escitalopram (Lexapro) 10 mg/day and has continued to smoke cigarettes. The nurse midwife admits her to the labor and delivery unit for observation.

KEY TERMS

Abortifacient: drug used to terminate pregnancy

Eclampsia: characterized by the onset of potentially fatal grand mal seizures; occurs in some pregnant patients with preeclampsia

Galactagogues: a category of herbs known to induce lactation or stimulate the production of breast milk

Organogenesis: formation of organs during the first 3 to 8 weeks after conception (embryonic stage of development)

Oxytocics: drugs that initiate uterine contractions, thus inducing childbirth

Preeclampsia: pregnancy-associated hypertension with proteinuria and/or manifestations of end-organ failure

Preterm labor: uterine contractions with cervical changes before 37 weeks of gestation, resulting in birth

Prostaglandins: chemical mediators with hormonelike effects that help initiate uterine contractions

Teratogenic: causing abnormal embryonic or fetal development

Tocolytics: drugs used to stop preterm labor

Uterotonics: drugs to control postpartum bleeding

INTRODUCTION

Drug use before and during pregnancy and lactation requires special consideration. People who are able to become pregnant may ingest drugs that cause fetal harm before they know they are pregnant. In general, patients who are pregnant or lactating should avoid or minimize the use of medications whenever possible. This chapter discusses drugs related to pregnancy and lactation, including infertility drugs, vaccines, tocolytics (drugs used to stop preterm labor), **oxytocics** (drugs used to initiate uterine contractions), uterotonics (drugs used to stop postpartum hemorrhage), and selected teratogenic drugs (agents causing abnormal embryonic or fetal development). Description of many of these drugs appears elsewhere in the text.

DRUG THERAPY FOR INFERTILITY

Infertility applies to (1) individuals younger than age 35 years who have been unable to conceive after at least 12 months of regular sexual intercourse without the use of contraception as well as (2) those older than age 35 years old after 6 months of regular intercourse without the use of contraception. In females, the most common cause is an ovulation disorder. Other causes include blocked fallopian tubes or tubal abnormalities, endometriosis, pelvic adhesions, uterine abnormalities, hormonal imbalances, and advanced female age. In males, causes include absence of sperm, declining sperm counts, testicular abnormalities, and ejaculatory dysfunction. Factors such as implantation, uterine and hormonal environment, and embryo integrity may also play a role; they are critical to fetal viability and a normally progressing pregnancy.

Drug therapy is an integral part of treating infertility. Drugs prescribed for a female experiencing infertility increase follicular maturation and promote ovulation. It is necessary to take the total dose at the same time each day to enhance effects of a particular medication. Also, coitus every other day enhances fertility due to increased sperm counts.

Table 6.1 presents the routes and dosage ranges for the infertility drugs, including their prototypes, indicated as such in the table and following section with the ⓟ icon.

Clomiphene Citrate

ⓟ **Clomiphene citrate** is an ovarian stimulator and selective estrogen receptor modulator. This drug increases the amount of follicle-stimulating hormone (FSH) and luteinizing hormone (LH) secreted by the pituitary gland, thus inducing ovulation for those who have infrequent or absent menstrual periods. Healthcare providers use it for the treatment of ovulatory failure in these patients who have tried to become pregnant but have failed. Ovulation occurs 5 to 10 days after the course of clomiphene treatment has been completed. Prior to beginning the drug regimen, the nurse instructs the patient about taking their basal temperature 5 to 10 days following administration. An incremental rise in temperature is an indication that ovulation has recently occurred.

Clomiphene is a mixture of zuclomiphene and enclomiphene. Metabolized by the liver, the drug has a half-life of 5 days. It is excreted in the feces and urine.

Possible adverse effects of clomiphene include ovarian enlargement, hot flashes, breast pain and tenderness, and uterine bleeding. Some patients have reported visual disturbances, abdominal discomfort, and headaches with clomiphene. Contraindications include liver disease, thyroid or adrenal disease, intracranial lesions, ovarian cysts, and abnormal uterine bleeding.

Letrozole

ⓟ **Letrozole** (Femara) is an aromatase inhibitor that is now recommended as first-line therapy over clomiphene to patients with anovulatory infertility related to polycystic ovary syndrome (PCOS). It works by blocking the conversion of testosterone and androstenedione to estradiol and estrone, which reduces the negative estrogenic feedback in the pituitary gland and increases follicle-stimulating hormone (FSH) production. The advantages of this medication over clomiphene include (1) fewer follicles produced and lower estradiol levels, and (2) a shorter half-life resulting in a reduced antiestrogen effect on the endometrium and cervical mucus. Despite the potential benefits of this medication for anovulatory infertility, the FDA has not approved the use of aromatase inhibitors in the treatment of infertility.

Menotropin

ⓟ **Menotropin** (Menopur) is a gonadotropin given to patients who have been diagnosed with anovulation. The drug stimulates FSH and LH to promote the development and maturation of ovarian follicles. Administration is subcutaneous, given in alternating sides of the abdomen. Following its administration, the patient receives human chorionic gonadotropin (hCG) (see later discussion). Menotropin is well absorbed and excreted in the urine.

During menotropin therapy, it is necessary to monitor both hCG and serum estradiol measurements. The adverse effects and contraindications of menotropin are similar to those of clomiphene citrate.

TABLE 6.1
DRUGS AT A GLANCE: Infertility Drugs*

Drug	Routes and Dosage Ranges
Clomiphene citrate (Clomid, Serophene)	50 mg PO once daily for 5 d; begin on the 5th day of the cycle if progestin-induced bleeding is scheduled or spontaneous uterine bleeding occurs prior to therapy; therapy may be initiated at any time if there has been no recent uterine bleeding; subsequent doses may be increased to 100 mg once daily for 5 d only if ovulation does not occur at the initial dose; max dosage: 100 mg PO once daily for 5 d for six cycles; discontinue if ovulation does not occur after three courses of treatment or if ovulatory responses occur but pregnancy is not achieved
Letrozole (Femara; Letrozole)	2.5 mg PO once daily for 5 d; begin on day 3, 4, or 5 following menstruation or progestin induced bleeding; increase to 5 mg daily for 5 d in subsequent cycles if ovulation does not occur; maximum dosage is 7.5 mg daily
Menotropin (Menopur; Menopur)	225 IU Sub-Q once beginning on cycle day 2 or 3; dosage adjustments may occur once every 2 d or by >150 IU; maximum daily dose should not exceed 450 IU and dosing should not extend beyond 20 d
Follitropin alfa (Gonal-F, Gonal-F RFF; Gonal-F, Gonal-F Pen)	75 IU Sub-Q daily; dose adjustment up to 37.5 IU after 14 d; if necessary, it can be increased every 7 d (max dosage: 300 IU); if response to follitropin is appropriate, hCG is given 1 d following the last dose; do not exceed 35 d of treatment
Follitropin beta (Follistim AQ; Puregon)	50 IU (cartridge) Sub-Q or 50 IU (vials) Sub-Q or IM for the first 7 d; increase by 25–50 IU at weekly intervals; if response to follitropin is appropriate, hCG is given 1 d following the last dose
Human chorionic gonadotropin (hCG) (Novarel; Pregnyl; Pregnyl)	5,000–10,000 units IM 1 d following menotropins or follitropins
Leuprolide (Eligard, Lupron Depot; Eligard, Lupron, Lupron Depot)	3.75 mg IM every 28 d for up to 24 mo or 11.25 mg every 3 mo for up to 24 mo

*Use of infertility drugs during pregnancy is not recommended.

Follitropins

Follitropin alfa (Gonal-F, Gonal-F RFF) and follitropin beta (Follistim AQ) are drugs used to induce ovulation and thus promote fertility. Administration is subcutaneous, in calibrated syringes provided by the manufacturer. It is important that the drugs not be shaken before administration. After receiving follitropins, as with menotropins, patients should also receive hCG (see following discussion)—1 day after the last dose of follitropin.

The adverse effects of the follitropins are similar to those of clomiphene. Contraindications include hypersensitivity to follitropins, as well as the presence of tumors in the ovary, breast, uterus, pituitary gland, or hypothalamus. It is necessary to monitor serum estradiol levels to determine the medication response.

Human Chorionic Gonadotropin

Human chorionic gonadotropin (Novarel, Pregnyl), or hCG, is a human formulation of hCG that is derived from the urine of pregnant people. It is used as a replacement for LH to stimulate ovulation following administration of menotropin or follitropin.

Adverse effects of hCG include arterial thrombosis, edema, depression, rupture of ovarian cysts, and ovarian hyperstimulation. Contraindications include neoplasms or known hypersensitivity to the hormone.

Leuprolide

Leuprolide (Eligard, Lupron Depot) is a gonadotropin-releasing hormone analogue that has an unlabeled use in the treatment of infertility. Administered subcutaneously or intramuscularly, it prevents premature ovulation and enhances the production of a larger quantity of quality eggs.

Potential adverse effects of leuprolide include hot flashes, headache, depression, insomnia, and vaginitis.

NCLEX Success

1. A female patient diagnosed with anovulation receives a prescription for menotropin to be administered subcutaneously. When providing education about medication administration, the nurse should teach the patient to:
   A. massage the area prior to administering the drug
   B. administer the drug at a 90-degree angle
   C. alternate the sides of the abdomen for the injection sites
   D. take human chorionic gonadotropin before the menotropin

DRUGS USED IN PREGNANCY

During pregnancy, the pregnant parent and fetus undergo physiologic changes that influence drug effects. In pregnant patients, physiologic changes alter drug pharmacokinetics (Table 6.2). In general, drug effects are less predictable because plasma volume expansion decreases plasma drug concentrations, and increased metabolism by the liver and increased elimination by the kidneys shorten the duration of drug actions and effects.

Maternal–Placental–Fetal Circulation

Drugs ingested during pregnancy reach the fetus through the maternal–placental–fetal circulation, which is completed about the 4th or 5th week after conception. On the maternal side, arterial blood pressure carries blood and drugs to the placenta. In the placenta, maternal and fetal blood are separated by a few thin layers of membrane, which drugs can readily cross.

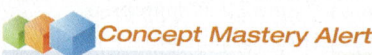
Concept Mastery Alert
Maternal arterial blood pressure delivers blood and drugs to the placenta. Diffusion takes place in the placenta.

Placental transfer begins about the 5th week after conception. After drugs enter the fetal circulation, relatively large amounts are pharmacologically active because the fetus has low levels of serum albumin and thus low levels of drug binding. Most drug molecules are transported to the fetal liver, where they are metabolized. Metabolism occurs slowly because the liver is immature in quantity and quality of drug-metabolizing enzymes. Drugs metabolized by the fetal liver are excreted by fetal kidneys into amniotic fluid. Excretion also is slow and inefficient due to immature development of fetal kidneys. Other drug molecules are transported directly to the heart, which then distributes them to the brain and coronary arteries. Drugs enter the fetal brain easily because the blood–brain barrier is poorly developed. Approximately half of the drug-containing blood is then transported through the umbilical arteries to the placenta, where it reenters the maternal circulation. The pregnant parent can metabolize and excrete some drug molecules for the fetus.

Drug Effects on the Fetus

Drug effects are determined mainly by the type and amount of drug, duration of exposure, and level of fetal growth and development during exposure. The fetus is sensitive to drug effects because it is small, has few plasma proteins that can bind drug molecules, and has a weak capacity for metabolizing and excreting drugs. In addition, the fetus is exposed to any drugs circulating in maternal blood. Molecular size, weight, and lipid solubility determine which substances (chemicals, drugs, and antibodies) are readily absorbed into the fetal circulation from the maternal circulation. When drugs are taken on a regular schedule, fetal blood usually contains 50% to 100% of the amount in maternal blood. This means that any drug that stimulates or depresses the central nervous, cardiovascular, respiratory, or other body system in the pregnant parent has the potential to stimulate or depress those systems in the fetus. In some cases, fetotoxicity occurs.

TABLE 6.2
Pregnancy: Physiologic and Pharmacokinetic Changes

Physiologic Change	Pharmacokinetic Change
Increased plasma and subsequent blood volume, up to 50% in a normal pregnancy Increased cardiac output (30%–50%) and increased blood flow to the uterus, kidneys, skin, and breasts	After it is absorbed into the bloodstream, a drug (especially if water soluble) is distributed and "diluted" more than in the nonpregnant state. Drug dosage requirements may increase. However, this effect may be offset by other pharmacokinetic changes of pregnancy
Increased weight (average 25 lb) and body fat	Drugs (especially fat-soluble ones) are distributed more widely. Drugs that are distributed to fatty tissues stay in the body longer because they are slowly released from storage sites into the bloodstream
Changes in protein binding, decreased serum albumin. Also, many plasma protein–binding sites are occupied by hormones and other endogenous substances that increase during pregnancy	The decreased capacity for drug binding leaves more free drug available for therapeutic or adverse effects on the patient and for placental transfer to the fetus. Thus, a given dose of a drug may produce greater effects than it would in the nonpregnant state
During most of a pregnancy, increased kidney blood flow and glomerular filtration rate secondary to increased cardiac output	Increased excretion of drugs by the kidneys, especially those excreted primarily unchanged in the urine (e.g., lithium, penicillins)
In late pregnancy, kidney blood flow may decrease when the patient assumes a supine position, secondary to the increased size and weight of the uterus	Decreased kidney blood flow may result in delayed excretion and prolonged effects of renally excreted drugs
Increased hormones (e.g., estrogen, progesterone) induce drug-metabolizing enzymes in the liver	Increased metabolism and clearance of many drugs

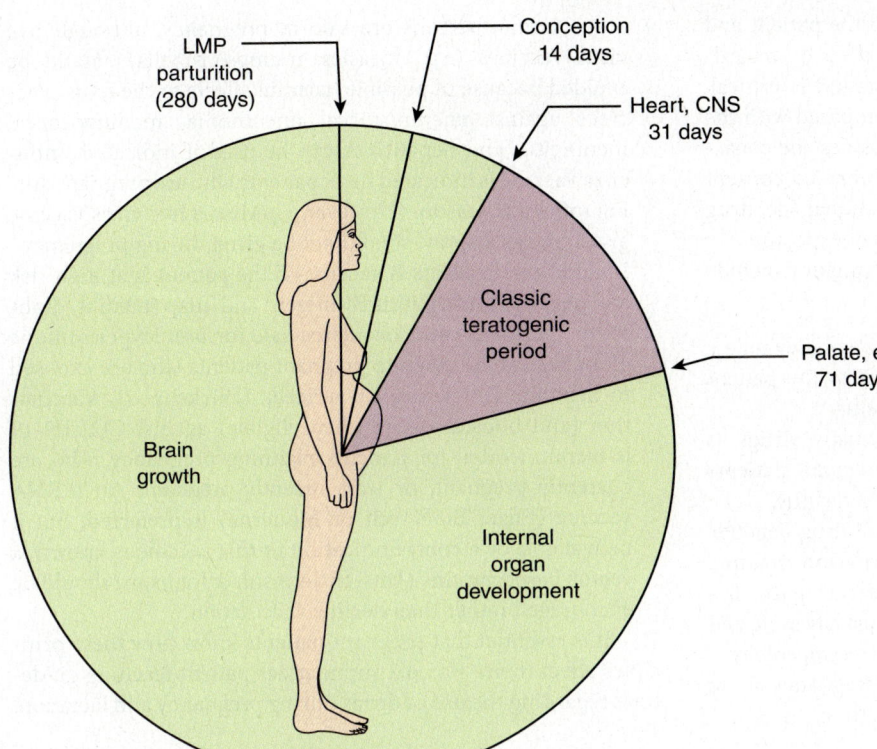

Figure 6.1. The gestational clock showing the classic teratogenic risk assessment. (Adapted from Niebyl, J. (1999). Drugs and related areas in pregnancy. In J. Sciarra (Ed.), *Obstetrics and gynecology*. Wolters Kluwer.)

Drugs that may be **teratogenic** (causing abnormal embryonic or fetal development) are a major concern. Drug-induced teratogenicity is most likely to occur when drugs are taken during the first 3 months of pregnancy, during **organogenesis** (formation of embryonic organs during the first 3 to 8 weeks after conception) (Fig. 6.1). Malformations that occur during the preembryonic period (1st and 2nd week of pregnancy postconception) rarely result in a viable fetus (the fetal stage starts after completion of week 8 of embryonic life). During the embryonic and fetal stages, teratogenic insult and timing result in the targeting of specific organ growth during organogenesis and subsequent maturation and refinement of an organ's physiologic purpose. For drugs taken during the second and third trimesters, adverse effects are usually manifested in the neonate (birth to 1 month) or infant (1 month to 1 year) as growth retardation, respiratory problems, infection, or bleeding. It should be emphasized, however, that drugs taken at any time during pregnancy can affect the baby's brain because brain development continues throughout pregnancy and after birth.

Concept Mastery Alert

Drugs that are potentially harmful to a fetus are considered *teratogenic*. Potentially teratogenic substances include alcohol, morphine, cocaine, salicylates, coumarin anticoagulants, sedatives, tetracyclines, thiazides, tobacco smoke, and large doses of vitamin K.

For 40 years, the U.S. Food and Drug Administration required manufacturers to assign pregnancy categories identifying potential risk for causing birth defects. Healthcare professionals sometimes made the wrong decisions about drugs based on these somewhat simplistic categories. The new system includes pregnancy information, risk summary, and clinical considerations, as well as data that should allow for better-informed prescribing decisions (see Chapter 2). Box 6.1 provides a list of teratogenic drugs.

Principles of Drug Therapy in Pregnancy

Before administering a drug to a pregnant patient, it is the responsibility and obligation of all healthcare providers, including nurses, to conduct a risk–benefit assessment—a compre-

BOX 6.1   Selected Teratogenic Drugs

- Angiotensin-converting enzyme (ACE) inhibitors (e.g., captopril) (second and third trimesters)
- Angiotensin II receptor blockers (ARBs; e.g., losartan)
- Antibacterials (e.g., tetracycline, tigecycline)
- Anticoagulant (e.g., warfarin)
- Antiepileptics (e.g., carbamazepine, valproate)
- Antineoplastics (e.g., ibritumomab, idarubicin, ifosfamide, irinotecan, methotrexate)
- Antithyroid agents (e.g., propylthiouracil)
- Antiviral (e.g., ribavirin)
- Benzodiazepine (e.g., alprazolam, diazepam, lorazepam, temazepam, triazolam)
- Bisphosphonates (e.g., pamidronate, zoledronic acid)
- Female sex hormones (e.g., estrogens, injectable progestins, oral contraceptives)
- Male sex hormones (e.g., androgens, anabolic steroids)
- Opioid analgesics (with prolonged use or high doses at term)
- Retinoids (e.g., acitretin, isotretinoin, and several topical preparations)
- Statin cholesterol-lowering drugs (e.g., atorvastatin)

hensive analytic comparison of the benefits to the patient and the risks to the fetus. Inclusion of family in a decision regarding drug exposure during pregnancy and lactation is critical. Ideally, the risk to the fetus should be small compared with the potential patient benefit. It is necessary to consider the consequences with and without drug therapy and informed consent should be obtained. Important factors are gestational age; drug route, dosage, and concentration; and duration of exposure.

General guidelines for drug therapy in pregnancy include the following:

- It is important that no drug be used during pregnancy unless it is clearly needed and the potential benefit to the patient outweighs the risk of potential harm to the fetus.
- However, although the teratogenicity of many drugs is unknown, most medications required by pregnant patients can be used safely, and most children are born healthy.
- When drug therapy is necessary, the choice of drug depends on the stage of pregnancy and available drug information. During the first trimester, for example, an older drug that has not been associated with teratogenic effects is usually preferred over a newer drug of unknown fetotoxicity or teratogenicity.
- It is important to give any drug used during pregnancy at the lowest effective dose for the shortest possible time.

- Some immunizations are safe in pregnancy, although live virus vaccines (e.g., measles, mumps, rubella) should be avoided because of possible harmful effects to the fetus. Vaccines against pneumococcal pneumonia, meningococcal meningitis, and hepatitis A can be used if indicated. Influenza vaccine is indicated in all patients who are pregnant during influenza season. (However, FluMist, a live virus vaccine given by nasal spray, should *not* be given during pregnancy.) In addition, hepatitis B vaccine (if the patient is at high risk and negative for hepatitis B antigen) and Tdap (tetanus, diphtheria, pertussis) are considered safe for use. Hyperimmune globulins can be given to pregnant patients who are exposed to hepatitis B, tetanus, or varicella (chickenpox). Vaccination (and booster doses when eligible) against COVID-19 is recommended for patients planning pregnancy, who are currently pregnant, or were recently pregnant. An mRNA vaccine (Pfizer/BioNTech or Moderna) is preferred, but if unavailable or a contraindication to this vaccine is known, a vector-based vaccine (Janssen/Johnson & Johnson) should be encouraged rather than decline vaccination.

It is essential that pregnant patients know how these principles affect them. Box 6.2 summarizes patient teaching guidelines regarding the use of drugs during pregnancy and lactation.

BOX 6.2 — *Patient Teaching Guidelines: Drug Use During Pregnancy and Lactation*

- Systemic drugs ingested by the pregnant person reach the fetus and may interfere with fetal growth and development. Safety during pregnancy has not been established for most drugs, and all drugs are relatively contraindicated. Drug use must be cautious and minimal to avoid harming the fetus.
- Use drugs only when necessary and very cautiously. If a sexually active person is not using effective contraception and takes drugs, there is a high risk that potentially harmful agents may be ingested before pregnancy is suspected or confirmed.
- Lifestyle or nontherapeutic drugs associated with problems during pregnancy include alcohol, caffeine, and cigarette smoking. Avoid alcohol when trying to conceive and throughout pregnancy; no amount is considered safe. Caffeine should be limited to no more than 200 to 300 mg/day. Smokers should quit if possible to avoid the effects of nicotine, carbon monoxide, and other chemicals on the fetus.
- Herbal supplements should be used with caution; their effects during pregnancy are unknown.
- To prevent the need for drug therapy, follow a healthy lifestyle (adequate nutrition, exercise, rest, and sleep; avoid alcohol and smoking) and avoid infection (use good personal hygiene, avoid contact with people known to have infections, maintain indicated immunizations).
- Inform any healthcare provider from whom treatment is sought if there is a possibility of pregnancy.
- Many drugs are excreted in breast milk and reach the nursing infant. The infant's healthcare provider should be informed about the nursing parent's medications and consulted about potential drug effects on the infant. Before taking over-the-counter medications, consult a healthcare provider.
- Recommendations for nontherapeutic drugs include the following:
    - Use alcohol in moderation and withhold nursing temporarily after consumption (2 hours per drink). The effects of alcohol on the baby are directly related to the amount of alcohol the nursing parent consumes. Moderate to heavy drinking (two or more drinks per day) can interfere with the ability to breast-feed, harm the baby's motor development, and slow the baby's weight gain.
    - Caffeine is considered compatible with breast-feeding. However, avoid large amounts because infants may be jittery and have difficulty sleeping.
    - Cigarette smoking is not an absolute contraindication but is strongly discouraged. Nicotine and an active metabolite are concentrated in milk, and the amounts reaching the infant are proportional to the number of cigarettes smoked by the nursing parent. The risk of sudden infant death syndrome (SIDS) is greater when smoking or when the baby is around secondhand (passive) smoke. Maternal smoking and passive smoke exposure may also increase respiratory and ear infections in infants.
    - Most illicit drugs (e.g., cocaine, heroin, marijuana, methamphetamine, phencyclidine) are contraindicated. Birthing parents with opioid dependence who are enrolled in a supervised methadone maintenance program may be allowed to breast-feed.

NCLEX Success

2. The nurse is providing immunization education to a pregnant patient. The patient should receive which of the following vaccines during cooler seasonal temperatures?
   A. rubella
   B. mumps
   C. influenza
   D. tetanus

Unfolding Patient Stories: Danielle Young Bear • Part 1

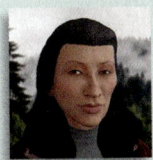

Danielle Young Bear is a 32-year-old construction worker who made a clinic appointment because she is experiencing a persistent cough and fatigue. She has a history of chronic lower back pain, and she visited the clinic 1 year ago with spasms caused by an injury. Danielle has followed guidance from a traditional Native American healer using herbal medicine. During that visit, she was given a prescription for pain medicine. Upon review of her current medications, you find that Danielle takes cyclobenzaprine, ibuprofen, and willow bark. While the nurse is providing education on the medications, the patient states that she is pregnant. What drug exposure risks during pregnancy should the nurse consider? (Danielle Young Bear's story continues in Chapter 16.)

Care for Danielle and other patients in a realistic virtual environment: **vSim** for Nursing (thepoint.lww.com/vSimPharm). Practice documenting these patients' care in DocuCare (thepoint.lww.com/DocuCareEHR).

FETAL THERAPEUTICS

Although the major concern about drugs ingested during pregnancy is adverse effects on the fetus, a few drugs are given to the pregnant patient for therapeutic effects on the fetus. These include digoxin for fetal tachycardia or heart failure, levothyroxine for hypothyroidism, penicillin for exposure to maternal syphilis and group B *Streptococcus* (GBS), and prenatal betamethasone to promote surfactant production, thus improving fetal lung function and decreasing respiratory distress syndrome in preterm infants. Also, pregnant patients who are rhesus factor (Rh)-negative receive Rh immune globulin (RhoGAM) for antenatal and postpartal prevention of sensitization to the Rh factor and hemolytic disease of the newborn.

MATERNAL THERAPEUTICS

Thus far, the main emphasis on drug use during pregnancy has related to actual or potential adverse effects on the fetus. Despite the general principle that drug use should be avoided whenever possible, pregnant patients may require drug therapy for immunizations, various illnesses, increased nutritional needs, pregnancy-associated problems, chronic disease processes, treatment of preterm labor, induction of labor, pain management during labor, and prevention of postpartum hemorrhage.

To meet the increased nutritional needs of pregnancy, healthcare providers order prenatal vitamins and mineral supplements for pregnant patients. Folic acid supplementation is especially important to prevent neural tube congenital anomalies, primarily spina bifida. Such abnormalities occur early in pregnancy, often before someone realizes they are pregnant. For this reason, the American College of Obstetricians and Gynecologists (ACOG) recommends that individuals who wish to become pregnant ingest 400 or 600 mcg of folic acid daily, either from food and/or a supplement.

The use of natural herbs as a supplement and as treatment for common ailments has greatly increased in popularity. Although herbs are natural, some may be poisonous. Not all herbs are safe for consumption during pregnancy and lactation. Box 6.3 summarizes information on the use of herbs in pregnancy.

BOX 6.3 Use of Herbs During Pregnancy

- Some herbs may contain ingredients that are contraindicated in pregnancy and lactation. Many herbs can cause miscarriage, preterm birth, and uterine contractions, which induce labor.
- As remedies, herbs are not subjected to rigorous testing and evaluation because they are not prescription drugs. Consequently, the quality and strength of such supplements may vary significantly, reducing safety for use during pregnancy and lactation.
- The U.S. Food and Drug Administration urges pregnant and lactating people to discuss the use of herbs or essential oils with their healthcare providers. Many may take herbal supplements without informing their obstetricians or nurse midwives, thus complicating and increasing the likelihood of drug interactions.
- In an effort to make herbal supplements safe, some organizations specializing in herbal remedies have performed extensive testing and evaluations to devise a safety rating scale for the general population and pregnant and breast-feeding people. However, the safety ratings can often be controversial and vague. Some herbs may be deemed safe when used orally in amounts found in food but unsafe or contraindicated when used in medicinal or concentrated amounts, especially in pregnancy.
- These herbs may be unsafe during pregnancy: black cohosh, blue cohosh, dong quai, ephedra, goldenseal, passion flower, pau d'arco, pennyroyal, roman chamomile, saw palmetto, and yohimbe.
- These herbs are likely safe during pregnancy:
  - Red raspberry leaf—helps tone uterus, increase milk production, decrease nausea, and ease labor pains
  - Peppermint leaf—relieves nausea, vomiting, and flatulence
  - Ginger root—relieves nausea and vomiting
  - Slippery elm bark—decreases nausea and relieves heartburn
- Oats and oat straw—reduces anxiety and restlessness.

> **Clinical Application 6.1**
> - What issues relating to teratogenic substances are of concern in Ms. Ross' pregnancy?

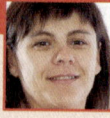

Management of Pregnancy-Associated Symptoms

Anemias

Two types of anemia are common during pregnancy. One is physiologic anemia (often defined as a hemoglobin below 11 g/dL or hematocrit below 33%), which results from expanded blood volume. The second is iron deficiency anemia, which is often related to long-term nutritional deficiencies.

Experts recommend an increase in iron consumption to about 27 to 30 mg/day. This is readily met by most prenatal vitamins and is adequate for nonanemic patients. Patients with iron deficiency anemia should receive additional iron supplementation of 40 to 200 mg/day until anemia is corrected.

Constipation

Elevated progesterone levels cause smooth muscle relaxation and decrease peristalsis, leading to constipation. Preferred treatment is to increase exercise and intake of fluids and high-fiber foods. If a laxative is required, a bulk-producing agent such as psyllium (Metamucil) is the most physiologic for the pregnant parent and safest for the fetus because it is not absorbed systemically. A stool softener such as docusate (Colace) or an occasional saline laxative (milk of magnesia) may also be used.

Mineral oil should be avoided because it interferes with absorption of fat-soluble vitamins. Reduced absorption of vitamin K can lead to bleeding in newborns. Castor oil, all strong laxatives, and excessive amounts of any laxative should be avoided because they can cause uterine contractions and initiate labor.

Gastroesophageal Reflux Disease

Gastroesophageal reflux disease (GERD), of which heartburn (pyrosis) is the main symptom, is very common in pregnant patients, especially as gestation increases. Hormonal changes relax the lower esophageal sphincter, and the growing fetus increases abdominal pressure. These developments allow gastric acid to pass into the esophagus and cause discomfort and esophagitis. In addition, GERD may trigger asthma attacks in pregnant patients with asthma.

Nonpharmacologic interventions include eating small meals; not eating for 2 to 3 hours before bedtime; avoiding caffeine, gas-producing foods, and constipation; and sitting in an upright position. For patients who do not obtain adequate relief with these measures, drug therapy may be needed. Pharmacologic management should start with antacids followed by sucralfate (Carafate). Because little systemic absorption occurs, the drugs are unlikely to harm the fetus if used in recommended doses. A histamine (H_2) receptor antagonist such as cimetidine (Tagamet) may also be effective. Proton pump inhibitors such as omeprazole (Prilosec) are thought to be safe, but some clinicians reserve them for patients for whom H_2 blockers are ineffective.

Gestational Diabetes Mellitus

Gestational diabetes mellitus (GDM) is glucose intolerance that first occurs during pregnancy. Pregnant patients at high risk for developing gestational diabetes (BMI > 30; age older than 40 years; family history of diabetes; being Hispanic, Native American, Asian, or African American; or previous birth of a large baby) may be screened as early as the first prenatal visit. If early testing is not performed, universal screening may be done between 24 and 28 weeks of gestation because of the maternal peripheral resistance of insulin due to hormones after the 24th week. The criterion for a diagnosis of GDM is based on the results of two or more elevated levels of the 100-g oral glucose tolerance test: fasting plasma glucose level of more than 95 mg/dL, 1-hour glucose level of more than 180 mg/dL, 2-hour glucose level of more than 155 mg/dL, and 3-hour glucose level of more than 140 mg/dL.

Patients with GDM are at higher risk for complications of pregnancy and possible fetal harm. Poor glycemic control, primarily hyperglycemia in early gestation resulting in fetal hyperinsulinemia, increases the likelihood of structural defects in the fetus, particularly during organogenesis. Congenital anomalies in the fetus often involve the heart and the central nervous system (CNS), leading to multiorgan malformations. Hyperinsulinemia increases the amount of growth factor causing macrosomia. Additionally, hyperinsulinemia interferes with the production of surfactant, which contributes to fetal lung maturity. Lack of surfactant results in respiratory distress syndrome in the neonate. Infants of patients with GDM who had been under close diabetic monitoring during pregnancy may have complications of hypoglycemia, hyperbilirubinemia, hypocalcemia, and polycythemia.

The goal of treatment during pregnancy is to keep blood glucose levels as near normal as possible because even mild hyperglycemia can be detrimental to the fetus; it stimulates the fetal pancreas to secrete high levels of insulin.

Insulin (see Chapter 41) does not cross the placenta and has a long history of safe usage. Thus, it is the drug of choice for treatment of diabetes during pregnancy. For patients who are unable or unwilling to take insulin, oral antidiabetic agents such as metformin or glyburide may be reasonable alternatives.

When the pregnancy ends, blood glucose levels usually return to a normal range within a few weeks. Patients may breastfeed, and those with hypoglycemia are safe during lactation.

Patients with GDM should be counseled that recurrence in future pregnancies is strong and that GDM is predictive of an increased risk of development of type 2 diabetes.

NCLEX Success

3. A nurse knows that teaching was successful when expectant parents give which of the following rationales for administering folic acid supplements?
   A. prevent hydrocele
   B. increase absorption
   C. prevent neural tube deformity
   D. decrease blood glucose

Nausea and Vomiting

Nausea and vomiting often occur during early pregnancy due to high levels of hCG and estrogen. Low blood sugar, as well as magnesium deficiency, can exacerbate nausea and vomiting. Ginger may be suggested initially to help control nausea and vomiting symptoms; however, pregnant patients may require antiemetic medications, if nausea and vomiting are severe and threaten maternal and fetal nutritional or metabolic status (hyperemesis gravidarum).

Treatment with pyridoxine (vitamin B6) has been shown to improve mild to moderate nausea with minimal side effects. When pyridoxine alone fails to improve nausea and vomiting, a combination of doxylamine–pyridoxine (Bonjesta) may be used. If drug therapy is unsuccessful in controlling nausea and vomiting, or weight loss and electrolyte imbalance persists, total parenteral nutrition may be necessary until oral fluids are tolerated.

Hypertensive Disorders in Pregnancy

Hypertensive disorders in pregnancy include preeclampsia and eclampsia, conditions that endanger the lives of the pregnant parent and fetus. **Preeclampsia** is manifested by hypertension and proteinuria, or hypertension and significant end-organ dysfunction with or without proteinuria after 20 weeks of gestation in a previously normotensive patient. Preeclampsia most often occurs during a first pregnancy, but it may affect people with chronic hypertension, diabetes mellitus, or multiple fetuses.

Management of hypertension in pregnancy varies. Outpatient observation, with frequent monitoring of patient and fetus, may be sufficient. Antihypertensive therapy is recommended for patients with severe hypertension (systolic blood pressure greater than 160 mm Hg or diastolic blood pressure greater than 110 mm Hg). Drug therapy for severe preeclampsia includes oral nifedipine (Procardia) (see Chapter 28), intravenous (IV) hydralazine or labetalol (Trandate) (see Chapter 26) for blood pressure control, as well as magnesium sulfate (see Chapter 53) for the prevention of seizures.

> **! Quality and Safety Alert: Safety**
>
> Magnesium sulfate is considered a high-alert medication and requires special precautions for administration and monitoring because of potentially severe adverse effects.

Safety measures include a unit protocol that standardizes drug concentration, flow rate, type of infusion pump, and frequency and type of maternal–fetal assessment data to be documented (serum magnesium levels, respiratory status, reflexes, uterine activity, urine output, fetal heart rate). This therapy reduces perinatal deaths and severe maternal hypertension.

If not effectively treated, preeclampsia may progress to **eclampsia**, which is characterized by potentially fatal grand mal seizures. Maternal complications can occur in up to 70% of pregnant patients with eclampsia including hemolysis, elevated liver enzymes, and low platelets (HELLP) syndrome and disseminated intravascular coagulation, cardiopulmonary arrest, and perinatal death.

Overdoses of magnesium sulfate may lead to hypotension, muscle paralysis, respiratory depression, and cardiac arrest. Close monitoring for signs of hypermagnesemia is necessary, and serum levels may be drawn in patients who have clinical signs of magnesium toxicity (Table 6.3). Calcium gluconate, the antidote for magnesium sulfate, should be readily available for use if hypermagnesemia occurs. Administration is slow IV push over 2 to 5 minutes. Neonates born to parents who received magnesium sulfate require assessment for hypermagnesemia and respiratory depression at birth.

TABLE 6.3

Magnesium Levels With Associated Signs and Symptoms of Toxicity[*]

Magnesium Value (mEq/L)	Signs and Symptoms
8–12	Loss of deep tendon reflexes
15	Respiratory distress
5–10	Electrocardiographic changes
25	Cardiac arrest

[*]Normal adult values for magnesium, 1.5 to 2 mEq/L; therapeutic serum magnesium level, 4 to 7 mEq/L.

Clinical Application 6.2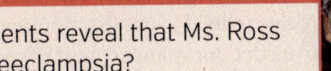

- What assessments reveal that Ms. Ross is at risk for preeclampsia?
- Why would administration of antiepileptic drugs be appropriate for Ms. Ross?
- The protein in Lauren's 24-hour urine collection is 500 mg. Her blood pressure continues to be high, with evidence of hyperreflexia (3+ reflexes). A magnesium sulfate drip is initiated with a loading dose of 6 g over 20 minutes per infusion pump. Oxytocin (Pitocin) infusion is started to induce labor. What are critical nursing assessments in this situation?

Management of Selected Infections in Pregnancy

Group B Streptococcus

An estimated 50% of pregnant patients are infected with group B *Streptococcus* (GBS). Although rarely serious in adults, GBS can cause sepsis, meningitis, and pneumonia in the newborn if the birthing parent does not receive intrapartum antibiotic prophylaxis. Potential outcomes for the parent include urinary tract infection (UTI), chorioamnionitis, postcesarean wound infection, and postpartum endometritis.

Because of the potentially serious consequences of infection with GBS, pregnant patients should have a rectovaginal culture at 36 to 37 $^6/_7$ weeks of gestation. A positive culture indicates infection that should be treated with an intravenous antibiotic that is effective against GBS. Penicillin (see Chapter 18) is the drug of choice, but alternative antibiotics can be prescribed for patients with a penicillin allergy.

Clinical Application 6.3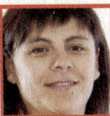

- Explain the risk associated with perinatal GBS.

Human Immunodeficiency Virus

Human immunodeficiency virus (HIV) infection in patients who are pregnant requires antiretroviral drug therapy. This helps prevent transmission to the fetus/newborn. Almost all HIV infections that are transmitted to a fetus/newborn are transmitted perinatally, either in utero, during labor and delivery, or in breast milk. The goal of treatment is to reduce the viral load as much as possible, which reduces the risk of transmission to the fetus/newborn. Antiretroviral drug therapy for the pregnant parent reduces perinatal transmission to less than 1% to 2%. In general, highly active antiretroviral therapy, or HAART, is safe, with recommended dosage the same as for nonpregnant patients (see Chapter 23).

When labor starts, the HIV-positive pregnant patient should receive IV zidovudine. The dosage is 2 mg/kg infused over 1 hour and then 1 mg/kg/h, until the umbilical cord is clamped.

Urinary Tract Infections

UTIs commonly occur during pregnancy and may include asymptomatic bacteriuria, cystitis, and pyelonephritis. Asymptomatic bacteriuria should be treated in pregnant patients because of its association with cystitis and pyelonephritis. If untreated, symptomatic cystitis occurs in approximately 30% to 40% of pregnant patients. Asymptomatic bacteriuria and UTIs are also associated with increased preterm births and infants with low birth weights. Hospitalization and intravenous antibiotics may be needed for management of pyelonephritis.

Influenza

Influenza poses a substantial risk for the pregnant patient and the fetus. Serious complications include bacterial pneumonia and dehydration, which can be fatal. Pregnant people are more likely to be hospitalized with influenza-related complications than nonpregnant people. Anyone who is pregnant or might be pregnant during the influenza season should receive the inactivated influenza vaccine. The influenza vaccine provides immunity to the fetus because the vaccine crosses the placenta. The immunity protects infants until they are old enough to be vaccinated.

Tetanus, Diphtheria, and Pertussis

The tetanus–diphtheria–pertussis (Tdap) vaccine, licensed in 2005, is the first vaccine for adolescents and adults that protects against all three diseases—tetanus, diphtheria, and pertussis. A single dose of the Tdap vaccine is recommended for all pregnant patients (in each pregnancy). If not given during pregnancy, it may be administered immediately postpartum. Administration of the Tdap, rather than the tetanus–diphtheria–toxoid vaccine (Td), is preferable because the prevalence of pertussis in the United States has been increasing.

NCLEX Success

4. A patient has been diagnosed with gestational diabetes. What effect does maternal hyperglycemia have on the fetus?
   A. It results in fetal hyperinsulinemia.
   B. It produces seizures in the newborn.
   C. It increases the mother's risk of preterm labor.
   D. It decreases the birth weight.

DRUGS THAT ALTER UTERINE MOTILITY: TOCOLYTICS

Drugs given to reduce the strength and frequency of uterine contractions, thus helping inhibit labor and maintain the pregnancy, are called **tocolytics**. Uterine contractions with cervical changes before 37 weeks of gestation are considered **preterm labor**. Preterm labor may occur spontaneously, or premature rupture of membranes, infection, preeclampsia, multiple gestation, cigarette smoking, or alcohol may precipitate it. Drug therapy is most effective when the cervix is minimally dilated and amniotic membranes are intact. Tocolytics do not reduce the number of preterm births, but they may postpone birth long enough to reduce problems associated with prematurity (e.g., respiratory distress, bleeding in the brain, infant death) and allow for neuroprotection (reduce likelihood of cerebral palsy). The goal of treatment is to delay birth long enough for antenatal administration of a corticosteroid such as betamethasone (Celestone Soluspan) to the pregnant patient to improve pulmonary maturity and function in fetal lungs by the increased production of surfactant. First-line tocolytics include nonsteroidal anti-inflammatory drugs (NSAIDs), calcium channel blockers, and beta-agonists. Magnesium sulfate may also be used as a tocolytic and for its neuroprotective effects. Table 6.4 presents route and dosage information for the tocolytics.

> ### ! Quality and Safety Alert: Evidence-Based Practice
>
> Cigarette smoking during pregnancy is the most modifiable risk factor associated with adverse pregnancy outcomes, including preterm birth, neonatal growth restriction, and sudden infant death syndrome. In addition, smoking and exposure to secondhand smoke increase the risk of infertility, placental abruption, preterm premature rupture of membranes, and placenta previa. Pregnant patients should be asked regularly about tobacco usage, including cigarettes, smokeless tobacco, and e-cigarettes, and provided pregnancy-tailored counseling on cessation. A common strategy for smoking cessation is the "5 As": ask about and document smoking status, advise patients who smoke to stop smoking and avoid secondhand smoke, assess their readiness to quit smoking, assist those who want to quit, and arrange for proper smoking cessation strategies. Nicotine replacement and bupropion are reasonable drug options that may be added to cessation counseling for pregnant or breast-feeding patients who are otherwise unable to quit. Reinforcing success and providing ongoing support increase maternal success with smoking cessation.

Nonsteroidal Anti-Inflammatory Drugs

The NSAID **indomethacin** (Indocin, Tivorbex) acts as a tocolytic by inhibiting uterine prostaglandins that initiate the uterine contractions of normal labor. Maternal adverse effects include nausea and vomiting, heartburn, headache, dizziness, and increased bleeding problems. Fetal adverse effects include constriction of the ductus arteriosus and oligohydramnios (decreased amniotic fluid). Because of these concerns, administration is not recommended after 32 weeks of gestation and for

TABLE 6.4
DRUGS AT A GLANCE: Tocolytics

Drug	Route and Dosage
ⓟ Indomethacin (Indocin, Tivorbex; 🍁 AURO-Indomethacin, MINT-Indomethacin)	50–100 mg PO or rectally and then 25 mg PO every 4–6 h
ⓟ Nifedipine (Procardia, Procardia XL, Adalat CC, Afeditab CR; 🍁 Adalat XL, Nifedipine ER)	20–30 mg PO, then 10–20 mg PO every 3–8 h for 48 h; max 180 mg/d
ⓟ Terbutaline sulfate	0.25 mg Sub-Q every 20–30 min for four doses
ⓟ Magnesium sulfate	IV infusion loading dose 6 g over 20 min; maintenance dose 2 g/h, according to contraction frequency and maternal toxicity

longer than 48 hours. There is a **BOXED WARNING** ◆ for this NSAID because of the increased risk of adverse cardiovascular events and gastrointestinal (GI) bleeding.

Nifedipine

ⓟ **Nifedipine** (Procardia, Procardia XL, Adalat CC) is a calcium channel blocking drug that decreases uterine contractions and lowers blood pressure by blocking calcium movement into muscle cells. A common adverse effect is maternal hypotension, which may reduce blood flow between the placenta and the uterus and thus compromise the fetus. Prolonged events of this nature can lead to adverse fetal outcomes, and severe adverse reactions have occurred when nifedipine is used in conjunction with IV magnesium sulfate. Pregnant patients with cardiovascular disease or who are hemodynamically unstable should not receive nifedipine.

Terbutaline Sulfate

ⓟ **Terbutaline sulfate** is a beta-adrenergic agent that inhibits uterine contractions by reducing intracellular calcium levels. Adverse maternal effects may include tachycardia and palpitations, tremors, hypokalemia, hyperglycemia, and pulmonary edema. Terbutaline sulfate crosses the placenta, producing fetal tachycardia and neonatal hypoglycemia. Contraindications include hyperthyroidism and diabetes, as well as placenta previa or placental abruption. There is a **BOXED WARNING** ◆ advising against prolonged administration (longer than 48 to 72 hours) because of the potential for serious maternal heart problems and death.

Magnesium Sulfate

ⓟ **Magnesium sulfate**, which has neuromuscular blocking activity, has long been given intravenously to help prevent preterm birth. This agent also offers neuroprotective properties to the neonate when administered before 32 weeks of gestation. Adjuvant use includes treatment for severe preeclampsia and eclampsia. Guidelines for administration of the drug are the same in tocolysis as in hypertension in pregnancy. In pregnant patients with abnormal kidney function, it is necessary to decrease the dosage or use an alternative treatment. Contraindications include myasthenia gravis and known cardiac compromise or conduction defects.

NCLEX Success

5. A patient is ordered to receive indomethacin for treatment of preterm labor. The nurse understands the teaching was successful when the patient states which of the following as adverse effects? (Select all that apply.)
   A. ductus arteriosus constriction
   B. polyhydramnios
   C. oligohydramnios
   D. ductus venosus constriction

DRUGS USED DURING LABOR AND DELIVERY AT TERM

Labor usually begins spontaneously and proceeds through delivery of the newborn and placenta. If labor does not occur spontaneously, it may be induced using an oxytocic, a drug that stimulates uterine contractions. Drugs often used during labor, delivery, and the immediate postpartum period include prostaglandins as well.

Labor Induction

Common reasons for labor induction include postterm pregnancy, intrauterine growth restriction, maternal hypertension or diabetes, and premature rupture of membranes. Labor can also be initiated for the termination of a pregnancy with administration of an **abortifacient** drug.

Prostaglandins

Prostaglandins have three significant uses in pregnancy: to promote cervical ripening so the cervix becomes thinner, which facilitates labor and induces delivery of the full-term infant; to promote uterine contractility for the expulsion of the fetus and placenta in an abortion; and to increase uterine contractility and decrease uterine bleeding in the postpartum period. The prostaglandin used for the third use is carboprost tromethamine (Hemabate), and it will be discussed with uterotonic medications later in the chapter (including Table 6.6). Table 6.5 summarizes the routes of administration and dosage information for prostaglandin medications.

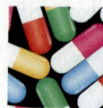

TABLE 6.5
DRUGS AT A GLANCE: Prostaglandins

Drug	Routes and Dosages
Dinoprostone (Cervidil, Prepidil, Prostin E_2; Cervidil, Prepidil, Prostin E_2)	0.5 mg inserted into cervical canal; repeated every 6 h; maximum dose 1.5 mg in 24 h; 10 mg vaginal insert placed in posterior fornix of vagina; remove in 12 h; not for VBAC
Misoprostol (Cytotec)	Intravaginally 25 mcg (1/4 of a 100-mcg tablet) every 3–6 h; not for VBAC; for postpartum hemorrhage, 600–1,000 mg rectally, 600–1,000 mg orally, or 800 mg sublingual

VBAC, vaginal birth after cesarean.

Dinoprostone (Cervidil, Prepidil, Prostin E_2) is a synthetic prostaglandin E_2 that stimulates uterine contractions, such as the ones in labor. The drug is available as an endocervical gel, a vaginal insert, and a vaginal suppository. The first two forms enhance cervical ripening so the fetus can pass easily through the birth canal. The vaginal suppository is an abortifacient.

Adverse effects of dinoprostone include back pain, abnormal uterine contractions, GI upset, diarrhea, and fever. Contraindications include hypersensitivity to prostaglandins, as well as previous cesarean section, uterine surgery, cephalopelvic disproportion, fetal distress, and vaginal bleeding. Administration to patients with asthma, glaucoma, or ruptured membranes warrants caution. Oxytocin may be initiated 30 minutes after removal of the Cervidil vaginal insert or 6 to 12 hours after final dose of Prepidil endocervical gel. A **BOXED WARNING** indicates that the medication should be used only with strict adherence to the recommended dosages and by medically trained personnel who can provide immediate care if needed.

Misoprostol (Cytotec), a synthetic prostaglandin E_1, inhibits gastric acid secretion and increases bicarbonate to protect the lining of the stomach. An unlabeled use of the drug is to increase cervical ripening and induce labor. If the course of treatment changes and oxytocin is to be given, it is essential to wait 4 hours from the last administration of misoprostol before starting oxytocin. The nurse assesses for hyperstimulation of the uterus and monitors for a nonreassuring fetal heart rate. There is a **BOXED WARNING** related to the risk of uterine rupture and induced abortion if administered for gastric ulcer prevention in an unknown pregnant woman. Contraindications include prior cesarean section or uterine surgery.

Oxytocics

Oxytocin (Pitocin), a synthetic form of oxytocin, is the most commonly used **oxytocic** drug. Use of this manufactured hormone induces labor or augments weak, irregular uterine contractions during labor. Physiologic doses produce a rhythmic uterine contraction–relaxation pattern that approximates the normal labor process. It also activates oxytocin and is contraindicated in the presence of fetal distress or unfavorable fetal positions and presentations, a hypertonic uterus, cephalopelvic disproportion, and obstetrical emergencies where surgical intervention is favored, such as prolapse of the umbilical cord or placenta previa. Table 6.6 summarizes the dosage and route of administration for oxytocin.

> **! Quality and Safety Alert: Safety**
> Oxytocin is considered a high-alert medication and requires special precautions for administration and monitoring because of potentially severe adverse effects.

TABLE 6.6
DRUGS AT A GLANCE: Oxytocics and Uterotonics

Drug	Routes and Dosage
Oxytocin (Pitocin; Oxytocin for injection)	Induction/augmentation: IV by infusion pump, 0.5–1 milliunits/min, in 30- to 60-min intervals gradually increased by 1–2 milliunits/min until desired contractions Postpartum hemorrhage: infusion of 30 units in 500 mL of IV fluids; 10–40 units added to 500–1,000 mL of IV fluids infused at a rate need to sustain uterine contraction and control uterine atony; 10 units IM after delivery of placenta
Methylergonovine (Methergine)	0.2 mg IM after delivery of the placenta or neonate's anterior shoulder, or during postpartum; may be repeated every 2–4 h 0.2 mg PO 3–4 times daily; max 7 d
Carboprost tromethamine (Hemabate; Hemabate)	250 mcg IM every 15–90 min, depending on uterine response; maximum 8 doses

Maternal adverse effects include cardiac dysrhythmias, hypertension, nausea, vomiting, excessive uterine stimulation, and water intoxication. Close monitoring of uterine activity and fetal response is essential. If a labor and delivery nurse is not available to monitor the fetal–maternal effects of oxytocin, it is necessary to suspend the infusion. There is a BOXED WARNING ◆ regarding the appropriate use of the medication for medical rather than elective induction of labor.

Pain Management

During early labor, pain occurs with uterine contractions. During later stages of labor, pain occurs with perineal stretching.

Analgesics

Intravenous systemic analgesics are commonly used to control pain during labor and delivery. These medications include opioids such as morphine, synthetic opioids such as fentanyl (Sublimaze), and opioid-antagonists such as butorphanol and nalbuphine (see Chapter 49). They may prolong labor and cause sedation and respiratory depression in the mother. These medications also cross the placenta and may result in alterations in fetal heart rate patterns and neonatal respiratory depression. If neonatal respiratory depression occurs, naloxone (Narcan) can be given.

Regional analgesia may be more effective than IV analgesics for pain management. Epidural analgesia involves administration of an opioid such as fentanyl, and an anesthetic, such as ropivacaine or bupivacaine, through a catheter placed in the epidural space. With regional anesthesia, the mother is alert and comfortable. The neonate is rarely depressed. For a cesarean section, spinal anesthesia is commonly used due to its rapid onset of effect using anesthetics like with epidural administration. A long-acting form of morphine, Duramorph, or other opioid medication can also be added to the spinal anesthesia to provide pain relief for approximately 24 hours. Possible adverse effects include maternal hypotension and urinary retention (bladder distention). No significant effects on the fetus or neonate have been reported.

Anesthetics

Local anesthetics are less commonly used to control discomfort and pain due to their short duration. They are injected by physicians for regional anesthesia in the pelvic area. Lidocaine or bupivacaine (see Chapter 50) are commonly used. Fetal bradycardia may briefly occur after administration but is usually not significant.

Clinical Application 6.4

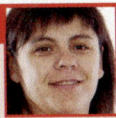

- An oxytocin (Pitocin) infusion begins to induce Ms. Ross' labor. What effect might magnesium sulfate have on her labor progress?

Uterotonics for Postpartum Hemorrhage

Uterotonics are drugs used to stop postpartum hemorrhage. After delivery of the placenta, oxytocin is the drug of choice for prevention or control of postpartum uterine bleeding. It is delivered IV through a bolus rate using an infusion pump. The drug reduces uterine bleeding by contracting the uterine muscle. It also plays a role in the letdown of breast milk to the nipples during lactation.

In the event of postpartum hemorrhage, other drugs (uterotonics) may be indicated for immediate use, such as Ⓟ **carboprost tromethamine** (Hemabate). This drug is a prostaglandin F₂ alpha agent that stimulates the uterus to contract. Contraindications include known allergy to prostaglandins, acute pelvic inflammatory disease, and active pulmonary, hepatic, kidney, or cardiac disease. Caution is warranted in asthma; hypertension; hypotension; anemia; uterine abnormalities; and diseases of the heart, kidneys, or liver. The use of antiemetic and antidiarrheal drugs reduces GI upset. There is a BOXED WARNING ◆ that the medication should be used only with strict adherence to the recommended dosages and by medically trained personnel who can provide immediate care if needed. Table 6.6 provides route and dosage information for carboprost.

Ⓟ **Methylergonovine** (Methergine) is an ergot derivative that increases the strength, duration, and frequency of the uterine contractions. Indications for use include the treatment of postpartum atony and hemorrhage as well as for uterine stimulation during the second stage of labor after delivery of the anterior shoulder. Contraindications include known allergy to methylergonovine and hypertension. It is important to monitor patients for hypertension, headache, dizziness, palpitations, and GI upset. Table 6.6 provides route and dosage information for methylergonovine.

Misoprostol (Cytotec), which is used for cervical ripening, may also be used for the management of postpartum hemorrhage.

Tranexamic acid (TXA; Cyklokapron, Lysteda; see Chapter 9), an antifibrinolytic drug, may be given concurrently with oxytocin, or prophylactically after clamping of the umbilical cord, in management of postpartum hemorrhage. Use of tranexamic acid has been shown to reduce the risk of death from postpartum hemorrhage without an increase in adverse effects.

Clinical Application 6.5

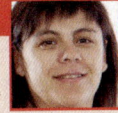

- Why is Ms. Ross at high risk for postpartum hemorrhage?
- What preventive measure is taken immediately after delivery of the placenta?

LACTATION

Lactation Induction

Metoclopramide (Reglan) stimulates the hormone prolactin after delivery, thus inducing lactation. The galactagogue, or lactation inducing, effect of this drug is considered an off-label use of metoclopramide. The prolactin-stimulating effect is dose related, with 10 to 15 mg two to three times a day recommended. Higher doses of the drug in the postpartum period have been associated with depression, and use in patients with a history of depression warrants caution.

The herbs fenugreek, fennel, milk thistle, and anise are examples of **galactagogues**, herbs thought to induce lactation or stimulate the production of breast milk.

Drug Use During Lactation

Antidepressants such as selective serotonin reuptake inhibitors (SSRIs) and serotonin and norepinephrine reuptake inhibitors (SNRIs) disturb the serotonin balance and are first-line choices for pharmacologic management of depression in lactating patients. Although antidepressants have been detected in human milk, the amount is very low to undetectable. For mothers with severe depression, the benefits often outweigh the risks, and pharmacologic treatment is recommended.

Box 6.4 presents a list of medications that are contraindicated during lactation. For a summary of patient teaching guidelines regarding the use of drugs during lactation, as well as pregnancy, see Box 6.2.

Lactation and Birth Control

Exclusive breast-feeding (no formula supplementation) may cause a patient to have an absence of menstrual periods. The potential for ovulation is reduced but does not offer total protection against pregnancy. The use of birth control during lactation is safe for the newborn. The concern is related to the quantity of milk production due to the presence of additional hormones in the maternal system.

Progesterone (progestin)-only contraceptives are the contraceptive of choice because they are unlikely to cause a decrease in milk production. These include several types: the "mini-pill," implant (Nexplanon), injection (Depo-Provera), and intrauterine devices (Kyleena, Liletta, Mirena, Skyla). These are good choices for patients exclusively breast-feeding because of the already decreased fertility with continuous lactation. Estrogen-containing contraceptives such as the vaginal ring (NuvaRing) and the transdermal patch (Xulane) have been associated with decreasing breast milk production.

BOX 6.4 *Selected Drugs That Are Contraindicated or Not Recommended During Lactation*

Angiotensin receptor blockers (ARBs; e.g., losartan)
Antibacterials (e.g., tigecycline, sulfamethoxazole/trimethoprim during newborn period)
Antidepressants (e.g., brexanolone, bupropion, desvenlafaxine, doxepin)
Antiepileptics (e.g., topiramate, zonisamide)
Antifungals (e.g., itraconazole, terbinafine)
Antihistamines (e.g., clemastine)
Antimanic agent (e.g., lithium)
Antipsychotics (e.g., clozapine)
Antivirals (e.g., famciclovir)
Benzodiazepine antianxiety and sedative/hypnotic drugs (e.g., alprazolam, diazepam, triazolam)
Beta-adrenergic blockers (e.g., atenolol)
Diuretics (e.g., amiloride, bumetanide, furosemide)
Nonbenzodiazepine sedative/hypnotics (e.g., ramelteon)
Opioid analgesics (e.g., codeine, hydromorphone)
Proton pump inhibitors (e.g., rabeprazole)
Retinoids (e.g., isotretinoin)
Statin cholesterol-lowering drugs (e.g., atorvastatin, simvastatin)

THE NURSING PROCESS

A concept map outlines the nursing process related to drug therapy considerations in this chapter. Additional nursing implications related to the disease process should also be considered in care decisions.

Assessment
- Assess each patient for possible pregnancy.
- If the patient is known to be pregnant, assess for gestational age; use of prescription, over-the-counter, herbal, nontherapeutic, and illegal drugs; and acute or chronic health problems.
- For labor (preterm, spontaneous, or induced), assess for length of gestation, uterine contractions, vaginal bleeding or discharge, cervical dilatation, fetal heart rate patterns, maternal vital signs, and length of labor.

Outcomes of Therapy

The patient will
- Avoid unnecessary drug ingestion.
- Use nonpharmacologic measures when possible.
- Obtain optimal care during pregnancy, labor and delivery, and the postpartum period.
- Avoid behaviors that may lead to complications of pregnancy and labor and delivery.
- Breastfeed safely and successfully, if desired.

Nursing Interventions
- Use nondrug measures to prevent or minimize the need for drug therapy during pregnancy.
- Promote/provide optimal prenatal care.
- Assist patients with chronic health problems to manage the disorder effectively and decrease risks of harm to self and baby.
- Help patients and families cope with complications of pregnancy and newborn attachment.

Evaluation
- Observe and interview actions taken to promote reproductive and general health and compliance with instructions for promoting and maintaining a healthy pregnancy and exclusive breast-feeding.
- Interview regarding ingestion of therapeutic and nontherapeutic drugs during prepregnancy, pregnancy, and lactating states.
- Observe and interview regarding health status of birthing parent and neonate.

Visit thePoint® at http://thePoint.lww.com/Frandsen13e for answers to NCLEX Success questions (in Appendix A), answers to Clinical Application Case Studies (in Appendix B), and more!

REFERENCES AND RESOURCES

American College of Obstetricians and Gynecologists. (2018). ACOG committee opinion #751. *Obstetrics & Gynecology, 132*(3), e131–e137.

American College of Obstetricians and Gynecologists. (2020). ACOG committee opinion #797. *Obstetrics & Gynecology, 135*(2), e51–e72.

American Pregnancy Association. (2021). *Herbs and pregnancy.* https://americanpregnancy.org/healthy-pregnancy/is-it-safe/herbs-and-pregnancy/

Anawalt, B. D., & Page, S. T. (2022). Causes of male infertility. *UpToDate.* Lexi-Comp, Inc. Retrieved March 19, 2022.

Auerbach, M., & Landy, H. L. (2022). Anemia in pregnancy. *UpToDate.* Lexi-Comp, Inc. Retrieved March 19, 2022.

August, P. (2022). Treatment of hypertension in pregnant and postpartum women. *UpToDate.* Lexi-Comp, Inc. Retrieved March 19, 2022.

August, P., & Sibai, B. M. (2022). Preeclampsia: clinical features and diagnosis. *UpToDate.* Lexi-Comp, Inc. Retrieved March 19, 2022.

Bakker, R., Pierce, S., & Myers, D. (2017). The role of prostaglandins E1 and E2, dinoprostone, and misoprostol in cervical ripening and the induction of labor: A mechanistic approach. *Archives of Gynecology and Obstetrics, 296*(2), 167–179.

Belfort, M. A. (2022). Postpartum hemorrhage: medical and minimally invasive management. *UpToDate.* Lexi-Comp, Inc. Retrieved March 19, 2022.

Berghella, V. (2022). Management of the third stage of labor: prophylactic drug therapy to minimize hemorrhage. *UpToDate.* Lexi-Comp, Inc. Retrieved March 19, 2022.

Berghella, V., & Hughes, B. L. (2022). COVID-19: Overview of pregnancy issues. *UpToDate*. Lexi-Comp, Inc. Retrieved March 19, 2022.

Blackburn, S. (2018). *Maternal, fetal, & neonatal physiology* (5th ed.). Elsevier.

Briggs, G. G., Towers, C. V., & Forinash, A. B. (2022). *Drugs in pregnancy and lactation* (12th ed.). Wolters Kluwer Health/Lippincott Williams & Wilkins.

Byrne, J. J., Saucedo, A. M., & Spong, C., Y. (2020). Evaluation of drug labels following the 2015 pregnancy and lactation labeling rule. *JAMA Network Open, 3*(8), e2015094.

Durnwald, C. (2022). Gestational diabetes mellitus: Glycemic control and maternal prognosis. *UpToDate*. Lexi-Comp, Inc. Retrieved March 19, 2022.

Durnwald, C. (2022). Gestational diabetes mellitus: Screening, diagnosis and prevention. *UpToDate*. Lexi-Comp, Inc. Retrieved March 19, 2022.

Fauser, B. (2022). Overview of ovulation induction. *UpToDate*. Lexi-Comp, Inc. Retrieved March 19, 2022.

Garner, C. D. (2022). Nutrition in pregnancy. *UpToDate*. Lexi-Comp, Inc. Retrieved March 19, 2022.

Hale, T. W. (2021). *Hale's medications & mothers' milk*. Springer Publishing Company.

Hooton, T. M., & Gupta, K. (2022). Urinary tract infections and asymptomatic bacteriuria in pregnancy. *UpToDate*. Lexi-Comp, Inc. Retrieved March 19, 2022.

Jamieson, D. J., & Rasmussen, S. A. (2022). Seasonal influenza and pregnancy. *UpToDate*. Lexi-Comp, Inc. Retrieved March 19, 2022.

Kahrilas, P. J. (2022). Medical management of gastroesophageal reflex disease in adults. *UpToDate*. Lexi-Comp, Inc. Retrieved March 19, 2022.

Kuohung, W., & Hornstein, M. (2022). Overview of infertility. *UpToDate*. Lexi-Comp, Inc. Retrieved March 19, 2022.

Kuohung, W., & Hornstein, M. (2022). Causes of female infertility. *UpToDate*. Lexi-Comp, Inc. Retrieved March 19, 2022.

Kuohung, W., & Hornstein, M. (2022). Treatments for female infertility. *UpToDate*. Lexi-Comp, Inc. Retrieved March 19, 2022.

Lockwood, C. L., & Magriples, U. (2022). Prenatal care: Patient education, health promotion, and safety of commonly used drugs. *UpToDate*. Lexi-Comp, Inc. Retrieved March 19, 2022.

Norwitz, E. R. (2022). Eclampsia. *UpToDate*. Lexi-Comp, Inc. Retrieved March 19, 2022.

Norwitz, E. R. (2022). Preeclampsia: Management and prognosis. *UpToDate*. Lexi-Comp, Inc. Retrieved March 19, 2022.

Pierce, S., Bakker, R., Myers, D. A., & Edwards, R. K. (2018). Clinical insights for cervical ripening and labor induction using prostaglandins. *American Journal of Perinatology Reports, 8*(4), e307–e314.

Ricci, S. S. (2022). *Essentials of maternity, newborn, and women's health nursing* (5th ed.). Wolters Kluwer Health/Lippincott Williams & Wilkins.

Roberts, V., & Myatt, L. (2022). Placental development and physiology. *UpToDate*. Lexi-Comp, Inc. Retrieved March 19, 2022.

Robinson, J. N., & Norwitz, E. R. (2022). Preterm birth: Risk factors, interventions for risk reduction, and maternal prognosis. *UpToDate*. Lexi-Comp, Inc. Retrieved March 19, 2022.

Rodriguez-Thompson, D. (2021). Cigarette and tobacco products in pregnancy: Impact on pregnancy and the neonate. *UpToDate*. Lexi-Comp, Inc. Retrieved March 19, 2022.

Rodriguez-Thompson, D. (2022). Tobacco and nicotine use in pregnancy: Cessation strategies and treatment options. *UpToDate*. Lexi-Comp, Inc. Retrieved March 19, 2022.

Simhan, H. N., & Caritis, S. (2022). Inhibition of acute preterm labor. *UpToDate*. Lexi-Comp, Inc. Retrieved March 19, 2022.

Simpson, K. R., Creehan, P. A., O'Brien-Abel, N., Roth, C. K., & Rohan, A. J. (2021). *Perinatal nursing* (5th ed.). Wolters Kluwer Health/Lippincott Williams & Wilkins.

Smith, J. A., & Fox, K. A. (2022). Nausea and vomiting of pregnancy: Treatment and outcome. *UpToDate*. Lexi-Comp, Inc. Retrieved March 19, 2022.

UpToDate. (2022). *Drug information*. Lexi-Comp, Inc. Retrieved March 19, 2022.

Wambach, K., & Spencer, B. (2021). *Breastfeeding and human lactation* (6th ed.). Jones & Bartlett, LLC.

Yawetz, S. (2022). Immunizations during pregnancy. *UpToDate*. Lexi-Comp, Inc. Retrieved March 19, 2022.

CHAPTER 7

Pharmacology and Female Health

LEARNING OBJECTIVES

After studying this chapter, you should be able to:

1. Describe the fundamental workings of the menstrual cycle.
2. Identify the signs and symptoms associated with common female reproductive health problems.
3. Evaluate the benefits and risks associated with postmenopausal hormone replacement therapy.
4. Identify the prototype drug for the estrogens, progestins, and estrogen–progestin combinations.
5. Describe the estrogens in terms of action, use, adverse effects, contraindications, and nursing implications.
6. Describe the progestins in terms of action, use, adverse effects, contraindications, and nursing implications.
7. Describe the estrogen–progestin combinations in terms of action, use, adverse effects, contraindications, and nursing implications.
8. Implement the nursing process in patients taking estrogens, progestins, and estrogen–progestin combinations.

CLINICAL APPLICATION CASE STUDY

Fifty-two-year-old Paula Bigelow has been reporting vaginal dryness, hot flashes, and night sweats for the past 6 months. She reports that her last normal menstrual period was over 1 year ago.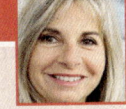

KEY TERMS

Estrogen: hormone produced primarily by the ovaries and secondarily by the adrenal cortex that promotes growth of specific body cells and development of most female secondary sexual characteristics

Menopause: permanent end of menstrual periods, which usually occurs in females 48 to 55 years of age

Progesterone: hormone produced in the ovaries and adrenal cortex that prepares the lining of the uterus for pregnancy

Progestin: synthetic form of progesterone that is similar to the hormone produced naturally by the body most often used in combination with an estrogen in contraceptive products

INTRODUCTION

This chapter focuses on drug therapy in the healthcare of nonpregnant females. To understand the management of drugs discussed in this chapter, it is important to recognize how estrogens and progestins regulate female physiologic processes.

OVERVIEW OF THE EFFECTS OF ESTROGENS AND PROGESTINS

To adequately understand the pharmacologic effects of estrogens and **progestins** (synthetic progesterone), it is important to understand the main effects of female reproductive hormones and the menstrual cycle. **Estrogen** and **progesterone** are female sex hormones produced primarily by the ovaries and secondarily by the adrenal cortex in nonpregnant females. Small amounts of estrogens are also synthesized in the liver, kidney, brain, skeletal muscle, testes, and adipose tissue.

The main function of the estrogens is to promote growth in tissues related to female reproduction and sexual characteristics. Three ovarian estrogens known as endogenous estrogens (estradiol, estrone, and estriol) are secreted in significant amounts. Estradiol is the major estrogen because it exerts more estrogenic activity than the other two estrogens combined.

In nonpregnant females, between puberty and **menopause** (permanent end of menstrual periods, which usually occurs between 48 and 55 years of age), estrogens are secreted in a monthly cycle called the menstrual cycle. When the endometrial lining of the uterus loses its hormonal stimulation, it is discharged vaginally as menstrual flow.

During pregnancy, the placenta in conjunction with the fetus produces large amounts of estrogen, causing enlargement of the uterus and breasts, growth of glandular tissue in the breasts, and relaxation of ligaments and joints in the pelvis. All these changes are necessary for the growth and birth of the fetus.

In general, progesterone has different effects on lipid metabolism compared with estrogen. That is, progesterone decreases high-density lipoprotein (HDL) cholesterol and increases low-density lipoprotein (LDL) cholesterol, both of which increase the risk of cardiovascular disease. Physiologic progesterone increases insulin levels but does not usually impair glucose tolerance. However, long-term administration of potent synthetic exogenous progestins, such as norgestrel, may decrease glucose tolerance and make diabetes mellitus more difficult to control.

In nonpregnant females, progesterone is secreted by the corpus luteum during the last half of the menstrual cycle, which occurs after ovulation. When fertilization does not take place, the estrogen and progesterone levels decrease, and menstruation occurs.

If the ovum is fertilized, progesterone acts to maintain the pregnancy by maintaining the endometrial lining of the uterus, preparing the breasts for lactation, and decreasing uterine contractility.

The menstrual cycle consists of the follicular phase (days 1 to 14) and the luteal phase (days 15 to 28). Hormones in the hypothalamus, pituitary gland, and ovary regulate this cycle. The usual length of a complete menstrual cycle is 28 days, and the first day of menstrual bleeding is day 1.

COMMON FEMALE REPRODUCTIVE HEALTH CONDITIONS

Deficiencies in endogenous sex hormones result in the absence of normal sexual development. In females with deficiencies of these hormones, primary sex organ maturity will not occur, and secondary sexual characteristics will not develop; normal growth and development of the adolescent will not occur, and reproduction is not possible. Assuming that the sexual organs and reproductive system are mature, endogenous sex hormone levels that drop after puberty will result in decreased secondary sexual characteristics. The ability to reproduce and carry a pregnancy to term is reduced.

In addition, normal and aberrant changes in hormone levels across the lifespan can lead to conditions associated with the reproductive system. The clinical manifestations are briefly discussed in the following sections. Drug therapy may be helpful.

Premenstrual Syndrome

Premenstrual syndrome (PMS) is characterized by physical, emotional, and behavioral symptoms that occur during the last half of the menstrual cycle and resolve with menses. The term PMS is used for those who experience these symptoms at a severe level that interferes with activities of daily living and personal relationships. A more severe, sometimes disabling, variant of PMS is premenstrual dysphoric disorder (PMDD), which can interfere greatly with work, school, social activities, and relationships. PMDD can disrupt daily life and destroy relationships and now appears in the *Diagnostic and Statistical Manual of Mental Health Disorders* (American Psychiatric Association [APA], 2013).

Clinical Manifestations

Signs and symptoms of PMS vary, with the most common being irritability and dysphoria. Clinical manifestations include the following symptoms:

- Physical: bloating, abdominal pain, headache, back pain, and breast tenderness
- Emotional: agitation, irritability, anxiety, and depression
- Behavioral: outbursts of anger, confusion, social withdrawal, and oversensitivity to insignificant events

The American College of Obstetrician and Gynecologists (ACOG) criteria for diagnosis of PMS consists of having at least one of the above emotional and one of the physical symptoms occurring 5 days before menses for each of three previous menstrual cycles (ACOG, 2000).

People with PMDD experience extreme symptoms including emotional disorders of agitation, anger, extreme mood shifts, difficulty concentrating, irritability, anxiety, and depression can cause extreme mood shifts, anger, anxiety, difficulty concentrating, depression, and feeling overwhelmed. It is important to distinguish PMDD from other medical and psychiatric conditions. According to the American Psychiatric Association (APA), PMDD is characterized by experiencing at least five or more common symptoms the week before menses with symptoms improving with the onset of menses and the symptoms gone in the weeks after menses. At least one of five or more symptoms must include change in mood, irritability or anger or impaired interpersonal relationships, depression or hopelessness or self-deprecation, or anxiety or tension (APA, 2013).

Drug Therapy

Antidepressants have proven effective in the treatment of PMS and PMDD, and a selective serotonin reuptake inhibitor (SSRI) or a serotonin and norepinephrine reuptake inhibitor (SNRI) may be ordered. Oral contraceptives containing drospirenone or any progestin provide additional options but are generally considered second-line therapy. If anxiety or insomnia is the main symptom, a benzodiazepine such as alprazolam (Xanax) may be useful, but monitoring is necessary because drug dependency may develop.

Endometriosis

Endometriosis is defined as the growth of endometrial tissue outside the uterine cavity (Zondervan et al., 2020). This tissue can be attached to ovaries, the fallopian tubes, the outside of the uterus, the bowels, and the retrovaginal septum.

Endometriosis is one of the most common gynecologic problems in the United States, affecting an estimated 11% of females. Risk factors include family history of endometriosis, increasing age, short menstrual cycles with longer flow, young menarche, high-fat diet, and few or no pregnancies.

Clinical Manifestations

Chronic pelvic pain is a classic symptom of endometriosis. Other characteristic indications include menorrhagia, dysmenorrhea, dyspareunia, fatigue, and abdominal pain. Infertility is also associated with endometriosis, especially in severe cases.

Drug Therapy

Drug therapy to manage the symptoms of endometriosis includes the use of nonsteroidal anti-inflammatory agents; hormonal contraceptives, including a low-dose oral contraceptive and a hormonal intrauterine device; and GnRH agonists. No data support one treatment or treatment combination over another. The treatment choice is based on symptom severity, response to treatment, contraceptive needs, and cost.

Menopause

Menopause is a normal physiologic process in aging resulting in the absence of menses for 1 year, with the average age at 51.

Menopause is related to deficiencies of endogenous sex hormones and a reduction in the number of ovarian follicles. Elevated follicle-stimulating hormone (FSH) levels (30 mIU/mL or higher) often signal menopause or ovarian failure. A decline in estrogen leads to elevated FSH levels as the anterior pituitary continues to release FSH with no effects. The decrease in estrogen levels also result in no luteinizing hormone (LH) surge and subsequently no ovulation. The absence of ovulation results in the decline of estrogen levels and the cessation of menses.

Clinical Manifestations

As a result of insufficient levels of circulating estrogen, secondary sexual characteristics diminish; there is a decrease in skin elasticity, body hair, and breast and subcutaneous tissue. The uterus and ovaries decrease in size, and the vagina becomes atrophic. Dyspareunia, urinary stress incontinence, and urinary tract infections may occur. Decreased estrogen results in vasomotor symptoms of "hot flushes" or "hot flashes," and night sweats may occur. Long-term estrogen deficiency causes an imbalance in bone remodeling, which may lead to osteoporosis. Cardiovascular risk factors increase as total cholesterol and LDL increase and HDL decreases.

Palpitations, headaches, and dizziness may be present, and postmenopausal people may exhibit insomnia, irritability, anxiety, and depression.

Drug Therapy

Hormone replacement therapy (HRT) with estrogen is the most effective treatment available for relief of menopausal symptoms, most importantly vasomotor symptoms. The U.S. Food and Drug Administration (FDA) recommends the use of HRT only with symptoms severe enough to warrant its use, at the lowest dose and for the shortest duration possible, to ease the menopausal transition. Although alternate drug therapies are available, none are as effective as estrogen. The combination of the selective estrogen receptor modulator bazedoxifene (Duavee) with conjugated estrogens (Premarin) is available in the United States for the treatment of postmenopausal vasomotor symptoms and the prevention of osteoporosis. This fixed-dose combination drug is appropriate for those who have an intact uterus who do not require a progestin. (Estrogen is discussed in detail later in the chapter.)

Other Drug Therapy That Alters the Reproductive Cycle

Exogenous estrogens and progestins can be taken at various stages in the reproductive cycle. When exogenous estrogens and progestins are administered for therapeutic purposes, they produce the same effects as endogenous hormones. Multiple preparations of estrogens and progestins are available for various purposes and in several forms. Clinical indications, routes of administration, and dosages are presented in the Drugs at a Glance tables.

> ### Clinical Application 7.1
> - Mrs. Bigelow has her FSH level measured, as ordered by her healthcare provider. Assuming Mrs. Bigelow has completed menopause, would the nurse expect the FSH levels to be high or low? Why?

ESTROGENS

Exogenous estrogens are used to treat female health disorders when endogenous estrogen levels are low or absent. **Conjugated estrogen** (Premarin), the prototype estrogen, is the most commonly used oral estrogen.

Pharmacokinetics

Conjugated estrogen and some synthetic derivatives of natural estrogens (e.g., ethinyl estradiol, the most widely used synthetic steroidal estrogen) are chemically modified to be effective with oral administration. After oral administration, these estrogens are well absorbed and are released slowly over several hours. Degradation occurs very slowly in the liver, allowing for high intrinsic potency. Ethinyl estradiol reaches peak plasma levels within 2 hours. It is 98% bound to plasma proteins, and its half-life varies from 6 to 20 hours. Extensive first-pass metabolism occurs in the liver, where further metabolism and conjugation occur; excretion of the conjugates is in bile and urine.

Transdermal estradiol patches (e.g., Climara, Menostar, Vivelle-Dot) allow for absorption of estrogen through the skin to the bloodstream. The transdermal route bypasses the liver; thus, less estrogen is received. With this route, patients experience less nausea and vomiting than with the oral route. Serum levels produced through transdermal application more closely mimic premenopausal estrogen levels compared with serum levels with oral estrogens. This form of estrogen reaches peak plasma levels within 4 hours, and its half-life is approximately 4 hours.

Action

Estrogens circulate in the bloodstream to target cells, where they enter cells and combine with receptor proteins in cell cytoplasm. After transport of the estrogen–receptor complex to the cell nucleus, this complex interacts with DNA to produce RNA and new DNA. These substances stimulate cell reproduction and production of various proteins. Estrogen primarily influences the reproductive system, although it also affects the skeletal, metabolic, and coagulation systems, as well as the skin and subcutaneous tissues.

Hormonal contraceptives that include estrogen act by several mechanisms. First, they inhibit hypothalamic secretion of GnRH, which inhibits pituitary secretion of FSH and LH. When these gonadotropic hormones are absent, ovulation and, therefore, conception cannot occur. Second, the drugs produce cervical mucous that resists penetration of spermatozoa into the upper reproductive tract. Third, the drugs interfere with endometrial maturation and reception of ova that are released and fertilized. These overlapping mechanisms make the drugs highly effective in preventing pregnancy.

Use

Indications for use of exogenous estrogens include birth control, menopause, and as replacement therapy in deficiency states.

Birth Control

Females 12 to 45 years of age use widely an estrogen, combined with a progestin, to control fertility. If pregnancy does occur, estrogens are contraindicated because their use during pregnancy has been associated with the occurrence of vaginal cancer in female offspring and possible harmful effects on male offspring. Use of birth control pills also includes treatment of menstrual disorders such as amenorrhea and dysmenorrhea.

At least 26 birth control pills can be used in specified combinations as emergency contraception (EC). It is recommended that the first dose of EC be taken within 120 hours of unprotected intercourse followed by a second dose of birth control pills 12 hours later.

Menopause

Healthcare providers prescribe estrogens to relieve symptoms of estrogen deficiency during menopause and to prevent or treat osteoporosis. Such use is usually called estrogen replacement therapy (ERT). When prescribers order estrogen for patients with an intact uterus, they also order a progestin to prevent unwanted thickening of the lining of the uterus and to decrease the risk of uterine cancer, a possible result of using estrogen alone. Both drug therapies are commonly referred to as HRT or menopausal hormone therapy (MHT), terms used to describe the administration of one or more female hormones during menopause.

Replacement Therapy in Deficiency States

Deficiency states usually result from hypofunction of the pituitary gland or the ovaries and may occur anytime during the life cycle. The most common time for this deficiency occurs in middle age and the use of replacement therapy must be evaluated based on health history and risk factors. For people who menstruate who are between approximately 12 and 45 years of age, prescribers may order an estrogen occasionally for menstrual disorders, including amenorrhea and abnormal uterine bleeding due to estrogen deficiency.

Other Uses of Estrogens

Estrogens may be used in the treatment of moderate to severe vasomotor and atrophic symptoms associated with menopause, prevention of postmenopausal osteoporosis, and palliative treatment for metastatic breast carcinoma and advanced androgen-dependent prostatic cancer. Treatment of abnormal uterine bleeding caused by hormonal imbalance, in the absence of organic pathology, requires an intravenous injection. Table 7.1 presents dosage information for the various estrogens.

The short-term use (1 to 2 years) of estrogens (sometimes synthetic) in postmenopausal patients may be indicated for management of menopausal symptoms. Note that the long-term use of estrogen-only therapy and estrogen–progestin combinations is no longer recommended for most people because of potentially serious adverse effects.

Patient-Related Variables and Estrogens

Patient-related variables specific to the use of estrogens include the following:

- Age:
  - Little information exists about the effects of estrogens in children, and the drugs are not generally indicated for use in the pediatric age group.
  - Because estrogens cause epiphyseal closure, caution is warranted with their use before completion of bone growth and attainment of adult height.
  - When it is necessary to give hormonal contraceptives to adolescents, they should receive the smallest effective doses.
- Reproduction, pregnancy, and lactation:
  - Estrogens are contraindicated in pregnancy and breast-feeding.
  - Patients taking estrogen should use barrier methods of contraception to avoid pregnancy.
  - Patients with abnormal or undiagnosed vaginal bleeding should not take estrogen.

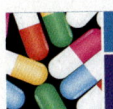

TABLE 7.1
DRUGS AT A GLANCE: Estrogens

Drug	Menopausal Symptoms	Female Hypogonadism	Prevention of Osteoporosis	Other
P Conjugated estrogens, equine (Premarin; 🍁 Premarin, C.E.S) synthetic conjugated (Congest)	PO 0.3–1.25 mg daily for 21 d followed by 7 d without the drug	PO 2.5–7.5 mg daily in divided doses, cyclically 20 d on and 10 d off the drug	PO 0.625 mg daily for 21 d and then 7 d without the drug	Dysfunctional uterine bleeding: IM or IV for emergency use, 25 mg, repeated in 6–12 h if necessary Atrophic vaginitis: topical, 2.4 g of vaginal cream inserted daily
Esterified estrogens (Menest; 🍁 Estragyn)	PO 0.3–1.25 mg daily	PO 2.5–7.5 mg daily in divided doses, cyclically 20 d on and 10 d off the drug		Breast cancer (inoperable, progressing): PO 10 mg three times a day for at least 3 mo in selected postmenopausal females
Estradiol cypionate (Depo-Estradiol)	IM 1–5 mg every 3–4 wk			
Estradiol, micronized (Estrace, Gynedol, Innofem, Estring, Vagifem; 🍁 Estrace, Estring, Vagifem), vaginal tablet, or vaginal cream (Estring, vaginal ring)	PO 0.5–2 mg daily for 3 wk and then 1 wk off or daily Monday through Friday, none on Saturday or Sunday as prescribed		PO 0.5 mg daily for 23 d and no drug for 5 d each month	Atrophic vaginitis: cream, 2–4 g daily for 2 wk, then 1–2 g daily for 2 wk, then 1 g one to three times weekly; vaginal ring (Estring), 1 every 3 mo
Estradiol transdermal system (Alora, Climara, Esclim, Menostar, Vivelle-Dot EstroGel, Elestrin, Divigel, Evamist; 🍁 Climara, Depo-Estradiol, Estradot, Menostar, Oesclim)	Climara: 0.025–0.1 mg/d topically to skin every week Menostar: 0.014 mg/d applied topically each week. Vivelle-Dot: 0.025–0.1 mg/d topically to skin two times per week Estrasorb (topical lotion; 1.74 g/pouch): two pouches applied topically to legs every day EstroGel (topical gel; 1.25 g/pump): one pump applied topically every day Evamist (topical spray; 1.53 mg/spray): one spray applied topically everyday		Climara: 0.025–0.1 mg/d topically to skin every week Menostar: 0.014 mg/d applied topically each week Vivelle-Dot: 0.025–0.1 mg/d topically to skin two times per week	
Estropipate (Ogen, Ortho-Est)	PO 0.625–5 mg daily, cyclically	PO 1.25–7.5 mg daily for 3 wk, followed by a rest period of 8–10 d. Repeat as needed	PO 0.625 mg daily for 25 d and no drug for 6 d each month	Ovarian failure: same dosage as for female hypogonadism Atrophic vaginitis: topical, 1–2 g vaginal cream daily

> **Quality and Safety Alert: Safety**
>
> Females who take a daily dose of a conjugated estrogen and medroxyprogesterone acetate regimen need education regarding the importance of breast self-examinations and recommendations for clinical breast examinations and mammography screening. It is essential that nurses teach patients to notify their healthcare providers if a breast lump is detected, because HRT must be discontinued until diagnostic procedures are complete.

- Abnormal kidney function and hepatic impairment:
  - Estrogen use has been associated with fluid retention and dilated kidneys, especially when used in higher doses. Patients with abnormal kidney function require close evaluation and management.
  - Advanced impairment may be a contraindication.
  - Impaired liver function may lead to impaired estrogen metabolism, with resultant accumulation which may cause an increase in adverse effects.
- Specific healthcare environments:
  - The home care nurse should teach or assist patients to take the drugs as prescribed and encourage patients to keep appointments for follow-up supervision and blood pressure monitoring.
  - The home care nurse should teach postmenopausal patients about nonhormonal strategies for preventing osteoporosis and cardiovascular disease.
  - The home care nurse should educate patients that when taking estrogen during a critical illness, there is an increased risk of thromboembolic disorders such as thrombophlebitis, deep vein thrombosis, and pulmonary embolism, which can result in limited mobility.

Adverse Effects

The most significant risk associated with estrogens are an increased risk of cardiovascular complications, such as stroke, heart attack, hypertension, thromboembolic and thrombotic disease, thrombophlebitis, retinal thrombosis, pulmonary embolism, and certain cancers. Other adverse effects of conjugated estrogens include menstrual disorders, such as breakthrough bleeding, dysmenorrhea, and amenorrhea, due to the hormonal imbalance that may occur with estrogen use. GI upset (nausea, vomiting, abdominal cramps, and bloating) may occur. Central nervous system adverse reactions such as migraine headache, dizziness, and mental depression may be caused or aggravated in some people who take estrogen, though the mechanism of action is unknown. Edema and weight gain may occur due to fluid retention. Gallbladder disease is common with estrogen use. Postmenopausal females who take estrogen are two to four times more likely to require surgery for gallbladder disease than those who do not take estrogen.

The FDA has issued a **BOXED WARNING** ◆ regarding estrogen use; supervised use at the lowest dose for the shortest duration should be prescribed. Estrogens are associated with the following:

- An increased risk of endometrial cancer. Estrogens should not be used alone in females with an intact uterus.
- An increased risk of thromboembolic events such as myocardial infarction, stroke, deep vein thrombosis, and pulmonary embolism. Estrogens (with or without progestins) should not be used for the prevention of cardiovascular disease.
- An increased risk of dementia in postmenopausal females. Estrogens should not be used for the prevention of dementia.
- An increased risk of breast cancer development in females taking estrogen–progestin combinations.

Contraindications

Estrogens have a wide variety of reported adverse reactions and effects on body tissues, and thus, many contraindications. It is important to avoid using estrogens in the following situations:

- Known or suspected pregnancy, because teratogenic effects that interfere with fetal development may result.
- Thromboembolic disorders, such as thrombophlebitis, deep vein thrombosis, or pulmonary embolism.
- Known or suspected cancers of breast or genital tissues, because the drugs may stimulate tumor growth. (An exception is the use of estrogens for treatment of metastatic breast cancer in females at least 5 years postmenopause.)
- Undiagnosed vaginal or uterine bleeding.
- Fibroid tumors of the uterus.
- Active liver disease, including liver cancer and impaired liver function.
- History of cerebrovascular disease, coronary artery disease, thrombophlebitis, hypertension, or conditions predisposing to these disease processes.
- Tobacco use, which leads to a greater risk of thromboembolic disorders in patients who take estrogen supplements, possibly because of increased platelet aggregation with estrogen ingestion and cigarette smoking. Estrogen also increases hepatic production of blood clotting factors. The FDA has issued a **BOXED WARNING** ◆ regarding the risk for serious cardiovascular events in smokers who use oral contraceptives; the risk increases with age, so oral contraceptives should not be used in smokers age 35 years and over.
- Family history of breast or reproductive system cancer.

Nursing Implications

An important nursing implication associated with estrogen use is identifying factors that contraindicate use of the drug in high-risk patients. The following information is essential in identifying such patients:

- Assessment of medical and social history. The nurse assesses for menopausal symptoms, cardiovascular disease (hypertension, hyperlipidemia, and cerebral vascular risk), gynecologic history (menstrual history, last menstrual period, and age at menopause), cancer history, and history of smoking.
- Assessment of family history of menopause, osteoporosis, cardiovascular disease, cerebrovascular disease, cognitive disease, and allergy status.
- Assessment of blood pressure, weight, height, pregnancy status, and lipid values. A clinical breast examination with a mammogram and pelvic examination are essential.

BOX 7.1 Drug Interactions: Estrogens

Drugs That Decrease the Effects of Estrogen
- Anticonvulsants, such as carbamazepine, oxcarbazepine, phenytoin, and topiramate:
  Induce enzymes that accelerate the metabolism of estrogens
- Barbiturates, rifampin, ritonavir, and tetracyclines:
  Induce enzymes that accelerate inactivation of estrogens

BOX 7.2 Patient Teaching Guidelines for Estrogens, Progestins, and Estrogen–Progestin Combinations

- Take your weight weekly, and report sudden weight gain to your healthcare provider. (Such weight gain may be due to fluid retention and edema.)
- Report any unusual vaginal bleeding immediately to your healthcare provider.
- Discuss the increased thromboembolic risk associated with smoking while using estrogens or progestins.
- Know the warning signs that may occur if a thromboembolism should develop—think ACHES [[severe] abdominal pain, chest pain, headache, eye changes, severe leg pain]. Seek medical attention immediately if such symptoms occur.
- If taking estrogen for long periods, have a physical examination at least annually. Have your blood pressure checked, as well as a breast and pelvic examination. Adverse conditions may occur when these drugs are taken for long periods. Your healthcare provider needs to monitor for adverse drug effects such as high blood pressure, gallbladder disease, and blood clotting disorders.
- If taking these medications for contraception, use a backup birth control method, and call your healthcare provider if you fail to take medications as prescribed or if an intrauterine device or a subdermal implant comes out of its own accord.

Preventing Interactions

Several drugs interact with estrogens, decreasing their effect (Box 7.1). With corticosteroids and estrogen, increased therapeutic effects and a risk of toxicity of the corticosteroids occur. Use of ropinirole with estrogen may require a dosage adjustment of the estrogen. Estrogens have a decreased effect on tamoxifen, sulfonylurea antidiabetic drugs, and anticoagulants, especially warfarin. St. John's wort increases the breakdown of estrogen, which may decrease the effectiveness of birth control pills.

Administering the Medication

Choice of preparation depends on the reason for use, desired route of administration, and duration of action. Although dosage needs vary with patients and the health conditions for which the drugs are prescribed, a general rule is to use the smallest effective dose for the shortest effective time. Estrogens are often given cyclically. In one regimen, the drug is taken for 3 weeks and then omitted for 1 week; in another, it is omitted the first 5 days of the month. These regimens more closely resemble normal secretion of estrogen and avoid prolonged stimulation of body tissues. It is necessary to give naturally occurring, nonconjugated estrogens (estradiol, estrone) intramuscularly because they are rapidly metabolized if administered orally. Administration of nonsteroidal synthetic preparations is usually oral or topical. Estrogen can be taken with food or at bedtime to decrease nausea, a common adverse reaction.

Transdermal estradiol (e.g., Climara, Menostar, Vivelle-Dot) allows for absorption of estrogen through the skin to the bloodstream. Depending on the preparation, patients apply the patches weekly or biweekly. The total amount of drug absorbed and the resulting plasma drug concentrations from transdermal estrogen can increase during exposure to heat; the nurse should advise patients to avoid exposing the patch to the sun for long periods of time.

Assessing for Therapeutic Effects

The therapeutic effects of estrogen vary depending on the reason for use. When treatment of menopausal symptoms is the goal, it is essential to assess for the decrease in hot flashes, vaginal dryness, and night sweats. When amenorrhea is the target, the occurrence of menstruation indicates that the hormone is working. When female hypogonadism is the treatment goal, the occurrence of menstruation and the presence of breast enlargement, axillary and pubic hair, and other secondary sexual characteristics indicate proper actions of the medication. When prevention of osteoporosis is the objective, the therapeutic effect includes the absence of bone fractures.

Assessing for Adverse Effects

The nurse assesses for the adverse effects of estrogen through the use of a history and physical examination. A careful assessment with each visit regarding the new onset of abdominal pain, chest pain, headache, vision change, and leg pain is essential in the early recognition of a potential blood clot. The nurse should ensure that blood pressure, glucose, lipid panel, pelvic examination (with Papanicolaou [Pap] smear), and mammography are monitored routinely based on patient age.

Patient Teaching

Box 7.2 presents patient teaching guidelines for estrogens.

Clinical Application 7.2

- Mrs. Bigelow receives a diagnosis of menopause. She asks about hormone replacement therapy. What additional information does the nurse need to provide the best information?
- Mrs. Bigelow has no absolute contraindications to hormone replacement therapy, and her healthcare provider prescribes Prempro 0.625/2.5 mg every day. What instructions would the nurse provide to Mrs. Bigelow to ensure that she completely understands the risks, benefits, and adverse effects of the hormone replacement therapy?

NCLEX Success

1. A nurse practitioner prescribes estrogen replacement therapy to relieve severe menopausal symptoms of hot flashes or flushes, which are the result of
   A. insufficient gonadotropin secretion
   B. vasomotor instability
   C. high levels of estrogen
   D. decreased progesterone

PROGESTINS

Progestins are used for a range of contraceptive and noncontraceptive purposes either alone or in combination with estrogens. The choice of preparation varies with use. **Medroxyprogesterone acetate** (Provera), a synthetic progestin and a progesterone derivative, is the prototype progestin.

Pharmacokinetics

Oral administration of medroxyprogesterone acetate and other progestins results in rapid absorption, and the drug can reach a maximum concentration in 1 to 2 hours. During the first 6 hours, half-life is about 2 to 3 hours; thereafter, half-life extends to 8 to 9 hours. Prompt degradation occurs in the liver, and metabolites are excreted primarily in the urine. Rapid absorption is also a characteristic of intramuscular progestins, which have a half-life of just a few minutes. Long-acting forms can maintain effective concentrations for 3 to 6 months; maximum concentrations can be achieved in 24 hours with a half-life of about 10 weeks. Gel preparations have sustained-release properties, and absorption is prolonged with half-lives of 1 to 2 days.

Action

Medroxyprogesterone acetate and other progestins diffuse freely into cells, where they bind to progesterone receptors. The progestins act primarily on the endometrial lining of the uterus by changing it from a proliferative endometrium into a secretory endometrium. They also suppress the release of pituitary hormones, which inhibit ovulation. Finally, they inhibit spontaneous uterine contractions.

Use

Progestin-only pills are one option for those who cannot or prefer not to use estrogen-containing contraceptives. Implantable intrauterine devices (IUDs) or subdermal implants are types of long-acting reversible contraceptives. Healthcare providers use progestins to prevent hyperplasia of the endometrial lining of the uterus in patients taking endogenous estrogen. In addition, progestins suppress ovarian function in dysmenorrhea, endometriosis, endometrial cancer, and uterine bleeding. These uses of progestins are extensions of the physiologic actions of progesterone on the neuroendocrine control of ovarian function and on the endometrium.

Progestin-only preparations are administered by a variety of routes. Etonogestrel (Nexplanon), a progestin-only preparation, is dispensed in a 4-mm rod implanted subdermally in the inner upper arm for long-acting reversible contraception. In addition, the progestin levonorgestrel is used as an EC. The EC is most effective if taken within 72 hours of unprotected intercourse but may be taken up to 120 hours after unprotected intercourse. Two-dose regimens for EC are equally as effective. Table 7.2 presents dosage information for the progestins.

> **! Quality and Safety Alert: Safety**
>
> The *etonogestrel implant* is one of the most effective contraceptives available. It has an efficacy equal to or better than that of sterilization but without the risks of invasive surgery.

For approximately 20 to 25 years, postmenopausal females with an intact uterus took progestins in combination with estrogen for long-term HRT. In HRT, the purpose of a progestin is to prevent endometrial cancer, which can occur with unopposed estrogenic stimulation. However, as previously stated, this combination currently is not recommended for long-term use because evidence has indicated that the adverse effects outweigh the beneficial effects.

> **Quality and Safety Alert: Evidence-Based Practice**
>
> The Women's Health Initiative (WHI), a large-scale randomized controlled trial examining the use of oral conjugated equine estrogen among postmenopausal females, has provided much information regarding female health. The most recent findings suggest that the timing of estrogen therapy initiation determines the coronary risk. Manson et al. report that when estrogen was started in females with an oophorectomy within the last 10 years of menopause or at an earlier age (less than 60 years), there was a 32% reduction in mortality (2020). Further findings confirm that estrogen therapy is not indicated for older females with longer menopause onset.

Patient-related variables specific to the use of medroxyprogesterone acetate and other progestins include the following:

- Age:
  - Progestins are not intended for use in children.
  - The use of progestins in patients ages 65 years and older is contraindicated due to an increased risk of dementia.
- Reproduction, pregnancy, and lactation:
  - Progestins are contraindicated in pregnancy and breastfeeding.
  - Long-term use for pregnancy prevention increases the risk of osteoporosis.
  - Female patients without a uterus should not use progestins.
- Abnormal kidney function and hepatic impairment:
  - Patients with abnormal kidney function require close evaluation and management because progestin metabolites are predominately excreted in urine.
  - Progestin use in patients with advanced abnormal kidney function is contraindicated.
  - Metabolism of progestins occurs primarily in the liver. Therefore, impaired liver function or liver disease prohibits its use.

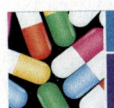

TABLE 7.2
DRUGS AT A GLANCE: Progestins

Drug	Routes and Dosage Ranges for Various Indications			
	Menstrual Disorders	**Endometriosis**	**Cancer**	**Contraception**
Medroxyprogesterone acetate (Provera, Depo-Provera, Depo-SubQ Provera 104; ✤ Depo-Provera, Provera)	Dysfunctional uterine bleeding: PO 2.5–10 mg daily for 5–10 d, beginning on 16th or 21st day of cycle	SubQ 104 mg/0.65 mL every 3 mo	Endometrial: IM 400–1,000 mg weekly until improvement and then 400 mg mo	Depo-Provera 150 mg IM every 12 wk; Depo-SubQ Provera 104 mg IM every 12 wk
Etonogestrel (Nexplanon) (Subdermal implant)				68 mg in a 4-mm rod implanted subdermally. Daily release of etonogestrel is 60–70 mcg initially and gradually reduces to 25–30 mcg over 3 y
Levonorgestrel (Next Choice, New Day, Take Action)				Emergency contraception: two-dose regimen PO 0.75 mg, dose repeated in 12 h; single dose regimen PO 1.5 mg; most effective when taken within 72 h of unprotected intercourse but may be taken up to 120 h after unprotected intercourse
Megestrol acetate (Megace ES; ✤ Megace OS, Megestrol)			Endometrial: PO 40–320 mg daily in 4 divided doses for at least 2 mo; Breast: PO 160 mg daily in 4 divided doses for at least 2 mo; Cachexia with HIV: PO initially 800 mg/d; normal range 400–800 mg/d (suspension only) or 625 mg/d ES suspension	
Norethindrone (Errin, Jencycla, Ortho Micronor, Camila, Jolivette, Nor-Q-D, Nora-BE)	Pregnancy prevention: PO 0.35 mg/d			
Progesterone (Crinone, Endometrin; ✤ Crinone, Endometrin; [vaginal gel], Prometrium)	Amenorrhea and dysfunctional uterine bleeding: IM 5–10 mg for 6–8 consecutive days; Secondary amenorrhea: 4% gel, 45 mg every other day; Other infertility: 90 mg vaginally daily in females requiring progesterone supplementation			

(Continued on page 108)

TABLE 7.2

DRUGS AT A GLANCE: Progestins (Continued)

Drug	Routes and Dosage Ranges for Various Indications			
	Menstrual Disorders	Endometriosis	Cancer	Contraception
Depot medroxyprogesterone acetate IM (Depo-Provera, Provera; 🍁 Depo-Provera, Provera)				
Depot medroxyprogesterone acetate SubQ (Depo-SubQ Provera)				
Levonorgestrel-releasing intrauterine device (Mirena, Kyleena; 🍁 Jaydess, Kyleena, Mirena)				Provides contraception for 5 y
Levonorgestrel-releasing intrauterine device (Liletta, Skyla)				Provides contraception for 3 y

Adverse Effects

The most significant risk associated with progestins is an increased risk of cardiovascular complications, such as stroke, heart attack, hypertension, thromboembolic and thrombotic disease, thrombophlebitis, retinal thrombosis, and pulmonary embolism. Other adverse effects include the following:

- Irregular vaginal bleeding (common; decreases during the first year of use). Amenorrhea may occur.
- Weight gain and fluid retention (common).
- Ophthalmic disorders, such as sudden, partial, or complete loss of vision.
- An increased risk of migraines and mental depression.
- Possible skin conditions, such as rash, acne, alopecia, and hirsutism (unwanted female hair growth).
- GI upset, with nausea and vomiting.
- Bone loss. A **BOXED WARNING** ◆ stipulates that some forms of medroxyprogesterone acetate cause calcium loss in bones, leading to weak bones and possible bone breakage.

Nurses should be aware that the FDA has recognized some of these problems and issued a **BOXED WARNING** ◆ for the progestins, stating that the drugs:

- Should not be used in pregnancy
- Should not be used in combination with estrogen for the prevention of cardiovascular disease or dementia
- Are associated with an increased risk of thromboembolic events, such as myocardial infarction, stroke, deep vein thrombosis, and pulmonary embolism in females taking estrogen–progestin combination therapy
- Are associated with an increased risk of dementia in post-menopausal females

Contraindications

Contraindications to progestins include allergies to the drugs, pregnancy or suspected pregnancy, and breast-feeding. Other contraindications are a history of active cardiovascular disease; thrombophlebitis; thromboembolic disorders; cerebral hemorrhage; kidney disease; hepatic disease; and carcinoma of the breast, ovaries, or endometrium. A final contraindication is undiagnosed vaginal bleeding. A history of depression warrants caution.

Nursing Implications

Nursing implications associated with progestins are very similar to those associated with estrogens. The following information is essential in identifying those for whom progestin therapy is contraindicated:

- Assessment of medical and social history. The nurse assesses for menopausal symptoms, cardiovascular disease (hypertension, hyperlipidemia, and cerebral vascular risk), gynecologic history (menstrual history, last menstrual period, and age at menopause), cancer history, and history of smoking.
- Assessment of family history of menopause, osteoporosis, cardiovascular disease, cerebrovascular disease, cognitive disease, and allergy status.
- Assessment of blood pressure, weight, height, with lipid panel, clinical breast examination with age-appropriate mammogram, pelvic examination, and Pap smear.

Preventing Interactions

Progestin use often alters liver function and endocrine function tests. It is essential when laboratory testing is indicated that healthcare providers be aware that progestins are being used. No reports of drug–drug, drug–food, or drug–herb interactions concerning progestin have appeared.

Administering the Medication

Progestins can be administered through a variety of routes. Oral, intramuscular, subcutaneous, intravaginal, intrauterine, and subdermal and transdermal preparations of the drug are available. To reduce the GI effects of the oral preparations, it is necessary to take them with food or at bedtime. For treatment of dysfunctional uterine bleeding and amenorrhea, cyclic administration of the drug is often warranted.

Assessing for Therapeutic Effects

When given for menstrual disorders, such as abnormal uterine bleeding, amenorrhea, dysmenorrhea, premenstrual discomforts, and endometriosis, the nurse observes for relief of symptoms.

> **Clinical Application 7.3**
> - Mrs. Bigelow has been taking Prempro 0.625/2.5 mg every day for 1 month. She calls the office when you are on duty. She is complaining of left leg pain and swelling that have been occurring off and on for 4 days. What is the nursing intervention?

Assessing for Adverse Effects

The nurse observes for breakthrough bleeding and provides reassurance to affected patients. The nurse assesses for irregular vaginal bleeding, a major reason that some do not want to take progestin-only contraceptives. The nurse ensures that lipid panels are assessed; decreased HDL and increased LDL cholesterol may occur, increasing the risk of cardiovascular disease and possibly leading to discontinuation of the progestin. In patients with a history of depression, discontinuation of the drug is essential at the first sign or indication of recurring depression.

Patient Teaching

Box 7.2 presents patient teaching guidelines for progestins. In addition to these guidelines, patients who have an intact uterus should take both estrogen and progestin; the progestin component (e.g., Provera) prevents endometrial cancer, an adverse effect of estrogen-only therapy. Combined estrogen–progestin therapy may increase blood sugar levels in patients with diabetes. This effect is attributed to progestin and is unlikely to occur with estrogen-only therapy. Patients with diabetes should report increased blood glucose levels. Take progestins with food or at bedtime to decrease nausea, a common adverse reaction.

> **NCLEX Success**
>
> 2. Postmenopausal patients with an intact uterus taking estrogen for hormone replacement therapy require progestin because
>   A. progestins enhance the effects of estrogen
>   B. combination therapy provides osteoporosis prevention
>   C. progestin opposes the effects of estrogen on the endometrium
>   D. uterine cancer is increased

ESTROGEN–PROGESTIN COMBINATIONS

The most effective and widely used contraceptives are estrogen–progestin combinations. For contraception, the prototype hormonal combination is ethinyl estradiol–norethindrone (Ortho-Novum). For HRT, the prototype drug is **conjugated estrogen–medroxyprogesterone** (Prempro).

Several varieties of progestins are part of combined oral contraceptives. The progestin component may determine the choice of a combination contraceptive product. Progestins have progestational, estrogenic, and androgenic qualities. These qualities vary depending on the type of the progestin and are an important consideration in the management of the adverse effects associated with hormonal contraceptives. Progestational qualities have an influence on the suppression of ovulation and reduction in menstrual bleeding. Estrogenic qualities may be associated with headache, breast tenderness, or fluid retention. Androgenic qualities are often associated with acne or hirsutism. Progestins with minimal androgenic activity are desogestrel and norgestimate; those with intermediate activity include norethindrone and ethynodiol, and those with high androgenic effects include norgestrel.

Pharmacokinetics

Absorption of ethinyl estradiol is good with oral administration, and it reaches peak plasma levels within 2 hours. It is 98% bound to plasma proteins, and its half-life varies from 6 to 20 hours. The estrogen undergoes extensive first-pass metabolism, additional metabolism, and conjugation in the liver; the conjugates are then excreted in bile and urine.

Action

The estrogen component of combined oral contraceptives prevents pregnancy by inhibiting ovulation; it prevents the formation of the follicle by suppressing FSH and LH and stabilizing the endometrium. The progestin component thins the endometrium, slows sperm transport, thickens cervical mucous, and suppresses the LH surge.

Use

The primary use of estrogen–progestin contraceptives is to prevent pregnancy. Four different types of hormonal contraceptives are common: monophasic contraceptives, which contain fixed amounts of both estrogen and progestin components; biphasics, which contain either fixed amounts of estrogen and varied amounts of progestin; triphasics, which contain three different doses of estrogen and progestin; and quadriphasics, which contain four different doses of estrogen and progestin (Table 7.3). Biphasic, triphasic, and quadriphasic preparations mimic normal variations of hormone secretion, decrease the total dosage of hormones, and may decrease adverse effects. These contraceptives are dispensed in containers with color-coded tablets that must be taken in the correct sequence. Dispensers with 28 tablets contain 7 inactive or placebo tablets of a third color. Several combination products and alternative dosage forms are available to help individualize treatment and promote adherence.

TABLE 7.3

Estrogen–Progestin Combinations Used as Contraceptives

Trade Names	Estrogen	Progestin
Monophasics		
Aubra EQ, Aviane-28, Delyla, Falmina, Lessina-28, Lutera, Sronyx, Vienva	Ethinyl estradiol 20 mcg	Levonorgestrel 0.1 mg
Altavera, Chateal, Kurvelo, Levora, Marlissa, Portia-28, Seasonique; 🍁 Aviane-28, Portia, Seasonale, Seasonique	Ethinyl estradiol 30 mcg	Levonorgestrel 0.15 mg
Junel Fe 1/20, Larin 1/20, Loestrin 1/20, Loestrin Fe 1/20, Microgestin Fe 1/20; 🍁 MinEstrin	Ethinyl estradiol 20 mcg	Norethindrone 1.0 mg
Junel Fe 1.5/30, Junel 21 1.5/30, Larin Fe 1.5/30, Loestrin 21 1.5/30, Loestrin Fe 1.5/30, Microgestin Fe 1.5/30; 🍁 Loestrin 1.5/30	Ethinyl estradiol 30 mcg	Norethindrone 1.5 mg
Ortho-Novum 1/35, Nortrel 1/35, Ortho-Novum 1/35 Brevicon 1/35, Ortho 1/35; 🍁 Select 1/35	Ethinyl estradiol 35 mcg	Norethindrone 1.0 mg
Alyacen, Aranelle, Balziva-28	Ethinyl estradiol 35 mcg	Norethindrone 0.4 mg
Necon 0.5/35, Nortrel 0.5/35	Ethinyl estradiol 35 mcg	Norethindrone 0.5 mg
Cryselle, Elinest, Low-Ogestrel	Ethinyl estradiol 30 mcg	Norgestrel 0.3 mg
Ogestrel	Ethinyl estradiol 50 mcg	Norgestrel 0.5 mg
Kelnor 1/35, Zovia 1/35E	Ethinyl estradiol 35 mcg	Ethynodiol diacetate 1.0 mg
Kelnor 1/50	Ethinyl estradiol 50 mcg	Ethynodiol diacetate 1.0 mg
Apri; 🍁 Apri, Freya, Marvelon	Ethinyl estradiol 30 mcg	Desogestrel 0.15 mg
Yasmin, Syeda, Zarah; 🍁 Zamine, Yasmin (all also approved for PMDD)	Ethinyl estradiol 30 mcg	Drospirenone 3.0 mg
Gianvi, Yaz, Nikki; 🍁 Yaz, Mya (all also approved for PMDD)	Ethinyl estradiol 20 mcg	Drospirenone 3.0 mg
Beyaz, Safyral; 🍁 Yaz Plus (all also approved for PMDD)	Ethinyl estradiol 20 mcg	Drospirenone 3.0 mg and 0.45 mg levomefolate calcium
Estarylla, Ortho-Cyclen, Sprintec, Tri-Cyclen; 🍁 Cyclen, Tri-Cyclen	Ethinyl estradiol 35 mcg	Norgestimate 0.25 mg
Extended-Cycle Monophasics		
Amethyst (taken continuously for 1 y)	Ethinyl estradiol 20 mcg	Levonorgestrel 0.09 mg
Altavera, Chateal, Kurvelo, Quasense; 🍁 Seasonale (taken continuously for 84 d, then low-dose estrogen pills for 7 d)	Ethinyl estradiol 30 mcg	Levonorgestrel 0.15 mg
Lutera, Orsythia, Sronyx (taken continuously for 84 d, then low-dose estrogen pills for 7 d)	Ethinyl estradiol 20	Levonorgestrel 0.10 mg
Biphasics		
Necon 10/11	Ethinyl estradiol 35 mcg	Norethindrone 0.5 mg/1 mg
Azurette, Kariva, Mircette	Ethinyl estradiol 20/10 mcg	Desogestrel 0.15 mg
Lo Loestrin Fe	Ethinyl estradiol 10	Norethindrone 1 mg
Extended-Cycle Biphasics		
LoSeasonique (taken continuously for 84 d, then low-dose estrogen pills for 7 d)	Ethinyl estradiol 20/10 mcg	Levonorgestrel 0.15 mg
Seasonique (taken continuously for 84 d, then low-dose estrogen pills for 7 d)	Ethinyl estradiol 30/10 mcg	Levonorgestrel 0.15 mg

TABLE 7.3

Estrogen–Progestin Combinations Used as Contraceptives (Continued)

Trade Names	Estrogen	Progestin
Triphasics		
Velivet, Caziant, Cyclessa; 🍁 Marvelon, Apri, Freya	Ethinyl estradiol 25 mcg	Desogestrel 0.1/0.125/0.15 mg
Necon 7/7/7, Dasetta 7/7/7	Ethinyl estradiol 35 mcg	Norethindrone 0.5/0.75/1.0 mg
Aranelle, Leena, Tri-Norinyl; 🍁 Lolo, Brevicon	Ethinyl estradiol 35 mcg	Norethindrone 0.5/1.0/0.5 mg
Estrostep Fe, Tri-Legest Fe	Ethinyl estradiol 20/30/35 mcg	Norethindrone 1.0 mg
Ortho Tri-Cyclen, Tri-Sprintec	Ethinyl estradiol 35 mcg	Norgestimate 0.18/0.215/0.25 mg
Ortho Tri-Cyclen Lo, Tri-Lo-Sprintec; 🍁 Tri-Cyclen Lo	Ethinyl estradiol 25 mcg	Norgestimate 0.18/0.215/0.25 mg
Enpresse, Lutera, Sronyx, Trivora-28	Ethinyl estradiol 30/40/30 mcg	Levonorgestrel 0.05/0.075/0.125 mg
Quadriphasic		
Natazia	Estradiol valerate 3/2/2/1 mg	Dienogest 0.0/2.0/3.0/0.0 mg
Extended-Cycle Quadriphasic		
Quartette (taken 91 d, repeat)	Ethinyl estradiol 20/25/30/10 mcg	Levonorgestrel 0.15/0.15/0.15/0
Ortho Evra transdermal patch (Xulane; 🍁 Evra)	Ethinyl estradiol 750 mcg	Norelgestromin 6 mg
NuvaRing vaginal insert (NuvaRing vaginal insert; 🍁 NuvaRing)	Ethinyl estradiol 2.7 mg	Etonogestrel 11.7 mg

Healthcare providers also use oral contraceptive preparations to treat menstrual disorders (e.g., amenorrhea, dysmenorrhea). The FDA has approved some oral contraceptives for the treatment of acne, such as Ortho Tri-Cyclen, Estrostep, and Yaz. Prescribers order Yaz and Beyaz for treatment of PMDD. Continuous-dosing oral contraceptives, which include Seasonale and Seasonique, are useful in the treatment of menorrhagia, metrorrhagia, endometriosis, and PMS. Such continuous-dosing oral contraceptives provide birth control protection for 3 consecutive months while suppressing ovarian function and reducing uterine bleeding; withdrawal bleeding occurs only four times per year.

Table 7.4 presents dosage information for noncontraceptive estrogen–progestin combinations.

Patient-related variables specific to the use of estrogen–progestin contraceptives include the following:

- Age:
  - Estrogen–progestin combinations are contraindicated during pregnancy and breast-feeding.
  - Estrogen–progestin contraceptives are contraindicated in smokers aged 35 years and older due to the increase of thromboembolism.
- Reproduction, pregnancy, and lactation:
  - Estrogen–progestin contraceptives are contraindicated for use in patients with reproductive cancers.
  - Estrogen-containing contraceptives in patients who have had jaundice during pregnancy may cause a reoccurrence of jaundice.
- Abnormal kidney function and hepatic impairment:
  - Oral contraceptives are associated with fluid retention and dilated kidneys due to increased renin–angiotensin–aldosterone system activity. Patients with abnormal kidney function require close evaluation and management.
  - Severe abnormal kidney function may be a contraindication to oral contraceptive use.
  - Hepatic impairment is an absolute contraindication, due to the metabolism of combined oral contraceptives in the liver.
  - Any patient in whom jaundice develops when taking estrogen should stop taking the drug and notify the prescriber.

Adverse Effects

Adverse effects of oral contraceptives may include the GI effects of nausea and vomiting. Taking the drugs with food or at bedtime minimizes nausea. Cardiovascular effects of thromboembolism, myocardial infarction, stroke, and hypertension may also occur. Earlier oral contraceptives, which contained larger amounts of estrogen than those currently used, did cause these problems, and they are much less common in most people who take low-dose preparations. However, for smokers 35 years of age and older, there is an increased risk of myocardial infarction and other cardiovascular disorders, even with low-dose pills. Also, gallbladder disease is more likely in those who use oral contraceptives or estrogen–progestin HRT than in those who do not take hormones. Researchers attribute this to increased concentration of cholesterol in bile acids, which leads to decreased

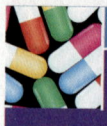

TABLE 7.4
DRUGS AT A GLANCE: Estrogen–Progestin Combinations Used for Noncontraceptive Purposes

Drug	Routes and Dosage Ranges for Various Indications	
	Menopausal Symptoms	**Prevention of Osteoporosis**
ⓟ Conjugated estrogens/medroxyprogesterone acetate (Prempro, Premphase; 🍁 Premplus)	PO 0.3/1.5 mg–0.625/2.5 mg daily	PO 0.3/1.5 mg–0.625/2.5 mg daily
Conjugated estrogens/medroxyprogesterone acetate (Premphase)	PO 0.625/5.0 mg daily	PO 0.625/5.0 mg daily
Estradiol/norethindrone (Activella, Amabelz; 🍁 Estalis)	PO 0.05 mg/0.1 every day; PO 1 mg/0.5 mg every day	PO 0.05 mg/0.1 every day; 1 mg/0.5 mg every day
Ethinyl estradiol/norethindrone acetate (FemHRT; 🍁 FemHRT)	PO 2.5 mcg/0.5 mg every day; PO 5 mcg/1 mg every day	PO 2.5 mcg/0.5 mg every day; PO 5 mcg/1 mg every day
Estradiol/drospirenone (Angeliq; 🍁 Angeliq)	PO 5 mcg/1 mg every day	PO 5 mcg/1 mg every day
Estradiol/levonorgestrel (Climara Pro; 🍁 Climara Pro)	Transdermal 0.045 mg/0.015 weekly	
Estradiol/norethindrone (CombiPatch; 🍁 Activella, Estalis)	Transdermal 0.05 mg/0.14 mg twice a week; transdermal 0.05 mg/0.25 mg twice a week	
Estradiol/progesterone (Bijuva)	PO 1 mg/100 mg every day	

solubility and increased precipitation of stones. Finally, edema, weight gain, and headache are other adverse effects that may be associated with combined oral contraceptives.

The FDA has issued the following **BOXED WARNING** ◆ regarding the use of oral contraceptives:

- Cigarette smoking increases the risk of cardiovascular adverse effects, especially in females 35 years of age and older.
- Possibility of broken bones and osteoporosis, especially after menopause, from loss of stored calcium from bones with the use of Depo-Provera and Depo-SubQ Provera. There is a greater risk of bone loss with long-term use.
- Risks of thromboembolic events increase with use of the Ortho Evra transdermal patch due to the higher levels of estrogen that are circulated into the blood.

Quality and Safety Alert: Evidence-Based Practice

Several studies have examined the risk of venous thromboembolism with hormone contraceptives. The results have been conflicting. No large prospective randomized studies have compared varying amounts of estrogen and progestin or routes of administration with the risk of venous thromboembolism. A systematic review and meta-analysis of venous thromboembolism among oral contraceptive users found that certain progestins did increase the risk. Increased venous thromboembolism risks were found among those monophasic [30 mcg of ethinyl estrogen] oral contraceptives containing the progestins; cyproterone acetate, desogestrel, drospirenone, and gestodene compared to levonorgestrel [Dragoman et al., 2018]. Providing appropriate health education regarding the adverse thromboembolic effects associated with hormonal contraception is essential. In patients 35 years of age or older, it is important to obtain a careful health history to assess for cardiovascular risk factors. Careful assessment and monitoring of blood pressure are essential, and elevations warrant discontinuation of hormonal contraception. Finally, hormonal contraception is contraindicated in people 35 years of age or older who use tobacco products.

Contraindications

Despite the decreased estrogen dosage, combined oral contraceptives are associated with several contraindications. These include cigarette smoking, age 35 years and older, a history of thromboembolic problems, and concurrent cirrhosis or active viral hepatitis, diabetes mellitus, hypertension, or migraine with aura. When estrogen is contraindicated, it is permissible to use a progestin-only contraceptive.

Yasmin, Yaz, and Beyaz contain the progestin drospirenone, which increases serum potassium. Therefore, contraindications to these oral contraceptives include abnormal kidney function, liver, or adrenal insufficiency; use of potassium-sparing diuretics, potassium supplements, angiotensin-converting enzyme inhibitors, angiotensin II receptor agonists, and heparin; and continuous, long-term use of nonsteroidal anti-inflammatory drugs.

Nursing Implications

It is necessary to assess each patient's need and desire for contraception, as well as willingness to comply with the prescribed regimen. Assessment includes determining a patient's knowledge about birth control, both pharmacologic and nonpharmacologic, and identifying patients in whom hormonal contraceptives are contraindicated or who are at increased risk for adverse drug effects. Adherence involves the willingness to take the drugs as prescribed and to have breast and pelvic examinations and blood pressure measurements every 6 to 12 months. The goal of effective oral contraceptive use is the prevention of pregnancy with the lowest effective dose of hormones.

Preventing Interactions

Several medications may reduce the effectiveness of oral contraceptives (i.e., increase the likelihood of pregnancy; Box 7.3). These include medications for tuberculosis and HIV as well as anticonvulsants. Patients should notify all healthcare providers who prescribe medications that they are taking a birth control pill. Use of an additional or alternative method of birth control is necessary (1) if a dose is missed or (2) if the oral contraceptive cannot be taken because of illness or infection.

> **Quality and Safety Alert: Safety**
>
> It is essential to add a different method of birth control while taking certain medications for the remainder of that reproductive cycle.

As previously mentioned, St. John's wort increases the breakdown of estrogen, which can decrease the effectiveness of birth control pills.

Administering the Medication

Numerous preparations are available, with different components and different doses of components, so that a preparation can be chosen to meet individual needs. Most oral contraceptives contain an estrogen and a progestin. The estrogen dose is usually 30 to 35 mcg. Smaller amounts (e.g., 20 mcg) may be adequate for small or underweight patients; larger amounts (e.g., 50 mcg) may be needed for large or overweight patients. Effects of estrogen components are similar when prescribed in equipotent doses, but progestins differ in progestogenic, estrogenic, antiestrogenic, and androgenic activity. Consequently, adverse effects may differ to some extent, and a patient may be able to tolerate one contraceptive better than another.

BOX 7.3 Drug Interactions: Oral Contraceptives

Drugs That Decrease the Effects of Oral Contraceptives

- Anticonvulsants, such as carbamazepine, hydantoins (ethotoin, mephenytoin, phenytoin), and succinimides:
  Induce hepatic cytochrome P450, resulting in increased metabolism
- Barbiturates such as phenobarbital, primidone, griseofulvin:
  Increase metabolism
- Benzodiazepines, rifampin, St. John's wort:
  Activate the hepatic enzyme cytochrome P450, resulting in increased metabolism
- Topiramate:
  Decreases contraceptive efficacy and increases breakthrough bleeding

---

Clinical Application 7.4

- Mrs. Bigelow has her FSH level measured, as ordered by her healthcare provider, and the levels are within normal range. After completion of her history, physical examination, and diagnostic tests, her healthcare provider begins her on hormonal contraceptives for menstrual regulation. She is on the second cycle of pills when she calls reporting irregular bleeding and requests a new pill. What is the nurse's best response?

Assessing for Therapeutic Effects

When taken correctly, estrogen–progestin contraceptive preparations are nearly 100% effective in preventing pregnancy. Therapeutic effects of oral contraceptives include the prevention of pregnancy with regulation of menses with shorter, lighter flow and reduction in ovarian cyst formation. Improvements in hemoglobin may occur due to decreased menstrual flow or if females are taking oral contraceptives with added iron.

Assessing for Adverse Effects

It is crucial to monitor for adverse drug effects such as high blood pressure, gallbladder disease, and blood clotting disorders, which may be associated with oral contraceptive use. The assessment of weight, blood pressure, regularity of menses (occurring only on the withdrawal pills), absence of chest pain, abdominal pain, headache, vision changes, and leg pain indicates an absence of adverse effects of the oral contraceptives.

Patient Teaching

It is essential that the patient seek information about the use of oral contraceptives. The nurse should be sure that the patient understands that oral contraceptives are very effective at preventing pregnancy but *do not* prevent transmission of sexually transmitted infections (e.g., human immunodeficiency virus [HIV], *Chlamydia*, gonorrhea). Box 7.2 presents teaching guidelines for patients taking contraceptives.

Unfolding Patient Stories: Rachel Heidebrink • Part 1

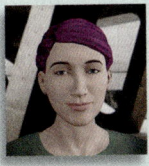

Rachel Heidebrink, a 22-year-old who sustained a fracture to the right greater trochanter in a motorcycle accident and had right hip hemiarthroplasty, developed a pulmonary embolism on postoperative day 1. The patient is on an oral estrogen–progestin combination for contraception. What actions should the nurse take when considering the diagnosis and adverse effects of the medication? (Rachel Heidebrink's story continues in Chapter 9.)

Care for Rachel and other patients in a realistic virtual environment: **vSim** *for Nursing* (thepoint.lww.com/vSimPharm). Practice documenting these patients' care in DocuCare (thepoint.lww.com/DocuCareEHR).

NCLEX Success

3. Patient teaching for a patient who will be using the transdermal patch Ortho Evra should include which of the following? (Select all that apply.)
   A. Apply to skin daily.
   B. Apply to clean and dry skin.
   C. Apply the patch on the same day of the week each week for 3 weeks.
   D. Apply the patch the first day of the menstrual cycle initially.
   E. Use a backup method for birth control the first 2 weeks of using the patch.
   F. Use a backup method for birth control the first 3 weeks of using the patch.

4. When oral contraceptives are contraindicated in a patient with liver disease, what other birth control option would be safe?
   A. Ortho Evra (contraceptive patch)
   B. Depo-Provera (injectable progestin)
   C. barrier method (condoms)
   D. Nexplanon (subdermal implant)

5. After patient teaching of the warning signs associated with combination hormonal contraception, what statement would result in the nurse providing additional education?
   A. "Breakthrough bleeding is a sign of a uterine abnormality."
   B. "I should immediately go to the emergency department if I get a sudden, severe headache that is not relieved with rest or analgesic."
   C. "Severe leg pain and swelling should immediately be reported."
   D. "Cardiovascular problems are the most severe adverse effect associated with oral contraceptives."

THE NURSING PROCESS

A concept map outlines the nursing process related to drug therapy considerations in this chapter. Additional nursing implications related to the disease process should also be considered in care decisions.

Assessment
- Periodic monitoring is needed throughout the drug therapy. A thorough health history is needed to determine conditions in which the drugs are used (i.e., pregnancy prevention, menopause, premenstrual syndrome).
- Assess for contraindications to drug therapy (i.e., allergies to drug components, current pregnancy and lactation status, history of seizure disorders, thrombophlebitis, cardiovascular disease, hepatic disease, kidney disease, osteoporosis, undiagnosed vaginal bleeding or pelvic disease, reproductive cancers, smoking, age, etc).
- Assess attitudes regarding the use of hormone use.
- Obtain baseline vital signs including, height, weight, body mass index (BMI), heart rate and blood pressure. It is important to continue to monitor these at subsequent visits.
- Assist with or complete a thorough physical examination including assessment of heart, lungs, abdomen, breasts, and pelvis before beginning treatment and annually during treatment.
- Monitor laboratory results, including urinalysis, kidney function tests, hemoglobin, Pap smear results, and sexually transmitted infection results.

Outcomes of Therapy
The patient will
- Use the drugs only as directed.
- Avoid preventable adverse drug effects.
- Monitor for adverse drug effects and report those immediately if they occur.
- Adhere to monitoring and follow-up examinations/procedures.

Nursing Interventions
- Educate the patient regarding the proper use of the drug therapy and the adverse drug effects.
- Administer the drug as prescribed to prevent adverse effects (i.e., IM injection with Depo-Provera).
- Schedule the patient at the minimum an annual examination and follow-up as recommended.
- Monitor laboratory results and ensure that patients schedule follow-up appointments.

Evaluation
- Interview and observe for accurate drug administration.
- Interview and observe for the effectiveness of the drug and the patient for response to the drug.
- Interview and observe for adverse effects for the drug.
- Compare follow-up blood pressure, BMI, and pertinent laboratory results to baseline values for acceptable levels.
- Evaluate the patient satisfaction of the drug therapy.

Visit thePoint® at http://thePoint.lww.com/Frandsen13e for answers to NCLEX Success questions (in Appendix A), answers to Clinical Application Case Studies (in Appendix B), additional information on pathophysiology, and more!

REFERENCES AND RESOURCES

American College of Obstetricians and Gynecologists (ACOG). (2000). ACOG Practice Bulletin: Number 15. *Obstetrics & Gynecology, 95*(4), 1–9.

American Psychiatric Association. (2013). *Diagnostic and statistical manual of mental disorders* (5th ed.). American Psychiatric Publishing.

Britton, L. E., Alspaugh, A., Greene, M. Z., & McLemore, M. R. (2020). An evidence-based update on contraception. *American Journal of Nursing, 120*(2), 22–33.

Dragoman, M. V., Tepper, N. K., Fu, R., Curtis, K. M., Chou, R., & Gaffield, M. E. (2018). A systematic review and meta-analysis of venous thrombosis risk among users of combined oral contraception. *International Journal of Gynecology & Obstetrics, 141*(3), 287–294.

Gudipally, P. R., & Sharma, G. K. (2020). *Premenstrual syndrome.* https://www.ncbi.nlm.nih.gov/books/NBK560698/

Karch, A. (2019). *Focus on nursing pharmacology* (8th ed.). Wolters Kluwer.

Kim, J. E., Chang, J. H., Jeong, M. J., Choi, J., Park, J. Y., Chaewon Baek, C., Shin, A., Park, S. M., Kang, D., & Choi, J.-Y. (2020). A systematic review and meta-analysis of effects of menopausal hormone therapy on cardiovascular diseases. *Scientific Reports, 10*(20631). doi.org/10.1038/s41598-020-77534-9

Manson, J. E., Bassuk, S. S., Kaunitz, A. M., & Pinkerton, J. V. (2020). The Women's Health Initiative trials of menopausal hormone therapy: Lessons learned. *Menopause, 27*(8), 918–928.

Mehta, J., Kling, J. M., & Manson, J. E. (2021). Risks, benefits, and treatment modalities of hormonal replacement therapy: Current concepts. *Frontiers in Endocrinology, 12,* 564781. doi.org/10.3389/fendo.2021.564781

Mishra, S., Elliot, H., & Marwaha, R. (2021). *Premenstrual dysphoric disorder.* https://www.ncbi.nlm.nih.gov/books/NBK532307/

Norris, T. L. (2019). *Porth's pathophysiology: Concepts of altered health states* (10th ed.). Wolters Kluwer.

Ricci, S. S. (2020). *Essentials of maternity, newborn, and women's health nursing.* Wolters Kluwer.

Trussell, J., Raymond, E. G., & Cleland, K. (2018). *Emergency contraception: A last chance to prevent unintended pregnancy.* http://ec.princeton.edu/questions/ec-review.pdf

Yonkers, K. A., & Simoni, M. K. (2018). Premenstrual disorders. *American Journal of Gynecology, 18*(1), 68–74. doi:10.1016/j.ajog.2017.05.045

Zondervan, K. T., Phil, D., Becker, C. M., & Missmer, S. A. (2020). Endometriosis. *New England Journal of Medicine, 382*(13), 1244–1256. doi:10.1056/NEJMra1810764

CHAPTER 8

Pharmacology and Male Health

LEARNING OBJECTIVES

After studying this chapter, you should be able to:

1. Discuss common male reproductive problems in terms of clinical considerations and manifestations.
2. Describe the androgens in terms of prototype, mechanism of action, indications for use, major adverse effects, and nursing implications.
3. Identify potential consequences of abusing androgens and anabolic steroids.
4. Discuss the phosphodiesterase type 5 inhibitors in terms of prototype, mechanism of action, indications for use, major adverse effects, and nursing implications.
5. Describe the 5-alpha reductase inhibitors in terms of prototype, mechanism of action, indications for use, major adverse effects, and nursing implications.
6. Describe the alpha-adrenergic blockers in terms of prototype, mechanism of action, indications for use, major adverse effects, and nursing implications.
7. Implement the nursing process for males who have reproductive disorders.

CLINICAL APPLICATION CASE STUDY

Phillip Johnson, a 52-year-old veterinarian, is seen in the clinic for hypertension control. He has a one-pack per day history of cigarette smoking and has begun walking to reduce his weight. For 5 years, he has been taking hydrochlorothiazide and atenolol to lower his blood pressure, which is well controlled. He has no other chronic health problems.

However, Mr. Johnson reports significant erectile dysfunction that has progressed over the past 9 months. This has significantly distressed him and his wife and has caused considerable marital discord.

KEY TERMS

Anabolic steroids: synthetic drugs with increased anabolic activity and decreased androgenic activity compared with testosterone

Androgen: male sex hormones, primarily testosterone, secreted by the testes in males, the ovaries in females, and the adrenal cortex in both males and females

Benign prostatic hypertrophy (BPH): benign enlargement of the prostate gland; also known as benign prostatic hyperplasia

Erectile dysfunction (ED): difficulty in initiating or maintaining penile erection that is satisfactory for sexual relations

Erectogenic: capable of causing an erection

Ergogenic: increase in muscular work capacity caused by drugs that enhance athletic performance

Testosterone: male sex hormone; secreted by the Leydig cells in the testes

INTRODUCTION

This chapter explores the drugs used to manage disorders and conditions that affect male reproductive health. To understand the drugs discussed in this chapter, an overview of the main disorders of male reproduction and clinical manifestations are described.

OVERVIEW OF REPRODUCTIVE HEALTH PROBLEMS IN MALES

This chapter highlights three conditions related to reproductive health common to males: androgen deficiency, erectile dysfunction, and benign prostatic hypertrophy.

Clinical Considerations

Androgen Deficiency

Lack of sufficient **testosterone**, the primary male sex hormone, can result in congenital or acquired hypogonadism in the male. Causes include genetic diseases, head or testicular trauma, alkylating agents, tumors, and radiation injury.

- Primary hypogonadism results from a testicular disorder. Common diseases that can cause primary hypogonadism are mumps, testicular inflammation, and trauma.
- Secondary hypogonadism results from a problem in the hypothalamus or the pituitary gland, areas of the brain that signal the testicles to produce testosterone, such as thyroid disorders, Cushing syndrome, or estrogen-secreting tumors. Chronic diseases (e.g., metabolic syndrome, diabetes) can lead to secondary hypogonadism.

Erectile Dysfunction

Erectile dysfunction (ED) is defined as difficulty initiating or maintaining penile erection that is satisfactory for sexual relations. ED is common in males with systemic disorders such as hypertension, ischemic heart disease, and diabetes and is associated with thyroid conditions, prostate cancer, and spinal cord injuries. Several research studies indicate that ED is a powerful predictor and risk factor of coronary artery disease, especially in males with no symptoms or history of cardiovascular disease and those older than 60 years of age. In addition, several drugs (antidepressants, antihypertensive agents, antipsychotics, diuretics, histamine receptor antagonists) and lifestyle factors (alcohol, tobacco, or cocaine use, obesity) have been known to cause the condition. Low testosterone levels rarely lead to ED but may reduce sex drive. Psychologic factors may also play a role, and these include sexual performance anxiety, relationship conflicts, and cultural and religious taboos.

Benign Prostatic Hypertrophy

Benign prostatic hypertrophy (BPH), also known as benign prostatic hyperplasia, is benign enlargement of the prostate gland.

It is thought that BPH is a normal element of the male aging process. Causes include changes in hormone balance and cell growth. Testosterone undergoes reduction to form the more potent androgen DHT, which has greater affinity for androgen receptors than testosterone. During the formation and growth of an embryo, DHT plays a critical role in the formation of the male external genitalia, whereas in the adult, DHT acts as the primary androgen in the prostate and in hair follicles.

Clinical Manifestations

Androgen Deficiency

Signs and symptoms of **androgen** deficiency in adult males include ED, infertility, decreased beard and body hair growth, decreased muscle mass, breast development (gynecomastia), and loss of bone mass (osteoporosis). Hypogonadism can also cause mental and emotional changes. As testosterone decreases, some males may experience symptoms similar to those of menopause in females, including fatigue, decreased sex drive, difficulty concentrating, and hot flashes.

To confirm a diagnosis of hypogonadism, it is necessary to perform laboratory tests. Serum testosterone is decreased. To determine the cause, it is also necessary to measure hormone levels in the serum: FSH, LH, prolactin, thyroid hormone, and estradiol. If normal or elevated FSH and LH serum levels are present with a low testosterone level and the testes are nonresponsive to hormonal stimulation, a primary hypogonadism is present. If FSH and LH are low along with the testosterone level, a secondary hypogonadism is present.

Erectile Dysfunction

The main clinical manifestation of ED is the consistent inability to attain or maintain an erection satisfactory for sexual activity. An associated symptom may be reduced sexual desire.

Benign Prostatic Hypertrophy

Clinical manifestations of BPH result from the obstruction of the urethra from the enlargement of the prostate gland, causing reduction in outflow of urine.

Males may experience urinary frequency, hesitancy, urgency, dribbling, and decrease force of the urinary stream. Nocturia, postvoid leakage, urinary stones, or infection can also occur.

On physical examination, a midline mass above the symphysis pubis, which likely represents an incompletely emptied bladder, may be visible. On digital rectal examination, rubbery enlargement of the prostate is present. Excretory urography may indicate emptying and filling defects in the bladder, urinary tract obstruction, calculi or tumors, and hydronephrosis.

Drug Therapy

Table 8.1 outlines the drugs used to maintain male reproductive health, which include the androgens and **anabolic steroids**, the phosphodiesterase type 5 (PDE5) inhibitors and prostaglandins, and the 5-alpha reductase inhibitors and the alpha$_1$-adrenergic blockers (Box 8.1).

ANDROGENS AND ANABOLIC STEROIDS

When clinicians use male sex hormones or androgens from exogenous sources for therapeutic purposes, the effects are the same as those of naturally occurring hormones. These effects include inhibition of endogenous sex hormones and sperm formation through negative feedback of pituitary LH and FSH. Anabolic steroids are synthetic drugs with increased anabolic activity and decreased androgenic activity compared with endogenous testosterone. They were developed during attempts to modify testosterone so that its tissue-building and growth-stimulating effects could be retained while the drug's masculinizing effects could be eliminated or reduced.

Prescribers may order male sex hormones for females to antagonize or reduce the effects of female sex hormones.

TABLE 8.1 Drugs Administered for Maintenance of Male Reproductive Health

Drug Class	Prototype	Other Drugs in the Class
Androgens	Testosterone	Methyltestosterone, Danazol*
Phosphodiesterase type 5 inhibitors	Sildenafil (Viagra, Revatio)	Avanafil (Stendra), Tadalafil (Cialis), Vardenafil (Levitra)
Prostaglandins		Alprostadil (Caverject aqueous, Caverject powder, Edex powder, Muse)
5-Alpha reductase inhibitors	Finasteride (Proscar)	Dutasteride (Avodart)
Alpha$_1$-adrenergic blockers	Tamsulosin (Flomax)	Alfuzosin (Uroxatral, Xatral), Doxazosin (Cardura), Silodosin (Rapaflo), Terazosin

*Used in females.

BOX 8.1 Effects of Testosterone on Body Tissues

Fetal Development

Large amounts of chorionic gonadotropin are produced by the placenta during pregnancy. Chorionic gonadotropin is similar to luteinizing hormone (LH) from the anterior pituitary gland. It promotes development of the interstitial or Leydig cells in fetal testes responsible for androgen production, which then secrete testosterone. Testosterone production begins in the 2nd month of fetal life. When present, testosterone promotes development of male sexual characteristics (e.g., penis, scrotum, prostate gland, seminal vesicles, and seminiferous tubules) and suppresses development of female sexual characteristics. In the absence of testosterone, the fetus develops female sexual characteristics.

Testosterone also provides the stimulus for the descent of the testes into the scrotum. This normally occurs after the 7th month of pregnancy, when the fetal testes are secreting relatively large amounts of testosterone. If the testes do not descend before birth, administration of testosterone or gonadotropic hormone, which stimulates testosterone secretion, produces descent in most cases.

Adult Development

Little testosterone is secreted in male children until 11 to 13 years of age. At the onset of puberty, testosterone secretion increases rapidly and remains at a relatively high level until about 50 years of age, after which it gradually declines.

The testosterone secreted at puberty acts as a growth hormone to produce enlargement of the penis, testes, and scrotum until approximately 20 years of age. The prostate gland, seminal vesicles, seminiferous tubules, and vas deferens also increase in size and functional ability. Under the combined influence of testosterone and follicle-stimulating hormone (FSH) from the anterior pituitary gland, sperm production is initiated and maintained throughout reproductive life. It affects various parts of the body.

- Skin. Testosterone increases skin thickness and activity of the sebaceous glands. Acne in the male adolescent is attributed to the increased production of testosterone.
- Voice. The larynx enlarges and deepens the voice of the adult male.
- Hair. Testosterone produces the distribution of hair growth on the face, limbs, and trunk typical of the adult man. In males with a genetic trait toward baldness, large amounts of testosterone cause alopecia (baldness) of the scalp.
- Skeletal muscles. Testosterone and its effects on protein metabolism are largely responsible for the larger, more powerful muscles of males. Testosterone helps the body retain nitrogen, form new amino acids, and build new muscle protein. At the same time, it slows the loss of nitrogen and amino acids formed by the constant breakdown of body tissues. Overall, testosterone increases protein anabolism (buildup) and decreases protein catabolism (breakdown).
- Bone. Testosterone makes bones thicker and longer. After puberty, more protein and calcium are deposited and retained in bone matrix causing a rapid rate of bone growth. The height of a male adolescent increases rapidly and then stops as epiphyseal closure occurs, when the cartilage at the end of the long bones in the arms and legs becomes bone, preventing further lengthening.

Anterior Pituitary Function

- High blood levels of testosterone decrease secretion of FSH and LH from the anterior pituitary gland. This, in turn, decreases testosterone production.

Thus, administration of androgenic or anabolic steroids to females causes suppression of menstruation and atrophy of the endometrial lining of the uterus.

Several dosage forms of androgens are available. They differ mainly in route of administration and pharmacokinetics. **Testosterone** is the prototype.

Pharmacokinetics

Like endogenous testosterone, the drug molecules are highly bound (98%) to plasma proteins and serum half-life varies (e.g., 8 days for intramuscular [IM] testosterone cypionate, 9 hours for oral fluoxymesterone). Testosterone is extensively metabolized in its first pass through the liver, so that nearly half of a dose is lost before it reaches the systemic circulation. About 90% of a dose is excreted in urine as conjugates of testosterone and its metabolites; the remainder is excreted in feces.

Action

Like other steroid drugs, testosterone penetrates the cell membrane and binds to receptor proteins in the cell cytoplasm. The steroid–receptor complex is then transported to the nucleus, where it activates ribonucleic acid (RNA) and deoxyribonucleic acid (DNA) production and stimulates cellular synthesis of protein.

Use

With testosterone, the most clear-cut indication for use is to treat androgen deficiency states (e.g., hypogonadism, cryptorchidism, impotence, oligospermia) in males of all ages. In postpubertal males who become androgen deficient, the hormone reestablishes and maintains masculine characteristics and functions. Table 8.2 gives route and dosage information for testosterone and other androgens and anabolic steroids.

Patient-related variables specific to the use of testosterone and other androgens and anabolic steroids include the following:

- Age:
  - The main indication for testosterone use in male children is for established sex hormone deficiencies; the hormone stimulates the development of masculine characteristics.
  - Virilization has been reported in children who were secondarily exposed to topical testosterone gel and solution; children should avoid contact with application sites in males using topical testosterone.
  - Sodium and water retention associated with testosterone may aggravate hypertension and other cardiovascular disorders in older adults.
  - Older males taking testosterone may be at greater risk for prostatic hyperplasia, prostate cancer, fluid retention, and transaminase elevations.

TABLE 8.2

DRUGS AT A GLANCE: Androgens

Drug	Routes and Dosage Ranges	
	Hypogonadism	Other
Testosterone cypionate (Depo-Testosterone; Andriol, Androderm, Axiron, Testim)	50–200 mg IM every 2–4 wk	
Testosterone enanthate (Xyosted; Andriol, Androderm, Axiron, Testim)	50–200 mg IM every 2–4 wk	
Testosterone gel (AndroGel 1%; AndroGel)	Apply 5 g (50 mg of drug) once daily in morning to skin of shoulders and upper arms or abdomen	
Testosterone pellets	150–80 mg sub-Q every 3–6 mo	Delayed puberty: lower dosage range sub-Q, for a limited duration (e.g., every 3 mo for 2–3 doses)
Testosterone transdermal systems (Androderm; Andriol, Androderm, AndroGel, Axiron)	Apply two systems (dose of 5 mg) nightly to back, abdomen, upper arm, or thigh	Transdermal preparations not recommended for use in children
Methyltestosterone		Cryptorchidism: 30 mg PO daily; buccal tablets, 15 mg PO daily
Danazol (Cyclomen)		Endometriosis: 800 mg PO daily in two divided doses for 3–9 mo Fibrocystic breast disease: 100–400 mg PO daily in two divided doses for 3–6 mo

- Reproduction, pregnancy, and lactation:
  - Testosterone is a component of female to male therapy for transgender males. Treatment may cause temporary or permanent infertility, and although menstruation may be suppressed, ovulation may occur. To avoid unwanted pregnancy, educate transgender males having sex with males to consider contraception.
  - Testosterone is teratogenic to the fetus so it should not be used during pregnancy.
  - The drug is present in breast milk.
- Abnormal kidney function and hepatic impairment:
  - Testosterone may cause fluid retention.
  - Use with caution in patients with hepatic impairment.

Quality and Safety Alert: Safety

Because testosterone can cause epiphyseal closure, it is essential to examine a child's hands and wrists using radiography every 6 months to detect bone maturation and to check that there is no loss of height if receiving testosterone therapy.

Stimulation of skeletal growth should continue for approximately 6 months after testosterone therapy stops. If premature puberty occurs (e.g., precocious sexual development, enlarged penis), it is necessary to stop the drug. Testosterones may cause or aggravate acne. Scrupulous skin care and other antiacne treatment may be necessary, especially in adolescent boys.

Adverse Effects

Common adverse effects from testosterone include acne, change in sex drive, hair loss, headache, bitter taste or mouth irritation, or gum tenderness. Additionally, hypercalcemia, jaundice, and edema may occur. Virilizing or masculinizing effects may vary. In adult males with adequate secretion of testosterone, adverse effects include priapism, increased sexual desire, reduced sperm count, and prostate enlargement. In prepubertal boys, adverse effects may involve premature development of sex organs and secondary sexual characteristics, such as enlargement of the penis and pubic hair. Priapism may occur. In females, adverse effects include hirsutism, deepening of the voice, and menstrual irregularities.

Contraindications

Contraindications to testosterone include pregnancy (because of possible masculinizing effects on a female fetus), preexisting liver disease, and disorders of the prostate. (Males with an enlarged prostate may have additional enlargement, and males with prostate cancer may experience tumor growth.)

Nursing Implications

Preventing Interactions

Some medications interact with testosterone, decreasing its effects (Box 8.2). Androgens may increase effects of cyclosporine and warfarin, apparently by slowing their metabolism and increasing their concentrations in the blood. Avoid these combinations,

BOX 8.2 Drug Interactions: Testosterone

Drugs That Decrease the Effects of Testosterone
- Barbiturates
  Increase enzyme induction and rate of metabolism
- Calcitonin
  Decreases calcium retention, thus antagonizing the calcium-retaining effects of androgens

when possible. If they are necessary, the nurse monitors serum creatinine and cyclosporine levels (for cyclosporine) and prothrombin time or international normalized ratio (INR) (for warfarin). High-fat meals decrease the effects of testosterone.

Concept Mastery Alert

Concurrent use of androgens with sulfonylureas is to be avoided if possible because androgens increase the effect of sulfonylureas. If simultaneous use is required, smaller sulfonylurea doses may be necessary, and blood glucose levels are to be monitored closely. Patients are to be assessed for signs of hypoglycemia.

Administering the Medication

Naturally occurring androgens are given by injection because they are metabolized rapidly by the liver if given orally. Some esters of testosterone have been modified to slow the rate of metabolism and thus prolong action. For example, IM testosterone cypionate and testosterone enanthate have slow onsets of action and last 2 to 4 weeks. As a result of first-pass metabolism, doses as high as 400 mg/day may be needed to produce adequate blood levels for full replacement therapy.

Several transdermal formulations of testosterone are available. They have a rapid onset of action and last approximately 24 hours. A topical gel (a 10-g dose delivers 100 mg) produces normal serum testosterone levels within 4 hours after application, and absorption of testosterone into the blood continues for 24 hours. Steady-state serum concentrations occur by the 2nd or 3rd day of use. When the gel is discontinued, serum testosterone levels remain in the normal range for 24 to 48 hours but decrease to pretreatment levels within about 5 days.

Assessing for Therapeutic and Adverse Effects

The nurse assesses for return of sex hormone levels, development of masculine characteristics in boys, and return of libido in adult males.

The nurse should assess for adverse effects, including hypersensitivity reaction, changes in sexual drive or masculinization, hair loss, changes in taste, oral irritation, and/or gum tenderness. The nurse also monitors serum calcium and observes for signs of hypercalcemia (e.g., kidney stones, polyuria, abdominal pain, nausea, vomiting, depression).

Patient Teaching

Box 8.3 presents patient teaching information for androgens.

BOX 8.3 Patient Teaching Guidelines for Androgens

General Considerations

- Be aware that use by athletes for body building is inappropriate and, if not prescribed by a licensed prescriber, is illegal.
- Continue medical supervision as long as the drugs are being taken.
- Weigh self once or twice weekly and record the amount. An increase may indicate fluid retention and edema.
- Practice frequent and thorough skin cleansing to decrease acne, which is most likely to occur in females and children.
- Keep all appointments for laboratory testing and follow-up care.
- As with all drugs, keep these medications in the original container, tightly closed, and out of reach of children.

Self-Administration

- Take oral preparations before or with meals, in divided doses.
- For buccal preparations, adhere to the following guidelines:
  - Take in divided doses.
  - Place the tablet between the cheek and gum and allow to dissolve (do not swallow).
  - Avoid eating, drinking, or smoking while the tablet is in place.
- For transdermal systems, adhere to the following guidelines:
  - Apply two Androderm systems nightly to clean, dry skin on the back, abdomen, upper arm, or thigh. Do not apply to the scrotum. Rotate sites, with 7 days between applications to a site. Press firmly into place for adherence.
  - Apply the prescribed amount of gel to clean, dry, intact skin of the shoulders and upper arms or the abdomen (do not apply to the genital area), once daily, preferably in the morning. Wash hands after application and allow sites to dry before dressing. After application, wait at least 1 hour and preferably 4 to 6 hours before showering or swimming.

Other Drugs in the Class

Danazol is a synthetic testosterone with weak androgenic activity. Clinicians may use the drug in females to prevent or treat endometriosis or fibrocystic breast disease. Danazol is seldom prescribed continuously beyond 6 months because it produces the same androgenic adverse effects as other androgens, which are of particular concern in females. Although some drug literature still lists metastatic breast cancer and some types of anemia as indications for use of androgens, newer drugs have largely replaced them for these purposes. In breast cancer, androgens are second-line hormonal agents, after antiestrogens (e.g., tamoxifen). In anemia associated with kidney failure, synthetic erythropoietin is more effective and more likely to be used. Administration of danazol is oral, and metabolism occurs in the liver. The route of excretion is unknown. A issued by the U.S. Food and Drug Administration (FDA) states that danazol is contraindicated in pregnancy and that a pregnancy test should be administered prior to the start of therapy. In addition, a nonhormonal method of contraception should be used during treatment. The warning also states that use of the drug is associated with the risk of a thromboembolic event and/or intracranial hypertension.

Methyltestosterone is a synthetic formulation of testosterone that can be used in adolescent males with delayed puberty to produce puberty. The drug is less extensively metabolized by the liver and more suitable for oral administration.

Abuse of Androgens and Anabolic Steroids

Drugs used to enhance athletic performance are termed **ergogenic** (causing an increase in muscular work capacity). Androgens and anabolic steroids are widely abused in attempts to enhance muscle development, muscle strength, and athletic performance.

 Quality and Safety Alert: Safety

Because of their abuse potential, androgens and anabolic steroids are schedule III controlled substances.

Although nonprescription sales of the drugs are illegal, they can be obtained. Athletes are considered a high-risk group because some start taking the drugs at a young age and continue for years. The use of performance-enhancing drugs in nonathletes is also on the rise Although steroids have a reputation for being dangerous to adult athletes, they are considered even more dangerous for teens because teens are still growing, and long-term effects may be as serious as those that occur with use of other illegal drugs.

Quality and Safety Alert: Safety

Anabolic steroids can stop bone growth and damage the heart, kidneys, and liver of adolescents.

In addition to those who take steroids to enhance athletic performance, some males take the drugs to produce a more muscular and impressive appearance. Steroid abusers usually take massive doses and often take several drugs or combine injectable and oral drugs for maximum effects. The large doses produce potentially serious adverse effects in several body tissues:

- Cardiovascular disorders include hypertension, decreased high-density blood lipoproteins, and increased low-density

lipoproteins, all of which promote heart attacks and strokes.
- Liver disorders include benign and malignant neoplasms, cholestatic hepatitis and jaundice, and peliosis hepatis, a disorder in which blood-filled cysts develop in the liver and may lead to hemorrhage or liver failure.
- Central nervous system disorders include aggression, hostility, combativeness, and dependence characterized by preoccupation with drug use, inability to stop taking the drugs, and withdrawal symptoms similar to those that occur with alcohol, cocaine, and narcotics. In some cases, psychosis may develop.
- Reproductive system disorders include decreased testicular function (e.g., decreased secretion of endogenous testosterone, decreased formation of sperm), testicular atrophy, and impotence in males. They include amenorrhea in females.
- Metabolic disorders include atherosclerosis-promoting changes in cholesterol metabolism and retention of fluids, with edema and other imbalances. Fluid and electrolyte retention contribute to the increased weight associated with drug use.
- Dermatologic disorders include moderate to severe acne in both sexes, depending on drug dosage.

Many of these adverse effects persist several months after the drugs are stopped and may be irreversible.

Androstenedione and DHEA, androgens produced by the adrenal cortex, are also available as over-the-counter (OTC) dietary supplements. They are marketed as safe, natural, alternative androgens for building muscles. These products, which have weak androgenic activity, act mainly as precursors to produce sex hormones.

DHEA is available alone as oral capsules or tablets and in a topical cream with vitamins and herbs. Contraindications to DHEA include prostate cancer or BPH as well as estrogen-responsive breast or uterine cancer, because DHEA may stimulate growth of the cancerous tissues. It is important that patients older than 40 years of age be aggressively screened for hormonally sensitive cancers before taking DHEA.

Adverse effects of DHEA include aggressiveness, hirsutism, insomnia, and irritability. Whether large doses of the OTC products can produce some of the serious adverse effects associated with standard anabolic steroids is unknown.

NCLEX Success

1. Four patients in an endocrine clinic are ordered to begin androgen therapy. The nurse reviews each patient's current medications and identifies which patient as able to begin androgen therapy without the risk of a known drug interaction?
   A. patient 1, taking cyclosporine
   B. patient 2, taking warfarin
   C. patient 3, taking sulfonylureas
   D. patient 4, taking heparin

2. A 19-year-old female athlete presents for her first prenatal visit and tells the nurse she has been on androgen therapy to improve her distance running. She asks the nurse if she can continue taking the androgens to maintain her "competitive edge." The nurse should instruct her that she
   A. can continue taking androgens because the drugs pose no risk to the fetus
   B. can continue taking androgens, but a higher dose will be required due to increased drug metabolism during pregnancy
   C. can continue taking androgens until the third trimester, when they must be discontinued because androgens cause an increased risk of premature rupture of membranes
   D. must stop taking androgens immediately, because they pose a risk to the fetus; she should discuss this with her healthcare provider at today's visit

3. Which of the following statements by a male patient taking transdermal androgens indicates that teaching has been adequate? (Select all that apply.)
   A. "I need to weigh myself once or twice weekly and record the amount."
   B. "I should wash my face and body thoroughly to decrease the risk of acne."
   C. "The patch systems should be applied nightly to skin on my back, abdomen, upper arm, or thigh."
   D. "I should apply the patch systems in the morning to the same site each and every day."

Clinical Application 8.1
- Mr. Johnson asks a nurse if he can take the "little blue pill that will improve his ED" (sildenafil). How should the nurse respond?

PHOSPHODIESTERASE TYPE 5 INHIBITORS

Prescribers commonly order PDE5 inhibitors as the first-line treatment for ED. These drugs do not cause an erection but help maintain the erection resulting from sexual stimuli by enhancing the vasodilatory effect of endogenous nitric oxide, increasing blood flow to the penis. The prototype PDE5 inhibitor is **sildenafil** (Viagra).

Pharmacokinetics

Sildenafil is significantly protein bound and is rapidly absorbed by the oral route. The drug is metabolized in the liver and is primarily excreted in the feces and to a lesser extent by the kidneys. The onset of action is 20 to 60 minutes, with a duration of up to 4 hours.

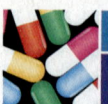

TABLE 8.3
DRUGS AT A GLANCE: Phosphodiesterase Type 5 Inhibitors

Drug	Routes and Dosage Ranges (Adult Males)
Sildenafil (Viagra, Revatio; ✦ AG-Sildenafil, Jamp-Sildenafil, Viagra)	Erectile dysfunction (Viagra): PO 25–100 mg 1 h before sexual activity; reduce dose with age older than 65 y, concurrent use of CYP3A4 inhibitors,* and abnormal kidney function or hepatic impairment
Avanafil (Stendra)	PO 100–200 mg 30 min before anticipated sexual activity, reduced dose with age older than 65 y, hepatic impairment, and concurrent use of CYP3A4 inhibitors*
Tadalafil (Cialis; ✦ Adcirca, Cialis)	PO 2.5–20 mg 2 h or more before anticipated sexual activity, PO 2.5–5 mg once daily, reduced dose with age older than 65 y, abnormal kidney function or hepatic impairment, and concurrent use of CYP3A4 inhibitors*
Vardenafil (Levitra; ✦ Levitra, Staxyn)	PO 5–20 mg 1 h before sexual activity, reduced dose with age older than 65 y, hepatic impairment, and concurrent use of CYP3A4 inhibitors*

*CYP3A4 inhibitors include azole antifungals, erythromycin, and saquinavir.

Action

Sildenafil improves erectile function by inhibiting the enzyme responsible for the breakdown of cyclic guanosine monophosphate (cGMP), a vasodilatory neurotransmitter in corporal tissues of the penis. This causes a vasodilatory effect in the smooth muscle of the corpus cavernosum that allows for a harder and longer-lasting erection.

Use

Sildenafil is used for the treatment of ED in males healthy enough for sexual activity. The FDA has also approved the drug for the treatment of pulmonary arterial hypertension in adult males and children. The drug should not be administered to females. Table 8.3 gives route and dosage information for sildenafil and other PDE5 inhibitors.

Patient-related variables specific to the use of sildenafil and other PDE5 inhibitors include hepatic impairment, as caution is warranted with the use of sildenafil. Patients with cirrhosis or other significant liver dysfunction should start with a lower dose to minimize worsening of the hepatic impairment.

Adverse Effects

Adverse reactions to sildenafil commonly include headache, facial flushing, dyspepsia, nasal congestion, and dizziness. Rarely, clinicians have reported nonarteritic ischemic optic neuropathy (NAION) due to obstruction of blood flow to the optic nerve, resulting in irreversible loss of vision in one or both eyes. Sudden auditory impairment and hearing loss accompanied by dizziness and tinnitus have been reported. Hearing loss is usually unilateral affecting high frequencies and may be reversible. Priapism is rare and usually associated with excessive dosing or concurrent use with another **erectogenic** drug (capable of causing an erection).

Contraindications

Concurrent use of organic nitrates in any form or the use of the drug riociguat should be avoided. Contraindications to sildenafil also include a known hypersensitivity to the drug. In addition, males who are not healthy enough to engage in sexual activity should not take sildenafil.

> **! Quality and Safety Alert: Safety**
>
> Prescribers should not order it for males who also take organic nitrates, commonly used to treat angina, because the sildenafil–nitrate combination can cause severe hypotension resulting in dizziness, syncope, heart attack, or stroke.

Nursing Implications

Preventing Interactions

Sildenafil, like other PDE5 inhibitors, is primarily metabolized by the cytochrome P450 (CYP) enzyme CYP3A4. Many medications interact with sildenafil, increasing or decreasing its effects (Box 8.4). In addition, several herbs and foods increase the drug's effects including grapefruit juice, saw palmetto, and yohimbine. Fatty foods decrease the effects of sildenafil.

Administering the Medication

Administration is generally oral. It is important not to take sildenafil more than once in a 24-hour period. A recent high-fat meal may delay drug action.

> **BOX 8.4 Drug Interactions: Sildenafil**
>
> **Drugs That Increase the Effects of Sildenafil**
> - Alcohol
>   *Increases the risk of orthostatic hypotension, tachycardia, dizziness, and headache*
> - Alpha-adrenergic blockers, antihypertensive drugs, cytochrome P450 3A4 inhibitors (e.g., azole antifungals, erythromycin, saquinavir, protease inhibitors)
>   *Increase risk of hypotension*

Assessing for Therapeutic and Adverse Effects

The nurse should assess that the patient reports the ability to initiate or maintain a penile erection for satisfactory sexual relations. Additionally, the nurse assesses for signs of adverse effects, including headache, facial flushing, dyspepsia, nasal congestion, and dizziness. Patients with symptoms of NAION or sudden decrease or loss of hearing should discontinue sildenafil and seek immediate medical care. Although rare, persistent priapism requires prompt medical treatment to avoid permanent penile damage. Because ED is a strong predictor of coronary artery disease, it is recommended that a cardiovascular assessment be completed in a noncardiac patient who presents with ED.

Patient Teaching

Box 8.5 contains patient teaching guidelines for sildenafil and other drugs for ED.

Other Drugs in the Class

Three other FDA-approved PDE5 inhibitors have similar effectiveness and safety profiles. Avanafil (Stendra), the newest PDE5 inhibitor, is a fast-acting and highly selective member of the class. The drug reaches its peak in 30 minutes, with a duration of 6 hours. Meals do not affect absorption rate or peak levels. Absorption and metabolism of the drug occurs in the liver through the CYP450 system. Excretion takes place in the feces through the bile. Adverse effects, common to other PDE5 inhibitors, include headache, flushing of the face, nasal congestion, and back pain.

BOX 8.5 **Patient Teaching Guidelines for Sildenafil and Other Drugs Used to Treat Erectile Dysfunction**

General Considerations
- Keep appointments for laboratory testing and follow-up care.
- As with all drugs, keep these medications in the original container, tightly closed, and out of reach of children.

Self-Administration
- Do not take any phosphodiesterase type 5 (PDE5) inhibitor with nitrates because a serious and potentially life-threatening drop in blood pressure may occur.
- Do not take sildenafil more than once a day.
- Avoid consuming a high-fat meal before taking sildenafil or vardenafil.
- Seek immediate medical attention for an erection lasting 4 hours or longer.
- Do not use intraurethral alprostadil without using a condom if your partner is pregnant.
- If symptoms of nonarteritic ischemic optic neuropathy or a sudden decrease or loss of hearing occurs while taking PDE5 inhibitors, discontinue the drug and seek medical attention.

Tadalafil (Cialis) has a longer half-life, which gives males the option of taking the drug up to 12 hours before sexual intercourse or as a lower dose, once-a-day daily medication. The drug reaches its peak in 2 hours, with a duration of 24 to 36 hours. Meals do not affect absorption rate or peak levels. Adverse effects, which may linger because of this longer-acting drug, include back and muscle pain.

Vardenafil (Levitra) has a time to peak effect of 1 hour and a duration of action of 4 hours. As with sildenafil, a high-fat meal delays absorption and reduces peak levels. The drug is available in an oral disintegrating tablet.

> **Quality and Safety Alert: Safety**
>
> Vardenafil is the only PDE5 inhibitor that prolongs the QT interval and should not be used with other drugs with similar effect, particularly class I and II antidysrhythmic drugs (see Chapter 27).

Like sildenafil, vardenafil reduces blood pressure and to a lesser degree increases the risk of light sensitivity, blurred vision, and loss of blue–green color discrimination.

ADJUVANT MEDICATIONS USED TO TREAT ERECTILE DYSFUNCTION

Clinicians consider adjuvant drugs second-line therapy in the management of ED and generally reserve them for patients who manifest insufficient response to or adverse effects from PDE5 inhibitors. Alprostadil is a synthetic enzyme that causes relaxation of cavernosal smooth muscle and dilation of cavernosal arterioles leading to increased penile blood flow. It is a prostaglandin, specifically a prostaglandin E_1.

Administration of alprostadil occurs in two ways: either as an injection into the penis or as a pellet inserted into it (via the urethral opening at the end of the penis). Box 8.6 presents notes about administering the drug. Intracavernosal alprostadil (Caverject) relaxes trabecular smooth muscle and dilates cavernosal arteries, resulting in penile engorgement and reduced venous outflow. Intraurethral alprostadil (Muse) is less efficacious than the intracavernosal drug (60% or less). Administration by either route can produce dose–response improvements in frequency of an erection sufficient for intercourse. The onset of action is immediate, following injection, and erection should not last longer than 1 hour with proper dosing (determined in a provider's office).

Intracavernosal injection of alprostadil is associated with a burning sensation, prolonged erection, and priapism, and long-term use is associated with penile fibrosis. Caution is warranted in patients concurrently receiving anticoagulants due to risk of bleeding and in patients at risk for priapism (e.g., sickle cell anemia or trait, multiple myeloma, leukemia). Intraurethral use of the drug is associated with penile pain and minor urethral bleeding. Discharge instruction in the technique for administration should be provided as well as counseling regarding possible adverse effects. Experts do not recommend alprostadil for concurrent use with other vasoactive agents.

BOX 8.6 Adjuvant Medications Used to Treat Erectile Dysfunction: Alprostadil

Intracavernosal Injection (Caverject Aqueous, Caverject Powder, Edex Powder)

- Injection may occur along the dorsolateral aspect of the proximal third of the penis, avoiding visible veins.
- It is necessary to rotate injection sites from one side of the penis to the other and change injection site with each dose.
- Self-injection may occur no more than three times per week and only once in 24 hours.
- To determine dose adequate for achieving satisfactory erection without causing priapism, it is important to have an initial injection in provider's office.

Intraurethral Administration (Muse)

- Prior to introducing pellet into urethra, it is important to void; residual urine in urethra aids in dispersing the medication.
- Intraurethral administration may occur no more than two times in 24 hours.
- To determine dose adequate for achieving satisfactory erection without causing priapism, the patient should visit the provider.

Clinical Application 8.2

- After an evaluation, the nurse practitioner suspects that Mr. Johnson's ED may result from the combination of obesity and antihypertensive medications. He receives a prescription for lisinopril, an angiotensin-converting enzyme inhibitor, which he will take along with hydrochlorothiazide. What patient teaching guidelines should the nurse discuss with Mr. Johnson and his wife?

5-ALPHA REDUCTASE INHIBITORS

The 5-alpha reductase inhibitors and the alpha$_1$-adrenergic blockers are the two major drug classes used to treat BPH. Each class works differently to enhance urination in males, and both classes of drugs can be prescribed simultaneously for management of BPH. Each class will be discussed separately.

Finasteride (Proscar), the prototype 5-alpha reductase inhibitor, represents this drug class and is used to treat BPH. The other drug in the class and used to treat BPH is dutasteride (Avodart).

Pharmacokinetics

Finasteride is well absorbed as an oral drug. It is 90% bound to plasma proteins. The onset of action is rapid, with a duration of 5 to 7 days. The half-life is 5 to 7 hours. Finasteride may take 3 to 6 months to reach maximum effects. The drug crosses the blood–brain barrier and has been found in semen.

Action

Finasteride acts by inhibiting 5-alpha reductase, the enzyme responsible for converting testosterone to 5-alpha DHT, one of its active metabolites. This inhibits the metabolism of testosterone, causing decreased proliferation of prostatic cells, which reduces the enlargement of the prostate gland and mechanical obstruction to the urethra.

Use

Prescribers order finasteride mainly to treat BPH. However, the drug is also available in smaller doses as Propecia, which is indicated for the prevention of male pattern baldness. Table 8.4 gives route and dosage information for finasteride.

Patient-related variables specific to the use of finasteride include the following:

- Age:
  - Children should not take the drug.
  - Older adults are prone to the hypotensive and hypothermic adverse effects from the vasodilation produced by finasteride.
- Reproduction, pregnancy, and lactation:
  - Females of childbearing age, particularly those who are pregnant or lactating, should not take the drug.
  - In animal reproduction studies, utero exposure to finasteride may lead to abnormal development of the male genital tract. Limited data are available regarding the effects of the drug in humans during pregnancy.
  - Poor seminal quality and male infertility have been reported and may be reversable with the drug is discontinued.
- Abnormal kidney function and hepatic impairment:
  - Caution is necessary when administering finasteride to patients with abnormal kidney function or hepatic impairment.

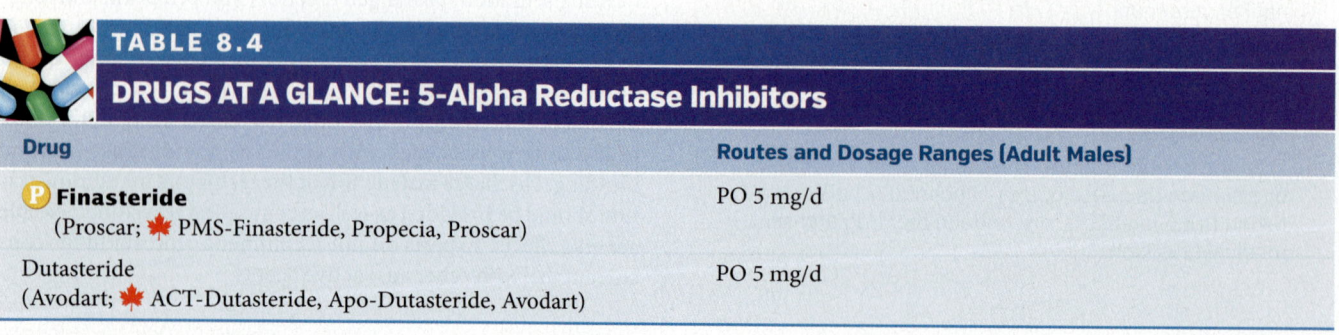

TABLE 8.4
DRUGS AT A GLANCE: 5-Alpha Reductase Inhibitors

Drug	Routes and Dosage Ranges (Adult Males)
Finasteride (Proscar; PMS-Finasteride, Propecia, Proscar)	PO 5 mg/d
Dutasteride (Avodart; ACT-Dutasteride, Apo-Dutasteride, Avodart)	PO 5 mg/d

Adverse Effects and Contraindications

Adverse effects of finasteride include various sexual dysfunctions, such as impotence, gynecomastia, reduced libido, and ejaculatory disorders. Dysfunction is usually transient. The drug may decrease sperm production, adversely affecting fertility.

Contraindications include known sensitivity to finasteride. Children and females of childbearing age, and those who are pregnant or lactating, should not take the drug.

Nursing Implications

Preventing Interactions

Concurrent use of finasteride has led to few drug and herb interactions. Use of the drug with testosterone reduces the effects of both finasteride and testosterone. Anticholinergics may decrease the effects of finasteride. The herb saw palmetto may increase the effects of the drug.

Administering the Medication

People may take finasteride once a day around the same time each day, without regard to food.

Quality and Safety Alert: Safety

Pregnant caregivers, nurses, or pharmacists should not handle the crushed drug, which can be absorbed and may be harmful to a male fetus.

Assessing for Therapeutic Effects

The nurse assesses for improved urinary function with patient voiding in sufficient amounts with no palpable bladder distention. Patients should report less urinary frequency, hesitancy, urgency, dribbling, nocturia, and an improved force of the urinary stream.

Quality and Safety Alert: Evidence-Based Practice

In a meta-analysis of 11 eligible randomized controlled studies, Zhang et al. (2019) evaluated the role of combination therapy (alpha$_1$-adrenergic blockers and PDE5 inhibitors) in patients for lower urinary tract symptoms secondary to benign prostatic hyperplasia. All relevant qualified data were pooled and reviewed comparing combination therapy to treatment without PDE5 inhibitors in 855 patients. Patients receiving combination therapy had better improvement in international prostate symptom scores, maximum urinary flow rate, and international index of erectile function compared to those without PDE5 inhibitors. The combination therapy was also well tolerated in patients.

Using evidence-based drug therapy to manage lower urinary tract symptoms secondary to benign prostatic hyperplasia can significantly improve quality of life and decrease the economic burden and treatment failure associated with management.

Assessing for Adverse Effects

The nurse should take a thorough sexual history in patients taking finasteride, including information regarding the presence of ED, infertility, gynecomastia, reduced libido, and ejaculatory disorders, such as decreased volume of ejaculate. The effect of the drug on sexual dysfunction may be difficult to assess in older males who report these disorders with increasing age and other health conditions.

Patient Teaching

Box 8.7 presents patient teaching guidelines for finasteride and other drugs used to treat BPH.

Quality and Safety Alert: Safety

People taking a 5-alpha reductase inhibitor should avoid donating blood because the blood could be administered to a pregnant person.

BOX 8.7 Patient Teaching Guidelines for Treatment of Benign Prostatic Hypertrophy

General Considerations

- Note that the maximum benefit from the medication is achieved in 6 to 12 months.
- Make sure to keep appointments for laboratory testing and follow-up care.
- Keep these medications in the original container, tightly closed, protected from light, and out of reach of children.
- Report a sulfa allergy before beginning tamsulosin therapy; a cross-allergic reaction has been reported.
- Seek medical care immediately if you are unable to void, if you pass bloody urine, or if you develop a fever.

Self-Administration

- Take oral preparations without regard to meals.
- Do not take other prescription or OTC medications without consulting your healthcare provider.
- Be careful when changing positions because dizziness may occur when standing up.
- If you are sexually active and able to become pregnant, use a barrier contraceptive to prevent pregnancy.
- Take terazosin at bedtime to reduce the adverse effects.
- Note that a decrease in libido and volume of ejaculate may occur; this is usually reversible when the drug is stopped.
- If you are having surgery, including dental surgery, tell the surgeon or dentist that you are taking tamsulosin. If you need to have eye surgery at any time during or after your treatment, be sure to tell your surgeon that you are taking or have taken tamsulosin.
- Do not drive a car, operate machinery, or perform dangerous tasks until you know how tamsulosin affects you. This medication may make you drowsy or dizzy.

Other Drugs in the Class

Dutasteride (Avodart) is the only other 5-alpha reductase inhibitor and has a stronger ability than finasteride to reduce the levels of DHT, causing the prostate to decrease in size. Symptoms may improve after 3 months of therapy. However, it may take 6 months or longer to determine the full benefit of the drug. People who are pregnant or may become pregnant should not handle dutasteride capsules for fear of causing harmful effects in male fetuses. A combination of the dutasteride and tamsulosin is available under the trade name of Jalyn. Females should not use Jalyn.

ALPHA$_1$-ADRENERGIC BLOCKERS

The alpha$_1$-adrenergic blockers are recommended over the PDE5 inhibitors for initial monotherapy for the treatment of BPH. Alpha$_1$-adrenergic blockers provide immediate therapeutic benefits, while PDE5 inhibitors require long-term treatment (6 to 12 months) before symptom improvement.

Ⓟ Tamsulosin (Flomax) is the prototype of the anti-BPH drugs. Other drugs in the class are used to treat hypertension (see Chapter 26), nasal congestion (see Chapter 31), and ophthalmic hyperemia (see Chapter 59).

Pharmacokinetics

Tamsulosin is well absorbed and is highly protein bound. The drug is extensively metabolized by the cytochrome P450 enzyme system, mainly by CYP3A4 and CYP2D6. It is excreted by the kidneys.

Action

Tamsulosin works by relaxing the muscles in the prostate and bladder neck, enhancing the ability to urinate. Blockage of alpha$_1$-adrenergic receptors decreases vascular smooth muscle contraction, influencing the activity of genitourinary smooth muscle.

Use

Prescribers order tamsulosin to improve urination and reduce complications in males with BPH. Females are also prescribed tamsulosin for ureteral calculi expulsion. Table 8.5 contains route and dosage information for tamsulosin and other alpha$_1$-adrenergic receptor blockers used to treat BPH.

Patient-related variables specific to the use of tamsulosin and other alpha$_1$-adrenergic receptor blockers include the following:

- Reproduction, pregnancy, and lactation:
  - Ejaculation failure, retrograde ejaculation, and decreased ejaculation has been associated with the drug's use.
  - Tamsulosin in the second and third trimester of pregnancy is not associated with adverse maternal or infant outcomes.
- Abnormal kidney function and hepatic impairment:
  - Tamsulosin should be used with caution in people with a CrCl <10 mL/minute although no dosage adjustment may likely be necessary.

Adverse Effects

Tamsulosin may cause adverse effects, including postural hypotension, weakness, sleepiness, difficulty falling or staying asleep, stuffy or runny nose, sore throat, and blurred vision. The drug may also lead to abnormal ejaculation due to inhibition of alpha$_{1A}$-adrenergic receptors on the vas deferens.

Contraindications

Contraindications to tamsulosin include a known hypersensitivity to the drug.

> **❗ Quality and Safety Alert: Safety**
>
> Evidence shows that a complication during cataract surgery may occur in patients taking tamsulosin. This problem is associated with the drug's effect on alpha$_1$ blockade of the dilator muscle of the iris, limiting dilation of the eye. It is important that patients are instructed to inform healthcare providers of taking tamsulosin prior to eye surgery because specific surgical procedures can be used to minimize risk.

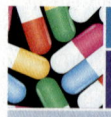

TABLE 8.5
DRUGS AT A GLANCE: Alpha$_1$-Adrenergic Blockers

Drug	Routes and Dosage Ranges (Adult Males)
Ⓟ **Tamsulosin** (Flomax; 🍁 APO-Tamsulosin CR, Flomax CR, Sandoz-Tamsulosin)	PO 0.4 mg 30 min after a meal to max of 0.8 mg/d
Alfuzosin (Uroxatral; 🍁 Apo-Alfuzosin, Sandoz-Alfuzosin, Xatral)	PO 10 mg/d to max of 10 mg/d
(Cardura; 🍁 Apo-Doxazosin, Teva-Doxazosin) Doxazosin XL (Cardura XL)	PO 1–8 mg/d to max of 8 mg/d PO extended release: 4–8 mg/d to max of 8 mg/d
Silodosin (Rapaflo; 🍁 Rapaflo, Sandoz Silodosin)	PO 8 mg/d
Terazosin (🍁 Apo-Terazosin, Dom-Terazosin, Pms-Terazosin)	PO start with 1 mg at bedtime to 1–5 mg/d to max of 20 mg/d

Nursing Implications

Preventing Interactions
The cytochrome P450 enzyme system is essential for the metabolism of many medications, including tamsulosin. Thus, the risk for drug interactions exists with tamsulosin, increasing its effects (Box 8.8).

Administering the Medication
Patients should take tamsulosin 30 minutes after eating at the same mealtime daily because fasting alters bioavailability and peak concentration. They should swallow capsules intact; it is essential not to open, crush, or chew the capsules.

Assessing for Therapeutic Effects
The nurse assesses for improved urinary function demonstrated by decreased urinary frequency, hesitancy, urgency, dribbling, nocturia, and improved force of the urinary stream. The patient should report a decrease in the pain associated with BPH as tamsulosin relaxes the smooth muscle in the bladder neck and the prostate, decreasing the resistance to urinary flow.

Assessing for Adverse Effects
The nurse assesses for orthostatic hypotension, difficulty with sleep, blurred vision, nasal congestion, sore throat, weakness, headache, sleepiness, difficulty falling or staying asleep, stuffy or runny nose, sore throat, and blurred vision.

Patient Teaching
Box 8.7 contains patient education guidelines for tamsulosin and other drugs used to treat BPH.

Other Drugs in the Class

Alfuzosin (Uroxatral) is classed as a nonreceptor subtype selective alpha$_1$-adrenergic blocker also used to treat BPH. The drug can be uroselective due to accumulation of drug in prostatic tissue. It has a strong safety profile and is well tolerated.

Doxazosin (Cardura) is effective and widely used as a treatment for symptoms associated with BPH. The drug has a rapid onset of action (1 to 2 weeks). Maximal plasma concentrations are achieved within 1 to 4 hours. With the longer 22-hour half-life of doxazosin, the drug can be taken in the morning or evening, with no difference in the incidence of adverse effects. However, it generally needs to be initiated at bedtime to reduce the postural light-headedness experienced soon after starting the drug. Major adverse effects include hypotension, dizziness, headache, nasal congestion, and fatigue. Sexual dysfunction is not commonly associated with drug use.

Silodosin (Rapaflo) produces similar short-term symptom reduction as other drugs in the class but causes greater risk of adverse effects, including sexual side effects (i.e., abnormal ejaculation). Patients should take the drug with meals. The drug is contraindicated in individuals with a creatinine clearance less than 30 mL/minute. Terazosin has an efficacy profile similar to doxazosin, as well as a similar adverse effect profile. The drug's main variation is a shorter 12-hour half-life, which may be attributed to the increased incidence of hypotension, headache, dizziness, nasal congestion, and fatigue if the drug is administered in the morning. Consequently, experts recommend that terazosin be given at bedtime.

The combination of a 5-alpha reductase inhibitor and an alpha$_1$-adrenergic blocker may be more effective in males with large prostates when monotherapy has been ineffective.

BOX 8.8 — Drug Interactions: Tamsulosin

Drugs That Increase the Effects of Tamsulosin
- Cimetidine
  Decreases clearance
- Other alpha blocker medications (e.g., alfuzosin, doxazosin, prazosin, terazosin); anticoagulants (e.g., warfarin); and phosphodiesterase type 5 inhibitors (e.g., avanafil, sildenafil, tadalafil, vardenafil)
  Increase the risk of orthostatic hypotension

NCLEX Success

4. In which of the following males would the use of sildenafil be contraindicated?
   A. 52-year-old with type 1 diabetes
   B. 58-year-old with unstable angina
   C. 69-year-old with asthma
   D. 74-year-old with cirrhosis

5. A 66-year-old patient recently diagnosed with benign prostatic hypertrophy is started on tamsulosin 0.4 mg PO daily. Which of the following if stated by the patient indicates that patient teaching has been successful? (Select all that apply.)
   A. "I should swallow the capsule whole and not chew it."
   B. "The best time to take the medication is in the morning."
   C. "This medication should make it easier for me to urinate and the dribbling of urine should improve."
   D. "I can take this medication even with my allergy to penicillin."
   E. "I should change positions slowly after taking tamsulosin as it could lower my blood pressure."
   F. "I should take the capsule 30 minutes after eating at the same mealtime daily."
   G. "I need to make sure that I tell my eye doctor that I am taking tamsulosin."
   H. "I should not expect improvement in my urinary symptoms for 6 to 12 months."

THE NURSING PROCESS

A concept map outlines the nursing process related to drug therapy considerations in this chapter. Additional nursing implications related to the disease process should also be considered in care decisions.

Assessment
- Periodic monitoring is needed throughout drug therapy.
  - Assess for conditions in which the drugs are used (e.g., deficiency states, erectile dysfunction [ED], benign prostatic hypertrophy [BPH]).
  - Assess attitude toward taking male sex hormones or drugs to improve sexual function or urinary flow.
  - Assess willingness to adhere to instructions for taking the drugs and follow-up procedures.
  - Assess for conditions that increase risks of adverse effects or are contraindications (e.g., pregnancy, kidney or liver disease, concurrent drugs).
- With androgens, check laboratory reports of liver function tests, serum electrolyte levels, and serum lipid levels. Assess weight and blood pressure regularly. For children, check radiograph examination reports of bone growth status initially and approximately every 6 months while androgens are being taken.
- With ED, assess risk factors for the development of the condition and current drugs.
- With BPH, assess urinary function, urine stream caliber and force, any symptoms of urinary hesitancy, and difficulty starting urination.

Outcomes of Therapy

The patient will
- Use the drugs only as directed.
- Avoid preventable adverse drug effects.
- Adhere to monitoring and follow-up procedures.
- Develop prevention and self-care measures to avoid ED (e.g., limitation or avoidance of alcohol and other drugs, smoking cessation, regular exercise and rest, stress reduction) or support interventions to decrease symptoms of BPH.
- Report healthy sexual functioning or improved urinary patterns of elimination based on cause of drug therapy.
- Avoid preventable complications with concomitant nitrate use in patients taking sildenafil.

Nursing Interventions
- Assist patients to use the drugs correctly (see Boxes 8.3, 8.5, and 8.7). Consider psychological counseling and therapy, as indicated. Demonstrate problem-solving skills regarding solutions to problems that occur.
- With androgen use, assist patient to reduce sodium intake if edema develops and record weight and blood pressure at regular intervals. Participate in school or community programs to inform children, parents, coaches, athletic trainers, and others of the risks of inappropriate use of androgens, anabolic steroids, and related dietary supplements.
- With ED, consider lifestyle modification and review of medication profile.
- With BPH, report any changes of urinary function, urine stream caliber and force, any symptoms of urinary hesitancy, or difficulty starting urination.

Evaluation
- Interview and observe for relief of symptoms and compliance with instructions for drugs prescribed.
- Interview and observe for adherence with instructions for taking prescribed drugs.
- Interview and observe for therapeutic and adverse drug effects.
- With androgen use, observe athletes and other males for increased weight and behavioral changes that may indicate drug abuse with androgens.
- With BPH, observe for adequate urinary elimination.

Visit **thePoint** at **http://thePoint.lww.com/Frandsen13e** for answers to NCLEX Success questions (in Appendix A), answers to Clinical Application Case Studies (in Appendix B), and more!

REFERENCES AND RESOURCES

American College of Obstetricians and Gynecologists (ACOG) Committee on Gynecologic Practice and Committee on Health Care for Underserved Women. (2021). ACOG Committee Opinion No. 823: Health care for transgender and gender diverse individuals. *Obstetrical Gynecology, 37*(3), e75–e88. doi:10.1097/AOG.0000000000004294

Aydin, C., & Senel, E. (2020). Impotence literature: scientometric analysis of erectile dysfunction articles between 1975 and 2018. *Andrologia, 52*(2), 13520. https://doi.org/10.1111/and.13520

Barnes, H., Brown, Z., Burns, A., & Williams, T. (2019). Phosphodiesterase 5 inhibitors for pulmonary hypertension. *Cochrane Database Systematic Review, 1*(1). doi: 10.1002/14651858.CD012621.pub2

Burnett, A. L., Nehra, A., Breau, R. H., Culkin, D. J., Faraday, M. M., Hakim, L. S., Heidelbaugh, J., Khera, M., McVary, K. T., Miner, M. M., Nelson, C. J., Sadeghi-Nejad, H., Seftel, A. D., & Shindel, A. W. (2018). Erectile dysfunction: AUA guideline. *The Journal of Urology, 200*(3), 633–641.

Dubin, J. M., Fantus, R. J., & Halpern, J. A. (2021). Testosterone replacement therapy in the era of telemedicine. *International Journal of Impotence Research*, 1–6. Advance online publication. https://doi.org/10.1038/s41443-021-00498-5

Hall, J. E., & Hall, M. E. (2020). *Guyton and Hall textbook of medical physiology* (14th ed.). Elsevier.

Hinkle, J. H., Cheever, K. H., & Overbaugh, K. J. (2021). *Brunner & Suddarth's textbook of medical-surgical nursing* (15th ed.). Wolters Kluwer.

Jindan, L., Xiao, W., & Liping, X. (2022). Evolving role of silodosin for the treatment of urological disorders—A narrative review. *Drug Design, Development, and Therapy, 16*, 2861–2884.

Jung, J. H., Kim, J., MacDonald, R., Reddy, B., Kim, M. H., & Dahm, P. (2017). Silodosin for the treatment of lower urinary tract symptoms in men with benign prostatic hyperplasia. *Cochrane Database of Systematic Reviews*, (11), CD012615. doi: 10.1002/14651858.CD012615.pub2

Lippincott advisor. (2022). Retrieved from http://advisor.lww.com

Manna, S., Gray, M., Kaul, V. F., & Wanna, G. (2019). Phosphodiesterase-5 (PDE-5) Inhibitors and ototoxicity: A systematic review. *Otology & Neurology, 40*(3), 276–283.

Mulhall, J. P., Giraldi, A., Hackett, G., Hellstrom, W. J. G., Jannini, E. A., Rubio-Aurioles, E., Trost, L., & Hassan, T. A. (2018). The 2018 revision to the process of care model for evaluation of erectile dysfunction. *Journal of Sexual Medicine, 15*(9), 1280–1292.

Norris, T. L. (2018). *Porth's pathophysiology: Concepts of altered health status* (10th ed.). Wolters Kluwer.

Zaami, S., Di Trana, A., Garcia-Algar, O., Marinelli, E., & Busardo, F. P. (2022). Editorial: Psychiatric and pharmacotoxicological insights on appearance and performance enhancing drugs. *Frontiers in Psychiatry, 13*. https://doi.org/10.3389/fpsyt.2022.918482

Theriault, B., Morin, F., & Cloutier, J. (2020). Safety and efficacy of Tamsulosin as medical expulsive therapy in pregnancy. *World Journal of Urology, 38*(9), 2301–2306. https://doi.org/10.1007/s00345-019-03022-z

Tucker, R. (2022). *2023 Lippincott's pocket drug for nurses*. Wolters Kluwer.

Zhang, J., Li, X., Yang, B., Wu, C., Fan, Y., & Li, H. (2019). Alpha-blockers with or without phosphodiesterase type 5 inhibitor for treatment of lower urinary tract symptoms secondary to benign prostatic hyperplasia: A systematic review and meta-analysis. *World Journal of Urology, 37*(1), 143–153. https://doi.org/10.1007/s00345-018-2370-z

Clinical Judgment in Practice: Section 2: Drug Therapy Throughout the Lifespan

A 3-year-old child is brought to the emergency department by the father. The child has a fever and cold symptoms. The father states that the child has been ill for 4 days. You are the nurse assigned to their care, and upon initial assessment, the child's temperature is 101.8°F axillary. The child's pulse is 120 and respirations 32 with substernal retractions. The child has wheezes in the right and left lower lobes of the lungs. During an interview with the child's father, you learn that the parents administered aspirin and hot water with cinnamon and honey for the previous 4 days. This morning the parents noted that their child was sleepier than normal, and the child had vomited the breakfast of oatmeal and milk. To prepare for the pediatrician's examination of the child, the child is weighed by the nurse assistant. The child is 30 lbs.

Step 1: Recognize Cues
Identify the relevant and important information from different sources, such as the medical history or subjective and objective data.

Answer: The child's temperature is 101.8°F axillary, pulse 120, and respirations 32. Wheezing is auscultated in the right and left lower lobes of the lungs. The nurse calculates the weight in kilograms. The child's weight is 36.63 kg. The child's sodium level is 123 mEq/L.

The father states that the child has been ill for 4 days. The child vomited this morning. The child is sleeping more than normal.

Step 2: Analyze Cues
Organize and link the recognized cues to the patient's clinical presentation.

Answer: You know that the administration of aspirin to children during a viral illness can lead to a potentially fatal condition called Reye syndrome. Signs and symptoms of Reye syndrome are related to swelling in the brain and liver. Reye syndrome is known as acute toxic-metabolic encephalopathy. The symptoms of Reye syndrome range from lethargy to coma. The child's sodium level is 123 mEq/L. As the sodium level decreases, the child is at risk for the development of seizures. At present, the ALT and AST are within normal limits. The child's elevated temperature should be treated with acetaminophen or ibuprofen. The dosage should be calculated according to the child's weight of 36.63 kg. The wheezing in the right and left lower lobes may be related to the development of asthma or pneumonia. A temperature of 101.8°F axillary is above normal and may be a viral or bacterial infection. An increased respiratory rate and bilateral substernal retractions are related to the closed lower lung airways.

Step 3: Prioritize Hypotheses
Evaluate hypotheses and rank them according to priority, such as urgency, likelihood, risk, difficulty, and/or time. Cluster your findings to generate a list of problems (actual or potential) you believe the patient is experiencing or may experience and determine the level of urgency. Which problem is of the greatest concern?

Answer: You prioritize the needs of the patient. In regard to the administration of aspirin, it places the child at risk for the development of Reye syndrome. The child's liver enzymes and electrolytes are monitored every 4 hours. In addition, the child's mental status should be monitored. The child's family will require patient teaching on the risk of administering aspirin to a child with a viral infection.

Due to the labored respirations with substernal retractions, you anticipate the child is to receive a respiratory treatment of albuterol.

The child's temperature should be reduced, so you anticipate that the primary care provider will prescribe acetaminophen. The temperature of 101.8°F axillary should be treated with acetaminophen 160 mg every 4 hours. According to the oral dosing in UpToDate, a child weighing 24 to 35 lbs should be administered 160 mg. Due to the child's vomiting, the child is dehydrated. The BUN is 28 mg/dL. You know the normal range for your hospital is 6 to 24 mg/dL. You anticipate IV fluids are to be ordered.

Step 4: Generate Solutions
Identify expected outcomes and use hypotheses to define a set of interventions for the expected outcomes.

Answer: You prioritize the care of the child: To resolve the child's dehydration, replacement of parenteral fluids is required. You anticipate that an IV of D_5NS will be ordered. You also anticipate the restriction of food and fluids until the nausea and vomiting is resolved. The child's electrolytes and liver enzymes must be monitored to determine the development of Reye syndrome and resolution of dehydration. To resolve the labored breathing, substernal retractions, and improve alveolar gas exchange, you anticipate respiratory treatments with albuterol and budesonide will be ordered by the pediatric healthcare provider and administered by the respiratory therapist. You will assess the child's pulmonary status every hour.

Step 5: Take Actions
Implement the solutions that address the highest priorities.

Answer: *You draw electrolytes and liver enzymes every 6 hours as ordered and communicate the laboratory results to the pediatric healthcare provider. You start an IV of D_5NS at 45 mL/hour. You assess the child's fluid volume, including the skin turgor and urine output. You administer acetaminophen 240 mg suppository. The respiratory therapist administers an albuterol nebulizer treatment followed by a budesonide nebulizer treatment. In 1 hour following administration of the nebulizer treatments with albuterol and budesonide, you assess the child's respiratory status. You assess lung sounds before and after the breathing treatments. Four hours after the administration of IV fluids, you draw a chemistry panel, AST, and ALT (liver enzymes).*

Step 6: Evaluate Outcomes
Compare observed outcomes against expected outcomes.

Answer: *One hour following the administration of the acetaminophen suppository, you assess the child's temperature. It is 98.4°F axillary. The respiratory rate is 32 with diminished substernal retractions. The lung sounds have increased wheezing per auscultation. The child has an improvement in the lung sounds, which is evidenced by the increased wheezing. Prior to the nebulizer treatment, the child had diminished lung sounds. Following the administration of IV D_5NS at 45 mL/hour for 4 hours, the serum sodium level is 127 mEq/L and the liver enzymes are within normal limits. The child's skin turgor is good, and the child is voiding at least 30 mL on average every hour. Twelve hours following administration of IV fluids, acetaminophen for fever, and respiratory treatments, the child's activity level has increased. The child is no longer lethargic, and the electrolytes and liver enzymes are within normal limits. You educate the parents on the risk of administering aspirin during a viral infection. The parents understand to administer either acetaminophen or ibuprofen for fever control. On the 2nd day of the child's hospitalization the child was able to tolerate clear liquids without nausea and vomiting. The child's temperature has been below 99°F axillary for 24 hours. The lungs sounds are clear without wheezing. The child no longer is noted with substernal retractions. The child is to be discharged tomorrow, and the parents are able to administer the inhalers with the use of a spacer.*

SECTION 3

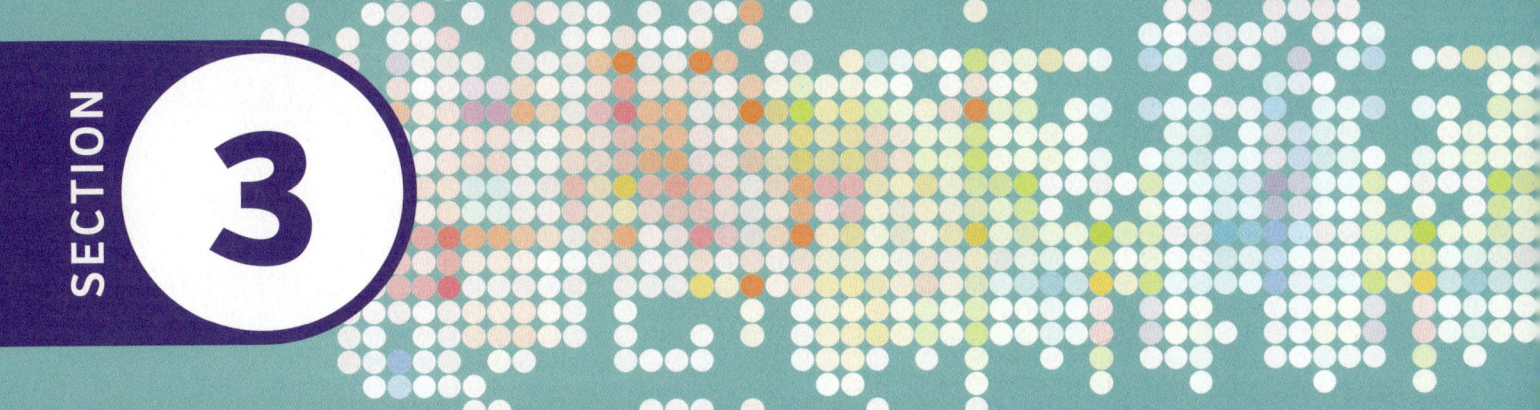

Drugs Affecting the Hematopoietic and Immune Systems

Chapter 9 Drug Therapy for Coagulation Disorders
Chapter 10 Drug Therapy for Dyslipidemia
Chapter 11 Drug Therapy for Hematopoietic Disorders
Chapter 12 Drug Therapy: Immunizations
Chapter 13 Drug Therapy to Decrease Immunity
Chapter 14 Drug Therapy for the Treatment of Cancer

CHAPTER 9

Drug Therapy for Coagulation Disorders

LEARNING OBJECTIVES

After studying this chapter, you should be able to:

1. Compare and contrast heparin and warfarin in terms of indications for use, onset and duration of action, route of administration, blood tests used to monitor effects, and nursing process implications.
2. Discuss antiplatelet agents in terms of indications for use and effects on blood coagulation.
3. Discuss direct thrombin inhibitors in terms of indications and contraindications for use, routes of administration, and major adverse effects.
4. Discuss direct factor Xa inhibitors in terms of indications and contraindications for use, routes of administration, and major adverse effects.
5. Describe thrombolytic agents in terms of indications and contraindications for use, routes of administration, and major adverse effects.
6. Identify the prototype drug for each drug class.
7. Describe systemic hemostatic agents for treating overdoses of anticoagulant and thrombolytic drugs.
8. Implement the nursing process in the care of patients receiving anticoagulant, antiplatelet, and thrombolytic agents.

CLINICAL APPLICATION CASE STUDY

Andrew Oliver, age 45 years, works as a mental health counselor. He presents to a small community emergency department with an acute anterior ST-elevation myocardial infarction. Within 20 minutes of arrival, he receives alteplase by continuous intravenous (IV) infusion over 3 hours. He also simultaneously receives an IV bolus of heparin and is started on a heparin drip. You are the nurse assigned to his care.

KEY TERMS

Embolus: object that migrates through the circulation until it lodges in a blood vessel, causing occlusion; may be a thrombus, fat, air, amniotic fluid, a bit of tissue, or bacterial debris

Fibrinolysin: enzyme that breaks down the fibrin meshwork that stabilizes blood clots; also referred to as plasmin

Hemostasis: prevention or stoppage of blood loss from an injured blood vessel and is the process that maintains the integrity of the vascular compartment

Heparin-induced thrombocytopenia (HIT): immune-mediated adverse effect that leads to thrombogenesis resulting in a decrease in platelet count associated with heparin administration in patients with detectable HIT antibodies

Plasmin: enzyme that breaks down the fibrin meshwork that stabilizes blood clots; also referred to as fibrinolysin

Plasminogen: inactive protein found in many body tissues and fluids

Thrombogenesis: formation of a blood clot

Thrombolysis: breakdown or dissolution of blood clots

Thrombosis: formation of a blood clot

Thrombus: blood clot

INTRODUCTION

Anticoagulant, antiplatelet, and thrombolytic drugs are used in the prevention and management of thrombotic and thromboembolic disorders. **Thrombogenesis** (or **thrombosis**), the formation of blood clots, is a normal body defense mechanism to prevent blood loss. Thus, this process may be lifesaving when it occurs as a response to hemorrhage; however, it may be life threatening when it occurs at other times, because the **thrombus**, or blood clot, can obstruct a blood vessel and block blood flow to tissues beyond the clot either at the site of clot formation or to another part of the body. To aid understanding of drug therapy for thrombotic disorders, this chapter provides a brief discussion of normal hemostasis, endothelial functions in relation to blood clotting, platelet functions, and blood coagulation.

OVERVIEW OF COAGULATION DISORDERS

Hemostasis is the process that maintains the integrity of the vascular compartment. It involves activation of several mechanisms, including vasoconstriction, formation of a platelet plug (a cluster of aggregated platelets), sequential activation of clotting factors in the blood (Fig. 9.1), and growth of fibrous tissue (fibrin) into the blood clot to make it more stable and to repair the tear (opening) in the damaged blood vessel. Overall, normal hemostasis is a complex process involving numerous interacting activators and inhibitors, including endothelial factors, platelets, and blood coagulation factors.

When a blood clot is being formed, **plasminogen**, an inactive protein present in many body tissues and fluids, is bound to fibrin and becomes a component of the clot. After the outward blood flow is stopped and the tear in the blood vessel is repaired, plasminogen is activated by plasminogen activator (produced by endothelial cells or the coagulation cascade) to produce plasmin. **Plasmin** (also called **fibrinolysin**) is an enzyme that breaks down the fibrin meshwork that stabilizes the clot; this fibrinolytic or thrombolytic action dissolves the clot.

Normally, thrombi are constantly being formed and dissolved, but the blood remains fluid, and flow is not significantly obstructed. If the balance between thrombogenesis and **thrombolysis**, dissolution of blood clots, is upset, thrombotic or bleeding disorders ensue. Thrombosis may occur in both arteries and veins. Arterial thrombosis is usually associated with atherosclerotic plaque, hypertension, and turbulent blood flow. These conditions damage arterial endothelium and activate platelets to initiate the coagulation process. Arterial thrombi cause disease by obstructing blood flow. If the obstruction is incomplete or temporary, local tissue ischemia (deficient blood supply) occurs. If the obstruction is complete or prolonged, local tissue death (infarction) occurs.

Venous thrombosis is usually associated with venous stasis. When blood flows slowly, thrombin and other procoagulant substances present in the blood become concentrated in local areas and initiate the clotting process. With a normal rate of blood flow, these substances are rapidly removed from the blood, primarily by Kupffer cells in the liver. A venous thrombus is less cohesive than an arterial thrombus, and an **embolus** can easily become detached and travel to other parts of the body. This embolus may be a thrombus, fat, air, amniotic fluid, tissue, or bacterial debris.

Venous thrombi cause disease by two mechanisms. First, thrombosis causes local congestion, edema, and perhaps inflammation by impairing normal outflow of venous blood (e.g., thrombophlebitis, deep vein thrombosis [DVT]). Second, embolization obstructs the blood supply when the embolus becomes lodged. The pulmonary arteries are common sites of embolization.

Thrombotic disorders occur much more often than bleeding disorders and are emphasized in this chapter. Bleeding disorders may result from excessive amounts of drugs that inhibit clotting.

Clinical Manifestations

Clinical manifestations of thrombosis vary depending on the size and location (arterial or venous system) of the thrombus. Symptoms are the result of decreased perfusion to an area due to the restriction or cessation of blood flow. Arterial blood clots in the cerebral, pulmonary, or cardiac system can produce a cerebrovascular accident, pulmonary embolism (PE), or myocardial infarction, respectively. Venous blood clots may lead to DVT; classic symptoms include leg swelling and pain on palpation in the calf or thigh. However, half of all affected patients do not have any symptoms of DVT.

Drug Therapy

Drugs given to prevent or treat thrombosis alter some aspect of the blood coagulation process (Table 9.1; see Fig. 9.1). Anticoagulant drugs, which prevent formation of new clots and extension of already existing clots, do not dissolve clots that have already formed. Widely used in thrombotic disorders, they are more effective in preventing venous thrombosis than arterial thrombosis. Antiplatelet drugs are used to prevent arterial

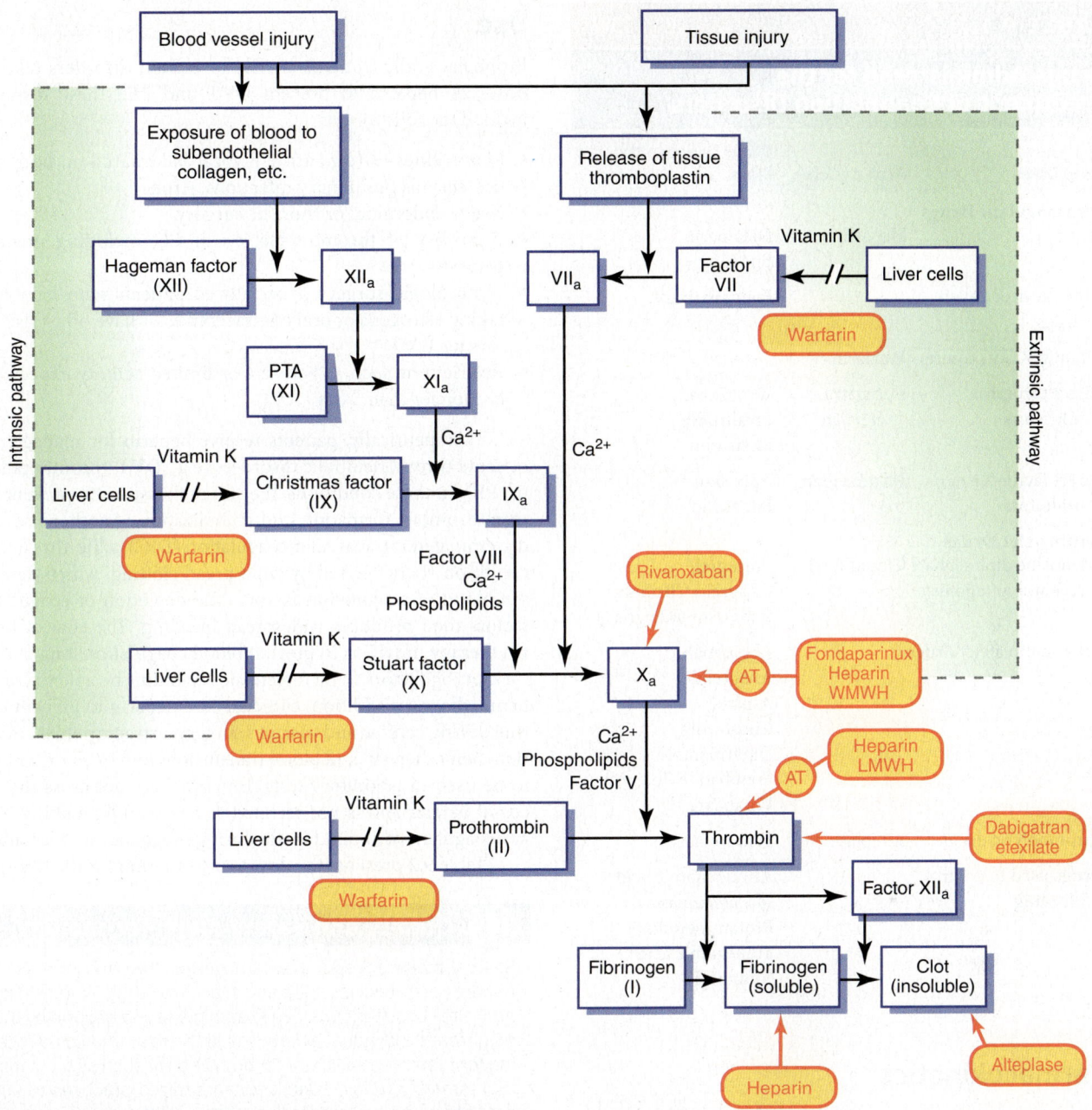

Figure 9.1. Details of the intrinsic and extrinsic clotting pathways. The sites of action of some of the drugs that can influence these processes are shown in *red*.

thrombosis. Thrombolytic drugs are used to dissolve thrombi and limit tissue damage in selected thromboembolic disorders.

> **! Quality and Safety Alert: Teamwork and Collaboration**
>
> Both the American College of Cardiology and the American Heart Association recommend that hospitals establish multidisciplinary teams to develop institution-specific written protocols, based on established clinical practice guidelines, for the triage and management of patients who present with symptoms indicative of acute myocardial ischemia. Additionally, a team-based approach to patient assessment and preliminary management helps to ensure that a patient receives essential care within the ideal 10 minutes after presentation of first medical contact.

ANTICOAGULANT DRUGS

There are four types of anticoagulants: heparins, vitamin K antagonists, direct thrombin inhibitors (DTIs), and direct factor Xa inhibitors.

HEARINS

Heparin is a pharmaceutical preparation of the natural anticoagulant produced primarily by mast cells in pericapillary connective tissue, and it is the prototype anticoagulant. Endogenous heparin is found in various body tissues, most abundantly in the liver and lungs. Exogenous heparin is obtained from bovine lung or porcine intestinal mucosa and standardized in units of biologic activity. See later in this chapter for a discussion of low-molecular-weight heparins (LMWHs).

TABLE 9.1

Drugs Administered for the Treatment of Coagulation Disorders

Drug Class	Prototype(s)	Other Drugs in the Class
Anticoagulant Drugs		
Heparins	Heparin	Dalteparin
		Enoxaparin
Other anticoagulant drugs		Fondaparinux
Vitamin K antagonists	Warfarin	
Direct thrombin inhibitors	Dabigatran etexilate	Argatroban
		Bivalirudin
		Desirudin
Direct factor Xa inhibitors	Rivaroxaban	Apixaban
		Edoxaban
Antiplatelet Drugs		
Adenosine diphosphate receptor antagonists	Clopidogrel	Prasugrel
		Ticagrelor (Brilinta)
		Cangrelor (Kengreal)
Other antiplatelet drugs		Abciximab
		Anagrelide
		Aspirin
		Cilostazol
		Dipyridamole
		Eptifibatide (Integrilin)
		Vorapaxar
Thrombolytic drugs	Alteplase	Tenecteplase
Drugs used to control bleeding		Aminocaproic acid
		Idarucizumab
		Protamine sulfate
		Tranexamic acid
		Vitamin K

Pharmacokinetics

Heparin must be given intravenously or subcutaneously because the gastrointestinal (GI) tract does not absorb the drug. After IV injection, the drug acts immediately. After subcutaneous injection, heparin acts within 20 to 30 minutes. Metabolism takes place in the liver and the reticuloendothelial system. Excretion, primarily in the form of inactive metabolites, occurs in the urine. Hemodialysis does not remove it.

Action

Heparin combines with antithrombin III (a natural anticoagulant in the blood) to inactivate clotting factors IX, X, XI, and XII; inhibit the conversion of prothrombin to thrombin; and prevent thrombus formation (see Fig. 9.1). After thrombosis has developed, heparin can inhibit additional coagulation by inactivating thrombin, preventing the conversion of fibrinogen to fibrin, and inhibiting factor XIII (fibrin-stabilizing factor). Other effects include inhibition of factors V and VIII and platelet aggregation.

Use

Prophylactically, patients at risk for certain disorders take low doses of heparin to prevent DVT and PE. These disorders include the following:

- Major illnesses (e.g., acute myocardial infarction, heart failure, serious pulmonary infections, stroke)
- Major abdominal or thoracic surgery
- A history of thrombophlebitis or PE, including pregnant patients
- Gynecologic surgery, especially in patients who have been taking estrogens or oral contraceptives or have other risk factors for DVT
- Restrictions such as bed rest or limited activity expected to last longer than 5 days

Therapeutically, patients receive heparin for management of acute thromboembolic disorders (e.g., DVT, thrombophlebitis, PE). In these conditions, the aim of therapy is to prevent further thrombus formation and embolization. Another use is in disseminated intravascular coagulation (DIC), a life-threatening condition characterized by widespread clotting, which depletes the blood of coagulation factors. The depletion of coagulation factors then produces widespread bleeding. The goal of heparin therapy in DIC is to prevent blood coagulation long enough for clotting factors to be replenished and thus be able to control hemorrhage. In addition, clinicians use heparin to prevent clotting during cardiac and vascular surgery, extracorporeal circulation, hemodialysis, and blood transfusions and in blood samples to be used in laboratory tests. Heparin does not cross the placental barrier and is not secreted in breast milk, making it the anticoagulant of choice for use during pregnancy and lactation.

Table 9.2 presents the dosage information for the heparins.

> **! Quality and Safety Alert: Technology**
>
> Several major adverse events have resulted from the use of heparin, and it is classified as a high-alert drug. Nurses demonstrate consistent practice in administrating heparin by their heightened individual awareness of the risks and by advocating for systems to account for human error such as bar coding and "smart" pumps. Effective standardized practices to support safety and quality include special safeguards to reduce the risk of errors that may harm the patient.

Patient-related variables specific to the use of heparin include the following:

- Age:
  - When children take heparin for systemic anticoagulation, weight is the basis for determination of dosage (approximately 50 units/kg).
  - Premature infants should not take heparin solutions containing benzyl alcohol as a preservative; metabolic acidosis and fatal reactions have resulted.
  - Older adults are more likely than younger adults to experience bleeding and other complications associated with this therapy.
- Reproduction, pregnancy, and lactation:
  - Preservative-free heparin solutions should be used during pregnancy.

TABLE 9.2

DRUGS AT A GLANCE: Anticoagulants

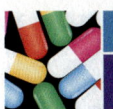

Drug	Indications for Use	Routes and Dosage Ranges (Adults, Unless Specified)
Heparins		
ⓟ **Heparin**	Prevention and management of thromboembolic disorders (e.g., DVT, PE, atrial fibrillation with embolization)	Adults: IV injection, 5,000 units initially, followed by 5,000–10,000 units every 4–6 h, to a maximum dose of 25,000 units/d; IV infusion, 5,000 units (loading dose), then 15–25 units/kg/h DIC, IV injection, 50–100 units/kg every 4 h; IV infusion, 20,000–40,000 units/d at initial rate of 0.25 units/kg/min, then adjusted according to aPTT; Sub-Q 10,000–12,000 units every 8 h, or 14,000–20,000 units every 12 h Low-dose prophylaxis, Sub-Q 5,000 units 2 h before surgery, then every 12 h until discharged from hospital or fully ambulatory Children: DIC, IV injection, 25–50 units/kg every 4 h; IV infusion, 50 units/kg initially, followed by 100 units/kg every 4 h or 20,000 units/m^2 over 24 h
Dalteparin (Fragmin; 🍁 Fragmin)	Prophylaxis of DVT in patients having abdominal or hip replacement surgery	Abdominal surgery, Sub-Q 2,500 IU 1–2 h before surgery and then once daily for 5–10 d after surgery Hip replacement surgery (3 options), Sub-Q 2,500 IU within 2 h before surgery and the evening of surgery (4–8 h after surgery) and then 5,000 IU once daily for 5–10 d; Sub-Q 2,500 IU 4–8 h after surgery and then 5,000 IU at least 6 h after postsurgical dose once daily for 5–10 d; Sub-Q 2,500 IU within 2 h before surgery and then Sub-Q 2,500 IU 4–8 h after surgery and then 5,000 IU once daily for 5–10 d
Enoxaparin (Lovenox; 🍁 Lovenox, Lovenox HP, Lovenox with Preservative)	Prevention and management of DVT and PE Management of unstable angina, to prevent or treat myocardial infarction	DVT prophylaxis in patients having hip or knee replacement surgery, Sub-Q 30 mg twice daily, with first dose within 12–24 h after surgery and continued until risk of DVT diminished or until adequately anticoagulated on warfarin Abdominal surgery, Sub-Q 40 mg once daily with first dose given 2 h before surgery, for 7–10 d DVT/PE management, outpatients, Sub-Q 1 mg/kg every 12 h; inpatients, 1 mg/kg every 12 h or 1.5 mg/kg every 24 h Moderate to high risk of thromboembolic disorders, Sub-Q 40 mg once daily; continue for length of hospital stay or until patient is fully ambulatory and risk of VTE has diminished Non–ST-elevation acute coronary syndromes, 1 mg/kg every 12 h in conjunction with recommended antiplatelet (i.e., PO aspirin 100–325 mg once daily) ST-elevation myocardial infarction between 15 min before or 30 min after fibrinolytic therapy, <75 y single IV bolus of 30 mg plus 1 mg/kg Sub-Q every 12 h with first Sub-Q dose given with IV bolus (maximum dose 100 mg for first 2 doses only); ≥75 y no IV bolus, Sub-Q 0.75 mg/kg every 12 h (maximum 75 mg for first 2 doses only)
Fondaparinux (Arixtra; 🍁 Arixtra)	Prevention of DVT following hip fracture surgery or knee or hip replacement Treatment of acute DVT or PE	Sub-Q 2.5 mg daily, with first dose 6–8 h after surgery and continuing for 5–9 d <50 kg, Sub-Q 5 mg once daily 50–100 kg, Sub-Q 7.5 mg once daily >100 kg, Sub-Q 10 mg once daily
Vitamin K Antagonist		
ⓟ **Warfarin** (Coumadin, Jantoven; 🍁 Apo-Warfarin, Coumadin, Taro-Warfarin)	Long-term prevention or management of venous thromboembolic disorders, including DVT, PE, and embolization associated with atrial fibrillation and prosthetic heart valves. May also be used after myocardial infarction to decrease reinfarction, stroke, venous thromboembolism, and death	PO 2–5 mg/d for 2–3 d, then adjusted according to the INR; average maintenance daily dose, 2–5 mg

(Continued on page 142)

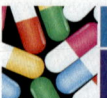

TABLE 9.2

DRUGS AT A GLANCE: Anticoagulants (Continued)

Drug	Indications for Use	Routes and Dosage Ranges (Adults, Unless Specified)
Direct Thrombin Inhibitors		
ⓟ Dabigatran etexilate (Pradaxa; ❋ Pradaxa)	Decrease the risk of stroke and systemic embolism with nonvalvular atrial fibrillation	PO 150 mg twice daily; in severe kidney failure, 75 mg twice daily
Argatroban (Argatroban)	Thrombosis prophylaxis or management in heparin-induced thrombocytopenia; adjunct to PTCA	IV continuous infusion 2 mcg/kg/min
Bivalirudin (Angiomax; ❋ Angiomax)	Patients with unstable angina undergoing PTCA; acute coronary syndrome; used concomitantly with aspirin therapy	IV bolus dose of 0.75 mg/kg followed by 4-h infusion at rate of 1.75 mg/kg/min
Desirudin (Iprivask)	Prophylaxis of DVT in patients having hip replacement surgery	Sub-Q, 15 mg every 12 h; first dose should be given 5–15 min before surgery and may be administered for up to 12 d postsurgery
Direct Factor Xa Inhibitors		
ⓟ Rivaroxaban (Xarelto; ❋ Xarelto)	Prophylaxis of DVT, which may lead to PE in patients having knee or hip replacement surgery Treatment and secondary prevention of DVT Stroke prevention in nonvalvular atrial fibrillation	PO 10 mg once daily; may be administered for up to 12 d postsurgery for knee replacement and 35 d postsurgery for hip replacement PO 15 mg twice daily with food for 21 d; followed by 20 mg once daily with food PO 20 mg once daily with evening meal with creatinine clearance >50 mL/min or 15 mg once daily with evening meal with creatinine clearance 15–50 mL/min
Apixaban (Eliquis; ❋ Eliquis)	Prophylaxis of DVT in patients having hip or knee replacement surgery Stroke prevention with atrial fibrillation Treatment of DVT and/or PE	PO 2.5 mg twice daily for 35 d with hip replacement; for 12 d for knee replacement. 5 mg twice daily or 2.5 mg twice daily with any two ≥80 y, body weight ≤60 kg, or serum creatinine ≥1.5 mg/dL DVT and PE treatment: PO 10 mg twice daily for 7 d; followed by 5 mg twice daily
Edoxaban (Savaysa; ❋ Lixiana)	Prevention of venous thromboembolic disease and stroke prevention in patients with nonvalvular atrial fibrillation Treatment of DVT and/or PE	Prevention: PO 60 mg d Treatment: after 5 d of parenteral anticoagulant in hemodynamically stable patients: ≤60 kg, PO 30 mg once daily >60 kg, PO 60 mg once daily

aPTT, activated partial thromboplastin time; DIC, disseminated intravascular coagulation; DVT, deep vein thrombosis; INR, international normalized ratio; PE, pulmonary embolism; PTCA, percutaneous transluminal coronary angioplasty or atherectomy.

- Abnormal kidney function and hepatic impairment:
  - The half-life of heparin may increase in people with abnormal kidney function or hepatic impairment; heparin dosage adjusted according to activated partial thromboplastin time (aPTT).
- Specific healthcare environments:
  - Critically ill patients have a high risk of DVT and PE as well as a higher morbidity and mortality. Effective prevention and treatment of thrombosis is necessary and typically includes LMWHs.

Adverse Effects

Hemorrhage is the major side effect of heparin therapy, hypersensitivity to the drug has occurred, and local irritation with subcutaneous injections of heparin can cause erythema and mild pain. **Heparin-induced thrombocytopenia (HIT)** (type II) is a potentially life-threatening complication of heparin administration, leading to a decrease in platelet count and detectable HIT antibodies. This condition occurs in 1% to 3% of people receiving heparin at therapeutic levels for 4 to 14 days, sometimes sooner in those who have previously received heparin. HIT is one of the most common immune-mediated adverse drug reactions. All patients exposed to any heparin at therapeutic or prophylactic doses or minute amounts in heparin flushes or on heparin-coated catheters, as well as those receiving LMWH, are at risk. If HIT occurs, it is necessary to discontinue all heparin and manage anticoagulation with a DTI such as argatroban.

Contraindications

Contraindications include GI ulcerations (e.g., peptic ulcer disease, ulcerative colitis), intracranial bleeding, dissecting aortic aneurysm, blood dyscrasias, severe kidney or liver disease, severe hypertension, polycythemia vera, and recent surgery of the eye, spinal cord, or brain.

Nursing Implications

Preventing Interactions

Many medications interact with heparin, increasing or decreasing its effect (Box 9.1). Some herbs and foods increase the effects of the drug including chamomile, garlic, ginger, ginkgo, ginseng, and high-dose vitamin E. No herbs or foods that decrease the effects of heparin have been identified.

Administering the Medication

Traditional anticoagulants have two major limitations: a narrow therapeutic window of adequate anticoagulation without bleeding and a highly variable individual dose–response that requires monitoring by laboratory testing. Prescribers use aPTT, which is sensitive to changes in blood clotting factors, except factor VII, to regulate heparin dosage. Thus, normal or control values of aPTT indicate normal blood coagulation, and therapeutic values of adequate anticoagulation indicate low levels of clotting factors and delayed blood coagulation. During heparin therapy, the aPTT should be maintained at approximately 1.5 to 2.5 times the control or baseline value. The normal control value is 25 to 35 seconds; therefore, therapeutic values of adequate anticoagulation are 45 to 70 seconds, approximately. With continuous IV infusion, blood for the aPTT may be drawn at any time; with intermittent administration, blood for the aPTT should be drawn approximately 1 hour before a dose of heparin is scheduled. It is not necessary to monitor aPTT with low-dose standard heparin given subcutaneously for prophylaxis of thromboembolism or with the LMWHs (e.g., enoxaparin).

The nurse should be aware that heparin has disadvantages: parenteral injection is necessary, and the drug has a short duration of action, which means that there is a need for frequent administration.

Assessing for Therapeutic Effects

The nurse assesses for the absence or reduction of signs and symptoms of thrombotic disorders (e.g., less edema and pain with DVT, less chest pain and respiratory difficulty with PE, absence of uncontrolled bleeding). It is also necessary to ensure that aPTT values are within the therapeutic range.

Assessing for Adverse Effects

The nurse assesses the patient for signs of overt bleeding or HIT. Protamine sulfate, which is discussed in more detail later in this chapter, is an antidote for standard heparin and LMWHs. Protamine is typically given for bleeding that may not respond to merely withdrawing the heparin or when hemorrhaging is present.

Patient Teaching

Education related to bleeding risk is essential for patients receiving heparin. The nurse reinforces instructions for safe use of the drug and related anticoagulants, reminding patients to obtain laboratory tests, and teaching how to observe for signs and symptoms of bleeding. Additional patient teaching guidelines for anticoagulants, including heparins, are outlined in Box 9.2.

Other Drugs in the Class

LMWHs are synthetic heparins, have smaller molecular structures, and efficiently inactivate factor Xa via antithrombin. The drugs are as effective as IV heparin in treating thrombotic disorders and provide a more predictable anticoagulant response at recommended doses. The drugs do not cross the placenta. Indications for their use include prevention or management of thromboembolic complications associated with surgery or ischemic complications of unstable angina and myocardial infarction. The currently available LMWHs, dalteparin (Fragmin) and enoxaparin (Lovenox), are not interchangeable (unit for unit) with standard heparin or another LMWH.

LMWHs are typically given subcutaneously in fixed or weight-based dosing without monitoring of blood coagulation. These characteristics simplify outpatient anticoagulant therapy and safety. Enoxaparin may be administered intravenously in specific situations but should not be given intramuscularly. The drugs are also associated with less thrombocytopenia than is standard heparin. However, monitoring of platelet counts during therapy is necessary. With significant bleeding, protamine sulfate may be considered, although it does not completely neutralize LMWHs; clinical bleeding may be reduced. The Institute for Safe Medication Practices (ISMP) classifies the LMWHs as high-alert drugs because there is a possible risk of significant harm when the drugs are used in error.

Fondaparinux (Arixtra) indirectly and selectively inhibits factor Xa by mechanisms identical to LMWHs but without affecting thrombin activity. As a synthetic pentasaccharide, the drug binds to antithrombin and is administered for pro-

---

BOX 9.1 *Drug Interactions: Heparin*

Drugs That Increase the Effects of Heparin

- Alteplase, direct thrombin inhibitors, platelet inhibitors
  Increase the risk of bleeding
- Antithrombin
  Increases pharmacologic effects
- Cephalosporins
  Lead to potential coagulopathies and risk of bleeding
- Penicillins (parenteral)
  Lead to altered platelet aggregation and increased risk of bleeding
- Warfarin
  May prolong and possibly invalidate the PT; if receiving both heparin and warfarin, draw blood for the PT at least 5 hours after the last IV heparin dose

Drugs That Decrease the Effects of Heparin

- Antihistamines, digoxin, nicotine, nitroglycerin (IV), tetracycline
  Decrease the anticoagulant effect

IV, intravenous; PT, prothrombin time.

BOX 9.2 Patient Teaching Guidelines for Anticoagulants

General Considerations

- Anticoagulant drugs are given to people who have had, or who are at risk of having, a heart attack, stroke, or other problems from blood clots. For home management of deep vein thrombosis, which usually occurs in the legs, you are likely to be given heparin injections for a few days, followed by warfarin for long-term therapy. These medications help prevent the blood clot from getting larger, traveling to your lungs, or recurring later.
- All anticoagulants can increase the risk of bleeding, so you need to take safety precautions to prevent injury.
- To help prevent blood clots from forming and decreasing blood flow through your arteries, you need to reduce risk factors that contribute to cardiovascular disease. This can be done by a low-fat, low-cholesterol diet (and medication if needed) to lower total cholesterol to below 200 mg/dL and low-density lipoprotein cholesterol to below 130 mg/dL; weight reduction if overweight; control of blood pressure if hypertensive; avoidance of smoking; stress reduction techniques; and regular exercise.
- To help maintain a steady level of anticoagulation with warfarin, do not change your intake of foods that are high in vitamin K, which decreases the effects of warfarin. These foods include broccoli, brussels sprouts, cabbage, cauliflower, chives, collard greens, kale, lettuce, mustard greens, peppers, spinach, tomatoes, turnips, and watercress.
- To help prevent blood clots from forming in your leg veins, avoid or minimize situations that slow blood circulation, such as wearing tight clothing, crossing the legs at the knees, prolonged sitting or standing, and bed rest. For example, on automobile trips, stop and walk around every 1 to 2 hours; on long plane trips, exercise your feet and legs at your seat and walk around when you can.
- Following instructions regarding these medications is extremely important. Too little medication increases your risk of problems from blood clot formation; too much medication can cause bleeding.
- While taking any of these medications, you need regular medical supervision and periodic blood tests. The blood tests can help your healthcare provider regulate drug dosage and maintain your safety.
- Notify your healthcare provider if you suddenly stop tobacco smoking, because this may result in a reduced clearance of warfarin. A dosage change may be necessary.
- With enoxaparin, you need an injection, usually every 12 hours. You or someone close to you may be instructed in injecting the medication, or a home care nurse may do the injections, if necessary.
- Avoid taking other drugs without the healthcare provider's knowledge and consent, inform any healthcare provider (including dentists) that you are taking an anticoagulant drug before any invasive diagnostic tests or treatments are begun, and keep all appointments for continuing care.
- With warfarin therapy, avoid walking barefoot; avoid contact sports; use an electric razor; avoid injections when possible; and carry an identification card, necklace, or bracelet (e.g., MedicAlert) stating the name of the drug and the healthcare provider's name and telephone number.
- A routine blood test is necessary to ensure that your warfarin dose is appropriate. The results of this test determine your daily dose of warfarin. Once the warfarin dose stabilizes, the blood tests are done less often (e.g., every 2 weeks).
- Report any sign of bleeding (e.g., excessive bruising of the skin, blood in urine or stool). If superficial bleeding occurs, apply direct pressure to the site for 3 to 5 minutes or longer if necessary.

Self-Administration

- With enoxaparin, wash hands and cleanse the skin to prevent infection; inject deep under the skin, around the navel, upper thigh, or buttocks; and change the injection site daily. If excessive bruising occurs at the injection site, rubbing an ice cube over an area before the injection may be helpful.
- With warfarin, the prescriber may set a dosing schedule that could vary from one day to the next. Do not rely on memory but keep a written record of the date and the amount of medication taken.

---

phylaxis of DVT in people undergoing hip or knee surgery. It is administered subcutaneously and has a longer half-life than LMWHs, necessitating only a once-daily dose. The ISMP classifies fondaparinux as a high-alert drug because there is a possible risk of significant harm when the drug is used in error. Fondaparinux has no effect on prothrombin time, aPTT, platelet aggregation, or bleeding time, so it does not require routine coagulation monitoring. As with other anticoagulants, bleeding is a concern particularly in patients with kidney dysfunction, because fondaparinux is primarily eliminated by the kidneys. Currently, no agent for reversal of fondaparinux is available.

Clinical Application 9.1

- To regulate the amount of heparin Mr. Oliver receives, his aPTT is measured. What is the therapeutic value for aPTT?

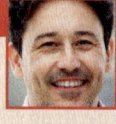

VITAMIN K ANTAGONISTS

Warfarin (Coumadin) is the most used oral anticoagulant and is the prototype vitamin K antagonist. Table 9.2 presents dosage information for warfarin.

Pharmacokinetics

Warfarin is well absorbed after oral administration. Administration with food may delay the rate but not the extent of absorption. The drug is highly bound to plasma proteins (98%), mainly albumin. Metabolism takes place in the liver. Excretion, primarily as inactive metabolites, occurs in the kidneys. Abnormal kidney function does not affect drug metabolism but may decrease excretion of the drug.

Action

Warfarin acts in the liver to prevent synthesis of vitamin K–dependent clotting factors (i.e., factors II, VII, IX, and X).

Similar to vitamin K in structure, warfarin therefore acts as a competitive antagonist to hepatic use of vitamin K. Conversely, vitamin K serves as the antidote for warfarin. Warfarin has no effect on circulating clotting factors or on platelet function, so the anticoagulant effects do not occur for 3 to 5 days after warfarin is started because clotting factors already in the blood follow their normal pathway of elimination.

Use

Warfarin is most useful in long-term prevention or management of venous thromboembolic disorders, including DVT, PE, and embolization associated with atrial fibrillation and prosthetic heart valves. In addition, warfarin therapy after myocardial infarction may decrease reinfarction, stroke, venous thromboembolism, and death. The smaller doses used now are equally effective as ones used formerly, with similar antithrombotic effects and decreased risks of bleeding.

Patient-related variables specific to the use of warfarin include the following:

- Age:
  - In children, informing others of use of warfarin in the child's environment (e.g., teachers, babysitters, healthcare providers) is necessary.
  - In older adults, warfarin metabolism may be altered so a lower dose of warfarin is usually required to produce a therapeutic effect.
- Reproduction, pregnancy, and lactation:
  - Warfarin is contraindicated during pregnancy because it crosses the placenta, has potential teratogenic effects, and causes fetal anticoagulation, which may lead to fatal fetal hemorrhage.
  - Exposure to warfarin during early pregnancy can cause embryopathy; fetal bleeding, including intracranial hemorrhage, can occur with exposure later in pregnancy.
- Abnormal kidney function and hepatic impairment:
  - Warfarin is more likely to cause bleeding in patients with hepatic disease because of decreased synthesis of vitamin K and decreased plasma proteins.
  - Only the liver eliminates warfarin; thus, the drug may accumulate in people with hepatic impairment, and dosage adjustment may be necessary.
- Specific healthcare environments:
  - For home management of DVT, warfarin may be self-administered, but a nurse usually visits, performs a fingerstick international normalized ratio (INR), and notifies the prescriber, who then prescribes the appropriate dose of warfarin. Periodic office or clinic visits are needed for blood tests and other follow-up care.

Adverse Effects

The primary adverse effect associated with warfarin therapy is hemorrhage. Additionally, nausea, vomiting, abdominal pain, alopecia, urticaria, dizziness, and joint or muscle pain may occur.

Contraindications

Contraindications to warfarin include GI ulcerations, blood disorders associated with bleeding, pregnancy, severe kidney or liver disease, severe hypertension, and recent surgery of the eye, spinal cord, or brain. Caution is warranted in patients with mild hypertension, kidney or hepatic disease, alcoholism, history of GI ulcerations, drainage tubes (e.g., nasogastric tubes, indwelling urinary catheters), or occupations with high risks of traumatic injury. The U.S. Food and Drug Administration (FDA) has issued a **BOXED WARNING** for warfarin because of the risk of its causing major or fatal bleeding.

Nursing Implications

Preventing Interactions

Many medications interact with warfarin, increasing or decreasing its effect (Box 9.3). In addition, many herbs and food interact with warfarin. Herbs and foods that increase the effects of warfarin include angelica, cat's claw, chamomile, chondroitin, cranberry juice, feverfew, garlic, ginkgo, goldenseal, grape seed extract, green tea, psyllium, and turmeric. Herbs that decrease the effects of warfarin include ginseng and St. John's wort. Since vitamin K is the antidote for warfarin, any food that contains vitamin K can reduce the effects of warfarin, increasing the risk of clot formation. Foods high in vitamin K include broccoli, brussels sprouts, cabbage, cauliflower, chives, collard greens, kale, lettuce, mustard greens, peppers, spinach, tomatoes, turnips, and watercress.

Administering the Medication

Vitamin K antagonists such as warfarin have a narrow therapeutic window of adequate anticoagulation without bleeding and a highly variable individual dose–response that requires monitoring by laboratory testing. Accurate drug administration, close monitoring of blood coagulation tests, safety measures to prevent trauma and bleeding, and avoiding interacting drugs are necessary.

> **! Quality and Safety Alert: Safety**
>
> When warfarin therapy begins, daily evaluation of INR is necessary until a stable daily dose is reached [the dose that maintains the prothrombin time [PT] and INR within therapeutic ranges and does not cause bleeding]. A therapeutic PT value is approximately 1.5 times control, or 18 seconds. Thereafter, a patient's INR values require checking every 2 to 4 weeks for the duration of oral anticoagulant drug therapy. If a prescriber changes the warfarin dose, more frequent INR measurements are necessary until a stable daily dose is again established. The nurse should administer warfarin after ensuring that laboratory values are within therapeutic parameters.

> **! Quality and Safety Alert: Safety**
>
> Institutions often have a protocol for the therapeutic range of INR. In the absence of a protocol, the nurse should hold the dose if the INR is above 3.0 and notify the healthcare provider.

Assessing for Therapeutic Effects

As with heparin, the nurse assesses for the absence or reduction of signs and symptoms of thrombotic disorders (e.g., less edema and pain with DVT, less chest pain and respiratory difficulty with PE, absence of uncontrolled bleeding, hematuria, or blood in the stools). It is also necessary to ensure that PT and INR values are within the therapeutic range.

Assessing for Adverse Effects

The nurse assesses for signs of bleeding, including excessive bruising of the skin, bleeding from IV sites or the gum line, and blood in the urine or stool.

BOX 9.3 Drug Interactions: Warfarin

Drugs That Increase the Effects of Warfarin

- Acetaminophen (high dose), allopurinol, amiodarone
  Increase the anticoagulant effect
- Alteplase, androgens, aspirin and other nonsteroidal anti-inflammatory drugs, azithromycin, bismuth subsalicylate, carbamazepine, chloral hydrate, chloramphenicol, cimetidine, ciprofloxacin and other quinolone antibiotics, cisapride, clarithromycin, clofibrate, cotrimoxazole, direct thrombin inhibitors, heparin, macrolide antibiotics, omeprazole, pravastatin, propranolol, quinidine, ranitidine, ritonavir, sertraline, simvastatin, sulfinpyrazone, sulfonamide, tamoxifen, tetracyclines, thyroid hormones, tricyclic antidepressants, vancomycin, vitamin E
  Increase the risk of bleeding
- Antithrombin
  Increases the pharmacologic effect
- Cephalosporins
  Result in potential coagulopathies and risk of bleeding

Drugs That Decrease the Effects of Warfarin

- Chlordiazepoxide, haloperidol, intravenous lipid emulsions (contains soybean oil), isotretinoin, meprobamate, spironolactone
  Cause effects by various mechanisms
- Chlorthalidone
  May diminish warfarin's ability to cause blood clots to form
- Ethchlorvynol, trazodone
  Cause effects by unknown mechanism
- Etretinate
  May induce anticoagulant's hepatic microsomal enzyme

Quality and Safety Alert: Safety

As the antidote for warfarin, vitamin K may be ordered if the INR level is 5 or more and signs of bleeding are present. Additionally, prothrombin complex concentrate (PCC), human (Kcentra), is used for urgent warfarin reversal with major or life-threatening hemorrhage.

Patient Teaching

The nurse reinforces instructions for safe use of warfarin, assists patients to obtain required laboratory tests, and teaches how to observe for signs and symptoms of bleeding. Additional patient teaching guidelines for anticoagulant medications, including vitamin K antagonists, are outlined in Box 9.2.

Clinical Application 9.2

- Mr. Oliver's prescriber adds warfarin to his treatment regimen. The order is for warfarin 5 mg PO daily and for evaluation of baseline PT and INR. The nurse administers the warfarin and reviews the order for the blood work for the next morning. What therapeutic INR value indicates that the warfarin dosage is appropriate?

Unfolding Patient Stories: Rachel Heidebrink • Part 2

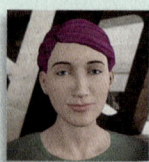

Think back to Chapter 7, where you met Rachel Heidebrink, who underwent a right hemiarthroplasty for a fracture to the right greater trochanter sustained in a motorcycle accident. She is diagnosed with a pulmonary embolism (PE) on postoperative day 1. How would the nurse explain the effect of heparin for the management of a PE and why the route of administration begins with an intravenous loading dose followed by a continuous infusion? What nursing assessments and interventions ensure the safe administration of intravenous heparin? How would the nurse explain the combination of oral and intravenous anticoagulant therapy?

Care for Rachel and other patients in a realistic virtual environment: **vSim** *for Nursing* (thepoint.lww.com/vSimPharm). Practice documenting these patients' care in DocuCare (thepoint.lww.com/DocuCareEHR).

NCLEX Success

1. The nurse is reviewing the laboratory results of a hospitalized patient receiving intravenous heparin therapy for pulmonary embolism. The activated partial thromboplastin time (aPTT) is 38 seconds (control 28 seconds). The nurse should
   A. not give the next dose because the level is too high
   B. continue the present order because the level is appropriate
   C. notify the healthcare provider that the aPTT is low and anticipate orders to increase the dose
   D. request an order for warfarin now that the patient is heparinized

2. In explaining the use of warfarin to a female patient, the nurse is correct in telling her which of the following regarding warfarin? (Select all that apply.)
   A. Warfarin is a vitamin K antagonist.
   B. Warfarin does not cross the placenta.
   C. Warfarin is used for long-term anticoagulation therapy.
   D. Warfarin is metabolized by the liver.

3. In developing a safe plan of care, the nurse recognizes that which of the following agents is the antidote for heparin?
   A. protamine zinc
   B. vitamin K
   C. protamine sulfate
   D. vitamin D

4. Which of the following assessment findings are positive outcomes in a patient receiving warfarin for the management of pulmonary embolism? (Select all that apply.)
   A. report of absence of chest pain
   B. respiratory rate of 18/min with no use of accessory muscles
   C. absence of uncontrolled bleeding
   D. international normalized ratio serum level of 3.2
   E. prothrombin time serum level of 18 seconds
   F. presence of hematuria

DIRECT THROMBIN INHIBITORS

DTIs have benefits compared with agents such as heparin and warfarin, including the inhibition of both circulating and clot-bound thrombin. Other advantages of DTIs include a more predictable dose–response anticoagulant effect, inhibition of thrombin-induced platelet aggregation, and the lack of production of immune-mediated thrombocytopenia. Heparin and warfarin are indirect inhibitors of thrombin. The DTIs exert their effect by interacting directly with the thrombin molecule without the need of a cofactor, such as heparin cofactor II or antithrombin. As such, they inhibit thrombin's ability to convert soluble fibrinogen to fibrin and to activate the fibrin-generating factors V, VIII, and IX. Because thrombin also stimulates platelets, DTIs also have antiplatelet activity.

Both parenteral and oral DTIs are available. The original prototype of the bivalent type, hirudin, is not commercially available; however, its discovery led to the development through recombinant technology of parenteral derivatives, bivalirudin, desirudin, argatroban, and one oral DTI, dabigatran. In this discussion, the only oral DTI, **dabigatran etexilate** (Pradaxa), serves as the prototype. Table 9.2 presents dosage information for the DTIs.

Pharmacokinetics

Dabigatran etexilate is an inactive prodrug that is rapidly hydrolyzed to dabigatran, its active form, in the body by plasma and hepatic esterases. The drug is excreted in the urine, and the systemic elimination is proportional to the glomerular filtration rate. Typically, the elimination half-life is 12 to 17 hours, which may take longer in older adults and those with kidney failure.

Action

As an inactive prodrug, dabigatran etexilate lacks anticoagulant activity. With conversion to the active form in the body, dabigatran has been shown to specifically and reversibly inhibit both free and fibrin-bound thrombin, the key enzyme in the coagulation cascade, thereby inhibiting coagulation. DTIs have no known antagonists. Given orally, the drug peaks in 1 hour.

Use

Dabigatran etexilate is used to prevent strokes and systemic embolization in individuals with nonvalvular atrial fibrillation. In addition, it is given for the treatment and prevention of DVT and PE. Therapeutic drug monitoring is not necessary.

Patient-related variables specific to the use of dabigatran etexilate and other direct thrombin inhibitors include the following:

- Age:
  - Dabigatran etexilate is identified in the Beers Criteria as a potentially inappropriate medication for older adults.
  - No dosage adjustment of dabigatran etexilate is needed in older patients with normal kidney function.
  - The drug should be used with caution in older adults who have a creatinine clearance less than 30 mL/min or in those aged 75 years or older.
- Reproduction, pregnancy, and lactation:
  - The drug should be used with caution in pregnancy and lactation.
- Abnormal kidney function and hepatic impairment:
  - Because dabigatran etexilate is cleared by the kidneys, it accumulates in patients with abnormal kidney function, and dosage adjustments may be required based on creatinine clearance calculations.
  - The use of the drug is not recommended in patients receiving hemodialysis.
  - Information from the drug's registry has suggested cholestatic liver injury as a rare adverse effect but has yet to be supported by current research studies.

Adverse Effects

The most common adverse effects associated with the administration of dabigatran etexilate are bleeding, dyspepsia, abdominal pain, gastritis, and anemia. The FDA has issued a **BOXED WARNING ◆** concerning the increased risk of blood clots in and around the spinal column when stopping the use of dabigatran etexilate.

> **! Quality and Safety Alert: Safety**
>
> After reports of severe liver injury in patients treated with dabigatran etexilate, Health Canada, a federal agency focused on maintaining and enhancing the health of Canadians, reviewed and concluded that there may be a link between the drug and liver injury and is working with the drug's manufacturer to update safety information regarding the apparent link between the drug and liver injury. Manufacturer administration of PRADAXA in patients with moderate hepatic impairment (Child-Pugh B) showed a large intersubject variability but no evidence of a consistent change in exposure or pharmacodynamics.

Contraindications

Contraindications include a known hypersensitivity to any of the components of dabigatran etexilate and in patients with active pathologic bleeding or with a mechanical prosthetic heart valve.

Nursing Implications

The ISMP classifies dabigatran etexilate as a high-alert drug because of the possible risk of significant harm that results when it is used in error.

Preventing Interactions

Many medications interact with dabigatran etexilate, altering its effect (Box 9.4).

Herbs that increase the effects of dabigatran etexilate include alfalfa, anise, bilberry, omega-3 fatty acids, and vitamin E. No herbs are known to decrease the drug's effects. No foods decrease the drug's bioavailability, although the drug's peak plasma concentration is delayed 2 hours if taken with food.

Administering the Medication

The drug capsules should be administered intact with a full glass of water without regard to meals. If the capsules are open or chewed, absorption is increased, and the risk of adverse drug effects is enhanced.

> **BOX 9.4 Drug Interactions: Dabigatran Etexilate**
>
> **Drugs That Increase the Effects of Dabigatran Etexilate**
> - Anticoagulants, apixaban, aspirin, antiplatelet agents (especially clopidogrel), collagenase, dasatinib, deferasirox, deoxycholic acid, edoxaban, hemin, limaprost, nonsteroidal anti-inflammatory agents, pentosan polysulfate sodium, prostacyclin analogues, salicylates, sugammadex, sulfinpyrazone, thrombolytics, tibolone, ticagrelor, vorapaxar
>   *Increase the risk of bleeding*
> - Amiodarone, clarithromycin, dronedarone, ketoconazole P-glycoprotein/ABCB1 inhibitors, quinidine, verapamil
>   *May increase serum concentration*
>
> **Drugs That Decrease the Effects of Dabigatran Etexilate**
> - Antacids, atorvastatin, lumacaftor, P-glycoprotein/ABCB1 inducers, proton pump inhibitors
>   *May decrease serum concentration*
> - Estrogen derivatives, progestins
>   *May decrease the anticoagulant effects*

Assessing for Therapeutic Effects

The nurse assesses for the absence of signs and symptoms of thrombotic disorders, including HIT, and for laboratory values within normal range. A therapeutic range has not been established for tests of anticoagulant activity.

Assessing for Adverse Effects

The most common adverse effect associated with the administration of dabigatran etexilate is bleeding; therefore, assessing for signs of bleeding is a priority. Additionally, the nurse assesses for other adverse effects, including GI and hematologic effects. The anticoagulant effects of dabigatran can be reversed by idarucizumab (Praxbind).

Patient Teaching

Patients need to understand that stopping the drug without provider instruction could increase the risk of blood clots. Patients should notify other healthcare providers about taking dabigatran etexilate, particularly with spinal or epidural procedures that increase the risk of bleeding around the spine, because paralysis may occur. Additional general patient teaching guidelines for anticoagulants, including the DTIs, are outlined in Box 9.2.

Other Drugs in the Class

In comparison to heparin, which binds only circulating thrombin, DTIs such as bivalirudin and desirudin block circulating thrombin and clot-bound thrombin. Bivalirudin is given intravenously as a specific and reversible DTI approved for the treatment of patients with unstable angina undergoing percutaneous transluminal coronary angioplasty (PTCA), as an anticoagulant in patients undergoing PTCA, and as an alternative to heparin in patients with or at risk of developing HIT. Desirudin has been shown to be more effective than enoxaparin in preventing DVT following total hip replacement. Desirudin is administered subcutaneously, and highly protein bound drugs do not modify its effects.

Argatroban is indicated for HIT, is eliminated in the liver, and can be used in people with kidney failure with replacement therapy. Administered intravenously, argatroban is very short acting due to its reversible binding to thrombin.

DIRECT FACTOR XA INHIBITORS

Direct factor Xa inhibitors inactivate circulating and clot-bound factor Xa. Unlike fondaparinux, which acts indirectly, this class of drugs binds directly and, by doing so, inhibits the production of thrombin. These direct oral anticoagulants, along with dabigatran, are at least as effective as the vitamin K antagonists but are associated with less life-threatening bleeding. Currently, three orally acting direct factor Xa inhibitors are approved, rivaroxaban, apixaban, and edoxaban; no direct factor Xa inhibitors are available for intravenous infusion. **P Rivaroxaban** serves as the prototype.

Pharmacokinetics

Rivaroxaban is rapidly absorbed and is highly bound to protein. The drug undergoes partial metabolism by CYP3A4 (an isozyme of the cytochrome P450 system) and is excreted in the urine (36% as unchanged drug) and feces (7% as unchanged drug). Peak plasma levels are reached in 2 to 4 hours, and the half-life is 5 to 9 hours.

Actions

Rivaroxaban inhibits platelet activation and formation of fibrin clotting by inhibition of factor Xa in both intrinsic and extrinsic coagulation pathways.

Use

Rivaroxaban is used in the treatment and secondary prevention of venous thromboembolism and in stroke prevention in patients with nonvalvular atrial fibrillation.

Patient-related variables specific to the use of rivaroxaban and other direct factor Xa inhibitors include the following:

- Age:
  - The safety of rivaroxaban in children has not been established.
  - According to the Beers Criteria (see Chapter 5), dosage adjustment is indicated in older adults with creatinine clearance between 30 and 50 mL/min.
  - Rivaroxaban is a potentially inappropriate medication in older adults (Beers Criteria) with a creatinine clearance less than 30 mL/min because of increased risk of bleeding.
- Reproduction, pregnancy, and lactation:
  - The safety of rivaroxaban during pregnancy and postpartum has not been established.
  - Patients planning to become pregnant should have an alternate anticoagulant considered prior to conception.
  - Until safety data are available, rivaroxaban and other direct acting oral anticoagulants are not recommended for use in patients who are breast-feeding (ACOG, 2018).

- Abnormal kidney function and hepatic impairment:
  - Rivaroxaban is metabolized in the kidney and the liver. Therefore, the drug should not be used in individuals with a creatinine clearance of less than 15 mL/min; with delayed excretion of the drug, there may be increased risk of bleeding.
  - Rivaroxaban should not be used in individuals with moderate to severe hepatic impairment.
- Specific healthcare environments:
  - Individuals who are critically ill may have complications necessitating the use of rivaroxaban, including treatment and secondary prevention of venous thromboembolism and for stroke prevention in patients with atrial fibrillation.
  - Critically ill patients have a high risk of DVT and PE, as well as an increased risk of bleeding in the presence of other coexisting conditions, particularly those involving the kidneys or liver.
  - In the home care setting, rivaroxaban use following knee or hip surgery for the prevention of venous thrombosis or management of nonvalvular atrial fibrillation has become common practice as the drug requires no INR monitoring.

Adverse Effects

Bleeding is the most common adverse effect of rivaroxaban, and this risk increases if the drug is taken with other agents that alter hemostasis. Intracranial, gastric, and retinal bleeding has been reported. Additionally, the possibility of spinal or epidural hematoma exists in patients undergoing epidural anesthesia or spinal puncture with procedures or trauma that can lead to permanent paralysis. Dosage adjustment is recommended with anticipated procedures involving the spine.

Contraindications

Contraindications to rivaroxaban include a known hypersensitivity to the drug. Benefits of therapy in pregnancy should outweigh risks.

Nursing Implications

Preventing Interactions

Numerous drugs interact with rivaroxaban, increasing or decreasing its effect (Box 9.5). Alfalfa, anise, bilberry, and grapefruit juice increase the effects of rivaroxaban. Conversely, St. John's wort may decrease the drugs effect.

Administering the Medication

Rivaroxaban is generally given at a fixed dose. Although 10-mg tablets can be administered without regard to food, 15- and 20-mg tablets should be taken with food. The drug should be administered with the evening meal for nonvalvular atrial fibrillation.

Assessing for Therapeutic Effects

The nurse should assess for the absence of DVT or other unanticipated clotting. No routine monitoring of INR or other coagulation parameters is required.

> **BOX 9.5** **Drug Interactions: Rivaroxaban**
>
> **Drugs That Increase the Effects of Rivaroxaban**
> - Anticoagulants, apixaban, aspirin, antiplatelet agents, collagenase, dasatinib, edoxaban, hemin, ibrutinib, limaprost, nonsteroidal anti-inflammatory agents, pentosan polysulfate sodium, prostacyclin analogues, salicylates, sugammadex, thrombolytics, tibolone, tipranavir, vorapaxar, vitamin E
>   *Increase the risk of bleeding*
> - Clarithromycin, osimertinib
>   *May increase serum concentration*
>
> **Drugs That Decrease the Effects of Rivaroxaban**
> - Bosentan, CYP3A4 inducers, deferasirox, estrogen derivatives, fusidic acid, nevirapine, progestins, siltuximab
>   *May decrease serum concentration*
> - Estrogen derivatives, progestins
>   *May decrease the anticoagulant effects*

Assessing for Adverse Effects

As with all anticoagulants, the nurse should observe for signs of bleeding, for any change in baseline kidney or hepatic function that could enhance the risk of bleeding, and for concurrent administration of drugs known to interact with rivaroxaban.

Patient Teaching

Education related to bleeding risk is essential for patients receiving rivaroxaban. The nurse reinforces instructions for safe use of the drug and related anticoagulants and teaching how to observe for signs and symptoms of bleeding. Patients should notify other healthcare providers about taking rivaroxaban, particularly before spinal or epidural procedures that increase the risk of bleeding around the spine, because paralysis may occur. Additional patient teaching guidelines for anticoagulants, including rivaroxaban, are outlined in Box 9.2.

Other Drugs in the Class

Apixaban (Eliquis) and edoxaban (Savaysa) are additional oral direct factor Xa inhibitors. A major advantage of these drugs is fixed dosing, less variability in drug effect for a given dose, and the lack of required monitoring. Although the overall risks of bleeding are similar to vitamin K antagonists, the risks for intracranial bleeding are less with the direct factor Xa inhibitors. These drugs carry the same risks in spinal or epidural procedures as rivaroxaban; the risk of paralysis may occur. As with rivaroxaban, and other anticoagulants, premature discontinuation of the direct factor Xa inhibitors without adequate alternative anticoagulation increases the risk of thrombosis. All drugs in the class pose a risk of hemorrhage and are classified as high-alert drugs by the ISMP because the drugs carry a heightened risk of causing significant patient harm when used in error. No drug that reverses the effects of the direct factor Xa inhibitors is currently available, and the drugs are not removed with dialysis. Should a patient experience hemorrhaging, oral activated charcoal may be given if the timing of administration would prove beneficial.

> **Quality and Safety Alert: Evidence-Based Practice**
>
> About one third of the patients with deep vein thrombosis (DVT) have a pulmonary embolism (PE). Clinical practice guidelines for the initial treatment of DVT and PE, issued by the American Society of Hematology (Ortel et al., 2020), strongly recommend the use of thrombolytics (e.g., alteplase, tenecteplase) followed by anticoagulation for patients who have a PE with hemodynamic compromise versus anticoagulation alone. For most stable patients with proximal DVT, anticoagulation with a direct oral anticoagulant (e.g., dabigatran, argatroban, bivalirudin, desirudin) is suggested over a vitamin K antagonist (e.g., warfarin). The guideline does not recommend a specific direct oral anticoagulant over another as factors such as cost, concomitant medication, and kidney function would need to be considered.

ANTIPLATELET DRUGS

Antiplatelet drugs prevent one or more steps in the prothrombotic activity of platelets. As described previously, platelet activity is very important in both physiologic hemostasis and pathologic thrombosis. Arterial thrombi, which are composed primarily of platelets, may form on top of atherosclerotic plaque and block blood flow in the artery. They may also form on heart walls and valves and embolize to other parts of the body.

Drugs used clinically for antiplatelet effects act by a variety of mechanisms to inhibit platelet activation, adhesion, aggregation, or procoagulant activity. These include drugs that block platelet receptors for thromboxane A_2, adenosine diphosphate (ADP), glycoprotein (GP) IIb/IIIa, and phosphodiesterase. Figure 9.2 describes the mechanism of action of some of the antiplatelet drugs. Aspirin, a cyclo-oxygenase inhibitor that has potent antiplatelet effects, is briefly discussed in this chapter and well described in Chapter 16.

ADENOSINE DIPHOSPHATE RECEPTOR ANTAGONISTS

The antiplatelet drug **clopidogrel** (Plavix) is the prototype ADP receptor antagonist and is in a class of drugs called thienopyridines. Clopidogrel and the other ADP receptor antagonists, prasugrel, ticagrelor, and cangrelor, have antiplatelet effects similar to aspirin and inhibit the ADP receptor on the surface of platelets. Clopidogrel has three shortcomings: delayed onset of action, irreversible inhibitory effects on platelets with no reversing agent or antidote, and significant individual variability in platelet response.

Pharmacokinetics

Clopidogrel is rapidly absorbed after oral administration and undergoes extensive first-pass metabolism in the liver. Clopidogrel is a prodrug and is converted to its active form by hepatic CYP2C19 (an isozyme of the cytochrome P450 system). To a lesser extent, activation of the drug also occurs via CYP3A4 enzymes. Platelet inhibition may occur 2 hours after a single dose, but the onset of action is slow, so that an initial loading dose is usually administered. The drug has a half-life of about 8 hours. The drug is excreted in the urine and feces.

Action

Clopidogrel irreversibly blocks the ADP receptor on platelet cell surface. Effective dose-dependent prevention of platelet aggregation can be seen within 2 hours of a single oral dose, but the onset of action is slow, so that a loading dose of 300 to 600 mg is usually administered. Platelet inhibition essentially lasts for the lifespan of the platelet (7 to 10 days). With repeated doses of 75 mg/d, maximum inhibition of platelet aggregation is achieved within 4 to 6 days. Platelet aggregation progressively returns to baseline from 4 to 10 days after discontinuing clopidogrel.

Use

Indications for use include reduction of myocardial infarction, stroke, and vascular death in patients with atherosclerosis and in those after placement of coronary stents. Specific uses include prevention of vascular ischemic events in patients with symptomatic atherosclerosis or with acute coronary syndrome (ACS) (with or without ST-segment elevation). The absolute risk reduction from clopidogrel and other ADP receptor antagonists is greater in patients at higher cardiovascular risk, particularly in patients with ACSs or those who have had a coronary stent implanted. In ACS, clopidogrel is given with aspirin (dual antiplatelet therapy). Patients may also take clopidogrel in conjunction with aspirin to prevent thrombosis following placement of an intracoronary stent.

People with atrial fibrillation who are unable to take vitamin K antagonists take clopidogrel instead. Adding clopidogrel to aspirin in people with atrial fibrillation reduces the rate of major vascular events compared with aspirin alone but is asso-

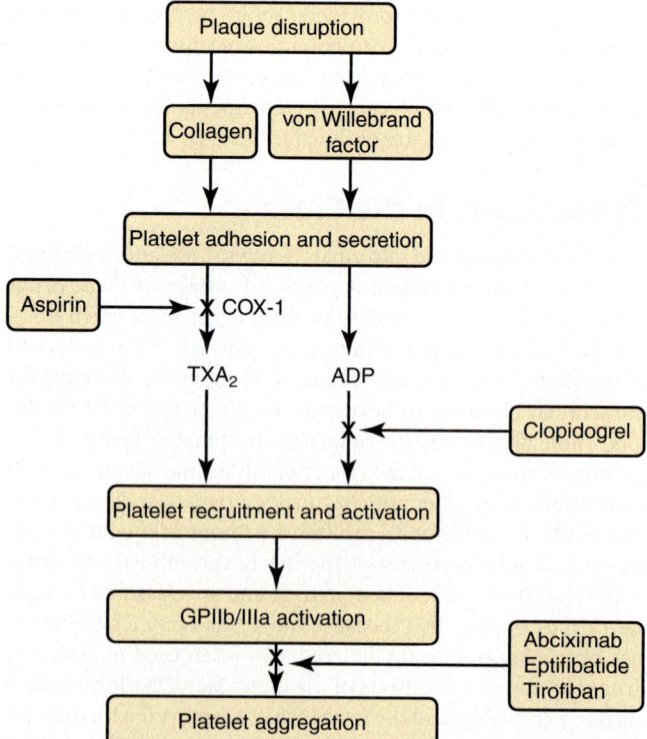

Figure 9.2. Details of the site of action of antiplatelet drugs on the process of platelet aggregation.

ciated with a greater risk of bleeding. Prescribers also order clopidogrel as an alternative antiplatelet drug for patients who cannot tolerate aspirin. Table 9.3 presents dosages for clopidogrel and other antiplatelet drugs.

Patient-related variables specific to the use of clopidogrel and other antiplatelet drugs include the following:

- Age:
  - Older adults are more likely than younger ones to experience bleeding and other complications of antiplatelet drugs.
  - Clopidogrel is commonly used to prevent thrombotic stroke in older adults but can increase the risk of hemorrhagic stroke.
  - A safe loading dose for clopidogrel in patients 75 years of age and older has not yet been established.
- Reproduction, pregnancy, and lactation:
  - If possible, clopidogrel should be discontinued 5 to 7 days prior to labor or delivery due to increased risk of maternal bleeding.
  - Data regarding fetal safety are limited, so the drug should be used only when strictly needed and for the shortest duration possible.
  - It is unknown if the drug is present in breast milk.
- Abnormal kidney function and hepatic impairment:
  - Because clopidogrel is metabolized in the liver, it may accumulate in people with hepatic impairment. Caution is necessary.

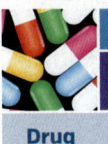

TABLE 9.3
DRUGS AT A GLANCE: Antiplatelets

Drug	Indications for Use	Routes and Dosage Ranges (Adults, Unless Specified)
Clopidogrel (Plavix; Plavix)	Reduction of atherosclerotic events (ACS, stroke, vascular death) in patients with atherosclerosis documented by recent stroke, recent myocardial infarction, or established peripheral artery disease	Adults: PO 300 mg or 600 mg loading dose; followed by 75 mg once daily for up to 12 mo in combination with aspirin Children ≤24 mo: PO 0.2 mg/kg/dose once daily possibly with aspirin >2 y: PO 1 mg/kg/dose once daily not to exceed adult dose possibly with aspirin
Aspirin (Ascriptin, Bayer, Ecotrin; Asaphen, Entrophen, Novasen, Praxis)	Prevention of myocardial infarction Treatment of ACS	Prevention of thromboembolic disorders in patients with prosthetic heart valves or TIAs: PO 81–325 mg once daily Treatment of ACS: PO initial 162–325 mg; followed by PO 81–325 mg once daily
Abciximab (ReoPro; ReoPro)	Used with PTCA to prevent rethrombosis of treated arteries. Intended for use with aspirin and heparin	IV bolus injection, 0.25 mg/kg 10–60 min before starting PTCA, then a continuous IV infusion of 0.125 mcg/kg/min (maximum 10 mcg/min) for up to 12 h
Anagrelide (Agrylin; Agrylin)	Essential thrombocythemia, to reduce the elevated platelet count, the risk of thrombosis, and associated symptoms	PO 0.5 mg four times daily or 1 mg twice daily initially, then titrate to lowest dose effective in maintaining platelet count <600,000/mm^3
Cangrelor (Kengreal)		IV 30 mcg/kg bolus prior to PTCA followed immediately by an infusion of 4 mcg/kg/min continued at least for 2 h or for duration of the PTCA, whichever is longer
Cilostazol	Intermittent claudication, to increase walking distance (before leg pain occurs)	PO 100 mg twice daily, 30 min before or 2 h after breakfast and dinner; reduce to 50 mg twice daily with concurrent use of fluconazole, itraconazole, erythromycin, or diltiazem
Dipyridamole (Persantine)	Prevention of thromboembolism after cardiac valve replacement, given with warfarin	PO 25–75 mg three times per day, 1 h before meals
Dipyridamole and aspirin (Aggrenox; Aggrenox)	Reduction of stroke risk in patients with previous TIA or thrombotic event	PO 1 capsule (200 mg extended-release dipyridamole/25 mg aspirin) twice daily
Eptifibatide (Integrilin; Integrilin, eptifibatide injection)	Acute coronary syndrome, including patients who are to be managed medically and those undergoing PTCA	IV bolus injection, 180 mcg/kg, followed by continuous infusion of 2 mcg/kg/min. See manufacturer's instructions for preparation and administration
Prasugrel (Effient; Effient)	Acute coronary syndrome	PO: adults ≥60 kg: loading dose: 60 mg; maintenance dose: 10 mg once daily (in combination with aspirin 81–325 mg/d)

(Continued on page 152)

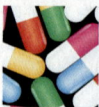

TABLE 9.3
DRUGS AT A GLANCE: Antiplatelets (Continued)

Drug	Indications for Use	Routes and Dosage Ranges (Adults, Unless Specified)
Tirofiban (Aggrastat; Aggrastat)	Acute coronary syndrome, with heparin, for patients who are to be managed medically or those undergoing PTCA Acute myocardial infarction Pulmonary embolism	IV infusion, loading dose: 25 mcg/kg over 5 min, then 0.15 mcg/kg/min for up to 18 h. Patients with abnormal kidney function (creatinine clearance ≤60 mL/min) should receive the same loading dose followed by 0.075 mcg/kg/min for up to 18 h. See manufacturer's instructions for preparation and administration
Ticagrelor (Brilinta; Brilinta)	Reduction of thrombosis in patients with coronary artery disease	PO initial 180 mg as loading dose; followed by 90 mg twice daily, 12 h after loading dose in combination with aspirin
Vorapaxar (Zontivity; Zontivity)	Reduction of thrombosis in patients with a history of myocardial infarction or with peripheral arterial disease	PO 2.08 mg once daily in combination with aspirin and/or clopidogrel

ACS, acute coronary syndrome; PTCA, percutaneous transluminal coronary angioplasty or atherectomy; TIA, transient ischemic attack.

Adverse Effects

The most common adverse effects associated with clopidogrel are pruritus, rash, purpura, and diarrhea. Thrombotic thrombocytopenic purpura, hemorrhage, and severe neutropenia have also occurred. People with variant forms of CYP2C19 may be poor or ultrarapid metabolizers of clopidogrel. Ultrarapid metabolizers of clopidogrel may have an increased risk of bleeding. With poor metabolizers, the benefits of the drug may not be adequate (see Quality and Safety Alert: Safety). The updated 2022 Clinical Pharmacogenetics Implementation Consortium Dosing Guidelines for clopidogrel continue to recommend an alternative antiplatelet therapy (e.g., prasugrel, ticagrelor) for CYP2C19 poor or intermediate metabolizers if there are no contraindications.

> ### ! Quality and Safety Alert: Safety
> The FDA has issued a **BOXED WARNING** concerning the use of clopidogrel in the 2% to 14% of the U.S. population who are reduced metabolizers of the drug. As a result of genetic variations in CYP2C19 function, the drug may be less effective in altering platelet activity in these individuals. These "poor metabolizers" may remain at risk for heart attack, stroke, and cardiovascular death, and alternate dosing of the clopidogrel or the use of other antiplatelet drugs should be considered. Genomic testing is available to determine if a patient is a poor metabolizer, although it is not routinely recommended at this time.

Contraindications

Contraindications to clopidogrel include hypersensitivity to the drug or any other component. It should not be used in patients with active bleeding in conditions such as intracranial hemorrhage or peptic ulcer disease.

Nursing Implications

Preventing Interactions

Many medications interact with clopidogrel, increasing or decreasing its effect (Box 9.6). Certain herbs and foods increase the effects of clopidogrel, including garlic, ginkgo biloba, ginger, green tea, horse chestnut, and St. John's wort; use of grapefruit may decrease the effects of the drug.

Administering the Medication

Patients take clopidogrel once daily without regard to food intake. Although the drug may be effective 2 hours after a single dose, the onset of action is slow, and an initial loading dose is usually administered. The FDA has approved a 300-mg tablet as a loading dose for appropriate patients. The effect of the drug is apparent as soon as 2 hours after the 300-mg dose.

> ### BOX 9.6 Drug Interactions: Clopidogrel
>
> **Drugs That Increase the Effects of Clopidogrel**
> - Aspirin, nonsteroidal anti-inflammatory drugs, platelet inhibitors, thrombolytics
>   *Increase the risk of bleeding*
> - Atorvastatin
>   *May affect antiplatelet activity*
> - Barbiturates, carbamazepine, rifampin, rifapentine
>   *Enhance antiplatelet effect*
> - Rifabutin
>   *May increase metabolism of clopidogrel*
>
> **Drugs That Decrease the Effects of Clopidogrel**
> - Amiodarone, dalfopristin, delavirdine, diltiazem, quinupristin, Vaprisol, zafirlukast
>   *Affect CPY34A enzymes, which play a role in clopidogrel metabolism*
> - Clarithromycin, erythromycin, ketoconazole, verapamil
>   *Reduce antiplatelet activity*
> - Omeprazole, lansoprazole
>   *May lead to inadequate platelet response*
> - Selective serotonin reuptake inhibitors
>   *May increase the risk of bleeding*

BOX 9.7 Patient Teaching Guidelines for Antiplatelet Drugs

General Considerations

- Antiplatelet drugs are given to people who have had, or who are at risk of having, a heart attack, stroke, or other problems from blood clots. For prevention of a heart attack or stroke, you are most likely to be given an antiplatelet drug (e.g., aspirin, clopidogrel).
- All antiplatelet drugs can increase your risk of bleeding, so you need to take safety precautions to prevent injury.
- Following instructions regarding these medications is extremely important. Too little medication increases your risk of problems from blood clot formation; too much medication can cause bleeding.
- While taking any of these medications, you need regular medical supervision and periodic blood tests. The blood tests can help your healthcare provider regulate drug dosage and maintain your safety.
- Avoid taking other drugs without the healthcare provider's knowledge and consent, inform any healthcare provider (including dentists) that you are taking an antiplatelet drug before any invasive diagnostic tests or treatments are begun, and keep all appointments for continuing care. This drug should be withheld 5 to 7 days prior to a planned surgical procedure.
- Report any sign of bleeding (e.g., excessive bruising of the skin, blood in urine or stool) to your healthcare provider. If superficial bleeding occurs, apply direct pressure to the site for 3 to 5 minutes or longer if necessary. In addition, notify your prescriber promptly if you develop fever, chills, or a sore throat.

Self-Administration

- Take aspirin with food or after meals, with 8 oz of water, to decrease stomach irritation. However, stomach upset is uncommon with the small doses used for antiplatelet effects. Do not crush or chew coated tablets (long-acting preparations).
- Take cilostazol 30 minutes before or 2 hours after morning and evening meals for better absorption and effectiveness.
- Take clopidogrel (Plavix) without regard to food.

Clinicians have demonstrated that dual antiplatelet therapy with aspirin and clopidogrel reduces stent thrombosis following percutaneous coronary intervention. It is recommended that patients who receive implants with a bare-metal stent or a drug-eluting stent take dual antiplatelet therapy for at least 12 months. If well tolerated, dual antiplatelet therapy can be continued for another 18 months.

Assessing for Therapeutic Effects

The nurse assesses for the absence of vascular ischemic events (e.g., pain, cyanosis, coolness of extremities). In addition, the nurse ensures that hemoglobin and hematocrit levels are within normal limits.

Assessing for Adverse Effects

The nurse assesses for common adverse effects, including pruritus, rash, purpura, and diarrhea; thrombotic thrombocytopenic purpura and hemorrhage; and severe neutropenia. No antidote exists for the effects of clopidogrel and the ADP receptor antagonist, prasugrel.

Patient Teaching

The nurse instructs patients to take medication as directed and not to double the medication if a dose is missed. Additional patient teaching guidelines are outlined in Box 9.7.

Other Drugs in the Class

Prasugrel (Effient) is an antiplatelet drug that has demonstrated improved cardiac outcome compared with clopidogrel for ACSs involving percutaneous coronary intervention. Also, this agent is used to reduce thrombotic cardiovascular events, including stent thrombosis. Although the drug requires hepatic conversion to an active metabolite, similar to clopidogrel, it is about 10 times more potent and has a more rapid onset of action, increasing the risk of bleeding. However, unlike clopidogrel, this activation is a rapid single-step process, and the TRITON-TIMI 38 trial demonstrated that individuals who are poor metabolizers of CYP2C19 had different clinical responses to prasugrel in comparison to clopidogrel.

Ticagrelor (Brilinta) and cangrelor (Kengreal) differ from clopidogrel and prasugrel in that the receptor blockade they cause is reversible. Both ticagrelor and cangrelor are effective and relatively safe when compared to clopidogrel. These drugs are used to reduce the rate of cardiovascular death, myocardial infarction, and stroke in patients with a history of myocardial infarction or ACS.

Cangrelor (Kengreal), the only intravenous ADP receptor antagonist, is administrated as an adjunct to PTCA to prevent a myocardial infarction during the procedure. The drug is administered intravenously prior to PTCA and continued throughout the duration of the procedure. Should ongoing use of an ADP receptor antagonist be required postprocedure, an oral ADP receptor antagonist is initiated. Cangrelor may also be administered in patients requiring repeat coronary revascularization and stent thrombosis in patients not currently receiving an ADP receptor antagonist or a GP IIb/IIIa inhibitor. Platelet inhibition occurs within 2 minutes, and no antiplatelet effect is observed an hour after discontinuation because of the drug's short half-life.

Ticagrelor also decreases the rate of stent thrombosis in individuals requiring a stent for the treatment of ACS. The most recent data suggest that ticagrelor has broader applicability of use in individuals with ACS as compared to prasugrel. (However, prasugrel seems to be better tolerated.) Ticagrelor may be administered without regard to meals, and for patients unable to swallow the tablets whole, the drug may be crushed and mixed with water to create a suspension for oral or nasogastric use. Ample water should be given after a suspension is used. Adverse effects of ticagrelor include increased uric acid levels and dyspnea. The FDA has issued a **BOXED WARNING** ◆ regarding the use of ticagrelor; the drug increases the risk of bleeding, including significant and possibly fatal hemorrhage. If possible, bleeding should be managed without the discontinuing of ticagrelor because the risk of cardiovascular events increases if it is discontinued. The chances of hemostasis with platelet transfusion are not known and may be limited. However, with life-threatening or serious bleeding, platelet transfusion may be required.

OTHER ANTIPLATELET DRUGS

Thromboxane A$_2$ Inhibitors

Aspirin exerts pharmacologic actions by inhibiting synthesis of prostaglandins. In this instance, it acetylates cyclo-oxygenase, the enzyme in platelets that normally synthesizes thromboxane A$_2$, a prostaglandin product that causes platelet aggregation. Thus, aspirin prevents formation of thromboxane A$_2$, thromboxane A$_2$–induced platelet aggregation, and thrombus formation. A single dose of 300 to 600 mg or multiple doses of 30 mg (e.g., daily for several days) of the drug inhibit the cyclo-oxygenase in circulating platelets almost completely. These antithrombotic effects persist for the life of the platelet (7 to 10 days). Aspirin may be used long term for prevention of myocardial infarction or stroke and in patients with prosthetic heart valves. It is also used for the immediate treatment of suspected or actual acute myocardial infarction, for transient ischemic attacks (TIAs), and for evolving thrombotic strokes. Adverse effects are uncommon with the small doses used for antiplatelet effects. However, there is an increased risk of bleeding, including hemorrhagic stroke. Because approximately 85% of strokes are thrombotic, the benefits of aspirin or other antiplatelet agents are thought to outweigh the risks of hemorrhagic strokes (approximately 15%). No antidote exists for the effects of aspirin because it produces irreversible platelet effects; platelet transfusion may be required. Further discussion of aspirin is found in Chapter 16.

Nonsteroidal anti-inflammatory drugs (NSAIDs), including ibuprofen and many other aspirin-related drugs, inhibit cyclo-oxygenase reversibly. Their antiplatelet effects subside when the drugs are eliminated from the circulation, and the drugs usually are not used for antiplatelet effects. However, patients who take an NSAID daily (e.g., for arthritis pain) may not need to take additional aspirin for antiplatelet effects. Acetaminophen does not affect platelets in usual doses (see Chapter 16).

Glycoprotein IIb/IIIa Receptor Antagonists

Despite significant pharmacodynamics differences between the three GP IIb/IIa antagonists, no evidence to date suggests significant differences in clinical outcomes. Abciximab (ReoPro) is a monoclonal antibody that prevents the binding of fibrinogen, von Willebrand factor, and other molecules to GP IIb/IIIa receptors on activated platelets. This action inhibits platelet aggregation. This drug is used with PTCA or removal of atherosclerotic plaque to prevent rethrombosis of treated arteries. It is used with aspirin and heparin and is contraindicated in patients who have recently received an oral anticoagulant or IV dextran. Other contraindications include active bleeding, thrombocytopenia, history of a serious stroke, surgery or major trauma within the previous 6 weeks, uncontrolled hypertension, or hypersensitivity to drug components.

Eptifibatide (Integrilin) and tirofiban (Aggrastat) inhibit platelet aggregation by preventing activation of GP IIb/IIIa receptors on the platelet surface and the subsequent binding of fibrinogen and von Willebrand factor to platelets. Antiplatelet effects occur during drug infusion and stop when the drug is stopped. The drugs are indicated for ACS (e.g., unstable angina, myocardial infarction) in patients who are to be treated medically or by angioplasty or atherectomy. Drug half-life is approximately 2.5 hours for eptifibatide and 2 hours for tirofiban; the drugs are cleared mainly by kidney excretion. With tirofiban, plasma clearance is approximately 25% lower in older adults and approximately 50% lower in patients with severe abnormal kidney function (creatinine clearance less than 30 mL/min). The drugs are contraindicated in patients with hypersensitivity to any component of the products; current or previous bleeding (within previous 30 days); a history of thrombocytopenia after previous exposure to tirofiban; a history of stroke within 30 days or any history of hemorrhagic stroke; major surgery or severe physical trauma within the previous month; severe hypertension (systolic blood pressure greater than 180 mm Hg with tirofiban or greater than 200 mm Hg with eptifibatide, or diastolic blood pressure greater than 110 mm Hg with either drug); a history of intracranial hemorrhage, neoplasm, arteriovenous malformation, or aneurysm; a platelet count less than 100,000/mm^3; serum creatinine 2 mg/dL or above (for the 180-mcg/kg bolus and the 2-mcg/kg/min infusion) or 4 mg/dL or above (for the 135-mcg/kg bolus and the 0.5-mcg/kg/min infusion); or dependency on dialysis (eptifibatide).

Bleeding is the most common adverse effect, with most major bleeding occurring at the arterial access site for cardiac catheterization. If bleeding occurs and cannot be controlled with pressure, the drug infusion and heparin should be discontinued. These drugs should be used cautiously if given with other drugs that affect hemostasis (e.g., warfarin, thrombolytics, other antiplatelet drugs).

Phosphodiesterase-3 Enzyme Inhibitor

Cilostazol inhibits phosphodiesterase, an enzyme that metabolizes cyclic adenosine monophosphate (cAMP). This inhibition increases intracellular cAMP, which then inhibits platelet aggregation and produces vasodilation. The inhibition of platelet aggregation induced by various stimuli (e.g., thrombin, ADP, collagen, arachidonic acid, epinephrine, shear stress) is reversible. The drug is highly protein bound (95% to 98%), mainly to albumin; extensively metabolized by hepatic cytochrome P450 enzymes; and excreted in urine (74%) and feces. Cilostazol and its two active metabolites accumulate with chronic administration and reach steady state within a few days.

The drug is indicated for the management of intermittent claudication. Symptoms usually improve within 2 to 4 weeks but may take as long as 12 weeks. The most common adverse effects are diarrhea and headache. The FDA has issued a **BOXED WARNING** ◆ for the use of cilostazol because it is contraindicated in patients with heart failure of any severity.

Other Agents

Anagrelide inhibits platelet aggregation induced by cAMP phosphodiesterase, ADP, and collagen. However, it is indicated only to reduce platelet counts for patients with **essential**

thrombocythemia (a chronic blood disorder characterized by excessive numbers of platelets). Doses to reduce platelet production are smaller than those required to inhibit platelet aggregation.

Dipyridamole inhibits platelet adhesion, but its mechanism of action is unclear. It is used for prevention of thromboembolism after cardiac valve replacement and is given with warfarin. The combination of dipyridamole and aspirin is indicated for prevention of stroke in those who have had stroke precursors (TIAs) or a previously completed thrombotic stroke.

THROMBOLYTIC DRUGS

The purpose of giving thrombolytic agents is to dissolve thrombi. These drugs stimulate conversion of plasminogen to plasmin, a proteolytic enzyme that breaks down fibrin, the framework of a thrombus. The main use of thrombolytic agents is for management of acute, severe thromboembolic disease, such as myocardial infarction, PE, and iliofemoral thrombosis.

The goal of thrombolytic therapy is to reestablish blood flow as quickly as possible and prevent or limit tissue damage. In coronary circulation, restoration of blood flow reduces morbidity and mortality by limiting myocardial infarction size. In cerebral circulation, rapid thrombus dissolution minimizes neuronal death and brain infarction that produce irreversible brain injury. For people with massive PE, the goal of fibrinolytic therapy is to restore pulmonary artery perfusion. Drugs with shorter half-lives increase the risk of rethrombosis or infarction. Anticoagulant drugs, such as heparin and warfarin, and antiplatelet agents are given following thrombolytic therapy to decrease reformation of a thrombus. Thrombolytic drugs are also used to dissolve clots in arterial or venous cannulas or catheters.

Alteplase is the prototype recombinant tissue plasminogen activator (rtPA). However, tenecteplase is the thrombolytic of choice in the United States and Canada; it is just as effective as alteplase but results in a decreased risk of noncerebral bleeding.

Pharmacokinetics

Administration of alteplase is by IV infusion. Metabolism occurs predominately in the liver. Following discontinuation of the infusion, more than 50% of the drug is cleared, with more than 80% clearance within 10 minutes. Excretion takes place in the urine.

Action

Alteplase is a protein that lyses unwanted fibrin blood clots by catalyzing the conversion of plasminogen to plasmin.

Use

Indications for alteplase include lysis of acute coronary arterial thromboembolism associated with evolving transmural myocardial infarction or acute pulmonary thromboembolism. Clinicians also considered it as first-line therapy for the treatment of acute ischemic stroke in selected people.

Table 9.4 presents dosage information for alteplase and other thrombolytic drugs.

Patient-related variables specific to the use of alteplase and other thrombolytic drugs include the following:

- Age:
  - Caution is warranted in older patients (65 to 80 years of age).
  - Alteplase is not recommended in people older than 80 years of age.
- Reproduction, pregnancy, and lactation:
  - Whether alteplase crosses the placenta or is excreted into breast milk is unknown.
- Abnormal kidney function and hepatic impairment:
  - Caution is necessary in patients with severe hepatic impairment.

TABLE 9.4

DRUGS AT A GLANCE: Thrombolytics

Drug	Indications for Use	Routes and Dosage Ranges (Adults, Unless Specified)
Alteplase (Activase, Cathflo Activase; ✻ Activase rtPA, Cathflo Activase)	Acute ischemic stroke Acute myocardial infarction Acute PE	Ischemic stroke: IV infusion, 0.9 mg/kg total dose administered (not to exceed 90 mg), with 10% of the total dose administered as an initial IV loading dose over 1 min, and the remainder administered over 60 min Myocardial infarction or PE: IV infusion, 100 mg over 3 h (1st hour, 60 mg with a bolus of 6–10 mg over 1–2 min initially; 2nd hour, 20 mg; 3rd hour, 20 mg) Myocardial infarction: accelerated IV infusion, 100 mg total dosage administered as a 15-mg IV bolus, followed by 50 mg IV infused over 30 min, and then 35 mg IV infused over the next 60 min. IV infusion, 100 mg over 3 h (1st hour, 60 mg with a bolus of 6–10 mg over 1–2 min initially; 2nd hour, 20 mg; 3rd hour, 20 mg)
Tenecteplase (TNKase; ✻ TNKase)	Acute myocardial infarction	IV bolus dose based on weight, 30 mg (for <60 kg) not to exceed 50 mg (>90 kg)

PE, pulmonary embolism.

Adverse Effects

As with other anticoagulants and antiplatelet agents, bleeding is the main adverse effect of alteplase. To minimize this risk, it is important to select recipients carefully, avoid invasive procedures when possible, and omit anticoagulant or antiplatelet drugs (except for aspirin) while thrombolytics are being given. The major risk of rtPA therapy is symptomatic brain hemorrhage, and when rtPA treatment is chosen, the prescriber should obtain informed consent signed by the patient, if appropriate, by a family member, or through emergency consent protocols. There is a 3% mortality rate and a 6% to 8% risk of symptomatic hemorrhage associated with its use. In rtPA overdose, aminocaproic acid serves as an antidote.

Contraindications

Due to an increased risk of bleeding, alteplase is contraindicated in patients with uncontrolled severe hypertension, aneurysm, arteriovenous malformation, known coagulopathy or internal bleeding, intracranial or intraspinal surgery or trauma within the past 3 months, intracranial mass, recent major surgery, or current use of oral anticoagulants. Alteplase can increase the risk of cerebral embolism in people with atrial fibrillation or atrial flutter.

Quality and Safety Alert: Evidence-Based Practice

The likelihood of improved neurologic outcomes is greater with earlier treatment of an acute ischemic stroke with intravenous recombinant tissue plasminogen activator (rtPA) or mechanical thrombectomy. In 2018, the American Heart Association (AHA)/American Stroke Association (ASA) Guidelines for the Early Management of Patients with Acute Ischemic Stroke supported the previous recommended upper time limit of 3 to 4.5 hours after onset of symptoms. In a review of six clinical trials of patients who underwent mechanical thrombectomy, results further suggested that the therapeutic benefit of thrombolytic treatment is greatest when given very early after ischemic stroke and declines throughout the first 4.5 hours after onset. Prompt treatment of acute ischemic stroke can maximize a patient's return to baseline neurologic function. Teaching of high-risk patients should emphasize the importance of seeking professional help as soon as neurologic symptoms develop to increase the magnitude of benefit from early treatment.

Nursing Implications

Only experienced personnel in an emergency department, a critical care unit, or diagnostic/interventional setting with cardiac and other monitoring devices in place should perform thrombolytic therapy. It is necessary to minimize intramuscular injections in patients who are receiving systemic thrombolytic therapy, because bleeding, bruising, or hematomas may develop.

The nurse assesses patients for cardiac dysrhythmias, including sinus bradycardia, premature ventricular contractions, and ventricular tachycardia resulting from reperfusion following coronary thrombolysis. Any evidence of bleeding must be promptly identified and reported.

Preventing Interactions

Many medications interact with alteplase, increasing its effect (Box 9.8). Cat's claw, dong quai, evening primrose, feverfew, garlic, ginkgo, ginseng, green tea, horse chestnut, and red clover increase the effects of alteplase. No herbs or foods appear to decrease its effect.

Administering the Medication

Before a thrombolytic agent is begun, it is essential to check INR, aPTT, platelet count, and fibrinogen to establish baseline values and to determine whether a blood coagulation disorder is present. Two or three hours after thrombolytic therapy is started, the nurse must ensure that the fibrinogen level is measured to determine that fibrinolysis is occurring. Alternatively, the nurse can check INR or aPTT for increased values because the breakdown products of fibrin exert anticoagulant effects. During and following alteplase administration, the nurse monitors blood pressure frequently and ensures that it is well controlled. The ISMP lists alteplase as a high-alert drug because of its potential risk of causing significant harm when used in error.

Administration is IV as a bolus injection or infusion. The nurse administers all infusions using an IV infusion device. Alteplase must be reconstituted as indicated and not shaken.

Assessing for Therapeutic Effects

The goal is to minimize total ischemic time and restore blood flow. Therapeutic effects include the following:

- For cardiac revascularization—stabilization of the patient, reversal of symptoms, stabilization of cardiac rhythm, decrease of the ST-segment elevations by 50% of the initial height, and absence of bleeding complications
- For cerebral revascularization—stabilization of the patient, reversal of symptoms, normal mentation, and absence of bleeding complications

Assessing for Adverse Effects

The nurse assesses for evidence of bleeding. In addition, it is necessary to determine that the condition leading to initiation of thrombolytic therapy is reversed and that there is a return of function. If bleeding does occur, it is most likely from a venipuncture or invasive procedure site, and local pressure may control it. If bleeding cannot be controlled or involves a vital organ, it is necessary to stop the thrombolytic drug and replace fibrinogen with whole blood plasma or cryoprecipitate. Giving aminocaproic acid or tranexamic acid may also be appropriate. When the drugs are used in acute myocardial infarction, cardiac dysrhythmias may occur when blood flow is reestablished. Therefore, antidysrhythmic drugs should be readily available.

BOX 9.8 **Drug Interactions: Alteplase**

Drugs That Increase the Effects of Alteplase

- Aspirin or other salicylates, abciximab, cilostazol, clopidogrel, dalteparin, dipyridamole, enoxaparin, eptifibatide, fondaparinux, heparin, nonsteroidal anti-inflammatory drugs, tinzaparin, tirofiban, warfarin

Increase the risk of bleeding

Patient Teaching

The nurse instructs patients and significant others regarding the purpose of the drug, the underlying condition, and the increased risk of bleeding. Patients should take special care brushing their teeth to reduce bleeding at the gum line. Discharge planning emphasizes managing the complications of the underlying disease (myocardial infarction or stroke) and seeking timely professional help if symptoms recur.

Other Drugs in the Class

All the available agents are effective with recommended uses. Thus, the choice of a thrombolytic agent depends mainly on risks of adverse effects and costs. All the drugs may cause bleeding. Tenecteplase (TNKase) is the other rtPA drug used mainly in acute myocardial infarction to dissolve clots obstructing coronary arteries and reestablish perfusion of tissues beyond the thrombotic area. The most common adverse effect is bleeding, which may be internal (e.g., intracranial, GI, genitourinary) or external (e.g., venous or arterial puncture sites, surgical incisions). Tenecteplase causes less noncerebral bleeding than alteplase, is easier to administer, and lacks antigenicity.

> ### Clinical Application 9.3
>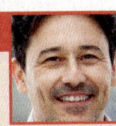
> - Before providing care for Mr. Oliver, the nurse reviews his chart (medical diagnosis and medication orders).
> - What is the main reason why patients such as Mr. Oliver receive alteplase and heparin?
> - What laboratory values should be obtained before a thrombolytic is administered?
> - For what adverse effects should the nurse monitor?
> - What nursing assessments and patient care goals are necessary in this case?

DRUGS USED TO CONTROL BLEEDING

Anticoagulant, antiplatelet, and thrombolytic drugs profoundly affect hemostasis, and their major adverse effect is bleeding. As a result, systemic hemostatic agents (antidotes) may be needed to prevent or treat significant bleeding episodes. Antidotes should be used cautiously because overuse can increase risks of recurrent thrombotic disorders. Table 9.5 presents the dosage information for the drugs used to control bleeding.

Reversal of Heparin and Low-Molecular-Weight Heparins

Protamine sulfate is an antidote for standard heparin and LMWHs. Because heparin is an acid and protamine sulfate is a base, protamine neutralizes heparin activity. Protamine dosage depends on the amount of heparin administered during the previous 4 hours. Each milligram of protamine neutralizes approximately 100 units of heparin or dalteparin and 1 mg of enoxaparin. The FDA has issued a **BOXED WARNING ◆** with the use of protamine sulfate because of the risk of severe hypotension, cardiovascular collapse, noncardiogenic pulmonary edema, catastrophic pulmonary vasoconstriction, and pulmonary hypertension with its use. A single dose should not exceed 50 mg because of the risk of severe hypotension, cardiovascular collapse, noncardiogenic pulmonary edema, catastrophic pulmonary vasoconstriction, and pulmonary hypertension with its use. The drug is given by slow IV infusion over at least 10 minutes (to prevent or minimize adverse effects of hypotension, bradycardia, and dyspnea). Its effects occur immediately and last for approximately 2 hours. A second dose may be required because heparin activity lasts approximately 4 hours. Severe hypotensive and anaphylactoid reactions may result from protamine administration. Thus, the drug should be given in settings with equipment and personnel for resuscitation and management of anaphylactic shock.

Reversal of Vitamin K Antagonists

Vitamin K (Mephyton) is an antidote for warfarin overdosage. An oral dose of 10 to 20 mg usually stops minor bleeding and returns the INR to a normal range within 24 hours. INR serum levels less than 5 with no significant bleeding may be managed with withholding of the warfarin based on protocols; INR levels greater than 5 may require the use of oral vitamin K. Decisions about management of a patient with an INR above the therapeutic range are based on the degree of elevation of the INR serum level, the clinical status of the patient with regard to bleeding, thrombogenic potential, as well as risk factors such as age and presence of concurrent disease.

Urgent reversal of warfarin overdosage in adults with acute major bleeding or in need of emergent surgery can be accomplished with PCC (Kcentra). The drug, collected from pooled human plasma, contains therapeutic levels of all four vitamin K–dependent coagulation factors (II, VII, IX, and X) and the antithrombotic proteins C and S. Dosing is based on the most current predose INR value and body weight. The drug should be administered concurrently with vitamin K to maintain factor levels once the effects of PCC have diminished. Resumption of anticoagulation should occur once the risk of thromboembolism outweighs the risk of acute bleeding. Unlike plasma, PCC does not require blood group typing or thawing, so it can be administered more quickly than frozen plasma and when administered at recommended doses provides a significantly lower volume than plasma.

The FDA has issued a **BOXED WARNING ◆** with the use of PCC because reversal of an anticoagulant state in patients being treated with vitamin K antagonist therapy may predispose the patient to a thromboembolic complication. Benefits of reversal must be weighed against potential risk of a subsequent thromboembolic event.

Reversal of Oral Direct Thrombin Inhibitors

Idarucizumab (Praxbind), a humanized monoclonal antibody fragment, is the antidote for dabigatran, currently the only oral DTI. The drug reverses the anticoagulant effects of dabigatran for uncontrolled or life-threatening bleeding or for emergency surgery or procedures. In adults, the drug is given intravenously, administered as two separate doses no more than 15 minutes apart. The

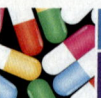

TABLE 9.5
DRUGS AT A GLANCE: Drugs Used to Control Bleeding

Drug	Indications for Use	Dosage (Adults, Unless Specified)
Aminocaproic acid (Amicar)	Control bleeding caused by overdoses of thrombolytic agents or bleeding disorders caused by hyperfibrinolysis (e.g., cardiac surgery, blood disorders, hepatic cirrhosis, prostatectomy, neoplastic disorders); antidote for rtPA	PO, IV infusion, 5 g initially, followed by 1.0 to 1.25 g/h for 8 h or until bleeding is controlled; maximum dose, 30 g/24 h
Idarucizumab (Praxbind; ✷ Praxbind)	Antidote for dabigatran etexilate (Pradaxa) Control life-threatening bleeding with overdosage of dabigatran Prevention or decrease of bleeding if emergency surgery is required	IV 5 g, administered as two separate 2.5-g doses no more than 15 min apart
Protamine sulfate	Treatment of heparin overdosage	Depends on the amount of heparin given within the previous 4 h
Prothrombin complex concentrate, human (✷ Beriplex P/N, Octaplex)	Urgent reversal of warfarin overdosage in adults with acute major bleeding or in need of urgent surgery	Individualize dosing based on patient's current predose INR value and body weight INR 2 to <4: 25 units/kg; not to exceed 2,500 units INR 4–6: 35 units/kg; not to exceed 3,500 units INR >6: 50 units/kg; not to exceed 5,000 units Administer vitamin K concurrently to maintain vitamin K–dependent clotting factor levels once the effects of prothrombin complex concentrate have diminished
Tranexamic acid (Cyklokapron, Lysteda; ✷ Cyklokapron, GD-Tranexamic Acid, Tranexamic Acid Injection BP)	Control bleeding caused by overdoses of thrombolytic agents Prevent or decrease bleeding from tooth extraction in patients with hemophilia	PO 25 mg/kg 3–4 times daily, starting 1 d before surgery, or IV 10 mg/kg immediately before surgery, followed by 25 mg/kg PO 3–4 times daily for 2–8 d
Vitamin K (Mephyton; ✷ AquaMEPHYTON, Mephyton)	Antidote for warfarin overdosage	PO 2.5–10 mg (rarely up to 25–50 mg) in a single dose, may repeat 12–48 h if needed, or IV, Sub-Q 2.5–10 mg (rarely up to 25–50 mg) in a single dose, measure INR after 6–8 h. Repeat dose if needed

drug's half-life is about 45 minutes in individuals with normal kidney function and the duration of the effect is about 24 hours. However, if coagulation parameters reelevate within 12 hours of administration, a second dose may be considered. Reversing the effects of dabigatran will subject a patient to an elevated risk of thrombosis, so it is necessary to resume anticoagulant therapy after 24 hours of administering idarucizumab, as appropriate.

Reversal of Thrombolytic Agents

Aminocaproic acid (Amicar) and tranexamic acid (Cyklokapron) are used to stop bleeding caused by overdoses of thrombolytic agents. Aminocaproic acid also may be used in other bleeding disorders caused by hyperfibrinolysis (e.g., in cardiac surgery, blood disorders, hepatic cirrhosis, prostatectomy, neoplastic disorders). Tranexamic acid also is used for short periods (2 to 8 days) in patients with hemophilia to prevent or decrease bleeding from tooth extraction or menorrhagia.

Depending on the indication for administration, aminocaproic acid may be infused as a loading dose over 15 to 60 minutes to reduce the risk of hypotension and dysrhythmias with a rapid bolus. A continuous infusion may be required. Tranexamic acid can be administered orally or intravenously. Tablets should be swallowed whole. A rapid IV bolus can be given, but the drug is usually administered diluted and administered intravenously over 5 to 30 minutes. Dosage of the drug should be reduced in the presence of moderate or severe abnormal kidney function.

NCLEX Success

5. A patient who received a copy of their genomic testing and is classed as a "poor metabolizer" of clopidogrel asks the nurse what it means. The nurse, understanding the variant response to CYP2C19, would be most correct in stating which of the following?

    A. "You metabolize the medication differently than some individuals and may not receive the same benefit from drug therapy."
    B. "You lack the CPY2C19 isozyme, so you will not need to take clopidogrel."
    C. "You will be prescribed less of the medication than is normally necessary."
    D. "You are at a higher risk of bleeding from the drug, so you must be extra careful."

THE NURSING PROCESS

A concept map outlines the nursing process related to drug therapy considerations in this chapter. Additional nursing implications related to the disease process should also be considered in care decisions.

Assessment
- Assess risk factors, history, or disease associated with thromboembolism, such as smoking, immobility, obesity, oral contraceptives, recent surgery, prosthetic heart valve, atrial fibrillation, and heart failure.
- Assess for signs and symptoms of thrombotic and thromboembolic disorders, such as DVT, pulmonary embolism, and disseminated intravascular coagulation (DIC).

Outcomes of Therapy
The patient will
- Receive or take anticoagulant and antiplatelet drugs correctly.
- Be monitored closely for therapeutic and adverse drug effects, especially when drug therapy is started and when changes are made in drugs or dosages.
- Use nondrug measures to decrease venous stasis and prevent thromboembolic disorders. Act to prevent trauma from falls and other injuries.
- Avoid or report adverse drug reactions.
- Verbalize or demonstrate knowledge of safe management of anticoagulant drug therapy.
- Keep follow-up appointments for tests of blood coagulation and drug dosage regulation.
- Avoid preventable bleeding episodes.

Nursing Interventions
- For patients who cannot ambulate safely because of weakness, sedation, or other conditions, keep the call light within reach, keep bed rails elevated, and assist in ambulation. Provide an electric razor for shaving.
- Avoid intramuscular injections, venipunctures, and arterial punctures when possible. Avoid inserting nasogastric tubes or indwelling urinary catheters if possible.
- Provide appropriate teaching (see Box 9.2).

Evaluation
- Interview and observe for relief of symptoms and compliance with instructions for which anticoagulants are prescribed.
- Interview and observe for accurate drug administration.
- Observe for signs and symptoms of thromboembolic disorders or bleeding.
- Evaluate blood coagulation tests for therapeutic ranges.
- Observe and interview regarding adverse drug effects.

Visit thePoint at http://thePoint.lww.com/Frandsen13e for answers to NCLEX Success questions (in Appendix A), answers to Clinical Application Case Studies (in Appendix B), additional information on pathophysiology, and more!

REFERENCES AND RESOURCES

American College of Obstetricians and Gynecologists (ACOG) (2018). ACOG Practice Bulletin No. 196: Thromboembolism in pregnancy. *Obstetrics and Gynecology, 132*(1), e1–e17. 10.1097/AOG.0000000000002706

Arnett, D. K., Blumenthal, R. S., Albert, M. A., Buroker, A. B., Goldberger, Z. D., Hahn, E. J., Himmelfarb, C. D., Khera, A., Lloyd-Jones, D., McEvoy, J. W., Michos, E. D., Miedema, M. D., Muñoz, D., Smith Jr., S. C., Virani, S. S., Williams Sr., K. A., Yeboah, J., & Ziaeian, B. (2019). 2019 ACC/AHA Guideline on the Primary Prevention of Cardiovascular Disease: A Report of the American College of Cardiology/American Heart Association Task Force on Clinical Practice Guidelines. *Journal of the American College of Cardiology, 74*(10), e177–e232.

CPIC. (2022). *Clinical Pharmacogenetics Implementation Consortium (CPIC) Dosing Guideline for Clopidogrel and CYP2C19.* Retrieved October 28, 2022, from https://cpicpgx.org/guidelines/guideline-for-clopidogrel-and-cyp2c19/

Lawson, J. S., & the ACC/AHA Writing Committee (2021). 2021ACC/AHA/SCAI guideline for coronary artery revascularization. *Journal American College of Cardiology, 79*(2), e21–e129.

Lippincott advisor. (2022). http://advisor.lww.com

Merchant, R.A., Topjain, A.A., Panchal, A.R., Cheng, A., Aziz, K., Berg, K. M., Lavonas, E. J., Magid, D. J. (2020). Part 1: Executive Summary: 2020 American Heart Association Guidelines for Cardiopulmonary Resuscitation and Emergency Cardiovascular Care. On behalf of the Adult Basic and Advanced Life Support, Pediatric Basic and Advanced Life Support, Neonatal Life Support, Resuscitation Education Science, and Systems of Care Writing Groups. *Circulation, 142*(16), suppl 2. S336. https://doi.org/10.1161/CIR.0000000000000929

Oakes, M. C., Reese, M., Colditz, G. A., Stoll, C. R. T., Hardi, A., Arnold, L. D., & Frolova, A. I. (2023). Efficacy of postpartum pharmacologic thromboprophylaxis: A systematic review and meta-analysis. *Obstetrics and Gynecology, 141*(4), 697–710. https://doi.org/10.1097/AOG.0000000000005122

Ortel, T.L., Neumann, I., Ageno, W., Beyth, R., Clark, N.P., Cuker, A., Hutten B. A., Jaff M. R., Manja V., Schulman, S., Thurston, C., Vedantham, S., Verhamme, P., Witt, D. M., Florez, I. D., Izcovich, A., Nieuwlaat, R., Ross, S., Schünemann, H. J., ... Zhang, Y. (2020). American Society of Hematology 2020 guidelines for management of venous thromboembolism: Treatment of deep vein thrombosis and pulmonary embolism. *Blood Advances, 4*(19): 4693–4738. https://doi.org/10.1182/bloodadvances.2020001830

Powers, W. J., Rabinstein, A. A., Ackerson, T., Adeoye, O. M., Bambakidis, N. C., Becker, K., Biller, J., Brown, M., Demaerschalk, B. M., Hoh, B., Jauch, E. C., Kidwell, C. S., Leslie-Mazwi, T. M., Ovbiagele, B., Scott, P. A., Sheth, K. N., Southerland, A. M., Summers, D. V., Tirschwell, D.L., & on behalf of the American Heart Association Stroke Council. (2019). 2019 Update to the 2018 Guidelines for the Early Management of Patients With Acute Ischemic Stroke: A Guideline for Healthcare Professionals From the American Heart Association/American Stroke Association. *Stroke, 50*(12), e344–e418. https://doi.org/10.1161/STR.0000000000000211

Tomaselli, G. F., Mahaffey, K. W., Cuker, A., Dobesh, P. P., Doherty, J. U., Eikelboom, J. W., Florido, R., Hucker, W., Mehran, R., Messé, S. R., Pollack Jr., C. V., Rodriguez, F., Sarode, R., Siegal, D., Wiggins, B. I., & Writing Committee. (2020). 2020 ACC Expert Consensus Decision Pathway on Management of Bleeding in Patients on Oral Anticoagulants: A Report of the American College of Cardiology Task Force on Expert Consensus Decision Pathways. *Journal of the American College of Cardiology, 76*(5), 594–622. 10.1016/j.jacc.2020.04.053

CHAPTER 10

Drug Therapy for Dyslipidemia

LEARNING OBJECTIVES

After studying this chapter, you should be able to:

1. Recognize the role of dyslipidemia in atherosclerotic cardiovascular disease.
2. Educate patients regarding lifestyle modification strategies to prevent or reduce dyslipidemia.
3. Identify the prototype drug from each drug class used to treat dyslipidemia.
4. Describe the classes of dyslipidemic drugs in terms of their mechanism of action, indications for use, major adverse effects, and nursing implications.
5. Implement the nursing process in the care of patients with dyslipidemia.

CLINICAL APPLICATION CASE STUDY

Edward Watkins, a 62-year-old man, has had elevated cholesterol and triglyceride levels at his two previous visits to the nurse practitioner. He has tried diet modification and increasing exercise; however, he remains overweight, and his lipid values remain elevated. His latest laboratory findings at this visit are total serum cholesterol 239 mg/dL, low-density lipoprotein (LDL) cholesterol 162 mg/dL, high-density lipoprotein (HDL) cholesterol 40 mg/dL, and triglycerides 220 mg/dL. His nurse practitioner decides to prescribe atorvastatin 10 mg PO once daily and gemfibrozil 600 mg PO twice a day.

KEY TERMS

Dyslipidemia: abnormal lipid levels in the blood; associated with atherosclerosis and its many pathophysiologic effects (e.g., myocardial ischemia and infarction, stroke, peripheral arterial occlusive disease)

Lipid profile: a panel of blood tests used to find abnormalities in lipids that measures three levels of cholesterol and a measurement of triglycerides

Lipoproteins: specific proteins in plasma that transport blood lipids; contain cholesterol, phospholipid, and triglyceride bound to protein. They vary in density and amounts of lipid and protein

INTRODUCTION

The focus of this chapter is on the management of **dyslipidemia**, a disorder of lipoprotein metabolism that causes abnormal lipid levels in the blood.

OVERVIEW OF DYSLIPIDEMIA

Blood lipids, which include cholesterol, phospholipids, and triglycerides, are derived from the diet or synthesized by the liver and intestine. **Lipoproteins** that carry lipids in blood vary in density and amounts of lipid and protein and are transported by binding to specific proteins in plasma. Elevated blood lipids, particularly cholesterol and triglycerides, are a major risk factor for atherosclerosis and cardiovascular disorders such as coronary artery disease and stroke.

For further details on blood lipids, metabolic syndrome, and types of blood lipid disorders, visit thePoint* (http://thePoint.lww.com/Frandsen13e)

Clinical Manifestations

A **lipid profile** consists of a total cholesterol, high-density lipoprotein (HDL) cholesterol, low-density lipoprotein (LDL) cholesterol, and triglycerides. For accurate interpretation, blood samples for laboratory testing of triglycerides should be drawn after the patient has fasted for 12 hours. Fasting does not appear to be required for cholesterol testing. However, because triglycerides require fasting and guidelines for interpreting nonfasting levels for evaluating cardiovascular risk have not been established, fasting is recommended prior to tests for a lipid profile. Normal lipid levels in adults and children are outlined in Table 10.1. Of the types of dyslipidemias most often described, hypercholesterolemia is usually emphasized; however, hypertriglyceridemia is also associated with most types of hyperlipoproteinemia.

In the past, the total cholesterol to HDL cholesterol ratio has been used to predict the risk of developing atherosclerosis (total cholesterol value divided by the value of the HDL cholesterol). Currently, the recommendations from the American College of Cardiology and the American Heart Association (ACC/AHA) do not target fixed LDL and HDL cholesterol goals but focus on calculating and reducing cardiovascular risk.

Screening

Evidence indicates that atherosclerotic lesions can begin in childhood. Identifying lipoprotein and cholesterol disorders in children might provide an opportunity for early cardiovascular risk reduction interventions and promote healthy lifestyle modifications. Recommendations from the National Heart, Lung, and Blood Institute (2012) support selective screening of children with a fasting lipid profile at age 2 who have a family history (first-degree relatives) of premature atherosclerotic cardiovascular disease (ADCVD) (by age 55 in males or by age 65 in females), have a parent with dyslipidemia, have any other risk factors or high-risk conditions, or have no available family history. If a new family history is identified or a high-risk condition develops as a child grows, a fasting lipid profile is advised. The National Heart, Lung, & Blood Institute and the American Academy of Pediatrics ((NHLBI/AAP) recommend that universal lipid screening should begin between ages 9 and 11 and again between 17 and 21 years of age. A screening lipid profile in children and adolescents can be done nonfasting.

In the absence of risk factors for ASCVD, middle-aged adults should be screened for dyslipidemia at least every 1 to 2 years. With known ASCVD risk and increasing age, frequency of testing should be based on current treatment guidelines, individual clinical circumstances, and the provider's best judgment.

Management

Management of dyslipidemia is guided by serum levels of cholesterol and triglycerides.

Overall, the most effective blood lipid profile for prevention or management of arteriosclerotic cardiovascular disease and its sequelae is high HDL cholesterol, low LDL cholesterol, and low total cholesterol; a low triglyceride level is also desirable. Treatment goals for patients with lipid abnormalities should be personalized by levels of risk. Therapeutic lifestyle changes are recommended to lower serum cholesterol levels for all age groups, particularly in patients who already have cardiovascular disease or diabetes mellitus.

TABLE 10.1

Plasma Cholesterol and Triglyceride Levels in Adults and Children

	Adults	Children (>3 Years of Age)
Total serum cholesterol (mg/dL)	Desirable = <200 Borderline = 200–239 Undesirable = 240 or above	Desirable = <170 Borderline = 170–199 Undesirable = 200 or above
LDL cholesterol (mg/dL)	Desirable = <130 Borderline = 130–159 Undesirable = 160 or above	Desirable = 110–129 Undesirable = >130 or above
HDL cholesterol (mg/dL)	Desirable = 40 or above* Undesirable = <40	Desirable level = >45 Borderline = 35–45 Undesirable = <35
Triglycerides (mg/dL)	Desirable = <150 Borderline = 150–199 Undesirable = 200 or above	Desirable = <125 Undesirable = >125 or above

*If the HDL cholesterol level is 60 mg/dL or above, one risk factor for coronary heart disease can be subtracted in adults when calculating risk.

Lifestyle Changes

Primary prevention of cardiovascular risk factors associated with dyslipidemia should begin in all healthy children older than 2 years and continue for life. Establishing a healthy lifestyle at an early age can prevent the development of risk factors associated with myocardial infarction and stroke that would necessitate drug therapies later in life. Guidelines of the ACC/AHA (2018) continue to support recommendations regarding the importance of lifestyle management in the treatment of dyslipidemia. Strategies that promote risk reduction of lifestyle factors include an emphasis on balanced nutrition and exercise. In healthy children and adolescents or those with dyslipidemia older than age 2, the use of the evidence-based Cardiovascular Health Integrated Lifestyle Diet, or CHILD 1, is recommended. Within appropriate age-, sex-, and activity-based requirements for growth and nutrition, intake of total fat can be safely limited to 25% to 30% of total calories, saturated fat intake to 8% to 10% of calories, and dietary cholesterol to 300 mg. High dietary fiber intake from foods (not supplements) is encouraged.

In adults, modification of total fat intake is recommended. Intake of total fat can be safely limited to 25% to 30% of total calories, saturated fat intake to 7% of calories, and dietary cholesterol to 200 mg with only enough calories to reach or maintain a healthy weight. LDL cholesterol–lowering macronutrients should be increased in the diet and include 2 g/day of plant stanols/sterols (e.g., margarine spreads [Benecol], stanol-fortified orange juice, cereals, granola bars) and 10 to 25 g/day of soluble fiber (e.g., psyllium preparations, oat bran, pectin, fruits, and vegetables). If patient is overweight or has obesity, a reduced-calorie diet consisting of fruits and vegetables (five or more servings/day), grains (six or more servings/day, one third of those as whole grains), fish, and lean meats is recommended. Additional focus on managing modifiable risk factors such as hypertension, diabetes, obesity, and cigarette smoking further reduces dyslipidemia and the development of ASCVD.

In children older than 5 years of age, 1 hour of daily moderate to vigorous activity is recommended. There is no evidence that increasing physical activity in healthy children is harmful. In adults, an increase in physical activity, including an emphasis on regular moderate-intensity aerobic exercise (usually 30 minutes at least three times weekly), will promote enhanced cardiovascular health and promote weight loss. In addition to aerobic activity, muscle-strengthening activity is recommended at least 2 days a week.

Support for patients who smoke in their cessation efforts is critical. In addition to numerous other benefits, HDL levels are higher in nonsmokers. If the patient is perimenopausal, hormone replacement therapy can raise HDL and lower LDL.

Herbs and Foods

A limited number of herbs and foods are reported to have evidence-based effects on cholesterol levels. Flaxseed and flaxseed ligans have shown to produce a decrease in LDL cholesterol. However, absorption of all medications may be decreased when taken with flax, resulting in a less than therapeutic effect. In addition, red yeast rice reduces total and LDL cholesterol although dosage standardization is a concern, and information about long-term safety is unavailable. Soy may show a small benefit in reducing LDL cholesterol though intake of soy proteins may have other beneficial vascular effects.

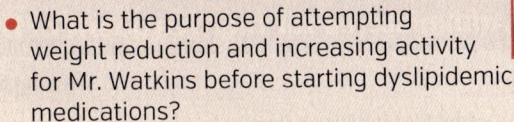

Clinical Application 10.1

- What is the purpose of attempting weight reduction and increasing activity for Mr. Watkins before starting dyslipidemic medications?
- How would the nurse interpret the current laboratory values of Mr. Watkins?

Drug Therapy

Therapeutic lifestyle changes (including dietary modification, physical activity, and smoking cessation) have been the cornerstone of population-based interventions to manage dyslipidemia. However, making the commitment is often insufficient to achieve recommended treatment targets. When lifestyle changes alone do not reduce blood lipids, dyslipidemic drugs are used in the management of patients with elevated blood lipids. Several organizations have released guidelines for the treatment of dyslipidemia and have placed different emphasis on the importance of targeting individual blood lipid levels (i.e., total cholesterol, LDL cholesterol, HDL cholesterol, triglycerides) and benchmark levels of cardiac risk to improve morbidity and mortality. Guidelines from 2013 for treatment of dyslipidemia released by the ACC/AHA updated the previous Adult Treatment Panel III recommendations of the National Cholesterol Education Program (NCEP). The recent 2018 ACC/AHA guidelines recommend using a lower-risk benchmark and standards for individuals who take dyslipidemic drugs and provide a calculator for a 10-year risk estimate for myocardial infarction or stroke. In these guidelines, treatment considerations to manage cardiovascular risk are more meaningful than targeting optimization of blood lipid levels. The U.S. Preventive Services Task Force recommends using statins to prevent cardiovascular disease.

Dyslipidemic drugs are used to decrease blood lipids, prevent, or delay the development of atherosclerotic plaque, promote the regression of existing atherosclerotic plaque, and reduce morbidity and mortality from ASCVD.

Clinical data suggest that drug therapy may be efficacious even for those with mild to moderate elevations of LDL cholesterol, particularly with preexisting cardiovascular disease. Dyslipidemic drugs act by altering the production, absorption, metabolism, or removal of lipids and lipoproteins. Depending on cardiovascular risk, drug therapy is initiated after 6 months of dietary and other lifestyle changes fail to decrease dyslipidemia to an acceptable level. It is also recommended for patients with signs and symptoms of coronary heart disease, a strong family history of coronary heart disease or dyslipidemia, or other risk factors for atherosclerotic vascular disease (e.g., hypertension, diabetes mellitus, cigarette smoking). Several drug classes, including hydroxymethylglutaryl-coenzyme A (HMG-CoA) reductase inhibitors or statins, fibric acid derivatives, bile acid sequestrants, cholesterol absorption inhibitors, and nicotinic acid are available, but none is effective in all types of dyslipidemia, so drug selection is based on the type of dyslipidemia and its severity. To lower cholesterol using a single drug, a statin is preferred. To lower cholesterol and triglycerides, a statin, a

TABLE 10.2

Drugs Administered for the Treatment of Dyslipidemia

Drug Class	Prototype	Other Drugs in the Class
HMG-CoA reductase inhibitors (statins)	Atorvastatin (Lipitor)	Fluvastatin (Lescol XL) Lovastatin (Altoprev) Pitavastatin (Livalo, Zypitamag) Pravastatin Rosuvastatin (Crestor) Simvastatin (Zocor, FloLipid)
Bile acid sequestrants	Cholestyramine (Prevalite)	Colesevelam (Welchol) Colestipol (Colestid)
Fibrates	Fenofibrate (Tricor)	Gemfibrozil (Lopid)
Cholesterol absorption inhibitor	Ezetimibe (Zetia)	
PCSK9 inhibitors	Alirocumab (Praluent)	Evolocumab (Repatha)
Miscellaneous dyslipidemic agent		Niacin

cholesterol absorption inhibitor, gemfibrozil, or a fibrate may be used. To lower triglycerides, gemfibrozil, ezetimibe, or a cholesterol absorption inhibitor may be given. Alternatively, in specific clinical situations (triglyceride level greater than 500 mg/dL), the vitamin niacin may be used. Categories of drugs are described in upcoming sections. Table 10.2 and the Drugs at a Glance tables list individual drugs used in the treatment of dyslipidemia. Figure 10.1 shows the sites of action of dyslipidemic drugs.

NCLEX Success

1. A person with type 1 diabetes mellitus and hypertension has the following lipid profile: total serum cholesterol 288 mg/dL, low-density lipoprotein (LDL) cholesterol 200 mg/dL, high-density lipoprotein (HDL) cholesterol 48 mg/dL, and triglycerides 200 mg/dL. How would you evaluate the results of the lipid profile? (Select all that apply.)
    A. LDL cholesterol is elevated.
    B. HDL cholesterol is within normal limits.
    C. Triglyceride level is elevated.
    D. Total cholesterol is within normal limits.

2. A 48-year-old patient visits their healthcare provider for an annual checkup. The patient is otherwise in good health, but assessment findings reveal the new onset of a slight increase in blood pressure and a total serum cholesterol of 240 mg/dL. What can the nurse anticipate as the preferred treatment for this patient?
    A. a low-lipid diet and an exercise program
    B. a low-lipid diet and a cholesterol synthesis inhibitor
    C. an exercise program and a fibrate
    D. a statin and beta blocker medication

HMG-COA REDUCTASE INHIBITORS

 Atorvastatin (Lipitor), one of the most widely used drugs in the United States, is the prototype of the class of drugs called the hydroxymethylglutaryl-coenzyme A (HMG-CoA) reductase inhibitors or statins. By decreasing production of cholesterol, the statins decrease total serum cholesterol, LDL cholesterol, very-low-density lipoproteins (VLDL) cholesterol, and triglycerides. They reduce LDL cholesterol within 2 weeks and reach maximal effects in approximately 4 to 6 weeks. HDL cholesterol levels remain unchanged or may increase.

Atorvastatin and other statins are useful for treating dyslipidemia and are an overall tool in the primary prevention of cardiovascular disease. Several clinical trials have supported the beneficial effects of statins in female patients with coronary artery disease. In addition, studies have suggested that atorvastatin may possess some benefits that other statins do not. Research has focused on multiple outcomes, including intimal thickness, results of imaging studies, mortality, incidence of stroke, and progression of lesions. Multiple studies have shown that statins reduce cardiovascular events primarily, if not exclusively, by lowering LDL, a causal factor for vascular disease. LDL cholesterol may also be a potent biomarker of statin benefit.

Quality and Safety Alert: Safety

Atorvastatin demonstrates the most favorable benefit-cost ratio of the four commonly used statin drugs, particularly in younger adults with low or medium cardiovascular risk.

Pharmacokinetics

Atorvastatin is rapidly absorbed following oral administration and undergoes extensive first-pass metabolism by the liver, which results in low levels of drug available for general circulation. Peak effect occurs in 1 to 2 hours. Food decreases the rate and extent of absorption. Metabolism occurs in the liver and is not dependent on kidney function for its metabolism. With atorvastatin, 80% to 85% of drug metabolites excreted in feces and the remaining products excreted in urine.

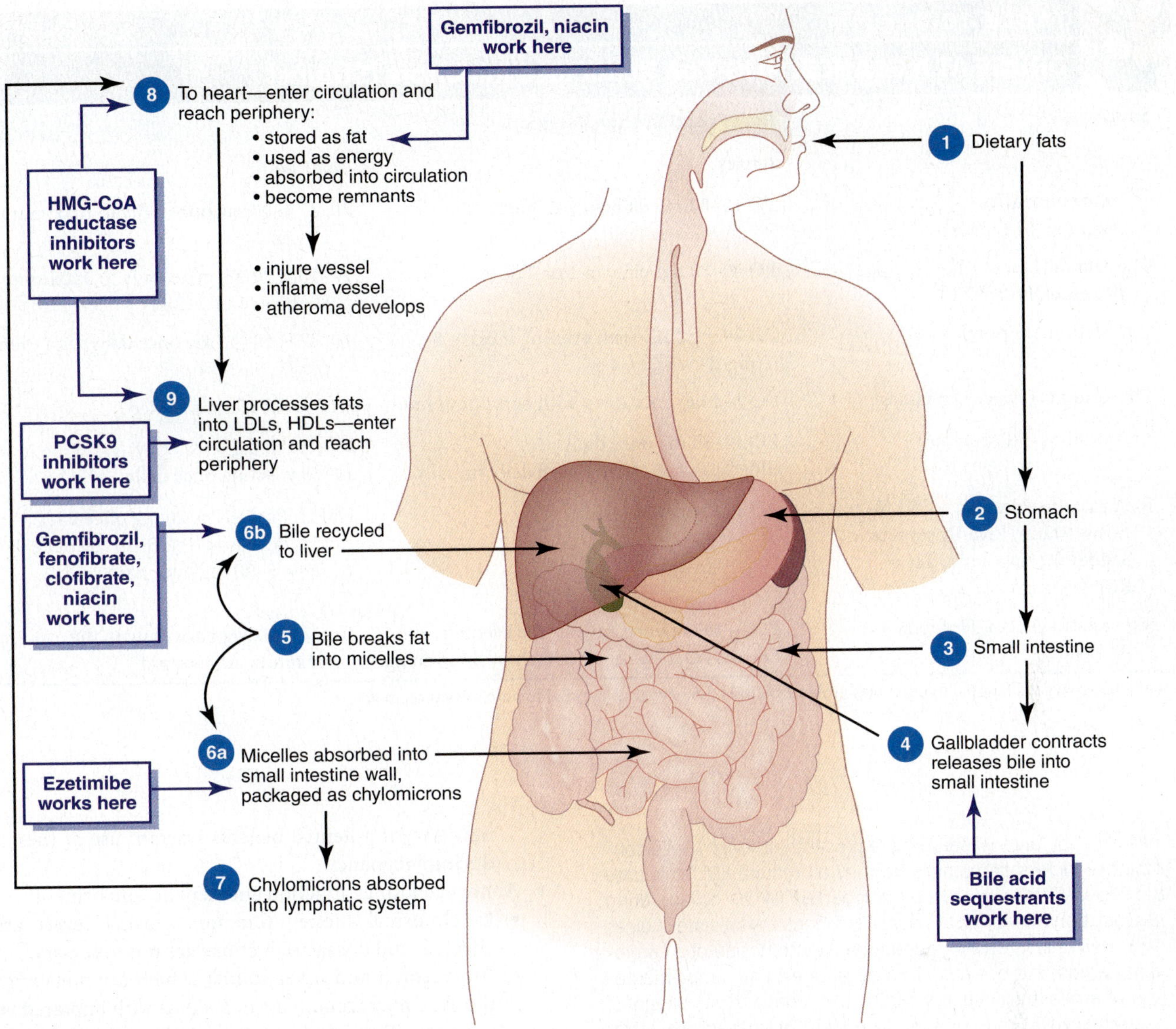

Figure 10.1. Sites of action of dyslipidemic drugs.

Action

The statins inhibit an enzyme (HMG-CoA reductase) required for hepatic synthesis of cholesterol. In part, metabolism involves one or more hepatic cytochrome P450 enzymes (including CYP2D6), leading to an increased risk of drug interactions and problems with certain foods (e.g., grapefruit juice). Additionally, some of the variability in the response to statins and associated adverse effects statins may relate to genetic differences in the rate of drug metabolism. For example, a CYP2D6 functional deficiency is present in about 7% of Caucasians and African Americans, and this deficiency is rare in people of Asian descent.

Use

Atorvastatin and the other statins are indicated for the treatment of hypercholesterolemia and reducing cardiovascular events in people with multiple risk factors. The statins are the most powerful drug class for reduction of LDL cholesterol. They result in an 18% to 55% decrease in LDL levels, as well as a 5% to 15% increase in HDL levels and a 7% to 30% decrease in triglycerides.

Table 10.3 presents dosage information for atorvastatin and other statins.

> **Quality and Safety Alert: Evidence-Based Practice**
>
> Over the past century, evidence has shown that LDLs are the major risk factor for arteriosclerotic cardiovascular disease. The American Heart Association and American College of Cardiology (AHA/ACC) updated the 2018 Cholesterol Guideline to emphasize percentage reduction in LDLs as a goal of therapy and underscore the importance of long-term monitoring of treatment effectiveness (Grundy, and the Guideline Writing Committee, 2019). At any level of LDL, the likelihood of a myocardial infarction is increased in the presence of known cardiovascular risk factors, such as cigarette smoking and hypertension (see Chapter 28). Evidence from multiple studies regarding statins has demonstrated that the frequency of myocardial infarctions can be significantly reduced by lowering LDL even when

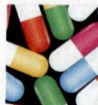

TABLE 10.3

DRUGS AT A GLANCE: HMG-CoA Reductase Inhibitors (Statins)

Drug	Routes and Dosage Ranges	
	Adults	**Children**
ⓟ **Atorvastatin** (Lipitor; ✦ Lipitor)	PO 10–80 mg daily in a single dose	*10–17 y*: 10 mg once daily to maximum of 20 mg/d
Fluvastatin (Lescol XL; ✦ Lescol, Lescol XL)	PO 40–80 mg daily in 1 or 2 doses	*10–16 y*: 20 mg once daily to maximum of 80 mg in 1 or 2 doses
Lovastatin (Altoprev)	PO 20 mg daily with evening meal to 80 mg/d	*10–17 y*: 10–40 mg once daily with evening meal
Pitavastatin (Livalo, Zypitamag)	PO 1–4 mg once daily with or without food	*<18 y*: not recommended
Pravastatin (✦ Pravachol)	PO 40–80 mg once daily Elderly, PO 40–80 mg once daily initially	*8–13 y*: 20 mg once daily *14–18 y*: 40 mg once daily
Rosuvastatin (Crestor; ✦ RAN-Rosuvastatin, Riva-Rosuvastatin, Sandoz-Rosuvastatin, Teva-Rosuvastatin)	PO 5–40 mg once daily	HoFH: *PO 7–17 y*: 20 mg once daily HeFH: *PO 8 to <10 y*: 5–10 mg once daily *10–17 y*: 5–20 mg once daily
Simvastatin (Zocor, FloLipid; ✦ Zocor)	PO 5–40 mg once daily in the evening Elderly, PO 5–40 mg once daily in the evening	*10–17 y*: 10 mg once daily in the evening to maximum of 40 mg/d

HeFH, heterozygous familial hypercholesterolemia; HoFH, homozygous familial hypercholesterolemia.

---

inflammation and risk factors are present. Although these contributory factors are important, they all require LDL to initiate the lesion. These guidelines, supported by 10 collaborating organizations, continue to advocate for healthy lifestyle choices over the lifespan as the foundation for arteriosclerotic cardiovascular disease risk reduction at all ages. Early implementation of a healthy lifestyle in youth can reduce development of risk factors and may prevent the need for subsequent statin therapy. Adherence to drug therapy and a healthy lifestyle and percentage change in LDL level should be assessed at 4 to 12 weeks after beginning a statin initiation or dosage adjustment and should be repeated every 3 to 12 months as needed.

Patient-related variables specific to the use of atorvastatin and other statins include the following:

- Age:
  - Statins are considered first-line therapy in the treatment of dyslipidemia in children. As with adults, management of children with dyslipidemia focuses on lifestyle modifications.
  - Adverse effects of statins in older adults are the same as in younger adults. However, the potential for aches, pains, or weakness from muscle issues can lead to safety concerns, such as falls.
  - Often, older adults take many drugs that can interact with statins and lead to adverse effects.
- Reproduction, pregnancy, and lactation:
  - Statins are potentially teratogenic and can cause or increase the risk of congenital anomalies. Careful consideration is necessary if potential benefits warrant use of these drugs during pregnancy.
- Abnormal kidney function and hepatic impairment:
  - In abnormal kidney function, plasma levels are not affected, and dosage reductions are not necessary.
  - Atorvastatin and other statins, which are metabolized in the liver, may accumulate in patients with impaired hepatic function. Thus, they are contraindicated in patients with active liver disease or unexplained elevations of serum aspartate aminotransferase or alanine aminotransferase.
  - These drugs should be used cautiously, in reduced dosages, for patients who ingest substantial amounts of alcohol or who have a history of liver disease.

Adverse Effects

Statins are usually well tolerated; the major adverse effects limiting statin use are the development of muscle symptoms, a condition known as statin-associated muscle syndromes. Muscle syndromes associated with statins include myopathies, myalgias, myositis, and muscle injury. Myopathies are important adverse effects and can range from discreet muscle pain to rhabdomyolysis. Statins can injure muscle tissue, resulting in muscle ache, pain, or weakness. Factors that increase the risk of rhabdomyolysis include advanced age, frail or small body frame, high dosage of statins, concomitant use of drugs that interfere with CPY3A4 including fibrates, hypothyroidism, and multiple systemic diseases such as abnormal kidney function secondary to diabetic nephropathy. Other more common adverse symptoms are usually mild and transient and include nausea, constipation, diarrhea, abdominal cramps or pain, headache, and skin rash. Hepatic dysfunction has been a source of concern, although the actual risk appears to be small.

Quality and Safety Alert: Safety

When patients who can become pregnant are treated with drug therapy for dyslipidemia, adequate patient education is critical to minimize complications associated with pregnancy. The absolute risk of teratogenicity with the use of statins appears to be relatively small; however, the use of birth control measures with statin use is essential. Careful consideration should be given if potential benefits warrant use of the drug class during pregnancy despite potential risks. The nurse advocates in the patient's care and promotes informed decision-making.

Contraindications

Limited data in early studies suggested that statins are potentially teratogenic. Statins are contraindicated with impaired hepatic function. Additional contraindications include lactation, because the drugs are secreted in breast milk, and hypersensitivity to statins.

Nursing Implications

The statins are the most effective dyslipidemic agents for improving clinical outcomes when used for primary and secondary prevention of cardiovascular disease. The choice and use of statins are based on several factors, including the degree of dyslipidemia, a specific drug's actions, drug interactions, the presence of abnormal kidney function or liver impairment, and cost.

Preventing Interactions

Many medications interact with atorvastatin, increasing or decreasing its effect (Box 10.1).

Administering the Medication

Because the bulk of cholesterol synthesis appears to occur at night, administration of statins normally takes place in the evening or at bedtime. However, atorvastatin has a long half-life, and evidence suggests that the drug can be given without regard to time of day. There is no definitive global recommendation for the entire class; thus, the timing of administration of statins should be based on manufacturer recommendations.

Assessing for Therapeutic Effects

The nurse monitors lipid response to therapy, looking for decreased levels of total serum cholesterol, LDL cholesterol, and triglycerides, as well as increased levels of HDL cholesterol. Effects occur in 1 to 2 weeks, with maximum effects in 4 to 6 weeks.

Assessing for Adverse Effects

Common adverse effects include nausea, diarrhea, abdominal pain, dyspepsia, and elevated liver function tests. The nurse monitors for signs or symptoms of muscle pain or weakness, mainly during the first months of therapy and when dosages are adjusted upward. If unexplained severe muscle symptoms, fatigue, or cola-colored urine develop, the statin should be held, and the prescriber notified to address the possibility of rhabdomyolysis.

Patient Teaching

In addition to contraceptive counseling, education should focus on the importance of monitoring liver function on a regular basis. Liver function tests are recommended before starting a statin, at 12 weeks after starting the drug, at every increase in dose, and then periodically. The nurse monitors patients with increased serum aminotransferases until the abnormal values resolve. If the increases are more than three times the upper limit of normal levels and persist, it is necessary to reduce the dose or change the drug.

See additional teaching guidelines presented in Box 10.2.

Other Drugs in the Class

Table 10.3 lists the other statins. Absorption following oral administration varies depending on the drug. Lovastatin and pravastatin are poorly absorbed, and fluvastatin has the highest rate of absorption. Most of the statins undergo extensive first-pass metabolism by the liver, which results in low levels of drug available for general circulation.

Patients may take pravastatin or simvastatin with or without food in the evening. They may take fluvastatin on an empty stomach or at bedtime. It is important to avoid taking them with grapefruit juice. Note that concurrent use of cimetidine, ranitidine, and omeprazole increases the effects of fluvastatin.

BOX 10.1 Drug Interactions: Atorvastatin

Drugs That Increase the Effects of Atorvastatin

- Magnesium- and aluminum-containing antacids
  Interfere with absorption; administer atorvastatin 2 hours before or after antacids
- Amiodarone and colchicine
  Decrease metabolism
- Azole antifungals
  Increase the risk of myopathy; it is recommended that statin therapy be interrupted temporarily if systemic azole antifungals are needed
- Cyclosporine, CYP3A inhibitors, diltiazem, fibric acid derivatives, niacin, and verapamil
  Increase the risk of severe myopathy or rhabdomyolysis
- Erythromycin, macrolide antibiotics, nefazodone, and protease inhibitors
  Decrease elimination

Drugs That Decrease the Effects of Atorvastatin

- Cholestyramine
  Decreases rate of bioavailability; administer atorvastatin at least 4 hours after this bile acid sequestrant
- Colestipol
  Decreases plasma levels

BOX 10.2 Patient Teaching Guidelines for Dyslipidemic Drugs

- Reducing low-density lipoprotein (LDL or "bad cholesterol") can improve blood flow in your arteries and decrease your risk for a heart attack or stroke.
- Healthiest blood cholesterol levels in adults are low total cholesterol (less than 200 mg/dL), low LDL (less than 130 mg/dL), and high-density lipoprotein (HDL) (greater than 35 mg/dL). High levels of blood triglycerides, another type of fat, are unhealthy.
- Dyslipidemic drugs are given to lower high concentrations of fats (total cholesterol, LDL cholesterol, and triglycerides) in your blood.
- The goal of management is to prevent heart attack, stroke, and peripheral arterial disease. If you already have heart and blood vessel disease, the drugs can improve your symptoms, activity level, and quality of life.
- Eating a low-fat diet is often the first step in treating high cholesterol or triglyceride levels and may be prescribed for 6 months or longer before drug therapy is begun.
- The diet should be continued when drug therapy is prescribed. It is important to reduce saturated fat intake (from meats, dairy products). Eating a bowl of oat cereal daily can help lower cholesterol by 5% to 10%. Dietitians or nutritionists can assist in developing guidelines that fit your needs and lifestyle.
- Overeating or gaining weight may decrease or cancel the lipid-lowering effects of the drugs.
- Other lifestyle changes that help improve cholesterol levels include regular aerobic exercise (raises HDL), losing weight (raises HDL, lowers LDL, lowers triglycerides), and not smoking (HDL levels are higher in nonsmokers).
- As an adult, have measurements of total cholesterol and HDL cholesterol at least once ever every 5 years. People with a personal or family history of dyslipidemia or other risk factors for cardiovascular disease should be tested more often.
- Home monitoring of cholesterol levels or regular orders to have your cholesterol level drawn will be part of your treatment plan.
- If you are taking a statin and plan or become pregnant, it is important to notify your prescriber as soon as possible as the drugs can cause or increase the risk of congenital anomalies.

NCLEX Success

3. A 36-year-old female patient has been taking atorvastatin 20 mg PO daily for 6 months to treat mild dyslipidemia. At a clinic appointment, she tells the nurse that she is 6 weeks pregnant. The nurse counsels the patient that it is likely that her midwife will counsel her

   A. to increase the dose of prenatal vitamins
   B. to change to a different statin medication
   C. to take her atorvastatin every other day
   D. about discontinuing the drug during pregnancy

BILE ACID SEQUESTRANTS

Cholestyramine (Prevalite), the prototype bile acid sequestrant, has the ability to reduce LDL cholesterol. It has little or no effect on HDL cholesterol and either no effect or an increased effect on triglyceride levels. There is no evidence that cholestyramine can be used as monotherapy, but it can play a role as an add-on drug with statins in combination therapy.

Pharmacokinetics

Cholestyramine is not absorbed when taken orally. Therefore, the drug is excreted in feces essentially unchanged.

Action

Cholestyramine binds bile acids in the intestinal lumen, causing the bile acids to be excreted in feces, preventing recirculation to the liver. Loss of bile acids stimulates hepatic synthesis of more bile acids from cholesterol. As more hepatic cholesterol is used to produce bile acids, more serum cholesterol moves into the liver to replenish the supply, thereby lowering serum cholesterol (primarily LDL). LDL cholesterol levels decrease within a week of starting cholestyramine and other bile acid sequestrants and reach maximal reductions within a month. When the drugs are stopped, pretreatment LDL cholesterol levels return within a month.

Use

Cholestyramine reduces LDL cholesterol levels (15% to 30%) and also produces a minimal elevation in HDL cholesterol (3% to 5%). Table 10.4 presents dosage information for cholestyramine and other bile acid sequestrants.

Patient-related variables specific to the use of cholestyramine and other bile acid sequestrants include the following:

- Age:
  - These drugs are safe and moderately effective in children and adolescents ages 6 to 18 years and decrease both total cholesterol and LDL cholesterol levels. A modest elevation in triglyceride levels has been reported.
  - Children do not tolerate the reported gastrointestinal (GI) adverse effects well.
  - Cholestyramine and other bile acid sequestrants are effective in older adults, although these individuals do not tolerate the adverse effects well.
- Reproduction, pregnancy, and lactation:
  - Lipid concentrations increase during pregnancy as required for normal fetal development. Should lipid concentration increase greater than expected, dietary intervention may be introduced and bile acid sequestrants may be recommended as needed.

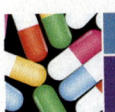

TABLE 10.4
DRUGS AT A GLANCE: Bile Acid Sequestrants

Drug	Routes and Dosage Ranges	
	Adults	**Children**
P Cholestyramine (Prevalite; ✦ Olestyr, PMS-Cholestyramine, Questran, Novo-Cholamine)	PO tablets, 4 g once or twice daily initially, gradually increased at monthly intervals to 8–16 g daily in 2 divided doses. Maximum daily dose, 24 g PO powder, 4 g 1–6 times daily	240 mg/kg/d in 3 divided doses
Colesevelam (Welchol; ✦ Lodalis)	PO 3.75 g daily in 1 or 2 doses with meals. Maximum daily dose, 4.375 g	
Colestipol (Colestid, Colestid Flavored; ✦ Colestid)	PO tablets, 2 g once or twice daily initially, gradually increased at 1- to 2-mo intervals, up to 16 g daily PO granules, 5 g daily initially, gradually increased at 1- to 2-mo intervals, up to 30 g daily in single or divided doses	

- Although cholestyramine is not absorbed systemically, the drug may interfere with maternal vitamin absorption and require more than regular prenatal supplementation.
- Since cholestyramine is not systemically absorbed, it is not thought to be present in breast milk.
- Abnormal kidney function and hepatic impairment:
  - Extended use of cholestyramine in patients with abnormal kidney function requires caution because the drug releases chloride. This effect can increase the risk of hyperchloremic metabolic acidosis.
  - Cholestyramine can further raise serum cholesterol. Therefore, its use in people with primary biliary cirrhosis warrants caution.

Adverse Effects

Cholestyramine is not absorbed systemically, so the main adverse effects are GI ones (abdominal fullness, flatulence, diarrhea, and constipation). Constipation is especially common, and a bowel program may be necessary to control this problem.

Contraindications

Cholestyramine is contraindicated in people with complete biliary obstruction, because bile is not secreted into the intestine. The drug can bind with vitamin K; thus, use in individuals with any coagulopathy requires caution.

Nursing Implications

Preventing Interactions

Cholestyramine may decrease absorption of many oral medications (e.g., digoxin, folic acid, glipizide, propranolol, tetracyclines, thiazide diuretics, thyroid hormones, fat-soluble vitamins, and warfarin). Apparently, no drugs significantly affect cholestyramine. Herbs and foods that increase the effects of cholestyramine include fibers such as oat bran and pectin. No herbs and foods seem to decrease the effects of cholestyramine.

In a patient who is taking cholestyramine in addition to other drugs, dosage of the interactive drug may need to be changed when the bile acid sequestrant is added or withdrawn. Also, because cholestyramine binds bile acids, cholestyramine may interfere with normal fat digestion and absorption and, therefore, may prevent absorption of the fat-soluble vitamins A, D, E, and K.

Administering the Medication

It is necessary to mix cholestyramine powder with water or other fluids, soups, cereals, or fruits such as applesauce and to follow with more fluid. The nurse ensures that the drug is not taken in a dry form. It is essential that cholestyramine not be given with other drugs; to minimize altered absorption, people should take the other drugs 1 hour before or 4 to 6 hours after cholestyramine.

Assessing for Therapeutic Effects

The nurse observes for decreased levels of total serum cholesterol, LDL cholesterol, and triglycerides and increased levels of HDL cholesterol. Maximum effects occur in approximately 1 month.

Assessing for Adverse Effects

The most common adverse effect is constipation. Other conditions relate to GI effects: abdominal discomfort or pain, nausea, vomiting, flatulence, diarrhea, anorexia, and steatorrhea. Increased bleeding tendencies may result from vitamin K malabsorption.

Patient Teaching

The nurse assesses the adequacy of levels of fat-soluble vitamins A, D, E, and K; supplementation may be required. Good dental hygiene is important because holding the mixture in the mouth can damage the teeth. Some products may contain aspartame or sugar, so caution is necessary in patients with phenylketonuria or diabetes mellitus.

Also, the nurse teaches patients that these drugs are used mainly to reduce LDL cholesterol further in those who are already taking a statin drug. The inhibition of cholesterol synthesis by a statin drug makes bile acid–binding drugs more effective. In addition, the combination increases HDL cholesterol and can further reduce the risk of cardiovascular disorders. Box 10.2 contains additional patient teaching information.

Other Drugs in the Class

In patients with elevated LDL cholesterol, colesevelam (Welchol) and colestipol (Colestid) may be used along with diet modifications to reduce serum cholesterol. Colesevelam is also used as an adjunct agent to improve glycemic control in adults with type 2 diabetes mellitus (see Chapter 41). Like cholestyramine, colesevelam and colestipol are not absorbed systemically but may interfere with absorption of fat-soluble vitamins A, D, E, and K. These drugs are not expected to be excreted in breast milk, but they may affect vitamin levels in nursing infants. Some products may contain phenylalanine. Patients who take the granular form of colestipol should not swallow the granules dry. Patients who take the tablet form of either drug should swallow tablets whole, without cutting, crushing, or chewing. The adverse effects profile and interactions are similar for all bile acid sequestrants.

Clinical Application 10.2

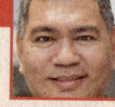

- Why is the combination of atorvastatin and gemfibrozil prescribed for Mr. Watkins?
- A nurse is counseling Mr. Watkins about his medication. He asks when he will need to have his laboratory work completed. What is the nurse's response?
- When educating Mr. Watkins about his new medication, the nurse teaches him about common adverse effects. What should be included in teaching about the adverse effects of atorvastatin? What signs and symptoms of complications does the nurse discuss with him?

FIBRATES

Fibrates are derivatives of fibric acid and are similar to endogenous fatty acids. The first fibrate to be developed, clofibrate, has essentially been replaced by other fibrates and is not discussed. Therefore, 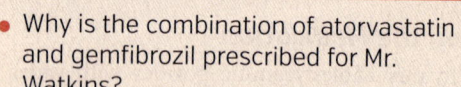 **fenofibrate** (Tricor) serves as the prototype in this discussion.

Pharmacokinetics

Fenofibrate is administered orally and is highly protein bound, primarily to albumin. Time to peak effect is 6 to 8 hours. Metabolism occurs in the liver and excretion is by urinary elimination.

Action

Fenofibrate and other fibrates increase the oxidation of fatty acids in liver and muscle tissue. Thus, they decrease hepatic production of triglycerides, decrease VLDL cholesterol, and increase HDL cholesterol.

Use

Fibrates are the most effective drugs for reducing serum triglyceride values, and their main indication for use is high serum triglycerides (greater than 500 mg/dL); they may result in a 20% to 50% decrease in triglyceride levels. They are also helpful for patients with low HDL cholesterol levels (10% to 20% increase). Additionally, fibrates are the drug of choice for hypertriglyceridemia associated with diabetes, gout, gastritis, or ulcer disease. There are no specific recommendations for use of these drugs in patients who are critically ill; drug interactions and adverse effects may restrict their use in critical illness.

Table 10.5 presents dosage information for the fibrates.

Patient-related variables specific to the use of fenofibrate and other fibrates include the following:

- Age:
  - Published studies of the use in children are limited. Thus, the safety and efficacy of fibrates in children are unclear.

TABLE 10.5 DRUGS AT A GLANCE: Fibrates

Drug	Routes and Dosage Ranges	
	Adults	**Children**
Fenofibrate (Antara, Fenoglide, Fibricor, Lipofen, Tricor, Triglide, Trilipix; Lipidil EZ, Lipidil Supra)	Antara (micronized) 30–90 mg once daily Fenofibrate (micronized) PO 43–130 once daily with meals Fenoglide 40–120 mg once daily Fibricor 35–105 mg once daily Tricor 48–145 mg once daily Triglide 160 mg once daily Trilipix 45–135 mg once daily	Fenofibrate (micronized) PO 67 mg/d/20 kg body weight with meals
Gemfibrozil (Lopid)	PO 1,200 mg daily, in 2 divided doses, 30 min before morning and evening meals	Safety and efficacy data limited

- Caution is warranted with fenofibrate dosage determination for older adults and lower starting dosages are recommended (67 mg/day).
- Reproduction, pregnancy, and lactation:
  - In pregnant patients who develop very severe hypertriglyceridemia and are at risk for pancreatitis, fenofibrate beginning in the second trimester may be ordered.
- Abnormal kidney function and hepatic impairment:
  - Since fibrates are excreted mainly by the kidneys, they accumulate in the serum of patients with abnormal kidney function.
  - Fenofibrate is contraindicated in patients with severe abnormal kidney function, and the recommended starting dose is 67 mg/day in patients with a creatinine clearance of less than 50 mL/minute. It is necessary to evaluate the effects of this dose on kidney function and to check triglyceride levels before increasing this dose.
  - Fibrates may cause a reversible elevated serum creatinine.
  - Patients with diabetes require close monitoring because kidney disease is a serious complication in this population.
  - Fibrates may cause hepatotoxicity.
  - Hepatitis (hepatocellular, chronic active, and cholestatic) has reportedly occurred after use of fenofibrate from a few weeks to several years.
  - It is necessary to monitor liver function during the first year of drug administration.
  - Discontinuation of the drug is warranted if elevated enzyme levels persist at more than three times the normal limit.
- Specific healthcare environments:
  - Because liver enzyme tests are recommended, patients who are housebound may need assistance in obtaining blood tests (e.g., lipids, liver function tests).

Adverse Effects

The main adverse effects are GI discomfort and diarrhea, which may occur less often with fenofibrate than with other fibrates. Fibrates may also increase cholesterol concentration in the biliary tract and formation of gallstones. Abnormal elevations of serum aminotransferases have occurred with both gemfibrozil and fenofibrate, but they usually subside after the drug is discontinued.

Contraindications

Contraindications include a hypersensitivity to fibrates, hepatic or (severe) abnormal kidney function, preexisting gallbladder disease, primary biliary cirrhosis, or persistent liver function abnormalities of unknown origin.

Nursing Implications

Preventing Interactions

Fenofibrate and other fibric acid derivatives may enhance the hypoprothrombinemic effect of warfarin-type oral anticoagulants, increasing the risk of bleeding. Patients receiving warfarin concurrently require a substantially decreased dosage of warfarin because fibrates displace warfarin from binding sites on serum albumin. Other drug–drug interactions are outlined in Box 10.3. No herbal interactions have been identified.

> **BOX 10.3 Drug Interactions: Fenofibrate**
>
> **Drugs That Increase the Effects of Fenofibrate**
> - Statins
>   *Increase the risk of severe myopathy or rhabdomyolysis*
> - Cyclosporine
>   *Mechanism for increase is unknown*
>
> **Drugs That Decrease the Effects of Fenofibrate**
> - Bile acid sequestrant drugs
>   *Decrease absorption; to avoid, take fenofibrate about 1 hour before or 4 to 6 hours after the bile acid sequestrant.*

Administering the Medication

It is necessary to give fenofibrate with food to increase drug absorption.

Assessing for Therapeutic Effects

The nurse assesses for decreased levels of total serum cholesterol, LDL cholesterol, and triglycerides and increased levels of HDL cholesterol. With fibrates, effects occur in approximately 1 month.

Assessing for Adverse Effects

GI disturbances as well as elevated liver function tests are common. Reportedly, hypersensitivity reactions, myopathy, rhabdomyolysis, blood dyscrasias, hepatotoxicity, cholelithiasis, cholestatic jaundice, pancreatitis, and reduced libido also occur, although these effects are rare. Risk of myopathy increases with concomitant use of statins.

Patient Teaching

The nurse instructs patients to report signs and symptoms of adverse effects to the healthcare provider. Throughout drug therapy, patients should have periodic blood tests. See Box 10.2 for general patient teaching information.

Other Drugs in the Class

Unlike fenofibrate, gemfibrozil is absorbed better on an empty stomach, so should be given about 30 minutes before the morning and evening meal.

CHOLESTEROL ABSORPTION INHIBITOR

Ezetimibe (Zetia) is the prototype of the newest class of dyslipidemic drugs, which act in the small intestine to inhibit absorption of cholesterol and decrease the delivery of intestinal

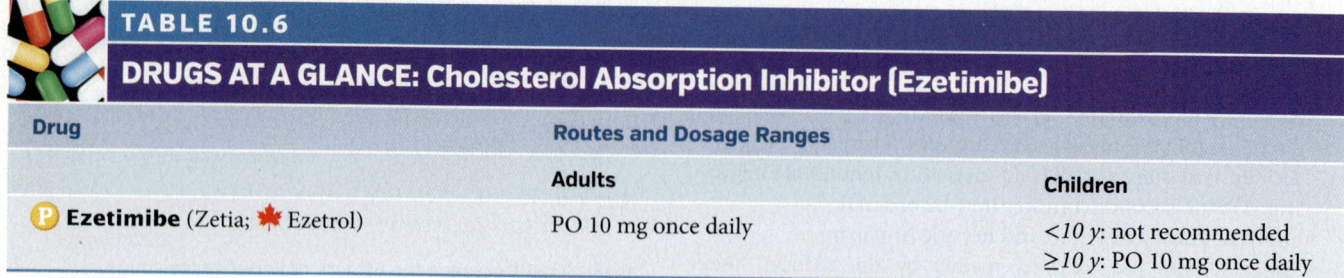

TABLE 10.6 DRUGS AT A GLANCE: Cholesterol Absorption Inhibitor (Ezetimibe)

Drug	Routes and Dosage Ranges	
	Adults	**Children**
ⓟ Ezetimibe (Zetia; ✣ Ezetrol)	PO 10 mg once daily	*<10 y:* not recommended *≥10 y:* PO 10 mg once daily

cholesterol to the liver, resulting in reduced hepatic cholesterol stores and increased clearance of cholesterol from the blood. This distinct mechanism is complementary to that of HMG-CoA reductase inhibitors, producing synergistic cholesterol-lowering effects when these drugs are used in combination. Ezetimibe reduces total cholesterol and triglycerides and increases HDL cholesterol.

Pharmacokinetics

Ezetimibe is significantly protein bound, is metabolized in the small intestine and liver, and is excreted predominately in feces. The time to peak effect is 4 to 12 hours.

Action

Ezetimibe blocks biliary and dietary cholesterol absorption at the brush border of the intestine without affecting absorption of fat-soluble vitamins and triglycerides.

Use

Ezetimibe is used together with dietary management for treatment of primary dyslipidemia. The drug may result in a 14% to 17% decrease in LDL levels. It can be used as monotherapy on in combination with a statin. When given as monotherapy (without a statin), ezetimibe does not require dosage reduction in geriatric patients. Table 10.6 presents dosage information for the drug.

Patient-related variables specific to the use of ezetimibe include the following:

- Age:
  - Safety and efficacy in children younger than 10 years of age have not been established.
- Reproduction, pregnancy, and lactation:
  - Ezetimibe has not been extensively studied in pregnancy so may have risks associated with its use.
- Abnormal kidney function and hepatic impairment:
  - Dosage adjustment of ezetimibe is necessary in patients with mild hepatic impairment. The drug is not recommended in patients with moderate to severe hepatic impairment.

Adverse Effects

The most common adverse effects of ezetimibe include headache, diarrhea, hypersensitivity reactions such as rash, and nausea.

Contraindications

Contraindications include pregnancy and lactation. Additional contraindications are hypersensitivity to ezetimibe or concomitant use with a statin in people with active hepatic disease.

Nursing Implications

The nurse instructs patients to maintain a low-cholesterol diet during ezetimibe therapy. Patients should report side effects to their healthcare providers.

Preventing Interactions

Some medications interact with ezetimibe, increasing or decreasing its effect (Box 10.4). Apparently, no herbs interact with this drug.

Administering the Medication

Ezetimibe may be administered with or without food. The patient takes the drug:

- At the same time each day
- At night if used in combination with a statin (ezetimibe may be given at the same time as a statin)
- Either 2 hours before or 4 hours after bile sequestrants to prevent altered absorption

Assessing for Therapeutic Effects

The nurse monitors lipid response to therapy with ezetimibe. Desired results include decreases in total cholesterol, LDL cholesterol, and triglycerides, with increases in HDL cholesterol. A therapeutic response occurs within 2 weeks of initiation of therapy and lasts as long as the drug is continued.

Assessing for Adverse Effects

The nurse observes for headache, dizziness, fatigue, diarrhea, and abdominal pain.

BOX 10.4 *Drug Interactions: Ezetimibe*

Drugs That Increase the Effects of Ezetimibe
- Cyclosporine
  Increases blood levels

Drugs That Decrease the Effects of Ezetimibe
- Bile acid sequestrant drugs
  Mechanism for decrease is unknown

Patient Teaching

The nurse instructs patients to report signs and symptoms of adverse effects to the healthcare provider. Throughout drug therapy, patients should have periodic blood tests. See Box 10.2 for general patient information.

PCSK9 INHIBITORS

PCSK9 inhibitors are fully humanized monoclonal antibodies that inactivate a protein in the liver called proprotein convertase subtilisin/kexin 9 (PCSK9) that regulates the lifespan of the cholesterol clearing receptors on the liver. The inhibition of PCSK9 significantly lowers LDL cholesterol levels. Ⓟ **Alirocumab** (Praluent) serves as the prototype of this class of drugs.

Pharmacokinetics

Alirocumab is administered subcutaneously every 2 to 4 weeks, and at recommended dosages, median times to maximum serum concentrations are 3 to 7 days. Following subcutaneous injection, the drug is distributed primarily in the circulatory system. As a protein, the drug degrades to small peptides and individual amino acids. At low concentrations, the drug is eliminated through binding to the PCSK9 receptors; at higher concentrations, it is eliminated principally through nonsaturable proteolysis.

Action

Unlike statins that lower cholesterol by inhibiting the synthesis of cholesterol, the PCSK9 inhibitors promote modulation of the receptor that clears cholesterol, thereby prolonging the receptor activity and promoting the clearance of cholesterol.

Use

Alirocumab is indicated in adults with ASCVD or familial hypercholesterolemia who require additional lowering of LDL cholesterol when diet and maximally tolerated statin therapy have not produced the desired therapeutic response.

The ability of alirocumab to reduce LDL cholesterol in patients with a history of statin intolerance has been supported in recent randomized clinical trials. Results indicate that cardiovascular events could be decreased with PCSK9 inhibitors. Table 10.7 presents dosage information for the alirocumab and the other PCSK9 inhibitors. These drugs may result in a 60% to 70% reduction in LDL levels.

Patient-related variables specific to the use of alirocumab and evolocumab include the following:

- Age:
  - Safety and efficacy in children and adolescents have not been established.
  - There is no reported need for dosage adjustments in older adults.
- Reproduction, pregnancy, and lactation:
  - No data are available about the use of PCSK9 inhibitors in pregnancy.
- Abnormal kidney function and hepatic impairment:
  - No adjustment to dosage is required in patients with mild to moderate abnormal kidney function or hepatic impairment. No data are available for use in individuals with severe abnormal kidney function or hepatic impairment.
- Specific healthcare environments:
  - Patients who are housebound may need assistance in obtaining serum lipid blood tests or instructed on home-monitoring techniques.
  - Patients should be advised to notify their healthcare provider of adverse effects or pregnancy and seek emergency treatment should signs of allergic reaction occur.
  - Patients should be supported to maximize lifestyle modification, including diet, exercise, and smoking cessation, to reduce cholesterol while taking alirocumab.

Adverse Effects

Alirocumab appears to be well tolerated, with injection site reactions the most common adverse effect. In addition, nasopharyngitis, itching, influenza, muscle pain, diarrhea, and serious allergic reactions have been reported with use of the drug.

Contraindications

Contraindications include known hypersensitivity to the drug or a component to the formulation. Limited information is available regarding additional contraindications.

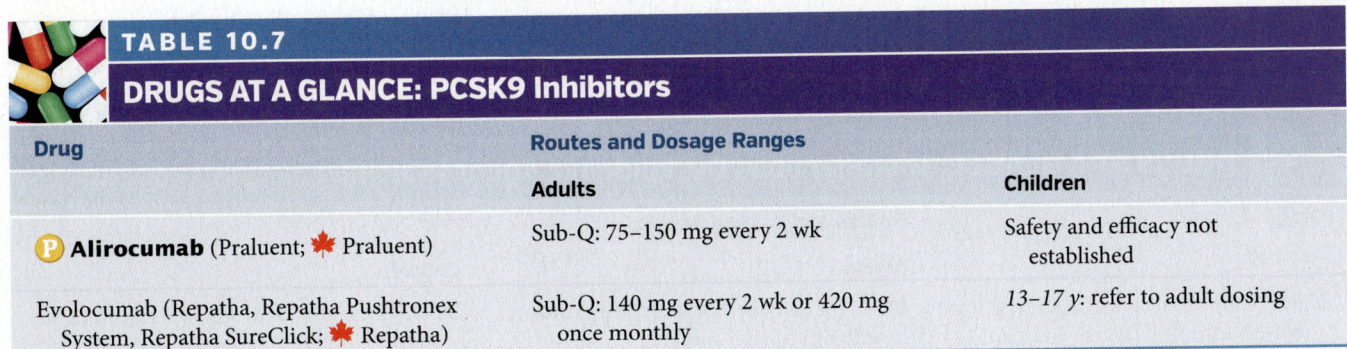

TABLE 10.7 DRUGS AT A GLANCE: PCSK9 Inhibitors		
Drug	**Routes and Dosage Ranges**	
	Adults	**Children**
Ⓟ **Alirocumab** (Praluent; 🍁 Praluent)	Sub-Q: 75–150 mg every 2 wk	Safety and efficacy not established
Evolocumab (Repatha, Repatha Pushtronex System, Repatha SureClick; 🍁 Repatha)	Sub-Q: 140 mg every 2 wk or 420 mg once monthly	13–17 y: refer to adult dosing

Nursing Implications

Preventing Interactions

No interactions have been reported that increase or decrease the therapeutic or adverse effects of the drug.

Administering the Medication

The drug should be administered by subcutaneous injection into the upper arm, abdomen, or thigh. The injection site should be rotated with each injection, and other drugs should not be given at the same injection site at the same time. The prefilled syringe or pen should be warmed to room temperature for 30 to 40 minutes before use. Note that it may take 20 seconds to inject the drug subcutaneously.

Assessing for Therapeutic Effects

The nurse monitors lipid response to therapy, looking for decreased levels of LDL cholesterol. Maximum effects begin in approximately 1 week; monitoring should occur within 4 to 8 weeks of initiation or dosage adjustment.

Assessing for Adverse Effects

The nurse should determine that no injection site reactions are present. In addition, it is necessary to observe that the patient manifests no signs or symptoms of influenza, cough, muscle pain, diarrhea, or allergic reaction to the drug.

Patient Teaching

Patients (and providers) need to read patient information and instructions each time the patient administers alirocumab in case new information is available. The nurse provides guidance to patients and caregivers regarding the proper subcutaneous injection technique, including aseptic technique and how to use the prefilled syringe or pen correctly. Patient instruction regarding discarding needles and syringes in a puncture-resistant disposal container is necessary. Patients should notify their healthcare provider if they become pregnant while taking alirocumab. Box 10.2 contains general patient teaching information.

Other Drugs in the Class

The only other drug currently approved as a PCSK9 inhibitor is evolocumab (Repatha). To date, the indications and drug profile of evolocumab appear similar to alirocumab. As further clinical trials proceed, the benefit of one drug over another in the class may be identified. Because evolocumab is administered as a 420-mg dose, three separate 140-mg injections consecutively within a 30-minute period must be administered. Both drugs in the class are expensive, possibly limiting use in patients who might benefit from a PCSK9 inhibitor.

MISCELLANEOUS DYSLIPIDEMIC AGENT

Niacin (nicotinic acid) is a vitamin that is no longer recommended as a dyslipidemic agent except in patients with high triglyceride levels (greater than 500 mg/dL) who have not been able to achieve the desired response or do not tolerate other drug therapy. For decreasing LDL cholesterol, other drugs (evolocumab or ezetimibe) are more effective when added to statin therapy. Although niacin does significantly increase HDL cholesterol, there is no evidence that the increase leads to improved patient outcomes. Serious concerns have been raised about the safety and efficacy of this vitamin in combination with statin therapy. Some formulations of sustained-release over-the-counter (OTC) niacin have been associated with an increased risk of hepatotoxicity. Niacin also increases blood glucose, causing possible problems with glucose control for people with diabetes. Poor tolerability often limits the use of niacin; the high doses required for dyslipidemic effects result in adverse effects. Niacin commonly causes skin flushing, pruritus, and gastric irritation, and it may lead to tachycardia, hypotension, dizziness, hyperglycemia, hyperuricemia, elevated liver aminotransferases, and hepatitis.

Table 10.8 presents dosage information for this oral drug.

COMBINATION THERAPY USED TO TREAT DYSLIPIDEMIA

When monotherapy is not effective in attaining target LDL cholesterol levels, combination therapies with lipid-lowering drugs that have different mechanisms of action are recommended. In general, the drug combinations that are most effective in reducing total and LDL cholesterol are (1) a statin with a cholesterol absorption inhibitor or a bile acid sequestrant or (2) niacin with a bile acid sequestrant. When a goal of therapy is to increase the level of HDL cholesterol, a fibrate, cholesterol absorption inhibitor, or niacin may be used. However, because niacin is no longer recommended except in specific situations, drug therapy

TABLE 10.8
DRUGS AT A GLANCE: Miscellaneous Dyslipidemic Agent (Niacin)

Drug*	Routes and Dosage Ranges	
	Adults	Children
Niacin (immediate release) (Niacor, Slo-Niacin; ❋ Niaspan, Niaspan FCT, Niodan)	PO 1–6 g daily, in 3 or 4 divided doses, with or just after meals	PO 55–87 mg/kg/d, in 3 or 4 divided doses, with or just after meals

*Do not substitute the immediate-release for the extended-release preparation.

may be more successful and better controlled with administration of individual drugs in combination. However, a fibrate–statin combination should be avoided because of increased risks of severe myopathy, and a niacin–statin combination increases the risks of hepatotoxicity. Adverse reactions from combination statin and cholesterol absorption inhibitor therapy are reported to be similar to those from statins alone. Combination preparations are not intended for initial therapy. The adverse effects and contraindications associated with individual drugs also apply when they are used in combination. All combinations, like individual preparations, should be used in conjunction with a cholesterol-reducing diet.

NCLEX Success

4. John Jones, a 47-year-old teacher, now takes cholestyramine, and the nurse teaches him about the medication and its use. The nurse should be concerned if, after the teaching session, Mr. Jones states
    A. "I should take the medicine with a full glass of water when I take my other medications"
    B. "I am taking this medication to decrease my LDL cholesterol level"
    C. "I should swallow the tablets whole"
    D. "I may need to supplement my intake of the fat-soluble vitamins A, D, E, and K"

5. The nurse practitioner adds cholestyramine to statin therapy in a patient with markedly elevated serum levels of LDL cholesterol. Which of the following if stated by the patient indicates that patient teaching has been successful? (Select all that apply.)
    A. "I need to mix the powder with water or other fluids before I take it."
    B. "I should wait 1 hour after I eat to take the medication."
    C. "I need to maintain good oral hygiene as the medication can damage my teeth."
    D. "If I notice an increased bleeding tendency, I need to notify the nurse practitioner."
    E. "I might have some GI effects, including constipation or abdominal pain."

THE NURSING PROCESS

A concept map outlines the nursing process related to drug therapy considerations in this chapter. Additional nursing implications related to the disease process should also be considered in care decisions.

Assessment
- Assess risk factors, history, or disease associated with atherosclerotic vascular disease, such as smoking, immobility, obesity, hypertension, or diabetes mellitus; signs and symptoms of an elevated serum cholesterol (>200 mg/100 mL) or triglycerides (>150 mg/100 mL); or both.

Outcomes of Therapy

The patient will
- Take lipid-lowering drugs as prescribed, decrease dietary intake of saturated fats and cholesterol, lose weight if obese and maintain the lower weight, have periodic measurements of blood lipids, avoid preventable adverse drug effects, receive positive reinforcement for efforts to lower blood lipid levels, and report feeling less anxious and more in control as risks of atherosclerotic cardiovascular disease are decreased.
- Begin primary prevention strategies in childhood with healthful eating habits (e.g., avoiding excessive fats, meat, and dairy products; obtaining adequate amounts of all nutrients, including dietary fiber; avoiding obesity), exercise, and avoiding cigarette smoking.

Nursing Interventions
- Help patients control risk factors. Weight loss often reduces blood lipids and lipoproteins to a normal range.
- Support measures to increase blood flow to tissues, including exercise, limiting time with legs in dependent position, and use of compression hose; provide appropriate teaching related to drug therapy (see Box 10.2).
- The most effective measures for preventing dyslipidemia and atherosclerosis are those related to a healthful lifestyle (e.g., diet low in cholesterol and saturated fats, weight control, exercise). Refer patients to a nutritionist. Overeating or gaining weight may decrease or cancel the lipid-lowering effects of the drugs.
- Secure counseling for smoking cessation for those who smoke, with patient understanding of the harm of exposure to second-hand smoke.
- Encourage adult patients to have their serum cholesterol level measured at least once every 5 years or as instructed by their health care provider. Adults and children with a personal or family history of dyslipidemia or other risk factors should be tested more often.
- Help patients and family members understand the desirability of lowering high blood lipid levels before serious cardiovascular diseases develop.

Evaluation
- Observe for decreased blood levels of total and LDL cholesterol and triglycerides with drug therapy; observe for increased levels of HDL cholesterol.
- Observe and interview regarding compliance with instructions for drug, diet, exercise, and other therapeutic and behavioral modification measures.
- Observe and interview regarding adverse drug effects.
- Validate the patient's ability to identify foods high and low in cholesterol and saturated fats.

Visit thePoint® at http://thePoint.lww.com/Frandsen13e for answers to NCLEX Success questions (in Appendix A), answers to Clinical Application Case Studies (in Appendix B), additional information on etiology and pathophysiology, and more!

REFERENCES AND RESOURCES

American Academy of Pediatrics. (1992). National Cholesterol Education Program: Report of the expert panel on blood cholesterol levels in children and adolescents. *Pediatrics, 89*, 525–584.

Daniels, S. R. (2020). Guidelines for screening, prevention, diagnosis and treatment of dyslipidemia in children and adolescents. In K. R. Feingold, B. Anawalt, A. Boyce, G. Chrousos, W. W. de Herder, K. Dhatariya, K. Dungan, J. M. Hershman, J. Hofland, S. Kalra, G. Kaltsas, C. Koch, P. Kopp, M. Korbonits, C. S. Kovacs, W. Kuohung, B. Laferrère, M. Levy, E. A. McGee, … D. P. Wilson (Eds.). *Endotext* [Internet]. MDText.com, Inc.; 2000. https://www.ncbi.nlm.nih.gov/books/NBK395579/

Grundy, S. M., Bailey, A. L., Stone, N. J., Beam, C., Birtcher, K. K., Blumenthal, R. S., Braun, L. T., de Ferranti, S., Faiella-Tommasino, J., Forman, D. E., Goldberg, R., Heidenreich, P. A., Hlatky, M. A., Jones, D. W., Lloyd-Jones, D., Lopez-Pajares, N., Ndumele, C. E., Orringer, C. E., Peralta, C. A., …; Guideline Writing Committee for the 2018 Cholesterol Guidelines. (2019). 2018 Cholesterol clinical practice guidelines: Synopsis of the 2018 American Heart Association/American College of Cardiology/Multisociety Cholesterol Guideline. *Annals of Internal Medicine, 170*(11), 779–783. https://doi.org/10.7326/M19-0365

Lee, J. W., Lim, H., Kim, J. H., & Kim, H. S. (2021). Reassessment of inclusion criteria in the 2013 the American College of Cardiology and the American Heart Association cholesterol guidelines for cardiovascular disease prevention. *Journal of Clinical Neurology (Seoul, Korea), 17*(1), 86–95. https://doi.org/10.3988/jcn.2021.17.1.86

Lippincott Advisor. (2022). http://advisor.lww.com

Malakar, A. K., Choudhury, D., Halder, B., Paul, P., Uddin, A., & Chakraborty, S. (2019). A review on coronary artery disease, its risk factors, and therapeutics. *Journal of Cellular Physiology, 234*(10), 16812–16823. https://doi.org/10.1002/jcp.28350

National Heart, Lung, and Blood Institute. (2012). *Expert panel on integrated guidelines for cardiovascular health and risk reduction in children and adolescents* (NIH Publication No. 12-7486). National Institutes of Health.

National Institutes of Health Expert Panel. (2001). *Third report of the National Cholesterol Education Program (NCEP) Expert Panel on detection, evaluation, and treatment of high blood cholesterol in adults (Adult Treatment Panel III)* (NIH Publication No. 01-3670). National Institutes of Health.

Norris, T. L. (2019). *Porth's pathophysiology: Concepts of altered health states* (10th ed.). Wolters Kluwer.

Pang, J., Chan, D. C., & Watts, G. F. (2020). The knowns and unknowns of contemporary statin therapy for familial hypercholesterolemia. *Current Atherosclerosis Reports, 22*(11), 64–64. https://doi.org/10.1007/s11883-020-00884-2

Pavlovic, J., Franco, O. H., Kavousi, M., Ikram, M. K., Deckers, J. W., Ikram, M. A., & Leening, J. G. (2020). Recommendations and associated levels of evidence for statin use in primary prevention of cardiovascular disease: A comparison at population level of the ESC, ACC/AHA, USPSTF, and CCS guidelines. *European Heart Journal, 41*(2).

Rosenson, R. S., & Baker, S. K. (2022). *Statin muscle-related adverse effects. UpToDate*. Lexi-Comp, Inc.

Stone, N. J., Robinson, J. G., Lichtenstein, A. H., Bairey Mertz, C. N., Blum, C. B., Lloyd-Jones, D. M., Eckel, R. H., Goldberg, A. C., Gordon, D., Levy, D., Lloyd-Jones, D. M., McBride, P., Schwartz, J. S., Shero, S. T., Smith Jr., S. C., Watson, K., Wilson, P. W. F.; American College of Cardiology/American Heart Association Task Force on Practice Guidelines. (2014). 2013 ACC/AHA guideline on the treatment of blood cholesterol to reduce atherosclerotic cardiovascular risk in adults: A report of the American College of Cardiology/American Heart Association Task Force on practice guidelines. *Circulation, 129*, S1–S45.

Ware, A. L., Young, P. C., Weng, C., Presson, A. P., Minich, L. L. A., & Menon, S. C. (2018). Prevalence of coronary artery disease risk factors and metabolic syndrome in children with heart disease. *Pediatric Cardiology, 39*(2), 261–267. https://doi.org/10.1007/s00246-017-1750-2

Writing Committee, Cholesterol Clinical Practice Guidelines. (2019). 2018 AHA/ACC/AACVPR/AAPA/ABC/ACPM/ADA/AGS/APhA/ASPC/NLA/PCNA guideline on the management of blood cholesterol: Executive summary. A report of the American College of Cardiology/American Heart Association Task Force on Clinical Practice Guidelines. *Circulation, 139*, e1046–e1081.

Volpe, M., & Patrono, C. (2021). The cardiovascular benefits of statins outweigh adverse effects in primary prevention: results of a large systematic review and meta-analysis. *European Heart Journal, 42*(44), 4518–4519. https://doi.org/10.1093/eurheartj/ehab647

Yebyo, H. G., Aschmann, H. E., & Puhan, M. A. (2019). Finding the balance between benefits and harms when using statins for primary prevention of cardiovascular disease: A modeling study. *Annals of Internal Medicine, 170*(1), 1–10. doi:10.7326/M18-1279

CHAPTER 11

Drug Therapy for Hematopoietic Disorders

LEARNING OBJECTIVES

After studying this chapter, you should be able to:

1. Briefly describe hematopoietic and immune functions.
2. Identify common clinical manifestations of inadequate erythropoiesis and diminished host defense mechanisms.
3. Discuss characteristics of erythropoiesis-stimulating agents in terms of the prototype, mechanism of action, indications for use, adverse effects, principles of therapy, and nursing implications.
4. Describe the characteristics of colony-stimulating factors in terms of the prototype, mechanism of action, indications for use, adverse effects, principles of therapy, and nursing implications.
5. Discuss interferons in terms of the prototype, mechanism of action, indications for use, adverse effects, principles of therapy, and nursing implications.
6. Implement the nursing process in the care of patients who take drugs to enhance hematopoietic and immune system function.

CLINICAL APPLICATION CASE STUDY

Alice Paul is a 76-year-old woman who is being treated with chemotherapy for inoperable liver cancer. She receives a combination chemotherapy regimen every 6 weeks. She is in the oncologist's office for routine laboratory work 10 days after chemotherapy and complains of severe fatigue. The results of her blood work are as follows: hemoglobin 10.9 g/dL, hematocrit 32%, white blood cell (WBC) count 2,000 cells/mm^3, absolute neutrophil count (ANC) 800 cells/mm^3, and platelet count 120,000/μL.

KEY TERMS

Biologic response modifiers: intrinsic and extrinsic substances in the body that enhance the body's response to infection; for example, interferons, monoclonal antibodies, interleukin-2, and types of colony-stimulating factors

Cytokines: small proteins released by cells that specifically affect cell-to-cell communication; these include colony-stimulating factors, interleukins, and interferons, which are involved in numerous physiologic responses, including hematopoiesis, cellular proliferation and differentiation, inflammation, wound healing, and cellular and humoral immunity

Erythropoiesis: production of red blood cells

Erythropoietin: hormone secreted by the kidneys that stimulates bone marrow production of red blood cells

Hematopoiesis: formation of blood cells

Immunocompetence: normal immune system function

Immunodeficiency: inadequate or impaired immune function

Immunostimulants: drugs that stimulate immune function to fight infection and disease

Neutropenia: low neutrophil count

Pegylation: process of modifying an interferon by treatment with polyethylene glycol

INTRODUCTION

Hematopoiesis is the formation of blood cells. Adequate blood cell production supports normal immune system function, or **immunocompetence**. These are vital processes in the human body's ability to fight harmful invaders. Inadequate or impaired hematopoiesis or immune function (**immunodeficiency**) leads to high risks of infection and cancer. Efforts to enhance a person's own body systems to fight disease include the development of drugs to stimulate hematopoiesis and immune function. People take these drugs to restore normal function or to increase the ability of the immune system to eliminate potentially harmful invaders. This chapter discusses several drugs that affect hematopoietic function and the immune system.

OVERVIEW OF HEMATOPOIESIS AND IMMUNE FUNCTION

Hematopoietic and immune blood cells originate in bone marrow in stem cells, which are often called pluripotent stem cells because they are capable of becoming different types of cells. As these stem cells reproduce, some cells are exactly like the original cells and are retained in the bone marrow to maintain a continuing supply. However, most reproduced stem cells differentiate to form other types of cells. The early offspring are committed to become a particular type of cell, and a committed stem cell that produces a cell type in a specific cell line is called a colony-forming unit (CFU). Figure 11.1 illustrates the process of hematopoiesis in red and white cells.

Hematopoietic growth factors or **cytokines** control the reproduction, growth, and differentiation of stem cells and CFUs. Cytokines are small proteins released by cells that specifically affect cell-to-cell communication. They also initiate the processes required to produce fully mature cells. Overall, cytokines are involved in numerous physiologic responses, including hematopoiesis, cellular proliferation and differentiation, inflammation, wound healing, and cellular and humoral immunity.

To understand the effects of drug therapy to enhance hematopoiesis or immune function, it is necessary to appreciate the physiologic effects of the endogenous hematopoietic cytokines. **Erythropoiesis** is the production of red blood cells. **Erythropoietin**, a hormone secreted by the kidneys, stimulates bone marrow production of red blood cells. Colony-stimulating factor (CSF) is a substance that stimulates the production of red blood cells and granulocytes. Interferons are natural substances that fight infection. They are made up of white blood cells and other cells. The three main types of interferons are interferon-alfa, interferon-beta, and interferon-gamma. Interleukins (ILs) produce cytokines, which act on nonhematopoietic cells. For further essential details on the physiologic effects of the endogenous cytokines, visit thePoint (http://thePoint.lww.com/Frandsen13e).

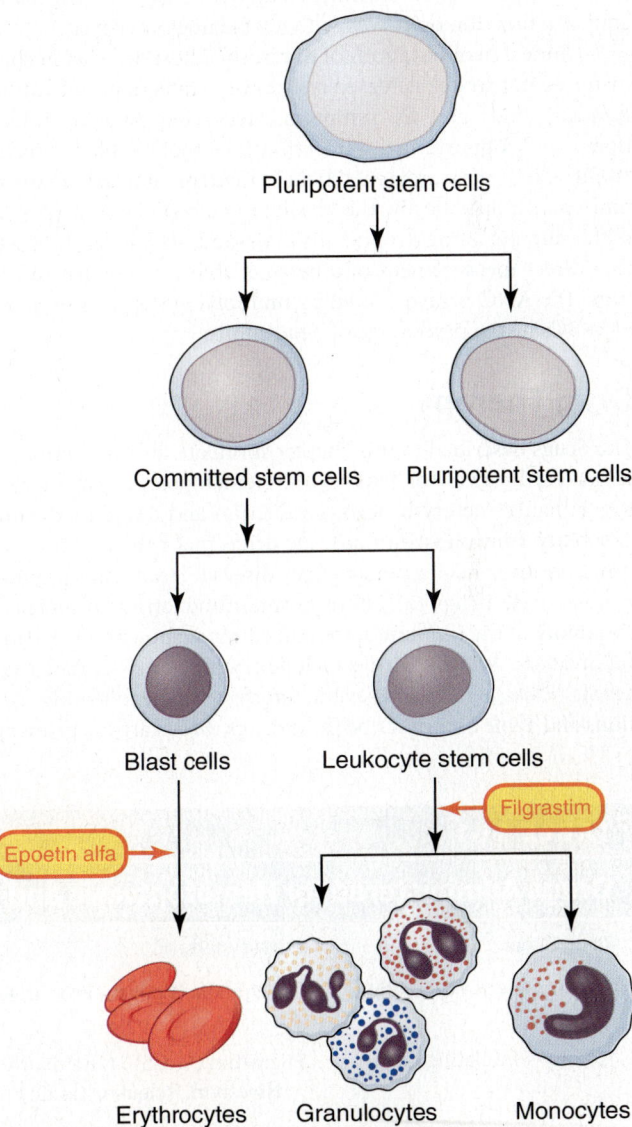

Figure 11.1. Hematopoietic and immune blood cell development. Formation, development, and differentiation of erythrocytes and leukocytes, with the site of effects of selected prototype drugs.

Clinical Manifestations

As red blood cells (RBCs) or white blood cells (WBCs) decrease, conditions related to inadequate hematopoiesis or poor immune function develop. Clinical manifestations of inadequate erythropoiesis include anemia. This results in a decrease in the oxygen-carrying capacity of blood and consequently a decreased oxygen availability to the tissues. A compensatory increase in heart rate and cardiac output initially increases cardiac output, offsetting the lower oxygen-carrying capacity of the blood. However, the oxygen demand becomes greater than the supply, and clinical manifestations are directly attributable to tissue hypoxia. Muscle weakness and easy fatigability are common. In severe anemia, the skin is usually pale to a waxy pallor, and cyanosis is typically absent. Headache, irritability, light-headedness, slowed thought processes, and depression are common central nervous system effects. (However, children appear to have a remarkable ability to function quite well with low hemoglobin levels.)

Clinical manifestations of diminished host defense mechanisms demonstrate decreased resistance to infections, including frequent colds and flu symptoms, recurring parasitic infections, and opportunistic infections. Complete blood (cell) count (CBC) measurements include **neutropenia** (low neutrophil count). Specifically, the absolute neutrophil count (ANC) is the number of neutrophils in the blood, which can be used as a direct measurement of a person's ability to combat infection. The ANC is determined by multiplying the total number of WBCs by the percentage of neutrophils.

Drug Therapy

The drugs described in this chapter stimulate the production of either erythrocytes or leukocytes. Hematopoietic growth factors enhance the erythrocyte production and oxygen-carrying capability. **Immunostimulants** are drugs that enhance immune function; they help a person fight disease. Healthcare providers use these drugs to restore normal function or to increase the ability of the immune system to eliminate potentially harmful invaders. Available drugs include erythropoiesis-stimulating agents (ESAs), CSFs, and several interferons. The following sections and Table 11.1 describe these drugs, which are the primary focus of this chapter. The section on *Adjuvant Medications* briefly discusses two ILs. Other chapters also discuss drugs with immunostimulant properties. These include traditional immunizing agents (see Chapter 12); levamisole, which restores functions of macrophages and T cells and is used with fluorouracil in the treatment of intestinal cancer (see Chapter 14); and antiviral drugs used in the treatment of acquired immunodeficiency syndrome (AIDS; see Chapter 23).

Most hematopoietic and immunostimulant drugs are synthetic versions of endogenous cytokines. Manufacturers use molecular biology–associated techniques to delineate the type and sequence of amino acids and to identify the genes responsible for producing the substances. Technicians then insert these genes into bacteria (usually *Escherichia coli*) or yeasts capable of producing the substances exogenously. Exogenous drug preparations have the same mechanisms of action as the endogenous products. Thus, CSFs bind to receptors on the cell surfaces of immature blood cells in the bone marrow and increase the number, maturity, and functional ability of the cells.

In cancer, the exact mechanisms by which interferons and ILs exert antineoplastic effects are unknown. However, their immunostimulant effects are thought to enhance activities of immune cells (i.e., natural killer [NK] cells, T cells, B cells, and macrophages), induce tumor cell antigens (which make tumor cells more easily recognized by immune cells), or alter the expression of oncogenes (genes that can cause a normal cell to change to a cancer cell).

All these drugs may produce adverse effects so that patients may not feel better when taking the drug. The combination of injections and adverse effects may lead to nonadherence in taking the drugs as prescribed.

ERYTHROPOIESIS-STIMULATING AGENTS

The hematopoietic growth factor **P epoetin alfa** (Epogen, Procrit, Retacrit) is the prototype recombinant form of human erythropoietin that helps the body produce more RBCs. The clinical benefit of treatment of anemia with an ESA is to reduce

TABLE 11.1

Drugs Administered for Hematopoiesis and Immunostimulation

Drug Class	Prototype(s)	Other Drugs in the Class
Erythropoiesis-stimulating agents	Epoetin alfa (Epogen, Procrit, Retacrit)	Darbepoetin alfa (Aranesp) Epoetin beta (Mircera)
Colony-stimulating factors	Filgrastim (G-CSF) (Granix, Neupogen, Nivestym, Releuko, Zarxio)	Pegfilgrastim (G-CSF) (Fulphila, Neulasta, Neulasta Onpro, Nyvepria, Udenyca, Ziextenzo) Sargramostim (GM-CSF) (Leukine)
Interferons	Interferon alfa-2b (Intron A)	Peginterferon alfa-2a (Pegasys) Interferon alfa-n3 (Alferon N) Interferon beta-1a (Avonex, Rebif) Interferon beta-1b (Betaseron) Interferon gamma-1b (Actimmune)

G-CSF, granulocyte colony-stimulating factor; GM-CSF, granulocyte–macrophage colony-stimulating factor.

the need and cost of blood transfusions, lessen the risk of infectious diseases from transfusions, and potentially enhance the overall quality of life as anemia is relieved. Although ESAs have been used to treat anemia associated with a variety of conditions, evidence indicates that the patients who benefit consistently from ESAs are prescribed epoetin alfa or another ESA for chemotherapy-associated anemia or those with anemia due to chronic kidney disease.

Pharmacokinetics

Both subcutaneous and intravenous (IV) administrations lead to good absorption (digestive enzymes would destroy the drug if it were given orally). The distribution is unknown, and metabolism occurs in the plasma. Excretion of a small amount occurs in the kidneys. The onset of action is 11 to 14 days.

Action

Epoetin alfa induces erythropoiesis by stimulating erythroid progenitor cells. This causes the release of reticulocytes from the bone marrow, leading to an increase in hemoglobin and hematocrit levels.

Use

Experts recommend epoetin alfa as a treatment option for cancer patients with chemotherapy-associated anemia who have a hemoglobin level that has decreased below 10 g/dL. Another use for the drug is in the prevention and treatment of anemia associated with chronic kidney disease and anemia caused by zidovudine therapy in patients with human immunodeficiency virus (HIV).

Clinical practice guidelines for use of ESAs from the American Society of Hematology and the American Society of Clinical Oncology advise that ESAs are indicated for the treatment of symptomatic anemia in patients with nonmyeloid neoplasms who are receiving chemotherapy. ESAs should be started when the hemoglobin is ≤10 g/dL. In addition, the prescriber should consider the patient's risk of thromboembolism (Loprinzi & Patnaik, 2022). Deep vein thrombosis (DVT) prophylaxis is recommended in perisurgery patients due to the increased risk of DVT. The U.S. Food and Drug Administration (FDA) has issued a **BOXED WARNING** ◆ directing prescribers that treatment of anemia with an ESA in patients with cancer who are not receiving chemotherapy offers no benefit and may cause serious harm.

Table 11.2 presents route and dosage information for the ESAs.

Patient-related variables specific to the use of epoetin alfa include the following:

- Age:
  - In premature infants, administration of epoetin alfa has an increased risk of retinopathy.
  - Premature infants should not receive epoetin alfa from multidose vials because they contain benzyl alcohol, which can be fatal. Single-dose vials do not contain benzyl alcohol.

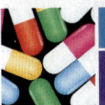

TABLE 11.2

DRUGS AT A GLANCE: Erythropoiesis-Stimulating Agents

Drug	Routes and Dosage Ranges
Epoetin alfa (Epogen, Procrit, Retacrit; Eprex)	Cancer chemotherapy: Adults, 150–300 units/kg Sub-Q three times weekly 1 mo to 12 y, 600 units/kg IV, Sub-Q once a week Cancer chemotherapy: Children ≥5 y and adolescents: 600 units/kg/dose IV once weekly Chronic kidney disease: Adults, 50–100 units/kg IV, Sub-Q three times weekly to achieve or maintain hemoglobin level of no more than 12 g/dL 1 mo to 12 y, 50 units/kg IV, Sub-Q three times a week Chronic kidney disease: Children ≥16 y 50 units/kg/dose IV or Sub-Q 3 times weekly Anemia due to zidovudine in patients infected with HIV: Adults, 100 units/kg IV or Sub-Q 3 times a week; withhold dose if Hb exceeds 12 g/dL Anemia due to zidovudine in patients infected with HIV: Infants ≥3 mo; children and adolescents ≤17 y 50–400 units/kg/dose IV or Sub-Q 2–3 times per day
Darbepoetin alfa (Aranesp; Aranesp)	Chronic kidney disease on dialysis: Adults, 0.75 mcg/kg IV/Sub-Q once weekly, adjusted to achieve and maintain hemoglobin level no more than 12 g/dL Chronic kidney disease on dialysis: Children <18 y, 0.45 mcg/kg IV/Sub-Q once weekly or 0.75 mcg/kg every 2 wk Chronic kidney disease not on dialysis: Children <18 y, 0.45 mcg/kg IV/Sub-Q once weekly or 0.75 mcg/kg every 2 wk Chronic kidney disease not on dialysis: Adults, Sub-Q, IV 0.45 mcg/kg once weekly; If hemoglobin dose not increase by >1 g/dL after 4 wk, increase the dose by 25% Cancer chemotherapy: Adults, 2.25 mcg/kg once weekly or 500 mcg once every 3 wk until completion of chemotherapy
Epoetin beta (Mircera)	Chronic kidney disease (on dialysis): Adults, IV (preferred) 0.6 mcg/kg once every 2 wk adjusted to achieve or maintain hemoglobin level of no more than 11 g/dL Chronic kidney disease (not on dialysis): Adults, IV, Sub-Q 0.6 mcg/kg once every 2 wk adjusted to achieve or maintain hemoglobin level of no more than 10 g/dL

- Older adults may be at greater risk of adverse effects, especially if large doses are used or if hemoglobin is increased quickly or raised above acceptable limits.
- Reproduction, pregnancy, and lactation:
  - Recombinant erythropoietin does not cross the human placenta.
  - Polyhydramnios and intrauterine growth retardation have been reported in use with females who have iron deficiency anemia with chronic kidney disease.
  - Multidose formulations containing benzyl alcohol should not be administered during pregnancy.
  - Endogenous erythropoietin is found in breast milk.
- Specific healthcare environments:
  - In patients with critical illness, maintenance of acceptable hemoglobin levels will reduce the risk of DVT and improve health-related outcomes.
  - In the home care setting, the nurse may need to teach patients or caregivers how to accurately administer the drug and provide assistance in obtaining appropriate laboratory tests (e.g., CBC, platelet count, tests of kidney or hepatic function) to monitor the responses to the drug.

Adverse Effects

The most common adverse effect of epoetin alfa is hypertension; raising the hemoglobin slowly minimizes this. Other adverse effects include headache, nausea, vomiting, diarrhea, and arthralgias.

> **Quality and Safety Alert: Safety**
>
> Epoetin alfa increases risks of myocardial infarction and stroke, especially if it is used to achieve hemoglobin levels greater than 12 g/dL. Epoetin alfa should be administered at the lowest dose effective in raising hemoglobin levels sufficiently to avoid the need for blood transfusion. Regular monitoring of hemoglobin is necessary until the level stabilizes.

Contraindications

Contraindications to epoetin alfa include known hypersensitivity to the drug or to albumin (or other cell-derived products from mammals). In addition, people with uncontrolled hypertension should not take epoetin alfa because it may further increase blood pressure.

Nursing Implications
Preventing Interactions

Lenalidomide, pomalidomide, and thalidomide enhance the risk of thrombus formation. No herbal or food interactions have been reported with epoetin alfa.

Administering the Medication

For patients with chronic kidney disease on hemodialysis, the nurse gives epoetin alfa by bolus injection at the end of dialysis. For other patients with an IV line, IV administration is appropriate. For patients without an IV line or who are ambulatory, subcutaneous administration is suitable. The vial should not be shaken. Retacrit should not be diluted. The nurse ensures that the remainder of a multidose vial is discarded 21 days after opening. It is also recommended that iron supplements be administered with epoetin alfa.

> **Quality and Safety Alert: Safety**
>
> A multidose vial of epoetin alfa is not appropriate for use in children because of the risk of medication error.

Assessing for Therapeutic Effects

The nurse observes for increased RBCs, hemoglobin, and hematocrit; increased energy and exercise capacity; and improved quality of life. Therapeutic effects depend on the dose and the patient's underlying condition. The goal is usually to achieve and maintain a hemoglobin level of no more than 12 g/dL. With epoetin alfa, it is necessary to measure iron stores (transferrin saturation and serum ferritin) before and periodically during treatment. The nurse ensures that hemoglobin levels are measured twice weekly until stabilized and maintenance drug doses are established.

Assessing for Adverse Effects

The nurse ascertains that blood pressure remains within a safe range and also assesses for headache, nausea, vomiting, diarrhea, or joint pain. Because there is an increased risk of myocardial infarction and stroke, assessment of mental status changes and chest pain or decreased cardiac perfusion is necessary.

> **Quality and Safety Alert: Safety**
>
> It is important to assess for signs of deep vein thrombus formation (e.g., swelling, pain, and redness of the affected limb) in patients taking epoetin alfa.

Patient Teaching

> **Quality and Safety Alert: Safety**
>
> Epoetin alfa is not effective unless sufficient iron is present; therefore, patient teaching may need to emphasize the importance of taking an iron supplement.

Box 11.1 presents additional patient teaching guidelines for this drug.

Other Drugs in the Class

Darbepoetin alfa (Aranesp) is another ESA used in the prevention or treatment of anemia associated with several conditions, including chronic kidney disease and myelosuppressive (depressed bone marrow function) anticancer chemotherapy. Epoetin alfa and darbepoetin are similarly effective in achieving and maintaining target hemoglobin levels. Darbepoetin is a relatively long-acting agent compared to epoetin alfa's shorter-acting duration. The absorption of this drug is slow via the subcutaneous route, and in kidney disease, peak plasma levels occur in adults in about 48 hours (36 hours in children). In cancer, the time to peak plasma levels is 74 hours (49 hours in chil-

BOX 11.1 Patient Teaching Guidelines for Hematopoietic Drugs and Immunostimulants

General Considerations

- Help your body maintain immune mechanisms and other defenses by healthy lifestyle habits, such as a nutritious diet, adequate rest and sleep, and avoidance of tobacco and alcohol.
- Practice meticulous personal hygiene and avoid people and circumstances in which you are exposed to infection.
- With interferons, report the occurrence of depression or thoughts of suicide, dizziness, hives, itching, chest tightness, cough, difficulty breathing or wheezing, or visual problems. These symptoms may require that the drug be stopped or the dosage reduced. In addition, avoid pregnancy (use effective contraceptive methods), avoid prolonged exposure to sunlight, wear protective clothing, and use sunscreens.

Self- or Caregiver Administration

- Take the drugs as prescribed. Although this is important with all medications, it is especially important with these. Obtaining beneficial effects and decreasing adverse effects depend largely on how the drugs are taken.
- It is possible to administer several of these medications at home, even though they are given by injection. If you are going to self-inject a medication at home, allow sufficient time to learn and practice the techniques under the supervision of a healthcare provider. Correct preparation and injection are necessary to increase beneficial effects and decrease adverse effects. Be sure to dispose of needles and syringes properly.
- Use correct techniques to prepare and inject the medications. Instructions for mixing the drugs should be followed exactly.
  - With epoetin alfa, follow these instructions:
    - Do not freeze or shake the drug vial.
    - Obtain appropriate laboratory tests to monitor the responses to the drug.
    - Take an iron supplement, if instructed, to ensure absorption of the drug.
    - Consume foods that contain vitamin C (e.g., fruit juice, strawberries, cantaloupe) to increase the absorption of iron.
  - With filgrastim, follow these instructions:
    - Take acetaminophen (e.g., Tylenol, others), if desired, to decrease bone pain.
    - Notify your prescriber if pain is not relieved, especially if taking high-dose IV therapy, because opioids may be necessary.
    - Recognize that dosage modification may be necessary if your WBC count is greater than 100,000 cells/mm^3.
  - With interferons, follow these instructions:
    - Store the drug in the refrigerator.
    - Do not freeze or shake the drug vial.
    - Do not change brands (changes in dosage may result).
    - Take at bedtime to reduce some common adverse effects (e.g., flulike symptoms such as fever, headache, fatigue, anorexia, nausea, and vomiting).
    - Take acetaminophen (e.g., Tylenol, others), if desired, to prevent or decrease fever and headache.
    - Maintain a fluid intake of 2 to 3 quarts daily.
  - With ILs, follow these instructions:
    - Store the drug in the refrigerator.
    - Do not freeze or shake the drug vial.
    - Do not use if solution is discolored or if it contains particles.
    - Do not breast-feed while taking this drug.
    - Take acetaminophen (e.g., Tylenol, others), if desired, to prevent or decrease fever and headache.
    - Maintain a fluid intake of 2 to 3 quarts daily.
    - Report any of the following to your prescriber: shortness of breath, edema, chest pain, unusual fatigue or weakness, and irregular heartbeat.

dren). Hemoglobin levels increase after 2 to 6 weeks of therapy with darbepoetin. Studies indicate that a patient with cancer-related anemia and hemoglobin of 10 g/dL or less feels better and requires fewer blood transfusions with use of the drug. No significant interactions have reportedly occurred with this drug.

Epoetin beta (Mircera) is used in the treatment of anemia associated with chronic kidney disease in adults—whether or not they require dialysis. The FDA has issued a **BOXED WARNING** ◆ for epoetin beta, reporting that it is not indicated and is not recommended for treatment of chemotherapy-induced anemia. Researchers terminated a study because more deaths occurred in patients taking epoetin beta than in those taking another ESA. This drug is also not indicated as a substitute for RBC transfusions in patients who need immediate correction of anemia. The adverse effects profile for epoetin beta is similar to that of other ESAs, with hypertension being the most common effect. As with all ESAs, an adequate intake of iron is required for drug effectiveness, and an iron supplement is usually necessary.

Clinical Application 11.1

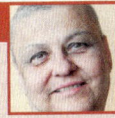

- What is the significance of Mrs. Paul's laboratory results?

Quality and Safety Alert: Evidence-Based Practice

Sinha et al. (2019) conducted a study to determine the efficacy, tolerability, and safety of darbepoetin alfa for the treatment of anemia in Indian patients with chronic kidney disease. Darbepoetin alfa is a long-acting erythropoiesis stimulating glycoprotein that has a threefold longer half-life than epoetin alfa. Patients with a hemoglobin less than 10 g/dL who had been receiving epoetin alfa were switched to darbepoetin alfa. The dosage and frequency of the darbepoetin alfa was lower than the epoetin alfa. Results revealed that in patients with chronic kidney disease who were undergoing dialysis, administration of darbepoetin alfa was equally as effective as the more frequent administration of epoetin alfa.

NCLEX Success

1. Which of the following drugs will enhance the outcome of therapy with epoetin alfa?
   A. iron
   B. potassium
   C. antacids
   D. analgesics

GRANULOCYTE COLONY-STIMULATING FACTORS

The drug **filgrastim** (Neupogen) is the prototype G-CSF used to stimulate blood cell production by the bone marrow in patients with bone marrow transplantation or chemotherapy-induced neutropenia. This drug can help prevent infection by reducing the incidence, severity, and duration of neutropenia associated with several chemotherapy regimens. Healthcare providers also use it to collect stem cells for transplantation. Experts believe that filgrastim promotes the growth of arterioles around blocked areas in coronary arteries. It may be more effective than drugs that stimulate capillary growth, because arterioles are larger and can carry more blood.

Pharmacokinetics

Filgrastim is completely absorbed. The duration of action of the drug is 4 days. It is systemically degraded, and the nature of its excretion is unknown. There is no evidence of drug accumulation over a period of 11 to 20 days. Filgrastim crosses the placenta and can enter breast milk.

Action

Filgrastim stimulates the production, maturation, and activation of neutrophils within bone marrow.

Use

Indications for filgrastim include (1) preventing infection in patients with neutropenia induced by cancer chemotherapy or bone marrow transplantation or (2) mobilizing stem cells from bone marrow to peripheral blood, where they can be collected and reinfused after chemotherapy that depresses bone marrow function. Most patients who take the drug have fewer days of fever, infection, and antimicrobial drug therapy. In addition, by promoting bone marrow recovery after a course of cytotoxic antineoplastic drugs, filgrastim also may allow for higher doses or more timely administration of subsequent antitumor drugs. Table 11.3 presents route and dosage information for the CSFs.

Patient-related variables specific to the use of filgrastim include the following:

- Age:
  - In pediatric clinical trials, filgrastim produced a greater incidence of subclinical spleen enlargement, but it is unknown if this affects growth and development or has long-term consequences.
  - Older adults may have a greater risk for adverse effects. They also are more likely to develop infections and may have less pronounced signs and symptoms.
- Reproduction, pregnancy, and lactation:
  - During pregnancy, a preservative-free solution should be used.
  - Filgrastim can be detected in breast milk, and concentrations are increased for at least 3 days following maternal filgrastim administration. Adverse effects have not been observed in breast-fed infants.
- Specific healthcare environments:
  - In the home care setting, the nurse needs to assess patients for signs of infection and teach them measures to reduce exposure to infection.
  - The nurse must also assess the patient's ability to administer the drug and to obtain appropriate laboratory tests (e.g., CBC, platelet count, tests of kidney or hepatic function) (see Box 11.1).

 Quality and Safety Alert: Safety

Patients should not receive filgrastim within 24 hours before or 24 hours after cytotoxic chemotherapy because it may act as a growth factor for any tumor, particularly of the myeloid type.

Quality and Safety Alert: Safety

Patients in a hospital setting are most vulnerable to infection, particularly nosocomial organisms, especially if their neutrophil count falls below 500/mm^3.

Adverse Effects and Contraindications

The most common adverse effects of filgrastim are drowsiness, fatigue, flulike symptoms, nausea, and bone pain. Contraindications include a known sensitivity to the drug and *E. coli*–derived proteins.

Nursing Implications

Preventing Interactions

No medications reportedly increase or decrease the effects of filgrastim. Likewise, no herbs or foods appear to increase or decrease the drug's effects.

Administering the Medication

The nurse administers filgrastim by subcutaneous or IV injection according to indication per the manufacturer's recommendation (Table 11.3):

- For cancer chemotherapy: subcutaneous bolus injection, IV infusion over 15 to 30 minutes, or continuous subcutaneous or IV infusion
- For bone marrow transplantation: IV infusion over 4 hours or by continuous IV or subcutaneous infusion
- For collection of stem cells: as a bolus or a continuous infusion
- For chronic neutropenia: subcutaneous injection

It is important not to shake a vial of filgrastim and to use it only once.

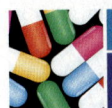

TABLE 11.3
DRUGS AT A GLANCE: Colony-Stimulating Factors

Drug	Routes and Dosage Ranges
P Filgrastim (G-CSF) (Granix, Neupogen, Nivestym, Releuko, Zarxio, Nivestym; 🍁 Grastofil, Neupogen, Nivestym)	Myelosuppressive chemotherapy: 5 mg/kg/d Sub-Q injection, IV infusion over 15–30 min, or continuous Sub-Q or IV infusion, up to 2 wk until ANC reaches 10,000/mm³ Bone marrow transplantation: 10 mcg/kg/d IV infusion initially at least 24 h after chemotherapy and >24 h after bone marrow infusion, then titrated according to neutrophil count (5 mcg/kg/d if ANC over 1,000/mm³ for 3 consecutive days; stop drug if over 1,000/mm³ for 3 d; if ANC drops below 1,000/mm³, restart filgrastim at 5 mcg/kg/d; if ANC drops below 1,000/mm³ during 5 mcg/kg/d dose, increase to 10 mcg/kg/d). Collection of peripheral stem cells: 10 mcg/kg/d Sub-Q for 6–7 d, with collection on the last 3 d of drug administration Severe, chronic neutropenia: 5 or 6 mcg/kg Sub-Q, once or twice daily, depending on clinical response and ANC
Pegfilgrastim (G-CSF) (Neulasta, Neulasta Onpro, Fulphila, Nyvepria, Udenyca, Ziextenzo; 🍁 Neulasta)	6 mg Sub-Q once per chemotherapy cycle; do not give between 14 d before and 24 h after cytotoxic chemotherapy Children for chemotherapy-induced neutropenia: <10 kg: Sub-Q: 0.1 mg/kg (0.01 mL/kg) 10–20 kg: Sub-Q: 1.5 mg (0.15 mL) 21–30 kg: Sub-Q: 2.5 mg (0.25 mL) 31 to <45 kg: Sub-Q: 4 mg (0.4 mL) ≥45 kg: Sub-Q: 6 mg (0.6 mL)
Sargramostim (GM-CSF) (Leukine; 🍁 Leukine)	Acute myeloid leukemia: Adults ≥55 y, 250 mcg/m²/d IV infusion over 4 h, starting on day 11 or 4 d following induction chemotherapy after bone marrow infusion for maximum of 42 d Bone marrow reconstitution: 250 mcg/m²/d IV infusion over 2 h, starting 2–4 h after bone marrow infusion and continuing for 21 d Children: ≥5 mo to <2 y: IV 250 mcg/m²/d infused over 4 h once daily; begin on day 0 of bone marrow transplantation and administer first dose after marrow infusion completed and continue for 21 d; discontinue if ANC > 20,000/mm³ >2 y and adolescents IV 250 mcg/m²/d infused over 2 h; begin 2 to 4 h after the marrow infusion and at least 24 h after chemotherapy; do not initiate until the post marrow infusion ANC <5,000/mm³ and continue until >1,500/mm³ for 3 d Graft failure or delay: 250 mcg/m²/d IV infusion over 2 h for 14 d; course of treatment may be repeated after 7 d of therapy if engraftment has not occurred Mobilization of stem cells: 250 mcg/m²/d Sub-Q or IV over 24 h

ANC, absolute neutrophil count; G-CSF, granulocyte colony-stimulating factor; GM-CSF, granulocyte–macrophage colony-stimulating factor.

Assessing for Therapeutic Effects

The nurse assesses for a decreased incidence of infection and a maintenance of the ANC within a target range of 1,500 to 10,000 cells/mm³.

Assessing for Adverse Effects

The nurse observes for drowsiness, fatigue, flulike symptoms, nausea, and bone pain. In addition, it is necessary to assess for erythema at subcutaneous injection sites.

> **Quality and Safety Alert: Safety**
>
> The nurse should check the ANC and report to the prescriber if it is 10,000 cells/mm³ or greater.

Patient Teaching

The nurse teaches the patient and family about accurate drug preparation and injection techniques as well as proper disposal of needles and syringes. Box 11.1 contains additional patient teaching guidelines.

Other Drugs in the Class

Pegfilgrastim (Fulphila, Neulasta, Neulasta Onpro, Nyvepria, Udenyca, Ziextenzo) and sargramostim (Leukine) are hematopoietic growth factors similar to filgrastim. They are used to treat patients who undergo bone marrow transplantation for Hodgkin disease, non-Hodgkin lymphoma, or acute lymphoblastic leukemia. With the administration of both of these medications, it is important to note that after transplantation, it takes 2 to 4 weeks for the engrafted bone marrow cells to mature and begin producing blood cells. During this time, patients have virtually no functioning granulocytes and are at high risk for infection. The administration of pegfilgrastim or sargramostim with lithium increases the production of WBCs, increasing the risk of a stroke or heart attack. Pegfilgrastim helps reduce the incidence, severity, and duration of neutropenia associated with several chemotherapy regimens and restore, promote, or accelerate bone marrow function. For information on administration of sargramostim to patients with cancer who have had bone marrow transplantation, see Table 11.3. The nurse should ensure that CBCs are performed twice weekly during therapy; the neutrophil count should not exceed approximately 20,000/mm³.

The most common adverse effects of pegfilgrastim are drowsiness, fatigue, flulike symptoms, nausea, and bone pain. Adverse effects of sargramostim include bone pain, fever, headache, muscle aches, generalized maculopapular skin rash, and fluid retention (peripheral edema, pleural effusion, pericardial effusion). Bone pain occurs in approximately 33% to 50% of patients; other effects occur in more than 10% of patients. Pleural and pericardial effusions are more likely at doses greater than 20 mcg/kg/d.

NCLEX Success

2. The nurse is administering filgrastim to a patient who has received a bone marrow transplant. Which laboratory parameter should the nurse monitor to determine if the drug is effective?
   A. hemoglobin
   B. basophils
   C. hematocrit
   D. neutrophils

3. The nurse is caring for a patient who is undergoing chemotherapy for cancer. The physician orders filgrastim. What should the nurse explain is the expected outcome after filgrastim administration?
   A. fewer infections
   B. decreased anemia
   C. longer life expectancy
   D. less nausea and vomiting

INTERFERONS

Interferons, called alfa, beta, or gamma, according to specific characteristics, are **biologic response modifiers** that bind to specific cell surface receptors and alter intracellular activities. Biologic response modifiers are intrinsic and extrinsic substances that enhance the body's response to infection. In viral infections, these immunostimulants induce enzymes that inhibit protein synthesis and degrade viral RNA. As a result, viruses are less able to enter uninfected cells, reproduce, and release new viruses. In addition to their antiviral effects, interferons also have antiproliferative and immunoregulatory activities. They can increase expression of major histocompatibility complex molecules, augment the activity of NK cells, increase the effectiveness of antigen-presenting cells in inducing the proliferation of cytotoxic T cells, aid the attachment of cytotoxic T cells to target cells, and inhibit angiogenesis (formation of blood vessels). (The recent development of more effective drugs has replaced the interferons as the standard of treatment for certain conditions.)

Synthetically produced interferons have the same capabilities as endogenous interferons. Thus, indications include treatment of viral infections and certain cancers. Ⓟ **Interferon alfa-2b** (Intron A) is the prototype for this class of drugs and is a product of recombinant DNA technology using *E. coli*.

Pharmacokinetics

Interferon alfa-2b is about 80% absorbed and widely distributed but does not cross the blood–brain barrier. There is minimal hepatic metabolism. Excretion is primarily kidney. Peak onset of action is 3 to 12 hours. The elimination half-life is approximately 2 to 3 hours.

Action

Interferon alfa-2b has both antiviral and antineoplastic activities. It exerts its cellular activities by binding to specific membrane receptors on the cell surface, enhancing immune response and inhibiting viral replication in virus-infected cells. The drug enhances the overall function of the immune system by increasing phagocytic activity of macrophages and monocytes, which augments cytotoxicity against cancer cells. Additionally, it suppresses the growth and reproduction of similar cells by cell division.

Use

Indications for use of interferon alfa-2b in adults 18 years of age and older include hairy cell leukemia, chronic hepatitis B and C, AIDS-related Kaposi sarcoma, condylomata acuminata (genital warts), malignant melanoma, and lymphoma (follicular). Table 11.4 presents route and dosage information for the interferons.

Patient-related variables specific to the use of interferons include the following:

- Age:
  - In children, interferons are used for the treatment of hemangiomas, hepatitis B, and chronic hepatitis C.
  - Multiuse vials should not be used in children because they contain benzyl alcohol, which could increase the risk of neurologic conditions.
- Reproduction, pregnancy, and lactation:
  - Adverse fetal effects have been reported in animal reproduction studies.
  - It is unknown if interferon is excreted in breast milk. The manufacturer recommends discontinuing nursing.
- Abnormal kidney function and hepatic impairment:
  - Hepatic enzymes may become elevated during treatment, especially in patients with preexisting liver disease. This increase may require discontinuation of the drug.
- Specific healthcare environments:
  - In the home care setting, the nurse must provide patient teaching on drug preparation and administration.
  - The following laboratory tests are required for monitoring drug response: CBC, platelet count, BUN, creatinine, AST, and ALT.

Adverse Effects

In the majority of patients, flulike symptoms (e.g., fever, chills, fatigue, muscle aches, headache, tachycardia) develop within 1 to 2 hours of administration of interferon alfa-2b and last up to 24 hours. Other symptoms include chest pain and alopecia. Adverse hematologic effects include neutropenia, anemia, and thrombocytopenia. The FDA has issued a **BOXED WARNING** ◆ for

TABLE 11.4

DRUGS AT A GLANCE: Interferons

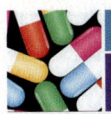

Drug	Routes and Dosage Ranges
(P) Interferon alfa-2b	Hairy cell leukemia: induction and maintenance, 2 million IU/m^2 Sub-Q, IM three times weekly up to 6 mo Kaposi sarcoma: induction and maintenance, 30 million IU/m^2 Sub-Q, IM three times weekly Lymphoma (follicular): 5 million IU/m^2 Sub-Q three times weekly up to 18 mo Malignant melanoma: 20 million IU/m^2 IV for 5 consecutive days per week for 4 wk (induction), followed by 10 million IU/m^2 Sub-Q three times weekly for 48 wk (maintenance) Hepatitis B: 5 million international units Sub-Q, IM daily or 10 million IU three times weekly (total of 30–35 million IU/wk) for 16 wk; children and adolescents: 3 million units/m^2/dose Sub-Q 3 times per week for 1 week; then 6 million units/m^2 3 times per week; maximum dose 10 million units; total duration of therapy 16–24 wk Hepatitis C: 3 million IU Sub-Q, IM three times weekly for 16 wk to 24 mo Condylomata acuminata: 1 million IU/lesion (maximum of 5 lesions) three times weekly for 3 wk; a second course could be administered in 12–16 wk Hemangioma: 3 million units/m^2/d (second-line therapy)
Interferon alfa-3n (Alferon N)	Condylomata acuminata: 250,000 IU/wart (maximum of 10 lesions) two times weekly for maximum 8 wk
Peginterferon alfa-2a (Pegasys; 🍁 Pegasys)	Chronic hepatitis B: Sub-Q, 180 mcg (1 mL) once weekly for 48 wk Chronic hepatitis C: Sub-Q, 180 mcg once weekly for 24 wk for viral genotypes 2 and 3; for 48 wk for viral strains 1 and 4; Children and Adolescents: 5 years and older: 180 mcg/dose in combination with ribavirin; maximum dose 180 mcg/dose; maximum dose 180 mcg/dose for 48 wk
Peginterferon alfa-2b	1 mcg Sub-Q once weekly for 1 y
Interferon beta-1a (Avonex, Rebif; Rebif Rebidose; 🍁 Avonex, Rebif)	Avonex, 30 mcg IM once per week Rebif, 8.8 mcg Sub-Q for 2 wk, then 22 mcg for 2 wk, and then 44 mcg; give all doses three times weekly, with at least 48 h between doses
Interferon beta-1b (Betaseron, Extavia; 🍁 Betaseron)	0.25 mg Sub-Q every other day
Interferon gamma-1b (Actimmune)	50 mcg/m^2 Sub-Q three times weekly; max dose 50 mcg/m^2; children and adolescents; body surface area ≤0.5 m^2 1.5 mcg/kg/dose Sub-Q 3 times weekly; maximum dose 50 mcg/m^2

all interferon alfa products because they can cause or aggravate fatal or life-threatening neuropsychiatric, ischemic, autoimmune, and infectious disorders. In addition, interferon alfa drugs should be discontinued in patients who develop severe decreases in neutrophil or platelet counts. Persistently severe or worsening effects usually lead to permanent discontinuation of interferon alfa. In many cases, these disorders resolve after the drug is stopped.

Contraindications

Contraindications to interferon alfa-2b include known sensitivity to the drug as well as signs and symptoms of liver disease (e.g., jaundice, ascites, bleeding disorders, or decreased serum albumin), autoimmune hepatitis, a history of autoimmune disease, or posttransplantation immunosuppression.

Nursing Implications

Preventing Interactions

Interferon should not be combined with myelosuppressive agents. Other medications interact with interferon alfa-2b, increasing its effects (Box 11.2). Apparently, no herbs interact with this drug.

Administering the Medication

The nurse may administer interferon alfa-2b intravenously, subcutaneously, intramuscularly, or intralesionally, as ordered. When administration is three times weekly, it should occur on a regular schedule (e.g., Monday, Wednesday, and Friday), at about the same time of day, at least 48 hours apart, per manufacturer's recommendation. To treat condylomata intralesionally, it is important to inject the drug into the base of each wart with a small-gauge needle. For large warts, injections may occur at several points per the manufacturer's recommendation.

Assessing for Therapeutic Effects

With parenteral interferons, the nurse observes for improvement in signs and symptoms. With hairy cell leukemia, hematologic tests may improve within 2 months, but optimal effects may require 6 months of drug therapy. With Kaposi sarcoma, skin lesions may resolve or stabilize over several weeks. With chronic hepatitis, liver function tests may improve within a few weeks.

| BOX 11.2 | Drug Interactions: Interferon Alfa-2b |

Drugs That Increase the Effects of Interferon Alfa-2b
- Bowel-cleansing phosphate and sulfate preparations, iopamidol, metrizamide, and other iodinated contrast media
  Increase the risk of seizure activity
- Clozapine
  Increases the risk and/or severity of hematologic toxicity
- Deferiprone, zidovudine
  Increase the risk of severe bone marrow toxicity
- Leflunomide
  Increases the risk of infections

Assessing for Adverse Effects

The nurse observes for acute flulike symptoms with interferon alfa-2b and assesses patient response through evaluation of liver function tests and WBC, RBC, and platelet values.

Patient Teaching

The nurse teaches the patient about accurate drug preparation and injection techniques as well as proper disposal of needles and syringes. The nurse also educates the patient that flulike symptoms occur within 1 to 2 hours of administration and may last up to 24 hours and be dose limiting; they may be relieved by acetaminophen.

Box 11.1 contains other patient teaching guidelines.

Other Drugs in the Class

Peginterferon alfa has largely replaced the older preparations of interferon alfa for some clinical uses. **Pegylation** is a process of modifying an interferon by treatment with polyethylene glycol, changing the pharmacokinetics of interferons so that they act longer and can be given less often. Peginterferons also produce steady blood levels, whereas unpegylated interferons provide fluctuating levels.

Peginterferon alfa-2a (Pegasys), in combination with ribavirin, with or without an antihepaciviral, is recommended only for certain genotypes of chronic hepatitis C, particularly in settings where newer interferon-free regimens are not accessible because of cost. Interferon alfa-3n (Alferon N) is used to treat condylomata acuminata in adults. Its side effect profile, particularly the flulike symptoms, is similar to that of other interferons.

Interferon beta-1a (Avonex, Rebif) and interferon beta-1b (Betaseron) are used for multiple sclerosis, an autoimmune neurologic disorder in which the drug slows progression of neurologic dysfunction, prolongs remissions, and reduces the severity of relapses. Flulike symptoms are common adverse effects.

Interferon gamma-1b (Actimmune) is used to treat chronic granulomatous disease, which involves impaired phagocytosis of ingested microbes and frequent infections. Drug therapy reduces the incidence and severity of infections.

> **! Quality and Safety Alert: Safety**
>
> A pregnancy if either parent is taking ribavirin (Chapter 23) may result in a child with congenital anomalies. Therefore, patient teaching must include the use of birth control measures to prevent pregnancy during treatment and for at least 6 months after stopping the drug.

ADJUVANT MEDICATIONS USED TO STIMULATE THE IMMUNE SYSTEM: INTERLEUKINS

Note that ILs are listed as high-alert medications by the Institute for Safe Medication Practices because the drug class has heightened risk of causing significant patient harm when used in error.

Aldesleukin (Proleukin) is a recombinant DNA version of IL-2. It activates cellular immunity, produces tumor necrosis factor (IL-1) and interferon gamma, and inhibits tumor growth. Its uses include treatment of metastatic kidney cancer and metastatic melanoma skin cancer. The FDA has issued a **BOXED WARNING** for aldesleukin, citing numerous concerns. Only patients with normal cardiac and pulmonary functions should receive the drug, and administration should occur in a hospital setting with critical care expertise and beds under supervision of an oncologist. Aldesleukin administration has been associated with capillary leak syndrome, which is characterized by a loss of vascular tone and extravasation of plasma proteins and fluid into the extravascular space. This results in hypotension and reduced organ perfusion that may be severe and can result in death. Development of moderate to severe lethargy should be a sign to withhold the drug. Finally, aldesleukin is associated with impaired neutrophil count with an increased risk of sepsis and bacterial endocarditis. Because few nurses are likely to give this drug, this chapter omits details about administration and patient monitoring.

Oprelvekin (Neumega) is recombinant IL-11, which stimulates platelet production. This drug is used to prevent severe thrombocytopenia and reduce the need for platelet transfusions in adults with nonmyeloid cancer receiving myelosuppressive chemotherapy and who are at high risk for thrombocytopenia. The drug should be discontinued at least 2 days prior to the next planned chemotherapy cycle. The FDA has issued a **BOXED WARNING** for oprelvekin because of the risk for allergic or hypersensitivity reactions, including anaphylaxis. The drug should be permanently discontinued in any patient developing an allergic or hypersensitivity reaction. Subcutaneous injections of the drug should be rotated among sites. The patient should be educated regarding signs of a hypersensitivity reaction, including wheezing, chest tightness, rash, itching, fever, and swelling of the face, lips, tongue, or throat. Dilutional anemia, severe fluid overload, and dysrhythmias have been reported.

> ### Clinical Application 11.2
>
> - Mrs. Paul has a great risk of infection, with a low WBC count and low ANC. What should the nurse teach the patient about preventing infection?
>
>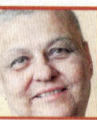

NCLEX Success

4. A patient with cancer was administered interferon alfa-2b today. After returning home, the patient calls the clinic and reports symptoms of fever, chills, fatigue, and muscle aches. What medication should the clinic nurse instruct the patient to take?
   A. aspirin
   B. codeine
   C. ibuprofen
   D. acetaminophen

5. Which of the following, if expressed by a patient taking interleukins, indicate that patient teaching was successful? (Select all that apply.)
   A. "I should store the medication in the refrigerator."
   B. "I should not use the medication if it is discolored."
   C. "I need to drink additional fluids while taking the medication."
   D. "I need to shake the medication to mix it well before taking."
   E. "I should not take acetaminophen if I have a fever or headache."
   F. "Shortness of breath and edema are side effects that I will need to learn to live with."

Clinical Application 11.3

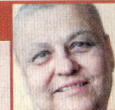

- Epoetin alfa is prescribed for Mrs. Paul's anemia. What dietary considerations should the nurse communicate to Mrs. Paul?

THE NURSING PROCESS

A concept map outlines the nursing process related to drug therapy considerations in this chapter. Additional nursing implications related to the disease process should also be considered in care decisions.

Assessment
- Assess the patient's status in relation to conditions for which hematopoietic and immunostimulant drugs are used (e.g., infection, neutropenia, cancer).
- Assess nutritional status and functional abilities.
- Assess adequacy of support systems and coping mechanisms.
- Assess baseline values of laboratory and other diagnostic test reports to aid monitoring of responses to hematopoietic and immunostimulant drug therapy.

Outcomes of Therapy
The patient will
- Participate in interventions to prevent or decrease infection.
- Remain afebrile during immunostimulant therapy.
- Experience increased immunocompetence as indicated by increased white blood cell (WBC) count (if initially leukopenic) or tumor regression.
- Experience relief or reduction of disease symptoms.
- Maintain nutritional level, appropriate appetite, and functional level of independence as able.
- Learn to self-administer medications accurately when indicated.

Nursing Interventions
- Support patient and others to practice and promote good hand hygiene techniques and sterile technique and to avoid contact with infected people.
- Encourage patients to participate in self-care and decision-making when feasible and engage with family members and significant others when feasible.
- Promote adequate nutrition, rest, sleep, and exercise.
- Inform patients about diagnostic test results, planned changes in therapeutic regimens, and evidence of progress.
- Use isolation procedures when indicated, usually when the neutrophil count is less than 500/mm^3.
- Monitor the complete blood (cell) count (CBC) and other diagnostic test reports for normal or abnormal values, reporting test results to prescribers when indicated. It is essential that darbepoetin and epoetin be stopped when the hemoglobin level approaches 12 g/dL and filgrastim and sargramostim be stopped when WBC counts normalize.
- Schedule drug administration, diagnostic tests, and other elements of care to conserve patients' energy.
- Assist patients or caregivers in learning how to prepare and inject darbepoetin alfa, epoetin alfa, filgrastim, or an interferon, when indicated.

Evaluation
- Compare current CBC reports with baseline values for changes toward normal levels (e.g., WBC count 5,000–10,000/mm^3).
- Compare weight and nutritional status with baseline values for maintenance or improvement.
- Observe and interview for decreased numbers or severity of disease symptoms and signs of infection.
- Observe for increased energy and ability to participate in ADLs.
- Observe and interview outpatients regarding adherence to follow-up care.
- Observe and interview regarding the mental and emotional status of the patient and family members.

Visit thePoint® *at* http://thePoint.lww.com/Frandsen13e *for answers to NCLEX Success questions (in Appendix A), answers to Clinical Application Case Studies (in Appendix B), additional information on pathophysiology, and more!*

REFERENCES AND RESOURCES

American Association for the Study of Liver Diseases/Infectious Diseases Society of America. *Recommendations for testing, managing, and treating hepatitis C.* Retrieved September 13, 2022, from https://www.aasld.org/sites/default/files/2022-07/PracticeGuidelines-HCV-November2018.pdf

Hinkle, J. L., Cheever, K. H., & Overbaugh, K. (2021). *Brunner & Suddarth's textbook of medical-surgical nursing* (15th ed.). Wolters Kluwer.

Loprinzi, C. L., & Patnaik, M. M. (2022). Role of erythropoiesis-stimulating agents in the treatment of anemia in patients with cancer. *UpToDate.* Lexi-Comp, Inc.

Norris, T. L. (2019). *Porth's pathophysiology: Concepts of altered health states* (10th ed.). Wolters Kluwer.

Sinha, S. D., Bandi, V. K., Bheemareddy, B. R., Thakur, P. J., Chary, S., Mehta, K., Pinnamareddy, V. K., Pandey, R., Sreepada, S., & Durugka, S. (2019). Efficacy, tolerability, and safety of darbepoetin alfa injection for the treatment of anemia associated with chronic kidney disease (CKD) undergoing dialysis: A randomized, phase II trial. *BMC Nephrology, 20*(1), N-PAG-N-PAG. https://doi.org/10.1186/s12882-019-1209-1

Spengler, U. (2022). Principles of interferon therapy in liver disease and the induction of autoimmunity. *UpToDate.* Lexi-Comp, Inc.

UpToDate. (2022). *Drug information.* Lexi-Comp, Inc.

CHAPTER 12

Drug Therapy: Immunizations

LEARNING OBJECTIVES

After studying this chapter, you should be able to:

1. Describe active and passive immunity and the agents that produce them.
2. Identify immunizations recommended for children and adolescents.
3. Identify immunizations recommended for adults.
4. Explain the indications for use, adverse effects, and contraindications of individual immunizing agents.
5. Teach parents (and their children) about the importance of immunizations to public health.
6. Inform people about recommended immunizations and record keeping.

CLINICAL APPLICATION CASE STUDY

Cynthia Williams, a 26-year-old college student, brings her 15-month-old son Riley to a family practice clinic for a well-child visit. Ms. Williams says that Riley has had his previous immunizations at the county health department every 2 months until the age of 6 months but that he has not had any immunizations since then.

KEY TERMS

Active immunity: antigenic immune response with antibody formation to an infection through administration of a vaccine or toxoid or through natural exposure to the disease

Antigenicity: ability of an antigen to bind specifically with certain products to promote better antibody formation

Immunization: bolstering a person's immune system by inducing antibody formation, thereby providing active protection against a specific infectious disease

Passive immunity: temporary state of immunity produced in a person who is susceptible to an infectious organism by administering serum-containing antibodies to the disease

Toxoids: altered bacterial toxins that are administered to stimulate antitoxin production and protect against the harmful effects of the toxin

Vaccines: microorganisms or components of microorganisms that are administered to stimulate antibody production against the microorganism prior to a natural infection

INTRODUCTION

Immunization, which involves bolstering a person's immune system by inducing antibody formation, thereby providing active protection against a specific infectious disease, has greatly improved human health and life expectancy. Immunizations are one of the key factors in reducing mortality and improving life expectancy in the United States over the past century. For greater than 70 years, immunizations have led to the elimination or near elimination of several vaccine-preventable diseases in the United States. Sustaining a well-developed vaccine delivery system and adequate surveillance of disease and of vaccine coverage can continue to significantly decrease the incidence of deaths, disabilities, and illness. The nurse plays a pivotal role in this process of assessing, teaching, administering immunizations, and evaluating patients who have received them for adverse effects.

OVERVIEW OF IMMUNIZATION

Types of Immunity

There are two main types of immunity. **Active immunity** is an antigenic immune response with antibody formation to an infection through administration of a vaccine or toxoid or through natural exposure to the disease. It results from administering a dead or weakened microorganism or piece of the microorganism to a person. The person's immune system responds by producing immunoglobulins (antibodies) specific for that microorganism, providing protection against disease with later exposure. **Passive immunity** is a temporary state of immunity produced in a person who is susceptible to an infectious organism by administering serum-containing antibodies to the disease. Passive immunity results from parenteral administration of immune serum containing disease-specific antibodies to a nonimmune person. Because passive immunity is only temporary, the person still needs a vaccine against a specific disease to develop antibodies that provide long-term immunity. Preparations used for immunization are biologic products prepared by pharmaceutical companies and are regulated by the U.S. Food and Drug Administration (FDA). The widespread use of these products in the United States has dramatically decreased the incidence of many infectious diseases, such as polio, influenza, pneumococcal disease, and hepatitis B.

Kinds of Immunizing Agents

Agents for Active Immunity

The biologic products used for active immunity are vaccines and toxoids. For maximum effectiveness, both of these products must be given before exposure to the pathogenic microorganism. Administration by the recommended route helps ensure the desired immunologic response.

Vaccines are suspensions of microorganisms or their antigenic products that have been killed (inactivated) or attenuated (weakened or reduced in virulence) so they can induce antibody formation while preventing infection altogether or causing only a very mild form of it. Many vaccines produce long-lasting immunity. Attenuated live vaccines produce active immunity, usually lifelong, that is similar to that produced by natural infection. There is a small risk that live vaccines may produce disease in people with severely impaired immune function, but this risk is very low with new vaccines developed using recombinant DNA technology.

Toxoids are bacterial toxins or products that have been modified to destroy toxicity while retaining antigenic properties (i.e., ability to induce antibody formation). Immunization with toxoids is not permanent, and scheduled repeat doses (boosters) are required to maintain immunity.

Additional components, such as aluminum or calcium phosphate, are added to some vaccines and toxoids, to slow absorption and increase **antigenicity** (ability of an antigen to bind specifically with certain products to promote better antibody formation). Products containing aluminum can only be given intramuscularly because greater tissue irritation occurs with subcutaneous injections of the immunizing agent.

In general, vaccines and toxoids are quite safe, and risks of the diseases they prevent are significantly greater than the risks of the vaccines. However, risks and benefits of vaccination are always considered individually, because no vaccine is completely effective or completely safe. People may still develop a disease after being immunized against it, but symptoms are usually less severe, and complications are fewer than if they had not been immunized. Adverse vaccine effects are usually mild and of short duration. The FDA evaluates vaccine safety before and after a vaccine is marketed; however, some adverse effects become apparent only after a vaccine is used in a large population.

Agents for Passive Immunity

Immune serums are the biologic products used for passive immunity. They act rapidly to provide temporary immunity lasting about 1 to 3 months in people exposed to or experiencing an infectious disease. The goal of therapy is to prevent or modify the disease process (i.e., decrease the incidence and severity of symptoms).

Immune globulin (IG) products are made from the serum of people with high concentrations of the specific antibody or immunoglobulin required. These products may consist of whole serum or only contain the immunoglobulin portion of serum in which the specific antibodies are concentrated. Immunoglobulin fractions are preferred over whole serum because they are more likely to be effective in disease prevention. All plasma used to prepare these products is screened for hepatitis B surface antigen. Hyperimmune serums are available for cytomegalovirus, hepatitis B, rabies, rubella, tetanus, and varicella zoster (shingles).

BOXED WARNING ◆ IG products can increase a patient's risk for the development of thrombosis. Risk factors that can contribute to thrombosis with IG include increased age, prolonged immobilization, hypercoagulability, past history of venous or arterial thrombosis, the use of estrogens, indwelling central vascular catheters, hyperviscosity, and cardiovascular disease. Administer the minimum dose for patients at risk for thrombosis, and monitor for signs and symptoms of thrombosis or hyperviscosity. The patient should be well hydrated.

INDIVIDUAL IMMUNIZING AGENTS

Box 12.1 provides information about current recommendations for immunizations. Table 12.1 lists vaccines and toxoids that are used routinely in the United States, and Table 12.2 lists immune serums that are used regularly in this country.

BOX 12.1 Recommended Immunizations by Age Group

Healthy Children and Adolescents (0 to 18 years)

- **Rotavirus vaccine** [either RV1 (Rotarix) or RV5 (RotaTeq)]
  - With Rotarix, a 2-dose series at 2 and 4 months is recommended; for RotaTeq, a 3-dose series is recommended at 2, 4, and 6 months. (If any dose in the series is either RotaTeq or unknown, default to 3-dose series.)
  - Catch-up vaccination: Do not start the series on or after age 15 weeks; the maximum age for the final doses is 8 months.
- **Diphtheria, tetanus, and pertussis vaccine**
  - A 5-dose series of DTaP (Daptacel or Infanrix) at ages 2, 4, 6, and 15 through 18 months and 4 through 6 years. DT given if child is allergic to pertussis vaccine.
- **Pneumococcal vaccine**
  - Four-dose series (PCV13, Prevnar 13) for healthy young children, at 2, 4, and 6 months and 12 through 15 months. Single dose if 6 to 18 years old and never vaccinated.
- **Chickenpox vaccine** (e.g., Varivax)
  - Two-dose series with the first dose at 12 to 15 months and the second dose at 4 to 6 years. Also recommended for adolescents who have never had chickenpox or been vaccinated with a single dose; 2 doses of vaccine are required for full immunity.
- *Haemophilus influenzae* **type b (Hib) conjugate vaccine**
  - Six weeks (minimum age) for 3-dose series PRP-T (ActHIB) or PRP-T (Hiberix) or 2-dose series PRP-OMP (PedvaxHIB).
  - A 2- or 3-dose Hib vaccine primary series and a booster dose (dose 3 or 4 depending on vaccine used in primary series) are administered at age 12 through 15 months to complete a full Hib series.
- **Measles, mumps, rubella, vaccine**
  - Two-dose series with first dose at ages 12 through 15 months and the second dose at 4 to 6 years.
- **Hepatitis A vaccine**
  - Two-dose series with the first dose between 1 and 2 years of age and the second dose at least 6 months after.
  - A hepatitis B (Hep B) monovalent vaccine should be given to all newborns within 24 hours of birth, with the second dose at age 1 to 2 months and the third dose at least 8 weeks after second dose and at least 16 weeks after first dose.
- **Human papillomavirus (HPV) vaccine (Gardasil 9)**
  - For all adolescents 11 or 12 years of age (can be given as early as 9 years) or up to 26 years of age if not received earlier. All vaccines are most effective if given before the person becomes sexually active.
- **Meningococcal vaccine**
  - Administration at 11 or 12 years of age with a booster dose at age 16 years. If not received earlier, 2 doses at least 8 weeks apart are recommended for adolescents up to age 21.
  - Two serogroup B meningococcal (MenB) vaccines are recommended in patients between 16 and 23 years of age for short-term protection against meningitis, with a preference for administration between ages 16 and 18 years.
- **COVID-19 vaccine**
  - For all children older than 5 years in 2-dose series of Pfizer-BioNTech; children 12 years and older also receive a booster of Pfizer-BioNTech at least 2 months after initial series.
- **Annual flu vaccination**
  - For all children older than 6 months.
  - Infants younger than 2 years of age and all children with underlying medical conditions should receive the trivalent inactive vaccine (TIV).
  - Combination vaccines are recommended for use in children who need multiple vaccines at a single visit (see Box 12.2 for available combination vaccines).

Adults

- **Chickenpox vaccine**
  - For nonpregnant adults who never had the disease or vaccine; a second dose of vaccine for adults who previously received a single dose.
- **Human papillomavirus (HPV) vaccine**
  - For females up to age 26 years, males up to age 21 years, and males 22 to 26 years who have sex with males, if not previously received.
- **Tdap vaccine booster**
  - 1 dose Tdap, then Td or Tdap booster every 10 years.
  - 1 dose Tdap each pregnancy; 1 dose Tdap during each pregnancy perferabley in early part of gestatonal weeks 27-36 1 dose Td/Tdap for wound management.
- **Two serogroup B meningococcal (MenB) vaccines**
  - Recommended in adults up to age 23 for short-term protection against meningitis, if not previously received.
- **Pneumococcal vaccine PPSV23 (Pneumovax)**
  - For all adults older than 65 years or/and adults younger than 65 years with certain chronic health conditions. Maximum is 2 doses in a lifetime.
  - The pneumococcal vaccine (PCV13) Prevnar is recommended for all adults older than 65 years and for adults younger than 65 years with immunocompromised who are at high risk for pneumococcal disease.
- **Herpes zoster vaccine (Shingrix)**
  - Two-dose series given 2 to 6 months apart to prevent herpes zoster (shingles) in adults aged 50 years and older.
- **Annual flu vaccination**
  - For all adults. People with underlying medical conditions should receive TIV.
- **COVID-19 vaccine**
  - For all adults in 2-dose series of Pfizer-BioNTech and Moderna given 4 to 8 weeks apart or a onetime Johnson & Johnson vaccine. A monovalent Johnson & Johnson booster is available in limited situations. Adults also receive a booster of either Pfizer-BioNTech or Moderna vaccine at least 2 months after initial series.

Use

Clinical indications for vaccines and toxoids include the following:

- Routine immunization of children against diphtheria, *Haemophilus influenzae* type b infection, hepatitis A and B, influenza, measles (rubeola), mumps, pertussis, pneumococcal infection, poliomyelitis, rotavirus, rubella (German measles), tetanus, COVID-19 (age 5 and older), and varicella (chickenpox).
- Postexposure prophylaxis with hepatitis A vaccine or IG effectively prevents infection with hepatitis A virus (HAV)

TABLE 12.1

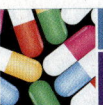

DRUGS AT A GLANCE: Vaccines and Toxoids for Active Immunity

Name/Characteristics	Indications for Use	Routes and Dosage Ranges Adults	Children
Vaccines			
COVID-19 (Pfizer-BioNTech, Moderna, Johnson & Johnson)	Effective against serious illness, hospitalizations, and death from SARS-CoV-2 infections	18+ y Pfizer-BioNTech 2-dose series 3–8 wk apart or Moderna 2-dose series 4–8 wk apart or Johnson & Johnson 1 dose with either Pfizer or Moderna booster 2 mo after first dose of J & J	Pfizer-BioNTech recommended 5+ y 2-dose series 3–8 wk apart 12–17 y Pfizer-BioNTech booster at least 5 mo after series 5–11 y no booster recommended
***H. influenzae* type b (Hib)** (ActHIB, PedvaxHIB, Hiberix; ✱ ActHIB, Hiberix) May be given at the same time as DTaP; measles, mumps, rubella (MMR); injected polio vaccine (IPV)	Prevention of H. *influenza* B; Routine immunization: ActHIB, Hiberix 3-dose series at 2, 4, 6, and booster 12–15 mo PedvaxHIB, 2-dose series at 2, 4, and booster 12–15 mo	Adults who are recipients of a successful hematopoietic stem cell transplant: revaccinate with a 3-dose regimen beginning 6–12 mo after the transplant, regardless of vaccination history. Doses should be administered ≥4 wk apart	0.5 mL IM at 2, 4, and 12–15 mo of age Administer IM; shake well prior to administration; administered within 24 h of reconstitution
Herpes zoster (Shingrix; ✱ Shingrix) Not indicated for prevention or treatment of chickenpox or treatment of shingles; duration of protection unknown	(contraindicated) Prevention of herpes zoster in adults 50 y and older	Adults ≥50 y: IM 0.5 mL administered as a 2-dose series at 0 and 2–6 mo If the primary series is delayed or interrupted, the series does not need to be restarted. If the interval between dose 1 and 2 is <4 wk, then the second dose should be repeated	
Hepatitis A (HepA) (Havrix, Vaqta; ✱ Avaxim, HAVRIX, VAQTA) More than 90% effective within 4 wk after first dose; contraindicated during febrile illness, immunosuppression; Havrix and Vaqta are interchangeable	Hepatitis A virus disease prevention; All children at age 1 y; workers in day care centers, laboratories, food-handling establishments; men who have sex with men; IV drug users; military personnel and travelers to areas where hepatitis A is endemic; community residents during an outbreak; people with chronic liver disease (e.g., hepatitis B or C, cirrhosis) or who receive transfusions for clotting disorders	Havrix (1,440 units in 1 mL), 1 mL IM initially and 6–12 mo later (2 doses) VAQTA (50 units/mL), IM in deltoid, 1 mL initially and 6–12 mo later (2 doses)	Havrix (360 or 720 units in 0.5 mL), 1–18 y, 360 units IM initially, then 1 and 6–12 mo later (2 doses) VAQTA (25 units/0.5 mL), 25 units IM initially and 6–18 mo later

(Continued on page 196)

TABLE 12.1
DRUGS AT A GLANCE: Vaccines and Toxoids for Active Immunity (Continued)

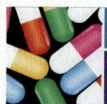

Name/Characteristics	Indications for Use	Routes and Dosage Ranges	
		Adults	**Children**
Hepatitis B (HepB) (Engerix-B, Recombivax HB, Heplisav-B; ❋ Engerix-B, Recombivax HB) Approximately 96% effective in children and young adults and 88% in adults older than 40 y; duration of protection unknown; serum antibody levels can be obtained	Hepatitis B disease prevention; All infants and children up to age 18; people with occupational exposure to blood (healthcare and emergency workers); household contacts or sexual partners of people with hepatitis B infection; people with HIV, kidney failure with replacement therapy, on hemodialysis; people with multiple sexual partners; men who have sex with men; IV drug users; residents and staff of institutions for developmentally disabled people; residents of correctional facilities	18 y and older Heplisav-B 0.5 mL IM 2 doses 1 mo apart 20 y and older Engerix-B, 1 mL IM initially, then 1 and 6 mo later (3 doses); predialysis and dialysis patients, 2 mL IM initially and 1, 2, and 6 mo later (4 doses) Recombivax HB, 1 mL IM initially and 1 and 6 mo later (3 doses); predialysis and dialysis patients, 1 mL IM initially and 1 and 6 mo later (3 doses)	Neonates to 18 y Engerix-B, Recombivax-HB: 0.5 mL per dose IM for a total of 3 doses given as follows: Ideally the first dose is administered at birth, the second dose at 1-2 months, and a final third dose at 6 months up to 18 months of age; minimum age for the third dose is 24 weeks.
Human papillomavirus (HPV) (Gardasil 9; ❋ Gardasil, Cervarix) Because HPV is a common sexually transmitted infection, the vaccine is most effective when taken before becoming sexually active	Gardasil, prevention of diseases caused by HPV types 6, 11, 16, and 18 (cervical, vaginal, and vulvar cancer; genital warts) in people ages 9–26 Cervarix, prevention of HPV types 16 and 18; recommended for females from ages 9–26 Gardasil 9, prevention of HPV types 6, 11, 16, 18, 31, 33, 45, 52, and 58; recommended for people from ages 9–26	0.5 mL IM initially, 2 mo after first dose, and 6 mo after first dose (3 doses) Gardasil 9, 0.5 mL IM initially and 6–12 mo after first dose (2 doses)	9 y and older; same as adults Routine vaccination at 11–12 y 2-dose schedule, minimum interval between first and second doses is 5 mo 3-dose schedule, minimum interval between first and second doses is 4 wk; minimum interval between the second and third dose is 12 wk; minimum interval between first and third dose is 5 mo
Influenza (IIV4) inactivated (Afluria; Fluad, Fluarix, Flublok, Flucelvax, FluLaval, Fluzone, Fluzone High-Dose, FluMist [LAIV4] live attenuated; ❋ Agriflu, Fluzone, Fluzone High Dose, Agriflu, Fluad, Fluad Pediatric, FluLaval Tetra, Fluviral, Quadrivalent Influvac) Formulated annually to include current strains; provides protective antibody concentrations for about 6 mo	Influenza A disease prevention; Annual immunization for all people older than 6 mo of age Do not administer LAIV4 live attenuated vaccine to immunocompromised patients or those with egg allergies, cochlear implants, or asplenia, or children 2–4 y with asthma	0.5 mL IM in a single dose; immunization, then 1 dose each season	6–35 mo, 0.25 mL IM, 1 dose if previously vaccinated; 2 doses at least 1 mo apart if first vaccination 3–8 y, 0.5 mL IM, 1 dose if previously vaccinated 6 mo to 8 y, 2 IM doses of inactivated influenza vaccine (administered a minimum of 4 wk apart) if first vaccination 9 y and older, 0.5 mL IM in a single dose

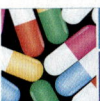

TABLE 12.1
DRUGS AT A GLANCE: Vaccines and Toxoids for Active Immunity (Continued)

Name/Characteristics	Indications for Use	Routes and Dosage Ranges	
		Adults	**Children**
Measles, mumps, and rubella (MMR) (M–M–R II; 🍁 M–M–R II, Priorix) Preferred and more commonly used than single immunizing agents; contains live, attenuated viruses that cause measles, mumps, and rubella; protects more than 95% of recipients for many years	Measles, mumps, and rubella prevention; Immunization at 12–15 mo and a second dose at 4–6 y	0.5 mL IM	Same as adults
Meningococcal group ACWY vaccine (MenACWY-D) (Menactra), **(MenACWY-CRM)** (Menveo), **(MenACWY-TT)** (MenQuadfi)	Meningococcal disease prevention; Short-term protection against meningitis adolescents are priority recipients. 2 y and older should receive a 2-dose primary series if immunocompromised, asplenic, or HIV+	Same as children	MenACWY-CRM > 2 mo MenACWY-D > 9 mo MenACWY-TT > 2 y 11–12 y should get first dose with a booster at 16 y with minimum interval of at least 8 wk
Meningococcal group B vaccine (MenB-FHbp) (Trumenba; 🍁 Trumenba) **(MenB-4C)** (Bexsero)	Short-term protection against meningitis, with a preference for administration between ages 16 and 18	10–25 y (Bexsero) 0.5 mL IM as a 2-dose series at least 1 mo apart 10–25 y (Trumenba) 0.5 mL IM as a 2-dose series at least 1 mo apart; or 0.5 mL IM initially, then 1–2 and 6 mo as a 3-dose series	Same dose series as adults
Pneumococcal conjugate vaccine 13-valent (PCV 13) (Prevnar 13) Contains 13 *Streptococcus pneumoniae* antigens conjugated to a protein to increase antigenicity	Prevention of systemic pneumococcal infections (e.g., bacteremia, meningitis, pneumonia, sinusitis, otitis media) in young children and 2–18 y children with certain medical conditions		Birth–6 mo, 0.5 mL IM at 2, 4, 6, and 12–15 mo (4 doses) 7–11 mo, 0.5 mL IM initially, at least 4 wk later, and after 1 y birthday (3 doses) 12–59 mo, 0.5 mL IM initially and at least 2 mo later (2 doses) 6–18 y, 0.5 mL IM in a single dose
Pneumococcal conjugate vaccine 15-valent (PCV 15) (Vaxneuvance) **20-valent (PCV 20)** (Prevnar 20) Contains 15 or 20 *Streptococcus pneumoniae* antigens conjugated to a protein to increase antigenicity **Or pneumococcal 23 polysaccharide (PPSV 23)** (Pneumovax 23; Pneumo 23)	Pneumococcal disease prevention; Adults who have chronic conditions that cause increased risk of pneumococcal infection and older adults	At risk adults age 18–64 y single dose 0.5 mL IM PCV15 followed by PPSV23 OR single dose PCV20 Healthy adults ≥65 single dose 0.5 mL IM PCV15 followed by PPSV23 or single dose 0.5 mL IM PCV20	

(Continued on page 198)

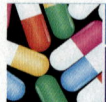

TABLE 12.1
DRUGS AT A GLANCE: Vaccines and Toxoids for Active Immunity (Continued)

Name/Characteristics	Indications for Use	Routes and Dosage Ranges	
		Adults	**Children**
Poliomyelitis, inactivated (IPV) (IPOL; ✷ Imovax Polio)	Polio disease prevention; Routine immunization of infants; immunization of adults not previously immunized and at risk for exposure (e.g., healthcare or laboratory workers)	0.5 mL Sub-Q monthly for 2 doses, then a third dose 6–12 mo later. Incompletely vaccinated: adults with at least 1 previous doses of OPV, <3 doses of IPV, or a combination of OPV and IPV equaling <3 doses, administer at least one 0.5 mL dose of IPV. Additional doses to complete the series may be given if time permits. Completely vaccinated and at increased risk of exposure: one 0.5 mL dose	0.5 mL Sub-Q at 2, 4, and 6–18 mo and 4–6 y of age (4 doses) or at 2 and 4 mo (2 doses)
Rabies vaccine (HDCV PCECV) (Imovax Rabies, RabAvert; ✷ Imovax Rabies) Immunity develops in 7–10 d and lasts 1 y or longer	Rabies disease prevention; Preexposure immunization in people at high risk for exposure (e.g., veterinarians, animal handlers); postexposure prophylaxis in people who have been bitten by potentially rabid animals or who have skin scratches or abrasions exposed to animal saliva (e.g., animal licking of wound), urine, or blood	Preexposure, 1.0 mL IM for 3 doses, 1 mL on days 0, 7, and 21 or 28; then, booster doses (1 mL) every 2–5 y based on antibody titers. Postexposure, 1 mL IM for immunocompetent 4 doses 1 mL on days 0, 3, 7, 14; immunocompromised IM 5 doses 1 mL each on days 0, 3, 7, 14, 28; in addition, patients should receive rabies immune globulin with the first dose (day 0). After the initial dose, other doses are given 3, 7, 14, and 28 d later	Same as adults
Rotavirus (RV) (RotaTeq; Rotarix; ✷ RotaTeq, Rotarix) Can be given with most other childhood vaccines; adverse effects are usually mild (e.g., diarrhea); a few cases of intussusception have been reported after administration of RotaTeq	Prevention of rotavirus gastroenteritis in infants between 6 and 32 wk of age	Individual doses administered orally	RotaTeq: infants 6–32 wk of age: oral 2 mL per dose for 3 dose, the first given at 6–12 wk of age, followed by subsequent doses at 4–10 wk intervals. Administer all doses by 32 wk of age. Rotarix: infants 6–24 wk of age: oral 1 mL per dose for 2 doses, the first dose given at 6 wk of age, followed by the second dose given ≥4 wk later. The 2 series should be completely by 24 wk of age

TABLE 12.1
DRUGS AT A GLANCE: Vaccines and Toxoids for Active Immunity (Continued)

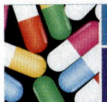

Name/Characteristics		Indications for Use	Routes and Dosage Ranges Adults	Children
Varicella (VAR) (Varivax; ✺ Varilrix, Varivax III) Contains live, attenuated varicella virus; contraindicated in hematologic or lymphatic malignancy, immunosuppression, febrile illness, or pregnancy	(contraindicated)	Varicella prevention; Immunization of children 12 mo and older; immunization of adults who have not had chickenpox	0.5 mL Sub-Q, followed by a second dose of 0.5 mL 4–8 wk after the first dose	12–15 mo, 0.5 mL Sub-Q followed by a second dose at 4–6 y of age
Toxoids				
Diphtheria, tetanus toxoids, and acellular pertussis (DTaP) (Daptacel, Infanrix; ✺ Adacel, Boostrix)		Routine immunization of infants and children 6 y and younger; prevention of tetanus, diphtheria, and pertussis infections	Not recommended for adults	Infants and children 6 y and younger, 0.5 mL IM for 2 doses at least 4 wk apart, followed by a booster dose 1 y later and when the child starts school
Tetanus, reduced diphtheria, acellular pertussis (Tdap) (Adacel, Boostrix)		Routine immunization of older children; primary immunization of adults; prevention of tetanus in previously immunized people who sustain a potentially contaminated wound	Adolescents single dose 0.5 mL IM at age 11–12 y Pregnant patients dose during each pregnancy Adults 0.5 mL booster dose of either Tdap or Td every 10 or 5 y after a dirty wound	Older than 6 y, same as adult
(Pediatric type) (DT) contains a larger amount of diphtheria antigen than "tetanus and diphtheria toxoids, adult type (Td)"		Routine immunization in children in whom pertussis vaccine is contraindicated (those who have adverse reactions to initial doses of DTaP vaccine)	Not recommended for use in adults	
Tetanus and diphtheria toxoids (adult type) (Td) (TDVax, Tenivac; ✺ Td Absorbed) Contains a smaller amount of diphtheria antigen than "diphtheria and tetanus toxoids, pediatric type (DT)"	C	Tetanus and diphtheria prevention; Primary immunization or booster doses in adults and children older than 6 y	Adults previously not immunized should receive 2 primary doses of 0.5 mL each given at an interval of 8 wk; third (reinforcing) dose of 0.5 mL 6–8 mo later Booster dose every 10 y thereafter	Older than 6 y, same as adults
Tetanus toxoid Protects about 100% of recipients for 10 y or more; for primary immunization of infants and children 6 y of age or older, usually given in combination (e.g., DTaP or DT); for primary immunization of adults usually given or alone or combined with diphtheria toxoid (e.g., Td adult type)	C	Tetanus prevention; Prophylaxis, 0.5 mL IM if wound contaminated and no booster dose was received for 5 y; 0.5 mL if wound is clean and no booster dose was received for 10 y	Primary immunization in adults not previously immunized, 0.5 IM mL for 3 doses: initially, 4–8 wk later, then at 6–12 mo; then, 0.5-mL booster dose every 10 y	Same as adults

TABLE 12.2

DRUGS AT A GLANCE: Immune Serums for Passive Immunity

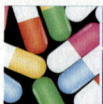

Serum/Characteristics	Indications for Use	Routes and Dosage Ranges
CMV immune globulin, intravenous, human (CMV-IGIV) (CytoGam; ✹ CytoGam) Contains antibodies against CMV	Prevention of CMV infection in the heart, kidney, liver, lung, and pancreas transplant recipients	Post transplantation: infusion, 150 mg/kg IV within 72 h; then 100–150 mg/kg at 2, 4, 6, and 8 wk; and then 50–100 mg/kg at 12 and 16 wk
Hepatitis B immune globulin, human (HBIG) (HepaGam B, Hyper HEP B S/D, Nabi-HB; ✹ Hyper HEP B S/D) Solution of immunoglobulins that contains antibodies to HBsAg	To prevent hepatitis after exposure; neonates born to HBsAg-positive or unknown-status mothers are given HBIG and the first dose of hepatitis B vaccine within 12 h of birth	Adults and children 0.06 mL/kg (usual adult dose, 3–5 mL) IM as soon as possible after exposure, preferably within 7 d; repeat dose in 1 mo
Immune globulin (human) (IG; IGIM) (Asceniv, Bivigam, Carimune NF, Gammagard, Hizentra, Privigen, GamaSTAN S/D, Hizentra, Privigen, Xembify; ✹ Cutaquig, Cuvitru, GamaSTAN S/D, Gammagard S/D, Gamunex, Hizentra, IGIVnex, Iveegam Immuno, Octagam, Panzyga) Given IM only; commonly called "gamma globulin"; obtained from pooled plasma of normal donors; consists primarily of IgG, which contains concentrated antibodies; produces adequate serum levels of IgG in 2–5 d	Antiviral prophylaxis; To decrease the severity of hepatitis A, measles, and varicella after exposure; to treat immunoglobulin deficiency	Adults and children Exposure to hepatitis A: 0.02 mL/kg IM Exposure to measles: 0.25 mL/kg IM within 6 d of exposure Exposure to varicella: 0.6–1.2 mL/kg IM Exposure to rubella (pregnant patients only): 0.55 mL/kg IM Immunoglobulin deficiency: 1.3 mL/kg IM initially and then 0.6 mL/kg every 3–4 wk
Immune globulin intravenous (IGIV) (Bivigam, Carimune NF, Gammagard, Hizentra, Privigen; ✹ GamaSTAN S/D, Hizentra, Privigen) Given IV only; provides immediate antibodies; half-life about 3 wk; mechanism of action in ITP is unknown; **BOXED WARNING** ◆ —IGIV has been associated with thrombosis, kidney dysfunction and failure, and death; it should be used cautiously in patients with abnormal kidney function or at risk for developing the condition	Immunodeficiency syndrome; idiopathic thrombocytopenic purpura (ITP)	See manufacturers' instructions
Rabies immune globulin (HRIG) (HyperRAB S/D, Imogam Rabies HT; ✹ HyperRAB S/D, Imogam Rabies Pasteurized) Gamma globulin obtained from plasma of people hyperimmunized with rabies vaccine; not useful in treatment of clinical rabies infection	Postexposure prevention of rabies, in conjunction with rabies vaccine	Adults and children 20 units/kg IM (half the dose may be injected around the wound) as soon as possible after possible exposure (e.g., animal bite)
$Rh_o(D)$ immune globulin (human) (HyperRHO S/D Full Dose, MICRhoGAM, RhoGAM, WinRho SDF; ✹ HyperRHO S/D Full Dose, HypRho-D, WinRho SDF) Prepared from fractionated human plasma; a sterile concentrated solution of specific immunoglobulin (IgG) containing anti-$Rh_o(D)$	To prevent sensitization in a subsequent pregnancy to the $Rh_o(D)$ factor in an Rh-negative mother who has given birth to an Rh-positive infant by an Rh-positive father	*Obstetric use*: administer according to the manufacturer's labeling Inject contents of 1 vial IM for every 15 mL fetal packed red cell volume within 72 h after delivery, miscarriage, or abortion. Consult package instructions for blood typing and drug administration procedures

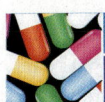

TABLE 12.2
DRUGS AT A GLANCE: Immune Serums for Passive Immunity (Continued)

Serum/Characteristics	Indications for Use	Routes and Dosage Ranges
Tetanus immune globulin (human) (HyperTET S/D; ✳ HyperTET S/D) Solution of globulins from plasma of people hyperimmunized with tetanus toxoid. Tetanus toxoid (Td) should also be given to initiate active immunization if minor wound and more than 10 y since Td, if major wound and more than 5 y since Td, or if Td primary immunization series was incomplete	To prevent tetanus in patients with wounds possibly contaminated with *Clostridium tetani* and whose immunization history is uncertain or incomplete. Treatment of tetanus infection	Adults and children Prophylaxis, 250 units IM as a single dose in conjunction with a tetanus toxoid containing vaccine. Treatment of clinical disease, 3,000–6,000 units IM in a single dose
Varicella-zoster immune globulin (human) (VZIG) (VariZIG; ✳ VariZIG) The globulin fraction of human plasma; antibodies last 1 mo or longer	Postexposure to chickenpox or shingles, to prevent or decrease severity of infections in children under 15 y of age who have not been immunized or who are immunodeficient because of illness or drug therapy. Infants born to mothers who develop varicella 5 d before or 2 d after delivery and premature infants of <28 wk of gestation	IM 125 units/10 kg up to a maximum of 625 units within 48 h after exposure if possible; may be given up to 96 h after exposure. Minimal dose, 125 units

CMV, cytomegalovirus; HBsAg, hepatitis B surface antigen; IgG, immunoglobulin G.

---

when administered within 2 weeks of exposure. Preexposure prophylaxis through the administration of hepatitis A vaccine or IG provides protection for unvaccinated persons traveling in high or intermediate HAV endemic areas.

- Routine immunization of adolescents and adults against diphtheria, tetanus, human papillomavirus, meningococcal meningitis, COVID-19, and pertussis; varicella, if immunity not established; as well as influenza annually.
- Immunization of prepubertal females or females of childbearing age against rubella.
- Immunization of people at high risk for serious morbidity or mortality from a chronic condition. For example, pneumococcal vaccine is recommended in people 65 years of age and older, as well as in people younger than 65 years of age with chronic diseases.
- Immunization of adults and children at high risk for a particular disease. For example, pneumococcal vaccine is recommended for people older than 2 years of age who have chronic respiratory disease or have had a splenectomy. Also, administration of quadrivalent human papillomavirus (HPV) vaccine is recommended in young adolescents to prevent genital warts and the risk of cervical cancer.

> ⚠ **Quality and Safety Alert: Safety**
>
> Rubella during the first trimester of pregnancy is associated with a high incidence of congenital anomalies in the newborn.

> ⚠ **Quality and Safety Alert: Safety**
>
> Tetanus prophylaxis in wound management Centers for Disease Control and Prevention/Advisory Committee on Immunization Practices [CDC/ACIP] is as follows:
> - Assess the type of wound and provide appropriate wound care.
> - Clean wounds contaminated with dirt, feces, soil, and saliva; clean puncture wounds from crushing, tears, burns, and frostbite. Wounds containing necrotic or gangrenous area should be debrided.
> - Tetanus toxoid: For children age less than 7 years, DTaP [DT if pertussis vaccine is contraindicated]; for children age ≥7 years and adults, Td is preferred to tetanus toxoid alone; Tdap may be preferred if the patient has not previously been vaccinated with Tdap or if tetanus vaccine is indicated for a pregnant woman.
> - For patients with HIV or severe immunodeficiency with contaminated wounds, administer tetanus immunoglobulin regardless of history of tetanus immunization.

Patient-related variables specific to the use of immunizing agents include the following:

- Age:
  Children
  - By 4 to 6 years of age, children should have received vaccinations against previously listed diseases, for example,

| BOX 12.2 | Combination Vaccines Used for Routine Childhood Immunizations |

DTaP-IPV (Kinrix, Quadracel)
DTaP-Hep B-IPV (Pediarix)
DTaP-IPV-Hib (Pentacel)
DTaP-IPV-Hib-HepB (Vaxelis)
Hep A-Hep B (Twinrix)
MMR-Var (ProQuad)

diphtheria, measles (rubeola), mumps, pertussis, and varicella (chickenpox).
- Because some vaccines are administered more than once, a child may receive more than 20 injections by 2 years of age. Two strategies that studies indicate are effective at increasing immunization rates are the use of combination vaccines and the administration of multiple vaccines (in separate syringes and at different sites) at one visit whenever feasible.
- Several combination vaccines are now available (Box 12.2), and others continue to be developed.
- Annual influenza vaccine is recommended for children and infants older than 6 months of age.
- Children's healthcare providers should implement the recommended childhood immunization schedule issued in January of each year by the Centers for Disease Control and Prevention (CDC).
- Providers should also refer to current guidelines about immunizations for children with chronic illnesses (e.g., asthma, heart disease, diabetes) or immunosuppression (e.g., from cancer, organ transplantation, or human immunodeficiency virus [HIV] infection).

Adolescents, young adults, and middle-aged adults
- Young adults who are healthcare workers, sexually active, or belong to a high-risk group should receive varicella vaccine (or a second dose if they previously received a single dose), hepatitis A and hepatitis B vaccines if not previously received, and Tdap, as well as measles–mumps–rubella (MMR) if they are not pregnant and rubella titer is inadequate or if proof of immunization is unavailable.
- In adults ≤25 years of age, routine vaccination for meningococcal group B disease is recommended when there is increased risk of serogroup B meningococcal disease or during serogroup B meningococcal disease.
- Middle-aged adults should maintain immunizations against tetanus–diphtheria with one booster dose of Tdap and influenza vaccine annually. High-risk groups (e.g., those with chronic illness and healthcare providers) should receive the hepatitis B vaccine series (if not previously received).

Older adults
- Adults born after 1956 should have at least one dose of MMR vaccine unless they have had either the vaccine or each of the three diseases.
- Older adults become more susceptible to some diseases, and influenza, pneumococcal infections, tetanus, and shingles can be especially serious in this population.
- The varicella-zoster virus, the same virus that causes chickenpox, can cause shingles later in life. An additional varicella vaccine to prevent zoster infections (shingles) is available for adults 60 years and older who have had chickenpox.

- Recommended immunizations for older adults 65 years of age and older include a Td or Tdap booster every 10 years, annual influenza vaccine, and a one-time administration of pneumococcal vaccine at 65 years of age.
- A second dose of pneumococcal vaccine may be given at 65 years of age if the first dose was given 5 years previously.
- As with younger adults, immunization for most other diseases is recommended for older adults at high risk for exposure due to occupation or travel.
- Reproduction, pregnancy, and lactation:
  - An up-to-date measles, mumps, and rubella vaccine is recommended 1 month or more before pregnancy if a pregnant person did not get the vaccine as a child.
  - Live vaccines are not recommended during pregnancy.
  - A pregnant person should be vaccinated against pertussis and flu.
  - A pregnant person should receive COVID-19 vaccine due to the severity of SARS-CoV-2 in pregnancy (Box 12.3).
  - Some people may need other vaccines before, during, or after they become pregnant. If the pregnant person works in a lab or travels to another country, hepatitis A, B, meningococcal, and other vaccines recommended for travel may be administered.

 Quality and Safety Alert: Safety

The recommended influenza vaccine should ideally be administered in September or October. Earlier administration of the influenza vaccine in July or August will result in a decrease in immunity.

- Patients with immunosuppression and cancer:
  - Compared with healthy people who are immunocompetent, patients with immunosuppression usually have an adequate, but reduced, antibody response to immunization, and require individualized immunizations.
  - In general, patients with diabetes mellitus or chronic pulmonary, kidney, or hepatic disorders who are not receiving

| BOX 12.3 | *Vaccinating Against COVID-19* |

- COVID-19 vaccines currently approved or authorized by the FDA *are effective* in preventing serious outcomes of coronavirus disease (COVID-19), including severe disease, hospitalization, and death.
- COVID-19 primary series vaccination is recommended for everyone ages 5 years and older in the United States for the prevention of COVID-19.
- A primary mRNA COVID-19 vaccine series is recommended for people ages 5 years and older who are moderately or severely immunocompromised, followed by a booster dose in those ages 12 years and older.
- A booster dose of COVID-19 vaccine is recommended for everyone ages 12 years and older. Timing of a booster dose varies based on COVID-19 vaccine product and immunocompetence.
- Efforts to increase the number of people in the United States who are *up to date* with their COVID-19 vaccines remain critical to preventing illness, hospitalizations, and deaths from COVID-19.

immunosuppressant drugs may receive both live attenuated and killed vaccines and toxoids to induce active immunity. However, they may need higher doses or more frequent administration to achieve adequate immunity.
- Patients with active malignant disease or HIV infections may receive killed vaccines or toxoids but not live vaccines (an exception is people with leukemia who have not received chemotherapy for at least 3 months).
- For children with HIV infection, most routine immunizations (DtaP, inactivated polio vaccine, MMR, *H. influenzae* type b [Hib], influenza) are recommended. MMR is not recommended in children with severe immunosuppression from HIV. Varicella vaccine is recommended only for children with no evidence of immunosuppression. Pneumococcal vaccine is recommended for HIV-infected people older than 2 years of age.
- When patients on immunosuppressive radiation or chemotherapy receive vaccines, it is important to administer them at least 2 weeks before the start of a treatment or 3 months after treatment is completed.
- Healthcare providers may give immune serum, which provides passive temporary immunity, to immunocompromised people or those with HIV infections who are exposed to an infectious disease, such as rubella or varicella, to impart passive immunity and reduce the risk of a person developing a serious infection.
- Patients receiving a systemic corticosteroid in high doses (e.g., prednisone 20 mg or equivalent daily) or for longer than 2 weeks should wait at least 3 months before receiving a live-virus vaccine.
- Short-term use (less than 2 weeks) or low to moderate doses (less than 20 mg of prednisone daily) of corticosteroids are not contraindications to immunizations.
- Long-term alternate-day therapy with short-acting agents, maintenance physiologic replacement doses, and the use of topical, inhaled, or intra-articular injections of corticosteroids are not contraindications.

> **Quality and Safety Alert: Safety**
> Patients with active malignant disease should not receive live vaccines.

Clinical Application 12.1
- Ms. Williams asks if Riley, who is getting over a cold and has some clear nasal discharge, should wait before having his scheduled immunizations. What is the nurse's best response?
- Ms. Williams reports the last time she had any immunizations was at 14 years of age. Based on her age and sex, what vaccines do authorities recommend?

Adverse Effects

Mild reactions to vaccines, such as injection site soreness and redness, fever, and muscle aches, are common, whereas severe and serious reactions, such as anaphylaxis or serum sickness, are rare. Adverse reactions to individual immunizing agents include the following:

- DTaP: soreness, erythema, edema at injection sites, anorexia, nausea, severe fever, encephalopathy, and seizures
- Hib vaccine: pain and erythema at injection sites
- Hepatitis B vaccine: injection site soreness, erythema, induration, fever, and anaphylaxis
- Influenza vaccine: via injection—pain, induration, and erythema at injection sites and flulike symptoms such as chills, fever, malaise, muscle aches; via intranasal spray—runny nose, headache, cough, sore throat, and irritability in children
- COVID-19 vaccine: pain, erythema and swelling at injection site and tiredness, headache, muscle pain, chills, fever, and nausea
- MMR vaccine: mild symptoms of measles—cough, fever up to 39.4°C (102°F), headache, malaise, photophobia, skin rash, sore throat, febrile seizures, arthralgia (joint pain), and anaphylaxis in recipients who are allergic to eggs
- Pneumococcal vaccine: local effects—soreness, induration, and erythema at injection sites; systemic effects—chills, fever, headache, muscle aches, nausea, photophobia, and weakness
- Polio vaccine: soreness at injection sites, fever, and anaphylaxis
- Varicella vaccine: early effects—transient soreness or erythema at injection sites; late effect—a mild, maculopapular skin rash with a few lesions
- Immune globulin intravenous (IGIV): chills, dizziness, dyspnea, fever, flushing, headache, nausea, urticaria, vomiting, tightness in chest, pain in chest, hip, or back, kidney dysfunction, acute kidney disease, and death

Contraindications

Contraindications to most vaccines and toxoids include the following:

- Acute febrile illness
- Immunosuppressive drug therapy
- Immunodeficiency states such as congenital immunodeficiency or active HIV disease
- Hematologic cancers (leukemia or lymphoma) or generalized malignancy
- Pregnancy

Nursing Implications

Preventing Interactions

Immunosuppressant drug therapy and interferon administration may interfere with vaccine response to live vaccines. Antiviral drugs may also interfere with the immune response to a live viral vaccine and should not be given 48 hours before and for 14 days after viral vaccine administration. Likewise, passive immunization with IG for exposure to a viral infection (e.g., measles, hepatitis A, varicella) can likewise interfere with active immunity, and it is necessary to delay administration of the viral vaccine for 2 to 6 months or more, depending on the person's immune status.

Measles vaccine can interfere with the response to tuberculosis (TB) skin testing. Patients should have the TB skin test either simultaneously with the measles vaccine, or they should delay it for 4 to 6 weeks after the test.

Quality and Safety Alert: Safety

Measles vaccine can also interfere with the activity of meningococcal vaccine, and it is essential to separate these two vaccines by at least a month.

Quality and Safety Alert: Safety

Salicylates may increase the risk of Reye syndrome with administration of the varicella vaccine.

Administering the Medication

Following package insert instructions for storing, reconstituting, and safely administering combination vaccines is essential for effectiveness of all immunizations. To maintain effectiveness of vaccines and other biologic preparations, the nurse helps ensure that immunization products are stored properly according to the manufacturer's instructions. Most products require refrigeration at 2°C to 8°C (35.6°F to 46.4°F). The nurse reconstitutes vaccines only with the supplied diluent and then uses them within the time frame recommended after reconstitution to maintain vaccine effectiveness.

Box 12.4 summarizes administration considerations for immunizations.

Assessing for Therapeutic Effects

Most vaccines take about 2 weeks for full antibody response and protection against the disease. A fourfold increase in immunoglobulin titer levels indicates an adequate antibody response. It is necessary to obtain antibody titer levels during pregnancy to determine immunity to viral infections such as measles and rubella because the fetus may be affected by active maternal infection during the pregnancy.

BOX 12.4 Administering Immunizing Agents

Accurate administration includes the following:
- Reading the package insert and check the expiration date on all biologic products (e.g., vaccines, toxoids, human immune serums).
- Following instructions for administering each vaccine.
- Checking the patient's temperature before giving a vaccine.
- Giving intramuscular (IM) human immune serum globulin with an 18- to 20-gauge needle, preferably in the gluteal muscles. If the dose is 5 mL or more, divide it and inject it into two or more IM sites. Follow manufacturer's instructions for preparation and administration of intravenous (IV) formulations.
- Having aqueous epinephrine 1:1,000 readily available before administering any vaccine.
- After administration of an immunizing agent in a clinic or office setting, having the patient stay in the area for at least 30 minutes.
- Providing patients with a Vaccine Information Statement (VIS).

Assessing for Adverse Effects

Careful screening of people for contraindications and observing vaccine precautions minimize serious adverse vaccine events.

Quality and Safety Alert: Safety

By law, healthcare providers must report potentially serious adverse effects using the Vaccine Adverse Event Reporting System (VAERS).

Quality and Safety Alert: Evidence-Based Practice

The Global Health Security Agenda was developed in February 2014 to "prevent, detect, and effectively respond to infectious disease threats, whether naturally occurring or caused by accidental or intentional release of dangerous pathogens." One key objective is to improve the global community's capacity to prevent, detect, and respond to public health. Its surveillance of immunization laws across countries assists researchers to examine epidemiology data and provide a justification for immunization policies. This process assists in global health security (Ghedamu & Meier, 2019).

Patient Teaching

The nurse ensures that the patient or parent receives current vaccine information about the benefits and risks of immunization—a Vaccine Information Statement (VIS)—for each vaccine dose given. Current VIS forms for all recommended vaccines, along with indications, contraindications, and the timing of immunizations doses, are available for download at the CDC website (see "References and Resources"). Box 12.5 presents additional patient teaching information.

NCLEX Success

1. A nurse is explaining to a parent how vaccines work. Vaccines provide which of the following?
   A. active immunity
   B. passive immunity
   C. innate immunity
   D. nonspecific immunity

2. The nurse is caring for a patient with severe immunosuppression. This condition is a contraindication to which of the following?
   A. all injectable immunizations
   B. the use of live bacterial or viral vaccines
   C. the use of immune globulins for passive immunity
   D. annual influenza vaccine

3. A child is receiving an immunization. The nurse should inform the parents that common aftereffects may include which of the following?
   A. skin rash and itching
   B. redness and soreness at the injection site
   C. muscle weakness and difficulty in walking
   D. nausea, vomiting, and diarrhea

BOX 12.5 Patient Teaching Guidelines for Immunizations

- Appropriate vaccinations should be maintained for adults as well as for children. Consult the Centers for Disease Control and Prevention (CDC) website or a healthcare provider for current information because recommendations for particular groups may change.
- Maintain immunization records for yourself and all members of your family. This is important because immunizations are often obtained at different places and over a period of many years. Written, accurate, up-to-date records help to prevent diseases and reduce unnecessary immunizations.
- If a healthcare provider recommends an immunization and you do not know whether you have had the immunization or the disease, it is probably safer to be immunized than to risk having the disease. Immunization after a previous immunization or after having the disease usually is not harmful.
- Most vaccines can cause fever and soreness at the site of injection. Acetaminophen (e.g., Tylenol) can be taken two to three times daily for 24 to 48 hours if needed to decrease fever and discomfort. Routine premedication with acetaminophen is not recommended. Lower antibody levels may occur, and it may not be necessary.
- Patients who receive a rubella (German measles) or a varicella (chickenpox) immunization must avoid becoming pregnant (i.e., use effective contraception) for 3 months afterward.
- If skin lesions develop after receiving live varicella vaccine (to prevent chickenpox), avoid skin contact with newborns, people who are pregnant, and anyone whose immune system is impaired. Skin lesions from a newly immunized person may transmit the vaccine virus to susceptible close contacts.
- After receiving a vaccine, stay in the area for approximately 30 minutes. If an allergic reaction is going to occur, it will usually do so within that time.

KEEPING UP-TO-DATE WITH IMMUNIZATION RECOMMENDATIONS

Recommendations regarding immunizations change periodically as additional information and new immunizing agents become available. Experts review and update vaccine recommendations in the United States on a frequent basis. Consequently, healthcare providers need to update their knowledge of vaccine recommendations at least annually. The best source of information for current recommendations is the CDC. The most current immunization schedules for all age groups are available at the CDC website (see "References and Resources" for website addresses). The main source of CDC recommendations is the Advisory Committee on Immunization Practices, which consists of experts appointed to advise the CDC on strategies to eliminate vaccine-preventable diseases. Information on vaccines needed for travel to foreign countries (e.g., Japanese encephalitis, typhoid, yellow fever) is also available at the CDC website and is frequently updated.

Other sources of information about immunizations include the American Academy of Pediatrics and the American Academy of Family Physicians. Local health departments may also be a source of information about immunizations, whether routine or necessary for foreign travel. Immunization sources can also provide information on new vaccine releases, vaccine availability, and usage of specific vaccines.

Unfolding Patient Stories: Juan Carlos • Part 1

Juan Carlos, a 52-year-old male with diabetes type 2, hypertension, and hyperlipidemia, is seen at the clinic for his annual checkup. According to age and health status, what vaccinations are recommended for him? What factors should the nurse consider if Juan's immunizations are not up-to-date? How would the nurse intervene if cultural factors, past experiences, or apprehension cause a reluctance to receive vaccinations? (Juan Carlos' story continues in Chapter 41.)

Care for Juan and other patients in a realistic virtual environment: **vSim** for Nursing (thepoint.lww.com/vSim-Pharm). Practice documenting these patients' care in DocuCare (thepoint.lww.com/DocuCareEHR).

NCLEX Success

4. A nurse is caring for a 74-year-old male patient. The nurse recognizes that he would most likely have a decreased immune response to the influenza vaccine if he is taking which of the following medications?
   A. levothyroxine
   B. prednisone
   C. metoprolol
   D. lovastatin

5. A nurse is preparing to administer an unfamiliar vaccine. To obtain current information and provide patient teaching about vaccine recommendations and contraindications, it is best to do which of the following?
   A. Ask a coworker about the vaccine (when and how it should be administered).
   B. Use a drug guide to look up the vaccine information.
   C. Access an internet search engine to find vaccine information.
   D. Obtain vaccine information and a Vaccine Information Statement (VIS) from the Centers for Disease Control and Prevention (CDC) website.

Clinical Application 12.2

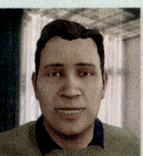

Ms. Williams does not have a personal immunization record for Riley. When administering the immunizations, the nurse records Riley's immunization information on both the clinic record and on a personal immunization record. Is there any way that the nurse can obtain Riley's previous vaccine record?

THE NURSING PROCESS

A concept map outlines the nursing process related to drug therapy considerations in this chapter. Additional nursing implications related to the disease process should also be considered in care decisions.

Assessment
- Determine the patient's previous history of diseases for which immunizing agents are available (e.g., measles, influenza).
- Ask the patient about previous immunization history and any adverse effects experienced.
- Determine whether the patient has any conditions that contraindicate administration of immunizing agents (e.g., malignancy, pregnancy, immunosuppressive drug therapy).
- For pregnant women not known to be immunized against rubella, a serum antibody titer should be measured to determine resistance or susceptibility to the disease.
- For patients with wounds, assess the type of wound and determine how, when, and where it was sustained. Such information may reveal whether tetanus immunization is needed.
- For patients exposed to infectious diseases, assess the extent of exposure (e.g., household or brief, casual contact) and when it occurred.

Outcomes of Therapy

The patient will
- Avoid diseases for which immunizations are available and recommended.
- Obtain recommended immunizations for self and children.
- Keep immunization appointments and maintain immunization records.

Nursing Interventions
- Provide information about the availability of immunizing agents.
- Assist patients in developing a system to maintain immunization records for themselves and their children.
- For someone exposed to rubeola, administration of measles vaccine within 48 hours can help prevent the disease.
- For someone with a puncture wound or a dirty wound, administration of tetanus immune globulin will prevent tetanus, a life-threatening disease.
- For someone with an animal bite, wash the wound immediately with large amounts of soap and water, then seek prompt health care. Administration of rabies immune globulin and vaccine may be needed to prevent rabies, a life-threatening disease.
- Explain to the patient that contracting rubella or undergoing rubella immunization during pregnancy, especially during the first trimester, may cause severe birth defects in the infant.

Evaluation
- Appraise patient's knowledge of and compliance with immunization schedules.
- Check immunization records when indicated.
- Interview and observe for adverse drug effects following administration of immunizing agents.

Visit thePoint® *at* **http://thePoint.lww.com/Frandsen13e** *for answers to NCLEX Success questions (in Appendix A), answers to Clinical Application Case Studies (in Appendix B), and more!*

REFERENCES AND RESOURCES

American Academy of Pediatrics (AAP). (2022). *Homepage.* http://www.aap.org

Centers for Disease Control and Prevention. *COVID-19.* https://www.cdc.gov/coronavirus/2019-ncov/

Centers for Disease Control and Prevention. (2022). *Recommendations and guidelines: Advisory Committee on Immunization Practices (ACIP).* https://www.cdc.gov/vaccines/hcp/acip-recs/

Centers for Disease Control and Prevention. (2022). *Travelers' health.* http://www.cdc.gov/travel

Centers for Disease Control and Prevention. (2020). *Tetanus.* https://www.cdc.gov/tetanus/clinicians.html#wound-management

Centers for Disease Control and Prevention. (2022). *Vaccines and immunizations. Immunization schedules.* http://www.cdc.gov/vaccines/recs/schedules

Ghedamu, T. S., & Meier, B. M. (2019). Assessing national public health law to prevent infectious disease outbreaks. Immunization law as a basis for global health security. *Journal of Law, Medicine, and Ethics, 47,* 412–426.

Meites, E., Szilagyi, P. G., Chesson, H. W., Unger, E. R., Romero, J. R., & Markowitz, L. E. (2019). Human Papillomavirus vaccination for adults: Updated recommendations of the advisory committee on immunization practices. *Morbidity and Mortality Weekly Report, 68*(32), 698–702.

Nelson, N. P., Link-Gelles, R., Hofmeister, M. G., Romero, J. R., Moore, K. L., Ward, J. W., & Schillie, S. F. (2018). Update: Recommendations of the advisory committee on immunization practices for use of hepatitis A vaccine for postexposure prophylaxis and for preexposure prophylaxis for international travel. *Morbidity and Mortality Weekly Report, 67*(43), 1216–1220.

Norris, T. L. (2018). *Porth's pathophysiology: Concepts of altered health states* (10th ed.). Wolters Kluwer.

UpToDate. (2022). *Drug information.* Lexi-Comp, Inc.

Vaccine Adverse Event Reporting System (VAERS). (2022). *Homepage.* http://www.vaers.hhs.gov

CHAPTER 13

Drug Therapy to Decrease Immunity

LEARNING OBJECTIVES

After studying this chapter, you should be able to:

1. Understand the clinical manifestations of allergic and immune disorders as well as transplant rejection reactions and graft versus host disease.
2. Discuss characteristics and uses of major immunosuppressant drugs in autoimmune disorders and organ transplantation.
3. Describe the cytotoxic immunosuppressant agents in terms of prototype, action, use, adverse effects, contraindications, and nursing implications.
4. Discuss the conventional antirejection agents in terms of prototype, action, use, adverse effects, contraindications, and nursing implications.
5. Describe the adjuvant drugs in terms of prototypes, indications and contraindications for use, major adverse effects, and administration.
6. Implement the nursing process in the care of patients receiving immunosuppressant drugs.

CLINICAL APPLICATION CASE STUDY

Sam Jones, a 35-year-old mechanic with type 1 diabetes mellitus and kidney failure with replacement therapy, received a kidney transplant from a living donor 2 years ago. To prevent organ rejection, he is currently taking cyclosporine, mycophenolate mofetil, and prednisone daily. He has monthly appointments at the nephrology clinic and has serum trough levels for cyclosporine measured before each visit. A month ago, Mr. Jones was hospitalized and received four infusions of muromonab-CD3 for an acute organ rejection reaction.

KEY TERMS

Autoantigens: protein complexes on a person's own tissue that stimulate an abnormal immune reaction

Autoimmune disorder: conditions associated with an abnormal immune response to self-antigens (autoantigens) on body tissue, resulting in ongoing inflammation and damage to body tissues

Checkpoint therapy: immunologic checkpoint blockade that uses monoclonal antibodies to either activate or antagonize immunologic pathways

Cytotoxic: causing cell death

Graft rejection reaction: activated immunologic response by the recipient to graft donor organ cells resulting in graft tissue damage and loss of graft organ function

Graft versus host disease: complication of bone marrow or stem cell transplantation in which activated T cells in donor bone marrow attack host tissues, producing inflammatory changes in the skin, liver, and gastrointestinal tract; this can also occur infrequently with a blood transfusion

Immunosuppression: suppression of the immune system

Monoclonal antibodies: immunoglobulins that are therapeutically replicated in laboratory cells to react with specific cell antigens to alter the immune response to an antigen

Murine antibodies: immunoglobulins created in mouse cells for use as therapeutic treatment for human diseases

Polyclonal antibodies: mixtures of antibodies (immunoglobulin A [IgA], plus IgD, IgE, IgG, and IgM) produced by several clones of B lymphocytes

INTRODUCTION

The immune response, normally a protective process, recognizes and destroys potentially harmful outside substances, helping the body defend itself against disease. However, disease processes can also develop when the immune system perceives a harmless substance, such as an antigen or the person's own body tissues, as foreign and tries to eliminate them. This inappropriate activation of the immune response is a major factor in allergic conditions (e.g., allergic asthma) and autoimmune disorders (e.g., rheumatoid arthritis, Crohn disease, psoriasis). **Autoimmune disorders** are conditions associated with an abnormal immune response to self-antigens (autoantigens) on body tissue, resulting in ongoing inflammation and damage to body tissues. These disorders occur when a person's immune system loses its ability to differentiate self from nonself. As a result, an immune response against host tissues occurs.

An appropriate, but undesirable, immune response also occurs when foreign tissue from another organism is transplanted into the body. With transplant therapy, if the immune response is not suppressed, a **graft rejection reaction** occurs in which the body reacts to the implanted cells as with other antigens and attempts to destroy the foreign tissue. It is an activated immunologic response by the recipient to graft donor organ cells resulting in graft tissue damage and loss of graft organ function. Although numerous advances have been made in transplantation technology, the ability to modulate the immune response remains a major factor in determining the success or failure of transplant therapy.

Immunosuppression is the suppression of the immune system. Immunosuppressant drugs are used to decrease an undesirable immune response by interfering with the production or function of immune cells and cytokines that contribute to tissue inflammation and damage. Drugs used therapeutically as immunosuppressants constitute a diverse group, some of which also are used for other purposes. Drug groups that are used to reduce the immune response include corticosteroids (see Chapter 17) and some **cytotoxic** (causing cell death) antineoplastic drugs (see Chapter 14). Healthcare providers use these drugs, discussed here in relation to their effects in modulating the body's response to autoimmune disorders or organ transplantation, to treat inflammatory autoimmune disorders or to prevent or treat transplant rejection reactions. The nursing management of patients receiving these drugs is the main focus of this chapter. To aid in the understanding of immunosuppressant drugs, descriptions of selected inflammatory autoimmune disorders, tissue transplantation, and rejection reactions appear below.

OVERVIEW OF ALTERED IMMUNE FUNCTION

Autoantigens are protein complexes on a person's own tissue that stimulate an abnormal immune reaction. In healthy people, the immune system's ability to inherently differentiate between cell surface proteins on its own cells, or self-antigens, and antigens on foreign cells provides protection against disease. However, in people who have received an organ transplant, this protective mechanism must be altered to avoid damage to the transplant and organ rejection. Drug therapy to suppress the body's ability to recognize self from nonself is a major part of transplantation protocols.

Tissue and organ transplantation involves replacing diseased host tissue with healthy donor tissue. The goal of such treatment is to save and enhance the quality of the recipient's life. Skin grafts and kidney and liver transplants are more commonly performed; heart, lung, intestine, and pancreas transplants are increasing in frequency. The use of biologic agents, which stimulate the production of hematopoietic stem cells from bone marrow and mobilize them into circulating blood (see Chapter 11), has helped to improve the availability of stem cells for transplant, reducing the need for bone marrow transplants.

Although many factors affect graft survival, including the degree of matching between donor tissues and recipient tissues, drug-induced immunosuppression is a major part of transplantation protocols. The goal is to provide adequate immunosuppression while minimizing adverse effects on normal body tissue. If immunosuppression is inadequate, a graft rejection reaction will occur with solid organ transplantation, and **graft versus host disease** (GVHD) will develop with bone marrow/stem cell transplantation. GVHD is a complication of bone marrow or stem cell transplantation in which activated T cells in donor bone marrow attack host tissues, producing inflammatory changes in the skin, liver, and gastrointestinal (GI) tract; this also occurs infrequently with a blood transfusion. If immunosuppressive drug therapy is excessive, serious infection may occur, some malignancies such as lymphomas and skin cancers may develop, and organ damage related to the proliferation of activated lymphocytes in normal body cells may result. Information about altered immune function pathophysiology can be found on thePoint®.

Clinical Manifestations

Allergic Disorders

Allergic asthma is characterized by increased production of IgE in response to inhaled allergens. The IgE–allergen complexes trigger inflammation, producing airway edema and increasing mucous production. People use immunosuppressants to reduce the airway edema and excessive vascular permeability that accompany this type of asthma (see Chapter 33).

Immune Disorders

Crohn disease is a chronic, recurrent, inflammatory bowel disorder that can affect any area of the GI tract. The chronic inflammation is attributed to a mixture of inflammatory mediators (e.g., IL-1 and IL-6, TNF-alpha) produced by overactivated macrophages in the lining of the bowel, which contribute to GI ulceration, bleeding, and diarrhea. The goal of treatment is to decrease inflammation and promote healing of bowel lesions.

Psoriasis, a hyperproliferative skin disorder, is characterized by an abnormal overproduction of skin cells, forming plaque lesions. Activated T lymphocytes producing cytokines are believed to stimulate the abnormal growth of the affected skin cells with accompanying inflammation from tissue infiltration of neutrophils and monocytes. Some medications (e.g., beta-adrenergic blockers, lithium) may precipitate or aggravate psoriasis.

Psoriatic arthritis is a type of arthritis associated with psoriasis that is similar to rheumatoid arthritis. It may be characterized by extensive and disabling joint damage, especially in the hand and finger joints.

Rheumatoid arthritis occurs when an abnormal immune response leads to chronic inflammation and damage of joint cartilage and bone. It is thought to involve the activation of T lymphocytes, release of inflammatory cytokines, and formation of antibodies in the joint tissue as well as other organs. Research in recent years has delineated the roles of TNF-alpha and IL-1 in the pathophysiology of rheumatoid arthritis. Symptoms may include fatigue, loss of energy, lack of appetite, low-grade fever, muscle and joint aches, and stiffness. Joints frequently become red, swollen, painful, and tender.

Rejection Reactions With Solid Organ Transplantation

Rejection reactions may be either acute or chronic. Acute reactions may occur from 10 days to a few months after transplantation and mainly involve cellular immunity and proliferation of T lymphocytes. Characteristics include signs of organ failure and inflammation of blood vessels, leading to arterial narrowing or obliteration. Treatment with immunosuppressant drugs is usually effective in ensuring short-term survival of the transplant but does not prevent chronic rejection. Chronic reactions, which occur after months or years of normal function, are caused by both cellular and humoral immunity and do not respond to increasing immunosuppressive drug therapy. Characteristics include fibrosis of blood vessels and progressive failure of the transplanted organ.

Rejection reactions produce both general manifestations of inflammation and specific organ manifestations, depending on the organ involved. With kidney transplantation, for example, acute rejection reactions produce fever, flank tenderness over the graft organ site, and symptoms of kidney failure (e.g., increased serum creatinine, decreased urine output, edema, weight gain, hypertension). Chronic kidney rejection reactions are characterized by a gradual increase in serum creatinine levels over 4 to 6 months. Along with observing for symptoms of decline in organ function, periodic organ tissue biopsies are often required to diagnose a chronic organ rejection process.

Bone Marrow/Stem Cell Transplantation and Graft Versus Host Disease

With bone marrow/stem cell transplantation, the donor marrow or stem cells, which contain T lymphocytes, develop an active immune response against antigens on the host's tissues, producing GVHD. Tissue damage is produced directly by the action of cytotoxic T cells and indirectly through the release of inflammatory mediators (e.g., complement) and cytokines (e.g., TNF-alpha and ILs).

Acute GVHD occurs in up to 50% of patients. It presents within 100 days of transplant. Signs and symptoms include delayed recovery of blood cell production in the bone marrow, skin rash, liver dysfunction (indicated by increased alkaline phosphatase, aminotransferases, and bilirubin), and diarrhea. The skin reaction is usually a pruritic maculopapular rash that begins on the palms and soles and may progress to cover the entire body. Liver involvement can lead to bleeding disorders and the development of hepatic encephalopathy.

Chronic GVHD occurs when symptoms persist or occur 100 days or more after transplantation. It is characterized by abnormal humoral and cellular immunity, severe skin disorders, and liver disease. Chronic GVHD appears to be an autoimmune disorder in which activated donor T cells continue to respond to the recipient's surface proteins as if they are foreign antigens.

Drug Therapy

Immunosuppressant drugs compose several groups of pharmacologic agents, with often overlapping mechanisms and sites of action (Table 13.1; Fig. 13.1). Older groups of immunosuppressant drugs often depress the immune system of the recipient nonspecifically. Therapeutic use of these drugs increases the risk of serious infections with bacteria, viruses, fungi, or protozoa. In addition, most cytotoxic immunosuppressant drugs that slow the proliferation of activated lymphocytes also produce damage to rapidly dividing cells in other tissues (e.g., mucosal cells, intestinal cells, hematopoietic stem cells).

As a result, serious, life-threatening complications can occur with the use of immunosuppressant agents. For example, patients with autoimmune disorders or organ transplants, who are receiving long-term immunosuppressant drug therapy, are at increased risk for serious infections, cancer (especially lymphoma), hypertension, kidney and hepatic disease, and metabolic bone disease. The Institute for Safe Medication Practices considers immunosuppressants to be members of a high-alert drug class in community healthcare because these drugs have a heightened risk of causing significant patient harm when used in error. The U.S. Food and Drug Administration (FDA) has issued numerous **BOXED WARNING** ◆ for these drugs.

TABLE 13.1

Drugs Administered to Suppress Immunity

Drug Class	Prototype(s)	Other Drugs in the Class
Cytotoxic Immunosuppressive Agents		
	Mycophenolate mofetil IV (CellCept, CellCept Intravenous) Mycophenolate sodium PO (Myfortic)	Azathioprine (Azasan, Imuran) Leflunomide (Arava) Methotrexate (Otrexup, Rasuvo, RediTrex, Xatmep)
Conventional Antirejection Agents		
	Cyclosporine (Gengraf, Neoral, SandIMMUNE)	Everolimus (Zortress, Afinitor) Sirolimus (Rapamune) Tacrolimus (Prograf)
Janus Kinase Inhibitor		
	Ruxolitinib (Jakafi)	Abrocitinib (Cibinqo) Baricitinib (Olumiant) Fedratinib (Inrebic) Pacritinib (Vonjo) Tofacitinib (Xeljanz, Xeljanz XR) Upadacitinib (Rinvoq)
Adjuvant Medications Used to Suppress Immune Function		
Antibody preparations		*Monoclonal* Alirocumab (Praluent) Alemtuzumab (Campath, Lemtrada) Basiliximab (Simulect) Bevacizumab (Avastin, Mvasi) Bezlotoxumab (Zinplava) Cetuximab (Erbitux) Ipilimumab (Yervoy) Nivolumab (Opdivo) Omalizumab (Xolair) Panitumumab (Vectibix) Rituximab (Rituxan, Truxima) Trastuzumab (Herceptin, Kanjinti, Ogivri) *Polyclonal* Antithymocyte globulin (Atgam, Thymoglobulin) Others
Tumor necrosis factor-alpha–blocking agents	Infliximab (Avsola, Remicade, Inflectra, Renflexis)	Adalimumab (Humira, Humira Pediatric Crohn's Start, Humira Pen) Certolizumab (Cimzia, Cimzia Prefilled, Cimzia Starter Kit) Etanercept (Enbrel, Enbrel Mini, Enbrel SureClick) Golimumab (Simponi, Simponi Aria) Leflunomide (Arava)
Interleukin-blocking agents	Anakinra (Kineret)	Tocilizumab (Actemra, Actemra ACTPen) Ustekinumab (Stelara) Ixekizumab (Taltz)
Fusion protein inhibitors	Abatacept (Orencia, Orencia ClickJect)	Belatacept (Nulojix)

Newer drug groups modify the immune response more specifically in response to excessive levels of cytokines and T-cell activity that cause tissue damaging inflammation and autoimmune reactions. These drugs, called immunomodulators or biologic response modifiers, are part of the growing number of drugs with more specific immunosuppressive actions that have been developed through monoclonal antibody cloning technology (see later discussion). Most are used in combination with older immunosuppressants for synergistic effects with lower doses that minimize drug toxicities, whereas some are replacing the older, nonspecific immunosuppressants.

Immunosuppressants discussed here are cytotoxic immunosuppressant agents, conventional antirejection agents, and adjuvant medications, including antibody preparations, cytokine inhibitors, and corticosteroids.

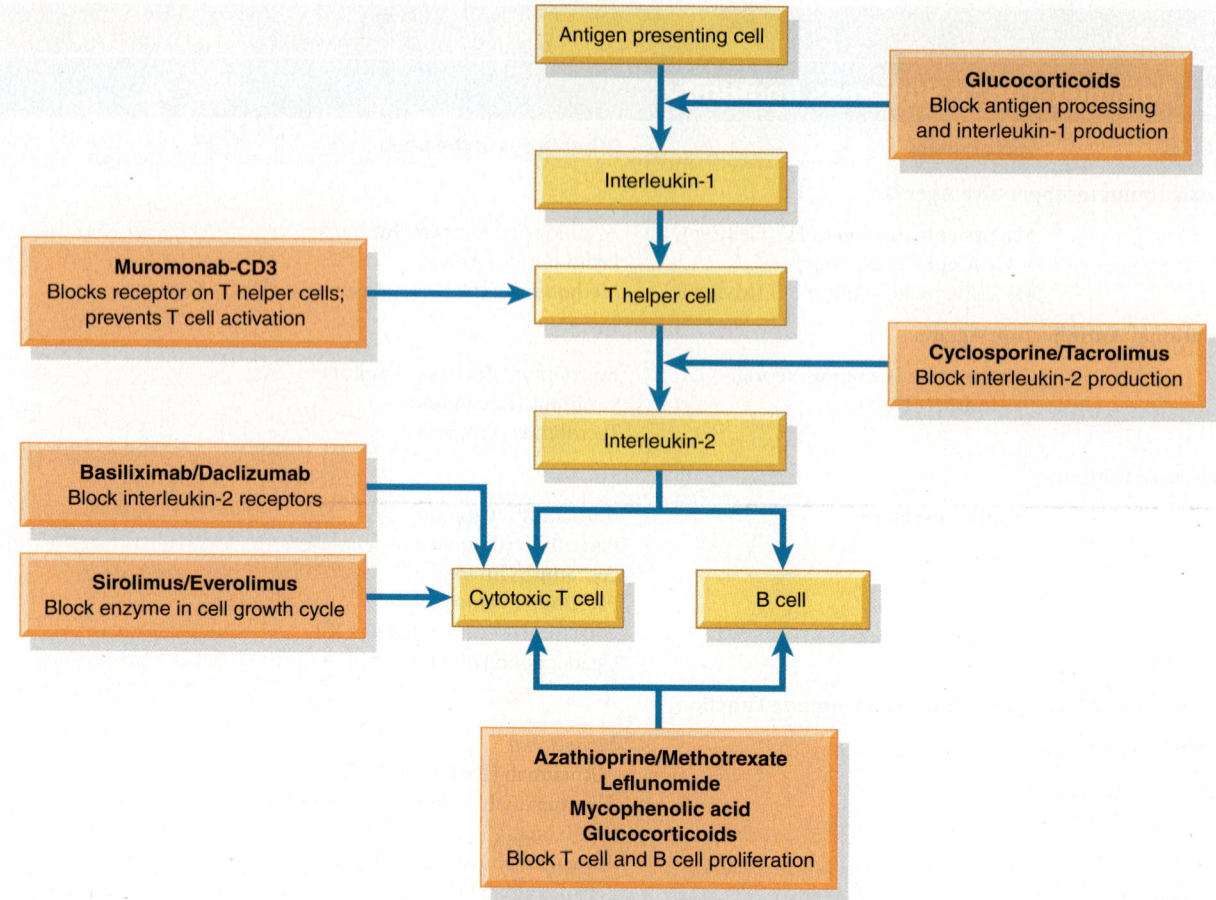

Figure 13.1. Activity of immunosuppressant drugs. Available immunosuppressants inhibit the immune response by blocking that response at various sites.

CYTOTOXIC IMMUNOSUPPRESSIVE AGENTS

The pharmacologic prophylaxis for GVHD is a combination of a calcineurin inhibitor, such as cyclosporine or tacrolimus, plus the antimetabolite methotrexate or mycophenolate mofetil. Cytotoxic immunosuppressive drugs damage or kill dividing cells, such as immunologically competent lymphocytes. Healthcare providers use these drugs primarily in cancer chemotherapy (see Chapter 14). However, in smaller doses, some cytotoxic drugs also exhibit immunosuppressive activities and are useful in the treatment of autoimmune disorders and the prevention of rejection reactions in organ transplantation. Since azathioprine is no longer widely used, ⓟ **mycophenolate mofetil** (CellCept) is the prototype in this discussion. Mycophenolate sodium (Myfortic) has similar properties to mycophenolate mofetil. Corticosteroids are combined with immunosuppressant agents as a front-line therapy for the treatment of clinical GVHD. It is unclear how the mechanism of action of the two drug classes provides prophylactic effects. Methylprednisolone possesses a 6-alpha-methyl group that blocks the specific binding of the corticosteroid to transcortin. Transcortin is a protein that transports steroids in the plasma. Methylprednisolone is bound to albumin. The lack of transcortin binding leads to a greater penetration of the cytotoxic immunosuppressive agent into the bronchial alveolar fluids, providing a greater therapeutic advantage in treating pulmonary inflammation.

Mycophenolate plus cyclosporine or tacrolimus is effective in the prevention of acute GVHD and is associated with a reduction in mucositis and an increase in blood forming cells that facilitate transplant recovery.

Pharmacokinetics

Mycophenolate mofetil is a prodrug that, after oral or intravenous (IV) administration, is rapidly broken down to mycophenolic acid, the active component. Metabolism to an active metabolite occurs in the liver, finally resulting in inactive metabolites. Excretion takes place in the urine. The distribution of mycophenolate sodium (Myfortic) possesses a delayed release.

Action

Mycophenolate is an antimetabolite agent that interferes with the production of cellular deoxyribonucleic acid (DNA) and ribonucleic acid and thus blocks cellular reproduction, growth, and development. As its active component, mycophenolic acid inhibits an enzyme needed for DNA synthesis and reduces the proliferation of lymphocytes. Mycophenolate mofetil's half-life is 17.9 ± 6.5 hours orally and 16.6 ± 5.8 hours parenterally, whereas mycophenolate sodium has a delayed release with a half-life of 8 to 16 hours.

Use

Uses of mycophenolate mofetil include the prophylaxis of organ rejection after cardiac, hepatic, and kidney transplants, as well as immunosuppression after other solid organ transplant procedures involving the lung, pancreas, and small intestine. Mycophenolate sodium, an oral formulation, has received FDA approval for use after kidney transplant to prevent organ rejection. Table 13.2 gives route and dosage information for mycophenolate and other cytotoxic immunosuppressant agents.

Patient-related variables specific to the use of mycophenolate include the following:

- Age:
  - Children who experience postoperative delayed graft function do not require dosage adjustments. Children with impaired kidney function taking mycophenolate warrant close observation for adverse effects.
  - Older patients should be prescribed mycophenolate cautiously due to the possibility of increased hepatic, kidney, or cardiac dysfunction. Patients aged 65 years or older may be at increased risk of certain infections, GI hemorrhage, and pulmonary edema.
- Reproduction, pregnancy, and lactation:
  - The FDA has issued a **BOXED WARNING** ◆ for mycophenolate mofetil regarding the risk of fetal loss and malformations. People of reproductive capability who are sexually active must use contraception. A negative pregnancy test for such patients is required prior to starting therapy. Contraceptive counseling is recommended prior to treatment and for several months after stopping treatment.
  - Mycophenolate has been used as an immunosuppressant in patients undergoing uterine transplantation. Mycophenolate is then discontinued and changed to a different agent prior to embryo transfer.
  - It is unknown if mycophenolate is present in breast milk. The decision to breast-feed should consider the risk of infant exposure.
- Abnormal kidney function and hepatic impairment:
  - In the immediate posttransplant period, no dosage adjustment is necessary for any degree of kidney dysfunction.
  - Increased monitoring of hepatic function is required for patients with hyperbilirubinemia and/or hypoalbuminemia.
- Specific healthcare environments:
  - In the home care setting, patients may be taking mycophenolate and other immunosuppressant drugs. The home care nurse must assess the environment for potential sources of infection, assist patients and other members of the household to understand the patient's susceptibility to infection, and teach ways to decrease risks of infection.
  - The home care nurse may need to assist with setting up a medication schedule and scheduling clinic visits for monitoring and follow-up care.
  - The home care nurse also assesses the patient's ability to safely self-administer the medications as prescribed,

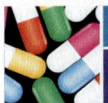

TABLE 13.2
DRUGS AT A GLANCE: Cytotoxic Immunosuppressive Agents

Drug	Routes and Dosage Ranges	
	Adults	**Children**
ⓟ **Mycophenolate mofetil/mycophenolate sodium** (CellCept, CellCept IV, Myfortic; 🍁 ACH-Mycophenolate, APO-Mycophenolate, CellCept, CellCept IV)	Kidney transplantation: PO, IV 1 g twice daily Cardiac and hepatic transplantation: PO, IV 1.5 g twice daily Delayed-release (Myfortic), PO 720 mg twice daily	Mycophenolate mofetil (kidney, heart, or liver transplant): Suspension: Infants ≥ 3 mo, children, adolescents: 600 mg/m²/dose daily PO: maximum daily dose: 2,000 mg/d Delayed-release tablets: BSA 1.25 to <1.5 m² 750 mg PO twice daily BSA ≥ 1.5 m² 1,000 mg PO twice daily
Azathioprine (Azasan, Imuran; 🍁 Apo-Azathioprine, Imuran, TEVA Azathioprine)	PO, IV 3–5 mg/kg/d initially; may be able to decrease to 1–3 mg/kg/d	Solid organ transplantation: 3–5 mg/kg/dose PO or IV beginning at the time of transplant; maintenance: 1–3 mg/kg/dose once daily
Leflunomide (Arava; 🍁 ACCEL-Leflunomide, APO-Leflunomide, Arava)	PO 100 mg once daily for 3 d and then 20 mg once daily	Juvenile idiopathic arthritis (alternative agent) <20 kg 10 mg PO every other day 20–40 kg 10 mg PO once daily >40 kg 20 mg PO once daily
Methotrexate (Otrexup, Rasuvo, RediTrex, Xatmep; 🍁 JAMP-Methotrexate, Metoject)	PO 7.5 mg/wk as single dose, or 2.5 mg every 12 h for 3 doses once weekly	Acute lymphoblastic leukemia (ALL) <1 y: 4,000–5,000 mg/m² over 24 h every 7 days for 2 doses ALL (immature B cell) 500 mg/m² over 30 min IV followed by 4,500 mg/m² over 23.5 h to complete a total dose of 5,000 mg/m² over 24 h on days 1, 15, 29, and 43 ALL (immature T cell) 100 mg/m² and then escalate dose by 50 mg/m² every 10 days for 5 doses total in combination with vincristine and pegaspargase Graft vs. host disease: Children and adolescents: 15 mg/m²/dose on day 1 and 10 mg/m²/dose on days 3 and 6 after allogeneic transplant (in combination with cyclosporine and prednisone)

monitors for adverse drug effects, and observes for signs of drug toxicity. Drug interactions with drugs from multiple prescribers as well as drug–nutrient and drug–herbal interactions can impact the patient's response to immunosuppressant drug therapy.

Adverse Effects

Common GI adverse effects of mycophenolate include nausea, vomiting, and diarrhea. The most serious risks associated with the use of this drug and some other immunosuppressant drugs are infection and increased risk of malignancy. Latent infections with the tuberculosis bacillus or hepatitis B virus may become active infections during immunosuppressant therapy.

Contraindications

Mycophenolate is contraindicated in patients who have displayed hypersensitivity to the medication. Use cautiously when administered with medications that cause CNS depression because the combination may result in increased CNS depression symptoms. Also use cautiously in patients with active peptic ulcer disease.

Nursing Implications

Preventing Interactions

Several drugs can increase and decrease the effects of mycophenolate, increasing or decreasing its effects (Box 13.1). Herbal preparations such as alfalfa, echinacea, ginseng, and bee venom, which potentially stimulate immune function, may interfere with mycophenolate and other immunosuppressant drug activity; thus, it is necessary to avoid them during therapy.

Administering the Medication

Quality and Safety Alert: Safety

Immunosuppressant drugs such as mycophenolate must be handled with care to avoid direct contact with skin or mucous membranes. Such contacts have produced teratogenic effects in animals. Patients should swallow oral tablets or capsules whole, without crushing or altering them, and should avoid inhaling the powder from the capsules. Caregivers should use caution to avoid direct contact when handling the drug.

Some mycophenolate preparations contain phenylalanine. Patients who are PKU positive must not be prescribed these formulations.

For best absorption, it is important to take oral mycophenolate on an empty stomach. To ensure correct dosing, it is important to measure the oral solution carefully using an accurate measuring device.

Assessing for Therapeutic Effects

After organ transplant, the absence of signs and symptoms of a rejection reaction is evidence of the therapeutic effects of mycophenolate immunosuppressive therapy. (Inflammatory changes in the organ tissue along with laboratory evidence of organ impairment usually accompany acute rejection reactions.) Periodic organ tissue biopsy is used to evaluate for signs of chronic rejection reaction.

BOX 13.1 Drug Interactions: Mycophenolate Mofetil

Drugs That Increase the Effects of Mycophenolate Mofetil
- Acyclovir, ganciclovir, probenecid, and salicylates
  Decrease excretion

Drugs That Decrease the Effects of Mycophenolate Mofetil
- Antacids containing magnesium, aluminum, and calcium; cholestyramine
  Decrease absorption as drug binds with mycophenolate

Assessing for Adverse Effects

A primary focus for nursing assessment is evidence of signs of infection, including fever, chills, sore throat, headache, swollen glands, cough, and urinary burning or frequency. Following organ transplant surgery, patients often take prophylactic antimicrobials for the first 3 to 6 months to prevent opportunistic infections. Wound healing may be slower during cytotoxic drug therapy with suppression of the normal inflammatory response.

Nursing care includes assessment of GI symptoms, oral intake, elimination pattern, fluid and electrolyte balance, and weight changes. Skin assessment for signs of rash, bruising, petechiae, and color changes such as pallor or jaundice of the skin or sclera offers important clues to allergic or hematologic complications and hepatotoxicity. Laboratory monitoring of the complete blood count (CBC), kidney function tests, and liver function tests performed prior to therapy and periodically during treatment limits the potential for bone marrow suppression and potential hepatotoxicity. The CBC is monitored weekly for the first month, twice monthly at months 2 and 3, and then monthly throughout the first year.

Clinical Application 13.1

- At his office visit, Mr. Jones tells the nurse that he has been regularly attending his son's Little League baseball games at a local park. What self-care measures related to his long-term need for immunosuppressive drug therapy should the nurse recommend?

Patient Teaching

The nurse should advise patients not to donate blood during and for 6 weeks after treatment. Individuals of reproductive age should receive counseling regarding pregnancy prevention and planning and the importance of consulting a healthcare provider if there is a possibility of pregnancy. Males should not donate sperm during therapy or for at least 90 days following mycophenolate discontinuation. Female partners of male patients should use highly effective contraception during and for 3 months after treatment.

Box 13.2 lists additional patient teaching guidelines for the cytotoxic immunosuppressant drugs.

Quality and Safety Alert: Safety

Mixing the drug with orange or apple juice improves taste; do not use grapefruit juice because it inhibits the metabolism of cyclosporine.

BOX 13.2 Patient Teaching Guidelines for Cytotoxic Immunosuppressant Drugs and Antirejection Drugs

General Considerations

- People taking medications that suppress the immune system are at high risk for development of infections. As a result, patients, caregivers, and others in the patient's environment need to wash their hands often and thoroughly, practice meticulous personal hygiene (e.g., take good care of the mouth, gums, and skin), avoid contact with people who have any infections, and practice other methods of preventing infection. Although infections often develop from the patient's own body flora or reactivation of a latent infection, other potential sources include water or soil around live plants, and raw fruits and vegetables. Attention to environmental cleansing as well as good personal and hand hygiene is required with immunosuppressant therapy.
- Understand that lifelong drug treatment to prevent potential organ rejection is required after transplant therapy. Obtain complete instructions about all the medications used to prevent rejection, including the purpose and activity of the drug; dose; route of administration (e.g., oral, injection); frequency and timing, potential adverse effects, and their management; and signs of complications and drug toxicity. Poor adherence and missed medication doses are an important cause of organ rejection and need for a subsequent transplant.
- Report adverse drug effects (e.g., signs or symptoms of infection such as sore throat or fever, decreased urine output if taking cyclosporine, easy bruising or bleeding if taking methotrexate) to a healthcare provider. If you have had a transplant, know the signs of transplant rejection.
- Try to maintain healthy lifestyle habits, such as eating a nutritious diet, getting adequate rest and sleep, and avoiding tobacco and alcohol. These measures enhance immune mechanisms and other body defenses.
- Carry identification that lists the drugs being taken; the dosage; the prescriber's name, address, and telephone number; and instructions for emergency treatment. Use of a MedicAlert bracelet is recommended in case of an accident or other emergency.
- Inform all healthcare providers that you are taking immunosuppressant drugs.
- Maintain regular supervision by a healthcare provider. This is extremely important for evaluating health status, evaluating drug responses and indications for dosage change, detecting adverse drug reactions, and having blood tests or other monitoring tests when indicated.
- Take no other drugs, prescription or nonprescription, without notifying the prescriber who is managing immunosuppressant therapy. Immunosuppressant drugs may influence reactions to other drugs, and other drugs may influence reactions to the immunosuppressants. Thus, taking other drugs may decrease therapeutic effects or increase adverse effects. In addition, some vaccinations should be avoided while taking immunosuppressant drugs.
- People of reproductive capability who are sexually active should practice effective contraceptive techniques during immunosuppressive drug therapy. With methotrexate, use contraception during and for at least 3 months (males) or one ovulatory cycle (females) after stopping the drug. With mycophenolate, effective contraception should be continued for 6 weeks after the drug is stopped. With sirolimus, effective contraception must be used before, during, and for 12 weeks after drug therapy.
- Wear protective clothing and use sunscreens to decrease exposure of skin to sunlight and risks of skin cancers. Also, methotrexate and sirolimus increase sensitivity to sunlight and may increase sunburn. Have cancer screening for early detection if you take immunosuppressant drugs.

Self-Administration

- Follow instructions about taking the drugs to achieve beneficial effects and decrease adverse effects. If unable to take a medication, report to the prescriber or other healthcare provider; do not stop unless advised to do so. For transplant recipients, missed doses may lead to transplant rejection; for patients with autoimmune diseases, missed doses may lead to acute flare-ups of symptoms. Take medications at approximately the same time each day to maintain consistent drug levels in the blood.
- With cyclosporine oral solution, use the same solution consistently. The available cyclosporine solutions (Neoral, Gengraf, SandIMMUNE) are not equivalent and cannot be used interchangeably. If a change in formulation is necessary, the dispensing pharmacy should consult the prescriber.
- Measure oral cyclosporine solution with the dosing syringe provided; add to orange or apple juice that is at room temperature (avoid grapefruit juice) into a glass container, stir well, and drink at once (do not allow diluted solution to stand before drinking). The amount of fluid should be large enough to increase palatability, especially for children, but small enough to be consumed quickly. Rinse the glass with more juice to ensure that the total dose is taken. Do not rinse the dosing syringe with water or other cleaning agents. Take on a consistent schedule regarding time of day and meals. These are the manufacturer's recommendations.
- Take mycophenolate on an empty stomach; food decreases drug absorption by approximately 40%. Do not crush mycophenolate tablets and do not open or crush the capsules.
- Take sirolimus consistently with or without food; do not mix or take the drug with grapefruit juice. Grapefruit juice inhibits metabolism and increases adverse effects. If also taking cyclosporine, take the sirolimus 4 hours after a dose of cyclosporine.
- If taking the oral solution, use the syringe that comes with the medication to measure and withdraw the dose from the bottle. Empty the dose into a glass or plastic container with at least 2 oz (1/4 cup or 60 mL) of water or orange juice. *Do not use any other liquid to dilute the drug*. Stir the mixture vigorously, and drink it immediately. Refill the container with at least 4 oz (1/2 cup or 120 mL) of water or orange juice, stir vigorously, and drink at once.
- Take tacrolimus with food to decrease stomach upset.
- If giving or taking an injected drug, be sure you understand how to mix and inject the medication correctly. With etanercept, for example, rotate injection sites, give a new injection at least 1 in from a previous injection site, and do not inject the medication into areas where the skin is tender, bruised, red, or hard. When possible, practice the required techniques and perform at least the first injection under supervision of a qualified healthcare professional.

Other Drugs in the Class

Healthcare providers have long used methotrexate (Otrexup, Rasuvo, RediTrex, Xatmep) for the treatment of cancer (higher doses), as well as for the treatment of autoimmune disorders, such as severe rheumatoid arthritis, juvenile rheumatoid arthritis, and severe psoriasis (lower doses). The use of methotrexate in combination with cyclosporine is the most widely used regimen in the prevention of GVHD after bone marrow transplantation.

Excretion of methotrexate is mainly in the urine, so the drug's half-life is prolonged in patients with abnormal kidney function, with risks of accumulation to toxic levels and additional kidney damage. However, the risks are less with the small doses used for the treatment of rheumatoid arthritis than for the high doses used in cancer chemotherapy. To decrease these risks, it is important to document adequate kidney function using the drug. Patients should be well hydrated.

The lower doses of methotrexate used for autoimmune disorders and transplant therapy reduce the incidence and severity of adverse effects. Oral mucositis can occur with methotrexate therapy, interfering with nutritional intake and contributing to the risk of infection. However, even in the low doses used in rheumatoid arthritis and psoriasis, methotrexate may cause hepatotoxicity. Prior to and during therapy, monitoring the CBC, kidney function, and liver function is essential. Liver function tests help guide methotrexate dosage. In general, dosage reduction is warranted if bilirubin is between 3 and 5 mg/dL, or aspartate aminotransferase is above 180 IU/L, and the drug should be omitted if bilirubin is above 5 mg/dL. Many clinicians recommend serial liver biopsies for patients on long-term, low-dose methotrexate.

Administration of methotrexate is weekly for rheumatoid arthritis or psoriasis, and patients should keep an accurate record of the date and time of each dose. To reduce gastric upset, they may take the drug with food. However, daily dosing for cytotoxic immunosuppressants should be consistent with regard to time and food (i.e., at the same time of day, with the same meal).

> **! Quality and Safety Alert: Safety**
>
> It is necessary to follow individual manufacturer's instructions for reconstituting and administering IV preparations of methotrexate—in consultation with a pharmacist as needed.

Leflunomide (Arava), an anti-inflammatory immunosuppressant, is useful only in the treatment of adults with rheumatoid arthritis. Authorities do not recommend the drug for children younger than 18 years of age. Contraindications include the presence of active hepatitis B or C infection or if the alanine aminotransferase level is greater than two times normal. With leflunomide, hepatotoxicity is a concern; hence, it is essential to obtain liver function tests before starting therapy. Also, patients should have kidney function tests, as well as liver function tests, every month for the first 6 months and then every 6 to 8 weeks thereafter. The FDA has issued a **BOXED WARNING ◆** for leflunomide regarding the risk of fetal loss and malformations. Patients of reproductive capability who are sexually active must use contraception. A negative pregnancy test for such patients is necessary prior to starting therapy. Contraceptive counseling for all patients is recommended prior to treatment and for several months after stopping treatment.

Azathioprine (Azasan, Imuran) is occasionally part of a maintenance immunosuppressive regimen following transplant, although cyclosporine or tacrolimus is used more commonly. Healthcare providers use azathioprine after organ transplant in children, as well as for the treatment of psoriasis, psoriatic arthritis, systemic lupus erythematosus, immune thrombocytopenia, inflammatory bowel disease, and other inflammatory disorders, but safety data are limited. Azathioprine has a high potential for toxicity, so regular assessments for adverse effects are critical. The FDA has issued a **BOXED WARNING ◆** for chronic immunosuppression with azathioprine because the drug increases the risk of malignancy.

CONVENTIONAL ANTIREJECTION AGENTS

 Cyclosporine (Neoral, Gengraf, SandIMMUNE), the first antirejection drug used to prevent transplant rejection reactions, is the prototype antirejection agent. Cyclosporine and related drugs are fungal metabolites with strong immunosuppressive effects. By selectively inhibiting proliferation of helper T cells and expression of cytokines, these antirejection drugs reduce the activity of other immune cells involved in graft rejection. Consequently, they are widely used in transplant therapy to prevent or reduce the graft rejection response.

Pharmacokinetics

Absorption of cyclosporine is highly variable. After oral administration, absorption is rather poor. The drug is highly bound to plasma proteins, and approximately 50% is distributed in erythrocytes, so drug levels in whole blood are higher than those in plasma. Peak plasma levels occur 4 to 5 hours after a dose. Metabolism of cyclosporine involves the CYP3A4 liver enzyme system, and elimination occurs mainly in the bile.

Action

Cyclosporine inhibits calcineurin, a protein needed for the synthesis of IL-2 and the subsequent proliferation of T cells and B cells. The drug binds with calcineurin on T lymphocytes and interferes with the production of IL-2. As previously described, activated T cells produce a cytokine, IL-2, which, in turn, inhibits signaling through the T-cell receptor. This action activates other lymphocytes, amplifying the immune response and producing the damaging inflammatory changes in tissue that occur with organ rejection and autoimmune disease.

Use

Healthcare providers use cyclosporine to prevent rejection reactions and prolong graft survival after solid organ transplantation (e.g., kidney, liver, heart, lung) or to treat chronic rejection in patients previously treated with other immunosuppressive agents. The drug inhibits both cellular and humoral immunity but affects T lymphocytes significantly more than B lymphocytes. With cyclosporine-induced deprivation of IL-2, T cells stimulated by the graft antigen are unable to multiple and differentiate, and graft organ destruction is inhibited. In addition to its use in solid organ transplantation, cyclosporine is useful in the prevention and treatment of GVHD, a complication of bone marrow transplantation. In GVHD, T lymphocytes from the transplanted marrow of the donor mount an immune response against the tissues of the recipient. Cyclosporine may inhibit donor T-cell activity, reducing the risk of GVHD. Other indications for use include treatment of psoriasis and rheumatoid arthritis.

Cyclosporine dosing is weight based in both adults and children, with higher doses given immediately before and after the transplant and then tapered over several months to minimize adverse effects and avoid excessive immunosuppression. Table 13.3 outlines the routes and dosages for cyclosporine and related drugs.

Patient-related variables specific to the use of cyclosporine include the following:

- Age:
  - Children as young as 6 months of age may receive cyclosporine in its oral form. Experience with this drug indicates that children require relatively high doses because they metabolize the drug rapidly.
  - Due to an increased incidence of infection and a greater risk of malignancy, older adults must be monitored carefully during antirejection drug therapy. Doses are individualized, considering age, function, and concurrent conditions. More frequent assessment and therapeutic blood level monitoring are essential in older adults after organ transplantation because of the increased risk of organ toxicity.
- Reproduction, pregnancy, and lactation:
  - Cyclosporine is an acceptable immunosuppressant for use in kidney or heart transplantation recipients who are planning to become pregnant.
  - Contraception may be considered for female patients on a stable, low maintenance dose who are greater than or equal to 1 year following transplantation.
  - Cyclosporine crosses the placenta.
  - Cyclosporine is not associated with teratogenic effects, but maternal use may result in low birth weight infants.
  - The manufacturer of cyclosporine recommends the discontinuation of breast-feeding.
- Abnormal kidney function and hepatic impairment:
  - There are no dosage adjustments in abnormal kidney function or hepatic impairment. Patients with solid organ

TABLE 13.3

DRUGS AT A GLANCE: Conventional Antirejection Agents

Drug	Routes and Dosage Ranges	
	Adults	Children
Cyclosporine (Gengraf, Neoral, SandIMMUNE; ❖ Cyclosporine, Neoral, SandIMMUNE IV)	Solid organ transplantation, rejection prophylaxis: Oral dose is dependent on the type of transplant; refer to institutional guidelines 5–6 mg/kg/d or 1/3 of the oral dose as a single dose, infused over 2–6 h Cyclosporine (manufacturer labeling for newly transplanted patients: Kidney: 9 ± 3 mg/kg/d in 2 divided doses Liver: 8 ± 4 mg/kg/d in 2 divided doses Heart: 7 ± 3 mg/kg/d in 2 divided doses	Solid organ transplantation, rejection prophylaxis: Oral dose is dependent on the type of transplant; refer to institutional guidelines 5–6 mg/kg/d or 1/3 of the oral dose as a single dose, infused over 2–6 h Cyclosporine (manufacturer labeling for newly transplanted patients: Kidney: 9 ± 3 mg/kg/d in 2 divided doses Liver: 8 ± 4 mg/kg/d in 2 divided doses Heart: 7 ± 3 mg/kg/d in 2 divided doses
Everolimus (Zortress, Afinitor, Afinitor Disperz; ❖ Afinitor, Afinitor Disperz)	Liver transplantation rejection prophylaxis Zortress/Afinitor: PO 1 mg tablet once daily (in combination with tacrolimus and corticosteroid)	Kidney transplantation rejection prophylaxis ≥1 y and adolescents: Initial 0.8 mg/m^2/dose twice daily (maximum single dose: 1/5 mg) to maintain concentration at 3–6 ng/mL
Sirolimus (Rapamune; ❖ Rapamune)	PO 6 mg as soon after kidney transplantation as possible and then 2 mg daily	Adolescents <40 kg: Loading dose: PO 3 mg/m^2 as loading dose and then 1 mg/m^2 daily ≥40 kg: Loading dose: PO 6 mg on day 1; maintenance: 2 mg once daily
Tacrolimus (Prograf, Astagraf XL, Envarsus XR, Prograf; ❖ Advagraf, Envarsus, Prograf, Sandoz Tacrolimus)	IV infusion, 25–50 mcg/kg/d, starting 6 h after transplantation or later, until the patient can tolerate oral drug; PO 150–200 mcg/kg/d, in 2 divided doses every 12 h, with the first dose 8–12 h after stopping the IV infusion	IV 50–100 mcg/kg/d; PO 200–300 mcg/kg/d

transplants commonly use cyclosporine, but the risk of nephrotoxicity increases as a result. To reduce toxicity and increase efficacy, attention must be given to dosage, other adverse effects, and potential drug interactions. Monitoring serum blood levels can help reduce this risk, and nephrotoxicity usually subsides after decreasing the dosage or stopping the drug. In kidney transplant recipients, when serum creatinine and blood urea nitrogen levels remain elevated, an evaluation of the patient and tissue biopsy is often necessary to differentiate cyclosporine-induced nephrotoxicity from a transplant rejection reaction.

- Specific healthcare environments:
  - In critically ill patients, the use of immunosuppressants during critical illness requires individualized risk versus benefit decision-making. It is necessary to balance the need to prevent transplant organ rejection against the risk of infection and associated drug toxicities, which may lead to loss of the engrafted organ.
  - In the home care setting, managing chronic rejection and minimizing drug toxicities is challenging because transplant recipients are living longer and multiple organ transplants and retransplants occur. Promoting correct medication use is critical to maintain therapeutic blood levels after transplantation and prevent organ rejection. Due to the variable bioavailability of cyclosporine when taken orally, patients should consistently take the drug at the same time each day. In addition to monitoring medication use, the home care nurse provides self-care teaching, monitors for sources of infection, obtains and monitors blood work, and implements health maintenance measures.

Adverse Effects

Nephrotoxicity, hirsutism, gingival hypertrophy, hypertension, and hyperlipidemia are significant adverse effects of cyclosporine. The FDA has issued a **BOXED WARNING** ◆ for cyclosporine regarding risks of hypertension and nephrotoxicity. After solid organ transplantation, with the need to continue lifelong immunosuppression to avoid graft rejection, serious infection is an ongoing concern.

Because transplant recipients are living longer, this has led to the recognition of long-term adverse effects associated with immunosuppressant drug therapy. For example, patients have an increased risk of developing a malignancy. The incidence of malignancy is unknown, but after 10 years of immunosuppression, authorities often estimate it to be 20% or more. Patients who have had kidney transplants are approximately three times more likely to develop cancer than those of the general population. The risk factors are based on the extent, duration, and type of immunosuppression. The most common malignancies in transplant recipients are skin cancers and lymphomas, and solid organ tumors may also occur. Regular screening tests for breast, cervical, colon, and prostate cancer, along with annual skin examinations, are recommended. The FDA has issued a **BOXED WARNING** ◆ limiting all long-term use of antirejection drugs to prescribers experienced in transplant therapy because of the increased risk of infections and certain malignancies such as lymphoma and skin cancer.

Contraindications

Contraindications to cyclosporine include the combined use of antirejection drugs that have the same mechanism of action and toxicities (e.g., tacrolimus and cyclosporine). Prescribers usually avoid such use after organ transplant.

Nursing Implications

Preventing Interactions

Numerous potential drug interactions affect the blood levels of cyclosporine, increasing or decreasing its effects (Box 13.3). Because these drugs are metabolized mainly by CYP3A4 enzymes and have a low therapeutic index, any drugs that increase or decrease levels of these enzymes have the potential to alter blood levels of cyclosporine. The herb St. John's wort may reduce this drug's therapeutic effects.

Administering the Medication

It is necessary to initiate antirejection drugs several hours prior to the transplant procedure. Administration is by IV infusion only until the patient can take the drug by the oral route. The risk of a severe allergic reaction is significantly higher following IV administration. Dilution of an oral cyclosporine solution should follow package instructions. Do not administer cyclosporine oral solution from a plastic or Styrofoam cup. Neoral oral solution may be diluted with room temperature orange juice or apple juice. SandIMMUNE oral solution may be diluted with milk, chocolate milk, or orange juice. Avoid changing diluents and mix them thoroughly. The solution and diluent should be drunk immediately. Mix in a glass container and rinse container with more diluent to ensure that the total dose is administered. Do not rinse the syringe before or after use. Rinsing will result in dosage variation.

To improve bioavailability, cyclosporine preparations were once prepared in alcohol and olive oil for oral administration and in alcohol and castor oil for IV administration. Anaphylactic reactions, attributed to the castor oil, have occurred with the IV formulation. Neoral and Gengraf are oral microemulsion formulations that are better absorbed than oral SandIMMUNE. These different drug formulations are not equivalent in their absorption and cannot be used interchangeably.

BOX 13.3 *Drug Interactions: Cyclosporine*

Drugs That Increase the Effects of Cyclosporine

- Aminoglycoside antibiotics and amphotericin B
  Increase nephrotoxic effects
- Azithromycin, fluconazole, and related antifungals; macrolide antibiotics
  Increase blood levels and toxic effects

Drugs That Decrease the Effects of Cyclosporine

- Carbamazepine, phenytoin, and rifampin
  Decreases therapeutic effects

Assessing for Therapeutic Effects

The nurse monitors for organ function and signs of rejection with solid organ transplants, assesses serum blood levels, and monitors and manages adverse drug effects. Cyclosporine has a very narrow therapeutic index; therefore, prescribers use serum drug levels to regulate cyclosporine dosing, and close monitoring is necessary. Blood levels measured 2 hours after a dose are used for dosage adjustments. Subtherapeutic levels may lead to organ transplant rejection, whereas high levels increase adverse effects.

Assessing for Adverse Effects

Acute nephrotoxicity can occur, progressing to chronic nephrotoxicity and kidney failure. It is essential to monitor kidney function tests (serum creatinine and blood urea nitrogen) and urine protein throughout cyclosporine therapy. To check for hepatotoxicity, it is necessary to conduct liver function tests (bilirubin, alanine aminotransferase, and aspartate aminotransferase) regularly. Periodic monitoring of fasting lipid levels (cholesterol, high- and low-density lipoproteins, and triglycerides) should also occur.

Patient Teaching

Box 13.2 presents patient teaching information for the conventional antirejection drugs.

Other Drugs in the Class

Everolimus (Zortress, Afinitor) reduces T-cell activation to decrease the immune response after kidney transplant and rejection. This drug, generally combined with cyclosporine and prednisone, allows lower posttransplant doses of both cyclosporine and the steroid; this minimizes adverse effects. Everolimus is available only as an oral formulation, and patients should take the drug consistently, with or without food, to maintain consistent therapeutic blood levels. The drug has been associated with an increased incidence of angioedema, early kidney graft thrombosis, delayed wound healing, elevated lipid levels, new-onset diabetes, and an increased risk of nephrotoxicity and proteinuria when combined with cyclosporine. It is necessary to obtain therapeutic blood levels of both cyclosporine and everolimus to minimize the risks of kidney toxicity when the drugs are used concurrently.

> **! Quality and Safety Alert: Safety**
>
> Use of an alcohol-free dexamethasone mouthwash prior to administration of everolimus will reduce the incidence and severity of stomatitis. Instruct the patient to swish and spit the mouthwash before taking the drug.

Sirolimus is an immunosuppressant used to prevent organ rejection in kidney transplants. Often, it is given concomitantly with a corticosteroid and cyclosporine. Sirolimus may have synergistic effects with cyclosporine because it has a different mechanism of action, and prescribers may order both drugs in combination. However, because the two drugs are metabolized by the same liver CYP3A4 enzymes, cyclosporine can increase blood levels of sirolimus, potentially to toxic levels. Consequently, it is essential that the drugs not be given at the same time; patients should take sirolimus 4 hours after a dose of cyclosporine.

Extensive metabolism of sirolimus occurs in the liver, and the drug may accumulate in the presence of hepatic impairment. If this occurs, reducing the maintenance dose by 35% may be warranted; changing the loading dose is not necessary. Monitoring using serum drug levels in patients who are likely to have altered drug metabolism due to age, concurrent disease, or other drugs is important. Use of sirolimus in children after kidney transplant to reduce the risk of nephropathy from cyclosporine or tacrolimus allows these other drugs to be given at lower doses or discontinued. Contraindications to use of sirolimus include recent lung and liver transplantation due to an increased incidence of delayed healing and graft failure in the transplanted organs. The FDA has issued a **BOXED WARNING** ◆ that use of sirolimus in patients receiving lung or liver transplants has been associated with increased morbidity and mortality.

Tacrolimus is similar to cyclosporine in its mechanisms of action, pharmacokinetic characteristics, and adverse effects. It prevents transplant rejection by inhibiting proliferation of T lymphocytes. Some transplant centers now use tacrolimus rather than cyclosporine, mainly because cyclosporine is given with corticosteroids. Using tacrolimus may allow corticosteroids to be reduced or stopped, thereby decreasing the adverse effects of long-term corticosteroid therapy. Tacrolimus, like cyclosporine, is not well absorbed orally, so it is necessary to give higher oral doses than IV doses to obtain similar blood levels. With IV administration, onset of action is rapid, but with oral administration, onset varies. It is essential that patients take the oral drug on a consistent time schedule because its bioavailability may vary. Dosing of tacrolimus is individualized according to clinical response, adverse effects, and serum blood levels.

Metabolism of tacrolimus takes place in the liver and intestine, and excretion of the several metabolites occurs in bile and urine. Dosage reduction is necessary with impaired liver or kidney function. It is essential to give the drug at the lowest effective dose because it may cause nephrotoxicity.

> ### Clinical Application 13.2
>
> - Mr. Jones calls the nephrology clinic to report shortness of breath and fatigue. Despite a decrease in appetite, he reports his weight has increased by 2 kg over the last week. The nurse recognizes that he is most likely experiencing which adverse effects from one of his immunosuppressant medications?

JANUS KINASE INHIBITOR

 Ruxolitinib (Jakafi) is classified as a Janus kinase inhibitor that is administered orally for acute treatment to prevent GVHD. It is also an antineoplastic agent used to treat polycythemia vera. New Janus kinase inhibitors have been approved and several are under investigation. These medications have targeted molecules with simple chemical structures as compared to similar therapeutic agents that are made by recombinant DNA, such as the monoclonal antibodies (see later discussion). They are used to treat rheumatoid arthritis, psoriatic arthritis, spondyloarthritis, and atopic dermatitis. The FDA has issued a **BOXED WARNING** ◆ for all Janus kinase inhibitors that their use should be avoided in patients with serious infections.

Pharmacokinetics

The onset of action is approximately 1.5 weeks or 1 to 11 days. With chronic GVHD, the median time is 3 weeks. Ruxolitinib is rapidly absorbed. The protein binding is 97% to albumin. Metabolism is in the liver with the CYP3A4 isoenzyme (it is also metabolized minimally by CYP2C9). The half-life is approximately 3 hours, with a peak of action in 1 to 2 hours. It is excreted primarily in the kidneys and 22% in the feces.

Action

Ruxolitinib selectively inhibits Janus kinases, mediating the signals of cytokine and growth factors that are responsible for hematopoiesis and immune function.

Use

Ruxolitinib is used for acute treatment of steroid-refractory acute GVHD in adult and pediatric patients. It is also used to treat polycythemia vera and myelofibrosis in adults. Table 13.4 outlines the routes and dosages for ruxolitinib.

Patient-related variables specific to the use of ruxolitinib include the following:

- Reproduction, pregnancy, and lactation:
    - Use of ruxolitinib in pregnant patients is not recommended.
    - Breast-feeding should be discontinued during ruxolitinib treatment and for 2 weeks after final dose of ruxolitinib.
- Abnormal kidney function and hepatic impairment:
    - The dosage of ruxolitinib is reduced in the presence of abnormal kidney function or hepatic impairment.

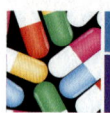

TABLE 13.4
DRUGS AT A GLANCE: Janus Kinase Inhibitor

Drug	Routes and Dosage Ranges	
	Adults	**Children**
Ⓟ Ruxolitinib (Jakafi; ✣ Jakafi)	PO 5 mg twice daily; increase dose to 10 mg twice daily after at least 3 d of treatment if ANC and platelets are not decreased by >50% compared to first day of ruxolitinib therapy CrCl: 15–59 mL/min and any platelet count: 5 mg once daily ESRD: CrCl <15 mL/min on dialysis and any platelet count: 5 mg once after dialysis ESRD: CrCl <15 mL/min not requiring dialysis: avoid use Stage 4 hepatic impairment and any platelet count: 5 mg once daily	Children ≥12 y: PO 5 mg twice daily; consider increasing the dose to 10 mg twice daily after at least 3 d of treatment if ANC and platelets are not decreased by >50% compared to first day of ruxolitinib therapy CrCl: 15–59 mL/min and any platelet count: 5 mg once daily ESRD: CrCl <15 mL/min on dialysis and any platelet count: 5 mg once after dialysis ESRD: CrCl <15 mL/min not requiring dialysis: avoid use Stage 4 hepatic impairment and any platelet count: 5 mg once daily
Abrocitinib (Cibinqo; ✣ Cibinqo)	Atopic dermatitis: PO 100 mg once daily; for significant response in after 12 wk increase dose to 200 mg once daily; discontinue with adequate treatment response	Safety and efficacy not established
Baricitinib (Olumiant; ✣ Olumiant)	Rheumatoid arthritis: PO 2 mg once daily COVID-19: Hospitalized patient with significant oxygen requirements: PO 4 mg once daily for 14 days Alopecia areata: PO 2 mg once daily; may increase to 4 mg once daily	COVID-19: Children 2–9 y: PO 2 mg once daily for 14 days or until hospital discharge; 9 y and adolescents: PO 4 mg once daily for 14 days or until hospital discharge
Fedratinib (Inrebic; ✣ Inrebic)	Myelofibrosis: PO 400 mg once daily for patients with a baseline platelet count ≥50,000/mm³	Safety and efficacy not established
Pacritinib (Vonjo)	Myelofibrosis: PO 200 mg twice daily	Safety and efficacy not established
Tofacitinib (Xeljanz, Xeljanz XR; ✣ AURO Tofacitinib, PMS-Tofacitinib, TARO-Tofacitinib, Xeljanz, Xeljanz XR)	Ankylosing spondylitis, psoriatic arthritis, rheumatoid arthritis: IR tablet PO 5 mg twice daily; ER tablet PO 11 mg once daily	Juvenile idiopathic arthritis, polyarticular course: 10 to <20 kg: PO (1 mg/mL): 3.2 mg twice daily 20 to <40 kg: PO 1 mg/mL): 4 mg twice daily ≥40 kg: PO (1 mg/mL): 5 mg twice daily
Upadacitinib (Rinvoq; ✣ Rinvoq)	Atopic dermatitis: PO 15 mg twice daily may increase to 30 mg Psoriatic arthritis: PO 15 mg once daily Rheumatoid arthritis: PO 15 mg once daily Ulcerative colitis: Induction PO 45 mg once daily for 8 wk; maintenance 15 mg once daily may increase to 30 mg once daily	Atopic dermatitis: Children ≥12 y and adolescents weighing ≥40 kg: PO 15 mg once daily; may increase to 30 mg once daily if adequate response

Adverse Effects

The central nervous system adverse effects include dizziness, headache, fatigue, and insomnia. Increased serum cholesterol is noted, as well as hypertriglyceridemia. Hematologic adverse effects include anemia, thrombocytopenia, and neutropenia. In postmarketing administration, the rate of hepatitis B exacerbation was reported.

Contraindications

There are no contraindications indicated in the manufacturer's labeling. The intake of grapefruit juice will increase the effect of ruxolitinib, and patients should be instructed to eliminate it from the diet.

Nursing Implications

Preventing Interactions

Immunosuppressant and corticosteroid agents interact with ruxolitinib. In addition, chemotherapeutic agents will increase immune suppression.

Administering the Medication

Ruxolitinib is administered orally without regard to food intake. For patients who have an inability to swallow, it can be administered through a nasogastric tube measuring 8 Fr or larger. The tablet should be suspended in 40 mL of water, stirred for 10 minutes, and administered within 6 hours of dispersion. Administer with the appropriate size syringe, and flush the NG tube with 75 mL of water. Administration is the same for pediatric patients. Do not administer with grapefruit juice due to an increase of serum drug levels or potential toxicity. Prior to initiation of ruxolitinib therapy, the patient should receive a tuberculin skin test; if the test is positive, the medication should not be given. Administering this drug in a patient with a positive tuberculin test decreases the immune response and increases the patient's risk of the development of active tuberculosis.

Assessing for Therapeutic and Adverse Effects

The CBC should be assessed at baseline and every 2 to 4 weeks. In patients with stage 3 to 4 liver GVHD, the CBC may be assessed more frequently. In addition, lipid levels should be monitored every 8 to 12 weeks. Perform period skin assessments to assess for the development of skin infections.

Other Drugs in the Class

Uses for other drugs in the Janus kinase inhibitor class of immunosuppressants are listed in Table 13.4. Abrocitinib has been shown to result in lymphoma and other malignancies. Baricitinib, tofacitinib, and upadacitinib also have a high rate of all malignancies except skin cancer. Patients with current or previous tobacco use who are receiving baricitinib, tofacitinib, or upadacitinib are at highest risk. The FDA has issued a **BOXED WARNING ◆** for fedratinib that serious and fatal encephalopathy, including Wernicke, has occurred in patients being treated with fedratinib. Pacritinib has the potential to impair male fertility.

ADJUVANT MEDICATIONS USED TO SUPPRESS IMMUNE FUNCTION

A significant number of adjuvant medications are used as immunosuppressants. Table 13.5 summarizes indications for use and dosages for these drugs.

Corticosteroids

Corticosteroids are potent anti-inflammatory agents that suppress the systemic immune response. Chapters 17 and 33 contain information about specific agents, including effects of therapeutic doses of corticosteroids. Used in a wide variety of inflammatory and allergic disorders, pharmacologic doses of corticosteroids block the production of IL-1, relieving signs and symptoms of inflammation by decreasing the accumulation of lymphocytes and macrophages and reducing levels of other cell-damaging cytokines. Corticosteroids, used in pharmacologic doses, suppress inflammation by suppressing activation and growth of lymphoid T cells and decreasing the formation and function of antibodies by B cells. For patients with transplanted tissues, corticosteroids are usually given with other agents to prevent acute graft rejection. Increasingly, in autoimmune disease, healthcare providers use biologic response modifiers, combined with a cytotoxic immunosuppressant (or alone), as primary therapy. These disease-modifying anti-inflammatory drugs, known as DMARDs, more specifically address the underlying autoimmune tissue process and can slow the destructive changes. Currently, prescribers order corticosteroids for episodic use during acute exacerbations of autoimmune disease and then taper or discontinue them as soon as possible.

The important adverse effects of corticosteroids have led many transplant centers to try to minimize or eliminate the use of these drugs as part of chronic immunosuppressive therapy when possible. Methods such as gradually tapering doses after transplant to no more than 10 mg daily in adults and using alternate-day therapy in children are strategies used to minimize the long-term adverse effects of corticosteroids.

Antibody Preparations

Antibody (immunoglobulin) preparations are produced in the laboratory or derived from animals injected with human lymphoid tissue to stimulate an immune response. Healthcare providers use such preparations in inflammatory autoimmune disorders, transplantation rejection reactions, and cancer treatment to block cell receptors that are part of the abnormal inflammation or cell proliferation process. The antibodies produced may be monoclonal or polyclonal. This section discusses several drugs.

Monoclonal antibodies, which originate from a single B-cell source, are immunoglobulins that are therapeutically replicated in laboratory cells to react with specific cell antigens to alter the immune response to an antigen. The isolation and cloning of individual B lymphocytes result in the production of biologically identical antibody molecules. To produce a monoclonal antibody, the human antigen to which the desired antibody will respond is first injected into a mouse or hamster. The animal mounts an immune response in which its B lymphocytes

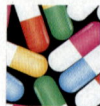

TABLE 13.5

DRUGS AT A GLANCE: Adjuvant Medications Used as Immunosuppressants

Drug	Routes and Dosage Ranges	
	Adults	**Children**
Antibody Preparations		
Monoclonal Antibodies		
Alirocumab (Praluent; 🍁 Praluent)	Hyperlipidemia: Sub-Q 75 mg once every 2 wk (maximum dose: 150 mg every 2 wk)	Safety and efficacy not established
Alemtuzumab (Campath, Lemtrada; 🍁 Lemtrada, MabCampath)	Campath (IV): progressively increase to a maintenance of 30 mg/dose three times weekly on alternate days for a total duration of therapy of up to 12 wk Lemtrada (IV): 12 mg daily for 5 consecutive days (total 60 mg), followed 12 mo later by 12 mg daily for 3 consecutive days (total 36 mg); total duration of therapy, 24 mo	Off-label use: Aplastic anemia: Children ≥2 y of age and adolescents (<50 kg): IV 0.2 mg/kg/dose for 10 d (maximum dose: 10 mg/dose) Children ≥2 y of age and adolescents (≥50 kg): IV 10 mg for 10 d
Basiliximab (Simulect; 🍁 Simulect)	20 mg IV within 2 h before transplantation and 20 mg 4 d after transplantation (total of 2 doses)	2–15 y, IV 12 mg/m² up to a maximum of 20 mg for 2 doses, as for adults
Bevacizumab (Avastin Mvasi; 🍁 Avastin, Mvasi, Zirabev)	Varies with disease process and concurrent chemotherapy IV: 5–15 mg/kg every 2–3 wk until disease progression or unacceptable toxicity	Safety and efficacy not established
Bezlotoxumab (Zinplava)	IV, 10 mg/kg as a single dose during antibacterial therapy	Primary CNS tumor: IV 10 mg/kg/dose every 2 wk
Cetuximab (Erbitux; 🍁 Erbitux)	IV, initial loading dose, 400 mg/m² infused over 120 min; maintenance dose, 250 mg/m² infused over 60 min weekly until disease progression or unacceptable toxicity	Safety and efficacy not established
Ipilimumab (Yervoy; 🍁 Yervoy)	IV, melanoma (unresectable or metastatic) 3 mg/kg every 3 wk for maximum of 4 doses; melanoma (adjuvant therapy) IV, 10 mg/kg every 3 wk for 4 doses, followed by 10 mg/kg every 12 wk for up to 3 y	Colorectal cancer: Children ≥12 y and adolescents: IV 1 mg/kg/dose every 3 wk in combination with nivolumab for up to 4 doses Melanoma: Children ≥12 y and adolescents: IV 3 mg/kg every 3 wk for maximum of 4 doses
Nivolumab (Opdivo; 🍁 Opdivo)	IV, 240 mg once every 2 wk or 480 mg every 4 wk until disease progression or unacceptable toxicity	Children ≥12 y or older IV <40 kg: 3 mg/kg once every 2 wk until disease progression or unacceptable toxicity
Panitumumab (Vectibix; 🍁 Vectibix)	After IV 6 mg/kg Administer with an infusion pump over 60 minutes every 14 days using a low-protein-binding 0.2- or 0.22-micrometer in-line filter. Don't give by IV push or bolus. For doses greater than 1,000 mg, infuse over 90 minutes.	Safety and efficacy not established
Omalizumab (Xolair; 🍁 Xolair)	150–375 mg Sub-Q every 2–4 wk based on body weight and pretreatment total serum IgE levels	Children: 6–12 y: Sub-Q 75–375 mg every 2–4 wk Children: ≥12 y: Sub-Q 150–375 mg every 2–4 wk Dose and frequency based on body weight and pretreatment total serum IgE levels
Rituximab (Rituxan, Truxima; 🍁 Rituxan)	Varies with disease process and combination regimens; IV infusion: usual starting dose 375 mg/m²; additional cycles may vary	Autoimmune hemolytic anemia: infants ≥4 mo, children, and adolescents; IV infusion, 375 mg/m² once weekly for 2–4 doses Chronic ITP: children and adolescents; IV infusion, 375 mg/m² once weekly for 4 doses Posttransplant lymphoproliferative disorder: infants ≥11 mo, children, and adolescents; IV infusion, 375 mg/m² once weekly for 3–4 doses

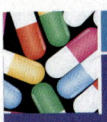

TABLE 13.5

DRUGS AT A GLANCE: Adjuvant Medications Used as Immunosuppressants (Continued)

Drug	Routes and Dosage Ranges	
	Adults	**Children**
Trastuzumab (Herceptin, Kanjinti, Ogivri; 🍁 Herceptin)	Varies with concurrent chemotherapy; IV, initial loading dose, 4 mg/kg infused over 90 min, followed by; maintenance dose, 2 mg/kg infused over 30 min weekly for total of 12–18 wk	Safety and efficacy not established
Polyclonal Antibodies		
Antithymocyte globulin (Atgam, equine; Thymoglobulin, rabbit; 🍁 Thymoglobulin)	Atgam, IV: 15 mg/kg/d for 14 d then every other day for 14 d (total of 21 doses) Thymoglobulin: 1.5 mg/kg/d IV for 7–14 d	Atgam: kidney transplant rejection; children and adolescents; IV, 10–15 mg/kg once daily for 14 d, up to total of 21 doses in 28 d, if needed Aplastic anemia: IV, 10–20 mg/kg once daily for 8–14 d; up to total of 21 doses in 28 d, if needed
Tumor Necrosis Factor-Alpha–Blocking Agents		
Infliximab (Avsola, Remicade, Inflectra, Renflexis; 🍁 Inflectra, Remicade, Remsima, Renflexis)	IV infusion, 3–5 mg/kg initially, 2 and 6 wk later and then every 8 wk	≥3 y and adolescents: IV 5–10 mg/kg/dose
Adalimumab (Humira, Humira Pediatric Crohn's Start, Humira Pen; 🍁 Abrilada, Amgevita SureClick, Hadlima, Humira)	Sub-Q 160 mg every other week then 80 mg/d 15 then 40 mg every other week beginning day 29	≥6 y: 40 kg, Sub-Q 80 mg every other week then 40 day 15; 40 kg, Sub-Q 160 mg then 40 mg/d 15; 40 mg beginning week
Certolizumab (Cimzia, Cimzia Prefilled, Cimzia Starter Kit; 🍁 Cimzia)	Sub-Q 400 mg every 2 wk for 3 doses then every 4 wk	Safety and efficacy not established
Etanercept (Enbrel, Enbrel Mini, Enbrel SureClick; 🍁 Enbrel, Brenzys, Erelzi)	Sub-Q 25 mg twice weekly, 72–96 h apart	≥2 y, 4–17 y, Sub-Q 0.8 mg/kg once weekly up to a maximum of 50 mg per dose
Golimumab (Simponi, Simponi Aria; 🍁 Simponi, Simponi IV)	IV, ankylosing spondylitis, psoriatic arthritis, rheumatoid arthritis 2 mg/kg at weeks 0, 4, and every 8 wk Sub-Q, ulcerative colitis 200 mg at week 0 then 100 mg at week 2, followed by 100 mg every 4 wk	Juvenile idiopathic arthritis, psoriatic arthritis ≥2 y and adolescents: IV 80 mg/m^2/dose at weeks 0, 4, and then every 8 wk thereafter Ulcerative colitis: ≥6 y and adolescents: Induction: <45 kg: 90 mg/m^2 (maximum dose: 200 mg/dose) at week 0 followed by 45 mg/m^2 week 2 (maximum dose: 100 mg/dose) Induction: ≥45 kg: 200 mg/dose at week 0 followed by 100 mg at week 2 Maintenance beginning at week 6 <45 kg: 45 mg/m^2 every 4 wk (maximum dose: 100 mg/dose) ≥45 kg: 100 mg every 4 wk
Leflunomide (Arava; 🍁 Arava, Mylan-Leflunomide)	Sub-Q: 50 mg once a month IV: 2 mg/kg at weeks 0, 4, and then every 8 wk thereafter	Juvenile idiopathic arthritis: 20 kg: PO 10 mg every other day 20–40 kg: PO 10 mg once a day >40 kg: PO 20 mg once daily

(Continued on page 224)

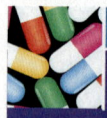

TABLE 13.5
DRUGS AT A GLANCE: Adjuvant Medications Used as Immunosuppressants (Continued)

Drug	Routes and Dosage Ranges	
	Adults	**Children**
Interleukin-Blocking Agents		
Anakinra (Kineret; 🍁 Kineret)	100 mg Sub-Q once daily	Safety and efficacy not established
Ixekizumab (Taltz; 🍁 Taltz)	160 mg (two 80 mg injections) Sub-Q at week 0, followed by 80 mg at weeks 2, 4, 6, 8, 10, and 12, then 80 mg every 4 wk	Safety and efficacy not established
Tocilizumab (Actemra, Actemra ACTPen; 🍁 Actemra) (given with or without methotrexate)	8 mg/kg IV, diluted in 100 mL normal saline infused over 1 h every 4 wk	<25 kg, IV: 8 mg/kg dilute in 50 mL normal saline infused over 1 h every 2–4 wk
Ustekinumab (Stelara; 🍁 Stelara)	Sub-Q by weight <100 kg, 45-mg dose >100 kg, 90-mg dose Initial dose repeated in 4 wk then every 12 wk thereafter	Children ≥12 y may be dosed by weight but FDA approval not received
Fusion Protein Inhibitors		
Abatacept (Orencia, Orencia ClickJect; 🍁 Orencia)	IV, according to body weight, initially at 2 and 4 wk after initial dose then every 4 wk; weight below 60 kg, 500 mg; 60–100 kg, 750 mg; above 100 kg, 1,000 mg	IV, according to body weight, initially at 2 and 4 wk after initial dose then every 4 wk; <75 kg, 10 mg/kg; 75–100 kg, 750 mg; more than 100 kg, 1,000 mg
Belatacept (Nulojix)	IV infusion over 30 min; initially 10 mg/kg before transplant; repeated in 96 h and then at weeks 2, 4, 8, and 12; 5 mg/kg at week 16 and every 4 wk thereafter	Safety and efficacy not established

are stimulated to produce a specific antibody against that antigen. These B lymphocytes are then recovered from the animal's spleen and fused with immortal myeloma cells (a cell line that can live forever in culture). This produces an antibody-secreting hybridoma, a cellular "antibody factory" able to produce large amounts of the desired identical antibody. The antibodies can then be isolated from the culture and prepared for clinical use. Because the antibodies are proteins and would be destroyed if taken orally, immunoglobulins must always be given by parenteral injection.

Because monoclonal antibodies are derived from one single cell line or clone, they can be designed to suppress the specific components of the immune system that cause tissue damage in particular disorders. These antibodies can block cellular growth receptors or inhibit proinflammatory cytokines that mediate inflammatory tissue damage associated with autoimmune disorders or transplant organ rejection. The generic names of drugs of the monoclonal antibodies end in "-mab," which identifies their origin and classification.

Older animal-derived IgA preparations (e.g., antithymocyte globulin [ATG], muromonab-CD3) are themselves antigenic. They usually elicit human antibodies against the animal cells within 2 weeks; hence, their use is appropriate only for short periods. **Murine antibodies** are immunoglobulins created in mouse cells for use as therapeutic treatment for human diseases. Basiliximab is an example of a mouse–human monoclonal antibody. The mouse-derived antibodies have parts of human antibodies added by recombinant DNA technology and are less likely to elicit an immune response. However, because antibodies are proteins, there is a risk of hypersensitivity reactions with administration of all biologic antibody products.

Polyclonal antibodies are mixtures of antibodies (IgA, IgD, IgE, IgG, and IgM) produced by several clones of B lymphocytes. Polyclonal immune globulin preparations contain a mixture of immunoglobulins. Each lymphocyte clone produces structurally and functionally different antibodies, even though a single antigen induces the humoral immune response.

Monoclonal Antibodies

Immunoglobulin monoclonal antibodies are known as mAbs. This classification of drugs is used to treat immunologic diseases. They also reverse drug effects and treat cancer. More than 500 mAbs have been developed. The action of mAbs is to modulate immunity, destroy cells, and neutralize infectious agents. The mAbs recruit proteins and immune cells to kill target cells. Some act through sequestration of plasma proteins or drugs, others block the physiologic interaction with the ligand receptors.

Monoclonal antibodies represent several drug classes that mimic the antibodies produced by the body as part of the immune response to invaders. When a monoclonal antibody attaches to a cell, it can make the cancer cell more visible to the immune system, block growth signals, stop new blood vessels from growing, deliver radiation or chemotherapy to cancer cells, or block the inflammatory process and subsequent destructive changes. **Checkpoint therapy** is an immunologic checkpoint blockade that uses monoclonal antibodies to either activate or antagonize immunologic pathways. The use of antibodies and other techniques circumvents the defenses that tumors use to suppress the immune system. Select monoclonal antibody drugs are presented to familiarize the nurse with the role these medications play to alter or enhance the immune response.

Alirocumab (Praluent) is a human monoclonal IgG antibody that binds to the proprotein convertase kexin type 9. Proprotein convertase kexin type 9 binds to the low-density lipoprotein receptors (LDLRs) to promote LDLR degradation. LDLRs clear the circulating LDL; by decreasing these receptors, the LDL cholesterol levels are decreased. Severe hypersensitivity reaction has been observed with the use of alirocumab.

Quality and Safety Alert: Evidence-Based Practice

Wang et al. (2021) evaluated the effects of alirocumab on cardiovascular events, CV mortality, and all-cause mortality. A total of 13 randomized control studies with 24,815 patients were included. Alirocumab considerably lowered the incidence of CV events when compared to the control group. Treatment with alirocumab has been associated with a decrease in all-cause mortality.

Basiliximab (Simulect) is a humanized IgG monoclonal antibody that acts as IL-2 receptor antagonist. By binding to IL-2 receptors on the surface of activated lymphocytes, it inhibits lymphocyte proliferation and cytokine production, critical components of the cellular immune response involved in rejection reactions. Uses include prevention of rejection of kidney transplants. Prescribers order the drug to be given in combination with cyclosporine and a corticosteroid. Common adverse effects include constipation, diarrhea, edema, fever, headache, hypertension, infection, nausea, and vomiting.

Alemtuzumab (Campath, Lemtrada) is a humanized monoclonal IgG antibody that binds to CD52, a protein present on the surface of mature T and B cells. Healthcare providers use Campath to treat B-cell chronic lymphocytic leukemia, and the drug is available in the United States only through a restricted distribution program. Lemtrada is available for the treatment of relapsing forms of multiple sclerosis (MS).

The FDA recommends that, because of its safety profile, Lemtrada be used to treat MS after inadequate response to at least two drugs. After treatment with alemtuzumab, these CD52-bearing T and B lymphocytes are targeted for destruction, which are believed to be the key mediators of the inflammatory process that causes MS. The FDA has issued a **BOXED WARNING** for alemtuzumab because of numerous risks associated with the development of serious and sometimes fatal autoimmune conditions (Lemtrada), bone marrow suppression (Campath), life-threatening infusion reactions (Campath, Lemtrada), and the development of malignancies, including thyroid cancer, melanoma, and lymphoproliferative disorders (Lemtrada). Prescribers may order antiemetics with alemtuzumab to prevent associated nausea and vomiting. In addition, antihistamines and/or antipyretics may be warranted. Concurrent antiviral drug prophylaxis is necessary.

Bevacizumab (Avastin) is a humanized monoclonal antibody that is classified as a vascular endothelial growth factor receptor inhibitor. This drug blocks growth signals and may prevent tumors from developing blood supplies, thus keeping them small. In a tumor that has already developed a blood vessel network, bevacizumab could cause the vessels to die and tumors to shrink. This drug is useful for (1) first- or second-line treatment with standard chemotherapy agents to treat certain metastatic or recurrent lung, kidney, ovarian, and colorectal cancers and for (2) treatment of glioblastoma multiforme. The FDA has issued a **BOXED WARNING** for bevacizumab because GI perforation has occurred in patients receiving the drug. It should be permanently discontinued if GI perforation occurs.

Bezlotoxumab (Zinplava) is a monoclonal antibody administered for the secondary prevention of *Clostridioides difficile* infection. It is used in conjunction with an antibacterial agent. Bezlotoxumab binds to the *C. difficile* toxin B to neutralize it and prevent the toxic effects.

Cetuximab (Erbitux) and panitumumab (Vectibix) are epidermal growth factor receptor inhibitors. These drugs are useful as monotherapy or in combination with select standard chemotherapy agents to treat certain recurring metastatic colorectal cancers. They attach to epidermal growth factor receptors on cancer cells that accept a certain growth signal; blocking this signal may slow or stop the cancer from growing. Only certain patients with genetic mutations (wild-type KRAS) benefit from treatment; those with colorectal tumors harboring a KRAS mutation demonstrate little or no positive effect from treatment. Clark and Sanoff (2023) recommend testing serum vitamin D levels and supplementing vitamin D to improve cancer-related outcomes in patients diagnosed with metastatic colorectal cancer treated with bevacizumab, cetuximab, or both.

Prior to the administration of cetuximab, the patient should receive an H_1 antagonist, such as diphenhydramine, IV 30 to 60 minutes prior to the first dose and subsequently based on assessment for skin rash or hypersensitivity reaction. Panitumumab must be administered with an infusion pump. During the infusion, the patient should be assessed for allergic skin reactions and hypersensitivity.

Ipilimumab (Yervoy) is a recombinant human IgG immunoglobulin monoclonal antibody that uses immunologic checkpoint blockade (checkpoint therapy) to bind to cytotoxic T-lymphocyte–associated antigen 4, antagonizing the immunosuppressive receptor and thereby enhancing T-cell activation and proliferation. The drug is useful in the treatment of unresectable or metastatic melanoma or as an adjuvant treatment for cutaneous melanoma with regional lymph node involvement. In melanoma, the drug may also indirectly mediate T-cell immune responses against tumors. Ipilimumab was the first treatment to demonstrate enhanced survival from melanoma. The FDA has issued a **BOXED WARNING** ◆ for ipilimumab because severe and fatal immune-mediated adverse effects, such as enterocolitis, dermatitis, neuropathy, and endocrinopathy, may occur.

> **Quality and Safety Alert: Safety**
>
> Ipilimumab used in combination with nivolumab can result in immune-mediated pneumonitis. Frequent pulmonary assessments are indicated when these two medications are combined.

Nivolumab (Opdivo) is an immunoglobulin monoclonal antibody that inhibits cell death of the PD-1 activity to block the ligands PD-L1 and PD-L2 from binding. This action inhibits the immune response. Nivolumab is administered for the treatment of metastatic colorectal, head and neck, and hepatocellular cancer, and Hodgkin lymphoma. It is also administered as adjunctive therapy for melanoma. Adrenal insufficiency may require hormone replacement with corticosteroid therapy.

Omalizumab (Xolair) is a humanized monoclonal antibody that selectively binds to human IgE, reducing sensitivity to inhaled or ingested allergens. IgE is commonly involved in type I hypersensitivity reactions that manifest the most prevalent allergic responses. The drug is used to treat allergic asthma not relieved by inhaled corticosteroids. Chapter 33 contains a further discussion of omalizumab, including dosage, route, and frequency of administration. Because of the risk of anaphylaxis, the FDA has issued a **BOXED WARNING** ◆ for omalizumab. Administration should occur only in a healthcare setting under direct medical supervision by a provider who can initiate treatment of life-threatening anaphylaxis.

Rituximab (Rituxan) is a monoclonal antibody directed against the protein CD20 antigen on the surface of B cells. The drug destroys B cells, so it is effective in treating diseases that are distinguished by overactive, dysfunctional, or extremely numerous B cells. This includes autoimmune disorders and cancers of the white blood cells, such as leukemias and lymphomas. When rituximab attaches to this protein on the B cells, it makes the cells more visible to the immune system, which can then attack. Immunizations should be administered 4 weeks or more before the start of therapy.

Ibritumomab (Zevalin), which is approved for non-Hodgkin lymphoma, combines a monoclonal antibody with radioactive particles. The drug attaches to receptors on cancerous blood cells and delivers a low level of radiation over a longer period helping to protect most of the surrounding healthy cells. Severe cytopenia can result, so blood counts should be monitored; severe cytopenia requires the discontinuation of ibritumomab.

Trastuzumab (Herceptin) is approved as an adjuvant for the treatment of early-stage breast cancer and gastric metastatic cancer that is human epidermal growth factor receptor 2 positive. The drug contains an antibody that attaches to the human epidermal growth factor receptor 2 receptors on cancer cells. The cancer cells then ingest the antibody, which releases a few molecules of chemotherapy, damaging the cancer cells. Chapter 14 contains a further discussion of trastuzumab. The FDA has issued a **BOXED WARNING** ◆ for trastuzumab because its use can result in subclinical and clinical cardiac failure. The risk is increased with anthracycline-containing chemotherapy. Left ventricular function should be assessed with the administration of trastuzumab. The patient should also be assessed within 24 hours of administration for pulmonary toxicity. Monitor the patient for dyspnea and hypotension. The medication should be discontinued with signs and symptoms of anaphylaxis, angioedema, interstitial pneumonitis, or acute respiratory distress syndrome.

Polyclonal Antibodies

ATG (Atgam, Thymoglobulin) is a nonspecific immune globulin preparation used for immunosuppression. Healthcare providers use ATG equine (Atgam), which is obtained from horse serum, to treat rejection reactions after kidney transplants and aplastic anemia in patients who are not considered candidates for bone marrow transplantation. They also use ATG rabbit (Thymoglobulin) to treat these rejection reactions. ATG contains antibodies that destroy lymphoid tissues and decrease the number of circulating T cells, thereby suppressing acute cellular and humoral immune responses. In addition to its high concentration of antibodies against T lymphocytes, the preparation contains low concentrations of antibodies against other blood cells.

With Atgam, potential recipients must have skin tests before administration to determine if they are allergic to horse serum. Because there is a high risk of anaphylactic reactions in recipients previously sensitized to horse serum, patients with positive skin tests require desensitization before drug therapy is begun. It is essential that emergency equipment for airway and allergy management be immediately available when ATG is administered. The FDA has issued a **BOXED WARNING** ◆ for ATG urging that its use be restricted to experienced prescribers.

Cytokine Inhibitors

Two major cytokines in chronic, inflammatory autoimmune disorders are TNF-alpha and IL-1. Knowledge of the role of these cytokines in autoimmune disease along with advances in monoclonal antibody production has led to the development of biologic agents directed against TNF and IL-1. Several monoclonal cytokine-inhibiting antibodies, which either block receptors for or reduce production of these cytokines, are used therapeutically in disorders such as rheumatoid arthritis, Crohn disease, and psoriasis to suppress inflammation and promote tissue healing.

Tumor Necrosis Factor-Alpha–Blocking Agents

The TNF-alpha–blocking agents act more rapidly than cytotoxic immunosuppressants (e.g., methotrexate) for autoimmune disorders and greatly improve the quality of life for patients with rheumatoid arthritis and Crohn disease. However, their use is also associated with significant risks of serious infections, especially with opportunistic organisms. Tuberculosis characterized by increased extrapulmonary and/or disseminated disease may occur. Other serious infections include pneumococcal infections, necrotizing fasciitis, *Pneumocystis* pneumonia, and systemic fungal infections such as aspergillosis and cryptococcosis.

P Infliximab (Remicade) is a humanized IgG monoclonal antibody used to treat rheumatoid arthritis and Crohn disease. The drug inhibits TNF-alpha from binding to its receptors and thus neutralizes its actions. Its ability to neutralize TNF-alpha accounts for its anti-inflammatory effects. Adverse effects of infliximab include formation of autoimmune antibodies and hypersensitivity reactions. Infections reportedly developed in approximately 21% of patients in clinical trials. In addition, dyspnea, hypotension, and urticaria have occurred.

It is important (1) to administer infliximab in settings in which personnel and supplies (e.g., epinephrine, antihistamines, corticosteroids) are available for the treatment of hypersensitivity reactions and (2) to discontinue the drug if severe reactions occur. The drug may aggravate heart failure.

Adalimumab (Humira) is a recombinant monoclonal antibody that binds to TNF-alpha receptor sites and prevents endogenous TNF-alpha from binding to the sites and exerting its injurious effects. Used to treat moderate to severe rheumatoid arthritis, the drug reduces the elevated levels of TNF-alpha in synovial fluid that are thought responsible for pain and joint destruction. Common adverse effects include injection site reactions, upper respiratory tract infections, headache, nausea, and skin rash.

Certolizumab (Cimzia), a TNF-alpha monoclonal antibody, is used for treating refractory Crohn disease. As with the other TNF-alpha blockers, risk of infection and allergic reactions are the major adverse effects of this drug. In addition, caution is advised when using certolizumab in patients with heart failure. Other common adverse effects include upper respiratory or bladder infection, rash, GI upset, headache, and injection site reactions.

Etanercept (Enbrel) is a synthetic TNF receptor that binds with TNF and prevents it from binding with its "normal" receptors on cell surfaces. This action inhibits TNF activity in inflammatory and immune responses. The drug is indicated for the treatment of moderate to severe rheumatoid arthritis in adults and children. In this condition, the TNF increases in joint synovial fluid are considered important in joint inflammation and destruction. Etanercept may be effective in combination with methotrexate in patients who do not respond adequately to methotrexate alone. Common adverse effects include headache, injection site reactions, and infections.

Limited information is available about the use of many of the newer immunosuppressants in children. The FDA has approved three TNF-alpha blockers—etanercept, infliximab, and adalimumab—for use in children 4 to 17 years of age who have severe juvenile rheumatoid arthritis that has not responded to conventional therapy.

Interleukin-Blocking Agents

P Anakinra (Kineret) is a recombinant IL-receptor antagonist. The drug binds to the IL-1 receptor and thereby blocks the inflammatory effects of IL-1. Indications for use include moderate to severe rheumatoid arthritis in adults. It may be used alone or in combination with cytotoxic immunomodulators but not with TNF-alpha–blocking agents or the fusion protein inhibitor abatacept because of increased risk of infection when these biologic agents are combined. Common adverse effects include headache, injection site reactions (redness, bruising, inflammation, pain), infection, nausea, diarrhea, decreased white blood cells, sinusitis, and flulike symptoms.

Tocilizumab (Actemra), a humanized monoclonal antibody that blocks IL-6 receptors, is used in adults and children with severe rheumatoid arthritis that has not responded to conventional immunosuppressants. IL-6, an inflammatory cytokine, is found in higher-than-normal concentrations in joints of patients with rheumatoid arthritis and contributes to chronic inflammation and joint destruction in the disorder. Tocilizumab may be combined with methotrexate. Common adverse effects include upper respiratory infection, hyperlipidemia, hypertension, leukopenia, and elevated liver enzymes. Screening for tuberculosis prior to treatment and monitoring of lipid levels and liver enzymes every 3 months during therapy is recommended.

Ustekinumab (Stelara) is a monoclonal antibody used to treat psoriasis. It blocks IL-12 and IL-23, reducing the inflammatory response and overactivity of T cells. Common adverse effects include headache, infection, lymphocytosis, and a first-dose reaction characterized by chills, fever, muscle aches, and nausea.

Ixekizumab (Taltz) is another monoclonal antibody used to treat adults with moderate to severe plaque psoriasis who are candidates for systemic therapy or phototherapy. This humanized IgG4 monoclonal antibody selectively binds with the IL-17A cytokine and inhibits its interaction with the IL-17 receptor. Ixekizumab inhibits the release of proinflammatory cytokines and chemokines.

Fusion Protein Inhibitors

P Abatacept (Orencia) is a fusion protein inhibitor synthesized from an IgG antibody fused to a cell protein that binds to antigen-presenting molecules. This action prevents the activation of T lymphocytes and the production of inflammatory cytokines. It inhibits activation of T lymphocytes in synovial membranes of joints affected by rheumatoid arthritis and decreases inflammation and structural joint destruction. Abatacept may be used alone or with other antirheumatoid arthritis drugs except anakinra and TNF-alpha–blocking agents. Common adverse effects include dizziness, headache, infections, and nausea. Evidence does not suggest the need for dose adjustment in the presence of liver or kidney disease.

Belatacept (Nulojix), a fusion protein inhibitor, is approved for use in the prevention of acute organ rejection after kidney transplantation. The drug binds to a receptor protein on antigen-presenting cells and inhibits the costimulatory signal required for T-cell activation. This prevents T-cell activation and cytokine production, thus reducing the risk of transplant organ rejection. There is an increased risk of lymphoma in people who develop Epstein–Barr virus infection during belatacept therapy. Because of that risk, the FDA has issued a **BOXED WARNING** ◆ that limits belatacept use to people who test positive for Epstein–Barr virus prior to transplant. Authorities do not recommend the drug for use after liver transplant because of increased risk of graft loss and associated mortality. Adverse effects include anemia, peripheral edema, hypertension, vomiting, diarrhea, constipation, fever, bladder and kidney infection, and leukopenia.

Clinical Application 13.3

- What are the specific teaching points to be covered with Mr. Jones regarding proper self-administration of his medication (cyclosporine, mycophenolate, and prednisone)?

NCLEX Success

1. The nurse should instruct the patient taking cyclosporine or tacrolimus that toxic levels of the drug may be reached if taken with which of the following beverages that inhibit metabolism of the drugs?
    A. orange juice
    B. coffee
    C. grapefruit juice
    D. milk

2. A nurse is caring for a patient who is taking immunosuppressant drugs. The most critical information to teach the patient is ways to do which of the following?
    A. to decrease infection
    B. to avoid weight gain
    C. to maintain a good fluid intake
    D. to increase rest and decrease exercise

3. A patient in an outpatient clinic is taking mycophenolate after a kidney transplant. Which of the following over-the-counter products is likely to interfere with the activity of this immunosuppressant?
    A. diphenhydramine, used for itchy mosquito bites
    B. acetaminophen, used for a tension headache
    C. magnesium/aluminum hydroxide, used for heartburn
    D. benzocaine/dextromethorphan throat lozenges, used for throat irritation

4. A patient is taking leflunomide for rheumatoid arthritis, and the provider monitors the patient's laboratory results on a regular basis. Which of the following laboratory findings indicates that the patient is experiencing an adverse effect?
    A. increased red blood cell count
    B. decreased creatinine
    C. increased white blood cell count
    D. decreased liver enzymes

5. Monoclonal antibodies are engineered to specifically target a certain antigen, such as one found on cancer cells. Which of the following actions by monoclonal antibodies have demonstrated effectiveness in cancer therapy? (Select all that apply.)
    A. Make the cancer cell more visible to the immune system.
    B. Block growth signals.
    C. Increase growth of new blood vessels.
    D. Deliver radiation or chemotherapy to cancer cells.

THE NURSING PROCESS

A concept map outlines the nursing process related to drug therapy considerations in this chapter. Additional nursing implications related to the disease process should also be considered in care decisions.

Assessment

- Assess for signs and symptoms of current infection or factors predisposing patients to potential infection, environmental factors that predispose to infection, nutritional status, and baseline values of laboratory and other diagnostic test results to aid monitoring of responses to immunosuppressant drug therapy.
- Assess adequacy of support systems for transplant recipients and autoimmune conditions.
- Assess patients after transplant for surgical wound healing, signs of organ rejection, and adverse effects of immunosuppressant drugs.
- Assess patients with autoimmune disorders (e.g., rheumatoid arthritis, Crohn's disease) for manifestations of the disease process and responses to drug therapy.

Outcomes of Therapy

The patient will
- Receive appropriate care before and after tissue or organ transplantation, including prevention or early recognition and treatment of rejection reactions.
- Verbalize essential information about immunosuppressant drugs and take according to treatment plan.
- Participate in interventions to prevent infection while immunosuppressed.
- Recognize adverse drug effects and seek treatment promptly.
- Keep appointments for follow-up care.
- Maintain diagnostic test values within acceptable limits.
- Demonstrate appropriate coping strategies in self and support systems.

Nursing Interventions

- Support patient and others to practice and promote good hand hygiene techniques and sterile technique and to avoid contact with infected people.
- Encourage patients to participate in self-care and decision-making when feasible and engage with family members and significant others when feasible.
- Use protective isolation techniques according to institutional policies after transplantation and/or when the neutrophil count is less than 500 per mm^3.
- Teach patient to report fever and other signs of infection immediately.
- Assist patient to maintain adequate nutrition, rest, sleep, and exercise patterns.
- Inform patient about diagnostic test results, changes in therapeutic regimen, and evidence of progress.
- Monitor renal function (creatinine, BUN), liver function (serum bilirubin, AST, ALT, alkaline phosphatase, albumin), CBC, and other diagnostic test results related to organ function throughout drug therapy.
- Consult multidisciplinary healthcare team members on the patient's behalf when indicated.
- Assist patients in learning strategies to manage day-to-day activities during long-term immunosuppression.

Evaluation

- Interview and observe for accurate drug administration.
- Interview and observe for personal hygiene practices and infection-avoiding maneuvers.
- Interview and observe for therapeutic and adverse drug effects with each patient contact.
- Compare current CBC and other reports with baseline values for acceptable levels, according to the patient's condition.
- Observe and assess outpatients regarding ability to comply and cope with follow-up care.
- Observe and assess outpatients regarding ability to recognize adverse effects that require prompt medical intervention.
- Interview and observe for organ function and absence of rejection reactions in posttransplantation patients.

Visit thePoint® at http://thePoint.lww.com/Frandsen13e for answers to NCLEX Success questions (in Appendix A), answers to Clinical Application Case Studies (in Appendix B), additional information on pathophysiology, and more!

REFERENCES AND RESOURCES

Bentata, Y. (2020). Mycophenolates: The latest modern and potent immunosuppressive drugs in adult kidney transplantation: What we should know about them. *Artificial Organs, 44,* 561–576.

Chao, N. J. (2022). Clinical manifestations, diagnosis, and grading of acute graft-versus-host disease. *UpToDate.* Wolters Kluwer.

Clark, J. W. & Sanoff, H. K. (2023). Systemic therapy for nonoperable metastatic colorectal cancer: Selecting the initial therapeutic approach. *UpToDate.* Lexi-Comp, Inc.

Hinkle, J. L., Cheever, K. H., & Overbaugh, K. J. (2021). *Brunner and Suddarth's textbook of medical-surgical nursing* (15th ed.). Wolters Kluwer.

Justiz-Vaillant, A. A., Modi, P., & Mohammadi, O. (2022). Graft versus host disease. StatPearls. https://www.ncbi.nlm.nih.gov/books/NBK538235/#:~:text=Acute%20GVHD%20can%20occur%20in,to%2080%25%20%5B7%5D

Lippincott Advisor. (2022). *Drug information.* Wolters Kluwer.

Manis, J. P. (2022). Overview of therapeutic monoclonal antibodies. *UpToDate.* Wolters Kluwer.

Vierling, J. M. (2022). Liver transplantation in adults: Overview of immunosuppression. *UpToDate.* Wolters Kluwer.

Wang, W., Feng, Z., & Bai, J. (2021). Effects of alirocumab on cardiovascular events and all-cause mortality: A systematic review and meta-analysis. *Reviews in Cardiovascular Medicine, 23*(3), 873–881. doi:10.3108/j.rcm2203093

UpToDate. (2023). *Drug information.* Lexi-Comp, Inc.

Zeiser, R. (2022). Prevention of graft-versus-host disease. *UpToDate.* Wolters Kluwer.

CHAPTER 14

Drug Therapy for the Treatment of Cancer

LEARNING OBJECTIVES

After studying this chapter, you should be able to:

1. Describe the clinical considerations and manifestations of cancer development.
2. Describe the major types of antineoplastic drugs in terms of mechanism of action, indications for use, and the nursing process.
3. Discuss adverse effects of cytotoxic antineoplastic drugs and their prevention or management.
4. Apply patient education regarding the administration of some anticancer drugs.
5. Understand how to implement assessment and nursing interventions in the care of patients undergoing drug therapy for cancer, including how to teach and promote efforts to prevent cancer.

CLINICAL APPLICATION CASE STUDY

Annette D'Angelo is a 64-year-old retired schoolteacher. Six months ago, she had her annual gynecologic visit and received a clean bill of health. Recently, she noticed abdominal bloating and felt extremely full after meals. She went to the emergency department with nausea and vomiting, and the physician diagnosed a bowel obstruction. In surgery, Ms. D'Angelo had a total hysterectomy and salpingo-oophorectomy with bowel resection. During the procedure, the surgeon placed an intraperitoneal catheter and port to allow the administration of intraperitoneal chemotherapy directly into the abdominal cavity. Ms. D'Angelo was found to have stage IV epithelial carcinoma of the ovary and fallopian tube and will require chemotherapy and radiation therapy.

KEY TERMS

Alopecia: hair loss

Cell cycle: series of intracellular events occurring from one cell division to the next

Chemotherapy: the treatment of cancer with an antineoplastic drug or with a combination of these drugs that are typically given in cycles

Mucositis: inflammation and erosion of oral mucous membranes

Mutation: abnormal structural change in the genetic material of a cell

Myelosuppression: bone marrow depression

Neutropenia: low neutrophil count

Oncogenes: genes that have the potential to cause a normal cell to become cancerous

Palliation: alleviation of pain and symptoms without expecting to eliminate the cause

Protooncogenes: genes that have the potential to change into active oncogenes

Remission: period when symptoms of a disease have subsided

Thrombocytopenia: low platelet count

Tumor lysis syndrome: life-threatening condition that occurs when large numbers of cancer cells are killed or damaged simultaneously and release their intracellular contents into the bloodstream

Tumor suppressor genes (also called antioncogenes): these genes inhibit unrestrained cell growth; when they are inactivated, the mutant abnormal cells may be allowed to proliferate

INTRODUCTION

The term *cancer* is used to describe many disease processes with the common characteristics of uncontrolled cell growth, invasiveness, and metastasis as a result of intracellular genetic changes that allow new cells to grow in an unregulated manner. Oncology is the study of cancer and its treatment. Drugs used in oncologic disorders include cytotoxic medications that kill, damage, or slow the growth of cancer cells as well as those that prevent or treat adverse drug effects. **Chemotherapy** is the treatment of cancer with an antineoplastic drug or with a combination of these drugs that are typically given in cycles. It is a major treatment modality for cancer, along with surgery and radiation therapy. Chu and DeVita (2021) have stated that chemotherapy for the treatment of cancer is used in four main clinical settings:

1. Primary induction treatment for advanced disease, which involves administration to patients who have cancer with no other effective approach to treatment.
2. Neoadjuvant treatment for localized disease, which involves the use of surgery and radiation as well as chemotherapy. Neoadjuvant chemotherapy is the administration of systemic therapy before surgery. The goal of this therapy is to reduce the morbidity and mortality and ultimately increase the chances for complete resection of the cancer.
3. Adjuvant treatment, which involves surgery and/or radiation.
4. Direct instillation of chemotherapy in the affected region of the body.

Major groups of anticancer drugs include traditional cytotoxic agents (e.g., alkylating agents, antimetabolites, antitumor antibiotics, plant alkaloids); newer cytotoxic "biologic targeted therapies" (e.g., monoclonal antibodies, growth factor inhibitors); and hormone inhibitors, which are not cytotoxic. In addition, several drugs play a role in ameliorating the adverse effects of cytotoxic drugs (e.g., cytoprotectants), including some immunostimulants.

This chapter describes the characteristics of cancer etiology, pathophysiology, clinical manifestations, and the drugs used in the treatment of this disease. A nurse who has additional training in chemotherapy use administers these drugs. The focus of this chapter is on the nursing management of patients receiving the medication and not on dosing and administration of individual drugs. The general considerations for chemotherapy management are outlined for each major drug group.

OVERVIEW OF CANCER

Normal cells reproduce in response to a need for tissue growth or repair and stop reproduction in response to growth regulation signals. The **cell cycle** is a series of intracellular events occurring from one cell division to another. It is the interval between the "birth" of a cell and its subsequent division into two daughter cells. This cycle involves the orderly stages of growth as well as protein, deoxyribonucleic acid (DNA), and ribonucleic acid (RNA) synthesis (Fig. 14.1). Newly formed daughter cells may then enter the resting phase (G_0) or proceed through the reproductive cycle to form more new cells. Normal cells regulated by normal growth genes are well differentiated in appearance and function, and they have a characteristic life span.

In contrast, malignant cells have lost the normal genetic regulation that controls cell growth, invading normal tissues and taking blood and nutrients away from these tissues. In hyperplasia, these cells grow in an uncontrolled fashion without regard to growth regulation signals (e.g., contact with other cells) that stop the growth

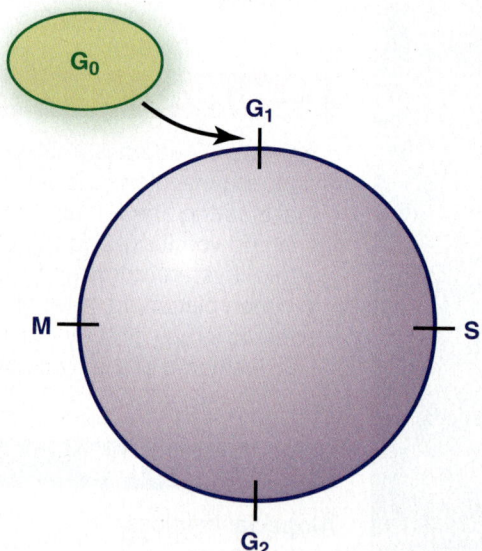

Figure 14.1. Normal cell cycle. The normal cell cycle (the interval between the birth of a cell and its division into two daughter cells) involves several phases. During the resting phase (G_0), cells perform all usual functions except replication–that is, they are not dividing but are capable of doing so when stimulated. Different types of cells spend different lengths of time in this phase, after which they either reenter the cell cycle and differentiate or die. During the first active phase (G_1), ribonucleic acid (RNA) and enzymes required for production of deoxyribonucleic acid (DNA) are developed. During the next phase (S), DNA is synthesized for chromosomes. During G_2, RNA is synthesized, and the mitotic spindle is formed. Mitosis occurs in the final phase (M). The resulting two daughter cells may then enter the resting phase (G_0) or proceed through the reproductive cycle.

of normal cells. In dysplasia, a buildup of extra cells changes how the tissue is organized. Also, malignant cells are undifferentiated, having lost the structural and functional characteristics of the cells from which they originated. In addition, they lack cell adhesion; hence, as well as invading normal tissue, malignant cells enter blood and lymph vessels, circulate through the body, and can produce additional neoplasms at sites distant from the primary tumor.

Clinical Considerations

A malignant cell develops from a damaged normal cell, beginning with a random **mutation** (abnormal structural change in the genetic material of a cell) that occurs in conjunction with acquired damage to genes that regulate normal cell growth. Usually, body defenses (e.g., an immune response) destroy a mutated cell if the DNA damage cannot be repaired by normal cell enzymes. However, if the mutated cell eludes destruction by the immune system and additional mutations develop without repair or apoptosis (programmed cell death) during succeeding cell divisions, malignant transformation may occur. Underlying the failure to repair or destroy these abnormal cells is damage to genes that regulate cell growth; the cells have lost their ability to effectively regulate cell growth. Additional changes allow cells with progressively more malignant characteristics to survive despite their abnormalities. It often takes years for malignant cells to be able to grow into a clinically detectable neoplasm.

Cancer is a heterogeneous disease and has multiple causes, such as environmental factors (tobacco) and genetic factors that may combine to contribute to the progression of malignancy. Tumor cells develop in epithelial, connective, lymph, or nerve tissue. Genetic causes of cancer include mutation of genes, abnormal activation of genes that regulate cell growth and mitosis, and damage to **tumor suppressor genes**. Tumor suppressor genes, also called antioncogenes, inhibit unrestrained cell growth. When they are inactivated, the mutant abnormal cells may be allowed to proliferate.

Abnormal genes, called **oncogenes**, have the potential to cause a normal cell to become cancerous. Oncogenes are mutations of normal growth-regulating genes, called **protooncogenes**, which are present in all body cells. Protooncogenes are genes that have the potential to change into active oncogenes. When protooncogenes are exposed to carcinogens and genetically altered to become oncogenes, they may stimulate cell growth continuously, allowing abnormal, disordered, and unregulated cell replication (Fig. 14.2). The unregulated cell growth and proliferation promoted by oncogenes contribute to neoplastic transformation of the cell. Tumors of the breast, colon, lung, and bone have all been linked to activation of oncogenes.

Abnormal tumor suppressor genes (i.e., absent, damaged, mutated, or inactivated) may be inherited or result from exposure to carcinogens. When a tumor suppressor gene inside a cell is inactivated, abnormal cells can begin unregulated cell growth. One tumor suppressor gene, p53, is present in virtually all normal tissues. When cellular DNA is damaged, the p53 gene allows time for DNA repair and restricts proliferation of cells with abnormal DNA. Mutations of the p53 gene, a common genetic change in cancer, are associated with more than 90% of small cell lung cancers and more than 50% of breast and colon cancers. Mutant p53 proteins can also form complexes with normal p53 proteins and inactivate the function of the normal suppressor gene.

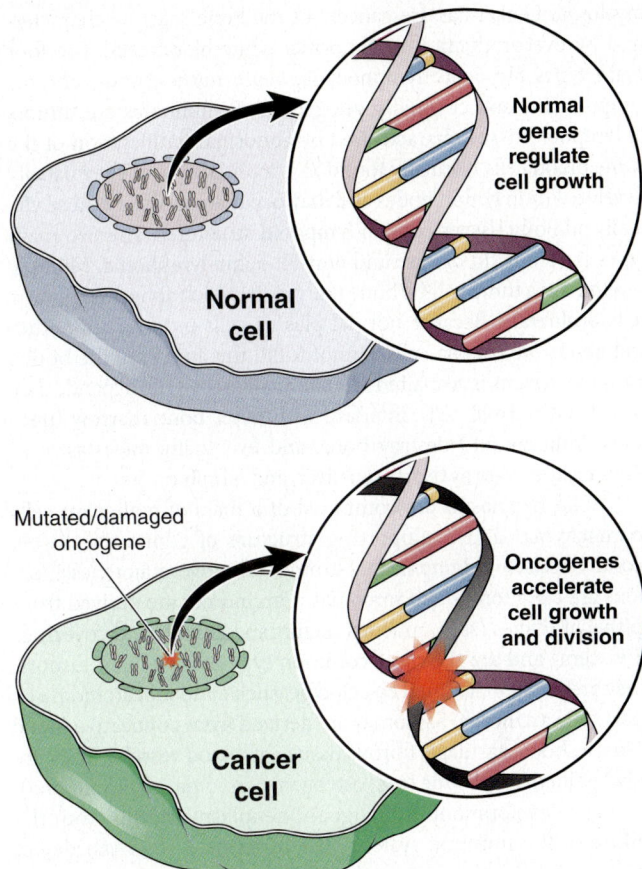

Figure 14.2. A mutated oncogene is a cancer cell. It is irregularly shaped and possesses a break in the DNA, leading to the loss of differentiation and rapid cell growth.

Thus, activation of oncogenes and inactivation of antioncogenes probably both play roles in cancer development. Multiple genetic abnormalities are characteristic of cancer cells and may occur concurrently or sequentially. Overall, evidence indicates that neoplastic transformation is a progressive process involving both a series of cellular mutations and damage to growth-regulating genes, which allows abnormal cells to replicate without normal immune destruction. Malignancy probably results from a combination of genetic and environmental factors experienced over a person's lifetime, including random cell mutations, exposure to carcinogens, and host genetic or tissue characteristics that increase susceptibility to cancer development.

Once a cancer develops, factors influencing its continued growth include blood and nutrient supply, immune response, and hormonal stimulation (e.g., in tumors of the breast, uterus, ovary, and prostate). Malignant tumors can form new blood vessels, a process called angiogenesis, to support their growth and escape immune destruction as a result of their similarity to other normal cells.

Types of Malignant Neoplasms

Malignant neoplasms are classified according to the type of tissue involved and other characteristics. Except for the acute leukemias, they are considered chronic diseases.

Hematologic malignancies involve the bone marrow and lymphoid tissues; they include leukemias, lymphomas, and multiple myeloma. Leukemias are cancers of the bone marrow characterized by overproduction of abnormal white blood cells. The four main types are acute lymphocytic, acute myelogenous, chronic lymphocytic, and chronic myelogenous. Lymphomas are tumors of lymphoid tissue characterized by abnormal proliferation of the white blood cells normally found in lymphoid tissue. They usually develop within lymph nodes and may occur anywhere, because virtually all body tissues contain lymphoid structures. The two main types are Hodgkin disease and non-Hodgkin lymphoma. Multiple myeloma is a tumor of the bone marrow in which abnormal plasma cells proliferate. Because normal plasma cells produce antibodies and abnormal plasma cells cannot fulfill this function, the body's immune system is impaired. As the malignant cells expand, they crowd out normal cells, interfere with other bone marrow functions, infiltrate and destroy bone, and eventually metastasize to other tissues, such as the spleen, liver, and lymph nodes.

Solid neoplasms are composed of a mass of malignant cells (parenchyma) and a supporting structure of connective tissue, blood vessels, and lymphatics (stroma). The two major classifications are carcinomas and sarcomas. Carcinomas are derived from epithelial tissues (skin, mucous membrane, linings and coverings of viscera) and are the most common type of malignant tumors. They are further classified by cell type, such as adenocarcinoma or basal cell carcinoma. Sarcomas are derived from connective tissue (muscle, bone, cartilage, fibrous tissue, fat, blood vessels). They are subclassified by cell type (e.g., osteogenic sarcoma, angiosarcoma).

The development of malignant neoplasms results from the failure of the immune system. The immune system can detect abnormal cells and destroy them. If a patient is immunocompromised, the risk of malignant neoplasm growth increases (Hinkle et al., 2021).

Grading and Staging of Malignant Neoplasms

When a malignant neoplasm is identified, it is further "graded" according to the degree of malignancy and "staged" according to tissue involvement. Grades 1 and 2 are similar to the normal tissue of origin and show cellular differentiation. Grades 3 and 4 are unlike the normal tissue of origin, less differentiated, and more malignant. Staging indicates whether the neoplasm is localized or metastasized and which organs are involved. These characteristics assist in treatment decision making. For example, localized tumors are usually amenable to surgery, radiation, or chemotherapy combined with radiation (concurrent) therapy, whereas metastatic disease requires systemic chemotherapy.

Clinical Manifestations

Clinical manifestations vary according to the location and extent of the disease process. There are few effects initially. However, local effects occur as the tumor grows; it becomes large enough to cause pressure, distort or affect blood supply in surrounding tissues, interfere with organ function, or obstruct ducts and organ outlets. Systemic conditions such as cachexia, anorexia, and weight loss result from the effects of the growing tumor's increasing overall metabolic demands and altering glucose utilization at the cellular level. Other symptoms and signs may include anemia, malnutrition, pain, immunosuppression, infection, hemorrhagic tendencies, thromboembolism, and hypercalcemia, as well as various symptoms related to impaired function of affected organs and tissues.

Drug Therapy

Chemotherapy is most often used to indicate the use of traditional cytotoxic antineoplastic drugs for the treatment of cancer. Except for hormone inhibitors that slow the growth of cancer cells stimulated by hormones, the purpose of all antineoplastic drugs is to damage or kill cancer cells (i.e., be cytotoxic). The goal of treatment with cytotoxic antineoplastic drugs is cure, **remission** (period when symptoms of a disease have subsided), or **palliation** (alleviation of pain and symptoms without expecting to eliminate the cause). In hematologic malignancies such as leukemias, drug therapy is the treatment of choice because the disease is disseminated and must be treated systemically rather than locally, with surgery or radiation. In solid tumors, drug therapy may be used, before (neoadjuvant) or after (adjuvant) surgery or radiation therapy and when there is metastasis that is not surgically resectable.

Antineoplastic drugs are also sometimes used in the treatment of nonmalignant conditions. For example, smaller doses of methotrexate are used as an immunosuppressant for treating the inflammation of rheumatoid arthritis and psoriasis.

Traditional chemotherapeutic drugs share common general characteristics (Box 14.1). Most chemotherapy regimens contain a combination of drugs with actions at different places in the cell cycle process of cell growth and replication (Fig. 14.3), destroying a greater number of cancer cells and reducing the risk of the emergence of drug resistance. Drug resistance may emerge when (1) cancer cells overexpress target genes that prevent the drugs being absorbed by the malignant cells, (2) tumor cells are able to inactivate the drug, or (3) apoptosis that occurs in tumor cells is defective. Oncologists order many newer drugs for use after initial cytotoxic drug therapy to prevent drug resistance from affecting the tumor response.

When administering chemotherapy agents, the prescriber will calculate the dosages utilizing the body surface area method. Chemotherapy administration usually occurs in cycles, depending on the type of cancer and which drugs are used. Cyclic administration involves taking the drugs for a specific period, with a recovery period following each treatment cycle. The recovery period allows time for the patient to produce new, healthy cells to replace the normal rapidly dividing cells that have been affected by the drugs. Chemotherapy is often continued as long as it is effective and does not produce unacceptable toxicity or until there is no longer any evidence of malignancy. Table 14.1 outlines the drugs used in cancer treatment.

CYTOTOXIC ANTINEOPLASTIC DRUGS USED TO TREAT CANCER

The consequences of inappropriate or erroneous chemotherapy may be fatal for patients (from the disease or from the treatment); thus, medical oncologists experienced in use of cancer drugs manage chemotherapy regimens.

 Quality and Safety Alert: Safety

Because of the toxicity of these drugs, nurses who administer intravenous (IV) cytotoxic chemotherapy receive special training and are certified in handling and administering the chemotherapy drugs safely and accurately.

BOX 14.1 Characteristics of Cytotoxic Antineoplastic Drugs

- Most of these drugs kill malignant cells by interfering with cell replication, with the supply and use of nutrients (e.g., amino acids, purines, pyrimidines), or with the genetic materials in the cell nucleus (DNA or RNA).
- The drugs act during the cell's reproductive cycle. Some, called cell cycle specific, act mainly during specific phases such as DNA synthesis or formation of the mitotic spindle. Others act during any phase of the cell cycle and are called cell cycle nonspecific.
- The drugs are most active against rapidly dividing cells, both normal and malignant. Commonly damaged normal cells are those of the bone marrow, the lining of the gastrointestinal tract, and the hair follicles. Healthy cells usually recover fairly soon. However, malignant cells have lost normal genetic growth regulation and continue to actively divide in an unregulated way; thus, more of them are susceptible to the effects of cytotoxic drugs.
- Each drug dose kills a specific percentage of cells. To achieve a cure, all malignant cells must be killed or reduced to a small number that can be killed by the person's immune system.
- Most cytotoxic antineoplastic drugs are potential teratogens, and pregnancy should be avoided during drug therapy and for several months after the therapy stops.
- Weight-based dosing is used to individualize dosing with all cytotoxic drugs due to their potential to cause significant toxicities to normal cells as well as cancer cells.
- Oncologists combine various cytotoxic drugs with different cell cycle activities and different organ toxicities in treatment plans called "regimens" to more effectively kill the cancer cells while minimizing damage to normal tissues.
- Most cytotoxic drugs are water soluble rather than lipid soluble; thus, they do not cross cell membranes readily and must be administered by intravenous injection or infusion.
- Many of the cytotoxic drugs are prodrugs that are metabolized by liver enzymes to active metabolites, which then have cytotoxic activity affecting protein, DNA, or RNA synthesis or cell division.
- Because cytotoxic drugs are primarily metabolized in the liver and then excreted in urine, they can also have toxic effects on the liver and kidney, especially at higher doses.
- Many cytotoxic antineoplastic drugs have U.S. Food and Drug Administration (FDA)-issued **BOXED WARNING** ◆ about potentially serious adverse effects, and all have special precautions for safe usage.

This chapter focuses on the overall nursing considerations for caring for patients receiving chemotherapy, not the administration of particular drugs. Therefore, information is not presented in a prototype format.

Pharmacokinetics

Most cytotoxic drugs are water soluble rather than lipid soluble and require administration by intravenous (IV) injection or infusion. Some, such as cyclophosphamide, are better absorbed and are available as oral formulations. A few, such as methotrexate, are also given intrathecally. The nitrosoureas (e.g., carmustine, lomustine) are unique in being lipid soluble and able to cross the blood–brain barrier; hence, they are widely used in the treatment of brain tumors. Carmustine is also formulated as a dissolving wafer, which can be implanted in the brain tissue at the time of surgical tumor resection.

Liposomal preparations of some cytotoxic drugs (e.g., doxorubicin) use a lipid membrane to encase the drug molecules. Liposomal preparations can increase drug concentration in malignant tissues that are more permeable, allowing the lipid vesicle to more easily concentrate in the tumor, while lowering the concentration in normal tissues that are less permeable, thereby increasing effectiveness and decreasing toxicity (e.g., cardiotoxicity).

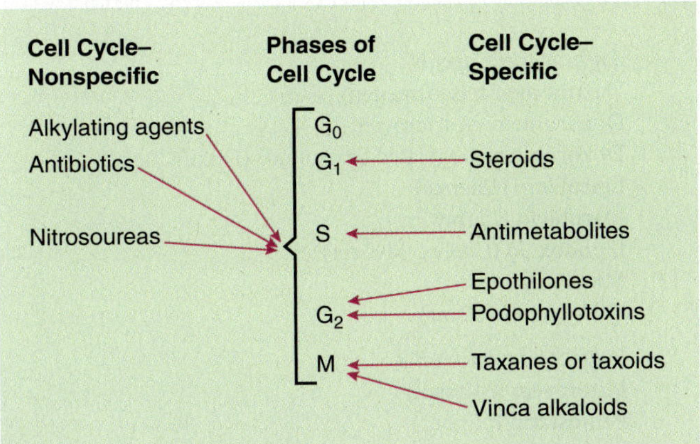

Action

Cytotoxic antineoplastic drugs are usually classified in terms of their mechanisms of action (alkylating agents, antimetabolites) or their sources (plant alkaloids, antibiotics).

Alkylating Drugs

Alkylating drugs include nitrogen mustard derivatives, nitrosoureas, platinum compounds, and triazenes. Before these drugs are administered, it is important to assess liver function.

- Nitrogen mustard derivatives are cell cycle–nonspecific agents, causing cross-linking of DNA and RNA and interfering with subsequent cell division. These agents exert biologic activity by covalently binding to macromolecules of DNA, RNA, and proteins. This activity interrupts the cell's DNA ability to replicate and transcribe leading to cell death or impairing cell function (Clowse & McCune, 2023). The most widely used alkylating drug, a nitrogen mustard derivative, is Ⓟ **cyclophosphamide**. This prodrug begins to act when it is converted metabolically. Cyclophosphamide prevents cell division through the cross-linking of DNA strands, resulting in decreased DNA synthesis. Cyclophosphamide causes an increase in antidiuretic hormone, thus impairing the kidney's ability to excrete water. When a patient experiences chemotherapy-induced nausea the stimulation of antidiuretic hormone release is exacerbated, thus increasing the risk of abnormal kidney function. The urologic toxicity of cyclophosphamide is hemorrhagic cystitis.

Figure 14.3. Cell cycle effects of cytotoxic antineoplastic drugs.

Cell Cycle–Nonspecific	Phases of Cell Cycle	Cell Cycle–Specific
Alkylating agents	G_0	
Antibiotics	G_1	Steroids
Nitrosoureas	S	Antimetabolites
		Epothilones
	G_2	Podophyllotoxins
	M	Taxanes or taxoids
		Vinca alkaloids

TABLE 14.1

Drugs Administered for the Treatment of Cancer

Drug Class	Prototype(s)	Other Drugs in the Class
Alkylating Drugs		
	Cyclophosphamide (nitrogen mustard derivative)	*Nitrogen mustard derivatives* Bendamustine (Bendeka, Treanda) Busulfan (Busulfex, Myleran) Chlorambucil (Leukeran) Estramustine (Emcyt) Ifosfamide (Ifex) Melphalan (Evomela, Alkeran) *Nitrosoureas* Carmustine (BiCNU, Gliadel) Lomustine (Gleostine) Procarbazine (Matulane) Streptozocin (Zanosar) Thiotepa (Tepadina) *Platinum compounds* Carboplatin (Paraplatin) Cisplatin Oxaliplatin *Triazene* Dacarbazine
Antimetabolites		
	Antifolate Methotrexate (Otrexup, Rasuvo, RedTrex, Trexall, Xatmep) *Purine antagonist* Mercaptopurine (Purinethol, Purixan) *Pyrimidine* Fluorouracil (5-FU)	*Antifolate* Pemetrexed (Alimta) Pralatrexate (Folotyn) *Purine antagonist* Cladribine (Mavenclad) Clofarabine (Clolar) Cytarabine (Cytosar) Thioguanine (Tabloid) *Pyrimidine* Azacitidine (Vidaza) Capecitabine (Xeloda) Decitabine Floxuridine Gemcitabine (Infugem) Nelarabine (Arranon) *Miscellaneous* Asparaginase (Erwinaze) Hydroxyurea (Hydrea, Droxia) Rasburicase (Elitek)
Antitumor Antibiotics		
	Daunorubicin	*Anthracycline agents* Dactinomycin (Cosmegen) Doxorubicin (Adriamycin) Doxorubicin (pegylated liposomal) (Doxil) Epirubicin (Ellence) Idarubicin (Idamycin) Lipodox 50 (Caelyx, Myocet) Mitoxantrone Valrubicin (Valstar)
	Bleomycin (Blenoxane) (polypeptide antibiotic)	*Polypeptide antibiotics* Mitomycin (Mitosol) Pentostatin (Nipent)

TABLE 14.1
Drugs Administered for the Treatment of Cancer (Continued)

Drug Class	Prototype(s)	Other Drugs in the Class
Plant Alkaloids		
	Vincristine sulfate (Vincasar PFS)	*Camptothecins* Irinotecan (Camptosar) Topotecan (Hycamtin) *Podophyllotoxins* Etoposide (Toposar, VePesid) *Taxanes* Cabazitaxel (Jevtana) Docetaxel (Docefrez, Taxotere) Paclitaxel (nanoparticle albumin bound) (Abraxane) Paclitaxel (conventional) (Apo-Paclitaxel) *Vinca alkaloids* Vinblastine Vinorelbine
Antimicrotubules		
Epothilone B analogs		Eribulin mesylate (Halaven) Ixabepilone (Ixempra kit)
Biologic Antineoplastic Drugs		
Monoclonal antibodies	Alemtuzumab (Campath, Lemtrada)	Bevacizumab (Avastin) Blinatumomab (Blincyto) Cetuximab (Erbitux) Dinutuximab (Unituxin) Ibritumomab tiuxetan (Zevalin, Tiuxetan) Ipilimumab (Yervoy) Nivolumab (Opdivo) Obinutuzumab (Gazyva) Ofatumumab (Arzerra) Panitumumab (Vectibix) Pembrolizumab (Keytruda) Pertuzumab (Perjeta) Rituximab (Riabni, Rituxan, Ruxience, Truxima) Tositumomab (Bexxar) Trastuzumab (Herceptin)
Growth factor and tyrosine kinase inhibitors	Erlotinib (Tarceva)	Afatinib (Gilotrif) Axitinib (Inlyta) Bosutinib (Bosulif) Cabozantinib (Cabometyx, Cometriq) Ceritinib (Zykadia) Dabrafenib (Tafinlar) Dasatinib (Sprycel) Everolimus (Afinitor Disperz, Zortress) Ibrutinib (Imbruvica) Imatinib (Gleevec) Lapatinib (Tykerb) Lenvatinib (Lenvima) Nilotinib (Tasigna) Palbociclib (Ibrance) Pazopanib (Votrient) Ponatinib (Iclusig) Regorafenib (Stivarga) Sorafenib (NexAVAR) Sunitinib (Sutent) Temsirolimus (Torisel) Trametinib (Mekinist)

(Continued on page 238)

TABLE 14.1

Drugs Administered for the Treatment of Cancer (Continued)

Drug Class	Prototype(s)	Other Drugs in the Class
Proteasome inhibitor	Bortezomib (Velcade)	Carfilzomib (Kyprolis) Ixazomib (Ninlaro)
Antineoplastic Hormone Inhibitors		
	Antiestrogens Tamoxifen (Soltamox) *Aromatase inhibitors* Anastrozole (Arimidex) *Antiandrogens* Flutamide (Eulexin)	Fulvestrant (Faslodex) Toremifene (Fareston) Exemestane (Aromasin) Letrozole (Femara) Abiraterone (Zytiga) Bicalutamide (Casodex) Enzalutamide (Xtandi) Nilutamide (Nilandron)
	Gonadotropin-releasing hormone agonists Leuprolide acetate (Eligard, Lupron Depot)	Goserelin (Zoladex) Triptorelin (Trelstar, Trelstar Mixject)
Cytoprotectant Drugs (see Chapter 11)		Amifostine (Ethyol) Dexrazoxane Epoetin alfa (Epogen, Procrit, Retacrit) Filgrastim (Granix, Neupogen, Nivestym, Releuko, Zarxio) Leucovorin Mesna (Mesnex) Palifermin (Kepivance) Sargramostim (Leukine)

- Nitrosoureas are highly lipid-soluble agents that interfere with DNA replication and RNA synthesis, and they may inhibit essential enzymatic reactions in cancer cells. Carmustine (BiCNU, Gliadel Wafer) and lomustine (Gleostine) are both cell cycle nonspecific. These features allow them to enter the brain and cerebrospinal fluid more readily than other antineoplastic drugs, which make them useful for treating lymphomas and brain tumors.
- Platinum compounds are cell cycle–nonspecific agents that are effective throughout the life cycle of the cell. **(P) Carboplatin** (Paraplatin) is the prototype of the platinum compound chemotherapy agents. They cross-link with DNA, inhibiting DNA, RNA, and protein synthesis. Cisplatin is the most widely used of the platinum compounds.
- Triazene compounds are cell cycle–nonspecific agents with antitumor and mutagenic properties. They interfere with DNA replication, RNA transcription, and protein synthesis. The drugs are effective for metastatic malignant melanoma, Hodgkin disease, and various sarcomas. The most widely used drug in the class is **(P) dacarbazine**. It is widely used for the treatment of metastatic melanoma.

Antimetabolites

Antimetabolites are drugs that are similar to metabolites or nutrients needed by cells for reproduction. Folate antagonists, purine antagonists, pyrimidine analogs, and miscellaneous antimetabolites are commonly prescribed individually or in combination with other chemotherapy agents.

- Folate antagonists such as **(P) methotrexate** (Otrexup, Rasuvo, RedTrex, Trexall, Xatmep) interfere with DNA synthesis, repair, and cellular replication, thus inhibiting the formation of folates.
- Purine antagonists such as **(P) mercaptopurine** (Purinethol, Purixan) inhibit DNA and RNA synthesis. This action occurs in the S phase of the cell cycle.
- Pyrimidine analogs such as **(P) fluorouracil** also affect DNA and RNA synthesis. The incorporation of fluorouracil into the tumor cell RNA, replacing uracil, means that cell growth is then affected.

Miscellaneous antimetabolites include asparaginase, hydroxyurea (Droxia, Hydrea), and rasburicase (Elitek). Asparaginase reduces the asparagine source that provides the destructive action of leukemia cells, thus inhibiting cell function. Hydroxyurea stops the cell cycle at the G_1/S phase and reduces G_1 phase to stop DNA repair. Rasburicase converts uric acid to allantoin: uric acid is increased in some malignancies.

These drugs are all most effective against rapidly growing tumors. Individual drugs vary in their effectiveness with different kinds of cancer.

Antitumor Antibiotics

Two types of antitumor antibiotics are noted as anthracycline agents and polypeptide agents. **(P) Daunorubicin** binds to DNA so that DNA and RNA transcription is blocked. They are active in all phases of the cell cycle, and their cytotoxic effects are similar to those of the alkylating agents. **(P) Bleomycin**

(Blenoxane) inhibits DNA, RNA, and protein synthesis in susceptible cells, preventing cell division. Mitomycin (Mitosol) causes DNA cross-linking and inhibits DNA synthesis.

Plant Alkaloids

Plant alkaloids include several types of drugs.

- Camptothecins (also called DNA topoisomerase inhibitors) inhibit an enzyme required for DNA replication and repair.
- Podophyllotoxin, etoposide acts by delaying the transit of cells from the S phase and can arrest cells in the late S phase or early G_2 phase of the cell cycle and prevent mitosis. These medications are topoisomerase II inhibitors, which cause DNA strand breakage.
- Taxanes are antimicrotubular agents that promote microtubule assembly and inhibit the weakening of microtubules. They inhibit depolymerization of microtubules, stopping the cell cycle and the tumor cell proliferation.
- Vinca alkaloids are also antimicrotubular agents, with **vincristine sulfate** as the prototype. Vinblastine and vinorelbine are the other drugs in the class. They are cell cycle–specific agents that interfere with cell mitosis. Despite having similar structures, they have different antineoplastic activities and adverse effects.

> **! Quality and Safety Alert: Safety**
>
> - Vincristine is dispensed in a minibag or other flexible plastic container (NOT IN A SYRINGE).
> - Vincristine should not be delivered to the patient at the same time with any medications intended for central nervous system (CNS) administration.
> - Vincristine is contraindicated in patients with demyelinating Charcot-Marie-Tooth syndrome.
> - There is a risk of dyspnea if vincristine is administered with mitomycin C.
> - Gastrointestinal (GI) toxicity and necrosis can occur if vincristine is administered with mitomycin C.

Use

Certain combinations of cytotoxic drugs with different cytotoxic activities in the cell cycle and different organ toxicities are most effective in certain types of cancer. Hence, concurrent administration of multiple drugs based on the patient's type of malignancy may be necessary. However, when both cytotoxic and hormone inhibitor drug therapies are required, concurrent administration is not appropriate, because hormone antagonists decrease malignant cell growth and cytotoxic agents are most effective when the cells are actively dividing. Patients with breast cancer usually receive a hormone-inhibiting drug before a cytotoxic drug in metastatic disease and after chemotherapy when used for adjuvant treatment.

Weight-based dosing is used to individualize dosing of all cytotoxic drugs to minimize toxicity of normal cells. In addition, some cytotoxic drugs have a cumulative maximum dose that can be given for cancer treatment without risk of irreversible vital organ damage (e.g., heart failure with doxorubicin, pulmonary fibrosis with carmustine and bleomycin). Table 14.2 provides route and dosage information for some cytotoxic antineoplastic drugs.

Patient-related variables specific to the use of cytotoxic chemotherapy agents include the following:

- Age:
  - Childhood cancer is rare but is one of the leading causes of disease-related death in individuals aged 1 to 19 years. Within that age group, mortality is higher in males. Also, mortality is greater in adolescents than in young children.
  - The most common childhood cancers include acute leukemias, central nervous system (CNS) tumors, germ cell tumors, lymphomas, neuroblastoma, retinoblastoma, sarcomas, thyroid cancer, and Wilms tumor.
  - Pediatric oncologists should design, order, and supervise chemotherapy for children. To determine dosage of cytotoxic drugs, prescribers should use body surface area, because this takes overall size into account.

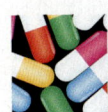

TABLE 14.2
DRUGS AT A GLANCE: Cytotoxic Antineoplastic Drugs

Drug	Routes and Dosage Ranges*	Clinical Uses	Adverse Effects
Alkylating Drugs			
Nitrogen Mustard Derivatives			
Cyclophosphamide (Procytox)	Induction therapy, PO 1–5 mg/kg/d; IV 40–50 mg/kg in divided doses over 2–5 d or 10–15 mg/kg every 7–10 d or 3–5 mg/kg twice weekly Maintenance therapy, PO 1–5 mg/kg daily	Hodgkin disease; non-Hodgkin lymphomas; leukemias; cancer of head and neck, breast, lung, or ovary; multiple myeloma; neuroblastoma	Bone marrow depression, nausea, vomiting, alopecia, hemorrhagic cystitis, hypersensitivity reactions, secondary leukemia, or bladder cancer
Bendamustine (Belrapzo, Bendeka, Treanda; Treanda)	IV 100 mg/m² on days 1 and 2 of a 21-d treatment cycle up to 8 cycles	Chronic lymphocytic leukemia, Hodgkin lymphoma, and multiple myeloma	Peripheral edema, fatigue, skin rash, weight loss, and lymphocytopenia

(Continued on page 240)

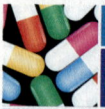

TABLE 14.2
DRUGS AT A GLANCE: Cytotoxic Antineoplastic Drugs (Continued)

Drug	Routes and Dosage Ranges*	Clinical Uses	Adverse Effects
Busulfan (Busulfex, Myleran; ❋ Busulfex, Myleran)	60 mg/kg or 1.8 mg/m²/d; usual range 4–8 mg/d; titrate dose to maintain WBC ≥ 15,000/mm³	Chronic lymphocytic leukemia	Edema, tachycardia, hypertension, thrombosis, hepatic venoocclusive disease, nausea, vomiting, stomatitis, hypomagnesemia, hyperglycemia, hypocalcemia, hypophosphatemia, neutropenia, and thrombocytopenia
Chlorambucil (Leukeran; ❋ Leukeran)	US labeling: PO 1 mg/kg/d for 3–6 wk or 0.4 mg/kg pulsed doses administered intermittently, biweekly, or monthly (increased by 0.1 mg/kg/dose until response or toxicity is seen) Canadian labeling: 0.15 mg/kg/d until WBC is 10,000/mm³, interrupt treatment for 4 wk, then may resume at 0.1 mg/kg/dose until response or toxicity is seen	Chronic lymphocytic leukemia, Hodgkin and non-Hodgkin lymphomas	Bone marrow depression, hepatotoxicity, and secondary leukemia
Estramustine (Emcyt)	PO 140 mg (1 h before or 2 h after meals). Do not administer with milk	Metastatic castration-resistant prostate cancer	Edema, nausea, vomiting, leukopenia, thrombocytopenia, and increased bilirubin
Ifosfamide (Ifex; ❋ Ifex)	IV 1.2 g/m²/d for 5 consecutive days. Repeat every 3 wk or after white blood cell and platelet counts return to normal after a dose	Germ cell testicular cancer	Bone marrow depression, hemorrhagic cystitis, nausea and vomiting, alopecia, CNS depression, and seizures
Melphalan (Alkeran, Evomela; ❋ Alkeran)	PO 6 mg/d for 2–3 wk, then 28 drug-free days, then 2 mg daily IV 16 mg/m² every 2 wk for 4 doses and then every 4 wk	Multiple myeloma and ovarian cancer	Bone marrow depression, nausea and vomiting, and hypersensitivity reactions
Nitrosoureas			
Ⓟ Carmustine (BiCNU, Gliadel; ❋ BiCNU)	IV 150–200 mg/m² every 6 wk Wafer, implanted in brain after tumor resection	Hodgkin disease, non-Hodgkin lymphomas, multiple myeloma, and brain tumors	Bone marrow depression, nausea, and vomiting
Lomustine (Gleostine; ❋ CeeNU)	PO 130 mg/m² every 6 wk	Hodgkin disease and brain tumors	Nausea and vomiting and bone marrow depression
Procarbazine (Matulane; ❋ Matulane)	PO 100 mg/m² days 1–7 every 21 d	Hodgkin lymphoma	Edema, flushing, alopecia, diaphoresis, hepatic insufficiency, jaundice, hypersensitivity, herpes virus, hearing loss, polyuria, and arthralgia
Streptozocin (Zanosar; ❋ Zanosar)	Daily schedule: 500 mg/m² for 6 d every 6 wk Weekly schedule: 1,000 mg/m² once weekly; if therapeutic response not achieved after 2 wk may increase dose to 1,500 mg/m² weekly	Pancreatic islet carcinoma metastasis	Glucose intolerance, bone marrow suppression, extravasation of tissue, and increased lactate dehydrogenase

TABLE 14.2
DRUGS AT A GLANCE: Cytotoxic Antineoplastic Drugs (Continued)

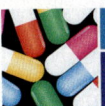

Drug	Routes and Dosage Ranges	Clinical Uses	Adverse Effects
Thiotepa (Tepadina; 🍁 Tepadina)	Bladder cancer: intravesical: 60 mg in 30–60 mL NS retained for 2 h once weekly for 4 wk Intercavity: 0.6–0.8 mg/kg Ovarian and breast cancer: IV 0.3–0.4 mg/kg every 1–4 wk	Bladder cancer Breast cancer Ovarian cancer	Dizziness, fatigue, alopecia, contact dermatitis, anemia, bleeding, leukopenia, thrombocytopenia, dysuria, urinary retention, and asthma
Platinum Compounds			
ⓟ Carboplatin (Paraplatin)	IV infusion 360 mg/m² on day 1 every 4 wk	Palliation of ovarian cancer and endometrial cancer	Bone marrow depression, nausea and vomiting, and nephrotoxicity
Cisplatin	IV 100 mg/m² once every 4 wk	Advanced carcinomas of testes, bladder, and ovary	Nausea, vomiting, anaphylaxis, nephrotoxicity, bone marrow depression, ototoxicity, and peripheral neuropathy
Oxaliplatin	IV infusion 85 mg/m² every 2 wk	Advanced colon cancer (with 5-fluorouracil and leucovorin)	Anaphylaxis, anemia, increased risk of bleeding or infection, and cold-induced acute neurotoxicities
Triazene			
ⓟ Dacarbazine	Hodgkin lymphoma: 375 mg/m² on days 1 and 15 every 4 wk Metastatic malignant melanoma: 250 mg/m² over 30 min once daily on days 1–5 every 3 wk	Hodgkin lymphoma Metastatic malignant melanoma	Infusion site pain Alopecia Nausea and vomiting Severe myelosuppression
Antimetabolites			
Miscellaneous			
Asparaginase (Erwinaze)	IM or IV 25,000 units/m² three times/wk (Mon., Wed., and Fri.) for 6 doses	Acute lymphocytic leukemia	Hypersensitivity reactions, including anaphylaxis
Hydroxyurea (Hydrea, Droxia, Siklos; 🍁 Apo-Hydroxyurea, Mylan-Hydroxyurea, Hydrea)	PO 15 mg/kg/d as a single dose; if blood counts are acceptable, may increase by 5 mg/kg/d Droxia (sickle cell anemia): 15 mg/kg/d as a single dose orally: monitor blood counts every 2 wk Canadian labeling: PO 20–30 mg/kg daily Solid tumors: 80 mg/kg as a single dose every 3rd day	Chronic myelogenous leukemia (CML), melanoma, ovarian cancer, and head and neck cancer Sickle cell anemia	Bone marrow depression, nausea, vomiting, and peripheral neuritis
Rasburicase (Elitek; 🍁 Fasturtec)	0.2 mg/kg/d for up to 5 d	Secondary tumor lysis	Peripheral edema, headache, rash, hypophosphatemia, nausea, and vomiting
Antifolates			
ⓟ Methotrexate (Otrexup, Rasuvo, Rheumatrex, Trexall, Xatmep; 🍁 ACH-Methotrexate, Metoject, PMS-Methotrexate)	Intrathecal: 15 mg/d one of early intensification phase. Repeat in 4 wk CNS prophylaxis: 15 mg/d on days 1, 8, 15, 22, and 29 PO 20 mg/m² on days 36, 43, 50, 57, and 64 Choriocarcinoma: PO, IM 15 mg/m² daily for 5 d	Leukemias; non-Hodgkin lymphomas; osteosarcoma; choriocarcinoma of testes; cancers of breast, lung, head, and neck	Bone marrow depression, nausea, vomiting, mucositis, diarrhea, fever, and alopecia

(Continued on page 242)

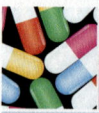

TABLE 14.2
DRUGS AT A GLANCE: Cytotoxic Antineoplastic Drugs (Continued)

Drug	Routes and Dosage Ranges	Clinical Uses	Adverse Effects
Pemetrexed (Alimta; ✽ Alimta, Taro-Pemetrexed)	IV 500 mg/m² on day 1 of each 21-d cycle (in combination with cisplatin)	Malignant pleural mesothelioma; non–small cell lung cancer; bladder, cervical, ovarian, thymic cancers	Fatigue, rash, nausea, anorexia, anemia, stomatitis, and pharyngitis
Purines			
Ⓟ Mercaptopurine (Purinethol (Purixan); ✽ Purinethol)	PO 1.5–2.5 mg/kg/d (100–200 mg for average adult)	Acute and chronic leukemias; lymphoblastic lymphoma	Bone marrow depression, nausea, vomiting, and mucositis
Cladribine (Mavenclad; ✽ Mavenclad)	IV infusion 0.09 mg/kg/d for 7 consecutive days	Hairy cell leukemia, Acute myeloid leukemia, T-cell large granular lymphocytic leukemia	Bone marrow depression, nausea, and vomiting
Clofarabine (Clolar; ✽ Clolar)	52 mg/m²/d for 5 d every 2–6 wk CrCl 30–60 reduce dose by 50%	Acute lymphoblastic leukemia, Acute myeloid leukemia	Tachycardia, nausea, vomiting, thrombocytopenia, anemia, leukopenia, neutropenia, and somnolence
Cytarabine (✽ PMS, Cytarabine)	IV 100 mg/m²/d continuous infusion for 7 d or 200 mg/m²/d continuous infusion (as 100 mg/m² over 12 h every 12 h) for 7 d	Acute myeloid leukemia	Bone marrow depression, nausea, vomiting, anaphylaxis, mucositis, and diarrhea
Thioguanine (Tabloid; ✽ Lanvis)	PO 2 mg/kg/d. May increase to 3 mg/kg/d if no response after 4 wk	Acute myeloid leukemia, acute lymphoblastic leukemia	Hyperuricemia, fluid retention, splenomegaly, stomatitis, anemia, ascites, and esophageal varices
Pyrimidines			
Ⓟ Fluorouracil (5-FU)	IV: dosage is depended on cancer staging and cancer type Topical: apply to skin cancer lesion two times per day for 2–6 wk	Carcinomas of the anus, bladder, breast, cervix, colon, esophageal, penis, stomach, and pancreas; solar keratoses and basal cell carcinoma; Children: Hepatoblastoma, nasopharyngeal carcinoma	Bone marrow depression, nausea, vomiting, and mucositis; pain, pruritus, and burning at site of application
Azacitidine (Vidaza; ✽ NAT-Azacitidine, REDDY-Azacitidine, Vidaza)	Sub-Q, initial cycle: 75 mg/m²/d for 7 d and then every 4 wk; dose can be increased to 100 mg/m²/d Treatment for a minimum of 6 cycles	Acute myeloid leukemia Myeloid dysplastic syndrome	Chest pain, peripheral edema, nausea, vomiting, and bone marrow depression
Capecitabine (Xeloda; ✽ ACH-Capecitabine, SANDOZ Capecitabine TARO-Capecitabine, TELVA-Capecitabine, Xeloda)	PO 1,250 mg/m² twice daily for 2 wk, every 21 d (can be given in combination with docetaxel)	Anal, biliary tract, breast, colon, esophageal, gastric, pancreas, and ovarian cancer	Diarrhea, edema, vomiting, and hyperbilirubinemia
Decitabine	15 mg/m² over 3 h every 8 h for 3 d (134 mg/m²/cycle) every 6 wk for at least 4 cycles	Acute myeloid leukemia Myeloid dysplastic syndrome	Chest pain, peripheral edema, nausea, vomiting, bone marrow depression, diarrhea, and hyperbilirubinemia
Floxuridine	0.5 g administered as a continuous hepatic intra-arterial infusion with an infusion pump	Colorectal cancer Hepatic metastasis	Diarrhea, stomatitis, bone marrow depression, cholecystitis, jaundice

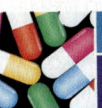

TABLE 14.2
DRUGS AT A GLANCE: Cytotoxic Antineoplastic Drugs (Continued)

Drug	Routes and Dosage Ranges*	Clinical Uses	Adverse Effects
Gemcitabine (Infugem)	IV 1,250 mg/m² on days 1 and 8 of 21 day cycle; given with paclitaxel	Breast cancer; Biliary, pancreatic, kidney, head and neck cancer; Ovarian cancer	Fever, flulike symptoms, headache, cough, myelosuppression, alopecia
Nelarabine (Arranon; ✱ Atriance)	IV 1,500 mg/m² on days 1, 3, and 5 repeated every 21 d	T-cell leukemia; Lymphoma	Dizziness, headache, paresthesia, somnolence, constipation, thrombocytopenia
Antitumor Antibiotics			
Ⓟ Bleomycin	IV, IM, sub-Q 0.25–0.5 units/kg once or twice weekly	Squamous cell carcinoma, Hodgkin and non-Hodgkin lymphomas, and testicular carcinoma	Pulmonary toxicity, mucositis, alopecia, nausea, vomiting, hypersensitivity reactions, and hypotension
Ⓟ Daunorubicin (✱ Cerubidine)	IV <60 y 45 mg/m² daily for 3 d; ≥60 y 30 mg/m² daily for 3 d; After course in each age group, then administer days 1 and 2 in combination with cytarabine	Acute leukemias and lymphomas	Cardiac failure, alopecia, red urine discoloration, bone marrow depression, and hyperuricemia
Dactinomycin (Cosmegen; ✱ Cosmegen)	IV 15 mcg/kg/d for 5 d and repeated every 2–4 wk	Rhabdomyosarcoma, Wilms tumor, choriocarcinoma, testicular carcinoma, and Ewing sarcoma	Bone marrow depression, nausea, and vomiting. Extravasation may lead to tissue necrosis
Doxorubicin conventional (Adriamycin)	Adults, IV 60–75 mg/m² every 21 d; Children, IV 30 mg/m² daily for 3 d, repeated every 4 wk	Acute leukemias; lymphomas; carcinomas of breast, lung, and ovary, multiple myeloma, osteosarcoma, uterine sarcoma, and others	Bone marrow depression, alopecia, mucositis, gastrointestinal (GI) upset, and cardiomyopathy. Extravasation may lead to tissue necrosis
Doxorubicin (pegylated liposomal) (Doxil; ✱ Caelyx)	IV infusion 20 mg/m², once every 3 wk	AIDS-related Kaposi sarcoma and multiple myeloma	Bone marrow depression, nausea, vomiting, fever, and alopecia
Epirubicin (Ellence; ✱ PMS-Epirubicin)	IV infusion 100–120 mg/m² every 3–4 wk	Breast cancer, soft tissue carcinoma	Cardiotoxicity, decreased left ventricular ejection fraction, atrioventricular block, and bradycardia
Idarubicin (Idamycin PFS)	IV injection 12 mg/m²/d for 3 d, with cytarabine	Acute myeloid leukemia	Congestive heart failure, headache, alopecia, nausea, vomiting, dark yellow urine, seizure, and peripheral neuropathy
Mitomycin (Mutamycin)	IV 20 mg/m² every 6–8 wk	Metastatic carcinomas of stomach and pancreas, gastric, hepatocellular, vulvar cancer (advanced)	Bone marrow depression, nausea, and vomiting. Extravasation may lead to tissue necrosis
Mitoxantrone	IV infusion 12 mg/m² on days 1–3, for induction of remission in leukemia	Acute nonlymphocytic leukemia and prostate cancer	Bone marrow depression, heart failure, and nausea
Pentostatin (Nipent)	IV 4 mg/m² every other week	Hairy cell leukemia unresponsive to interferon alfa	Bone marrow depression, hepatotoxicity, nausea, and vomiting
Valrubicin (Valstar)	Intravesically 800 mg once weekly for 6 wk	Bladder cancer	Dysuria, urgency, frequency, bladder spasms, and hematuria

(Continued on page 244)

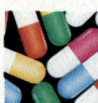

TABLE 14.2
DRUGS AT A GLANCE: Cytotoxic Antineoplastic Drugs (Continued)

Drug	Routes and Dosage Ranges	Clinical Uses	Adverse Effects
Plant Alkaloids			
Camptothecins			
Irinotecan (Camptosar)	IV infusion 125 mg/m² over 90 min on days 1, 8, 15, and 22 of a 6-wk treatment cycle (may adjust upward to 150 mg/m²)	Metastatic cancer of colon or rectum, recurrent glioblastoma	Bone marrow depression and diarrhea
Topotecan (Hycamtin; 🍁 TEVA-Topotecan)	IV infusion 1.5 mg/m² daily for 5 consecutive days every 21 d	Advanced ovarian cancer and small cell lung cancer, cervical cancer	Bone marrow depression, nausea, vomiting, and diarrhea
Podophyllotoxins			
Etoposide (Toposar; 🍁 VePesid, GEN-Etoposide)	IV 50–100 mg/m²/d for 5 d PO 100–200 mg/m²/d for 5 d Administer daily doses >200 mg in 2 divided doses	Small cell lung cancer and testicular cancer Non-Hodgkin lymphoma, non–small cell lung cancer, small cell lung cancer, and testicular cancer	Bone marrow depression, allergic reactions, nausea, vomiting, and alopecia
Antimicrotubule/Taxane Derivatives			
Cabazitaxel (Jevtana; 🍁 Jevtana)	Premedicate with IV diphenhydramine 25 mg, dexamethasone 8 mg, and ranitidine 50 mg 30 min before cabazitaxel IV 25 mg/m² once every 3 wk (in combination with prednisone)	Prostate cancer	Fatigue, diarrhea, bone marrow depression, alopecia, mucosal inflammation, febrile neutropenia, and increased AST, ALT, and bilirubin
Docetaxel	IV infusion 60–100 mg/m² every 3 wk	Advanced breast cancer and non–small cell lung cancer	Bone marrow depression, nausea, vomiting, hypersensitivity reactions, and peripheral neuropathy
Paclitaxel (nanoparticle albumin bound) (Abraxane)	Breast cancer: IV 260 mg/m² every 3 wk Non–small cell lung cancer: IV 100 mg/m² on days 1, 8, and 15 of each 21-d cycle (in combination with carboplatin) Pancreatic adenocarcinoma, biliary cancer: IV 125 mg/m² on days 1, 8, and 15 of a 28-d cycle (in combination with gemcitabine)	Metastatic breast cancer, locally and advanced or metastatic non–small cell lung cancer, and metastatic pancreatic adenocarcinoma Metastatic biliary cancer	ECG abnormality, peripheral edema, peripheral neuropathy, alopecia, nausea, vomiting, bone marrow depression, oral candidiasis, keratitis, and increased serum creatinine
Paclitaxel (conventional)	Premedicate with PO dexamethasone 20 mg at 12 and 6 h prior to the dose, IV diphenhydramine 50 mg 30–60 min prior to dose, and IV famotidine Breast cancer: 175 mg/m² over 3 h every 3 wk for 4 cycles (administer sequentially following an anthracycline-containing regimen) Non–small cell lung cancer: IV 135 mg/m² over 24 h every 3 wk with cisplatin Ovarian: 135 or 175 mg/m² 3 h every 3 wk (if previously untreated, combine with cisplatin)	Breast cancer, non–small cell lung cancer, and ovarian cancer	ECG abnormality, peripheral edema, peripheral neuropathy, alopecia, nausea, vomiting, bone marrow depression, and increased serum creatinine

TABLE 14.2
DRUGS AT A GLANCE: Cytotoxic Antineoplastic Drugs (Continued)

Drug	Routes and Dosage Ranges*	Clinical Uses	Adverse Effects
Antimicrotubule/Vinca Alkaloid			
ⓟ Vincristine sulfate (Vincasar PFS)	Adults: IV 1.4 mg/m² weekly Children: IV 2 mg/m² weekly	Hodgkin and other lymphomas, acute leukemia, neuroblastoma, and Wilms tumor	Peripheral neuropathy. Extravasation may lead to tissue necrosis
Vinblastine	Adults: IV 3.7–11.1 mg/m² (average 5.5–7.4 mg/m²) weekly Children: IV 2.5–7.5 mg/m² weekly	Metastatic testicular carcinoma, Hodgkin disease, and choriocarcinoma	Bone marrow depression, nausea, and vomiting. Extravasation may lead to tissue necrosis
Vinorelbine	IV injection 30 mg/m² once weekly	Non–small cell lung cancer	Bone marrow depression and peripheral neuropathy. Extravasation may lead to tissue necrosis
Antimicrotubule: Epothilone B Analog			
Eribulin mesylate (Halaven; 🍁 Halaven)	IV ¼ mg/m² on days 1 and 8 of a 21-d treatment cycle	Breast cancer and liposarcoma	Fatigue, weight loss, constipation, nausea, vomiting, weakness, dyspnea, fever, cough, and increased ALT
Ixabepilone (Ixempra kit)	IV infusion 40 mg/m² over 3 h, every 3 wk	Advanced breast cancer	Bone marrow suppression, peripheral neuropathy, nausea, vomiting, diarrhea, mucositis, and hypersensitivity

AIDS, acquired immunodeficiency syndrome; ALT, alanine aminotransferase; AST, aspartate aminotransferase; CNS, central nervous system; ECG, electrocardiogram; WBC, white blood (cell) count.
*Dosages may vary significantly or change often, according to use in different types of cancer and in different combinations.

- Special efforts are necessary to maintain nutrition, organ function, psychological support, growth and development, and other aspects of health status during and after therapy.
- Chemotherapy-induced nausea and vomiting (CINV) impacts the quality of life in children receiving chemotherapy (Sherani et al., 2021).
- Research has led to the adoption of a triple therapy regimen of antiemetic prophylaxis in pediatric patients with cancer; a 5-HT3 antagonist (granisetron, ondansetron, tropisetron, or palonosetron), dexamethasone, and neurokinin-1 antagonist (aprepitant) (Di Lorenzo, 2023).
- Alternative and complementary therapy for the treatment of CINV includes ginger or other herbal supplements for functional dyspepsia or other motility disorders. Hypnotherapy may benefit children who experience anticipatory nausea and vomiting prior to chemotherapy administration.
- Long-term follow-up care is important for childhood cancer survivors because they have an increased risk of health problems. For example, children who receive an anthracycline drug (e.g., doxorubicin) are at increased risk for cardiotoxic effects (e.g., heart failure) during treatment or after receiving the drug. Efforts to reduce cardiotoxicity include using alternative drugs (if effective), giving smaller cumulative doses of the anthracycline and observing patients closely so that early manifestations can be recognized and treated before heart problems occur. Children also are at increased risk for developing cancers in later life (e.g., leukemia) (LaCasce & Ng, 2021). In addition, long-term survivors of Hodgkin lymphoma may develop an impairment in the growth of soft tissues or bones, thyroid dysfunction, gonadal dysfunction, cardiopulmonary toxicity, second malignancies, or the impairment of overall health (McClain & Kamdar, 2022).
- Increasing age is a risk factor for development of cancer, and the number of new cancer cases is about 10 times greater in people 65 years of age and older. Although older adults are more likely to have chronic cardiovascular, kidney, and other disorders (comorbidities) that increase their risks of serious adverse effects, it is important to consider several factors besides age when treating older adults for cancer.
- Physiologic age-related changes that may add to the challenge of managing cancer include decreased kidney function, reduced hepatic blood flow, and diminished cardiac reserve. For example, older adults with impaired kidney function are more sensitive to the neurotoxic effects of vincristine and need reduced dosages of some drugs (e.g., cyclophosphamide, methotrexate). Creatinine clearance (CrCl) must be monitored in these patients because serum creatinine is not

a reliable indicator of kidney function due to older adults' decreased muscle mass. Older adults also must be assessed for signs and symptoms of toxicity of chemotherapy agents due to diminished metabolism and elimination of drugs. In patients with liver metastasis, drug metabolism will be greatly affected because most antineoplastic drugs are metabolized by the liver. Thus, decreased liver blood flow and decreased liver size can lead to drug accumulation due to decreased clearance, resulting in increased toxicity.

Quality and Safety Alert: Patient-Centered Care

The Multinational Association of Supportive Care in Cancer (MASCC) updated the antiemetic guidelines for CINV for adults. The first-line therapy is metoclopramide. The second-line therapy is levomepromazine (methotrimeprazine) and olanzapine. Third-line therapy includes tropisetron and levosulpiride (Davis et al., 2021).

Quality and Safety Alert: Evidence-Based Practice

Herrstedt et al. (2022) examined the prevention of CINV in older patients. The authors examined studies and variables to determine evidence-based recommendations for the prophylaxis of CINV in the past 40 years. The prevention of CINV has improved with the use of $5-Ht_3$-receptor antagonists and NK_1-receptor antagonists. None of the guidelines examined provided significant recommendations for older patients receiving chemotherapy. In treating CINV with older adult patients, the lowest dose of olanzapine should be administered. Further research needs to be directed toward CINV treatment in the older adult population.

- Reproduction, pregnancy, and lactation:
  - Cytotoxic drugs are potentially embryotoxic, teratogenic, and carcinogenic.
  - Patients who are sexually active and able to become pregnant should use effective contraception.
  - Cytotoxic chemotherapy agents result in intrauterine growth restriction, prematurity, and low birth weight infants.
  - Cytotoxic chemotherapy is not recommended for use in breast-feeding.
- Abnormal kidney function and hepatic impairment:
  - The alkylating drugs may be nephrotoxic. These effects usually subside when the drug is stopped. For example, cisplatin, an alkylating agent, has multiple active metabolites that are renally excreted, causing kidney tubular damage. When a patient already has significant kidney dysfunction, oncologists avoid using this drug.
  - The antimetabolites may also be nephrotoxic. Methotrexate use in patients with impaired kidney function may lead to accumulation of toxic amounts or additional kidney damage. Evaluation of the patient's kidney status should take place before and during methotrexate therapy. If significant abnormal kidney function occurs, it is necessary to discontinue the drug or to reduce the dosage until kidney function improves. In patients who receive high doses of methotrexate for treatment of osteosarcoma, the drug may cause kidney damage resulting in acute kidney disease. Nephrotoxicity is attributed to precipitation of methotrexate and a metabolite in kidney tubules. Reducing abnormal kidney function involves monitoring kidney function closely, ensuring adequate hydration, alkalinizing the urine, and measuring serum drug levels. With mercaptopurine, dosage reduction is necessary to prevent nephrotoxicity. With irinotecan, dosage reduction is necessary in patients with moderate abnormal kidney function (CrCl, 20–39 mL/minute).
  - Caution is warranted with many other drugs when used in patients with abnormal kidney function. Cytarabine is detoxified mainly by the liver. However, patients with abnormal kidney function may have more central nervous system–related adverse effects, and dosage reduction may be necessary. Gemcitabine has resulted in mild proteinuria and hematuria during clinical trials, and hemolytic–uremic syndrome has been reported in a few patients. Signs of this syndrome may include anemia, elevated bilirubin and reticulocyte counts, and kidney failure. If this condition occurs, it is essential to stop gemcitabine immediately; hemodialysis may be required. Bleomycin is rarely associated with nephrotoxicity, but its elimination half-life is prolonged in patients with a CrCl of less than 35 mL/minute. Asparaginase often increases blood urea nitrogen; acute kidney disease and fatal abnormal kidney function have been reported. Procarbazine may cause more severe adverse effects if given to patients with impaired kidney function. Hospitalization is recommended for the first course of treatment.
  - Some antineoplastic drugs are hepatotoxic, and the liver is the site of the metabolism of many. Patients with metastatic cancer often have impaired liver function, and their risk of further impairment or accumulation of toxic drug levels increases. It is necessary to monitor hepatic function with most drugs. However, abnormal values for the usual liver function tests (e.g., serum aspartate aminotransferase [AST] and alanine aminotransferase [ALT], bilirubin, alkaline phosphatase) may indicate liver injury but do not indicate decreased ability to metabolize drugs. Dosage reduction may be necessary in some cases. The following paragraphs describe the hepatic effects of selected cytotoxic chemotherapy drugs and precautions to reduce hepatotoxicity.
  - Alkylating drugs may lead to hepatotoxicity.
  - Antimetabolites also have hepatotoxic effects. Methotrexate may cause acute hepatotoxicity (increased serum ALT and AST, hepatitis) as well as chronic hepatotoxicity (fibrosis and cirrhosis). Chronic toxicity is potentially fatal. It is more likely to occur after prolonged use (e.g., 2 years or longer) and after a total dose of at least 1.5 g. It is essential that liver function tests be closely monitored in patients with preexisting liver damage or impaired hepatic function. Gemcitabine has increased serum ALT and AST in most patients during clinical trials. Mercaptopurine causes hepatotoxicity, especially with higher doses (above 2.5 mg/kg/d) and in combination with doxorubicin. Encephalopathy and fatal liver necrosis have occurred. It is essential to stop the drug if signs of hepatotoxicity (e.g.,

jaundice, hepatomegaly) occur. Serum aminotransferases, alkaline phosphatase, and bilirubin should be monitored weekly initially and then monthly.
- Antitumor antibiotics may be hepatotoxic as well. Daunorubicin (liposomal formulation) requires dosage reduction according to serum bilirubin (e.g., bilirubin 1.2–3 mg/dL, three fourths the normal dose; bilirubin above 3 mg/dL, one half the normal dose). Doxorubicin toxicity increases with impaired hepatic function. It is necessary to perform liver function tests before drug administration and to reduce the dosage of both regular and liposomal formulations according to the serum bilirubin. Idarubicin is not appropriate for patients with a serum bilirubin above 5 mg/dL.
- Some plant alkaloids have hepatic effects. Irinotecan may cause abnormal liver function tests in patients with liver metastases. Paclitaxel may cause more toxicity in patients with impaired hepatic function. Hospitalization is recommended for the first course of therapy. Topotecan is cleared from plasma more slowly in patients with hepatic impairment. Vinblastine and vincristine may cause more toxicity with hepatic impairment, and dosage should be reduced 50% for patients with a direct serum bilirubin value above 3 mg/dL.
- Asparaginase is hepatotoxic in most patients; it may increase preexisting hepatic impairment and hepatotoxicity of other medications. Signs of liver impairment, which usually subside when the drug is discontinued, include (1) increased AST, ALT, alkaline phosphatase, and bilirubin and (2) decreased serum albumin, cholesterol, and plasma fibrinogen. Procarbazine may cause increased hepatotoxicity in cases of impaired hepatic function.
- Specific healthcare environments:
  - Critical care: Cytotoxic drug treatment is often significantly dose reduced or discontinued in critically ill patients with compromised perfusion to the liver and kidneys, which can increase toxicity.
  - Palliative care: Chemotherapy, which can alleviate pain or obstruction in critically ill patients with advanced cancer, is used on a case-by-case basis with consideration of therapeutic benefits versus the risks of treatment toxicities.
  - Home care: Although administration of cytotoxic drug therapy occurs most frequently in a clinic or hospital setting, people often self-administer oral cytotoxic drugs, and some give themselves IV infusions at home. All cytotoxic drugs are hazardous substances and require special handling and disposal, according to safety guidelines, in the home. The home care nurse may be involved in a wide range of activities associated with antineoplastic drug therapy, including administering the anticancer drugs, administering other drugs to prevent or manage adverse effects, and assessing patient and family responses to therapy.

Quality and Safety Alert: Patient-Centered Care

Psychosocial issues that may affect treatment include access to care, financial and transportation issues, functional status, need for independence, and social support.

Quality and Safety Alert: Patient-Centered Care

A major nursing role involves teaching about the disease process, managing pain and other symptoms, providing information about the specific anticancer drugs being given, preventing or managing adverse drug effects, preventing infection, maintaining adequate food and fluid intake, and ensuring self-care measures. Referral to palliative care early in the disease trajectory has resulted in improved quality of life, cost of care, and even survival in patients with metastatic cancer.

Adverse Effects

Common adverse effects of the cytotoxic chemotherapy agents include **alopecia** (hair loss), anemia, bleeding, fatigue, **mucositis** (inflammation and erosion of oral mucous membranes), nausea and vomiting, **neutropenia** (low neutrophil count), **myelosuppression** (bone marrow depression), and **thrombocytopenia** (low platelet count). The dose-limiting toxicity for most of the cytotoxic drugs is myelosuppression.

The administration of irinotecan may cause diarrhea. Early forms of diarrhea may be associated with cholinergic symptoms. The administration of atropine can prevent these cholinergic symptoms. Loperamide should be administered with late forms of diarrhea, which is life threatening.

Quality and Safety Alert: Safety

When cytotoxic drugs are combined, it is essential to monitor the complete blood (cell) count before and after each treatment to allow time for bone marrow recovery before the next treatment.

Other problems may include damage to the heart, liver, lungs, kidneys, or nerves. In general, adverse effects depend on the specific drugs used and the patient's health status. Baseline liver and kidney function testing is necessary before all cytotoxic drug treatment, and the presence of preexisting disease may contraindicate use of a drug that is associated with serious liver or kidney toxicity. Box 14.2 describes the adverse effects of treatment with antineoplastic drugs.

With treatment of leukemias and lymphomas, a serious, life-threatening adverse effect called **tumor lysis syndrome** may occur. This condition develops when large numbers of cancer cells are killed or damaged simultaneously and release their intracellular contents into the bloodstream. As a result, hyperkalemia, hyperphosphatemia, hyperuricemia, hypomagnesemia, hypocalcemia, and acidosis develop. Signs and symptoms depend on the severity of the metabolic imbalances but may include GI upset, fatigue, altered mental status, hypertension, muscle cramps, paresthesias (numbness and tingling), tetany, seizures, electrocardiographic changes (e.g., dysrhythmias), cardiac arrest, reduced urine output, and acute kidney disease. To prevent or minimize tumor lysis syndrome, aggressive hydration with IV normal saline, alkalinization with IV sodium bicarbonate, and administration of allopurinol (e.g., 300 mg daily for

BOX 14.2 Complications of Chemotherapy and Their Management

Complications of anticancer drug therapy range from minor to life threatening. Vigilant efforts toward prevention or early detection and treatment are needed.

- **Nausea** and **vomiting** commonly occur and are treated with antiemetics (see Chapter 38). With traditional cytotoxic chemotherapy, the drugs are most effective when started before drug administration and continued on a regular schedule for 24 to 48 hours afterward. An effective regimen is a serotonin receptor antagonist (e.g., ondansetron) and a corticosteroid (e.g., dexamethasone), given orally or intravenously. Other measures include a benzodiazepine (e.g., lorazepam) for anticipatory nausea and vomiting and limiting oral intake for a few hours. Guidelines have not been developed for managing nausea and vomiting with the biologic antineoplastic drugs.
- **Anorexia** interferes with nutrition. Well-balanced meals, with foods the patient is able and willing to eat, and nutritional supplements, to increase intake of protein and calories, are helpful.
- **Fatigue** is often caused or aggravated by anemia and can be treated with administration of erythropoietin. Alternating periods of activity and rest and an adequate diet may also be helpful.
- **Alopecia** (hair loss) occurs with cyclophosphamide, doxorubicin, methotrexate, and vincristine. Counsel patients taking these drugs that hair loss is temporary and that hair may grow back a different color and texture; suggest the purchase of wigs, hats, and scarves before hair loss is expected to occur; and instruct patients to use a mild shampoo and avoid rollers, permanent waves, hair coloring, and other treatments that damage the hair.
- **Mucositis** (also called stomatitis) often occurs with the antimetabolites, antibiotics, plant alkaloids, and growth factor/tyrosine kinase inhibitors. It usually lasts 7 to 10 days and may interfere with nutrition; lead to oral ulcerations, infections, and bleeding; and cause pain. Nurse or patient interventions to minimize or treat this mucositis include the following:
  - Brush the teeth after meals and at bedtime with a soft toothbrush and floss once daily. Stop brushing and flossing if the platelet count drops below 20,000/mm³ because gingival bleeding is likely. Teeth may then be cleaned with soft, sponge-tipped or cotton-tipped applicators.
  - Rinse the mouth several times daily, especially before meals (to decrease unpleasant taste and increase appetite) and after meals (to remove food particles that promote growth of microorganisms). One suggested solution is 1 tsp of table salt and 1 tsp of baking soda in 1 quart of water. Commercial mouthwashes are not recommended, because their alcohol content causes drying of oral mucous membranes.
  - Encourage the patient to drink fluids. Systemic dehydration and local dryness of the oral mucosa contribute to the development and progression of mucositis. Pain and soreness contribute to dehydration. Fluids usually tolerated include tea, carbonated beverages, ices (e.g., popsicles), and plain gelatin desserts. Fruit juices may be diluted with water, ginger ale, Sprite, or 7 Up to decrease pain, burning, and further tissue irritation. Drinking fluids through a straw may be more comfortable, because this decreases contact of fluids with painful ulcerations.
  - Encourage the patient to eat soft, bland, cold, nonacidic foods. Although individual tolerances vary, it is usually better to avoid highly spiced or rough foods.
  - Remove dentures entirely or for at least 8 hours daily because they may irritate oral mucosa.
  - Inspect the mouth daily for signs of inflammation and lesions.
  - Give medications for pain. Local anesthetic solutions, such as viscous lidocaine, can be taken a few minutes before meals. Because the mouth and throat are anesthetized, swallowing and detecting the temperature of hot foods may be difficult, and aspiration or burns may occur. Doses should not exceed 15 mL every 3 hours or 120 mL in 24 hours. If systemic analgesics are used, they should be taken 30 to 60 minutes before eating.
  - For oral infections resulting from mucositis, local or systemic antimicrobial drugs are used. Fungal infections with *Candida albicans* can be treated with antifungal tablets, suspensions, or lozenges. Severe infections may require systemic antibiotics, depending on the causative organism as identified by cultures of mouth lesions.
- **Infection** is common because the disease and its treatment lower host resistance to infection.
  - If fever occurs, especially in a patient with neutropenia, possible sources of infection are usually cultured, and antibiotics are started immediately.
  - Severe neutropenia can be prevented or its extent and duration minimized by administering filgrastim or sargramostim to stimulate the bone marrow to produce leukocytes. A protective environment may be needed to decrease exposure to pathogens.
  - Instruct the patient to avoid exposure to infection by avoiding crowds, anyone with a known infection, and contact with fresh flowers, soil, animals, or animal excrement. Frequent and thorough hand hygiene by the patient and everyone involved in their care is necessary to reduce exposure to pathogenic microorganisms.
  - The patient should take a bath daily and put on clean clothes. In addition, the perineal area should be washed with soap and water after each urination or defecation.
  - When venous access devices are used, take care to prevent them from becoming sources of infection. For implanted catheters, inspect and cleanse around exit sites according to agency policies and procedures. Use strict sterile technique when changing dressings or flushing the catheters. For peripheral intravenous lines, the same principles of care apply, except that sites should be changed every 3 days or if signs of phlebitis occur.
  - Avoid indwelling urinary catheters when possible. When they are necessary, cleanse the perineal area with soap and water at least once daily and provide sufficient fluids to ensure an adequate urine output.
  - Help the patient maintain a well-balanced diet. Oral hygiene and analgesics before meals may increase food intake. High-protein, high-calorie foods and fluids can be given between meals. Nutritional supplements can be taken with or between meals. Provide fluids with high nutritional value (e.g., milkshakes or nutritional supplements) if the patient can tolerate them and has an adequate intake of water and other fluids.
- **Bleeding** may be caused by thrombocytopenia and may occur spontaneously or with minor trauma. Precautions

BOX 14.2 Complications of Chemotherapy and Their Management (Continued)

should be instituted if the platelet count drops to 50,000/mm³ or below. Measures to avoid bleeding include giving oprelvekin to stimulate platelet production and prevent thrombocytopenia; avoiding trauma, including venipuncture and injections, when possible; using an electric razor for shaving; checking skin, urine, and stool for blood; and, for platelet counts less than 20,000/mm³, stopping brushing and flossing the teeth.

- **Extravasation.** Several drugs (called vesicants) cause severe inflammation, pain, ulceration, and tissue necrosis if they leak into soft tissues around veins. Thus, efforts are needed to prevent extravasation or to minimize tissue damage if it occurs.
  - Identify patients at risk for extravasation, including those who are unable to communicate (e.g., patients who are sedated, infants), have vascular impairment (e.g., from multiple attempts at venipuncture), or have obstructed venous drainage after axillary node surgery.
  - Be especially cautious with the anthracyclines (e.g., doxorubicin) and the vinca alkaloids (e.g., vincristine). Choose peripheral IV sites carefully, avoiding veins that are small or located in an edematous extremity or near a joint. Inject the drugs slowly (1–2 mL at a time) into the tubing of a rapidly flowing IV infusion, for rapid dilution and detection of extravasation. Observe the venipuncture site for swelling and ask the patient about pain or burning. After a drug has been injected, continue the rapid flow rate of the IV fluid for 2 to 5 minutes to flush the vein.
  - If using a central IV line, do not give the drug unless patency is indicated by a blood return. Using a central line does not eliminate the risk of extravasation.
  - When extravasation occurs, the drug should be stopped immediately. Techniques to decrease tissue damage include aspirating the drug (about 5 mL of blood, if able) through the IV catheter before it is removed, elevating the involved extremity, and applying warm (with dacarbazine, etoposide, vinblastine, and vincristine) or cold (with daunorubicin and doxorubicin) compresses. Nurses involved in cytotoxic chemotherapy must know the procedure to be followed if extravasation occurs so that it can be instituted immediately.

- **Hyperuricemia** from rapid breakdown of malignant cells can lead to kidney damage. Risks of nephropathy can be decreased by high fluid intake, high urine output, alkalinizing the urine with sodium bicarbonate, and giving allopurinol to inhibit uric acid formation.

- **Hand–foot syndrome** (also called palmar–plantar erythrodysesthesia or erythema) is a sunburn type of skin reaction with redness, tenderness, and possibly peeling, numbness, and tingling of palms and soles. It is associated with some traditional cytotoxic drugs (e.g., capecitabine, doxorubicin, fluorouracil) and some growth factor/tyrosine kinase inhibitors (e.g., lapatinib, sorafenib, sunitinib). It is attributed to leakage of drug from capillaries into the palms and soles; heat and friction increase leakage. Management efforts involve decreasing heat and friction (e.g., minimizing exposure of hands and feet to hot water), avoiding increased pressure (e.g., from long walks, squeezing small implements in cooking, gardening), or applying ice packs for 15 or 20 minutes at a time. Acetaminophen may be taken for discomfort.

- **Complications of intraperitoneal chemotherapy with cytotoxic agents:** With the administration of intraperitoneal cisplatin, the risk of nephrotoxicity is noted, and the clinician must pay attention to the patient's hydration status. This risk is increased with CINV. The nurse monitors the patient's albumin level and assesses for ascites and peripheral edema. Hypersensitivity reactions are noted with a few patients receiving cytotoxic chemotherapy, particularly cisplatin or carboplatin. If a hypersensitivity reaction occurs, the patient should receive IP normal saline. Assess the patient for abdominal pain due to the infusion of abdominal fluids. Low-grade pain is treated with acetaminophen or nonsteroidal anti-inflammatory drugs (NSAIDs). Assess the ability to flush the access port. Inability to access the port or infuse the drug requires a fluoroscopic examination (Markman & Olawaiye, 2021).

---

adults and 10 mg/kg/d for children) to reduce uric acid levels are necessary. Treatment of hyperkalemia may include IV dextrose and regular insulin (to drive potassium into cells) or Kayexalate to eliminate potassium in feces. Treatment of hyperphosphatemia may include administration of aluminum hydroxide or another phosphate-binding agent. Maintenance of urine pH of 7 or higher prevents kidney failure due to precipitation of uric acid crystals in the kidneys. Hemodialysis may be necessary if the other measures are ineffective in maintaining urinary elimination.

Contraindications

There are several contraindications to the use of cytotoxic antineoplastic drugs.

- Generally, pregnancy and lactation preclude their use.
- Myelosuppression may be a factor.

Quality and Safety Alert: Safety

Use of the cytotoxic agents that cause bone marrow suppression is not appropriate in people with a white blood count less than 2,000 cells/mm³, a neutrophil count less than 1,500 cells/mm³, and/or platelet count less than 50,000/mm³.

Hematologic monitoring before and after each treatment is necessary to limit the risk of infection and serious bleeding.

- The taxanes, paclitaxel, and docetaxel can produce severe peripheral neuropathy involving the sensory nerve fibers. It is called a dying-back process, affecting the distal nerve and then the Schwann cells and neuronal cells (Lee, 2019). In the event of severe neuropathy or the neutrophil count is less than 500 mm³ for 1 week or longer, hematopoietic growth factor (granulocyte colony-stimulating factor) should be initiated.

- As previously stated, specific cytotoxic drugs may lead to certain adverse effects, and these drugs may be contraindicated in individual patients. Severe hepatic or abnormal kidney function is also a contraindication to the use of specific cytotoxic agents that cause significant toxicities to the liver and kidney, respectively.

Nursing Implications

The nurse should be aware that each antineoplastic drug is used in the schedule, route, and dosage judged to be most effective for a particular type of cancer. With combinations of drugs, it is necessary to adhere to the recommended schedule precisely because safety and effectiveness may be schedule dependent.

Preventing Interactions

Interactions involving changes in hepatic metabolism are the most common reason for cytotoxic drug interactions. Cytochrome P450 (CYP) 3A4 enzymes in the liver metabolize several cytotoxic drugs, including taxanes, vinca alkaloids, and irinotecan. Drugs that inhibit these enzymes such as the azole antifungals, erythromycins, and protease inhibitors may increase blood levels and toxicities of a cytotoxic drug. CYP3A4 enzyme inducers, on the other hand (e.g., carbamazepine, griseofulvin, phenytoin, St. John's wort), can decrease blood levels and cytotoxic drug effects. In addition, use of noncancer drugs that have the same toxicities can cause drug interactions. Antimicrobials with kidney toxicity, such as amphotericin B and aminoglycosides, can increase the nephrotoxicity of cisplatin and carboplatin. The chemotherapy nurse and a pharmacist should evaluate the potential for drug interactions.

Administering the Medication

A certified chemotherapy nurse administers IV cytotoxic drugs. The nurse verifies free flow of IV fluid into the vein and assesses adequate blood return. Peripheral infusion of cytotoxic drugs occurs through a newly initiated IV catheter in a large, upper extremity vein. Whenever possible, veins of the antecubital fossa, wrist, dorsum of the hand, and the arm where an axillary lymph node dissection has been performed are ones to avoid. Insertion of an indwelling central venous catheter is often appropriate for patients who have poor peripheral venous access, who require many doses of chemotherapy, or who require continuous infusions. When multiple drugs are given, administration of the drug most likely to cause venous irritation takes place first. Some of the cytotoxic drugs given by IV infusion are potential tissue irritants or vesicants and cause tissue necrosis if they leak outside the vein into surrounding tissue (extravasation).

Intraperitoneal chemotherapy with cisplatin or paclitaxel requires premedication with diphenhydramine, cimetidine, dexamethasone, ondansetron or its equivalent, and aprepitant. CINV increases the risk of kidney toxicity associated with the administration of cisplatin. Before accessing the IP port, a topical anesthetic, commonly liposomal lidocaine, is applied 30 minutes before the procedure. The chemotherapy is administered into the IP port with a 19- or 20-gauge right-angle needle. The chemotherapy is mixed with 1 L of warmed (37 degree) normal saline. The patient is placed in a supine or semi-Fowler position. The bed should be no higher than 30 degrees. The treatment is infused under gravitational flow. A second liter of saline is instilled as tolerated. During the infusion of the second liter of fluids, the patient is repositioned from side to side every 15 minutes for 1 hour to help disperse the infusate. After administration, the port and catheter are flushed with at least 10 mL of heparin 100 units/mL. The needle is removed and a pressure dressing is applied. The dressing can be removed after 12 hours (Markman & Olawaiye, 2021).

> **Clinical Application 14.1**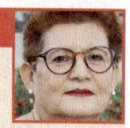
>
> - It is 2 weeks since Ms. D'Angelo's surgery. She is scheduled to begin her chemotherapy.
> - Her chemotherapy regimen is as follows:
>   - Cycle length: 21 days
>   - Total cycles: 6 cycles
>   - Paclitaxel 135 mg/m^2 IV-dilute in 500 mL NS or D5W administered over 24 hours (Day 1)
>   - Cisplatin 100 mg/m^2 IP (Day 2)
>   - Paclitaxel 60 g/m^2 IP (Day 8)
> - What patient teaching will you provide to Ms. D'Angelo?
> - What interventions should be implemented before, during, and after the administration of cisplatin and paclitaxel?
> - What interventions should be implemented with the administration of intraperitoneal chemotherapy?

> **Clinical Application 14.2**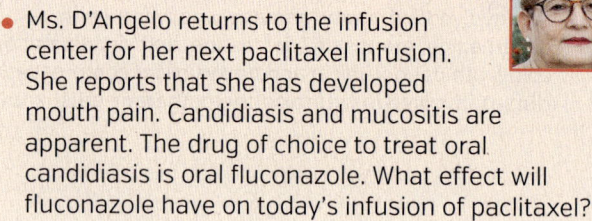
>
> - Ms. D'Angelo returns to the infusion center for her next paclitaxel infusion. She reports that she has developed mouth pain. Candidiasis and mucositis are apparent. The drug of choice to treat oral candidiasis is oral fluconazole. What effect will fluconazole have on today's infusion of paclitaxel?

Established infusion guidelines aid nurses who administer these drugs and increase the safety of both patients and nurses. These guidelines include the following:

- Ensure appropriate orders (e.g., be sure the prescriber is qualified to write chemotherapy orders; do not accept verbal or telephone orders).
- Do not give injectable drugs unless certified to administer chemotherapy.
- If handling a powdered form of a drug, avoid inhaling the powder.
- Do not prepare the drugs in eating areas (to decrease risk of oral ingestion).
- Ensure adequate hydration before and after administration, frequent voiding, and use of a protective medication (e.g., mesna) to help prevent hemorrhagic cystitis.

> **Quality and Safety Alert: Safety**
>
> - Check all IV drug preparations for appropriate dilution, dosage that corresponds to the prescriber's order, absence of precipitates, expiration dates, and so forth.
> - Avoid direct contact with solutions for injection by wearing gloves, face shields, and protective clothing (e.g., disposable, liquid-impermeable gowns).
> - Dispose of contaminated materials (e.g., needles, syringes, ampules, vials, IV tubing, and bags) in puncture-proof containers labeled "Warning: Hazardous Material."
> - Wear gloves when handling patients' clothing, bed linens, or excreta. Blood and body fluids are contaminated with drugs or metabolites for about 3 to 5 days after a dose.
> - Wash hands thoroughly after exposure or potential exposure and after removing gloves.

Assessing for Therapeutic Effects

The nurse helps evaluate treatment effects by assessing for:

- Absence of or reduction in tumor size on physical examination, radiograph, computed tomography scan, magnetic resonance imaging scan, or bone scan
- Laboratory testing, which demonstrates decrease in malignant cells, normalization of serum chemistry levels, and decrease in abnormal tumor serum (tumor marker) protein levels
- Improved functional status, appetite, weight gain, and energy
- Decrease in cancer-related symptoms (e.g., pain, fatigue, dyspnea, cough, anorexia, nausea, vomiting)

Assessing for Adverse Effects

The nurse assesses for the many adverse effects the cytotoxic drugs have on body tissues. Box 14.2 summarizes common adverse effects of these drugs and their management.

Patient Teaching

Box 14.3 presents patient teaching guidelines for anticancer drugs.

BOX 14.3 *Patient Teaching Guidelines for Drugs Used for the Treatment of Cancer*

- There are many different chemotherapy drugs, and the ones used for a particular patient depend on the type of malignancy, its location, and other factors. Some are taken orally at home; many are given intravenously, in outpatient clinics, by nurses who are specially trained to administer the medications and monitor your condition. The medications are usually given in cycles such as every few weeks.
- The goal of chemotherapy is to be as effective as possible with tolerable side effects. Particular side effects vary with the medications used; some increase risks of infection, and some cause anemia, nausea, or hair loss. All of these can be managed effectively, and several medications can help prevent or minimize side effects. In addition, some helpful activities are listed below.
- Keep all appointments for chemotherapy, blood tests, and checkups. This is extremely important. Chemotherapy effectiveness depends on its being given on time; blood tests help to determine when the drugs should be given and how the drugs affect your body tissues.
- Do everything you can to avoid infection, such as avoiding other people who have infections and washing your hands frequently and thoroughly. If you have a fever, chills, sore throat, or cough, notify your oncologist.
- Try to maintain or improve your intake of nutritious food and fluids; this will help you feel better and maintain your weight at a more optimal level to promote healing. A dietitian can be helpful in designing a diet to meet your needs and preferences.
- If your chemotherapy may cause bleeding, decrease the likelihood by shaving with an electric razor, avoiding aspirin and other nonsteroidal anti-inflammatory drugs (including over-the-counter Advil, Aleve, and others), and avoiding injections, cuts, and other injuries when possible. If you notice excessive bruising, bleeding gums when you brush your teeth, or blood in your urine or bowel movement, notify your oncologist immediately.
- If hair loss is expected with the medications you take, use wigs, scarves, and hats. Purchase them before starting chemotherapy, if possible. Hair loss is temporary; your hair will grow back!
- Inform any other physician, dentist, or healthcare provider that you are taking chemotherapy before any diagnostic test or treatment begins. Some procedures may be contraindicated or require special precautions.
- If you are sexually active and able to become pregnant, use effective contraceptive measures during and a few months after chemotherapy.
- Although specific instructions vary depending on the drugs you are taking, the following are a few precautions with some commonly used drugs:
  - With cyclophosphamide, take the tablets on an empty stomach. If severe stomach upset occurs, take with food. Also, drink 2 or 3 quarts of fluid daily, if possible, and urinate often, especially at bedtime. If blood is seen in the urine or signs of cystitis occur (e.g., burning with urination), report to a healthcare provider. The drug is irritating to the bladder lining and may cause cystitis. High fluid intake and frequent emptying of the bladder help to decrease bladder damage.
  - With doxorubicin, the urine may turn red for 1 to 2 days after drug administration. This discoloration is harmless; it does not indicate bleeding. Also, report to a healthcare provider if you have edema, shortness of breath, and excessive fatigue. Doxorubicin may need to be stopped if these symptoms occur.
  - With fluorouracil, drink plenty of liquids while taking.
  - With methotrexate, avoid alcohol, aspirin, and prolonged exposure to sunlight.
  - With oxaliplatin, avoid exposure to cold during, and for 3 to 5 days after, drug administration. This helps prevent or minimize nerve damage that may cause numbness, tingling, and pain in the throat or hands. Swallowing and daily activities that require hand grasping may be impaired.
  - With vincristine, eat high-fiber foods, such as whole cereal grains, if you are able, to prevent constipation. Also, try to maintain a high fluid intake. A stool softener or bulk laxative may be prescribed for daily use.

NCLEX Success

1. A patient is receiving a cytotoxic drug that will likely result in bone marrow depression. When providing education for the patient and family members or caregivers, which of the following teaching considerations should be the priority for the nurse?
   A. Wash hands often, and avoid people with colds, flu, or other infections.
   B. Do not expect fatigue and weakness, which are uncommon.
   C. Expect gastrointestinal upset. More nausea and vomiting may occur when the blood cell counts are low.
   D. Take acetaminophen for fever.

2. In explaining antineoplastic therapy to a family member of a patient who is to receive treatment with a cytotoxic drug, which of the following explanations is most accurate?
   A. Antineoplastic therapy damages both malignant and nonmalignant cells.
   B. It causes few adverse effects.
   C. It stimulates growth of cancer cells.
   D. It must be given daily.

3. A patient with chronic lymphocytic leukemia is beginning to receive an oral cyclophosphamide. Which of the following instructions is most accurate? (Select all that apply.)
   A. Administer the drug with food only with gastric upset.
   B. Take the drug on an empty stomach.
   C. Take the drug at bedtime.
   D. Administer the drug 1 hour before a meal or 2 hours afterward.

ADJUVANT MEDICATIONS USED TO TREAT CANCER

Biologic Antineoplastic Drugs

Two factors promoting carcinogenesis are (1) failure of the immune system to eliminate mutant and malignant cells and (2) failure of growth-regulating processes to control the proliferation of premalignant and malignant cells. Biologic agents target cellular differences between the malignant and normal cells. By doing this, they stimulate the immune system to fight cancer cells and inhibit their growth and proliferation.

Treatment of cancer with biologic agents continues to expand, as more of these agents are designed to interact with proteins overexpressed on the surface of cancer cells. The ability to test individual tumor tissues for the presence of altered cell surface proteins and growth factors has become feasible. Thus, these drugs inhibit malignant cell growth and in some cases stimulate the immune system to destroy tumor cells. Biologic drugs are useful both alone and combined with cytotoxic drug treatment, reducing the adverse effects of traditional cytotoxic chemotherapy. Others, such as imatinib, which is used for chronic myeloid leukemia (it targets the tyrosine kinase enzyme involved in leukemia cell growth), are effective as monotherapy treatment for malignancy.

Biologic antineoplastic drugs include immunotherapy drugs and drugs that "target" biologic processes of malignant cells. Some immunologic anticancer drugs are discussed in Chapter 11 (e.g., interferon alfa for acquired immunodeficiency syndrome [AIDS]-related Kaposi sarcoma, selected leukemias, malignant melanoma, and non-Hodgkin lymphoma and interleukin-2 for kidney cancer). Newer biologic agents (targeted therapies) are commonly used to treat lung, colorectal, breast, and hematologic malignancies in older adults. Table 14.3 presents the route and dosage information of biologic agents used in cancer treatment plus the use and adverse effects information for the currently approved biologic antineoplastic drugs—the monoclonal antibodies, tyrosine kinase inhibitors, and proteasome inhibitors.

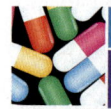

TABLE 14.3
DRUGS AT A GLANCE: Biologic Antineoplastic Drugs

Drug	Routes and Dosage Ranges	Clinical Uses	Adverse Effects
Monoclonal Antibodies			
P **Alemtuzumab** (Campath, Lemtrada; ✲ Lemtrada, MabCampath)	IV infusion, initially, 3 mg/d as a 2-h infusion. Increase to 10 mg/d and then to 30 mg/d as tolerated maintenance and 30 mg/d three times weekly on alternate days for up to 12 wk	B-cell chronic lymphocytic leukemia	Allergic infusion reactions (dyspnea, fever, chills, skin rash), immunosuppression, hypotension, hypertension, peripheral edema, nausea, vomiting, diarrhea, and mucositis
Bevacizumab (Avastin; ✲ Avastin)	IV infusion 5 mg/kg once every 14 d until disease progression is detected	Breast, cervical, colorectal, and kidney cell cancer; refractory glioblastoma, non–small cell lung cancer, epithelial ovarian, fallopian, primary peritoneal cancer, and endometrial cancer	Heart failure, hemorrhage, hypertension, diarrhea, leukopenia, pain, dyspnea, dermatitis, stomatitis, and vomiting

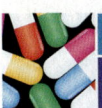

TABLE 14.3
DRUGS AT A GLANCE: Cytotoxic Antineoplastic Drugs (Continued)

Drug	Routes and Dosage Ranges	Clinical Uses	Adverse Effects
Blinatumomab (Blincyto; Blincyto)	Premedicate with dexamethasone 20 mg IV 1 h prior to the first dose of each cycle, prior to first dose of each cycle Cycle 1: IV 9 mcg daily administered as a continuous infusion on days 1–7 followed by 28 mcg daily as a continuous infusion on days 8–28 of a 6-wk treatment cycle Cycles 2–5: 28 mcg daily administered as a continuous infusion on days 1–28 of a 6-wk cycle	Acute lymphoblastic leukemia (B-cell precursor), Philadelphia chromosome negative	Peripheral edema, neurotoxicity, skin rash, hypokalemia, hypomagnesemia, hyperglycemia, nausea, constipation, infection, bone marrow depression, and hypersensitivity
Cetuximab (Erbitux; Erbitux)	IV infusion, initially, 400 mg/m^2 over 2 h; maintenance, 250 mg/m^2 over 1 h once weekly	Metastatic colorectal cancer and head and neck squamous cell cancer	Anemia, leukopenia, infusion reaction, nausea, diarrhea, stomatitis, vomiting, dyspnea, and fever
Dinutuximab (Unituxin; Unituxin)	Children: premedicate with IV morphine 50 mcg/kg, diphenhydramine 0.5–1 mg/kg/dose and acetaminophen 10–15 mg/kg/dose prior to infusion IV 17.5 mg/m^2 d for 4 consecutive days for a maximum of 5 cycles (in combination with sargramostim, isotretinoin)	Neuroblastoma	Hypotension, pain, urticarial, proteinuria, increased ALT and AST, vomiting, diarrhea, bone marrow depression, increased serum creatinine, and fever
Ibritumomab tiuxetan (Zevalin; Zevalin)	Premedicate with PO acetaminophen 650 mg and diphenhydramine 50 mg Administer with rituximab IV 250 mg/m^2 at 50 mL per hour on day 1; days 7, 8, 9 250 mg/m^2 at 100 mL/h Y-90 3.2 mg/2 L	Non-Hodgkin lymphoma	Severe or fatal infusion reaction and severe bone marrow depression
Ipilimumab (Yervoy; Yervoy)	IV 3 mg/kg every 3 wk for a maximum of 4 doses	Melanoma, unresectable or metastatic, hepatocellular carcinoma, kidney cancer	Anemia, diarrhea, decreased hemoglobin, weight loss, and increased ALT and AST
Nivolumab (Opdivo; Opdivo)	IV 3 mg/kg once every 2 wk	Hodgkin lymphoma, melanoma, non–small cell lung cancer, and kidney cancer	Peripheral edema, malaise, skin rash, hyponatremia, hyperkalemia, increased TSH, hypocalcemia, increased serum cholesterol, diarrhea, and increased creatinine
Obinutuzumab (Gazyva; Gazyva)	Premedicate with acetaminophen, antihistamine, and glucocorticoid 30–60 min prior to treatment IV 100 mg on day 1 followed by 900 mg on day 2 and followed by 1,000 mg weekly for 2 doses (days 8 and 15) Cycle 2–6: 1,000 mg on day 1 every 28 d for 5 doses	Chronic lymphocytic leukemia and follicular lymphoma	Hypophosphatemia, hypocalcemia, hyperkalemia, hyponatremia, hypoalbuminemia, hypokalemia, bone marrow depression, increased AST and ALT, musculoskeletal pain, and increased serum creatinine

(Continued on page 254)

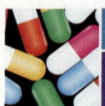

TABLE 14.3

DRUGS AT A GLANCE: Cytotoxic Antineoplastic Drugs (Continued)

Drug	Routes and Dosage Ranges	Clinical Uses	Adverse Effects
Ofatumumab (Arzerra, Kesimpta; Kesimpta)	Premedicate with acetaminophen, antihistamine, and corticosteroid 30–120 min prior to treatment IV cycle 1 (cycle is 28 d): 300 mg on day 1; followed by 1,000 mg on day 8 Subsequent cycles: 1,000 mg on day 1 every 28 d; continue for at least 3 cycles	Chronic lymphocytic leukemia	Fatigue, skin rash, diarrhea, nausea, bone marrow depression, infection, pneumonia, and infusion reaction
Panitumumab (Vectibix; Vectibix)	IV infusion, 6 mg/kg over 60 min every 14 d. Doses over 1,000 mg should be given over 90 min	Metastatic colorectal cancer	Infusion reactions, skin rash, pulmonary fibrosis, nausea, vomiting, and diarrhea; 90% of patients receiving panitumumab have developed severe dermatologic adverse effects
Pembrolizumab (Keytruda; Keytruda)	Adults: IV infusion 200–400 mg once every 3–6 weeks Children: ≥2 years-adolescents IV 2 mg/kg/dose (maximum dose: 200 mg/dose); administer once every 3 wk until disease progression, unacceptable toxicity, or in patients without disease progression for up to 24 months	Metastatic breast, cervical, cutaneous squamous cell, esophageal, gastric, non–small cell lung, kidney, urothelial cancers Children: Hodgkin lymphoma, Merkel cell carcinoma, primary mediastinal large B-cell lymphoma	Exfoliative dermatologic conditions, Stevens-Johnson syndrome, Myocardial infarction, myocarditis, pericarditis, vasculitis, hypo/hyperthyroidism, adrenocortical insufficiency, colitis, neutropenia, thrombocytopenia, pancytopenia, hepatoxicity, cerebral hemorrhage, uveitis, pneumonitis
Pertuzumab (Perjeta; Perjeta)	IV 840 mg over 60 min followed by a maintenance dose of 420 mg over 30–60 min every 3 wk for 3–6 cycles; may be administered	Metastatic breast cancer	Bone marrow depression, alopecia, upper respiratory infection, fatigue, weakness, diarrhea, nausea, and vomiting; possible decreased left ventricular ejection fraction and congestive heart failure; evaluate cardiac function prior and during treatment
Rituximab (Riabni, Rituxan, Ruxience, Truxima; Rituxan, Rituxan SC)	IV infusion 375 mg/m² once weekly for 4–8 doses Chronic lymphocytic leukemia: IV 375 mg/m² given on the day prior to fludarabine/cyclophosphamide then 500 mg/m² on day 1 every 28 d of a cycles 2–6	Non-Hodgkin lymphoma and chronic lymphocytic leukemia	Hypersensitivity reactions, peripheral edema, fever, rash, fatigue, nausea, diarrhea, weight gain, bone marrow depression, cough, and increased ALT
Tositumomab (iodine 131–tositumomab) (Bexxar; Bexxar)	IV infusion over 60 min. If administered with iodine 131, infuse over 20 min	Non-Hodgkin lymphoma	Fever, chills, nausea, vomiting, skin rash, headache, cough, infection, and pain
Trastuzumab (Herceptin; Herceptin)	IV infusion 4 mg/kg initially and then 2 mg/kg once weekly	Metastatic breast and gastric cancer (HER2+)	Cardiotoxicity (dyspnea, edema, heart failure)
Kinase Inhibitors			
P Erlotinib (Tarceva; Tarceva, APO-Tarceva, PMS-Erlotinib; Teva-Erlotinib)	Non–small cell lung: PO 150 mg once daily Pancreatic: PO 100 mg once daily	Non–small cell lung cancer and pancreatic cancer	Dyspnea, edema, thrombosis, fatigue, alopecia, skin rash, increased ALT and AST, bone marrow depression, and infection

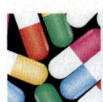

TABLE 14.3
DRUGS AT A GLANCE: Cytotoxic Antineoplastic Drugs (Continued)

Drug	Routes and Dosage Ranges	Clinical Uses	Adverse Effects
Afatinib (Gilotrif; ✦ Gilotrif)	PO 40 mg once daily	Non–small cell lung cancer, metastatic	Acne, weight loss, hypokalemia, increased ALT and AST, epistaxis, cystitis, and conjunctivitis
Axitinib (Inlyta; ✦ Inlyta)	PO 5 mg twice	Kidney cancer	Hypertension, fatigue, voice disorder, headache, palmar–plantar erythrodysesthesia, skin rash, decreased serum bicarbonate, proteinuria, increased AST and ALT, and increased alkaline phosphatase
Bosutinib (Bosulif; ✦ Bosulif)	PO 500 mg once daily	Philadelphia chromosome-positive chronic myelogenous leukemia	Edema, fatigue, headache, hypophosphatemia, bone marrow depression, increased ALT and AST, arthralgia, cough, dyspnea, and fever
Cabozantinib (Cabometyx, Cometriq; ✦ Cabometyx)	Hepatocellular and kidney cancer: PO 60 mg once daily Thyroid cancer (medullary, metastatic): PO 140 mg once daily (do not exceed 180 mg)	Kidney cancer Metastatic medullary thyroid cancer Hepatocellular carcinoma Thyroid cancer	GI perforation, hypertension, fatigue, voice disorder, headache, palmar–plantar erythrodysesthesia, skin rash, decreased serum bicarbonate, proteinuria, increased AST and ALT, and increased alkaline phosphatase
Ceritinib (Zykadia; ✦ Zykadia)	PO 750 mg once daily	Non–small cell lung cancer	Nausea, vomiting, skin rash, fatigue, diarrhea, decreased hemoglobin, and increased AST and ALT
Dabrafenib (Tafinlar; ✦ Tafinlar)	PO 150 mg every 12 h	Metastatic melanoma, solid tumors, thyroid cancer	Peripheral edema, rash, alopecia, hyperglycemia, hypophosphatemia, bone marrow depression, increased AST and ALT, and increased alkaline phosphatase
Dasatinib (Sprycel; ✦ Sprycel)	PO 100–140 mg daily	Chronic myelogenous leukemia and acute lymphoblastic leukemia	Anemia, diarrhea, dyspnea, edema, fever, infection, nausea, pain, and skin rash
Everolimus (Afinitor, Afinitor Disperz, Zortress; ✦ Afinitor Disperz)	PO 10 mg daily	Breast, neuroendocrine tumors, lung, pancreatic, and kidney cancer	Fatigue, edema, hypertension, diabetes mellitus, and increased serum creatinine
Ibrutinib (Imbruvica; ✦ Imbruvica)	CLL: PO 420 mg once daily Mantle cell carcinoma: PO 500 mg once daily	Chronic lymphocytic leukemia, Mantle cell carcinoma	Edema, fatigue, increased uric acid, infection, urinary tract infection, arthropathy, fever, atrial fibrillation, and increased serum creatinine
Imatinib (Gleevec) (Apo-Imatinib; ✦ ACT-Imatinib, Gleevec, Teva-Imatinib)	Adults: PO 400–800 mg/d Children: 3 y and older, PO 260–340 mg/m^2/d	Philadelphia chromosome-positive chronic myeloid leukemia and gastrointestinal stromal tumors	Dyspnea, edema, heart failure, hemorrhage, nausea, vomiting, diarrhea, neutropenia, and thrombocytopenia
Lapatinib (Tykerb; ✦ Tykerb)	PO 1,250 mg (5 tablets) once daily on days 1–21, with capecitabine PO 2,000 mg/m^2/d (in 2 doses, 12 h apart) on days 1–14 in a repeating 21-d cycle	Advanced breast cancer	Diarrhea, dyspnea, insomnia, nausea, vomiting, and stomatitis

(Continued on page 256)

TABLE 14.3

DRUGS AT A GLANCE: Cytotoxic Antineoplastic Drugs (Continued)

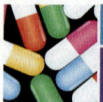

Drug	Routes and Dosage Ranges	Clinical Uses	Adverse Effects
Lenvatinib (Lenvima; ❋ Lenvima)	Endometrial cancer: PO 20 mg once daily in combination with pembrolizumab Kidney cancer: PO 18 mg once daily in combination with everolimus Thyroid cancer: 24 mg once daily	Endometrial, kidney, and thyroid cancer	Hypertension, fatigue, headache, voice disorder, increased thyroid-stimulating hormone, proteinuria, hemorrhage, arthralgia, abnormal kidney function, and cough
Nilotinib (Tasigna; ❋ Tasigna)	PO 400 mg BID	Chronic myeloid leukemia	QT prolongation and sudden death, peripheral edema, hyperglycemia, pruritus, night sweats, nausea, vomiting, neutropenia, increased ALT and AST, and limb pain
Palbociclib (Ibrance; ❋ Ibrance)	PO 125 mg once daily for 21 d, followed by a 7-d rest	Breast cancer	Bone marrow depression, fatigue, peripheral neuropathy, nausea, vomiting, and alopecia
Pazopanib (Votrient; ❋ Votrient)	PO 800 mg once daily	Kidney cancer and soft tissue sarcoma	Hypertension, edema, cardiac insufficiency, QT prolongation, hair discoloration, increased ALT and AST, and diarrhea
Ponatinib (Iclusig; ❋ Iclusig)	PO 45 mg once daily	Philadelphia chromosome–positive, acute lymphoblastic leukemia, and chronic myeloid leukemia	Bone marrow depression, increased ALT and AST, fever, urinary tract infection, hypertension, peripheral edema, congestive heart failure, and arterial ischemia; monitor for evidence of arterial occlusion, heart failure, hepatotoxicity, and venous thromboembolism
Regorafenib (Stivarga; ❋ Stivarga)	PO 160 mg daily for the first 21 d of a 28-d schedule	Colorectal cancer and locally advanced, unresectable, or metastatic gastrointestinal stromal tumor	Hypertension, fatigue, alopecia, headache, palmar–plantar erythrodysesthesia, skin rash, decreased serum bicarbonate, proteinuria, increased AST and ALT, and bone marrow depression
Sorafenib (NexAVAR; ❋ NexAVAR)	PO 400 mg twice daily	Hepatocellular cancer, kidney cancer, and thyroid cancer	Hypertension, fatigue, voice disorder, peripheral sensory neuropathy, hypoalbuminemia, hypophosphatemia, increased thyroid-stimulating hormone, hypocalcemia, bone marrow depression, increased ALT and AST, myalgia, limb pain, dyspnea, and cough
Sunitinib (Sutent; ❋ Sutent)	Pancreatic neuroendocrine tumor: 37.5 mg once daily Gastrointestinal stromal tumor and kidney cancer: 50 mg once daily for 4 wk of a 6-wk treatment cycle (4 wk on, 2 wk off)	Pancreatic neuroendocrine tumor, gastrointestinal stromal tumor, and kidney cancer	Hypertension, decreased left ventricular ejection fraction, peripheral edema, chest pain, fatigue, mouth pain, skin discoloration, increased uric acid, and increased AST and ALT, serum alkaline phosphatase, and serum bilirubin
Temsirolimus (Torisel; ❋ Torisel)	IV 25 mg once daily	Kidney cancer	Edema, chest pain, headache, insomnia, hyperglycemia, hypercholesterolemia, hypophosphatemia, bone marrow depression, increased alkaline phosphatase, increased serum AST, mucositis, nausea, vomiting, dyspnea, and cough

TABLE 14.3

DRUGS AT A GLANCE: Cytotoxic Antineoplastic Drugs (Continued)

Drug	Routes and Dosage Ranges	Clinical Uses	Adverse Effects
Trametinib (Mekinist; ✦ Mekinist)	PO 2 mg once daily	Melanoma, thyroid cancer	Hypertension, cardiomyopathy, decreased left ventricular ejection fraction, dermatitis, rash, palmar–plantar erythrodysesthesia, hypoalbuminemia, diarrhea, stomatitis, abdominal pain, increased ALT and AST, and hematuria
Proteasome Inhibitors			
ⓟ Bortezomib (Velcade; ✦ ACT Bortezomib, PMS-Bortezomib)	IV injection, 1.3 mg/m², twice weekly for 2 wk, followed by a 10-d rest period	Multiple myeloma	Edema, nausea, vomiting, diarrhea, anemia, neutropenia, thrombocytopenia, and peripheral neuropathy
Carfilzomib (Kyprolis; ✦ Kyprolis)	Cycle 1: IV 20 mg/m² over 10 min on days 1 and 2. If tolerated, increase dose to 27 mg/m² over 10 min on days 8, 9, and 16 of a 28-d cycle Cycles 2–12: IV 27 mg/m² over 10 min on days 1, 2, 8, 9, 15, and 16 of a 28-d treatment cycle Cycle 13 and beyond: 56 mg/m² over 30 min on days 1, 2, 15, and 16 of a 28-d treatment cycle. Continue until disease progression or unacceptable toxicity	Multiple myeloma	Edema, hypertension, chest wall pain, fatigue, insomnia, peripheral neuropathy, hypokalemia, hypomagnesemia, nausea, vomiting, increased AST and creatinine, and bone marrow depression
Ixazomib (Ninlaro; ✦ Ninlaro)	PO 4 mg once weekly on days 1, 8, and 15 d of a 28-d cycle in combination with lenalidomide and dexamethasone	Multiple myeloma	Peripheral edema, peripheral neuropathy, skin rash, diarrhea, constipation, nausea, vomiting, bone marrow depression, eye disease, and upper respiratory tract infection

ALT, alanine aminotransferase; AST, aspartate aminotransferase; TSH, thyroid-stimulating hormone.

Monoclonal Antibodies

Monoclonal antibodies, which may be used alone or in combination with traditional cytotoxic antineoplastic drugs and other treatment modalities, have become an integral part of treatment plans for a variety of cancers. Metabolic pathways for many of the monoclonal antibodies are incompletely identified, but experts believe that the drugs are processed mainly in the reticuloendothelial system.

The monoclonal antibodies act in various ways:

- ⓟ **Alemtuzumab** (Campath, Lemtrada), blinatumomab (Blincyto), ipilimumab (Yervoy), and rituximab (Riabni, Rituxan, Ruxience, Truxima) bind to an antigen on both normal T and B lymphocytes and malignant lymphoid cells to activate antibody- and complement-mediated cytotoxicity. The malignant lymphoid cells are more susceptible to immune destruction, and the normal lymphocytes can later repopulate in the bloodstream.
- Obinutuzumab (Gazyva) and ofatumumab (Arzerra, Kesimpta) are monoclonal antibodies that bind to the antigen CD20 to activate an antibody-dependent response, causing tumor cell death.
- Bevacizumab (Alymsys, Avastin, Mvasi, Zirabev), cetuximab (Erbitux), ibritumomab (Zevalin Y-90), and trastuzumab (Herceptin) all bind to growth factor receptors found on blood vessels, colorectal cancer cells, and breast cancer cells, respectively, to prevent intracellular growth factors from becoming activated and stimulating cell growth. Inhibition of microvascular growth assists in retarding the growth of metastatic tissue. In addition, cetuximab binds to the epidermal growth factor (EGF) receptor to block the binding of EGF. The blockage prevents the phosphorylation and activation of receptor-associated kinases and apoptosis results.
- Panitumumab (Vectibix) is a recombinant human immunoglobulin G2 that binds to the EGF receptor, which inhibits the binding of EGF. EGF blocks phosphorylation and tyrosine

kinase activation to stop cell growth and proliferation. Pertuzumab (Perjeta) has a similar action, but it targets the human epidermal growth factor receptor 2 protein (HER2). It is combined with trastuzumab for a greater human epididymis 2, or HER2, inhibition.

- Dinutuximab (Unituxin) is administered to children who have been diagnosed with a neuroblastoma. This monoclonal antibody binds to the disialoganglioside GD2, which is abundant or highly expressed in a neuroblastoma. The binding to GD2 allows for cell lysis and complement-dependent cytotoxicity.
- Like ibritumomab, the tositumomab radioconjugate (Bexxar) is a monoclonal antibody conjugated with a radioisotope that targets receptors on B lymphocytes.
- Nivolumab (Opdivo) is a G4 monoclonal antibody. Monoclonal antibodies are used in cancer treatment. Nivolumab inhibits cell death by binding with programmed death receptor 1 (PD-1), thus blocking its L1 and L2 ligands. The negative PD-1 receptor signaling and then disrupts the T-cell cytotoxic response. By blocking the T-cell cytotoxic response, tumor-specific T cells enter the tumor to induce programmed tumor cell death.

Fewer adverse effects are associated with monoclonal antibody therapy than those of cytotoxic drugs. However, although some adverse effects are rare, they are serious (e.g., heart failure, bleeding problems, electrolyte imbalances) and vary depending on the drug.

Significant drug interactions with the monoclonal antibodies are few. Enzymes in the liver do not metabolize the monoclonal antibodies; hence, they do not compete with other drugs for these enzymes. However, when combined with cytotoxic agents in the same treatment regimen, dosage reductions are often advisable.

Administration of monoclonal antibodies is by IV infusion because all preparations would be destroyed by GI enzymes if taken orally. The infusion occurs over a given period, generally 90 to 120 minutes initially, in a monitored healthcare setting. Premedication may be necessary, and frequent observation of the patient for signs of a hypersensitivity infusion reaction is important. In cases of acute hypersensitivity (urticaria, hypotension, dyspnea, wheezing), it is essential that the infusion be stopped and emergency measures implemented promptly (oxygen, epinephrine, bronchodilators, IV diphenhydramine, and dexamethasone). Mild infusion reactions require slowing or temporarily stopping the infusion and administering IV diphenhydramine 50 mg and acetaminophen 650 to 1,000 mg orally.

> **Quality and Safety Alert: Safety**
>
> When tositumomab radioconjugate (Bexxar) is given, radiation safety precautions (careful body fluid precautions, good handwashing, and limiting intimate contact time) are necessary for a week after dosing.

Clinical Application 14.3

- Ms. D'Angelo's oncologist has determined that she requires a different medication because of the adverse effects of paclitaxel. She will be started on bevacizumab and carboplatin. What are the actions of bevacizumab and carboplatin?

Growth Factor and Tyrosine Kinase Inhibitors

Growth factors such as EGF (which stimulates the growth of epithelial cells in the skin and other organs) and platelet-derived growth factor (which stimulates the proliferation of vascular smooth muscle and endothelial cells) bind to transcellular membrane receptors and initiate intracellular events that result in cell growth. EGF, which is normally produced in the kidneys and salivary glands, is found in almost all body fluids. When EGF binds to the external portion of the EGF receptor, also called the tyrosine kinase receptor, it sends signals to intracellular kinase enzymes stimulating cell proliferation and angiogenesis. Intracellular tyrosine kinases play an important role in the proliferation and differentiation of cells; thus, blocking these receptors can decrease intracellular protein synthesis and lead to cell death (Fig. 14.4).

 Erlotinib (Tarceva) is a growth inhibitor that blocks the tyrosine kinase portion of the EGF receptor, inhibiting cell proliferation and inducing cell death. The action and use of other EGF inhibitors that are similar to erlotinib are described further. Axitinib (Inlyta) inhibits the vascular endothelial receptors to promote cell death in kidney cancer tumor growth. Bosutinib (Bosulif), dasatinib (Sprycel), and imatinib inhibit the kinase BCR-ABL and the proto-oncogene c-KIT. Both growth factors are significant in the development of chronic myelogenous leukemia. Cabozantinib (Cometriq) slows the advancement of medullary thyroid cancer. Cabozantinib (Cabometyx) is effective in treating advanced kidney cancer. Both of these drugs are strong CYP3A4 inhibitors and inducers. It may require 2 to 3 days to adjust the dosage when administered with another medication that is metabolized by CYP3A4. The U.S. Food and Drug Administration (FDA) has issued a **BOXED WARNING** for Cometriq because it may cause GI perforation. Therefore, it is important to instruct the patient about the signs and symptoms of this condition. Ceritinib (Zykadia) is an inhibitor of anaplastic lymphoma kinase, which is active in the pathogenesis of non–small cell lung cancer. The patient will require a 5-HT$_3$RA to prevent nausea and vomiting. Dabrafenib is commonly administered with trametinib to inhibit the mitogen-activated protein kinase pathway leading to oncogene homolog B1 (BRAF) V600 melanoma cell death. BRAF V600 is a mutation of metastatic melanoma. Ibrutinib irreversibly inhibits Bruton tyrosine kinase (BTK), which is a factor of the B-cell receptor that is integral in the survival of cancerous B cells. Ibrutinib decreases B-cell proliferation through the inhibition of BTK. Mechanistic target of rapamycin (mTOR) is another type of kinase inhibitor. Everolimus (Afinitor) is a macrolide immunosuppressant in this subclass of kinase inhibitors. Its action decreases the lipoma volume in kidney angiomyolipomas. Temsirolimus (Torisel), another mTOR inhibitor, binds to the protein FKBP-12, halting the G$_1$ phase of the tumor cell in the treatment of kidney cancer.

Lapatinib (Tykerb), another kinase inhibitor, is an oral agent administered for advanced and metastatic breast cancer. Some breast tumors have a strong expression of HER2, and this drug affects the expression of the EGF (ErbB1) and HER2.

Lenvatinib (Lenvima) is a tyrosine kinase inhibitor used to treat unresectable hepatocellular cancer, advanced kidney cancer, and thyroid cancer. It is a vascular endothelial growth factor (VEGF) inhibitor. It blocks the VEGF receptors 1, 2, and 3; fibroblast growth factor receptors 1, 2, 3, and 4; and platelet-derived

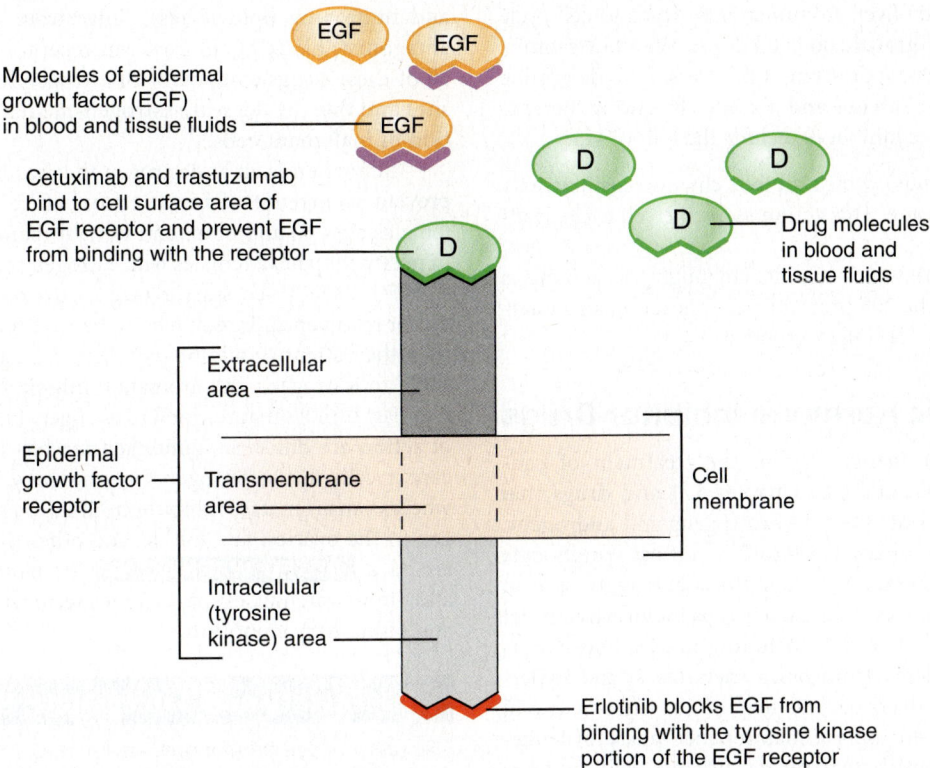

Figure 14.4. Actions of selected biologic targeted drugs. These drugs prevent epidermal growth factor (EGF) from combining with its receptors and thereby prevent or decrease cell growth. Cetuximab and trastuzumab bind with the extracellular portion of the EGF receptor. Erlotinib blocks the intracellular (tyrosine kinase) portion of the EGF receptor.

growth factor receptor (PDGFR); KIT; and RET to slow the rate of cancer advancement. Pazopanib (Votrient) inhibits the same factors as lenvatinib along with fibroblast growth factor receptor, interleukin-2 receptor–inducible T-cell kinase, leukocyte-specific protein tyrosine kinase, and transmembrane glycoprotein receptor tyrosine kinase to treat kidney cancer or soft tissue sarcoma. Nilotinib targets BCR-ABL kinase, c-KIT, and PDGFR in the treatment of chronic myeloid leukemia. The action of this medication has a stronger effect than imatinib. Prior to the administration of nilotinib, a patient should have a baseline ECG and another 7 days after the first dose. The FDA has issued a BOXED WARNING ◆ for nilotinib alerting patients who take the drug that they may be prone to the development of a prolonged QT interval. Nilotinib should not be administered to patients with hypokalemia or hypomagnesemia. It is also a strong inhibitor of CYP3A4. Also, it is important to instruct the patient to take the medication 1 hour before a meal or 2 hours after a meal. In addition, the patient should not consume grapefruit or grapefruit juice.

The drugs pazopanib (Votrient), ponatinib (Inclusig), regorafenib (Stivarga), sorafenib (NexAVAR), and sunitinib (Sutent) are kinase inhibitors with multiple targets. They reduce tumor growth by various actions to block tumor angiogenesis. They are BCR-ABL inhibitors used to treat acute lymphoblastic leukemia and chronic myeloid leukemia.

Common adverse effects of the tyrosine kinase inhibitors include leukopenia, thrombocytopenia, skin rashes, and diarrhea. Skin care, maintaining adequate hydration and nutrition, and monitoring for signs of dehydration and electrolyte imbalances are priorities with use of these antineoplastic drugs.

With the tyrosine kinase inhibitors, drugs also metabolized by the CYP3A4 liver enzyme system may affect tyrosine kinase inhibitors. Enzyme inhibitors (azole antifungals, erythromycin, protease inhibitors) and grapefruit juice may increase blood levels, whereas CYP3A4 enzyme inducers (rifampin, carbamazepine, phenytoin, St. John's wort) may decrease blood levels. An increase or decrease in dosage may be necessary with concurrent administration of inducers or inhibitors, respectively.

Self-administration of the oral tyrosine kinase inhibitors generally occurs in the home setting.

> **! Quality and Safety Alert: Safety**
>
> Tyrosine kinase inhibitors must be handled as hazardous substances and stored securely in the original labeled container. No crushing or cutting of tablets should occur. If the patient is unable to swallow the oral formulation whole or has a feeding tube, it is necessary to dissolve the tablet in water in accordance with individual manufacturer's instructions and ingest it immediately.

Proteasome Inhibitors

Proteasomes are enzyme complexes in the cytoplasm and nucleus of all body cells, both normal and malignant. These enzymes regulate intracellular protein activity. **Bortezomib** (Velcade) inhibits proteasomes, affecting multiple proteins within cells. Experts believe it has multiple mechanisms of cytotoxicity (e.g., preventing formation of new blood vessels in tumors and accelerating death of malignant cells). The drug is moderately protein bound (83%) and is metabolized by several CYP450 enzyme systems in the liver. Administration leads to cell cycle arrest, delayed tumor growth, and cell death. With bortezomib, which can cause myelosuppression, it is necessary to determine the blood cell count at baseline and periodically during therapy.

Other proteasome inhibitors include the following:

- Carfilzomib (Kyprolis), which inhibits chymotrypsin activity of the 20S proteasome. This action stops the cell cycle, leading to apoptosis.
- Ixazomib (Ninlaro), which inhibits chymotrypsin activity of beta-5 subunit of the 20S proteasome. This action also interrupts the cell cycle, leading to apoptosis.

Antineoplastic Hormone Inhibitor Drugs

The main hormonal agents used in the treatment of cancer are the corticosteroids (see Chapter 17) and drugs that block the production of activity of estrogens and androgens. Pharmacologic doses of corticosteroids suppress lymphocyte production, causing lymphocyte apoptosis and regression of lymphoid tissue. Other uses for these drugs include treatment of the complications of cancer, including nausea and vomiting, intracerebral edema from brain metastases, and hypercalcemia. However, adverse effects may occur. Chronic use of oral glucocorticoids during the maintenance phase of leukemia treatment can contribute to the development of long-term adverse effects such as osteoporosis, myopathy, hypertension, glucose intolerance, cataracts, and decreased growth rate in children. Hence, intermittent long-term therapy with glucocorticoids is generally used to maximize cytotoxic effects on lymphoid tissue while minimizing adverse long-term consequences. Prednisone and dexamethasone are the preparations most commonly used for cancer treatment. Sex hormone–blocking drugs are used mainly to control tumor growth and relieve symptoms. They are not cytotoxic, and adverse effects are usually mild.

Sex hormones act as growth factors in some malignancies (e.g., estrogens in breast cancer, testosterone in prostate cancer). Surgical removal of the ovaries or testes, which produce hormones, or therapy with hormone receptor–blocking drugs may be effective in decreasing hormonal stimulation and slowing the growth of hormone-dependent cancers. Removal of the ovaries is most likely in premenopausal females with breast cancer and the testes in males with prostate cancer. Currently used drugs interfere with hormone production or hormone action at the cellular level (Fig. 14.5).

The main hormone inhibitor drugs are the antiestrogens, aromatase inhibitors, antiandrogens, and gonadotropin-releasing hormone (GnRH) analogs. Chapter 7 and Table 14.4 describe these drugs.

Antiestrogens

 Tamoxifen (Soltamox) and toremifene (Fareston) are selective estrogen receptor modulators (SERMs) used in the treatment of breast cancer. One estrogen receptor antagonist, fulvestrant (Faslodex), may also be useful. These drugs, which bind to estrogen receptors in both normal and malignant cells, are effective only in the treatment of tumors with estrogen receptors. SERMs block some estrogen receptors while activating others (increasing bone mineral density and improving lipid levels). Fulvestrant is a pure estrogen antagonist, blocking all estrogen receptors. In breast cancer, all of these drugs compete with estrogen for receptor binding sites and thereby decrease estrogen-mediated growth stimulation of malignant cells.

Tamoxifen is an antiestrogen that has been widely used to prevent recurrence of breast cancer after surgical excision in females ages 40 and older and to treat metastatic breast cancer in postmenopausal females with estrogen receptor–positive disease. It is usually necessary to take the drug for 5 years to prevent tumor recurrence. Tamoxifen can be continued for 10 years, and then the patient should be switched to an aromatase inhibitor. Both antiestrogens and aromatase inhibitors block the growth of breast tumors that respond to estrogen, but their mechanisms of action are different. Tamoxifen inhibits the ability of breast cancer cells to use estrogen for growth by blocking receptors, whereas an aromatase inhibitor inhibits the production of estrogen in the ovaries, fat, muscle, and other tissues. The FDA has issued a **BOXED WARNING** ◆ for tamoxifen that serious and life-threatening events include uterine malignancies, stroke, and pulmonary embolism.

> **! Quality and Safety Alert: Safety**
>
> Sexually active premenopausal females who take tamoxifen should use effective nonhormonal barrier contraception during therapy and for 2 months after the drug is discontinued.

Aromatase Inhibitors

 Anastrozole (Arimidex), exemestane (Aromasin), and letrozole (Femara) are aromatase inhibitors used to prevent or treat recurrence of estrogen-responsive breast cancer in postmenopausal females. Aromatase is an enzyme that catalyzes the production of estrogen in the ovaries of premenopausal females and in fat, liver, and muscle cells of postmenopausal or females who have had an oophorectomy. Thus, inhibiting aromatase reduces estrogen levels in the blood and target tissues, including the breast.

> **! Quality and Safety Alert: Evidence-Based Practice**
>
> The efficacy of aromatase inhibitors in breast cancer prevention has been reported. In clinical trials, aromatase inhibitors versus tamoxifen resulted in reduced breast cancer recurrence, particularly in years 0 to 1. Tamoxifen alone has been found to reduce breast cancer recurrence during years 2 to 4. Aromatase inhibitors alone revealed a lower recurrence rate in years 0 to 1 [Pritchard, 2023].

Tumors may become resistant to tamoxifen because of mutations in receptors that alter drug binding. Letrozole, following tamoxifen, is the current standard of care, and exemestane is also used (instead of tamoxifen) for metastatic breast cancer in postmenopausal females.

Antiandrogens

Antiandrogen therapy, known as androgen deprivation therapy (ADT), is the treatment for advanced prostate cancer. The methods for ADT include estrogens to suppress testosterone,

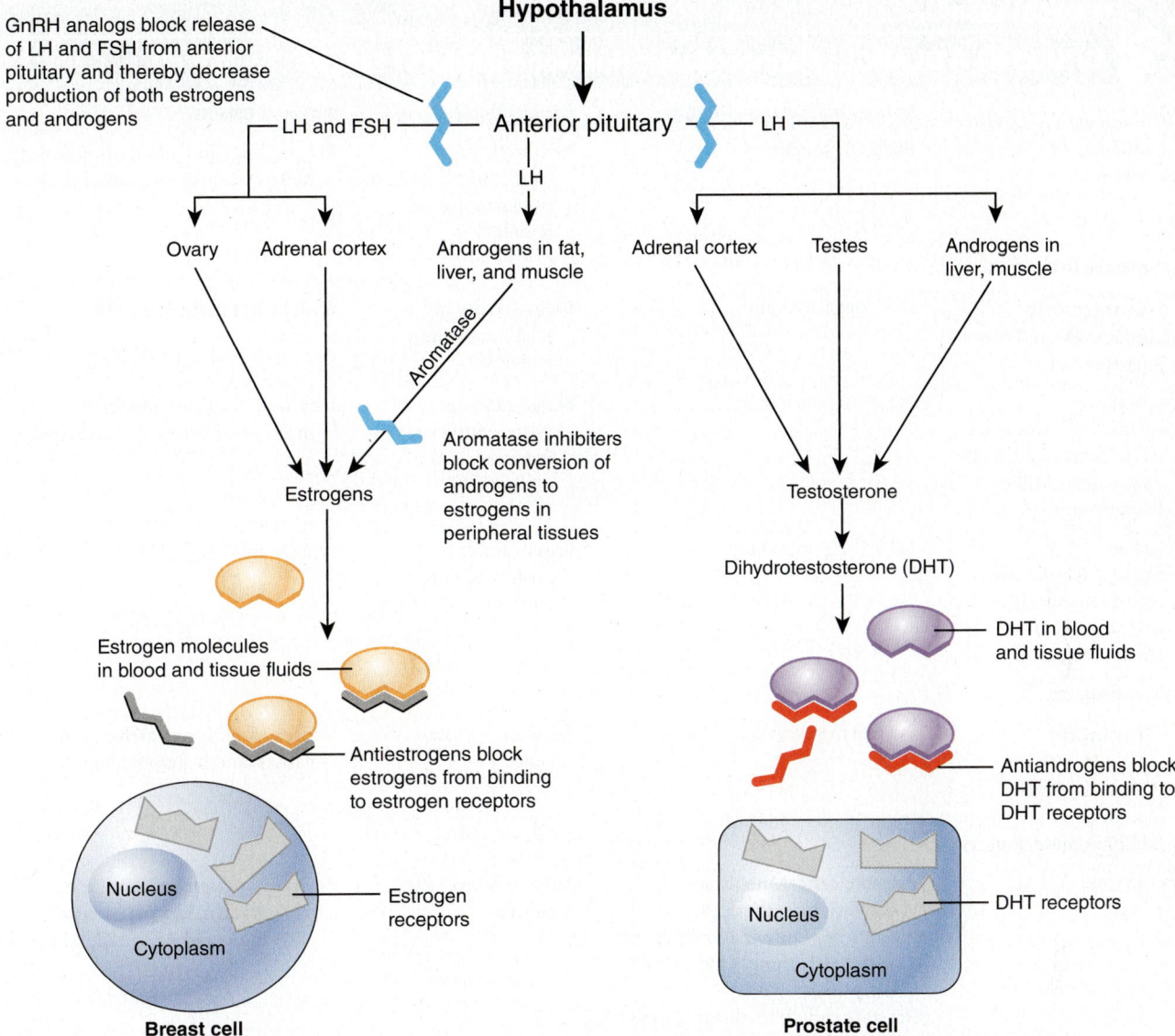

Figure 14.5. Actions of hormone inhibitor drugs. Drugs used to treat breast cancer block the production of estrogens (e.g., gonadotropin hormone–releasing hormone [GnRH] analogs, aromatase inhibitors) or prevent estrogens from binding to receptors in breast cancer cells (antiestrogens). Drugs used to treat prostate cancer block the production of androgens (e.g., GnRH analogs) or prevent DHT, the active from of testosterone, from binding to receptors in prostate cancer cells (antiandrogens). FSH, follicle-stimulating hormone; LH, luteinizing hormone.

TABLE 14.4
DRUGS AT A GLANCE: Antineoplastic Hormone Inhibitor Drugs

Drug	Routes and Dosage Ranges	Clinical Uses	Adverse Effects
Antiestrogens			
ⓟ Tamoxifen (Soltamox; ✳ Apo-Tamox, Mylan-Tamoxifen, Nolvadex-D, Teva-Tamoxifen, PMS-Tamoxifen)	PO 20 mg daily for 5 y (premenopausal) PO 20 mg daily for 2–3 y (postmenopausal)	Breast cancer, after surgery or radiation; prophylaxis in high-risk females; and treatment of metastatic disease	Hot flashes, nausea, vomiting, vaginal discharge, and risk of endometrial cancer in females who have not had a hysterectomy
Fulvestrant (Faslodex; ✳ Faslodex, TEVA-Fulvestrant)	IM 250 mg once monthly (one 5-mL or two 2.5-mL injections)	Advanced breast cancer in postmenopausal females	GI upset, hot flashes, and injection site reactions

(Continued on page 262)

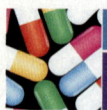

TABLE 14.4

DRUGS AT A GLANCE: Antineoplastic Hormone Inhibitor Drugs (Continued)

Drug	Routes and Dosage Ranges	Clinical Uses	Adverse Effects
Toremifene (Fareston)	PO 60 mg once daily	Metastatic breast cancer in postmenopausal females	QT prolongation, hot flashes, nausea, hypercalcemia, and tumor flare
Aromatase Inhibitors			
ⓟ Anastrozole (Arimidex; ❋ ACT-Anastrozole)	PO 1 mg once daily	Breast cancer in postmenopausal females	Nausea, hot flashes, and edema
Exemestane (Aromasin; ❋ Aromasin, ACT-Exemestane, APO-Exemestane, MED-Exemestane)	PO 25 mg once daily	Breast cancer in postmenopausal females	Hot flashes, nausea, depression, insomnia, anxiety, dyspnea, pain
Letrozole (Femara; ACH-Letrozole, Apo-Letrozole, Bio-Letrozole, Femara, JAMP-Letrozole)	PO 2.5 mg once daily	Breast cancer in postmenopausal females	Nausea and hot flashes
Antiandrogens			
ⓟ Flutamide (Eulexin; ❋ PMS-Flutamide, Teva-Flutamide, NU-Flutamide, Euflex)	PO 250 mg every 8 h	Advanced prostatic cancer	Nausea, vomiting, diarrhea, hot flashes, and hepatotoxicity
Abiraterone (Yonsa, Zytiga)	Prostate cancer metastatic, castration resistant PO 1,000 mg daily in combination with prednisone 5 mg twice daily Prostate cancer metastatic, high risk castration sensitive PO 1,000 mg once daily with 5 mg prednisone once daily	Advanced prostatic cancer	Edema, hypertension, hot flash, hyperglycemia, hypernatremia, UTI, Increased ALT, AST, bilirubin
Bicalutamide (Casodex; ❋ ACH-Bicalutamide, ACT Bicalutamide, Casodex, Com-Bicalutamide)	PO 500 mg once daily (with goserelin or leuprolide)	Advanced prostatic cancer	Nausea, vomiting, diarrhea, hot flashes, pain, and breast enlargement
Enzalutamide (Xtandi)	Prostate cancer, castration resistant: PO 160 mg once daily until disease progression or acceptable toxicity Prostate cancer metastatic, castration sensitive: PO 160 mg once daily until disease progression or acceptable toxicity	Advanced prostatic cancer	Hypertension, peripheral edema, neutropenia, dizziness, fatigue, arthralgia
Nilutamide (Nilandron; ❋ Anandron)	PO 300 mg daily for 30 d and then 150 mg daily	Advanced breast cancer in postmenopausal females	Diarrhea, GI bleeding, heart failure, and hyperglycemia

TABLE 14.4
DRUGS AT A GLANCE: Antineoplastic Hormone Inhibitor Drugs (Continued)

Drug	Routes and Dosage Ranges	Clinical Uses	Adverse Effects
Gonadotropin-Releasing Hormone Agonists			
Leuprolide acetate (Eligard, Lupron Depot; ✦ Eligard, Lupron Depot)	Prostate cancer, advanced: IM Lupron Depot 7.5 mg every month or Lupron Depot 22.5 mg (3 mo); 22.5 mg every 12 wk or Lupron Depot 30 mg (4 mo); 30 mg every 16 wk or Lupron Depot 45 mg (6 mo); 45 mg every 24 wk Sub-Q Eligard: 7.5 mg monthly or 22.5 mg every 3 mo or 30 mg every 4 mo or 45 mg every 6 mo Leuprolide acetate 5 mg/mL solution 1 mg/d	Prostate cancer	Vasodilation, emotional lability, mood changes, headache, skin rash, seborrhea, weight gain, local injection site reaction, bone pain, neuropathy, hematuria, and ureteral or bladder outlet obstruction
Goserelin (Zoladex; ✦ Zoladex, Zoladex LA)	Advanced prostate cancer: sub-Q implant 28 d, 3.6 mg every 28 wk Sub-Q implant 12 wk: 10.8 mg every 12 wk Canadian labeling: same as above Breast cancer: sub-Q 3.6 mg every 28 d	Prostate cancer Breast cancer	Hot flashes, transient increase in bone pain, peripheral edema, and vasodilation
Triptorelin (Trelstar, Trelstar Mixject; ✦ Decapeptyl, Trelstar)	IM 3.75 mg every 4 wk or 11.25 mg every 12 wk or 22.5 mg every 24 wk	Advanced prostatic cancer	Increased serum glucose, decreased hemoglobin and red blood cells, increased serum alkaline, musculoskeletal pain, and increased blood urea nitrogen

surgical orchidectomy, or medical castration. Additional systemic therapies include abiraterone and prednisone with ADT, enzalutamide or apalutamide with ADT, docetaxel with ADT, or triplet therapy. Triplet therapy combines ADT with docetaxel plus a second agent, abiraterone or darolutamide (Lee & Smith, 2022).

Abiraterone (Yonsa, Zytiga), bicalutamide (Casodex), enzalutamide (Xtandi), **flutamide** (Eulexin), and nilutamide (Nilandron) are antiandrogens used to treat advanced prostate cancer. The drugs bind to androgen receptors in cells of the prostate gland and thereby block the effects of the active form of testosterone, dihydrotestosterone, on malignant prostate cell growth. Antiandrogens are also able to block the effects of adrenal testosterone production, which accounts for about 10% of testosterone and is not affected by the GnRH analogs.

All of the androgen receptor antagonists are administered orally. Abiraterone is used for metastatic prostate cancer and should be combined with a GnRH analog. Nilutamide is approved specifically for use in prostate cancer after surgical orchiectomy to reduce bone pain, slow progression, and increase survival time.

Gonadotropin-Releasing Hormone Agonists

Leuprolide acetate (Eligard, Lupron Depot) is a synthetic version of the hypothalamic luteinizing hormone (LH) and GnRH that acts as an inhibitor of gonadotropin secretion. The action results in the suppression of ovarian and testicular function. A decrease in LH and follicle-stimulating hormone (FSH) results, with a subsequent decrease in estrogen in females and testosterone in males. In the treatment of advanced prostate cancer, leuprolide reduces testosterone to castration levels. It is important to monitor prostate-specific antigen and testosterone levels, as well as to check the injection site for hypersensitivity reactions. The nurse should instruct the patient to report hematuria and diminished urinary output.

The synthetic LH preparation goserelin (Zoladex, Zoladex LA) is administered for the treatment of breast cancer and prostate cancer. It inhibits the anterior pituitary secretion of gonadotropin. In the initial phase of treatment, the levels of LH and FSH are increased, and a sustained suppression of the pituitary gonadotropins results. The ultimate effect of goserelin will result in an inhibition of GnRH. Long-term administration to males decreases serum testosterone at or below castration levels. Goserelin raises blood glucose levels, so it is important to instruct the patient on blood glucose monitoring. Also, males have an increased risk of myocardial infarction. It should be noted that significant bone pain will occur in the first week of therapy. Continuing therapy will result in bone loss; thus, it is necessary to monitor bone density.

The agent triptorelin (Trelstar, Trelstar Mixject) is administered for prostate cancer. It reduces testosterone levels in males and LH and FSH in females. The reduction in testosterone in males results in castration. The patient must be instructed to notify the prescriber of rash or hives.

Cytoprotectant Drugs

Cytoprotectant agents reduce the adverse effects of cytotoxic drugs, some of which can be severe, debilitating, or life threatening (see Box 14.2). Severe adverse effects of cytotoxic drugs may also limit drug dosage or frequency of administration, thereby limiting the effectiveness of chemotherapy. Several cytoprotective drugs are available to protect body tissues from one or more adverse effects and allow for a more optimal dose and schedule of cytotoxic agents. To be effective, it is necessary to time administration in relation to administration of the cytotoxic agent. Table 14.5 lists cytoprotective agents and their clinical uses.

NCLEX Success

4. A patient is prescribed fulvestrant. What is the action of this drug?
   A. Fulvestrant is highly cytotoxic to both cancer cells and normal cells.
   B. Fulvestrant blocks estrogen receptors and decreases estrogen-mediated growth stimulation.
   C. Fulvestrant boosts the immune response to increase the effectiveness of other chemotherapy agents.
   D. Fulvestrant stops cancer cell maturation in the G_1 phase of the cell cycle.

5. Hormone inhibitor drugs are most effective in which of the following?
   A. treating breast or prostate cancer
   B. preventing hematologic malignancies
   C. treating thyroid and pituitary tumors
   D. protecting normal cells from cytotoxic drugs

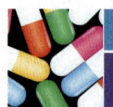

TABLE 14.5
DRUGS AT A GLANCE: Cytoprotectant Drugs

Drug	Routes and Dosage Ranges	Clinical Use
Amifostine (Ethyol)	IV infusion 910 mg/m² once daily within 30 min of starting chemotherapy	Reduction of cisplatin-induced kidney toxicity
Dexrazoxane (✽ Zinecard)	IV 10 times the amount of doxorubicin (e.g., dexrazoxane 500 mg/m² per doxorubicin 50 mg/m²) and then give doxorubicin within 30 min of completing dexrazoxane dose	Reduction of doxorubicin-induced cardiomyopathy in females with metastatic breast cancer who have received a cumulative dose of 300 mg/m² and need additional doxorubicin
Epoetin alfa (Epogen, Procrit, Retacrit; ✽ Eprex)	Sub-Q 150–300 units/kg three times weekly, adjusted to maintain desired hematocrit	Treatment of chemotherapy-induced anemia
Filgrastim (Granix, Neupogen, Nivestym, Zarxio; ✽ Grastofil, Neupogen)	Sub-Q, IV 5 mcg/kg/d, at least 24 h after cytotoxic chemotherapy, up to 2 wk or an absolute neutrophil count of 10,000/mm³	Treatment of chemotherapy-induced neutropenia
Leucovorin (✽ Lederle Leucovorin)	"Rescue," PO, IV, IM 15 mg every 6 h for 10 doses, starting 24 h after methotrexate begun Colorectal cancer, IV 20 mg/m² or 200 mg/m², followed by 5-fluorouracil, daily for 5 d, repeated every 28 d	"Rescue" after high-dose methotrexate for osteosarcoma Advanced colorectal cancer, with 5-fluorouracil
Mesna (Mesnex; ✽ Uromitexan)	IV, 20% of ifosfamide dose for 3 doses (at time of ifosfamide dose, then 4 h and 8 h after ifosfamide dose)	Prevention of cyclophosphamide and ifosfamide-induced hemorrhagic cystitis
Palifermin (Kepivance; ✽ Kepivance)	IV bolus, 60 mcg/kg daily for 6 total doses 3 consecutive days before and 3 d after high-dose chemotherapy (4th dose at least 1 d before stem cell infusion)	Prevent oral mucositis in hematologic malignancies before stem cell transplant
Sargramostim (Leukine)	IV infusion, 250 mcg/m²/d until absolute neutrophil count is above 1,500/mm³ for 3 d, up to 42 d	Myeloid reconstitution after bone marrow transplant; to decrease chemotherapy-induced neutropenia

THE NURSING PROCESS

A concept map outlines the nursing process related to drug therapy considerations in this chapter. Additional nursing implications related to the disease process should also be considered in care decisions.

Assessment

- Assess the patient's condition before chemotherapy is started and often during treatment. Useful information includes the type, grade, and stage of the tumor, as well as the signs and symptoms of cancer. General manifestations include anemia, malnutrition, weight loss, pain, and infection. Specific manifestations depend on the organs affected.
- Assess for other diseases and organ dysfunctions (e.g., cardiac, pulmonary, renal, hepatic) that can influence individual response to chemotherapy.
- Assess emotional status, coping mechanisms, family relationships, financial resources, and social support mechanisms. Anxiety and depression are common features during cancer diagnosis and treatment.
- Assess laboratory test results before chemotherapy to establish baseline data and during chemotherapy to monitor drug effects.
  - **Blood tests for tumor markers** (tumor-specific antigens on cell surfaces). Alpha-fetoprotein is a fetal antigen normally present during intrauterine and early postnatal life but absent in adulthood. Increased amounts may indicate hepatic or testicular cancer. Carcinoembryonic antigen (CEA) is secreted by several types of malignant cells (e.g., colorectal cancer). A rising level may indicate tumor progression; levels that are elevated before surgery and disappear after surgery indicate adequate tumor excision. If CEA levels rise later, it probably indicates tumor recurrence. With chemotherapy, falling CEA levels indicate effectiveness. Other tumor markers are immunoglobulins (elevated levels may indicate multiple myeloma) and prostate-specific antigens (elevated levels may indicate prostatic cancer).
  - **CBC** to check for anemia, leukopenia, and thrombocytopenia because most cytotoxic antineoplastic drugs cause bone marrow depression. It is necessary to perform a CBC and white blood cell differential before each cycle of chemotherapy to determine dosage and frequency of drug administration, to monitor bone marrow function so fatal bone marrow depression does not occur, and to assist in planning nursing care. For example, the patient is very susceptible to infection when the leukocyte count is low, and bleeding is likely when the platelet count is low.
  - **Other tests.** These include tests of kidney and liver function, serum calcium, uric acid, and others, depending on the organs affected by the cancer or its treatment.

Outcomes of Therapy

The patient will
- Receive assistance in coping with the diagnosis of cancer.
- Experience reduced anxiety and fear.
- Receive chemotherapy accurately and safely.
- Experience reduction of tumor size, shift towards normal laboratory values, or other therapeutic effects of chemotherapy.
- Experience minimal bleeding, infection, nausea and vomiting, and other consequences of chemotherapy.
- Maintain adequate food and fluid intake and body weight.

Nursing Interventions

- Strengthen host defenses by promoting a healthful lifestyle (e.g., good nutrition, adequate rest and exercise, stress management techniques, avoiding or minimizing alcohol and tobacco use).
- For patients receiving cytotoxic anticancer drugs, try to prevent or minimize the incidence and severity of adverse reactions.
- Provide supportive care to patients and families. Physiologic care includes pain management, comfort measures, and assistance with nutrition, hygiene, ambulation, and other activities of daily living as needed. Psychological care includes allowing family members or significant others to be with the patient and participate in care when desired and keeping patients and families informed.

Evaluation

- Monitor drug administration for accuracy.
- Observe and interview for therapeutic effects of chemotherapy.
- Compare current laboratory reports with baseline values for changes toward normal values.
- Compare weight and nutritional status with baseline values for maintenance or improvement.
- Observe and interview for adverse drug effects and interventions to prevent or manage them.
- Observe and interview for effective pain management and other symptom control.

Visit thePoint® *at* **http://thePoint.lww.com/Frandsen13e** *for answers to NCLEX Success questions (in Appendix A), answers to Clinical Application Case Studies (in Appendix B), and more!*

REFERENCES AND RESOURCES

Chu, E., & DeVita, V. T. (2021). *Physicians' cancer chemotherapy drug manual 2021*. Jones & Bartlett Learning.

Clowse, M. B., & McCune, W. J. (2023). General toxicity of cyclophosphamide in rheumatic disease. *UpToDate*. Lexi-Comp, Inc.

Davis, M., Hui, D., Davies, A., Ripamonti, C., Capela, A., DeFeo, G., DelFabbro, E., & Bruera, E. (2021). MASCC antiemetics in advanced cancer updated guideline. *Supportive Care in Cancer, 29*, 8097–8107. doi:10.1007/s00520-021-06437-w

Di Lorenzo, C. (2023). Approach to the infant or child with nausea and vomiting. In *UpToDate*. Lexi-Comp, Inc.

Hesketh, P. J. (2022). Prevention and treatment of chemotherapy-induced nausea and vomiting in adults. In *UpToDate*. Lexi-Comp, Inc.

Hinkle, J. L., Cheever, K. H., & Overbaugh, K. J. (2021). *Brunner & Suddarth's textbook of medical-surgical nursing* (15th ed.). Wolters Kluwer.

Konstantinopoulos, P. A., & Bristow, R. E. (2022). Patient selection and approach to neoadjuvant chemotherapy for new diagnosed advanced ovarian cancer. *UpToDate*. Lexi-Comp, Inc.

LaCasce, A. S., & Ng, A. H. (2021). Second malignancies after treatment of classic Hodgkin lymphoma. In *UpToDate*. Lexi-Comp, Inc.

Lee, E. Q. (2019). Overview of neurologic complications of non-platinum chemotherapy. In *UpToDate*. Lexi-Comp, Inc.

Lee, R. J., & Smith, M. R. (2022). Initial systemic therapy for advanced, recurrent, and metastatic noncastrate (castration sensitive) prostate cancer. *UpToDate*. Lexi-Comp, Inc.

Markman, M., & Olawaiye, A. (2021). Intraperitoneal chemotherapy for treatment of ovarian cancer. *UpToDate*. Lexi-Comp, Inc.

McClain, K. L., & Kamdar, K. (2022). Overview of Hodgkin lymphoma in children and adolescents. In *UpToDate*. Lexi-Comp, Inc.

Norris, T. L. (2019). *Porth's pathophysiology: Concepts of altered health states* (10th ed.). Wolters Kluwer.

Pritchard, K. I. (2023). Adjuvant endocrine therapy for non-metastatic, hormone receptor-positive breast cancer. In *UpToDate*. Lexi-Comp, Inc.

Runowicz, C. D., & Brewer, M. (2022). Chemotherapy of ovarian cancer in pregnancy. *UpToDate*. Lexi-Comp, Inc.

Sherani, F., Boston, C., & Mba, N. (2019). Latest update on prevention of acute chemotherapy-induced nausea and vomiting in pediatric cancer patients. *Oncology Reports, 21*(89), 1–9. doi:10.1007/s11912-019-0840-0

UpToDate. (2023). *Drug information*. Lexi-Comp, Inc.

Clinical Judgment in Practice: Section 3: Drugs Affecting the Hematopoietic and Immune Systems

A 29-year-old patient has developed chronic kidney failure due to polycystic kidney disease. The patient is dialyzed three times per week. The patient's glomerular filtration rate is 12 mL/min/1.73 m^2. The patient has been placed on the transplant list. At 12:00 p.m. January 29, the patient is notified that a kidney match has become available. The patient's kidney transplant surgery was completed successfully. Following surgery, the patient's blood pressure was 160/80, pulse 92, and respirations 24. The nephrologist has ordered dialysis until the transplanted kidney begins to work effectively. In preparation for discharge, the nursing staff and transplant coordinator must plan and implement patient teaching. The primary care nurse begins the patient teaching by reviewing the teaching plan with the patient. Following 2 days of dialysis, the transplanted kidney begins to work effectively. The glomerular filtration rate is 94 mL/min/1.73 m^2.

The serum creatinine level is 0.8 mg/dL. Regarding the patient teaching plan, the patient states, "I am anxious to learn about the medications I will be taking so I maintain a healthy kidney." The nephrologist informs the patient and nursing staff that the patient will be tentatively scheduled for discharge in 2 days. The patient weighs 58 kg and is receiving mycophenolate mofetil 870 mg orally twice per day, prednisone 116 mg orally in two divided doses, and cyclosporine 91 mg orally twice per day.

Step 1: Recognize Cues
Identify the relevant and important information from different sources, such as the medical history or subjective and objective data.

Answer: The patient states, "I am anxious to lean about the medications I will be taking so I maintain a healthy kidney." The patient is tentatively scheduled for discharge in 2 days.

Step 2: Analyze Cues
Organize and link the recognized cues to the patient's clinical presentation.

Answer: You link the statement from the patient and preparation for discharge to develop a teaching plan so the patient will understand all of the information that is vital to their health.

Step 3: Prioritize Hypotheses
Evaluate hypotheses and rank them according to priority, such as urgency, likelihood, risk, difficulty, and/or time. Cluster your findings to generate a list of problems (actual or potential) you believe the patient is experiencing or may experience and determine the level of urgency. Which problem is of the greatest concern?

Answer: You prioritize that patient teaching for the care of the kidney transplant patient is implemented to promote the health and independence of the patient during discharge.

Step 4: Generate Solutions
Identify expected outcomes and use hypotheses to define a set of interventions for the expected outcomes.

Answer: You prioritize the following teaching plan:
- What are the actions, indications for use, adverse effects, drug–herbal–food interactions, and administration guidelines with all antirejection medications.
- What are the interventions and rationales for the prevention of infection?
- What signs and symptoms should be reported to the physician/nephrologist?
- Identify the vaccines that are safe to be administered following a kidney transplant and in combination with antirejection medications.

Step 5: Take Actions
Implement the solutions that address the highest priorities.

Answer: You provide the following specific teaching to prepare the patient for discharge and self-care.

Mycophenolate:
The combination of mycophenolate, prednisone, and cyclosporine is to prevent the rejection of the newly transplanted kidney. These drugs prevent rejection by suppressing your immune system. Graft versus host disease is the rejection of the transplanted kidney, and the addition of prednisone and cyclosporine with the mycophenolate is the treatment for graft versus host disease. Due to the immunosuppressive effects of the medication, you will be more prone to infections. It is important to keep the home clean and free of mold that can contribute to infections. Also, you may want to wear a mask to prevent infection when in contact with other people. Nausea, vomiting, and diarrhea are

adverse effects of mycophenolate. Mycophenolate should not be combined with the herbal preparations alfalfa, echinacea, ginseng, and bee venom due to the increase of immunosuppression. When taking oral mycophenolate, do not crush or chew the tablet. It is to be swallowed whole, and for best absorption, take it on an empty stomach. The following symptoms should be reported to the prescriber: signs of infection, fever chills, sore throat, headache, swollen glands, cough, urinary burning or frequency. Your healthcare provider may require blood work to be drawn. A complete blood count is monitored weekly for the first month, twice monthly for months 2 and 3, and then monthly throughout the first year.

Prednisone:
Prednisone enhances immunosuppression. The administration of prednisone may require a tapering dosage. Follow the administration guidelines of the prescriber. As with the other immunosuppressant medications, protect from getting an infection.

Cyclosporine:
Cyclosporine activates the white blood cells to increase the immune response by damaging the inflammatory changes in the tissue that occur with organ rejection. Cyclosporine prevents rejection reactions and prolongs the survival of the transplanted kidney. Adverse effects include kidney insufficiency, increased tissue of the gums known as gingival hyperplasia, and increased blood cholesterol known as hyperlipidemia. The combination of St. John's wort may reduce the therapeutic effect of cyclosporine. Dilution of an oral cyclosporine solution should follow package instructions. Do not administer cyclosporine oral solution from a plastic or Styrofoam cup. Neoral oral solution may be diluted with room temperature orange juice or apple juice. Sandimmune oral solution may be diluted with milk, chocolate milk, or orange juice. Avoid changing diluents and mix them thoroughly. The solution and diluent should be drunk immediately. Mix in a glass container and rinse the container with more diluent to ensure the total dose is administered. Do not rinse the syringe before or after use. Rinsing will result in dosage variation.

You also provide the following general patient teaching points:

- The administration of antirejection medications is a lifelong treatment to prevent potential organ rejection that is required after the kidney transplant.
- Carry identification of kidney transplant and medication list.
- Maintain a healthy lifestyle by eating a nutritious diet, getting adequate rest and sleep, and avoiding alcohol and tobacco.
- Maintain regular visits with the healthcare provider and obtain laboratory testing as prescribed.
- Wear protective sun screen to decrease exposure to sun and possible skin cancer development.
- Do not consume grapefruit or grapefruit juice due to its inhibitory effects with immunosuppressant medications.
- Avoid getting an infection by wearing a mask in crowded places, practicing good hygiene habits with proper and frequent handwashing, and avoiding contact with people who are suffering from infectious diseases.
- Consult your healthcare provider about the vaccines to be administered to protect from infection. It is recommended that an annual influenza A and B booster be administered. A COVID-19 vaccine is also recommended. Live vaccines such as measles, mumps, rubella, oral polio, varicella intranasal influenza, and other live vaccines should not be administered.

Step 6: Evaluate Outcomes
Compare observed outcomes against expected outcomes.

Answer: You have implemented the teach back method to evaluate the patient's understanding of the patient teaching regarding the antirejection agents and self-care following discharge. The patient was able to accurately teach back all aspects of the teaching plan that you implemented. In addition, the patient verbalized the need to call the transplant team if any questions arise. The patient was able to report the signs and symptoms of infection.

SECTION 4

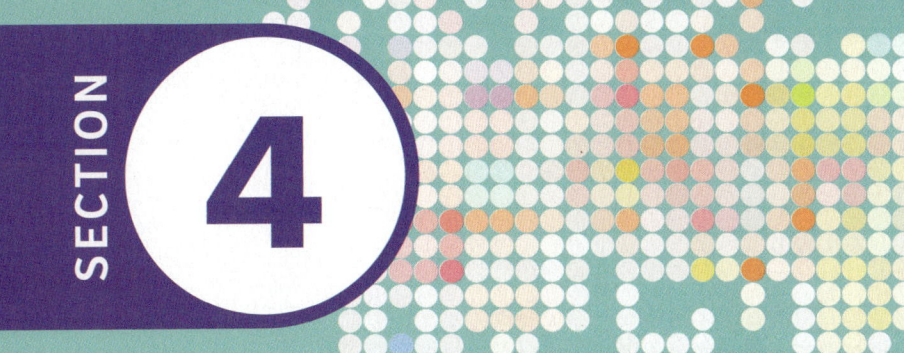

Drugs Affecting Inflammation and Infection

Chapter 15 Inflammation, Infection, and the Use of Antimicrobial Agents

Chapter 16 Drug Therapy to Decrease Pain, Fever, and Inflammation

Chapter 17 Drug Therapy With Corticosteroids

Chapter 18 Drug Therapy With Beta-Lactam Antibacterial Agents

Chapter 19 Drug Therapy With Aminoglycosides and Fluoroquinolones

Chapter 20 Drug Therapy With Tetracyclines, Sulfonamides, and Urinary Antiseptics

Chapter 21 Drug Therapy With Macrolides and Miscellaneous Anti-Infective Agents

Chapter 22 Drug Therapy for Tuberculosis and *Mycobacterium avium* Complex Disease

Chapter 23 Drug Therapy for Viral Infections

Chapter 24 Drug Therapy for Fungal Infections

Chapter 25 Drug Therapy for Parasitic Infections

CHAPTER 15

Inflammation, Infection, and the Use of Antimicrobial Agents

LEARNING OBJECTIVES

After studying this chapter, you should be able to:

1. Describe the characteristics of inflammation.
2. Describe, in general, the groups of drugs used to treat inflammation.
3. Identify the common microorganisms that cause infection and their key characteristics.
4. Discuss the characteristics of infection and methods of infection control.
5. Discuss ways to minimize emergence of drug-resistant microorganisms.
6. List ways to increase the benefits and decrease the risks associated with antimicrobial drug therapy.
7. Apply the nursing process in the care of patients receiving antimicrobial therapy.

CLINICAL APPLICATION CASE STUDY

Alisa Warren, a 25-year-old woman with early-onset rheumatoid arthritis, is a social worker in a pediatric hospital. She has a heavy caseload, and her lunch often consists of a soda, chips, and a sweet roll from the snack machine. She and her partner spend most evenings watching movies and television because her pain prevents her from participating in many activities. Recently, her practitioner prescribed methylprednisolone, a corticosteroid, to help manage the inflammation associated with the arthritis.

KEY TERMS

Antibacterial: ability to kill bacteria or interfere with the ability of bacteria to grow and replicate

Antibiotic: antimicrobial drug that has the ability to kill or inhibit bacterial growth and replication

Antibiotic resistance: ability of certain bacteria to survive and multiply in the presence of antibiotics

Anti-infective: agent or substance with antibacterial, antiviral, and antifungal properties

Anti-inflammatory agent: drug indicated when the inflammatory response is inappropriate, abnormal, or persistent or destroys tissue

Antimicrobial agent: drug used to prevent or treat infections caused by pathogenic (disease-producing) microorganisms such as bacteria, fungi, viruses, and parasites

Bacteria: single-celled microorganisms that do not have a nuclei and reproduce by fission or splitting

Bactericidal: agent that kills bacteria

Bacteriostatic: agent that inhibits bacterial growth and replication

Broad spectrum: effective against a wide range of bacteria

Colonization: presence and growth of microorganisms on host tissues

Community-acquired infection: infection caused by microorganisms that originated in a setting outside of a healthcare facility

Community-acquired pneumonia: pneumonia contracted by a person outside of a healthcare facility

Detection of antigens: technique to identify pathogens that uses features of culture and serology but reduces the time required for diagnosis

Empiric therapy: drug therapy undertaken prior to obtaining a definite diagnosis

Fungi: plantlike microorganisms that live as parasites on living tissue or as saprophytes on decaying organic matter

Healthcare-associated pneumonia: pneumonia that has been acquired in other healthcare facilities, such as nursing homes

Hospital-acquired infection: infection acquired from microorganisms in hospitals and other healthcare facilities

Inflammation: immunologic response to allergy, infection, or injury that increases the migration of leukocytes and blood flow to assist in repairing tissues

Opportunistic: microorganisms in normal flora that become pathogenic under conditions that are favorable for their (over)growth

Penicillin-binding proteins: bacterial proteins that function in cell wall synthesis and serve as target sites for penicillin to bind

Serology: method of identifying infectious agents by measuring the antibody level (titer) in the serum of an infected host

Susceptibility: vulnerability of the bacteria to an antibiotic's effects

Viruses: intracellular parasites that survive only in living tissues

INTRODUCTION

This chapter is an introduction to the pathophysiologic effects of inflammation and infection. Readers should note that the format of this chapter is different from that of previous chapters. This chapter presents an overview of the anti-inflammatory and antimicrobial therapy to allow an understanding of a broad classification of the drugs involved and their impact on decreasing inflammation associated with infection and the infective process.

To help prevent inflammation caused by allergy, injury, or infection, the nurse should be familiar with **anti-inflammatory agents**, drugs indicated when the inflammatory response is inappropriate, abnormal, or persistent or destroys tissue. The anti-inflammatory agents administered to reduce the inflammatory process include aspirin, nonsteroidal anti-inflammatory drugs (NSAIDs), and corticosteroids. Healthcare providers use medicines known as **antimicrobial agents** to prevent or treat infections caused by pathogenic (disease-producing) microorganisms such as bacteria, fungi, viruses, and parasites. Antimicrobial agents treat inflammation resulting from infectious processes with antimicrobial drugs.

Most microorganisms live in equilibrium with the human host and do not cause disease; however, even beneficial bacteria may cause infections in certain conditions. When the balance is upset and infection occurs, characteristics of the infecting microorganisms and the adequacy of host defense mechanisms are major factors in determining the severity of the infection and the person's ability to recover. In addition, overuse of antimicrobial agents may lead to serious infections caused by drug-resistant microorganisms. To help prevent infectious diseases and participate effectively in antimicrobial drug therapy, the nurse must be knowledgeable about microorganisms, host responses to microorganisms, and antimicrobial drugs.

OVERVIEW OF INFLAMMATION

To adequately understand the pharmacologic treatment of inflammation, it is important to understand the causes, clinical considerations, and manifestations of inflammation. This will make it easier to understand the drug therapy associated with the treatment of inflammation, as addressed in Chapters 16 and 17.

Inflammation is the cellular response of the body to tissue damage and injury. The cells and tissues of the body are killed or injured by chemical, physical, or infectious agents. If inflammation is caused by an infectious agent, the localizing effects increase the risk of the spread of infection (Fig. 15.1).

The body's autoimmune response can also produce an inflammatory process. There are three stages of acute inflammation. The first stage of acute inflammation is the immunologic response of the body that produces increased migration of leukocytes and flow of blood to the cells and tissues affected to help repair the tissues. As the leukocytes invade, there is a slowing of the blood flow and

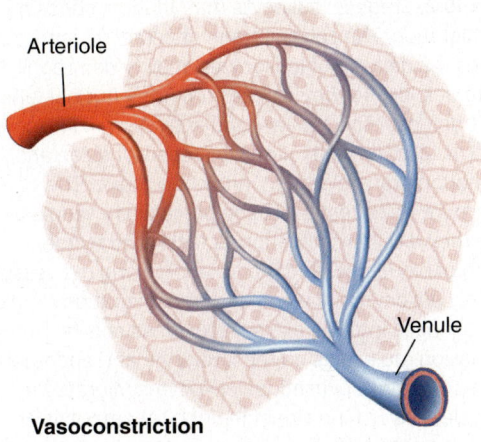

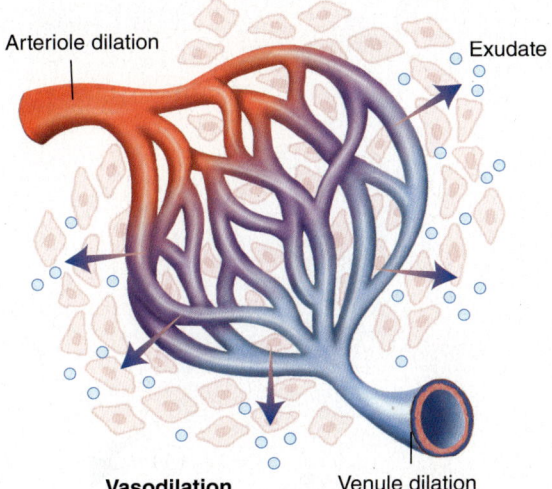

Figure 15.1. Stage 1: vascular stage. The vascular stage of acute inflammation, which is characterized by changes in the small blood vessels at the site of injury. It begins with vasoconstriction followed rapidly by vasodilation. Vasodilation results in an increase in capillary blood flow, causing heat and redness, which are two of the cardinal signs of inflammation. This is accompanied by an increase in vascular permeability with outpouring of protein-rich fluid (exudate) into the extravascular spaces. The loss of proteins reduces the capillary osmotic pressure and increases the interstitial osmotic pressure. This, coupled with an increase in capillary pressure, causes a marked outflow of fluid and its accumulation in the tissue spaces, producing the swelling, pain, and impaired function that represent the other cardinal signs of acute inflammation. As fluid moves out of the vessels, stagnation of flow and clotting of blood occur. This aids in localizing the spread of infectious microorganisms.

margination, which is the adhesion of the leukocytes to the wall of the blood vessels. In the second stage, the leukocytes then transmigrate from the vascular space to the extravascular tissue. They travel to the tissue injury site by chemotaxis (Fig. 15.2).

In the third stage of acute inflammation, opsonization facilitates phagocytosis. During opsonization, a substance coats the foreign antigens, producing inflammation that makes the antigens more susceptible to the macrophages and leukocytes, which in turn increases phagocytic activity. The two opsonins are complement factor C3b and antibodies (Fig. 15.3).

For an in-depth discussion of the phases of acute inflammation and the pathophysiology of acute and chronic inflammation, visit thePoint® http://thePoint.lww.com/Frandsen13e.

Clinical Manifestations

The clinical manifestations of acute inflammation are pain, redness, and swelling. Breaks in the integumentary system result in the drainage of exudate. In the event of a viral or bacterial infection associated with the inflammation, fever and general malaise sometimes occur. In chronic inflammation, tissue destruction and scarring may develop. The development of scarring replaces the connective or parenchymal tissue, resulting in diminished mobility or function. As previously stated, granulomas may occur because of an uncontrolled acute inflammatory process.

Drug Therapy

Aspirin, NSAIDs, and corticosteroids are administered to decrease inflammation (see Chapters 16 and 17). Aspirin and NSAIDs block the synthesis of prostaglandin in the central and peripheral nervous systems. The anti-inflammatory response produced by the administration of corticosteroids occurs through the inhibition of interleukin-1, cytokines, and the tumor necrosis factor. Corticosteroids also impair phagocytosis by preventing phagocytic cells from leaving the bloodstream. They decrease the amount of lymphocytes, fibroblasts, and collagen needed for tissue repair.

> **Clinical Application 15.1**
> - Now that Ms. Warren has been given a corticosteroid to decrease the inflammation of her joints, what is she at risk for developing?

OVERVIEW OF MICROORGANISMS

Microorganisms that cause infectious disease include bacteria, viruses, fungi, and parasites. **Bacteria** are single-celled microorganisms without nuclei that reproduce by fission or splitting. They are classified according to whether they are aerobic (require oxygen) or anaerobic (cannot live in the presence of oxygen), their ability to retain Gram stain (gram positive) or to reject Gram stain (gram negative), and their shape (e.g., cocci, rods). **Antibiotics** are antimicrobial drugs used to treat bacterial infections.

Viruses are intracellular parasites that survive only in living tissues. They are officially classified according to their structure but are more commonly described according to origin and the disorders or symptoms they produce. Human pathogens include adenoviruses, herpesviruses, and retroviruses (see Chapter 23).

Fungi are plantlike microorganisms that live as parasites on living tissue or as saprophytes on decaying organic matter. Approximately 50 species are pathogenic in humans (see Chapter 24). Parasites are microorganisms in the animal kingdom that infect other animals. Parasites that infect human hosts include arthropods, protozoa, and helminths (see Chapter 25).

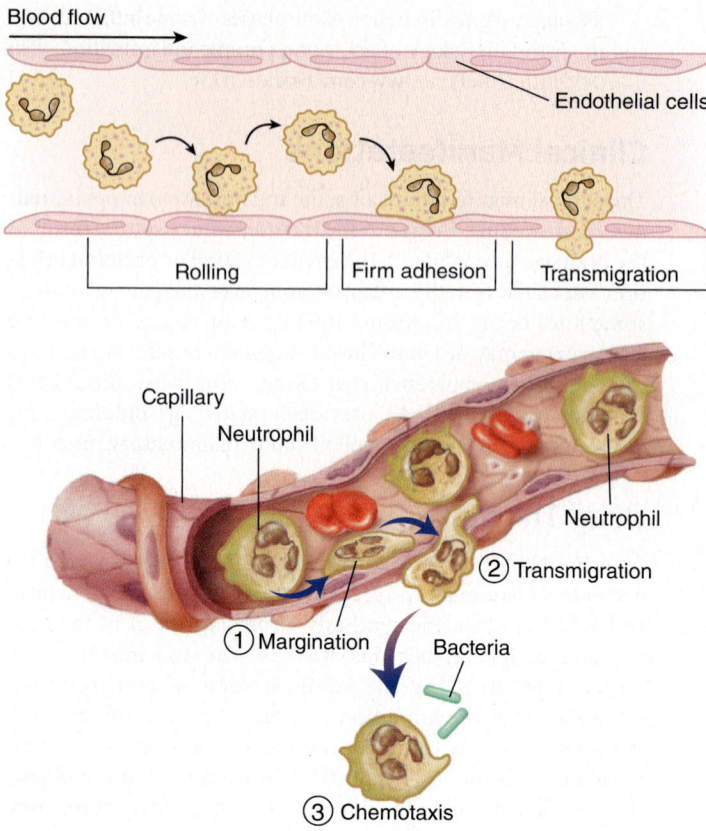

Figure 15.2. Stage 2: leukocyte margination, adhesion, and transmigration. The cellular stage of acute inflammation involves the delivery of leukocytes, mainly neutrophil, to the site of injury so they can perform their normal functions of host defense. The delivery and activation of leukocytes can be divided into the following steps: adhesion and margination, transmigration, and chemotaxis. The recruitment of leukocytes to the precapillary venules, where they exit the circulation, is facilitated by the slowing of blood flow and margination along the vessel surface. Leukocyte adhesion and transmigration from the vascular space into the extravascular tissue is facilitated by adhesion molecules on the leukocyte and endothelial surfaces. After extravasation, leukocytes migrate in the tissues toward the site of injury by chemotaxis or locomotion oriented along a chemical gradient.

Colonization is the presence and growth of microorganisms on host tissues. The microorganisms do not necessarily cause tissue injury or elicit an immune response in the human body. The human body also has sterile areas, in which microorganisms do not live. Sterile areas that do not communicate directly with the external environment include organs such as the heart and liver, the musculoskeletal system, and body fluids such as urine. Areas typically populated by microorganisms include the skin, upper respiratory tract, and colon.

Infection begins with colonization by microorganisms. Infections occur when microorganisms invade a host, attach to host cell receptors, and multiply in sufficient numbers to cause injury, causing clinical signs and symptoms indicative of an infection.

The infection of a microorganism stimulates the body's immune response. In many instances, this immune response is sufficient to contain an infection. However, most microorganisms have characteristics that allow them to adapt to ensure their survival, and these adaptations help protect them from normal body defense mechanisms.

Box 15.1 describes common bacterial pathogens of humans. Accurate assessment and documentation of symptoms can aid in early detection and diagnosis of infectious disease.

Key Characteristics of Common Microorganisms

Antimicrobial drugs are an important intervention to treat infections that could otherwise cause significant injury and harm to the human host. To understand antimicrobial drug use, it is

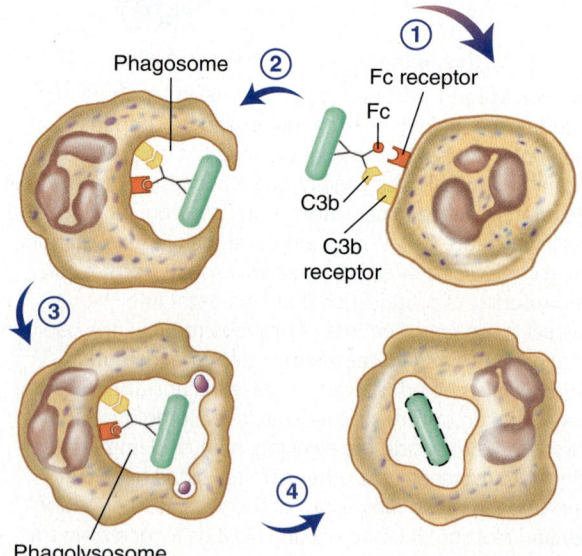

Figure 15.3. Stage 3: opsonization and phagocytosis. Once at the site of injury, the products generated by tissue injury trigger a number of leukocyte responses, including phagocytosis and cell killing. Opsonization of microbes (1) by complement factor C3b and antibody facilitates recognition by neutrophil C3b and the antibody Fc receptor. Receptor activation (2) triggers intracellular signaling and actin assembly in the neutrophil, leading to formation of pseudopods that enclose the microbe within a phagosome. The phagosome (3) then fuses with an intracellular lysosome to form a phagolysosome into which lysosomal enzymes and oxygen radicals (4) are released to kill and degrade the microbe.

BOX 15.1 Common Bacterial Pathogens

Gram-Positive Bacteria

Staphylococci

Staphylococcus aureus bacteria are part of the normal microbial flora of the skin and upper respiratory tract and also are common pathogens. Some people carry (are colonized with) *S. aureus* in the anterior nares. The bacteria are spread mainly by direct contact with people who are infected or who are carriers. The hands of healthcare workers are considered a major source of indirect spread and hospital-acquired infections. The bacteria also survive on inanimate surfaces for long periods of time.

S. aureus organisms can cause skin infections such as boils and carbuncles. When burns or surgical wounds become contaminated with *S. aureus*, they often produce endotoxins that destroy erythrocytes, leukocytes, platelets, fibroblasts, and other human cells. These bacteria may also cause infections of the respiratory tract and urinary tract. Many strains when ingested also produce enterotoxins that cause food poisoning.

High-risk groups for staphylococcal infections include newborns, older adults, and people who are malnourished or have obesity or who have diabetes. In children, staphylococcal infections of the respiratory tract are most common in those younger than 2 years of age. In adults, staphylococcal pneumonia often occurs in people with chronic lung disease or as a secondary bacterial infection after influenza, which destroys the ciliated epithelium of the respiratory tract and thereby aids bacterial invasion.

Staphylococcus species, non-*aureus* (SSNA) describes a group of bacteria that are also part of the normal microbial flora of the skin and mucosal surfaces and are common pathogens. The most common member of this group involved in infections is *Staphylococcus epidermidis*.

Infections due to SSNA are often associated with treatment devices such as intravascular catheters, prosthetic heart valves, cardiac pacemakers, orthopedic prostheses, cerebrospinal fluid shunts, and peritoneal catheters. SSNA infections include endocarditis, bacteremia, and other serious infections and are especially hazardous to immunocompromised patients. Treatment usually requires removal of any infected medical device as well as appropriate antibiotic therapy.

Streptococci

Certain streptococci are part of the normal microbial flora of the throat and nasopharynx in many healthy people. These bacteria do not usually cause disease unless the mucosal barrier is damaged by trauma, previous infection, or surgical manipulation, which allows the bacteria to enter the bloodstream and other parts of the body where they colonize and cause an infection.

Streptococcus pneumoniae bacteria, often called "pneumococci," are common. They cause pneumonia, sinusitis, otitis media, and meningitis. Pneumococcal pneumonia usually develops when the mechanisms that normally expel inhaled microorganisms (i.e., the mucociliary blanket and cough reflex) are impaired by viral infection, smoking, immobility, or other insults. When *S. pneumoniae* reach the alveoli, they proliferate, cause acute inflammation, and spread rapidly to involve one or more lobes. Alveoli fill with proteinaceous fluid, neutrophils, and bacteria.

Older adults have high rates of illness and death from pneumococcal pneumonia, which can often be prevented by pneumococcal vaccine (see Chapter 12). Pneumococcal sinusitis and otitis media usually follow a viral illness, such as the common cold, which injures the protective ciliated epithelium and fills the air spaces with nutrient-rich tissue fluid, in which the pneumococci thrive. *S. pneumoniae* is a common pathogen in bacterial sinusitis. In young children, upper respiratory tract infections may be complicated by acute sinusitis. Many children have repeated episodes of pneumococcal otitis media by 6 years of age, which may result in reduced hearing acuity. Pneumococcal meningitis may develop from sinus or middle ear infections or an injury that allows pneumococcal bacteria from the nasopharynx to enter the meninges. *S. pneumoniae* infection is a common cause of bacterial meningitis in adults. Other potential secondary complications include septicemia, endocarditis, pericarditis, and empyema.

Streptococcus pyogenes (beta-hemolytic streptococcus) bacteria are often part of the normal flora of the skin and oropharynx that may become pathogenic in other body regions. The bacteria spread from person to person by direct contact with oral or respiratory secretions. They cause severe streptococcal pharyngitis ("strep throat"), scarlet fever, and rheumatic fever. Endocarditis and glomerulonephritis may occur as sequelae following untreated or inadequately treated streptococcal pharyngitis.

Enterococci

Enterococci are normal flora in the human intestine but are also found in soil, food, water, and animals. Although the genus *Enterococcus* contains approximately 12 species, the main pathogens are *Enterococcus faecalis* and *Enterococcus faecium*. Most enterococcal infections occur in hospitalized patients, especially those in critical care units. Risk factors for hospital-acquired infections include serious underlying disease, prior surgery, abnormal kidney function, and the presence of urinary or vascular catheters. These bacteria, especially *E. faecalis*, are usually secondary invaders in urinary tract or wound infections. Enterococci may also cause endocarditis, which occurs most often in people with underlying heart disease, such as an injured valve. When the bacteria reach a heart valve, they multiply and release emboli of foreign particles into the bloodstream. Symptoms of endocarditis include fever, heart murmurs, enlarged spleen, and anemia. This infection is diagnosed by isolating enterococci from blood cultures. If not treated promptly and appropriately, enterococcal endocarditis may be fatal.

Gram-Negative Bacteria

Bacteroides

Bacteroides are anaerobic bacteria normally found in the digestive, respiratory, and genital tracts. They are the most common bacteria in the colon. *Bacteroides fragilis*, the major human pathogen, causes intra-abdominal and pelvic abscesses (e.g., after surgery or trauma that allows fecal contamination of these tissues), brain abscesses (e.g., from bacteremia or spread from a middle ear or sinus infection), and bacteremia, which may spread the bacteria throughout the body.

(Continued on page 276)

BOX 15.1 Common Bacterial Pathogens (Continued)

Escherichia coli

E. coli inhabit the intestinal tract of humans. They are normally nonpathogenic in the intestinal tract where they serve a beneficial role by synthesizing vitamins and by competitively discouraging growth of potential pathogens. In other parts of the body, however, they act as pathogens.

E. coli cause most urinary tract infections. They also cause pneumonia and sepsis in immunocompromised hosts and meningitis and sepsis in newborns. *E. coli* pneumonia often occurs in debilitated patients after colonization of the oropharynx. In healthy people, the normal gram-positive bacteria of oral cavities attach to material that coats the surface of oral mucosa and prevents transient *E. coli* from establishing residence. People who are debilitated or with severe illness produce an enzyme that destroys the material that allows gram-positive flora to adhere to oral mucosa. This allows *E. coli* (and other gram-negative enteric bacteria) to compete successfully with the normal gram-positive flora and colonize the oropharynx. Then, droplets of the oral flora are aspirated into the respiratory tract, where impaired protective mechanisms allow survival of the aspirated bacteria.

E. coli also cause enteric gram-negative sepsis, which is acquired from the normal enteric bacterial flora. When *E. coli* and other gram-negative bacteria reach the bloodstream of healthy people, host defenses eliminate the organisms; however, when the organisms reach the bloodstream of people with severe illnesses or immunocompromised status, the host is unable to mount adequate defenses and sepsis occurs. In newborns, *E. coli* are the most common gram-negative bacteria causing hospital-acquired septic shock and meningitis.

E. coli often cause diarrhea and dysentery. One strain, called O157:H7, causes hemorrhagic colitis, a disease characterized by severe abdominal cramps, copious bloody diarrhea, and hemolytic uremic syndrome (hemolytic anemia, thrombocytopenia, and acute kidney injury), which occurs most often in children. The main reservoir of this strain is the intestinal tract of animals, especially cattle, and several epidemics have been associated with ingestion of undercooked ground beef. Other sources include contaminated water and milk and person-to-person spread.

Klebsiella

Klebsiella bacteria, which are normal bowel flora, may infect the respiratory tract, urinary tract, bloodstream, burn wounds, and meninges, most often as opportunistic infections in debilitated persons. *Klebsiella pneumoniae* are a common cause of pneumonia, especially in people with pulmonary disease, bacteremia, and sepsis.

Proteus

Proteus bacteria are normally found in the intestinal tract and in decaying matter. They most often cause urinary tract and wound infections but may infect any tissue, especially in debilitated people. Infection often occurs with antibiotic therapy, which decreases drug-sensitive bacteria and allows drug-resistant *Proteus* bacteria to proliferate.

Pseudomonas

Pseudomonas bacteria are found in water, soil, skin, and intestines. They are found in the stools of some healthy people and possibly 50% of inpatients. *Pseudomonas aeruginosa*, the species most often associated with human disease, can cause infections of the respiratory tract, urinary tract, wounds, burns, meninges, eyes, and ears. Because of its resistance to many antibiotics, it can cause severe infections in people receiving antibiotic therapy for burns, wounds, and cystic fibrosis. *P. aeruginosa* colonizes the respiratory tract of most patients with cystic fibrosis and infects approximately 25% of burn patients. Infection is more likely to occur in hosts who are very young or very old or who have an impaired immune system. Sources of infection include catheterization of the urinary tract, trauma or procedures involving the brain or spinal cord, and contamination of respiratory ventilators.

Serratia

Serratia marcescens bacteria are found in infected people, water, milk, feces, and soil. They cause serious hospital-acquired infections of the urinary tract, respiratory tract, skin, burn wounds, and bloodstream. They also may cause hospital epidemics and produce drug-resistant strains. High-risk patients include newborns and patients who are debilitated or immunosuppressed.

Salmonella

Approximately 1,400 *Salmonella* species have been identified; several are pathogenic to humans. The bacteria cause gastroenteritis, typhoid fever, septicemia, and a severe, sometimes fatal type of food poisoning, in which diarrhea usually begins several hours after ingesting contaminated food and may continue for days, along with nausea, vomiting, headache, and abdominal pain. The primary reservoir is the intestinal tract of many animals. Humans become infected through ingestion of contaminated water or food. Water becomes polluted by introduction of feces from any animal excreting salmonellae. Infection via food usually results from ingestion of contaminated meat or by hands transferring organisms from an infected source. In the United States, undercooked poultry and eggs are common sources.

Shigella

Shigella species cause gastrointestinal problems ranging from mild diarrhea to severe bacillary dysentery. Humans, who seem to be the only natural hosts, become infected after ingestion of contaminated food or water. Effects of shigellosis are attributed to loss of fluids, electrolytes, and nutrients and to the ulceration that occurs in the colon wall.

important to have a basic understanding of the microorganisms they target. The following sections provide information about microorganisms and how they interact with human hosts.

Normal Flora

Normal skin flora includes staphylococci, streptococci, diphtheroids, and transient environmental microorganisms. The upper respiratory tract contains staphylococci, streptococci, pneumococci, and diphtheroids, as well as *Haemophilus influenzae*. The external genitalia contain skin organisms, and the vagina contains lactobacilli, *Candida*, and *Bacteroides*. The colon contains *Escherichia coli*, *Klebsiella*, *Enterobacter*, *Proteus*, *Pseudomonas*, *Bacteroides*, clostridia, lactobacilli, streptococci, and staphylococci.

Normal flora protects the human host in a variety of ways. For example, normal bowel flora synthesizes vitamin K and vitamin B complex. The intestinal flora also plays a role in digestion. Furthermore, by competing with potential pathogens for nutrients and by preventing adhesion and growth of pathogens, beneficial microorganisms interfere with the ability of potential pathogens to cause infections.

In certain instances, normal flora can become pathogenic. For example, microorganisms that are part of the normal flora and nonpathogenic in one area of the body may be pathogenic in other parts of the body; for example, *E. coli* is part of the normal intestinal flora, but it is a common cause of urinary tract infections.

Host Defense Mechanisms

Although the numbers and virulence of microorganisms help determine whether a person acquires an infection, another major factor is the host's ability to defend itself against the would-be invaders.

Major defense mechanisms of the human body are intact skin and mucous membranes, various **anti-infective** (having antibacterial, antiviral, and antifungal properties) secretions, mechanical movements, phagocytic cells, and the immune and inflammatory processes. The skin prevents penetration of foreign particles, and its secretions and normal bacterial flora inhibit growth of pathogenic microorganisms. Secretions of the gastrointestinal, respiratory, and genitourinary tracts (e.g., gastric acid, mucus) kill, trap, or inhibit growth of microorganisms. Coughing, swallowing, and peristalsis help remove foreign particles and pathogens trapped in mucus, as does the movement of cilia. Phagocytic cells in various organs and tissues engulf and digest pathogens and cellular debris. The immune system produces lymphocytes and antibodies. The inflammatory process is the body's response to injury by microorganisms, foreign particles, chemical agents, or physical irritation of tissues. Inflammation localizes, destroys, dilutes, or removes the injurious agents so tissue healing can occur (see previous discussion).

Many factors impair host defense mechanisms and predispose the host to infection by disease-producing microorganisms. These factors include:

- Breaks in the skin and mucous membranes related to trauma, inflammation, open lesions, or insertion of prosthetic devices, tubes, and catheters for diagnostic or therapeutic purposes
- Impaired blood supply
- Neutropenia and other blood disorders
- Malnutrition
- Poor personal hygiene
- Suppression of normal bacterial flora by antimicrobial drugs
- Suppression of the immune system and the inflammatory response by immunosuppressive drugs, cytotoxic antineoplastic drugs, and adrenal corticosteroids
- Diabetes and other chronic diseases
- Advanced age

> **Quality and Safety Alert: Evidence-Based Practice**
>
> The World Health Organization funded a study by Chu et al. (2020) to investigate the optimum distance for avoiding person-to-person transmission of Sars CoV_2 and COVID-19 and to assess face mask usage and eye protection in the prevention of these viruses. The researchers performed a systematic review and meta-analysis and identified 172 observational studies across 16 countries and continents, with a total of 25,697 patients. Virus transmission was lower with physical distancing of 1 m (3.28 ft) or more. Face mask use with N95 and other masks with respirators resulted in a large reduction in infection. The optimum use of face masks, respirators, and eye protection in public and healthcare facilities assisted in the prevention of person-to-person transmission of Sars CoV_2 and COVID-19.

Clinical Application 15.2

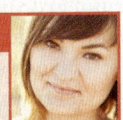

- Which alteration in Ms. Warren's defense mechanisms places her at risk for developing an infection?
- What intervention is primary in preventing the transmission of infection?

NCLEX Success

1. A college student is seen in the campus health center with a sore throat. Examination of the throat reveals redness and swelling but no sign of infection. Which of the following is an accurate description of the inflammatory process?

   A. A granuloma will develop if the inflammation is unresolved.
   B. The student is not at risk for the development of an infection.
   C. There is an influx of leukocytes to the throat.
   D. Scarring will result from phagocytic action.

Opportunistic Pathogens

Opportunistic microorganisms are usually normal endogenous or environmental flora and nonpathogenic. However, they become pathogens under conditions that are favorable for their (over) growth, such as in hosts whose defense mechanisms are impaired. Opportunistic infections are likely to occur in people with severe burns, cancer, human immunodeficiency virus (HIV) infection, indwelling intravenous or urinary catheters, and antibiotic or corticosteroid drug therapy. Opportunistic bacterial infections, often caused by drug-resistant microorganisms, are usually serious and may be life-threatening. Fungi of the *Candida* genus, especially *Candida albicans*, may cause life-threatening bloodstream or deep tissue infections, such as abdominal abscesses. Viral infections may cause fatal pneumonia in people with kidney or cardiac disorders, in those with HIV infection, and in those who have received bone marrow transplants.

> **Clinical Application 15.3**
> - Although Ms. Warren realizes that she has an increased risk of infection, she enjoys her work. What factors other than the administration of corticosteroid medications place her at risk for contracting an infection?
> - What teaching can a nurse provide to decrease Ms. Warren's risk of infection?

Laboratory Identification of Pathogens

Laboratory tests of infected fluids or tissues can identify the pathogen that is responsible for an infection. Bacteria and fungi can be differentiated by simple microscopy. In this test, a specimen is applied to a slide and examined under a microscope. Various dyes, such as Gram stain, and solutions, such as potassium hydroxide, are often applied to help differentiate or further classify microorganisms.

In some cases, there are insufficient microbes in a specimen to identify a causative organism. To obtain a sufficient amount of microbes, laboratory personnel resort to culturing microorganisms from a specimen sample. Culture involves growing a microorganism in the laboratory. Identification of some microorganisms (e.g., intracellular pathogens such as chlamydiae and viruses) requires different techniques. **Serology** identifies infectious agents indirectly by measuring the antibody level (titer) in the serum of an infected host. A tentative diagnosis can be made if the antibody level against a specific pathogen rises during the acute phase of the disease and falls during convalescence. The **detection of antigens** is a technique to identify pathogens that uses features of culture and serology but reduces the time required for diagnosis. Microbial deoxyribonucleic acid (DNA) and ribonucleic acid can also be used to identify pathogenic microorganisms. Examples of these tests include DNA probe hybridization and polymerase chain reaction, which can detect whether DNA for a specific organism is present in a sample.

Community-Acquired Versus Hospital-Acquired Infections

Infections are often categorized as community acquired or hospital acquired. **Community-acquired infections** are infections caused by microorganisms that originated in a community setting outside of a healthcare facility. One type of common community-acquired infection is **community-acquired pneumonia** (CAP), which is an infection of the lung parenchyma, in which the patient does not acquire the infection in a healthcare facility. Globally, CAP is the leading cause of morbidity and mortality. In contrast, **hospital-acquired infections** are infections acquired from microorganisms in hospitals and other healthcare facilities. A hospital-acquired pneumonia is contracted in the hospital. Ventilator-associated pneumonia is pneumonia that is acquired more than or equal to 48 hours after endotracheal intubation. **Health care-associated pneumonia** is acquired in other health care facilities, such as nursing homes. As a general rule, community-acquired infections are less severe and easier to treat. Hospital-acquired infections are usually more severe and difficult to manage because they are often caused by microorganisms that are less susceptible to the effects of antimicrobial drugs. These microorganisms are discussed in the next section.

Antibiotic-Resistant Microorganisms

Antibiotic resistance is the ability of certain bacteria to survive and multiply despite antibiotic therapy. Bacteria that have this ability to live in the presence of antibiotics are said to be antibiotic resistant.

Infections that are often associated with high rates of resistance include lower respiratory tract infections and those infections associated with cystic fibrosis or osteomyelitis. These infections are often difficult to treat because they tend to recur, involve multiple or resistant organisms, or, in the case of osteomyelitis, involve anatomic locations where antibiotics do not penetrate well. The increasing prevalence of antibiotic-resistant bacteria is a major public health concern (Box 15.2). Infections caused by antibiotic-resistant organisms often require more

---

BOX 15.2 *Antibiotic-Resistant Staphylococci, Streptococci, and Enterococci*

Methicillin-Resistant and Vancomycin-Intermediate/Vancomycin-Resistant *Staphylococcus* Species

Penicillin-resistant staphylococci developed in the early days of penicillin use because these bacteria produced beta-lactamase enzymes (penicillinases) that destroyed penicillin. Methicillin was one of five drugs developed to resist the action of beta-lactamase enzymes; however, eventually, strains of *Staphylococcus aureus* became resistant to these drugs as well. The mechanism of resistance in methicillin-resistant *Staphylococcus aureus* (MRSA) is alteration of penicillin-binding proteins (PBPs). PBPs, the target sites of penicillins and other beta-lactam antibiotics, are proteins required for maintaining integrity of bacterial cell walls. Beta-lactam antibiotics bind to these PBPs and produce defective bacterial cell walls, which kill the bacteria. MRSA have an additional altered PBP. Methicillin cannot bind effectively to this PBP, and so it is unable to inhibit bacterial cell wall synthesis except with very high drug concentrations. Consequently, minimum inhibitory concentrations (MICs) of methicillin increased to high levels that were difficult to achieve.

The term "MRSA" is commonly used but misleading because the bacteria are widely resistant to many antibiotics other than just methicillin. MRSA frequently colonize nasal passages of healthcare workers and are increasingly a cause of hospital-acquired infections, especially in critical care units. In addition, the incidence of methicillin-resistant *Staphylococcus epidermidis* (MRSE, often reported as

BOX 15.2 *Antibiotic-Resistant Staphylococci, Streptococci, and Enterococci* (Continued)

methicillin-resistant *Staphylococcus* species, non-*aureus* [SSNA]) isolates is increasing.

A major reason for concern about infections caused by MRSA and MRSE is that bacteria are now developing resistance to vancomycin, an antibiotic previously used extensively to treat or prevent infections caused by *S. aureus*, *S. epidermidis*, and enterococci. Options to treat these infections are limited, and measures to reduce the incidence and prevent spread of methicillin- and vancomycin-resistant organisms are paramount.

Penicillin-Resistant *Streptococcus pneumoniae* (Pneumococci)

Penicillin has long been the drug of choice for treating pneumococcal infections caused by *S. pneumoniae* (e.g., CAP, bacteremia, meningitis, and otitis media). However, penicillin-resistant strains and multidrug-resistant strains are increasingly identified. Risk factors include frequent antibiotic use and prophylactic use of antibiotics. After resistant strains have developed, they spread to others, especially in areas where people are in close contact such as in daycare centers and hospital settings.

S. pneumoniae are thought to develop resistance to penicillin by decreasing the ability of their PBPs to bind with penicillin. Bacteria displaying high-level penicillin resistance may also be cross-resistant to drugs from the same or similar antibiotic classes. To decrease the spread of resistant *S. pneumoniae*, the Centers for Disease Control and Prevention (CDC) has proposed:

- Improved surveillance to delineate prevalence by geographic area and assist clinicians in choosing appropriate antimicrobial therapy.
- Rational use of antibiotics to reduce exposures to drug-resistant pneumococci. For example, prophylactic antibiotic therapy for otitis media may increase colonization and infection of young children with drug-resistant organisms.
- Pneumococcal vaccination for people older than 2 years of age with increased risk of pneumococcal infection and for all people older than 65 years of age.

Vancomycin-Resistant Enterococci

Enterococci are a component of normal intestinal flora that can act as pathogens if they infect other areas of the body. Vancomycin is an antibiotic that was commonly used to treat these bacteria; however, in large part to the widespread use of vancomycin to treat other drug-resistant staphylococcal infections such as MRSA and MRSE, vancomycin-resistant *Enterococcus* (VRE) have emerged. Additionally, some strains of enterococci have developed additional resistance to other antibiotics. The incidence of multidrug-resistant enterococci and VRE has increased in recent years.

To decrease the spread of VRE, the CDC recommends avoiding or minimizing the use of vancomycin in routine surgical prophylaxis, empiric therapy for febrile patients with neutropenia (unless the prevalence of MRSA or MRSE is high), systemic or local prophylaxis for intravascular catheter infection or colonization, selective decontamination of the gastrointestinal tract, eradication of MRSA colonization, primary treatment of antibiotic-associated colitis, and routine prophylaxis for very low-birth-weight infants or patients on continuous ambulatory peritoneal dialysis. Thorough hand hygiene and environmental cleaning are also important, because VRE can survive for long periods on hands, gloves, stethoscopes, and environmental surfaces. Personnel must remove or change gloves after contact with patients known to be colonized or infected with VRE. Ideally, designated stethoscopes are restricted for use only with VRE-infected patients. If stethoscopes must be used for both VRE-infected and uninfected patients, it is important to thoroughly clean them between patients.

---

toxic and expensive drugs, leading to prolonged illness or hospitalization and increased mortality rates.

Interestingly, antibiotic overuse can contribute to antibiotic resistance. Resistant organisms are especially likely to emerge in critical care units and large hospitals where patients with serious illness often require extensive antibiotic therapy. The constant presence of antibiotics provides an environment conducive to the survival of the fittest bacteria, which is facilitated by killing of microorganisms that might ordinarily serve to keep these bacteria in check. Furthermore, because pathogenic microorganisms are often spread by contaminated hands or objects, patients in critical care units are more at risk for infection with antibiotic-resistant organisms resulting from person-to-person transmission by healthcare workers or equipment.

Resistant organisms and the antibiotics to which they develop resistance vary in geographic areas, communities, and hospitals according to the use of particular antibiotics. Nationally, resistant bacterial strains of major concern include penicillin-resistant *Streptococcus pneumoniae*, methicillin-resistant *Staphylococcus aureus* (MRSA) and methicillin-resistant *Staphylococcus epidermidis* (MRSE), vancomycin-resistant enterococcus (VRE), extended-spectrum beta-lactamase (ESBL)-producing gram-negative bacilli, and multidrug-resistant tuberculosis (MDR-TB). All of these organisms are resistant to multiple antibiotics. A CAP caused by drug-resistant *S. pneumoniae* is difficult to treat. Risk factors associated with this CAP are age of 65 years or older and a history of immunosuppressive illness or therapy, alcohol use disorder, and medical comorbidities. Use of beta-lactam, macrolide, or fluoroquinolone therapy in the past 3 to 6 months increases the prevalence of *S. pneumoniae* CAP. Drug-resistant organisms are described in Box 15.2, and MDR-TB is discussed in Chapter 22. Viruses and fungi also develop resistance to antimicrobial drugs, as discussed in Chapters 23 and 24, respectively.

 Quality and Safety Alert: Safety

Patients receiving antibiotics must be closely monitored for evidence of improvement. Failure to improve within 24 to 36 hours could indicate antibiotic resistance.

NCLEX Success

2. When a female who is taking an antibiotic develops a thick, white, curdlike vaginal discharge with pruritus, the nurse suspects that the patient has a vaginal yeast infection. What would explain this development?
   A. A drug for a fungal infection should have been prescribed instead of a drug for bacterial infection.
   B. The antibiotic has altered the normal vaginal environment.
   C. The antibiotic that was prescribed was not effective.
   D. Yeast infections are side effects of antibiotics.

Clinical Application 15.4

- Despite taking care to prevent an infection, Ms. Warren becomes ill and develops a fever with other signs and symptoms of an infection. The family nurse practitioner asks her what infectious illnesses her assigned patients have had and whether she has had direct contact with these patients. The nurse also asks if any of her friends or family members have been ill. What rationale underlies the nurse's questions?

Mechanisms of Antibiotic Resistance in Bacteria

Bacterial resistance to antimicrobial drugs may be either intrinsic or acquired.

The five main processes of intrinsic mechanisms of resistance are outlined below:

1. Bacteria may inactivate the antibiotic. For example, some bacteria produce enzymes that change the chemical structure of certain antibiotics, thus rendering them ineffective.
2. Bacteria may modify target sites for the antibiotic. For example, **penicillin-binding proteins** (PBPs) are bacterial proteins that function in cell wall synthesis. Penicillin typically binds to these bacterial proteins. By altering the PBPs, the bacteria prevent the antibiotic from recognizing and engaging this target.
3. Bacteria may alter metabolic pathways or substitute the usual enzymes needed to carry out activities involved with growth and reproduction. In doing this, bacteria develop resistance to antibiotics that exert their effect by interfering with enzymes needed for growth and reproduction.
4. Bacteria may alter their cell wall structure to reduce permeability. This confers resistance to antibiotics that must enter the bacterial cell to attach to a target.
5. Some bacteria have the ability to pump drug molecules out of the cell (efflux). By removing the antibiotic, the bacteria prevent the antibiotic from engaging the target site and exerting an effect.

The mechanisms of acquired resistance include genetic alterations. The three processes of acquired resistance are as follows:

1. In gene transfer, bacteria are in close approximation to then transfer to genetic content. For example, bacteria with inherent mechanisms for antibiotic resistance may transfer genetic content material that confers this antibiotic resistance to other species of bacteria. When these genetically altered bacteria replicate, the resistance is passed on to subsequent generations of bacteria.
2. In transfer mutations, the mutations often develop during bacterial replication. If the mutation provides antibiotic resistance, the mutated bacteria can continue to multiply and thus produce billions of copies of resistant microorganisms.
3. Selective pressure, or natural selection, refers to the survival of the fittest bacteria. When antibiotic therapy is initially begun, the weakest bacteria are killed first while the strongest bacteria, which are best able to withstand the effects of antibiotic therapy, remain. If antibiotic therapy is stopped prematurely before these more resistant microorganisms are overcome, the more resistant organisms predominate. These mechanisms explain why, when a new antibiotic is used, resistance may rapidly appear and be disseminated to multiple bacteria.

Clinical Manifestations

The clinical manifestations of infections are outlined in Box 15.2.

Drug Therapy

Several terms are used to describe drugs that are used to treat infections caused by microorganisms. Anti-infective, like antimicrobial, is a general descriptive term that designates agents with **antibacterial**, antiviral, and antifungal properties. Antibacterial is a term that designates agents that kill bacteria or interfere with the ability of bacteria to grow and replicate. An antibiotic is a drug that has the ability to kill or inhibit bacterial growth and replication; therefore, an antibiotic is an antibacterial drug. Antibiotics are used to treat bacterial infections.

Both antiviral and antifungal drugs are agents that have the ability to destroy or inhibit the replication of viruses or fungi, respectively. Antiviral drugs are used to treat viral infections, and antifungal drugs are used to treat fungal infections.

Additional terms are used to describe the properties of antibacterial drugs. **Broad-spectrum** antibiotics are antibacterial drugs that are effective against a wide range of bacteria (e.g., both gram-positive and gram-negative bacteria), whereas narrow-spectrum antibiotics are those that are effective against a limited range or a specific type of bacteria. Generally, a narrow-spectrum antibiotic is preferred over a broad-spectrum antibiotic when possible because broad-spectrum drugs are more likely to kill some normal flora, which disrupts the microbial balance. As a result, the patient is at greater risk for an opportunistic infection when taking a broad-spectrum antibiotic. The action of an antibacterial drug is usually described as **bactericidal** (kills the bacteria) or **bacteriostatic** (inhibits growth of the bacteria). Whether a drug is bactericidal or bacteriostatic often depends on its concentration at the infection site and the sensitivity of the bacteria to the drug. Because successful treatment with bacteriostatic antibiotics depends on the ability of the host's immune system to eliminate the inhibited bacteria, bactericidal drugs are preferred in serious infections, especially in people with impaired immune function.

Antimicrobials are among the most frequently used drugs worldwide. Their success in saving lives and decreasing severity and duration of infectious diseases has encouraged their extensive use. Unfortunately, these same attributes have led to antibiotic overuse, misuse, or abuse. Inappropriate use of antibiotics is responsible for unnecessary adverse drug effects, emergence of drug-resistant microorganisms, and increases in healthcare costs. All healthcare professionals should note that the goal of treatment with antibiotics is to eradicate the causative microorganism and return the host to full physiologic functioning. This differs from the goal of most drug therapy, which is to relieve signs and symptoms rather than cure the underlying disorder.

Guidelines to promote appropriate use of antimicrobial drugs include the following:

- Avoid the use of antibacterial drugs to treat viral infections; antibacterial drugs are ineffective in viral infections.
- Give antibacterial drugs only when a significant bacterial infection is diagnosed or strongly suspected or when there is an established indication for prophylaxis.
- Use a narrow-spectrum antibacterial drug instead of a broad-spectrum drug, whenever possible, in order to decrease the risk of a superinfection.
- Collect specimens (e.g., sputum, urine) for culture and Gram stain before giving the first dose of an antibiotic. For best results, specimens must be collected accurately and taken directly to the laboratory. If analysis is delayed, contaminants may overgrow pathogenic microorganisms.
- Minimize antimicrobial drug therapy for fever unless other clinical manifestations or laboratory data indicate infection.
- Follow recommendations of the Centers for Disease Control and Prevention (CDC) for prevention and treatment of infections, especially those caused by drug-resistant organisms (e.g., gonorrhea, penicillin-resistant streptococcal infections, MRSA, VRE, MDR-TB).
- Consult infectious disease physicians, infection control nurses, and infectious disease pharmacists about local patterns of drug-resistant organisms and treatment of complicated infections.

Box 15.3 presents patient teaching guidelines for antimicrobials.

BOX 15.3 Patient Teaching Guidelines for Antimicrobial Drugs

General Considerations

- Wash hands often and thoroughly, especially before preparing food or eating and after exposure to body secretions (e.g., urine, feces, sputum, nasal secretions), to prevent infection and avoid spreading an infection to others.
- Eat a balanced diet and get adequate fluid intake, rest, and exercise. This helps the body fight infection, prevents further infection, and increases the effectiveness of antimicrobial drugs by optimizing body processes.
- Take all prescribed doses of an antimicrobial drug to prevent recurrence of the infection. Also, stopping antimicrobial drugs when symptoms are relieved can lead to the development of antibiotic-resistant microorganisms that cause infections that are more severe and harder to treat.
- Report any problems that occur when taking an antimicrobial drug so that adverse effects can be identified and managed through interventions or through substitution by another equally effective antimicrobial drug.
- Discard all discontinued antimicrobial drugs. These drugs are carefully selected to treat specific illnesses, so taking inadequate amounts of an inappropriate drug can cause greater harm than benefit.
- Report any other drugs being taken to the prescriber to avoid drug interactions that could have harmful consequences.
- Report any drug allergies to all healthcare providers and wear a medical identification emblem that lists allergens to ensure that the antimicrobial drug ordered is safe for you.
- Notify the prescriber if you are pregnant because some antimicrobial drugs can cause problems for the developing fetus.
- Be aware that antibiotics are not indicated for treatment of viral infections. If an antibiotic is not indicated, taking it may result in more harm than good.

Self-Administration

- Take antimicrobial drugs at evenly spaced intervals around the clock, unless instructed otherwise, to maintain adequate blood levels.
- Ask if the antimicrobial drug can be taken with food. Food may decrease drug absorption for some oral antimicrobials; therefore, these are taken on an empty stomach, approximately 1 hour before or 2 hours after meals.
- Store most liquid preparations in the refrigerator to ensure that the medicine remains stable and is evenly dispersed in solution. Also, check expiration dates and discard any medication that remains after all prescribed doses have been taken.
- Take the medications with a full glass of water to help tablets and capsules dissolve better in the stomach and decrease stomach irritation.
- Report nausea, vomiting, diarrhea, skin rash, recurrence of symptoms for which the antimicrobial drug was prescribed, or signs of new infection (e.g., fever, cough, sore mouth, drainage) to a healthcare professional. These problems may indicate adverse effects of the drug, lack of therapeutic response to the drug, or another infection. Any of these requires evaluation and may indicate changes in drug therapy.

Empiric Therapy

Because laboratory tests used to definitively identify causative organisms and to determine their antibiotic **susceptibility** (vulnerability to an antibiotic's effects) usually require 48 to 72 hours, the prescriber usually initiates treatment with an antimicrobial drug that is likely to be effective. Drug therapy undertaken prior to obtaining a definite diagnosis is called **empiric therapy**. Empiric therapy is based on an informed estimate of the most likely pathogen(s) given the patient's signs and symptoms and the site of infection, as well as knowledge of communicable diseases currently infecting other people in the community. For example, urinary tract infections are often caused by *E. coli*; thus, an antibiotic that is effective against this microorganism is indicated.

Culture and Sensitivity Studies

The culture identifies the causative microorganism. The sensitivity study is the laboratory test to determine the susceptibility of an antimicrobial agent in the treatment of the causative microorganism. Once a specific microorganism is identified by laboratory culture, it is important to determine susceptibility, which is the vulnerability of the bacteria to the effects of an antibiotic. Susceptibility tests determine which drugs are likely to be effective against the organism. Laboratory reports indicate whether the organism is susceptible (S) or resistant (R) to the tested drugs. Susceptibility refers to the bacteria or fungus' inability to grow in the presence of one or more antimicrobial agents. Resistance refers to the antimicrobial's inability to kill the bacteria or fungus. It is then possible to "match the drug to the bug."

> **Concept Mastery Alert**
>
> Culturing bacteria helps identify the causative organism. To determine which antibiotic agents would be effective for the causative organism, a susceptibility test is performed.

One indication of susceptibility is the minimum inhibitory concentration (MIC). The MIC is the lowest concentration of an antibiotic that prevents visible growth of microorganisms. Some laboratories report MIC instead of, or in addition to, S (susceptibility) or R (resistance).

Susceptible organisms have low or moderate MICs that can be attained by giving usual doses of an antimicrobial agent. For the drug to be effective, its serum and tissue concentrations should usually exceed the MIC of an organism for a certain period. By how much and for how long drug concentrations need to exceed the MIC depend on the drug class and the bacterial species. Some antibiotics may be given for shorter lengths of time as a result of a post-antibiotic effect, a persistent effect of an antimicrobial on bacterial growth after brief exposure of the organisms to a drug.

Resistant organisms have high MICs and may require higher concentrations of drug than can be achieved in the body. In some cases, the minimum bactericidal concentration (MBC) is reported, indicating no growth of the organism in the presence of a particular antibiotic. The MBC is especially desirable for infected hosts with impaired immune functions.

> **NCLEX Success**
>
> 3. When a patient fails to respond to an antibiotic, the nurse suspects antibiotic resistance. Which mechanism of resistance does the nurse recognize as an example of acquired antibiotic resistance?
>   A. Alterations are made in the bacterial cell wall structure to make it less permeable.
>   B. Bacteria exchange genetic content that transfers resistance from one bacterial strain to another.
>   C. Efflux is used to extrude bacteria from within the bacterial cell.
>   D. Metabolic pathways are altered so bacteria targeting a specific enzyme of the metabolic pathway are ineffective.
>
> 4. A patient who is taking an antibiotic for an infection shows no signs of improvement. When a laboratory report indicates that the causative organism is not susceptible to the prescribed antibiotic, what is the priority nursing intervention? (Select all that apply.)
>   A. Notify the pharmacist to provide a different antibiotic.
>   B. Notify the prescriber of the culture report.
>   C. Stop the current antibiotic and use the susceptible antibiotic.
>   D. Inform the patient that the antibiotic is ineffective.
>   E. Notify the prescriber of the sensitivity report.
>
> 5. What is the best action a nurse can take to prevent infection?
>   A. Instruct patients with respiratory illnesses on proper pulmonary hygiene.
>   B. Recommend influenza and pneumococcal vaccines to patients older than 65 years of age.
>   C. Teach a patient the importance of adequate nutrition and rest.
>   D. Wash hands before and after each patient contact.

A patient's response to antimicrobial therapy cannot always be correlated with the MIC of an infecting pathogen. Thus, reports of drug susceptibility testing must be applied in the context of the site of infection, the characteristics of the drug, and the clinical status of the patient.

Patterns of Antibiotic Resistance

Over time, patterns of antibiotic resistance change in the community and in healthcare facilities; therefore, continuing efforts must be made to identify which antibiotics are most effective. Bacteria that are resistant to certain antibiotics are typically susceptible to others. Infectious disease specialists and laboratory personnel are helpful resources to identify resistance patterns and trends in these instances, and this information may be considered when deciding empiric therapy.

Ability to Penetrate Infected Tissues

Several antimicrobials are effective in urinary tract infections because they concentrate in the urine. However, the choice of an effective antimicrobial drug may be limited in infections of the brain, eyes, gallbladder, or prostate gland because many drugs are unable to reach therapeutic concentrations in these tissues. For infection in these areas, the prescriber will consider the ability of the drug to penetrate the affected region rather than deciding therapy based solely on susceptibility testing.

Toxicity and Risk-to-Benefit Ratio

In general, the least toxic drug is used; however, for serious infections, drugs with an increased risk of toxicity may be necessary. In these instances, the prescriber will weigh the benefits of treatment versus the risks of adverse effects when determining therapy.

Cost

It is always necessary to take the cost of the medication into account. If a less expensive drug is likely to be effective in a given infection, it is recommended instead of a more expensive agent. For hospitals and nursing homes, personnel costs relating to preparation and administration are also important to consider. For example, for the patient who cannot swallow tablets, a liquid preparation may be less expensive to prepare than a tablet that needs to be crushed.

Combination Therapy

Antimicrobial drugs are often used in combination. Indications for combination therapy may include the following:

- Infections caused by multiple microorganisms (e.g., abdominal and pelvic infections).
- Hospital-acquired infections, which may be caused by many different organisms.
- Serious infections in which a combination of antimicrobial drugs is synergistic.
- Likely emergence of drug-resistant organisms if a single drug is used (e.g., in tuberculosis).
- Fever or other signs of infection in patients whose immune system is suppressed. Combinations of antibacterial plus antiviral and/or antifungal drugs may be needed.

Nursing Considerations

In addition to drug therapy, the nurse should be aware of and take the following precautions to help patients avoid the spread of infection:

- Implement isolation procedures appropriately, when indicated.
- To prevent spread of respiratory infections, teach patients to cough into the bend of their elbow instead of covering their mouth or nose with hands or tissues. Advise patients to avoid crowds when they are ill.
- To prevent the likelihood that patients will acquire infections, advise them to avoid crowds during influenza season (approximately November through February) and when other communicable diseases are spreading through the local community. Recommend an annual influenza vaccine and pneumococcal vaccine (see Chapter 12) to high-risk populations (e.g., people with chronic diseases such as diabetes and heart, lung, or kidney problems; older adults; healthcare personnel who are likely to be exposed).
- Assist or instruct patients at risk about pulmonary hygiene measures to prevent accumulation or promote removal of respiratory secretions. These measures include ambulating, turning, coughing and deep breathing exercises, and incentive spirometry.
- Use sterile technique when changing any dressing. If a wound is not infected, sterile technique helps prevent infection. If the wound is already infected, sterile technique avoids introducing new bacteria. Remove dressings with clean gloves, discard them in a moisture-proof bag, and wash hands before putting on sterile gloves to apply the new dressing.
- To minimize the spread of infections, adhere to current established guidelines published by the CDC for isolation precautions to prevent transmission of infectious agents in healthcare settings. Visit the CDC website for the latest information on standard precautions and transmission-based precautions.
- For patients with infections, monitor temperature for increased or decreased fever and monitor the WBC count for changes.
- For patients receiving antimicrobial therapy, maintain an adequate fluid intake to assist with kidney clearance to decrease drug toxicity.
- Assist the patient with hand hygiene, maintaining nutrition and fluid balance, getting adequate rest, and handling secretions correctly. These measures help the body to fight the infection, prevent further infection, and enhance the effectiveness of antimicrobial medications.
- Assist patients in using antimicrobial drugs safely and effectively.
- Instruct patient on all aspects of medication administration.

> **Quality and Safety Alert: Evidence-Based Practice**
>
> Jennifer Wyeth is the lead infection prevention and control nurse at the Frimley Health National Foundation Trust in the United Kingdom. In a 2019 article, she addresses the current global crisis caused by antimicrobial resistance. She states no new antimicrobial agents have been developed since the 1980s, in large part because it is not a profitable endeavor. Thus, it is important that nurses and the entire healthcare team take the initiative to promote strategies to prevent the development and spread of infections. Basic standard body substance precautions must be implemented, including the use of personal protective equipment, respiratory hygiene, sharps safety, safe and aseptic injection practices, and maintenance of sterile instruments and devices. The healthcare team must adhere to strict hand hygiene and instruct patients and families on such practice. In addition, when healthcare environments are renovated and remodeled, the institution must pay attention and adhere to the most current health building codes and guidelines.

THE NURSING PROCESS

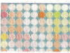

A concept map outlines the nursing process related to drug therapy considerations in this chapter. Additional nursing implications related to the disease process should also be considered in care decisions.

Assessment
- Assess for inflammation and infection.
- Understand that the general signs and symptoms of infection are the same as for inflammation. Local signs of inflammation include redness, heat, edema, and pain; systemic signs include fever and leukocytosis.
- Assess for signs and symptoms of inflammation. Inflammation is the normal response to any injury; infection requires the presence of a microorganism. The two often occur together. Inflammation may weaken the tissue, allowing microorganisms to invade and cause infection. Infection (tissue injury by microorganisms) stimulates inflammation.
- Assess for the presence of factors that increase the risk of infection.
- Assess culture and sensitivity reports for appropriate antibacterial therapy.
- Assess for drug allergies. If the patient has allergies, assess for specific signs and symptoms.
- Assess baseline kidney and hepatic function.

Outcomes of Therapy

The patient will
- Adhere to anti-inflammatory medication regimen as ordered.
- Receive antimicrobial drugs accurately when given by healthcare providers or caregivers.
- Take drugs as prescribed and for the length of time prescribed when self-administered as an outpatient.
- Experience decreased inflammation, fever, white blood cell (WBC) count, and other signs and symptoms of infection.
- Be monitored regularly for therapeutic and adverse drug effects.
- Receive prompt recognition and treatment of potentially serious adverse effects.
- Verbalize and practice measures to prevent future infections.
- Be safeguarded against hospital-acquired infections by healthcare providers.

Evaluation
- Evaluate the patient's adherence to medication administration.
- Evaluate for adverse drug effects.
- Evaluate for decreasing signs and symptoms of infection and inflammation.
- Evaluate patient's understanding of patient teaching regarding antimicrobial medications and anti-inflammatory agents.

Visit thePoint at http://thePoint.lww.com/Frandsen13e for answers to NCLEX Success questions (in Appendix A), answers to Clinical Application Case Studies (in Appendix B), additional information on pathophysiology, and more!

REFERENCES AND RESOURCES

Centers for Disease Control and Prevention. (2021a). *Standard precautions for all patient care.* Retrieved from https://www.cdc.gov/infectioncontrol/basics/standard-precautions.html

Centers for Disease Control and Prevention. (2021b). *Transmission-based precautions.* Retrieved from https://www.cdc.gov/infectioncontrol/basics/transmission-based-precautions.html

Chu, D., Akl, E. A., Duda, S., Solo, K., Yaacoub, S., & Schunemann, H. J. (2020). Physical distancing, face masks, and eye protection to prevent person-to-person transmission of SARS-CoV-2 and COVID-19; a systemic review and meta-analysis. *The Lancet, 395*, 1973–1987.

Norris, T. L. (2019). *Porth's pathophysiology: Concepts of altered health states.* Wolters Kluwer.

Pierce, V. M. (2021). Overview of antibacterial susceptibility testing. *UpToDate.* Wolters Kluwer.

Ramirez, J. A. (2021). Overview of community-acquired pneumonia in adults. *UpToDate.* Wolters Kluwer.

Wyeth, J. (2019). The importance of infection control in tackling the antimicrobial resistance crisis. *British Journal of Nursing, 28*(5), 284–286. doi:10.12968/bjon.2019.28.5.284

CHAPTER 16

Drug Therapy to Decrease Pain, Fever, and Inflammation

LEARNING OBJECTIVES

After studying this chapter, you should be able to:

1. Discuss the role of prostaglandins in the etiology of pain, fever, and inflammation.
2. Identify the major manifestations of fever and inflammation.
3. List and describe two common disorders that specifically produce inflammation.
4. Identify the prototype and describe the action, use, adverse effects, contraindications, and nursing implications for the salicylates.
5. Identify the action, use, adverse effects, contraindications, and nursing implications for acetaminophen.
6. Identify the prototype and describe the action, use, adverse effects, contraindications, and nursing implications for the propionic acid derivatives.
7. Identify the prototype and describe the action, use, adverse effects, contraindications, and nursing implications for the oxicam derivatives.
8. Identify the prototype and describe the action, use, adverse effects, contraindications, and nursing implications for the acetic acid derivatives.
9. Identify the prototype and describe the action, use, adverse effects, contraindications, and nursing implications for the selective COX-2 inhibitors.
10. Identify the prototype and describe the action, use, adverse effects, contraindications, and nursing implications for the mitotic agent.
11. Identify the prototype and describe the action, use, adverse effects, contraindications, and nursing implications for uricosuric medications.
12. Implement the nursing process in the care of patients undergoing drug therapy for pain, fever, and inflammation.

CLINICAL APPLICATION CASE STUDY

Audrey Mason is a 72-year-old retired physical education teacher who is being seen by her primary care provider for bilateral hip and knee pain. She has been taking a minimum of eight 325-mg aspirins per day without pain relief. Her physician orders x-rays of her hips and knees, which reveal osteoarthritis in both joints. She begins taking ibuprofen (Motrin) 600 mg three times per day. In addition, she receives a diagnosis of degenerative joint disease related to osteoarthritis and a referral to an orthopedic surgeon. The surgeon schedules Mrs. Mason for a right total knee replacement in 1 month. Because she has a body mass index (BMI) of 30, the surgeon places her on a calorie reduction diet.

KEY TERMS

Antiprostaglandin: drug that inhibits the synthesis of prostaglandins

Antipyretic: drug that has the ability to lower body temperature

Arachidonic acid: phospholipid released in the cell membrane in response to cellular injury

Cyclooxygenase: enzyme that produces prostaglandins from arachidonic acids

Hyperuricemia: elevated levels of uric acid in the blood resulting from accelerated generation of uric acid through purine metabolism or impaired kidney excretion of uric acid

Nonsteroidal anti-inflammatory drug (NSAID): medication that inhibits the synthesis of prostaglandins; used to prevent and treat mild to moderate pain and inflammation

Prostaglandin: chemical mediator found in most body tissues; helps regulate many cell functions and participate in the inflammatory response as well as initiate uterine contractions in labor

Reye syndrome: potentially fatal disease characterized by encephalopathy and fatty liver accumulations; associated with the use of aspirin and NSAIDs after viral infections such as chickenpox or influenza in children and adolescents

Salicylism: toxic effects of a salicylate drug; may occur with an acute overdose or with chronic use of therapeutic doses, especially the higher doses taken for anti-inflammatory effects

Tophi: deposits of uric acid crystals in the joints, kidneys, and soft tissues

Uricosuric: drug that increases urinary excretion of uric acid

INTRODUCTION

This chapter provides an introduction to the pharmacologic care of the patient who is experiencing pain, fever, or inflammation. The pharmacologic agents administered for inflammation can also diminish fever and relieve pain. Acetaminophen decreases fever and relieves pain, but it does not reduce inflammation. Other topics of discussion include osteoarthritis and gout, allowing the nurse to apply knowledge of disease that produces inflammation and the related administration of anti-inflammatory agents to reduce pain. The drugs discussed in this chapter include aspirin (acetylsalicylic acid), acetaminophen, and the nonsteroidal anti-inflammatory drugs (NSAIDs), as well as those drugs used to prevent or treat gout.

Aspirin, acetaminophen, and NSAIDs can also be called **antiprostaglandins** because they inhibit the synthesis of prostaglandins. **Prostaglandins** are chemical mediators found in most body tissues; they help regulate many cell functions and participate in the inflammatory response. They are formed when cellular injury occurs and phospholipids in cell membranes respond by releasing **arachidonic acid**. **Cyclooxygenase** (COX) enzymes then metabolize arachidonic acid to produce prostaglandins, which act briefly in the area where they are produced and are then inactivated. The enzyme COX-1 is normally synthesized continuously and is present in all tissues and cell types, especially in platelets and endothelial cells as well as in the gastrointestinal (GI) tract and the kidneys. Prostaglandins produced by COX-1 are important in numerous homeostatic functions and have protective effects on the stomach and kidneys. In the stomach, prostaglandins decrease gastric acid secretion, increase mucous secretion, and regulate blood circulation. In the kidneys, they help maintain adequate blood flow and function. In the cardiovascular system, they help regulate vascular tone (i.e., vasoconstriction and vasodilation) and platelet function. Drug-induced inhibition of these prostaglandins results in the adverse effects associated with aspirin and related nonselective NSAIDs, especially gastric irritation, ulceration, and bleeding. Inhibition of COX-1 activity in platelets may be more responsible for GI bleeding than inhibition of COX-1 activity in gastric mucosa.

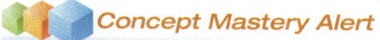

Concept Mastery Alert

COX-1 enzymes are continuously present in all tissues, not just at the time of inflammation. They secrete a cytoprotective mucus.

COX-2 is also normally present in several tissues (e.g., brain, bone, kidneys, GI tract, female reproductive system). However, it is thought to occur in small amounts or to be inactive until stimulated by pain and inflammation. In inflamed tissues, COX-2 is induced by inflammatory chemical mediators such as interleukin-1 (IL-1) and tumor necrosis factor alpha (TNF-alpha). In the GI tract, trauma and *Helicobacter pylori* infection, a common cause of peptic ulcer disease, also induce COX-2. Overall, prostaglandins produced by COX-2 are associated with pain and other signs of inflammation. Inhibition of COX-2 results in the therapeutic effects of analgesia and anti-inflammatory activity. The COX-2 inhibitor drugs are NSAIDs designed to selectively inhibit COX-2 and relieve pain and inflammation with fewer adverse effects than those that inhibit both COX-1 and COX-2, especially stomach damage. However, with long-term use, adverse effects still occur in the GI, kidney, and cardiovascular systems.

As indicated in Table 16.1 and Figure 16.1, prostaglandins exert various and opposing effects in different body tissues.

TABLE 16.1
Prostaglandins

Prostaglandin	Locations	Effects
PGD_2	Airways, brain, mast cells	Bronchoconstriction
PGE_2	Brain, kidneys, vascular smooth muscle, platelets	Bronchodilation Gastroprotection Increased activity of the GI smooth muscle Increased sensitivity to pain Increased body temperature Vasodilation
PGF_2	Airways, eyes, uterus, vascular smooth muscle	Bronchoconstriction Increased activity of the GI smooth muscle Increased uterine contraction (e.g., menstrual cramps)
PGI_2 (prostacyclin)	Brain, endothelium, kidneys, platelets	Decreased platelet aggregation Gastroprotection Vasodilation
PGA_2 (thromboxane A_2)	Kidneys, macrophages, platelets, vascular smooth muscle	Increased platelet aggregation Vasoconstriction

GI, gastrointestinal.

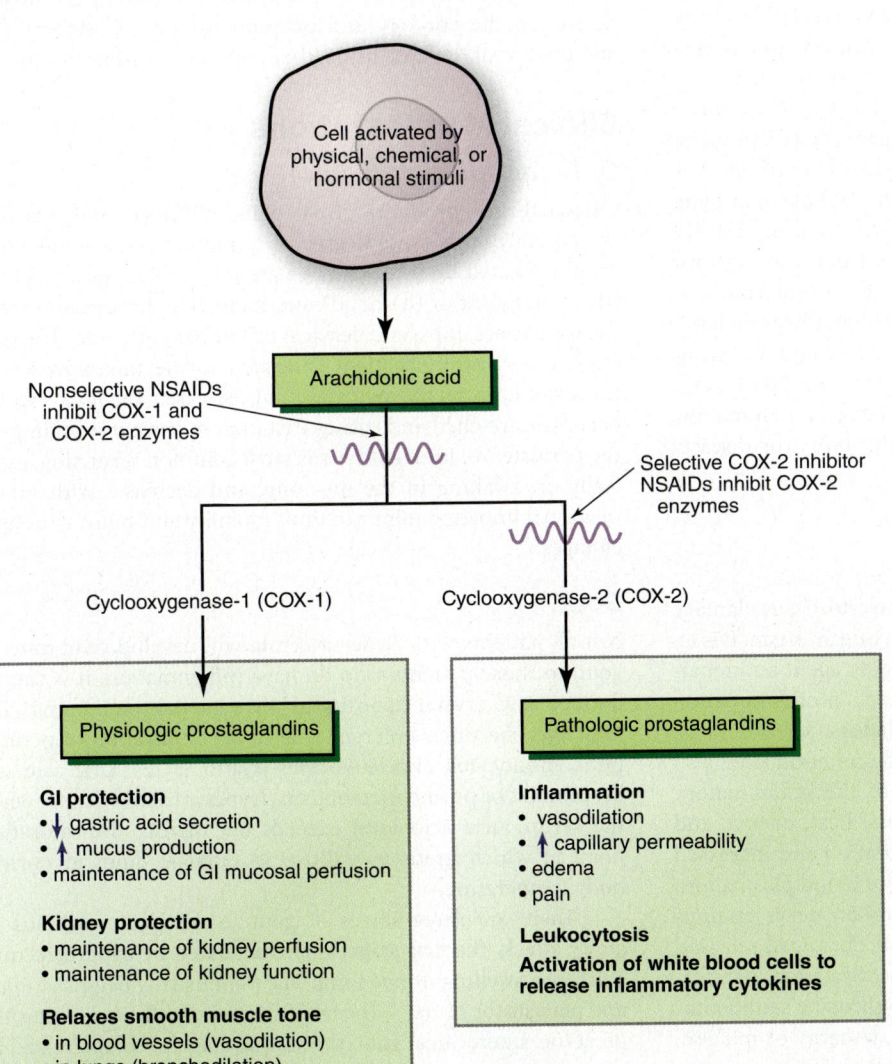

Figure 16.1. Metabolic pathways for arachidonic acid result in production of physiologic and pathologic (i.e., inflammatory) prostaglandins. Nonselective and selective nonsteroidal anti-inflammatory drugs (NSAIDs) inhibit production of prostaglandins by inhibiting steps in the arachidonic acid pathway. GI, gastrointestinal.

OVERVIEW OF PAIN, FEVER, AND INFLAMMATION

To adequately understand the administration of aspirin, acetaminophen, and NSAIDs, it is important to understand the role prostaglandins play in mediating pain, fever, and inflammation.

Pain

Pain is the sensation of discomfort, hurt, or distress. It is a common human ailment and may occur with tissue injury and inflammation. Prostaglandins sensitize pain receptors and increase the pain associated with other chemical mediators of inflammation and immunity, such as bradykinin, histamine, and leukotriene (Box 16.1).

Fever

Fever is an elevation of body temperature above the normal range. Body temperature is controlled by a regulating center in the hypothalamus. Normally, there is a balance between heat production and heat loss so that a constant body temperature is maintained. When there is excessive heat production, mechanisms to increase heat loss are activated. As a result, blood vessels dilate, more blood flows through the skin, sweating occurs, and body temperature usually stays within normal range.

Fever occurs when the set point of the hypothalamus is raised in response to the presence of pyrogens (fever-producing agents). Endogenous pyrogens include cytokines such as IL-1, IL-6, and tumor necrosis factor (see Box 16.1). Exogenous pyrogens include bacteria and their toxins or other by-products. The upward adjustment of the hypothalamic set point in response to the presence of a pyrogen is mediated by prostaglandin E_2 (see Table 16.1). The body responds to the higher hypothalamic set point by vasoconstriction of blood vessels and shivering, raising the core body temperature to the higher set point. Fever may accompany conditions such as dehydration, inflammation, infectious processes, some drug use, brain injury, or diseases involving the hypothalamus.

Inflammation

Inflammation is the normal body response to tissue damage from any source, and it may occur in any tissue or organ. It is an attempt by the body to remove the damaging agent and repair the damaged tissue. The signs and symptoms of inflammation are the work of a variety of chemical mediators (see Box 16.1). Prostaglandin E_2 and others induce inflammation and also enhance the effects of other mediators of the inflammatory response. Local manifestations are redness, heat, edema, and pain. Redness and heat result from vasodilation and increased blood supply. Edema results from leakage of blood plasma into the area. Pain occurs when pain receptors on nerve endings are stimulated by heat, edema, and pressure; chemicals released by the damaged cells; and prostaglandins. Systemic manifestations include leukocytosis, increased erythrocyte sedimentation rate, fever, headache, loss of appetite, lethargy or malaise, and weakness. Both local and systemic manifestations vary according to the cause and extent of tissue damage. In addition, inflammation may be acute or chronic. See Chapter 15 for more information.

Inflammation may be a component of virtually any illness. Inflammatory conditions affecting organs or systems are often named by adding the suffix "itis" to the involved organ or system (e.g., hepatitis). Inflammation may be important in the pathology of disorders (not previously identified as inflammatory conditions) such as heart disease and Alzheimer disease. Anti-inflammatory drugs are indicated when the inflammatory response is inappropriate, abnormal, or persistent or destroys tissue.

Table 16.2 lists the medications administered in the reduction of pain, fever, and inflammation.

OVERVIEW OF DISORDERS THAT PRODUCE INFLAMMATION

Osteoarthritis and gout are two common disorders that specifically produce inflammation. *Osteoarthritis* produces inflammation and degradation of the cartilage, bone, and synovium. *Gout* is an arthritic condition characterized by an overproduction of uric acid or an inability to excrete uric acid, resulting in **hyperuricemia** (elevated levels of uric acid in the blood). For further details on the etiology and pathophysiology of osteoarthritis and gout, visit thePoint http://thePoint.lww.com/Frandsen.

Clinical Manifestations

Osteoarthritis

Osteoarthritis produces joint pain, stiffness, and instability, possibly with some degree of immobility. The joints commonly affected by osteoarthritis are the carpometacarpal joint (the distal joint of the hand) and metatarsophalangeal joint of the feet, knees, hips, and cervical or lumbar vertebrae. The pain experienced by the patient is related to the inflammation of the synovium. As the synovial fluid increases, the joint capsule becomes stretched and causes irritation to the nerve endings of the periosteum. Joint stiffness is most common on arising, especially on awaking in the morning, and decreases with movement. An impaired joint can limit mobility and cause structural changes.

Gout

Not all patients with hyperuricemia will develop symptoms of gout; in those patients who do have inflammation, it is caused by uric acid crystal deposits in the synovial joint lining. The joint then becomes enlarged due to the infiltration of neutrophils, monocytes, and leukocytes (Gaffo, 2022). Uric acid is a by-product of purine metabolism. Hyperuricemia occurs when the serum uric acid level exceeds 6.8 mg/dL, the saturation point at which urate crystallizes in biologic fluids at normal body temperature.

There are three stages of gout. Acute gouty arthritis or gouty attack, the first stage, is characterized by hyperuricemia, pain, and swelling of one joint. The pain usually begins at night and persists for 10 days. The most commonly affected joint is the great toe. Intercritical gout, the second stage, is characterized by a symptom-free period of several years followed by the recurrence of symptoms. Chronic tophaceous gout, the third stage, is

BOX 16.1 Chemical Mediators of Inflammation and Immunity

Bradykinin is a kinin in body fluids that becomes physiologically active with tissue injury. When tissue cells are damaged, white blood cells (WBCs) increase in the area and ingest damaged cells to remove them from the area. When the WBCs die, they release enzymes that activate kinins. The activated kinins increase and prolong the vasodilation and increased vascular permeability caused by histamine. They also cause pain by stimulating nerve endings for pain in the area. Thus, bradykinin may aggravate and prolong the erythema, heat, and pain of local inflammatory reactions. It also increases mucous gland secretion.

Complement is a group of plasma proteins essential for normal inflammatory and immunologic processes. More specifically, complement destroys cell membranes of body cells (e.g., red blood cells, lymphocytes, platelets) and pathogenic microorganisms (e.g., bacteria, viruses). The system is initiated by an antigen–antibody reaction or by tissue injury. Components of the system (called C1 through C9) are activated in a cascade type of reaction in which each component becomes a proteolytic enzyme that splits the next component in the series. Activation yields products with profound inflammatory effects. C3a and C5a, also called anaphylatoxins, act mainly by liberating histamine from mast cells and platelets, and their effects are therefore similar to those of histamine. C3a causes or increases smooth muscle contraction, vasodilation, vascular permeability, degranulation of mast cells and basophils, and secretion of lysosomal enzymes by leukocytes. C5a performs the same functions as C3a and also promotes movement of WBCs into the injured area (chemotaxis). In addition, it activates the lipoxygenase pathway of arachidonic acid metabolism in neutrophils and macrophages, thereby inducing formation of leukotrienes and other substances that increase vascular permeability and chemotaxis.

In the immune response, the complement system breaks down antigen–antibody complexes, especially those in which the antigen is a microbial agent. It enables the body to produce inflammation and localize an infective agent. More specific reactions include increased vascular permeability, chemotaxis, and opsonization (coating a microbe or other antigen so it can be more readily phagocytized).

Cytokines may act on the cells that produce them, on surrounding cells, or on distant cells if sufficient amounts reach the bloodstream. Thus, cytokines act locally and systemically to produce inflammatory and immune responses, including increased vascular permeability and chemotaxis of macrophages, neutrophils, and basophils. Two major types of cytokines are interleukins (produced by leukocytes) and interferons (produced by T lymphocytes or fibroblasts). IL-1 mediates several inflammatory responses, including fever; IL-2 (also called T-cell growth factor) is required for the growth and function of T lymphocytes. Interferons are cytokines that protect nearby cells from invasion by intracellular microorganisms, such as viruses and rickettsiae. They also limit the growth of some cancer cells.

Histamine is formed (from the amino acid histidine) and stored in most body tissue, with high concentrations in mast cells, basophils, and platelets. Mast cells, which are abundant in skin and connective tissue, release histamine into the vascular system in response to stimuli (e.g., antigen–antibody reaction, tissue injury, and some drugs). After it is released, histamine is highly vasoactive, causing vasodilation (increasing blood flow to the area and producing hypotension) and increasing permeability of capillaries and venules (producing edema). Other effects include contracting smooth muscles in the bronchi (producing bronchoconstriction and respiratory distress), GI tract, and uterus; stimulating salivary, gastric, bronchial, and intestinal secretions; stimulating sensory nerve endings to cause pain and itching; and stimulating movement of eosinophils into injured tissue. Histamine is the first chemical mediator released in the inflammatory response and immediate hypersensitivity reactions (anaphylaxis).

When histamine is released from mast cells and basophils, it diffuses rapidly into other tissues. It then acts on target tissues through both histamine-1 (H_1) and histamine-2 (H_2) receptors. H_1 receptors are located mainly on smooth muscle cells in blood vessels and the respiratory and GI tracts. When histamine binds with these receptors, resulting events include contraction of smooth muscle, increased vascular permeability, production of nasal mucus, stimulation of sensory nerves, pruritus, and dilation of capillaries in the skin. H_2 receptors are also located in the airways, GI tract, and other tissues. When histamine binds to these receptors, there is increased secretion of gastric acid by parietal cells in the stomach mucosal lining, increased mucous secretion and bronchodilation in the airways, contraction of esophageal muscles, tachycardia, inhibition of lymphocyte function, and degranulation of basophils (with additional release of histamine and other mediators) in the bloodstream. In allergic reactions, both types of receptors mediate hypotension (in anaphylaxis), skin flushing, and headache. The peak effects of histamine occur within 1 to 2 minutes of its release and may last as long as 10 minutes, after which it is inactivated by histaminase (produced by eosinophils) or N-methyltransferase.

Leukotrienes, like prostaglandins, are derived from arachidonic acid metabolism. Leukotrienes, identified as LTB_4, LTC_4, LTD_4, and LTE_4, mediate inflammation and immune responses. LTB_4 plays a role in chemotaxis, mediating the aggregation of leukocytes at sites of injury. LTC_4, LTD_4, and LTE_4 produce smooth muscle contractility, bronchospasm, and increased vascular permeability.

Nitric oxide (NO) is synthesized by a variety of cells by the enzyme NO synthase from the amino acid arginine. It readily diffuses across cell membranes, where it reacts with a wide variety of molecules and is inactivated. NO inhibits aggregation of platelets, preventing formation of blood clots. NO relaxes smooth muscles in blood vessels, producing vasodilation. It inhibits inflammation in the walls of blood vessels. NO also plays a role in protecting against invading microbes. Helper T lymphocytes, active in the inflammatory response, secrete NO. NO also enhances the killing of phagocytized microbes within the lysosomes of cells.

Platelet-activating factor (PAF), like prostaglandins and leukotrienes, is derived from arachidonic acid metabolism and has multiple inflammatory activities. It is produced by mast cells, neutrophils, monocytes, and platelets. Because these cells are widely distributed, PAF effects can occur in virtually every organ and tissue. Besides causing platelet aggregation, PAF activates neutrophils, attracts eosinophils, increases vascular permeability, causes vasodilation, and causes IL-1 and TNF-alpha to be released. PAF, IL-1, and TNF-alpha can induce each other's release.

TABLE 16.2

Medications Administered for Pain, Fever, and Inflammation

Drug Class	Prototype	Other Drugs in the Class
Salicylate	Aspirin (acetylsalicylic acid)	Magnesium salicylate (Doans Pills) Salsalate
Nonnarcotic analgesic antipyretic	Acetaminophen (Tylenol, paracetamol)	
Nonsteroidal anti-inflammatory drugs (NSAIDs)		
Propionic acid derivatives	Ibuprofen (Motrin)	Diflunisal Fenoprofen (Fenortho, Nalfon) Flurbiprofen Ketoprofen Meclofenamate sodium Mefenamic acid Nabumetone Naproxen sodium (Aleve, Anaprox) Oxaprozin (Daypro) Tolmetin sodium
Oxicam derivatives	Meloxicam (Anjeso)	Piroxicam (Feldene)
Acetic acid derivatives	Indomethacin (Indocin, Tivorbex)	Diclofenac potassium (Cambia, Zorvolex) Etodolac (Lodine) Ketorolac Nabumetone Sulindac
Selective COX-2 inhibitor	Celecoxib (CeleBREX)	

COX-2, cyclooxygenase-2.

characterized by the presence of solid deposits of urate crystals, known as **tophi**, in the joints and elsewhere (Fig. 16.2). In the kidneys, urate deposits may form kidney stones or cause other damage (Perez-Ruiz, 2020). After the first attack of acute gouty arthritis, up to 10 years may pass before permanent damage to the joints and kidneys occurs.

Drug Therapy

Medications used in the treatment of osteoarthritis include aspirin, acetaminophen, and NSAIDs (see Table 16.2). As previously mentioned, all of these medications produce an analgesic effect and reduce fever. However, only aspirin and the NSAIDs reduce inflammation. As the medications are discussed, their properties will be explained in detail, identifying their use and implications for administration (see Fig. 16.3).

The treatment of gout involves the administration of NSAIDs and corticosteroids (see Chapter 17) to reduce inflammation as well as **uricosuric** agents to increase the elimination of uric acid. Table 16.3 lists the antigout medications and uricosuric agents. These drugs will be discussed later in this chapter.

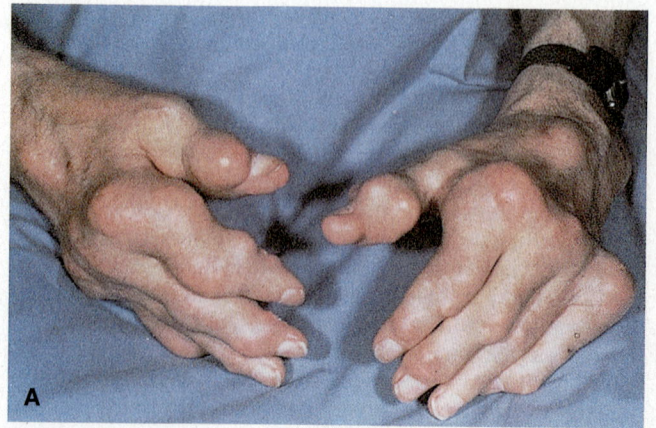
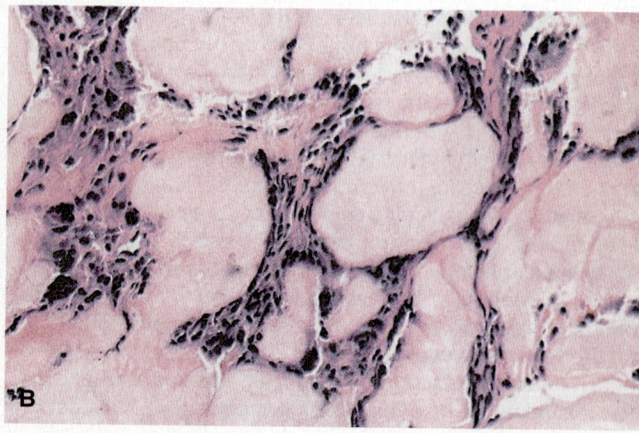

Figure 16.2. **A.** Gouty tophi projections. **B.** Tophi: Jellylike projections under the skin.

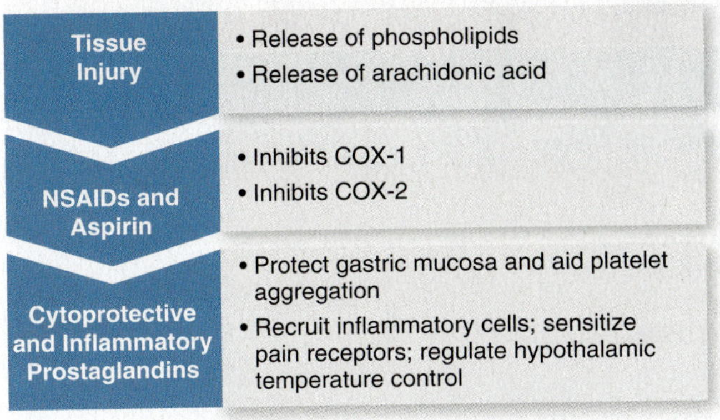

Figure 16.3

Tissue Injury
- Release of phospholipids
- Release of arachidonic acid

NSAIDs and Aspirin
- Inhibits COX-1
- Inhibits COX-2

Cytoprotective and Inflammatory Prostaglandins
- Protect gastric mucosa and aid platelet aggregation
- Recruit inflammatory cells; sensitize pain receptors; regulate hypothalamic temperature control

Figure 16.3. Tissue injury and the action of nonsteroidal anti-inflammatory agents.

Clinical Application 16.1

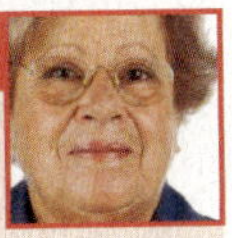

- In an education session with Mrs. Mason, the nurse employed by Mrs. Mason's insurance provider is instructing her about the clinical manifestations of osteoarthritis. What information should the nurse provide?

NCLEX Success

1. A home care nurse is visiting an 88-year-old patient who is taking acetaminophen for arthritic knee pain. Which of the following patient teaching statements is most appropriate to implement?
   A. "Acetaminophen will only relieve pain but not the inflammation from arthritis."
   B. "Acetaminophen is appropriate for the treatment of inflammation from arthritis."
   C. "Your primary healthcare provider should consider a prescription of acetaminophen/hydrocodone (Vicodin)."
   D. "The acetaminophen should be administered on an empty stomach."

Quality and Safety Alert: Evidence-Based Practice

Oladosu et al. (2020) states that incomplete pain relief after the administration of NSAIDs is common, but it is unknown whether malabsorption or increased drug metabolism contributes to the diminished effects of NSAIDs. This pilot study examined the pain assessment data of women with dysmenorrhea. Also, hypermetabolism of serum naproxen was analyzed. The preliminary findings suggest that poor drug absorption contributes to reduced pain relief.

SALICYLATES

The salicylates, of which **aspirin** is the prototype, relieve pain by acting both centrally and peripherally to block the transmission of pain impulses. They act peripherally to prevent the sensation of pain receptors to various chemical substances released by damaged cells. These agents are also **antipyretic** and reduce fever by acting on the hypothalamus to decrease its response to pyrogens and resetting the body temperature at a lower level. In addition, these drugs diminish inflammation by preventing prostaglandins from increasing the pain and edema produced by other substances released by damaged cells.

Aspirin and other salicylates also have the ability to suppress platelet aggregation. Low-dose aspirin is indicated for patients who have experienced an ischemic stroke, transient ischemic attack, angina, and acute myocardial infarction (or any myocardial infarction), reducing the risk of death and/or a recurrent event (level A recommendations). This indication stems from its antiplatelet activity and resultant effects on blood coagulation (i.e., decreased clot formation). Immediate-release aspirin, 75 to 100 mg/day, is used for primary prevention of myocardial infarction or stroke in healthy adults. High-dose aspirin, 4 to 8 g/day in 4 to 5 divided doses, is effective in reducing inflammation in rheumatoid disorders.

Pharmacokinetics

Aspirin is administered orally or rectally with an onset of action of 5 to 30 minutes orally and 1 to 2 hours rectally. The oral preparation peaks in 15 to 120 minutes, and the duration of action is 3 to 6 hours. The rectal preparation peaks in 4 to 5 hours, and the duration of action is 6 to 8 hours. The drug is metabolized in the liver and has a half-life of 15 minutes to 12 hours. Excretion takes place in the urine. The drug crosses the placenta and enters the breast milk.

Action

The ability of aspirin to inhibit prostaglandins produces the inflammatory effects needed for analgesia and antirheumatic effects. Its antipyretic effects are less well understood. Authorities believe that the drug acts on the thermoregulatory center of the hypothalamus, thus blocking the effects of the endogenous pyrogens and inhibiting the synthesis of prostaglandins. Aspirin also has antiplatelet effects. At low doses, it blocks the synthesis of thromboxane A_2 to inhibit platelet aggregation; this lasts for the life of the platelet.

Use

As an analgesic agent, aspirin is used to relieve mild to moderate pain. As an antipyretic agent, it is used only in adults. As an anti-inflammatory agent, it is used to decrease inflammation in patients with osteoarthritis, juvenile rheumatoid arthritis, and spondyloarthropathies. In addition, aspirin is used for its antiplatelet effects to reduce the risk of transient ischemic attacks and strokes as well as the risk of death from myocardial infarction. A 75- to 81-mg dose of aspirin is given preoperatively to patients undergoing coronary artery bypass graft surgery and continued during surgery. A 325-mg loading dose is given postoperatively 6 hours after extubation. A 325-mg dose of aspirin is then continued indefinitely. Table 16.4 presents specific dosage information for aspirin and other salicylates. In the event a patient is pregnant and diagnosed with polycythemia vera, which is uncommon during childbearing years, they will require a low-dose aspirin regimen throughout pregnancy despite known adverse effects to the fetus. Pregnant patients at

TABLE 16.3

Medications Administered for Gout

Drug Class	Prototype	Other Drugs in the Class
Mitotic agent	Colchicine (Colcrys, Mitigare)	
Uricosuric	Allopurinol (Zyloprim)	Febuxostat (Uloric) Pegloticase (Krystexxa) Probenecid Rasburicase (Elitek)

risk for preeclampsia should be administered 81 to 162 mg of aspirin once daily, beginning at 12 to 16 weeks' gestation and continued until delivery.

Patient-related variables specific to the use of aspirin include the following:

- Age:
  - Aspirin is not recommended for use in children to reduce fever due to the association with **Reye syndrome**, a life-threatening illness characterized by encephalopathy, hepatic damage, and other serious problems. This syndrome usually occurs after a viral infection, such as influenza or chickenpox, during which aspirin was given for fever.
  - Aspirin may be prescribed for children to reduce inflammation or for antiplatelet effects.
  - Aspirin is safe in therapeutic doses for analgesic and antipyretic use. It is also usually safe in the low doses prescribed for prevention of myocardial infarctions and cerebrovascular accidents.
- Reproduction, pregnancy, and lactation:
  - Low-dose aspirin has been evaluated to improve live births in patients diagnosed with antiphospholipid syndrome who have experienced recurrent pregnancy loss. Aspirin is initiated prior to pregnancy and is continued throughout the pregnancy unless heparin or low-molecular weight heparin is prescribed.
  - Salicylate is present in umbilical cord and newborn serum following maternal use of aspirin. The amount and associated fetal outcomes are dependent on maternal dosage.
  - In most cases, aspirin should be avoided at 20 weeks' gestation.
  - Low-dose aspirin is recommended in pregnant patients at risk for preeclampsia.
  - Salicylic acid is present in breast milk, but the amount is dependent on the maternal dose.
- Abnormal kidney function and hepatic impairment:
  - Aspirin is nephrotoxic in high doses, and protein binding of aspirin is reduced in patients with kidney failure, which

TABLE 16.4

DRUGS AT A GLANCE: Salicylates

Drug	Routes and Dosage Ranges	
	Adults	**Children**
(P) Aspirin (acetylsalicylic acid; ✦ Asaphen)	Pain, fever: PO 325–650 mg every 4 h PRN; usually single dose, 650 mg Osteoarthritis or rheumatoid arthritis: PO 2–6 g/d in divided doses Acute rheumatic fever: PO 5–8 g/d, in divided doses Prophylaxis of myocardial infarction, transient ischemic attack, and cerebrovascular accident: PO 81–325 mg/d Transient ischemic attack: PO 1,300 mg/d in divided doses (650 mg twice a day or 325 mg four times a day) Acute myocardial infarction: PO 162–325 mg or rectal suppository 600 mg Pregnant women with polycythemia vera: PO 75 mg daily during pregnancy Preeclampsia prevention 81–162 mg beginning at 12–16 weeks' gestation	**Do not administer to children with chickenpox or influenza.** **Recommended daily doses by weight:** 24–35 lb (10.6–15.9 kg), 162 mg; 36–47 lb (16–21.4 kg), 243 mg; 48–59 lb (21.5–26.8 kg), 324 mg; 60–71 lb (26.9–32.3 kg), 405 mg; 72–95 lb (32.4–43.2 kg), 486 mg; 96 lb or above (43.3 kg or above), 648 mg Pain, fever: PO 10–15 mg/kg every 4 h, up to 60–80 mg/kg/d Juvenile rheumatoid arthritis: PO 90–130 mg/kg/d, divided doses, every 6–8 h; target plasma salicylate level, 150–300 mg/mL Acute rheumatic fever: PO 100 mg/kg/d, divided doses, for 2 wk, then 75 mg/kg/d for 4–6 wk
Magnesium salicylate (Doans Pills)	PO 650 mg three to four times per day	Older than 2 y of age: PO 50–75 mg/kg/d divided in 4–6 doses (maximum 3.6 g/d)
Salsalate	Osteoarthritis or rheumatoid arthritis: PO 20 mg/d or 10 mg twice daily	Dosage not established

means that blood levels of the active drug are higher than they would be otherwise.
- Aspirin can also decrease the blood flow in the kidneys by inhibiting the synthesis of prostaglandins that dilate kidney blood vessels.
- In patients who depend on prostaglandins to maintain an adequate kidney blood flow, the prostaglandin-blocking effects of aspirin result in constriction of kidney arteries and arterioles, decreased kidney blood flow, decreased glomerular filtration rate, and retention of salt and water.

Adverse Effects

GI adverse effects of aspirin include nausea, dyspepsia, heartburn, and epigastric discomfort. Decreased platelet aggregation results in GI blood loss and hemorrhage. In addition, petechiae and bruising may also occur. Aspirin toxicity occurs at levels above 300 mcg/mL. Acute toxicity results in respiratory alkalosis, hyperpnea, tachypnea, hemorrhage, confusion, pulmonary edema, seizures, tetany, metabolic acidosis, fever, coma, and cardiovascular collapse. Kidney and respiratory failure occurs with doses of 20 to 25 g in adults and 4 g in children. **Salicylism**, toxicity due to salicylates that may be associated with chronic use, is characterized by dizziness, tinnitus, difficulty hearing, and mental confusion.

Contraindications

Aspirin is contraindicated in patients with a known sensitivity to aspirin; in those who are allergic to tartrazine, due to a cross-sensitivity; and in those with a known risk of bleeding. The U.S. Food and Drug Administration (FDA) has issued a **BOXED WARNING** ◆ stating that children or teenagers should not take aspirin to treat chickenpox or flulike symptoms because of the risk of Reye syndrome.

Aspirin should be administered cautiously to patients with impaired kidney function. It is a salicylate that crosses the placenta entering the fetal circulation placing the fetus at risk for adverse effects such as intrauterine growth retardation, salicylate toxicity, increased risk of bleeding, and neonatal acidosis. Low birth weight, increased intracranial bleeding, and stillbirth have been reported in infants born to a patient with impaired kidney function who took aspirin late in pregnancy.

Nursing Implications

Preventing Interactions

Alcohol and ginkgo increase the effects of aspirin. Box 16.2 lists the medications that interact with aspirin by increasing or decreasing its effects.

Administering the Medication

Aspirin should be taken with a full glass of water or other fluid and with food or just following food. Administering the medication with food decreases gastric irritation. Although the crushing of tablets or capsules results in faster absorption, this

---

BOX 16.2 Drug Interactions: Aspirin

Drugs That Increase the Effects of Aspirin
- Acidifying agents (e.g., vitamin C)
  Acidify urine and thereby decrease the urinary excretion rate of salicylates
- Anticoagulants, oral
  Increase the risk of bleeding; patients taking anticoagulants should not take aspirin
- Angiotensin-converting enzyme inhibitors, beta-adrenergic blockers
  Decreased antihypertensive effects
- Codeine, hydrocodone, and oxycodone
  Have additive analgesic effects due to mechanism of action
- Corticosteroids
  Have additive gastric irritation and possible ulcerogenic effects

Drugs That Decrease the Effects of Aspirin
- Alkalinizing agents (e.g., sodium bicarbonate)
  Increase the rate of kidney excretion
- Ibuprofen
  Competes with aspirin for COX-1 inhibition
  Negates the cardioprotective benefits of low-dose aspirin
- Misoprostol
  Prevents aspirin-induced gastric ulcers

---

action destroys the long-acting feature and increases the risk of adverse effects and toxicity.

The dose of aspirin given depends mainly on the condition being treated. Low doses (325 mg initially and 75 to 81 mg daily) are used for the drug's antiplatelet effects in preventing arterial thrombotic disorders such as myocardial infarction and stroke. Because aspirin is highly protein bound, lower-than-average doses are needed for patients with low serum albumin levels, because a larger proportion of each dose is free to exert pharmacologic activity. Larger doses are needed for anti-inflammatory effects (maximum daily dosage, 8,000 mg) than for analgesic and antipyretic effects (325 to 650 mg every 4 hours). In general, patients taking low-dose aspirin to prevent myocardial infarction or stroke should continue to take the aspirin if their prescribers order a COX-2–inhibiting NSAID because the COX-2 inhibitors have little effect on platelet function.

Assessing for Therapeutic Effects

If aspirin is given for pain, the nurse uses a pain scale to assess the intensity of the patient's pain, which should decrease. If the drug is given for fever, the nurse records the patient's temperature every 2 to 4 hours and should see a reduction in temperature. If the drug is given for inflammation, the nurse assesses for signs of inflammation, which should decrease. Patients receiving aspirin as a preventive agent for myocardial infarction or transient ischemic attack should be without chest pain or confusion.

Assessing for Adverse Effects

The nurse assesses the patient for bleeding tendencies, GI irritation, nausea, vomiting, and diarrhea, which all may result from aspirin use. The skin is assessed for signs of decreased coagulation. The nurse performs a thorough pulmonary and integumentary assessment, looking for signs of hypersensitivity to aspirin, including dyspnea, bronchospasm, and rash.

Toxicity: Recognition and Management

Salicylate intoxication (salicylism) may occur with an acute overdose or with chronic use of therapeutic doses, especially the higher doses taken for anti-inflammatory effects. Chronic ingestion of large doses saturates a major metabolic pathway, thereby slowing drug elimination, prolonging the serum half-life, and causing drug accumulation. The therapeutic serum level of salicylate is 100 to 300 mcg/mL for the treatment of arthritis and rheumatic fever. Toxicity occurs at levels above 300 mcg/mL.

As previously stated, salicylism is characterized by dizziness, tinnitus, difficulty hearing, and mental confusion. Additional manifestations include nausea, vomiting, fever, fluid and electrolyte deficiencies, visual changes, drowsiness, hyperventilation, and other conditions. Severe central nervous system (CNS) dysfunction (e.g., delirium, stupor, coma, seizures) indicates life-threatening toxicity.

Treatment of Overdose

In mild salicylate toxicity, stopping the drug or reducing the dose is usually sufficient. In severe salicylate overdose, treatment is symptomatic and aimed at preventing further absorption from the GI tract, increasing urinary excretion, and correcting fluid, electrolyte, and acid–base imbalances. When the drug may still be in the GI tract, gastric lavage and activated charcoal help reduce absorption. Intravenous (IV) sodium bicarbonate produces an alkaline urine in which salicylates are more rapidly excreted, and hemodialysis effectively removes salicylates from the blood. IV fluids are indicated when high fever or dehydration is present. The specific content of IV fluids depends on the serum electrolyte and acid–base status.

Patient Teaching

Box 16.3 presents patient teaching guidelines for aspirin.

Other Drugs in the Class

Magnesium salicylate is a less potent prostaglandin than aspirin. It can cause acid–base imbalances. As with all salicylates, the patient should be taught the risk of GI bleeding. The drug is well absorbed and peaks in 20 minutes.

Salsalate is a salicylate with antipyretic, analgesic, antirheumatic, and anti-inflammatory properties. It is indicated for relief of pain and fever as well as treatment of rheumatic fever, rheumatoid arthritis, and osteoarthritis. It is absorbed in the small intestine rather than in the stomach and is reported to cause fewer GI adverse effects than aspirin. Onset, peak, and duration of action are similar to aspirin. The drug is metabolized in the liver and excreted in the urine.

BOX 16.3 Patient Teaching Guidelines for Aspirin

- Keep aspirin out of the reach of children.
- Do not overadminister the medication due to the risk of toxicity.
- Take the medication with food or after meals to prevent stomach upset.
- Do not crush or chew enteric-coated or sustained-release tablets.
- Know that aspirin is as effective as more costly medication.
- Watch for bleeding, ringing in the ears, or diminished hearing.
- Understand that fever is one way the body fights infection. Taking the medication for fever is not usually recommended unless the fever is high or is accompanied by other symptoms.
- Avoid aspirin for approximately 2 weeks before and after major surgery or dental procedures to decrease the risk of excessive bleeding. If pregnant, do not take aspirin for approximately 2 weeks before the estimated delivery date.
- Inform a healthcare provider if you have ever had an allergic reaction (e.g., asthma, difficulty breathing, hives), severe GI symptoms (e.g., ulcer, bleeding), or rash or other skin disorder after taking aspirin.
- Avoid and minimize ingestion of alcohol due to gastric irritation and risk of bleeding.
- Use aspirin cautiously if you are on a low-sodium diet; one aspirin tablet contains 553 mg of sodium.

Clinical Application 16.2

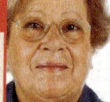

- Mrs. Mason is taking eight 325-mg aspirin tablets per day without adequate pain relief. She is at risk for what adverse effects associated with aspirin?

NCLEX Success

2. An automobile worker visits an occupational health nurse. The worker has pain in the right hand due to repetitive movements and has been taking aspirin 650 mg every 2 hours. Which of the following symptoms is indicative of salicylate toxicity?

   A. ringing in the ears
   B. halos around lights
   C. edema
   D. dysrhythmia

NONNARCOTIC ANALGESIC ANTIPYRETIC: ACETAMINOPHEN

Acetaminophen (also called APAP, an abbreviation of *N*-acetyl-*p*-aminophenol) is a nonprescription drug commonly used as an aspirin substitute because it does not cause nausea, vomiting, or GI bleeding, and it does not interfere with blood

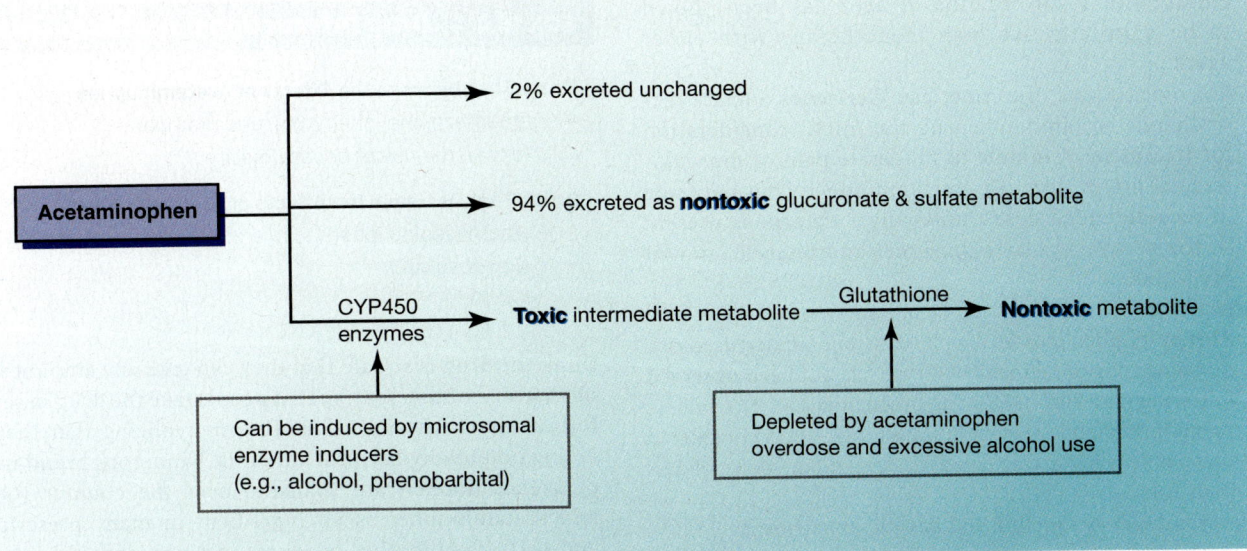

Figure 16.4. Metabolic pathway for acetaminophen. CYP450, cytochrome P450.

clotting. It is equivalent to aspirin in analgesic and antipyretic effects; however, it does not have the anti-inflammatory activity of aspirin.

Pharmacokinetics

Acetaminophen is well absorbed with oral administration, and peak plasma concentrations are reached within 30 to 120 minutes. Duration of action is 3 to 4 hours. Acetaminophen is metabolized in the liver (Fig. 16.4). Approximately 94% is excreted in the urine as nontoxic glucuronate and sulfate conjugates, and 2% is excreted unchanged. The remaining 4% is metabolized by cytochrome P450 enzymes to a toxic metabolite, which is normally inactivated by conjugation with glutathione and excreted in the urine. With usual therapeutic doses, a sufficient amount of glutathione is available in the liver to detoxify acetaminophen.

Action

To reduce fever, acetaminophen acts directly on the hypothalamus to increase vasodilation and sweating. To diminish pain, it acts via an unknown mechanism of action.

Use

Acetaminophen is used to reduce fever and decrease minor pain. The drug is sometimes given to children and patients at risk for seizures who are receiving the diphtheria, pertussis, and tetanus immunization to reduce pain and fever; this is an unlabeled use. Table 16.5 presents specific dosage for acetaminophen.

Patient-related variables specific to the use of acetaminophen include the following:

- Age:
  - Acetaminophen is usually the drug of choice for pain or fever in children.
  - Children seem less susceptible to liver toxicity than adults, apparently because they form less of the toxic metabolite during metabolism of acetaminophen.
  - Toxicity has occurred when parents or caregivers have given the liquid concentration intended for children to infants. The concentrations are different and cannot be given interchangeably.
  - Alternating acetaminophen and ibuprofen (which has antipyretic properties; see subsequent discussion) every 4 hours over a 3-day period to control fever in young

TABLE 16.5

DRUGS AT A GLANCE: Acetaminophen

Drug	Routes and Dosage Ranges	
	Adults	**Children**
P Acetaminophen (Tylenol; ❋ Abenol, Apo-Acetaminophen, Atasol, Novo-Gesic)	PO or rectal suppository: 325–650 mg every 4–6 h Extended release: 1,300 mg every 8 h IV injection: Ofirmev 1,000 mg administered in a 100-mL vial over 15 min	Recommended doses by age: PO, 0–3 mo, 40 mg; 4–11 mo, 80 mg; 12–23 mo, 120 mg; 2–3 y, 160 mg; 4–5 y, 240 mg; 6–8 y, 320 mg; 9–10 y, 400 mg; 11 y, 480 mg Rectal: 3–11 mo, 80 mg every 6 h; 12–36 mo, 80 mg every 4 h; 3–6 y, 120 mg every 4–6 h; 6–12 y, 325 mg every 4–6 h

children (6 to 36 months of age) has been shown to be more effective than monotherapy with either agent.
- For older adults, the American Geriatrics Society recommends acetaminophen be the initial consideration for treatment of middle to moderate pain of musculoskeletal origin (level B). Acetaminophen is usually safe in recommended doses, unless liver damage is present or the person regularly consumes an excessive amount of alcohol.
- Reproduction, pregnancy, and lactation:
  - Acetaminophen crosses the placenta, but an increased risk of major congenital malformations has not been observed following maternal use during pregnancy.
  - Acetaminophen is present in breast milk but is considered acceptable with a calculated relative infant dose of less than 10%.
- Abnormal kidney function and hepatic impairment:
  - Acetaminophen can cause fatal liver necrosis in overdose because it forms a metabolite that can destroy liver cells.
  - The hepatotoxic metabolite is formed more rapidly when drug-metabolizing enzymes in the liver have been stimulated by ingestion of alcohol, cigarette smoking, and drugs such as antiseizure medications and others.
  - Patients who smoke, consume large quantities of alcohol, and take antiseizure medications are at high risk for hepatotoxicity with usual therapeutic doses.

Adverse Effects

Hepatotoxicity and kidney failure are the most common adverse effects of acetaminophen. Hypersensitivity reactions marked by rash and fever may occur in patients who have developed an allergy to the drug. Myocardial damage may develop in patients when doses of 5 to 8 g/day are ingested over several weeks or when 4 g/day have been ingested over 1 year.

Contraindications

Contraindications to acetaminophen use include known hypersensitivity to the drug. Caution is necessary with administration in impaired hepatic and kidney function. The drug crosses the placenta and enters the breast milk; therefore, caution is also required in pregnancy and lactation.

Nursing Implications

Preventing Interactions

Medications that increase or decrease acetaminophen effects are listed in Box 16.4. Herbal supplements that increase the effects of acetaminophen are willow root, meadow root, and ginkgo.

Administering the Medication

Acetaminophen is administered orally or by rectal suppository. Acetaminophen should be given with food to reduce GI upset. It is important that the recommended dosage not be exceeded. The recommended maximum daily dose of acetaminophen is 4 g for adults; additional amounts constitute an overdose. Ingestion of an overdose may be accidental or intentional. One contributing factor may be that some people

> **BOX 16.4 Drug Interactions: Acetaminophen**
>
> **Drugs That Increase the Effects of Acetaminophen**
> - Carbamazepine, phenytoin, and rifampin
>   *Increase the risk of hepatotoxicity*
>
> **Drugs That Decrease the Effects of Acetaminophen**
> - Carbamazepine, phenytoin, and rifampin
>   *Delay absorption*

think the drug is so safe that they can take any amount without harm. Another may be that people take the drug in several formulations without calculating or realizing that they are taking potentially harmful amounts. Numerous brand names of acetaminophen are available over the counter (OTC), and acetaminophen is an ingredient in many prescription and OTC combination products (e.g., oxycodone and acetaminophen [Percocet], as well as OTC cold, flu, headache, and sinus remedies). It is necessary to measure infant doses using a dropper and child doses using a household teaspoon or 5-mL syringe. The nurse should caution parents and caregivers to ask the healthcare provider or prescriber for written instructions on giving acetaminophen to their children, to read the labels of all drug products very carefully, and to avoid giving children acetaminophen from multiple sources. The FDA also recommends limiting the duration of use (5 days or less in children, 10 days or less in adults, and 3 days in both adults and children when used to reduce fever) unless directed by a physician.

> **Quality and Safety Alert: Safety**
>
> For patients who regularly consume an excessive amount of alcohol, short-term ingestion of usual therapeutic doses of acetaminophen may cause hepatotoxicity, and it is recommended that these persons ingest no more than 2 g daily. The FDA has issued a warning advising people who ingest three or more alcoholic drinks daily to avoid acetaminophen or to ask a physician before taking even small doses.

Assessing for Therapeutic Effects

When administering acetaminophen as an antipyretic agent, the nurse assesses for reduced fever. The nurse records the patient's temperature every 2 to 4 hours. When administering the drug as an analgesic, the nurse assesses for decreased pain.

Assessing for Adverse Effects

The most common and severe adverse effect associated with acetaminophen use is hepatotoxicity and hepatic failure; therefore, the nurse assesses for jaundice. It is also important to assess urinary output, blood urea nitrogen, and creatinine because of the risk of kidney toxicity. In addition, it is critical to assess for a rash or fever because these are the first signs of a hypersensitivity reaction. The nurse assesses a patient who has a past history of myocardial damage and takes acetaminophen daily for chest pain and dyspnea. If the patient develops a rash, they should stop taking the drug.

Toxicity: Recognition and Management

Acetaminophen poisoning may occur with a single large dose (possibly as little as 6 g, but usually 10 to 15 g) or with chronic ingestion of excessive doses (5 to 8 g/day for several weeks or 3 to 4 g/day for 1 year). Potentially fatal hepatotoxicity is the main concern and is most likely with doses of 20 g or more. Metabolism of acetaminophen produces a toxic metabolite that is normally inactivated by combining with glutathione. In overdose situations, the supply of glutathione is depleted and the toxic metabolite accumulates and directly damages liver cells (see Fig. 16.4). Acute kidney injury may also occur.

Early symptoms (12 to 24 hours after ingestion) of toxicity are nonspecific (e.g., anorexia, nausea, vomiting, diaphoresis) and may not be considered serious or important enough to report or seek treatment. At 24 to 48 hours, symptoms may subside, but tests of liver function (e.g., aspartate aminotransferase, alanine aminotransferase, bilirubin, prothrombin time) begin to show increased levels. Later manifestations may include jaundice, vomiting, and CNS stimulation with excitement and delirium, followed by vascular collapse, coma, and death. Peak hepatotoxicity occurs in 3 to 4 days; recovery in nonfatal overdoses occurs in 7 to 8 days.

It is important to obtain plasma acetaminophen levels when an overdose is known or suspected, preferably within 4 hours after ingestion and every 24 hours for several days. Minimal hepatotoxicity is associated with plasma levels of less than 120 mcg/mL at 4 hours after ingestion or less than 30 mcg/mL at 12 hours after ingestion. With blood levels greater than 300 mcg/mL at 4 hours after ingestion, about 90% of patients develop liver damage.

Treatment of Overdose

Gastric lavage is recommended if acetaminophen overdose is detected within 4 hours after ingestion, and activated charcoal can be given to inhibit absorption. In addition, the specific antidote is acetylcysteine, a mucolytic agent given by inhalation in respiratory disorders. Acetylcysteine may be given orally or intravenously (dosages are listed with other antidotes in Chapter 2). The drug supplies cysteine, a precursor substance required for the synthesis of glutathione. The synthesized glutathione combines with a toxic metabolite and decreases hepatotoxicity. Acetylcysteine is most beneficial if given within 8 hours of acetaminophen ingestion but may be helpful within 36 hours. It does not reverse damage that has already occurred.

Patient Teaching

Box 16.5 presents patient teaching guidelines for acetaminophen.

NONSTEROIDAL ANTI-INFLAMMATORY DRUGS

Nonsteroidal anti-inflammatory drugs (NSAIDs) are medications used to prevent and treat mild to moderate pain and inflammation. NSAIDs inhibit the synthesis of prostaglandins.

As discussed in the introduction to this chapter, the mechanism of action of NSAIDs involves the blocking of COX enzymes. These drugs are classified into two types or "generations." First-generation NSAIDs block both COX-1 and COX-2, and second-generation NSAIDs block only COX-2. Both first- and second-generation NSAIDs have the potential to cause serious cardiovascular thrombotic events. All NSAIDs are contraindicated in the setting of coronary artery bypass graft surgery. The nonsteroidal anti-inflammatory agents ibuprofen and indomethacin are used initially in treating patent ductus arteriosus.

> **BOX 16.5 Patient Teaching Guidelines for Acetaminophen**
>
> - Do not exceed the recommended dosage, and do not take any other medications containing acetaminophen.
> - Inform the healthcare provider if a rash or fever develops.
> - For better absorption, chew "chewable" tablets and do not swallow them whole.

PROPIONIC ACID DERIVATIVES

The propionic acid derivatives are NSAIDs that inhibit prostaglandin synthesis in both the central and peripheral nervous systems. The prototype is **ibuprofen** (Motrin, Advil).

Pharmacokinetics

Ibuprofen is 80% absorbed in the GI tract. Its onset of action is 1 hour, producing antipyretic effects, reaching a peak in 1 to 2 hours. The duration of action is 6 to 8 hours. Ibuprofen is metabolized in the liver and eliminated in the urine. A small amount of the medication is eliminated in biliary excretion.

Action

Ibuprofen blocks prostaglandin synthesis and modulates T-cell production. It inhibits the inflammatory cells by the process of chemotaxis to destroy the cells of inflammation. A first-generation NSAID, it blocks COX-1 and COX-2 but is more selective with COX-1.

Use

Ibuprofen is used to relieve mild to moderate pain, including dysmenorrhea (painful menstruation). It is also used to treat inflammation related to rheumatoid arthritis and osteoarthritis. In addition, it is effective in reducing fever. During initial attacks of acute gout, NSAIDs such as ibuprofen may be administered. Table 16.6 gives dosage information for ibuprofen and the other propionic acid derivatives.

Patient-related variables specific to the use of ibuprofen include the following:

- Age:
  - For children older than 6 months of age, ibuprofen is recommended for reduction of fever.

- The FDA has approved ibuprofen for the treatment of patent ductus arteriosus in neonates who do not respond to conventional treatment.
- Older adults taking ibuprofen on a long-term basis are evaluated for GI blood loss, kidney dysfunction, edema, hypertension, and drug–drug or drug–drug disease interactions. A gastroprotective agent is recommended for patients at risk for upper GI bleeding.
- Reproduction, pregnancy, and lactation:
  - NSAIDs may delay or prevent rupture of ovarian follicles. Discontinue use of NSAIDs in patients having difficulty conceiving or undergoing investigation of fertility.
  - The use of NSAIDs close to conception may increase the risk of miscarriage.
  - NSAIDs should be avoided beginning at 20 weeks' gestation.
  - Ibuprofen is considered compatible with breast-feeding.

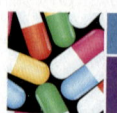

TABLE 16.6
DRUGS AT A GLANCE: Propionic Acid Derivatives

Drug	Routes and Dosage Ranges	
	Adults	**Children**
Ibuprofen (Motrin, Advil)	Osteoarthritis, rheumatoid arthritis: PO 300–600 mg three or four times per day; maximum 3,200 mg/d Pain, dysmenorrhea: PO 400 mg every 4–6 h PRN; maximum 3,200 mg/dL IV 400–800 mg every 6 h Migraine: PO 400 mg at onset of headache	6 mo to 12 y: fever, initial temperature 39.2°C (102.5°F) or less, PO 5 mg/kg every 6–8 h; initial temperature above 39.2°C (102.5°F), PO 5–10 mg/kg every 6–8 h; maximum dose 40 mg/kg/d Juvenile arthritis: PO 20–40 mg/kg/d, in three or four divided doses
Diflunisal	Osteoarthritis and rheumatoid arthritis: PO 500–1,000 mg/d in two divided doses, increased to a maximum of 1,500 mg/d if necessary Pain: PO 500–1,000 mg initially and then 250–500 mg every 8–12 h	Not recommended for children <12 y of age
Fenoprofen (Fenortho, Nalfon)	Osteoarthritis and rheumatoid arthritis: PO 400–600 mg three to four times per day; maximum dose 3,200 mg/d Pain: 200 mg every 4–6 h as needed	Dosage not established
Flurbiprofen (ophthalmic)	Osteoarthritis, rheumatoid arthritis: PO 200–300 mg/d in two, three, or four divided doses Inhibition of intraoperative miosis: (ophthalmic) 1 drop every 30 min, beginning 2 h before surgery (total of four drops)	Dosage not established
Ketoprofen	Pain, dysmenorrhea: PO 25–50 mg every 6–8 h PRN Osteoarthritis, rheumatoid arthritis: PO 150–300 mg/d in three or four divided doses Extended release: 200 mg once daily Maximum: 300 mg/d for regular formulation; 200 mg/d for extended release; 100–150 mg/d for patients with impaired kidney function	Do not give to children <16 y unless directed by a physician
Meclofenamate sodium	Inflammatory disease: PO 200–400 mg/d in 3–4 divided doses; maximum 400 mg/d Dysmenorrhea: PO 100 mg three times per day starting at the onset of menstrual flow	Dosage not established
Mefenamic acid (✣ Ponstan)	Pain: PO 500 mg and then 250 mg every 6 h not to exceed 1-wk administration Dysmenorrhea: PO 500 mg beginning at the onset of menstrual bleeding followed by 250 mg every 6 h. Do not exceed 3 d	Adolescents ≥14 y same as adult dosing
Nabumetone (Relafen, Relafen DS)	Arthritis: PO initial 1,000 mg as a single dose; adjust dose according to the patient response up to 2,000 mg/d 1–2 divided doses Patients <50 kg dose should be <1,000 mg/d	Dosage not established

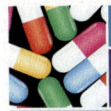

TABLE 16.6
DRUGS AT A GLANCE: Propionic Acid Derivatives (Continued)

Drug	Routes and Dosage Ranges	
	Adults	**Children**
Naproxen sodium (Aleve, Naprosyn, Anaprox, Apo-Napro-Na)	Naproxen: PO 250–500 mg twice daily Gout: PO 750 mg initially and then 250 mg every 8 h until symptoms subside Maximum: 1,250 mg/d Naproxen sodium, pain, dysmenorrhea, acute tendonitis; bursitis: PO 550 mg every 12 h or 275 mg every 6–8 h Maximum: 1,375 mg/d OA, RA, AS: PO 275–550 mg twice a day Acute gout: PO 825 mg initially and then 275 mg every 8 h until symptoms subside Controlled release (Naprelan): 750–1,000 mg once daily	Juvenile arthritis (naproxen only): PO 10 mg/kg/d in two divided doses. Oral suspension (125 mg/5 mL) twice daily according to weight: 13 kg (29 lb), 2.5 mL; 25 kg (55 lb), 5 mL; 39 kg (84 lb), 7.5 mL OTC preparation not recommended for children <12 y
Oxaprozin (Daypro)	PO 600–1,200 mg once daily Maximum: 1,800 mg/d or 26 mg/kg/d, whichever is lower, in divided doses	6–16 y 22–31 kg: 600 mg once daily 32–54 kg: 900 mg once daily ≥55 kg: 1,200 mg once daily

- Abnormal kidney function and hepatic impairment:
  - Ibuprofen can cause or aggravate abnormal kidney function, even though it is eliminated mainly by hepatic metabolism. By inhibiting prostaglandins that dilate kidney blood vessels, it can decrease the blood flow in the kidneys.
  - In patients who depend on prostaglandins to maintain an adequate kidney blood flow, the prostaglandin-blocking effects of ibuprofen result in constriction of kidney arteries and arterioles, decreased kidney blood flow, decreased glomerular filtration rate, and retention of salt and water.
  - People at highest risk for abnormal kidney function from the use of ibuprofen and related drugs are those with pre-existing abnormal kidney function, those older than 50 years of age, those taking diuretics, and those with hypertension, diabetes, or heart failure.
  - Measures to prevent or minimize kidney damage include avoiding nephrotoxic drugs when possible, treating the disorders that increase risk of kidney damage, stopping the ibuprofen if abnormal kidney function occurs, monitoring kidney function, reducing dosage, and maintaining hydration.
  - Ibuprofen is metabolized in the liver, requiring that the dosage of the medication be decreased in patients with hepatic problems. The maximum daily dosage of ibuprofen in patients with hepatitis is 2 g.

> **Quality and Safety Alert: Safety**
>
> It is important for the home care nurse to instruct the patient about all aspects of administration of ibuprofen. Because the medication is available in OTC preparations with many trade names, patients may not realize that they are taking an ibuprofen-containing drug. Overdosing may occur.

Adverse Effects

Ibuprofen can cause kidney damage by other mechanisms, including a hypersensitivity reaction that leads to acute kidney injury, manifested by proteinuria, hematuria, and pyuria. Biopsy reports usually indicate inflammatory reactions such as glomerulonephritis or interstitial nephritis.

The GI adverse effects of ibuprofen are many: dry mouth, gingival hyperplasia, dyspepsia, heartburn, nausea, epigastric pain, constipation, and GI ulceration with occult blood loss. The genitourinary effects include nephrotoxicity, elevated blood urea nitrogen and creatinine, and edema. The respiratory adverse effects include dyspnea, bronchospasm, hemoptysis, and pharyngitis. In addition, anaphylactic reactions may also occur. The FDA has issued a **BOXED WARNING** stating that NSAIDs cause an increased risk of serious cardiovascular thrombotic events, including stroke or myocardial infarction.

Contraindications

The FDA has issued a **BOXED WARNING** stating that ibuprofen is contraindicated for the treatment of perioperative pain after coronary artery bypass graft. Ibuprofen is contraindicated in patients with a known allergy to NSAIDs and salicylates. Allergic reactions are more common in patients with rhinitis, asthma, chronic urticaria, and nasal polyps.

Nursing Implications
Preventing Interactions

Herbs and foods that increase the effects of ibuprofen include alcohol, garlic, ginger, ginkgo, and feverfew. Medications that interact with ibuprofen, increasing or decreasing its effects are listed in Box 16.6.

> **BOX 16.6 Drug Interactions: Ibuprofen**
>
> **Drugs That Increase the Effects of Ibuprofen**
> - Anticoagulants
>   *Increase the risk of bleeding*
> - Codeine, oxycodone, and hydrocodone
>   *Have an additive analgesic effect*
> - Corticosteroids
>   *Have additive gastric irritant and possible ulcerogenic effects*

Administering the Medication

Ibuprofen is administered orally, and the total daily dose should not exceed 3,200 mg. When administered intravenously, it should be diluted in a concentration of 4 mg/mL or less using 0.9% sodium chloride, 5% dextrose, or lactated Ringer's. The dilution remains stable for 24 hours. Prior to the administration of the IV preparation, the patient should be well hydrated. Researchers have reported that the rapid infusion of ibuprofen intravenously was safe and effective in treating pain. The maximum total serum amount of IV ibuprofen was twice that of oral ibuprofen.

Assessing for Therapeutic Effects

When ibuprofen is administered for pain, the nurse assesses the patient for diminished pain as reported on a pain scale. When the drug is administered for fever, the nurse records the patient's temperature every 2 to 4 hours and assesses for reduced temperature. When the drug is administered for inflammation, the nurse notes anti-inflammatory effects, particularly in the joints related to arthritis, and assesses for decreased inflammation.

Assessing Adverse Effects

The nurse assesses the patient for dyspepsia or GI bleeding, including hemoptysis or melena. Complete blood count and clotting times are assessed for signs of anticoagulation. In addition, the nurse assesses for signs and symptoms of hypersensitivity to ibuprofen, including rash and bronchospasm.

Patient Teaching

Box 16.7 presents patient teaching guidelines for ibuprofen.

Other Drugs in the Class

Several other propionic acid derivatives are available.

> **BOX 16.7 Patient Teaching Guidelines for Ibuprofen**
>
> - Take this drug with food or liquid to decrease gastric irritation.
> - Drink 2 to 3 quarts of fluid daily when taking this drug regularly.
> - Report any signs of bleeding (e.g., nosebleed, vomiting blood, bruising, blood in the urine or stool), difficulty breathing, severe stomach upset, swelling, or weight gain to your healthcare provider.

Diflunisal and fenoprofen have the same action as the prototype drug ibuprofen. Diflunisal requires adequate albumin levels for sufficient drug distribution. Fenoprofen's peak serum level is decreased when administered with food, but the administration with food decreases stomach upset. Flurbiprofen and ketoprofen have the same action in providing anti-inflammatory response. Meclofenamate sodium, mefenamic acid, and naproxen are used to treat inflammatory disease processes and dysmenorrhea. Oxaprozin and nabumetone are similar to other drugs in the propionic derivative class. Patients who have taken nabumetone and who have a history of asthma, aspirin intolerance, or rhinitis are at increased risk of an anaphylactic reaction.

> **Clinical Application 16.3**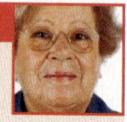
> - When teaching Mrs. Mason about ibuprofen, what is necessary to say about the action of the medication?
> - What are the adverse reactions of ibuprofen?
> - What specific patient teaching should be provided to Mrs. Mason?

OXICAM DERIVATIVES

Oxicam derivatives are another type of NSAID. The prototype is Ⓟ **meloxicam** (Anjeso).

Pharmacokinetics

Meloxicam is metabolized by the liver and excreted in the feces and urine. The onset of action is 1 hour, and peak serum concentrations occur in 5 to 6 hours. The drug crosses the placenta and enters breast milk.

Action

Meloxicam is a COX-1 and COX-2 inhibitor, producing anti-inflammatory, analgesic, and antipyretic effects. It is more selective for COX-2 inhibition in the brain, kidney, ovary, uterus, cartilage, bone, and sites of inflammation.

Use

Meloxicam is administered for the treatment of osteoarthritis and rheumatoid arthritis. Table 16.7 gives the dosage information for meloxicam and a related drug.

Patient-related variables specific to the use of meloxicam include the following:

- Age:
  - In children aged 2 years or older, meloxicam is used to treat the signs and symptoms of pauciarticular or polyarticular juvenile rheumatoid arthritis.
  - Children aged 2 years or older are at greater risk of abdominal pain, diarrhea, fever, headache, and vomiting.
  - Older adults are at greater risk for GI bleeding.
- Reproduction, pregnancy, and lactation:
  - Meloxicam may delay or prevent rupture of ovarian follicles; this may be associated with infertility.

TABLE 16.7
DRUGS AT A GLANCE: Oxicam Derivatives

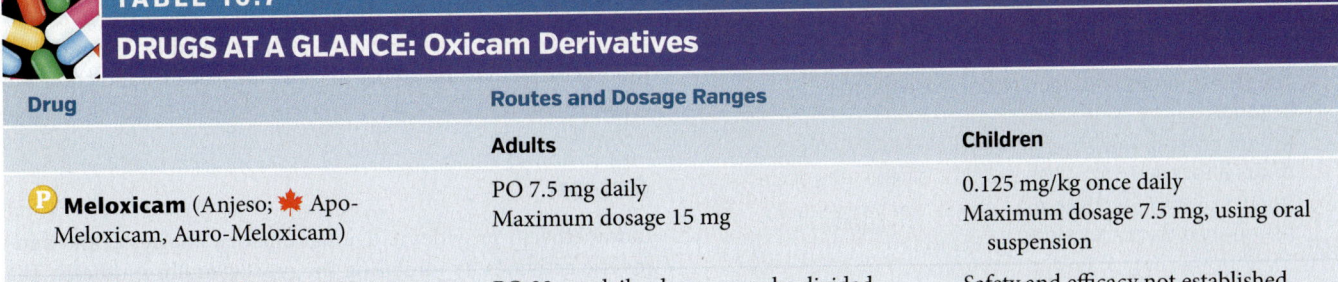

Drug	Routes and Dosage Ranges	
	Adults	**Children**
ⓟ **Meloxicam** (Anjeso; 🍁 Apo-Meloxicam, Auro-Meloxicam)	PO 7.5 mg daily Maximum dosage 15 mg	0.125 mg/kg once daily Maximum dosage 7.5 mg, using oral suspension
Piroxicam (Feldene; 🍁 Apo-Piroxicam)	PO 20 mg daily; dosage may be divided	Safety and efficacy not established

- Meloxicam may increase the risk of miscarriage due to the cyclooxygenase-2 inhibition.
- Congenital anomalies have been observed with in utero exposure to meloxicam.
- Abnormal kidney function and hepatic impairment:
  - Use of meloxicam in patients with creatinine clearance less than 20 mL/min has not been studied and is not recommended in these patients.
  - Patients undergoing hemodialysis should receive a maximum of 7.5 mg/day.

Adverse Effects

Meloxicam is associated with several adverse effects. Respiratory effects include dyspnea, hemoptysis, bronchospasm, pharyngitis, and rhinitis. Hematologic effects consist of bleeding, platelet inhibition, and decreased hemoglobin and hematocrit, along with bone marrow depression and edema. GI effects include nausea, dyspepsia, diarrhea, vomiting, and diarrhea. The FDA has issued a **BOXED WARNING** ◆ stating that patients who take meloxicam are at risk for cardiovascular events and GI bleeding. In addition, headache, dizziness, drowsiness, and insomnia may occur.

Contraindications

Meloxicam should not be administered to patients with a known aspirin allergy. It is also contraindicated postoperatively in patients who have just undergone coronary artery bypass surgery.

Nursing Implications

Preventing Interactions

Some medications interact with meloxicam, increasing its effects (Box 16.8). As with all NSAIDs, alcohol, garlic, ginseng, and ginger increase the risk of bleeding. Giving meloxicam with lithium increases the risk of lithium toxicity.

Administering the Medication

Administration of meloxicam with food or fluids reduces gastric irritation. It is necessary to shake the oral suspension gently before use.

Assessing for Therapeutic Effects

When giving meloxicam for pain, the nurse assesses the pain level using a pain scale to determine that analgesic effects are attained. When giving it for fever, the nurse records the patient's temperature every 2 to 4 hours to check for diminished body temperature. When giving it for inflammation, the nurse assesses for diminished redness and swelling.

Assessing for Adverse Effects

The nurse assesses the patient for signs and symptoms of hypersensitivity reactions such as shortness of breath and bronchospasm. It is also necessary to assess for hemoptysis as well as blood in the stool or urine. In addition, the nurse must assess for signs and symptoms of cardiovascular events.

Patient Teaching

Box 16.9 presents patient teaching guidelines for meloxicam.

Other Drugs in the Class

Piroxicam (Feldene) is similar to meloxicam in terms of pharmacokinetics. It is metabolized predominantly by CYP2C9. Patients who are poor CYP2C9 metabolizers have reduced metabolism and increased serum levels.

NCLEX Success

3. A prescriber in an orthopedic care practice orders meloxicam for the treatment of osteoarthritis. Which of the following medications when combined with meloxicam places the patient at greatest risk?
   A. antimicrobials
   B. lithium
   C. selective serotonin inhibitors
   D. hydrochlorothiazide

BOX 16.8 Drug Interactions: Meloxicam

Drugs That Increase the Effects of Meloxicam

- Angiotensin-converting enzyme inhibitors and diuretics
  Increase the risk of kidney failure
- Aspirin and anticoagulants
  Increase the risk of gastrointestinal bleeding

> **BOX 16.9 Patient Teaching Guidelines for Meloxicam**
>
> - Take these drugs with food to decrease gastric irritation.
> - Do not operate machinery until you know how these drugs affect you. Dizziness and drowsiness may occur.
> - Report sore throat, dyspnea, edema, and tarry stools to your healthcare provider.

ACETIC ACID DERIVATIVES

The prototype NSAID of the acetic acid derivative group is **indomethacin** (Indocin, Tivorbex). The acetic acid derivatives have strong anti-inflammatory effects and more severe adverse effects than the propionic acid derivatives.

Pharmacokinetics

With oral administration of indomethacin, the onset of action is 30 minutes, with a peak in 1 to 2 hours and a duration of action of 4 to 6 hours. With IV administration, onset of action is immediate, with an unknown peak and a duration of action of 15 to 30 minutes. The drug is metabolized in the liver and has a half-life of 4.5 to 6 hours. It is excreted by the kidneys. Indomethacin has the ability to cross the placenta and enter the breast milk.

Action

Indomethacin provides anti-inflammatory, analgesic, and antipyretic activities by inhibiting the prostaglandin synthesis. The exact mechanism is unknown, but it inhibits COX-1 and COX-2. It is mainly a selective COX-1 inhibitor.

Use

Indomethacin is administered to relieve pain associated with rheumatoid arthritis, osteoarthritis, ankylosing spondylitis, bursitis, tendonitis, and gouty arthritis. During initial attacks of acute gout, the drug may be given. Parenteral, but not oral, administration is used to produce closure of patent ductus arteriosus in premature infants who weigh 500 to 1,750 g. Table 16.8 gives dosage information for indomethacin and the other acetic acid derivatives.

TABLE 16.8 DRUGS AT A GLANCE: Acetic Acid Derivatives

Drug	Routes and Dosage Ranges	
	Adults	**Children**
Indomethacin (Indocin, Tivorbex; Apo-Indomethacin, Sandoz-Indomethacin)	PO, rectal suppository: 75 mg/d initially, increased by 25 mg/d at weekly intervals to a maximum of 150–200 mg/d, if necessary Acute gouty arthritis, acute painful shoulder: PO 75–150 mg/d in three or four divided doses until pain and inflammation are controlled (e.g., 3–5 d for gout; 7–14 d for painful shoulder), then discontinued	In special circumstances, such as juvenile rheumatoid arthritis, children older than 2 y of age may receive the drug. Initial dose is 2 mg/kg/d in divided doses, not to exceed 4 mg/kg/d Premature infants with patent ductus arteriosus: IV 0.1–0.25 mg/kg every 12 h for a total of three doses
Diclofenac potassium (Cambia, Zorvolex; Apo-Diclo, Apo-Diclo SR Voltaren, Voltaren XR, Cambia, Zipsor)	Osteoarthritis: PO 100–150 mg/d in divided doses (e.g., 50 mg two or three times or 75 mg twice or 100 mg once daily) Rheumatoid arthritis: PO 150–200 mg/d in two, three, or four divided doses Ankylosing spondylitis: PO 100–125 mg/d in four or five divided doses (e.g., 25 mg four or five times daily) Pain, dysmenorrhea: (diclofenac potassium only) PO 50 mg three times daily Acute migraine: 50-mg packet mixed in 30–60 mL water as a single dose at the onset of a headache (Cambia) Mild to moderate pain: 25-mg liquid capsule PO four times daily Actinic keratosis topical: cover lesion with gel and smooth into skin; do not cover with dressing (Solaraze) Transdermal patch: apply to the most painful area two times daily (Flector) Ophthalmic: 1 drop to the affected eye starting 24 h after cataract surgery for 2 wk	Dosage not established Off-label use: juvenile idiopathic arthritis in children ≥3 y 2–3 mg/kg/d in divided doses

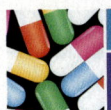

TABLE 16.8
DRUGS AT A GLANCE: Acetic Acid Derivatives (Continued)

Drug	Routes and Dosage Ranges	
	Adults	**Children**
Etodolac (Lodine; ❋ Taro-Etodolac)	Pain: 200–400 mg PO every 6–8 h Osteoarthritis: 600–1,200 mg/d PO in 2–4 divided doses Rheumatoid arthritis: 500 mg PO twice daily	PO extended release 20–30 mg: 400 mg once daily 31–45 kg: 600 mg once daily 46–80 kg: 800 mg once daily >60 kg: 1,000 mg once daily
Ketorolac	Single dose: IV 30 mg, IM 60 mg Multiple dose: IM or IV 30 mg every 6 h PRN to a maximum of 120 mg/d PO 20 mg as the first dose for patients who received 60 mg IM or 30 mg IV as a single dose or 30 mg in a multiple dose followed by 10 mg every 4–6 h to a maximum of 40 mg/d Older adults (>65 y), those with abnormal kidney function, those with weight <50 kg (110 lb; IV, IM 15 mg every 6 h to a maximum of 60 mg/d) Itching from allergic conjunctivitis: ophthalmic Acular PF: for cataract surgery, 1 drop every four times daily after surgery and continue for 2 wk Acular LS: 1 drop four times daily PRN for burning and stinging for up to 4 d after surgery Pain and photophobia: use for 3 d	Use one single-dose injection 1 mg/kg IM up to a maximum of 30 mg or 0.5 mg/kg IV up to a maximum of 15 mg
Nabumetone (Relafen DS) (Apo-Nabumetone, Mylan-Nabumetone, Teva-Nabumetone)	PO 1,000–2,000 mg/d in one or two doses	Dosage not established
Sulindac (❋ Apo-Sulin, Teva-Sulindac)	PO 150–200 mg twice a day; maximum of 400 mg/d Acute gout, acute painful shoulder: PO 200 mg twice a day until pain and inflammation subside (e.g., 7–14 d), then reduce dosage or discontinue	Dosage not established

Patient-related variables specific to the use of indomethacin include the following:

- Age:
  - The FDA has approved IV indomethacin for treatment of patent ductus arteriosus in premature infants. The ductus arteriosus joins the pulmonary artery to the aorta in the fetal circulation. If the ductus reopens, the drug is repeated in 12 to 24 hours. Indications that the ductus has reopened would be the signs and symptoms of heart failure such as dyspnea and a heart murmur.
  - The Beers Criteria indicate that indomethacin is an inappropriate medication for the older adult population and should be avoided. When an older adult must take indomethacin, it is necessary to use the lowest recommended dose and frequency.
- Reproduction, pregnancy, and lactation:
  - Indomethacin may delay or prevent rupture of ovarian follicles; this may be associated with infertility.
  - Indomethacin may increase the risk of miscarriage due to the cyclooxygenase-2 inhibition.
  - Congenital anomalies have been observed with in utero exposure to indomethacin.
- Abnormal kidney function and hepatic impairment:
  - In patients with abnormal kidney function, caution is required. Severe abnormal kidney function is a contraindication.
  - In patients with hepatic impairment, caution is necessary. Dosage reduction is appropriate.

Adverse Effects

Indomethacin and all acetic acid derivatives result in a risk of GI bleeding and bleeding ulcer. Abdominal pain, distention, vomiting, and transient ileus may occur. CNS adverse effects include headache, dizziness, somnolence, and insomnia. Patients are at risk for abnormal kidney function and decreased clotting time. With IV preparations, the most severe respiratory adverse effect is pulmonary hemorrhage.

Contraindications

Indomethacin should not be administered to patients with a known history of salicylate hypersensitivity. Patients with a past history of GI bleeding should not take the drug. It should not be administered postoperatively to patients who have just had a coronary artery bypass graft. The parenteral formulations are contraindicated in infection, bleeding, thrombocytopenia, coagulation defects, and necrotizing enterocolitis. As stated earlier, indomethacin is contraindicated in severe abnormal kidney function.

Nursing Implications

Preventing Interactions

Certain drugs interact with indomethacin (Box 16.10). The administration of alcohol, feverfew, garlic, ginger, and ginkgo also increases the bleeding potential.

Administering the Medication

Administering oral indomethacin after meals or with an antacid decreases GI irritation. Patients with gouty arthritis should not take the sustained-release preparation. Patients with a history of proctitis or rectal bleeding should not use rectal suppositories. IV administration requires dilution of 1 mg with 1 mL of sterile water or normal saline. It is necessary to administer the dose over 5 to 10 seconds. Good IV access is imperative to prevent extravasation of the drug into the tissues. The oral preparation of indomethacin must be stored in a light-protected container.

Assessing for Therapeutic Effects

Before administering indomethacin, the patient must be assessed for salicylate allergy, which can cause bronchospasm, dyspnea, and rash. After the drug has had time to work, it is imperative to assess for diminished pain and inflammation. The nurse observes the patient's mobility in response to diminished inflammation. When administering indomethacin for gout, inflammation is generally relieved in 24 to 36 hours.

Assessing for Adverse Effects

A careful assessment of the cardiac and CNS effects is imperative. The nurse assesses for bleeding, vomiting, and abdominal pain. The FDA has issued a **BOXED WARNING** for indomethacin, stating that an increased risk of adverse cardiovascular thrombotic effects, including myocardial infarction and cerebrovascular accident, has been noted with the drug. Because of the risk of hypersensitivity, the nurse assesses for dyspnea, bronchospasm, and hemoptysis. In addition, if the patient complains of abdominal pain that is indicative of transient ileus, the nurse notifies the physician immediately.

BOX 16.10 Drug Interactions: Indomethacin

Drugs That Increase the Effects of Indomethacin
- Phenytoin, salicylates, sulfonamides, and sulfonylureas
  Result in displacement of protein-binding activities
- Salicylates, anticoagulants, and lithium
  Increase the risk of bleeding

> **! Quality and Safety Alert: Safety**
>
> Assessment for GI pain, rapid pulse, and diaphoresis is essential in patients who receive ketorolac. These symptoms are indicative of GI perforation.

Patient Teaching

Box 16.11 lists patient teaching guidelines for indomethacin.

Other Drugs in the Class

Several other acetic acid derivatives deserve mention.

Diclofenac reversibly inhibits COX-1 and COX-2 to produce an anti-inflammatory response. It is readily absorbed by the GI tract, with 50% to 60% reaching the systemic circulation. The nonsteroidal effects are well distributed to the synovial fluid and easily pass into the breast milk. The drug is more than 99% bound to albumin and undergoes first-pass metabolism. Two thirds of elimination of diclofenac is in the urine, and one third is in the feces. The half-life of the transdermal preparation is 12 hours, whereas that of the oral preparation is 1 to 2 hours. The transdermal formulation is administered to relieve acute pain. The topical preparation is used to treat actinic keratosis. The ophthalmic preparation is administered to relieve photosensitivity following refractive surgery.

Etodolac possesses the same mechanism of action as diclofenac. Etodolac is administered for the treatment of pain, osteoarthritis, and rheumatoid arthritis. Diclofenac is administered for ankylosing spondylitis, dysmenorrhea, gout, migraine, pain, osteoarthritis and rheumatoid arthritis.

Ketorolac, an injectable NSAID often used for pain, is contraindicated in patients at risk for excessive bleeding. Thus, this drug should not be administered during labor and delivery, before or during any major surgery, with suspected or confirmed cerebrovascular bleeding, or to patients who are

---

BOX 16.11 Patient Teaching Guidelines for Indomethacin

- For parents or caregivers of an infant being treated for patent ductus arteriosus:
  - Be sure you receive information about and understand the action, adverse effects, and therapeutic effects of indomethacin.
- Understand the administration guidelines for indomethacin.
- Administer the oral preparation with food or immediately after a meal.
- If necessary, take the medication with an antacid to decrease gastric irritation.
- Report adverse effects such as chest pain, weakness, or disorientation to your healthcare provider.
- Do not operate machinery due to dizziness or somnolence.
- Report sore throat, fever, rash, weight gain, or tarry stools to your healthcare provider.

currently taking aspirin or other NSAIDs. The FDA has issued a BOXED WARNING ◆ for ketorolac; the drug places the patient at risk for GI irritation, inflammation, ulceration, bleeding, and perforation. Parenteral ketorolac reportedly compares with morphine and other opioids in analgesic effectiveness for moderate or severe pain. However, its use is limited to 5 days because it increases the risk of bleeding. Hematomas and wound bleeding have been reported with postoperative use. Intranasal formulation is administered for the treatment of acute, severe migraine.

Sulindac is used for inflammatory disorders, including ankylosing spondylitis and acute painful shoulder due to bursitis or tendonitis. The therapeutic response of sulindac is usually noted in 1 week. The drug is 90% absorbed and 98% bound to albumin.

Nabumetone is administered for rheumatoid and osteoarthritis. It blocks prostaglandin synthesis through the inhibition of COX. Prior to administering nabumetone, a baseline hemoglobin and hematocrit should be assessed. The patient should be instructed to report any signs or symptoms of abdominal pain or black tarry stools.

SELECTIVE COX-2 INHIBITOR: CELECOXIB

Celecoxib (CeleBREX) is the only selective COX-2 inhibitor on the market in the United States. The selective COX-2 inhibitors etoricoxib and parecoxib, which are available in the United Kingdom and other countries, are not available in the United States. COX-2 inhibitors were designed to selectively block production of prostaglandins associated with pain and inflammation without blocking those associated with protective effects on gastric mucosa, kidney function, and platelet aggregation. Thus, they produce less gastric irritation and abnormal kidney function than aspirin and other NSAIDs.

Pharmacokinetics

Celecoxib, which is administered orally, has a slow onset of action. The drug reaches its peak in 3 hours. It is highly protein bound (97%), and the serum half-life is 11 hours. It is metabolized by the cytochrome P450 enzymes in the liver to inactive metabolites that are then excreted in the urine. A small amount is excreted unchanged in the urine. Celecoxib crosses the placenta and enters the breast milk.

Action

COX-2 is activated with inflammation. Celecoxib inhibits the COX-2 enzyme to decrease inflammation. It does not affect the COX-1 enzyme, thus protecting the lining of the GI tract and not inhibiting clotting factors.

Use

Celecoxib is administered for acute and long-term treatment of juvenile rheumatoid arthritis, rheumatoid arthritis, osteoarthritis, and ankylosing spondylitis. It is used to treat acute pain and primary dysmenorrhea. In addition, the drug is given in familial adenomatous polyposis to reduce the number of colorectal polyps. Unlabeled uses include the treatment of acute pain, ankylosing spondylitis, juvenile idiopathic arthritis, osteoarthritis, primary dysmenorrhea, and rheumatoid arthritis. Table 16.9 presents specific dosage information for celecoxib.

Patient-related variables specific to the use of celecoxib include the following:

- Age:
  - Celecoxib is recommended only for children aged 2 years and older to treat juvenile rheumatoid arthritis.
  - In children, the median peak serum concentration is 3 hours. The range of peak serum concentration is 3 to 6.2 hours.
- Reproduction, pregnancy, and lactation:
  - Celecoxib may delay or prevent rupture of ovarian follicles; this may be associated with infertility.
  - Celecoxib may increase the risk of miscarriage due to the cyclooxygenase-2 inhibition.
  - Congenital anomalies have been observed with in utero exposure to celecoxib.
  - Celecoxib is present in breast milk; however, administration is acceptable when the relative infant dose is less than 10%.
- Abnormal kidney function and hepatic impairment:
  - In patients with significant abnormal kidney function, celecoxib is contraindicated.
  - In patients with hepatic impairment, the dosage of celecoxib should be reduced by 50%.

TABLE 16.9

DRUGS AT A GLANCE: Celecoxib

Drug	Routes and Dosage Ranges	
	Adults	**Children**
Celecoxib (CeleBREX; ACT Celecoxib, AG-Celecoxib)	PO 100 mg two times daily may be increased to 200 mg/d two times daily Acute pain, dysmenorrhea: 400 mg and then 200 mg two times daily Familial adenomatous polyposis: 400 mg two times daily Ankylosing spondylitis: 200 mg/d after 6 wk, a trial of 400 mg/d may be tried for 6 wk; if no effect is seen, another therapy is recommended	Children older than 2 y of age PO 10 or 25 kg or less: 50-mg capsule BID More than 25 kg: 100-mg capsule BID

Adverse Effects

The CNS adverse reactions of celecoxib include headache, dizziness, somnolence, and insomnia. Some patients have noted ophthalmic changes with administration of the drug. Patients taking celecoxib are at increased risk for myocardial infarction and cerebrovascular accident. The FDA has issued a **BOXED WARNING** ◆ for celecoxib concerning its cardiac and vascular risks. Dermatologic adverse effects include rash, pruritus, sweating, dry mucous membranes, and stomatitis.

Dyspepsia and GI bleeding can occur with the administration of prolonged high doses of celecoxib, but the risk is not as profound as the COX-1 and COX-2 inhibitors. Anaphylactic reactions can also occur if the patient is allergic to celecoxib or has an aspirin or NSAID-related allergy.

Contraindications

Celecoxib is contraindicated in patients who have a known allergy to sulfonamides, NSAIDs, and aspirin. It is also contraindicated in patients with abnormal kidney function. It should not be administered to patients with perioperative pain or to those who have just undergone coronary artery bypass graft surgery.

Nursing Implications

Preventing Interactions

The administration of anticoagulants or aspirin with celecoxib increases the risk of bleeding. Patients taking lithium and celecoxib are at risk for lithium toxicity. Celecoxib combined with alcohol or smoking increases the patient's risk of GI bleeding.

Administering the Medication

When administering celecoxib, the nurse should be certain to administer it 2 hours before or after an antacid to ensure absorption. Prior to administering celecoxib, assess the patient for allergic reactions to NSAIDs. The medication must be stored in a light-protected container.

Assessing for Therapeutic Effects

The nurse assesses for diminished pain and swelling associated with inflammation. The joints are assessed for redness, heat, and stiffness. Mobility should increase with the administration of celecoxib.

Assessing for Adverse Effects

The nurse assesses the patient for signs and symptoms of chest pain, shortness of breath, confusion, or numbness of the extremities. These symptoms are indicative of cardiac events such as myocardial infarction or cerebrovascular accident. Also, it is necessary to assess for dyspepsia, GI irritation, and GI bleeding as well as CNS depression and ophthalmic changes. Finally, the nurse assesses for anaphylactic reactions, including sore throat, itching, weight gain, and edema.

> **BOX 16.12** *Patient Teaching Guidelines for Celecoxib*
>
> - Take the medication with food or meals to prevent gastric upset.
> - Do not operate machinery if you have central nervous system depression.
> - Report sore throat, rash, itching, weight gain, swelling of feet and ankles, and changes in vision to your health care provider.

Patient Teaching

Box 16.12 presents patient teaching guidelines for celecoxib.

> **NCLEX Success**
>
> 4. A 76-year-old patient is taking celecoxib for arthritic back pain. When administering celecoxib, which of the following patient teaching points is most important?
>   A. Any chest pain should be reported to the prescriber immediately.
>   B. Celecoxib can be administered with warfarin.
>   C. Increased mobility should be reported to the prescriber.
>   D. Celecoxib can be administered with aspirin during periods of infection.

ANTIGOUT MEDICATION: THE MITOTIC AGENT COLCHICINE

 Colchicine (Colcrys, Mitigare), the prototype agent for the treatment and prevention of gout, is the most commonly administered antigout medication.

> **⚠ Quality and Safety Alert: Safety**
>
> Colchicine has a narrow therapeutic index. The drug accumulates, leading to severe and potentially fatal adverse effects.

Pharmacokinetics

Colchicine is absorbed rapidly in the GI tract, with a slow onset of action; it reaches its peak in 1 to 2 hours. The drug is metabolized in the liver and has a half-life of 26 to 31 hours. It is primarily eliminated in the feces, with a smaller amount excreted in the urine. Colchicine crosses the placenta and enters the breast milk.

Action

Colchicine inhibits the migration of WBCs into the body tissues containing urate crystals. The phagocytic action of the drug decreases the inflammatory reaction to the urate crystals deposited in the tissues.

Use

Colchicine is administered for the treatment and prophylaxis of acute gout in adults. An off-label use of colchicine is ordered for patients with acute or recurrent pericarditis. Table 16.10 gives specific dosage information for this drug.

Patient-related variables specific to the use of colchicine include the following:

- Age:
  - Colchicine is only administered to children 4 years of age and older to treat familial Mediterranean fever.
  - In older adults, colchicine is administered cautiously; the dosage should be reduced by half in people 70 years of age and older.
- Reproduction, pregnancy, and lactation:
  - Colchicine should not be discontinued in patients with Mediterranean fever who are planning to become pregnant.
  - Colchicine dosage should be reduced in patients planning to become pregnant who are being treated for musculoskeletal diseases.
  - Colchicine crosses the placenta and is present in breast milk.
  - Colchicine is compatible with breast-feeding.
- Abnormal kidney function and hepatic impairment:
  - For mild to moderate abnormal kidney function, a regular dosage of colchicine is administered. If the creatinine clearance is less than 30 mL/min, a dosage adjustment is not necessary, but the drug should not be given more than once every 2 weeks.
  - For patients on dialysis, 0.6 mg is given as a single dose no more than once every 2 weeks.
  - In mild to moderate hepatic impairment, colchicine should be administered cautiously. The patient should be assessed closely for adverse effects.
  - In severe hepatic impairment, the dosage should be the same, but the drug should not be given more than once every 2 weeks.

Adverse Effects

GI adverse effects are the most common due to the absorption and elimination in the GI tract. These GI conditions include nausea, vomiting, and abdominal pain and dyspepsia. Hematologic adverse effects such as bone marrow depression and aplastic anemia may occur. Hepatotoxicity is also an adverse effect of colchicine. Other adverse effects include peripheral neuropathy, alopecia, rash, purpura, dermatoses, myopathy, muscle pain, and weakness.

Contraindications

Colchicine is contraindicated in patients who have a known hypersensitivity to the medication. It should not be administered concurrently with cyclosporines or ranolazine or with a strong to moderate CYP3A4 inhibitor in the presence of hepatic impairment or abnormal kidney function. It is administered cautiously in pregnancy or in the presence of abnormal kidney function or hepatic impairment.

Nursing Implications

Preventing Interactions

Several medications, when combined with colchicine, result in toxicity and severe adverse effects. Agents that increase the serum level of colchicine and the risk of toxicity are atazanavir, clarithromycin, indinavir, itraconazole, ketoconazole, nefazodone, nelfinavir, ritonavir, saquinavir, telithromycin, diltiazem, erythromycin, fluconazole, and verapamil. In addition, colchicine should not be combined with grapefruit juice or alcohol. The serum concentration of colchicine will be increased. It also decreases cyanocobalamin (vitamin B_{12}) absorption. Administration of colchicine with tea will reduce effectiveness.

Administering the Medication

It is necessary to administer colchicine with food to reduce gastric distress.

Assessing for Therapeutic Effects

Therapeutic effects occur within 24 to 48 hours after oral administration. The nurse assesses for decreased pain, swelling, and inflammation of affected joints. Edema may not decrease for several days.

Assessing for Adverse Effects

The nurse assesses for severe GI adverse effects such as vomiting and diarrhea, which may lead to an alteration in fluid and electrolytes with dehydration. The nurse also assesses for numbness, tingling, or muscle weakness. In addition, bone marrow depression is assessed and liver enzymes are monitored.

Patient Teaching

Box 16.13 presents patient teaching guidelines for the mitotic agent colchicine.

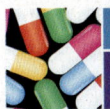

TABLE 16.10

DRUGS AT A GLANCE: Colchicine

Drug	Routes and Dosage Ranges	
	Adults	Children
ⓟ Colchicine (Colcrys, Mitigare; ✦ JAMP-Colchicine, PMS-Colchicine, Sandoz Colchicine)	Acute gout: PO 1.2 mg at the first sign of gout flare Prophylaxis of gout flares: PO 0.6 mg/d to a maximum of 1.2 mg/d	Familial Mediterranean fever: Children 4–6 years: PO 0.3–1.8 mg/day in 1–2 divided doses; titrate by increasing or decreasing dose in 0.3 mg/day based on efficacy; maximum dose: 2.4 mg/day Children >6–12 years: PO 0.9–1/8 mg/day in 1–2 divided doses: titrate by increasing to decreasing dose in 0.3 mg/day based on efficacy; maximum dose: 2.4 mg/day Children >12 years and adolescents: PO 1.2–2.4 mg/day in 1–2 divided doses; titrate by increasing or decreasing the dose in 0.3 mg/day based on efficacy; maximum dose: 2.4 mg/day

> **BOX 16.13 Patient Teaching Guidelines for Colchicine**
>
> - Take colchicine at the onset of acute gouty symptoms.
> - For acute gouty flare-ups, take one dose and the second dose 1 hour later.
> - Do not drink grapefruit juice or alcohol.
> - Be aware that GI adverse effects are common with colchicine; call your prescriber if the abdominal pain is too severe.
> - Report severe diarrhea and muscle weakness to your healthcare provider.
> - Understand that the resulting bone marrow depression may cause fatigue, increased risk of bleeding, or increased risk of infection.
> - See your primary health provider with persistent gouty attacks.
> - Follow a low-purine diet by avoiding beer, alcohol, organ and game meats, sardines, anchovies, scallops, asparagus, spinach, and peas.

URICOSURIC AGENTS

Several uricosuric agents are used to reduce serum uric acid levels. **Allopurinol** (Zyloprim), a xanthine oxidase inhibitor, is the prototype uricosuric drug.

Pharmacokinetics

Allopurinol is absorbed in the GI tract, with an onset of action of 24 to 48 hours and a peak of action of 2 to 6 hours. The drug's half-life is 1 to 3 hours. It is metabolized as an active metabolite oxypurinol and is eliminated slowly in the urine. It is also excreted in the breast milk.

Action

Allopurinol inhibits the enzyme that is responsible for the conversion of purines to uric acid. This action reduces the purines to uric acid and thus reduces the uric acid production to decrease the serum and urinary uric acid levels. The result of this action is the reduction of the symptoms of gout.

Use

Allopurinol and uricosuric agents are administered for the management of the signs and symptoms of primary and secondary gout or stages of gout. Allopurinol is also given in acute and chronic tophaceous gout to reduce uric acid concentrations. Other indications include leukemia, lymphoma, and malignancies that result in elevated serum uric acid levels. Table 16.11 gives the specific dosage information for these drugs.

Patient-related variables specific to the use of allopurinol include the following:

- Age:
  - Allopurinol is not routinely administered to children, except to those with hyperuricemia secondary to cancer and chemotherapy treatment.
  - When administering allopurinol IV, it is essential to ensure that the child is hydrated to maintain a neutral or slightly alkaline urine output.
  - In older adults, the initial dose of allopurinol is 100 mg/day, which can be increased until the desired uric acid level is obtained.
  - Older adults receiving allopurinol must maintain fluid intake to produce a urine output of at least 2,000 mL/day.
- Reproduction, pregnancy, and lactation:
  - Allopurinol crosses the placenta.
  - Breast-feeding is not recommended with the administration of allopurinol.
- Abnormal kidney function and hepatic impairment:
  - The dosage of allopurinol is reduced based on the patient's creatinine clearance. See Table 16.11 for specific dosage information.
  - In patients with hepatic impairment, allopurinol is administered cautiously. The dosage does not need to be adjusted, but it is important to monitor liver function.

Adverse Effects

Allopurinol has several adverse effects. CNS adverse effects include drowsiness, headache, and vertigo. Hematologic adverse effects are agranulocytosis, aplastic anemia, and bone marrow depression. The most common GI effects are nausea, vomiting, diarrhea, abdominal pain, and indigestion. Hepatotoxicity and abnormal kidney function are risk factors with the use of allopurinol.

Contraindications

Patients with a known hypersensitivity to allopurinol should not take allopurinol. Also, patients with a family history or history of idiopathic hemochromatosis should not receive the drug.

Nursing Implications

Preventing Interactions

Several medications, including azathioprine, mercaptopurine, cyclophosphamide, cyclosporine, and thiazide diuretics, increase the risk of uricosuric-associated toxicity. The administration of ampicillin and amoxicillin with allopurinol increases the risk of developing a rash. Anticoagulation effects are increased when combined with warfarin and aspirin. Alcohol combined with allopurinol decreases the excretion of uric acid.

Administering the Medication

It is necessary to administer allopurinol after meals to ensure absorption.

Assessing for Therapeutic Effects

The nurse assesses for decreased pain, inflammation, and joint swelling. In patients with tophi (see Fig. 16.2), it is important to assess for increased joint mobility and decrease in tophi prominence. It is vital to assess serum uric acid levels. The normal serum uric acid level is 3.0 to 7.0 mg/dL.

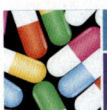

TABLE 16.11
DRUGS AT A GLANCE: Uricosuric Agents

Drug	Routes and Dosage Ranges	
	Adults	**Children**

Allopurinol (Zyloprim, Aloprim; ✦ Apo-Allopurinol, Apo-Allopurinol A)	Gout and hyperuricemia: PO 100–800 mg/k/d in divided doses, depending on the severity of the disease (200–300 mg/d is the usual dose)
	Maintenance: establish dose that maintains serum uric acid levels within normal limits
	Hyperuricemia: PO 200–300 mg/d; adjust the dose based on urate levels
	Prevention of uric acid nephropathy in certain malignancies: PO 600–800 mg/d for 203 d with a high fluid intake; maintenance dose as above
	Recurrent calcium oxalate stones: PO 200–300 mg/d; adjust dose based on 24-h urinary urate determinations
	Parenteral administration: IV 200–400 mg/m²/d as a continuous infusion or at 6-, 8-, or 1-h intervals
	Dosage based on creatinine clearance:
	  140 mL/min—400 mg
	  120 mL/min—350 mg
	  100 mL/min—300 mg
	  80 mL/min—250 mg
	  60 mL/min—200 mg
	  40 mL/min—150 mg
		Secondary hyperuricemia associated with various malignancies:
		6–10 y: PO 300 mg/d; adjust dose based on serum uric acid levels
		<6 y: PO 150 mg/d; adjust dose after 48 h of treatment based on serum uric acid level
		Parenteral: 200 mg/m²/d IV as continuous infusion or at 6-, 8-, or 12-h intervals

Febuxostat (Uloric; ✦ Uloric, MAR-Febuxostat)	PO 40 mg/d; if serum uric acid level is not <6 mg/dL in 2 wk, dosage should be increased to 80 mg/d	Safety and efficacy not established
Pegloticase (Krystexxa)	IV 8 mg every 2 wk	Safety and efficacy not established
Probenecid	PO 0.25 g BID for 1 wk; then 0.5 g BID; maintenance, continue dosage that maintains the normal serum uric acid levels. When no attacks occur for 6 mo or longer, decrease the dose to 0.5 g every 6 mo	Safety and efficacy not established
Rasburicase (Elitek; ✦ Fasturtec)	Hyperuricemia associated with malignancy IV 0.2 mg/kg once daily for up to 5 d (use beyond 5 d or more than one course is not recommended)	IV 0.2 mg/kg once daily for up to 5 d (use beyond 5 d or more than one course is not recommended)

Assessing for Adverse Effects

The nurse assesses for diminished urine output or cloudy urine, which may be indicative of the development of uric acid kidney stones. It is also important to assess for GI effects such as nausea, vomiting, diarrhea, and abdominal pain. The nurse assesses for bruising, bleeding, and anemia. Finally, the nurse assesses aspartate aminotransferase and alanine aminotransferase levels for hepatotoxicity and creatinine clearance for abnormal kidney function.

Patient Teaching

Box 16.14 presents patient teaching guidelines for the uricosuric medications, including allopurinol.

Other Drugs in the Class

Febuxostat (Uloric) is the first medication for the treatment of gout to be developed in approximately 45 years. A chemically

> **BOX 16.14** *Patient Teaching Guidelines for Allopurinol*
>
> - Take fluid to yield at least 2,000 mL of urine output per day.
> - Report decreased urine output or cloudy urine, which could be indicative of uric acid stone formation, to your healthcare provider.
> - Report any rashes or skin eruptions to your healthcare provider.
> - Do not drive or operate machinery until the central nervous system effects are known.
> - Maintain appointments for serum uric acid levels, liver enzymes, and creatinine clearance to be drawn.

engineered nonpurine agent, it selectively inhibits xanthine oxidase. Clinical studies have indicated that it is more effective in lowering serum uric acid levels than allopurinol. The most common adverse effect is hepatotoxicity. It is also necessary to assess patients who take febuxostat for the development of cardiovascular events such as myocardial infarction.

Pegloticase (Krystexxa) is a uric acid–specific uricosuric medication. Prior to the IV administration of pegloticase, all other antihyperuricemic medications should be discontinued. The patient should be premedicated with corticosteroids and antihistamines. Pegloticase has a high rate of anaphylactic reactions. It is important to observe the patient carefully for rash, wheezing, and bronchospasm.

Rasburicase (Elitek) has the ability to enzymatically degrade uric acid. It is administered for hyperuricemia associated with malignancy. Rasburicase can result in methemoglobinemia. Methemoglobin is a transformation product of oxyhemoglobin, which then enters the circulating blood.

 Quality and Safety Alert: Safety

In Canada, a safety alert was issued for febuxostat in which data suggested a link between a drug reaction and rash with eosinophilia and systemic symptoms. In addition, many patients who experienced serious skin reactions with febuxostat also reported similar skin reactions while using allopurinol. Each patient who receives febuxostat should be assessed for the development of a rash. The nurse should inform the physician if a rash develops and suggest that a complete blood count be obtained.

Probenecid increases the urinary excretion of uric acid. This uricosuric action means that it can be used therapeutically to treat hyperuricemia and gout. It is not effective in acute attacks of gouty arthritis but prevents hyperuricemia and tophi associated with chronic gout. Probenecid may cause acute gout until serum uric acid levels are within the normal range; concomitant administration of colchicine prevents this effect. (Probenecid also is used with penicillin, most often in treating sexually transmitted diseases. It increases blood levels and prolongs the action of penicillin by decreasing the rate of urinary excretion.)

Unfolding Patient Stories: Danielle Young Bear • Part 2

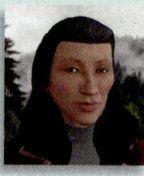

Recall Danielle Young Bear, the 32-year-old construction worker you met in Chapter 6, who is being seen at the clinic for persistent cough and fatigue who also has a history of chronic lower back pain and spasms. Danielle requests a nonnarcotic, inexpensive medication. Compare and contrast the actions and side effects of acetaminophen, aspirin, and ibuprofen for managing pain and inflammation. Which of these would you recommend? Why? If you don't recommend one of these, what do you recommend? Provide your rationale.

Care for Danielle and other patients in a realistic virtual environment: *vSim for Nursing* (thepoint.lww.com/vSimPharm). Practice documenting these patients' care in DocuCare (thepoint.lww.com/DocuCareEHR).

NCLEX Success

5. A patient is being treated with colchicine for acute gouty flare-up. Which of the following statements indicates the need for increased patient education?

   A. "I am going to stop taking the colchicine because of the diarrhea I am having."
   B. "The gastrointestinal effects are difficult to deal with, but I know they will decrease my gouty symptoms."
   C. "I will continue my colchicine just as it has been prescribed for me."
   D. "The diarrhea I am experiencing can result in dehydration. If I have lethargy, I will call my prescriber."

THE NURSING PROCESS

A concept map outlines the nursing process related to drug therapy considerations in this chapter. Additional nursing implications related to the disease process should also be considered in care decisions.

Assessment
- Assess for signs and symptoms of pain, site of pain, type and duration of pain, and factors that relieve or increase pain.
- Assess for limitation in activity or mobility.
- In patients with gout assess for abdominal pain, joint pain, redness, swelling, and limitation in mobility.
- Assess for fever (thermometer readings above 99.6°F or 37.3°C). Signs and symptoms include hot, dry skin, flushed face, reduced urine output, and dehydration.
- Assess the use of OTC analgesic, antipyretic, or anti-inflammatory agents.
- Assess for allergic reactions to aspirin or NSAIDs.
- Assess for history of peptic ulcer disease, GI bleeding, hepatic and kidney disease.

Outcomes of Therapy
The patient will
- Experience relief of discomfort with minimal adverse drug effects.
- Experience increased mobility and activity tolerance.
- Inform healthcare providers if taking aspirin, an NSAID, or acetaminophen regularly.
- Self-administer the drugs safely.
- Avoid overuse of the drugs.

Nursing Interventions
- Implement measures to prevent or minimize pain, fever, and inflammation.
- Treat the disease processes (e.g., infection, arthritis) or circumstances (e.g., impaired blood supply, lack of physical activity, poor positioning or body alignment) thought to be causing pain, fever, or inflammation.
- Treat pain as soon as possible; early treatment may prevent severe pain and anxiety and allow the use of milder analgesic drugs. Use distraction, relaxation techniques, or other nonpharmacologic techniques along with drug therapy, when appropriate.
- With acute musculoskeletal injuries (e.g., sprains), think RICE: Rest, Ice, Compression, Elevation to decrease pain, swelling, and inflammation. Cold therapy should be applied for 20 minutes every 3 to 4 hours for 48 hours.
- Assist patients to drink 2 to 3 L of fluid daily when taking an NSAID regularly. This strategy decreases gastric irritation and helps to maintain good kidney function. With long-term use of aspirin, fluids help prevent precipitation of salicylate crystals in the urinary tract. With antigout drugs, fluids help prevent precipitation of urate crystals and formation of urate kidney stones. Fluid intake is especially important initially when serum uric acid levels are high and large amounts of uric acid are being excreted.
- Provide appropriate teaching for any drug therapy.

Evaluation
- Interview and observe regarding relief of symptoms.
- Interview and observe regarding mobility and activity levels.
- Interview and observe regarding safe, effective use of the drugs.
- Select drugs appropriately.

Visit thePoint® *at* http://thePoint.lww.com/Frandsen13e *for answers to NCLEX Success questions (in Appendix A), answers to Clinical Application Case Studies (in Appendix B), additional information on etiology and pathophysiology, and more!*

REFERENCES AND RESOURCES

Gaffo, A. L. (2022). Clinical manifestations and diagnosis of gout. *UpToDate*. Wolters Kluwer.

Hinkle, J. H., Cheever, K. H., Overbaugh, K. (2021). *Brunner & Suddarth's textbook of medical-surgical nursing* (15th ed.). Wolters Kluwer.

Lippincott Advisor. (2022). *Drug information*. Wolters Kluwer.

Norris, T. L. (2019). *Porth's pathophysiology: Concepts of altered health states* (10th ed.). Wolters Kluwer.

Oladosu, F. A., Tu, F. F., Garrison, E. F., Dillane, K. E., Roth, G. E., Hellman, K. M. Low serum naproxen concentrations are associated with minimal pain relief: a preliminary study in women with dysmenorrhea. *Pain Medicine.* 2020;21(11):3102-3108. https://doi.org/10.1093/pm/pnaa133

Perez-Ruiz, F. (2020). Pharmacologic urate-lowering therapy and treatment of tophi in patients with gout. *UpToDate.* Wolters Kluwer.

UpToDate. (2022). *Drug information.* Lexi-Comp, Inc.

CHAPTER 17

Drug Therapy With Corticosteroids

LEARNING OBJECTIVES

After studying this chapter, you should be able to:

1. Understand the physiologic effects of endogenous corticosteroids.
2. Identify the characteristics of adrenal cortex disorders.
3. Describe the action and the clinical indications for use of exogenous corticosteroids.
4. Understand the contraindications and adverse effects of corticosteroids as well as the nursing implications of their use.
5. Analyze how other drugs and substances as well as other factors may affect the need for corticosteroids.
6. Apply the nursing process when a patient is administered a corticosteroid.

CLINICAL APPLICATION CASE STUDY

Emma Mae Thompson is a 65-year-old woman who lives alone. Since she was 15 years old, she has smoked one pack of unfiltered cigarettes per day. When she was diagnosed with chronic obstructive pulmonary disease (COPD) 5 years ago, she quit smoking. She takes albuterol sulfate one inhalation per nebulizer every 12 hours and beclomethasone dipropionate 160 mcg every 12 hours. Recently, she was treated for pneumonia. Mrs. Thompson's physician prescribes prednisone orally in a tapering dose, according to the following schedule:

Day 1: 10 mg before breakfast, 5 mg before lunch, 5 mg before supper, 10 mg at bedtime
Day 2: 5 mg before breakfast, 5 mg before lunch, 5 mg before supper, 10 mg at bedtime
Day 3: 5 mg before breakfast, 5 mg before lunch, 5 mg before supper, 5 mg at bedtime
Day 4: 5 mg before breakfast, 5 mg before supper, 5 mg at bedtime
Day 5: 5 mg before breakfast, 5 mg at bedtime
Day 6: 5 mg before breakfast

KEY TERMS

Addison disease: primary adrenocortical insufficiency with inadequate production of cortisol and aldosterone

Addisonian crisis: condition that mimics hypovolemic and septic shock; also known as adrenocortical insufficiency

Aldosterone: mineralocorticoid hormone secreted by the adrenal cortex to increase sodium reabsorption by the kidneys and indirectly regulate blood levels of potassium, sodium, and bicarbonate; also regulates pH, blood volume, and blood pressure

Corticosteroid: steroid hormone produced by the adrenal cortex; examples include androgens, glucocorticoids, and mineralocorticoids

Cortisol: the main glucocorticoid secreted as part of the body's response to stress

Cushing disease: adrenocortical hyperfunction; may result from excessive corticotropin or primary adrenal tumor

Glucocorticoid: adrenal cortical hormone that protects the body against stress and affects protein and carbohydrate metabolism

Immunosuppression: suppression of the immune system

Mineralocorticoid: steroid hormone released by the adrenal cortex to promote sodium and water retention and potassium excretion

Negative feedback mechanism: when the output of a system affects the stimulus for the system (e.g., hormone secretion produces an effect that shuts off the stimulus for further hormone secretion)

Steroid: lipid-soluble hormone produced by the gonadal organs or the adrenal cortex

INTRODUCTION

This chapter provides an introduction to the **corticosteroids**, also known as the **glucocorticoids** or **steroids**. These lipid-soluble hormones are produced by the gonadal organs or the adrenal cortex, part of the adrenal glands. These hormones affect almost all body organs and are extremely important in maintaining homeostasis when secreted in normal amounts. Disease results from inadequate or excessive secretion. Exogenous corticosteroids are used as drugs in a variety of disorders. Their use must be closely monitored, because they have profound therapeutic and adverse effects. To understand the effects of corticosteroids used as drugs (exogenous corticosteroids), it is necessary to understand the physiologic effects and other characteristics of the endogenous hormones.

PHYSIOLOGY OF ENDOGENOUS CORTICOSTEROIDS

Corticosteroid secretion is controlled by the hypothalamus, the anterior pituitary, and adrenal cortex (the hypothalamic–pituitary–adrenal, or HPA, axis). Various stimuli (e.g., low plasma levels of corticosteroids, pain, anxiety, trauma, illness, being placed under anesthesia) activate the system. These stimuli cause the hypothalamus of the brain to secrete corticotropin-releasing hormone or factor (known as CRH or CRF), which stimulates the anterior pituitary gland to secrete corticotropin, and corticotropin then stimulates the adrenal cortex to secrete corticosteroids.

The rate of corticosteroid secretion is usually maintained within relatively narrow limits but changes according to need. When plasma corticosteroid levels rise to an adequate level, secretion of corticosteroids slows or stops. The mechanism by which the hypothalamus and anterior pituitary "learn" that no more corticosteroids are needed is called a **negative feedback mechanism** (Fig. 17.1).

This negative feedback mechanism is normally very important, but it does not work during stress responses. The stress response activates the sympathetic nervous system (SNS) to produce more epinephrine and norepinephrine and the adrenal cortex to produce as much as 10 times the normal amount of **cortisol** (the main glucocorticoid secreted as part of the body's response to stress). The synergistic interaction of these hormones increases the person's ability to respond to stress. However, the increased SNS activity continues to stimulate cortisol production and overrules the negative feedback mechanism. Excessive and prolonged corticosteroid secretion damages body tissues.

Corticosteroids are secreted directly into the bloodstream. Cortisol is approximately 90% bound to plasma proteins, and this high degree of protein binding slows cortisol movement out of the plasma, so that it has a relatively long plasma half-life of 60 to 90 minutes. The remaining 10% is unbound and biologically active. In contrast, aldosterone is only 60% bound to plasma proteins and has a short half-life of 20 minutes. In general, protein binding functions as a storage area from which the hormones are released as needed. This promotes more consistent blood levels and more uniform distribution to the tissues.

The adrenal cortex produces approximately 30 steroid hormones, which are divided into glucocorticoids, mineralocorticoids, and adrenal sex hormones. Chemically, all corticosteroids are derived from cholesterol and have similar chemical structures. However, despite their similarities, slight differences cause them to have different functions.

Glucocorticoids

Although the term "corticosteroids" actually refers to all secretions of the adrenal cortex, it is most often used to designate the glucocorticoids, which are important in metabolic, inflammatory, and immune processes. Glucocorticoids include cortisol, corticosterone, and cortisone. Cortisol accounts for at least 95% of glucocorticoid activity; corticosterone and cortisone account for a small amount of activity. Glucocorticoids are secreted cyclically, with the largest amount being produced in the early morning and the smallest amount during the evening hours (in people with a normal day–night schedule). At the cellular level, glucocorticoids account for most of the characteristics and physiologic effects of the corticosteroids (Box 17.1). The chronic use of the glucocorticoids will produce adverse effects that include suppression of the hypothalamic–pituitary–adrenal axis, Cushing disease, increased susceptibility to infections, and mental status changes.

Mineralocorticoids

Mineralocorticoids are a class of steroid hormone released by the adrenal cortex to promote sodium and water retention and potassium excretion. They play a vital role in the maintenance

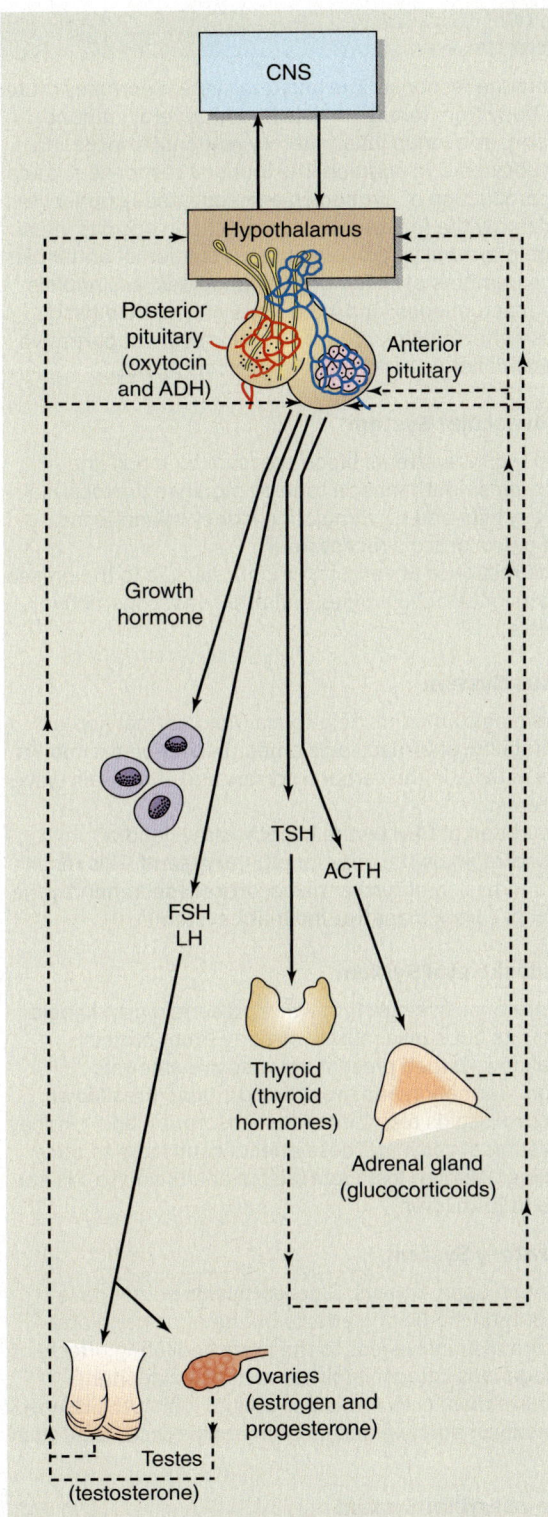

Figure 17.1. Control of hormone production by the hypothalamic–pituitary target cell feedback mechanism. Hormone levels from the target glands regulate the release of hormones from the anterior pituitary through a negative feedback system. The *dashed line* represents feedback control. ACTH, adrenocorticotropic hormone; ADH, antidiuretic hormone; CNS, central nervous system; FSH, follicle-stimulating hormone; LH, luteinizing hormone; TSH, thyroid-stimulating hormone. [From Norris, T. L. (2019). *Porth's pathophysiology: Concepts of altered health states* (10th ed., Fig. 40.3, p. 1183). Wolters Kluwer Health | Lippincott Williams & Wilkins.]

of fluid and electrolyte balance through their influence on salt and water metabolism. **Aldosterone** is the main mineralocorticoid and is responsible for approximately 90% of mineralocorticoid activity. Aldosterone is secreted by the adrenal cortex to increase sodium reabsorption by the kidneys and indirectly regulates blood levels of potassium, sodium, and water retention and potassium excretion. Characteristics and physiologic effects of mineralocorticoids are summarized in Box 17.2.

Adrenal Sex Hormones

The adrenal cortex secretes male (androgens) and female (estrogens and progesterone) sex hormones. Compared with the effect of hormones produced by the testes and ovaries, the adrenal sex hormones have an insignificant effect on normal body function. Adrenal androgens, secreted continuously in small quantities by both sexes, are responsible for most of the physiologic effects exerted by the adrenal sex hormones. They increase protein synthesis (anabolism), which increases the mass and strength of muscle and bone tissue; they affect development of male secondary sex characteristics; and they increase hair growth and libido in women. Excessive secretion of adrenal androgens in women causes masculinizing effects (e.g., hirsutism, acne, breast atrophy, deepening of the voice, amenorrhea). Female sex hormones are secreted in small amounts and normally exert few physiologic effects. Excessive secretion may produce feminizing effects in men (e.g., breast enlargement, decreased hair growth, voice changes).

OVERVIEW OF ADRENAL CORTEX DISORDERS

Disorders of the adrenal cortex involve increased or decreased production of corticosteroids, especially cortisol as the primary glucocorticoid and aldosterone as the primary mineralocorticoid. These disorders include the following:

- **Primary adrenocortical insufficiency** (**Addison disease**) is associated with destruction of the adrenal cortex by disorders such as tuberculosis, cancer, or hemorrhage; with atrophy of the adrenal cortex caused by autoimmune disease or prolonged administration of exogenous corticosteroids; and with surgical excision of the adrenal glands. In primary adrenocortical insufficiency, there is inadequate production of both cortisol and aldosterone.
- **Secondary adrenocortical insufficiency**, produced by inadequate secretion of corticotropin, is most often caused by prolonged administration of corticosteroids. This condition is largely a glucocorticoid deficiency; mineralocorticoid secretion is not significantly impaired.
- **Congenital adrenogenital syndromes and adrenal hyperplasia** result from deficiencies in one or more enzymes required for cortisol production. Low plasma levels of cortisol result in excessive corticotropin secretion, which then leads to excessive adrenal secretion of androgens and hyperplasia (abnormal increase in number of cells).
- **Androgen-producing tumors** of the adrenal cortex, which are usually benign, produce masculinizing effects.
- **Adrenocortical hyperfunction** (**Cushing disease**) may result from excessive corticotropin or a primary adrenal

> **BOX 17.1** **Effects of Glucocorticoids on Body Processes and Systems**

Carbohydrate Metabolism

- ↑ Formation of glucose (gluconeogenesis) by breaking down protein into amino acids. The amino acids are then transported to the liver, where they are acted on by enzymes that convert them to glucose. The glucose is then returned to the circulation for use by body tissues or storage in the liver as glycogen.
- ↓ Cellular use of glucose, especially in muscle cells. This is attributed to a ↓ effect of insulin on the proteins that normally transport glucose into cells and by ↓ numbers and functional capacity of insulin receptors.
- Both the ↑ production and ↓ use of glucose promote higher levels of glucose in the blood (hyperglycemia) and may lead to diabetes. These actions also increase the amount of glucose stored as glycogen in the liver, skeletal muscles, and other tissues.

Protein Metabolism

- Breakdown of protein into amino acids (catabolic effect); ↑ rate of amino acid transport to the liver and conversion to glucose.
- ↓ Rate of new protein formation from dietary and other amino acids (antianabolic effect).
- The combination of ↑ breakdown of cell protein and ↓ protein synthesis leads to protein depletion in virtually all body cells except those of the liver. Thus, glycogen stores in the body are ↑ and protein stores are ↓.

Lipid Metabolism

- ↑ Breakdown of adipose tissue into fatty acids; the fatty acids are transported in the plasma and used as a source of energy by body cells.
- ↑ Oxidation of fatty acids within body cells.

Inflammatory and Immune Responses

- ↓ Inflammatory response. Inflammation is the normal bodily response to tissue damage and involves three stages. First, a large amount of plasmalike fluid leaks out of capillaries into the damaged area and becomes clotted. Second, leukocytes migrate into the area. Third, tissue healing occurs, largely by growth of fibrous scar tissue. Normal or physiologic amounts of glucocorticoids probably do not significantly affect inflammation and healing, but large amounts of glucocorticoids inhibit all three stages of the inflammatory process.
- More specifically, corticosteroids stabilize lysosomal membranes (and thereby prevent the release of inflammatory proteolytic enzymes); ↓ capillary permeability (and thereby ↓ leakage of fluid and proteins into the damaged tissue); ↓ the accumulation of neutrophils and macrophages at sites of inflammation (and thereby impair phagocytosis of pathogenic microorganisms and waste products of cellular metabolism); and ↓ production of inflammatory chemicals, such as interleukin-1, prostaglandins, and leukotrienes, by injured cells.
- ↓ Immune response. The immune system normally protects the body from foreign invaders, and several immune responses overlap inflammatory responses, including phagocytosis. In addition, the immune response stimulates the production of antibodies and activated lymphocytes to destroy the foreign substance. Glucocorticoids impair protein synthesis, including the production of antibodies; ↓ the numbers of circulating lymphocytes, eosinophils, and macrophages; and ↓ amounts of lymphoid tissue. These effects help account for the immunosuppressive and antiallergic actions of the glucocorticoids.

Cardiovascular System

- Help regulate arterial blood pressure by modifying vascular smooth muscle tone by modifying myocardial contractility and by stimulating kidney mineralocorticoid and glucocorticoid receptors
- ↑ The response of vascular smooth muscle to the pressor effects of catecholamines and other vasoconstrictive agents

Nervous System

- Physiologic amounts help to maintain normal nerve excitability; pharmacologic amounts ↓ nerve excitability, slow activity in the cerebral cortex, and alter brain wave patterns.
- ↓ Secretion of CRH by the hypothalamus and of corticotropin by the anterior pituitary gland. This results in suppression of further glucocorticoid secretion by the adrenal cortex (negative feedback system).

Musculoskeletal System

- Maintain muscle strength when present in physiologic amounts but cause muscle atrophy (from protein breakdown) when present in excessive amounts.
- ↓ Bone formation and growth and ↑ bone breakdown. Glucocorticoids also ↓ intestinal absorption and ↑ kidney excretion of calcium. These effects contribute to bone demineralization (osteoporosis) in adults and to ↓ linear growth in children.

Respiratory System

- Maintain open airways. Glucocorticoids do not have direct bronchodilating effects but help maintain and restore responsiveness to the bronchodilating effects of endogenous catecholamines, such as epinephrine.
- Stabilize mast cells and other cells to inhibit the release of bronchoconstrictive and inflammatory substances, such as histamine.

Gastrointestinal System

- ↓ Viscosity of gastric mucus. This effect may ↓ protective properties of the mucus and contribute to the development of peptic ulcer disease.

↑, increase/increased; ↓, decrease/decreased.

---

tumor. Adrenal tumors may be benign or malignant. Benign tumors often produce one corticosteroid normally secreted by the adrenal cortex, but malignant tumors often secrete several corticosteroids.

- **Hyperaldosteronism** is a rare disorder caused by adenoma (a benign tissue from glandular tissue) or hyperplasia of the adrenal cortex cells that produce aldosterone. It is characterized by hypokalemia, hypernatremia, hypertension, thirst, and polyuria.

> **BOX 17.2** **Effects of Mineralocorticoids on Body Processes and Systems**
>
> - The overall physiologic effects are to conserve sodium and water and eliminate potassium. Aldosterone increases sodium reabsorption from kidney tubules, and water is reabsorbed along with the sodium. When sodium is conserved, another cation must be excreted to maintain electrical neutrality of body fluids; thus, potassium is excreted. This is the only potent mechanism for controlling the concentration of potassium ions in extracellular fluids.
> - Secretion of aldosterone is controlled by several factors, most of which are related to kidney function. In general, secretion is increased when the potassium level of extracellular fluid is high, the sodium level of extracellular fluid is low, the renin–angiotensin system of the kidneys is activated, or the anterior pituitary gland secretes corticotropin.
> - Inadequate secretion of aldosterone causes hyperkalemia, hyponatremia, and extracellular fluid volume deficit (dehydration). Hypotension and shock may result from decreased cardiac output. Absence of mineralocorticoids causes death.
> - Excessive secretion of aldosterone produces hypokalemia, hypernatremia, and extracellular fluid volume excess (water intoxication). Edema and hypertension may result.

DRUG THERAPY WITH EXOGENOUS CORTICOSTEROIDS

Exogenous corticosteroids, or glucocorticoids, are administered to treat disorders of the adrenal cortex or endocrine system. The administration of corticosteroids decreases the inflammatory symptoms and alters the immune response produced by nonendocrine disorders. Hydrocortisone, a short-acting corticosteroid and an exogenous equivalent of endogenous cortisol, was once considered the prototype corticosteroid drug. Now, **P prednisone**, an intermediate-acting corticosteroid, is the prototype corticosteroid. Table 17.1 lists the glucocorticoids and mineralocorticoids.

Pharmacokinetics

The rate of absorption of corticosteroids depends on the route of administration. Oral administration results in rapid absorption by the gastrointestinal (GI) tract, with rapid distribution to the intestines, muscles, liver, and kidneys. The corticosteroid is metabolized by the liver by cytochrome P450 3A4 enzymes, and the medication is conjugated to inactive metabolites. About 25% of the metabolites are excreted in the bile and then in the feces. The other 75%, which enter the circulation, are excreted in the kidneys. Plasma binding affects metabolism of corticosteroids, which means that patients with serum albumin levels less than 3.5 g/dL are prone to increased effects of corticosteroids and symptoms of hypercorticism.

The administration of exogenous corticosteroids suppresses the HPA axis. As a result, secretion of corticotropin decreases, causing atrophy of the adrenal cortex and decreased production of endogenous adrenal corticosteroids.

Action

Like endogenous glucocorticoids, exogenous corticosteroids act at the cellular level by binding to drug receptors in target tissues. The lipid-soluble drugs easily diffuse through the cell membranes of target cells. Inside the cell, they bind with receptors in intracellular cytoplasm. The drug–receptor complex then moves to the cell nucleus, where it interacts with DNA to stimulate or suppress gene transcription.

Corticosteroids can increase or decrease the transcription of many genes to alter the synthesis of proteins. These proteins regulate many physiologic effects, such as the transportation of proteins. Metabolic effects do not occur for at least 45 to 60 minutes because of the time required for protein synthesis. Several hours or days may be needed for full production of proteins.

Because the genes vary in different types of body cells, corticosteroid effects also vary, depending on the specific cells being targeted. For example, suprapysiologic concentrations of glucocorticoids induce the synthesis of lipolytic and proteolytic enzymes and other specific proteins in various tissues. Overall, corticosteroids have multiple mechanisms of action and effects (Fig. 17.2), including the following:

- **Inhibiting arachidonic acid metabolism.** Normally, when a body cell is injured or activated by various stimuli, the enzyme phospholipase A_2 causes the phospholipids in cell membranes to release arachidonic acid. Free arachidonic acid is then metabolized to produce proinflammatory prostaglandins (see Chapter 16) and leukotrienes. At sites of tissue injury or inflammation, corticosteroids induce the synthesis of proteins that suppress the activation of phospholipase A_2. This action, in turn, decreases the release of arachidonic acid and the formation of prostaglandins and leukotrienes.
- **Strengthening or stabilizing biologic membranes.** Two biologic membranes are especially important in inflammatory processes. Stabilization of cell membranes inhibits the release of arachidonic acid and production of prostaglandins and leukotrienes, as described above. Stabilization of lysosomal membranes inhibits release of bradykinin, histamine, enzymes, and perhaps other substances from lysosomes. (Lysosomes are intracellular structures that contain inflammatory chemical mediators and enzymes that destroy cellular debris and phagocytized pathogens.) This reduces capillary permeability and thus prevents leakage of fluid into the injured area and development of edema. It also reduces the chemicals that normally cause vasodilation and tissue irritation.
- **Inhibiting the production of interleukin-1, tumor necrosis factor, and other cytokines.** This action also contributes to the anti-inflammatory and immunosuppressant effects of corticosteroids.
- **Impairing phagocytosis.** The drugs inhibit the ability of phagocytic cells to leave the bloodstream and move into the injured or inflamed tissue.
- **Impairing lymphocytes.** The drugs inhibit the ability of these immune cells to increase in number and perform their functions.
- **Inhibiting tissue repair.** The drugs inhibit the growth of new capillaries, fibroblasts, and collagen needed for tissue repair.

TABLE 17.1

Adrenal Corticosteroid Drugs

Drug Class	Prototype	Other Drugs in the Class
Glucocorticoid	Prednisone (Deltasone, predniSONE, Intensol, Rayos)	Beclomethasone (QVAR RediHaler, Beconase AQ, QNASL)
		Betamethasone (betamethasone acetate and sodium phosphate) (Celestone, Soluspan, Betamethasone)
		Budesonide (Pulmocort, Rhinocort Allergy, Entocort EC, Uceris)
		Cortisone acetate
		Dexamethasone (TaperDex 12 Day; TaperDex 6 Day, TaperDex 7 Day, TopiDex, ZCort 7 Day)
		Flunisolide
		Fluticasone (Arnuity Ellipta, Flovent Diskus, Flovent HFA); fluticasone topical
		Hydrocortisone (Ala Cort, Ala Scalp, Anucort, Anusol, Colocort, Cortef, Cortenema, Cortifoam, Nutracort, Solu-Cortef)
		Methylprednisolone (Depo-Medrol, MedrolSOLU-Medrol)
		Mometasone (Asmanex, Asmanex HFA, Sinuva, Elocon)
		Prednisolone (Pred Forte, Pred Mild)
		Triamcinolone (Kenalog, Oracort, Triderm)
		Triamcinolone (nasal) acetonide (GoodSense Nasal Allergy Spray, Nasacort Allergy); Nasacort Allergy (all over-the-counter)
		Triamcinolone (systemic; intralesional) (Kenalog, Kenalog 80, P-Care K40, P-Care K80, Pod-Care 100K, Pro-C-Dure 5, Pro-C-Dure 6, Zilretta)
		Triamcinolone (topical) (Trianex, Triderm)
Mineralocorticoid	Fludrocortisone	

Use

Corticosteroids are administered to control symptoms but do not cure underlying disease processes. They are extensively used to treat many different disorders. Except for replacement therapy in deficiency states, the use of corticosteroids is largely empiric. Because the drugs affect virtually every aspect of inflammatory and immune responses, they are used in the treatment of a broad spectrum of diseases with an inflammatory or immunologic component.

Table 17.2 presents information about routes of administration and dosage ranges.

General Indications

The corticosteroids discussed in this chapter are used to treat potentially serious or disabling disorders, including the following:

- Allergic or hypersensitivity disorders, such as allergic reactions to drugs, serum and blood transfusions, and dermatoses with an allergic component.
- Collagen disorders, such as systemic lupus erythematosus, scleroderma, and periarteritis nodosa. Collagen is the basic structural protein of connective tissue, tendons, cartilage, and bone, and it is, therefore, present in almost all body tissues and organ systems. The collagen disorders are characterized by inflammation of various body tissues. Signs and symptoms depend on which body tissues or organs are affected and the severity of the inflammatory process.
- Dermatologic disorders that may be treated with systemic corticosteroids include acute contact dermatitis, erythema multiforme, herpes zoster (prophylaxis of postherpetic neuralgia), lichen planus, pemphigus, skin rashes caused by drugs, and toxic epidermal necrolysis. Corticosteroid preparations that are applied topically in dermatologic disorders are discussed in Chapter 61.
- Endocrine disorders, such as adrenocortical insufficiency and congenital adrenal hyperplasia (see Chapter 45 for additional information). Corticosteroids are given to replace or substitute for the natural hormones (both glucocorticoids and mineralocorticoids) in cases of insufficiency and to suppress corticotropin when excess secretion causes adrenal hyperplasia. These conditions are rare and account for a small percentage of corticosteroid use.
- GI disorders, such as ulcerative colitis and regional enteritis (Crohn disease).
- Hematologic disorders, such as idiopathic thrombocytopenic purpura or acquired hemolytic anemia.
- Hepatic disorders characterized by edema, such as cirrhosis and ascites.
- Neoplastic disease, such as acute and chronic leukemias, Hodgkin disease, other lymphomas, and multiple myeloma (see later discussion).

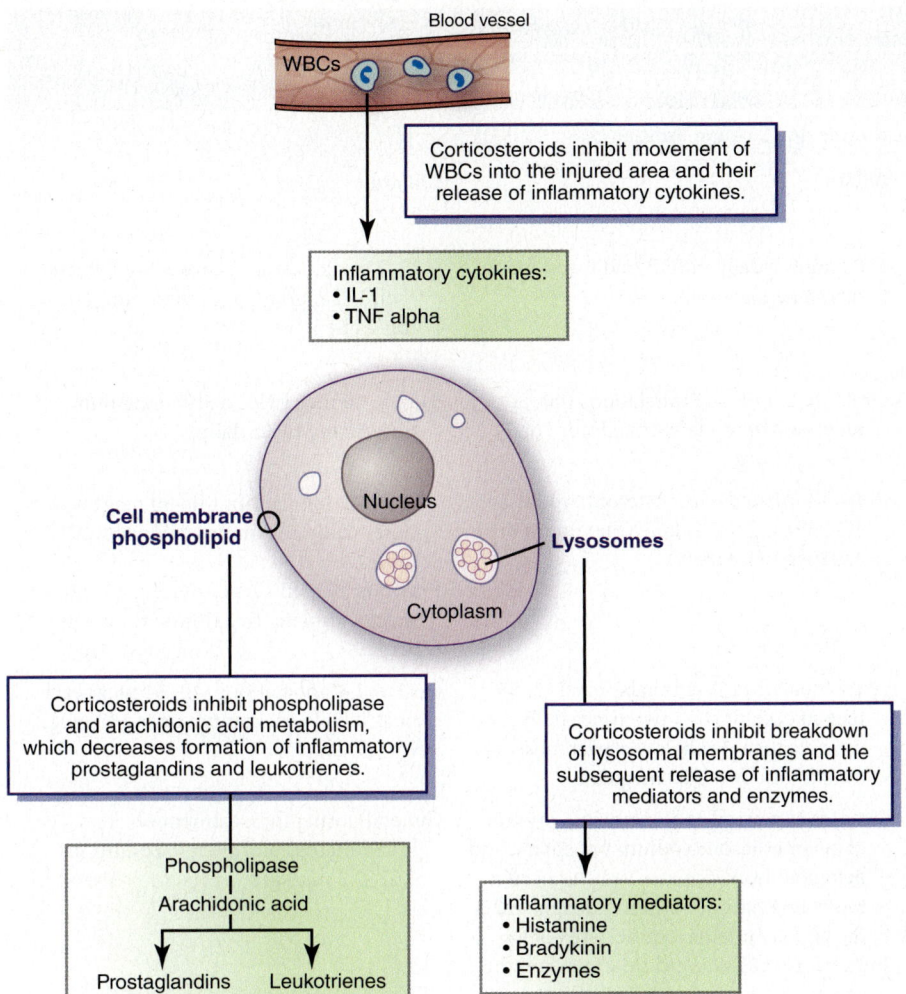

Figure 17.2. Inflammatory processes and anti-inflammatory actions of corticosteroids. Cellular responses to injury include the following: phospholipid in the cell membrane is acted on by phospholipase to release arachidonic acid, metabolism of arachidonic acid produces the inflammatory mediators prostaglandins and leukotrienes, lysosomal membrane breaks down and releases inflammatory chemicals (e.g., histamine, bradykinin, intracellular digestive enzymes), and white blood cells (WBCs) are drawn to the area and release inflammatory cytokines (e.g., interleukin-1 [IL-1] alpha). Overall, corticosteroid drugs act to inhibit the release, formation, or activation of various inflammatory mediators. TNF, tumor necrosis factor.

- Neurologic conditions, such as cerebral edema, brain tumor, acute spinal cord injury (see later discussion), and myasthenia gravis.
- Ophthalmic disorders, such as optic neuritis, sympathetic ophthalmia, and chorioretinitis. Corticosteroid preparations that are applied topically in ophthalmologic disorders are discussed in Chapter 59.
- Organ or tissue transplants and grafts (e.g., kidney, heart, bone marrow). Corticosteroids suppress cellular and humoral immune responses (see Chapter 13) and help prevent rejection of transplanted tissue. Drug therapy is usually continued as long as the transplanted tissue is in place.
- Kidney disorders characterized by edema, such as the nephrotic syndrome.
- Respiratory disorders, such as asthma, status asthmaticus, COPD, and inflammatory disorders of nasal mucosa (rhinitis).
- Rheumatic disorders, such as ankylosing spondylitis, acute and chronic bursitis, acute gouty arthritis, rheumatoid arthritis, and osteoarthritis.
- Shock. Corticosteroids are clearly indicated only for shock resulting from **addisonian crisis** (also known as adrenal or adrenocortical insufficiency), which may mimic hypovolemic or septic shock. Kaufman (2022) states that the rationale for administering glucocorticoids in patient with sepsis and septic shock is based on data, which suggests that critical illness invokes a state of adrenal insufficiency. However, it is very rare that critically ill patients will experience absolute adrenal insufficiency. The use of corticosteroids in septic shock has been highly controversial, and some older randomized studies and meta-analyses have indicated that corticosteroids are not beneficial in treating septic shock. However, in some newer meta-analysis studies, the use of systemic corticosteroids did shorten the duration of shock. The established guidelines for the use of glucocorticoids in patients with sepsis include the following:
- Adult patients with septic shock should not be administered glucocorticoid therapy as initial therapy.
- Therapy should be started if the systolic blood pressure is less than 90 mm Hg for more than 1 hour following fluid and vasopressor resuscitation.
- If hydrocortisone therapy is initiated, only hydrocortisone in less than 400 mg divided doses should be administered.
- In patients diagnosed with primary adrenal insufficiency that results in adrenal crisis, the treatment is begun with 1 to 3 L of 0.9% saline solution of dextrose 5% with 0.9% saline. In addition, hydrocortisone 100 mg IV bolus is administered followed by 50 mg IV every 6 hours or 200 mg/24 hours continuous IV infusion for the first 24 hours. Once the patient is stabilized, the administration of oral glucocorticoids is begun (Nieman, 2022a, 2022b).

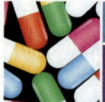

TABLE 17.2

DRUGS AT A GLANCE: Adrenal Corticosteroid Medications

Drug	Routes and Dosage Ranges	
	Adults	**Children**
Glucocorticoids		
ⓟ **Prednisone** (predniSONE, Deltasone, Intensol, Rayos; 🍁 Apo-Prednisone, Teva-PredniSONE, Winpred)	5–60 mg PO daily initially, adjusted for maintenance	0.25–2 mg/kg/dose PO every 6–48 h, and then 1–2 mg/kg/24 h (maximum 60 mg/24 h)
Beclomethasone (QVAR RediHaler, Beconase AQ, QNASL; 🍁 QVAR)	Oral inhalation: 1–2 inhalations (40–80 mcg) two times daily (maximum daily dose 320 mcg)	5–11 y: 40 mcg twice daily (maximum dose 80 mg twice daily)
	Previous inhaled corticosteroid: initial dose 40–160 mcg twice daily (maximum dose 320 mcg twice daily)	≥12 y: 1–2 inhalations (40–80 mcg) two times daily (maximum daily dose 320 mcg) Previous inhaled corticosteroid: 40–160 mcg twice daily (maximum dose 320 mcg)
Beclomethasone (Beconase AQ, QNASL, QNASL Children's; 🍁 Apo-Beclomethasone, Mylan-Beclo AQ, Rivanase AQ)	Nasal inhalation: 1–2 inhalations (42–84 mcg in each nostril) two times daily; as maintenance, 1 inhalation each nostril (maximum dose 320 mcg daily)	6–11 y: 1–2 inhalations (42–84 mcg) each nostril daily (maximum dose 168 mcg)
Betamethasone (betamethasone acetate and sodium phosphate) (Celestone, Soluspan Betamethasone; 🍁 Celestone, Soluspan)	Dosages expressed as a combined amount of betamethasone sodium phosphate and betamethasone acetate; 1 mg equivalent to betamethasone sodium phosphate 0.5 mg and betamethasone acetate 0.5 mg Initial dose 0.25–9 mg/d IM (based on the severity of disease and patient response	General dosing for treatment of inflammatory and allergic conditions: 0.02–0.3 mg/kg/d
Betamethasone acetate and sodium phosphate (Celestone Soluspan; Betaject, Celestone Soluspan)	0.25–9 mg IM daily; 0.25–2 mL intra-articular injection	
Budesonide (Pulmicort, Pulmicort Flexhaler; 🍁 Pulmicort Nebuamp, Pulmicort Turbuhaler, TEVA-Budesonide)	Oral inhalation: 360 mcg twice daily; maximum dose 720 mcg twice daily Maintenance: 200–400 mcg twice daily or 400 mcg once daily	*National Asthma Education and Prevention Program (NAEPP 2007):* 5–11 y Low dose: 180–400 mcg/d Medium dose: >400–800 mcg/d High dose: >800 mcg/d Children ≥12 y: Refer to adult dosing
Budesonide (Rhinocort Allergy; 🍁 Mylan-Budesonide AQ, Rhinocort Aqua, Rhinocort Turbuhaler)	Nasal inhalation: one spray (32 mcg) in each nostril once daily or twice daily	6–11 y: one spray in each nostril once daily (total dose 64 mcg/d) ≥12 y: Refer to adult dosing
Budesonide (Entocort EC; 🍁 Cortiment, Entocort)	Oral capsule Crohn disease or ulcerative colitis: 9 mg PO once daily in the morning, for up to 8 wk	Children ≥8 y and adolescents ≤17 y (weighing >25 kg) 9 mg daily in the morning for up to 8 wk and then 6 mg once daily for 2 wk
Budesonide (Uceris; 🍁 Entocort)	Rectal foam (Uceris) Initial: 2 mg twice daily for 2 wk Maintenance: 2 mg once daily for 4 wk Rectal enema (Entocort): initial 2 mg (one enema) once daily at night prior to bedtime for 4 wk	
Cortisone acetate	PO 25–300 mg daily, individualized for condition and response Physiologic replacement: PO 25–35 mg/d	

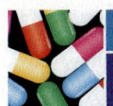

TABLE 17.2

DRUGS AT A GLANCE: Adrenal Corticosteroid Medications (Continued)

Drug	Routes and Dosage Ranges	
	Adults	**Children**
Dexamethasone (TaperDex 12 Day; TaperDex 6 Day, TaperDex 7 Day, TopiDex, ZCort 7 Day; 🍁 Apo-Dexamethasone, Dexamethasone Omega Unidose)	0.75–9 mg PO daily in 2–4 doses; higher range for serious diseases	0.08–0.3 mg/kg/d
Flunisolide	Oral inhalation: 2 inhalations (160 mcg) twice daily Maximum dose: 320 mcg twice daily	6–11 y: 80 mcg twice daily Maximum dose: 160 mcg twice daily ≥12 y: Refer to adult dosing
Flunisolide	Nasal inhalation: 2 sprays in each nostril twice daily; maximum daily dose 8 sprays in each nostril	6–14 y: 1 spray in each nostril three times daily or 2 sprays in each nostril two times daily; maximum daily dose 4 sprays in each nostril
Fluticasone (Arnuity Ellipta, Flovent Diskus, Flovent HFA; 🍁 APO-Fluticasone HFa, Lovent Diskus, Flovent HFA, PMS-Fluticasone HFA)	Oral inhalation: Arnuity Ellipta: 100 mcg once daily; maximum 100 mcg once daily Flovent HFA: 2 inhalations (88 mcg) two times daily (maximum daily dose 440 mcg inhaled two times daily)	<12 y: Not recommended
Fluticasone (Flonase Allergy Relief OTC; 🍁 Apo-Fluticasone, RATIO-Flonase, TEVA-Fluticasone)	Nasal inhalation: 200 mcg daily initially (2 sprays each nostril once daily or 1 spray each nostril twice daily). After a few days, reduce dosage to 100 mcg daily (1 spray each nostril once daily) for maintenance therapy.	4–11 y: 100 mcg daily (1 spray per nostril once daily). *Do not use more than 2 mo per year* ≥12 y: refer to adult dosing
Fluticasone topical (🍁 Cutivate)	Apply a thin film to affected area one to two times daily	≥3 mo: refer to adult dosing
Hydrocortisone (Ala Cort, Ala Scalp, Anucort, Anusol, Colocort, Cortef, Cortenema, Cortifoam, Nutracort, Solu-Cortef; 🍁 Barriere-HC, Cortenema, Cortifoam, Emo Cort, Hyderm, Hydroval, NOVO-Hydrocort, Prevex HC, SANDOZ Hydrocortisone, Sama HC)	Apply sparingly to skin two to four times daily	Same as adults
Hydrocortisone (A-Hydrocort, Cortef, Solu-Cortef; Cortef, Solu-Cortef)	Anti-inflammatory or immunosuppression IM, IV: initial 100–500 mg/dose at intervals of 2, 4, or 6 h PO: initial 20–240 mg/d Multiple sclerosis IM, IV: 800 mg/d for 1 wk, followed by 320 mg every other day for 1 mo PO: 200 mg/d for 1 wk, followed by 80 mg every other day for 1 mo *For adrenal insufficiency*, see Chapter 45	PO: 2.5–10 mg/kg/d or 75–300 mg/m²/d in 3–4 divided doses IM, IV: 0.56–8 mg/kg/d
Hydrocortisone (Cortenema; Cortenema)	100 mg enema rectally every night for 21 d or until optimal response	
Hydrocortisone acetate (Cortifoam; Cortifoam)	1 applicator rectally one to two times per day for 2–3 wk and then once every 2–3 d if needed	

(Continued on page 322)

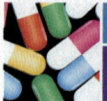

TABLE 17.2
DRUGS AT A GLANCE: Adrenal Corticosteroid Medications (Continued)

Drug	Routes and Dosage Ranges	
	Adults	**Children**
Methylprednisolone (Depo-Medrol, SOLU-Medrol; 🍁 Depo-Medrol, Medrol, SOLU-Medrol, Uni-MED)	4–48 mg daily PO initially, gradually reduced to lowest effective level 10–40 mg IM or IV initially, adjusted to condition and response Acute respiratory distress syndrome Early severe: (day 1–6 of onset) IV loading dose of 1 mg/kg over 30 min; followed by a slow taper • Days 1–14: 1 mg/kg/d in divided doses or as a continuous infusion • Days 15–21: 0.5 mg/kg/d in divided doses or as a continuous infusion • Days 22–25: 0.25 mg/kg/d in divided doses or as a continuous infusion • Days 26–28: 0.125 mg/kg/d in divided doses or as a continuous infusion Late persistent (day 7–14 of onset) IV loading dose of 2 mg/kg over 30 min, followed by a slow taper • Days 1–14: 2 mg/kg/d in divided doses or as a continuous infusion • Days 15–21: 1 mg/kg/d in divided doses or as a continuous infusion • Days 22–25: 0.5 mg/kg/d in divided doses or as a continuous infusion • Days 26–28: 0.25 mg/kg/d in divided doses or as a continuous infusion • Days 29–30: 0.125 mg bolus over 30 min	Infants and children: Not <0.5 mg/kg/24 h IM or IV
Methylprednisolone acetate (Depo-Medrol)	40–120 mg IM once daily	
Mometasone (Asmanex, Asmanex HFA, Propel, Propel MiniSDS, Sinuva, Elocon; 🍁 Asmanex Twisthaler, Mosaspray, Nasonex, SANDOZ Mometasone, Elocon PMS, TARO-Mometasone, TEVA-Mometasone)	Oral inhalation • Low-dose therapy: 110–220 mcg/d • Medium-dose therapy: >220–440 mcg/d • High-dose therapy: >440 mcg/d 2 sprays (100 mcg/spray) in each nostril once daily (200 mcg/d) Topical cream applied sparingly to affected area Topical lotion applied, a few drops to affected area	Oral inhalation Children 4–11 y: 110 mcg inhaler in the evening 2–11 y: 1 spray (50 mcg) in each nostril once daily (100 mcg/d) >12 y: same as adults Children >2 y to adolescents Topical cream applied sparingly to affected area Topical lotion applied a few drops to affected area
Prednisolone (Millipred; 🍁 Pediapred, PMS-Prednisolone)	5–60 mg PO daily initially, adjusted for maintenance	0.1–2 mg/kg/d PO in divided doses
Prednisolone (Pred Forte, Pred Mild; 🍁 Diopred, Minims Prednisolone, PMS-Prednisolone, Sod Phos Fort, Pred Forte, SANDOZ Prednisolone, TEVA-Prednisolone)	1–2 drops in conjunctival sac two to four times per day; during the initial 24–48 h, the dosing frequency may be increased if necessary. If signs and symptoms fail to improve after 2 d, reevaluate. Do not discontinue therapy prematurely; withdraw therapy with gradual tapering of dose in chronic conditions	Ophthalmic inflammation in children is an off-label use Prednisone acetate: 1% instill 1–2 drops into conjunctival sac three to six times daily

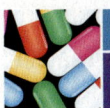

TABLE 17.2
DRUGS AT A GLANCE: Adrenal Corticosteroid Medications (Continued)

Drug	Routes and Dosage Ranges	
	Adults	**Children**
Triamcinolone acetonide (GoodSense Nasal Allergy Spray, Nasacort Allergy; Nasacort Allergy) (all over-the-counter; ✱ Apo-Triamcinolone AQ, Nasacort AQ)	Nasal inhalation: 2 sprays (110 mcg) in each nostril once daily (total dose 220 mcg/d); may increase to maximal daily dose of 440 mcg if indicated	2–6 y: 1 spray (55 mcg) in each nostril once daily ≥6 y: 2 sprays (110 mcg) in each nostril once daily (220 mcg/d) initially; reduce to 1 spray per nostril once daily (110 mcg/d)
Triamcinolone (Kenalog, Kenalog 80, P-Care K40, P-Care K80, Pod-Care 100K, Pro-C-Dure 5, Pro-C-Dure 6, Zilretta; ✱ Kenalog-10, Kenalog-40)	Intralesional: 1 mg initial dose; dose varies due to disease and lesion to be treated; may be treated weekly or less frequently Intra-articular: 2–20 mg every 3–4 wk as needed	Lowest possible dose to control disease
Triamcinolone (Trianex, Triderm; ✱ Aristocort, Aristocort R, Oracort, Triaderm)	Apply a thin film to affected areas two to four times per day	0.25%–0.5%: apply a thin film
Mineralocorticoid		
Fludrocortisone (✱ Florinef)	Chronic adrenocortical insufficiency: 0.1 mg PO daily Salt-losing adrenogenital syndromes: 0.1–0.2 mg daily	0.05–0.1 mg PO daily

NCLEX Success

1. A child has contracted a rash caused by poison ivy over a large portion of their arms and legs following a camping trip. The healthcare provider has prescribed oral prednisone, which is to be administered in a tapering dose over the next 10 days. What effect does the medication have on the rash?
   A. It decreases the accumulation of neutrophils and macrophages at the site, thus reducing inflammation.
   B. It eliminates the itching associated with the allergy.
   C. It increases the white blood cell count to assist in healing.
   D. It increases the protein metabolism to allow for the rejuvenation of tissue.

2. A patient is admitted to the emergency department in anaphylactic shock following numerous bee stings. The prescriber orders parenteral administration of corticosteroids. What effect is expected from the administration of these agents?
   A. decreased heart rate and blood pressure
   B. increased circulation to the lower extremities
   C. increased or restored cardiovascular responsiveness
   D. decreased production of aldosterone

Specific Uses

Corticosteroids are also commonly used for the following specific conditions.

Allergic Rhinitis

Allergic rhinitis (also called seasonal rhinitis, hay fever, and perennial rhinitis) is a common problem for which corticosteroids are given by nasal spray, once or twice daily. The drugs decrease mucus secretion and inflammation. Therapeutic effects usually occur within a few days with regular use. Systemic adverse effects are minimal with recommended doses but may occur with higher doses, including adrenocortical insufficiency from HPA suppression.

Arthritis

Corticosteroids are the most effective drugs for rapid relief of the pain, edema, and restricted mobility associated with acute episodes of joint inflammation. They are usually given on a short-term basis. When inflammation is limited to three or fewer joints, the preferred route of drug administration is by injection directly into the joint. Intra-articular injections relieve symptoms in approximately 2 to 8 weeks, and several formulations are available for this route. However, corticosteroids do not prevent disease progression and joint destruction. As a general rule, a joint should not be injected more often than three times yearly because of risks of infection and damage to intra-articular structures from the injections and from overuse when pain is relieved.

Asthma

Corticosteroids are commonly used in the treatment of asthma because of their anti-inflammatory effects. In addition, corticosteroids increase the effects of adrenergic bronchodilators to prevent or treat bronchoconstriction and bronchospasm. The drugs increase the number of beta-adrenergic receptors and increase or restore responsiveness of beta receptors to beta-adrenergic bronchodilating drugs. Research indicates that responsiveness to beta-adrenergic bronchodilators increases within 2 hours and that numbers of beta receptors increase within 4 hours.

In acute asthma or status asthmaticus unrelieved by inhaled beta-adrenergic bronchodilators, high doses of systemic corticosteroids are given orally or intravenously along with bronchodilators for approximately 5 to 10 days. Although these high doses suppress the HPA axis, the suppression lasts for only 1 to 3 days, and other serious adverse effects are avoided. Thus, systemic corticosteroids are used for short-term therapy, as needed, and not for long-term treatment. People who regularly use inhaled corticosteroids also require high doses of systemic drugs during acute attacks because aerosols are not effective. As soon as acute symptoms subside, it is necessary to taper the dose; people should take the lowest effective maintenance dose or discontinue the drug. In chronic asthma, inhaled corticosteroids are the drugs of first choice. This recommendation evolved from increased knowledge about the importance of inflammation in the pathophysiology of asthma and the development of aerosol corticosteroids that are effective with minimal adverse effects.

Inhaled drugs may be given alone or with systemic drugs. In general, inhaled corticosteroids can replace oral drugs when daily dosage of the oral drug has been tapered to 10 to 15 mg of prednisone or the equivalent. When a patient is being switched from an oral to an inhaled corticosteroid, the inhaled drug should be started during tapering of the oral drug, approximately 1 or 2 weeks before discontinuing or reaching the lowest anticipated dose of the oral drug. When a patient requires a systemic corticosteroid, coadministration of an aerosol allows smaller doses of the systemic corticosteroid. Although the inhaled drugs can cause suppression of the HPA axis and adrenocortical function, especially at higher doses, they are much less likely to do so than systemic drugs. However, the U.S. Food and Drug Administration (FDA) has issued a **BOXED WARNING** ◆ for people who are transferred from systemically active corticosteroids to flunisolide inhaler because deaths have occurred from adrenal insufficiency.

Clinical Application 17.1

- What is the purpose of administering prednisone to Mrs. Thompson?
- What is the purpose of tapering the dose?
- Could prednisone be discontinued without tapering the dose?

⚠ Quality and Safety Alert: Evidence-Based Practice

Lempp et al. (2022) conducted a study to assess if the use of inhaled corticosteroid therapy affects glycemic control in patients with chronic obstructive pulmonary disease (COPD) and diabetes mellitus type 2 (T2DM). Many studies have shown mixed results between the association of inhaled corticosteroids and worsening of glycemic control. In this study, inhaled corticosteroids did not impact glycemic control among patients with comorbid COPD and T2DM.

Cancer

Corticosteroids are commonly used in the treatment of lymphomas, lymphocytic leukemias, and multiple myeloma. In these disorders, corticosteroids inhibit cell reproduction and are cytotoxic to lymphocytes. In addition to their anticancer effects in hematologic malignancies, corticosteroids are beneficial in treatment of several signs and symptoms that often accompany cancer, although the mechanisms of action are unknown and drug/dosage regimens vary widely. Corticosteroids are used to treat anorexia, nausea and vomiting, cerebral edema and inflammation associated with brain metastases or radiation of the head, spinal cord compression, pain and edema related to pressure on nerves or bone metastases, graft versus host disease after bone marrow transplantation, and other disorders that occur in patients with cancer. Patients tend to feel better when taking corticosteroids, although the basic disease process may be unchanged.

Primary Central Nervous System Lymphomas

Formerly considered rare tumors of older adults, central nervous system (CNS) lymphomas are being diagnosed more frequently in younger patients. They are usually associated with chronic **immunosuppression** (suppression of the immune system) caused by immunosuppressant drugs or acquired immunodeficiency syndrome (AIDS). Many of these lymphomas are very sensitive to corticosteroids, and therapy is indicated when the diagnosis is established.

Other Central Nervous System Tumors

Corticosteroid therapy may be useful in both supportive and definitive treatment of brain and spinal cord tumors, and neurologic signs and symptoms often improve dramatically within 24 to 48 hours. Corticosteroids help relieve symptoms by controlling edema around the tumor, at operative sites, and at sites receiving radiation therapy. Some patients no longer require corticosteroids after surgical or radiation therapy, whereas others require continued therapy to manage neurologic symptoms. Adverse effects of long-term corticosteroid therapy may include mental changes ranging from mild agitation to psychosis and steroid myopathy (muscle weakness and atrophy) that may be confused with tumor progression. Mental symptoms usually improve if the drug dosage is reduced and resolve if the drug is discontinued; steroid myopathy may persist for weeks or months.

Chemotherapy-Induced Emesis

Corticosteroids have strong antiemetic effects; the mechanism is unknown. One effective regimen is a combination of an oral or intravenous (IV) dose of dexamethasone (10 to 20 mg) and a serotonin antagonist or metoclopramide given immediately before the chemotherapeutic drug. This regimen is the treatment of choice for chemotherapy with cisplatin, which is a strongly emetic drug.

Postoperative Nausea and Vomiting

Postoperative nausea and vomiting is a common complication during recovery from anesthesia. It is most common in women; there is also a high risk in children. Nausea and vomiting occur due to a variety of factors. For example, anxiety and fear play a role in their development. Stimulation of the vestibular system will induce nausea and vomiting. The high cortical centers communicate with the central pattern generator in the medulla. The antiemetic regimen to prevent postoperative nausea and vomiting includes the application of a scopolamine patch 2 hours prior to the induction of anesthesia, dexamethasone 4 to 8 mg IV after anesthetic induction, and ondansetron 4 mg IV at the conclusion of the surgery.

Chronic Obstructive Pulmonary Disease

Corticosteroids are more helpful in acute exacerbations of COPD than in stable disease. However, oral corticosteroids may improve pulmonary function and symptoms in some patients. As in asthma and rhinitis, the drugs decrease mucus secretion and inflammation. Lymphocytes are involved in the inflammatory response in both asthma and COPD. In patients with COPD, the CD8 cell numbers increase and lead to secretion of proinflammatory cytokines and cytotoxic molecules. The administration of the medication roflumilast, a phosphodiesterase 4 inhibitor, and corticosteroids decreases the degradation cyclic adenosine monophosphate to decrease the inflammatory activity (Ferguson & Make, 2022; Stoller, 2022). Note that inhaled corticosteroids can also be used. Although they produce minimal adverse effects, their effectiveness in COPD has not been clearly demonstrated.

Inflammatory Bowel Disease

Patients who suffer from Crohn disease or ulcerative colitis often require periodic corticosteroid therapy. In patients with active mucosal inflammation, oral prednisone, 40 mg daily, is usually given until symptoms subside. With severe disease, patients often require hospitalization, IV fluids for hydration, and parenteral corticosteroids until symptoms subside. Budesonide may be used for low-risk patients with Crohn disease. It inhibits protein synthesis, thus decreasing the formation of inflammatory cytokines. The oral capsule dissolves in the small intestine and acts locally before being absorbed into the bloodstream and transported to the liver for metabolism. It has fewer adverse effects than systemic corticosteroids but is also less effective and more expensive. The topical formulation is available in foam or enema to be administered in the proximal and splenic flexure to reduce colonic inflammation (Peppercorn & Cheifetz, 2022).

In ulcerative colitis, corticosteroids are usually used when aminosalicylates (e.g., mesalamine) are not effective or when symptoms are more severe. Initially, hydrocortisone enemas may be effective. If they are not, oral prednisone (20 to 60 mg daily) may be given until symptoms subside. In severe disease, oral prednisone may be required initially. After remission of symptoms is achieved, the dose can be tapered by 2.5 to 5 mg/day each week to a dose of 20 mg. Then, tapering may be slowed to 2.5 to 5 mg/day every other week. As in Crohn disease, patients with severe ulcerative colitis often require hospitalization and parenteral corticosteroids. One regimen uses IV hydrocortisone 300 mg/day or the equivalent dose of another drug. When the patient's condition improves, oral prednisone can replace the IV corticosteroid.

Spinal Cord Injury

High-dose corticosteroid therapy to treat spinal cord injury is a common practice in clinical settings, although controversy exists regarding its use. Data suggest that methylprednisolone may be effective in acute spinal cord injury when given in high doses within 8 hours of the injury. Methylprednisolone improves neurologic recovery, although it does not improve mortality, and its use is unlikely to result in normal neurologic function. In addition, severe adverse outcomes, including wound and systemic infections, GI hemorrhage, and pneumonia, have been reported.

Septic Shock

During critical illness, the body induces a state of absolute or relative adrenal insufficiency. The patient's illness affects cortisol levels and the function of the HPA activation, resulting in increased levels of cortisol. The impairment of HPA results in adrenocortical hyporesponsiveness and resistance to glucocorticoids. In patients with refractory shock with a blood pressure less than 90 mm Hg for more than 1 hour following fluid resuscitation and administration of vasopressor medication, hydrocortisone less than 400 mg/day in divided doses is recommended (Kaufman, 2022).

> **Quality and Safety Alert: Evidence-Based Practice**
>
> Ceccato et al. (2021) analyzed two observational cohorts of patients in the intensive care unit who were being treated for community acquired pneumonia to determine the effectiveness of hydrocortisone. The study concluded that corticosteroid treatment may benefit patients with community acquired pneumonia who have septic shock and/or are noted to possess a high inflammatory response requiring invasive mechanical ventilation.

Prevention of Acute Adrenocortical Insufficiency

Suppression of the HPA axis may occur with corticosteroid therapy and may lead to life-threatening inability to increase cortisol secretion when needed to cope with stress. It is most likely to occur with abrupt withdrawal of systemic corticosteroid drugs. The risk of HPA suppression is high with systemic drugs given for more than a few days, although patients vary in degree and duration of suppression with comparable doses, and the minimum dose and duration of therapy that cause suppression are unknown.

When corticosteroids are given for replacement therapy, adrenal insufficiency is lifelong, and drug administration must be continued (see Chapter 45). When the drugs are given for purposes other than replacement and then discontinued, the HPA axis usually recovers within several weeks to months, but recovery may take a year. Several strategies have been developed to minimize HPA suppression and risks of acute adrenal insufficiency, including the following:

- Administering a systemic corticosteroid during high-stress situations (e.g., moderate or severe illness, trauma, surgery) to patients who have received pharmacologic doses for 2 weeks within the previous year or who receive long-term systemic therapy (i.e., are steroid dependent).
- Giving short courses of systemic therapy for acute disorders, such as asthma attacks, and then decreasing the dose or stopping the drug within a few days.

- Gradually tapering the dose of any systemic corticosteroid. Although specific guidelines for tapering dosage have not been developed, higher doses and longer durations of administration in general require slower tapering, possibly over several weeks. The goal of tapering may be to stop the drug or to decrease the dosage to the lowest effective amount.
- Using local rather than systemic therapy when possible, alone or in combination with low doses of systemic drugs. Numerous preparations are available for local application, including aerosols for oral or nasal inhalation; formulations for topical application to the skin, eyes, and ears; and drugs for intra-articular injections.
- Using alternate-day therapy (ADT), which involves titrating the daily dose to the lowest effective maintenance level and then giving a double dose every other day (most commonly administered in the morning).

> **Concept Mastery Alert**
>
> If a patient is on a daily regimen of a corticosteroid and develops even a minor illness, the daily corticosteroid dosage should be increased. Typically, the stress of even a minor illness requires that the dose be doubled. When illness is more severe, greater increases in dosage are required.

Use in Special Populations

Patient-related variables specific to the use of prednisone include the following:

- Age:
  - Corticosteroids are used in children for the same conditions as in adults, most commonly asthma.
  - Children with severe asthma may require continual corticosteroid therapy.
  - For children with asthma who are prescribed inhaled corticosteroids, a moderate dosage is recommended.
  - Oral corticosteroids can result in growth impairment.
  - Use cautiously in older patients. The smallest dose should be prescribed with the shortest duration of administration.
- Reproduction, pregnancy, and lactation:
  - Prednisone is acceptable for use in patients with rheumatic and musculoskeletal disorders who are planning to become pregnant.
  - Prednisone is the preferred oral corticosteroid for the treatment of maternal conditions during pregnancy. It has been determined that placental enzymes limit passage to the embryo.
  - Prednisone administration is considered acceptable in patients who are breast-feeding.
- Abnormal kidney function and hepatic impairment:
  - No dosage adjustments are required with abnormal kidney function or hepatic impairment.
- Specific healthcare environments:
  - In patients with critical illness, adrenal insufficiency is the most clear-cut indication for use of a corticosteroid, and even a slight impairment of the adrenal response during severe illness can be lethal if corticosteroid therapy is not instituted (see Chapter 45).
  - In patients with COPD, some studies have found that the parenteral administration of methylprednisolone may be effective for the treatment of acute respiratory failure. If other medications do not produce adequate bronchodilation, IV corticosteroid therapy is a reasonable treatment choice in the first 72 hours of the illness. The nurse assesses the patient for pulmonary infection because corticosteroid therapy places the patient at increased risk for pulmonary infection.
  - In patients with nonacute respiratory distress syndrome, glucocorticoids can be administered. This treatment is recommended early in the disease process, most commonly in the first 14 days. Administering glucocorticoids to patients who are early in the disease or have less severe symptoms is not recommended. Studies examining the benefit of corticosteroid therapy revealed that improved gas exchange decreased the number of days patients with ARDS were on mechanically assisted ventilation (Siegel & Siemieniuk, 2022). The studies reviewed by Siegel revealed the importance of monitoring individual patients who are administered corticosteroids for signs and symptoms of infection.
  - Patients with AIDS require assessment and treatment for adrenal insufficiency, if indicated.
  - Corticosteroids improve survival and decrease risks of respiratory failure with pneumocystosis, a common cause of death in patients with AIDS. The recommended regimen is prednisone 40 mg twice daily for 5 days, then 40 mg once daily for 5 days, and then 20 mg daily until completion of treatment for pneumocystosis.
  - The effect of corticosteroids on risks of other opportunistic infections or neoplasms is unknown.
  - In the home care setting, corticosteroids are extensively used by all age groups, for a wide variety of disorders, and by most routes of administration. Because of potentially serious adverse effects, especially with oral drugs, it is extremely important that these drugs be used as prescribed.
  - Home care nurses teach, demonstrate, supervise, monitor, or do whatever is needed to facilitate correct use. They also must teach patients and caregivers interventions to minimize adverse effects of these drugs.

> **Quality and Safety Alert: Safety**
>
> When caring for a patient with COPD and a history of heart failure who takes a tapering dose of prednisone, it is necessary to instruct the patient to check their weight daily. The patient should also assess their extremities for edema. If the patient's weight increases, edema is evident, and shortness of breath develops, the patient should notify their primary health provider.

Clinical Application 17.2

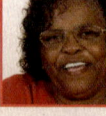

Mrs. Thompson states, "Since I have been taking this prednisone, the arthritis pain in my knees doesn't seem as bad."

- Why has her arthritic pain in her knees decreased with the administration of oral prednisone?
- What patient teaching is specific to the administration of prednisone?

NCLEX Success

3. A patient with cancer asks the nurse why a corticosteroid is given before chemotherapy. Which of the following is the nurse's best response?
   A. It will prevent the development of anemia related to the chemotherapy.
   B. It will prevent the development of hiccups, which is associated with chemotherapy.
   C. It will prevent nausea and vomiting that occur with chemotherapy.
   D. It will boost your immune system and prevent infection.

Adverse Effects

Administration of more than 5 mg daily of corticosteroids results in adverse reactions. Possible adverse effects include the following:

- **Adrenocortical insufficiency:** fainting, weakness, anorexia, nausea, vomiting, hypotension, shock, and death (if untreated)
- **Adrenocortical excess**
- **Cushingoid features:** "moon face" and buffalo hump due to the redistribution of fat
- **CNS effects:** vertigo, headache, paresthesias, insomnia, and seizures
- **Cardiovascular symptoms:** hypotension, shock, hypertension, heart failure, thromboembolism, thrombophlebitis, fat embolism, and cardiac dysrhythmias
- **Diminished immunity:** increased susceptibility to infection
- **Endocrine effects:** diabetes, hyperglycemia, and hypercholesterolemia; diminished T_3 and T_4 levels, resulting in hypothyroidism; and reduced growth because of altered synthesis of DNA
- **Fluid and electrolyte effects:** fluid retention, hypokalemia, and hypocalcemia
- **Integumentary effects:** reddened skin, thinner skin, stretch marks, skin tears, and delayed wound healing
- **Musculoskeletal effects:** hypocalcemia, which places the patient at risk for osteoporosis and fracture development, and serum hypocalcemia, which increases the release parathyroid hormone, increasing the loss of calcium from bone
- **Ocular effects:** cataracts and glaucoma
- **Reproductive effects:** amenorrhea or irregular menstrual cycles

Quality and Safety Alert: Patient-Centered Care

Evidence suggests that the administration of corticosteroids to patients receiving chemotherapy may result in hiccups. Healthcare providers must be cognizant of the effect oral steroids can have on the development of hiccups.

Contraindications

Corticosteroids are contraindicated in patients who experience allergic response to the medications. Patients with systemic fungal infections should not receive corticosteroids. Other contraindications include amebiasis, hepatitis B, vaccinia, varicella, and antibiotic-resistant infections. Also, patients who have been diagnosed with immunosuppression should not take corticosteroids. Patients receiving corticosteroids should not receive live virus vaccines, because of the risk of contracting the virus.

Caution is necessary when administering corticosteroids to patients with kidney disease, liver disease, hypothyroidism, recent GI surgery, peptic ulcer and inflammatory bowel disease, heart failure, thrombophlebitis, and diabetes.

Nursing Implications

Many factors have an effect on drug dosage, such as the specific drug to be given, the desired route of administration, the reason for use, expected adverse effects, and patient characteristics. In general, the patient should take the smallest effective dose for the shortest effective time. It is necessary to individualize the dosage according to the severity of the disorder being treated, whether the disease is acute or chronic, and the patient's response to drug therapy. For children, corticosteroid dosages should be calculated based on the severity of disease rather than the child's weight. If life-threatening disease is present, patients usually receive high doses until acute symptoms subside. Gradual dose reduction follows, until a maintenance dose is determined or the drug is discontinued. If life-threatening disease is not present, patients may still receive relatively high doses initially and then lower ones. Gradual reduction (tapering) over several days is necessary. With long-term corticosteroid therapy, periodic attempts to reduce dosage are desirable to decrease adverse effects. One way is to reduce the dose gradually until symptoms worsen, indicating the minimally effective dose.

Prescribers order physiologic doses (approximately 15 to 20 mg of hydrocortisone or its equivalent daily) to replace or substitute for endogenous adrenocortical hormone. They usually order pharmacologic doses (supraphysiologic amounts) for anti-inflammatory, antiallergic, antistress, and immunosuppressive effects.

Compared with hydrocortisone, newer corticosteroids are more potent on a weight basis but are equipotent in anti-inflammatory effects when given in equivalent doses. Statements of equivalency with hydrocortisone are helpful in evaluating new drugs, comparing different drugs, and changing drugs or dosages. However, dosage equivalents apply only to drugs given orally or intravenously.

Preventing Interactions

Many medications increase or decrease the therapeutic effects of corticosteroids (Box 17.3). Herbal interactions with corticosteroids are most often related to changes in sodium and potassium. Licorice (the root of glycyrrhiza glabra) increases the effects of corticosteroids, which may potentiate its effects; cautious use of licorice with corticosteroids is necessary.

Administering the Medication

Corticosteroids can be given by several different routes to produce local or systemic effects, depending on the clinical problem. If feasible, these drugs should be given locally rather than systemically to prevent or decrease systemic toxicity. Several formulations have been developed for oral inhalation in the treatment of asthma and for nasal inhalation in the treatment of allergic rhinitis. When these drugs must be given systemically, the oral route is preferred. Parenteral administration is

> **BOX 17.3** **Drug Interactions: Corticosteroids**
>
> **Drugs That Increase the Effects of Corticosteroids**
> - Estrogens, oral contraceptives, ketoconazole, macrolide antibiotics (e.g., erythromycin)
>   *Increase the effects of corticosteroids by inhibiting the enzymes that normally metabolize corticosteroids in the liver.*
> - Diuretics (e.g., furosemide and thiazides)
>   *Increase hypokalemia.*
>
> **Drugs That Decrease the Effects of Corticosteroids**
> - Antacids and cholestyramine
>   *Decrease the absorption of corticosteroids.*
> - Carbamazepine, phenytoin, rifampin
>   *Induce microsomal enzymes in the liver and increase the rate at which corticosteroids are metabolized or deactivated.*

indicated only for patients who are seriously ill or unable to take oral medications. For IM or IV injections, sodium phosphate or sodium succinate salts are used because they are most soluble in water. For intra-articular or intralesional injections, acetate salts are used because they have low solubility in water and provide prolonged local action.

Scheduling of drug administration is more important with corticosteroids than with most other drug classes. Most adverse effects occur with long-term administration of high doses. A major adverse reaction is suppression of the HPA axis and subsequent loss of adrenocortical function. Certain schedules are often recommended to prevent or minimize HPA suppression.

Corticosteroids can be given in relatively large, divided doses for approximately 48 to 72 hours in acute situations until the condition has been brought under control. After acute symptoms subside or 48 to 72 hours have passed, the dosage is tapered so that a slightly smaller dose is given each day until the drug can be discontinued completely (total period of use: approximately 1 week). Such a regimen may be useful in allergic reactions, contact dermatitis, exacerbations of chronic conditions (e.g., bronchial asthma), and stressful situations such as surgery.

Daily administration is required in cases of chronic adrenocortical insufficiency. The entire daily dose can be taken each morning, between 6:00 and 9:00 a.m. This schedule simulates normal endogenous corticosteroid secretion.

Stress Dosage Therapy

As previously stated, long-term use of pharmacologic doses (e.g., more than 5 mg of prednisone daily) of corticosteroids produces adverse reactions. For this reason, such corticosteroid therapy should be reserved for life-threatening conditions or severe, disabling symptoms that do not respond to treatment with more benign drugs or other measures. For people receiving chronic corticosteroid therapy, dosage must be increased during periods of stress or illness. Some common sources of stress for most people include surgery and anesthesia, infections, anxiety, and extremes of temperature. Note that events that are stressful for one patient may not be stressful for another. Some guidelines for corticosteroid dosage during stress include the following:

- During minor or relatively mild illness (e.g., viral upper respiratory infection, any febrile illness, strenuous exercise, gastroenteritis with vomiting and diarrhea, minor surgery), doubling the daily maintenance dose is usually adequate. After the stress period is over, it is appropriate to reduce the dosage abruptly to the usual maintenance dose.
- During major stress or severe illness, even larger doses are necessary. For example, a patient undergoing abdominal surgery may require 300 to 400 mg of hydrocortisone on the day of surgery. Gradual dose reduction to usual maintenance doses within approximately 5 days is sufficient if postoperative recovery is uncomplicated. As a general rule, it is better to administer excessive doses temporarily than to risk inadequate doses and adrenal insufficiency. The patient also may require sodium chloride and fluid replacement, antibiotic therapy if infection is present, and supportive measures if shock occurs.
- During acute stress situations of short duration, such as traumatic injury or invasive diagnostic tests (e.g., angiography), a single dose of approximately 100 mg of hydrocortisone immediately after the injury or before the diagnostic test is usually sufficient.
- Many chronic diseases that require long-term corticosteroid therapy are characterized by exacerbations and remissions. It is usually necessary to increase the dosage of corticosteroids during acute flare-ups of disease symptoms but can then decrease the dosage gradually to maintenance levels.

Alternate-Day Therapy

ADT, in which a double dose is taken every other morning, is usually preferred for other chronic conditions. This schedule allows rest periods so that adverse effects are decreased while anti-inflammatory effects continue. ADT seems to be as effective as more frequent administration in most patients with bronchial asthma, ulcerative colitis, and other conditions for which long-term corticosteroid therapy is prescribed. ADT is used only for maintenance therapy (i.e., clinical signs and symptoms are controlled initially with more frequent drug administration). ADT can be started after symptoms have subsided and stabilized.

Intermediate-acting glucocorticoids (e.g., prednisone, prednisolone, methylprednisolone) are the drugs of choice for ADT. Long-acting drugs (e.g., betamethasone, dexamethasone) are not recommended because of their prolonged suppression of adrenocortical function.

ADT has other advantages. It probably decreases susceptibility to infection and does not retard growth in children, as do other schedules.

ADT is not usually indicated in patients who have previously received corticosteroids on a long-term basis. First, these patients already have maximal HPA suppression, so a major advantage of ADT is lost. Second, if these patients begin ADT, recurrence of symptoms and considerable discomfort may occur on days when drugs are omitted. Patients with severe disease and very painful or disabling symptoms also may experience severe discomfort with ADT.

Assessing for Therapeutic Effects

The goal of corticosteroid therapy is usually to reduce symptoms to a tolerable level. Total suppression of symptoms may require excessively large doses and produce excessive adverse effects.

Because systemic corticosteroids can cause serious adverse reactions, indications for their clinical use should be as clear-cut as possible. Therapeutic effects depend largely on the reason for use.

Prescribers order hydrocortisone for the treatment of Addison disease. Following the parenteral administration of the medication, the nurse monitors the patient for activity tolerance, ability to move in bed, and restoration of fluid balance. Decreases in weakness, weight loss and anorexia, nausea and vomiting, hyperpigmentation, hypotension, hyponatremia, and hyperkalemia should be evident.

Prednisone is the drug of choice for nonendocrine disorders in which anti-inflammatory, antiallergic, antistress, and immunosuppressive effects are desired. The nurse assesses the patient for diminished inflammation. Inhaled corticosteroids also reduce inflammation and allergic responses and do not lead to the serious adverse effects of systemic corticosteroids.

Healthcare providers consider dexamethasone (parenteral or oral) the corticosteroid of choice for cerebral edema associated with brain tumors, craniotomy, or head injury, because it is thought to penetrate the blood–brain barrier more readily and achieve higher concentrations in cerebrospinal fluids and tissues. It also has minimal sodium- and water-retaining properties. With brain tumors, the drug is more effective in metastatic lesions and glioblastomas than astrocytomas and meningiomas. The therapeutic response to the medication is decreased intracranial pressure.

In patients treated for rheumatoid arthritis with corticosteroid agents, the nurse assesses for decreased pain and edema in the joints, increased mobility, and increased ability to perform activities of daily living.

Organ transplant recipients administered corticosteroids to prevent rejection of the transplanted tissues should have absence of signs and symptoms of rejections.

Assessing for Adverse Effects

The nurse assesses patients with adrenocortical insufficiency for fainting, weakness, anorexia, nausea, vomiting, hypotension, and shock. Patients with adrenocortical excess are assessed for fat accumulation on the face or dorsocervical fat, diabetes, nervousness, euphoria, anxiety, and behavioral changes.

Adrenocortical excess also leads to the musculoskeletal conditions, such as osteoporosis, fractures, muscle weakness and atrophy, and growth impairment in children. Cardiovascular effects include fluid and electrolyte changes, with fluid retention, edema, hypertension, heart failure, hypernatremia, hypokalemia, and metabolic acidosis. Ocular changes include increased intraocular pressure, glaucoma, and cataracts. The nurse assesses for increased susceptibility to infection and changes to the skin, including redness, thinning, stretch marks, and tissue injury. Females may experience menstrual irregularities, acne, and excessive facial hair.

Patient Teaching

Box 17.4 identifies patient teaching guidelines for corticosteroids.

BOX 17.4 — Patient Teaching Guidelines for Long-Term Corticosteroid Therapy

General Considerations

- Realize that in most instances, corticosteroids are used to relieve symptoms; they do not cure the underlying disease process. However, they can improve comfort and quality of life.
- Take the drug exactly as directed. Missing a dose or two, stopping the drug, changing the amount or time of administration, taking extra drug (except as specifically directed during stress situations), or any other alterations may result in complications. Some complications are relatively minor; several are serious or life threatening. When these drugs are being discontinued, the dosage is gradually reduced over several weeks. They must not be stopped abruptly.
- Wear a special medical alert bracelet or tag or carry an identification card stating the drug being taken; the dosage; the prescriber's name, address, and telephone number; and instructions for emergency treatment. If an accident or emergency situation occurs, healthcare providers must know about corticosteroid drug therapy to give additional amounts during the stress of the emergency.
- Report to all healthcare providers that corticosteroid drugs are being taken or have been taken within the past year. Current or previous corticosteroid therapy can influence treatment measures, and such knowledge increases the ability to provide appropriate treatment.
- Maintain regular medical supervision. This is extremely important so that the prescriber can detect adverse reactions, evaluate disease status, and evaluate drug response and indications for dosage change, as well as other responsibilities that can be carried out only with personal contact between the prescriber and the patient. Periodic blood tests, x-ray studies, and other tests may be performed during long-term corticosteroid therapy.
- Take no other drugs, prescription or nonprescription, without notifying the prescriber who is supervising corticosteroid therapy. Corticosteroid drugs influence reactions to other drugs, and some other drugs interact with corticosteroids to either increase or decrease their effects. Thus, taking other drugs can decrease the expected therapeutic benefits or increase the incidence or severity of adverse effects.
- Avoid exposure to infection when possible, including crowds and people known to have an infection. Wash hands frequently and thoroughly. These drugs increase the likelihood of infection, so preventive measures are necessary. If infection does occur, healing is likely to be slow.
- Practice safety measures to avoid accidents (e.g., falls and possible fractures due to osteoporosis, cuts or other

(Continued on page 330)

BOX 17.4 Patient Teaching Guidelines for Long-Term Corticosteroid Therapy (Continued)

injuries because of delayed wound healing, soft tissue trauma because of increased tendency to bruise easily).

- Weigh yourself frequently when starting corticosteroid therapy and at least weekly during long-term maintenance. An initial weight gain is likely to occur and is usually attributed to increased appetite. Later weight gains may be caused by fluid retention.
- Ask the prescriber about the amount and kind of activity or exercise needed. As a general rule, being as active as possible helps prevent or delay osteoporosis, a common adverse effect. However, increased activity may not be desirable for everyone.
- Follow instructions for other measures used in treatment of the particular condition (e.g., other drugs and physical therapy for rheumatoid arthritis). Such measures may allow smaller doses of corticosteroids and decrease adverse effects.
- Understand that the dosage may need to be temporarily increased with illness, surgery, or other stressful situations because corticosteroids impair the ability to respond to stress. Clarify with the prescriber predictable sources of stress and the amount of drug to be taken if the stress cannot be avoided.
- In addition to stressful situations, report sore throat, fever, or other signs of infection; weight gain of 5 lb or more in a week; or swelling in the ankles or elsewhere. These symptoms may indicate adverse drug effects, and changes in corticosteroid therapy may be indicated.
- Realize that muscle weakness and fatigue or disease symptoms may occur when drug dosage is reduced, withdrawn, or omitted (e.g., the nondrug day of alternate-day therapy). Although these symptoms may cause some discomfort, they should be tolerated if possible rather than increasing the corticosteroid dose. If severe, dosage or time of administration may have to be changed.
- Understand that dietary changes may be helpful in reducing some adverse effects. Decreasing salt intake may help decrease swelling. Eating high-potassium foods, such as citrus fruits and juices or bananas, may help prevent potassium loss. Adequate intake of calcium, protein, and vitamin D may help to prevent or delay osteoporosis, and vitamin may help to prevent excessive bruising.
- Anticipate that your prescriber will reduce your dose of oral corticosteroid, with the goal of stopping the drug entirely or continuing with a smaller dose. Long-term therapy should be used only when necessary because of the potential for serious adverse effects, and the lowest effective dose should be given.
- Understand that with local applications of corticosteroids, there is usually little systemic absorption and few adverse effects, compared with oral or injected drugs. When effective in relieving symptoms, it is better to use a local than a systemic corticosteroid. In some instances, combined systemic and local application allows administration of a lesser dose of the systemic drug.
- Be aware that commonly used local applications are applied topically for skin disorders, by oral inhalation for asthma, and by nasal inhalation for allergic rhinitis. Although long-term use is usually well tolerated, systemic toxicity can occur if excess corticosteroid is inhaled or if occlusive dressings are used over skin lesions. Thus, a corticosteroid for local application must be applied correctly and not overused.
- Know that corticosteroids are not the same as the steroids often abused by athletes and body builders. Those are anabolic steroids derived from testosterone, the male sex hormone.

Self- or Caregiver Administration

- Take an oral corticosteroid with a meal or snack to decrease GI upset.
- If taking the medication once a day or every other day, take before 9:00 a.m.; if taking multiple doses, take at evenly spaced intervals throughout the day.
- Report to the prescriber if unable to take a dose orally because of vomiting or some other problem. In some circumstances, the dose may need to be given by injection.
- If taking an oral corticosteroid in tapering doses, be sure to follow instructions exactly to avoid adverse effects.
- When applying a corticosteroid to skin lesions, do not apply more often than ordered and do not cover with an occlusive dressing unless specifically instructed to do so.
- With an intranasal corticosteroid, use on a regular basis (usually once or twice daily) for the best anti-inflammatory effects.
- With an oral inhalation corticosteroid, use on a regular schedule for anti-inflammatory effects. The drugs are *not* effective in relieving acute asthma attacks or shortness of breath and should not be used "as needed" for that purpose. Use metered-dose inhalers as follows (unless instructed otherwise by a healthcare provider):
  1. Shake canister thoroughly.
  2. Place canister between lips (both open and pursed lips have been recommended) or outside lips.
  3. Exhale completely.
  4. Activate canister while taking a slow, deep breath.
  5. Hold breath for 10 seconds or as long as possible.
  6. Wait at least 1 minute before taking additional inhalations.
  7. Rinse mouth after inhalations to decrease the incidence of oral thrush (a fungal infection).
  8. Rinse mouthpiece at least once per day.

Clinical Application 17.3

The home care nurse is visiting Mrs. Thompson. She says, "I am having itching in my vaginal area, and drinking citrus juices is painful." During the assessment, the nurse notices white patches in her mouth.
- What are the white patches in Mrs. Thompson's mouth?
- Why has she developed itching in the vaginal area?
- What is the cause of these symptoms?

NCLEX Success

4. A child is taking long-term systemic corticosteroids. What factor influences the child's diminished growth?
   A. hypokalemia
   B. fluid retention
   C. altered DNA synthesis
   D. increase in parathyroid hormone

5. A patient is being treated with long-term corticosteroid therapy. The patient's spouse has just received a diagnosis of terminal cancer. How is the spouse's diagnosis likely to affect the patient's treatment?
   A. The patient may need an increase in corticosteroids because of the stress.
   B. The patient may need a decrease in corticosteroids because of the increase in cortisol.
   C. The patient may need to be changed to a different corticosteroid because of the stress.
   D. The patient may need to be switched to a parenteral form of corticosteroid.

THE NURSING PROCESS

A concept map outlines the nursing process related to drug therapy considerations in this chapter. Additional nursing implications related to the disease process should also be considered in care decisions.

Assessment

With the initiation of corticosteroid therapy:
- For a patient receiving short-term corticosteroid therapy, assess the extent and severity of symptoms. This will be a baseline to evaluate the effectiveness of corticosteroid therapy.
- For a patient receiving long-term systemic corticosteroid therapy:
  - Assess for such conditions as diabetes mellitus, tuberculosis, and peptic ulcer disease, because corticosteroids may result in the development or exacerbation of these disorders. If one of these conditions is present, it is essential that corticosteroid therapy be altered and other medications given concomitantly.
  - Assess for signs and symptoms of infection. If acute infection is present, treatment with appropriate antibiotics either before corticosteroid drugs are started or concomitantly with corticosteroid therapy is necessary.
  - Assess for infection-related symptoms, which should decrease.
  - Assess for wound healing because corticosteroids impair healing.
- With previous or current corticosteroid therapy:
  - If corticosteroids have been prescribed in the past, assess the patient's past response to corticosteroids.
  - Assess the patient for significant sources of stress, such as hospitalization, diagnostic testing, infection, illness, and psychosocial problems.
  - Assess the type of systemic corticosteroid medication the patient is taking, the dosage and schedule of administration, the purpose for which the medication has been prescribed, and the length of time to be administered.
  - If the patient undergoes anesthesia and surgery, expect that he or she will commonly require higher doses of corticosteroids for several days. Specific regimens vary according to the type of anesthesia, surgical procedure, patient condition, prescriber preference, and other variables.
  - Expect that a patient undergoing an invasive diagnostic test may be given one extra dose of corticosteroid.
  - Assess for acute adrenal insufficiency.
  - Assess for signs and symptoms of adrenocortical excess and adverse drug effects.
  - Assess for signs and symptoms of the disease for which long-term corticosteroid therapy is given.

Outcomes of Therapy

The patient will
- Administer the drug correctly, and understand the adverse effects, including risk of infection.
- See a health care provider regularly to monitor for therapeutic and adverse drug effects.
- Seek the health care provider for strategies to cope with body image changes.
- Verbalize or demonstrate essential drug information.

Nursing Interventions

- Instruct the patient on the effects of steroid therapy.
- Assess for diminished inflammation.
- Assess for infection.
- Instruct on good handwashing.
- Instruct on the adverse effects of steroid therapy.
- Encourage activity to slow demineralization of bone.
- Instruct the patient to avoid stress and exposure to extreme temperatures.
- Instruct the patient to eat a diet high in protein, calcium, and vitamin D.
- Reverse or protective isolation is sometimes indicated for organ transplant patients receiving corticosteroid.
- Because long-term corticosteroid therapy weakens the skin and bones, there are risks of skin damage and fractures with even minor trauma; use care during ADLs and procedures.

Evaluation

- Interview and observe for relief of symptoms for which corticosteroids were prescribed.
- Interview and observe for accurate drug administration.
- Interview and observe for adverse drug effects on a regular basis.

Visit thePoint® *at* **http://thePoint.lww.com/Frandsen13e** *for answers to NCLEX Success questions (in Appendix A), answers to Clinical Application Case Studies (in Appendix B), and more!*

REFERENCES AND RESOURCES

Ceccato, A., Russo, A., Oscanoa, P., Tiseo, G., Gabamus, A., DiGiannatale, P., Nogas, S., Ciloniz, C., Menichetti, F., Niederman, M., Falcone, M., & Torres, A. (2021). Real-world corticosteroid use in sever pneumonia: A propensity-score-matched study. *Critical Care*, 25(1), 1–7. https://doi.org/10.1186/s13054-021-03840-x

Feinleib, J., Kwan, L. H., & Yamani, A. (2022). Postoperative nausea and vomiting. *UpToDate*. Lexi-Comp, Inc.

Ferguson, G. T., & Make, B. (2022). Management of refractory chronic obstructive pulmonary disease. *UpToDate*. Lexi-Comp, Inc.

Hesketh, P. J. (2022). Prevention and treatment of chemotherapy-induced nausea and vomiting in adults. *UpToDate*. Lexi-Comp, Inc.

Hinkle, J. H., Cheever, K. H., & Overbaugh, K. (2021). *Brunner & Suddarth's textbook of medical-surgical nursing* (15th ed.). Wolters Kluwer.

Kaufman, D. A. (2022). Glucocorticoid therapy in septic shock. *UpToDate*. Lexi-Comp, Inc.

Lempp, M. P., Sigler, M. A., Adesoye, A. A., Ponnuru, A., & DuVal, C. E. (2022). Assessment of glycemic control in veterans with chronic obstructive pulmonary disease, and type 2 diabetes mellitus on inhaled corticosteroid therapy. *Journal of Pharmacy Practice*, 35(1), 7–12. https://doi.org/10.1177/0897190020936870

Nieman, L. K. (2022a). Pharmacologic use of glucocorticoids. *UpToDate*. Lexi-Comp, Inc.

Nieman, L. K. (2022b). Treatment of adrenal insufficiency in adults. *UpToDate*. Lexi-Comp, Inc.

Norris, T. L. (2019). *Porth's Pathophysiology: Concepts of altered health status* (10th ed.). Wolters Kluwer.

Peppercorn, M. A., & Cheifetz, A. S. (2022). Overview of budesonide therapy in the treatment of inflammatory bowel disease in adults. *UpToDate*. Lexi-Comp, Inc.

Siegel, M., & Siemieniuk, R. (2022). Acute respiratory distress syndrome: Supportive care and oxygenation in adults. *UpToDate*. Lexi-Comp, Inc.

Stoller, J. K. (2022). COPD exacerbations: Management. *UpToDate*. Lexi-Comp, Inc.

UpToDate. (2022). *Drug Information*. Lexi-Comp, Inc.

CHAPTER 18

Drug Therapy With Beta-Lactam Antibacterial Agents

LEARNING OBJECTIVES

After studying this chapter, you should be able to:

1. Describe general characteristics of beta-lactam antibiotics.
2. Discuss the penicillins in relation to effectiveness, safety, spectrum of antibacterial activity, mechanism of action, indications for use, administration, observation of patient response, and teaching of patients.
3. Recognize the importance of questioning patients about allergies before the initial dose of all drugs, especially penicillins.
4. Describe characteristics of beta-lactamase inhibitor drugs.
5. Give the rationale for combining a penicillin and a beta-lactamase inhibitor drug.
6. Discuss the cephalosporins in relation to effectiveness, safety, spectrum of antibacterial activity, mechanism of action, indications for use, administration, observation of patient response, and teaching of patients.
7. Discuss the carbapenems in relation to effectiveness, safety, spectrum of antibacterial activity, mechanism of action, indications for use, administration, observation of patient response, and teaching of patients.
8. Discuss the one monobactam drug in relation to effectiveness, safety, spectrum of antibacterial activity, mechanism of action, indications for use, administration, observation of patient response, and teaching of patients.
9. Implement the nursing process when caring for patients receiving beta-lactam antibacterials.

CLINICAL APPLICATION CASE STUDY

Paul O'Brian, a 55-year-old professional musician who travels frequently, has no known drug allergies. He is being scheduled for the placement of a new cardiac pacemaker tomorrow. The physician orders that cefazolin be administered "on call" for the procedure (1 g IV).

KEY TERMS

Beta-lactamase: enzyme produced by some bacteria that attacks the beta-lactam ring rendering the drug ineffective and leading to a resistance to beta-lactam antibiotics

Cross-allergenicity: allergy to a drug of another class with a similar chemical structure

Extended-spectrum: bactericidal activity against a wide range of bacteria

Minimum inhibitory concentration: the lowest concentration of an antimicrobial drug that will inhibit the visible growth of a microorganism

Superinfection: infection after a previous infection; typically caused by microorganisms that are resistant to the antibiotics used previously

INTRODUCTION

This chapter discusses the pharmacologic care of the patient who is receiving a drug in the antibiotic class of beta-lactam antibacterials, specifically the penicillins, cephalosporins, carbapenems, and monobactams. Beta-lactam antibacterial drugs inhibit synthesis of bacterial cell walls by binding to proteins (penicillin-binding proteins; see Chapter 15) in bacterial cell membranes. This binding produces a defective cell wall that allows leakage of the intracellular contents, destroying the microorganisms. Beta-lactam antibacterial drugs are typically considered bactericidal.

Beta-lactam antibacterials derive their name from the beta-lactam ring that is part of their chemical structure. An intact beta-lactam ring is essential for the antibacterial activity of these drugs. Several Gram-positive and Gram-negative bacteria produce **beta-lactamases**, which are enzymes that disrupt the beta-lactam ring and inactivate the beta-lactam antibacterial drugs. This is the major mechanism by which microorganisms acquire resistance to these drugs. Penicillinase and cephalosporinase are beta-lactamase enzymes that act on penicillins and cephalosporins to render them resistant and ineffective. Patients receive beta-lactamase inhibitors concurrently with the beta-lactam antibacterial drugs to overcome this resistance.

Although a beta-lactam ring is common to all beta-lactam antibiotics, the characteristics of these drugs vary widely because of differences in their chemical structures. Because of these differences, the range of activity to particular bacteria is also different. The drugs may also differ in the routes of administration, susceptibility to beta-lactamase enzymes, and adverse effects. Table 18.1 lists the various types of beta-lactam antibiotics.

TABLE 18.1

Beta-Lactamase Antibacterials Administered for the Treatment of Infection

Drug Class	Prototype	Other Drugs in the Class
Penicillins	**Ampicillin**	Amoxicillin (Amoxil, Larotid) Carbenicillin indanyl sodium Penicillin G benzathine (Bicillin LA) Penicillin G procaine Penicillin V (Penicillin VK) Dicloxacillin Nafcillin Oxacillin Piperacillin Ampicillin–sulbactam (Unasyn) Amoxicillin–clavulanate (Augmentin) Piperacillin/tazobactam
Cephalosporins	**Cefazolin**	Cefadroxil Cephalexin Cefaclor Cefotetan Cefoxitin Cefprozil Cefuroxime Cefdinir Cefditoren Cefixime Cefotaxime Cefpodoxime Ceftazidime (Fortaz) Ceftibuten Ceftriaxone Cefepime (Maxipime) Ceftaroline (Teflaro) Ceftolozane–tazobactam (Zerbaxa) Ceftazidime–avibactam (Avycaz) Cefiderocol (Fetroja)
Carbapenems	**Imipenem–cilastatin** (Primaxin)	Ertapenem (Invanz) Meropenem (Merrem) Doripenem Meropenem–vaborbactam (Vabomere) Imipenem–relebactam (Recarbrio)
Monobactam	**Aztreonam** (Azactam)	

PENICILLINS

The penicillins are effective and safe, and they are among the most commonly prescribed antibacterials. The first antibiotic developed was penicillin, which was derived from the *Penicillium* mold. When penicillin was introduced, it was effective against many organisms. It was once necessary to give the drug parenterally because it was destroyed by gastric acid, and injections were painful. With extensive use, strains of drug-resistant staphylococci appeared. Scientists developed semisynthetic derivatives, formed by adding side chains to the penicillin nucleus, to increase gastric acid stability, beta-lactamase stability, and antimicrobial spectrum of activity, especially against Gram-negative microorganisms. As a class, penicillins usually are more effective in treating infections caused by Gram-positive bacteria than those caused by Gram-negative bacteria. However, their clinical usefulness varies significantly according to the subgroup or individual drug and microbial patterns of resistance.

Ampicillin is the prototype penicillin.

Pharmacokinetics

After absorption, ampicillin is widely distributed. Penetration into the cerebrospinal fluid (CSF) occurs only with inflamed meninges. The kidneys rapidly excrete ampicillin, largely as unchanged drug, and it produces high drug concentrations in the urine. It is present in breast milk, and the volume of distribution increases during pregnancy, when the half-life, generally 1 to 2 hours, is decreased.

Action

Ampicillin, like all penicillins, inhibits bacterial cell wall synthesis by binding to one or multiple penicillin-binding proteins.

Use

Clinical indications for use of ampicillin include bacterial infections caused by susceptible microorganisms. Healthcare providers use the drug in the treatment or prophylaxis of infective endocarditis. The drug's broad spectrum is often useful in skin, soft tissue, respiratory, gastrointestinal (GI), and genitourinary infections. The broad-spectrum coverage of ampicillin extends its activity against Gram-negative bacilli. Note that the incidence of resistance among streptococci, staphylococci, and other microorganisms continues to increase.

Table 18.2 provides route and dosage information for the individual penicillins.

TABLE 18.2 DRUGS AT A GLANCE: Penicillins

Drug	Routes and Dosage Ranges	
	Adults	Children
Penicillins G and V		
These drugs remain effective for a limited number of uses. They are the drugs of choice for the treatment of streptococcal pharyngitis, for prevention of recurrent attacks in patients who have had previous acute rheumatic fever due to group A *Streptococcus*, and for treatment of neurosyphilis.		
Penicillin G benzathine (Pfizerpen; Crystapen)	IM 1.2–2.4 million units in a single dose Prophylaxis of recurrent rheumatic fever, IM 1.2 million units every 3–4 wk Treatment of syphilis, IM 2.4 million units (1.2 million units in each buttock) as a single dose	IM 25,000–50,000 units/kg (maximum 2.4 million units) Prophylaxis of recurrent rheumatic fever, 25,000–50,000 units/kg times one dose q3–4wk (maximum 1.2 million units)
Penicillin G procaine	IV, IM 600,000–4.8 million units daily in 1 or 2 doses	IM 25,000–50,000 units/kg/d in divided doses every 12–24 h
Penicillin V (Apo-Pen VK, Novo-Pen-VK, Nu-Pen-VK)	PO 125–500 mg every 6–8 h	PO 125–250 mg twice daily
Penicillinase-Resistant (Antistaphylococcal) Penicillins		
Penicillinase-resistant penicillins are the drugs of choice for methicillin-susceptible *Staphylococcus aureus*. Although called "methicillin resistant," these staphylococcal microorganisms are also resistant to other antistaphylococcal penicillins.		
Dicloxacillin	PO 125–1,000 mg every 6 h	Not recommended in newborns ≤40 kg: 12.5–100 mg/kg/d divided every 6 h ≥40 kg: 125–500 mg every 6 h
Nafcillin	IM 500 mg every 4–6 h IV 500 mg–2 g every 4–6 h; maximum daily dose 18 g for serious infections	IM 25 mg/kg every 12 h IV 50–200 mg/kg/d in divided doses every 4–6 h

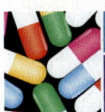

TABLE 18.2
DRUGS AT A GLANCE: Penicillins (Continued)

Drug	Routes and Dosage Ranges	
	Adults	**Children**
Oxacillin	IM, IV 250–2,000 mg every 4–6 h	≤40 kg: IM, IV 100–200 mg/kg/d in divided doses every 6 h >40 kg: same as adults

Aminopenicillins
The aminopenicillins are drugs of choice for prevention of bacterial endocarditis due to procedures that produce transient bacteremia. Ampicillin is excreted mainly by the kidneys; thus, it is useful in some urinary tract infections (UTIs). Because some is excreted in bile, it is useful in biliary tract infections not caused by biliary obstruction. It is used in the treatment of bronchitis, sinusitis, and otitis media.

Drug	Adults	Children
(P) Ampicillin (✶ Novo-Ampicillin)	PO, IM, IV 250–500 mg every 6 h. In severe infections, doses up to 2 g every 4 h may be given IV	Infants/children: PO 50–100 mg/kg/d in divided doses every 6 h (maximum dose 2–4 g/d) IM, IV 100–400 mg/kg/d in divided doses every 6 h (maximum dose 12 g/d)
Amoxicillin (Amoxil, Larotid; ✶ Apo-Amoxi, Mylan-Amoxicillin, Novamoxin, NPR-Amoxicillin, Nu-Amoxi, PHL-Amoxicillin, Pro-Amox-250, Pro-Amox-500)	PO 250–500 mg every 8 h or 500–875 mg every 12 h	3 mo or more: PO 20–30 mg/kg/d in divided doses every 12 h More than 3 mo: 20–50 mg/kg/d in divided doses every 8–12 h
Piperacillin (✶ Piperacillin for injection)	IM, IV 200–300 mg/kg/d in divided doses every q4–6 h. IM injections should not exceed 2 g/injection and use should be reserved for uncomplicated infections. Usual adult dosage, 3–4 g every 4–6 h; maximum daily dose 24 g	Infants/children/adolescents (non–FDA approved) ≥12 y IV 200–300 mg/kg/d in divided doses every 4–6 h; maximum daily dose 24 g/d

Penicillin–Beta-Lactamase Inhibitor Combinations
The beta-lactamase inhibitors display negligible antimicrobial activity but contain the beta-lactam ring. Coadministered with beta-lactam antibiotics, the inhibitors' sole function is to bind with the beta-lactamases (enzymes that degrade the beta-lactam ring) to prevent inactivation of the beta-lactam antibiotics.

Drug	Adults	Children
Ampicillin–sulbactam (Unasyn)	IM, IV 1.5–3 g q6h (maximum dose of 4 g/d of sulbactam)	1 y or older: IV 100–400 mg/kg/d in divided doses q6h (maximum 8 g ampicillin/d; 12 g Unasyn) Doses up to 300 mg/kg/d may be given for severe infections in infants older than 1 mo of age
Amoxicillin–clavulanate (Augmentin, Augmentin XR; ✶ Amoxi-Clav, Apo-Amoxi-Clav, Clavulin, Novo-Clavamoxin, ratio-Aclavulanate)	PO 250–1,000 mg every 8 h or 875 mg every 12 h	≥40 kg: same as adults <40 kg: 20–90 mg/kg/d in divided doses every 8–12 h
Piperacillin/tazobactam (Zosyn; ✶ AJ-PIP/TAZ, piperacillin, and tazobactam for injection)	IV 2.25–4.5 g every 6–8 h	≥40 kg: same as adults IV 80–100 mg/kg/d based on piperacillin component every 8 h

Quality and Safety Alert: Safety

Before prescribing ampicillin or other penicillins for streptococcal infections, clinicians should perform culture and susceptibility studies and be aware of local patterns of streptococcal susceptibility and resistance.

Patient-related variables specific to the use of ampicillin include the following:

- Age:
  - Use caution in neonates because immature kidney function slows drug elimination. Dosage should be based on age, weight, severity of the infection being treated, and kidney function.

- Older patients are susceptible to **superinfections** (infections after a previous infection, typically caused by microorganisms that are resistant to the antibiotics used earlier) when given any anti-infective agent.
- Reproduction, pregnancy, and lactation:
  - Ampicillin crosses the placenta.
  - Ampicillin is present in breast milk but considered acceptable to use at routine doses while breast-feeding.
- Abnormal kidney function and hepatic impairment:
  - Because ampicillin is excreted primarily by the kidneys, use caution with abnormal kidney function.
  - Ampicillin can be used in patients with hepatic impairment, as can almost all the penicillins.
  - Use caution when using amoxicillin–clavulanate (Augmentin) in patients with hepatic injury or destruction. No specific recommendations for dosage adjustment are available.
  - Contraindications include development of cholestatic jaundice and hepatic dysfunction with previous use of the drug. Cholestatic liver impairment usually subsides when the drug is stopped.

> **BOX 18.1   Drug Interactions: Ampicillin**
>
> **Drugs That Increase the Effects of Ampicillin**
> - Allopurinol
>   *Increases the incidence of skin rash*
> - Clavulanic acid
>   *Overcomes resistance in bacteria that secrete beta-lactamase*
> - Probenecid
>   *Inhibits the kidney tubular secretion*
> - Uricosuric drugs
>   *Block kidney excretion*
>
> **Drugs That Decrease the Effects of Ampicillin**
> - Chloroquine
>   *Decreases the serum concentration*
> - Fusidic acid
>   *Diminishes the therapeutic effect*
> - Tetracycline derivatives
>   *Diminish the therapeutic effect*

Adverse Effects

The most common adverse effects of ampicillin are hypersensitivity reactions, including rash and/or anaphylactoid reactions. Commonly reported GI adverse effects include abdominal pain, diarrhea, gastritis, and nausea and vomiting. Nephropathy, such as interstitial nephritis, although infrequent, has occurred with all penicillins. It is most often associated with high doses of parenteral penicillins and is attributed to hypersensitivity reactions.

In addition, high doses of penicillin G irritate the central nervous system (CNS). The adverse effects related to CNS toxicity include confusion, lethargy, twitching, dysphagia, seizures, and coma. The penicillinase-resistant penicillins, such as nafcillin, may result in hepatotoxicity. The extended-spectrum penicillins may lead to hypokalemia and hypernatremia.

Note that the FDA has issued a **BOXED WARNING** to alert healthcare providers that inadvertent IV administration of penicillin G benzathine may result in cardiopulmonary arrest and death. Long-acting repository forms have additives that decrease their solubility in tissue fluids and delay their absorption.

Contraindications

Contraindications include hypersensitivity or allergic reactions to any penicillin formulation. An allergic reaction to one penicillin means the patient is allergic to all drugs of the penicillin class. The potential for **cross-allergenicity**, also referred to as cross-sensitivity, is the allergy to a drug of another class with a similar chemical structure. The cephalosporins and carbapenems each possess the characteristic bicyclic core structure. This chemical unit is thought to be most responsible for beta-lactam hypersensitivity. Recent data suggest that the incidence is less than 1%, lower than previously thought.

Nursing Implications

Preventing Interactions

Many medications interact with ampicillin, increasing or decreasing its effects (Box 18.1). The administration of the herbal supplement khat decreases the absorption of ampicillin. In addition, ampicillin inhibits the kidney tubular secretion of methotrexate, which may lead to prolonged and higher drug concentrations of methotrexate.

Penicillins are often given concomitantly with aminoglycosides for serious infections, such as those caused by *Pseudomonas aeruginosa*. These drugs should not be admixed in a syringe, given in an IV solution, or administered via Y-site because the penicillin inactivates the aminoglycoside. If feasible, dose separation is ideal.

Administering the Medication

It is necessary to give oral ampicillin, like most oral penicillins, on an empty stomach, approximately 1 hour before or 2 hours after a meal. Patients should take the oral drug with a full glass of water, preferably to promote absorption and decrease inactivation, which may occur in an acidic environment. If need be, they may take it with food; however, the absorption rate decreases with food. Oral suspensions of the drug are stable for 7 days at room temperature and 14 days when refrigerated.

When diluted with 0.9% sodium chloride, ampicillin is stable for 8 hours for concentrations up to 30 mg/mL. It is stable for only 1 hour when diluted with dextrose-containing solutions for concentrations of 10 to 20 mg/mL. It is necessary to give IV penicillins for the full prescribed course of treatment to prevent complications such as rheumatic fever, endocarditis, and glomerulonephritis. IV concentrations should not exceed 30 mg/mL.

Assessing for Therapeutic Effects

When assessing for the therapeutic effects of ampicillin or any drug within the penicillin class, it is imperative to determine if the signs and symptoms of infection have decreased. For example, the nurse assesses whether the patient is afebrile, whether the pain at the site of infection has decreased, or whether there is improvement in the characteristics of the wound. It is not necessary to obtain drug levels when administering ampicillin or any of the antimicrobials in the penicillin class. However, blood levels of a penicillin need to be maintained above the **minimum inhibitory concentration** (MIC) of the microorganisms causing the infection. The MIC is the lowest concentration of an antimicrobial drug that will inhibit the visible growth of a microorganism. Thus, continuous or extended infusions may be beneficial with serious infections, especially those caused by relatively resistant organisms such as *Pseudomonas* or *Acinetobacter*.

Assessing for Adverse Effects

The nurse carefully assesses the characteristics of a rash, if present. It is necessary to distinguish, if possible, a hypersensitivity reaction from a nonallergic ampicillin rash. When administering ampicillin, it is recommended that serum creatinine and blood urea nitrogen (BUN) be monitored.

Patient Teaching

The nurse instructs patients to take oral penicillins for the full prescribed course of treatment to prevent complications. Box 18.2 outlines patient teaching guidelines for ampicillin and other oral penicillins.

Other Drugs in the Class

The **extended-spectrum** drugs (e.g., piperacillin, a derivative of ampicillin) and penicillin–beta-lactamase inhibitor combinations (e.g., Zosyn), which have bactericidal activity against a wide range of bacteria, are most likely to be used in critical care units for the treatment of respiratory diseases such as pneumonia, bloodstream, or other infections. Through chemical modification, these extended-spectrum drugs affect additional types of bacteria, typically Gram-negative bacteria. With cephalosporins, third- and fourth-generation drugs are commonly used and usually given by intermittent intravenous (IV) infusions every 8 or 12 hours.

Antistaphylococcal Penicillins and Aminopenicillins

The choice of a beta-lactam antibacterial depends on the organism causing the infection, severity of the infection, and other factors. Penicillin G or the aminopenicillin amoxicillin is the drug of choice in many infections. Other aminopenicillins like piperacillin (paired with beta-lactamase inhibitor tazobactam) are indicated in *Pseudomonas* infections. Antistaphylococcal penicillin is indicated in staphylococcal infections; the antistaphylococcal drugs of choice are nafcillin or oxacillin for IV use and dicloxacillin for oral use.

With intramuscular (IM) penicillins, it is necessary to inject them deep into large muscle masses to decrease tissue irritation. With IV penicillins, it is necessary to usually first dilute reconstituted penicillins in 50 to 100 mL of 5% dextrose or 0.9% sodium chloride injection and infuse them over 30 to 60 minutes to minimize vascular irritation and phlebitis. It should be noted that ticarcillin may cause decreased platelet aggregation.

Penicillin–Beta-Lactamase Inhibitor Combinations

Beta-lactamase inhibitors are drugs with a beta-lactam structure but minimal antibacterial activity. Newer agents have been developed, which are non–beta-lactam beta-lactamase inhibitors. They bind with and inactivate the beta-lactamase enzymes produced by many bacteria (e.g., *Escherichia coli*; *Klebsiella*, *Enterobacter*, and *Bacteroides* species; *Staphylococcus aureus*). When combined with a penicillin, the beta-lactamase inhibitor protects the penicillin from destruction by the enzymes and extends the penicillin's spectrum of antimicrobial activity. Thus, the combination drug may be effective in infections caused by bacteria that are resistant to a beta-lactam antibiotic alone.

Clavulanate, sulbactam, and tazobactam are the beta-lactamase inhibitors available in combinations with penicillins.

- Ampicillin–sulbactam is available as Unasyn, in vials with 1 g of ampicillin and 0.5 g of sulbactam or 2 g of ampicillin and 1 g of sulbactam.
- Amoxicillin and clavulanate is marketed as Augmentin, in 250-, 500-, and 875-mg tablets, each of which contains 125 mg of clavulanate.

BOX 18.2 *Patient Teaching Guidelines for Oral Penicillins*

General Considerations

- Do not take any penicillin if you have ever had an allergic reaction to penicillin in which you had difficulty breathing, swelling, or skin rash. However, some people call a minor stomach upset an allergic reaction, which is incorrect, and they are not given penicillin when that is the best antibiotic in a given situation.
- Complete the full course of drug treatment for greater effectiveness and prevention of secondary infection with drug-resistant bacteria.
- Follow instructions carefully about amount and frequency of dosing. Drug effectiveness depends on maintaining adequate blood levels. Penicillins often need more frequent administration than some other antibiotics, because they are rapidly excreted by the kidneys.

Self- or Caregiver Administration

- Take most penicillins on an empty stomach, 1 hour before or 2 hours after a meal. Penicillin V, amoxicillin, and Augmentin can be taken with food. (Take Augmentin with meals to increase absorption and decrease GI upset.)
- Take each dose with a full glass of water; do not take with orange juice or with other acidic fluids (they may destroy the drug).
- Take at even intervals, preferably around the clock.
- Shake liquid penicillins well, so they are mixed thoroughly, and measure the dose accurately.
- Discard liquid penicillin after 1 week if it is stored at room temperature or after 2 weeks if it is refrigerated. Liquid forms deteriorate and should not be taken after their expiration dates.
- Report skin rash, hives, itching, severe diarrhea, shortness of breath, fever, sore throat, black tongue, or any unusual bleeding to your healthcare provider. These symptoms may indicate an allergy to penicillin.

> **Quality and Safety Alert: Safety**
>
> Two 250-mg tablets are not equivalent to one 500-mg tablet.
> - Augmentin is also available as 1,000-mg extended-release tablets containing 62.5 mg of clavulanate. In addition, a chewable formulation is available as 200 mg of amoxicillin and 28.5 mg of clavulanate, as well as 400 mg of amoxicillin and 57 mg of clavulanate.
> - Piperacillin/tazobactam is marketed as Zosyn, an IV formulation. Patients with sepsis may require loading doses of 3.375 to 4.5 g over 30 minutes. Piperacillin–tazobactam may be given as an extended infusion over 4 hours to maximize the time blood levels of the drug are above the MIC of the organism.

NCLEX Success

1. A nurse is preparing to administer the first dose of piperacillin/tazobactam to a patient in an infusion clinic. The nurse should take which of the following precautions?
   A. Ask the patient about past allergic reactions to penicillins.
   B. Ask the patient about past allergic reactions to aminoglycosides.
   C. Mix the piperacillin/tazobactam with lidocaine to reduce pain of infusion.
   D. Instruct the patient to eat a snack to decrease stomach upset from piperacillin/tazobactam.

CEPHALOSPORINS

Cephalosporins are a widely used group of drugs derived from a fungus and closely related chemically to the penicillins. Cephalosporins are broad-spectrum agents with activity against both Gram-positive and Gram-negative bacteria. Compared with penicillins, these drugs are generally less active against Gram-positive organisms but more active against Gram-negative ones. Although technically cefoxitin and cefotetan are not cephalosporins, they are categorized with the cephalosporins because of their similarities to the group.

Classification

Cephalosporins are classified into five subgroups, or "generations," based on their pharmacology and spectrum of activity.

First-Generation Cephalosporins

The first cephalosporin, cephalothin, is no longer available for clinical use. However, it may be used to determine susceptibility to first-generation cephalosporins, which have essentially the same spectrum of antimicrobial activity. In general, first-generation cephalosporins have strong activity against Gram-positive bacteria and poor activity against Gram-negative bacteria. Therefore, these drugs are effective against streptococci, staphylococci (except methicillin-resistant *S. aureus* [MRSA]), *Shigella*, *E. coli*, *Proteus mirabilis*, *Klebsiella* spp., and *Bacteroides* species (except *Bacteroides fragilis*). They are not effective against *Enterobacter*, *Pseudomonas*, and *Serratia* species.

Often, healthcare providers use first-generation cephalosporins for surgical prophylaxis, especially with prosthetic implants, because Gram-positive organisms such as staphylococci cause most infections of surgical sites. Prescribers may also order them for treatment of infections caused by susceptible organisms in body sites where drug penetration and host defenses are adequate.

 Cefazolin, the prototype cephalosporin, is the drug of choice for surgical prophylaxis in most surgical procedures. Some advantages of cefazolin over other first-generation cephalosporins include less frequent dosing, higher blood levels after parenteral administration, and increased Gram-positive coverage. Cefazolin is also the drug of choice for methicillin-susceptible *S. aureus* (MSSA).

Second-Generation Cephalosporins

Second-generation cephalosporins are more active against some Gram-negative organisms and somewhat less active against Gram-positive cocci than the first-generation agents. Thus, they may be effective in infections resistant to other antibiotics, including infections caused by *Haemophilus influenzae*, *Klebsiella* species, *E. coli*, and some strains of *Proteus*. Because each of these drugs has a different antimicrobial spectrum, susceptibility tests must be performed for each drug rather than for the entire group, as may be done with first-generation drugs. Cefoxitin (Mefoxin) and cefotetan (Cefotan), for example, are active against *B. fragilis*, an anaerobic organism resistant to most drugs.

Often, other uses for second-generation cephalosporins also include surgical prophylaxis, especially for gynecologic and colorectal surgery. In the past, prescribers ordered the drugs empirically for treatment of intra-abdominal infections such as pelvic inflammatory disease, diverticulitis, and other infections caused by organisms inhabiting pelvic and colorectal areas (perhaps caused by penetrating wounds of the abdomen). This practice is no longer recommended because of the increasing resistance of *Bacteroides* species to these agents.

Third-Generation Cephalosporins

Third-generation cephalosporins further extend the spectrum of activity against Gram-negative organisms. In addition to activity against the usual enteric pathogens (e.g., *E. coli*, *Proteus*, and *Klebsiella* species), they are also active against several strains resistant to other antibiotics and to first- and second-generation cephalosporins. Thus, they may be useful in infections caused by unusual strains of enteric organisms such as the group *Enterobacterales* (which includes *Citrobacter*, *Serratia*, *Enterobacter*, *P. mirabilis*, and *E. coli*). Another difference is the ability of third-generation cephalosporins (ceftriaxone and cefuroxime) to penetrate inflamed meninges to reach therapeutic concentrations in CSF. Thus, they may be useful in meningeal infections caused by common pathogens, including *H. influenzae*, *Neisseria meningitidis*, and *Streptococcus pneumoniae*. Although some of the drugs are active against *Pseudomonas* organisms (ceftazidime), drug-resistant strains may emerge when this particular cephalosporin is used alone for treatment of pseudomonal infection.

Overall, cephalosporins gain Gram-negative activity and lose Gram-positive activity as they move from the first to the third generation. The second- and third-generation drugs are more active against Gram-negative organisms because they are more resistant to the beta-lactamase enzymes (cephalosporinases) produced by some bacteria to inactivate cephalosporins.

Fourth-Generation Cephalosporins

Fourth-generation cephalosporins have a greater spectrum of antimicrobial activity and greater stability against breakdown by beta-lactamase enzymes compared with third-generation drugs. Cefepime, the first fourth-generation cephalosporin to be developed, is active against both Gram-positive and Gram-negative organisms. With Gram-positive organisms, it is active against streptococci and staphylococci (except for methicillin-resistant staphylococci). With Gram-negative organisms, its activity against *P. aeruginosa* is similar to that of ceftazidime, and its activity against *Enterobacterales* is greater than that of third-generation cephalosporins. Moreover, cefepime retains activity against strains of *Enterobacterales* and *P. aeruginosa* that have acquired resistance to third-generation agents. A newer fourth-generation cephalosporin, cefiderocol (Fetroja), is a siderophore cephalosporin with Gram-negative activity. Cefiderocol uses bacterial iron-transport mechanisms to selectively bring the drug into the bacteria where it can exert its effects. Cefiderocol is typically reserved for multidrug-resistant organisms.

Fifth-Generation Cephalosporins

Ceftaroline (Teflaro) is an IV cephalosporin used for the treatment of community-acquired pneumonia and skin infections. It is the first cephalosporin to be considered active against resistant Gram-positive organisms, such as MRSA, vancomycin-resistant *S. aureus* (VRSA), vancomycin-insensitive *S. aureus* (VISA), and heteroresistant VISA. Because ceftaroline retains activity against VISA and VRSA, it is often used off-label in vancomycin failures.

Pharmacokinetics

After the cephalosporins are absorbed, they achieve therapeutic concentrations in most body fluids and tissues, with maximum concentrations in the liver and kidneys. However, many cephalosporins do not reach therapeutic levels in the CSF. Most third-generation cephalosporins achieve more consistent CSF penetration in those patients with inflamed meninges.

Cefazolin is distributed into most body tissues and crosses the placenta. The onset of action is rapid with both IV and IM administration. The drug peaks at the end of IV infusion and within 1 to 2 hours with IM injection. The duration of action is 6 to 12 hours. The drug, which is largely excreted unchanged via the kidneys, concentrates in the urine. Thus, metabolism is not hepatic. Therefore, no dosage adjustments are necessary with hepatic impairment.

Action

Cefazolin inhibits the third and last step of bacterial wall synthesis by binding to one or more penicillin-binding proteins.

Use

Cefazolin is a frequently used parenteral agent. It reaches a higher serum concentration, is more protein bound, and has a slower rate of elimination than other first-generation drugs. These factors prolong serum half-life, which means that cefazolin can be given less frequently.

Clinical indications for the use of the cephalosporins include surgical prophylaxis and treatment of infections of the respiratory tract, skin and soft tissues, bones and joints, urinary tract, brain and spinal cord, and bloodstream (septicemia). In infections caused by MRSA, cephalosporins are not clinically effective even if in vitro testing indicates susceptibility (except for the newest cephalosporin, ceftaroline). Infections caused by *Neisseria gonorrhoeae*, at one time susceptible to penicillin, are now treated with a third-generation cephalosporin such as ceftriaxone.

The particular drug used in surgical prophylaxis depends largely on the type of organism likely to be encountered in the operative area. First-generation cephalosporins, mainly cefazolin, are used for procedures associated with Gram-positive postoperative infections because of activity against streptococci and methicillin-susceptible staphylococci. Second-generation cephalosporins, mainly cefotetan and cefoxitin, are often used for abdominal procedures, especially gynecologic and colorectal surgery, in which enteric Gram-negative postoperative infections may occur. Third-generation cephalosporins should not be used for surgical prophylaxis because they are less active against staphylococci than cefazolin, and the Gram-negative organisms the third-generation cephalosporins are most useful against are rarely encountered in elective surgery.

Additionally, fourth- and fifth-generation cephalosporins are not typically used for surgical prophylaxis. Widespread usage for prophylaxis promotes emergence of drug-resistant organisms.

A single dose of a cephalosporin is usually sufficient, although repeat doses are necessary in patients undergoing a surgical procedure exceeding 2 to 4 hours or procedures involving major blood loss. (Postoperative doses are no longer recommended, with exceptions sometimes made for cardiac procedures. If cephalosporins are used, they should generally not be given more than 24 hours after surgery.) Blood levels need to be maintained above the MIC of the microorganisms causing the infection being treated for at least 40% to 50% of the dosing interval. Continuous or extended infusion strategies may be beneficial with serious infections, especially those caused by relatively resistant organisms such as *Pseudomonas* or *Acinetobacter*.

Table 18.3 provides important route and dosage information about cephalosporins.

> **Quality and Safety Alert: Patient-Centered Care**
>
> When used perioperatively, cephalosporins should be given within 60 minutes before the first skin incision is made so the drug has time to reach therapeutic serum and tissue concentrations.

Patient-related variables specific to the use of cefazolin include the following:
- Age:
  - Use with caution in neonates because immature kidney function slows elimination.
  - In children, dosage should be based on age, weight, severity of the infection, and kidney function.

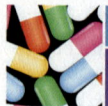

TABLE 18.3
DRUGS AT A GLANCE: Cephalosporins

Drug	Characteristics/Indications	Routes and Dosage Ranges Adults	Children
First Generation			
Cefazolin (cefazolin for injection)	Active against streptococci, staphylococci, *Neisseria*, *Salmonella*, *Shigella*, *Escherichia*, *Klebsiella*, *Listeria*, *Bacillus*, *Haemophilus influenzae*, *Corynebacterium diphtheriae*, *Proteus mirabilis*, and *Bacteroides* (except *B. fragilis*)	IM, IV 1–2 g every 8 h (maximum dose 12 g/d)	IM, IV 25–100 mg/kg/d in divided doses every 6–8 h (maximum dose 6 g/d)
Cefadroxil (Apo-Cefadroxil, PRO-Cefadroxil, Teva-Cefadroxil)	Active against streptococci such as *Streptococcus pyogenes*, staphylococci, *Escherichia*, *P. mirabilis*, and *Klebsiella* Prosthetic joint infection: active against *Staphylococcus* (oxacillin susceptible)	PO 1 g/d in a single or 2 divided doses for 10 d Prosthetic joint infection: 500 mg every 12 h	PO 30 mg/kg/d in a single dose or divided every 12 h
Cephalexin (Apo-Cephalex, Dom-Cephalexin, Keflex, PMS Cephalexin, Teva-Cephalexin)	Active against streptococci such as *Streptococcus pyogenes*, *Staphylococcus aureus*, *P. mirabilis*, *Klebsiella pneumoniae*, *H. influenzae*, and *Moraxella catarrhalis*	PO 250–500 mg every 6–8 h	>1 y to <15 y: PO 25–100 mg/kg/d in divided doses every 6–8 h (maximum dose 4 g/d)
Second Generation			
Cefaclor (Apo-Cefaclor, Ceclor, Novo-Cefaclor)	Active against streptococci and staphylococci	PO 200–500 mg every 8 h	PO 20–40 mg/kg/d in divided doses every 8–12 h for 7 d
Cefotetan (Cefotan)	Effective against most organisms except *Pseudomonas* Highly resistant to beta-lactamase enzymes	IV, IM 1–6 g/d in divided doses every 12 h Surgical prophylaxis, IV 1–2 g 30–60 min before surgery	IV, IM 20–40 mg/kg every 12 h (maximum 6 g/d)
Cefoxitin (Mefoxin; cefoxitin for injection)	The first cephamycin (derived from a different fungus than cephalosporins) Possible major clinical use: stems from increased activity against *B. fragilis*, an organism resistant to most other antimicrobial drugs	IV 1–2 g every 6–8 h Surgical prophylaxis, IV 1 or 2 g 30–60 min before surgery	IV 80–160 mg/kg/d in divided doses every 4–6 h. Do not exceed 12 g/d
Cefprozil (Apo-Cefprozil, Auro-Cefprozil)		PO 500 mg every 24 h for 10 d (administer >10 d for *Streptococcus pyogenes*)	Otitis media: ≥6 mo PO 7.5 mg/kg/dose Tonsillitis: 2–12 y PO 7.5 mg/kg/dose every 12 h (maximum dose 1,000 mg/d)
Cefuroxime (Zinacef; Apo-Cefuroxime, Auro-Cefuroxime, Ceftin, cefuroxime for injection, PRO-Cefuroxime)	Similar to other second-generation cephalosporins Penetrates CSF in the presence of inflamed meninges	PO 250–500 mg every 12 h for 10 d IV, IM 500 mg–1.5 g every 6–8 h Surgical prophylaxis, IV 1.5 g 30–60 min before initial skin incision	PO 20–30 mg/kg/d in two divided doses for 10 d IV, IM 75–150 mg/kg/d in divided doses every 6–8 h (maximum dose 6 g/d)

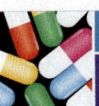

TABLE 18.3
DRUGS AT A GLANCE: Cephalosporins (Continued)

Drug	Characteristics/Indications	Routes and Dosage Ranges Adults	Children
Third Generation			
Cefdinir	Active against *H. influenzae*, *Streptococcus pneumoniae*, and *S. pyogenes*	PO 300 mg twice/d for 5–10 d or 600 g daily for 10 d	PO 7–14 mg/kg twice/d for 5–10 d
Cefditoren	Active against *Streptococcus pneumoniae*, *S. pyogenes*, and *M. catarrhalis*	PO 200–400 mg/d twice daily for 10 d	>12 y: refer to adult dosing
Cefixime (Suprax; ✦ Auro-Cefixime, Suprax)	Active against *Escherichia*, *P. mirabilis*, *H. influenzae*, *Streptococcus pneumoniae*, and *Klebsiella*	PO 400 mg daily in divided doses every 12–24 h	PO 8 mg/kg divided doses every 12–24 h
Cefotaxime (✦ cefotaxime sodium for injection, Claforan)	Activity against most Gram-positive and Gram-negative bacteria, including several strains resistant to other antibiotics. Recommended for serious infections caused by susceptible microorganisms	IV, IM 1–2 g every 4–12 h; maximum dose 12 g/d	IV, IM >50 kg: same as adults <50 kg to 12 y and age >1 mo: IV, IM 50–180 mg/kg/d, in divided doses every 6–8 h
Cefpodoxime	Active against *Streptococcus pyogenes*, *H. influenzae*, *K. pneumoniae*, *Staphylococcus aureus*, *P. mirabilis*, and *Staphylococcus saprophyticus*	PO 100–400 mg every 12 h for 10 d	PO ≥2 mo to <12 y 10 mg/kg/d divided every 12 h ≥12 y 100–400 mg every 12 h
Ceftazidime (Fortaz, Tazicef; ✦ ceftazidime for injection, Fortaz)	Active against Gram-positive and Gram-negative organisms. Especially effective against Gram-negative organisms, including *P. aeruginosa* and other bacterial strains resistant to aminoglycosides. Indicated for serious infections caused by susceptible organisms	IV, IM 500–2,000 mg every 8–12 h Cystic fibrosis: 90–150 mg/kg/d	Mild infections: IM, IV 30–50 mg/kg/d divided every 8 h (maximum dose 3,000 mg/d) Severe infections: 200 mg/kg/d divided every 8 h (maximum dose 6 g/d)
Ceftibuten	Active against *Streptococcus pneumoniae*, *S. pyogenes*, and *M. catarrhalis*	PO 400 mg daily for 10 d	6 mo to <12 y: 9 mg/kg/dose for 10 d (maximum dose 400 mg/d) ≥12 y: refer to adult dosing
Ceftriaxone (✦ ceftriaxone for injection)	First third-generation cephalosporin approved for once-daily dosing. Antibacterial activity against most Gram-positive and Gram-negative bacteria, including several strains resistant to other antibiotics	IV, IM 1–2 g every 12–24 h	Infants/children IM, IV 50–100 mg/kg/d in 1–2 divided doses (maximum dose 4 g/d) Meningitis, IV, IM 100 mg/kg/d, not to exceed 4 g daily, in divided doses every 12 h

(Continued on page 344)

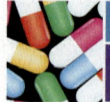

TABLE 18.3
DRUGS AT A GLANCE: Cephalosporins (Continued)

Drug	Characteristics/Indications	Routes and Dosage Ranges	
		Adults	**Children**
Fourth Generation			
Cefepime (Maxipime)	Indicated for use in sepsis; in severe infections of the lower respiratory and urinary tract, skin and soft tissue, and female reproductive tract; and in febrile neutropenic patients May be used as monotherapy for all infections caused by susceptible organisms. Higher doses should be used for serious infections due to *P. aeruginosa*	IV 1–2 g every 8–12 h IM 0.5–1 g every 12 h	IM, IV 50 mg/kg every 8–12 h, not to exceed recommended adult dose
Cefiderocol (Fetroja)	Indicated for complicated UTI included pyelonephritis. Typically reserved for infections caused by multidrug-resistant organisms including *P. aeruginosa*	2 g IV every 8 hours	
Fifth Generation			
Ceftaroline (Teflaro)	Active against *Streptococcus pyogenes, S. agalactiae, S. pneumoniae, H. influenzae, K. pneumoniae, Klebsiella oxytoca, Staphylococcus aureus* (including methicillin-susceptible and methicillin-resistant isolates), *P. mirabilis, Staphylococcus saprophyticus,* and *Escherichia coli*	Community-acquired pneumonia: IV 600 mg every 12 h for 5–7 d Skin infection: IV 600 mg every 12 h for 5–14 d	IV ≥ 2 mo to <2 y: 8 mg/kg/dose every 8 h for 5–14 d ≥2 y to <18 y: 12 mg/kg/dose every 8 h for 5–14 d
Cephalosporin–Beta-Lactamase Inhibitor Combinations			
Ceftolozane–tazobactam (Zerbaxa)	For treatment of intra-abdominal infections caused by *Enterobacter cloacae, Escherichia coli, Klebsiella oxytoca, K. pneumoniae, P. aeruginosa, B. fragilis, Streptococcus anginosus, S. constellatus,* and *S. salivarius*	IV 1.5 g every 8 h for 4–14 d	
Ceftazidime–avibactam (Avycaz)	Active against *Enterobacter cloacae, Escherichia coli, K. oxytoca, K. pneumoniae, P. aeruginosa, Enterobacter aerogenes,* and *Proteus*	IV 2.5 g every 8 h for 5–14 d Intra-abdominal infections: combine with metronidazole	

- In older adults, decreased kidney function, other disease processes, and concurrent drug therapies increase the risks of adverse effects.

Quality and Safety Alert: Safety

Specialized pediatric dosing references can provide guidance for dosing of most cephalosporins based on the child's age and weight.

- Reproduction, pregnancy, and lactation:
  - Although cephalosporins cross the placenta, they are generally considered compatible for use during pregnancy.
- Abnormal kidney function and hepatic impairment:
  - Cefazolin and all other parenteral cephalosporins, except ceftriaxone, require dosage adjustment in patients with abnormal kidney function. Usual doses may produce high and prolonged serum drug levels, and a lower dose or an increased period between doses is necessary.
  - Cefazolin is moderately dialyzable, and the normal dose or a supplemental dose should be administered after dialysis.

Quality and Safety Alert: Patient-Centered Care

With liquid suspensions for children, shaking to resuspend the medication and measuring with a measuring spoon or calibrated device to ensure safe dosing are necessary. Parents or caregivers should not use household spoons because they vary widely in capacity and may lead to incorrect dosing.

Adverse Effects

Adverse effects to cefazolin and the other cephalosporins are similar to those of most other antibiotics: abdominal pain, diarrhea, gastritis, nausea, and vomiting. Primarily, effects of particular importance are hypersensitivity reactions and superinfections.

Contraindications

A contraindication to the use of a cephalosporin is a previous severe anaphylactic reaction to a penicillin. Because cephalosporins are chemically similar to penicillins, there is a risk of cross-sensitivity. However, incidence of cross-sensitivity is low, especially in patients who have had delayed reactions (e.g., skin rash) to penicillins. Another contraindication is cephalosporin allergy. Immediate allergic reactions with anaphylaxis, bronchospasm, and urticaria occur less often than delayed reactions with skin rash, drug fever, and eosinophilia.

Nursing Implications

Preventing Interactions

Cephalosporins have been associated with a decrease in prothrombin activity, which may be due to depletion of vitamin K in the gut flora. It is necessary to monitor patients previously stabilized on anticoagulants. Box 18.3 outlines drug–drug interactions. There are no identified herbal interactions. How-

BOX 18.3 Drug Interactions: Cephalosporins

Drugs That Increase the Effects of Cephalosporins
- Aminoglycosides
  Increase the risk of nephrotoxicity
- Entecavir
  Leads to competitive inhibition of transporters in kidney tubules
- Furosemide
  Increases the risk of nephrotoxicity
- Nimodipine
  Increases the risk of nephrotoxicity
- Vancomycin
  Increases the risk of nephrotoxicity

ever, each gram of cefazolin has 46 mg (2 mEq) of sodium, which may have a negative effect on patients with heart failure.

Administering the Medication

To prevent complications, it is essential to administer cefazolin and other cephalosporins for the full prescribed course of treatment.

Quality and Safety Alert: Safety

It is important to avoid giving cephalosporins to people with life-threatening allergic reactions to penicillin (anaphylaxis, laryngeal swelling, angioedema, or hives).

The nurse should not mix ceftriaxone and IV solutions of calcium-containing salts or administer these drugs simultaneously, because of the potential for ceftriaxone–calcium precipitation. It is possible to minimize adverse effects by administering most oral cephalosporins with food or milk.

Assessing for Therapeutic Effects

It is important to assess for a decrease in signs and symptoms of infection, such as decrease in white blood cell count, decrease pain at the site of the infection, normal temperature, and wound healing.

Assessing for Adverse Effects

The nurse carefully evaluates any rash. If possible, it is necessary to distinguish a hypersensitivity reaction from a nonallergic cefazolin rash. Drug levels are not required when administering cefazolin or any of the cephalosporins. If the patient is experiencing abnormal kidney function, monitoring of serum creatinine and BUN is recommended, because adjustment for kidney dysfunction may be necessary.

Patient Teaching

The nurse instructs patients that cephalosporins, like all antibiotics, should be given for the full prescribed course of treatment to prevent complications. Box 18.4 outlines patient teaching guidelines.

BOX 18.4 Patient Teaching Guidelines for Oral Cephalosporins

General Considerations

- Inform your primary provider if you have ever had a severe allergic reaction to penicillin in which you had difficulty breathing, swelling, or skin rash. A small number of people are allergic to both penicillins and cephalosporins because the drugs are similar in chemical structure.
- Also, inform your primary provider if you have had a previous allergic reaction to a cephalosporin (e.g., Cefazolin). If you are not sure whether a new prescription is a cephalosporin, ask the pharmacist before having the prescription filled.
- Complete the full course of drug treatment for greater effectiveness and prevention of secondary infection with drug-resistant bacteria.
- Follow instructions about dosing frequency; effectiveness depends on maintaining adequate blood levels.

Self- or Caregiver Administration

- Take most oral drugs with food or milk to prevent stomach upset.
- Take cefpodoxime and cefuroxime (Zinacef) with food to increase absorption.
- Do not take cefaclor, cefdinir, or cefpodoxime with antacids containing aluminum or magnesium (e.g., Maalox, Mylanta) or with Pepcid, Tagamet, or Zantac. These drugs decrease absorption of these antibiotics and make them less effective. If necessary to take one of the drugs, take it 2 hours before or 2 hours after a dose of these antibiotics.
- Shake liquid preparations well to mix thoroughly and measure the dose accurately.
- Report the occurrence of diarrhea, especially if it is severe or contains blood, pus, or mucus. Cephalosporins can cause antibiotic-associated colitis, and the drug may need to be stopped.
- Inform your healthcare provider if you are breast-feeding. These drugs enter breast milk.

Other Drugs in the Class

Cefotetan may cause hypoprothrombinemia (by killing intestinal bacteria that normally produce vitamin K or a chemical structure that prevents activation of prothrombin) or platelet dysfunction. Treatment of bleeding may involve giving vitamin K but does not restore normal platelet function or normal bacterial flora in the intestines.

Two cephalosporin–beta-lactamase combinations are available in the United States. Ceftolozane–tazobactam has broad-spectrum capabilities against aerobic and facultative Gram-negative bacilli; it is effective against extended-spectrum *Enterobacterales*. The primary use of this drug combination is treatment of infections resulting from multidrug-resistant *P. aeruginosa*. It is also used to treat complicated intra-abdominal infections and urinary tract infections caused by *E. coli*, *Klebsiella*, *Proteus*, and *P. aeruginosa*. Ceftolozane binds to one or more penicillin-binding proteins to inhibit the final step of peptidoglycan synthesis to interrupt bacterial cell wall synthesis. Tazobactam covalently binds to plasmid-mediated and chromosomal bacterial beta-lactamases. It also irreversibly inhibits beta-lactamases, including penicillinases and cephalosporinases.

Ceftolozane is not metabolized, whereas tazobactam is hydrolyzed to an inactive metabolite. Both are excreted largely unchanged in the urine. Ceftolozane–tazobactam is administered intravenously over 60 minutes. If combined with probenecid, the serum concentration of ceftolozane–tazobactam is increased. Like most cephalosporin antibiotics, there is a risk of cross-reactivity with penicillin allergies. The drug is otherwise well tolerated.

 Quality and Safety Alert: Evidence-Based Practice

Patients with hematological malignancy who have undergone hematopoietic cell transplantation are prone to the development of multidrug-resistant *P. aeruginosa*. These patients are prone to increased risk of morbidity and mortality. Ceftolozane–tazobactam is a good option for the treatment of multidrug-resistant *P. aeruginosa*. Hakki and Lewis (2018) conducted a study to report the use of ceftolozane–tazobactam for invasive multidrug-resistant *P. aeruginosa* in patients who have been diagnosed with hematologic malignancy and have undergone hematopoietic cell transplantation. Treatment was successful while on ceftolozane–tazobactam. No participants died while on ceftolozane–tazobactam, and all patients remained alive 30 days following discontinuation of the drug combination.

Ceftazidime–avibactam, which is effective against carbapenem-resistant *Enterobacterales* (CRE), is indicated for intra-abdominal infections and urinary tract infections, including pyelonephritis. This drug combination is frequently used off-label to treat pneumonia, bacteremia, or other infections due to CRE. The mechanism of action of this drug is similar to that of other beta-lactam antibiotics. The avibactam component functions as a beta-lactamase inhibitor, which like tazobactam, inhibits the degradation of the ceftazidime by plasmid-mediated beta-lactamases.

NCLEX Success

2. A cardiac surgeon orders cefazolin 1 g IV "on call" to the operating room for a patient scheduled for a heart valve replacement. The surgery is scheduled for 7:00 a.m. the next morning. What is the rationale for giving the antibiotic at 6:30 a.m.? The last dose was administered more than 8 hours ago.
   A. The cefazolin must be given 60 minutes before the procedure for legal reasons.
   B. The cefazolin must be given within 60 minutes before the first skin incision to reach therapeutic concentrations.
   C. The cefazolin trough level will be checked at 6:00 a.m., which would allow the level to come back before administration of the "on call" dose.
   D. The last dose was administered yesterday.

3. Which of the following classes of cephalosporins have the best activity against Gram-positive organisms?
   A. first-generation cephalosporins
   B. second-generation cephalosporins
   C. third-generation cephalosporins
   D. fourth-generation cephalosporins

Clinical Application 18.1

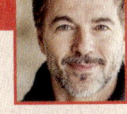

The nurse asks Mr. O'Brian if he has had an allergy to penicillin or cephalosporins. He denies any known allergies to drugs.
- Why is cefazolin the drug of choice for his cardiac pacemaker procedure?
- Before administering this medication, what factors should the nurse assess?
- Why did the nurse ask the patient about a penicillin allergy with the administration of a cephalosporin?

CARBAPENEMS

Carbapenems are broad-spectrum, bactericidal beta-lactam antimicrobials. The group consists of four drugs. **Imipenem–cilastatin (Primaxin)** is the prototype.

Pharmacokinetics

Imipenem–cilastatin, which is given parenterally, is distributed in most body fluids and body tissues. The drug has a rapid onset of action and peaks at the end of the infusion, and its duration is 6 to 8 hours. An enzyme (dehydropeptidase) in kidney tubules rapidly breaks down the imipenem component; therefore, the drug reaches only low concentrations in the urine. However, the cilastatin inhibits the destruction of imipenem, increasing the urinary concentration of imipenem and reducing its potential kidney toxicity. Recommended doses indicate the amount of imipenem; the solution contains an equivalent amount of cilastatin. (The drugs are available only in the combined form.)

Action

Like other beta-lactam drugs, imipenem–cilastatin and the other carbapenems inhibit synthesis of bacterial cell walls by binding with penicillin-binding proteins.

Use

Imipenem–cilastatin is effective in infections caused by a wide range of bacteria, including penicillinase-producing staphylococci, *E. coli*, *Proteus* species, *Enterobacter–Klebsiella–Serratia* species, *P. aeruginosa*, and *Enterococcus faecalis*. Its main use is in the treatment of infections caused by organisms resistant to other drugs. Considered to be a very broad-spectrum antibiotic, imipenem–cilastatin covers a range of Gram-negative and Gram-positive aerobes and anaerobes. It is used to treat infections of the lower respiratory tract, urinary tract, intra-abdominal infections, bone and joints, and skin and skin structures. It can also be used to treat polymicrobial infections (caused by multiple microorganisms), bacterial septicemia, and endocarditis.

Table 18.4 gives specific route and dosage information for carbapenems.

Patient-related variables specific to the use of imipenem–cilastatin include the following:

- Age:
  - The use of imipenem–cilastatin is appropriate in children, but the drug should not be given in children with CNS infections because of the risk of seizures.
  - Caution is warranted in neonates with all carbapenems because immature kidney function slows elimination.
  - In children, dosages are calculated based on age, weight, severity of infection, and kidney function.
  - In older adults, imipenem–cilastatin and other carbapenems are relatively safe, although decreased kidney function, other disease processes, and concurrent drug therapies increase the risks of adverse effects, requiring lower doses.
- Reproduction, pregnancy, and lactation:
  - Use the drug during pregnancy only if the benefit outweighs the risk to the fetus.
  - The drug is present in breast milk and the importance of breast-feeding to the patient and child should be considered.

TABLE 18.4

DRUGS AT A GLANCE: Carbapenems

Drug	Routes and Dosage Ranges	
	Adults	**Children**
Imipenem–cilastatin (Primaxin; imipenem and cilastatin for injection)	IV 250–1,000 mg every 6–8 h based on imipenem component (maximum dose 4 g/d) IM 500–750 mg every 12 h	>3 mo: noncentral nervous system infections IV 15–25 mg/kg every 6 h (maximum dose 4 g/d)
Ertapenem (Invanz; Invanz)	IV, IM 1 g once daily	3 mo–12 y: IV, IM 15 mg/kg twice daily (maximum dose 1 g/d)
Meropenem (Merrem; Meropenem for injection)	IV 1.5–6 g/d in divided doses every 8 h	≥3 mo: 10–40 mg/kg in divided doses every 8 h (maximum dose 6 g/d)
Doripenem	IV 500 mg every 8 h	Safety and efficacy not yet established
Carbapenem–Beta-Lactamase Inhibitor Combinations		
Meropenem–vaborbactam (Vabomere; Vabomere)	IV 4 g every 8 h (administer as a 3-hour infusion)	Safety and efficacy not yet established
Imipenem-relebactam (Recarbrio)	1 g IV every 6 h	Safety and efficacy not yet established

- Abnormal kidney function and hepatic impairment:
  - Dosage reduction of imipenem–cilastatin and all other carbapenems is typically necessary with abnormal kidney function, and caution is warranted in patients with creatinine clearance ≤20 mL per minute because of the increased risk of seizures.
  - Patients with severe abnormal kidney function (≤5 mL per minute) should not receive imipenem–cilastatin unless hemodialysis is initiated within 48 hours.
  - Imipenem–cilastatin may cause abnormalities in liver function test results (i.e., elevated alanine and aspartate aminotransferases, alkaline phosphatase), but hepatitis and jaundice rarely occur.
  - There are no specific recommendations or guidelines for dosage adjustment in patients with hepatic impairment.
- Specific healthcare environments:
  - The basic principles of IV care are an important component in administering this medication at home. Potential for secondary infections is a concern.

Adverse Effects

Adverse effects, including the risk of cross-sensitivity in patients with penicillin hypersensitivity and gastric disturbances, are similar to those of other beta-lactam antibiotics. In addition, there have been reports of CNS toxicity, including seizures. Seizures are more likely in patients with a preexisting seizure disorder or when recommended doses are exceeded; however, they have occurred in other patients as well.

Contraindications

Contraindications to imipenem–cilastatin include a hypersensitivity to carbapenems. There is a potential for cross-reactivity with patients that have a severe penicillin allergy due to the common beta-lactam ring. Patients with severe shock or atrioventricular block should not receive the IM formulation (containing lidocaine).

Nursing Implications
Preventing Interactions

Box 18.5 outlines drug–drug interactions with imipenem–cilastatin. There are no herbal interactions. All carbapenems may decrease the serum concentrations of divalproex. The drug may cause positive Coombs test results.

BOX 18.5 Drug Interactions: Imipenem–Cilastatin

Drugs That Increase the Effects of Imipenem–Cilastatin
- Cyclosporine
  May increase central nervous system effects
- Ganciclovir
  May lead to generalized seizures
- Probenecid
  Increases drug level and half-life

Administering the Medication

It is important to avoid administering imipenem–cilastatin and the other carbapenems to people with life-threatening allergic reactions to penicillin (anaphylaxis, laryngeal swelling angioedema, or hives). In addition, IM administration of imipenem–cilastatin is not recommended for people with severe or life-threatening infections such as endocarditis, shock, or septicemia. To prepare imipenem–cilastatin for IM injection, lidocaine, a local anesthetic, is added to decrease pain. The solution is contraindicated in people allergic to this type of local anesthetic. The IM formulation is not for IV use.

Assessing for Therapeutic Effects

When assessing for the therapeutic effects of imipenem–cilastatin, it is important to note if the signs and symptoms of the infection have improved. In the event of a lower respiratory infection, the lung sounds should be assessed for a decrease in rales. With joint infections, the nurse assesses whether the joint is cool to touch, whether pain in the joint decreased, and whether joint mobility has improved.

Assessing for Adverse Effects

Drug levels are not required when administering imipenem–cilastatin or any of the carbapenems. It is recommended that serum creatinine and BUN be monitored instead.

The nurse carefully assesses any rash. It is necessary to distinguish, if possible, a hypersensitivity reaction from a nonallergic imipenem–cilastatin rash.

Carbapenems generally resist cleavage by most beta-lactamases. Carbapenem-resistant strains of *P. aeruginosa* are arising due to the altered permeability to this class of drugs and specific changes that occur on the protein outer membranes.

Patient Teaching

Imipenem–cilastatin and the other carbapenems are typically used for illnesses that are considered critical. Therefore, patient teaching guidelines focus on instructing the patient and family about the purpose of the drug and the importance of reporting adverse effects.

Other Drugs in the Class

Ertapenem is administered for catheter-related infections of the blood and hospital-acquired ventilator-associated pneumonia (VAP) in patients with multiple drug-resistant organisms. Meropenem has an overall spectrum of activity similar to that of imipenem, although meropenem is less active against Gram-positive bacteria. The drug is often given in the treatment of febrile neutropenia, which frequently occurs in patients with hematologic malignancies and in cancer patients who take chemotherapeutic drugs that cause bone marrow suppression. The addition of vaborbactam with meropenem expands the activity of meropenem against CRE. Imipenem–relebactam (Recarbrio) is similar to meropenem–vaborbactam; the addition of the beta-lactamase inhibitor expands the activity of the imipenem against CRE. Imipenem–relebactam does have some increased coverage against imipenem resistance *P. aeruginosa*.

Monobactams

Currently, the only monobactam available for use is **aztreonam** (Azactam), which serves as the prototype of this class. Aztreonam is active against aerobic Gram-negative bacteria, including *Enterobacterales* and *P. aeruginosa*, and many strains that are resistant to multiple antibiotics. The coverage is similar to that of the aminoglycosides, but the drug does not cause kidney damage or hearing loss. Because Gram-positive and anaerobic bacteria are resistant to aztreonam, the drug's ability to preserve normal Gram-positive and anaerobic flora may be an advantage compared with other antimicrobial agents.

Pharmacokinetics

Aztreonam, which is given parenterally, is distributed in most body fluids and tissues, including the lungs, liver, kidney, bone, uterus, intestine, sputum, bile, pleural fluid, and synovial fluids. In addition, the drug also crosses the placenta and is excreted in breast milk. It is stable in the presence of beta-lactamase enzymes. Peak action occurs in 1 hour, with a duration of 4 to 12 hours; the onset of action depends on the organism and dose. Aztreonam is metabolized in the liver to inactive metabolites, which are excreted in the urine.

Action

Like other beta-lactam drugs, aztreonam inhibits synthesis of bacterial cell walls by binding with penicillin-binding proteins. However, aztreonam, because of its monobactam structure, has limited cross-allergenicity between itself and other beta-lactam antibiotics. It is generally considered safe to administer aztreonam to patients with a penicillin allergy.

Use

Aztreonam is effective in infections caused by *N. gonorrhoeae*, *H. influenzae*, and most *Enterobacter–Klebsiella–Serratia* species, and it is often active against *P. aeruginosa*. Although it is often considered to have similar coverage to aminoglycosides, extended-spectrum penicillins, and third-generation cephalosporins, aztreonam lacks Gram-positive coverage. Also, anaerobes are not susceptible to aztreonam. Indications for use include infections of the urinary tract, skin and skin structures, and lower respiratory tract. Other indications include intra-abdominal and gynecologic infections as well as Gram-negative septicemia. The FDA considers aztreonam solution for inhalation as an orphan drug for control of Gram-negative bacteria in the respiratory tracts of patients diagnosed with cystic fibrosis.

It should be noted that aztreonam may cause an elevation in hepatic enzymes; however, on discontinuation of the drug, most enzymes return to pretherapy levels. There are no specific recommendations or guidelines for dosage adjustment in patients with hepatic impairment.

Table 18.5 presents general route and dosage information for aztreonam.

Patient-related variables specific to the use of aztreonam include the following:

- Age:
  - Aztreonam can be used in children older than 1 month of age.
  - Some adverse effects occur more frequently in children, resulting from the severity of the illness being treated or the higher doses that are typically administered in pediatrics.
  - In children, dosages should be based on age, weight, severity of infection, and kidney function.
  - In older adults, decreased kidney function, other disease processes, and concurrent drug therapies increase the risks of adverse effects.
- Reproduction, pregnancy, and lactation:
  - Aztreonam crosses the placenta and is present in breast milk.
  - Risk–benefit considerations should be made before prescribing during pregnancy and lactation.
- Abnormal kidney function and hepatic impairment:
  - It is necessary to reduce the dosage of aztreonam in patients with abnormal kidney function.
  - Aztreonam is moderately dialyzable, and patients with life-threatening infections should receive a supplemental dose after each hemodialysis session.
- Specific healthcare environments:
  - Aztreonam use in critical illnesses is typically reserved for patients with severe penicillin allergy.
  - Monotherapy with aztreonam may lead to resistant *P. aeruginosa* infections. Combination therapy is often recommended.

Adverse Effects

In general, adverse effects of aztreonam are similar to those of other beta-lactam antibiotics, including possible hypersensitivity reactions. The most common adverse effects include rash, diarrhea, nausea, vomiting, and localized thrombophlebitis.

TABLE 18.5

DRUGS AT A GLANCE: Aztreonam

Drug	Routes and Dosage Ranges	
	Adults	**Children**
Aztreonam (Azactam)	For urinary tract infection: IM, IV 0.5–1 g every 8–12 h For moderate systemic infection: IM, IV 1 g every 8–12 h or IV 2 g every 8–12 h For meningitis: IV 2 g every 6–8 h	IM, IV 30 mg/kg every 6–8 h

Prolonged use may cause fungal or bacterial superinfections. *Clostridium difficile*–associated diarrhea and pseudomembranous colitis should be concerns with extended use.

Contraindications

Contraindications to aztreonam include a hypersensitivity to any component of aztreonam.

Nursing Implications

Preventing Interactions

Box 18.6 outlines drug–drug interactions for aztreonam. As yet, there are no identified herb or food interactions. Aztreonam and aminoglycosides, when used in combination, can demonstrate synergistic effects against some strains of organisms, specifically *P. aeruginosa* and some *Enterobacterales*. This synergy has also been seen with other beta-lactam antibiotics. There is a potential for false-positive reactions in urine glucose tests using Benedict solution, Clinitest, or Fehling solution.

Administering the Medication

Aztreonam may be administered intravenously or intramuscularly.

Assessing for Therapeutic Effects

When assessing the patient for the therapeutic effects of aztreonam, it is important to determine if the signs and symptoms of the infection have improved. The nurse assesses whether the white blood cell count has decreased. In the lower respiratory tract, the lung sounds should be assessed. Increased clear breath sounds are indicative of improvement in the respiratory status.

Improvement in urinary tract infection signs and symptoms include lack of burning or pain upon urination, a decrease in urinary frequency, and clear urine color. Wound infections should be assessed for decrease in wound drainage, decreased redness, and decrease swelling and pain.

Assessing for Adverse Effects

The nurse carefully assesses any rash. It is important to distinguish a hypersensitivity reaction from a nonallergic aztreonam rash, if possible. Drug levels are not required when administering aztreonam. Monitoring of serum creatinine, BUN, and liver function tests is recommended in patients taking aztreonam.

Patient Teaching

Aztreonam is typically used for illnesses that are considered critical. Therefore, patient teaching guidelines focus on instructing the patient and family about the purpose of the drug and importance of reporting adverse effects.

NCLEX Success

4. In acute kidney disease, doses of which of the following antibiotics must be reduced? (Select all that apply.)
   A. nafcillin
   B. cefazolin
   C. meropenem
   D. aztreonam

5. A nurse working in the neurointensive care unit is caring for a patient with a head injury who has been experiencing seizures and now has pneumonia caused by *Pseudomonas aeruginosa*. The physician has prescribed imipenem 1 g IV every 6 hours plus gentamicin for the pneumonia. Before administering the antibiotics, the nurse should do which of the following?
   A. Avoid mixing the imipenem and gentamicin in the same IV bag to prevent inactivation of the gentamicin.
   B. Remind the physician of the patient's seizures and inquire whether a different antibiotic might be safer.
   C. Suggest to the physician that imipenem is used to treat Gram-positive infections and will not be effective in this patient.
   D. Set the infusion pump to deliver the imipenem over 15 minutes.

BOX 18.6 Drug Interactions: Aztreonam

Drugs That Increase the Effects of Aztreonam
- Aminoglycosides
  Increase the risk of nephrotoxicity
- Furosemide
  May increase serum levels

Drugs That Decrease the Effects of Aztreonam
- Cefoxitin
  Induces the production of beta-lactamases
- Chloramphenicol
  May antagonize bactericidal activity

THE NURSING PROCESS

A concept map outlines the nursing process related to drug therapy considerations in this chapter. Additional nursing implications related to the disease process should also be considered in care decisions.

Assessment
- With all beta-lactam anti-infective agents (penicillins, cephalosporins, carbapenem, aztreonam), ask the patient if he or she has experienced a skin rash, hives, swelling, or difficulty breathing when the drug has been administered in the past.

Outcomes of Therapy

The patient will
- Take oral beta-lactam antibacterials as directed.
- Receive parenteral beta-lactam drugs by appropriate techniques to minimize tissue irritation.
- Receive prompt and appropriate treatment if hypersensitivity reactions occur.

Nursing Interventions
- After giving a penicillin parenterally in an outpatient setting, keep the patient in the area for at least 30 minutes. Anaphylactic reactions are more likely to occur with parenteral than oral use and within a few minutes after injection.
- In any patient care setting, keep emergency equipment and supplies readily available.
- Monitor patient response to beta-lactam drugs.
- Monitor dosages of beta-lactam drugs for patients with impaired kidney function.
- Provide patient teaching regarding drug therapy (see Boxes 18.2 and 18.4).

Evaluation
- Observe for improvement in signs of infection.
- Interview and observe for adverse drug effects.

Visit *thePoint* at http://thePoint.lww.com/Frandsen13e for answers to NCLEX Success questions (in Appendix A), answers to Clinical Application Case Studies (in Appendix B), and more!

REFERENCES AND RESOURCES

Hakki, M., & Lewis, J. S. (2018). Ceftolozane-tazobactam therapy for multi-drug resistant *Pseudomonas aeruginosa* infections in patients with hematologic malignancies and hematopoietic-cell transplant recipients. *Infection, 46*, 431–434. doi:10.1007/s15010-018-1125-5

Hinkle, J. L., Cheever, K. H., & Overbaugh, K. (2021). *Brunner & Suddarth's textbook of medical-surgical nursing* (15th ed.). Wolters Kluwer Health/Lippincott Williams & Wilkins.

Letourneau, A. R. (2022a). *Cephalosporins.* UpToDate.

Letourneau, A. R. (2022b). *Penicillin, antistaphylococcal penicillins, and broad-spectrum penicillins.* UpToDate.

Lippincott. (2022). *Nursing2023 drug handbook* (43rd ed.). Wolters Kluwer.

Lupia, T., Corcione, S., Mornese Pinna, S., & De Rosa, F. G. (2020). New cephalosporins for the treatment of pneumonia in internal medicine wards. *Journal of Thoracic Disease, 12*(7), 3747–3763. https://doi.org/10.21037/jtd-20-417

Norris, T. L. (2019). *Porth's pathophysiology: Concepts of altered health states* (10th ed.). Wolters Kluwer.

Tucker, R. (2021). *2022 Lippincott's pocket drug for nurses.* Wolters Kluwer.

CHAPTER 19

Drug Therapy With Aminoglycosides and Fluoroquinolones

LEARNING OBJECTIVES

After studying this chapter, you should be able to:

1. State the rationale for the increasing use of single daily doses of aminoglycosides.
2. Discuss the importance of measuring serum drug levels during aminoglycoside therapy.
3. Describe measures to decrease nephrotoxicity and ototoxicity with aminoglycosides.
4. Identify characteristics of aminoglycosides and fluoroquinolones in relation to effectiveness, safety, spectrum of antimicrobial activity, indications for use, administration, and observation of patient responses.
5. Recognize factors influencing selection and dosage of aminoglycosides and fluoroquinolones.
6. Describe characteristics, uses, adverse effects, and nursing process implications of aminoglycosides and fluoroquinolones.
7. Discuss principles of using aminoglycosides and fluoroquinolones in abnormal kidney function and critical illness.
8. Recognize the importance of the judicious use of aminoglycosides and fluoroquinolones to decrease the rate of antibiotic resistance.
9. Implement the nursing process in the care of patients receiving aminoglycosides and fluoroquinolones.

CLINICAL APPLICATION CASE STUDY

Edward Louis, an 84-year-old man, has a history of prostatitis and recurrent bacterial urinary tract infections. He is complaining of a fever, hesitancy, and dysuria.

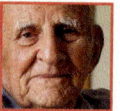

KEY TERMS

Concentration-dependent bactericidal effect: relation of bactericidal ability of a drug to its concentration the greater the concentration of the drug, the faster and the more extensive the killing of the bacteria. The goal is to maximize concentration of the drug

Extended-interval dosing: dosing regimen that provides once-daily administration of an aminoglycoside with demonstrated decreased nephrotoxicity and ototoxicity while maintaining therapeutic efficacy; also called pulse dosing

Nephrotoxicity: adverse effects on kidney function due to toxic effects of drugs and chemicals

Ototoxicity: adverse effects on the structures of the ear, especially the cochlea and auditory nerve

Peak level: highest concentration of a drug in the patient's bloodstream taken after the administration of a drug

Postantibiotic effect: persistent effect of an antimicrobial on bacterial growth after brief exposure of the organisms to a drug

Therapeutic index: range of concentration levels considered effective and safe

Trough level: lowest concentration of a drug in the patient's bloodstream taken just prior to administrating the next dose of a drug

INTRODUCTION

Healthcare practitioners have used the aminoglycosides to treat serious aerobic gram-negative infections extensively for many years. However, increasing rates of antibiotic resistance, which limit therapeutic options, have become a growing concern. Select aminoglycosides have shown stability in the face of the emergence of resistance. The quinolones are also older drugs originally used only for the treatment of urinary tract infections (see Chapter 20). Synthesis of the quinolones involves adding a fluorine molecule to the quinolone structure. This addition increases drug activity against gram-negative microorganisms, broadens the antimicrobial spectrum to include several other microorganisms, and allows the use of the drugs in treating systemic infections. General characteristics, mechanisms of action, indications for and contraindications to use, nursing process implications, and principles of therapy for the aminoglycosides and the fluoroquinolones are described in this chapter. Individual drugs and the prototype drugs, with routes of administration and dosage ranges, are presented in Table 19.1 and the Drugs at a Glance tables.

> **! Quality and Safety Alert: Teamwork and Collaboration**
>
> Reducing the risks for healthcare-associated infections and antimicrobial-resistant organisms requires a comprehensive and persistent effort by multiple members of the healthcare team. This includes procedures to prevent the spread of infection from patient to patient or staff to patient, as well as measures to reduce the overall use of antimicrobial agents. These efforts should be an absolute priority for hospitals and healthcare workers, with the resources and coordination provided to create change and protect patients.

AMINOGLYCOSIDES

Aminoglycosides are bactericidal agents with similar pharmacologic, antimicrobial, and toxicologic characteristics. They are frequently used for the treatment of serious infections caused by gram-negative aerobic microorganisms such as *Pseudomonas* and *Proteus* species, *Escherichia coli*, and *Klebsiella*, *Enterobacter*, and *Serratia* species as well as mycobacteria. Less commonly, aminoglycosides (in combination with other agents) have also been used in the treatment of select gram-positive infections. The drugs are not effective against gram-negative anaerobes. Aminoglycosides have shown relative stability against the development of resistant organisms compared with other antibiotic classes. Despite the relatively broad spectrum of activity of aminoglycosides, widespread clinical use is limited because of the availability of other less toxic agents with comparable effectiveness that do not require serum drug concentration monitoring. **Gentamicin**, the most widely used aminoglycoside, is the prototype. Patients often receive gentamicin in combination with other antibiotics for serious systemic infections in the clinical setting. Gentamicin and other aminoglycosides are typically not used as monotherapy because they demonstrate inadequate clinical effectiveness at most sites except in the treatment of lower urinary tract infections.

Maintenance doses are based on the level of serum drug concentrations. **Peak level** and **trough level** correspond to the highest and lowest concentrations of a drug in a person's bloodstream, respectively. They are particularly useful as a process of measuring drug concentrations at intervals to determine timing between dosages. This helps ensure a steady, consistent concentration of a drug in circulation. Since the aminoglycosides have a narrow **therapeutic index** (range of concentration levels considered effective and safe), obtaining peak and trough levels

TABLE 19.1
Drug Therapy With Aminoglycosides and Fluoroquinolones

Drug Class	Prototype(s)	Other Drugs in the Class
Aminoglycosides	Gentamicin	Amikacin Neomycin Paromomycin Plazomicin (Zemdri) Streptomycin Tobramycin
Fluoroquinolones	Ciprofloxacin (Cipro)	Levofloxacin Moxifloxacin Ofloxacin Delafloxacin (Baxdela)

of the drug minimizes the risk of adverse effects. Peak serum concentrations should be determined 30 to 60 minutes after drug administration (5 to 8 mcg/mL for gentamicin and tobramycin; 20 to 30 mcg/mL for amikacin). Measurement of both peak and trough levels helps maintain therapeutic serum levels without excessive toxicity. For gentamicin and tobramycin, peak levels above 10 to 12 mcg/mL and trough levels above 2 mcg/mL for prolonged periods have been associated with nephrotoxicity. For accuracy, it is necessary to draw blood samples at the correct times and to document the timing of drug administration and blood sampling accurately, based on institutional recommendations.

Pharmacokinetics

Gentamicin is poorly absorbed from the gastrointestinal (GI) tract. Thus, when given orally, the drug exerts local effects in the GI tract. It is rapidly and completely absorbed from intramuscular (IM) injection sites and reaches peak effects in 30 to 90 minutes if circulatory status is proficient. After intravenous (IV) administration, the peak effect occurs 30 minutes after a 30-minute infusion. Plasma half-life is 2 to 4 hours in patients with normal kidney function. The volume of distribution is increased by edema, ascites, and fluid overload, and it is decreased with dehydration.

After parenteral administration, gentamicin is widely distributed in extracellular fluid and reaches therapeutic levels in blood, urine, bone, inflamed joints, and pleural and ascitic fluids. Gentamicin accumulates in high concentrations in the proximal kidney tubules of the kidney, potentially leading to acute tubular necrosis. This damage to the kidney and kidney function from toxic effects is termed **nephrotoxicity**. Gentamicin also accumulates in high concentrations in the inner ear, damaging sensory cells in the cochlea (disrupting hearing) and the vestibular apparatus (disturbing balance). This damage to the inner ear is termed **ototoxicity**. Gentamicin is poorly distributed in the central nervous system, intraocular fluids, and respiratory tract secretions.

Action

Aminoglycosides penetrate the cell walls of susceptible bacteria and bind irreversibly to 30S and 50S ribosomal subunits, intracellular structures that synthesize proteins. As a result, the bacteria cell membrane becomes defective and cannot synthesize the proteins necessary for their function and replication.

Use

The major clinical use of gentamicin (most commonly with other antibacterial agents) is empiric therapy for serious infections caused by susceptible aerobic gram-negative organisms. Treatment of infections such as septicemia, respiratory tract infections, urinary tract infections, intra-abdominal infections, and osteomyelitis often involves gentamicin. In pseudomonal infections, patients may receive gentamicin concurrently with an antipseudomonal penicillin (e.g., piperacillin/tazobactam) for synergistic therapeutic effects. The penicillin-induced breakdown of the bacterial cell wall makes it easier for gentamicin to reach its site of action inside the bacterial cell. Researchers have demonstrated decreased mortality from combination antibiotic therapy in treatment of infections due to *Pseudomonas aeruginosa* and other multidrug-resistant gram-negative bacilli. Once a bacterial species has been identified and its susceptibilities to alternate agents are known, aminoglycosides are usually discontinued in favor of less toxic antibiotics in the completion of a treatment course.

Table 19.2 presents dosage information for gentamicin and the other aminoglycosides.

Patient-related variables specific to the use of gentamicin and other aminoglycosides include the following:

- Age:
  - Individualization of the dose is extremely critical in children and in older adults because of the low therapeutic index of gentamicin.
  - The risk of nephrotoxicity and ototoxicity may be increased in neonates because of their immature kidney function.
  - In older adults, decreased kidney function, other disease processes, and concurrent drug therapies increase the adverse effects, specifically aminoglycoside-induced nephrotoxicity and ototoxicity.
- Reproduction, pregnancy, and lactation:
  - Although serious adverse effects have not been reported for all aminoglycosides, several accounts of irreversible congenital deafness in children whose parent had taken streptomycin during pregnancy have been reported, so potential risk is a consideration.
  - The broad-spectrum effects of gentamicin are beneficial in the treatment of intra-amniotic infection of both the mother and fetus.
- Abnormal kidney function and hepatic impairment:
  - Dosage reduction of gentamicin and other aminoglycosides is essential with abnormal kidney function.
  - Gentamicin should be used with caution in severe hepatic disease, such as cirrhosis, because of the possibility of precipitating hepatorenal syndrome.

Adverse Effects

Gentamicin and other aminoglycosides result in similar adverse reactions. A **BOXED WARNING** ◆ issued by the U.S. Food and Drug Administration (FDA) alerts healthcare professionals that these drugs are nephrotoxic and ototoxic and must be used very cautiously in the presence of abnormal kidney function.

Nephrotoxicity occurs more frequently in patients with a history of abnormal kidney function. Extended duration of treatment with gentamicin may also contribute to nephrotoxicity. In most cases, nephrotoxicity is reversible on discontinuation of the drug. Ototoxicity (auditory or vestibular) may develop after extended use and is usually irreversible. Dizziness, vertigo, tinnitus, and hearing loss may be signs of ototoxicity and damage to the eighth cranial nerve. Peripheral neuropathy, including numbness, skin tingling, and muscle twitching, also occurs as a result of damage to the nerves. Therefore, the use of gentamicin in patients

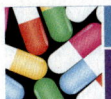

TABLE 19.2
DRUGS AT A GLANCE: Aminoglycosides

Drug	Characteristics	Routes and Dosage Ranges Adults	Children
Gentamicin (✽ Gentamicin Injection)	Effective against several gram-negative organisms, although some strains have become resistant Acts synergistically with antipseudomonal penicillins against *P. aeruginosa* and with ampicillin or vancomycin against enterococci	Conventional dosing: IM, IV 1–2.5 mg/kg/dose every 8–24 h depending on kidney function ODA dosing: 4–7 mg/kg/dose once daily	<5 y: IM, IV 2.5 mg/kg/dose every 8 h ≥5 y: IM, IV 2–2.5 mg/kg/dose every 8 h
Amikacin (✽ Erfa-Amikacin, VPI-Amikacin)	Retains a broader spectrum of antibacterial activity than other aminoglycosides because it resists degradation by most enzymes that inactivate gentamicin and tobramycin Major clinical use is in infections caused by organisms resistant to other aminoglycosides (e.g., *Pseudomonas*, *Proteus*, *E. coli*, *Klebsiella*, *Enterobacter*, *Serratia*), whether community or hospital acquired	IM, IV 15–20 mg/kg every 24 h, or 5 mg/kg every 8 h, or 7.5 mg/kg every 12 h Kidney dosing: 5–7.5 mg/kg/dose every 8–24 h	≥11 y: IM: 15 to 30 mg/kg/dose every 24 h *Neonates*: IM, IV 10 mg/kg initially and then 7.5 mg/kg every 12 h
Neomycin	Given orally or topically to prepare GI tract for surgery. Although poorly absorbed from the GI tract, toxic levels may accumulate in the presence of kidney failure Used topically, often in combination with other drugs, to treat infections of the eye, ear, and skin (burns, wounds, ulcers, dermatoses) When used for wound or bladder irrigations, systemic absorption may occur if the area is large or if drug concentration exceeds 0.1%	PO, suppression of intestinal bacteria (with erythromycin 1 g) 1 g given at 1 p.m., 2 p.m., and 11 p.m. the day before an 8 a.m. surgery; hepatic coma, 4–12 g daily in divided doses every 4–6 h for 5–6 d	
Paromomycin (✽ Humatin)	Effective in treating acute and chronic intestinal amebiasis	PO: 25–35 mg/kg/d divided every 8 h for 5–10 d	PO: 25–35 mg/kg/d divided every 8 h for 5–10 d
Plazomicin (Zemdri)	Used to treat complicated urinary tract infections and pyelonephritis caused by *Escherichia coli*, *Klebsiella pneumoniae*, *Proteus mirabilis*, and *Enterobacter cloacae* in patients who have limited or no other treatment options	IV: 15 mg/kg once daily for 4–7 d infused over 30 min; continue with appropriate oral drug therapy for a combined total of 7–10 d	Not approved for children and adolescents <18 y
Streptomycin (✽ Streptomycin)	May be used in a 4- to 6-drug regimen for treatment of multidrug-resistant tuberculosis	IM 15/kg/d or 1–2 g/d	IM 20–40 mg/kg/d in 2 divided doses, every 12 h (maximum dose 1 g/d)
Tobramycin (✽ Tobramycin)	Similar to gentamicin in antibacterial spectrum but may be more active against *Pseudomonas* organisms Often used with other antibiotics for septicemia and infections of burn wounds, other soft tissues, bone, the urinary tract, and the central nervous system	Conventional dosing: IM, IV 1–2.5 mg/kg/dose every 8–24 h depending on kidney function ODA dosing: 4–7 mg/kg/dose once daily	<5 y: IM, IV 2.5 mg/kg/dose every 8 h ≥5 y: 2–2.5 mg/kg/dose every 8 h

GI, gastrointestinal; IM, intramuscular; IV, intravenous; ODA, once-daily aminoglycoside.

with myasthenia gravis and other neuromuscular disorders warrants extreme caution, because increased muscle weakness may occur.

Contraindications

Contraindications include a hypersensitivity to aminoglycosides. Prescribers generally reserve aminoglycosides for infections that have not responded to less toxic drugs.

Nursing Implications

Dosage of aminoglycosides must be carefully monitored based on serum concentrations. Two major dosing schedules are used: one involving multiple daily doses (conventional dosing) and one involving **extended-interval dosing** (once-daily dosing or once-daily aminoglycosides [ODA]). The use of ODA dosing, unless contraindicated, has replaced the common multiple daily dosing in many people. The ODA method uses higher doses (e.g., 4 to 7 mg/kg) to produce high initial drug concentrations, with no repeat dosing until the serum concentration is quite low (typically 24 hours later). The rationale for this dosing approach is a potential increase in efficacy with a reduced incidence of nephrotoxicity. Most patients can be successfully treated using ODA. However, ODA is not appropriate for certain people. In general, the following circumstances contraindicate its use: age of 3 months or less and pregnancy or postpartum status. Extended-interval dosing of children older than 3 months may be a reasonable alternative in some situations and in patients in some age groups. The ODA dosing practice evolved from increased knowledge about the **concentration-dependent bactericidal effects** and **postantibiotic effects** of aminoglycosides. Concentration-dependent bactericidal effects mean that a large dose of aminoglycosides, with high peak serum concentrations, kills more microorganisms. Postantibiotic effects mean that aminoglycosides continue killing microorganisms even at low serum concentrations. Monitoring of random level (12-hour) serum evaluation in a single-dosing regimen replaces traditional peak and trough serum monitoring.

With the multiple-dose regimen, a patient receives an initial loading dose, based on patient weight and the desired peak serum concentration, to achieve therapeutic serum concentrations rapidly. If the patient has a body mass index of greater than or equal to 30 kg/m², adjusted body weight should be used because aminoglycosides are not significantly distributed in body fat.

Prescribers adjust dosages according to serum drug levels and creatinine clearance (CrCl). With conventional dosing, it is necessary to take gentamicin peak levels 30 minutes after the end of a 30-minute IV infusion or 1 hour after IM injection. The nurse ensures that trough levels are obtained immediately before the next dose is given. With ODA dosing, it is necessary to obtain a 12-hour random gentamicin level 12 hours after the start of the infusion.

Preventing Interactions

Many medications interact with gentamicin, increasing or decreasing its effects (Box 19.1). When patients who are taking agents that may lead to nephrotoxicity receive gentamicin, careful monitoring and caution are necessary.

BOX 19.1 Drug Interactions: Gentamicin

Drugs That Increase the Effects of Gentamicin
- Acyclovir, amphotericin B, carboplatin and cisplatin, cephalosporins, cyclosporine, ganciclovir, pamidronate, salicylates, and vancomycin
  Increase the risk of nephrotoxicity
- Arbekacin, loop diuretics
  Increase the risk of nephrotoxicity and ototoxicity

Drugs That Decrease the Effects of Gentamicin
- Penicillins
  Decrease serum concentrations

Caution is also warranted when administering diphenhydramine and chlorpheniramine with gentamicin, because gentamicin may mask symptoms of ototoxicity. In addition, ginger may increase the effect of gentamicin by masking these effects. No foods appear to increase the effect of the drug.

The nurse should not mix penicillins and aminoglycosides in a syringe or IV solution or administer them via a Y-site, because the penicillin inactivates the aminoglycoside. If feasible, dose separation is ideal.

Administering the Medication

The nurse uses only the IV route of administration, if possible, because IM injections may be erratic. If gentamicin is used concomitantly with a penicillin-class agent, it is necessary to administer the penicillin 1 hour before or after the gentamicin infusion. Gentamicin is available in an ophthalmic preparation, and concurrent administration of other ophthalmics should be spaced 10 minutes before or after the gentamicin preparation.

Quality and Safety Alert: Safety

The nurse demonstrates consistent practice in administering antibiotics that require peak and trough levels by checking, prior to administration, for the latest values and next order for peak and trough levels. Effective standardized practices help ensure safety and quality and reduce harm to the patient.

Assessing for Therapeutic Effects

The nurse assesses for response to drug therapy and ensures that signs and symptoms of the infection are resolving. It is important to observe for return to baseline vital signs and normalization of white blood count. The nurse assesses for absence of local signs of infection.

Assessing for Adverse Effects

Monitoring of gentamicin serum concentrations is crucial for both effectiveness and the avoidance of toxicity. Serum concentrations should be evaluated when the patient has received three or four doses for a conventional dosing regimen. Once the desired peak and trough have been achieved, periodic monitoring is necessary.

BOX 19.2 Patient Teaching Guidelines for Aminoglycosides

General Considerations

- Report changes in urinary patterns to your healthcare provider since aminoglycoside antibiotics may cause damage to the kidneys.
- Report any ringing in the ears or hearing loss since aminoglycosides can cause injury to the ears.
- Be aware that you may experience vertigo while on this medication. Drinking plenty of liquids if fluids are not restricted can help.
- Notify your provider before taking this drug if you plan to become pregnant or are actively breast-feeding.

Self-Administration

- If using a gentamicin ophthalmic preparation, do not take it by mouth. Wash hands before and after use. Administer any other ophthalmic preparations 10 minutes before or after gentamicin ophthalmic.

NCLEX Success

1. A critically ill patient is receiving gentamicin 1.5 mg/kg intravenously every 8 hours. The patient has recently stopped producing urine, and the most recent laboratory results indicate that the patient's creatinine level has risen from a normal value of 0.8 to 3.6 mg/dL. At the next scheduled time for administration of gentamicin, the nurse should
   A. administer half the prescribed dose
   B. hold the gentamicin and notify the provider
   C. administer gentamicin as prescribed
   D. draw a blood sample for testing the gentamicin trough level before the dose and then administer as prescribed

2. A provider writes an order for gentamicin 7 mg/kg intravenously every 24 hours and ampicillin 500 mg intravenously every 6 hours. The patient has a diagnosis of endocarditis. This is not an ideal antibiotic regimen for endocarditis because
   A. it is best to use multiple daily dosing of gentamicin for endocarditis
   B. the addition of gentamicin to ampicillin increases the risk of treatment failure in endocarditis
   C. the appropriate single daily dose of gentamicin is 15 mg/kg once daily
   D. streptomycin is the recommended aminoglycoside for use in endocarditis

Monitoring of kidney function is also essential; if signs of nephrotoxicity occur, it is necessary to discontinue treatment. In addition, patients with vertigo or tinnitus may demonstrate signs of vestibular injury; if ototoxicity occurs, treatment is discontinued. Other adverse effects to assess for include edema, skin itching, reddening of skin, and possible rash.

Patient Teaching

Patient teaching guidelines are outlined in Box 19.2.

Other Drugs in the Class

Of the other aminoglycosides, tobramycin and amikacin are the most frequently administered by IM or IV routes and carry the same risks of ototoxicity and nephrotoxicity as gentamicin. A **BOXED WARNING** exists for these drugs; neuromuscular blockage and respiratory paralysis have been reported following their use. The aminoglycosides are poorly absorbed from the GI tract. Thus, when given orally, they exert local effects on the GI tract.

In addition, streptomycin, neomycin, plazomicin (Zemdri), and paromomycin are used in specific situations. Specifically, neomycin is given orally to prepare the GI tract for surgery. Amikacin retains a broader spectrum of antibacterial activity because it resists degradation by most enzymes that inactivate gentamicin and tobramycin. Plazomicin is reserved for use in adults with complicated urinary tract infections who have limited or no other treatment options. Paromomycin is used in adults and children for the treatment of acute and chronic intestinal amebiasis. The drug acts directly on ameba and has antibacterial activity against normal and pathogenic organisms in the GI tract. Prolonged use may result in fungal or bacterial superinfection, including *Clostridium difficile*–associated diarrhea and pseudomembranous colitis. The drug is also administered as adjunct therapy in patients with hepatic coma. It should be administered orally with meals.

FLUOROQUINOLONES

Fluoroquinolones are synthetic drugs with activity against gram-negative and some gram-positive organisms. **P Ciprofloxacin** (Cipro) is the prototype. Newer fluoroquinolones have been developed with a broader spectrum of activity that provides improved coverage of gram-positive organisms and, in one case, anaerobes. Although the oral administration of fluoroquinolones has allowed ambulatory treatment of infections that previously required parenteral therapy and hospitalization, the extensive use of these antibiotics has led to antimicrobial resistance to the drug class.

Pharmacokinetics

Ciprofloxacin is well absorbed from the upper GI tract, like all quinolones; it achieves 70% bioavailability. Once absorbed, it achieves therapeutic concentrations in most body fluids. With immediate-release ciprofloxacin, concentrations peak in 30 minutes to 2 hours. Ciprofloxacin is partially metabolized in the liver; it forms four metabolites, which have limited activity. Hepatic conversion of ciprofloxacin to active metabolites is 10% to 20% of ciprofloxacin elimination. The kidneys are the main route of elimination, and approximately 30% to 60% of an oral dose is excreted unchanged in the urine. Additional excretion is achieved via the feces.

Action

Fluoroquinolones are bactericidal agents that cause cell death. Ciprofloxacin acts by interfering with enzymes required for synthesis of bacterial DNA and, therefore, necessary for bacterial growth and replication.

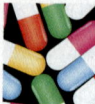

TABLE 19.3
DRUGS AT A GLANCE: Fluoroquinolones

Drug	Characteristics	Routes and Dosage Ranges for Adults
Ciprofloxacin (Cipro; ✤ ACT Ciprofloxacin, Cipro)	Effective in respiratory tract, urinary tract, gastrointestinal tract, and skin and soft tissue infections Used as one of 4–6 drugs in treatment of multidrug-resistant tuberculosis Used to treat anthrax infections and prophylaxis	PO 500–750 mg every 12 h UTI/pyelonephritis: extended-release tablets 500 mg to 1 g every 24 h IV 400 mg every 12 h PO 500 mg every 12 h
Delafloxacin (Baxdela)	Treatment of acute bacterial infections of skin and skin structure	PO 450 mg every 12 h for 5–14 d IV 300 mg every 12 h for 5–14 d
Levofloxacin (✤ Levaquin)	Indicated for treatment of bronchitis, cystitis, pneumonia, sinusitis, skin and skin structure infections, and pyelonephritis Used as anthrax prevention	PO, IV 250–750 mg once daily. Infuse 250–500 mg IV dose slowly over 60 min. Infuse 750 mg IV dose over 90 min PO, 750 mg once daily
Moxifloxacin (✤ Auro-Moxifloxacin)	Indicated for community-acquired pneumonia, sinusitis, bronchitis, skin and soft tissue infections, and intra-abdominal infections Used as anthrax prevention	PO, IV 400 mg once daily. Infuse IV dose slowly over 60 min PO, 400 mg once daily
Ofloxacin (✤ Apo-Oflox)	See ciprofloxacin, above	PO 200 mg every 12 h for 3–10 d

CDC, Centers for Disease Control and Prevention; UTI, urinary tract infection; IV, intravenous.

Use

Ciprofloxacin is the most potent fluoroquinolone against gram-negative bacteria. Ciprofloxacin and other fluoroquinolones are indicated to treat infections of the respiratory, genitourinary, and GI tracts, as well as infections of the bones, joints, skin, and soft tissues.

The FDA has recommended that use of the fluoroquinolones be limited to complicated infections in patients for whom drugs with lower toxicity profiles are not available for their treatment. Currently, ciprofloxacin is also recommended as first-line treatment for suspected *Bacillus anthracis* infections (anthrax) until culture and susceptibility results are available. The drug class also shows promise in the treatment of pulmonary tuberculosis. Table 19.3 presents important information about the fluoroquinolones.

Patient-related variables specific to the use of ciprofloxacin and other fluoroquinolones include the following:

- Age:
  - Ciprofloxacin and other fluoroquinolones are not routinely used as first-line therapy in children.
  - Ciprofloxacin has been approved for use in children with complicated urinary tract infections and pyelonephritis from *E. coli*.
  - Ciprofloxacin is recommended in children for the prophylaxis and treatment of anthrax exposure.
  - In older adults, decreased kidney function, other disease processes, and concurrent drug therapies increase the risks of adverse effects, necessitating close monitoring.
  - Older adults with normal kidney function should have an adequate fluid intake and urine output when taking fluoroquinolones to prevent drug crystals from forming in the urinary tract.
- Reproduction, pregnancy, and lactation:
  - Due to physiologic changes in pregnancy, serum concentrations of ciprofloxacin in pregnant patients may be lower than in nonpregnant patients.
  - Ciprofloxacin is recommended for the prophylaxis and treatment of pregnant patients with anthrax exposure.
  - Fluoroquinolones should be used during pregnancy for the treatment of other infections only if safer, effective drug therapy is not available.
- Abnormal kidney function and hepatic impairment:
  - Abnormal kidney function increases and prolongs serum drug levels so a decreased dosage may be required.

Quality and Safety Alert: Evidence-Based Practice

The U.S. Food and Drug Administration (FDA) issued a warning recommending that fluoroquinolones be avoided in patients with known aortic aneurysms or those with risk factors for aneurysm, as observational studies suggested an association between aortic aneurysm or dissection and systemic use of fluoroquinolones given by mouth or injection (2018). A retrospective analysis by Newton et al. (2021) expanded the concerns to all adults and not just high-risk individuals. The researchers reviewed filled prescriptions for fluoroquinolones or a comparable antibiotic from 2005 to 2017 for adults aged 18 to 64 in the United States. Of the 47,596,545 prescriptions reviewed, 9,053,961 were fluoroquinolones and 38,542,584 were a comparable antibiotic. Statistical analysis indicated that compared with other antibiotics, adults aged 35 years or older who took fluoroquinolones had an increased incidence of aortic aneurysm development within 90 days of starting the drug. This association was consistent across either sex or comorbidities.

These findings are consistent with recent international studies showing an increased risk of aortic aneurysm and dissection after fluoroquinolone use that led to the FDA to limit use of fluoroquinolones in high-risk patients. This retroactive study raises concerns regarding the safety of this class of drugs for use in the general population.

Adverse Effects

Ciprofloxacin and other fluoroquinolones carry risk of serious adverse effects. The most frequent adverse effects are GI side effects and include nausea, vomiting, and abdominal discomfort. Some patients experience dizziness and mild headache. Allergic and skin reactions have occurred. Photosensitivity can occur while taking ciprofloxacin with exposure to direct or indirect sunlight, and artificial light or sunlamps may also precipitate photosensitivity reactions. Tendon rupture and tendinitis are serious concerns with the fluoroquinolones. There is increasing concern for the risk of aortic aneurysm with the use of fluoroquinolones.

The FDA has expanded the **BOXED WARNING** ◆ for fluoroquinolones, alerting health professionals not only to the increased disabling risk of tendinitis and tendon rupture but also to the significant risk of peripheral neuropathy, central nervous system and cardiac effects, and dermatologic and hypersensitivity reactions. The risk is greater for people older than 60 years of age; those with heart, kidney, and lung transplants; and those taking corticosteroid medications. Adverse effects can occur up to weeks after beginning fluoroquinolones and may potentially be permanent. Discontinuation of the fluoroquinolone is necessary with the development of adverse effects. In addition, a **BOXED WARNING** ◆ exists for fluoroquinolones, including ciprofloxacin, because the drug class may exacerbate muscle weakness in persons with myasthenia gravis; its use should be avoided in patients with this condition. QT interval prolongation may occur, and the degree of severity varies by agent.

Contraindications

Contraindications include hypersensitivity and concurrent use of tizanidine. Current data have shown that ciprofloxacin crosses the placenta and is found in amniotic fluid and cord blood.

Nursing Implications

Preventing Interactions

Many medications interact with ciprofloxacin, increasing or decreasing its effects (Box 19.3). Fluoroquinolones have the potential to prolong the QT interval and may increase the risks of torsade de pointes and sudden death. Patients should not receive drugs such as the antidysrhythmic amiodarone, which prolong the QT interval, in conjunction with fluoroquinolones. Ciprofloxacin reduces theophylline clearance by 30%. Reportedly, fatal reactions have occurred after concurrent use of ciprofloxacin and theophylline.

Herbs and foods also interact with ciprofloxacin. Ciprofloxacin can chelate with cations, and drugs containing iron, multivitamins, calcium, magnesium, aluminum salt, and sucralfate may significantly reduce the absorption of ciprofloxacin. Therefore, patients should take oral ciprofloxacin 2 hours before or 6 hours after such agents. Patients should also avoid taking oral ciprofloxacin with dairy products or other calcium-containing foods. In addition, patients should not take didanosine and ciprofloxacin simultaneously. Enteral feedings should be discontinued for 1 to 2 hours prior to and after ciprofloxacin administration; enteral feedings decrease drug absorption by more than 30%. The use of dong quai and St. John's wort should also be avoided as these preparations also increase photosensitivity, intensifying the risk of sunburn or skin rash.

The nurse should also watch for severe hypoglycemia, which has developed in patients receiving concomitant glyburide and fluoroquinolones, including ciprofloxacin. Although most cases have affected patients with diabetes, severe cases of hyperglycemia have occurred in patients not previously diagnosed with the disease.

BOX 19.3 *Drug Interactions: Ciprofloxacin*

Drugs That Increase the Effects of Ciprofloxacin
- Fosphenytoin, ivabradine
  Possibly prolong QT interval
- Angiotensin-converting enzyme inhibitors, angiotensin II receptor blockers, spironolactone
  May enhance the dysrhythmogenic effect
- Probenecid
  May decrease excretion

Drugs That Decrease the Effects of Ciprofloxacin
- Aluminum-, calcium-, iron-, and magnesium-containing products, sucralfate, quinapril (contains magnesium)
  Impair absorption
- Didanosine, quinapril
  Decrease serum concentrations

Clinical Application 19.1

Mr. Louis is started on ciprofloxacin (Cipro) 500 mg orally every 12 hours, after exhausting all alternate drug treatment options.
- What patient teaching should the nurse provide?

Administering the Medication

Severe hypersensitivity reactions have occurred with the administration of fluoroquinolones. The nurse should discontinue the antibiotic immediately if skin rash or other signs or symptoms of hypersensitivity occur. To reduce the risk of irritation to the veins causing burning, swelling, and pain, the nurse administers the IV formulation over 60 minutes through a verified patent IV line. If administration through a nasogastric tube is necessary, the nurse crushes immediate-release tablets and mixes them with water. Enteral feedings reduce the serum concentration of ciprofloxacin, and the nurse gives tube feedings 1 hour before and 2 hours after administering the drug. Patients should take fluoroquinolones, like all antibiotics, for the full prescribed course of treatment to prevent complications.

Assessing for Therapeutic Effects

Assessing for factors that increase the risk of adverse effects is important; these include impaired kidney function, inadequate fluid intake, concomitant use of multivitamins or antacids, or frequent exposure to sunlight in the usual activities of daily living.

It is not necessary to take drug levels when administering ciprofloxacin or any of the fluoroquinolones. Serum creatinine and blood urea nitrogen (BUN) are recommended values to monitor when administering ciprofloxacin.

Assessing for Adverse Effects

The nurse assesses for nausea, diarrhea, vomiting, abdominal pain, headache, increased liver enzymes, and injection site reactions. It may be necessary to stop ciprofloxacin therapy if a harmful effect is severe enough. Any rash warrants careful evaluation, and if a hypersensitivity reaction occurs, the nurse discontinues the drug immediately and notifies the prescriber.

Patient Teaching

Patient teaching guidelines are outlined in Box 19.4.

Other Drugs in the Class

Other systemic fluoroquinolones include levofloxacin, moxifloxacin, delafloxacin, and ofloxacin. The mechanism of action, adverse effects profile, and interactions of these agents are similar to those of ciprofloxacin. Differences exist among individual fluoroquinolones regarding effectiveness in killing various bacterial species. Levofloxacin, moxifloxacin, and ofloxacin are effective in the treatment of community-acquired pneumonia, acute exacerbation of chronic bronchitis, acute bacterial sinusitis, and skin and skin structure infections. Delafloxacin is used for the treatment of acute bacterial skin and skin structure infections. Levofloxacin is also used to treat postexposure inhalational anthrax and prophylaxis and treatment of plague due to *Yersinia pestis*. Levofloxacin and ofloxacin are useful in the treatment of cystitis and urinary tract infection. Ofloxacin also is prescribed for urethral and cervical gonorrhea, urethritis and cervicitis due to *Chlamydia trachomatis*, and other infections of the urethra and cervix, including pelvic inflammatory disease.

Clinical Application 19.2

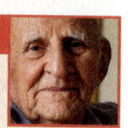

Mr. Louis returns to the clinic for a repeat urine culture and sensitivity on day 7 of antibiotic therapy.

- What assessment findings, if found by the nurse, indicate that treatment with ciprofloxacin has been successful?

BOX 19.4 Patient Teaching Guidelines for the Fluoroquinolones

General Considerations

- Avoid exposure to sunlight during and for several days after taking one of these drugs. Stop taking the drug and notify the prescriber if skin burning, redness, swelling, rash, or itching occurs. Sunscreen lotions do not prevent photosensitivity reactions.
- Be very careful if driving or doing other tasks requiring alertness or physical coordination. These drugs may cause dizziness, lightheadedness, or drowsiness.
- Report any episodes of fainting or decreased heart rate and report any history of prolonged QT syndrome.
- Report any increased tendon pain, jaundice, rash, or mood changes as these may indicate side effects from taking a fluoroquinolone.

Self-Administration

- Take levofloxacin solution and ofloxacin 1 hour before or 2 hours after meals on an empty stomach. Ciprofloxacin (Cipro) may be taken with food to decrease gastrointestinal upset. Levofloxacin tablets and moxifloxacin can be taken with or without regard to meals.
- Drink 2 to 3 quarts of fluid daily if you are able to help prevent kidney problems.
- Do not take antacids containing magnesium or aluminum (e.g., Mylanta or Maalox); any products containing iron, magnesium, calcium (e.g., Tums), or zinc (e.g., multivitamins); or sucralfate or buffered didanosine preparations at the same time or for several hours before or after a dose of the fluoroquinolone. (Consult product-specific information for individual drug recommendations.)

Unfolding Patient Stories: Harry Hadley • Part 1

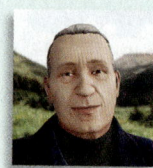

Harry Hadley was diagnosed 3 days ago with cellulitis in his right lower leg caused by a feral cat bite. A wound culture was obtained and oral augmentin was started. His infection has worsened, and he is admitted to the hospital for treatment with intravenous vancomycin. Culture results are positive for MRSA. How would the nurse respond when Harry questions why he was prescribed the augmentin 3 days ago instead of vancomycin? What are the spectra of organism coverage for augmentin and vancomycin? What drug resistance concerns should the nurse consider? Describe how the nurse evaluates wound culture and sensitivity findings and how the test determines the most effective anti-infective medication. (Harry Hadley's story continues in Chapter 61.)

Care for Harry and other patients in a realistic virtual environment: **vSim** *for Nursing* (thepoint.lww.com/vSimPharm). Practice documenting these patients' care in DocuCare (thepoint.lww.com/DocuCareEHR).

NCLEX Success

3. A patient from a nursing home arrives at the emergency department with acute pyelonephritis. The provider prescribes ciprofloxacin 500 mg PO twice daily. The patient has a history of seizures and bradycardia. The nurse should
   A. counsel the patient's caregiver to avoid administering the ciprofloxacin with the patient's anticonvulsant
   B. ask the provider to check blood levels of the patient's anticonvulsant(s) before giving the first dose of ciprofloxacin
   C. tell the provider about the patient's seizure and dysrhythmia history and inquire whether another type of antibiotic might be selected
   D. advise the patient's caregiver to discontinue the ciprofloxacin after the patient's fever is gone

4. A nurse reading a patient's chart notices that the patient is scheduled to receive ciprofloxacin 500 mg PO at 9:00 a.m. The medication administration record also indicates that Maalox 30 mL PO and hydrochlorothiazide 25 mg PO are due at 9:00 a.m. The nurse should
   A. administer all the medications as scheduled
   B. hold the Maalox until 11:00 a.m.
   C. ask the provider to discontinue hydrochlorothiazide because of increased risk of ototoxicity
   D. administer the Maalox and ciprofloxacin but hold the hydrochlorothiazide

5. An outpatient has just received a prescription for ciprofloxacin 500 mg PO twice daily for acute bronchitis. The nurse should teach the patient
   A. not to take ciprofloxacin with a meal
   B. to restrict fluid intake to avoid fluid overload
   C. to take ciprofloxacin with an antacid (e.g., Tums) to decrease the chance of stomach upset
   D. to avoid prolonged exposure to sunlight

THE NURSING PROCESS

A concept map outlines the nursing process related to drug therapy considerations in this chapter. Additional nursing implications related to the disease process should also be considered in care decisions.

Assessment

With aminoglycosides, assess for the presence of factors that predispose the patient to nephrotoxicity or ototoxicity.
- Check laboratory reports of renal function (e.g., serum creatinine, CrCl, BUN) for abnormal values.
- Assess for impairment of balance or hearing, including audiometry reports if available.
- Analyze current medications for drugs that interact with aminoglycosides, increasing the risk of nephrotoxicity or ototoxicity.

With fluoroquinolones, assess for the presence of factors that increase risks of adverse drug effects (e.g., impaired renal function, inadequate fluid intake, concomitant use of multivitamins or antacids, frequent or prolonged exposure to sunlight in usual activities of daily living).
- Assess laboratory tests (e.g., complete blood counts, tests of renal and hepatic function) for abnormal values.

Outcomes of Therapy

The patient will
- Receive aminoglycoside dosages that are individualized by age, weight, renal function, and serum drug levels.
- Have serum aminoglycoside levels monitored when indicated.
- Have renal function tests performed regularly during aminoglycoside and fluoroquinolone therapy.
- Receive adequate hydration during aminoglycoside and fluoroquinolone therapy.
- Be regularly monitored for adverse drug effects.

Nursing Interventions

- With aminoglycosides, weigh patients accurately (dosage is based on total body weight for nonobese patients and adjusted body weight for obese patients) and monitor laboratory reports of BUN, serum creatinine levels, serum drug levels, and urinalysis for abnormal values.
- Force fluids to at least 2,000 to 3,000 mL daily if not contraindicated. Keeping the patient well hydrated reduces risks of nephrotoxicity with aminoglycosides and crystalluria with fluoroquinolones.
- Avoid concurrent use of other nephrotoxic drugs when possible.
- Provide appropriate teaching (see Boxes 19.2 and 19.4).

Evaluation

- Interview and observe for improvement in the infection being treated.
- Interview and observe for adverse drug effects.

Visit thePoint® at http://thePoint.lww.com/Frandsen13e for answers to NCLEX Success questions (in Appendix A), answers to Clinical Application Case Studies (in Appendix B), and more!

REFERENCES AND RESOURCES

Bower, W. A., Schiffer, J., Atmar, R. L., Keitel, W. A., Friedlander, A. M., Liu, L., Yu, Y., Stephens, D. S., Quinn, C. P., Hendricks, K., & ACIP Anthrax Vaccine Work Group. (2019). Use of Anthrax Vaccine in the United States: Recommendations of the Advisory Committee on Immunization Practices, 2019. *Morbidity and Mortality Weekly Report Recommendations and Reports*, 68(4), 1–14. https://doi.org/10.15585/mmwr.rr6804a1

Centers for Disease Control and Prevention. Sexually Transmitted Diseases (STDs) Web site. Retrieved September 10, 2022, from http://www.cdc.gov/std

Cobussen, M., Haeseker, M. B., Stoffers, J., Wanrooij, V. H. M., Savelkoul, P. H. M., & Stassen, P. M. (2021). Renal safety of a single dose of gentamicin in patients with sepsis in the emergency department. *Clinical Microbiology and Infection*, 27(5), 717–723.

Food and Drug Administration. (2018). *Fluoroquinolone antibiotics: Safety communication—Increased risk of ruptures or tears in the aorta blood vessel in certain patients* [Posted 12/20/2018]. Retrieved September 12, 2022, from https://www.fda.gov/drugs/drug-safety-and-availability/fda-warns-about-increased-risk-ruptures-or-tears-aorta-blood-vessel-fluoroquinolone-antibiotics

Hinkle, J. H., Cheever, K. H., & Overbaugh, K. J. (2021). *Brunner & Suddarth's textbook of medical-surgical nursing* (15th ed.). Wolters Kluwer.

Lungu, I. A., Moldovan, O. L., Biriş, V., & Rusu, A. (2022). Fluoroquinolones hybrid molecules as promising antibacterial agents in the fight against antibacterial resistance. *Pharmaceutics, 14*(8), 1749. https://doi.org/10.3390/pharmaceutics14081749

Newton, E. R., Akerman, A. W., Strassle, P. D., & Kibbe, M. R. (2021). Association of fluoroquinolone use with short-term risk of development of aortic aneurysm. *JAMA Surgery, 156*(3), 264–272. doi:10.1001/jamasurg.2020.6165

St. Cyr, S., Barbee, L., Workowski, K. A., Bachmann, L. H., Pham, C., Schlanger, K., Torrone, E., Weinstock, H., Kersh, E. N., & Thorpe, P. (2020). Update to CDC's treatment guidelines for gonococcal infection. *Morbidity and Mortality Weekly Report Recommendations Report, 69*, 1911–1916.

CHAPTER 20

Drug Therapy With Tetracyclines, Sulfonamides, and Urinary Antiseptics

LEARNING OBJECTIVES

After studying this chapter, you should be able to:

1. Identify the prototype and describe the characteristics, action, use, adverse effects, contraindications, and nursing implications of the tetracyclines.
2. Identify the prototype and describe the characteristics, action, use, adverse effects, contraindications, and nursing implications of the sulfonamides.
3. Identify the prototype and describe the action, use, adverse effects, contraindications, and nursing implications for the adjuvant urinary antiseptic agents used in the treatment of urinary tract infections.
4. Implement the nursing process in the care of patients being treated with tetracyclines, sulfonamides, or urinary antiseptics.

CLINICAL APPLICATION CASE STUDY

Karen Parsons is a 19-year-old college student. She comes to the health clinic with complaints of urinary frequency and burning on urination. Her medication history includes ongoing, long-term treatment of acne with a tetracycline. She takes 250 mg of the drug orally daily. The physician diagnoses her with a urinary tract infection and prescribes trimethoprim–sulfamethoxazole (Bactrim) DS (160/800 mg), one tablet orally twice daily for 3 days.

KEY TERMS

Antimicrobial resistance: microbial resistance to drugs once successfully used to destroy microorganisms

Crystalluria: presence of crystals in the urine, indicating kidney irritation

INTRODUCTION

This chapter introduces the pharmacologic management of the patient experiencing an infection that is treated with tetracyclines or sulfonamides. These older, broad-spectrum, bacteriostatic drugs are rarely used for systemic infections because of **antimicrobial resistance** and the development of more effective or less toxic drugs. Such resistance occurs when the microbe develops resistance mechanisms to drugs once successfully used to destroy the microorganism. This discussion also introduces the urinary antiseptic agents administered for urinary tract infections (UTIs). Table 20.1 lists the drugs discussed in this chapter. The Drugs at a Glance tables present information about routes of administration and dosage ranges for both prototypes and other related drugs.

TETRACYCLINES

The tetracyclines are antibiotics, derived from chlortetracycline, that have been used to treat serious, life-threatening infections. The drugs in this class have similar pharmacologic properties. Tetracyclines are effective against both Gram-negative and Gram-positive microorganisms, but the older drugs are usually not drugs of choice. Like all antibiotic classes, the antimicrobial activities of tetracyclines are subject to both class-specific and intrinsic antibiotic-resistance mechanisms. However, resistant bacteria infrequently inactivate tetracyclines biologically or alter the drugs chemically, as with many other antibiotics. Rather, resistance develops primarily as the result of the bacteria's preventing accumulation of the drug inside the cell. Researchers have made chemical modifications that have resulted in semisynthetic drugs with activity against specific drug-resistant organisms.

Prescribers still order tetracyclines for bacterial infections caused by *Brucella* and *Vibrio cholerae*. The drugs also remain effective against rickettsiae, chlamydia, some protozoa, spirochetes, and others (see "Use" of tetracyclines). **P Tetracycline hydrochloride** is the prototype of this class.

Pharmacokinetics

Administration of tetracycline is oral, and the stomach absorbs 75% of the medication. Its peak of action is 2 to 4 hours. Tetracycline is widely distributed to the tissues, with 65% of the drug protein bound. It has the ability to cross the placenta and enter breast milk. Elimination of 50% to 60% of the drug occurs in the urine within 72 hours. Its half-life in patients with normal kidney function is 8 to 11 hours.

Action

Tetracycline penetrates microbial cells by passive diffusion and an active transport system. Intracellularly, it binds to the 30S ribosomes and possibly the 50S ribosomes and inhibits microbial protein synthesis. In patients with acne, it suppresses the growth of *Propionibacterium acnes* with sebaceous follicles, reducing the free fatty acid content in the sebum.

Use

Tetracycline is effective for treating *Mycoplasma*, *Chlamydia*, and *Rickettsia*. Healthcare providers administer it for the treatment of chronic bronchitis, gonorrhea, and syphilis in patients with a known allergy to penicillin. Combined with other drugs, it may be effective in the eradication of *Helicobacter pylori*, thus reducing the risk of duodenal ulcers. Tetracycline is also useful in treating small animal bites and Lyme disease. In addition, it may be useful as adjunctive therapy for acute intestinal amebiasis and acne vulgaris. Finally, prescribers order tetracycline when penicillin is contraindicated to treat infections caused by *Klebsiella*, *Neisseria gonorrhoeae*, *Treponema pallidum*, *Listeria monocytogenes*, *Clostridium*, *Bacillus anthracis*, *Fusobacterium fusiforme*, and *Actinomyces*.

Table 20.2 provides route and dosage information about tetracycline and related drugs.

TABLE 20.1

Drug Therapy With Tetracyclines, Sulfonamides, and Urinary Antiseptics

Drug Class	Prototype(s)	Other Drugs in the Class
Tetracyclines	**P Tetracycline** (Achromycin V)	Demeclocycline hydrochloride Doxycycline (Vibramycin, Oracea, Monodox) Minocycline hydrochloride (Minocin, Dynacin, Solodyn, Ximino) Eravacycline (Xerava) Omadacycline (Nuzyra) Sarecycline (Seysara) Tigecycline (Tygacil)
Sulfonamides	**P Trimethoprim–sulfamethoxazole** (Bactrim, Septra, others)	Mafenide acetate (Sulfamylon) Sulfadiazine Silver sulfadiazine (Silvadene) Sulfasalazine (Azulfidine)
Urinary antiseptics	**P Nitrofurantoin** (Macrobid, Macrodantin)	Phenazopyridine hydrochloride Trimethoprim

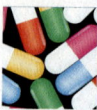

TABLE 20.2 DRUGS AT A GLANCE: Tetracyclines

Drug	Routes and Dosage Ranges	
	Adults	**Children**
ⓟ **Tetracycline hydrochloride** (Achromycin V; 🍁 Apo-Tetra, Nu-Tetra)	250–500 mg PO every 6 h	Older than 8 y: 25–50 mg/kg/d PO in four divided doses
Demeclocycline hydrochloride (Declomycin)	150 mg PO every 6 h or 300 mg every 12 h	Older than 8 y: 8–12 mg/kg/d PO in two to four divided doses
Doxycycline (Vibramycin, Oracea, Monodox; 🍁 Apprilon, Vibramycin)	100–200 mg/d PO/IV, in one to two divided doses	Older than 8 y: weight <45 kg: 2–5 mg/kg/d PO/IV in one to two divided doses (max dose 200 mg/d) Weight ≥45 kg: same as adults
Eravacycline (Xerava)	IV: 1 mg/kg every 12 h for 4–14 d	Not recommended for children
Minocycline hydrochloride (Minocin, Dynacin, Solodyn, Ximino; 🍁 Dom Minocycline, Sandoz Minocycline)	200 mg PO initially, then 100 mg every 12 h (max dose 400 mg/d) 200 mg IV initially, followed by 100 mg every 12 h Acne: 45–54 kg: 45 mg PO daily 55–77 kg: 65 mg PO daily 78–102 kg: 90 mg PO daily 103–125 kg: 115 mg PO daily 126–136 kg: 135 mg PO daily	Older than 8 y: 4 mg/kg PO initially, then 2 mg/kg every 12 h; 4 mg/kg IV, followed by 2 mg/kg every 12 h (max dose 400 mg/d)
Omadacycline (Nuzyra)	Pneumonia, community-acquired IV: loading dose infuse 200 mg over 60 min or 100 mg over 30 min through a dedicated IV line; in no dedicated line, flush with NS or D_5W before and after infusion of drug; maintenance dose: IV: 100 mg once daily or PO 300 mg once daily for 7–14 d Skin and skin structure infections: loading dose infuse 200 mg over 60 min or 100 mg over 30 min through a dedicated IV line; in no dedicated line, flush with NS or D_5W before and after infusion of drug or PO 450 mg once daily on days 1 and 2; maintenance dose: IV: 100 mg once daily or PO 300 mg once daily for 7–14 d	Not recommended for children
Sarecycline (Seysara)	Weight based 33–54 kg: PO 60 mg once daily 55–84 kg: PO 100 mg once daily 85–136 kg: PO 150 mg once daily	≥9 y: same as adults
Tigecycline (Tygacil; 🍁 Tygacil)	Community-acquired pneumonia: IV 100 mg initially; 50 mg maintenance dose every 12 h for 7–14 d Intra-abdominal infections: IV 100 mg initially; 50 mg maintenance dose every 12 h for 5–14 d Skin and skin structure infections: IV 100 mg initially; 50 mg maintenance dose every 12 h for 5–14 d	8–11 y: IV 1.2–2.0 mg/kg/dose every 2 h up to 50 mg/dose ≥12 y: IV 50 mg every 12 h

Patient-related variables specific to the use of tetracycline include the following:

- Age:
  - In children younger than 8 years of age, doxycycline is the only tetracycline that should be used because it interferes with enamel development to a lesser extent than other tetracyclines, which can cause a permanent yellow, gray, or brown discoloration. (In bone, tetracycline deposits form a stable compound in bone-forming tissue and may interfere with bone growth.)
  - In older adults receiving tetracyclines, kidney and hepatic function must be monitored.
- Reproduction, pregnancy, and lactation:
  - Tetracycline is generally contraindicated in pregnancy because it may cause fatal hepatic necrosis in the patient. If given, the drug may interfere with bone and tooth development in the fetus. However, in some disorders, the benefit to the patient may outweigh the risk of hepatic dysfunction; such disorders include rickettsial infections, ehrlichiosis, inhalational anthrax, and malaria.
  - Breast-feeding patients should not take the drug because it is secreted into breast milk.
  - The combination of oral contraceptives and tetracycline results in diminished contraceptive effects, requiring use of an additional form of birth control.
- Abnormal kidney function and hepatic impairment:
  - Tetracycline is contraindicated in patients with abnormal kidney function/failure.
  - Caution and monitoring are warranted when tetracycline is administered to patients with known hepatotoxicity.

Adverse Effects

Several adverse effects may occur following the administration of tetracycline. These include the following:

- Hypersensitivity such as rash, urticaria, serum sickness, or anaphylaxis. Maculopapular and erythematous rashes may also occur.
- Central nervous system (CNS) conditions such as intracranial hypertension (most severe CNS effect).
- Gastrointestinal (GI) conditions such as flatulence, diarrhea, nausea, vomiting, and epigastric distress (commonly reported). Esophagitis, pancreatitis, and staphylococcal enterocolitis may also occur.
- Superinfections:
- Candidal: sore throat; white patches on the oral mucosa; or a black, furry tongue
- GI: pseudomembranous colitis
- Other conditions such as increased pigmentation, photosensitivity reactions, azotemia, kidney and hepatic toxicity, as well as retardation of bone growth. Discoloration of the teeth and enamel hypoplasia may occur in children younger than 8 years of age.

Contraindications

Contraindications to tetracycline include kidney failure and known hypersensitivity to the drug. Other contraindications are young age (less than 8 years) and pregnancy; as previously stated, the drug causes permanent discoloration of teeth, defects in tooth enamel, and retardation of bone growth.

Nursing Implications

Preventing Interactions

Many medications interact with tetracycline hydrochloride, increasing or decreasing its effects (Box 20.1). Tetracycline also affects the action of several drugs. Administering oral anticoagulants with tetracycline enhances the effect of vitamin K. Digoxin combined with tetracycline leads to increased digoxin absorption, resulting in digoxin toxicity. Giving penicillins with tetracycline interferes with the bactericidal effects of the penicillins. In addition, certain herbs increase the effects of trimethoprim–sulfamethoxazole (TMP–SMZ) including garlic, ginseng, ginger, and St. John's wort. Foods that affect the action of tetracycline include dairy products, which decrease the absorption of the antibiotic.

Administering the Medication

It is important to obtain a culture and sensitivity prior to beginning therapy with tetracycline. Administration of the drug is oral. The medication is most effective when taken on an empty stomach. Patients should take the medication 1 hour before meals or 2 hours after meals. It is important not to take it with dairy products, antacids, or iron supplements. The combination of tetracycline with metallic ions such as aluminum, calcium, iron, or magnesium inhibits tetracycline absorption. If the patient has consumed dairy products, antacids, or iron supplements, it is necessary to withhold tetracycline for 2 hours.

 Quality and Safety Alert: Safety

Tetracycline and other tetra derivatives (metacycline, doxycycline) should never be used after the expiration date. The administration of outdated tetracycline may cause severe kidney damage due to a change in the drug's chemical structure over time.

Assessing for Therapeutic Effects

The nurse assesses for decreased signs and symptoms of the infection, such as decreased pain and fever.

BOX 20.1 Drug Interactions: Tetracycline

Drugs That Increase the Effects of Tetracycline
- Methoxyflurane
  Increases the risk of nephrotoxicity

Drugs That Decrease the Effects of Tetracycline
- Aluminum, antacids, bismuth subsalicylate, didanosine, ferrous sulfate, calcium, kaolin, laxatives, magnesium, pectin, zinc
  Decrease antibiotic absorption

Assessing for Adverse Effects

The nurse assesses for GI irritation, nausea, epigastric distress, diarrhea, and vomiting. The patient is also assessed for rash, anaphylaxis, and serum sickness. If a patient is exposed to sunlight, it is necessary to assess for sunburn or photosensitivity reactions. In addition, the nurse checks the patient's complete blood count for anemia and signs and symptoms of superinfection.

Patient Teaching

Box 20.2 identifies patient teaching guidelines for tetracycline.

Other Drugs in the Class

Doxycycline (Vibramycin), one of the most active tetracyclines, is used most often clinically because it possesses advantages over traditional tetracyclines and minocycline. The drug is less likely to cause photosensitivity and causes less tooth discoloration and bony growth retardation (it binds calcium to a lesser extent than tetracycline); thus, it is the only tetracycline recommended for use in children younger than 8 years of age. Also, doxycycline is one of the drugs (along with ciprofloxacin; see Chapter 19) recommended by the Centers for Disease Control and Prevention (CDC) for the treatment of *B. anthracis* (anthrax). People with inhalational anthrax should receive a multidrug regimen of either doxycycline or ciprofloxacin concurrently with at least one more recommended drug for 60 days following exposure. The drug is also useful for infections with *Chlamydia trachomatis* and in respiratory tract infections due to *Mycoplasma pneumoniae*. In addition, doxycycline is effective in treating gonorrhea in patients who are allergic to penicillin. Doxycycline is incompatible with allopurinol, barbiturates, erythromycin lactobionate, heparin, meropenem, nafcillin, penicillin, piperacillin, sulfonamides, and riboflavin.

Parenteral administration of doxycycline requires mixing with lactated Ringer's or dextrose 5% and lactated Ringer's. Slow infusion is necessary (range of 1 to 12 hours).

Demeclocycline hydrochloride is useful in the treatment of bacterial infections such as acne, pertussis, and UTIs caused by Gram-positive or Gram-negative organisms. An unlabeled use is for the treatment of chronic syndrome of inappropriate secretion of antidiuretic hormone. When administering demeclocycline, it is important to monitor the patient's blood urea nitrogen (BUN). Increases in the BUN are secondary to antianabolic effects. Demeclocycline is the tetracycline most likely to cause photosensitivity.

Eravacycline (Xerava), an intravenous (IV) agent, has shown promise in the treatment of serious infections caused by a broad range of aerobic and anaerobic Gram-negative and Gram-positive bacteria (the exception is complicated UTIs in adults). It is approved for use in the treatment of complicated intra-abdominal infections caused by *Staphylococcus aureus, Escherichia coli, Klebsiella pneumoniae, Klebsiella oxytoca, Enterococcus faecalis, Enterococcus faecium*, and others, even in patients with infections caused by extended-spectrum beta-lactamase–producing organisms.

Minocycline hydrochloride (Minocin) is a semisynthetic tetracycline derivative used to treat a variety of bacterial infections, including UTIs, respiratory infections, skin infections, and severe acne. The drug is also useful in the treatment of rickettsial infections and as an adjunct to amebicides in the management of acute intestinal amebiasis. Oral absorption is good; foods and fluids affect absorption of minocycline less than other tetracyclines. IV administration of minocycline requires slow infusion. Prolonged IV administration of minocycline may be associated with thrombophlebitis. The drug is stable in all IV solutions but is incompatible with calcium-containing solutions.

Omadacycline (Nuzyra), available both orally and intravenously, has been successful in the treatment of community-acquired pneumonia and bacterial skin and skin structure infections. Susceptible bacteria include methicillin-resistant *S. aureus* (MRSA), vancomycin-resistant *Enterococci*, penicillin-resistant *Streptococcus pneumoniae, Haemophilus influenzae*, and *E. coli*.

Sarecycline (Seysara) is used to treat acne vulgaris in patients who are at least 9 years of age. The drug is similar to tetracycline in terms of adverse-effect profile. Administer sarecycline with or without food. The drug should be taken with adequate fluids to reduce the risk of esophageal irritation and ulceration. To avoid interference with absorption, the drug should not be given at the same time as any iron-containing preparations (i.e., aluminum, calcium, or magnesium antacids).

Tigecycline (Tygacil), an IV tetracycline, is derived from minocycline. It is useful in the treatment of community-acquired bacterial pneumonia, complicated skin and skin structure infections, and complicated intra-abdominal infections. Because tigecycline is not affected by the two major mechanisms of tetracycline resistance, it may have activity against tetracycline-resistant organisms. The drug has a broad spectrum of coverage and has bacteriostatic activity against many Gram-positive pathogens including MRSA, vancomycin-resistant *Enterococcus*, and penicillin-resistant *Streptococcus pneumoniae*; some Gram-negative organisms (important exceptions are *Proteus, Pseudomonas, Providencia*, and *Morganella* species); anaerobes; and atypical species. The U.S. Food and Drug Administration (FDA) has issued a **BOXED WARNING** because of the increased risk of mortality in patients treated with tigecycline compared with other drugs used to treat serious infections.

BOX 20.2 Patient Teaching Guidelines for Tetracycline

- Take tetracycline around the clock because it inhibits but does not kill bacteria.
- Avoid sunlamps, tanning beds, and intense or prolonged exposure to sunlight.
- Wear sunscreen and protective clothing when in the sun.
- Report severe nausea, vomiting, diarrhea, skin rash, or perineal itching to your healthcare provider. These symptoms may require changing or stopping the drug.
- Take the drug on an empty stomach, at least 1 hour before or 2 hours after meals.
- Do not take the drug with or within 2 hours of consuming dairy products, antacids, or iron supplements.
- If you must take an antacid, take it at least 2 hours before or 4 hours after taking tetracycline.
- Take each dose with 8 oz of water.
- If you are taking an oral contraceptive, use another form of birth control for the duration of therapy. The effectiveness of oral contraceptives is decreased when combined with tetracycline.
- Never take outdated tetracycline due to the risk of severe reactions.

Clinical Application 20.1

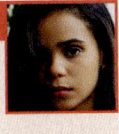

A nurse at the college health center who is interviewing Ms. Parsons about her recent health history asks about her sexual activity. Ms. Parsons replies that she has a new boyfriend with whom she has had sexual intercourse every day for the past 5 days. She says she is taking oral contraceptives. The nurse also gathers information regarding Ms. Parsons's sunbathing practices (the college is on the Gulf Coast). Ms. Parsons reports that she has been going to the beach daily.

- Based on the information gathered in the interview regarding the fact Ms. Parsons is sexually active, what instruction should the nurse provide related to the tetracycline she is taking?
- What teaching should the nurse at the health center provide related to the administration of tetracycline?
- Based on the fact that Ms. Parsons has been going to the beach daily, what is she at risk for developing?

NCLEX Success

1. A patient is admitted to the emergency department after opening an envelope containing a substance that experts have identified as anthrax. Which of the following medications is likely to be administered?
    A. tetracycline
    B. doxycycline
    C. amoxicillin–clavulanic acid combination
    D. neomycin

2. A patient receiving tetracycline should receive which of the following instructions regarding the medication?
    A. Take tetracycline with food.
    B. Take tetracycline in combination with antacids.
    C. Take the first dose and then obtain a test known as culture and sensitivity.
    D. Take tetracycline with a full glass of water.

SULFONAMIDES

Sulfonamides are bacteriostatic drugs that were once effective against a wide range of Gram-positive and Gram-negative bacteria. However, increasing resistance is making them less useful. It is important to document susceptibility with culture and sensitivity testing, but sulfonamides may be active against *Streptococcus pyogenes*, some staphylococcal strains, *H. influenzae*, *Nocardia*, *C. trachomatis*, and toxoplasmosis. The **trimethoprim-sulfamethoxazole** (TMP–SMZ) combination (Bactrim, Septra) is useful in UTIs due to *Enterobacteriaceae* and *Pneumocystis jirovecii* infection (in high doses), and it serves as the prototype. The combination of drugs demonstrates synergistic antimicrobial activity that is greater than the dose of either drug used alone. Other drugs in the class vary in extent of systemic absorption and clinical indications. Some sulfonamides are well absorbed and can be used in systemic infections; others are poorly absorbed and have more local effects. Table 20.3 summarizes key information about sulfonamides.

Pharmacokinetics

TMP–SMZ is rapidly and nearly completely absorbed in the GI tract, and the half-life of the medication is 6 to 11 hours. It enters the extracellular spaces, crosses the placental and blood–brain barriers, and appears in small amounts in breast milk. Metabolism occurs in the liver, and excretion takes place in the kidneys as metabolites and unchanged drug.

Action

TMP–SMZ and other sulfonamides act as antimetabolites of para-aminobenzoic acid (PABA), which microorganisms require to produce folic acid. In turn, folic acid is necessary for the production of bacterial intracellular proteins. Sulfonamides enter into the reaction instead of PABA, compete for the enzyme involved, and cause formation of nonfunctional derivatives of folic acid. Thus, sulfonamides halt multiplication of new bacteria but do not kill mature, fully formed bacteria. With the exception of the topical sulfonamides used in burn therapy, the presence of pus, serum, or necrotic tissue interferes with sulfonamide action because these materials contain PABA. Some bacteria can change their metabolic pathways to use precursors or other forms of folic acid and thereby develop resistance to the antibacterial action of sulfonamides. After resistance to one sulfonamide develops, cross-resistance to others is common.

Use

TMP–SMZ acts by inhibiting bacterial synthesis of essential nucleic acids and proteins. Uses include the treatment of *P. jirovecii* pneumonitis, severe UTIs, *Shigella* enteritis, and *Enterobacteriaceae*. Other organisms treated with TMP–SMZ are *Viridans streptococcus*, *Staphylococcus epidermidis*, *Salmonella*, *Klebsiella*, *Nocardia*, and *Pseudomonas*.

Quality and Safety Alert: Evidence-Based Practice

Drug resistance is an ongoing concern with antibiotics and leads to treatment failure with drug therapy. *S. aureus* resistance to methicillin (MRSA) emerged in the early 2000s, leading to the use of TMP–SMZ and clindamycin as the empirical management of *S. aureus*. Khamash et al. (2019) completed a retrospective observational study of bacterial cultures collected from patients younger than 18 years treated with TMP–SMZ for *S. aureus* infection from 2005 to 2017. Overall, 932 (38%) isolates were MRSA and 1,499 (62%) were methicillin-susceptible *S. aureus*. During this period, the proportion of methicillin-resistant samples declined from 41% to 27%, while TMP–SMZ and clindamycin resistance significantly increased. The greatest decline in resistance was in samples derived from community exposure. The study suggests that the trend in drug resistance to *S. aureus* infection in children continues to evolve, enhancing the importance of using antibiotic-susceptibility results in drug selection.

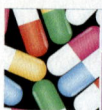

TABLE 20.3
DRUGS AT A GLANCE: Sulfonamides

Drug	Routes and Dosage Ranges	
	Adults	**Children**
ⓟ Trimethoprim–sulfamethoxazole (Bactrim, Septra, others; ❋ Apo-Sulfatrim)	UTI: one double-strength tablet PO twice daily for 3 d IV: 8–20 mg (TMP component)/kg/d divided dosing every 6–12 h (diluted and administered over 60–90 min)	UTI and otitis media: PO 8-mg/kg trimethoprim and 40-mg/kg sulfamethoxazole in two divided doses every 12 h for 10 d
Mafenide acetate (Sulfamylon)	Topical application to burned area, once or twice daily, in a thin layer	Same as adults
Sulfadiazine	2–8 g PO daily in divided doses every 6 h	>2 y: 100–200 mg/kg/d PO in divided doses every 6 h Neonate: 50 mg/kg every 12 h for 12 mo
Silver sulfadiazine (Silvadene; ❋ Dermazine, Flamazine)	Cover burned area with cream one to two times daily	Same as adults
Sulfasalazine (Azulfidine; ❋ PMS-Sulfasalazine, Salazopyrin)	Ulcerative colitis: 3–4 g PO daily in four divided doses initially; 2 g daily in divided doses for maintenance; max dose, 4 g Rheumatoid arthritis: maintenance, 2 g PO daily in divided doses, every 12 h	30–60 mg/kg/d PO in two to six divided doses initially, followed by 30 mg/kg/d in four divided doses; max daily dose, 2 g
Combination drug in which the dosage is based on trimethoprim component	Shigellosis: same dose as above for 5 d Severe UTI: IV 8–10 mg (trimethoprim component)/kg/d in two to four divided doses, up to 14 d *P. jirovecii* pneumonia: IV 15–20 mg (trimethoprim component)/kg/d in three or four divided doses, every 6–8 h up to 21 d; IV doses should be given over 60–90 min	Shigellosis: same dose as above for 5 d Severe UTI: IV 8–10 mg (trimethoprim component)/kg in two to four divided doses, every 6–8 h or every 12 h, up to 14 d *P. jirovecii* pneumonia: IV 15–20 mg (trimethoprim component)/kg/d in three or four divided doses, every 6–8 h up to 21 d

Patient-related variables specific to the use of TMP–SMZ and other sulfonamides include the following:

- Age:
  - Children younger than 2 months of age should not receive TMP–SMZ and other systemic sulfonamides.
  - If a fetus or young infant receives a sulfonamide by placental transfer, in breast milk, or by direct administration, the drug displaces bilirubin from binding sites on albumin. As a result, bilirubin may accumulate in the bloodstream (hyperbilirubinemia) and CNS (kernicterus), resulting in life-threatening toxicity.
  - In older adults, kidney function must be assessed because TMP–SMZ may cause abnormal kidney function.
  - Older people are also at greater risk of hyperkalemia due to the effects of aging on kidney function.
- Reproduction, pregnancy, and lactation:
  - Use of the drug during pregnancy increases the risk of congenital malformations.
  - Trimethoprim interferes with folic acid metabolism, decreasing patient levels. Adequate folic acid supplementation during pregnancy may decrease the risk of some congenital anomalies.
  - The drug should be avoided during the third trimester since it may cause kernicterus in the newborn.
- Abnormal kidney function and hepatic impairment:
  - Weight-based dosing recommendations in patients with abnormal kidney function guide the use of TMP–SMZ and other systemic sulfonamides.

Adverse Effects

TMP–SMZ has several adverse effects. These include the following:

- GI effects: abdominal pain, nausea, vomiting, diarrhea, anorexia, and pancreatitis
- Hematologic effects: aplastic anemia, agranulocytosis, eosinophilia, thrombocytopenia, and leukopenia
- Dermatologic effects: pruritus, urticaria, Stevens-Johnson syndrome, and skin photosensitivity
- Kidney effects: increased BUN and serum creatinine, kidney failure, and interstitial nephritis

Contraindications

Contraindications include a known hypersensitivity to any sulfa drug, trimethoprim, TMP–SMZ, or any other of the sulfonamides, salicylates, or megaloblastic anemia related to folate deficiency. The drug is also contraindicated in infants less than 2 months of age.

Nursing Implications

Culture and sensitivity testing should be completed prior to administering the drug. When administering TMP–SMZ, it is important to monitor potassium level as hyperkalemia may result particularly in the older adult and individuals with abnormal kidney function or hypoaldosteronism. The drug should be discontinued at the first sign of a rash.

Preventing Interactions

Trimethoprim and sulfamethoxazole both inhibit specific cytochrome P450 enzymes, leading to concurrent multiple drug and herb interactions, increasing or decreasing the effects of TMP–SMZ (Box 20.3). The drug inhibits warfarin metabolism and is associated with a threefold increased risk of GI bleeding when compared with other antibiotics. Other interactions include sulfonylureas (hypoglycemia), anticonvulsants (toxicity), and methotrexate (pancytopenia).

Administering the Medication

In general, TMP–SMZ is commonly administered orally, with or without food. It is important to take it with a full glass of water. In patients with severe pneumonia caused by *P. jirovecii*, the drug is administered parenterally.

> **Quality and Safety Alert: Safety**
>
> Parenteral TMP–SMZ must be diluted in D_5W (variable stability in normal saline). Parenteral TMP–SMZ drug combination should not be mixed with other drugs and IV lines must be flushed to remove any residual drug prior to administration. The drug should not be administered intramuscularly.

Assessing for Therapeutic Effects

If the patient is taking TMP–SMZ for treatment of a UTI, the nurse assesses for decreased symptoms of this infection, such as the elimination of pain when voiding, cloudy urine, and fever. If the patient is taking TMP–SMZ for treatment of *Pneumocystis* pneumonia, it is necessary to assess for resolution of symptoms including nonproductive cough, shortness of breath, or fever. If the drug is given for prophylaxis of pneumocystosis, the nurse observes for development of symptoms.

Assessing for Adverse Effects

The nurse assesses the patient's intake and output. If the intake is greater than the output, assessment of kidney function is necessary. The nurse also assesses for hyperkalemia, anemia, and changes in the complete blood count that are indicative of blood dyscrasias. In addition, it is necessary to assess for signs and symptoms of superinfection or hypersensitivity reactions. Septra, an IV form of TMP–SMZ, contains sodium metabisulfite, which may produce allergic reactions in some patients. It is necessary to assess for hives, skin redness, itching, wheezing, shortness of breath, and possible anaphylaxis.

Patient Teaching

Box 20.4 identifies patient teaching guidelines for TMP–SMZ.

Other Drugs in the Class

Mafenide (Sulfamylon) is a topical anti-infective agent administered for bacteriostatic treatment of Gram-negative and Gram-positive organisms such as *Pseudomonas aeruginosa* and other anaerobes that may be associated with second- and third-degree burns. The drug is absorbed rapidly, reaching its peak in 2 to 4 hours. Close monitoring of the patient's fluid and electrolyte status is necessary. Metabolic acidosis is a possibility. The nurse attempts to assess for signs and symptoms of allergic reaction; however, it is difficult to determine whether the reaction is due to allergy or severe burns.

Sulfadiazine is a short-acting sulfonamide that interferes with bacterial utilization of PABA. It inhibits folic acid biosynthesis that is required for the bacteria's growth. It is used in combination with pyrimethamine for the treatment of cerebral toxoplasmosis and chloroquine-resistant malaria. When this medication is used, it is imperative that the patient maintains a fluid intake that allows for an output of 1,500 mL of urine in 24 hours. Combination with pyrimethamine decreases the development of **crystalluria** (precipitation of drug crystals in

---

BOX 20.3 Drug Interactions: TMP–SMZ

Drugs That Increase the Effects of TMP–SMZ

- Alkalinizing agents such as sodium bicarbonate
  Increase the rate of urinary excretion, raising the levels of sulfonamides in the urinary tract and increasing effectiveness in UTIs
- Methenamine compounds such as urinary acidifiers
  Increase the risk of nephrotoxicity
- Salicylates, nonsteroidal anti-inflammatory agents, oral anticoagulants, phenytoin, methotrexate
  Increase the risk of nephrotoxicity by displacing sulfonamides from plasma protein binding sites
- Sulfonylureas
  Increase hypoglycemic reactions

BOX 20.4 Patient Teaching Guidelines for TMP–SMZ

- Take TMP–SMZ with 8 oz of water.
- Take the drug before or after meals.
- Drink a minimum of 2 to 3 L of fluid per day to reduce the formation of crystals and stones in the urinary tract.
- Be aware that the effectiveness of oral contraceptives is decreased when combined with TMP–SMZ, so another method of birth control should be used.
- Avoid sunlamps, tanning beds, and intense or prolonged exposure to sunlight.
- When in the sun, wear sunscreen and protective clothing.
- Inform your dentist or prescriber that you are taking a sulfonamide. Changes in laboratory values may occur as a result of taking the drug.
- If you have diabetes, monitor your blood sugar values, as reduced blood sugar levels can occur.

the urine) and stone formation. It is important to instruct the patient to consume fluids liberally and report any symptoms of blood dyscrasias, such as pallor, fever, or sore throat.

Silver sulfadiazine (Silvadene), a silver salt, has bactericidal effects on the bacterial cell wall and cell membrane that inhibit folic acid synthesis. It has antimicrobial activity against bacteria and yeast. This medication is indicated for the treatment of second- and third-degree burns. It is effective against *Pseudomonas*, *E. coli*, *Klebsiella*, *Proteus*, *Staphylococcus*, and *Streptococcus*. With large burn areas and prolonged use, patients may absorb significant amounts of silver sulfadiazine systemically. It is necessary to monitor for adverse effects of sulfonamides. Contraindications include pregnancy and age less than 1 month.

Sulfasalazine (Azulfidine) is used for ulcerative colitis and rheumatoid arthritis. The bacteriostatic action of the medication occurs in the intestine, where the intestinal flora converts the drug to two metabolites, one of which acts as an anti-inflammatory agent. It reduces *Clostridium* and *E. coli* in the stools. Sulfasalazine is contraindicated in patients who have an allergy to salicylates. The nurse instructs patients that taking this drug may make their urine yellow-orange.

> ### Clinical Application 20.2
> - What aspects of patient teaching should the nurse at the college health center provide to Ms. Parsons regarding the administration of sulfamethoxazole and trimethoprim?
> - The nurse should tell Ms. Parsons about which adverse effects?

ADJUVANT MEDICATIONS USED TO TREAT URINARY TRACT INFECTIONS: URINARY ANTISEPTICS

The adjuvant medications used to treat UTIs are trimethoprim and the urinary antiseptic agents. Urinary antiseptics may be bactericidal for sensitive organisms in the urinary tract because these drugs are concentrated in kidney tubules and reach high levels in urine. They are not used in systemic infections because they do not attain therapeutic plasma levels. The adjuvant medications include nitrofurantoin, phenazopyridine, and trimethoprim. Table 20.4 provides dosage information for the adjuvant urinary tract agents administered as adjunctive therapy for UTIs.

Nitrofurantoin

Ⓟ Nitrofurantoin (Macrobid, Macrodantin) is an anti-infective agent that is administered for the treatment and prophylaxis of UTIs. The drug is effective for UTIs caused by *E. coli*, *S. aureus*, *Enterobacter*, *Enterococcus*, and *Klebsiella*. Administration of nitrofurantoin with food aids in absorption and decreases the onset of adverse effects. The two formulations differ with regard to the size of crystals in the preparation. Older adults should not take the medication because of the risk of kidney, pulmonary, and hepatic toxicities. Contraindications include abnormal kidney function as well as pregnancy—in the first trimester, there is a risk of fetal malformations, and between week 38 and delivery, there is a risk of hemolytic anemia. Other significant adverse effects of nitrofurantoin include (1) nonspecific ST- and T-wave changes and bundle branch block and (2) CNS changes such as fever, malaise, depression, headache, lethargy, and vertigo. In addition, the nurse should inform patients that the drug may cause the urine to turn brown.

Although few drugs interact with nitrofurantoin, magnesium-containing antacids may reduce absorption and subsequent urinary secretion. Concurrent use of fluconazole may lead to hepatic and pulmonary toxicities.

Phenazopyridine

Phenazopyridine hydrochloride is a urinary analgesic administered to provide pain relief related to burning, urgency, frequency, and irritation of the lower urinary tract mucosa. The pain is a result of infection, trauma, cystoscopic examinations, surgery, or catheter insertion. Phenazopyridine, an azo dye, is a drug that acts directly on the urinary tract mucosa to provide

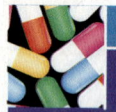

TABLE 20.4

DRUGS AT A GLANCE: Adjuvant Drugs for Urinary Tract Infections/Urinary Antiseptics

Drug	Routes and Dosage Ranges	
	Adults	**Children**
Ⓟ **Nitrofurantoin** (Macrobid, Macrodantin; ✽ Macrodantin, Macrobid)	Macrobid: 100 mg every 12 h for 7 d Macrodantin: 100 mg PO two times daily for 5 d Prophylaxis of recurrent urinary tract infection (UTI) in women Macrodantin: 50–100 mg PO at bedtime	Children older than 12 y: dual-release capsules: 100 mg every 12 h for 7 d Children 1 mo and older: macrocrystal capsules, 5–7 mg/kg/d PO in four divided doses for 7 d
Phenazopyridine hydrochloride (✽ Pyridium)	100–200 mg PO three times daily after meals	6–12 y: 12 mg/kg/d PO, in three divided doses after meals for 2 d
Trimethoprim	100 mg PO every 12 h for 10 d or 200 mg every 24 h for 10 d	4–6 mg/kg/d in divided doses every 12 h Otitis media: children ≥10 mg/kg/d PO in divided doses every 12 h for 10 d

analgesia. Metabolism occurs in the liver. It is necessary to administer the medication with food to decrease GI distress. The nurse should tell the patient that the urine will turn reddish orange. The FDA has issued a **BOXED WARNING** ◆ cautioning that if the patient's skin turns yellow, this must be reported to the healthcare provider immediately. This is a sign that phenazopyridine is accumulating in the patient's system. It is also necessary to report a sore throat, fever, bruising, or bleeding. Contraindications to phenazopyridine include abnormal kidney function and hepatitis.

Trimethoprim

Trimethoprim is a folate antagonist that is a urinary tract anti-infective. Most administered in combination with sulfamethoxazole or as an adjuvant agent with the sulfonamides (see Sulfonamides), it is also given singly. Prescribers order it for susceptible infections and UTIs. The CDC has recommended that trimethoprim be used (unlabeled use) in the treatment of *P. jirovecii* pneumonia. This drug inhibits folic acid reduction to tetrahydrofolate, thus interfering with the bacterial cell growth. Contraindications include a known folate deficiency, fragile X syndrome, and a creatinine clearance less than 15 mL/minute. Patient teaching should include taking the entire course of medication even if symptoms improve; having a sufficient fluid intake (2,000 to 3,000 mL/24 hours); and reporting symptoms such as sore throat, fever, bruising, or rash to the healthcare provider. Rash and pruritus are the most common adverse effects. There also have been occasional reports of nausea, vomiting, thrombocytopenia, and leukopenia.

NCLEX Success

3. A patient develops a urinary tract infection following the delivery of an infant. The nurse practitioner is considering prescribing trimethoprim–sulfamethoxazole. What assessment is necessary to make?

    A. if the patient is breast-feeding
    B. if the patient has been treated with the medication in the past
    C. if anyone in the patient's family has a known allergy to the drug
    D. if the patient is experiencing hematuria

4. A nurse practitioner has prescribed nitrofurantoin for a patient with a urinary tract infection. Which of the following cardiovascular adverse effects is this patient at risk for developing?

    A. inverted T wave
    B. widened QRS
    C. premature ventricular contraction (PVC)
    D. bundle branch block

5. A patient with a urinary tract infection is prescribed phenazopyridine by the healthcare provider. Which of the following adverse effects should the patient report immediately to the healthcare provider? (Select all that apply.)

    A. yellowing of the skin
    B. edema
    C. bruising
    D. malaise
    E. sore throat
    F. fever

Clinical Application 20.3

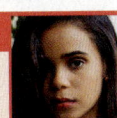

In addition to the sulfamethoxazole with trimethoprim, Ms. Parsons receives a prescription for phenazopyridine 200 mg three times per day.

- What patient teaching related to the administration of phenazopyridine does the nurse provide to Ms. Parsons?
- The nurse should teach Ms. Parsons that phenazopyridine will affect her urine in what way?
- What other patient teaching should Ms. Parsons receive?

THE NURSING PROCESS

A concept map outlining the nursing process related to drug therapy considerations in this chapter is found in the map below. General aspects of the nursing process in antimicrobial drug therapy, described in Chapter 15, apply to the patient receiving tetracyclines, sulfonamides, and urinary antiseptics. Additional nursing implications related to the disease process should also be considered in care decisions.

Assessment
- With tetracyclines, assess for conditions in which the drugs must be used cautiously or are contraindicated, such as impaired kidney or hepatic function.
- With sulfonamides, assess for signs and symptoms of disorders for which the drugs are used:
  - For UTIs, assess urinalysis reports for white blood cell and bacteria counts; urine culture reports for type of bacteria; and symptoms of dysuria, frequency, and urgency of urination.
  - For burns, assess the size of the wound, amount and type of drainage, presence of edema, and amount of eschar.
  - Ask patients specifically if they have ever taken a sulfonamide and, if so, whether they had an allergic reaction.
- With urinary antiseptics, assess for signs and symptoms of UTI.

Outcomes of Therapy
The patient will
- Receive or self-administer the drugs as directed.
- Experience relief of signs and symptoms of infection being treated.
- Receive prompt and appropriate treatment if adverse effects occur.

Nursing Interventions
- During tetracycline therapy for systemic infections, monitor laboratory tests of kidney function for abnormal values.
- During sulfonamide therapy, encourage sufficient fluids to produce a urine output of at least 1,500 mL daily. A high fluid intake decreases the risk of crystalluria.
- Avoid urinary catheterization when possible. If catheterization is necessary, use sterile technique. The urinary tract is normally sterile except for the lower third of the urethra.
  - A single catheterization may cause infection. With indwelling catheters, bacteria colonize the bladder and produce infection within 2 to 3 weeks, even with meticulous care.
  - When indwelling catheters must be used, measures to decrease UTI include using a closed drainage system; keeping the perineal area clean; forcing fluids, if not contraindicated, to maintain a dilute urine; and removing the catheter as soon as possible. Do not disconnect the system and irrigate the catheter unless obstruction is suspected. Never raise the urinary drainage bag above bladder level.
- Force fluids in anyone with a UTI unless contraindicated. Bacteria do not multiply as rapidly in dilute urine. In addition, emptying the bladder frequently allows it to refill with uninfected urine. This decreases the bacterial population of the bladder.
- Teach women to cleanse themselves from the urethral area toward the rectum after voiding or defecating to avoid contamination of the urethral area with bacteria from the vagina and rectum. Also, voiding after sexual intercourse helps cleanse the lower urethra and prevent UTI.
- Provide additional teaching related to any drug therapy (see Boxes 20.2 and 20.4).

Evaluation
- Interview and observe for administering medications as prescribed.
- Interview and observe for improvement in the infection being treated.
- Interview and observe for adverse drug effects.

Visit **thePoint** at **http://thePoint.lww.com/Frandsen13e** for answers to NCLEX Success questions (in Appendix A), answers to Clinical Application Case Studies (in Appendix B), and more!

REFERENCES AND RESOURCES

Hinkle, J. H., Cheever, K. H., & Overbaugh, K. J. (2021). *Brunner & Suddarth's textbook of medical-surgical nursing* (15th ed.). Wolters Kluwer.

Khamash, D. F., Voskertchian, A., Tamma, P. D., Akinboyo, I. C., Carroll, K. C., & Milstone, A. M. (2019). Increasing clindamycin and trimethoprim-sulfamethoxazole resistance in pediatric staphylococcus aureus infections. *Journal of the Pediatric Infectious Diseases Society, 8*(4), 351–353. https://doi.org/10.1093/jpids/piy062

May, D. B. (2022). Trimethoprim-sulfamethoxazole: An overview. *UpToDate*. Lexi-Comp, Inc.

Norris, T. L. (2018). *Porth's pathophysiology: Concepts of altered health states* (10th ed.). Wolters Kluwer.

Smith, C. A. (2021). Trimethoprim-sulfamethoxazole and hyperkalemia. *Nephrology Nursing Journal, 48*(2), 177–180.

CHAPTER 21

Drug Therapy With Macrolides and Miscellaneous Anti-Infective Agents

LEARNING OBJECTIVES

After studying this chapter, you should be able to:

1. Describe the characteristics and specific uses of macrolide anti-infective agents.
2. Identify the prototype and describe the action, use, adverse effects, contraindications, and nursing implications of macrolides.
3. Describe the action, use, adverse effects, contraindications, and nursing implications of miscellaneous anti-infective agents.
4. Implement the nursing process in the care of patients being treated with macrolides and miscellaneous anti-infective agents.

CLINICAL APPLICATION CASE STUDY

Juro Nikki, a 65-year-old man, has had chronic obstructive pulmonary disease for a number of years. He presents to the physician's office with a respiratory tract infection. He begins taking azithromycin, 500 mg for one dose and then 250 mg, orally daily for 4 days.

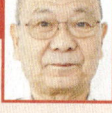

KEY TERMS

Gray syndrome: dangerous adverse condition that occurs in newborns who are given chloramphenicol; may lead to fatalities

Methicillin-resistant *Staphylococcus aureus*: microorganisms resistant to broad-spectrum antibiotics such as penicillin and erythromycin; frequently colonizes nasal passages of healthcare workers and is increasing as a cause of infection in healthcare facilities

Methicillin-sensitive *Staphylococcus aureus*: methicillin-susceptible strains of *Staphylococcus aureus*

Mycobacterium avium complex: caused by atypical mycobacteria; opportunistic infection that occurs mainly in people with advanced human immunodeficiency virus infection

Oxazolidinones: a class of antibiotics; active against aerobic Gram-positive bacteria by inhibiting protein synthesis

Staphylococcal species nonaureus: other strains of antibiotic-resistant staphylococci

Streptogramins: class of antibacterial drugs; produced by *Streptomyces graminofaciens* bacteria

Vancomycin infusion reaction/hypersensitivity infusion reaction: adverse reaction when dalbavancin or vancomycin is administered too quickly; characterized by hypotension, flushing, and skin rash

Vancomycin-resistant enterococci: pathogenic bacteria that are resistant to vancomycin

Vancomycin-resistant *Enterococcus faecium*: *Enterococcus faecium* that is resistant to vancomycin

INTRODUCTION

The drugs described in this chapter are heterogeneous in their antimicrobial spectra, characteristics, and clinical uses. Some are used often, and some are used only in specific circumstances. The drugs to be described in the following sections include the macrolides and miscellaneous anti-infective agents. The Drugs at a Glance tables present information about individual drugs and the prototype drugs, with routes of administration and dosage ranges.

MACROLIDES

The macrolides, which include erythromycin as well as azithromycin, clarithromycin, and fidaxomicin, have similar antibacterial spectra and mechanisms of action. Macrolides are widely distributed into body tissues and fluids and may be bacteriostatic or bactericidal, depending on drug concentration in infected tissues. They are effective against Gram-positive cocci, including group A streptococci, pneumococci, and most staphylococci. They are also effective against species of *Corynebacterium, Treponema, Legionella, Chlamydia, Neisseria,* and *Mycoplasma* as well as some anaerobic species of genera such as *Bacteroides* and *Clostridia*.

The prototype macrolide is ⓟ **erythromycin**. This drug is now used less often because of microbial resistance, numerous drug interactions, and the development of newer macrolides. Compared with erythromycin, the other drugs in the class (e.g., azithromycin, clarithromycin, fidaxomicin) have enhanced antibacterial activity, require less frequent administration, and cause less nausea, vomiting, and diarrhea (see Other Drugs in the Class). Macrolide antibiotics are especially useful as a treatment option for persons who are allergic to penicillin. Erythromycin is available in several preparations. Ophthalmic and topical preparations are discussed in Chapters 59 and 61, respectively.

Pharmacokinetics

The oral preparation of erythromycin has an onset of action in 1 to 2 hours and reaches its peak in 1 to 4 hours. The intravenous (IV) preparation has a more rapid onset of action, reaching a peak of action in less than 1 hour. Erythromycin is metabolized in the liver by the cytochrome P450 3A4 (CYP3A4) isoenzymes and is absorbed in the small intestine. It is excreted mainly in bile; approximately 20% is excreted in urine. Depending on the specific salt formulation used, food can have a variable effect on the absorption of oral erythromycin.

Action

Erythromycin enters the microbial cells and reversibly binds to the 50S subunits of ribosomes, thereby inhibiting microbial protein synthesis and leading to cell death. The medication has bacteriostatic or bacteriocidal activity against susceptible bacteria.

Use

Erythromycin is useful in the following ways:

- For prevention of rheumatic fever, gonorrhea, syphilis, pertussis, and chlamydial conjunctivitis in newborns (ophthalmic ointment)
- For treatment of other infections (e.g., Legionnaires disease, genitourinary infections caused by *Chlamydia trachomatis*, intestinal amebiasis caused by *Entamoeba histolytica*)

The drug is administered for upper respiratory infections caused by group A beta-hemolytic streptococci. It is used with sulfonamides for upper respiratory infections caused by *Haemophilus influenzae*. Prophylactically, erythromycin is administered to prevent alpha-hemolytic streptococcal endocarditis before dental or other procedures in patients who have valvular heart disease and are allergic to penicillin. Table 21.1 provides route and dosage information for erythromycin and other macrolides.

Patient-related variables specific to the use of erythromycin and other macrolides include the following:

- Age:
  - Erythromycin is a high-risk medication when used in neonates. It should be avoided due to the risk of hypertrophic pyloric stenosis unless treating *C. trachomatis* pneumonia.
- Reproduction, pregnancy, and lactation:
  - The effectiveness of oral contraceptives is decreased when combined with erythromycin. An alternative form of contraception should be used when taking anti-infective agents such as erythromycin or other macrolides.
  - Patient pregnancy status should be determined prior to administration as risk to the fetus has been reported.
  - Both oral and parenteral forms of erythromycin cross the placenta and enter breast milk.
  - The manufacturer of erythromycin recommends caution to be used when administered to a breast-feeding patient; erythromycin is considered compatible when used at the recommended dosage.
  - In some cases, the breast-fed infant may have a loss of appetite, rash, and somnolence when exposed to macrolide antibiotics. In addition, orange-red stool has been reported following erythromycin exposure.
- Abnormal kidney function and hepatic impairment:
  - Erythromycin should be used with caution in patients with hepatic impairment.
  - Erythromycin use has also been associated with cholestatic hepatitis.
- Specific healthcare environments:
  - For critically ill patients who need a macrolide antibiotic, one of the newer macrolides is preferred over erythromycin because these drugs have a broader spectrum of activity against several groups of microorganisms and fewer effects on the metabolism of other drugs.

Adverse Effects

Erythromycin may result in several adverse effects. Gastrointestinal (GI) effects include nausea, vomiting, diarrhea, cramping, anorexia, hepatotoxicity, and pseudomembranous colitis. If fever and jaundice occur after 1 to 2 weeks of drug administration, they subside after the drug is discontinued. Central nervous system (CNS) effects are reversible hearing loss, confusion, lability of emotions, and alterations in thought processes. Cardiac effects, with the IV form of the drug, include possible ventricular dysrhythmias. Allergic reactions include redness of the skin, rash, bronchospasm, or anaphylaxis.

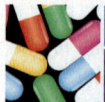

TABLE 21.1
DRUGS AT A GLANCE: Macrolides

Drug	Routes and Dosage Ranges	
	Adults	**Children**
ⓟ **Erythromycin** Erythromycin stearate Erythromycin lactobionate (E.E.S. 400, EES Granules, Ery-Tab, EryPed 200 or 400, Erythrocin)	250–500 mg PO every 6–12 h Severe infections: up to 4 g daily in divided doses Lactobionate: 15–20 mg/kg/d IV in divided doses q6h or 500 mg–1 g q6h to be infused over 30–60 minutes or may be given as a continuous infusion over 24 h (max dose 4 g/d) Severe infections: up to 4 g daily in divided doses	PO 30–50 mg/kg/d PO in divided doses every 6–12 h Lactobionate: 15–50 mg/kg/d IV in divided doses every 6 h, not to exceed 4 g/d
Azithromycin (✹ Apo-Azithromycin Z, Azithromycin for Injection, Dom-Azithromycin, PRO-Azithromycin, Zithromax)	Respiratory and skin infections: 500 mg PO as a single dose on day 1 and then 250 mg once daily for 2–5 d Extended-release suspension (Zmax): 2 g as a single dose; PO 1 g as a single dose Nongonococcal urethritis and cervicitis caused by *C. trachomatis*: 1 g as a single dose MAC: prevention, 1,200 mg PO once per week; treatment, 600 mg PO once daily; secondary prophylaxis, 500–600 mg daily in combination with ethambutol Bacterial sinusitis: Tri-Pak 500 mg PO daily for 3 d, or Zmax extended-release formula 2 g PO as a single dose CAP: IV 500 mg daily for at least 2 d followed by 500 mg PO daily for total of 7–10 d treatment	6 mo to 2 y, otitis media: 1-d regimen: PO 30 mg/kg as a single dose (maximum dosage 1,500 mg); 3-d regimen PO 10 mg/kg once daily for 3 d (maximum dosage 500 mg) 3-d regimen, pharyngitis/tonsillitis: PO 12 mg/kg (not to exceed 500 mg) once daily for 2–5 d
Clarithromycin (✹ ACT-Clarithromycin XL, APO-Clarithromycin, APO-Clarithromycin XL, Dom-Clarithromycin, PMS Clarithromycin)	PO 250–500 mg q12h or 1,000 mg daily for 7–14 d Prevention/treatment of MAC: 500 mg PO q12h or 1,000 mg XL daily; discontinue when CD4 count is >100 cells/mm³ Chronic maintenance: 500 mg daily plus ethambutol Bronchitis and CAP (extended-release): PO 250 mg every 12 h or 1,000 mg daily for 7 d Acute maxillary sinusitis: PO 1,000 mg daily for 14 d	PO 7.5 mg/kg, not to exceed 500 mg every 12 h Prevention/treatment of MAC: same as above
Fidaxomicin (Dificid; ✹ Dificid)	*C. difficile* diarrhea: PO 200 mg BID for 10 d	Safety and efficacy not established

CAP, community-acquired pneumonia; MAC, *Mycobacterium avium* complex.

Contraindications

Contraindications to erythromycin include a known hypersensitivity reaction to the drug or any macrolide. As previously stated, hepatic insufficiency requires careful use. The U.S. Food and Drug Administration (FDA) has issued a regarding erythromycin estolate, a Canadian preparation of erythromycin; administration to patients with known liver disease warrants caution. Patients who are breast-feeding should not take erythromycin because the drug is concentrated in the breast milk. This can alter the bowel flora of the infant and interfere with fever assessments. Also, people should not take erythromycin if they are concurrently using drugs highly dependent on CYP3A4 liver enzymes for metabolism.

Nursing Implications

Preventing Interactions

Many medications interact with erythromycin, increasing or decreasing its effects (Box 21.1). Also, both grapefruit juice and St. John's wort decrease absorption of the antibiotic.

> **❗ Quality and Safety Alert: Safety**
>
> Drugs that are processed in the liver and small intestine by cytochrome P450, such as erythromycin, exhibit increased serum blood levels with concurrent ingestion of grapefruit and other fruits such as Seville oranges, tangelos, pomelos, and Minneolas. Studies have shown that the juice from these fruits increased the drug's serum blood levels by 84%, increasing the risk of adverse effects, particularly related to heart rhythm.

BOX 21.1 Drug Interactions: Erythromycin

Drugs That Increase the Effects of Erythromycin
- Chloramphenicol
  Increases effectiveness against strains of resistant Staphylococcus aureus
- Streptomycin
  Increases effectiveness against Enterococcus in bacteremia, brain abscess, endocarditis, meningitis, and urinary tract infection

Drugs That Decrease the Effects of Erythromycin
- Antacids, calcium, magnesium, aluminum, zinc
  Decrease antibiotic absorption
- Etravirine, lincosamide antibiotics
  Decrease serum concentration of erythromycin
- Ethanol
  Decreases absorption of erythromycin

In addition, as stated previously, the CYP3A4 isoenzymes in the liver metabolize erythromycin. The drug interacts with other drugs metabolized by the same isoenzyme and interferes with the elimination of several drugs. As a result, the affected drugs are eliminated more slowly, their serum levels are increased, and they are more likely to cause adverse effects and toxicity unless the erythromycin dosage is reduced. In combination with potent inhibitors of CYP3A4 (e.g., fluconazole, diltiazem), erythromycin increases the risk of sudden cardiac death. A partial list of other interacting drugs from a variety of drug classes includes carbamazepine (Tegretol), cyclosporine, digoxin, disopyramide, lopinavir/ritonavir, lovastatin, nevirapine, pimozide, quinidine, rifampin, ritonavir, simvastatin, theophylline, triazolam, and warfarin.

Administering the Medication

Drinking 6 to 8 oz of water with the medication is important; adequate water intake aids medication absorption. The drug is taken on an empty stomach at evenly spaced intervals around the clock. Regular intervals help maintain therapeutic blood levels. People should not take erythromycin after taking antacids because antacids decrease the absorption of both the tablet and suspension form of erythromycin.

The nurse may administer the IV preparation of erythromycin without regard to meals. It is important to consult the manufacturer's instructions for dissolving, diluting, and administering the parenteral form of erythromycin to achieve therapeutic effects. The IV formulation has limited stability in the solution. Also, instructions differ for intermittent and continuous infusions. The nurse infuses the medication in a peripheral or central IV site every 6 hours over 30 to 60 minutes.

Assessing Therapeutic Effects

The nurse assesses for decreased pain, fever, and malaise. Both the local and systemic signs of the infection are decreased; the patient has decreased signs and symptoms of the specific infection for which erythromycin is being administered.

Assessing for Adverse Effects

The patient is assessed for hearing loss, which is reversible with discontinuation of the medication. The nurse also assesses for nausea, vomiting, and diarrhea. These symptoms may be severe and result in an alteration in acid–base balance. In addition, the nurse assesses for superinfection, as noted, with the development of pseudomembranous colitis. It is important to assess the patient's psychosocial responses that are adverse effects of erythromycin, such as crying, laughing, and altered thought processes. Finally, the nurse assesses for skin rash, urticaria, edema, dermatitis, and bronchospasm, which are indicative of an allergic reaction to erythromycin.

When administering the IV form of the drug, the nurse assesses the infusion site for phlebitis.

Patient Teaching

Box 21.2 identifies patient teaching guidelines for erythromycin.

Other Drugs in the Class

The macrolides azithromycin and clarithromycin are derivatives of erythromycin, and the structural modifications significantly alter their spectrum of activity as well as dosing and administration schedules.

The drugs are active against the atypical mycobacteria that cause **Mycobacterium avium complex** (MAC) disease. MAC disease (see Chapter 22) is an opportunistic infection that occurs mainly in people with advanced human immunodeficiency virus (HIV) infection. *Helicobacter pylori*, a pathogen implicated in peptic ulcer disease, is also susceptible to treatment with azithromycin or clarithromycin as part of a combination regimen (see Chapter 37).

BOX 21.2 Patient Teaching Guidelines for Erythromycin

- Take erythromycin around the clock because it inhibits but does not kill bacteria.
- Take erythromycin on an empty stomach, 1 hour before meals or 2 to 3 hours after meals.
- Do not drink grapefruit juice or consume Seville oranges, tangelos, pomelos, or Minneolas while taking erythromycin as juices from these fruits may cause disruption in heart rhythm (i.e., ventricular dysrhythmias).
- Do not take with or within 2 hours of consuming dairy products or antacids.
- Take each dose with 8 oz of water.
- Be aware that the effectiveness of oral contraceptives is decreased when combined with erythromycin.
- Understand that adverse effects may include stomach cramping, gastrointestinal discomfort, labile emotions, crying, laughing, and abnormal thinking.
- Report severe or watery diarrhea, nausea, vomiting, dark urine, yellowing of the eyes or skin, loss of hearing, itching, and rash to your prescriber.

Azithromycin is useful in the treatment of lower respiratory infections, pharyngitis, and tonsillitis caused by *Haemophilus ducreyi*, *H. influenzae*, *Moraxella catarrhalis*, and *Streptococcus pneumoniae*. Prescribers order the drug for children older than 6 months of age for otitis media. It is also effective for treatment of community-acquired pneumonia (CAP) caused by *S. pneumoniae* as well as for genital ulcer disease in men and pelvic inflammatory disease in women.

The onset of action of azithromycin is rapid, with a peak in 2.5 to 3.2 hours. The duration of action is 24 hours. The medication is metabolized in the liver and is distributed extensively to the tissues, skin, lungs, sputum, tonsils, and cervix. A minimal amount enters the cerebrospinal fluid (CSF). Major elimination of the drug is in the bile, with only 6% of excretion in the urine. The mechanism of action is the inhibition of RNA-dependent protein synthesis at the chain elongation step; the drug binds to the 50S ribosomal subunit to block the involved transpeptide. The parenteral form of azithromycin is stable in 5% dextrose and water; 5% dextrose and lactated Ringer solution, lactated Ringer solution, normal saline; and all 5% dextrose and saline IV fluids.

The adverse effects of azithromycin are similar to those of erythromycin. Caution is necessary with azithromycin in patients who have gonorrhea, syphilis, pseudomembranous colitis, and hepatic impairment and abnormal kidney function, as well as in patients who are lactating. Alfuzosin, amiodarone, and artemether combined with azithromycin can enhance QT elongations. Careful assessment of the cardiac status is crucial when these medications are combined. Close monitoring of the international normalized ratio (INR) and prothrombin time is necessary when azithromycin is administered with warfarin. To ensure adequate absorption, patients should take the oral medication on an empty stomach, 2 hours before or after the administration of aluminum- or magnesium-containing antacids.

Clarithromycin is a macrolide administered for bronchitis, sinusitis, otitis media, MAC, peptic ulcer disease, pertussis, pharyngitis, tonsillitis, and pneumonia. Prescribers also order the drug for prophylactic use in patients with underlying cardiac conditions who are undergoing invasive procedures that predispose them to infective endocarditis. It is also useful in skin infections caused by *Staphylococcus aureus* and *Streptococcus pyogenes* as well as in duodenal ulcers caused by *H. pylori*.

Absorption of clarithromycin is rapid, and the serum half-life is 3 to 7 hours. The drug is 42% to 50% protein bound, and it is widely distributed to all body tissues except the CNS. The metabolism of the medication takes place partially in the liver with CYP3A4 and is converted to the active metabolite. The elimination takes place in the urine, with 20% to 40% of the drug unchanged. (An additional 10% to 15% remains as the metabolite.) Clarithromycin binds to the 50S ribosome to inhibit protein synthesis. One of its metabolites is two times as active as the parent compound against certain organisms.

The adverse effects of clarithromycin are headache, rash, abnormal taste, nausea, vomiting, abdominal pain, and dyspepsia. People should not take the drug with ergot derivatives, pimozide, cisapride, astemizole, colchicine, or terfenadine because of the risk of increased levels of the medications and toxicity. Generally, people may take it with or without food; however, they should take the extended-release form on an empty stomach. As with the other macrolides, use of aluminum- or magnesium-containing antacids within 2 hours of administration of clarithromycin decreases absorption of the antibiotic.

Fidaxomicin (Dificid) is a macrolide antibiotic that is used to treat *Clostridium difficile*–associated diarrhea. The medication is able to block the RNA polymerase sigma subunit, leading to inhibited protein synthesis in *C. difficile* and eventual cell death. It is minimally absorbed and is widely distributed in the GI tract. Fidaxomicin is converted to a less effective metabolite, OP-118, and is primarily excreted in the feces. No dosage adjustment is necessary in patients with altered kidney or hepatic function. Researchers have observed no adverse effects in animal studies.

Clinical Application 21.1

The home care nurse is visiting Mr. Nikki to assess his lung status and medication regimen. Along with azithromycin, Mr. Nikki is taking omeprazole 20 mg orally daily for gastric reflux and 30 mL of Maalox at night. Since his myocardial infarction 6 months ago, he has been also taking warfarin 2 mg orally daily.

- The nurse is educating Mr. Nikki about all aspects of azithromycin. Identify all aspects of patient teaching that he should receive.
- What instructions does the nurse provide regarding the other medications Mr. Nikki is taking?
- What laboratory tests are important to monitor during the administration of azithromycin?

NCLEX Success

1. The nurse instructs a patient on the administration of clarithromycin. Which of the following patient teaching instructions is appropriate?
    A. Take the medication on an empty stomach.
    B. Take the medication with a calcium supplement.
    C. Take the medication with a glass of milk.
    D. Take the medication with cheese.

2. A teenage patient has been taking erythromycin for an upper respiratory tract infection for 5 days. At school, the teenager complains about being unable to hear the teacher and is sent to the school nurse's office. After assessing the patient's hearing with a tuning fork, the nurse determines that the patient's hearing is diminished. What is the most important nursing intervention?
    A. The nurse should notify the parents to call the primary care provider; this is an adverse effect of erythromycin.
    B. The nurse should inform the parents of a primary care provider who specializes in ear, nose, and throat surgery.
    C. The nurse should instruct the patient to stop taking the erythromycin and the hearing will improve.
    D. The nurse should call the primary care provider and inform the patient of a change in antibiotics.

3. A patient who had rheumatic fever as a child has an appointment for a tooth extraction. The dentist prescribes which of the following medications prior to the extraction?
   A. chloramphenicol
   B. vancomycin
   C. clarithromycin
   D. digoxin

MISCELLANEOUS ANTI-INFECTIVE AGENTS

The miscellaneous anti-infective agents have properties similar to those of other drug classes and may belong to new classes. To simplify the understanding of these medications, they are introduced in a summary format. The medications discussed in this section include chloramphenicol, clindamycin, dalbavancin, daptomycin, linezolid, metronidazole, oritavancin, quinupristin–dalfopristin, rifaximin, tedizolid, telavancin, tigecycline, and vancomycin. Table 21.2 summarizes route and dosage information for these antibacterial drugs.

Quality and Safety Alert: Patient-Centered Care

Prior to beginning therapy with anti-infective agents, it is necessary to review the prescriber's orders and culture the suspected site of infection. The culture and sensitivity report determines the anti-infective agent that is most effective in treating the infection. This is particularly important before starting vancomycin, quinupristin–dalfopristin, daptomycin, or linezolid. These drugs have relatively narrow spectra of activity, and it is critical to determine appropriate indications for their use to decrease the likelihood of resistance.

Chloramphenicol

Chloramphenicol is a broad-spectrum, bacteriostatic antibiotic that is active against most Gram-positive and Gram-negative bacteria, rickettsiae, chlamydiae, and treponemes. It acts by distributing well into body tissues and fluids, including CSF, but low drug levels are obtained in urine. It is metabolized in the liver and excreted in the urine.

Chloramphenicol is rarely used now to treat infections because of the effectiveness and low toxicity of alternative drugs.

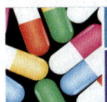

TABLE 21.2
DRUGS AT A GLANCE: Miscellaneous Anti-infective Agents

Drug	Routes and Dosage Ranges	
	Adults	**Children**
Chloramphenicol (🍁 Chloromycetin Succinate)	IV 50–100 mg/kg/d in divided doses every 6 h (max dose 4 g/d)	Meningitis (infants older than 30 d and children): 50–100 mg/kg/d in divided doses every 6 h Other infections (infants older than 30 d and children): 50–75 mg/kg/d in divided doses every 6 h (max daily dose 4 g)
Clindamycin hydrochloride (Cleocin; 🍁 Apo-Clindamycin, Ava-Clindamycin, Clindamycin-150 or 300, Dalacin C, Dalacin C Palmitate, Riva Clindamycin, Teva-Clindamycin)	PO 150–450 mg q6–8h (max dose 1.8 g/d) 1.2–2.7 g/d IM or IV 600–2,700 mg in 2–4 divided doses; max dose: 4.8 g/d	PO 8–40 mg/kg/d in divided doses q6–8h; up to 20 mg/kg/d in severe infections Neonates, 15–20 mg/kg/d in divided doses q6–8h 1 mo and older, IM, IV 20–40 mg/kg/d in divided doses q6–8h; up to 40 mg/kg/d in severe infections
Dalbavancin (Dalvance; 🍁 Xydalba)	Skin infections: single-dose regimen, 1,500 mg as a single dose Two-dose regimen: 1,000 mg as a single dose initially followed by 500 mg as a single dose 1 wk later Reduced dose with abnormal kidney function	Dosage and safety not established
Daptomycin (Cubicin RF; 🍁 Cubicin, Cubicin RF)	Skin/soft tissue infections: 4 mg/kg IV q24h for 7–14 d MSSA, MRSA, bacteremia, or right-sided endocarditis: 6 mg/kg/d for 2–6 wk	Safety and efficacy not established
Linezolid (Zyvox; 🍁 Apo-Linezolid, Linezolid injection, Sandoz-Linezolid, Zyvoxam)	VRE infections 600 mg PO or IV q12h for 10–28 d	≤11 y: 10 mg/kg PO or IV q8h ≥12 y: refer to adult dosing

(Continued on page 382)

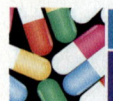

TABLE 21.2
DRUGS AT A GLANCE: Miscellaneous Anti-infective Agents (Continued)

Drug	Routes and Dosage Ranges	
	Adults	**Children**
Metronidazole (Flagyl; ✦ APO-MetroNIDAZOLE, Auro-MetroNIDAZOLE, PMS-MetroNIDAZOLE)	Anaerobic bacterial infection: 500 mg PO, IV q6–8 h, not to exceed 4 g/d Surgical prophylaxis and colorectal surgery: 500 mg IV infused over 30–60 min 0.5–1 h before surgery *C. difficile* colitis: 250–500 mg PO q6–8 h for 10–14 d	Anaerobic infections (older than 7 d and weight 1,200–2,000 g): 15 mg/kg/d PO, IV in divided doses q12h Anaerobic infections in children *older than* 7 d and weighing *more than* 2,000 g: 30 mg/kg/d in divided doses q12h ≥1 mo, 15–35 mg/kg/d PO in divided doses q8h; 30 mg/kg/d IV in divided doses q6h
Oritavancin (Kimyrsa, Orbactiv)	Skin infections: IV 1,200 mg as a single dose	Dosage and safety not established
Quinupristin–dalfopristin	Skin and skin structure infections: 7.5 mg/kg IV over 60 min q12h	Same as adults MRSA: IV 7.5 mg/kg/dose every 8 hours VP shunt infection: 7.5 mg/kg/dose q8h
Rifaximin (Xifaxan; ✦ Zaxine)	200 mg PO three times daily for 3 d	12 y and older: same as adults
Tedizolid phosphate (Sivextro)	Bacterial skin infection: IV 200 mg once daily for 6 d	Dosage and safety not established
Telavancin (Vibativ; ✦ Vibativ)	Skin infection: IV 10 mg/kg every 24 h for >5 days may extend 14 days Ventilator-associated bacterial pneumonia: IV 10 mg/kg every 24 h; the duration of administration varies based on disease severity and response to therapy; treatment is typically for 7 days reduced dose in abnormal kidney function	Dosage and safety not established
Tigecycline (Tygacil; ✦ Tygacil)	100 mg IV single dose initially; maintenance dose 50 mg q12h for 5–14 d	Dosage and safety not established
Vancomycin (Firvanq, Vancocin, Vancomycin HCl; ✦ JAMP-Vancomycin, PMS Vancomycin, Vancocin)	Antibiotic-associated pseudomembranous colitis: 100–500 mg PO q6h (PO dose not for treating systemic infections) 20–45 mg/kg/d IV in divided doses	Antibiotic-associated pseudomembranous colitis: 40 PO mg/kg/d in divided doses q6–8h (PO dose not for treating systemic infections) 1 mo and older, 10–15 mg/kg IV q6h

MRSA, methicillin-resistant *Staphylococcus aureus*; MSSA, methicillin-sensitive *Staphylococcus aureus*; VREF, vancomycin-resistant *Enterococcus faecium*.

However, it is still used in serious infections for which no adequate substitute drug is available. Specific infections include meningococcal, pneumococcal, or *Haemophilus pneumoniae* type b (Hib) meningitis in penicillin-allergic patients; anaerobic brain abscess; *Bacteroides fragilis* infections; and rickettsial infections and brucellosis when tetracyclines are contraindicated. In infections caused by **vancomycin-resistant enterococci** (VRE), pathogenic bacteria that are resistant to vancomycin, chloramphenicol is effective against some enterococcal strains.

Chloramphenicol is associated with several adverse effects. The FDA has issued a **BOXED WARNING** ◆ reporting the development of serious and fatal blood dyscrasias with chloramphenicol use. Irreversible bone marrow depression, which may lead to aplastic anemia, may appear weeks or months after therapy. A dose-related reversible bone marrow depression usually responds to discontinuation of the drug. Monitoring with a complete blood count, platelet count, reticulocyte count, and serum iron test every 2 days is essential. Experts recommend that patients be hospitalized to facilitate close monitoring. In addition, periodic measurements of serum drug levels are recommended when possible. Therapeutic levels are 5 to 20 mcg/mL. Discontinuation of therapy should occur as soon as possible, and use of the drug for trivial infections or for prophylaxis of infections should not take place. Also, because chloramphenicol concentrations may increase in patients with impaired kidney function, dose adjustments may be necessary. In addition, the patient may need an increase in dietary riboflavin, pyridoxine, and vitamin B_{12}. It is important to consult a dietician regarding dietary needs.

Neonates should not receive chloramphenicol because of the risk of **gray syndrome**, a dangerous and potentially fatal condition that occurs in newborns. Symptoms of gray syndrome begin 3 to 4 days after the drug is administered. Infants present with abdominal distention, progressive pallid cyanosis, vasomotor collapse, irregular respirations, and death. If drug therapy is stopped within a few hours of symptom onset of gray syndrome, affected infants will recover. Infants are also at risk for gray syndrome if their mothers are receiving chloramphenicol and are breast-feeding.

When administering chloramphenicol, the nurse reconstitutes the drug in 50 to 100 mL of 5% dextrose and water and infuses it over 15 to 30 minutes. Chloramphenicol combined with rifampin or phenobarbital results in accelerated hepatic metabolism of chloramphenicol.

Clindamycin

Clindamycin hydrochloride (Cleocin), a lincosamide, is similar to the macrolides in its mechanism of action and antimicrobial spectrum. Bacteriostatic in usual doses, this drug is effective against Gram-positive cocci, including group A streptococci, pneumococci, most staphylococci, and some anaerobes such as *Bacteroides* and *Clostridia*. Clindamycin enters microbial cells and attaches to 50S subunits of ribosomes, thereby inhibiting microbial protein synthesis.

Clindamycin is often used to treat infections caused by *B. fragilis*. Because these bacteria are usually mixed with Gram-negative organisms from the gynecologic or GI tracts, prescribers usually order that clindamycin be given with another drug, such as an aminoglycoside or a fluoroquinolone, to treat mixed infections. The drug may be useful as a penicillin substitute in patients who are allergic to penicillin and who have serious streptococcal, staphylococcal, or pneumococcal infections in which the causative organism is susceptible to clindamycin (including prevention of perinatal group B streptococcal disease). A topical solution is useful in the treatment of acne, and a vaginal cream is available. Clindamycin does not reach therapeutic concentrations in the CNS and cannot be used for treating meningitis.

Clindamycin is well absorbed with oral administration and reaches peak plasma levels within 1 hour after a dose. It is widely distributed in body tissues and fluids, except CSF, and it crosses the placenta. It is highly bound (90%) to plasma proteins. It is metabolized in the liver, and the metabolites are excreted in the bile and urine.

Adverse effects associated with clindamycin are many. It may be necessary to reduce the dosage in patients with severe hepatic failure to prevent accumulation and toxic effects. The FDA has issued a **BOXED WARNING** ◆ for clindamycin regarding the potential of severe and possible fatal colitis. If diarrhea develops in a patient receiving clindamycin, discontinuation of the drug is essential. With severe and persistent diarrhea, it is critical to check the stools for white blood cells, blood, mucus, and the presence of *C. difficile* toxin. It may be necessary to perform sigmoidoscopy to more definitively determine whether the patient has pseudomembranous colitis. The appearance of lesions on sigmoidoscopy means that the clindamycin should be stopped immediately. Although pseudomembranous colitis may occur with any antibiotic, it has often been associated with clindamycin therapy. Other adverse effects of clindamycin include nausea and vomiting.

Neonates and infants should receive clindamycin only if the drug is clearly indicated, and then, monitoring of liver and kidney function is necessary. Diarrhea and pseudomembranous colitis may occur with topical clindamycin for treatment of acne. Clindamycin should be used cautiously in patients with liver impairment because it is excreted by the liver.

People should take oral clindamycin with a full glass of water to avoid esophageal irritation. It is important *not* to refrigerate the reconstituted oral solution. When administering clindamycin intramuscularly, the nurse gives no more than 600 mg in one injection. To avoid pain, induration, and abscess formation, it is necessary to administer the medication into the deep tissues. When administering clindamycin intravenously, the nurse either dilutes 300 to 600 mg of the drug in 50 mL of IV fluid and gives it over 10 to 20 minutes, or the nurse dilutes 900 mg in 50 to 100 mL and administers it over 20 minutes. The dilution of the medication in IV fluids decreases the risk of phlebitis. The patient is at risk for cardiac arrest if the medication is administered as a bolus. Clindamycin must not be administered with erythromycin; the combination decreases the effects of clindamycin.

Dalbavancin

Dalbavancin (Dalvance) is a glycopeptide antibiotic. The drug binds to D-alanyl–D-alanine terminus in the nascent cell wall peptidoglycan, which prevents cross-linking and interferes with the cell wall synthesis. It has bactericidal action against *S. aureus* and *S. pyogenes* in skin and skin structure infections. Dalbavancin is 90% protein bound, primarily to albumin. It is excreted unchanged in the urine and as a hydroxyl metabolite in the feces. The drug possesses a half-life of 346 hours.

Administration of dalbavancin is by a single- or double-dose regimen. Infusion should be slow to prevent a **hypersensitivity infusion reaction**, characterized by hypotension, flushing, and skin rash. The nurse must assess the patient's hydration level with the administration of the drug. A reduced dose of the drug is recommended for patients with hepatic insufficiency or abnormal kidney function. Assessment of bilirubin, aspartate aminotransferase, and alanine aminotransferase (ALT) levels is necessary throughout the course of treatment. Any elevation in ALT requires discontinuation of the drug.

Daptomycin

Daptomycin (Cubicin) belongs to the lipopeptide class. It is a bactericidal agent effective only for Gram-positive infections caused by *S. aureus* (including oxacillin-resistant strains), *S. pyogenes*, group B streptococci, and *Enterococcus faecalis* (vancomycin-susceptible strains only). In combination with gentamicin, daptomycin is synergistic in killing staphylococci and enterococci. Indications are limited to the treatment of complicated skin and skin structure infections caused by the above organisms.

Available only for IV administration, daptomycin reaches target concentrations by the third daily dose. The drug is excreted primarily by the kidneys. Its mechanism of action is unique. Daptomycin kills bacteria by inhibiting synthesis of bacterial proteins, DNA, and RNA.

The most common adverse effects of daptomycin are constipation, nausea, diarrhea, and vomiting. Adverse musculoskeletal effects have occurred, primarily at increased serum creatine kinase (CK) levels. These effects are usually asymptomatic, but it is necessary to discontinue the drug in patients who develop muscle pain or weakness. Unexplained increases in serum CK levels associated with symptoms of myopathy should prompt discontinuation of daptomycin. Also, if daptomycin is combined with "statin" cholesterol-lowering medications, the risk of musculoskeletal adverse effects is greater. If possible, concomitant use of these "statins" should be avoided. In addition, no information regarding use in children or during pregnancy and lactation is available.

When administering daptomycin intravenously, the nurse mixes the daptomycin with normal saline or lactated Ringer solution and infuses it over 30 minutes. The drug is incompatible with dextrose-containing IV solutions.

Linezolid

Linezolid (Zyvox) is a member of the **oxazolidinone** class. It is active against aerobic Gram-positive bacteria. The drug exhibits bactericidal activity against most staphylococci, enterococci, and streptococci. It is indicated for healthcare-acquired and community-acquired pneumonia, complicated and uncomplicated skin and skin structure infections, and **vancomycin-resistant *Enterococcus faecium*** (VREF) infections. The drug is bacteriostatic against enterococci (including *E. faecalis* and *E. faecium*) and staphylococci (including methicillin-resistant strains) and bactericidal for most streptococci.

Linezolid acts by inhibiting protein synthesis by a unique mechanism. The drug binds to the bacterial 23S ribosomal RNA of the 50S subunit, thus preventing an essential component of the bacterial translation process. It is well absorbed orally, distributes widely, and undergoes hepatic elimination.

The FDA has issued a **BOXED WARNING** stating that linezolid should not be administered to patients who are currently taking selective serotonin reuptake inhibitors, serotonin–norepinephrine reuptake inhibitors, tricyclic antidepressants, or monoamine oxidase inhibitors. It is thought that linezolid inhibits the action of monoamine oxidase A, an enzyme responsible for breaking down serotonin in the brain. Thus, high levels of serotonin build up in the brain, causing toxicity. This buildup of serotonin is referred to as serotonin syndrome; affected patients present with muscle twitching, excessive sweating, shivering, shaking, fever, and diarrhea. The combination results in severe CNS reactions. It is necessary to discontinue the psychiatric agent prior to administration of the linezolid and closely monitor the patient for CNS adverse effects. The nurse assesses for mental status changes, muscle twitching, shivering, and lack of coordination.

Also, myelosuppression (bone marrow depression; e.g., anemia, leukopenia, pancytopenia, thrombocytopenia) is a serious adverse effect that may occur with prolonged linezolid therapy—longer than 2 weeks. Monitoring of the patient's complete blood count is necessary; if myelosuppression occurs, discontinuation of the drug is warranted. Myelosuppression usually improves with drug discontinuation. Pseudomembranous colitis may also occur. Mild cases usually resolve with drug discontinuation; moderate or severe cases may require fluid and electrolyte replacement and an antibacterial drug that is effective against *C. difficile* organisms. Hypertension may occur with the concomitant ingestion of linezolid and adrenergic drugs (e.g., dopamine, epinephrine); therefore, blood pressure and heart rate must be monitored. In addition, oral linezolid causes symptomatic hypoglycemia.

The effects of linezolid in pregnant patients and in children are largely unknown. Because linezolid is a weak monoamine oxidase inhibitor, patients should avoid food high in tyramine content (aged cheeses, fermented or air-dried meats, sauerkraut, soy sauce, tap beers, red wine) while taking the drug.

When administering the IV preparation of linezolid, the nurse infuses the drug over 30 to 120 minutes. It is important to infuse no other medications with linezolid sequentially and flush the line with 5% dextrose and water, normal saline, or lactated Ringer solution.

Metronidazole

Metronidazole (Flagyl) is effective against anaerobic bacteria, including Gram-negative bacilli such as *Bacteroides*, Gram-positive bacilli such as *Clostridia*, and some Gram-positive cocci. The drug is also effective against protozoa that cause amebiasis, giardiasis, and trichomoniasis (see Chapter 25). It achieves therapeutic concentrations in body fluids and tissues and can be used to treat anaerobic brain abscesses. Metronidazole is eliminated by the liver and kidneys.

Clinical indications for metronidazole include prevention or treatment of anaerobic bacterial infections (e.g., in colorectal surgery, intra-abdominal infections) and treatment of *C. difficile* infections associated with pseudomembranous colitis. As part of a combination regimen, the drug is also useful in treatment of infections caused by *H. pylori*. It is contraindicated during the first trimester of pregnancy and must be used with caution in patients with CNS or blood disorders. The safety and efficacy of metronidazole have been established in children only for the treatment of amebiasis, although the drug is used for other infections in pediatric patients without reported unusual adverse effects.

Metronidazole has several adverse effects. Dermatologic effects are skin rash, pruritus, and thrombophlebitis at the infusion site. CNS effects include seizures, peripheral paresthesias, ataxia, confusion, dizziness, and headache. The most common GI effects are nausea, vomiting, diarrhea, and metallic taste. The nurse tells the patient that consumption of alcohol when taking metronidazole will produce a disulfiram reaction, resulting in symptoms of flushing, headache, nausea, vomiting, and chest and abdominal pain.

Prior to administering metronidazole, the nurse must review the manufacturer's instructions, as metronidazole requires specific techniques for preparation and administration.

Oritavancin

Oritavancin (Kimyra, Orbactiv) is a glycopeptide used to treat acute bacterial skin and skin structure infections. Organisms susceptible to this anti-infective agent include several species of *Streptococcus* (*S. pyogenes*, *S. agalactiae*, *S. dysgalactiae*, *S. anginosus*) and *E. faecalis*. Oritavancin disrupts the bacterial cell wall membrane, leading to cell death. Significant adverse effects of oritavancin include tachycardia, hypersensitivity, headache, dizziness, and peripheral edema. Also, in the postmarketing phase of drug development, *C. difficile* diarrhea reportedly occurred.

Quinupristin–Dalfopristin

Quinupristin–dalfopristin belongs to a class of antimicrobials referred to as **streptogramins**, produced by the bacterium *Streptomyces graminofaciens*. Both components are active antimicrobials that affect bacterial ribosomes to decrease protein synthesis. The combination is bacteriostatic against *E. faecium* (including vancomycin-resistant strains) and bactericidal against **methicillin-sensitive *Staphylococcus aureus*** (MSSA). It is not active against *E. faecalis*. Quinupristin–dalfopristin is indicated for skin and skin structure infections caused by *S. aureus* or group A *Streptococcus*. The FDA has removed the approval of quinupristin–dalfopristin for the treatment of VREF. It has been established that linezolid is most effective. Quinupristin and dalfopristin is approved for treatment of complicated skin and soft tissue infections.

Quinupristin–dalfopristin undergoes biliary excretion and fecal elimination. The drug combination is a strong inhibitor of CYP3A4 enzymes and, therefore, interferes with the metabolism of drugs such as cyclosporine, antiretrovirals, carbamazepine, and many others. Toxicity may occur with the inhibited drugs.

When administering quinupristin–dalfopristin parenterally, the nurse mixes it in a minimum of 250 mL of 5% dextrose solution and infuses it over 60 minutes to decrease venous irritation. Medication toxicity may occur if it is administered in shorter infusion times. To decrease irritation, it may be necessary to use a central venous catheter for drug administration. The medication is not to be mixed with any other drug. The IV line should not be flushed with saline or heparin-containing solutions, which are incompatible with quinupristin–dalfopristin. The medication is compatible with anidulafungin, aztreonam, caspofungin, ciprofloxacin, fenoldopam, fluconazole, haloperidol, metoclopramide, and potassium chloride. When administering quinupristin–dalfopristin with these medications, the nurse must infuse them with 5% dextrose and water.

Rifaximin

Rifaximin (Xifaxan) is a structural analog of rifampin. The drug is used to prevent hepatic encephalopathy and to treat irritable bowel syndrome with diarrhea. Rifaximin is useful in infectious (traveler's) diarrhea caused by *Escherichia coli* but is not effective in diarrhea caused by *Campylobacter jejuni* (see Chapter 40). Whether rifaximin is effective to treat diarrhea caused by *Shigella* or *Salmonella* species is not known. Because of its very limited systemic absorption (97% eliminated in feces), rifaximin cannot be used to treat systemic infections, including infections caused by invasive strains of *E. coli*. Therefore, diarrhea occurring with fever or bloody stools requires treatment with alternative agents. After treatment with rifaximin begins, patients reporting worsening or persistent diarrhea for longer than 24 to 48 hours, fever, or blood in the stool should receive therapy with an alternative agent. Patients may take rifaximin before or after meals.

Adverse effects of rifaximin are flatulence, headache, abdominal pain, nausea, constipation, and vomiting. Prolonged use of rifaximin may result in bacterial or fungal superinfection. The patient may develop *C. difficile* or pseudomembranous colitis more than 2 months after the discontinuation of antibiotic therapy.

Tedizolid

Tedizolid (Sivextro) is an oxazolidinone antibiotic used for the treatment of acute bacterial skin and skin structure infections caused by *Enterococcus*, *Staphylococcus*, and *Streptococcus*. Organisms susceptible to the drug include Gram-positive types of *S. aureus* (including **methicillin-resistant *Staphylococcus aureus*** [MRSA] and MSSA isolates), *S. pyogenes*, *S. agalactiae*, *S. anginosus*, and *E. faecalis*. Tedizolid binds the 50S ribosome, preventing the formation of the 70S initiation complex, which is essential for bacterial translation and inhibits protein synthesis. The oral form is well absorbed and 70% to 90% protein bound. Metabolism occurs in the liver, where the drug is converted to phosphatases. Most excretion is in the feces (82%), and the remainder (18%) is in the urine.

Administration is oral or IV. The IV form should be 0.8 mg/mL in normal saline. Dosage adjustment is not required for abnormal kidney function or hepatic impairment. The manufacturer's labeling does not identify any contraindications to this medication. Drug–drug interactions with monoamine oxidase inhibitors may occur.

Telavancin

Telavancin (Vibativ) is a glycopeptide antibiotic that is administered for the treatment of complicated skin and skin structure infections caused by *E. faecalis* and certain species of *Streptococcus* (*S. pyogenes*, *S. agalactiae*, and *S. anginosus*). It is also administered for hospital-acquired and ventilator-associated bacterial pneumonia caused by *S. aureus*. The polymerization to telavancin blocks the polymerization and cross-linking of peptidoglycan. The drug then binds to D-alanine–D-alanine on the cell wall. Telavancin inhibits bacterial cell wall synthesis and also changes the cell's permeability.

The drug is administered IV and given every 24 hours for >5 days to 14 days. Telavancin is administered parenterally over 60 minutes. The line should be flushed before and after the medication is infused. The drug's adverse effects include a metallic taste, nausea, vomiting, increased serum creatinine, pruritus, and diarrhea. A prolonged QT interval is apparent on an electrocardiogram. In a , the FDA has reported that patients with preexisting moderate to severe abnormal kidney function (CrCl ≤ 50 mL/minute) who take telavancin have an increased chance of mortality.

> **! Quality and Safety Alert: Safety**
>
> Patients of childbearing age should have a serum pregnancy test prior to administration. Adverse outcome in the fetus can occur.

Tigecycline

Tigecycline (Tygacil) is a glycylcycline, a class of anti-infective agents that are structurally related to the tetracyclines and share many of the same properties. It is a derivative of minocycline but is not classified as a tetracycline. Healthcare providers use tigecycline for CAP, complicated intra-abdominal infections, and skin or skin structure infections. The drug has both bactericidal and bacteriostatic properties. It is effective in treating MRSA and vancomycin-sensitive *E. faecalis*. The drug is distributed extensively to the tissues and is highly protein bound. It is metabolized in the liver and excreted in the feces and urine. It acts by binding to the 30S ribosome of susceptible bacteria to inhibit protein synthesis.

The nurse administers tigecycline intravenously over 30 to 60 minutes in a dedicated IV line or a Y-site connection. The drug is incompatible with amphotericin B, chlorpromazine, diazepam, methylprednisolone, sodium succinate, and voriconazole.

Vancomycin

Vancomycin (Firvanq, Vancocin) is active only against Gram-positive microorganisms. Parenteral vancomycin has been used extensively to treat infections caused by MRSA and methicillin-resistant **staphylococcal species nonaureus** (SSNA, including *Staphylococcus epidermidis*) as well as endocarditis caused by *Streptococcus viridans* (in patients allergic to or with infections resistant to penicillins and cephalosporins) or *E. faecalis* (with an aminoglycoside).

S. pneumoniae remain susceptible to vancomycin, although vancomycin-tolerant strains have been identified. Prophylactic use of the drug for Gram-positive infections in patients who are at high risk for developing MRSA infections (e.g., those with diabetes, previous hospitalization, or MRSA in their nasal passages) and who require placement of long-term intravascular catheters and other invasive treatments or monitoring devices is extensive. Oral vancomycin is useful only to treat staphylococcal enterocolitis and pseudomembranous colitis caused by *C. difficile*.

Partly because of this widespread use, healthcare providers encounter VRE more often, especially in critical care units, and treatment options for infections caused by these organisms are limited. To decrease the spread of VRE, the Centers for Disease Control and Prevention (CDC) recommends limiting the use of vancomycin. Specific recommendations include avoiding or minimizing use in empiric treatment of febrile patients with neutropenia (unless the prevalence of MRSA or SSNA is high), in initial treatment for *C. difficile* colitis (metronidazole is preferred), and as prophylaxis for surgery, low birth weight infants, intravascular catheter colonization or infection, and peritoneal dialysis.

Vancomycin acts by inhibiting cell wall synthesis, thus altering bacterial cell membrane permeability and RNA synthesis. Excretion of vancomycin occurs in the kidneys; dosage reduction is required in abnormal kidney function. In bacterial colitis, administration of vancomycin is oral because the drug is not absorbed from the GI tract and acts within the bowel lumen. Elimination of large amounts of vancomycin in the feces occurs after oral administration.

For systemic infections, administration of the drug is IV, and it reaches therapeutic plasma levels within 1 hour after infusion. It is very important to give IV infusions slowly, over 1 to 2 hours, to avoid an adverse reaction characterized by hypotension, flushing, and skin rash. This reaction, sometimes called **vancomycin infusion reaction** or hypersensitivity infusion reaction, is attributed to histamine release. Close monitoring of serum drug levels of IV vancomycin is important. When administering IV vancomycin, the nurse dilutes 500-mg doses in 100 mL and 1-g doses in 200 mL of 0.9% NaCl or 5% dextrose injection and infuses it over at least 60 minutes.

Quality and Safety Alert: Evidence-Based Practice

In a 2019 study of linezolid versus daptomycin treatment for periprosthetic joint infections, both linezolid and daptomycin were effective in treating Gram-positive pathogens. Oe et al., found that daptomycin provided higher clinical success rates and fewer adverse effects. The patients in the study group had higher red blood cell counts and decreased C-reactive protein levels. Thus, the effectiveness of linezolid and daptomycin are equivalent to control infections, but daptomycin had significant decreases in C-reactive protein and inflammation of the joint.

Clinical Application 21.2

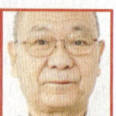

Mr. Nikko develops bloody diarrhea that is positive for *C. difficile* on culture. His prescriber now orders vancomycin 500 mg orally every 6 hours.
- What is the action of vancomycin?
- Why is vancomycin administered orally?

NCLEX Success

4. A nurse practitioner sees a 19-year-old college student in the student health center for severe diarrhea. The nurse diagnoses traveler's diarrhea based on the student's history, which included recent travel to Mexico. The student receives a prescription for rifaximin 200 mg orally three times daily for 3 days. Four days later, the student calls the office and reports the presence of a fever and unresolved diarrhea. Which of the following is the most appropriate information to communicate to the student?

   A. Advise the student to return to the clinic for further tests and a different antibiotic.
   B. Call the pharmacy and authorize one refill of rifaximin.
   C. Advise the student that it takes up to 48 to 72 hours after the completion of treatment for the diarrhea to completely resolve.
   D. Tell the student to continue drinking plenty of fluids and report back in 24 hours.

5. A recent nursing graduate is preparing to administer vancomycin to a patient intravenously. The nurse states that the patient reported experiencing flushing with the last dose of vancomycin. The nurse should

   A. infuse the vancomycin over 30 minutes to decrease the chance of a reaction
   B. hold the vancomycin dose until the physician's rounds the following morning
   C. dilute the vancomycin in 50 mL of normal saline solution and infuse over 60 minutes
   D. contact the nurse practitioner, report the reaction, and request an order for diphenhydramine pretreatment

THE NURSING PROCESS

A concept map outlines the nursing process related to drug therapy considerations in this chapter. Additional nursing implications related to the disease process should also be considered in care decisions.

Assessment
- Assess for infections that macrolides and the designated miscellaneous drugs are used to prevent or treat.
- Assess each patient for signs and symptoms of the specific current infection.
- Assess culture and susceptibility reports when available.
- Assess each patient for risk factors that increase risks of infection (e.g., immunosuppression) or risks of adverse drug reactions (e.g., impaired kidney or hepatic function).

Outcomes of Therapy

The patient will
- Take or receive macrolides and miscellaneous antimicrobials accurately, for the prescribed length of time.
- Experience decreased signs and symptoms of the infection being treated.
- Be monitored regularly for therapeutic and adverse drug effects.
- Verbalize and practice measures to prevent recurrent infection.

Nursing Interventions
- Use measures to prevent and minimize the spread of infection (see Chapter 15).
- Monitor for fever and other signs and symptoms of infection.
- Monitor laboratory reports for indications of the patient's response to drug therapy (e.g., white blood cell count, tests of kidney function).
- Encourage fluid intake to decrease fever and maintain good urinary tract function.
- Provide foods and fluids with adequate nutrients to maintain or improve nutritional status, especially if febrile and hypermetabolic.
- Assist patients to prevent or minimize infections with streptococci, staphylococci, and other gram-positive organisms.
- Provide appropriate patient teaching for any drug therapy (see accompanying display).

Evaluation
- Interview and observe for improvement in the infection being treated.
- Interview and observe for adverse drug effects.

Visit thePoint at http://thePoint.lww.com/Frandsen13e for answers to NCLEX Success questions (in Appendix A), answers to Clinical Application Case Studies (in Appendix B), and more!

REFERENCES AND RESOURCES

Graziani, A. L. (2022). Azithromycin and clarithromycin. *UpToDate.* Lexi-Comp, Inc.

Hansen, M. P., Scott, A. M., McCullough, A., Thorning, S., Aronson, J. K., Beller, E. M., Glasziou, P. P., Hoffmann, T. C., Clark, J., & Del Mar, C. B. (2019). Adverse events in people taking macrolide antibiotics versus placebo for any indication. *Cochrane Database of Systematic Reviews,* (1), CD011825. doi:10.1002/14651858.CD011825.pub2

Hinkle, J. H., Cheever, K. H., & Overbaugh, K. J. (2021). *Brunner & Suddarth's textbook of medical-surgical nursing* (15th ed.). Wolters Kluwer.

Murray, B. E., & Miller, W. R. (2022). Treatment of enterococcal infections. *UpToDate.* Lexi-Comp, Inc.

Oe, M. S. K., Hirata, M., Kawamura, H., Ueda, N., Nakamura, T., Iida, H., & Saito, T. (2019). Linezold versus daptomycin treatment for periprosthetic joint infections: A retrospective cohort study. *Journal of Orthopaedic Surgery and Research,* 34(114), 1–8. doi:10.1186-019-1375-7

Tucker, R. (2022). *2023 Lippincott's pocket drug guide for nurses.* Wolters Kluwer.

UpToDate. (2022). *Drug information.* Lexi-Comp, Inc.

CHAPTER 22

Drug Therapy for Tuberculosis and *Mycobacterium avium* Complex Disease

LEARNING OBJECTIVES

After studying this chapter, you should be able to:

1. Describe the characteristics of tuberculosis and *Mycobacterium avium* complex.
2. Describe the characteristics of latent, active, and drug-resistant tuberculosis.
3. Describe drug therapy for tuberculosis, including the rationale for multiple-drug therapy.
4. List the action, uses, adverse effects, contraindications, and nursing implications of first-line antitubercular drugs.
5. Describe how second-line antitubercular drugs are added to drug regimens to treat multidrug-resistant tuberculosis.
6. Describe the drugs used to prevent or treat *Mycobacterium avium* complex.
7. Discuss ways to increase adherence to antitubercular drug therapy regimens.
8. Implement the nursing process in the care of patients undergoing drug therapy for tuberculosis.

CLINICAL APPLICATION CASE STUDY

Jennifer Grant is a 27-year-old woman. While doing volunteer work in a foreign country, she is exposed to tuberculosis, and now she has a fever, productive cough, and night sweats. Her healthcare provider refers her to an infectious disease specialist at a local university hospital. Her sputum culture for acid-fast bacilli is positive for *Mycobacterium tuberculosis*, and her chest x-ray is consistent with tuberculosis. Ms. Grant is started on a once-daily regimen of isoniazid 300 mg for 6 months, rifampin 600 mg for 6 months, pyrazinamide 1,500 mg for 2 months, and ethambutol 1,200 mg for 2 months. She is an alert, cooperative patient. You are the nurse in the university hospital's infectious disease clinic where Ms. Grant is receiving follow-up care.

KEY TERMS

Directly observed therapy: method of medication administration where a nurse (or responsible adult) observes a patient taking a dose of antitubercular drug

Extensively drug-resistant tuberculosis: relatively rare type of multidrug-resistant tuberculosis that is resistant to isoniazid and rifampin plus resistant to any fluoroquinolone and at least one of three injectable second-line drugs (i.e., amikacin, kanamycin, or capreomycin)

Jaundice: yellow discoloration of the skin and of body tissues and fluids resulting from abnormally high levels of bilirubin in the blood; common symptom when drugs cause liver damage

Multidrug-resistant tuberculosis: tuberculosis that is resistant to at least one first-line antitubercular drug and at least isoniazid and rifampin

INTRODUCTION

Tuberculosis (TB) is an infectious disease that usually affects the lungs but may involve the lymph nodes, pleurae, bones, joints, kidneys, and the gastrointestinal (GI) tract. TB, which commonly occurs in many parts of the world, affects one third of the world's population. According to the World Health Organization (WHO) (2021), 1.5 million people died from TB in 2020. TB is the 13th leading cause of death worldwide and the second leading infectious killer after COVID-19. **Multidrug-resistant tuberculosis** (MDR-TB), a type of TB that is resistant to at least one first-line antitubercular drug and at least isoniazid and rifampin, remains a public health threat. Eight countries accounted for two thirds of new TB cases: India, China, Indonesia, the Philippines, Pakistan, Nigeria, Bangladesh, and South Africa. In 2020, the United States reported 7,174 TB cases. The COVID-19 pandemic likely interfered with TB reporting worldwide. TB remains a leading cause of death worldwide for people living with human immunodeficiency virus (HIV).

OVERVIEW OF TUBERCULOSIS AND *MYCOBACTERIUM AVIUM* COMPLEX DISEASE

Mycobacterium tuberculosis, the tubercle bacillus, is the cause of TB. In general, these bacilli multiply slowly, and they may lie dormant in the body for many years. *Mycobacterium avium* and *Mycobacterium intracellulare*, which may also cause lung disease, are different types of mycobacteria that resemble each other so closely that they are usually grouped together as *M. avium* complex (MAC). These atypical mycobacteria are found in water (including natural water sources, indoor water systems, pools, and hot tubs) and soil throughout the United States as well as in animals.

Clinical Considerations and Manifestations

There are four phases in the initiation and progression of TB.

1. **Transmission.** This occurs when an uninfected person inhales infected airborne droplets that are exhaled by an infected person. Major factors affecting transmission are the number of bacteria expelled by the infected person and the closeness and duration of the contact between the infected and the uninfected person.
2. **Primary infection.** Authorities estimate that 30% of people who are exposed to TB bacilli become infected and develop a mild, pneumonialike illness that is often undiagnosed. The initial infection occurs about 2 to 10 weeks after exposure. Within approximately 6 months of exposure, macrophages encapsulate the bacilli in calcified tubercles. The macrophages are unable to eliminate the bacteria completely. In the center of the calcified tubercle lies a caseous (cheesy) mass that contains small numbers of viable but dormant TB bacilli. The calcified tubercles, most commonly located in the upper lobes of the lungs, are visible on a chest radiograph.
3. **Latent TB infection.** The immune system is able to stop bacterial growth in most people who become infected with TB bacteria. The bacteria become inactive, although they remain alive in the body and can become active later. People with inactive or latent TB infection have no symptoms, do not feel sick, and do not spread TB to others. Active TB can develop years later if the latent infection is not effectively treated. In many people with latent TB, the infection remains inactive throughout their lives. In others, the TB bacteria become active and cause disease, usually when a person's immune system becomes weak as a result of disease, immunosuppressive drugs, or aging.
4. **Active TB.** About 5% to 10% of people develop active TB when they are first infected. People with latent TB develop active disease in two ways: further exposure to infected airborne droplets or reactivation of the latent TB because of weakened immune status. Although the lungs are the most common site for an active TB infection, the disease can spread to other parts of the body. Disseminated TB can infect the musculoskeletal system; the spine is the most common site, followed by the knees and hips. Other sites include the brain, liver, and kidneys.

Both new and reactivated infections of TB are more likely in people whose immune system is depressed by diseases such as HIV, diabetes mellitus, or cancer. Immunosuppression results from drugs used during cancer treatment and after organ transplantation. In people with both TB and HIV, TB progresses more rapidly, often involves extrapulmonary sites, is more severe, and is often fatal.

In addition to latent TB, a major concern among public health and infectious disease authorities is an increase in drug-resistant infections. Drug-resistant mutants of *M. tuberculosis* microorganisms may be present in any infected person. When infected people receive anti-TB drugs, the drugs do not kill or weaken the drug-resistant mutants. Instead, the resistant bacteria are able to reproduce in the presence of the drugs and to transmit the property of drug resistance to newly produced bacteria. Eventually, the majority of TB bacilli in the body are drug resistant. Once a drug-resistant strain of TB emerges, it can be transmitted to other people just like a drug-susceptible strain.

The emergence of drug-resistant TB organisms has long been attributed mainly to poor patient adherence to prescribed anti-TB drug therapy—that is, when previously infected patients do not take the drugs and doses prescribed for the length of time prescribed. However, drug-resistant strains can spread from one person to another, and there is increasing evidence that many drug-resistant infections are new infections, especially in people whose immune system is suppressed. Drug-resistant TB has been identified in many parts of the world, especially in India, China, and Russia and is a major concern in people infected with HIV. Most cases in the United States occur in those who are foreign-born. Factors contributing to the development of drug-resistant disease include delayed diagnosis and delayed determination of drug susceptibility (which can take several weeks). In addition, some countries lack adequate laboratory facilities or do not test TB bacteria for susceptibility to second-line anti-TB drugs. These delays in effective treatment allow rapid disease progression and rapid transmission to others, especially to those with impaired immune systems. Important causes of drug-resistant TB include failure to properly complete a full course of TB treatment; prescription of the wrong treatment by a healthcare provider (wrong dose or length of time); lack of availability of drugs for proper treatment; and poor quality drugs. Additional risk factors include redevelopment of TB after past treatment; immigration from an area where drug-resistant TB is common; and spending time with someone known to have drug-resistant TB (CDC, 2022).

MDR-TB is associated with rapid progression, with 4 to 16 weeks from diagnosis to death, and a high death rate (50% to 80%). It is also difficult and expensive to treat; most experts recommend 18 months of drug therapy. The cure rate is only about 50% or less for MDR-TB compared with a cure rate of 90% or more for drug-susceptible strains of TB. Authorities now describe some MDR-TB cases as **extensively drug-resistant tuberculosis** (XDR-TB), a relatively rare type of MDR-TB that is resistant to isoniazid and rifampin plus resistant to any fluoroquinolones and at least one of three injectable second-line drugs (i.e., amikacin, kanamycin, or capreomycin). XDR-TB was first reported in 2006 and is now reported on six continents (Heysell & Friedland, 2022). Some cases of TB are resistant to six or seven drugs, and there are essentially no effective drugs for their treatment.

Experts believe that the organisms that cause MAC are transmitted by inhalation of droplets of contaminated water; there is no evidence of spread to humans from animals or other humans. MAC rarely causes significant disease in immunocompetent people but causes an opportunistic pulmonary infection in approximately 50% of patients with advanced HIV infection.

The initial symptoms of TB are a low-grade temperature, weight loss, cough, fatigue, and night sweats. The cough may be nonproductive or productive. Pulmonary and systemic symptoms may be present for weeks to months. Hemoptysis may occur. Dyspnea and orthopnea become progressively worse as TB becomes more advanced. Symptoms are less pronounced in older adults. Extrapulmonary TB occurs in 20% of U.S. cases; it is more prevalent in patients with HIV disease (Hinkle et al., 2021).

Symptoms of MAC include a productive cough, weight loss, hemoptysis, and fever. As the disease becomes disseminated through the body, chronic lung disease develops, and the bacteria are found in the blood, bone marrow, liver, lymph nodes, and other body tissues.

Box 22.1 gives information about the tuberculin skin test reactions and TB blood tests, which may be useful in diagnosis.

BOX 22.1   *Guidelines for Interpretation of Tests for Tuberculosis*

Mantoux Skin Test

Intradermal injection of five tuberculin units of purified protein derived from *Mycobacterium tuberculosis*

When to Use (General)

- For people who are at high risk for acquiring tuberculosis (TB) because of exposure to someone with TB
- For people who are at high risk to progression from latent to active TB because of other medical conditions

How to Interpret Results

Induration: 5 mm or More

- Consider positive in:
  - People infected with HIV
  - People in recent contact with a person with TB
  - People with changes on chest radiograph consistent with prior TB
  - People with organ transplants
  - People who are immunosuppressed for other reasons (e.g., prednisone use)

Induration: 10 mm or more

- Consider positive in:
  - Recent immigrants from high-prevalence countries
  - People who inject drugs
  - Residents and employees of high-risk congregate settings (e.g., long-term care facilities or prisons)
  - Mycobacteriology laboratory personnel
  - People in high-risk clinical positions
  - Children younger than 4 years of age
  - Infants, children, and adolescents exposed to high-risk adults

Induration: 15 mm or More

- Consider positive in any person, including people with no known risk of TB

False-Positive Reactions Possible

- When a non-TB mycobacterial infection is present or when the patient has had previous bacillus Calmette-Guérin (BCG) vaccination (BCG, derived from *Mycobacterium bovis*, is used to vaccinate children against TB in many parts of the world.)

False-Negative Reactions Possible

- When the patient's weakened immune system is unable to react to the skin test
- When there has been a very recent TB infection (within 8 to 10 weeks of exposure)
- When live-virus vaccinations (e.g., measles or smallpox) have been given recently

Blood Test

Interferon gamma release assay (IGRA) measures the concentration of a substance (interferon gamma), which is released from white blood cells when the blood of a person infected with *M. tuberculosis* is mixed with antigens derived from *M. tuberculosis* (e.g., QuantiFERON-TB Gold)

When to Use

- The Centers for Disease Control and Prevention (CDC) states that this test can be used in place of tuberculin skin testing in all situations in which a tuberculin skin test is recommended.[a]

How to Interpret Results

- Positive: indicates a patient has been infected with TB
- Negative: indicates that infection with TB is unlikely
- Indeterminate: also possible

Major Advantages

- People need only a single visit for the test; results are available in 24 hours.
- People who have received previous BCG vaccinations do not have false-positive results.

[a]The IGRA does not determine whether there is latent TB or active disease.

> **Clinical Application 22.1**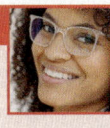
>
> - Identify the signs and symptoms of TB shown by Ms. Grant. Is her TB latent or active?

Drug Therapy

Drugs are used to treat both latent TB and active TB. Patients with latent TB cannot spread the disease to others, but treatment of the latent disease prevents progression of the disease to an active state. It is particularly important to treat latent TB in those patients who are at high risk for progression to active TB. Treatment of active TB prevents worsening of the disease in the individual patient and prevents spread of the disease to others. *It is essential to initiate drug therapy promptly and to complete the entire course of treatment.*

Four treatment regimens have been approved for latent TB. Fewer drugs are necessary to treat latent TB because fewer mycobacterial organisms are present. The drugs used in the four treatment regimens are INH, RIF, and rifapentine (Table 22.1).

The U.S. Food and Drug Administration (FDA) has approved 10 drugs for the treatment of active TB. However, the following discussion considers only the first-line anti-TB drugs, which are INH, RIF, and other rifamycins, ethambutol, and pyrazinamide. (Note that more drugs are necessary to treat active TB, because more mycobacterial organisms are present.) People with active TB need to take several drugs for 6 to 9 months.

Use of multiple drugs to treat TB is necessary to prevent the development of drug-resistant TB. TB regimens are modified for use with HIV, drug resistance, and pregnancy, as well as in children. Because drug susceptibility testing results can be delayed, treatment always begins empirically; it may be necessary to adjust the regimen when results are known (Table 22.2).

The Centers for Disease Control and Prevention (CDC) recently approved a shortened 4-month regimen of rifapentine, moxifloxacin, isoniazid, and pyrazinamide (CDC, 2022).

Second-line anti-TB drugs are also used in combination with other drugs when there is drug resistance to one of the first-line drugs or the patient is unable to tolerate use of a first-line drug. The second-line drugs are certain aminoglycoside antibiotics (amikacin, capreomycin sulfate [Capastat], kanamycin, and streptomycin); cycloserine (Seromycin); ethionamide (Trecator); para-aminosalicylic acid (Paser); and certain fluoroquinolones (most commonly used are moxifloxacin [Avelox] and levofloxacin [Levaquin]). Recently, two new anti-TB drugs have been developed (the first new anti-TB drugs in many years): bedaquiline (Sirturo) and delamanid (Deltyba). The FDA has licensed bedaquiline; delamanid has not yet been licensed by the FDA but is conditionally approved in Europe (Drew & Sterling, 2022). Second-line drugs also include other antibiotics (amoxicillin–clavulanate; imipenem–cilastatin; linezolid; meropenem).

Adequate drug therapy of patients with active TB usually produces improvement within 2 to 3 weeks, with decreased fever and cough, weight gain, improved well-being, and improved chest radiographs. Most patients have negative sputum cultures within 3 to 6 months. If the patient is symptomatic or if the culture is positive after 3 months, nonadherence or drug resistance must be considered. Cultures that are positive after 6 months often include drug-resistant organisms. The WHO (2020) prioritizes use of an all-oral regimen of 9 to 12 months when treating MDR-TB. The FDA approved a 6-month regimen consisting of bedaquiline, pretomanid, and linezolid (UpToDate, 2022). A longer regimen is used for more severe MDR-TB disease or the presence of advanced HIV infection. The longer regimen includes levofloxacin or moxifloxacin; bedaquiline and linezolid; and clofazimine and

TABLE 22.1
Treatment Regimens for Latent Tuberculosis

Drugs	Duration	Interval	Minimum Dosage
Isoniazid	9 mo	Daily (treatment for adults; persons living with HIV if antiretrovirals interact with RIF or RPT; children over age 2; pregnant women)	270 doses
		Twice weekly	76 doses
Isoniazid	6 mo	Daily	180 doses
		Twice weekly	52 doses
Isoniazid and rifapentine	3 mo	Once weekly • Treatment for persons 2 y or older and patients with HIV/AIDS and receiving antiretroviral treatment • Not recommended for children younger than 2 y of age; women who are pregnant or expect to become pregnant in the next 3 mo; and patients with presumed infection with isoniazid- or rifampin (RIF)-resistant TB	12 doses
RIF	4 mo	Daily	120 doses
INH and RIF	3 mo	Daily	90 doses

HIV/AIDS, human immunodeficiency virus/acquired immunodeficiency syndrome.

TABLE 22.2

Drug Regimens for Microbiologically Confirmed Pulmonary Tuberculosis Caused by Drug-Susceptible Organisms

Regimen	Intensive Phase			Continuation Phase				Regimen Effectiveness
	Drug*	Interval and Dose† (Minimum Duration)		Drugs	Interval and Dose†,‡ (Minimum Duration)	Range of Total Doses	Comments‡,§	
1	INH RIF PZA EMB	7 d/wk for 56 doses (8 wk), or 5 d/wk for 40 doses (8 wk)		INH RIF	7 d/wk for 126 doses (18 wk), or 5 d/wk for 90 doses (18 wk)	182–130	This is the preferred regimen for patients with newly diagnosed pulmonary tuberculosis	Greater
2	INH RIF PZA EMB	7 d/wk for 56 doses (8 wk), or 5 d/wk for 40 doses (8 wk)		INH RIF	Three times weekly for 54 doses (18 wk)	110–94	Preferred alternative regimen in situations in which more frequent DOT during continuation phase is difficult to achieve	
3	INH RIF PZA EMB	Three times weekly for 24 doses (8 wk)		INH RIF	Three times weekly for 54 doses (18 wk)	78	Use regimen with caution in patients with HIV and/or cavitary disease. Missed doses can lead to treatment failure, relapse, and acquired drug resistance	
4	INH RIF PZA EMB	7 d/wk for 14 doses then twice weekly for 12 doses¶		INH RIF	Twice weekly for 36 doses (18 wk)	62	Do not use twice-weekly regimens in HIV-infected patients or patients with smear-positive and/or cavitary disease. If doses are missed, then therapy is equivalent to once weekly, which is inferior	Lesser

*Other combinations may be appropriate in certain circumstances; additional details are provided in the section "Recommended Treatment Regimens."
†When DOT is used, drugs may be given 5 days per week and the necessary number of doses adjusted accordingly. Although there are no studies that compare five with seven daily doses, extensive experience indicates that this would be an effective practice. DOT should be used when drugs are administered <7 days per week.
‡Based on expert opinion, patients with cavitation on initial chest radiograph and positive cultures at completion of 2 months of therapy should receive a 7-month (31-week) continuation phase.
§Pyridoxine (vitamin B$_6$), 25 to 50 mg/day, is given with INH to all persons at risk of neuropathy (e.g., pregnant patients; breast-feeding infants; persons with HIV; patients with diabetes, alcohol use disorder, malnutrition, or chronic kidney disease; or patients with advanced age). For patients with peripheral neuropathy, experts recommend increasing pyridoxine dose to 100 mg/day.
¶Recommended time frame in the United States is to administer all doses for intensive phase within 3 months and for 4-month continuation phase within 6 months; 6-month regimen completed in 9 months.
DOT, directly observed therapy; EMB, ethambutol; HIV, human immunodeficiency virus; INH, isoniazid; PZA, pyrazinamide; RIF, rifampin.
From https//www.cdcgov/tb/topic/treatment/tbdisease.htm on September 9, 2022.

cycloserine as well as additional drugs if needed. The optimal approach to treatment of pregnant patients with MDR-TB is uncertain.

Diagnosis of drug-resistant TB is established by identification of the TB organism in sputum and by drug susceptibility testing showing resistance to one or more anti-TB drugs. WHO prioritizes the use of oral agents over injectable agents. Treatment of XDR-TB is with bedaquiline, pretomanid, and linezolid. An alternative is an intensive phase of five drugs continued for 5 to 7 months beyond sputum culture conversion; then a continuation phase for up to 24 months beyond culture conversion.

Clinical Application 22.2

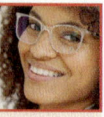

- Ms. Grant is taking isoniazid (INH), rifampin (RIF), pyrazinamide, and ethambutol. Why is she taking four drugs? How long will she continue to take these four drugs?

ISONIAZID

Isoniazid (INH), the most commonly used anti-TB drug and the prototype, is bactericidal, relatively inexpensive, and nontoxic. Although use by itself for treatment of latent TB is appropriate, use with other anti-TB drugs is essential for treatment of active TB.

Pharmacokinetics

INH is well absorbed from the GI tract, with peak serum concentrations occurring 1 to 2 hours after a 300-mg dose. Food slows absorption. The drug penetrates and reaches therapeutic concentrations in essentially all body fluids and cavities, including the cerebrospinal fluid (CSF). Its half-life is 1 to 4 hours. It is acetylated in the liver to acetylisoniazid, which is excreted by the kidneys. Metabolism of INH is genetically determined; some people are "slow acetylators," and others are "rapid acetylators." A person's rate of acetylation affects response to INH. If the rate is slow, INH is more likely to accumulate to toxic concentrations, and the development of peripheral neuropathy is more likely. However, there is no significant difference in the clinical effectiveness of INH. Liver or kidney impairment may slow elimination.

Action

INH is selective for mycobacteria, inhibiting formation of bacterial cell walls. The drug not only kills actively growing intracellular and extracellular organisms but also inhibits the growth of dormant organisms in macrophages and tuberculous lesions.

Use

It is appropriate to use INH alone or in combination with other anti-TB drugs in the treatment of latent TB. However, it is essential that it *always* be given in combination with other anti-TB drugs in the treatment of active TB. Table 22.3 gives route of administration and dosage information for INH.

For the treatment of TB in pregnancy, the initial regimen should be INH, RIF, and ethambutol for 2 months, followed by INH and RIF for 7 months. Box 22.2 contains more information about the use of anti-TB drugs in pregnancy.

Patient-related variables specific to the use of isoniazid include the following:

- Age:
  - If children are unable to swallow tablets, INH tablets may be crushed and mixed in soft food.
  - Vitamin B_6 (pyridoxine) is administered to breast-feeding infants or children at risk for INH-induced neuropathy.
  - The risk of INH-induced hepatitis is greater in adults above age 50.
- Reproduction, pregnancy, and lactation:
  - Treatment of latent TB can be delayed until after delivery if appropriate. TB causes adverse maternal and fetal outcomes. INH is used to treat active TB during pregnancy. The risk of maternal hepatotoxicity is increased.
  - Treatment of active TB with INH is not a contraindication for breast-feeding. Monitor the infant for jaundice. **Jaundice** is a yellow discoloration of the skin and of body tissues and fluids resulting from abnormally high levels of bilirubin in the blood; it is a common symptom when drugs cause liver damage.
- Abnormal kidney function and hepatic impairment:
  - No INH dosage adjustment is necessary for abnormal kidney function; however, caution is warranted when administering to patients with severe abnormal kidney function.

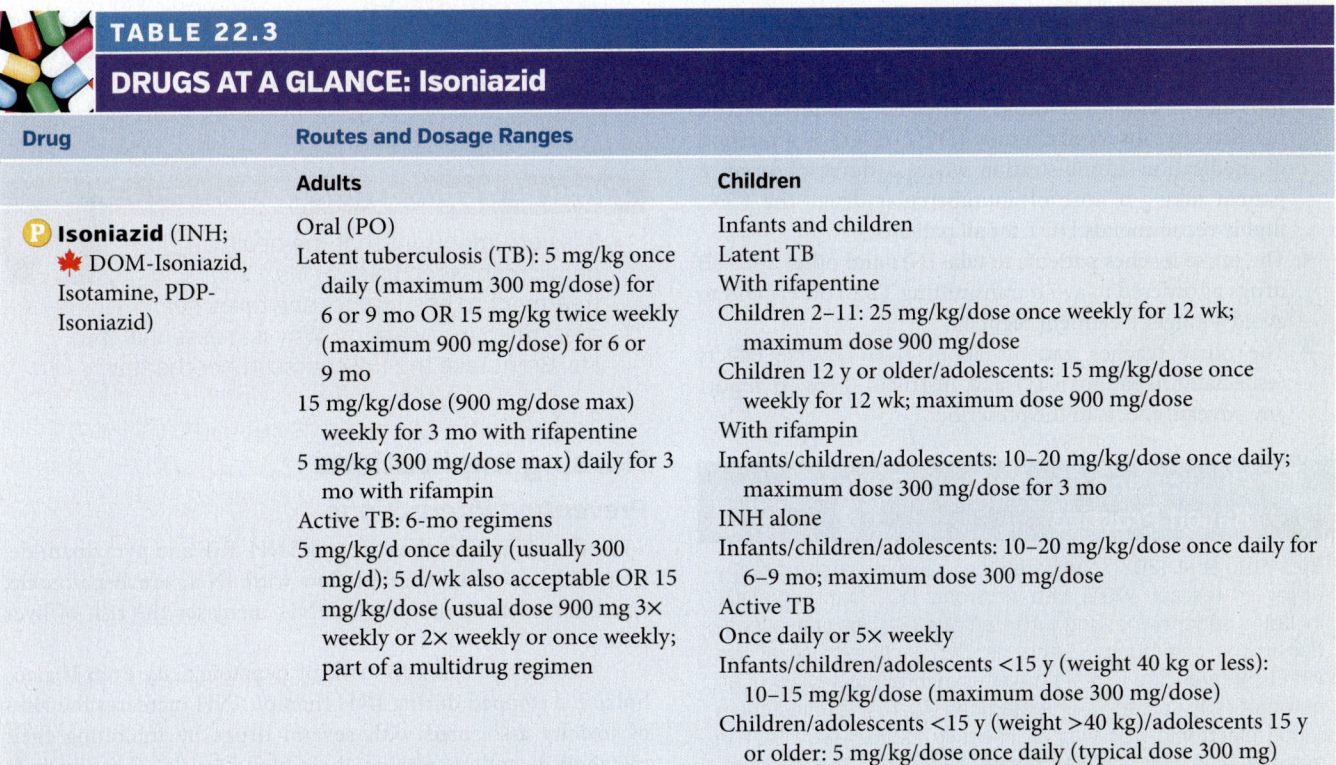

TABLE 22.3
DRUGS AT A GLANCE: Isoniazid

Drug	Routes and Dosage Ranges	
	Adults	**Children**
Isoniazid (INH; DOM-Isoniazid, Isotamine, PDP-Isoniazid)	Oral (PO) Latent tuberculosis (TB): 5 mg/kg once daily (maximum 300 mg/dose) for 6 or 9 mo OR 15 mg/kg twice weekly (maximum 900 mg/dose) for 6 or 9 mo 15 mg/kg/dose (900 mg/dose max) weekly for 3 mo with rifapentine 5 mg/kg (300 mg/dose max) daily for 3 mo with rifampin Active TB: 6-mo regimens 5 mg/kg/d once daily (usually 300 mg/d); 5 d/wk also acceptable OR 15 mg/kg/dose (usual dose 900 mg 3× weekly or 2× weekly or once weekly; part of a multidrug regimen	Infants and children Latent TB With rifapentine Children 2–11: 25 mg/kg/dose once weekly for 12 wk; maximum dose 900 mg/dose Children 12 y or older/adolescents: 15 mg/kg/dose once weekly for 12 wk; maximum dose 900 mg/dose With rifampin Infants/children/adolescents: 10–20 mg/kg/dose once daily; maximum dose 300 mg/dose for 3 mo INH alone Infants/children/adolescents: 10–20 mg/kg/dose once daily for 6–9 mo; maximum dose 300 mg/dose Active TB Once daily or 5× weekly Infants/children/adolescents <15 y (weight 40 kg or less): 10–15 mg/kg/dose (maximum dose 300 mg/dose) Children/adolescents <15 y (weight >40 kg)/adolescents 15 y or older: 5 mg/kg/dose once daily (typical dose 300 mg)

HIV, human immunodeficiency virus.

BOX 22.2 Treatment of Tuberculosis in Pregnancy

- Initial regimen: isoniazid (INH), rifampin (RIF), and ethambutol daily for 2 months followed by INH and RIF twice weekly for 7 months (total treatment 9 months)
  - INH: good safety record in pregnancy; breast-feeding should not be discouraged during treatment with INH; pregnant and breast-feeding patients who are receiving INH should take vitamin B_6 (pyridoxine) supplementation, and their breast-fed infants should also receive pyridoxine.
  - RIF: good safety record in pregnancy; breast-feeding should be discontinued.
- Ethambutol: may cause ophthalmic abnormalities in infants born to patients receiving ethambutol; drug should be used in pregnancy if the benefits outweigh the risks.
- Pyrazinamide: not recommended; effect on fetus is unknown.
- Antituberculosis drugs contraindicated in pregnancy: streptomycin, kanamycin, amikacin, capreomycin, fluoroquinolones

---

- Damage to the liver is a serious adverse effect of INH. This risk is compounded because INH is given concurrently with other anti-TB drugs, which also cause liver damage. The risk of INH-induced hepatitis worsens with daily alcohol consumption or chronic liver disease.
- The nurse assesses the patient monthly for symptoms of hepatitis (anorexia, nausea, fatigue, malaise, and jaundice).
- Use cautiously in patients with severe hepatic impairment.
- The FDA issued a **BOXED WARNING** for INH, stating severe and sometimes fatal hepatitis may occur, usually within the first 3 months of treatment, although it may develop even after many months of therapy.
- Liver function tests must be monitored. Discontinue INH if signs/symptoms of hepatotoxicity occur; if serum bilirubin is 3 mg/dL or more; or if liver enzymes are greater than 5 times the upper limit of normal.
- Black and Hispanic women are at greater risk for fatal hepatotoxicity from INH.
- Children are less at risk for hepatotoxicity, but monitoring is still indicated.
- Specific healthcare environments:
  - The home care nurse needs to ensure that patients take INH and other anti-TB drugs as directed. The nurse carries out **directly observed therapy** (DOT). DOT is a method of medication administration where a nurse observes a patient taking a dose of antitubercular drug. The CDC highly recommends DOT for all patients.
  - The nurse teaches patients to take INH and other anti-TB drugs as ordered to avoid transmitting TB to others and to avoid a longer treatment regimen.
  - The nurse teaches patients about INH adverse effects (especially hepatotoxicity) and instructs them to report any adverse effects to the prescriber.

! Quality and Safety Alert: Evidence-Based Practice

Burzynski et al. (2021) compared the use of in-person directly observed therapy (DOT) with electronic DOT. In-person DOT included patients meeting with staff at a TB clinic or at a location in the community. Electronic DOT included use of live video conferencing in real time or asynchronous review of an automatically uploaded time-stamped video. The researchers found electronic DOT was as effective as in-person DOT in assuring high levels of TB treatment adherence. The researchers recommend electronic DOT as a standard care option.

Adverse Effects

Potentially serious adverse effects of INH include hepatotoxicity and peripheral neuropathy. Manifestations of hepatotoxicity are symptoms of hepatitis or elevated liver enzymes. Indications of peripheral neuropathy may include numbness and tingling in the hands and feet. Those at high risk for peripheral neuropathy include pregnant patients; breast-feeding infants; and patients with HIV infection, diabetes, alcohol use disorder, malnutrition, chronic kidney disease, or advanced age. Preventing peripheral neuropathy requires concurrent administration of pyridoxine (vitamin B_6). Patients with risk factors should take 25 to 50 mg/day.

Contraindications

Contraindications to INH include a hypersensitivity to the drug, acute hepatic disease, or INH-induced liver damage. Caution is warranted in older adult patients, as well as in those people with chronic non–INH-related liver disease or alcohol use disorder, in those with seizure disorders (especially if taking phenytoin), and in those with severe abnormal kidney function.

Clinical Application 22.3

- It is very important that the health department keep track of Ms. Grant's treatment to ensure that she takes her prescribed medications. Why is it essential that Ms. Grant take the full course of her therapy?

Nursing Implications

Preventing Interactions

Some drugs increase the effects of INH. RIF and pyrazinamide, frequently given in combination with INH, are hepatotoxic, and their administration with INH increases the risk of liver injury.

Alcohol increases the risk of hepatotoxicity even if alcohol use is stopped during INH therapy. INH increases the risks of toxicity associated with several drugs by inhibiting their metabolism and increasing their blood levels. These include benzodiazepines (diazepam and triazolam), carbamazepine, metoprolol, and phenytoin. Concurrent use should be avoided when possible or blood levels of the drug whose metabolism is inhibited should be monitored. INH may enhance the adverse hepatic effects of acetaminophen. Antacids and food slow the absorption of INH.

Administering the Medication

Administration of INH is usually oral (PO), but an intramuscular (IM) form is also available. Regardless of the route, it is necessary to take liver enzymes prior to beginning administration and then monthly thereafter if risk factors for liver injury are present. Patients should take INH on an empty stomach, 1 hour before or 2 hours after a meal, with a full glass of water. Food delays absorption. However, people may take INH with food if it causes GI upset. Because INH is a weak monoamine oxidase inhibitor, a mild tyramine reaction is rare but possible. Consuming histamine-containing foods (skipjack, tuna, or tropical fish) with INH may cause a histamine reaction with headache, sweating, palpitations, itching, wheezing, and dyspnea.

Only patients who are unable to take the drug orally should receive INH parenterally. The nurse gives INH by deep injection into a large muscle mass at an approved site. It is necessary to rotate the site. Local pain and irritation may accompany the injection.

Assessing for Therapeutic Effects

If the patient is being treated with INH for latent TB, the nurse observes for signs and symptoms of active disease, such as fever, productive cough, positive sputum cultures, night sweats, fatigue, and malaise. If the patient is being treated for active TB, the nurse observes for clinical improvement, such as a decrease in the following symptoms—cough, sputum production, fever, night sweats, and fatigue; the nurse should also see an increased appetite and weight as well as an increasing feeling of well-being. Follow-up sputum smears and sputum cultures should be negative for acid-fast bacilli. It is necessary to obtain sputum cultures monthly until two consecutive cultures are negative. The appearance of the chest radiograph should also improve.

Assessing for Adverse Effects

The nurse frequently assesses for signs and symptoms of hepatotoxicity, including hepatitis (jaundice, anorexia, nausea, vomiting, and abdominal pain). The nurse reports their development to the healthcare provider promptly to prevent possible liver failure and death. Any increase in liver enzymes or bilirubin must be reported immediately. In addition, the nurse assesses for signs and symptoms of peripheral neuropathy (tingling, numbness, and paresthesias of the extremities).

Patient Teaching

Box 22.3 presents patient teaching guidelines for INH.

> **Clinical Application 22.4**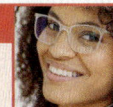
> - The nurse assesses Ms. Grant when she returns to the clinic for follow-up visits. For what adverse effects of INH does the nurse plan to monitor her?

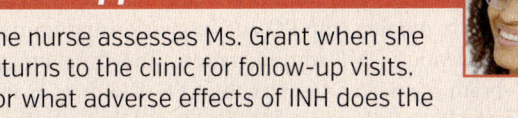

1. The nurse who is giving isoniazid (INH) anticipates an order for which one of the following vitamins, usually given with INH?
   A. vitamin B_3 (niacin)
   B. vitamin B_6 (pyridoxine)
   C. folic acid (folate)
   D. vitamin D (calcitriol)

2. The nurse should teach patients taking isoniazid to avoid alcohol because of the increased risk of
   A. central nervous system depression
   B. liver damage
   C. drug-resistant tuberculous organisms
   D. rapid drug metabolism

BOX 22.3 Patient Teaching Guidelines for Isoniazid

- If you have a positive tuberculin skin test and you are taking isoniazid (INH) to treat latent tuberculosis (TB), follow the drug regimen exactly for the length of time prescribed to prevent development of active TB. Treatment may last for months or years.
- If you are being treated for active TB, you should begin to feel better in about 2 to 3 weeks. If you do not, notify the healthcare provider who is managing the TB infection.
- When you take your INH every day, take the ordered dose of vitamin B_6 (pyridoxine) at the same time, so you do not forget to take your vitamin B_6. Vitamin B_6 helps prevent the adverse effects of leg numbness and tingling.
- Take INH on an empty stomach if possible, 1 hour before or 2 hours after a meal. If stomach upset occurs, take the drug with food.
- Take all other anti-TB drugs prescribed along with INH.
- Avoid alcoholic beverages while taking INH.
- INH can cause liver damage. Watch for the following signs and symptoms of liver damage (i.e., hepatitis): loss of appetite, nausea, yellowing of skin or eyes (jaundice), light-colored stools, dark urine, fatigue, and malaise. If such symptoms occur, stop taking INH and **immediately** report the symptoms to the healthcare provider who is managing the TB infection.
- If you begin to experience numbness, burning, or tingling of your arms or legs, notify the TB healthcare provider. These are the symptoms of another adverse effect of INH.
- The healthcare provider will order blood tests to check your liver function. Be sure to keep these appointments to have blood drawn. You may also need to have sputum cultures.

RIFAMYCINS

Rifamycins are a class of drugs that is bactericidal for the treatment of intracellular and extracellular TB organisms. 🅿 **Rifampin** (RIF; Rifadin) is the prototype rifamycin. RIF and INH are synergistic in combination, eliminating TB bacilli from sputum and producing clinical improvement faster than any other drug regimen, unless the causal bacteria are resistant to one or both drugs.

Pharmacokinetics

RIF is well absorbed orally and diffuses well into body tissues and fluids, with highest concentrations occurring in the liver, lungs, gallbladder, and kidneys. Peak serum concentration occurs in 2 to 4 hours with PO administration and immediately with intravenous (IV) administration. The drug crosses the blood–brain barrier and enters the CSF. The drug is metabolized in the liver and excreted primarily in bile; a small amount is excreted in urine. Its elimination half-life is approximately 3 to 4 hours, depending on the dose. Because it is a strong inducer of drug-metabolizing enzymes, its half-life becomes shorter with continued use.

Action

RIF is bactericidal for TB organisms. It kills mycobacteria by inhibiting synthesis of RNA and thereby causing production of defective, nonfunctional proteins.

Use

Healthcare providers use RIF to treat susceptible TB infections. Patients use it alone for latent TB and in combination with other anti-TB drugs for active TB. For the use of RIF in pregnancy, see Box 22.2. Home care considerations with RIF and the other rifamycins are the same as for INH.

RIF has important uses other than in the treatment of TB, including prophylaxis for people exposed to meningococcal meningitis as well as in the treatment of MAC. An unlabeled use is in the treatment of leprosy, which is caused by *Mycobacterium leprae*. The drug also has several other unlabeled uses: treatment of prosthetic valve endocarditis due to methicillin-resistant *Staphylococcus aureus* (MRSA), prophylaxis for exposure to *Haemophilus influenzae* infections and *Neisseria meningitidis*, and treatment of certain staphylococcal infections (including MRSA) when combined with another antistaphylococcal antibiotic to prevent resistance.

Table 22.4 gives route and dosage information for RIF and the other rifamycins.

Patient-related variables specific to the use of rifampin include the following:

- Reproduction, pregnancy, and lactation:
  - Rifampin may decrease the effectiveness of hormonal contraceptives.
  - Postnatal hemorrhages have been reported in infant and mother if the drug is administered in the last few weeks of pregnancy. Due to risks of untreated TB, rifampin is used when the risk of maternal disease is moderate to high. Increased risk of maternal hepatotoxicity requires temporary drug withdrawal in pregnant and postpartum patients.
  - The manufacturer recommends stopping breast-feeding or discontinuing the drug. Other experts report no contraindication to breast-feeding if treating drug-susceptible TB.
- Abnormal kidney function and hepatic impairment:
  - Rifampin doses of 600 mg or less per day require no adjustment based on kidney status.
  - No dosage adjustment is required for preexisting hepatic impairment. If new or worsening hepatic damage occurs during use, discontinue rifampin. Monitor for symptoms of hepatotoxicity.
- Specific healthcare environments:
  - In critically ill patients, RIF interacts with many nonnucleoside reverse transcriptase inhibitors (NNRTIs) and protease inhibitors (PIs), generally reducing the effectiveness of these antiretroviral drugs. RIF decreases blood levels and therapeutic effects of the anti-HIV drugs.
  - This effect is much less pronounced with rifabutin (see *Other Drugs in the Class*).

Adverse Effects

Adverse effects of RIF include GI upset, skin rashes, hepatotoxicity, and acute kidney injury. The drug causes a harmless red-orange discoloration of urine, tears, sweat, and other body fluids. It may stain soft contact lenses permanently. Prolonged use may result in bacterial or fungal superinfections, including pseudomembranous colitis or *Clostridium difficile*–associated diarrhea.

Contraindications

Contraindications to RIF include hypersensitivity to the drug (or other rifamycins). Caution is warranted in patients who have a history of liver disease, in those who are currently receiving medications known to cause harm to the liver (particularly pyrazinamide), in those with a history of alcohol use disorder, or in those who are receiving treatment for HIV.

Nursing Implications

Preventing Interactions

RIF has many interactions with other drugs. It induces hepatic cytochrome P4503A4 enzymes and accelerates the metabolism of numerous other drugs, thereby decreasing their serum concentrations, half-lives, and therapeutic effects. Use of RIF requires careful review of the patient's drug regimen for potential interactions.

Drugs that RIF affects include antiretroviral drugs (NNRTIs and PIs), benzodiazepines, corticosteroids, cyclosporine, estrogens, fluconazole, methadone, metoprolol, phenytoin, propranolol, oral contraceptives, oral sulfonylureas, theophylline, verapamil, and warfarin. The following examples illustrate the effects of RIF on other drugs. RIF may decrease the serum concentration of the NNRTIs efavirenz and nevirapine. The anti-TB drug also decreases the serum concentration of the PI ritonavir. RIF interacts with warfarin; a decreased anticoagulant

TABLE 22.4

DRUGS AT A GLANCE: Rifamycins

Drug	Routes and Dosage Ranges	
	Adults	**Children**
Rifampin (RIF; Rifadin; ❋ Rifadin, Rofact)	Oral (PO) or intravenous (IV) Latent tuberculosis (TB): 10 mg/kg/d (maximum 600 mg/d) for 4 mo Active TB: 10 mg/kg/d (maximum 600 mg/d) OR 10 mg/kg 5 d/wk (maximum 600 mg); initial intensive phase part of 4-drug regimen for 2 mo; continuation phase with INH for at least 4 mo	Oral (PO) or IV Latent TB: 15–20 mg/kg/d once daily (maximum 600 mg/d) for 4 mo Active TB: Infants/children/adolescents <15 y (weight 40 kg or less) 10–20 mg/kg/d (maximum 600 mg/d) OR 10–20 mg/kg 5 d/wk; maximum dose 600 mg Children/adolescents <15 y (weight >40 kg) or adolescents 15 y or older 10 mg/kg/dose daily or 5 d/wk; maximum dose 600 mg; initial intensive phase part of 4-drug regimen for 2 mo; continuation phase with INH for at least 4 mo
Rifapentine (Priftin)	Latent TB: once weekly for 3 mo in combination with isoniazid (maximum dose 900 mg) 25.1–32 kg: 600 mg 32.1–50 kg: 750 mg >50 kg: 900 mg Active TB: 6-mo regimen with INH initial phase, 600 mg PO twice weekly with an interval of not <72 h between doses; continuation phase, 600 mg PO once weekly for 4 mo; 4-mo regimen initial phase 1.2 g daily for 8 weeks with moxifloxacin, INH, and pyrazinamide; continuation phase 1.2 g daily for 9 weeks with moxifloxacin and INH	Latent TB: Children 2 years–adolescence once weekly for 3 mo 10–14 kg: 300 mg 14.1–25 kg: 450 mg 25.1–32 kg: 600 mg 32.1–50 kg: 750 mg >50 kg: 900 mg Active TB: 6-mo regimen: children 12 y or older and adolescents initial phase 600 mg twice weekly with 72 h or more between doses for 2 mo; continuation phase 600 mg once weekly for 4 mo 4-mo regimen: children 12 y or older and adolescents (weight 40 kg or greater) 1,200 mg once daily for 17 wk (119 total doses) with moxifloxacin, INH, and pyrazinamide
Rifabutin (Mycobutin; ❋ Mycobutin)*	Latent TB: 300 mg PO once daily for 4 mo Active TB: 300 mg PO once daily as part of a multidrug regimen Disseminated MAC in advanced HIV infection Prophylaxis: 300 mg PO once daily (150 mg twice daily if GI upset) Treatment: 300 mg PO once daily as adjunct therapy with clarithromycin or azithromycin (plus ethambutol)	Infants, children, adolescents Active TB: 10–20 mg/kg PO once daily (maximum dose 300 mg) MAC prophylaxis: 300 mg PO once daily Treatment (add-on therapy for severe infection): 10–20 mg/kg PO once daily (maximum 300 mg)

*Administered as alternative to rifampin.
GI, gastrointestinal; MAC, *Mycobacterium avium* complex.

effect occurs approximately 5 to 8 days after RIF is started and lasts for 5 to 7 days after RIF is stopped. Close monitoring of the prothrombin time and INR is essential with an increase of the dosage of warfarin as necessary. In addition, RIF decreases the effectiveness of oral contraceptives, and women who use these contraceptives and take RIF should use another method of birth control. Finally, concurrent administration with RIF with methadone may precipitate signs and symptoms of opiate withdrawal unless methadone dosage is increased.

Administering the Medication

The drug is taken on an empty stomach, either 1 hour before or 2 hours after a meal. However, if patients are unable to tolerate it on an empty stomach, they may take it with a meal and a large glass of water. Food may delay or reduce the peak of action.

RIF is available for IV administration. The nurse reconstitutes the drug with 10 mL of sterile water to yield 60 mg/mL. The nurse then adds this to D_5W 100 mL and infuses it over 30 minutes or adds this to D_5W 500 mL and infuses it over 3 hours. The infusion rate should range from 30 minutes to 3 hours depending on the dose and volume of IV solution. The final concentration should not exceed 6 mg/mL.

Assessing for Therapeutic Effects

If the patient is being treated with RIF for latent TB, the nurse observes for signs and symptoms of active disease. If the patient is being treated with the drug for active disease, the nurse observes for clinical improvement. Therapeutic effects are usually apparent with the first 2 to 3 weeks of drug therapy for active disease.

BOX 22.4 Patient Teaching Guidelines for the Rifamycins

- If you have a positive tuberculin skin test and you are receiving rifampin (RIF) or rifapentine to treat latent tuberculosis (TB), you should follow the drug regimen exactly for the length of time prescribed to prevent development of active TB. Treatment may last for months.
- If you are being treated for active TB, you should begin to feel better in about 2 to 3 weeks. If you do not, notify the healthcare provider who is managing the TB infection.
- Take RIF on an empty stomach, 1 hour before or 2 hours after a meal. If you cannot tolerate the drug on an empty stomach, take the drug with meals and with a full glass of water.
- If you are unable to swallow capsules, notify your prescriber and contact your pharmacist. RIF is available as an oral suspension.
- Take all other anti-TB drugs prescribed along with RIF.
- Avoid alcoholic beverages while taking RIF.
- RIF can cause liver damage. Watch for signs and symptoms of hepatitis: fever, loss of appetite, nausea, vomiting, yellowing of skin or eyes, light-colored stools, dark urine, and malaise. If such symptoms occur, stop taking RIF immediately and promptly report the symptoms to the healthcare provider who is managing the TB infection.
- The healthcare provider will order blood tests to check on liver function throughout your RIF therapy. Keep all appointments.
- RIF causes a red-orange discoloration of tears, saliva, urine, and other body secretions. Although the discoloration is harmless, it may permanently stain soft contact lenses. Consult an eye care professional; you may need to refrain from wearing your soft contact lenses.
- RIF decreases the effectiveness of oral contraceptives. Use a barrier type of contraception during RIF therapy.
- If you are taking rifabutin, report the following symptoms of uveitis (sensitivity to light, excessive tears, or eye pain) to the healthcare provider as soon as possible.
- Ask a medical professional for information about any drugs that you take that may interact with RIF and the other rifamycins. Learn about those signs and symptoms that indicate drug ineffectiveness and that need to be reported to the healthcare provider.

Assessing for Adverse Effects

The nurse assesses for GI adverse effects such as anorexia, epigastric distress, abdominal cramps, nausea, vomiting, and diarrhea. Even pseudomembranous colitis is possible. The nurse observes for hypersensitivity reactions such as fever, tachycardia, anorexia, and malaise; flushing, itching, and rash may also occur. RIF can also produce a flulike syndrome of fever, chills, and muscle aches.

The patient taking RIF must be observed for signs and symptoms of hepatotoxicity—increased serum liver enzymes and bilirubin, jaundice, anorexia, abdominal pain, nausea, and vomiting. Observation for these adverse effects is crucial if the patient already has liver damage, has liver disease, or is taking another drug that also causes hepatotoxicity. Any symptoms of hepatotoxicity must be reported immediately to the healthcare provider to prevent further liver damage, liver failure, or death.

Patient Teaching

Box 22.4 presents patient teaching guidelines for RIF and the rifamycins.

Other Drugs in the Class

Rifapentine (Priftin) and rifabutin (Mycobutin) are bactericidal first-line drugs for the treatment of TB. These drugs are similar to RIF in effectiveness, side effects, and enzyme activity. Like RIF, rifapentine and rifabutin cause a harmless red-orange discoloration of body fluids and permanent staining of soft contact lenses. Adverse effects of rifapentine and rifabutin include neutropenia, leukopenia, thrombocytopenia, hepatotoxicity, headache, fever, nausea, vomiting, and diarrhea. Rifapentine's additional adverse effects include hepatitis uveitis (an eye disorder with inflammation, pain, and impaired vision).

Patients must use rifapentine with at least one other drug, such as INH, to which the causative bacteria are susceptible. They may take it, in combination with INH, in a 3-month regimen for the treatment of latent TB. The major advantage of rifapentine is that it can be used in combination with INH in a once-weekly dosing regimen during the 4-month continuation phase of treatment for active TB. It is not recommended during pregnancy. Rifabutin is used for the treatment of MAC in people with advanced HIV disease and is substituted for RIF in patients with HIV disease. Like rifapentine, rifabutin decreases blood levels and therapeutic effects of the anti-HIV drugs (as well as many other drugs). However, this effect is much less pronounced with rifabutin. Rifabutin has no advantage over RIF in the treatment of TB, but it may be taken concurrently with INH for patients who need prophylaxis against both *M. tuberculosis* and *M. avium*.

Clinical Application 22.5

- The nurse teaches Ms. Grant about her medication. What adverse effect of RIF should the nurse include in patient teaching so that the patient does not become alarmed and stop taking the medication?

NCLEX Success

3. The nurse is reviewing a patient's medications and sees that the patient is receiving rifampin. The nurse's greatest concern about rifampin and its drug interactions is
   A. it decreases the metabolism of many other drugs
   B. it increases the metabolism of many other drugs
   C. it increases the risk for GI bleeding if given with warfarin
   D. it increases the risk of adverse effects from anti-seizure drugs

ADJUVANT FIRST-LINE ANTITUBERCULAR DRUGS

Several other drugs are used to treat TB. Table 22.5 contains route and dosage information for these drugs.

Pyrazinamide

Pyrazinamide is part of a multidrug anti-TB regimen used with INH, RIF, and ethambutol during the first 2 months, the initial phase, of treatment for active TB. This drug is bactericidal against actively growing mycobacteria in macrophages, but its exact mechanism of action is unknown. It is well absorbed from the GI tract and penetrates most body fluids and tissues, including macrophages containing tuberculous mycobacteria. It has a rapid onset and peaks in 2 hours. It is metabolized in the liver and excreted mainly by the kidneys. Its half-life is 9 to 10 hours.

The most common adverse effect of pyrazinamide is GI upset. Gout may also occur; pyrazinamide inhibits urate excretion, and this characteristic causes hyperuricemia in most patients and may cause acute attacks of gout. The most severe adverse effect is hepatotoxicity; a patient with preexisting liver impairment should not take the drug unless it is essential. Pyrazinamide enhances the hepatotoxic effect of RIF. The nurse must assess patients without liver impairment for symptoms of liver dysfunction every 2 weeks during the usual 8 weeks of therapy. If such symptoms occur, measurement of liver enzymes is necessary. If significant liver damage is indicated, it is essential to discontinue pyrazinamide.

Contraindications to pyrazinamide include a hypersensitivity to the drug, severe preexisting hepatic damage, or acute attacks of gout. Caution is warranted in patients with a history of alcohol use disorder. Weigh risks and benefits of the drug before use in pregnancy.

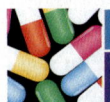

TABLE 22.5
DRUGS AT A GLANCE: Adjuvant First-Line Antitubercular Drugs*

Drug	Routes and Dosage Ranges†	
	Adults	**Children**
Pyrazinamide (✸ PDP-Pyrazinamide; Tebrazid)	Active tuberculosis (TB): oral (PO) initial 2-mo phase follow with continuation phase of 4–7 additional months (part of multidrug regimen) Daily therapy 40–55 kg: 1,000 mg 56–75 kg: 1,500 mg 76–90 kg: 2,000 mg Twice-weekly therapy 40–55 kg: 2,000 mg 56–75 kg: 3,000 mg 76–90 kg: 4,000 mg Three times/week 40–55 kg: 1,500 mg 56–75 kg: 2,500 mg 76–90 kg: 3,000 mg There is also a 4-mo regimen with moxifloxacin	Active TB: PO initial 2-mo phase follow with continuation phase of 4–7 additional months (part of multidrug regimen) Infants/children/adolescents (weight <40 kg): 35 mg/kg/dose once daily or 5× weekly; suggest 30–40 mg/kg/dose Children/adolescents (weight 40 kg or more): 40–55 kg 1,000 mg; 56–75 kg 1,500 mg; 76–90 kg 2,000 mg; given once daily or 5× weekly There are also 2×/week and 3×/week regimens
Ethambutol (Myambutol; ✸ Etibi)	Active TB Daily therapy: 40–55 kg: 800 mg 56–75 kg: 1,200 mg 76–90 kg: 1,600 mg Twice-weekly therapy: 40–55 kg: 2,000 mg 56–75 kg: 2,800 mg 76–90 kg: 4,000 mg Disseminated MAC in advanced HIV infection: 15 mg/kg once daily; given in combination with clarithromycin or azithromycin	Active TB Infants/children/adolescents <15 y (weight <40 kg) 20 mg/kg/dose PO once daily or 5× weekly Children/adolescents <15 y (weight 40 kg or more) or adolescents 15 y or older PO once daily or 5× weekly 40–55 kg: 800 mg 56–75 kg: 1,200 mg 76–90 kg: 1,600 mg MAC, secondary prophylaxis or treatment (if HIV exposed or infected) Infants and children, 15–25 mg/kg/d once daily (maximum 2.5 g/d) with clarithromycin (or azithromycin) for severe disease add rifabutin Adolescents, 15 mg/kg/dose daily with clarithromycin (or azithromycin) with or without rifabutin

*When treating active TB, pyrazinamide and ethambutol are part of a multidrug regimen.
†Twice-weekly therapy should always be administered using directly observed therapy (DOT). For three times weekly therapy, consult the literature.
HIV, human immunodeficiency virus; MAC, *Mycobacterium avium* complex.

Ethambutol

Ethambutol (Myambutol) is a tuberculostatic drug that inhibits synthesis of RNA and thus interferes with mycobacterial protein metabolism. It may be a component in a four-drug regimen for initial treatment of active TB that may be caused by drug-resistant organisms. When culture and susceptibility reports become available (usually after several weeks), it may be appropriate to stop ethambutol if the causative organisms are susceptible to INH and RIF or continue it if the organisms are resistant to either INH or RIF and susceptible to ethambutol. To achieve therapeutic serum levels, patients should take the total daily dose of ethambutol at one time. Mycobacterial resistance to the drug develops slowly.

Ethambutol is well absorbed from the GI tract, even when given with food. The drug has a rapid onset, peaks in 2 to 4 hours, and lasts 20 to 24 hours. It is metabolized in the liver and excreted primarily by the kidneys. (Dosage reduction is necessary with impaired kidney function.) The half-life is 3 to 4 hours.

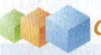

Concept Mastery Alert

It is important to educate a patient who has been prescribed ethambutol on the visual acuity adverse effect of the medication. Some patients taking this medication have developed optic neuritis, which is an inflammatory, demyelinating disorder of the optic nerve. A patient with optic neuritis will have a decrease in visual acuity and an inability to distinguish red from green. The patient teaching should include this information, and the patient should notify the prescriber promptly. Ethambutol should be discontinued if this disorder develops. The visual acuity should improve when the medication is discontinued. Ophthalmic abnormalities have been reported in infants born to patients receiving ethambutol.

NCLEX Success

4. A patient who is receiving ethambutol comes into the clinic for a follow-up visit. Which finding on the assessment indicates a serious adverse reaction to the drug?

   A. a sputum culture that is negative for acid-fast bacilli
   B. changes in visual acuity
   C. poor appetite and GI upset
   D. dizziness and hearing loss

FIRST-LINE DRUG COMBINATIONS USED TO TREAT TUBERCULOSIS

INH/RIF (Rifamate) and INH/RIF/pyrazinamide (Rifater) are combination products developed to increase convenience for patients and promote adherence to the prescribed drug therapy regimen for drug-susceptible TB. A tablet of Rifamate contains 150 mg of INH and 300 mg of RIF, and two tablets daily provide the recommended doses for a 6-month, short-course treatment regimen. A tablet of Rifater contains 50 mg of INH, 120 mg RIF, and 300 mg pyrazinamide and is FDA approved for the first 2 months of a 6-month, short-course treatment. Dosage depends on weight, with four tablets daily for patients weighing 44 kg or less, five tablets daily for those weighing 45 to 54 kg, and six tablets daily for those weighing 55 kg or more. Rifater not only reduces the number of pills a patient has to take each day but also prevents the patient from taking only one of the three medications, which can lead to MDR-TB.

SECOND-LINE DRUGS USED TO TREAT TUBERCULOSIS

The second-line anti-TB drugs are indicated for treatment of the following infections:

- Strains of *M. tuberculosis* that are resistant to first-line drugs
- TB when the patient has a hypersensitivity or inability to tolerate a first-line drug
- MDR-TB and XDR-TB

The second-line drugs are always used in combination regimens with first-line drugs. In many cases, the second-line drugs are less effective than the first-line drugs. Second-line drugs often have more frequent and severe adverse effects, and they may be more expensive as well. Little research exists on the use of the second-line drugs to treat latent TB in people exposed to MDR-TB. Healthcare providers have gained experience in the use of combinations of first-line and second-line drugs in the treatment of MDR-TB and XDR-TB

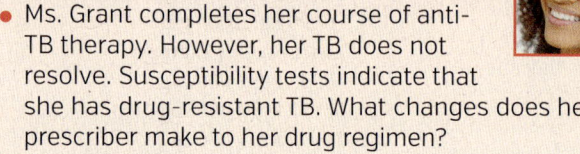

Clinical Application 22.6

- Ms. Grant completes her course of anti-TB therapy. However, her TB does not resolve. Susceptibility tests indicate that she has drug-resistant TB. What changes does her prescriber make to her drug regimen?

DRUGS USED TO TREAT *MYCOBACTERIUM AVIUM COMPLEX* DISEASE

The main drugs used in treatment of MAC disease in patients with HIV are the macrolides azithromycin and clarithromycin (see Chapter 21) as well as ethambutol and rifabutin (described earlier in this chapter). Other drugs include amikacin, fluoroquinolones, and streptomycin. Treatment of MAC begins with twice-daily administration of clarithromycin 500 mg or azithromycin 500 to 600 mg once daily. A second drug is also used, either ethambutol or rifabutin. Ethambutol is preferable because its use is associated with a lower relapse rate. Also, rifabutin interacts with clarithromycin, decreasing clarithromycin levels. In patients who are severely immunocompromised, rifabutin or a fluoroquinolone (levofloxacin or moxifloxacin) may also be used as a third drug.

The U.S. Public Health Service and the Infectious Disease Society of America recommend at least 12 months of therapy. In some patients whose immune status improves with antiretroviral therapy, MAC treatment can be discontinued. However, the experts have not yet determined an exact timeline for discontinuing the anti-MAC drugs, and close follow-up is necessary to prevent relapse.

SPECIAL STRATEGIES TO INCREASE ADHERENCE TO ANTITUBERCULAR DRUG REGIMENS

The complex drug regimens necessary to treat TB require special strategies to assist patients in adhering to their drug treatment plan. The combination of complex drug regimens administered over long periods of time and the risk of transmission of the disease to others if the patient does not adhere to the drug regimen presents the nurse with unique challenges. Strategies for successful drug treatment involve the nurse, the treating primary care provider, the family and friends of the patient, public health departments, and the community as a whole. The nurse has a role in each of the following strategies.

- Supporting the use of short-course regimens, intermittent drug administration, and DOT. Shorter regimens and intermittent drug administration, if possible, make adherence easier for patients. Fixed-dose combinations of drugs are useful; they reduce the number of pills needed. The CDC and other experts strongly recommend DOT to ensure patient adherence. Incentives and enablers also prove useful. These include assistance with transportation to the healthcare provider for follow-up evaluations and tokens or food coupons given to patients each time they appear at the healthcare facility for treatment or follow-up.
- Educating patients, family members, and patient contacts. This may be especially important with treatment of latent TB. Most people are more motivated to take medications and schedule follow-up care when they have symptoms than when they feel well and have no symptoms. It is essential to emphasize the importance of treatment for the future health of the individual person, significant others, and the community. In addition, the patient should receive information about common and potential adverse effects of drug therapy and what to do if they occur.
- Providing support services and resources. These require substantial financial resources and may include more workers to provide DOT at the patient's location, flexible clinic hours, and reduced waiting times and to assist patients with child care, transportation, or other social service needs that encourage them to initiate and continue treatment. Lack of these services (e.g., clinics far from patients' homes, with inconvenient hours, long waiting times, and unsupportive staff) may deter patients from seeking evaluation for a positive skin test, initiating treatment, or completing the prescribed treatment and follow-up care.
- Individualizing treatment regimens. Individualized treatment is necessary whenever possible to increase patient convenience and minimize disruption of usual activities of daily living.
- Promoting communication and continuity of care. With patients for whom English is not their first language, it is desirable to have a healthcare provider who speaks their language or who belongs to their ethnic group. This provider may be able to teach patients more effectively, elicit cooperation with treatment, administer DOT, and be a consistent support person.

NCLEX Success

5. A patient has not adhered to the drug regimen for tuberculosis. Which of the following is most effective to enhance adherence?
   A. explaining the importance of adherence
   B. having the patient's family administer the medication
   C. evaluating serum drug levels to determine adherence
   D. having nursing staff directly watch the patient take the medication

THE NURSING PROCESS

A concept map outlines the nursing process related to drug therapy considerations in this chapter. Additional nursing implications related to the disease process should also be considered in care decisions.

Assessment
- Assess for infections that macrolides and the designated miscellaneous drugs are used to prevent or treat.
- Assess each patient for signs and symptoms of the specific current infection.
- Assess culture and susceptibility reports when available.
- Assess each patient for risk factors that increase risks of infection (e.g., immunosuppression) or risks of adverse drug reactions (e.g., impaired kidney or hepatic function).

Outcomes of Therapy

The patient will
- Take or receive macrolides and miscellaneous antimicrobials accurately, for the prescribed length of time.
- Experience decreased signs and symptoms of the infection being treated.
- Be monitored regularly for therapeutic and adverse drug effects.
- Verbalize and practice measures to prevent recurrent infection.

Nursing Interventions
- Use measures to prevent and minimize the spread of infection (see Chapter 15).
- Monitor for fever and other signs and symptoms of infection.
- Monitor laboratory reports for indications of the patient's response to drug therapy (e.g., white blood cell count, tests of kidney function).
- Encourage fluid intake to decrease fever and maintain good urinary tract function.
- Provide foods and fluids with adequate nutrients to maintain or improve nutritional status, especially if febrile and hypermetabolic.
- Assist patients to prevent or minimize infections with streptococci, staphylococci, and other Gram-positive organisms.
- Provide appropriate patient teaching for any drug therapy (see accompanying display).

Evaluation
- Interview and observe for improvement in the infection being treated.
- Interview and observe for adverse drug effects.

Visit thePoint at http://thePoint.lww.com/Frandsen13e for answers to NCLEX Success questions (in Appendix A), answers to Clinical Application Case Studies (in Appendix B), and more!

REFERENCES AND RESOURCES

Burzynski, J., Mangan, J. M., Lam, C. K., Macaraig, M., Salerno, M. M., deCastro, B. R., Goswami, N. D., Lin, C. Y., Schluger, N. W., Vernon, A.; eDOT Study Team. (2021). In-person vs electronic directly observed therapy for tuberculosis treatment adherence: A randomized noninferiority trial. *JAMA Network Open, 5*(1), e2144210. doi:10.100jamanetworkopen20214-4210

Centers for Disease Control and Prevention. (2021). *Reported tuberculosis in the United States, 2020*. Retrieved August 31, 2022, from https://www.cdc.gov/tb/statistics/reports/2020

Centers for Disease Control and Prevention. (2022). *TB risk factors*. Retrieved September 1, 2022, from https://www.cdc.gov/tb/topic/basics/risk.htm

Currier, J. S. (2022). *Mycobacterium avium* complex (MAC) infections in persons with HIV. *UpToDate*. Retrieved November 10, 2022, from www.uptodate.com./contents/mycobacterim-avium-complex

Drew, R. H., & Sterling, T. R. (2022). Antituberculous drugs: An overview. *UpToDate*. Retrieved September 10, 2022, from www-uptodate-com./contents/antituberculous-drugs-an-overview

Heysell, S. K., & Friedland, G. (2022). Epidemiology of extensively drug-resistant tuberculosis. *UpToDate*. Lexi-Comp, Inc.

Hinkle, J. L., Cheever, K. H., & Overbaugh, K. J. (2021). *Brunner & Suddarth's textbook of medical-surgical nursing* (15th ed.). Wolters Kluwer.

Horsburgh Jr., C. R. (2022). Treatment of latent tuberculosis infection in nonpregnant adults without HIV infection. *UpToDate*. Lexi-Comp, Inc.

Lippincott Advisor. (2022). *Drug information*.

Lardizabal, A. A., & Reichman, L. B. (2022). *Adherence to tuberculosis treatment*. UpToDate.

Norris, T. L. (2019). *Porth's pathophysiology: Concepts of altered health states* (10th ed.). Wolters Kluwer Health/Lippincott Williams & Wilkins.

Schluger, N. W., Heysell, S. K., & Friedland, G. (2022). Treatment of drug-resistant pulmonary tuberculosis in adults. *UpToDate*. Lexi-Comp, Inc.

Sterling, T. R. (2022). Treatment of drug-susceptible pulmonary tuberculosis in nonpregnant adults without HIV infection. *UpToDate*.

UpToDate. (2022). *Drug information*. Lexi-Comp, Inc.

World Health Organization. (2021). *Tuberculosis*. Retrieved July 29, 2022, from http://www.who.int/news-room/fact-sheets/detail/tuberculosis

World Health Organization. (2020). WHO *consolidated guidelines on tuberculosis. Module 4: treatment-drug resistant tuberculosis treatment*.

CHAPTER 23

Drug Therapy for Viral Infections

LEARNING OBJECTIVES

After studying this chapter, you should be able to:

1. Identify the characteristics of viruses and common viral infections.
2. Identify the major clinical manifestations of common viral infections.
3. Identify the action, use, adverse effects, contraindications, and nursing implications for medications administered for the treatment of COVID-19 in hospital and home-based patient care.
4. Identify the prototype and describe the action, use, adverse effects, contraindications, and nursing implications for antiviral agents administered for herpes simplex and varicella–zoster virus.
5. Identify the prototype and describe the action, use, adverse effects, contraindications, and nursing implications for antiviral agents administered for cytomegalovirus.
6. Identify the prototype and describe the action, use, adverse effects, contraindications, and nursing implications of drugs administered for respiratory syncytial virus.
7. Identify the prototypes and describe their action, use, adverse effects, contraindications, and nursing implications of drugs administered for influenza.
8. Identify the prototype and describe the action, use, adverse effects, contraindications, and nursing implications for the nucleoside analog antiviral agents administered for hepatitis.
9. Identify the prototype and describe the action, use, adverse effects, contraindications, and nursing implications for the nucleoside reverse transcriptase inhibitors administered for human immunodeficiency virus (HIV).
10. Identify the prototype and describe the action, use, adverse effects, contraindications, and nursing implications for the nonnucleoside reverse transcriptase inhibitors administered for HIV.
11. Identify the prototype and describe the action, use, adverse effects, contraindications, and nursing implications for the protease inhibitors administered for HIV.
12. Identify the prototype and describe the action, use, adverse effects, contraindications, and nursing implications for the integrase strand transfer inhibitors administered for HIV.
13. Identify the prototype and describe the action, use, adverse effects, contraindications, and nursing implications for fusion protein inhibitors administered for HIV.
14. Identify the prototype and describe the action, use, adverse effects, contraindications, and nursing implications for CCR5 antagonists administered for HIV.
15. Identify the combination medications administered for HIV; describe the action, use, adverse effects, contraindications, and nursing implications.
16. Implement the nursing process in the care of the patient undergoing drug therapy for viral infections.

CLINICAL APPLICATION CASE STUDY

Ann Jackson is 30 years old. She calls her primary healthcare provider's office. She says that she has a cold sore under her nose on the right side. Since childhood, she has had occasional outbreaks of this infection. Her physician orders valacyclovir 2,000 mg orally once daily for 1 day.

KEY TERMS

Antiretroviral drugs: antiviral medications used in the treatment of retroviral infections such as HIV

Antiretroviral therapy (ART): several combinations of antiretroviral drugs used at one time to treat HIV/AIDS

COVID-19: a respiratory disease caused by SARS-CoV-2

Genital herpes: a herpesvirus that appears on the genitals

Hepatitis: liver inflammation due to a virus; five different viruses cause viral hepatitis—hepatitis A, B, C, D, and G

Herpesvirus: any virus belonging to the family of the Herpesviridae

Human immunodeficiency virus (HIV): an infection caused by a retrovirus that infects the immune system, leading to acquired immunodeficiency syndrome (AIDS). There are two types of HIV virus, HIV-1 and HIV-2; most infections in the United States are caused by HIV-1, and infections with HIV-2 occur mainly in Africa

Immunocompetent: having a normal immune response

Retrovirus: virus with an RNA genome that relies on reverse transcriptase to transform its genome from RNA to DNA (e.g., HIV)

Viral load: number of HIV RNA particles in the blood

INTRODUCTION

Viruses cause pneumonia, hepatitis, acquired immunodeficiency syndrome (AIDS), and other disorders that affect most body systems. Many potentially pathogenic viral strains exist, including more than 150 that infect the human respiratory tract. Viral infections vary from mild, localized diseases with few symptoms to severe systemic illnesses and death. Antiviral agents that possess a narrow spectrum of effect on the viral process have the ability to target the invading virus. Drug therapy for the treatment of viral infections is discussed. In addition, the antiretroviral agents used to treat HIV/AIDS are described in this chapter. Box 23.1 provides specific information about selected viruses and viral infections. For more details on the etiology and pathophysiology of viruses and viral infections, visit thePoint® at http://thePoint.lww.com/Frandsen13e.

OVERVIEW OF VIRUSES AND VIRAL INFECTIONS

Viruses, the infectious agents that cause viral infections, are intracellular parasites that gain entry to human host cells by binding to receptors on cell membranes. Methods of spread of viral infections include secretions from infected people, ingestion of contaminated food or water, breaks in the skin or mucous membranes, sexual contact, pregnancy, breast-feeding, and organ transplantation. Viruses replicate in the host with the use of metabolic processes.

Viruses induce antibodies and immunity. Antibodies are proteins that defend against microbial or viral invasion. Antibodies against infecting viruses can prevent the viruses from reaching the bloodstream or, if they are already in the bloodstream, prevent their invasion of host cells. Most adults possess immunity to some viral diseases because they have become infected earlier in their lives. However, patients who are immunocompromised have impaired or weakened immune systems and may develop the infection because of decreased immunity.

Clinical Manifestations of Viral Infections

Viral infection may occur without signs and symptoms of illness. If illness does occur, the clinical course is usually short and self-limited. Recovery occurs as the virus is eliminated from the body. Some viruses (e.g., herpesvirus) can survive in host cells for many years and cause a chronic, latent infection that periodically becomes reactivated. Also, autoimmune diseases may be caused by viral alteration of host cells so that lymphocytes recognize the host's own tissues as being foreign.

Symptoms usually associated with acute viral infections include fever, headache, cough, malaise, muscle pain, nausea and vomiting, diarrhea, insomnia, and photophobia. White blood cell counts usually remain normal. Other signs and symptoms vary with the type of virus and body organs involved.

Drug Therapy

Scientists have developed several vaccines (see Chapter 12) to prevent viral infections as well as numerous drugs to treat COVID-19, HIV, and other viral infections. Most of these antiviral drugs inhibit viral reproduction but do not eliminate viruses from tissues. In general, available drugs are expensive, relatively toxic, and effective in a limited number of infections. Some may be useful in treating an established infection if given promptly and in chemoprophylaxis if given before or soon after exposure. Protection conferred by chemoprophylaxis is immediate but lasts only while the drug is being taken. The remainder of this chapter describes the subgroups of antiviral drugs. Table 23.1 summarizes the medications used to treat viral infections.

BOX 23.1 Selected Viral Infections

Avian Influenza

Influenza A is most responsible for annual outbreaks of epidemics with varying intensity that can result in occasional pandemics. Influenza B commonly causes outbreaks every 2 to 4 years. Human influenza H1 and H3 subtypes circulate continuously. In recent years, the highly pathogenic H5N1 subtype of influenza A has been found in numerous countries. It occurs mainly in birds and poultry, but a few hundred human cases have been confirmed. Most human cases occur after exposure to infected poultry or surfaces contaminated with poultry droppings. Because human infection may cause respiratory failure and has a high mortality rate, the possibility that these viral strains might mutate so that they infect humans more easily is a major public health concern. This virus is considered the most likely cause of a future worldwide influenza epidemic. Other strains of influenza have been identified. They include H5N6, H9N2, H7, H7N9, H6N1, H10N8, and H10N7. The migration of birds has the potential to carry pathogens leading to public health hazards.

Coronaviruses

Coronaviruses can cause one third of community-acquired upper respiratory tract infections in children and adults. The viruses may cause diarrhea in infants and children. These viral infections are classified as a family within the Nidovirales order. The viruses replicate using a set of messenger RNAs. There are four generations: alpha, beta, gamma, and delta.

Severe Acute Respiratory Syndrome (SARS)

In 2003, the world experienced an outbreak of severe acute respiratory syndrome or SARS, the clinical manifestations of which included fever, lower respiratory track illnesses with cough and shortness of breath, and lung infiltrates. Some patients developed acute respiratory distress syndrome. Older adults with chronic disease possessed a potential for poor prognosis.

The treatment regimen for SARS was supportive care to assist with pulmonary instability, high-dose glucocorticoids, and ribavirin. Antiretroviral agents lopinavir and ritonavir were administered. Remdesivir was an experimental antiretroviral agent that has activity against SARS.

COVID-19

In 2019, Wuhan, a city in the Hubei Province of China, saw an outbreak of pneumonia cases. By February 2020, the outbreak spread globally and was designated as COVID-19 by the World Health Organization (WHO). Many variants and subvariants of COVID-19 have been identified since the onset of the pandemic. Similar to that of influenzae, the spread of COVID-19 occurs through direct contact with infected secretions or large airborne droplets, though COVID-19 is more easily transmitted than influenza viruses. Symptoms appear in 2 to 14 days following exposure, with a median time of 4 to 5 days from exposure with the development of symptoms. After the onset of symptoms, the viral RNA levels are elevated; thus, it is thought that viral transmission is more likely early in the viral disease. The following comorbid conditions increase the severity of the illness: cardiovascular disease, diabetes mellitus, hypertension, chronic lung disease, and chronic kidney disease. Additional risk factors include BMI of 30.0 or higher and liver disease. Older persons are also at greater risk for severe disease and death.

The clinical manifestations of COVID-19 include fever, fatigue, dry cough, anorexia, myalgia, dyspnea, and increased sputum production. COVID-19 testing is completed with a swab to test for SARS-CoV-2. A nasopharyngeal swab is used to collect secretions from deep within the upper respiratory tract. If the patient has a productive cough, an oropharyngeal swab should be used to collect sputum. If the patient is on mechanical ventilation, the patient should be tested by aspirating secretions from the lower respiratory tract.

Home care for patients with nonsevere infections includes antipyretics, analgesics, and adequate hydration. Good hand hygiene and disinfection of frequently touched surfaces is recommended. Also, the patient should wear a mask and isolate from other individuals in the home. The patient should quarantine for 5 days. Isolation can end after 5 days if the patient is fever free without the use of fever-reducing medications. Immunocompromised patients diagnosed with COVID-19 should isolate for 10 days and consult with their primary care provider before ending isolation. For patients with up-to-date COVID-19 vaccinations, quarantine is not necessary unless the onset of symptoms is noted. The patient should watch for symptoms for 10 days; if symptoms develop, the patient should get tested and isolate at home wearing a well-fitting mask.

Herpesvirus Infections

Cytomegalovirus Infection and Retinitis

Cytomegalovirus (CMV) infection is common, and most people become infected by adulthood. Infection is usually asymptomatic in healthy, **immunocompetent** adults. Like other **herpesviruses**, CMV can cause a primary infection and then remain latent in body tissues, probably for life. This means that the virus can be shed in secretions of an asymptomatic host and spread to others by contact with infected saliva, blood, urine, semen, breast milk, and cervical secretions. It also means that the virus may lead to an opportunistic infection when the host becomes immunosuppressed. During pregnancy, CMV is transmitted to the fetus across the placenta and may cause infection in the brain, inner ears, eyes, liver, and bone marrow. Learning and cognitive disabilities can result from congenital CMV infection. Children spread the virus to each other in saliva or urine, whereas adolescents and adults transmit the virus mainly through sexual contact.

Major populations at risk for development of active CMV infection are patients with cancer, who receive immunosuppressant drugs, and organ transplant recipients, who must receive immunosuppressant drugs to prevent their body's rejection of the transplanted organ. Patients with advanced HIV infection are also at risk, but the incidence has decreased with active **antiretroviral therapy** or ART.

Common manifestations of disease include pneumonitis, hepatitis, encephalitis, adrenal insufficiency, cellular necrosis and inflammation in various body tissues, gastrointestinal inflammation, and gastric ulcerations. In the eye, CMV infection produces retinitis, usually characterized by blurred vision and decreased visual acuity. Visual impairment is progressive and irreversible and, if untreated, may result in blindness. CMV retinitis may also indicate systemic CMV infection or may be entirely asymptomatic.

BOX 23.1 Selected Viral Infections (Continued)

Genital Herpes Infection

Genital herpes infection is caused by the herpes simplex virus (HSV) and produces recurrent, painful, blisterlike lesions on skin and mucous membranes. HSV is usually transmitted through direct contact with open lesions or secretions, including genital secretions. Primary infection occurs at a site of viral entry, where the virus infects epithelial cells, produces progeny viruses, and eventually causes cell death. After primary infection, latent virus may become dormant within sensory nerve cells. In response to various stimuli (e.g., intense sunlight, emotional stress, febrile illness, menstruation), latent virus may become reactivated and lead to viral reproduction and shedding.

In the fetus, HSV may be transmitted from an infected birth canal, and neonatal herpes is a serious complication of maternal genital herpes. Neonatal herpes usually becomes evident within the first week of life and may be manifested by the typical clusters of blisterlike lesions on skin or mucous membranes. Irritability, lethargy, jaundice, altered blood clotting, respiratory distress, seizures, or coma may also occur. Neonatal herpes carries a high mortality rate. In immunosuppressed patients, HSV infection may result in severe, systemic disease.

Herpes Zoster

Herpes zoster is caused by the highly contagious worldwide varicella–zoster virus. Most children in the United States are infected by early school age. The virus produces chickenpox on first exposure and is spread from person to person by the respiratory route or by contact with secretions from skin lesions. Recovery from the primary infection leaves latent infection in nerve cells. Reactivation of the latent infection (usually later in life) causes herpes zoster (more commonly known as "shingles"), a localized cluster of painful, blisterlike skin lesions. Over several days, the vesicles become pustules and then rupture and heal. Because the virus remains in sensory nerve cells, pain can persist for months after the skin lesions heal. Most cases of herpes zoster infection occur among older adult and immunocompromised patients. (vaccines to prevent herpes zoster are discussed in Chapter 12)

Human Immunodeficiency Virus Infection

Human immunodeficiency virus (HIV) infection is caused by a **retrovirus** that infects the immune system. Two types of HIV virus have been identified: HIV-1 and HIV-2. Most infections in the United States are caused by HIV-1; HIV-2 infections occur mainly in Africa. HIV binds to receptors on the surface of CD4+ cells (especially T lymphocytes or helper T cells). HIV entry and replication eventually results in cell death. Because CD4+ cells play major roles in regulating immune function, their destruction results in serious impairment of the immune system.

The initial phase of HIV infection is characterized by influenzalike symptoms (e.g., fever, chills, muscle aches) that may last several weeks. During this time, the virus undergoes rapid replication. The next phase is characterized by a dramatic decline in the rate of viral replication, attributed to a partially effective immune response. During this phase, no visible manifestations of HIV infection may be present. However, replication of HIV continues and antibodies may be detected in the serum. During this period, the person is seropositive (HIV+) and infectious but asymptomatic. Eventually, the immune system is substantially damaged and the rate of viral reproduction accelerates. The **viral load** is the number of HIV RNA particle in the blood. When viral load and immunodeficiency reach significant levels, the illness is termed acquired human immunodeficiency syndrome (AIDS) and serious opportunistic infections occur. With effective drug therapy, viral load decreases and the CD4+ cell count increases, so that HIV-infected people may live for many years without progression to AIDS.

HIV infection occurs in all age groups and can spread to a new host during any phase of infection. The virus is commonly spread by sexual intercourse, injection of intravenous drugs with contaminated needles, and mucous membrane contact with infected blood or body fluids and perinatally from mother to fetus. The virus is not spread through casual contact. Healthcare workers may be infected by needlestick injuries. They should be aware that postexposure prophylaxis is available and may significantly reduce the risk of transmission.

Respiratory Syncytial Virus Infection

Respiratory syncytial virus (RSV) is a highly contagious virus that is present worldwide and infects most children by school age. Epidemics of RSV infection often occur in nurseries, day care centers, and pediatric hospital units during winter months. RSV infects and destroys respiratory epithelium in the bronchi, bronchioles, and alveoli. It is spread by respiratory droplets and secretions, direct contact with an infected person, and contact with fomites, including the hands of caregivers.

RSV is the most common cause of bronchiolitis and pneumonia in infants and causes severe illness in those younger than 6 months of age. These infants usually have wheezing, cough, respiratory distress, and fever. The infection is usually self-limited and resolves in 1 to 2 weeks. Antiviral therapy with ribavirin is used in some cases. The mortality rate from RSV infection is low in children who are generally healthy but increases substantially in those with congenital heart disease or immunosuppression. In older children, RSV infection produces much milder disease but may be associated with acute exacerbations of asthma.

In adults, RSV infection causes colds and bronchitis, with symptoms of fever, cough, and nasal congestion. Infection occurs most often in those in close contact with children, including pediatric healthcare workers. In older adults, RSV infection may cause pneumonia requiring hospitalization. In immunocompromised patients, RSV infection may cause severe and potentially fatal pneumonia.

Viral Hepatitis

Viral hepatitis is characterized as an inflammation of the liver. There are several types of viral **hepatitis**, and new hepatitis viruses are still being identified. Worldwide, viral hepatitis has increased in recent years. All hepatitis viruses have similar effects on the liver, although they differ in some other characteristics. Vaccines are available to prevent hepatitis A and B (see Chapter 12).

Hepatitis A virus (HAV) is transmitted mainly by the fecal–oral route and close contact with an infected person; foodborne outbreaks also occur, usually from infected food handlers or contaminated produce in the United States. The virus survives for long periods in the environment (e.g., in water and soil) and on human hands and inanimate objects. It resists freezing, detergents, and acids but can be inactivated by chlorine and temperatures above 185°F.

(Continued on page 408)

BOX 23.1 Selected Viral Infections (Continued)

Hepatitis A

The HAV reproduces only in liver and gastrointestinal cells, from which viral particles are released into blood and bile. The average incubation period is 25 to 30 days. The patient is infectious during the incubation period and for 7 to 10 days after symptoms develop. In infected adults, about 70% develop symptoms, including fever and jaundice, that may last as long as 2 months. Most recover without treatment and develop immunity against future HAV infections; 10% to 20% require hospitalization. In children, many are asymptomatic or develop flulike or nonspecific symptoms without jaundice. However, even children with few or no symptoms may shed virus in their stools and be a source of community infection for as long as 6 months. The availability of hepatitis A vaccine has greatly decreased the number of reported cases. The vaccine is recommended for children and adults at increased risk of contracting the disease (e.g., travelers to certain countries, men who have sex with men, intravenous drug users, recipients of clotting factor replacement) and for persons with chronic liver disease.

Hepatitis B

Hepatitis B virus (HBV) can be transmitted by contact with contaminated blood and other body fluids (e.g., perinatally, during sexual contact with an infected person, by sharing needles during IV drug use, and by undergoing acupuncture, hemodialysis, tattooing, or ear and body piercing). The HBV can live up to 3 days on various surfaces that appear clean. The incubation period is 30 to 180 days. Increased hepatitis B surface antigens and liver enzymes (ALT, AST) occur before symptoms of HBV infection develop. After symptoms develop, antibodies to the viral antigens are produced and the presence of antigens and viral DNA in the patient's blood indicate that the patient is infectious.

Healthcare and public safety workers are at increased risk of developing HBV infection from injuries with contaminated equipment (e.g., contaminated needles) and from other exposures to infected body fluid. Any person exposed to infected body fluids should be evaluated for HBV infection; any person diagnosed with HBV infection should be evaluated for liver disease and for HIV infection. It is estimated that 70,000 Americans become infected with HBV every year and approximately 5,000 of them will die of the complications caused by the infection. Many Americans have chronic HBV infection; asymptomatic chronic carriers of HBV may transmit the infection to others. Hepatitis B can lead to cirrhosis, liver cancer, liver failure, and death.

Hepatitis C

Hepatitis C virus (HCV) can be transmitted by contact with contaminated blood or other body fluids. Persons at high risk of exposure include healthcare and public safety workers; IV drug users; those with multiple sex partners; those undergoing hemodialysis, tattoos, or body piercings; and those who received blood transfusions before 1990, when screening blood for HCV was started. In addition, the virus may be transmitted to infants during pregnancy and lactation.

The HCV incubation period is 14 to 80 days; infection is diagnosed by testing for viral DNA or antibodies. HCV infection affects people of all ages but is most often found among 20- to 39-year-olds. Infected persons can be asymptomatic for years, but most eventually develop chronic liver disease. In the United States, HCV infection is the leading cause of cirrhosis, liver cancer, and liver transplants. Effective drug therapy may cure HCV infection.

TABLE 23.1

Drugs Administered for the Treatment of Viral Infections

Drug Class/Type	Prototype	Other Drugs in the Class/Related Drugs
Drugs for Acute Severe Respiratory Syndrome Coronavirus 2 (SARS-CoV-2)		
		Remdesivir (Veklury) Tocilizumab (Actemra) Baricitinib (Olumiant)
Drug Therapy for Outpatient Management of Coronavirus 2 (SARS-CoV-2)		
		Nirmatrelvir and ritonavir
Drugs for Herpesvirus Infections		
Drugs for herpes simplex virus and varicella–zoster virus	Acyclovir (Zovirax)	Docosanol (Abreva) Famciclovir Penciclovir (Denavir) Trifluridine Valacyclovir (Valtrex)
Drugs for cytomegalovirus	Ganciclovir (Cytovene)	Cidofovir Foscarnet (Foscavir) Valganciclovir (Valcyte)
Drugs for Respiratory Syncytial Virus		
Antiviral agent	Ribavirin (Virazole)	
Monoclonal antibody	Palivizumab (Synagis)	

TABLE 23.1

Drugs Administered for the Treatment of Viral Infections (Continued)

Drug Class/Type	Prototype	Other Drugs in the Class/Related Drugs
Drugs for Influenza		
Adamantanes	Amantadine hydrochloride (Gocovri, Osmolex ER)	Rimantadine
Endonuclease inhibitor	Baloxavir marboxil (Xofluza)	Peramivir (Rapivab) Zanamivir (Relenza)
Drugs for Hepatitis B: Nucleoside Analogs		
	Lamivudine (Epivir, Epivir-HBV)	Adefovir dipivoxil (Hepsera) Entecavir (Baraclude) Ribavirin Tenofovir alafenamide (Vemlidy) Tenofovir disoproxil fumarate (Viread)
Drugs for Hepatitis C: Polymerase Inhibitors		
	Sofosbuvir (Sovaldi)	
Drugs for Hepatitis C: Antihepaciviral, Nucleoside		
	Ribavirin	
Antiretroviral Drugs		
Nucleoside/nucleotide reverse transcriptase inhibitors (NRTIs)	Zidovudine (Retrovir)	Abacavir sulfate (Ziagen) Abacavir, lamivudine, and zidovudine (Trizivir) Didanosine Dolutegravir and lamivudine (Dovato) Dolutegravir, abacavir, and lamivudine (Triumeq) Elvitegravir, cobicistat, emtricitabine, and tenofovir disoproxil fumarate (Stribild) Emtricitabine (Emtriva) Emtricitabine and tenofovir (Truvada) Emtricitabine, tenofovir, efavirenz (Atripla) Lamivudine (Epivir, Epivir-HBV) Stavudine Tenofovir disoproxil fumarate (Viread) Zidovudine and lamivudine (Combivir)
Nonnucleoside/nonnucleotide reverse transcriptase inhibitors (NNRTIs)	Efavirenz (Sustiva)	Delavirdine mesylate Etravirine (Intelence) Nevirapine (Viramune) Rilpivirine (Edurant)
Protease inhibitors (PIs)	Saquinavir mesylate (Invirase)	Atazanavir (Reyataz) Darunavir (Prezista) Fosamprenavir calcium (Lexiva) Indinavir sulfate (Crixivan) Lopinavir/ritonavir (Kaletra) Nelfinavir mesylate (Viracept) Ritonavir (Norvir) Tipranavir (Aptivus)
Integrase strand transfer inhibitors (INSTIs)	Raltegravir (Isentress, Isentress HD)	Dolutegravir (Tivicay)
Fusion protein inhibitors	Enfuvirtide (Fuzeon)	
CCR5 antagonists	Maraviroc (Selzentry)	
P450 inhibitor	Cobicistat (Tybost)	
Integrase inhibitor, reverse transcriptase inhibitor, nucleoside, reverse transcriptase inhibitor, nucleotide	ⓟ Bictegravir, emtricitabine, and tenofovir alafenamide (Biktarvy)	

DRUGS FOR COVID-19

COVID-19 is a respiratory disease caused by SARS-CoV-2. The virus spreads from person to person through respiratory droplets produced when an infected person talks, sneezes, or coughs. The viral infection can result in acute severe respiratory syndrome. The management of COVID-19's variants and subvariants is constantly evolving based on continued research. The discussion of medications used for the treatment of COVID-19 will not address the prototypes but instead will be presented with the specific medications used in the treatment of the viral illness caused by COVID-19.

In this section, the drug therapy discussed is based on treatment for hospitalized and home-based patient care. Patients who are admitted to the acute care facility and placed on oxygen are treated with medications that are identified in Figure 23.1: dexamethasone, remdesivir, tocilizumab, and baricitinib. These medications represent the steroid, antiretroviral, and immunomodulator drug classes. Each will be discussed here in regard to their action and use in the treatment of COVID-19. Dexamethasone is also discussed in Chapter 17. Tocilizumab and baricitinib are also discussed in Chapter 13. COVID-19 patients in the acute viral stage may be at risk for the development of thrombosis. The administration of anticoagulants may be prescribed.

UpToDate (2022a, 2022b) recommends early treatment with nirmatrelvir–ritonavir or sotrovimab (Chapter 13) for unvaccinated individuals or those with inadequate vaccine response. This population is at great risk for the development of severe disease. The care of all patients is based on symptom management. For patients experiencing a cough, over-the-counter cough suppressants such as benzonatate, guaifenesin, or dextromethorphan are available (Chapter 31). Metered-dose inhaled bronchodilators or glucocorticoids are commonly prescribed (Chapter 33). Chest pain related to acute COVID-19 can be treated with ibuprofen 400 to 600 mg orally every 8 hours as needed for 1 to 2 weeks. See Figure 23.1 for the selection of COVID-19–specific therapy. See Tables 23.1 and 23.2 for the specific medications and guidelines for dosages.

> **Quality and Safety Alert: Safety**
>
> Nebulizer treatments should not be used due to the risk of SARS-CoV-2 droplets expelled into the air placing others at risk for COVID-19 viral infection.

Drug Therapy for Acute Severe Respiratory Syndrome Coronavirus 2 (SARS-CoV-2)

As stated previously, the medications administered for this COVID-19 condition are dexamethasone, remdesivir, tocilizumab, and baricitinib. Remdesivir, tocilizumab, and baricitinib

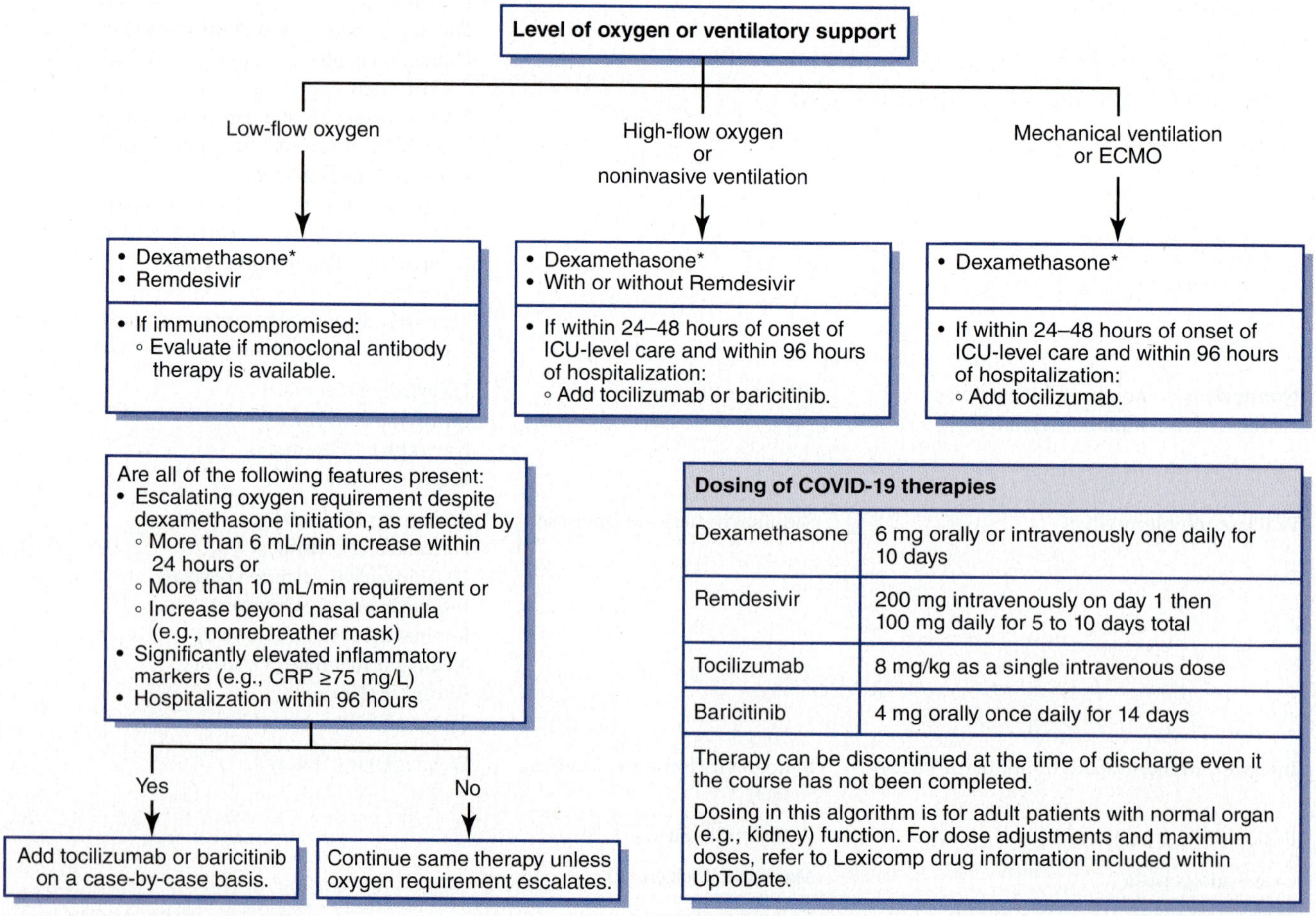

Figure 23.1. This algorithm covers the approach to COVID-19 therapy for patients requiring oxygen. (Reproduced with permission from: Anesi, G. L. COVID-19: Management of the intubated adult. In UpToDate, Post, T. W. (Eds.), *UpToDate*, Waltham, MA. Retrieved January 24, 2023. Copyright © 2023 UpToDate, Inc. and its affiliates and/or licensors. All rights reserved.)

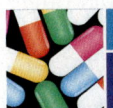

TABLE 23.2

DRUGS AT A GLANCE: Drugs for Acute Severe Respiratory Syndrome and Outpatient Management of Coronavirus 2 (SARS-CoV-2)

Drug	Route and Dosage Ranges
Remdesivir (Veklury; 🍁 Veklury)	Hospitalized patients: 200 mg IV as a single dose on day 1, followed by 100 mg once daily for 5 days or until hospital discharge; may extend to up to 10 days in certain patients (if no substantial improvement by day 5, on mechanical ventilation or extracorporeal membrane oxygenation). Initiate as soon as possible after the diagnosis of COVID-19; ideally within 72 hours of a positive SARS-CoV-2 test
Tocilizumab (Actemra; 🍁 Actemra)	8 mg/kg (patients >30 kg) or 12 mg/kg (patients <30 kg) IV as a single dose (maximum 800 mg/dose, in combination with glucocorticoids; if clinical improvement does not occur, a second dose may be given ≥8 hours after the first dose). Use remdesivir in combination with dexamethasone Use for COVID-19 is not recommended in the outpatient setting Nonhospitalized patients with rheumatoid arthritis: 200 mg IV as a single dose on day 1; followed by 100 mg once daily on days 2 and 3; initiate as soon as possible and within 7 days of symptom onset
Baricitinib (Olumiant; 🍁 Olumiant)	4 mg PO once daily in combination with remdesivir and/or corticosteroids COVID-19 with kidney impairment eGFR ≥ 60 mL/min 1.73 m²: no dosage adjustment eGFR > 30 to <60 mL/min 1.73 m²: 2 mg once daily eGFR 15 to <30 mL/min 1.73 m²: 1 mg once daily eGFR, 15 mL/min 1.73 m²: use is not recommended
Drug Therapy for Outpatient Management of Coronavirus 2 (SARS-CoV-2)	
Nirmatrelvir and Ritonavir (Paxlovid; 🍁 Paxlovid)	Nirmatrelvir 300 mg with ritonavir 100 mg PO, administered together, twice daily for 5 days eGFR ≥ 30 to <60 mL/min nirmatrelvir and ritonavir 100 mg twice daily eGFR < 30 mL/min: use is not recommended

will be discussed in detail. Dexamethasone is reviewed in Chapter 13; the therapeutic effects of the use of dexamethasone for COVID-19 will be discussed here.

Remdesivir

Remdesivir is a nucleotide analog that is active against severe acute respiratory syndrome coronavirus 2. It has been shown to reduce the risk of COVID-19–associated hospitalization.

Pharmacokinetics

Remdesivir is 88% to 93.6% protein bound with a half-life of 1 hour. It is eliminated in the urine and feces.

Action and Use

In SARS-CoV-2 RNA, dependent RNA polymerase is required for viral replication. Remdesivir inhibits this viral replication. Remdesivir triphosphate acts as an adenosine triphosphate analogue and competes for the SARS-CoV-2 RNA chains, resulting in RNA chain termination during the viral RNA replication.

Remdesivir is used for adult and pediatric patients 12 years and older who weigh 40 kg or greater, have laboratory-confirmed COVID-19, have mild to moderate symptoms, and are at high risk for progression to severe COVID-19.

Patient-related variables specific to the use of remdesivir include the following:

- Age:
  - Remdesivir is approved for administration in adult and pediatric patients aged 12 years and older with a body weight of 40 kg or higher.
- Reproduction, pregnancy, and lactation:
  - Studies have shown that pregnant and postpartum patients treated with remdesivir recovered in 28 days. The adverse effects were the same as for nonpregnant patients.
  - Remdesivir and the GS-441524 metabolite have been detected in breast milk.
  - According to the manufacturer, the decision to breast-feed while taking remdesivir should take the risk of exposure to the infant into consideration. The infant should be protected from exposure to SARS-CoV-2. The patient should consider expressing breast milk and the baby being fed by another individual.
- Abnormal kidney function and hepatic impairment:
  - There are no dosage adjustments in abnormal kidney function or hepatic impairment.
- Specific healthcare environments:
  - Nonhospitalized and hospitalized patients should be administered remdesivir in a healthcare facility. The patient should be monitored for signs and symptoms of infusion reaction.

Adverse Effects and Contraindications

Severe bradycardia and sinus bradycardia have been reported in patients receiving remdesivir. Hypersensitivity and infusion reactions include angioedema, bradycardia, dyspnea, fever, hypertension, hypotension, hypoxia, nausea, rash, tachycardia, and wheezing. Mild to moderate elevations in serum ALT and AST have been noted, but it is unknown if this is related to remdesivir or SARS-CoV-2.

The only contraindication to remdesivir is hypersensitivity to the drug.

Nursing Implications

Preventing Interactions

Any medication that is a CYP3A inducer may decrease the serum concentration of remdesivir. Medications identified that decreased levels of remdesivir include metamizole, rifabutin, rifapentine, carbamazepine, phenytoin, and primidone. Chloroquine and hydroxychloroquine decrease the effect of remdesivir, and the combination must be avoided. St. John's wort also decreases levels of remdesivir.

Administering the Medication

Remdesivir is only administered with normal saline. No other drugs or solution should be administered concurrently. Due to the irritating effect of the medication, the parenteral administration of remdesivir should be done over 30 to 120 minutes. It is important to assess the IV access. Remdesivir is an irritant and will cause tissue damage; thus, extravasation should be avoided.

> **Quality and Safety Alert: Safety**
>
> There are two formulations of IV remdesivir. The concentrated solution of remdesivir should be used only in adults and pediatric patients ≥12 years of age and weighing ≥40 kg. The Institute for Safe Medication Practices reports numerous medication errors related to the two formulations.

Assessing for Therapeutic Effects

It is important to assess the patient's pulmonary status when administering remdesivir. Within 5 days, patients administered remdesivir should have an increase in pulmonary outcomes, resulting in a decreased need for mechanical ventilation. The patient should have a decrease in dyspnea and improved lung function.

Assessing for Adverse Effects

The patient should be observed throughout the administration and 1 hour following the administration of remdesivir for signs and symptoms of infusion reaction and hypersensitivity. The patient's cardiac status should be assessed frequently throughout the infusion for signs and symptoms of bradycardia or tachycardia. In addition, the patient's blood pressure should be assessed due to the risk of hypotension. The nurse should also assess ALT and AST levels and report any elevation to the prescriber. In addition, the creatinine clearance should be monitored and any decrease in creatinine clearance should be reported to the prescriber.

> **BOX 23.2 Patient Teaching Guidelines for Antiviral Drugs**
>
> - Prevention is better than treatment, partly because medications used to treat viral infections may cause serious adverse effects. Thus, whenever possible, it is important to use techniques to prevent viral infections, such as limiting exposure with those infected with a viral illness.
> - Wash hands thoroughly for 20 seconds and do so frequently; this helps prevent most infections.
> - Do not touch your face.
> - Have immunizations against viral infections as indicated.
> - With genital herpes, avoid sexual intercourse when visible lesions are present and always wash hands after touching any lesion.
> - Understand that drugs may relieve symptoms but do not cure viral infections. For example, treatment of genital herpes does not prevent transmission to others, and treatment of cytomegalovirus (CMV) retinitis may not prevent disease progression.
> - Ask a healthcare provider for information about managing adverse drug effects.
> - If taking foscarnet or ganciclovir for CMV retinitis, have eye examinations approximately every 6 weeks.
> - If taking ganciclovir, maintain regular appointments for the assessment of the complete blood count and kidney function.
> - Administer antiviral agents for recurrent genital herpes lesions as soon as signs and symptoms begin.
> - Use gloves to apply topical antiviral ointment to lesions.

Patient Teaching

Box 23.2 identifies the patient teaching guidelines for antiviral drugs.

> **Quality and Safety Alert: Evidence-Based Practice**
>
> Tocilizumab is used for treating cytokine release syndrome, a highly fatal syndrome, in patients diagnosed with COVID-19. Kaya and Kavak (2021) conducted a retrospective study of 308 patients diagnosed with COVID-19 who were treated with tocilizumab. The median age of the patients in the study was 60 years. Seventy-five percent were male and 56.8% were female. Each patient had at least one comorbidity. Based on this and other studies, tocilizumab has been shown to be effective in treating COVID-19 in patients who are at risk for developing cytokine release syndrome.

Tocilizumab

Tocilizumab, sarilumab, or rituximab can be administered to patients with COVID-19 with markedly elevated inflammatory markers. The inflammatory markers are D-dimer, ferritin, and proinflammatory cytokines including interleukin (IL-6). These markers are associated with critical and fatal COVID-19. The use of tocilizumab, sarilumab, or rituximab blocks the inflammatory pathway and may prevent disease progression. In 2021, the FDA issued an emergency use authorization for tocilizumab for the treatment of hospitalized adults and pediatric patients aged 2 years and older with COVID-19 who are receiving systemic corticosteroids and require supplemental oxygen or extracorporeal membrane oxygenation (ECMO). Tocilizumab is not approved for outpatient use.

Pharmacokinetics

Tocilizumab has an onset of action of 4 hours with a volume of distribution of 8.75 L. The half-life is 11 to 13 days. The bioavailability is 95%. The patient may experience fever and hypotension a few hours after administration.

Action and Use

Tocilizumab is an antagonist of interleukin-6 receptor to decrease the inflammatory response of endogenous interleukin-6. This antagonistic effect leads to a reduction in cytokine and acute phase reactant production.

The labeled use of tocilizumab is severe cytokine release syndrome, giant cell arteritis, rheumatoid arthritis, and systemic sclerosis-associated interstitial lung disease. The use in COVID-19 is unlabeled by the FDA.

Patient-related variables specific to the use of tocilizumab include the following:

- Age:
  - Tocilizumab is administered to patients aged 2 years and older for COVID-19 in combination with dexamethasone.
- Reproduction, pregnancy, and lactation:
  - Tocilizumab may be considered for use in patients with rheumatic and musculoskeletal diseases who are planning to conceive.
  - Tocilizumab crosses the placenta. The lowest exposure to the fetus is the period of organogenesis. The greatest risk of exposure is in the third trimester.

Adverse Effects and Contraindications

The reported adverse effects are hypercholesterolemia, constipation, neutropenia, increased ALT and AST, and infusion reaction. Angioedema has been reported with infusion. Stevens-Johnson syndrome, constipation, diverticulitis, hepatic failure, and various infections have been reported in postmarketing of the drug.

The only reported contraindication of tocilizumab is hypersensitivity to the drug.

Nursing Implications

Preventing Interactions

Tocilizumab should be used cautiously in patients with diverticulitis, who are at risk for GI perforation. The FDA has issued a **BOXED WARNING** ◆ related to the development of potentially fatal infections. Patients have been reported to develop tuberculosis or the reactivation of latent tuberculosis. Some patients who test negative prior to therapy may develop active infection.

Administering the Medication

The diluted infusion solution should be at room temperature prior to the administration of the medication. The IV solution should be infused over 60 minutes utilizing a dedicated IV line. No other medications should be infused in the line. Tocilizumab should never be infused as an IV push or IV bolus. Assess the patient for infusion reaction.

Assessing for Therapeutic Effects

The assessment of pulmonary function should include chest x-rays and testing of pulmonary function. The outcome of care is an improvement in pulmonary function and diminished inflammation.

Assessing for Adverse Effects

Assessing for adverse effects includes monitoring HDL, AST, and ALT levels; assessing the patient for constipation and abdominal pain due to the risk of GI perforation; and assessing for infusion reaction, hypertension, and fever.

Patient Teaching

Tocilizumab is an interleukin-6 receptor inhibitor. It is not an antiviral or antiretroviral agent. Thus, the important patient teaching information will be in Chapter 13. Patient teaching interventions related to tocilizumab being used for COVID-19 include good hand hygiene to protect from infections. The patient should report any signs of abdominal pain.

Baricitinib (Olumiant)

In July 2021, baricitinib was issued emergency use authorization from the FDA for the treatment of COVID-19 in hospitalized patients aged 2 years and older. It no longer requires administration with remdesivir.

Pharmacokinetics

Baricitinib has a volume of distribution of 76 L. It is 50% plasma protein bound and 45% serum protein bound. The drug is metabolized in the liver by CYP3A4. The peak of action is 1 hour. The half-life is approximately 10 hours. Excretion in the urine is 75% and 20% in the feces. Approximately 15% of the drug remains unchanged.

Action and Use

The intracellular Janus kinase (JAK) enzymes are inhibited by baricitinib. The action of baricitinib's inhibition of JAK enzymes reduces the following serum immunoglobulins; IgG, IgM, IgA, and C-reactive protein. Baricitinib has an unlabeled use for the treatment of COVID-19 in hospitalized patients. The labeled use is treatment of rheumatoid arthritis.

Patient-related variables specific to the use of baricitinib include the following:

- Age:
  - The FDA recommends (2021) administering remdesivir in combination with baricitinib for children aged 2 to less than 9 years. It is also recommended in combination with remdesivir in adolescents. The duration of administration is 14 days.
- Reproduction, pregnancy, and lactation:
  - Use in pregnant patients with COVID-19 may be considered when the benefit for the improvement of COVID-19–related symptoms outweighs the risk to the fetus.

- It is unknown if baricitinib is present in breast milk, and breast-feeding is not recommended.
- Abnormal kidney function and hepatic impairment:
  - Adjust dosage with abnormal kidney function. Do not administer with eGFR less than 30 mL/minute/1.73 m².
  - Do not administer with severe hepatic impairment.

Adverse Effects and Contraindications

The FDA has reported that serious venous thrombosis, pulmonary embolism, and serious infections have been observed in COVID-19 patients treated with baricitinib.

Baricitinib is contraindicated with the administration of live vaccines.

Nursing Implications
Preventing Interactions

Myelosuppressive agents may decrease the therapeutic effects of baricitinib. Immunosuppressive agents may enhance the immunosuppressive effect of baricitinib. Patients receiving the COVID-19 vaccine less than 14 days before initiating drug therapy will need to be revaccinated at 2 to 3 months after therapy is completed.

Administering the Medication

Baricitinib may be administered with or without food. The tablets may be chewed or dispersed in a small amount of liquid. The container should be rinsed, and any residual medication should be administered to the patient. The administration of baricitinib through a gastronomy tube (G-tube) involves placing the tablets in water to disperse; ensure that the tablets can pass through the G-tube. For NG tube feeding, place the number of prescribed tablets in 30 mL of room temperature water and swirl the water to disperse the medication adequately; administer with a syringe in the NG tube. For tubes less than 12 French, hold the syringe horizontally and shake during the administration to avoid the tube from becoming clogged. Be sure to rinse the container and administer any remaining fluid to ensure that the adequate dosage is administered.

Assessing for Therapeutic Effects

The assessment of pulmonary function should include chest x-rays and testing of pulmonary function. Care outcomes should include improvement in pulmonary function and diminished inflammation.

Assessing for Adverse Effects

Assessing for adverse effects includes monitoring HDL, AST, and ALT levels, and assessing the patient for constipation and abdominal pain due to the risk of GI perforation.

Patient Teaching

Instruct the patient on the use of baricitinib in treating severe adult respiratory syndrome. Instruct the patient to report any signs and symptoms of abdominal discomfort.

Dexamethasone

As seen in Figure 23.1, dexamethasone is recommended for use in treating severely ill patients with COVID-19. The recommended dosage is 6 mg daily for 10 days or until discharge. Dexamethasone or other glucocorticoids should not be used for the prevention or treatment of mild to moderate COVID-19. Patients taking glucocorticoids are at risk for the development of hyperglycemia and the development of bacterial, fungal, or *Strongyloides* infections, and patients should be monitored for adverse effects (see Chapter 17).

Drug Therapy for Outpatient Management of Coronavirus 2 (SARS-CoV-2)

Nirmatrelvir and ritonavir (Paxlovid) are oral agents that prevent the advancement of severe respiratory disease in patients diagnosed with COVID-19.

Nirmatrelvir and Ritonavir (Paxlovid)

Nirmatrelvir and ritonavir have been approved for emergency use in adults. The drugs have not been studied in pediatric patients. However, the FDA has based its approval for use on patients aged 12 years and older weighing 40 kg or more.

Pharmacokinetics

The distribution of nirmatrelvir is 104.7 L. It is 69% protein bound with minimal metabolism. The half-life of elimination is 1/79 hours. The peak of action is 3 hours with excretion in the urine and feces. Ritonavir's distribution is 112.4 L, and it is 98% protein bound. Ritonavir is metabolized by CYP3A4 and minimally with CYP2D6. The half-life of elimination is 6.15 hours with a peak of action of 3.98 hours. It is primarily excreted in feces with minimal excretion in the urine.

Action and Use

Nirmatrelvir is a peptidomimetic inhibitor of SARS-CoV-2, resulting in the inhibition of viral replication. Ritonavir assists in increasing the plasma concentration of nirmatrelvir, an action that increases the action of nirmatrelvir.

Nirmatrelvir and ritonavir are used for the treatment of outpatient COVID-19. They are also used for HIV/AIDS, discussed later in the chapter.

Patient-related variables specific to the use of nirmatrelvir and ritonavir include the following:

- Age:
  - Nirmatrelvir and ritonavir are approved in children aged 12 years and older who weigh at least 40 kg.
- Reproduction, pregnancy, and lactation:
  - Nirmatrelvir and ritonavir are administered together. Nirmatrelvir has produced adverse effects in embryo–fetal development.
  - The use of nirmatrelvir and ritonavir should not be withheld from pregnant patients when the benefits outweigh the risk.
  - Lactation is not contraindicated.
- Abnormal kidney function and hepatic impairment:
  - A reduced dosage of nirmatrelvir is required with eFGR 30 to less than 60 mL/minute.
  - Nirmatrelvir is not recommended with eGFR less than 30 mL/minute.
  - Nirmatrelvir and ritonavir are not recommended in severe hepatic impairment.

Adverse Effects and Contraindications

Hypertension and cardiovascular adverse effects, including angioedema, have been reported. The GI adverse effect of diarrhea and myalgia of the neuromuscular system have also been documented. Nirmatrelvir and ritonavir may produce hypersensitivity reactions.

Nirmatrelvir and ritonavir are contraindicated with significant hypersensitivity to any component of either drug or any history of Stevens-Johnson syndrome. Any drug that is a strong inducer of CYP3A4 and that increases the metabolism of nirmatrelvir should not be administered.

Nursing Implications
Preventing Interactions

As stated previously, nirmatrelvir requires CYP3A4 to enhance metabolism. Any drug that is a strong CYP3A4 inducer should not be administered so that the action of nirmatrelvir remains sufficient.

Administering the Medication

Nirmatrelvir and ritonavir are coadministered orally. The tablets are administered whole. They should not be crushed or chewed. They can be administered with or without food.

Assessing for Therapeutic Effects

The outcome of care should include improvement of lung function, decreased shortness of breath, and decrease in viral symptoms.

Assessing for Adverse Effects

The assessment of fever, pulmonary function, and pain is required for patients with COVID-19 who are treated with nirmatrelvir/ritonavir. The patient should also be assessed for signs of hypersensitivity reaction, diarrhea, and myalgia.

Patient Teaching

Since nirmatrelvir/ritonavir is administered for outpatient treatment, the patient and family should have significant patient teaching regarding monitoring for improvement of COVID-19–related symptoms and adverse effects. If a dose of the medication is missed, administer the dose. Do not administer a double dose of the medication. If the patient's COVID-19 symptoms do not improve, contact the healthcare provider.

DRUGS FOR HERPESVIRUS INFECTIONS

Drugs for Herpes Simplex Virus and Varicella–Zoster Virus

A **herpesvirus** is any virus belonging to the family of the Herpesviridae. The herpesviruses include HSV, varicella–zoster virus (VZV), and CMV. There are two types of herpes viral infections: HSV-1 and HSV-2. HSV-1 causes fever blisters or cold sores on the lips, mouth, or face, and HSV-2 causes genital warts. **Ⓟ Acyclovir (Zovirax)**, the prototype antiviral agent used to combat the herpesviruses, is an oral, parenteral, and topical antiviral drug.

Pharmacokinetics

After oral administration, the body absorbs 15% to 30% of the acyclovir dosage, reaching a peak of action in 1.5 to 2 hours. The drug is distributed to the tissues of the lower levels of the central nervous system (CNS). It is 9% to 33% protein bound and has a half-life of 2 to 3.5 hours. Acyclovir crosses the placenta and enters breast milk. Excretion of unchanged drug occurs in the urine.

Action and Use

Following uptake by infected cells, acyclovir is converted to acyclovir monophosphate by the enzyme thymidine kinase. Acyclovir triphosphate inhibits DNA polymerase, thus interrupting viral DNA replication. This action reduces viral shedding and prevents formation of new lesions.

Immunocompromised patients take acyclovir for initial and recurrent cutaneous and mucosal HSV and VZV. Prescribers also order the drug for the treatment of **genital herpes** (a herpesvirus that appears on the genitals); it decreases viral shedding as well as the duration of skin lesions and pain. Acyclovir does not eliminate inactive virus in the body and thus does not prevent recurrence of the disease unless oral drug therapy is continued. However, prolonged or repeated courses of drug therapy may result in the emergence of acyclovir-resistant viral strains, especially in immunocompromised patients. In patients with an altered immune response, authorities recommend the intravenous (IV) form for severe genital herpes, and nonimmunocompromised patients should also receive IV preparations. Acyclovir is effective against the HSV. Parenteral acyclovir is used to treat viral encephalitis. It is administered orally for the treatment of HSV and VZV. Table 23.3 presents route and dosage information for acyclovir and other drugs used for HSV and VZV.

Patient-related variables specific to the use of acyclovir include the following:

- Age:
  - The half-life of acyclovir in neonates is 4 hours—longer than in adults.
  - The treatment of HSV gingivostomatitis is an off-label use of acyclovir in infants and children.
- Reproduction, pregnancy, and lactation:
  - Acyclovir crosses the placenta. There is no reported increased in congenital anomalies with exposure to acyclovir.
  - Acyclovir is recommended for treatment of genital herpes simplex in pregnant patients.
  - Acyclovir is present in breast milk, but it is compatible with breast-feeding.
- Abnormal kidney function and hepatic impairment:
  - There have been reports of kidney failure with acyclovir.
  - It is necessary to reduce the dosage of acyclovir in patients with altered kidney function according to the creatinine clearance (CrCl). In patients who are on hemodialysis, the half-life of acyclovir is approximately 5 hours.
  - No dosage adjustments are required in patients with hepatic impairment.

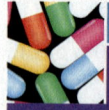

TABLE 23.3 DRUGS AT A GLANCE: Drugs for Herpes Simplex Virus (HSV) and Varicella-Zoster Virus (VZV)			
Drug	**Routes and Dosage Ranges**		
	Adults	**Children**	
Acyclovir (Zovirax; APO-Acyclovir, MYLAN-Acyclovir, TEVA-Acyclovir, Zovirax)	Genital herpes: 200 mg PO every 4 h, five times daily for 10 d for initial infection; 400 mg two times daily to prevent recurrence of chronic infection; 200 mg every 4 h five times daily for 5 d to treat recurrence Herpes zoster: 800 mg PO every 4 h five times daily for 7–10 d Chickenpox: 20 mg/kg PO (max dose 800 mg) four times daily for 5 d Mucosal and cutaneous HSV infections in ICH: 5 mg/kg IV infused over 1 h, every 8 h for 7 d VZV in ICH: 10 mg/kg IV infused over 1 h, every 8 h for 7 d HSV encephalitis: 10 mg/kg IV infused over 1 h, every 8 h for 10 d Topically to lesions every 3 h six times daily for 7 d	Younger than 12 y 10 or 20 mg/kg IV every 8 h for 7 or 10 d, depending on the condition being treated—chickenpox 2 y and older and weight 40 kg or less, 20 mg/kg PO four times daily for 5 d Weight above 40 kg, 800 mg PO four times daily for 5 d 12 y and older, topical, same as adults	
Docosanol (Abreva)	Topically to lesions five times daily for up to 10 d	Older than 12 y: adult dosage	
Famciclovir (ACT-Famciclovir, APO-Famciclovir, Famvir, PMS-Famciclovir, SANDOZ Famciclovir)	Herpes zoster: 500 mg PO every 8 h for 7 d Genital herpes: 125 mg PO twice daily for 5 d	Safety and efficacy not established	
Penciclovir (Denavir)	Topically every 2 h while awake for 4 d	Safety and efficacy not established	
Trifluridine (APO-Trifluridine, Viroptic)	Topically 1 drop in affected eye every 2 h: maximum dose 9 drops per day: when healing is complete, reduce dose to 1 drop every 4 h for 7 d: maximum dose drops per day	≥6 y: topically 1 drop in affected eye every 2 h: maximum dose 9 drops per day: when healing is complete, reduce dose to 1 drop every 4 h for 7 d: maximum dose drops per day	
Valacyclovir (Valtrex; APO-Valacyclovir, AURA-Valacyclovir, BIO-Valacyclovir, DOM-Valacyclovir, JAMP-Valacyclovir, MAR-Valacyclovir, SANDOZ-Valacyclovir, Valtrex)	Herpes labialis: 2 g PO twice daily for 1 d Herpes zoster: 1 g PO every 8 h for 7 d Recurrent genital herpes: PO 500 mg PO every 12 h daily for 5 d Reduce dosage with abnormal kidney function	Herpes labialis: adolescents, same as adults Safety not established	

ICH, immunocompromised host.

Adverse Effects and Contraindications

Acyclovir has minimal adverse effects. The most commonly reported adverse effects are malaise, headache, nausea, vomiting, and diarrhea. The parenteral form may lead to phlebitis at the injection site, hives, itching, rash, nausea, vomiting, elevated liver enzymes, and acute kidney injury. The parenteral form may result in encephalopathy, a rare but potentially serious adverse effect. Other serious drug-related effects include thrombocytopenia purpura and hemolytic uremic syndrome.

Contraindications to acyclovir include a known hypersensitivity to the drug, heart failure, kidney disease, and lactation. Caution is necessary in patients who are receiving nephrotoxic agents.

Nursing Implications
Preventing Interactions

The most significant interactions with acyclovir include increased serum concentrations with probenecid, drowsiness with zidovudine, and abnormal kidney function when combined with medications that cause kidney toxicity. Hydantoins and valproic acid combined with acyclovir lead to decreased antiepileptic effects, placing patients at risk for seizure activity. The use of acyclovir and theophylline results in theophylline toxicity.

Administering the Medication

With the topical preparation of acyclovir, it is important to wash the hands thoroughly prior to administration and apply with a gloved hand. It is crucial that the medication be prescribed and therapy started as soon as symptoms arise. With the oral medication, patients may take the drug without respect to food intake. With the parenteral form of acyclovir, it is necessary to infuse it over 1 hour to prevent kidney damage. The nurse ensures that the patient is well hydrated with 2 to 3 L of fluid per 24 hours. Acyclovir is incompatible with blood products and protein-containing solutions. In patients with a body mass index (BMI) of 30.0 or higher, it is essential to calculate acyclovir dosages according to ideal body weight.

Assessing for Therapeutic Effects

The nurse assesses for the healing of lesions, decreased pain, and itching. When administering acyclovir prophylactically for genital herpes, the nurse assesses for fewer recurrences.

Assessing for Adverse Effects

The nurse assesses for signs and symptoms of hypersensitivity to the acyclovir. With the topical drug, the nurse assesses for burning, stinging, and pruritus. With the parenteral drug, the nurse assesses for phlebitis at the injection site. It is also necessary to assess for confusion, coma, seizures, and tremors. In addition, the nurse assesses the aspartate aminotransferase (AST) and alanine aminotransferase (ALT) for elevations, as well as blood urea nitrogen (BUN) and serum creatinine for increases.

Patient Teaching

Box 23.2 identifies general patient teaching guidelines for the antiviral drugs.

Other Drugs in the Class

Docosanol (Abreva) is an over-the-counter topical antiviral agent that works in the early stages of intracellular events of viral entry into the target cells. This action of the drug makes viral entry into the cell difficult, thus preventing viral replication. Uses include the treatment of HSV of the face and lips. The patient should notify their primary healthcare provider if symptoms do not resolve in 10 days.

Famciclovir and valacyclovir (Valtrex) are oral agents with greater bioavailability than acyclovir and administered less frequently. Both medications are administered for the treatment of herpes simplex and herpes zoster infections. Dosage should be reduced in patients with decreased creatinine clearance. Famciclovir is metabolized to penciclovir, its active form and is excreted mainly in the urine. Valacyclovir is converted to acyclovir by intestinal and hepatic metabolism. It then inhibits DNA synthesis and viral replication.

Penciclovir (Denavir) is a topical drug used for the treatment of recurrent herpes labialis. The cold sore minimally absorbs the drug. The patient should apply the ointment every 2 hours for 4 days. If the lesion does not improve, it is important to notify the primary healthcare provider.

Trifluridine is an ophthalmic drug used to treat primary keratoconjunctivitis and recurring epithelial keratitis caused by type 1 or 2 HSV (see Chapter 59).

NCLEX Success

1. A patient in the intensive care unit is being administered remdesivir parenterally for the treatment of acute severe respiratory syndrome coronavirus 2 (SARS-CoV-2). Which of the following is a priority assessment during administration of remdesivir?
    A. heart rate
    B. lung sounds
    C. urine output
    D. respiratory rate

2. A patient experiences recurrences of herpes simplex, with an outbreak on the lips. Which medication can be applied in the early stages of the viral illness?
    A. docosanol
    B. valganciclovir
    C. Neosporin
    D. tobramycin

Clinical Application 23.1

- What is a cold sore? How does valacyclovir work to decrease Ms. Jackson's symptoms and ultimately heal the cold sore?
- What patient teaching does the nurse provide to Ms. Jackson?

Drugs for Cytomegalovirus

Cytomegalovirus (CMV) is a type of herpesvirus. The first agent developed for the treatment of CMV infection was 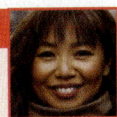 **ganciclovir**, the prototype. Prescribers use ganciclovir to treat CMV in immunocompromised patients, including those with AIDS and patients who have received transplants.

Pharmacokinetics

With oral administration, the onset of action of ganciclovir is 2 to 4 hours, and with IV administration, the onset of action is 1 hour. The drug is distributed widely to all tissues, including the cerebrospinal fluid (CSF) and eye tissue. The half-life is 1.7 to 5.8 hours, and in abnormal kidney function, the half-life is prolonged. It is excreted unchanged in the urine.

Action and Use

Like acyclovir, ganciclovir inhibits viral DNA synthesis. It is changed to a substrate that inhibits the binding of deoxyguanosine triphosphate to DNA polymerase.

The IV form of ganciclovir is for the treatment of CMV retinitis in immunocompromised patients. This preparation is also used for the treatment or prevention of CMV in transplant recipients. Patients take oral ganciclovir for the prevention of CMV if they have advanced HIV infection or are at risk for disease development. In 2009, the Centers for Disease Control and Prevention (CDC) identified an unlabeled use of intravitreal ganciclovir plus systemic foscarnet for the treatment of VZV in patients with progressive outer retinal necrosis in patients with HIV. Table 23.4 summarizes route and dosage information for ganciclovir and related drugs.

Patient-related variables specific to the use of ganciclovir include the following:

- Age:
  - Ganciclovir should be administered cautiously in older adults, who often have impaired organ function or concomitant diseases and use other drugs.
- Reproduction, pregnancy, and lactation:
  - Ganciclovir inhibits spermatogenesis in males and suppresses fertility in females.
  - Animal studies suggest that ganciclovir has the potential to cause congenital anomalies.
  - Breast-feeding is not recommended with ganciclovir.
- Abnormal kidney function and hepatic impairment:
  - Risk of toxicity is greater with ganciclovir because excretion of the drug occurs in the kidneys. Dose reduction, when indicated by decreased CrCl, may minimize these risks.
  - Reduce the dosage of ganciclovir according to the CrCl. Hemodialysis patients should receive ganciclovir following dialysis.
  - The IV dosage for dialysis patients is 1.25 mg/kg every 48 to 72 hours, with a maintenance dose of 0.625 mg/kg every 48 to 72 hours.

Adverse Effects and Contraindications

Adverse effects of ganciclovir include chills, fever, pruritus, anorexia, nausea, vomiting, anemia, leukopenia, neutropenia,

TABLE 23.4

DRUGS AT A GLANCE: Drugs for Cytomegalovirus (CMV)

Drug	Routes and Dosage Ranges	
	Adults	**Children**
Ganciclovir (Cytovene)	CMV retinitis: induction therapy, 5 mg/kg/dose IV every 12 h for 14–21 d; maintenance therapy, 5 mg/kg/dose as a single daily dose for 7 d/wk or 6 mg/kg/d for 5 d/wk Prevention of CMV disease in transplant patients: same as induction and maintenance therapy, but the induction course is 7–14 d	CMV CNS disease in HIV-exposed patients: 5 mg/kg/dose every 12 h plus foscarnet until symptoms improve followed by chronic suppression CMV retinitis: same as adult dose (slow infusion) Prevention of CMV in transplant patients: same as adult dose Neonatal congenital CMV: 6 mg/kg/dose every 12 h for 6 wk; if HIV positive, a longer duration of therapy is considered
Cidofovir (MAR-Cidofovir) Note: Probenecid must be administered with each dose (25–40 mg/kg/dose in children)	Induction therapy, 5 mg/kg IV once weekly for 2 consecutive weeks; maintenance therapy, 5 mg/kg IV every 2 wk. Administer 1 L of normal saline IV before each infusion over 1–2 h and 1 L at the start of the infusion or immediately following over 1–3 h	Induction therapy, 5 mg/kg/dose IV once weekly for 2 consecutive weeks; maintenance therapy, 5 mg/kg/dose IV once every 2 wk until consecutive negative adenovirus sample. Hydrate with 20 mL/kg of normal saline for 1 h before induction therapy followed by 2 h of maintenance fluid
Foscarnet (Foscavir; Vocarvi)	CMV retinitis: induction therapy, 60 mg/kg/dose IV every 8 h for 14–21 d or 90 mg/kg IV every 12 h for 14–21 d; maintenance therapy, 90–120 mg every 12 h for 2 wk, followed by 120 mg/kg daily for ≥2 wk Acyclovir-resistant HSV: 40 mg/kg/dose IV every 8–12 h for 14–21 d	CMV CNS disease: 60 mg/kg/dose IV every 8 h in combination with ganciclovir followed by 90–120 mg/kg/dose daily CMV retinitis: 60 mg/kg/dose IV every 8 h for 14–21 d with or without ganciclovir followed by 90–120 mg/kg/dose daily Acyclovir-resistant herpes simplex: 40–60 mg/kg/dose IV every 8 h until lesions heal Chickenpox not responding to acyclovir: 40–60 mg/kg/dose IV every 8 h for 7–10 d
Valganciclovir (Valcyte; APO-AURA-Valganciclovir, TEVA-Valganciclovir, Valcyte)	CMV retinitis: 900 mg PO twice daily for 21 d, then 900 mg PO once daily Prevention of CMV disease following kidney or heart transplant: 900 mg PO once daily beginning within 10 d of transplant; continue therapy until 100 d with heart or kidney transplant or 200 d for kidney transplant	1–3 mo, 16 mg/kg/dose PO every 12 h 4 mo to 16 y, dose in mg = 7 × body surface × CrCl (begin within 10 d of transplant and continue until 100 d posttransplant); doses should be rounded to the nearest 25-mg increment; max dose 900 mg/d

thrombocytopenia, neuropathy, retinal detachment, hematuria, and sepsis. There may be increases in BUN and serum creatinine. Ganciclovir causes granulocytopenia and thrombocytopenia in 20% to 40% of recipients, often during the first 2 weeks of therapy. The FDA has issued a recovery usually occurs within a week of stopping the drug. A second **BOXED WARNING** ◆ advises female and male patients of childbearing age to maintain contraceptive precautions during ganciclovir therapy and for a minimum of 90 days after drug therapy.

Patients should not receive ganciclovir if their neutrophil count is less than 500/mm^3 or their platelet count is below 25,000/mm^3. A known hypersensitivity to ganciclovir or any of the antiviral agents is also a contraindication. Caution is warranted in abnormal kidney function.

Nursing Implications
Preventing Interactions
Several drugs interact with ganciclovir. Imipenem combined with ganciclovir increases the risk of seizure activity. Amphotericin B, antineoplastic agents, didanosine, dapsone, pentamidine, probenecid, trimethoprim–sulfamethoxazole, and zidovudine administered with ganciclovir increase the risk of bone marrow suppression. Cyclosporine and ganciclovir result in nephrotoxicity. Mycophenolate, probenecid, and tenofovir increase the serum concentration of ganciclovir–valganciclovir. Sodium-containing foods combined with ganciclovir may lead to hypernatremia. Echinacea has a potential to stimulate the autoimmune response in patients with HIV.

Administering the Medication
Parenteral ganciclovir requires slow infusion, over at least 1 hour. Too rapid administration results in toxicity and excessive plasma levels. The medication is compatible with 5% dextrose and water, lactated Ringer, and normal saline. Administration using intramuscular, subcutaneous, or IV push is contraindicated. Ganciclovir is a hazardous medication, and it is necessary to use appropriate precautions for handling and disposal. The nurse checks the manufacturer's guidelines and does not allow the powder or the reconstituted medication to touch the skin. The nurse does not administer the drug to patients with a platelet count less than 25,000/mm^3 or a neutrophil count less than 500/mm^3.

Assessing for Therapeutic Effects
The nurse assesses the patient for improvement in vision and visual acuity related to retinitis. It is also important to assess for improvement in symptoms related to pneumonia, hepatitis, encephalitis, adrenal insufficiency, and gastrointestinal (GI) inflammation or ulcerations.

Assessing for Adverse Effects
The nurse assesses BUN, creatinine, CrCl, CBC, and platelet count for impaired kidney function and bone marrow depression. The nurse assesses for signs and symptoms of hypersensitivity reactions. It is important to assess for neuropathic changes such as pain and diminished sensation.

Patient Teaching
Box 23.2 identifies general patient teaching guidelines for the antiviral drugs.

Other Drugs in the Class
Cidofovir is an IV drug indicated for treatment of CMS retinitis in patients with AIDS. After conversion to cidofovir diphosphate, it suppresses CMV replication by selective inhibition of viral DNA synthesis. Serum creatinine level should be monitored. If the creatinine is greater than 1.5 mg/dL, it is important to discontinue therapy. The FDA has issued three **BOXED WARNING** ◆ for cidofovir. The drug has possible carcinogenic and teratogenic adverse effects. It may also be nephrotoxic, and prior to administration, the patient should receive 1 L of normal saline and oral probenecid. In addition, it places the patient at risk for neutropenia. Valganciclovir (Valcyte) is an oral drug administered for CMV retinitis and prevention of CMV infections following organ transplant. Administer the medications with a high-fat diet to enhance absorption. The FDA has issued a **BOXED WARNING** ◆ for valganciclovir; granulocytopenia (neutropenia), anemia, and thrombocytopenia may occur. If severe bone marrow depression occurs, it is essential that the drug be discontinued.

Foscarnet (Foscavir) is an IV drug administered for CMV retinitis, acyclovir-resistant HSV, and other CMV infections related to diminished immune response. The patient should be well hydrated throughout the infusion of the medication. In addition to the warning related to potential abnormal kidney function, the FDA has issued a **BOXED WARNING** ◆ regarding seizures with use of foscarnet, which may occur related to impaired kidney function, diminished serum calcium, and CNS conditions. It is important to use foscarnet cautiously in patients with kidney disease and to assess for signs of abnormal kidney function.

NCLEX Success

3. A patient receives a prescription for valganciclovir for the prevention of cytomegalovirus infections following organ transplantation. Which of the following nursing interventions should be implemented?
    A. Instruct the patient to take the medication following a meal high in fat.
    B. Instruct the patient to take the meal with large amounts of fluids.
    C. Instruct the patient to report abdominal pain.
    D. Instruct the patient to report diminished sense of hearing.

DRUGS FOR RESPIRATORY SYNCYTIAL VIRUS

RSV is a single-stranded RNA virus that causes respiratory tract illness in persons of all ages. The prototype drug used to treat RSV is **ribavirin** (Virazole), a synthetic nucleoside antiviral drug, is one of the few antiviral drugs that is indicated for use in children. Its main use is for the treatment of RSV infections.

The treatment for immunocompromised patients can include the administration of an intravenous immune globulin and/or glucocorticoids. The use of the combination treatment with ribavirin assists in reducing the lower respiratory tract infection, which can be fatal. The inhaled form of ribavirin is primarily used for the treatment of RSV. There is an oral form of ribavirin that has an off-label use in treating RSV. The accepted use of the oral form of ribavirin is the treatment of hepatitis C. This form will be presented in the section on Drug Therapy for Hepatitis C.

Pharmacokinetics

Ribavirin, which is inhaled systemically, has a slow onset of action. It reaches its peak of action in 60 to 90 minutes. The medication is metabolized at the cellular level, with a 9.5-hour half-life. It is excreted in the feces and urine.

Action and Use

Ribavirin inhibits the replication of RNA and DNA viruses to stop the influenza virus RNA polymerase activity. This action interferes with the elongation and initiation of RNA fragments, which stops protein synthesis.

Inhaled ribavirin may be effective in infants and children with severe RSV infection of the lower respiratory tract. Table 23.5 presents route and dosage information for ribavirin.

Patient-related variables specific to the use of ribavirin include the following:

- Age:
  - The FDA has issued a **BOXED WARNING** ◆ that sudden respiratory deterioration has been noted in infants during the initial aerosolized treatment. If this occurs, stop the administration.
  - The FDA has issued a **BOXED WARNING** ◆ that significant teratogenic and/or embryocidal effects have been reported.
- Reproduction, pregnancy, and lactation:
  - Ribavirin aerosolized inhalation treatments are contraindicated in pregnant patients. No pregnant individuals should be in the same room with a patient who is being administered ribavirin inhalation treatments.

Adverse Effects and Contraindications

Adverse effects include fatigue, insomnia, headache, anemia, nausea, and anorexia. Less than 1% of the population experiences hypotension, cardiac arrest, conjunctivitis, bronchospasm, apnea, and decline in respiratory function. Healthcare workers caring for children treated with RSV may report headache, conjunctivitis, nausea, rash, dizziness, chest pain, bronchospasm, pharyngitis, and rhinitis. The FDA has issued a **BOXED WARNING** ◆ for ribavirin; the drug causes significant teratogenic effects, according to animal studies. People who are pregnant or plan to become pregnant should not care for children receiving inhalation therapy or be in the room when it is being administered.

Contraindications to ribavirin include a known hypersensitivity to the drug or its components.

Nursing Implications

Preventing Interactions

There are no known drug or herb interactions with inhaled ribavirin. However, mixing the drug with other inhaled or aerosol medications is to be avoided.

Administering the Medication

Administration in a well-ventilated room is necessary; there should be six air exchanges per hour. Patients who are mechanically ventilated require monitoring for malfunction or obstruction of the expiratory valve, which could result in

TABLE 23.5

DRUGS AT A GLANCE: Drugs for Respiratory Syncytial Virus (RSV) Infection

Drug	Routes and Dosage Ranges	
	Adults	**Children**
Ⓟ **Ribavirin** (inhalation)* (Virazole)	Inhalation: 2 g over 2 h every 8 h Off-label use: RSV in hematopoietic cell or heart/lung transplant recipients	Inhalation, diluted to a concentration of 20 mg/mL for 12–18 h/d for 3–7 d
Ⓟ Palivizumab (Synagis) Monoclonal antibody	Not for adult use	Infants and children <24 mo: IM 15 mg/kg once monthly throughout RSV season, first dose administered prior to commencement of RSV season; if hospitalized at the start of RSV season, palivizumab should be given 48–72 h before discharge or promptly after discharge The American Association of Pediatrics recommends a maximum of 5 doses per season; if hospitalization occurs for breakthrough RSV infection, monthly prophylaxis should be discontinued for the remainder of the season

*Ribavirin for the treatment of hepatitis is found in Table 23.7.

high positive end-expiratory pressures. The nurse should know that when using an SPAG-2 unit for administration, it is important to discard solutions every 24 hours and when the liquid level is low.

Assessing for Therapeutic Effects

The nurse assesses respiratory status, including dyspnea, apnea, labored respirations, nasal flaring, contractions, shallow respirations, wheezing, rales, and rhonchi.

Assessing for Adverse Effects

The nurse assesses level of comfort; crying, grimacing, and anxiety could indicate pain. The level of activity may indicate increased fatigue. The nurse also assesses the airway for bronchospasm or alterations in pulmonary function, including cyanosis. In addition, the nurse assesses vital signs for hypotension and changes in cardiac status. In infants, it is important to assess for sudden deterioration of respiratory function at the initiation of oral inhalation of ribavirin. If deterioration in respiratory function is noted, stop the treatment and notify the prescriber. If the oral inhalation ribavirin is reinstated, the infant should be continuously monitored and coadministration of bronchodilators may be prescribed.

Patient Teaching

Box 23.2 identifies general patient teaching guidelines for antiviral drugs.

MONOCLONAL ANTIBODY FOR RESPIRATORY SYNCYTIAL VIRUS

 Palivizumab (Synagis) is a monoclonal antibody approved for the treatment of RSV. It is only approved for use in infants and children younger than 24 months of age.

Pharmacokinetics

The bioavailability of palivizumab in infants and children younger than 24 months of age without congenital heart disease is 70%. The half-life of the drug is 20 to 24.5 days, with a peak serum level in 3 to 5 days. Palivizumab concentrations are sufficient to inhibit RSV 2 days following administration. The excretion of palivizumab may increase in patients with chronic lung disease or in the presence of antipalivizumab antibodies.

Action and Use

Palivizumab exhibits neutralizing and fusion-inhibiting activity against RSV, thus inhibiting its replication.

Patient-related variables specific to the use of palivizumab include age. Specifically, palivizumab is used in pediatric patients who were born at less than 35 weeks of gestation. These infants should also be less than 6 months of age at the beginning of the RSV season. Palivizumab is not for adult use.

Adverse Effects and Contraindications

The reported adverse effects of palivizumab are skin rash, fever, antibody development, angioedema, dyspnea, hypotonia, pruritus, respiratory failure, unresponsiveness, urticaria, hypersensitivity reaction, injection site reaction, and thrombocytopenia.

Palivizumab is contraindicated in hypersensitivity reactions or hypersensitivity reaction to any humanized monoclonal antibodies.

Nursing Implications

Preventing Interactions

Palivizumab should not be combined with vitamins, minerals, or over-the-counter medications. The nurse should consult with the prescriber regarding specific drug interactions.

Administering the Medication

Administer undiluted palivizumab deep into intramuscular tissues in the anterolateral aspect of the thigh. Never administer palivizumab in the gluteal muscle due to risk of damage to the sciatic nerve.

Assessing for Therapeutic Effects

Assess pulmonary status for unlabored respirations and absence of retractions.

Assessing for Adverse Effects

Assess for injection reaction and hypersensitivity reaction. The infant or child's lung sounds should be auscultated for clarity.

Patient Teaching

Box 23.2 identifies general patient teaching guidelines for the antiviral drugs. In addition, the nurse instructs families about the risk of exposure with pregnancy and aspects of ribavirin administration.

> **Quality and Safety Alert: Evidence-Based Practice**
>
> At an Atlanta, Georgia, health center from 2012 to 2019, Rostad et al. (2021) conducted a retrospective case–control study of children with sickle cell disease (SCD) who have respiratory viral panels performed. The researchers identified 3,676 tests performed on 2,636 patients over the seven seasons. It was found that 6% of RSV-positive tests were among the 6.1% of the patients. The study revealed that RSV infections are common in children with SCD. In addition, younger children with SCD are at higher risk for the development of RSV. Thus, SCD patients have a higher risk of developing RSV than does the general population. Understanding the epidemiology and clinical outcomes of RSV in children with SCD will assist medical decision-making in this patient population.

> **Clinical Application 23.2**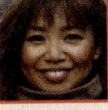
>
> Ms. Jackson's 1-year-old child, James, is admitted to the pediatric medical division with a diagnosis of respiratory syncytial virus. Ms. Jackson is pregnant with twins.
> - What precautions does the nurse need to take with Ms. Jackson and her child?
> - What patient teaching does the nurse provide to Ms. Jackson and her family?
> - What assessments does the nurse implement when caring for James?

> ### NCLEX Success
>
> 4. When caring for an infant receiving ribavirin, the nurse notes the fluid level is low in the SPAG-2 unit. What action should the nurse take?
>   A. Discard the remaining fluid and add more fluid.
>   B. Add 10 mL of normal saline to the SPAG-2 unit.
>   C. Discard the SPAG-2 unit.
>   D. Add sterile water to the SPAG-2 unit.

DRUGS FOR INFLUENZA

Influenza A or B virus is an acute respiratory illness. Two classes of drugs are used for the prophylaxis and treatment of influenza A. The first class is adamantanes, which includes **amantadine hydrochloride** (Gocovri, Osmolex ER). Amantadine is discussed further below as well as in Chapter 48 with regard to its use in the treatment of Parkinson disease. The second class is the neuraminidase inhibitors, which includes oseltamivir phosphate. Table 23.6 summarizes route and dosage information for the adamantanes and the neuraminidase inhibitors.

Adamantanes

Amantadine hydrochloride is a synthetic antiviral agent administered for the treatment of influenza A, an RNA virus. According to the CDC, amantadine hydrochloride is no longer recommended for the treatment or prophylaxis of influenza A; when used for this purpose, amantadine resistance has developed. Amantadine hydrochloride is not effective against influenza B. This chapter discusses amantadine because it may be used in the event of the reemergence of adamantane-susceptible strains of influenza A.

TABLE 23.6 DRUGS AT A GLANCE: Drugs for Influenza

Drug	Routes and Dosage Ranges	
	Adults	**Children**
Adamantanes		
Amantadine hydrochloride (Gocovri, Osmolex ER; PDP-Amantadine)	Influenza A prophylaxis: 200 mg PO daily or 100 mg PO twice daily for 10 d after exposure Uncomplicated influenza: same as above; continue 24–48 h after symptoms subside	Not recommended for age <1 y Influenza A prophylaxis: 1–9 y: 4.4–8.8 mg/kg/d PO in one or two divided doses not to exceed 150 mg/d Uncomplicated influenza: same as above; continue 24–48 h after symptoms subside
Rimantadine	Influenza A: prophylaxis, 100 mg PO twice daily; treatment, 100 mg PO twice daily start within 48 h of symptoms for 5–7 d	1–9 y, 5 mg/kg/d PO in divided doses (max dose: 150 mg/d) 10 y and older, same as adults
Neuraminidase Inhibitors		
Oseltamivir phosphate (Tamiflu; NAT-Oseltamivir, Tamiflu)	Prophylaxis, 75 mg PO daily for 10 d begin within 2 d after exposure Treatment, 75 mg PO twice daily for 5 d within 2 d of exposure	Birth to 1 y, consult manufacturer's recommendations Infants <1 y, weight-based dosing; 3 mg/kg/dose twice daily for 5 d 1–12 y Prophylaxis, ≤15 kg, 30 mg/d PO; 15–23 kg, 45 mg/d PO; 23–40 kg, 60 mg/d PO; >40 kg 75 mg/d; all for 10 d Treatment, 30–75 mg PO twice daily for 5 d
Peramivir (Rapivab; Rapivab)	IV 600 mg in a single dose	No dosage available in children
Zanamivir (Relenza Diskhaler; Relenza Diskhaler)	Prophylaxis, 2 inhalations per day for 28 d Treatment, 2 inhalations (10 mg total) every 12 h for 5 d (begin within 2 d of symptoms), first day 2 inhalations 2 h apart then every 12 h	Prophylaxis (5 y and older), same as adult Treatment (7 y and older), same as adult
Endonuclease Inhibitors		
Baloxavir marboxil (Xofluza)	40 to <80 kg: 40 mg PO as a single dose within 48 h of influenza symptoms >80 kg: 80 mg PO as a single dose within 48 h of influenza symptoms	Children >12 years of age, same as adult dosing

Pharmacokinetics

Amantadine is well absorbed, with an onset of action in 48 hours and a peak of action in 1 to 4 hours. It is distributed throughout the body fluids with the highest concentrations in the lung tissues. The medication is not metabolized, and 80% to 90% of the drug is eliminated unchanged in the urine.

Action and Use

Amantadine blocks the uncoating of the virus, thus preventing penetration in the host.

Uses for amantadine include prophylactic and symptomatic treatment of influenza A.

Patient-related variables specific to the use of amantadine include the following:

- Age:
  - Adjust dosage in older adults, according to the patient's kidney function. It may be necessary to administer amantadine in two divided doses.
- Reproduction, pregnancy, and lactation:
  - Adverse events have been noted in animal reproduction studies. Teratogenic events have been documented in humans.
  - Amantadine should not be used in the treatment of Parkinson disease in pregnant patients.
  - Amantadine is present in breast milk. The decision to breast-feed during therapy should consider the risk to the infant and related benefits to both infant and patient.
- Abnormal kidney function and hepatic impairment:
  - Reduce dosage in patients with impaired kidney function according to the CrCl.
  - Patients on hemodialysis should take amantadine 200 mg orally every 7 days.

Adverse Effects and Contraindications

Use of amantadine is associated with several adverse effects. CNS effects may include depression as well as dizziness, light-headedness, nervousness with anxiety, and inability to concentrate. Cardiovascular adverse effects include orthostatic hypotension and peripheral edema. Other adverse effects are anorexia, constipation, nausea, diarrhea, dry nose, and bluish mottling of the skin on the legs and hands.

Contraindications to amantadine include a known hypersensitivity to the medication.

Nursing Implications

Preventing Interactions

Anticholinergic agents administered during the course of amantadine therapy may enhance the anticholinergic effects such as urinary retention, dry mouth, narrow-angle glaucoma, and hypertension. Alcohol increases CNS depression.

Administering the Medication

Patients should take the first dose of amantadine early in the morning and the second dose in the early evening, 12 hours later. They should take the drug with a full glass of water or with food to prevent disruptive sleep patterns. It is necessary to store the medication at room temperature in a tightly closed, light-protected container. High-risk patients who have not been vaccinated previously with the influenza A vaccine can receive amantadine with the vaccine.

Assessing for Therapeutic Effects

The nurse assesses for a decrease in flulike symptoms such as decreased fever, malaise, pain, cough, and rhinitis.

Assessing for Adverse Effects

The nurse assesses the patient's mental status regarding alertness and ability to cope. Also, it is necessary to assess for dizziness and light-headedness as well as for pedal edema and signs of orthostatic hypotension with position changes.

Patient Teaching

Box 23.2 identifies general patient teaching guidelines for the antiviral drugs.

Other Drugs in the Class

Rimantadine is an oral drug used to control outbreaks of influenza A. The drug can be used in combination with oseltamivir or zanamivir but is not recommended in combination with amantadine. It reaches a peak of action in 6 hours. Rimantadine is metabolized in the liver and is excreted unchanged in the urine. The serum half-life is 25.4 hours, which may be prolonged with liver or abnormal kidney function.

Neuraminidase Inhibitors

The neuraminidase inhibitors are active against influenza A or B virus. The CDC recommends these antiviral medications be used for influenza because "on the basis of recent viral surveillance and resistance data, the greater than 99% of currently calculated influenza virus strains are sensitive to these medications." In this class, the prototype drug is **oseltamivir** (Tamiflu). The CDC recommends antiviral treatment of influenza or suspected influenza begin as soon as possible with baloxavir marboxil (Xofluza), oseltamivir, peramivir, and zanamivir. Baloxavir marboxil is an endonuclease inhibitor that will be discussed after the neuraminidase inhibitors.

Pharmacokinetics

Oseltamivir is well absorbed and distributed as oseltamivir carboxylate. The half-life of the drug is 1 to 3 hours. It is metabolized in the liver, and 90% is excreted in the urine with the remainder excreted in the feces.

Action and Use

Oseltamivir, in its active form oseltamivir carboxylate, inhibits the viral enzyme neuraminidase. This enzyme helps the newly formed virus to exit the host cell. By inhibiting this viral enzyme, oseltamivir carboxylate prevents new virus from infecting other cells.

Oseltamivir is an oral drug administered to adults and children 1 year or older who have contracted influenza A or B. The recipients of treatment must have been symptomatic for 2 days or less. Adults and children 1 year of age or older may also take it prophylactically. Table 23.6 gives route and dosage information for oseltamivir.

Patient-related variables specific to the use of oseltamivir include the following:

- Age:
  - There is limited information on administering oseltamivir to infants.
- Reproduction, pregnancy, and lactation:
  - Oseltamivir phosphate and oseltamivir carboxylate cross the placenta.
  - Oseltamivir is the preferred neuraminidase inhibitor for the treatment and prophylaxis of influenza during pregnancy.
  - No adverse effects have been noted with breast-feeding.
- Abnormal kidney function and hepatic impairment:
  - Use caution in patients with abnormal kidney function and hepatic impairment.

Adverse Effects and Contraindications

The adverse effects of oseltamivir are nausea, vomiting, abdominal pain, diarrhea, conjunctivitis, and epistaxis. Contraindications include a known hypersensitivity to the medication.

Patients who are breast-feeding should not take oseltamivir.

Nursing Implications
Preventing Interactions

Probenecid increases the serum concentration of oseltamivir. It is necessary to assess for thrombocytopenia if these drugs are administered together. People should not take oseltamivir 48 hours before receiving the influenza virus vaccine or for 2 weeks after receiving the vaccine.

Administering the Medication

According to the FDA, the manufacturer of the oral suspension of oseltamivir has changed the concentration from 12 to 6 mg/mL. The lower concentration allows for more accurate measurement because it does not become as frothy as the 12-mg concentration.

> **Quality and Safety Alert: Patient-Centered Care**
>
> People may take oseltamivir with food to improve tolerance and prevent GI upset. If necessary, adult capsules can be opened and the powder mixed in a sweetened liquid to make the drug more palatable (e.g., mixed with chocolate or strawberry syrup) to be administered to children.

Assessing for Therapeutic Effects

The nurse assesses for a decrease in flulike symptoms such as fever, malaise, pain, cough, and rhinitis.

Assessing for Adverse Effects

The nurse assesses the patient for GI upset, including nausea, vomiting, and diarrhea. It is also necessary to assess the nares for signs of bleeding and irritation as well as the conjunctiva for irritation, redness, and drainage.

Patient Teaching

Box 23.2 identifies general patient teaching guidelines for the antiviral drugs.

Other Drugs in the Class

Peramivir (Rapivab) is a parenteral antiviral agent that is given only to adults with influenza A or B. Geriatric patients with altered CrCl require a reduced dosage. Adverse effects are hypertension, insomnia, hyperglycemia, constipation, neutropenia, and increased AST, and proteinuria. During postmarketing of peramivir, users reported the following adverse effects: abnormal behavior, anaphylaxis, erythema, hallucinations, exfoliative dermatitis, skin rash, and Stevens-Johnson syndrome. When administering peramivir in the healthcare facility, the nurse must assess for wheezing, bronchospasm, and skin rash. It is also important to assess for neurologic abnormalities. In addition, it is necessary to obtain a baseline CBC and serum creatinine prior to the administration of the drug.

Zanamivir (Relenza) has a similar action to oseltamivir. Patients take the medication using a Diskhaler delivery system, which should be used cautiously in patients with chronic obstructive pulmonary disease and asthma because of the risk of bronchospasm. A rapid-acting inhaled bronchodilator should be available. It is important that the nurse instruct all patients about the use of the inhaler and report worsening respiratory symptoms or the occurrence of diarrhea, nausea, and vomiting. Zanamivir has an unlabeled use in H1N1 virus infection.

Endonuclease Inhibitor

 Baloxavir marboxil (Xofluza) is an endonuclease inhibitor that blocks influenza. It is approved for the treatment of influenza A viruses, including H7N9 and H5N1. It is active against influenza viruses that are resistant to oseltamivir.

Pharmacokinetics

Baloxavir is highly protein bound and metabolized completely, converted by UGT1A3 and CYP3A4 to an active metabolite. The medication's half-life is 79.1 hours. It reaches a peak in 4 hours. Eighty percent of the baloxavir is excreted in the feces with approximately 14% excreted in the urine.

Action and Use

Baloxavir marboxil is converted to baloxavir. Baloxavir is an inhibitor of the endonuclease activity of the polymerase acidic protein. The endonuclease activity is responsible for influenza virus replication.

Baloxavir has antiviral activity against both influenza A and B. It also has antiviral activity against virus strains that are currently resistant to other antiviral agents. Patient-related variables specific to the use of baloxavir marboxil include the following:

- Age:
  - Some children develop a gene mutation with the use of baloxavir, resulting in delayed symptom resolution.
- Reproduction, pregnancy, and lactation:
  - Due to a lack of research, the use of baloxavir is not recommended in pregnancy or lactation.

Adverse Effects and Contraindications

Adverse effects reported with the administration of baloxavir marboxil include diarrhea that may include melena, erythema, facial swelling, skin rash, urticaria, delirium, and eyelid edema. The medication is contraindicated in patients with a known hypersensitivity to antiviral agents.

Nursing Implications
Administering the Medication

Baloxavir marboxil should be administered within 48 hours of the onset of influenza symptoms. Patients weighing 40 to less than 80 kg should be administered a 40-mg single dose. Patients weighing 80 kg or greater should be administered 80 mg orally. There are no dosage adjustments for abnormal kidney function or hepatic impairment.

Assessing for Therapeutic and Adverse Effects

It is important to assess the patient for a decrease in influenza symptoms such as fever, cough, myalgia, and congestion. Assess the patient for diarrhea with blood, erythema, facial edema, and eyelid edema.

DRUGS FOR HEPATITIS B: NUCLEOSIDE ANALOGS

Hepatitis B is a double-stranded DNA virus. Drug therapy for HBV includes pegylated interferon and antiviral agents, particularly lamivudine. The goal of therapy is to reduce the risk of transmission to others and prevent long-term complications such as cirrhosis or hepatocellular carcinoma. The following section discusses the nucleoside analog **lamivudine** (Epivir, Epivir-HBV) as the prototype antiviral agent for HBV.

Pharmacokinetics

Lamivudine is rapidly absorbed in the GI tract, after which it is distributed with less than 36% of the drug bound by plasma protein. Approximately 4.2% of the drug is metabolized to a trans-sulfoxide metabolite. The half-life of the drug is 2 hours in children and 5 to 7 hours in adults. The drug is excreted unchanged in the urine.

Action

Incorporation of a monophosphate form of lamivudine into the viral DNA of HBV polymerase results in the termination of the DNA chain. The drug also inhibits the transcription of the viral RNA chain in HBV. In addition, as a cytosine analog, lamivudine inhibits HIV reverse transcriptase of the viral RNA chain.

Use

Prescribers order lamivudine for the treatment of chronic hepatitis B in patients who have evidence of hepatitis B viral replication and active inflammation of the liver. Patients with HIV may also take the drug when ART with a multidrug regimen is necessary. An unlabeled use is for postexposure to HIV as part of a multidrug regimen. Table 23.7 gives route and dosage information for lamivudine and the other antiviral agents used for hepatitis.

Patient-related variables specific to the use of lamivudine include the following:

- Age:
  - Pancreatitis is prevalent in children who take lamivudine. Monitor children closely; if signs and symptoms of pancreatitis develop, such as upper abdominal pain, back pain, and vomiting, discontinue the drug.
- Reproduction, pregnancy, and lactation:
  - Lamivudine has a high level of crossing the placental barrier. No increased risk has been noted in the first trimester. Maternal antiretroviral therapy may be associated with adverse pregnancy outcomes, including preterm delivery, stillbirth, low birth weight, and small for gestational age infants.
  - Breast-feeding is contraindicated in patients with hepatitis B due to risk of transmission to the infant.
- Abnormal kidney function and hepatic impairment:
  - Reduce dosage for abnormal kidney function according to the CrCl.

Adverse Effects and Contraindications

A main adverse effect of lamivudine is pancreatitis. Other adverse effects include nausea, vomiting, diarrhea, abdominal pain, neutropenia, myalgia, neuropathy, and musculoskeletal pain. In addition, patients have reported headache, fatigue, insomnia, cough, sinusitis, and infections of the ear, nose, and throat. The FDA has issued a **BOXED WARNING** ◆ for the nucleoside analogs stating that lactic acidosis and severe hepatomegaly with steatosis have been reported.

Contraindications to lamivudine include a known hypersensitivity to the drug or any of the components of the drug.

Nursing Implications
Preventing Interactions

Several drugs interact with lamivudine. Trimethoprim–sulfamethoxazole increases the serum level of lamivudine. Ganciclovir–valganciclovir may enhance the adverse effects of lamivudine. Ribavirin increases the hepatotoxic effects of lamivudine. In addition, administration of lamivudine and zidovudine increases the serum level of zidovudine. Zalcitabine and lamivudine result in the inactivation of both drugs.

Administering the Medication

Patients may take lamivudine with or without food.

Assessing for Therapeutic Effects

The nurse assesses for decreased malaise, myalgia, loss of appetite, and abdominal pain. If the patient had jaundice, the nurse assesses for diminished yellowing of the skin and sclera. It is necessary to palpate the liver and lymph nodes for decreased size. Monitoring AST and ALT for decreasing serum levels is important. The administration of lamivudine decreases the effects of hepatitis, leading to an improvement in the serum liver enzyme levels.

Assessing for Adverse Effects

The nurse assesses for abdominal pain, particularly in pediatric patients. Such pain may be indicative of pancreatitis. Also, the nurse assesses for GI effects such as nausea, vomiting, and diarrhea, as well as for headache, myalgia, and musculoskeletal pain. It is also necessary to assess for upper respiratory effects such as sinusitis and infections.

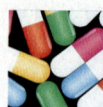

TABLE 23.7

DRUGS AT A GLANCE: Drugs for Hepatitis

Drug	Routes and Dosage Ranges	
	Adults	**Children**
Nucleoside Analogs		
ⓟ **Lamivudine** (Epivir, Epivir-HBV; 🍁 3TC, APO-Lamivudine, Apo-Lamivudine HBV, Heptovir)	100 mg PO daily	2–17 y, 3 mg/kg PO daily up to max 100 mg daily
Adefovir dipivoxil (Hepsera; 🍁 APO-Adefovir, Hepsera)	10 mg PO daily	Younger than 12 y, safety and efficacy have not been established
Entecavir (Baraclude; 🍁 ACCEL-Entecavir, APO-Entecavir, Auro-Entecavir, JAMP-Entecavir, MINT-Entecavir, PMS-Entecavir)	PO 1 mg CrCl 30–49 mL/min: decrease dose by 50% CrCl 10–29 mL/min: decrease dose by 70%	PO 10–11 kg: 0.15 mg once daily >11–14 kg: 0.2 mg once daily >14–17 kg: 0.25 mg once daily >17–20 kg: 0.3 mg once daily >20–23 kg: 0.35 mg once daily >23–26 kg: 0.4 mg oral solution once daily >26–30 ,g: 0.45 mg oral solution once daily >30 kg: 0.5 mg once daily
Ribavirin (🍁 Ibavyr)	<66 kg: 800 mg daily (400 mg in the a.m. and p.m.) 66–80 kg: 1,000 mg daily (400 mg in a.m. and 600 mg in p.m.) 81–105 kg: 1,200 mg daily (600 mg in a.m. and 600 mg in p.m.) >105 kg: 1,400 mg daily (600 mg in a.m. and 800 mg in p.m.)	<47 kg: 15 mg/kg/d in 2 divided doses 47–59 kg: 800 mg daily (400 mg in a.m. and p.m.) 60–73 kg: 1,000 mg daily (400 mg in a.m. and 600 mg in p.m.) >73 kg: 1,200 mg daily (600 mg in a.m. and p.m.)
Tenofovir alafenamide (Vemlidy; 🍁 Vemlidy)	PO 25 mg once daily	No dosage established
Tenofovir disoproxil fumarate (Viread; 🍁 Viread)	300 mg PO daily	Recommended only for ages 12 years and older; see adult dosing
Polymerase Inhibitors		
ⓟ Sofosbuvir (Sovaldi)	400 mg PO with or without food	Oral pellets 1 or more spoonful of sprinkles on a nonacidic soft food

Patient Teaching

Box 23.2 identifies general patient teaching guidelines for antiviral drugs. In addition, the nurse teaches the patient the signs of symptoms of lactic acidosis, including musculoskeletal pain.

Other Drugs in the Class

Adefovir dipivoxil (Hepsera) is a purine nucleotide analog administered for chronic hepatitis B, with active viral replication producing elevation in AST/ALT. The drug requires cautious use in kidney dysfunction. Entecavir (Baraclude) inhibits the HBV polymerase to reduce viral DNA levels. Ribavirin is an oral antiviral drug administered in combination with peginterferon alfa-2a or peginterferon alfa-2b for chronic hepatitis B. Tenofovir disoproxil fumarate (Viread) is useful for the treatment of chronic hepatitis B in patients with compensated or decompensated liver disease. It is also used in combination with other antiretrovirals for HIV infection. Tenofovir disoproxil fumarate has primarily replaced adefovir, because tenofovir is more potent and effective without the combination of other medications. Tenofovir alafenamide (Vemlidy) is also useful in the treatment of chronic hepatitis B in patient with compensated liver disease. It inhibits replication of HBV and inhibits HBV polymerase.

DRUGS FOR HEPATITIS C

Hepatitis C is both acute and chronic hepatitis. Acute hepatitis rarely causes hepatic failure and leads to chronic hepatitis. Chronic hepatitis C can lead to cirrhosis, hepatocellular carcinoma, and require liver transplant.

Polymerase Inhibitors

ⓟ **Sofosbuvir (Sovaldi)** is a polymerase inhibitor that treats patients infected with hepatitis C. Each patient diagnosed with hepatitis C should also be tested for HBV prior to initiating sofosbuvir therapy. For patients coinfected with hepatitis B and hepatitis C, fulminant hepatitis or hepatic failure may develop, or death may occur if hepatitis B is not treated.

Pharmacokinetics

Sofosbuvir is 65% protein bound. During metabolism, the liver pharmacologically forms the drug to an active nucleoside analog triphosphate GS-461203. The dephosphorylation results in the formation of the nucleoside inactive metabolite GS-331007. Sofosbuvir's half-life elimination is 0.4 hours. It reaches a peak in ½ to 2 hours and is 80% excreted in the urine, with 14% excreted in the feces.

Action and Use

Sofosbuvir is an antiviral agent used to treat hepatitis C. It inhibits HCV NS5B RNA-dependent RNA polymerase, which is essential for viral replication. It acts as a chain terminator.

Patient-related variables specific to the use of sofosbuvir include the following:

- Reproduction, pregnancy, and lactation:
  - When hepatitis C infection is detected during pregnancy, treatment should be deferred until after delivery.
  - The decision to breast-feed during therapy should consider the risk of exposure and the benefits to the infant.
- Abnormal kidney function and hepatic impairment:
  - No dosage adjustments related to abnormal kidney function.
  - Safety and efficacy have not been established in patients with decompensated cirrhosis.

Adverse Effects and Contraindications

Sofosbuvir is administered with ribavirin or peginterferon alfa. This section identifies the adverse effects reported with sofosbuvir combination therapy with ribavirin. The CNS adverse effects reported with sofosbuvir are fatigue, headache, insomnia, chills, and irritability. Pruritus and rash have been reported as dermatologic effects. Nausea, loss of appetite, and diarrhea are the gastrointestinal adverse effects. Six to twenty percent of patients developed anemia. Neutropenia is reported in less than 1% of patients. In postmarketing, patients have reported angioedema, bradycardia, and lactic acidosis. Sofosbuvir produces a rapid reduction in hepatitis C viral load during direct-acting therapy for hepatitis C and may lead to glucose metabolism with diabetes, resulting in potential hypoglycemia.

There are no reported contraindications with sofosbuvir; however, the contraindications noted with ribavirin or peginterferon alfa must be considered. Amiodarone administered with the sofosbuvir combination regimen can lead to fatal bradycardia with cardiac arrest.

Nursing Implications
Preventing Interactions

Amiodarone administered with the sofosbuvir combination regimen can lead to fatal bradycardia with cardiac arrest.

Administering the Medication

Administer sofosbuvir with or without food. In pediatric patients, the sofosbuvir pellets should be sprinkled in soft nonacidic foods such as pudding, mashed potatoes, or ice cream that are at or below room temperature.

Assessing for Therapeutic Effects

Assess for decreased ALT and AST levels.

Assessing for Adverse Effects

Assess for hypoglycemia in diabetic patients. Assess blood counts for anemia or neutropenia. Assess for signs and symptoms of fatigue. Assess for kidney and hepatic adverse effects.

Patient Teaching

See Box 23.2 for specific patient teaching guidelines for patients being administered antiviral agents. Diabetic patients must monitor blood sugar for hypoglycemia.

Antihepaciviral Nucleoside

P Ribavirin oral formulation is an antihepaciviral nucleoside administered for the treatment of hepatitis C. It also has off-label uses with chronic hepatitis E infection for immunocompromised patients who have received a solid organ transplant, been diagnosed with hematologic cancer, or who have HIV infection.

Pharmacokinetics

Ribavirin systemic is not protein bound. It is distributed in the erythrocytes and metabolized in the liver. The half-life is 44 hours with chronic hepatitis C infection. The peak of action is approximately 2 hours in children aged 3 years and older. In adults, it is 3 hours. The drug is primarily excreted in the urine and minimally in the feces.

Action and Use

Systemic ribavirin inhibits the replication of RNA and DNA viruses. It also inhibits viral RNA polymerase in the influenza virus. Systemic ribavirin is used to treat chronic hepatitis C.

Patient-related variables specific to the use of ribavirin systemic include the following:

- Age:
  - Administer with caution in older adults due to risk of anemia.
  - The combination of interferons for pediatric patients may result in decreased growth velocity.
  - Administration to neonates has resulted in fatal metabolic acidosis.
- Reproduction, pregnancy, and lactation:
  - Obtain a pregnancy test prior to initiating therapy and with ongoing treatment.
  - In utero exposure to ribavirin at doses one twentieth of the recommended human dose cause significant teratogenic and embryocidal events in animal studies.
  - Breast-feeding is not recommended if the infant is at risk of contracting hepatitis C.

Adverse Effects and Contraindications

Dermatologic adverse effects include alopecia, dermatitis, pruritus, and xeroderma. Growth retardation has been seen in children. Gastrointestinal adverse effects include abdominal pain, loss of appetite, dyspepsia, nausea, and vomiting. Hyperbilirubinemia was reported in 10% to 14% of patients. Arthralgia, dyspnea, and flulike symptoms have also been reported.

Ribavirin is contraindicated in patients who have reported hypersensitivity to the drug, in patients who are pregnant and their partners, and in patients diagnosed with thalassemia major and sickle cell anemia.

Nursing Implications
Preventing Interactions

A **BOXED WARNING** ◆ has been assigned to systemic ribavirin. Hemolytic anemia has been reported with ribavirin therapy. The anemia with ribavirin may become worse in patients with cardiac disease, potentially leading to fatal or nonfatal myocardial infarction.

Administering the Medication

Oral ribavirin should be administered with food. The capsule should not be opened, crushed, or broken. The drug should be handled with gloves and protective gown. In the event of the patient vomiting, the drug, eye, and face should be protected from contamination.

Assessing for Therapeutic Effects

Assess AST and ALT levels. In the event of increased hepatic insufficiency, the use of the drug should be discontinued.

Assessing for Adverse Effects

Assess the patient for signs and symptoms of hypersensitivity to the drug; the skin integrity for rash, hair loss, and itching; and GI function for nausea, pain, and vomiting.

Patient Teaching

See Box 23.2 for specific patient teaching guidelines for patients taking antiviral agents.

DRUGS FOR HUMAN IMMUNODEFICIENCY VIRUS (ANTIRETROVIRAL DRUGS)

The cycle of HIV, an infection of the immune system caused by a retrovirus, begins with the entry of the virus that binds to receptors on the surface of the CD4 cell, followed by reverse transcription, integration, replication, assembly, maturation, and budding. There are two types of HIV virus, HIV-1 and HIV-2. HIV can lead to AIDS.

To fight HIV, healthcare providers use a variety of **antiretroviral drugs** (medications used in the treatment of retroviral infections). The broad classifications of these drugs are the nucleoside and nucleotide reverse transcriptase inhibitors (NRTIs), nonnucleoside reverse transcriptase inhibitors (NNRTIs), protease inhibitors (PIs), and the integrase strand transfer inhibitors (INSTIs). Other drug classifications used to treat HIV include the fusion protein inhibitors and CCR5 antagonists (Fig. 23.2). In general, newer drugs and drug combinations are more effective for viral suppression. The selection of an antiretroviral regimen is determined from the results of drug resistance testing. The goal of ART is a reduction in morbidity and mortality. ART assists in improving patients' quality of life and suppressing conversion to AIDS. It is also important to educate patients about the prevention of HIV transmission and maternal–fetal transmission.

ART for the treatment of HIV/AIDS involves the use of several combinations of antiretroviral drugs. Combination therapy causes fewer serious adverse effects and is more convenient for patients, encouraging medication adherence. Combination therapy also assists in the prevention of drug resistance. The regimen usually consists of two NRTIs with an NNRTI or a PI. Authorities do not recommend using some of the older drugs for initial treatment but may suggest them when drug-resistant infections develop with the newer drugs. Patients often undergo genotypic or phenotypic testing for drug resistance to guide ART.

When administering antiretroviral agents, it is important to distinguish whether the patient has taken antiretroviral agents in the past. Patients who have received antiretroviral agents are *treatment experienced*, whereas those who have not received them are *treatment naive*. The most commonly prescribed antiretroviral drug classes used in initial therapy include nucleoside reverse transcriptase inhibitor combinations, INSTIs, bictegravir, PIs, and NNRTIs.

The U.S. Department of Health and Human Services recommends one of the following regimens for early management of HIV:

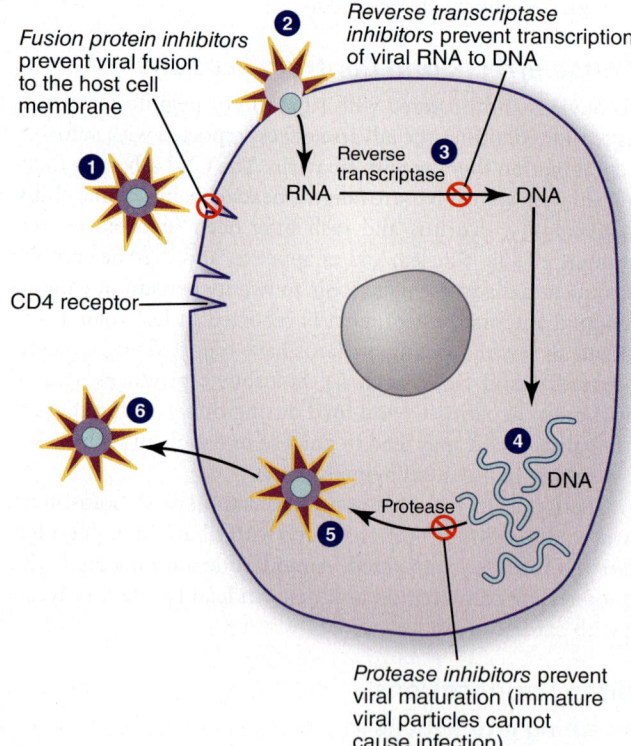

Figure 23.2. Human immunodeficiency virus (HIV) entry into cells and replication; actions of anti-HIV drugs. (1) The virus attaches to receptors (e.g., CD4 molecules) and coreceptors (CCR5 molecules) on the host cell membrane. (2) The virus becomes uncoated and releases its RNA into the host cell. (3) The enzyme reverse transcriptase converts RNA to DNA, which is necessary for viral replication. (4) The DNA codes for protein synthesis, which produces immature viral particles. (5) The enzyme protease assembles the immature viral particles into mature viruses. (6) Mature viruses are released from the host cell.

- Dolutegravir plus tenofovir and either emtricitabine or lamivudine
- Bictegravir, emtricitabine, and tenofovir alafenamide
- Ritonavir-boosted darunavir plus tenofovir and either emtricitabine or lamivudine

Combination ART is also important to prevent opportunistic infections in patients with HIV-1 or HIV-2.

- Dolutegravir with tenofovir alafenamide–emtricitabine or bictegravir–emtricitabine–tenofovir alafenamide are the recommended combinations.
- Tenofovir disoproxil fumarate and emtricitabine (Truvada) combine an NRTI and NNRTI. This combination drug interferes with HIV viral RNA-dependent DNA polymerase, resulting in the inhibition of viral replication.
- Tenofovir alafenamide and emtricitabine (Descovy) also combines reverse transcriptase inhibitor nucleoside and reverse transcriptase inhibitor nucleotide. It interferes with HIV viral RNA-dependent DNA polymerase activity, thus inhibiting viral replication.
- Abacavir and lamivudine (Epzicom) is a third NRTI combination. Abacavir is a guanosine analogue that through phosphorylation becomes carbovir triphosphate to inhibit viral replication. Lamivudine is a cytosine analog that inhibits HIV reverse transcription, thus inhibiting RNA-dependent DNA polymerase of reverse transcriptase.

Other regimens include INSTI raltegravir, elvitegravir/cobicistat, dolutegravir, PI of ritonavir-boosted lopinavir, or ritonavir-boosted darunavir. One of the newest combination medications for HIV is bictegravir, emtricitabine, and tenofovir alafenamide (Biktarvy). This medication combines drugs from the following broad classifications: integrase inhibitor, reverse transcriptase inhibitor, nucleoside, reverse transcriptase inhibitor, and nucleotide. It will be described in detail later in the chapter.

It is important to be familiar with the action, adverse effects, and nursing implications of each medication. The nurse must also educate patients and caregivers about administration of the medications and drug–drug interactions. For questions regarding any of the drugs, the nurse should contact a pharmacist or infection control physician.

Nucleoside Reverse Transcriptase Inhibitors

The NRTIs are structurally similar to DNA components (adenosine, cytosine, guanosine, and thymidine) and thus easily enter human cells and viruses in human cells. For example, **zidovudine** (Retrovir), the prototype, is able to substitute for thymidine. The drugs are more active in slowing the progression of acute infection rather than in treating chronically infected cells. Thus, they do not cure HIV infection or prevent transmission of the virus through sexual contact or blood contamination.

Pharmacokinetics

The oral preparation of zidovudine is quickly absorbed in the GI tract, reaching a peak of action in ½ to 1½ hours. The drug, which can cross the blood–brain barrier, is readily distributed to the CSF. It also crosses the placenta. Zidovudine is metabolized in the liver. It is 25% to 38% protein bound with a half-life of ½ to 3 hours. It is excreted in the urine; 72% to 74% is excreted as metabolites, with 14% to 18% excreted unchanged. (With the IV preparation, 45% to 60% is excreted as metabolites and 18% to 29% as unchanged drug.)

Action and Use

Like all NRTIs, zidovudine has the ability to incorporate into the DNA chains by viral reverse transcriptase. (HIV needs this enzyme to convert RNA to DNA and replicate.) Thus, the drug blocks the addition of further nucleotides and terminates viral replication.

Patients take zidovudine for the treatment of HIV infection—in combination with two or more other antiretroviral agents. Pregnant patients who are infected with HIV take the drug as monotherapy to prevent the transmission of HIV to the fetus. Should the patient not receive antiviral therapy during pregnancy, intravenous zidovudine is administered at the onset of labor. An unlabeled use is postexposure prophylaxis for HIV exposure with a multidrug regimen. Table 23.8 presents route and dosage information for zidovudine and other NRTIs.

Patient-related variables specific to the use of zidovudine include the following:

- Age:
  - Adverse cardiac effects have been associated with pediatric patients aged 7 to 16 years with perinatally acquired HIV.
- Reproduction, pregnancy, and lactation:
  - Viral suppression sustained below the limits of detection with ART and modification of therapy is recommended in patients of all genders who are living with HIV and planning pregnancy. The patient who will become pregnant must be informed of the potential risks and benefits of ART prior to conception and throughout the pregnancy.
  - No increased risk of overall teratogenic effects has been observed following first trimester exposure, according to the ART pregnancy registry.
  - To prevent maternal–fetal HIV transmission in neonates, experts recommend that zidovudine be given as soon as possible after birth—6 to 12 hours after delivery. It is necessary to continue the dose until the neonate is 6 weeks of age. Infants born to patients whose viral load (number of HIV RNA particles within the blood) is significantly below normal should receive zidovudine combined with nevirapine. If the infant develops a rash, there should be no dosage increase during the 14-day lead-in period.
  - Zidovudine has not been detected in the serum of breastfeeding infants exposed to breast milk.
- Abnormal kidney function and hepatic impairment:
  - For patients on hemodialysis or peritoneal dialysis and with a CrCl less than 15 mL/minute, the oral dose should be 100 mg every 6 to 8 hours or 300 mg daily. The IV dose should be 1 mg/kg every 6 to 8 hours.

Adverse Effects and Contraindications

Patients administered zidovudine have reported headache and malaise. Other significant adverse effects include

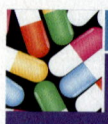

TABLE 23.8
DRUGS AT A GLANCE: Antiretroviral Drugs: Nucleoside Reverse Transcriptase Inhibitors (NRTIs)

Drug	Routes and Dosage Ranges	
	Adults	**Children**
Zidovudine (Retrovir; ✹ ALTI-Zidovudine, APO-Zidovudine, AZT, Retrovir [AZT])	300 mg PO twice daily or 200 mg PO three times per day; 1 mg/kg/dose IV every 4 h Prevention of maternal–fetal HIV transmission during labor and delivery (give when labor begins): 2 mg/kg IV as loading dose followed by a continuous IV infusion of 1 mg/kg/h until umbilical cord is clamped Cesarean section: begin 3 h before surgery Prevention of HIV following needlesticks: begin 2 h after exposure, 200 mg PO three times per day plus lamivudine 150 mg twice daily and a PI for high-risk exposure	Neonatal HIV: use in combination with other antiretroviral agents Premature infants <35 wk of gestational age, 2 mg/kg dose PO every 12 h or 1.5 mg/kg/dose IV every 12 h Infants <30 wk, increase dose to every 8 h at 4 wk of age Infants ≥30 wk, increase dose to every 8 h at 2 wk of age Full-term infants, 2 mg/kg/dose PO every 6 h or 1.5 mg/kg/dose every 6 h Prevention of maternal–fetal HIV transmission (zidovudine is used in neonates as monotherapy) 2 mg/kg/dose PO every 12 h or 1.5 mg/dose IV every 12 h; increase to every 8 h as follows: Preterm infants <30 wk, increase dose to every 8 h at 4 wk of age ≥30 wk, increase above dose to every 8 h at 2 wk of age Full-term infants 2 mg/kg PO every 6 h; alternate dosing <2.5 kg, 10 mg PO twice daily >2.5 kg, 15 mg PO twice daily 1.5 mg/kg IV every 6 h HIV: <6 wk, 2 mg/kg/dose PO every 6 h 6 wk to <12 y, 20 mg/m²/h IV continuous infusion 120 mg/m²/dose IV every 6 h ≥12 y, 1 mg/kg/dose IV intermittent infusion every 4 h around the clock
Abacavir sulfate (Ziagen; ✹ APO-Abacavir, MINT-Abacavir, Ziagen)	300 mg PO twice daily or 600 mg daily 1 mg/kg/dose IV every 4 h Hepatic impairment: 200 mg PO two times per day	3 mo to 16 y, 8 mg/kg PO twice daily, not to exceed 300 mg/dose
Abacavir and lamivudine (Epzicom; ✹ APO-Abacavir, APO-Lamivudine, Kivexa, Mylan Abacavir/Lamivudine, Teva-Abacavir/Lamivudine)	Abacavir 600 mg and lamivudine 300 mg PO daily	Children and adolescents weighing ≥25 kg: same as adult
Abacavir, lamivudine, and zidovudine (Trizivir; ✹ APO-Abacavir–Lamivudine–Zidovudine)	1 tablet PO twice daily; not recommended for patients who weigh <40 kg	<40 kg: not recommended ≥40 kg: PO 1 tablet twice daily
Didanosine (✹ Videx EC)	Videx <60 kg, 125 mg PO twice daily or 250 mg PO daily ≥60 kg, 200 mg PO twice daily or 400 mg PO daily Videx EC 25 kg to <60 kg, 250 mg PO daily ≥60 kg, 400 mg PO daily When taken with tenofovir, <60 kg and CrCl ≥60 mL/min, 200 mg once daily; ≥60 kg and CrCl ≥60 mL/min: 250 mg once daily	Videx 1 to <3 mo 50 mg/m² ≥3–8 mo 100 mg/m² PO twice daily >8 mo, 120 mg/m² PO twice daily (not to exceed adult dose) Videx EC ≥6 y 20 to <25 kg, 200 mg PO once daily 25 to <60 kg, 250 mg PO once daily ≥60 kg, 400 mg PO once daily

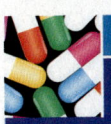

TABLE 23.8

DRUGS AT A GLANCE: Antiretroviral Drugs: Nucleoside Reverse Transcriptase Inhibitors (NRTIs) (Continued)

Drug	Routes and Dosage Ranges	
	Adults	**Children**
Dolutegravir and lamivudine (Dovato; ✦ Dovato) Combination antiretroviral agent: integrase inhibitor and reverse transcriptase inhibitor, nucleoside	Dolutegravir 50 mg and lamivudine 300 mg PO with or without food 2 h before or 6 h after cation-containing antacids or laxatives, oral supplements with iron or calcium	Safety and efficacy not studied
Dolutegravir, abacavir, and lamivudine (Triumeq, Triumeq PD; ✦ Triumeq) Combination drug: integrase inhibitor and reverse transcriptase inhibitor	Triumeq: Abacavir 600 mg, dolutegravir 50 mg, and lamivudine 300 mg Administer with or without food. If the patient is on concomitant therapy with efavirenz, fosamprenavir/ritonavir, tipranavir/ritonavir, carbamazepine, or rifampin and additional daily single-component dolutegravir tablet should be administered 12 h after Triumeq	Infants and Children weighing 10 -<25 kg: Trimeq PD tablets for oral suspension (abacavir 60 mg/dolutegravir 5 mg/lamivudine 30 mg per tablet) 10 -<14 kg: oral: 4 tablets daily 14 -<20 kg: oral 5 tablets once daily 20 -<25 kg: oral 6 tablets once daily Children and Adolescents weighing ≥25 kg: Trimeq (abacavir 600 mg/dolutegravir 50 mg/lamivudine 300 mg per tablet) oral one tablet once daily Oral administration with or without food. Administer 2 h before or 6 h after cation-containing antacids or laxatives, sucralfate, oral supplements containing iron or calcium at the same time if administered with food
Elvitegravir, cobicistat, emtricitabine, and tenofovir disoproxil fumarate (Stribild; ✦ Stribild)	Prior to initiation of therapy, the patient should be tested for hepatitis B. Hepatic function must be monitored closely Combination medication of: Elvitegravir: 150 mg Cobicistat: 150 mg Emtricitabine: 200 mg Tenofovir disoproxil fumarate: 300 mg One tablet PO daily	Children ≥12 y and weighing ≥35 kg one tablet PO once daily
Emtricitabine (Emtriva; ✦ Emtriva)	Capsules, 200 mg PO daily Solution, 240 mg PO daily	0–3 mo, 3 mg/kg/d PO 3 mo to 17 y, >33 kg, 200 mg PO once daily Solution, 6 mg/kg per PO per day
Emtricitabine and tenofovir (Truvada; ✦ Truvada)	Emtricitabine 200 mg and tenofovir 300 mg, one tablet PO daily	Not intended for children
Emtricitabine, tenofovir, and efavirenz (Atripla; ✦ Atripla)	Emtricitabine 200 mg, tenofovir disoproxil 300 mg, and efavirenz 600 mg; one tablet PO daily	Not intended for children
Lamivudine (Epivir, Epivir-HBV; ✦ 3TC, APO-Lamivudine, APO-Lamivudine HBV, Heptovir)	150 mg PO two times per day or 300 mg/d; PO as a single dose in combination with other antiretroviral agents	1–3 mo, 4 mg/kg PO twice daily 3 mo to 16 y, 4 mg/kg PO two times per day; max dose 150 mg two times daily
Stavudine	<60 kg, 30 mg PO every 12 h ≥60 kg, 40 mg PO every 12 h	Birth to 13 d, 0.5 mg/kg PO every 12 h ≥14 d and <30 kg, 1 mg/kg PO every 12 h ≥30 kg, same as adults
Tenofovir disoproxil fumarate (Viread; ✦ APO-Tenofovir, Auro-Tenofovir, JAMP-Tenofovir, MYLAN-Tenofovir Disoproxil, NAT-Tenofovir, PMS-Tenofovir, TEVA-Tenofovir, Viread)	300 mg PO daily with meals	≥12 y and ≥35 kg, same as adults
Zidovudine and lamivudine (Combivir; ✦ APO-Lamivudine–Zidovudine, Combivir, TEVA-Lamivudine/Zidovudine)	Zidovudine 300 mg and lamivudine 150 mg PO daily	Adolescents ≥30 kg, same as adults

nausea, vomiting, and anorexia. The FDA has issued a **BOXED WARNING** ◆ related to the adverse effects of granulocytopenia, aplastic or hemolytic anemia, pancytopenia with bone marrow hypoplasia, leukopenia, and lymphadenopathy with zidovudine. It is necessary to adjust the dosage in patients who develop anemia or neutropenia. Two other **BOXED WARNING** ◆ for zidovudine relate to lactic acidosis and severe hepatomegaly with steatosis and symptomatic myopathy and myositis. The risk of liver disease increases in females, during pregnancy, with patients who have a BMI of 30.0 or higher, and with prolonged use. If clinical or laboratory signs of lactic acidosis or hepatotoxicity develop, it is essential that the drug be discontinued.

Contraindications to zidovudine include a known hypersensitivity to the drug or history of lactic acidosis.

Nursing Implications
Preventing Interactions

Antiretroviral agents administered in combination with zidovudine result in an increased risk of lactic acidosis and hepatomegaly. Other drugs also have significant effects when taken with zidovudine. Clozapine increases the risk of agranulocytosis. If possible, patients should not receive clozapine and zidovudine together. Acyclovir and valacyclovir enhance CNS depression. Ribavirin enhances the development of anemia. Acetaminophen, ganciclovir, and interferon alfa enhance bone marrow suppression. Other medications interact with zidovudine, increasing or decreasing its effects (Box 23.3).

Administering the Medication

Patients may take oral preparation of zidovudine with or without food. They should take the drug around the clock to avoid variations in serum peak and trough levels. The nurse should mix the parenteral preparation in 5% dextrose and water or normal saline. Infusion should take place over ½ hour in neonates and 1 hour in children and adults. Zidovudine is incompatible with blood products and protein solutions.

Assessing for Therapeutic Effects

The nurse monitors the patient's CD4 and cell count for increase or decrease in viral load. An increase in the CD4 count indicates a decrease in viral load and the ability to fight viral infections. In addition, the nurse assesses the patient's clinical status for decrease in the development of opportunistic infections.

BOX 23.3 *Drug Interactions: Zidovudine*

Drugs That Increase the Effect of Zidovudine
- Divalproex, doxorubicin, fluconazole, flucytosine, indomethacin, methadone, pentamidine, probenecid, vincristine, valproic acid
  Decrease the metabolism of zidovudine, thus increasing serum levels, leading to toxicity

Drugs That Decrease the Effect of Zidovudine
- Protease inhibitors, rifamycin derivatives (excluding rifabutin)
  Decrease serum concentration

Assessing for Adverse Effects

The nurse assesses for malaise, CNS depression, and GI symptoms such as nausea, vomiting, and diarrhea, as well as for myalgia and hepatomegaly. The development of anemia usually occurs 2 to 4 weeks after the start of therapy. Neutropenia is most likely to occur in 6 to 8 weeks. It is important to obtain the patient's CBC as a baseline measure before therapy begins and then every 2 weeks from then on. In addition, the nurse assesses the hemoglobin, hematocrit, and granulocyte count for hematologic toxicity. If the hemoglobin level is less than 7.5 g/dL or the reduction is greater than 25% of the baseline value, it may be necessary to interrupt therapy and administer transfusions. This is also the case if the granulocyte count is less than 750/mm^3 or greater than 50% of the baseline measure.

Patient Teaching

Box 23.4 identifies general patient teaching guidelines for antiretroviral drugs. Because lactic acidosis may develop, the nurse teaches the patient the signs and symptoms of this condition, including musculoskeletal pain.

Other Drugs in the Class

Abacavir sulfate (Ziagen) inhibits the viral reverse transcriptase through competition with the natural DNA nucleoside and incorporation into viral DNA. It is contraindicated in moderate to severe hepatic impairment. Abacavir is administered in combination with other antiretroviral agents. The FDA has issued a **BOXED WARNING** ◆ stating that patients taking abacavir may have serious and sometimes fatal hypersensitivity reactions. Patients who test positive for *HLA-B*5701* allele are at greatest risk for hypersensitivity reactions. Patients may also be at risk for lactic acidosis.

Abacavir, lamivudine, and zidovudine (Trizivir) is used for HIV-1 treatment. The FDA has issued a **BOXED WARNING** ◆ stating that patients with the *HLA-B*5701* allele are prone to a hypersensitivity reaction. The medications in this HIV drug work synergistically to inhibit reverse transcriptase by way of DNA chain termination after the incorporation of the nucleoside analogue and delay the emergence of mutations.

Didanosine is an oral antiretroviral that is administered 30 minutes before meals or 2 hours after meals. The drug blocks the HIV replication in T cells and monocytes to block viral DNA synthesis and replication. Patients should not combine it with alcohol due to the increased risk of pancreatitis. It is necessary to reduce the drug dosage in abnormal kidney function.

Dolutegravir and lamivudine (Dovato) combine dolutegravir, an INSTI and lamivudine, a cytosine analog, to block the strand transfer step of retroviral DNA integration and inhibition of RNA and DNA polymerase activities of reverse transcriptase. The patient's CD4 count and viral DNA should be monitored closely.

Dolutegravir, abacavir, and lamivudine (Triumeq, Triumeq PD) have the same action as dolutegravir and lamivudine and also convert cellular enzymes to the active metabolite, carbovir triphosphate, to inhibit the activity of reverse transcriptase through competition with the dGTP substrate and incorporating in the viral DNA.

Elvitegravir, cobicistat, emtricitabine, and tenofovir disoproxil fumarate (Stribild) combine an integrase inhibitor,

BOX 23.4 Patient Teaching Guidelines for Antiretroviral Drugs

- Take all antiretroviral agents as prescribed.
- Inform the prescriber of any vitamins, herbs, or OTC medications.
- Birth control pills may not work with antiretrovirals.
- Do not stop the medication without informing the prescriber.
- If a missed dose is more than 8 hours, skip the missed dose and go back to the normal time.
- If symptoms worsen, call the physician or nurse practitioner.
- Wash hands frequently and thoroughly; this helps prevent most infections.
- Have immunizations against viral infections as indicated.
- Always practice safe sex, such as barrier methods during intercourse.
- In cases of intravenous drug use, use and promote the use of clean needles.
- Effective treatment of HIV infection requires close adherence to drug therapy regimens involving several drugs and daily doses. Missing as few as one or two doses can decrease blood levels of antiretroviral drugs and result in increased HIV replication and development of drug-resistant viral strains.
- Request information about adverse effects associated with the specific drugs you are taking and what you should do if they occur.
- Have regular blood tests, including viral load, CD4+ cell count, complete blood count, and others as indicated (e.g., tests of kidney and liver function).
- Keep your healthcare providers informed about all medications being taken; do not take any other drugs (including drugs of abuse, herbal preparations or products, vitamin/mineral supplements, nonprescription drugs) without consulting a healthcare provider. These preparations may make anti-HIV medications less effective or more toxic.
- These medications vary in their interactions with food and should be taken appropriately for optimal benefit. Unless otherwise instructed, take the drugs as follows:
    - Abacavir, Combivir, emtricitabine, famciclovir, fosamprenavir, Kaletra tablets, lamivudine, nevirapine, tenofovir, Trizivir, valacyclovir, and zidovudine with or without food. However, do not take abacavir or efavirenz with a high-fat meal.
    - Atripla, efavirenz, entecavir, or indinavir on an empty stomach or 1 hour before or 2 hours after a meal.
    - Atazanavir, darunavir, ganciclovir, Kaletra oral solution, nelfinavir, ritonavir, and tipranavir with food.
    - Saquinavir within 2 hours after a meal or with a full meal.
- To give nelfinavir to infants and young children, mix the oral powder with a small amount of water, milk, or formula (if necessary). Give the entire amount to the child, who must take it all to obtain the full dose. Do not use acidic foods or juices (e.g., applesauce, orange juice, apple juice) because they produce a bitter taste.

reverse transcriptase inhibitor, nucleoside, and NRTI. The combination medication is administered orally with food. It is used to treat HIV-1 in adult and pediatric patients aged 12 years and older. It is contraindicated with alfuzosin, carbamazepine, ergot derivatives, phenobarbital, phenytoin, rifampin, and sildenafil. The CD4, HIV RNA plasma levels, serum creatinine, serum phosphorous, and creatinine clearance should be monitored closely. The patient should be administered calcium and vitamin D supplements.

Emtricitabine (Emtriva) inhibits HIV-1 reverse transcriptase to inhibit HIV activity. Again, dosage reduction in abnormal kidney function is necessary. Prior to beginning therapy, it is important to check liver function and assess it periodically throughout treatment. The nurse also assesses patients with depression for suicidal ideation. In addition, the nurse instructs patients to avoid driving or operating machinery until their response to the medication is known.

Emtricitabine and tenofovir (Truvada) is a reverse transcriptase inhibitor, nucleoside, and reverse transcriptase nucleotide. Emtricitabine is a cytosine analogue. Tenofovir is an analog of adenosine 5 monophosphate. This combination interferes with HIV viral RNA-dependent DNA polymerase to inhibit viral replication.

Emtricitabine, tenofovir, and efavirenz (Atripla) add the NNRTI of HIV-1 to block the RNA-dependent and DNA-dependent polymerase to assist in blocking HIV-1 replication.

Stavudine is an NRTI that is administered in combination with other antiretroviral medications. The World Health Organization recommends 30 mg every 12 hours in all adult and adolescent patients regardless of their weight. Geriatric patients require close monitoring for peripheral neuropathy. The dosage of stavudine should be reduced in patients with abnormal kidney function.

Nonnucleoside Reverse Transcriptase Inhibitors

The NNRTIs inhibit viral replication in infected cells by directly binding to reverse transcriptase and preventing its function. NRTIs and NNRTIs inhibit reverse transcriptase by different mechanisms, and therefore, they may have synergistic antiviral effects. The prototype NNRTI is P **efavirenz** (Sustiva).

Pharmacokinetics

An oral drug, efavirenz is absorbed in the GI tract. Absorption is increased after consumption of a fatty meal. Its peak of action occurs in 3 to 5 hours. Efavirenz is approximately 99% protein bound, primarily to albumin. The drug is metabolized by the hepatic enzymes cytochrome P450 (CYP) enzymes CYP3A4 and CYP2B6, which convert it to inactivated hydroxylated metabolites. The serum half-life is 52 to 76 hours after a single dose and 40 to 55 hours after multiple doses. It is eliminated as metabolites in the feces (16% to 61%) and the urine (14% to 34%).

Action and Use

Efavirenz binds to reverse transcriptase to block RNA-dependent and DNA-dependent polymerase activities that includes HIV-1 replication. People take the medication in combination with other antiretroviral agents for HIV-1 infection. Table 23.9

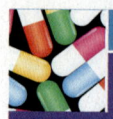

TABLE 23.9

DRUGS AT A GLANCE: Antiretroviral Drugs: Nonnucleoside Reverse Transcriptase Inhibitors (NNRTIs)

Drug	Routes and Dosage Ranges	
	Adults	**Children**
ⓟ Efavirenz (Sustiva; 🍁 Auro-Efavirenz, JAMP-Efavirenz, MYLAN-Efavirenz, Sustiva, TEVA-Efavirenz)	600 mg PO daily Dosage adjustments: with concomitant rifampin (if patient ≥50 kg), 800 mg PO daily; with concomitant voriconazole, efavirenz 300 mg PO daily and voriconazole 400 mg PO every 12 h	3.5–5 kg: 100 mg daily 5–7.5 kg: 150 mg daily 7.5–15 kg: 200 mg daily 15 to <20 kg: 250 mg daily 20 to <25 mg: 300 mg daily 25 to <32.5 kg: 350 mg daily 32.5 to <40 kg: 400 mg daily ≥40 kg: 600 mg once daily
Delavirdine mesylate	400 mg PO three times per day	≥16 y: same as adult dose
Etravirine (Intelence; 🍁 Intelence)	200 mg PO twice daily after meals	Not recommended
Nevirapine (🍁 APO-Nevirapine XR, Auro-Nevirapine, JAMP-Nevirapine, MYLAN-Nevirapine)	Initial, 200 mg twice daily for 14 d; maintenance, 200 mg PO twice daily (immediate-release tablets) in combination with additional antiretroviral medications; 400 mg PO once daily (extended-release tablets)	Immediate-release tablets, 150 mg/m^2/dose PO once daily for the first 14 d (max dose: 200 mg/d); increase dose to 150 mg/m^2/dose PO twice daily if no rash or untoward effects (max 400 mg/d)
Rilpivirine (Edurant; 🍁 Edurant)	PO 25 mg once daily	Children ≥12 y, refer to adult dosing

presents route and dosage information for efavirenz and the other NNRTIs.

Patient-related variables specific to the use of efavirenz include the following:

- Age:
  - According to current guidelines, efavirenz is not used in infants or children less than 3 years of age.
  - When administering the medication to children who cannot swallow, the capsules can be opened and mixed with grape jelly to improve peppery taste.
- Reproduction, pregnancy, and lactation:
  - The manufacturer recommends patients of reproductive potential undergo pregnancy testing prior to the initiation of efavirenz.
  - Efavirenz has a moderate level of transfer across the human placenta.
  - The HHS perinatal guidelines consider efavirenz an alternative ART for pregnant patients living with HIV who are antiretroviral naive, who have had ART therapy in the past but are restarting, or who require a new ART regimen. Patients who become pregnant while taking efavirenz in the first trimester do not have an increased risk of teratogenic effects. Efavirenz can be continued if viral suppression is sufficient.
  - Fetal neural tube defects have been reported with efavirenz, but the risk is not known to be greater than the general population.
  - Efavirenz is present in breast milk.
- Abnormal kidney function and hepatic impairment:
  - No dosage adjustments required in impaired kidney function.
  - Efavirenz is not recommended in moderate to severe hepatic impairment.

Adverse Effects and Contraindications

CNS adverse effects include dizziness, headache, insomnia, altered ability to concentrate, abnormal dreams, nervousness, and depression. Genitourinary adverse effects are kidney stone and hematuria. Patients may experience fever and fatigue, skin rash, erythema multiforme, Stevens-Johnson syndrome, and toxic epidermal necrolysis. In addition, patients may have increased levels of serum cholesterol, AST, and ALT.

Contraindications to efavirenz include a known hypersensitivity to the medication and suicidal ideation. Because the drug may cause undesired fetal effects, particularly in the first trimester, patients who are pregnant should not take it. Efavirenz is also contraindicated with breast-feeding.

Nursing Implications
Preventing Interactions

Taking efavirenz with a fatty meal will increase the medication's serum effects. The herbal supplement St. John's wort will decrease efavirenz antiretroviral activity. Many medications interact with efavirenz, increasing or decreasing its effects (Box 23.5).

Administering the Medication

Patients who experience CNS adverse effects, such as CNS depression, should take efavirenz at bedtime. They may take the medication on an empty stomach. Patients should not take efavirenz for 2 hours after consuming a high-fat meal. They should not discontinue efavirenz suddenly or without the consent of the prescriber.

BOX 23.5	**Drug Interactions: Efavirenz**

Drugs That Increase the Effect of Efavirenz
- Fluconazole, ritonavir
  Increase serum levels
- Alcohol
  Increases central nervous system depression

Drugs That Decrease the Effects of Efavirenz
- Rifampin, saquinavir
  Decrease serum levels

BOX 23.6	**Drug Interactions: Saquinavir**

Drugs That Increase Effects of Saquinavir
- Delavirdine, clarithromycin, indinavir, ketoconazole, ritonavir
  Increase serum levels

Drugs That Decrease the Effects of Saquinavir
- Carbamazepine, dexamethasone, phenobarbital, phenytoin, rifabutin, rifampin
  Decrease serum levels

Assessing for Therapeutic Effects

The nurse assesses the CD4 count for increased ability to fight against viral infections.

Assessing for Adverse Effects

The nurse assesses for skin rash and onset of Stevens-Johnson syndrome as well as for lack of concentration, increased nervousness, and impaired psychiatric effects. It is also necessary to assess for alterations in GI status such as nausea, vomiting, and diarrhea, as well as urinary output for bleeding and complaints of pain related to kidney stones. In addition, the nurse assesses the serum cholesterol, AST, and ALT values for possible increases.

Patient Teaching

Box 23.4 identifies general patient teaching guidelines for antiretroviral drugs. The nurse should teach patients to use barrier contraceptives when taking efavirenz, not to drive or operate machinery until the effects of the medication are known, and to notify the prescriber in the event of pregnancy.

Other Drugs in the Class

Delavirdine mesylate, etravirine (Intelence), and nevirapine are NNRTIs used in combination with additional antiretroviral agents to treat HIV. Delavirdine mesylate has life-threatening adverse effects when combined with CYP3A4 inducers. The drugs of greatest concern are dysrhythmic agents, clarithromycin, dapsone, rifabutin, benzodiazepines, calcium channel blockers, ergot derivatives, indinavir, saquinavir, quinidine, and warfarin. Administration of etravirine with antifungal agents will increase serum levels of etravirine and decrease the antifungal activity. Etravirine should be administered with food to increase absorption. Nevirapine is administered in combination with zidovudine to pregnant patients who are HIV positive to prevent transmission of HIV to the fetus. The ◆ BOXED WARNING ◆ issued by the FDA states that the most significant adverse effect of nevirapine is the abrupt onset of flu-like symptoms, abdominal pain, fever with or without a rash, and jaundice. These adverse effects may progress to hepatic failure and encephalopathy.

Rilpivirine (Edurant) is useful in treatment-naive patients whose viral load is less than 100,000 copies/mL and whose CD4 count is ≥200 cells/μL. It is administered alone or in combination with emtricitabine–tenofovir–disoproxil fumarate and rilpivirine–emtricitabine–tenofovir alafenamide. Caution is warranted in patients with long QT syndrome or torsade de pointes. It is important to avoid the use of rilpivirine in patients with reduced kidney function. During the administration of rilpivirine, it is necessary to monitor a patient's cholesterol levels because changes may occur (less than or equal to 48 weeks).

Protease Inhibitors

The PIs are antiretroviral drugs that exert their effects against HIV at a different phase of its life cycle than reverse transcriptase inhibitors. They inhibit the HIV enzyme protease, which is required to process viral protein precursors into mature particles capable of infecting other cells. Thus, PIs are active in both acutely and chronically infected cells. Compared with the NNRTIs and the integrase inhibitors, the PIs have a high genetic barrier to resistance. **Ⓟ Saquinavir mesylate** is the prototype PI. Note that other PIs have replaced saquinavir as the PI of choice because of increasing resistance and adverse effects. If saquinavir is administered, electrocardiogram (ECG) monitoring for long QT syndrome is necessary. Reportedly, diminished resistance results with lopinavir/ritonavir (Kaletra), atazanavir/ritonavir, and darunavir/ritonavir.

The PIs are most commonly administered in combination with the nucleosides. In addition, ritonavir is a PI, and cobicistat is a cytochrome P450 inhibitor. Each of these medications is administered in combination with other antiretroviral agents to boost antiretroviral activity. These agents are described as boosting agents. Pharmacokinetic boosting improves the plasma trough concentrations and increases the drug's half-life and maximum concentration.

Pharmacokinetics

Absorption of saquinavir mesylate is in the GI tract. However, absorption is enhanced when the drug is taken with a high-fat meal. It is 99% protein bound, and there is no distribution in the CSF. Saquinavir is metabolized by the liver enzyme CYP3A4 with extensive first-pass effect. The half-life is 13 hours. Saquinavir is excreted primarily in the feces (only 1% to 3% in the urine) within 5 days.

Action and Use

Saquinavir binds to the site of HIV-1 protease activity to prevent the cleavage of viral gag-pol polyproteins that are required for the maturation of the HIV virus. This action produces immature noninfectious viral particles.

The main purpose of using saquinavir is to reduce the viral load in HIV—in combination with other antiretroviral agents. Prescribers may also order it with colchicine for familial Mediterranean fever, gout prophylaxis, and gout flare-up and with phosphodiesterase-5 enzyme inhibitors for pulmonary hypertension or erectile dysfunction. Table 23.10

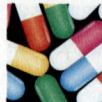

TABLE 23.10
DRUGS AT A GLANCE: Antiretroviral Drugs: Protease Inhibitors (PIs)

Drug	Routes and Dosage Ranges	
	Adults	**Children**
ⓟ Saquinavir mesylate	1,000 mg PO twice daily with ritonavir 100 mg in combination with a full meal	5 to <15 kg: 50 mg/kg/dose twice daily plus ritonavir 3 mg/kg/dose twice daily 15 to <40 kg: 50 mg/kg/dose twice daily plus ritonavir 2.5 mg/kg/dose twice daily ≥40 kg: 1,000 mg twice daily plus ritonavir 100 mg twice daily
Atazanavir (Reyataz; ✸MYLAN-Atazanavir, Reyataz, TEVA-Atazanavir)	Antiretroviral naive, 300 mg PO once daily plus ritonavir 100 mg; patients who do not tolerate ritonavir: 400 mg PO once daily Antiretroviral experienced, 300 mg PO once daily plus ritonavir 100 mg Pregnant patients, 300 mg PO once daily plus ritonavir 100 mg once daily	6–12 y Antiretroviral naive 15–24 kg, 150 mg PO once daily plus ritonavir 80 mg once daily 25–31 kg, 200 mg PO once daily plus ritonavir 100 mg PO once daily 32–38 kg, 250 mg once daily plus ritonavir 100 mg PO once daily ≥39 kg, 300 mg PO once daily plus 100 mg once daily Antiretroviral experienced 25–31 kg, 200 mg PO once daily plus ritonavir 100 mg PO once daily 32–38 kg, 250 mg once daily plus ritonavir 100 mg PO once daily ≥39 kg, 300 mg PO once daily plus 100 mg once daily
Darunavir (Prezista; ✸APO-Darunavir, Prezista)	Antiretroviral naive, 800 mg PO once daily with ritonavir 100 mg Antiretroviral experienced, if genotypic testing is not possible, 600 mg PO with ritonavir 100 mg once daily	≥6 y ≥20 to <30 kg, 375 mg PO twice daily with ritonavir 50 mg twice daily ≥30 to <40 kg, 450 mg PO twice daily with ritonavir 60 mg twice daily ≥40 kg, 600 mg PO twice daily with ritonavir 100 mg twice daily
Fosamprenavir calcium (Lexiva; ✸Telzir)	Unboosted regimen: 1,400 mg PO twice daily Ritonavir-boosted regimen, 1,400 mg PO plus ritonavir 100–200 mg once daily (not recommended in PI-experienced patients) Or 700 mg PO plus ritonavir 100 mg twice daily	Antiretroviral naive 2–5 y, 30 mg/kg/dose PO twice daily ≥6 y Unboosted regimen, 30 mg/kg/dose Ritonavir-boosted regimen, 18 mg/kg/dose plus 3 mg/kg/dose ritonavir PO twice daily (do not exceed adult dosage)
Indinavir sulfate	Unboosted regimen, 800 mg PO every 8 h Boosted regimen, 800 mg PO twice daily with ritonavir 100–200 mg When combined with other antiretroviral agents, consult manufacturer's recommendations	Safety and efficacy not established
Lopinavir/ritonavir (Kaletra; ✸Kaletra)	Antiretroviral naive or antiretroviral experienced, lopinavir 400 mg/ritonavir 100 mg PO twice daily Antiretroviral naive or antiretroviral experienced with efavirenz, fosamprenavir, nelfinavir, nevirapine, lopinavir 500 mg/ritonavir 125 mg twice daily, or lopinavir 533 mg/ritonavir 133 mg solution PO twice daily Once-daily dosing, lopinavir 800 mg/ritonavir 200 mg PO once daily	14 d to 6 mo, 16 mg/kg PO twice daily 6 mo to 18 y: <15 kg, 12 mg/kg PO twice daily 15–40 kg, 10 mg/kg PO twice daily >40 kg, lopinavir 400 mg/ritonavir 100 mg PO twice daily Combination therapy with efavirenz, fosamprenavir, nelfinavir, or nevirapine 6 mo to 18 y: <15 kg, 13 mg/kg PO twice daily 15–45 kg, 11 mg/kg PO twice daily >45 kg, same as adults

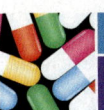

TABLE 23.10
DRUGS AT A GLANCE: Antiretroviral Drugs: Protease Inhibitors (PIs) (Continued)

Drug	Routes and Dosage Ranges	
	Adults	**Children**
Nelfinavir mesylate (Viracept; ❋Viracept)	750 mg PO three times per day or 1,250 mg PO twice daily	2–13 y: 45–55 mg/kg PO twice daily or 25–35 mg/kg PO three times daily not to exceed 2,500 mg/d (mix oral powder in milk or water/do not mix with acidic juices)
Ritonavir (Norvir; ❋Norvir)	600 mg PO twice daily; increase dose as follows: 300 mg twice daily for 1 d, 400 mg twice daily for 2 d, and 500 mg twice daily for 1 d. Then increase by 100 mg twice daily every 2–3 d to recommended dosage of 600 mg PO twice daily	>1 mo: 350–400 mg/m² PO twice daily; initial dose 250 mg/m² PO twice daily; titrate upward every 2–3 d by 50 mg/m² PO twice daily
Tipranavir (Aptivus; ❋Aptivus)	500 mg PO twice daily (administer with ritonavir 200 mg PO twice daily)	≥2 y: 14 mg/kg or 375 mg/m² PO twice daily; max 500 mg/dose (administer with ritonavir 6 mg/kg or 150 mg/m² twice daily)

summarizes route and dosage information for saquinavir and the other PIs.

Patient-related variables specific to the use of saquinavir include the following:

- Age:
  - The administration saquinavir and the other PIs in older adults warrant caution because of the risk of organ dysfunction.
- Reproduction, pregnancy, and lactation:
  - Saquinavir crosses the human placenta.
  - Maternal ART may be associated with adverse pregnancy outcomes including preterm delivery, stillbirth, low birth weight, and small for gestational age.
  - Monitor pregnant patients more frequently when ART is prescribed.
  - It is unknown if saquinavir is present in breast milk.
- Abnormal kidney function and hepatic impairment:
  - No dosage adjustment is necessary, but saquinavir should be administered cautiously in severe abnormal kidney function or kidney failure with replacement therapy.

Adverse Effects and Contraindications

Cardiovascular adverse effects include hypertension, hypotension, and chest pain. CNS adverse effects include back pain, fatigue, neuropathy, paresthesia, anxiety, depression, and suicidal ideation. Dermatologic adverse effects are pruritus, rash, and eczema. Hematologic adverse effects are thrombocytopenia, pancytopenia, and anemia. Elevations in creatinine kinase, AST and ALT, and bilirubin have occurred.

Contraindications to saquinavir include a known hypersensitivity to the drug. Other conditions that preclude its use are congenital or acquired prolongation of the QT interval, atrioventricular block, hepatic impairment, refractory hypokalemia, or hypomagnesemia.

Nursing Implications
Preventing Interactions

Medications that interact with saquinavir are found in Box 23.6. The use of ergot alkaloids with PIs increases the risk of ergot toxicity. St. John's wort and garlic decrease the antiretroviral activity of saquinavir. One quart per day of grapefruit juice will increase plasma concentrations of saquinavir, leading to the development of adverse drug effects.

Administering the Medication

Patients should take saquinavir with ritonavir. To ensure maximum bioavailability, the nurse should instruct patients to take saquinavir within 2 hours of a meal or on a full stomach. Patients should have an ECG prior to the start of therapy and 3 to 4 days after therapy is begun. It is also necessary to measure serum potassium, magnesium, triglycerides, and cholesterol before the initiation of therapy.

Assessing for Therapeutic Effects

The nurse assesses for an increase in T helper CD4 cells. The CD4 count is a measure of the ability to fight infections.

Assessing for Adverse Effects

The nurse assesses for ECG-related changes, specifically QT prolongation, as well as for signs and symptoms of peripheral neuropathy. In addition, the nurse assesses the mouth for signs of ulcerations related to increase gastric acid.

It is important to check laboratory results. The nurse assesses the CBC and bilirubin for anemia, thrombocytopenia, and pancytopenia; serum potassium and magnesium levels; and AST or ALT for elevation.

Patient Teaching

Box 23.4 presents patient teaching guidelines for antiretroviral drugs.

Other Drugs in the Class

Atazanavir (Reyataz), darunavir (Prezista), fosamprenavir (Lexiva), indinavir, lopinavir/ritonavir (Kaletra), nelfinavir mesylate (Viracept), ritonavir, and tipranavir (Aptivus) are other PI medications used either alone or in combination with other antiretroviral agents in treating HIV-naive or experienced patients. Atazanavir and darunavir are contraindicated in hypersensitivity due to the risk of Stevens-Johnson syndrome. Hyperlipidemia is a risk with these medications, so the cholesterol level should be monitored. Lopinavir/ritonavir has significant adverse effects, including hypertriglyceridemia, myocardial infarction, and GI toxicity. Lopinavir, in this combination, may be part of a multidrug antiretroviral regimen. Patients should take it with food. Monitoring for signs and symptoms of pancreatitis, onset of diabetes, and triglyceride elevation is necessary. The nurse should instruct the patient about blood glucose testing. It is also important to monitor amylase, triglycerides, inorganic phosphorus, thyroid function, and CBC. An adverse effect of ritonavir is a prolonged QT interval. Patients taking tipranavir have developed a loss of glycemic control, thus the blood glucose level should be monitored. The application of sunscreen is important due to photosensitivity.

CYTOCHROME P450 INHIBITOR

Cobicistat (Tybost) is a boosting agent administered with atazanavir or darunavir or other retroviral agent. The purpose in combining cobicistat with antiretroviral agents is based on its action to increase exposure of CYP3A4 substrates in atazanavir or darunavir. This action increases the antiretroviral activity of these antiretroviral agents.

NCLEX Success

5. Which of the following electrocardiographic changes warrant the discontinuation of saquinavir mesylate?
   A. prolongation of the QT interval
   B. inverted T wave
   C. elongated ST segment
   D. premature ventricular contraction

Integrase Strand Transfer Inhibitors

INSTIs block the action of integrase, a viral enzyme of HIV-1 essential for viral replication. The only member of this drug class approved by the FDA is **raltegravir** (Isentress, Isentress HD). This drug is comparable to efavirenz in terms of its ability to suppress HIV.

Pharmacokinetics

Raltegravir is absorbed by the GI tract. The rate of absorption is doubled if the drug is taken with a high-fat meal. It is 83% protein bound. Raltegravir is metabolized by hepatic glucuronidation mediated by UGT1A1. The serum half-life is 9 hours. The drug is eliminated in the feces and urine.

Action and Use

Raltegravir blocks HIV-1 integrase to prevent the formation of the HIV-1 provirus to decrease the viral load and increase the active CD4 cells. Specifically, after HIV reverse transcriptase enters CD4 T cells, the enzyme transcribes viral RNA into DNA. As the integrase combines with viral DNA and other cellular cofactors, it forms the preintegration complex. The integrase removes the nucleotide from the 3′ terminus to expose reactive hydroxyl groups. The preintegration complex enters the host cell nucleus, binding to host cell DNA. Integrase then nicks each strand of the host cell DNA, exposing 5′ phosphate groups to enable covalent bonding of host and viral DNA. When the strand transfer is complete, the host cell enzymes repair the gaps between the viral and host DNA.

Raltegravir is a first-line antiviral agent that is administered with tenofovir and emtricitabine to treatment-experienced adults. These patients must have evidence of viral replication and HIV-1 strains resistant to multiple antiretroviral drugs. Table 23.11 supplies information about the route of administration and dosage for raltegravir.

Patient-related variables specific to the use of raltegravir include the following:

- Abnormal kidney function and hepatic impairment:
  - With kidney failure with replacement therapy, the dosage should be administered after dialysis on dialysis days.
  - No dosage adjustments with hepatic impairment.
- Reproduction, pregnancy, and lactation:
  - Raltegravir has a high rate of transfer across the placenta.
  - No increased risk of overall teratogenic effects has been observed following first trimester exposure, according to data collected by ART.

Adverse Effects and Contraindications

Few adverse effects occur with raltegravir. The most common include headache, dizziness, nausea, diarrhea, vomiting, abdominal pain, fever, and rhabdomyolysis. Sometimes serum glucose level, hepatic enzymes, and lipase level increase, though researchers have found that patients show excellent tolerance and lack of effect on lipids.

Contraindications include a known hypersensitivity to the medication. The drug is not suitable for treatment-naive patients and patients who are breast-feeding.

Nursing Implications

Preventing Interactions

Some medications interact with raltegravir, increasing or decreasing its effects (Box 23.7). St. John's wort decreases the effects of raltegravir.

Administering the Medication

Patients may take raltegravir with or without meals.

Assessing Therapeutic and Adverse Effects

The nurse assesses for an increase in T helper CD4 cells. The CD4 count measures the ability to fight against infections.

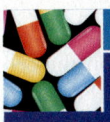

TABLE 23.11
DRUGS AT A GLANCE: Antiretroviral Drugs: Integrase Strand Transfer Inhibitors (INSTIs), Fusion Protein Inhibitors, and CCR5 Antagonists

Drug	Routes and Dosage Ranges	
	Adults	Children
Integrase Strand Transfer Inhibitors (INSTIs)		
ⓟ Raltegravir (Isentress, Isentress HD; ✦ Isentress, Isentress HD)	400 mg PO twice daily or 1,200 mg PO once daily	2 to <12 y 10 to <14 kg: 75 mg PO twice daily 14 to <20 kg: 100 mg PO twice daily 20 to <28 kg: 150 mg PO twice daily 28 to <40 kg: 200 mg PO twice daily ≥40 kg: 300 mg PO twice daily >12 y: see adults
Dolutegravir (Tivicay, Tivicay PD; ✦ Tivicay)	10, 25, or 50 mg PO 2 h before or 6 h after cation antacids	Same as adults
Fusion Protein Inhibitors		
ⓟ Enfuvirtide (Fuzeon; ✦ Fuzeon)	90 mg Sub-Q twice daily	6–16 y, 2 mg/kg Sub-Q twice daily
CCR5 Antagonists		
ⓟ Maraviroc (Selzentry; ✦ Celsentri)	300 mg PO twice daily	<16 y: safety and efficacy have not been established >16 y, same as adults
Cytochrome P450 Inhibitor		
Cobicistat (Tybost; ✦ Tybost)	PO 150 mg with food and atazanavir or darunavir	No dosage approved
Integrase Inhibitor, Reverse Transcriptase Inhibitor, Nucleoside, Reverse Transcriptase Inhibitor, Nucleotide		
ⓟ Bictegravir, emtricitabine, and tenofovir alafenamide (Biktarvy; ✦ Biktarvy)	Bictegravir 50 mg/emtricitabine 200 mg/tenofovir alafenamide 25 mg PO once daily	Pediatric patients weighing >25 kg PO bictegravir 50 mg/emtricitabine 200 mg/tenofovir alafenamide 25 mg once daily; in clinical trials, the youngest patients were 6 years of age

In addition, the nurse assesses for GI upset, headache, dizziness, fever, and rhabdomyolysis. It is necessary to monitor blood sugar, liver enzymes, and lipase levels for increases.

Patient Teaching

Box 23.4 presents patient teaching guidelines for antiretroviral drugs.

Fusion Protein Inhibitors

The drugs in this new class inhibit the HIV virus from binding to, fusing with, and entering the human cell. ⓟ **Enfuvirtide** (Fuzeon) is the only drug in this class. This drug is for use only by patients who have previously been treated with antiretroviral agents. ART-naive patients should not use it.

Pharmacokinetics

Following subcutaneous administration, enfuvirtide has a peak of action of 4 to 8 hours. The drug is 84% absorbed and distributed to the CSF in 2 to 18 hours. It is 92% protein bound. Enfuvirtide is metabolized by proteolytic hydrolysis in which it is catabolized into amino acids. The medication is not excreted; the amino acids are recycled.

Action and Use

Enfuvirtide inhibits the fusion of the membrane of the HIV-1 virus with that of the cell, thus preventing HIV from entering the cell. It is used in combination with other antiretrovirals in treating HIV-1. Table 23.11 gives route of administration and dosage information for enfuvirtide.

Patient-related variables specific to the use of enfuvirtide include reproduction, pregnancy, and lactation. Specifically, it should be noted that enfuvirtide has minimal to low transmission across the placenta. It is not known if enfuvirtide is present in breast milk.

BOX 23.7 Drug Interactions: Raltegravir

Drugs That Increase the Effects of Raltegravir
- Proton pump inhibitors
  Increase the serum concentration

Drugs That Decrease the Effects of Raltegravir
- Efavirenz, fosamprenavir, rifampin, tipranavir
  Decrease the serum concentration

Adverse Effects and Contraindications

The most commonly reported adverse effects to enfuvirtide are fatigue, insomnia, nausea, and diarrhea. Injection site reactions such as rash, pain, discomfort, redness, hypersensitivity, and nodule development may also occur. Researchers have reported bacterial pneumonia in 3% of patients who used enfuvirtide. Less than 10% of patients may have elevated serum creatine phosphokinase, myalgia, and limb pain.

Contraindications to enfuvirtide include a hypersensitivity to the drug and lactation.

Nursing Implications
Preventing Interactions

PIs increase serum enfuvirtide levels.

Administering the Medication

The nurse injects enfuvirtide subcutaneously into the upper arm, abdomen, or anterior thigh. Injection of the drug into blood vessels, navel, moles, scars, or other areas with changes to the skin should never occur. Rotation of injection sites and assessment of the sites for reactions is necessary. It is important not to inject enfuvirtide into large nerves that are close to the skin near the buttocks, elbow, knee, or groin.

Assessing for Therapeutic and Adverse Effects

The nurse assesses for an increase in T helper CD4 cells. The CD4 count measures the ability to fight against infections.

Also, the nurse assesses the injection site for signs of hypersensitivity such as rash, redness, nodules, or pain. The nurse also assesses for diarrhea, nausea, or other signs of GI distress. In addition, it is necessary to assess the serum creatine phosphokinase for elevation along with myalgia or limb pain. Finally, the nurse assesses pulmonary status, looking for cough, fever, or bacterial pneumonia.

Patient Teaching

The nurse instructs the patient or family about the proper technique for the administration of the enfuvirtide. Daily administration is necessary, and if a dose is missed, it is important to notify the primary care provider. Instruct the rotation of injection sites and assessment of site for changes. Box 23.4 provides general patient teaching guidelines for antiretroviral drugs.

CCR5 Antagonists

Currently, there is only one member of this antiretroviral class, **P maraviroc** (Selzentry). It blocks the receptor site to which the HIV needs to interact to enter the cell.

Pharmacokinetics

Maraviroc is absorbed in the GI tract. The drug has a slow onset of action, reaching a peak of action in ½ to 4 hours. Its half-life is 14 to 18 hours. Maraviroc is 76% protein bound. The drug is metabolized by the liver with the CYP3A enzyme to inactive metabolites. It is excreted in the urine (20%; 8% remains unchanged) and kidneys (76%; 25% remains unchanged).

Action and Use

Maraviroc binds to the human chemokine receptor on the cell membrane. This action prevents the interaction of HIV-1 and CCR5 that is needed for HIV to enter the cell and replicate.

People with HIV take maraviroc in combination with other antiretroviral agents for detectable CCR5-tropic HIV-1 possessing evidence of viral replication. They may have HIV-1 strains that are resistant to many other antiretroviral drugs. Those with a CrCl less than 30 mL/minute or with kidney failure with replacement therapy should not take maraviroc. Table 23.11 gives route of administration and dosage information for maraviroc.

Patient-related variables specific to the use of maraviroc include the following:

- Reproduction, pregnancy, and lactation:
  - Maraviroc has moderate transfer across the placenta.
  - It is not known if maraviroc is present in breast milk.
- Abnormal kidney function and hepatic impairment:
  - No dosage adjustment with abnormal kidney function or hepatic impairment.
  - If the patient is receiving a potent CYP3A4 inhibitor on intermittent hemodialysis, the use of maraviroc is contraindicated.

Adverse Effects and Contraindications

The most common adverse effects of maraviroc are fever; rash; upper respiratory infection with cough; vascular hypertension; and CNS depression with dizziness, anxiety, and depression. Other less significant adverse effects are lipodystrophy, pruritus, benign skin neoplasms, genital warts, elevated bilirubin, joint pain, conjunctivitis, and otitis media. The FDA has issued a **BOXED WARNING** ◆ for maraviroc, stating that it may lead to drug-induced hepatotoxicity with allergic features following 1 month of treatment. Allergic reactions such as pruritic rash, fever, eosinophilia, fever, increased IgE, and symptoms of hepatitis that can be life threatening may precede this condition.

Contraindications to maraviroc include severe abnormal kidney function and use of medications that are potent CYP3A4 inhibitors.

Nursing Implications
Preventing Interactions

Several medications interact with maraviroc, increasing or decreasing its effects (Box 23.8). St. John's wort decreases the effects of the drug.

BOX 23.8 Drug Interactions: Maraviroc

Drugs That Increase the Effects of Maraviroc
- Strong CYP3A4 inhibitors, atazanavir, darunavir, fosamprenavir calcium, indinavir sulfate, lopinavir/ritonavir, nelfinavir mesylate

Increase the serum concentration

Drugs That Decrease the Effects of Maraviroc
- Efavirenz, rifampin, carbamazepine, phenobarbital, phenytoin

Decrease the serum concentration

Administering the Medication

Patients may take maraviroc before meals, with meals, or after meals. However, high-fat foods enhance absorption.

Assessing for Therapeutic Effects

The nurse assesses for an increase in T helper CD4 cells. The CD4 count measures the ability to fight against infections.

Assessing for Adverse Effects

In addition, the nurse assesses the bilirubin, AST, and ALT levels for signs of hepatotoxicity. It is also necessary to assess the temperature for fever and monitor the IgE levels, which are indicative of the onset of hepatitis. The nurse also assesses for rash or other skin changes such as the development of neoplasms; for cough and upper respiratory infection; and the ear canal for otitis media or complaints of ear pain.

Patient Teaching

The nurse instructs the patient to use caution when changing positions due to possible drug-induced dizziness. The nurse also tells the patient to report rash, yellow skin or eyes, muscle pain, or fatigue. Additional general patient teaching guidelines are presented in Box 23.4.

COMBINATION MEDICATION FOR HIV-1: INTEGRASE INHIBITOR, REVERSE TRANSCRIPTASE INHIBITOR, NUCLEOSIDE, REVERSE TRANSCRIPTASE INHIBITOR, NUCLEOTIDE

Bictegravir, emtricitabine, and tenofovir alafenamide (Biktarvy) is one of the newest antiretroviral agent for the treatment of HIV-1 in adult and pediatric patients. Approved for use in the United States in February 2018, it is a once-a-day treatment for HIV-1. This combination medication increases the immune response and assists in fighting infections. In 8 to 24 weeks, the amount of HIV in the patient's system will be lowered or undetectable.

Pharmacokinetics

Bictegravir is 99% protein bound; tenofovir alafenamide is 80% protein bound; emtricitabine is only 4% protein bound. Bictegravir is metabolized by the CYP3A enzymes, and tenofovir alafenamide is converted intracellularly by hydrolysis. Bictegravir reaches a peak in 2 to 4 hours and has a 17.3-hour half-life. It is excreted in the feces and urine. Emtricitabine's half-life is 10.4 hours, with a peak in 1.5 to 2 hours. It is excreted in the feces and urine. Tenofovir alafenamide reaches a peak in 0.5 to 2 hours and has a half-life in 51 minutes. Tenofovir diphosphate's half-life is 150 to 180 hours. As with the other drugs, it is excreted in the feces and urine.

Action and Use

Bictegravir inhibits HIV integrase and binds to the integrase site to block the transfer strand of DNA integration. Emtricitabine and tenofovir alafenamide are converted intracellularly to tenofovir and is phosphorylated by cellular kinases to tenofovir diphosphate. This action interferes with HIV and HIV viral RNA-dependent DNA polymerase activities to inhibit viral replication.

Patient-related variables specific to the use of bictegravir include the following:

- Reproduction, pregnancy, and lactation:
  - Bictegravir crosses the placenta.
  - Pharmacokinetic studies on bictegravir are insufficient to determine dosage recommendations during pregnancy.
  - Emtricitabine is present in breast milk; excretion of bictegravir and tenofovir alafenamide is unknown.
- Abnormal kidney function and hepatic impairment:
  - Use is not recommended with CrCl less than 30 mL/minute.
  - Use in not recommended with severe hepatic impairment.

Adverse Effects and Contraindications

Bictegravir, emtricitabine, and tenofovir alafenamide combination has the ability to increase the creatinine clearance, low-density lipoprotein, amylase, as well as the ALT and AST. Diarrhea, nausea, abdominal pain, dyspepsia, flatulence, and vomiting are common gastrointestinal adverse effects.

Bictegravir, emtricitabine, and tenofovir alafenamide combination is contraindicated with dofetilide and rifampin.

Nursing Implications

Preventing Interactions

Aminoglycoside, acyclovir, and valacyclovir increase serum concentrations of tenofovir. Adefovir diminishes the effect of tenofovir. Do not combine with medications that induce CYP3A4 action.

Administering the Medication

Administer bictegravir, emtricitabine, and tenofovir alafenamide with or without food. Administer 2 hours before or 6 hours after aluminum or magnesium containing antacids. Administer with food with concomitant calcium or iron containing supplements or antacids; coadministration with or 2 hours after calcium or iron containing supplements or antacids is not recommended under fasting conditions.

Assessing for Therapeutic

The nurse assesses for an increase in T helper CD4 cells. The CD4 count measures the ability to fight against infections.

Assessing for Adverse Effects

Assess CD4 count, HIV RNA plasma levels, serum creatinine, urine glucose, and serum phosphorous. Patients with chronic kidney disease are at risk for increased kidney damage. Patients administered bictegravir, emtricitabine, and tenofovir alafenamide are at risk for bone loss and fracture; bone density should be monitored.

Patient Teaching

The general patient teaching guidelines presented in Box 23.4 may be useful.

THE NURSING PROCESS

A concept map outlines the nursing process related to drug therapy considerations in this chapter. Additional nursing implications related to the disease process should also be considered in care decisions.

Assessment
- Assess for signs and symptoms of viral infections and resolution of signs and symptoms following the administration of antiviral medications.
- Assess kidney and hepatic function.
- Assess viral hepatitis risk factors, exposure, and signs and symptoms of liver dysfunction.
- Assess baseline data to assist in monitoring response to drug therapy.
  - Vital signs, weight, and nutritional status
  - Signs and symptoms of disease and opportunistic infections associated with disease and immunosuppression
- CBC; CD4+; lymphocyte count; plasma levels of viral RNA; and BUN, AST, ALT, AST, and creatinine

Outcomes of Therapy
The patient will
- Receive or take antiviral drugs as prescribed.
- Be safeguarded against new or recurrent infection.
- Act to prevent spread of viral infection to others and recurrence in self.
- Avoid preventable adverse drug effects and drug interactions.
- Receive emotional support and counseling to assist in coping with HIV infection or genital herpes.

Nursing Interventions
- Follow recommended policies and procedures for preventing spread of viral infections.
- Assist patients in learning ways to control spread and recurrence of viral infections.
- Assist patients to maintain immunizations against viral infections.
- For patients receiving systemic antiviral drugs, monitor serum creatinine and other tests of kidney function, CBC, and fluid balance.
- For patients with HIV infection, help to schedule their drug therapy regimen as conveniently as possible (to promote adherence), monitor for changes in baseline data during each contact, prevent opportunistic infections (e.g., herpes infections) when possible, and manage adverse effects of drug therapy to promote quality of life.

Evaluation
- Observe for improvement in signs and symptoms of the viral infection for which a drug is given.
- Interview outpatients regarding their compliance with instructions for taking antiviral drugs.
- Interview and observe for use of infection control measures.
- Interview and observe for adverse drug effects.
- Observe the extent and severity of any symptoms in patients with HIV infection or viral hepatitis.

Visit thePoint° at http://thePoint.lww.com/Frandsen13e for answers to NCLEX Success questions (in Appendix A), answers to Clinical Application Case Studies (in Appendix B), additional information on etiology and pathophysiology, and more!

REFERENCES AND RESOURCES

Barr, F. E., & Graham, B. S. (2022). Respiratory syncytial virus infection: Treatment. *UpToDate.* Lexi-Comp, Inc.

Centers for Disease Control and Prevention. (2022a). *COVID-19 quarantine and isolation.* https://www.cdc.gov/coronavirus/2019-ncov/your-health/quarantine-isolation.html#anchor_1642600273484

Centers for Disease Control and Prevention. (2022b). *Opening and mixing oseltamivir capsules with liquids if a child cannot swallow capsules.* https://www.cdc.gov/flu/highrisk/mixing-oseltamivir-qa.htm

Centers for Disease Control and Prevention. (2022c). *What you should know about flu antiviral drugs.* https://www.cdc.gov/flu/treatment/whatyoushould.htm

Fletcher, C. V. (2022). Overview of antiretroviral agents used to treat HIV. *UpToDate.* Lexi-Comp, Inc.

Food and Drug Administration. (2021). *Fact sheet for healthcare providers: Emergency authorization for Actemra (tocilizumab).* https://www.fda.gov/media/150321/download

Friel, T. J. (2022). Epidemiology, clinical manifestations, and treatment of cytomegalovirus infection in immunocompetent adults. *UpToDate.* Lexi-Comp, Inc.

Gottlieb, G. S. (2022). Treatment of HIV-2 infection. *UpToDate.* Lexi-Comp, Inc.

Hinkle, J. L., Cheever, K. H., & Overbaugh, K. (2022). *Brunner & Suddarth's textbook of medical-surgical nursing* (15th ed.). Wolters Kluwer.

Kaya, S., & Kavak, S. (2021). *Efficacy of tocilizumab in COVID-19: Single-center experience.* BioMed Research International, 2021, 1–7. https://doi.org/10.1155/2021/1934685

Lok, A. (2022). Hepatitis B virus: Overview of management. *UpToDate.* Lexi-Comp, Inc.

McIntosh, K. (2022a). Coronaviruses. *UpToDate.* Lexi-Comp, Inc.

McIntosh, K. (2022b). COVID-19: Clinical features. *UpToDate.* Lexi-Comp, Inc.

McIntosh, K. (2022c). COVID-19: Epidemiology, virology, and prevention. *UpToDate.* Lexi-Comp, Inc.

McIntosh, K. (2022d). Middle East respiratory syndrome coronavirus: Treatment and prevention. *UpToDate.* Lexi-Comp, Inc.

McIntosh, K. (2022e). Severe acute respiratory syndrome (SARS). *UpToDate.* Lexi-Comp, Inc.

Mikkelsen, M. E., & Abramoff, B. (2022). COVID-19 evaluation and management of adults following acute viral illness. *UpToDate.* Lexi-Comp, Inc.

Norris, T. L. (2019). *Porth's pathophysiology concepts of altered health states* (10th ed.). Wolters Kluwer.

Rostad, C. A., Maillis, A. N., Lai, K., Bakshi, N., Jerris, R. C., Lane, P. A., Yee, M. E., & Yildirim, I. (2021). The burden of respiratory syncytial virus infections among children with sickle cell disease. *Pediatric Blood Cancer,* 68, e28759. https://doi.org/10.1002/pbc.28759

Sax, P. E. (2022a). Acute and early HIV infection: Treatment. *UpToDate.* Lexi-Comp, Inc.

Sax, P. E. (2022b). Selecting antiretroviral regimens for the treatment-naïve HIV infected patient. *UpToDate.* Lexi-Comp, Inc.

Stephenson, I. (2022). Avian influenza: Epidemiology, transmission, and pathogenesis. *UpToDate.* Lexi-Comp, Inc.

UpToDate. (2022a). *Drug information.* Lexi-Comp, Inc.

UpToDate. (2022b). *Practice changing update: Infectious diseases, treatment of COVID-19 in outpatients at risk for severe disease.* https://www-uptodate-com.proxy.library.maryville.edu/contents/covid-19-outpatient-evaluation-and-management-of-acute-illness-in-adults?search=covid%2019%20home%20treatment&source=search_result&selectedTitle=1~150&usage_type=default&display_rank=1

Wald, A. (2022). Treatment and prevention of herpes simplex virus type 1 in immunocompetent adolescents and adults. *UpToDate.* Lexi-Comp, Inc.

Zachary, K. C. (2022). Pharmacology of antiviral drugs for influenza. *UpToDate.* Lexi-Comp, Inc.

CHAPTER 24

Drug Therapy for Fungal Infections

LEARNING OBJECTIVES

After studying this chapter, you should be able to:

1. Describe the characteristics of fungi and fungal infections.
2. Discuss antibacterial drug therapy and immunosuppression as risk factors for development of fungal infections.
3. Identify the prototype and describe the action, use, adverse effects, contraindications, and nursing implications for polyenes.
4. Identify the prototype and describe the action, use, adverse effects, contraindications, and nursing implications for azoles.
5. Identify the prototype and describe the action, use, adverse effects, contraindications, and nursing implications for echinocandins.
6. Identify the prototype and describe the action, use, adverse effects, contraindications, and nursing implications for the pyrimidine analog.
7. Identify the prototype and describe the action, use, adverse effects, contraindications, and nursing implications for the miscellaneous antifungal agents.
8. Implement the nursing process when caring for patients undergoing drug therapy for fungal infections.

CLINICAL APPLICATION CASE STUDY

Maria Angelo, age 21, is receiving antibiotic therapy for a strep throat. Following the completion of the course of antibiotics, she begins complaining of vaginal itching. She also notices a cheesy yellow vaginal discharge. Her primary care provider diagnoses *Candida albicans* vaginal infection and prescribes fluconazole (Diflucan) 150 mg PO, one dose.

KEY TERMS

Candidiasis: infection either containing or caused by *Candida* fungi

Dermatophytes: fungal parasite that grows in or on the skin

Fungi: plantlike organisms that live as parasites on living tissue or as saprophytes on decaying organic matter

Immunocompromised: having an impaired or weakened immune system

Molds: fungi that are widely dispersed in the environment and either saprophytic or parasitic; multicellular organisms composed of colonies of tangled strands

Mycoses: disease induced by a fungus or resembling such a disease

Yeasts: unicellular fungi of the genus *Saccharomyces* or *Candida*

INTRODUCTION

This chapter introduces the pharmacologic care of the patient diagnosed with a fungal infection. Three broad classifications of antifungal agents are prescribed in the treatment of fungal infections. The first group discussed is the polyenes, which are administered for severe fungal infections. The second group is the azoles, which are the most commonly prescribed antifungal medications. The third group is the echinocandins, which have fungicidal activity against *Candida*, including azole-resistant organisms, and fungistatic activity against *Aspergillus*. This chapter also discusses antifungal agents used in the treatment of dermatophytic infections.

OVERVIEW OF FUNGAL INFECTIONS

Fungi are plantlike organisms (e.g., molds and yeasts) that are widely dispersed in the environment and are either saprophytic (i.e., obtain food from dead organic matter) or parasitic (i.e., obtain nourishment from living organisms). **Molds** are multicellular organisms composed of colonies of tangled strands. They form a fuzzy coating on various surfaces (e.g., the mold that forms on spoiled food, the mildew that forms in damp environments). **Yeasts** are unicellular organisms. Some fungi, called **dermatophytes**, can grow only at the cooler temperatures of body surfaces. Other fungi, termed dimorphic, can grow as molds outside the body and as yeasts in the warm temperatures of the body. As molds, these fungi produce spores that can persist indefinitely in the environment and can be carried by the wind to distant locations. When these mold spores enter the body, most often by inhalation, they rapidly become yeasts that can invade body tissues. Dimorphic fungi include a number of human pathogens such as those that cause blastomycosis, histoplasmosis, and coccidioidomycosis.

Structurally, fungi are larger and more complex than bacteria. They have a thick, rigid cell wall, of which glucan is one of the components. Glucan is formed by the fungal enzyme, glucan synthase. Fungi also have a cell membrane composed mainly of ergosterol, a lipid that is similar to cholesterol in human cell membranes. Within the cell membrane, structures are mostly the same as those in human cells (e.g., a nucleus, mitochondria, Golgi apparatus, ribosomes attached to endoplasmic reticulum, a cytoskeleton with microtubules and filaments).

Fungal infections may be mild and superficial or life threatening and systemic. Fungi that are pathogenic in humans exist in soil, decaying plants, and other environmental habitats. Some are even part of the endogenous human flora. For example, *Candida albicans* organisms are part of the normal microbial flora of the skin, mouth, gastrointestinal (GI) tract, and vagina. Growth of *Candida* organisms is normally restrained by intact immune mechanisms and bacterial competition for nutrients. When these restraining forces are altered (e.g., by suppression of the immune system, antibacterial drug therapy), fungal overgrowth and opportunistic infection can occur, leading to the fungal infection called **candidiasis**. Oral candidiasis causes mouth pain and pain on swallowing. Vulvovaginal candidiasis is associated with antibiotic, glucorticoid, or oral contraceptives causing vaginal itching and discharge. Dermatophytes cause superficial infections of the skin, hair, and nails. They obtain nourishment from keratin, a protein in skin, hair, and nails. Dermatophytic infections include tinea pedis (athlete's foot) and tinea capitis (ringworm of the scalp) (see Chapter 61).

Systemic or invasive **mycoses** include the endemic mycoses that can cause disease (e.g., blastomycosis, coccidioidomycosis, histoplasmosis, sporotrichosis) in healthy hosts who are exposed to them in the environment and the opportunistic mycoses (e.g., aspergillosis, candidiasis, cryptococcosis) that cause serious infection, mainly in immunosuppressed hosts. The fungi that cause endemic mycoses exist as molds in the environment; they grow in soil and decaying organic matter. Infection is acquired by inhalation of airborne spores from contaminated soil. Histoplasmosis, coccidioidomycosis, and blastomycosis usually occur as pulmonary disease but may be systemic. These infections often mimic common bacterial infections, and their severity is determined both by the extent of the exposure to the organism and by the immune status of the host. The fungi that cause opportunistic mycoses may be part of the normal body flora (e.g., *Candida* species) or exist in the environment (*Aspergillus, Cryptococcus*). Infection occurs after inhalation or inoculation of the fungus into body tissues.

Fungi may have characteristics that enhance their ability to cause disease. *Cryptococcus neoformans* organisms, for example, can become encapsulated, which allows them to evade the normal immune defense mechanism of phagocytosis. *Aspergillus* organisms produce protease, an enzyme that allows them to destroy structural proteins and penetrate body tissues.

Most fungal infections occur in healthy people but are more severe and invasive in **immunocompromised** hosts or those with an impaired or weakened immune system. Serious infections are increasing in incidence, largely because of human immunodeficiency virus (HIV) infections, the use of immunosuppressant drugs to treat patients with cancer or organ transplants, the use of indwelling intravenous (IV) catheters for prolonged drug therapy or parenteral nutrition, implantation of prosthetic devices, and widespread use of broad-spectrum antibacterial drugs.

Clinical Manifestations

The specific pathophysiologic changes associated with fungal infections relate to the causal fungus and the tissues in which it has been colonized. Detailed discussion of specific characteristics of selected fungal infections and pathophysiologic changes can be found on thePoint (http://thePoint.lww.com/Frandsen13e).

Drug Therapy

Development of drugs that are effective against fungal cells without being excessively toxic to human cells has been limited because fungal cells are similar to human cells. Most of the available drugs target the fungal cell membrane and produce potentially serious toxicities and drug interactions. In general, antifungal drugs disrupt the structure and function of fungal cell components (Fig. 24.1).

Polyenes (e.g., amphotericin B), azoles (e.g., fluconazole), the miscellaneous class triterpenoid (e.g., ibrexafungerp), and the miscellaneous agent griseofulvin act on ergosterol to disrupt the fungal cell membrane. Amphotericin B (and nystatin) binds

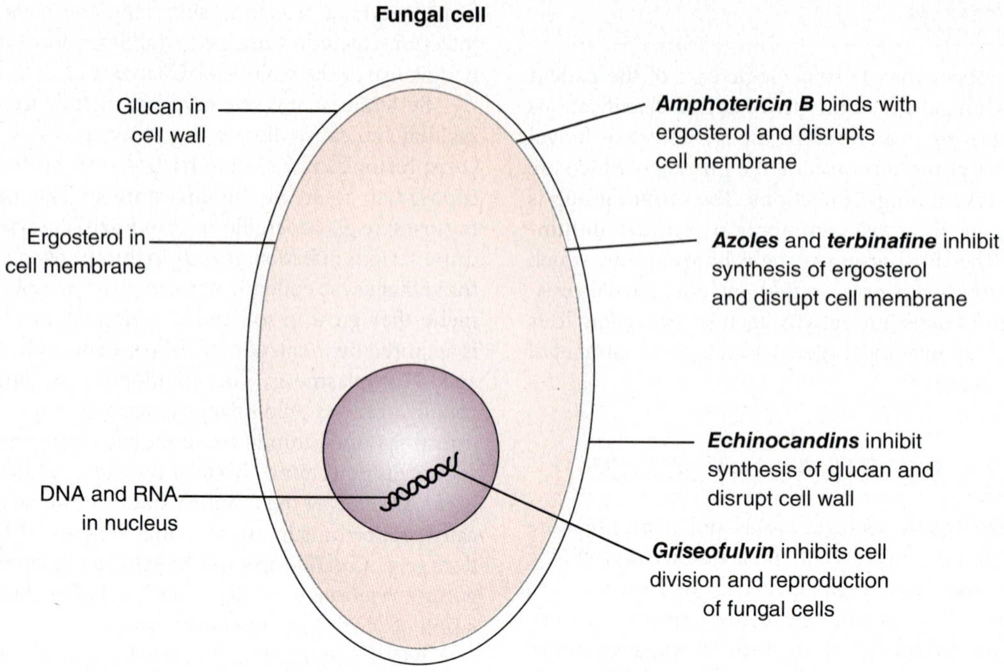

Figure 24.1. Actions of antifungal drugs on fungal cells.

- Glucan in cell wall
- Ergosterol in cell membrane
- DNA and RNA in nucleus
- **Amphotericin B** binds with ergosterol and disrupts cell membrane
- **Azoles** and **terbinafine** inhibit synthesis of ergosterol and disrupt cell membrane
- **Echinocandins** inhibit synthesis of glucan and disrupt cell wall
- **Griseofulvin** inhibits cell division and reproduction of fungal cells

to ergosterol and forms holes in the membrane, causing leakage of fungal cell contents and lysis of the cell. The azole drugs bind to an enzyme that is required for synthesis of ergosterol. This action causes production of a defective cell membrane, which also allows leakage of intracellular contents and destruction of the cell. Both types of drugs also affect cholesterol in human cell membranes, a characteristic considered mainly responsible for the drugs' adverse effects.

Echinocandins (e.g., caspofungin) disrupt fungal cell walls rather than fungal cell membranes. They inhibit glucan synthase, an enzyme required for synthesis of glucan. Glucan is a component of the fungal cell wall; its depletion leads to leakage of cellular contents and cell death. Because human cells do not contain cell walls, these drugs are less toxic than the polyene and azole antifungals.

Drugs for superficial fungal infections of the skin and mucous membranes are often applied topically. Numerous preparations are available, many without a prescription. Drugs for systemic infections are given intravenously or orally. Patients with HIV infection or severe neutropenia due to treatment with cytotoxic cancer drugs require aggressive treatment of fungal infections, because they are at high risk for developing life-threatening systemic mycoses. Selected antifungal drugs are further described in the following sections.

Table 24.1 summarizes the medications used in the treatment of fungal infections.

Clinical Application 24.1

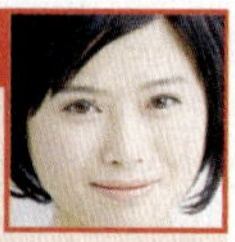

- Ms. Angelo is told that she has a *Candida* infection. What does the nurse tell her about the cause of the fungal infection?
- What symptoms does Ms. Angelo experience?

POLYENES

Amphotericin B deoxycholate, the prototype polyene, is active against most types of pathogenic fungi and is fungicidal or fungistatic, depending on the concentration in body fluids and the susceptibility of the causative fungus. Because of its toxicity, the drug is used only for serious fungal infections. It is usually given for 4 to 12 weeks. There are two additional formulations of amphotericin B. Amphotericin B lipid-based formulations include Abelcet and AmBisome.

Pharmacokinetics

Amphotericin B must be given intravenously for systemic infections. After the infusion is complete, the drug is rapidly taken up by the liver and other organs. It is then slowly released back into the bloodstream. Despite its long-term use, little is known about its distribution and metabolic pathways. Drug concentrations in most body fluids are higher in the presence of inflammation; concentrations in cerebrospinal fluid (CSF) are low with or without inflammation. The drug has an initial serum half-life of 24 hours, which represents redistribution from the bloodstream to tissues. This is followed by a second elimination phase, with a half-life of 15 days, which represents elimination from tissue storage sites. Most of the drug is thought to be metabolized in the tissues; some is excreted in the urine and can be detected for several weeks.

Lipid formulations (Abelcet, AmBisome) reach higher concentrations in diseased tissues than in normal tissues, so that larger doses can be given to increase therapeutic effects. At the same time, they cause less damage to normal tissues and decrease adverse effects. These products are much more expensive than the deoxycholate form. They are most likely to be used for patients with preexisting abnormal kidney function or

TABLE 24.1

Drugs Administered for Fungal Infections (Antifungal Agents)

Drug Class	Prototype	Other Drugs in the Class
Polyenes	Amphotericin B • Deoxycholate formulation • Lipid formulations (Abelcet, AmBisome)	Nystatin
Azoles	Fluconazole (Diflucan)	Butoconazole (Gynazole-1)* Clotrimazole Econazole (Ecoza, Spectazole)* Itraconazole (Sporanox, Tolsura) Ketoconazole Miconazole (Oravig) Oxiconazole (Oxistat)* Posaconazole (Noxafil) Sulconazole (Exelderm)* Terconazole (Terazol 3, Terazol 7)* Tioconazole (Vagistat-1 [OTC]) Voriconazole (Vfend, Vfend IV) Isavuconazole (Cresemba)
Echinocandins	Caspofungin (Cancidas)	Anidulafungin (Eraxis) Micafungin (Mycamine)
Miscellaneous antifungal agents for superficial mycoses	Griseofulvin	Ciclopirox (Loprox, Penlac)* Terbinafine (Lamisil) Tolnaftate (Tinactin)* Ibrexafungerp (Brexafemme)
Pyrimidine analog	Flucytosine (Ancobon)	

*Topical antifungal agents.

Action

Amphotericin B binds to the sterols within the fungal cell membrane, resulting in a change in the membrane's permeability. This action destroys the fungal cells and prevents them from reproducing. Depending on the concentration of the medication, it has either a fungicidal or fungistatic effect.

Use

Amphotericin B is reserved for patients with progressive and potentially fatal infections resulting from cryptococcosis, North American blastomycosis, systemic candidiasis, disseminated moniliasis, coccidioidomycosis, and histoplasmosis. It is also used for mucormycosis caused by the species of *Mucor*, *Rhizopus*, *Absidia*, *Conidiobolus*, and *Basidiobolus*; sporotrichosis; and aspergillosis. The drug is also given as an adjunctive agent in the treatment of American mucocutaneous leishmaniasis. A **BOXED WARNING** ◆ issued by the U.S. Food and Drug Administration (FDA) states that amphotericin B should be reserved for progressive or potentially fatal infections. It is not recommended for use in noninvasive disease due to the risk of toxicity.

Conditions in which other nephrotoxic drugs are routinely given (e.g., bone marrow transplant recipients) and when high doses are needed for difficult to treat infections. The lipid preparations differ in their characteristics and cannot be used interchangeably. Abelcet is used in the treatment of aspergillosis. AmBisome is used in the treatment of cryptococcal meningitis in HIV-infected patients. Patients who are febrile and neutropenic are given AmBisome for presumed fungal infections. Also, AmBisome is administered in the treatment of *Aspergillus*, *Candida*, or *Cryptococcus* when conventional amphotericin is not tolerated.

Table 24.2 presents specific information about the use of polyenes, including dosages for adults and children.

Patient-related variables specific to the use of amphotericin B include the following:

- Age:
  - Children require careful assessment of electrolytes due to magnesium wasting with the drug.
  - Children with serious fungal infections have been treated successfully with the drug, without unusual or severe adverse effects.
  - Older adults, with the impaired kidney and cardiovascular functions that usually accompany aging, are especially vulnerable to serious adverse effects and thus require close monitoring to reduce the incidence and severity of nephrotoxicity, hypokalemia, and other adverse drug reactions.
  - Lipid formulations of amphotericin B are less nephrotoxic than the conventional deoxycholate formulation and may be preferred for older adults.
- Reproduction, pregnancy, and lactation:
  - Amphotericin B crosses the placenta and enters the fetal circulation.

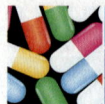

TABLE 24.2
DRUGS AT A GLANCE: Polyenes

Drug	Type of Infection Treated	Routes and Dosage Ranges Adults	Children
℗ Amphotericin B deoxycholate (✸ Fungizone IV)	Serious, systemic fungal infections (e.g., candidiasis, histoplasmosis) Cutaneous candidiasis Oral candidiasis	Dosage is individualized according to the disease severity Initial IV dose: 0.25 mg/kg/d. Gradually increase dosage to 0.5–1 mg/kg/d, infused over 2–6 h Topical: apply two to four times daily for 1–4 wk Oral suspension: 100 mg/mL, 1 mL swish and swallow four times per day	Same as for adults for IV, skin preparations, and oral suspension
Amphotericin B lipid complex (Abelcet; ✸ Abelcet)	Systemic infections in patients who do not tolerate Fungizone	IV 5 mg/kg/d	Same as adults
Liposomal amphotericin B (AmBisome; ✸ AmBisome)	Systemic infections in patients who do not tolerate Fungizone Empiric treatment of presumed fungal infections in febrile, neutropenic patients	IV 3–6 mg/kg/d	Same as adults
Nystatin (✸ PMS-Nystatin, Nyaderm, TEVA-Nystatin)	Candidiasis of skin, mucous membrane, and intestinal tract	Oral or intestinal infection: PO tablets 1–2 (500,000–1,000,000 units) three times daily; oral suspension 4–6 mL (400,000–600,000 units) four times daily; oral troches 1–2 (200,000–400,000 units) four to five times daily Topically to skin lesions, two to three times daily Intravaginally, 1 vaginal tablet once daily for 14 d	Oral suspension, older than 1 y: same as adults; infants, 2 mL (200,000 units) four times daily Oral troches, same as adults for children old enough to suck on the lozenge until it dissolves

- It is not known whether amphotericin B is present in breast milk; due to the potential for toxicity, the manufacturer does not recommend its use while breast-feeding.
- Abnormal kidney function and hepatic impairment:
  - Amphotericin B deoxycholate is nephrotoxic. Abnormal kidney function occurs in most patients (up to 80%) within the first 2 weeks of therapy but usually subsides with dosage reduction or drug discontinuation. Permanent impairment occurs in a few patients.
  - Recommendations to decrease nephrotoxicity include hydrating patients with a liter of 0.9% sodium chloride solution intravenously and monitoring serum creatinine and blood urea nitrogen (BUN) at least weekly. If the patient's BUN exceeds 40 mg/dL or serum creatinine exceeds 3 mg/dL, the drug should be stopped, or dosage should be reduced until kidney function recovers. Another strategy is to give a lipid formulation (e.g., Abelcet, AmBisome), which is less nephrotoxic.
  - For patients who already have abnormal kidney function or other risk factors for development of abnormal kidney function, a lipid formulation is indicated. Kidney function should still be monitored frequently.
- Although the main concern with amphotericin B is nephrotoxicity, monitoring of hepatic function during use is recommended.
- Specific healthcare environments:
  - In critically ill patients, lipid formulations may be preferred because they are less nephrotoxic.
  - In patients receiving home care, the nurse should assess immune function with the administration of amphotericin B.

Adverse Effects

Adverse effects of amphotericin B are often severe, with the most serious being multiple organ failure, respiratory arrest, and cardiac arrest. Other adverse effects include the following:

- GI: nausea, vomiting, dyspepsia, bleeding (GI)
- Genitourinary: hypokalemia, azotemia, kidney failure
- Hematologic: leukopenia, thrombocytopenia
- Electrolyte imbalances: hyperkalemia, hypomagnesemia, hyponatremia

Contraindications

Patients with a known allergy to amphotericin B and impairment of kidney function should not receive the drug.

Nursing Implications

Preventing Interactions

Many medications interact with amphotericin B, increasing or decreasing its effect (Box 24.1). Researchers have not reported that any herbs interact with the drug.

Administering the Drug

The pharmacy should reconstitute and prepare amphotericin B for IV administration. It is necessary to infuse the prepared solutions of amphotericin within 8 hours of reconstitution. The patient should receive a test dose to assess tolerance for the drug. Doubling maintenance doses and infusing them on alternate days is fine. Larger doses of the lipid preparations are recommended to achieve therapeutic effects similar to those of the deoxycholate preparation. When possible, it is best to administer amphotericin B through a separate IV line. When injecting it into an existing IV line, flushing of the line with a 5% dextrose solution should occur before and after administration both with deoxycholate and lipid formulations. Do not use an in-line filter with the lipid formulations.

Specific instructions for administration of the various forms of amphotericin B are as follows:

- IV form: give in 5% dextrose in water over 2 to 6 hours with the use of in-line filter. This drug should not be mixed with any other medications.
- Abelcet: give over 2 hours without the use of an in-line filter.
- Amphotericin cream or lotion: apply liberally to skin lesions and rub in gently.

Prior to beginning treatment, it is necessary to obtain a culture of the infection. However, treatment with amphotericin B should begin prior to return of the culture results. The nurse monitors injection sites for signs of phlebitis. The nurse administers aspirin, antihistamines, and antiemetics, which are used to manage adverse effects, prior to the administration of amphotericin B. It is essential to assess the sodium balance throughout the administration. By maintaining the serum sodium level within normal range, the patient has decreased symptoms of drug discomfort. Small doses of corticosteroids assist in diminishing chills related to drug administration.

Assessing for Therapeutic Effects

The nurse assesses for decrease in symptoms of the fungal infection. The administration of amphotericin B is consistent with the cure of infection. When the infection is controlled, the administration of amphotericin B continues with a maintenance dose for a period of time (Hinkle et al., 2021).

Assessing for Adverse Effects

The nurse assesses for severe chilling, headaches, malaise, nausea, vomiting, and generalized pain. It is necessary to monitor the patient's electrolytes for hypokalemia and hyponatremia. When administering amphotericin topically, the nurse assesses for a hypersensitivity reaction at the site of the application. IV administration of amphotericin is irritating to the injection and requires assessment for phlebitis and thrombophlebitis.

Patient Teaching

Box 24.2 identifies patient teaching guidelines for amphotericin B.

Other Drugs in the Class

Nystatin has the same mechanism of action as amphotericin B. However, it is used only for topical therapy of oral, intestinal, and vaginal candidiasis because it is too toxic for systemic use. Although given orally for oral or intestinal infections, the drug is not absorbed systemically and is excreted in the feces. With oral use, adverse effects include nausea, vomiting, and diarrhea; with vaginal application, adverse effects include local irritation and burning.

BOX 24.1 Drug Interactions: Amphotericin B

Drugs That Increase the Effects of Amphotericin B
- Antibiotics (nephrotoxic)
  Increase the risk of nephrotoxicity
- Antineoplastic agents
  Increase kidney toxicity, bronchospasm, and hypotension
- Cardiac glycosides
  Increase the risk of digitalis toxicity due to hypokalemia
- Corticosteroid, corticotropin, skeletal muscle relaxants
  Increase potassium depletion

Drugs That Decrease the Effects of Amphotericin B
- Clotrimazole, fluconazole, ketoconazole
  Increase resistance to fungal infection
- Flucytosine
  Increases flucytosine toxicity

BOX 24.2 Patient Teaching Guidelines for Amphotericin B

- Long-term use of amphotericin is necessary.
- You may not notice the effects of the medication for several weeks.
- Use good hygiene to prevent reinfection or spread of infection.
- The home should be kept meticulously clean and free of mold-producing substances, such as potted plants, fresh flowers, and adhesive nonslip bathtub appliques. The bathroom should be cleaned daily with bleach, and air conditioning and air filtration systems should be kept clean.
- You may experience side effects such as nausea and vomiting, so eat small, frequent meals.
- Be aware that topical administration of the medication may cause staining of clothes.
- Report skin irritations with the use of topical amphotericin.
- Report fever, chills, muscle aches, and headache.
- Report irritation at the injection site.

> **NCLEX Success**
>
> 1. When administering amphotericin B, what drug is administered to prevent the development of chilling, fever, malaise, and nausea?
>   A. aminophylline
>   B. ibuprofen
>   C. penicillin G
>   D. aspirin

AZOLES

The azoles are the largest group of commonly used antifungal agents. Many are used topically, and some are available without a prescription for dermatologic (see Chapter 61) or vaginal use (e.g., butoconazole, clotrimazole, miconazole, terconazole, tioconazole). It is necessary to obtain a prescription to use azoles for other indications.

Systemic azoles include ketoconazole, fluconazole, itraconazole, posaconazole, voriconazole, and isavuconazole. Although ketoconazole was the first azole developed, **ⓟ fluconazole** (Diflucan) is considered to be the prototype medication of the class. Fluconazole and other drugs in the class have a broader spectrum of fungal activity, are distributed more effectively, and have fewer adverse effects and drug interactions.

Pharmacokinetics

Fluconazole is administered orally or parenterally. The oral preparation has a slow onset of action with a peak of action in 1 to 2 hours and duration of action 2 to 4 days. The oral drug is well absorbed and reaches therapeutic levels in most body fluids and tissues, including the meninges. The IV preparation has a rapid onset of action, with a peak of action in 1 hour and the same duration of action 2 to 4 days. The azoles interact with cytochrome P450 (CYP) enzymes, which can potentially produce significant interactions with many other drugs (those in which there is a decrease in the metabolism and increase in the risk of toxicity with affected drugs).

Fluconazole is apparently a less potent inhibitor of CYP3A4 enzymes than ketoconazole and itraconazole. As a result, drug interactions with fluconazole are of lesser magnitude and usually occur only with dosages of 200 mg/day or more. However, fluconazole is a strong inhibitor of CYP2C9 enzymes. Fluconazole crosses the placenta and enters the breast milk. It is excreted in the urine.

Action

Fluconazole binds to sterols in the fungal cell membrane. This action changes the membrane's permeability, producing a fungicidal or fungistatic effect depending on the drug concentration and the fungal organism.

Use

Fluconazole and the other azoles discussed in this section are used systemically or both topically and systemically. Fluconazole is often the drug of choice for localized candidal infections (e.g., urinary tract infections, thrush) and is useful for systemic candidiasis. However, resistant strains of *Candida* organisms occur with extensive use of fluconazole. Fluconazole is also used for long-term suppression of cryptococcal meningitis in patients with acquired immunodeficiency syndrome (AIDS), after initial use of amphotericin B. It is used prophylactically in the prevention of candidiasis in patients with bone marrow transplants.

Table 24.3 provides detailed information about the use of azoles, including dosages for adults and children.

Patient-related variables specific to the use of fluconazole include the following:

- Age:
  - In children with *Candida* infections, the maximum daily dosage of fluconazole should not exceed 600 mg/day.
  - Older patients with *Candida* infections receiving fluconazole require monitoring of creatinine clearance and hepatic enzymes.
- Reproduction, pregnancy, and lactation:
  - Patients who may become pregnant and who are taking doses greater than 400 mg/day should use effective contraception during therapy and for 1 week after the final fluconazole dose.
  - Following exposure to fluconazole in the first trimester, malformations have been noted in infants when the maternal fluconazole doses were greater than 400 mg/day.
  - Fluconazole is present in breast milk. Serious adverse events in breast-feeding infants have not been reported. Fluconazole is considered compatible with breast-feeding.
- Abnormal kidney function and hepatic impairment:
  - The manufacturer recommends that in addition to 100% of the dose administered after dialysis on dialysis days, patients should receive a reduced dose according to their creatinine clearance on nondialysis days. In patients with a creatinine clearance of 50 mL/minute or less, the patient should take 50% of the recommended dose.
  - The azoles may cause hepatotoxicity, ranging from mild elevations in alanine aminotransferase (ALT) and aspartate aminotransferase (AST) to clinical hepatitis, cholestasis, hepatic failure, and death.
  - Fatal hepatic damage has occurred mainly in patients with serious underlying conditions, such as AIDS or malignancy, and with multiple concomitant medications.
  - The drugs are relatively contraindicated in patients with increased liver enzymes, active liver disease, or a history of liver damage with other drugs. They should be used only if expected benefits outweigh risks of liver injury.
- Specific healthcare environments:
  - Fluconazole penetrates tissues well, including CSF. In many critically ill patients, IV administration may be necessary, but the drug is well absorbed when administered orally (or by nasogastric tube).
  - In patients receiving home care, the nurse should educate the patient and family about measures to prevent the reinfection and spread of the fungal infection.

TABLE 24.3
DRUGS AT A GLANCE: Azoles

Drug	Type of Infection Treated	Routes and Dosage Ranges	
		Adults	**Children**
Fluconazole (Diflucan; ✱ DOM-Fluconazole, Apo-Fluconazole, Diflucan)	Oropharyngeal, esophageal, vaginal, and systemic candidiasis; Prevention of candidiasis after bone marrow transplantation; Cryptococcal meningitis	Oropharyngeal candidiasis, PO, IV 200 mg first day and then 100 mg daily for 2 wk; Esophageal candidiasis, PO, IV 200 mg first day and then 100 mg daily for at least 3 wk; Vaginal candidiasis, PO 150 mg as a single dose; Systemic candidiasis, PO, IV 400 mg first day and then 200 mg daily for at least 4 wk; Prophylaxis, PO, IV 400 mg once daily; Cryptococcal meningitis, PO, IV 400 mg first day and then 200–400 mg/d for 10–12 wk	Oropharyngeal candidiasis, PO, IV 6 mg/kg first day and then 3 mg/kg/d for at least 2 wk; Esophageal candidiasis, PO, IV 6 mg/kg first day and then 3 mg/kg/d for at least 3 wk; Systemic candidiasis, PO, IV 6–12 mg/kg/d; Cryptococcal meningitis, PO, IV 12 mg/kg first day and then 6 mg/kg/d for 10–12 wk
Clotrimazole	Oropharyngeal candidiasis	Treatment, PO 10 mg dissolved slowly five times per day for 14 d; Prophylaxis, PO 10 mg dissolved slowly three times daily for the duration of chemotherapy or until steroids are reduced to maintenance level	≥3 y: 10 mg troche dissolved slowly five times per day
Itraconazole (Sporanox, Tolsura; ✱ Sporanox)	Systemic fungal infections, including aspergillosis and in neutropenic and immunocompromised hosts; Onychomycosis; Tinea infections	Systemic infection, PO 200 mg once or twice daily for 3 mo; Blastomycosis, histoplasmosis, aspergillosis, IV 200 mg twice daily for 4 doses and then 200 mg/d; Onychomycosis, fingernail, PO 200 mg twice daily for 1 wk, no drug for 3 wk, and then repeat dosage for 1 wk; toenail, PO 200 mg once daily for 12 consecutive wk; Oral solution, 100–200 mg daily (10–20 mL), swish and swallow three times daily for 3–5 d; Tinea infections, PO 100–200 mg daily for 1–4 wk	Safety and efficacy not established. 3- to 16-y-old patients have been treated with 100 mg daily for systemic infections and 6-mo- to 12-y-old patients have been treated with 5 mg/kg once daily for 2 wk without serious or unusual adverse effects
Isavuconazole (Cresemba; ✱ Cresemba)	Treatment of invasive aspergillosis and mucormycosis in adults	Aspergillosis, IV, PO 372 mg (isavuconazole 200 mg) every 8 h for 6 doses and then 372 mg (isavuconazole 200 mg)/d, starting 12–24 h after the last loading dose; Mucormycosis, IV, PO 372 mg (isavuconazole 200 mg) every 8 h for 6 doses and then 372 mg (isavuconazole 200 mg)/d, starting 12–24 h after the last loading dose	Safety and efficacy not established
Ketoconazole (✱ Apo-Ketoconazole, Teva-Ketoconazole)	Candidiasis, histoplasmosis, and coccidioidomycosis; Cutaneous candidiasis; Tinea infections	PO 200 mg once daily, increased to 400 mg once daily if necessary in severe infections; Topically, once daily for 2–6 wk	2 y and older: PO 3.3–6.6 mg/kg/d as a single dose

(Continued on page 452)

TABLE 24.3
DRUGS AT A GLANCE: Azoles (Continued)

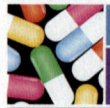

Drug	Type of Infection Treated	Routes and Dosage Ranges	
		Adults	Children
Posaconazole (Noxafil; Posanol)	Treatment of oropharyngeal candidiasis Prevention of invasive fungal infection	Prevention: PO 200 mg three times daily Oropharyngeal candidiasis PO 100 mg twice daily initially and then 200 mg once daily for 13 d	Adolescents ≥13 y: refer to adult dosing
Voriconazole (Vfend, Vfend IV; Apo-Voriconazole, Sandoz-Voriconazole, Teva-Voriconazole, Vfend)	Esophageal candidiasis Invasive aspergillosis Other serious fungal infections	Esophageal candidiasis, PO 200 mg every 12 h for weight of ≥40 kg; 100 mg every 12 h for weight <40 kg. Give at least 14 d or 7 d after symptoms resolve Aspergillosis and other serious infections, IV 6 mg/kg every 12 h for 2 doses (loading dose) and then 4 mg/kg every 12 h (maintenance dose)	Dosage not established except in off-label uses

Quality and Safety Alert: Patient-Centered Care

When administering azoles, it is necessary to check ALT, AST, and serum bilirubin before drug use, after several weeks of drug use, and every 1 to 2 months during long-term therapy. If ALT and AST increase to more than three times the normal range, the azole should be discontinued. Hepatotoxicity may be reversible if drug therapy is stopped.

Quality and Safety Alert: Evidence-Based Practice

In a review of literature related to the use of oral fluconazole in the treatment of vulvovaginal candidiasis, Paquette and Elwood (2019) explored the drug's use in pregnancy. Although the drug may be associated with spontaneous abortion, no evidence validated the drug's role in stillbirth or its uncertain link to congenital malformations. To ensure the safety of both patient and baby, it is important that the correct diagnosis is confirmed and the safest drug therapy be used for the appropriate length of time. The benefit should exceed the risk, but appropriate treatment should be initiated as indicated.

Adverse Effects

Although fluconazole is usually well tolerated, it may cause nausea, vomiting, diarrhea, abdominal pain, headache, and skin rash. In addition, elevation of liver enzymes and hepatic necrosis has reportedly occurred, and alopecia often occurs in patients receiving prolonged, high-dose treatment.

In April 2016, the FDA released an alert because of a study conducted in Denmark. Researchers found that the administration of fluconazole 400 to 800 mg/day for the treatment of a yeast infection during pregnancy increased the woman's risk of miscarriage. A single dose of 150 mg was not linked to birth-related abnormalities.

Contraindications

Fluconazole is contraindicated in patients who have experienced a hypersensitivity reaction to the azole medications.

Nursing Implications

Preventing Interactions

Azoles inhibit the metabolism of many drugs (by inhibiting CYP drug-metabolizing enzymes in the liver and small intestine, especially CYP3A4 enzymes), thus increasing the effects and possible toxicity of azoles. Many medications increase or decrease the effects of fluconazole (Box 24.3). Researchers have not identified any herbs that interact with fluconazole.

Although the main concern about azole drug interactions is increased toxicity of inhibited drugs, ketoconazole may be given with cyclosporine and tacrolimus to decrease dosages and costs of the immunosuppressant drugs. There may also be a reduced risk of fungal infections, which commonly occur in people with an impaired immune system.

The nurse should note that fluconazole is apparently a less potent inhibitor of CYP3A4 enzymes than ketoconazole and itraconazole. As a result, drug interactions with fluconazole are of lesser magnitude and usually occur only with dosages of 200 mg/day or more. However, fluconazole is a strong inhibitor of CYP2C9 enzymes, and concurrent administration of losartan, phenytoin, or warfarin results in greater risks of toxicity with the inhibited drugs.

Administering the Medication

When administering IV fluconazole, it is necessary to follow the manufacturer's recommendations. Until the medication is

> **BOX 24.3 Drug Interactions: Fluconazole**
>
> **Drugs That Increase the Effects of Fluconazole**
> - Benzodiazepines (alprazolam, midazolam, triazolam), calcium channel blockers (felodipine, nifedipine), cyclosporine, phenytoin, statins (atorvastatin, simvastatin), sulfonylureas, tacrolimus, theophylline, warfarin, vincristine, zidovudine
>   *Increase serum levels and toxic effects of these drugs due to inhibition of cytochrome P450*
>
> **Drugs That Decrease the Effects of Fluconazole**
> - Cimetidine, rifampin
>   *Decrease serum level of fluconazole*

> **BOX 24.4 Patient Teaching Guidelines for Fluconazole**
>
> - Implement hand hygiene and maintain environmental cleanliness.
> - The home should be kept meticulously clean and free of mold-producing substances, such as potted plants, fresh flowers, and adhesive nonslip bathtub appliques. The bathroom should be cleaned daily with bleach, and air conditioning and air filtration systems should be kept clean.
> - Have kidney function tests as ordered.
> - Have hepatic function tests as ordered.
> - To avoid experiencing side effects such as nausea and vomiting, eat small, frequent meals.
> - Report any skin eruption to the prescriber.
> - Report any changes in stool or urine to the prescriber.
> - Find out about adverse effects of the drug, and report any adverse effects to the prescriber.

prepared for administration, the nurse should not remove the overwrap of the package. The inner bag maintains the sterility of the medication. The nurse assesses the bag for minute leaks by squeezing it firmly. If any leaks are apparent, it is necessary to discard the medication. The nurse should never mix fluconazole with any other medications. Continuous infusion of fluconazole occurs at a maximum rate of 200 mg/hour. When administering the oral suspension, it is necessary to shake the elixir vigorously prior to pouring the dose. To decrease gastric upset, the nurse administers the medication with food.

Assessing for Therapeutic Effects

The patient who is treated for systemic mycoses should have a decrease in fever and malaise. There is also healing of skin and mucous membrane lesions. Treatment of intestinal candidiasis results in diminished diarrhea. The female patient who has experienced discomfort from vaginal candidiasis should have decreased burning and itching along with diminished vaginal discharge.

Assessing for Adverse Effects

The nurse must assess the skin for signs of skin rash. The GI assessment should include assessing for nausea, vomiting, diarrhea, and abdominal pain. All of the azoles cause hepatotoxicity with an elevation of the AST and ALT levels. Thus, it is necessary to assess hepatic enzymes every 1 to 2 months during therapy. Assessment of kidney function tests should occur weekly, with dosage reduction or discontinuation of the drug if kidney toxicity results. All of the azoles (with the exception of isavuconazole) may cause prolongation of the QTc interval.

Patient Teaching

Box 24.4 identifies patient teaching guidelines for fluconazole.

Other Drugs in the Class

Ketoconazole (Extina, Nizoral) has largely been replaced by the newer drugs, but it may still be used for long-term therapy because it is less expensive than other azoles. It may also be used with cyclosporine and tacrolimus because it increases blood levels of these immunosuppressant drugs and allows smaller dosages in patients with organ transplants.

Itraconazole (Sporanox, Tolsura) is a broad-spectrum antifungal with activity against *Candida*, *Cryptococcus*, and *Aspergillus*. It can be given orally or intravenously. Drug absorption may be decreased in patients with achlorhydria and in those receiving a concurrent antacid, histamine H_2 antagonist, or proton pump inhibitor. Serum levels should be measured to ensure adequate absorption. Drug concentrations are higher in visceral organs than in serum; little drug appears in urine or CSF. The oral capsule should be given with food to ensure maximal absorption. The oral solution should be given without food.

Usual doses may cause GI upset, and higher doses may cause hypokalemia, hypertension, edema, and heart failure. Itraconazole has many drug interactions. Drugs that increase the pH of gastric acid (e.g., antacids, histamine H_2 blockers, proton pump inhibitors) decrease absorption of itraconazole and should be given at least 2 hours after itraconazole. Drugs that induce drug-metabolizing enzymes (e.g., carbamazepine, phenytoin, rifampin) decrease serum levels of itraconazole. Itraconazole increases serum levels of cyclosporine, digoxin, oral sulfonylureas, and warfarin; it decreases serum levels of carbamazepine, phenytoin, and rifampin. The FDA has issued a **BOXED WARNING** ◆ about the risks of heart failure and drug interactions with itraconazole.

Posaconazole (Noxafil) and voriconazole (Vfend) are second-generation azoles. Both are well absorbed with oral administration. Posaconazole is used to treat *Candida*, *Cryptococcus*, *Aspergillus*, and *Mucor*. It is widely distributed, metabolized by the CYP3A4 enzymes, and eliminated in the feces. Acidic cola drinks and fruit juices increase absorption. Patients with severe vomiting and diarrhea should be monitored for breakthrough fungal infections. Voriconazole is used to treat *Candida*, *Cryptococcus*, and *Aspergillus*. It is widely distributed and metabolized by CYP2C9, CYP2C19, and CYP3A4 and eliminated renally. IV voriconazole should be used with caution in patients with CrCl < 50 mL/minute due to potential for accumulation of the IV vehicle sulfobutyl ether betacyclodextrin sodium. If possible, the oral formulation should be used in these patients. Transient visual disturbance is a common adverse effect, occurring in approximately 30% of recipients. Additional adverse effects such as torsades de pointes, cardiac arrest, and sudden death have been reported with voriconazole in critically ill individuals with comorbidities.

Isavuconazole (Cresemba), the newest of the azole antifungals, has a spectrum activity similar to that of the other azoles with respect to *Candida* species. It has slightly less activity against *Aspergillus* spp. compared to voriconazole but has similar *Mucorales* coverage compared to posaconazole. The drug is available in both IV and oral (PO) formulations; both are considered bioequivalent. Isavuconazole is considered to have fewer drug interactions compared to the other azole antifungals. Adverse reactions may include nausea, vomiting, diarrhea, headache, and abdominal pain. Unlike other azoles, the drug shortens the QTc interval. The clinical relevance of this is unknown.

Clinical Application 24.2

- Before Ms. Angelo takes fluconazole, what assessments should the nurse make?
- What is the action of fluconazole?
- Ms. Angelo returns to the primary care provider's office 2 weeks later. She has an active *Candida albicans* infection. The primary care provider prescribes fluconazole 200 mg PO for one dose and then 100 mg PO daily for 14 days. What adverse effects should the nurse tell the patient to watch for?

NCLEX Success

2. A patient who is being treated for a seizure disorder with phenytoin receives a diagnosis of candidiasis. The prescriber orders fluconazole. In regard to the drug interactions of fluconazole and phenytoin, which of the following is a priority related to the administration of the two medications?
   A. The dosage of phenytoin should be increased.
   B. The fluconazole will be ineffective with the phenytoin.
   C. The patient should be assessed for phenytoin toxicity.
   D. The fluconazole dosage will need to be increased.

3. A prescriber writes an order for fluconazole 250 mg IV per hour. Which of the following nursing interventions is most appropriate?
   A. Begin the IV infusion at 125 mg/hour and increase it to 250 mg/hour after 4 hours.
   B. Inform the prescriber that the maximum dose is 200 mg/hour IV.
   C. Administer the fluconazole at 250 mg/hour IV.
   D. Administer the fluconazole at 200 mg/hour IV.

4. A patient who is undergoing hemodialysis has received a diagnosis of a systemic *Candida* infection. Which of the following interventions should be implemented when administering fluconazole?
   A. Administer the full dose of fluconazole after dialysis.
   B. Administer the full dose of fluconazole before dialysis.
   C. Administer one half of the dose of fluconazole after dialysis.
   D. Administer one half of the dose of fluconazole before dialysis.

5. A patient is receiving a high dose of fluconazole intravenously. Which of the following laboratory values indicate the development of hepatic necrosis?
   A. creatinine clearance of 50 mL/minute
   B. blood urea nitrogen of 15 mg/dL
   C. aspartate aminotransferase of 10 units/L
   D. alanine aminotransferase of 200 units/L

ECHINOCANDINS

The echinocandins have fungal activity against *Candida*, including azole-resistant organisms, and fungistatic activity against *Aspergillus*. The prototype for this class of antifungals is **caspofungin** (Cancidas).

Pharmacokinetics

Caspofungin is highly bound to plasma albumin. It is metabolized in the liver and by the plasma to inactive metabolites. It is excreted in the urine and feces. Its half-life is 9 to 11 hours.

Action

Caspofungin inhibits the synthesis of the fungal cell wall, interfering with the reproduction and growth of susceptible fungi.

Use

Caspofungin is used to treat invasive aspergillosis in patients who do not tolerate other antifungal drugs. It is also used to treat *Candida* infections related to intra-abdominal, pleural space, or esophageal abscesses or peritonitis. In addition, it is given to febrile neutropenic patients who possess a suspected fungal infection.

Table 24.4 provides information about the use of echinocandins, including dosages.

Patient-related variables specific to the use of caspofungin include the following:

- Age:
  - Caspofungin is approved for use in children older than 3 months to treat candidemia and invasive candidiasis.
  - Dosage should be established based on body surface area rather than weight.
  - Both children and adults receiving rifampin or phenytoin with caspofungin require an increased dose. The combination

TABLE 24.4
DRUGS AT A GLANCE: Echinocandins

Drug	Type of Infection Treated	Routes and Dosage Ranges	
		Adults	**Children**
P **Caspofungin** (Cancidas; ❋ Cancidas)	Invasive aspergillosis Candidiasis	IV infusion over 1 h, 70 mg initially and then 50 mg daily Hepatic impairment, 70 mg initially and then 35 mg daily	Safety and efficacy not established in children younger than 3 mo of age Infants and children 3 mo to 17 y are administered 70 mg/m^2/dose on the first day and 50 mg/m^2/dose daily. The dosage may be increased to 70 mg/m^2/dose daily
Anidulafungin (Eraxis; ❋ Eraxis)	Treatment of candidemia, esophageal candidiasis, and other *Candida* infections	Candidemia, IV infusion 200 mg initially and then 100 mg daily Esophageal candidiasis, IV infusion 100 mg initially and then 50 mg daily	Dosage not established
Micafungin (Mycamine; ❋ Mycamine)	Treatment of esophageal candidiasis Prevention of *Candida* infections in patients undergoing hematopoietic stem cell transplantation	Treatment: IV infusion 100–150 mg daily Prevention: IV infusion 50 mg daily	Candidiasis, systemic: Duration of therapy should be individualized based on blood culture and resolution or symptoms: Infants <4 months: IV 10 mg/kg/dose once daily; dosage can be increased to 15 mg/kg/dose Infants >4 months, children, and adolescents: IV: initial 2 mg/kg/dose once daily; usual maximum dosage 100 mg/dose may increase to 4 mg/kg/dose if clinical condition does not improve

of rifampin or phenytoin with caspofungin leads to the inhibition of organic anion-transporting polypeptide-1 (OATP-1), producing caspofungin metabolism leading to its excretion.
- Reproduction, pregnancy, and lactation:
  - Based on animal studies, caspofungin may cause fetal harm.
  - It is not known if caspofungin is present in breast milk.
- Abnormal kidney function and hepatic impairment:
  - For hepatic insufficiency, dose reduction is recommended. It is not recommended with severe hepatic insufficiency.

Adverse Effects

Adverse effects of caspofungin include fever, headache, nausea, skin rash, vomiting, and phlebitis at the injection site.

Contraindications

Caspofungin is contraindicated in patients who have experienced a hypersensitivity reaction to the medication. It should not be administered with mannitol.

Nursing Implications

Preventing Interactions

Certain medications interact with caspofungin, increasing or decreasing its effects (Box 24.5). Researchers have not reported that any herbs interact with caspofungin.

Administering the Medication

It is essential to administer caspofungin intravenously, and the drug is incompatible with any other IV medication, including dextrose. The medication should be at room temperature prior to administration. It is necessary to reconstitute the 50- or 70-mg vials of caspofungin in 10.5 mL of normal saline or sterile water. The reconstituted medication yields 5 or 7 mg/mL, respectively. Reconstituted solutions are stable for 24 hours when stored at 25°C. The reconstituted medication is added to 250 mL of normal saline or half-normal saline. The nurse administers the IV fluids with the medication slowly over 1 hour.

Prior to administering the first dose of caspofungin, the nurse assesses baseline liver and kidney function along with electrolytes, complete blood count, and platelet count. During administration, the nurse assesses for hypersensitivity reactions and phlebitis at the infusion site. Concurrent administration with tacrolimus requires assessment of serum blood levels.

Assessing for Therapeutic Effects

The therapeutic effect of caspofungin is a decrease in the growth of fungi. The patient has decreased symptoms of malaise, fever, and GI symptoms.

BOX 24.5 **Drug Interactions: Caspofungin**

Drugs That Increase the Effects of Caspofungin
- Cyclosporine
  Increases serum effects (when cyclosporine and caspofungin are administered together)

Drugs That Decrease the Effects of Caspofungin
- Antiseizure medications (e.g., carbamazepine, phenytoin); antiviral medications used to treat human immunodeficiency virus (HIV) (e.g., efavirenz, nelfinavir, nevirapine); dexamethasone; rifampin
  Reduce blood levels and therapeutic effectiveness

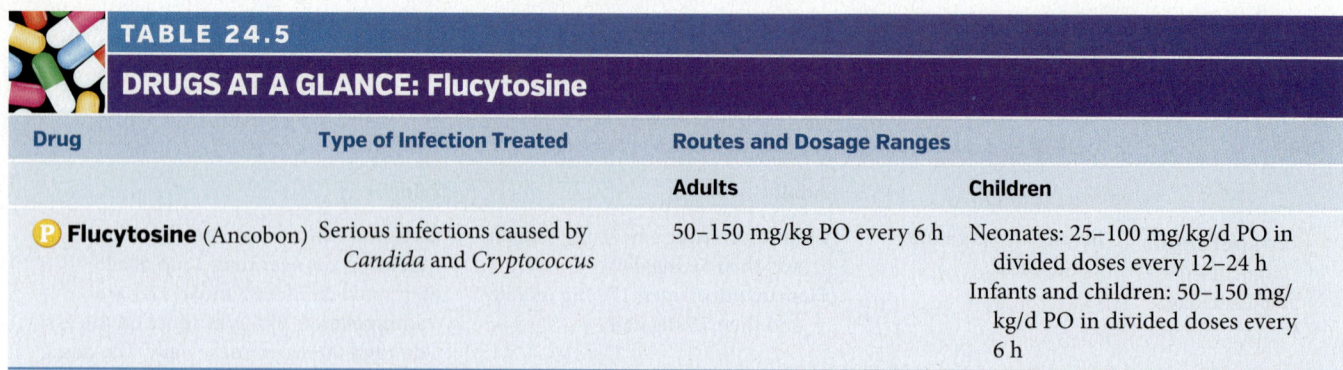

TABLE 24.5 DRUGS AT A GLANCE: Flucytosine

Drug	Type of Infection Treated	Routes and Dosage Ranges	
		Adults	**Children**
ⓟ Flucytosine (Ancobon)	Serious infections caused by *Candida* and *Cryptococcus*	50–150 mg/kg PO every 6 h	Neonates: 25–100 mg/kg/d PO in divided doses every 12–24 h Infants and children: 50–150 mg/kg/d PO in divided doses every 6 h

Assessing for Adverse Effects

When administering 50 mg daily of caspofungin, the nurse observes for nausea, vomiting, and phlebitis at the infusion site. When administering 50 to 70 mg, the nurse assesses for these adverse effects plus fever, headache, and abnormal laboratory reports (e.g., decreased white blood cells, hemoglobin and hematocrit, increased serum potassium, and liver aminotransferase enzymes). In addition, the nurse assesses for a histamine reaction, including facial edema, wheezing, dyspnea, chest tightness, skin eruptions, and itching. Patients suffering from any cardiovascular disease warrant assessment for increasing weight and peripheral edema.

Patient Teaching

Caspofungin is administered in the acute care setting. The patient should receive instruction about the histamine reaction to the medication and the necessity of reporting any cardiac symptoms.

Other Drugs in the Class

Anidulafungin (Eraxis) is a semisynthetic antifungal medication that inhibits glucan synthase, an essential component in the fungal cell wall. It is used to treat esophageal candidiasis and other *Candida* infections. It produces similar adverse effects as caspofungin and warrants cautious use with hepatic impairment.

Micafungin (Mycamine) is approved for adult and pediatric patients.

PYRIMIDINE ANALOG

ⓟ **Flucytosine**, the prototype pyrimidine analog, is an antifungal agent used to treat cryptococcosis, candidiasis, and chromomycosis. This drug is similar in structure to cytosine. As the fungal organism attempts to use flucytosine in place of cytosine to construct DNA, fungal cell division is interrupted.

> **Quality and Safety Alert: Patient-Centered Care**
>
> Safety alerts for the administration of flucytosine include the following:
> - The Institute for Safe Medication Practices (ISMP) states that flucytosine causes a significant risk of patient harm when used in error.
> - Flucytosine is associated with hematologic, kidney, and hepatic adverse effects. Assess complete blood count, blood urea nitrogen, creatinine, AST, and ALT.

Pharmacokinetics

Flucytosine is absorbed by the GI tract and distributed to the CSF, aqueous humor, joints, peritoneal fluid, and bronchial secretions. It is 3% to 4% protein bound and metabolized by the liver. The serum half-life with normal kidney function is 2 to 5 hours. In patients with anuria, the half-life ranges from 30 to 250 hours. In patients with kidney failure with replacement therapy, the serum half-life is 75 to 200 hours. Flucytosine is excreted in the urine, greater than 90% unchanged.

Action

Flucytosine affects the cell membrane of the fungus to cause fungal death. The exact mechanism is unknown.

Use

Flucytosine is used as an adjunctive agent with amphotericin B for the treatment of systemic fungal infections caused by *Candida* and *Cryptococcus*. Flucytosine is added to the therapy due to its anticandidal activity and ability to penetrate the CSF and brain tissue. It can be administered in combination with other antifungal agents for the treatment of chromomycosis and aspergillosis.

Table 24.5 presents specific information about the use of the pyrimidine analog flucytosine, including dosages for adults and children.

Patient-related variables specific to the use of flucytosine include the following:

- Age:
  - In children, flucytosine should be used in combination with amphotericin B or another antifungal drug because of the development of resistance.
- Reproduction, pregnancy, and lactation:
  - Flucytosine is metabolized to fluorouracil, which may cause adverse events if administered during pregnancy.
  - Although it is unknown if flucytosine is present in breast milk, a decision regarding continuing or discontinuing breast-feeding must take into account the significance of treatment to the patient.
- Abnormal kidney function and hepatic impairment:
  - The FDA has issued a **BOXED WARNING** ◆ indicating that flucytosine should be used with extreme caution in patients with abnormal kidney function.

- When administering flucytosine to patients with impaired kidney function, a reduced dosage is used at the beginning. For patients with a creatinine clearance of 20 to 40 mL/minute, an individual dose is administered every 12 hours. For those with a creatinine clearance of 10 to 20 mL/minute, an individual dose is administered every 24 hours. For those with a creatinine clearance of less than 10 mL/minute, an individual dose is administered every 24 to 48 hours.
- Patients receiving hemodialysis should be given 20 to 50 mg/kg following the dialysis treatment.
- Since hepatotoxicity and bone marrow toxicity appear to be related, hepatic and hematologic function should be monitored closely.
- The dose should be adjusted according to hepatic function and any signs and symptoms of hematologic toxicity.

Adverse Effects

Adverse effects of flucytosine include the following:

- GI: nausea, vomiting, diarrhea, duodenal ulcer, and GI bleeding.
- Bone marrow depression: after 10 to 26 days of therapy. Bone marrow depression and hepatotoxicity are related to the administration of higher doses.
- Dermatologic: rash, photosensitivity, pruritus, and urticaria.

Contraindications

Flucytosine is contraindicated in patients who have a known hypersensitivity to the medication or any component of the formulation.

Nursing Implication

Preventing Interactions

Certain medications interact with flucytosine, increasing or decreasing its effect (Box 24.6). No documented interactions between flucytosine and herbs exist. When the drug is given with food, the rate of absorption decreases.

Administering the Medication

It is necessary to perform a culture and sensitivity before the initiation of therapy and at intervals throughout the course of treatment.

When treating endocarditis, amphotericin B is administered in combination with flucytosine. The oral dosage of flucytosine is 25 mg/kg four times daily for at least 6 weeks after

BOX 24.6 Drug Interactions: Flucytosine

Drugs That Increase the Effects of Flucytosine
- Amphotericin B
  Increases serum levels of flucytosine

Drugs That Decrease the Effects of Flucytosine
- *Saccharomyces boulardii* (probiotic; Florastor)
  Flucytosine decreases the levels of Saccharomyces boulardii.

BOX 24.7 Patient Teaching Guidelines for Flucytosine

- Report any unusual bleeding such as bleeding of the gums or mouth.
- Take the entire course of treatment, which could be a minimum of 4 to 6 weeks.

valve replacement. When treating meningoencephalitis caused by cryptococcal fungi, the oral dosage of flucytosine is 25 mg/kg every 6 hours for 2 weeks. If the patient's clinical condition improves, the flucytosine and amphotericin B are discontinued, and the patient is started on fluconazole 400 mg/day. Administering the medication with food decreases the rate but not the extent of drug absorption.

Assessing for Therapeutic Effects

The patient has decreased symptoms of the fungal infection related to endocarditis and meningoencephalitis caused by *Candida* or *Cryptococcus*.

Assessing for Adverse Effects

The nurse assesses for dermatologic reactions such as rash, photosensitivity, pruritus, and urticaria. Baseline hepatic and kidney function is also assessed prior to beginning therapy and at frequent intervals throughout therapy due to the adverse effect of hepatotoxicity and kidney toxicity. It is necessary to check leukocyte and differential counts weekly as well as platelet counts to rule out bone marrow depression. In addition, the nurse assesses intake and output to determine any change in pattern or amount of urine output.

Patient Teaching

Box 24.7 identifies patient teaching guidelines for flucytosine.

MISCELLANEOUS ANTIFUNGAL AGENTS FOR SUPERFICIAL MYCOSES

The miscellaneous antifungal agents are administered for dermatophyte infections of the scalp and nails. **Griseofulvin** is the prototype for this class.

Pharmacokinetics

Griseofulvin is absorbed in the GI tract and metabolized in the liver. The serum half-life is 9 to 24 hours. The medication is excreted in the urine, feces, and perspiration.

Action

Griseofulvin disrupts the metaphase of cell division by binding to keratin, making it resistant to fungal invasion.

Use

Griseofulvin is used for the treatment of susceptible tinea infections of the skin, hair, and nails. Table 24.6 gives specific information about the use of miscellaneous antifungal agents, including dosages for adults and children.

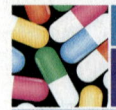

TABLE 24.6
DRUGS AT A GLANCE: Miscellaneous Antifungal Agents for Superficial Mycoses

Drug	Type of Infection Treated	Routes and Dosage Ranges	
		Adults	**Children**
Griseofulvin	Dermatophytosis (skin, hair, nails)	PO Microsize: 500–1,000 mg/d in single or divided doses Ultramicrosize: 375 mg/d in single or divided doses. Up to 750 mg/d have been used to eradicate tinea unguium and tinea pedis	Children >2 y PO Microsize: 10–20 mg/kg/d in single or divided doses; tinea capitis, 20–25 mg/kg/d for 8–12 wk Ultramicrosize: 7.3 mg/kg/d in single dose or 2 divided doses. Maximum dosage is 750 mg/d
Terbinafine (Lamisil; ✣ Apo-Terbinafine, Lamisil, JAMP-Terbinafine)	Tinea infections Onychomycosis of fingernails or toenails	Tinea infections, topically to skin, once or twice daily for at least 1 wk and no longer than 4 wk Onychomycosis, fingernail, PO 250 mg daily for 6 wk; toenail, PO 250 mg daily for 12 wk	
Ibrexafungerp (Brexafemme)	Vulvovaginal candidiasis	300 mg PO twice daily for 1 day	

Patient-related variables specific to the use of griseofulvin include the following:

- Age:
  - Safety has not been established in children 2 years of age and younger.
- Reproduction, pregnancy, and lactation:
  - The drug crosses the placenta and adverse effects have been observed in the fetus; use during pregnancy is contraindicated.
  - Patients of reproductive potential should use effective contraception during therapy (estrogen containing contraceptives may be less effective).
  - Males should avoid procreation for at least 6 months after therapy.
  - Griseofulvin is contraindicated during lactation.
- Abnormal kidney function and hepatic impairment:
  - Griseofulvin is contraindicated in patients with hepatic impairment.

Adverse Effects

Adverse effects of griseofulvin include the following:

- Central nervous system (CNS): dizziness, fatigue, headache, insomnia, and mental confusion
- Dermatologic: erythema, photosensitivity, and urticaria
- GI: sometimes gastric upset with nausea and vomiting
- Other: hepatotoxicity and proteinuria

Contraindications

Griseofulvin is contraindicated in patients with a known hypersensitivity reaction. It is also contraindicated with liver disease, porphyria, pregnancy, and lactation.

Nursing Implications

Preventing Interactions

Some medications interact with griseofulvin, increasing or decreasing its effect (Box 24.8). Substances that increase the effect of griseofulvin include alcohol and vitamin E.

Administering the Medication

It is necessary to administer griseofulvin with meals to decrease gastric upset. Greater absorption occurs when the drug is given with a high-fat meal. Storage in a tightly covered container at 15°C to 30°C is required.

Assessing for Therapeutic Effects

Tinea infections of skin (e.g., ringworm) improve in 3 to 8 weeks. Onychomycosis of toenails may require a year or more. The most effective therapeutic results are achieved when the patient has two to three consecutive negative cultures.

Assessing for Adverse Effects

The nurse assesses for safety related to CNS depression. The nurse also assesses for dermatologic reactions such as rash,

---

BOX 24.8 *Drug Interactions: Griseofulvin*

Drugs That Increase the Effects of Griseofulvin

- Estrogen
  Possible breakthrough bleeding

Drugs That Decrease the Effects of Griseofulvin

- Barbiturates and rifampin
  Decrease griseofulvin drug action

> **BOX 24.9 Patient Teaching Guidelines for Griseofulvin**
>
> - Avoid exposure to sunlight or extreme artificial light.
> - Know that oral contraceptive effects are diminished.

photosensitivity, or urticaria. The urine is assessed for evidence of protein and liver enzymes are checked for signs and symptoms of hepatotoxicity. Patients who are allergic to penicillin are monitored for hypersensitivity reactions.

Patient Teaching

Box 24.9 identifies patient teaching guidelines for griseofulvin.

Other Drugs in the Class

Terbinafine (Lamisil) is a broad-spectrum antifungal that inhibits an enzyme needed for synthesis of ergosterol, a structural component of fungal cell membranes. It has fungicidal activity against dermatophytes and has been used mainly for topical treatment of ringworm infections and oral treatment of onychomycosis. Therapeutic effects may not be evident until months after drug therapy is stopped, because of the time required for growth of healthy nail. The drug is metabolized to inactive metabolites and excreted in the urine.

Common adverse effects with oral terbinafine include headache, diarrhea, and abdominal discomfort, and with long-term use for onychomycosis, skin reactions and liver failure may also occur. Hepatotoxicity is uncommon but has occurred in people with and without preexisting liver disease and has led to liver transplant or death. Terbinafine is not recommended for patients with chronic or active liver disease, and serum ALT and AST should be checked before starting the drug. The FDA has issued a **BOXED WARNING** ◆ for this drug regarding the risk of hepatotoxicity.

Ibrexafungerp (Brexafemme) is a newer antifungal in the triterpenoid class. It is indicated for vulvovaginal candidiasis in adult and postmenarchal pediatric females. The drug works similar to other antifungals by blocking the formation of 1,3-β-D-glucan by inhibiting glucan synthase, which results in fungal cell wall damage. It is important to note that the activity is retained at a pH of 4.5 (normal vaginal pH). Ibrexafungerp is contraindicated in pregnancy, and pregnancy status of the patient should be verified prior to treatment.

THE NURSING PROCESS

A concept map outlines the nursing process related to drug therapy considerations in this chapter. Additional nursing implications related to the disease process should also be considered in care decisions.

Assessment

- Assess for superficial lesions of skin, hair, and nails, which are usually characterized by pain, burning, and itching. Some lesions are moist; others are dry and scaling.
- Assess warm, moist areas of the body; candidiasis occurs in such places. Skin lesions are likely to occur in perineal and intertriginous areas. They are usually moist, inflamed, pruritic areas with papules, vesicles, and pustules. Vaginal infection causes a cheesy vaginal discharge. Oral candidiasis has white patchy lesions on the buccal mucosa. Intestinal infection causes diarrhea. Systemic infection causes chills and fever, myalgia, arthralgia, and prostration.
- Assess for cough, fever, generalized malaise, and signs and symptoms of diminished pulmonary function. Blastomycosis, coccidioidomycosis, and histoplasmosis may be asymptomatic or mimic influenza, pneumonia, or tuberculosis, with cough, fever, malaise, and other pulmonary manifestations. Severe histoplasmosis may also cause fever, anemia, enlarged spleen and liver, leukopenia, and GI tract ulcers.
- Assess cognition and altered mental status. Cryptococcosis may involve the lungs, skin, and other body organs. In patients with AIDS or other immunosuppressant disorders, it often involves the CNS and produces mental status changes, headache, dizziness, and neck stiffness.
- Assess skin and lymph nodes. Sporotrichosis involves these areas. This infection usually produces small nodules that look like insect bites initially and ulcerations later. Nodules and ulcers also may develop in local lymphatic channels and nodes. The infection can spread to other parts of the body in immunocompromised patients.
- Assess for systemic mycoses producing severe symptoms that may be life-threatening. Confirmation involves recovery of organisms from specimens of body tissues or fluids.

Outcomes of Therapy

The patient will
- Take or receive systemic antifungal drugs as prescribed.
- Apply topical drugs accurately.
- Act to prevent recurrence of fungal infection.
- Avoid preventable adverse effects from systemic drugs.

Nursing Interventions

- Observe standard precautions while assessing or providing care to patients with skin lesions. Superficial infections (e.g., ringworm) are highly contagious and can be spread by sharing towels and hairbrushes. Systemic mycoses are not usually contagious.
- Decrease patient exposure to environmental fungi. For inpatients who are neutropenic or otherwise immunocompromised, do not allow soil-containing plants in the room and request regular cleaning and inspection of air-conditioning systems. For outpatients, assist to identify and avoid areas of potential exposure (e.g., soil contaminated by chicken, bird, or bat droppings; areas where buildings are being razed, constructed, or renovated). If exposure is unavoidable, instruct to spray areas with water to minimize airborne spores and to wear disposable clothing and a face mask. Patients working with landscaping are at risk for exposure to sporotrichosis; instruct to wear gloves and long sleeves. Implement measures for obese patients with skin candidiasis. Apply dry padding to intertriginous areas to help prevent irritation and candidal growth.
- Implement measures for patients with oropharyngeal ulcerations. Provide soothing oral hygiene, nonacidic fluids, and soft, bland foods.
- Implement measures for patients with systemic fungal infections. Monitor respiratory, cardiovascular, and neurologic status at least every 8 hours. Provide medications (e.g., analgesics, antihistamines, antipyretics, antiemetics) for patients receiving IV amphotericin B.

Evaluation

- Observe for relief of symptoms for which an antifungal drug was prescribed.
- Interview outpatients regarding their compliance with instructions for using antifungal drugs.
- Interview and observe for adverse drug effects with systemic antifungal agents.

Visit thePoint® *at* **http://thePoint.lww.com/Frandsen13e** *for answers to NCLEX Success questions (in Appendix A), answers to Clinical Application Case Studies (in Appendix B), additional information on etiology and pathophysiology, and more!*

REFERENCES AND RESOURCES

Cox, G. M. (2022). Clinical management and monitoring during antifungal therapy of the HIV-infected patient with cryptococcal meningoencephalitis. *UpToDate*. Lexi-Comp, Inc.

Hinkle, J. H., Cheever, K. H., & Overbaugh, K. (2021). *Brunner & Suddarth's textbook of medical-surgical nursing* (14th ed.). Wolters Kluwer.

Houšť, J., Spížek, J., & Havlíček, V. (2020). Antifungal drugs. *Metabolites, 10*(3), 106. https://doi.org/10.3390/metabo10030106

Kludjian, G., & Gallagher, J. (2021). Ibrexafungerp: A novel antifungal agent that is easier to pronounce than spell. *Contagion, 6*(4), 8–9.

Lewis, R. E. (2022). Pharmacology of echinocandins. *UpToDate*. Lexi-Comp, Inc.

Lippincott advisor. (2022). http://advisor.lww.com

Norris, T. L. (2018). *Porth's pathophysiology: Concepts of altered health states* (10th ed.). Wolters Kluwer.

Nursing 2022 drug handbook. (2021). Wolters Kluwer.

Paquette, V. C., & Elwood, C. (2019). The safety of oral fluconazole therapy in pregnancy. *Journal De L'association Medicale Canadienne, 191*(7), 178. https://doi.org/10.1503/cmaj.190079

UpToDate. (2022). *Drug information*. Lexi-Comp, Inc.

US Department of Health and Human Services (HHS) Panel on Opportunistic Infections in Adults and Adolescents with HIV. Guidelines for the prevention and treatment of opportunistic infections in adults and adolescents with HIV: Recommendations from the Centers for Disease Control and Prevention, the National Institutes of Health, and the HIV Medicine Association of the Infectious Diseases Society of America. Updated May 26, 2020. Retrieved March 6, 2022, from https://clinicalinfo.hiv.gov/sites/default/files/guidelines/documents/Adult_OI.pdf

CHAPTER 25

Drug Therapy for Parasitic Infections

LEARNING OBJECTIVES

After studying this chapter, you should be able to:

1. Describe the types of parasitic infections and their clinical manifestations.
2. Identify the prototype and describe the action, use, adverse effects, contraindications, and nursing implications for the amebicides.
3. Identify the prototype and describe the action, use, adverse effects, contraindications, and nursing implications for the antimalarial drugs.
4. Identify the prototype and describe the action, use, adverse effects, contraindications, and nursing implications for the anthelmintic drugs.
5. Identify the prototype and describe the action, use, adverse effects, contraindications, and nursing implications for the scabicides and pediculicides.
6. Implement the nursing process in the care of the patient being treated with antiparasitic agents.

CLINICAL APPLICATION CASE STUDY

Lacy Michelson, age 35 years, is a missionary. She has just returned from a 2-year stay in a developing country. She comes to the clinic with severe diarrhea, fever, chills, headache, and myalgia. Ms. Michelson receives a diagnosis of giardiasis and malaria as well as a prescription for chloroquine 500 mg daily by mouth for 3 weeks and metronidazole 250 mg three times a day by mouth for 7 days.

KEY TERMS

Larvae: developmental forms of a parasite

Parasite: a living organism that survives at the expense of another organism, called the host

INTRODUCTION

A **parasite** is a living organism that survives at the expense of another organism, called the host. The parasite gains nutrition from the host. Parasitic infestations are common human ailments worldwide. The effects of parasitic diseases on human hosts vary from minor to major and can be life threatening. Parasitic diseases discussed in this chapter are those caused by protozoa, helminths (worms), scabies, and pediculi (lice). There are currently no licensed vaccines to combat infection with any human parasite. Therefore, preventive measures, insecticide use, surveillance processes, and drug therapy are used to control parasitic infestations and any resulting diseases.

OVERVIEW OF PARASITIC INFECTIONS

Protozoa can infect the digestive tract and other body tissues, and resulting infections include amebiasis, giardiasis, malaria, and trichomoniasis. Helminths can also infect these sites, causing several infections. Scabies and pediculi affect the skin. Information on the etiology and pathophysiology of parasitic infections is located on thePoint.

Clinical Manifestations

Amebiasis may be with no symptoms. Affected people may have nausea, vomiting, diarrhea, abdominal cramping, and weakness. If the disease is severe, prolonged, and untreated, these people may experience symptoms from ulcerations of the colon or abscesses of the liver (hepatic amebiasis).

Giardiasis may be with no symptoms or produce diarrhea, abdominal cramping and distention, and flatulence. The clinical manifestations increase and decrease in intensity over months. If the infection is untreated, it may resolve spontaneously or progress to a chronic disease with anorexia, nausea, malaise, weight loss, and continued diarrhea with large, foul-smelling stools. Deficiencies of vitamin B_{12}, folate, and fat-soluble vitamins (see Chapter 35) may occur.

Malaria is an acute febrile illness that initially seems to resemble influenza in terms of its symptoms. In a nonimmune individual, symptoms appear a week or more (usually 10 to 15 days) after the infective mosquito bite. The first symptoms (fever, headache, chills, and vomiting) may be mild and difficult to identify as malaria. The characteristic paroxysms of chills, fever, and copious perspiration may not be present at the early stage of disease. If not treated within 24 hours, *Plasmodium falciparum* malaria can progress to severe illness, often leading to death. During acute malarial attacks, the cycles occur every 36 to 72 hours. Clinical symptoms occur because of the large parasite burden. Children with severe malaria often develop severe anemia, respiratory distress in relation to metabolic acidosis, and/or cerebral malaria. In adults, multiorgan involvement is also frequent. In malaria-endemic areas, people may develop partial immunity, allowing asymptomatic infections to occur.

Trichomoniasis affects women and men differently. Women usually have vaginal burning, itching, and foul-smelling yellow-gray, frothy discharge. Men may be with no symptoms or have symptoms of urethritis.

Helminthiasis involves worm infestations; helminths are most often found in the gastrointestinal (GI) tract. However, several types penetrate body tissues or produce **larvae** (developmental forms of parasites) that migrate to the blood, lymph channels, lungs, liver, and other body tissues. Hookworm, roundworm, and threadworm larvae migrate through the lungs and may cause symptoms of pulmonary congestion. Hookworms may cause anemia by feeding on blood from the intestinal mucosa; fish tapeworms may cause megaloblastic or pernicious anemia by absorbing folic acid and vitamin B_{12}. Large masses of roundworms or tapeworms may cause intestinal obstruction. The major symptom usually associated with pinworms is intense itching in the perianal area (pruritus ani).

Scabies is characterized by burrows produced by the mite that create visible skin lesions, most often between the fingers, around the nails, and on the elbows and wrists. The lesions may also involve skin that is usually covered by clothing; the buttocks, belt line, penis, and skin around the nipples are likely places for mites to burrow.

Pediculosis leads to pruritus, which is usually the major symptom of the disease. This symptom results from an allergic reaction to parasite secretions. In addition to the intense discomfort associated with pruritus, scratching is likely to cause skin excoriation with secondary bacterial infection and formation of vesicles, pustules, and crusts.

Clinical Application 25.1

- Ms. Michelson has received a diagnosis of a *Giardia* infection. What vitamin deficiency is she at risk for developing?
- What are the initial symptoms of giardiasis?

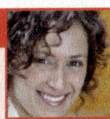

Drug Therapy

To combat parasitic diseases, healthcare professionals use antiparasitic drugs, including amebicides, antimalarials, other antiprotozoal agents, anthelmintics, scabicides, and pediculicides. Table 25.1 lists these drugs.

AMEBICIDES

Amebicides, or drugs used to treat amebiasis, are classified according to their site of action. The prototype **metronidazole** (Flagyl), a synthetic compound with amebicidal and trichomonacidal activity, is effective in both intestinal and extraintestinal amebiasis. Chloroquine is a tissue or extraintestinal amebicide because it acts in the bowel wall, liver, and other tissues. Chloroquine is discussed as an antimalarial agent because it is most commonly used for the prevention and treatment of malaria.

Tetracycline and doxycycline, which are antibacterial drugs (see Chapter 20), act against amebae in the intestinal lumen by altering the bacterial flora required for amebic viability. One of these drugs may be used with other amebicides in the treatment of all forms of amebiasis except with no symptoms of intestinal amebiasis.

Pharmacokinetics

Metronidazole is 80% absorbed by the GI tract, reaching a peak of action in 1 to 3 hours. The drug is widely distributed to the

TABLE 25.1

Drugs Administered for Parasitic Infections

Drug Class	Prototype	Other Drugs in the Class
Amebicide	Metronidazole (Flagyl)	Nitazoxanide (Alinia) Tinidazole
Antibacterial	Tetracycline	Doxycycline
Antimalarial	Chloroquine phosphate	Quinine Artemether/lumefantrine (Coartem) Atovaquone/proguanil (Malarone) Hydroxychloroquine (Plaquenil) Mefloquine Primaquine
Anthelmintic	Mebendazole (Emverm) Ivermectin (Stromectol)	Albendazole Triciabendazole
Scabicide/pediculicide	Permethrin	Crotamiton (Crotan) Lindane Malathion (Ovide) Spinosad (Natroba)

Action and Use

Metronidazole diffuses across the cell membrane of anaerobic and aerobic microorganisms to cause cell death. The biochemical mechanism of action of the drug is unknown. Indications include intestinal amebiasis, amebic liver abscess, trichomoniasis, and bacterial vaginosis. The U.S. Food and Drug Administration (FDA) has not approved this drug or any other amebicide for the prophylaxis of amebiasis. The FDA has issued a **BOXED WARNING** ♦ for metronidazole and tinidazole, stating that these drugs should be used only for indicated conditions because they have produced carcinogenicity in rats. Table 25.2 gives route and dosage information for metronidazole and other amebicides.

Patient-related variables specific to the use of metronidazole include the following:

- Age:
  - Prescribers should use the adjusted body weight in dosing children who have an increased body mass index.
- Reproduction, pregnancy, and lactation:
  - Metronidazole crosses the placenta. Cleft lip with or without cleft palate has been reported following the first trimester use of metronidazole. Also, there is an increased risk of congenital anomalies.
  - Metronidazole may be used to treat giardiasis in the second or third trimesters.
  - Bacterial vaginosis and vaginal trichomoniasis are associated with adverse pregnancy outcomes (such as premature membrane rupture and premature delivery). The Centers for Disease Control and Prevention (CDC) recommends metronidazole twice daily for the treatment of bacterial vaginosis in nonpregnant and pregnant patients diagnosed with bacterial vaginosis.

cerebrospinal fluid, bone, and cerebral and hepatic abscesses. Its half-life is 6 to 8 hours. Metronidazole is metabolized in the liver (30% to 60%), with most excreted in the urine (77%) and some in the feces (14%).

TABLE 25.2

DRUGS AT A GLANCE: Amebicides

Drug	Routes and Dosage Ranges	
	Adults	**Children**
ⓟ **Metronidazole** (Flagyl; ❋ Flagyl, PMS-Metronidazole)	Amebiasis: 750 mg PO for 5–10 d Giardiasis: 750 mg extended-release PO daily for 7 d Trichomoniasis: 2 g PO in 1 d or 250 mg PO three times per day for 7 d	Amebiasis: 35–50 mg/kg/d PO in three divided doses for 7–10 days
Nitazoxanide (Alinia)	*G. duodenalis* or *C. parvum*: 500 mg PO every 12 h for 3 d	1–3 y: 100 mg PO every 12 h for 3 d (increase duration to 14 d in HIV exposed or patients infected with cryptosporidia) 4–11 y: 200 mg PO every 12 h for 3 d (increase duration to 14 d in HIV exposed or patients infected with cryptosporidia) ≥12 y: refer to adult dosing
Tinidazole	Amebiasis: 2 g/d PO for 3 d Amebiasis, liver abscess: 2 g/d PO for 3–5 d Bacterial vaginosis: 2 g/d PO for 2 d or 1 g/d PO for 5 d Giardiasis: 2 g PO as single dose Trichomoniasis: 2 g PO as single dose	Intestinal amebiasis or amebiasis liver abscess (age >3 y): 50 mg/kg/d PO for 3–5 d (maximum 2 g/d)

- Metronidazole and its active hydroxyl metabolite are present in breast milk at the same concentrations as maternal plasma concentrations. The CDC guidelines for metronidazole state breast-feeding should be withheld for 12 to 24 hours after a single dose of 2 g.
- Abnormal kidney function and hepatic impairment:
  - Use with caution in abnormal kidney function or hepatic impairment due to potential drug accumulation.

Adverse Effects and Contraindications

The adverse effects of metronidazole include headache, dizziness, ataxia, darkening of urine, diarrhea, nausea, vomiting, and an unpleasant metallic taste. Contraindications include a known hypersensitivity to the drug.

Nursing Implications

Preventing Interactions

Concomitant use of metronidazole with barbiturates increases the metabolism of the antiamebic drug, thus decreasing its therapeutic effect. Administration of metronidazole with anticoagulants (e.g., warfarin) increases bleeding tendencies due to decreased vitamin K metabolism. Ingesting alcoholic beverages or alcohol-containing medications while taking metronidazole may cause tachycardia, warmth or redness under the skin, a tingly feeling, and nausea and vomiting. Also, disulfiram and alcohol combined with metronidazole may lead to a disulfiramlike reaction, with tachycardia, nausea, flushing, and vomiting. No herbal interactions with metronidazole reportedly occur.

Administering the Drug

Patients may take metronidazole with food to improve medication adsorption. It is important not to crush extended-release preparations. If the patient is unable to swallow regular metronidazole pills, it may be necessary to crush them.

Assessing for Therapeutic Effects

The nurse assesses patients with intestinal amebiasis for decreased abdominal pain and diarrhea. Stool specimens are assessed for amebic cysts and trophozoites periodically for 6 months. Also, the nurse checks the feces for increase in form that is indicative of diminished diarrhea stools and improved hydration.

Patients with trichomoniasis are assessed for decreased vaginal drainage and odor.

Assessing for Adverse Effects

It is necessary to assess for headache; diminished muscular coordination; GI upset, including metallic taste; and hypersensitivity reactions such as rash and bronchospasm.

Patient Teaching

Box 25.1 identifies patient teaching guidelines for antiparasitic drugs, including metronidazole.

Other Drugs in the Class

Nitazoxanide (Alinia) is a less commonly used drug. In *Cryptosporidium parvum* infection, it inhibits the growth of sporozoites and oocysts. In *Giardia duodenalis* infection, it inhibits the growth of trophozoites. Nitazoxanide is administered with food for the treatment of diarrhea.

Tinidazole, a chemical relative of metronidazole, is approved for the treatment of amebiasis, giardiasis, bacterial vaginosis, and trichomoniasis. Cytochrome P4503A4 enzymes in the liver metabolize the drug, and caution is warranted with use in people with impaired liver function. The most common adverse effects are a bitter metallic taste and nausea.

NCLEX Success

1. A patient with intestinal amebiasis has received a prescription for metronidazole. The patient later develops a cough and takes a prescription cough syrup. What adverse effect will the patient experience?
   A. edema
   B. bronchospasm
   C. flushing
   D. bradycardia

2. What assessment should the nurse implement when caring for a patient who is receiving metronidazole for intestinal amebiasis?
   A. diminished diarrhea
   B. hypomagnesemia
   C. increased temperature
   D. hyperkalemia

Clinical Application 25.2

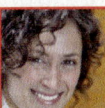

- What is the action of metronidazole (Flagyl)?
- What patient education should the nurse provide to Ms. Michelson?

ANTIMALARIALS

Antimalarials act at different stages in the life cycle of plasmodial parasites. Some drugs, such as **chloroquine phosphate**, are effective against erythrocytic forms and are therefore useful in preventing or treating acute attacks of malaria. Although these drugs do not prevent infection with the parasite, they do prevent clinical manifestations.

Widespread resistance in most malaria-endemic countries has led to decline in the use of chloroquine for the treatment of malaria caused by *P. falciparum*, although it remains effective in most regions for disease caused by *Plasmodium vivax*. Other drugs, such as primaquine, act against exoerythrocytic or tissue forms of the parasite to prevent initial infection and recurrent attacks or to cure some types of malaria. Combination drug therapy, administered concomitantly or consecutively, is common with antimalarial drugs.

Pharmacokinetics

Chloroquine is rapidly absorbed by the GI tract, and the drug is widely distributed and retained throughout the body tissues

> **BOX 25.1** **Patient Teaching Guidelines for Antiparasitic Drugs**
>
> **General Considerations**
>
> - Use measures to prevent parasitic infection or reinfection:
>   - Support public health measures to maintain a clean environment (i.e., sanitary sewers, clean water, regulation of food-handling establishments and food-handling personnel).
>   - When traveling to wilderness areas or to tropical or developing countries, check with the local health department about precautions needed to avoid parasitic infections.
>   - Practice good hand hygiene and other personal hygienic practices.
>   - When a family member or other close contact contracts a parasitic infection, be sure to complete prompt appropriate treatment and follow-up care.
>   - Avoid ingesting raw fish and undercooked meat.
>   - With vaginal infections, avoid sexual intercourse or use a condom.
>
> **Self- or Caregiver Administration**
>
> - Take the full course of the medication. For malaria prophylaxis, for example, take chloroquine at the same time each week, and set up a calendar with time and date of administration.
> - Take atovaquone/proguanil, chloroquine and related drugs, oral metronidazole, and tinidazole with or after meals. Food increases absorption of atovaquone and decreases gastrointestinal irritation with the other drugs.
> - Avoid alcoholic beverages while taking metronidazole or tinidazole and for 3 days after the drugs are stopped. Flushing, headache, nausea, sweating, and vomiting may occur if alcohol is ingested.
> - Be aware that metronidazole has an unpleasant metallic taste. Taking this drug will make your urine dark in color. Do not be alarmed.
> - Know that metronidazole is contraindicated in pregnancy. Let your healthcare provider/prescriber know if you think you could be pregnant before taking the medication.
> - Have an ophthalmic examination at the start of chloroquine use and every 3 months during drug therapy. Also have complete blood count studies as ordered.
> - Take or give most anthelmintics without regard to mealtimes or food ingestion. Mebendazole tablets should be chewed or crushed and mixed with food.
> - Have a culture for ova and parasites 3 weeks after initial mebendazole use. Eat frequent small meals and maintain excellent hydration if diarrhea develops. Report fever and severe diarrhea.
> - With a pinworm infection, adhere to the following instructions:
>   - Disinfect the toilet facilities after use.
>   - Launder bed linens, nightclothes, undergarments, and towels every day.
>   - Ensure family members are treated for pinworms because they are highly contagious.
>   - Follow strict handwashing and excellent hygienic practices.
> - Use pediculicides and scabicides as directed on the label or product insert, as instructions vary among preparations. Use gloves prior to applying permethrin cream rinse, cream, or lotion.
> - With pediculosis and scabies, wash bed linens, towels, undergarments, and clothes daily.
> - Inspect the head, genital area, and other parts of the body for lice and scabies to determine if they have been killed.
> - With permethrin administration, report stinging, tingling, skin numbness, rash, itching, and rash to the prescriber.

such as the central nervous system (CNS), eyes, cardiopulmonary system, liver, kidneys, and spleen. The peak of action is 1 to 2 hours with a serum half-life of 3 to 5 days. It is 55% protein bound and partially metabolized by the liver. Chloroquine is excreted by the kidneys. Small amounts of the drug are present in the urine for months following the discontinuation of drug therapy.

Action and Use

Chloroquine inhibits DNA and RNA polymerase, thus interfering with the metabolism and hemoglobin used by parasites. The drug also inhibits prostaglandin effects while concentrating within the parasitic acid vesicles. It raises the internal pH to inhibit parasitic growth. Uses of chloroquine include the suppression and chemoprophylaxis of malaria. Healthcare providers also use it for the treatment of acute malaria caused by *Plasmodium malariae*, *Plasmodium ovale*, and *P. falciparum*, as well as for extraintestinal amebiasis. Table 25.3 gives route and dosage information for chloroquine and the other antimalarial drugs.

Patient-related variables specific to use of chloroquine include the following:

- Reproduction, pregnancy, and lactation:
  - Chloroquine and its metabolites cross the placenta and can be detected in cord blood and the urine of newborns.
  - Chloroquine does not increase the risk of adverse fetal events when used for malaria prophylaxis.
  - Dosing of chloroquine is the same for pregnant and nonpregnant adults.

Adverse Effects

Adverse effects of chloroquine are usually mild because small doses are used for prophylaxis; administration of the larger doses required for the treatment of acute attacks occurs only for short periods. CNS changes include visual disturbances with retinal damage and difficulty to focus. Cardiovascular adverse effects include electrocardiogram changes with prolonged QRS intervals and hypotension. Other significant adverse effects are nausea, vomiting, diarrhea, loss of appetite, skin rash, pruritus, and hair loss. Reportedly, ototoxicity and muscle weakness may also occur.

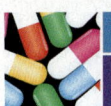

TABLE 25.3
DRUGS AT A GLANCE: Antimalarials

Drug	Routes and Dosage Ranges	
	Adults	**Children**
ⓟ **Chloroquine phosphate**	Prophylaxis: 500 mg/wk PO on the same day each week; start 1–2 wk prior to exposure; continue while in endemic area and for 4 wk after leaving the endemic area Treatment: 1 g PO, followed by 500 mg 6, 24, and 48 h after first dose Extraintestinal amebiasis: 1 g/d PO for 2 d followed by 500 mg/d for at least 2–3 wk	Prophylaxis: 8.3 mg/kg/wk PO on the same day each week (do not exceed 500 mg/dose); begin 1–2 wk prior to exposure; continue while in the endemic area and for 4 wk after leaving endemic area. Treatment: 16.7 mg/kg PO (maximum 1,000 mg), followed by 8.3 mg/kg (maximum 500 mg) 6, 24, and 48 h after first dose
Artemether/lumefantrine (Coartem)	25–35 kg: 3 tablets PO at hour 0 and hour 8 the 1st day and then 3 tablets twice daily on day 2 and day 3 (total of 18 tablets per treatment course) Patients ≥35 kg: 4 tablets at hour 0 and hour 8 the 1st day and then 4 tablets twice daily on day 2 and day 3 (total of 24 tablets per treatment course)	5–15 kg: 1 tablet PO at hour 0 and hour 8 the 1st day and then 1 tablet twice daily on day 2 and day 3 (total of 6 tablets per treatment course) 15–25 kg: 2 tablets PO at hour 0 and hour 8 the 1st day and then 2 tablets twice daily on day 2 and day 3 (total of 12 tablets per treatment course) 25–35 kg: 3 tablets at hour 0 and hour 8 on the 1st day and then 3 tablets twice daily on day 2 and day 3 (total of 18 tablets per treatment course) ≥35 kg: 4 tablets PO at hour 0 and hour 8 the 1st day and then 4 tablets twice daily on day 2 and day 3 (total of 24 tablets per treatment course)
Atovaquone/proguanil (Malarone; ✹ Malarone, Malarone Pediatric)	Prophylaxis: 250 mg/100 mg PO once daily; start 1–2 d prior to entering malaria-endemic area and continue throughout the stay and for 7 d after returning Acute treatment: 1 g/400 mg PO as a single dose, once daily for 3 consecutive days	Prophylaxis (begin 1–2 d prior to entering a malaria-endemic area; continue throughout the stay and for 7 d after returning; take as a single dose, once daily): 5–8 kg: 31.25/12.5 mg 9–10 kg: 46.8/18.75 mg 11–20 kg: 62.5/25 mg 21–30 kg: 125/50 mg 31–40 kg: 187.5/75 mg >40 kg: 250/100 mg PO Acute treatment: 5–8 kg: 125/50 mg 9–10 kg: 187.5/75 mg 11–20 kg: 250/100 mg 21–30 kg: 500/200 mg 31–40 kg: 750/300 mg >40 kg: 1 g/400 mg PO as a single dose once daily for 3 consecutive days
Hydroxychloroquine (Plaquenil; ✹ Plaquenil, APO-Hydroxychloroquine, JAMP-Hydroxychloroquine)	Prophylaxis: 400 mg once weekly for 2 wk before entering and 8 wk after leaving endemic area Treatment of acute disease: 800 mg PO initially, then 400 mg 6 h later, and 400 mg/d for 2 d (total of four doses)	Prophylaxis: 5 mg/kg PO once weekly for 2 wk before entering and 8 wk after leaving endemic area Treatment of acute disease: 13 mg/kg PO initially, then 6.5 mg/kg 6 h later, and 6.5 mg/kg/d PO for 24 and 48 h (total of four doses)
Mefloquine	Prophylaxis: 250 mg PO 1 wk before travel and then 250 mg weekly during travel and for 4 wk after leaving a endemic area Treatment: 1,250 mg (5 tablets) as a single dose	Prophylaxis: 1/4 tablet PO for 15–19 kg weight, 1/2 tablet for 20–30 kg, 3/4 tablet for 31–45 kg, and 1 tablet for above 45 kg, according to the schedule for adults
Primaquine (✹ Primaquine)	30 mg once daily in combination with chloroquine for 14 d For patients with intermediate G6PD activity may administer 45 mg once weekly for 8 weeks	0.39 mg/kg once daily for 14 d (maximum: 15 mg/d)
Quinine (Qualaquin; ✹ APO-Quinine, JAMP-Quinine)	648 mg PO every 8 h for 7 d in combination with doxycycline, tetracycline, or clindamycin	10 mg/kg/d PO in divided doses every 8 h for 3 to 7 d in combination with doxycycline, tetracycline, or clindamycin

Contraindications

Contraindications to chloroquine include a known hypersensitivity to 4-aminoquinoline compounds and the presence of retinal and visual field changes. Caution is necessary in porphyria, psoriasis, retinal disease, glucose-6-phosphate dehydrogenase (G-6-DP) deficiency, alcoholism, pregnancy, and lactation.

Nursing Implications

Preventing Interactions

Some medications interact with chloroquine, increasing or decreasing its effects (Box 25.2). When the drug is combined with alcohol, the risk of GI distress increases.

Administering the Medication

For malaria prophylaxis, it is necessary to take chloroquine on the same day each week. The nurse may set up a calendar to assist with adherence. For malaria treatment, it is necessary to take the drug as prescribed and at the same time each day. Chloroquine can be taken with food to reduce gastric distress. When administering chloroquine to children, it is essential to double-check the dosage because young people are especially sensitive to the 4-aminoquinoline compounds that the drug contains.

> **Concept Mastery Alert**
>
> Teach patients taking chloroquine to avoid foods that acidify their urine, such as cranberries, prunes, plums, cheeses, meats, fish, eggs, and grains. These foods might interact with antimalarials and increase excretion, thus decreasing the effect of the drug.

Assessing for Therapeutic and Adverse Effects

The nurse assesses for a decrease in signs and symptoms of malaria. Fever and chills usually subside in 24 to 48 hours. Blood smears for plasmodia are negative in 24 to 72 hours. Also, the nurse assesses for nausea, vomiting, diarrhea, pruritus, rash, headache, and visual changes.

Patient Teaching

Box 25.1 identifies patient teaching guidelines for antiparasitic drugs, including chloroquine phosphate.

BOX 25.2 Drug Interactions: Chloroquine

Drugs That Increase the Effects of Chloroquine
- Cimetidine
  May increase the plasma concentration

Drugs That Decrease the Effects of Chloroquine
- Magnesium trisilicate
  May reduce bioavailability
- Vitamin C
  Increases urinary excretion

Other Drugs in the Class

Quinine was once the primary antimalarial drug, but synthetic agents that cause fewer adverse reactions have largely replaced it. However, this drug may still be useful in the treatment of chloroquine-resistant *P. falciparum* malaria. Also, it relaxes skeletal muscles and may be effective in the prevention and treatment of nocturnal leg cramps.

Artemisinin-based combination therapies (ACTs) are used for the treatment of uncomplicated malaria to prevent or delay development of drug resistance. The artemisinin component has the most rapid parasite clearance times of any antimalarial drug. The drugs appear to act by binding iron and breaking down peroxide bridges, resulting in the generation of free radicals that damage parasite proteins. Artemether/lumefantrine (Coartem), a combination product, is the only ACT recommended by the World Health Organization (WHO) for the treatment of uncomplicated malaria in the United States.

People may take Coartem with a full meal for optimal absorption. It may be necessary (1) to crush the tablets and mix them in 5 to 10 mL of water and (2) to rinse the container and ingest the contents. If vomiting occurs, it is important to repeat the dosage in 2 hours. People with known QT prolongation should avoid taking Coartem. If people take this combination drug with grapefruit juice, the potential for QT prolongation is enhanced.

> **Quality and Safety Alert: Safety**
>
> Before prescribing primaquine, healthcare providers should screen patients for G-6-DP deficiency. This genetic disorder, which occurs most often in males, causes hemolysis of red blood cells and can lead to hemolytic anemia.

Atovaquone–proguanil (Malarone) is a combination product with adult and pediatric formulations. Uses include the prevention and treatment of malaria, including chloroquine-resistant strains. The constituent drugs inhibit two different pathways in plasmodial reproduction. Atovaquone blocks the parasite mitochondrial electron transport chain, and proguanil inhibits the folate pathway and appears to act by a direct mechanism as well. This activity enhances atovaquone's mitochondrial membrane toxicity, and the combination maintains exceptional clinical efficacy for worldwide treatment and prevention, even if antifolate resistance is present. Adverse effects include vomiting, diarrhea, abdominal pain, headache, and pruritus.

Hydroxychloroquine (Plaquenil) is a derivative of chloroquine with essentially the same actions and uses with fewer adverse effects. When used for nonsevere infections caused by *P. vivax* or *P. ovale*, administer in combination with primaquine. Other uses of this drug include treatment of rheumatoid arthritis and lupus erythematosus.

Mefloquine is used to prevent *P. falciparum* malaria, including chloroquine-resistant strains, and to treat acute malaria caused by *P. falciparum* or *P. vivax*. The FDA has issued a **BOXED WARNING** for mefloquine, warning that patients with major psychiatric disorders should not take the drug. Mefloquine can trigger neuropsychiatric adverse reactions that can persist after the drug has been discontinued. It should be administered with food and at least 8 oz of water on the same day each week.

Primaquine is most commonly used to prevent recurrent attacks of malaria caused by *P. vivax* and *P. ovale*. Also, it may prevent the initial occurrence of malaria. When used to prevent initial occurrence of malaria (causal prophylaxis), people should take primaquine concurrently with a suppressive agent (e.g., chloroquine, hydroxychloroquine) after they have returned from a malarious area. Primaquine is not effective for the treatment of acute attacks of malaria.

> **! Quality and Safety Alert: Evidence-Based Practice**
>
> In 2020, Daly, Minuti, and Khan searched the PubMed and Cochrane Library databases to identify randomized clinical trials, meta-analyses, systemic reviews, and observational studies of the epidemiology, diagnosis, and treatment of malaria from January 2016 through March 2022. They also reviewed relevant articles from the WHO. Their analysis concluded that approximately 2,000 cases of malaria are diagnosed in the United States annually. Most cases are among travelers returning from malaria-endemic countries. Preventing and treating malaria depends on the drug sensitivity of parasites. Intravenous artesunate is the first-line therapy to treat severe malaria.

NCLEX Success

3. Which of the following aspects of teaching is most important to provide to a patient who is taking chloroquine phosphate?
   A. Take chloroquine with vitamin C.
   B. Have frequent ophthalmologic examinations.
   C. Administer antacids to reduce gastric distress.
   D. Take chloroquine on an empty stomach.

> **Clinical Application 25.3**
>
> - When providing patient teaching to Ms. Michelson regarding the chloroquine, what is most important information that the nurse should impart?

ANTHELMINTICS

Anthelmintics are used for the treatment of helminthiasis. Ivermectin and benzimidazole are the two primary anthelmintic agents. There are three benzimidazoles, and **mebendazole** (Emverm) is the prototype of this class of medications. Albendazole and triclabendazole (Egaten) are the other anthelmintic agents. Most of these drugs act locally to kill or cause expulsion of parasitic worms from the intestines. Some of these medications act systemically against parasites that have penetrated various body tissues. The goal of anthelmintic therapy may be to eradicate the parasite completely or to decrease the magnitude of infestation ("worm burden").

Pharmacokinetics

Mebendazole is administered orally with a slow onset of action. The drug reaches peak of action in 2 to 4 hours. Approximately 2% to 10% is absorbed. It reaches its highest concentrations in the liver and muscle. Mebendazole is 95% protein bound and has an elimination half-life of 3 to 6 hours. The drug is metabolized extensively by the liver. It is excreted mostly in the feces and minimally in the urine.

Action

Mebendazole blocks glucose uptake by susceptible helminths. The drug depletes glycogen stores that the worms need for survival and reproduction, resulting in their death.

Use

Uses for mebendazole include the treatment of infections with *Enterobius vermicularis* (pinworm), *Trichuris trichiura* (whipworm), and *Ascaris lumbricoides* (roundworm), as well as *Ancylostoma duodenale* and *Necator americanus* (hookworms). Unlabeled uses of this drug are for infections with *Ancylostoma caninum* (eosinophilic enterocolitis), *Capillaria philippinensis* (capillariasis), *G. duodenalis* (giardiasis), *Mansonella perstans* (filariasis), and visceral larva migrans (toxocariasis). Table 25.4 presents route and dosage information for mebendazole and the other anthelmintics. The WHO recommends preventive therapy with mebendazole or other benzimidazoles in pregnant patients after the first trimester who live in area of soil-transmitted helminth infections. There is an increased risk of congenital anomalies when administered during the first trimester. Mebendazole is present in breast milk. Caution is necessary with lactation.

Adverse Effects

Dizziness, drowsiness, headaches, seizures, transient abdominal pain, diarrhea, nausea, and vomiting may occur with mebendazole. Hematologic effects such as agranulocytosis, anemia, leukopenia, and neutropenia sometimes take place. The hepatic enzymes alanine aminotransferase (ALT) and aspartate aminotransferase (AST) may be increased. Genitourinary effects include casts in the urine, glomerulonephritis, and hematuria. Finally, hypersensitivity reactions have reportedly occurred.

Contraindications

Contraindications to mebendazole include known hypersensitivity to the drug.

Nursing Implications

Preventing Interactions

Certain medications interact with mebendazole, increasing or decreasing its effects (Box 25.3). Serum levels of mebendazole may be increased with food.

Administering the Medication

Administering mebendazole involves chewing and swallowing the tablets or crushing them and mixing them with food, whether solid or liquid. Taking the drug with food increases its serum levels.

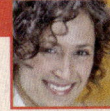

TABLE 25.4

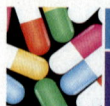

DRUGS AT A GLANCE: Anthelmintics

Drug	Routes and Dosage Ranges	
	Adults	**Children**
Mebendazole (Emverm; Vermox)	Trichuriasis, ascariasis, and hookworm: 100 mg PO morning and evening on 3 consecutive days Enterobiasis: 1 tablet PO once; repeat treatment if not cured in 3 wk	Children 2 y of age and older, same as adults Safety and efficacy have not been established in children younger than 2 y of age
Albendazole	Ascariasis (intestinal roundworm) 400 mg PO Enterobiasis (pinworms): 400 mg as a single dose; may repeat in 2 wk	Ascariasis: ≤2 y: 200 mg PO as a single dose; may repeat in 3 wk Ascariasis: >2 y and adolescents 400 mg PO as a single dose; may repeat in 3 wk Enterobiasis: ≤2 y: 200 mg PO as a single dose; may repeat in 3 wk Enterobiasis: >2 y and adolescents 400 mg PO as a single dose; may repeat in 3 wk
Triclabendazole (Egaten)	Fascioliasis: 10 mg/kg PO every 12 h for 2 doses; the 250-mg tablets are scored and divisible into two equal halves of 125 mg if the dose cannot be adjusted exactly round the dose upward	Fascioliasis: Children ≥6 y to adolescents: 10 mg/kg/dose every 12 h for 2 doses; round dose up to the nearest half (125 mg) or whole tablet (250 mg)
Ivermectin (Stromectol)	Strongyloidiasis: PO 200 mcg/kg as a single dose	Children ≥15 kg: refer to adult dosing

Assessing for Adverse Effects

The nurse assesses for CNS depression, dizziness, and seizure activity. The nurse also assesses for GI disorders, including nausea, vomiting, diarrhea, and alterations in fluid volume. In addition, the hepatic enzymes AST and ALT must be assessed for elevations leading to hepatic failure. Finally, the nurse assesses for blood in the urine and glomerulonephritis. Assessing for rash and alterations in pulmonary status related to hypersensitivity to the medication is also necessary.

Assessing for Therapeutic Effects

The nurse obtains a stool sample for culture for ova and parasites after 3 weeks of drug administration. A negative stool culture is the optimum outcome of drug therapy. There is a complete eradication of the parasite, and any "worm burden" is now nonexistent.

BOX 25.3 Drug Interactions: Mebendazole

Drugs That Increase the Effects of Mebendazole
- Metronidazole
  Enhances the toxic effect of mebendazole and the development of adverse effects

Drugs That Decrease the Effects of Mebendazole
- Aminoquinolines (antimalarials), carbamazepine, phenytoin
  Decrease the serum concentration

Patient Teaching

Box 25.1 identifies patient teaching guidelines for antiparasitic drugs, including mebendazole.

Other Drugs in the Class

Albendazole should be administered with a high-fat meal to increase absorption in treating systemic disease. It is effective in the treatment of ascariasis. The recommended dosage of albendazole is 400 mg as a single oral dose. Triclabendazole (Egaten) has increased absorption when administered with food. It should be used cautiously when combined with medications that result in QT prolongation.

Ivermectin (Stromectol), which is used for numerous parasitic infections, is most active against strongyloidiasis (caused by the roundworm *Strongyloides stercoralis*). Another use for this drug is in the oral treatment of resistant lice infestations. It has relatively few adverse effects but may cause nausea and vomiting.

NCLEX Success

4. A patient who has enterobiasis, which is caused by *Enterobius vermicularis*, is receiving treatment with mebendazole. Which of the following agents decreases the serum concentration of mebendazole?
   A. alcohol
   B. phenytoin
   C. ampicillin
   D. metronidazole

SCABICIDES AND PEDICULICIDES

Topical and oral medications are administered for the treatment of scabies as well as for head or pubic lice. **Permethrin**, a pediculicide, is a first-line treatment and the prototype for the treatment of lice and scabies, caused by *Pediculosis capitis* and *Sarcoptes scabiei*, respectively.

Pharmacokinetics and Action

After topical administration of permethrin, 2% is absorbed through the skin and metabolized in the liver by ester hydrolysis to inactive metabolites. The drug is then excreted in the urine. It inhibits the influx of sodium ions through the nerve cell membrane channels of the parasites to delay the repolarization, resulting in the paralysis or death of the lice or scabies.

Use

A single application of permethrin is useful in the treatment of infestation with *P. capitis* or *S. scabiei*. Prophylactic applications are effective during epidemics of lice. The CDC recommends permethrin as one of the drugs of choice for the treatment of pubic hair lice during pregnancy. Permethrin also is the recommended treatment for scabies during pregnancy. Permethrin is present in breast milk as noted in agricultural animals. It is unknown if permethrin is present in human breast milk. There is minimal systemic absorption, and thus, breast-feeding is not expected to result in infant exposure. Table 25.5 presents route and dosage information for permethrin and related drugs.

Adverse Effects and Contraindications

The most common adverse effects of permethrin are pruritus, rash of the scalp, erythema, burning, tingling, numbness or pain of the scalp, and edema. Contraindications include a known hypersensitivity to chrysanthemums, pyrethroid, or pyrethrin, as well as age less than 2 months.

Nursing Implications

Administering the Medication

> **! Quality and Safety Alert: Safety**
>
> When administering permethrin for head lice or scabies, wear gloves to prevent spreading the infection or infecting the caregiver. Follow administration directions included in Table 25.5.

Assessing for Therapeutic and Adverse Effects

The nurse assesses for lice or scabies. It is also necessary to assess the areas of application of permethrin for inflammation, pruritus, erythema, and rash. The nurse asks the patient if there is any burning, stinging, tingling, scalp numbness or pain, or edema.

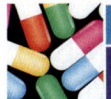

TABLE 25.5

DRUGS AT A GLANCE: Scabicides and Pediculicides

Drug	Routes and Dosage Ranges	
	Adults	**Children**
Permethrin	Head lice: apply large volume of cream, rinse to clean, damp hair to saturate hair and scalp; apply behind ears and at the base of the neck; leave on for 10 min before rinsing with water; repeat in 1 wk if lice and nits are present Scabies: apply cream head to toe; leave on 8–14 h before washing off with water; reapply in 1 wk if mites appear. Follow the previous steps if reapplication is needed	Same as adults
Crotamiton (Crotan)	Scabies: apply a thin layer and massage drug on the skin of the entire body from neck to the toes; repeat application in 24 h; may retreat if new lesions appear	Scabies: apply a thin layer on the skin of the entire body; apply once daily for 3 d followed by a cleansing bath after 48 h of the last application
Lindane	Head lice: rub lotion into affected area, leave in place for 12 h and then wash or shampoo (rub into the affected area for 4 min and rinse thoroughly) Scabies: apply to the entire skin except the face, neck, and scalp; leave in place for 24 h; then remove by shower	Not recommend for use in children <50 kg due to safety concerns >10 y: same as adults
Malathion (Ovide)	Head lice: apply to hair, rub in well to wet hair, then dry hair without covering or using a hair dryer; after 8–12 h, shampoo, rinse, and comb hair with a fine-toothed comb to remove dead lice and eggs; if necessary, repeat in 7–9 d	Contraindicated in neonates and infants ≥6 y: same as adults
Spinosad (Natroba)	Apply to dry scalp and rub in gently and then apply to hair; leave on for 10 min and then rinse with warm water and shampoo; repeat in 7 d if the first treatment is ineffective	≥6 mo: same as adults

Patient Teaching

Box 25.1 identifies patient teaching guidelines for antiparasitic drugs, including permethrin.

Other Drugs in the Class

Crotamiton (Crotan) lotion or cream is FDA-approved for the treatment of scabies in adults. Crotamiton should not be applied to the face, eyes, or mouth.

Lindane is a second-line drug for scabies and pediculosis. The FDA has issued a **BOXED WARNING** ◆ for lindane because neurologic toxicities, including seizures and death, have been reported even when it is taken as directed. The drug is also contraindicated in premature infants and individuals with known uncontrolled seizure disorders. Lindane is useful in people who cannot tolerate a safer, first-line drug for scabies; have hypersensitivity reactions to such a drug; or are resistant to treatment with such a drug. It is necessary to provide guidance about accurate use to individuals taking the drug.

Administration is topical, and absorption through intact skin is substantial. CNS toxicity has been reported with excessive use, especially in infants and children. The drug is available in a 1% concentration as a lotion and shampoo.

Malathion (Ovide) is a pediculicide used in the treatment of resistant head lice infestations, and pyrethrin preparations are available over the counter for the treatment of pediculosis. If required, a second application can be applied in 7 to 9 days.

Spinosad (Natroba), a pediculicidal and ovicidal drug, is useful for the treatment of head lice. It causes insect paralysis and death due to excitation of the CNS of the parasite. Topical administration results in no absorption.

NCLEX Success

5. A prescriber has ordered permethrin for an older patient who has received a diagnosis of scabies. What is the action of permethrin?
   A. It inhibits the influx of sodium through the nerve cell membranes to paralyze the parasite.
   B. It inhibits the influx of calcium through the nerve cell membranes to paralyze the parasite.
   C. It inhibits the influx of potassium through the nerve cell membranes to paralyze the parasite.
   D. It inhibits the influx of chloride through the nerve cell membranes to paralyze the parasite.

THE NURSING PROCESS

A concept map outlines the nursing process related to drug therapy considerations in this chapter. Additional nursing implications related to the disease process should also be considered in care decisions.

Assessment
- Assess for exposure to parasites (e.g., overcrowded housing, institutional resident, history of parasites in environment, geographic location [travel to area of poor sanitation, an underdeveloped country, or a tropical region], and personal hygiene) and use of prophylactic measures, as appropriate.
- With vaginal trichomoniasis, assess in relation to sexual activity; sexual partners need simultaneous treatment to prevent reinfection.
- With pubic (crab) lice, assess sexual activity; lice transmission may occur with sexual or other close contact and contact with infested bed linens.
- Assess for signs and symptoms. These vary greatly, depending on the type and extent of parasitic infestation.

Outcomes of Therapy
The patient will
- Experience relief of symptoms for which antiparasitic drugs were taken.
- Self-administer drugs accurately.
- Avoid preventable adverse effects.
- Act to prevent recurrent infestation.
- Keep appointments for follow-up care.

Nursing Interventions
- Use environmental health measures to avoid exposure to or prevent transmission of parasitic diseases.
- Follow-up with examination and possibly treatment of household and other close contacts of people with helminthiasis, amebiasis, trichomoniasis, scabies, and pediculosis.
- Teach those traveling regarding measures to decrease exposure to mosquito bites (e.g., wear long-sleeved, dark clothing; use an effective insect repellent such as DEET; sleep in well-screened rooms or under mosquito netting).
- Use effective personal hygiene and other health measures to avoid exposure, prevent transmission of parasitic disease, or reinfection.
- Ensure follow-up measures, such as testing of stool specimens; vaginal examinations; anal swabs, smears, and cultures.
- With vaginal infections, avoid sexual intercourse, or have the male partner use a condom.

Evaluation
- Interview and observe for relief of symptoms.
- Interview outpatients regarding compliance with instructions for taking antiparasitic drugs and measures to prevent recurrence of infestation.
- Interview and observe for adverse drug effects.
- Interview and observe regarding food intake or changes in weight.

Visit thePoint at http://thePoint.lww.com/Frandsen13e for answers to NCLEX Success questions (in Appendix A), answers to Clinical Application Case Studies (in Appendix B), additional information on etiology and pathophysiology of protozoal infections, and more!

REFERENCES AND RESOURCES

Centers for Disease Control and Prevention (CDC). (2023). *Parasites-Scabies: Medications*. Retrieved January 28, 2023, from https://www.cdc.gov/parasites/scabies/health_professionals/meds.html

Daly, J. (2022). Treatment of uncomplicated falciparum malaria in non-pregnant adults and children. *UpToDate*. Lexi-Comp, Inc.

Daly, J., Minuti, A., & Khan, N. (2022). Diagnosis, treatment, and prevention of malaria in the US: A review. *Journal of the American Medical Association, 328*(5), 460–471.

Guyton, A. C., & Hall, J. E. (2020). *Guyton & Hall textbook of medical physiology* (14th ed.). Elsevier.

Hinkle, J. H., Cheever, K. H., & Overbaugh, K. J. (2021). *Brunner & Suddarth's textbook of medical-surgical nursing* (15th ed.). Wolters Kluwer.

Leder, K., & Weller, P. F. (2022). Treatment and prevention of cryptosporidiosis. *UpToDate*. Lexi-Comp, Inc.

Leder, K., Weller, P. F., & Reddy, N. (2022). Ascariasis. *UpToDate*. Lexi-Comp, Inc.

Travassos, M., & Laufer, M. K. (2022). Antimalarial drugs: An overview. In *UpToDate*. Lexi-Comp, Inc.

Weller, P. F. (2022a). Anthelmintic therapies. *UpToDate*. Lexi-Comp, Inc.

Weller, P. F. (2022b). Antiprotozoal therapies. *UpToDate*. Lexi-Comp, Inc.

World Health Organization. (2020). *Tackling antimalarial drug resistance*. Retrieved January 28, 2023, from https://www.who.int/publications/m/item/WHO-UCN-GMP-2020.07

Clinical Judgment in Practice: Section 4: Drugs Affecting Inflammation and Infection

A 60-year-old patient is 2 weeks status post left knee arthroscopy. The sutures were removed on the 10th postoperative day. At that time, a 0.25-cm open area of the incision was noted with clear drainage. The patient is being seen in the orthopedic surgeon's office for a follow-up appointment. The patient reports that for the last week, the left knee pain had been a 3 out of 10 on a 10-point pain scale; however, over the past 24 hours, the pain has increased to an 8 out of 10. The patient also reports thick gray drainage that has saturated the 4 × 4 gauze every 2 hours for the past 24 hours. The nurse assesses the incision and notes that it is separated 0.50 cm with redness at the incision site. The patient's temperature is 102.4°F orally, pulse 110, respirations 20 and regular, and blood pressure is 96/68. The patient states that blood pressure is normally 120/80. One week prior, the patient returned to work, which required sitting at a desk for long periods with the knee bent. The patient's medication regimen includes naproxen 500 mg twice daily, enalapril maleate 25 mg daily, and metformin 500 mg extended release at 5 p.m. daily.

Step 1: Recognize Cues
Identify the relevant and important information from different sources, such as the medical history or subjective and objective data.

Answer: *Complaints of increased pain with a rating of 8/10 along with elevated temperature (102.4°F orally), rapid pulse (110), and low blood pressure (96/68). The increased drainage from the left knee incision since the orthopedic visit 4 days ago. The drainage is now gray and thick saturating 4 × 4s every 2 hours. The incision is reddened and open.*

Step 2: Analyze Cues
Organize and link the recognized cues to the patient's clinical presentation.

Answer: *You link the clustered symptoms to be associated with a wound infection and possible sepsis. The naproxen may mask the temperature due to its antipyretic effects. The patient's low blood pressure is a warning sign of septicemia.*

Step 3: Prioritize Hypotheses
Evaluate hypotheses and rank them according to priority, such as urgency, likelihood, risk, difficulty, and/or time. Cluster your findings to generate a list of problems (actual or potential) you believe the patient is experiencing or may experience and determine the level of urgency. Which problem is of the greatest concern?

Answer: *You prioritize a left knee postoperative infection with the risk of septicemia.*

Step 4: Generate Solutions
Identify expected outcomes and use hypotheses to define a set of interventions for the expected outcomes.

Answer: *The patient is 2 weeks postoperative, and the incision has opened with drainage that has increased in the past 4 days. In addition, the patient has an elevated temperature and tachycardia. Thus, you suspect a postoperative infection of the left knee. You anticipate the orthopedic surgeon will schedule the patient for surgical débridement of the left knee. Also, you recognize the need to culture the wound prior to surgery or the administration of an anti-infective medication. Since you are the orthopedic surgeon's surgical nurse and you anticipate the patient will need surgery in the afternoon, you assess the last time the patient ate or drank and report this to the anesthesia team. You inform the patient not to eat or drink anything because surgery will be scheduled. Also, you inquire if the patient is allergic to any medications, especially anti-infective agents.*

Step 5: Take Actions
Implement the solutions that address the highest priorities.

Answer: *As the preoperative nurse, you start an IV of lactated Ringer's at a rate of 125 mL/hour. Because the patient will have a peripherally inserted central catheter line postoperative for 1 month and receive 500 mg of vancomycin IV every 12 hours at home, you will need to provide patient education on the use of an electronic pump so the vancomycin can be infused over 1 hour. The home care nurse will need to assess the patient's kidney function and wound healing. The home care nurse will obtain vancomycin peak and trough levels as ordered.*

Step 6: Evaluate Outcomes
Compare observed outcomes against expected outcomes.

Answer: *The wound culture was positive for methicillin-resistant Staphylococcus aureus. The vancomycin peak is 45 mcg/mL, and the trough is 20 mcg/mL. Vital signs are 97.2°F orally, pulse 86, respirations 20, and blood pressure 120/76.*

SECTION 5

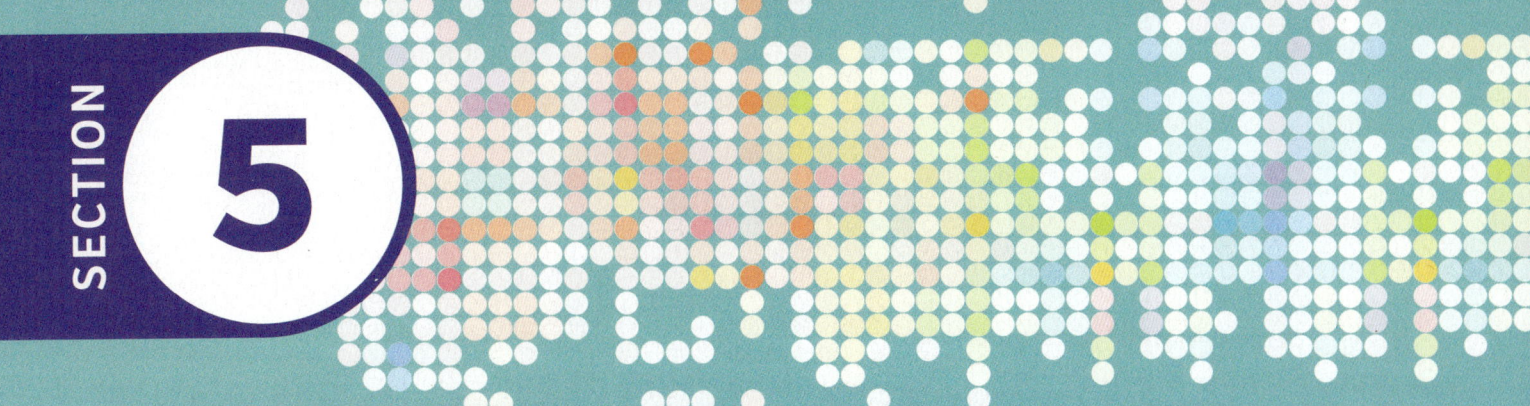

Drugs Affecting the Cardiovascular System

Chapter 26 Drug Therapy for Hypertension
Chapter 27 Drug Therapy for Dysrhythmias
Chapter 28 Drug Therapy for Coronary Heart Disease
Chapter 29 Drug Therapy for Shock and Hypotension
Chapter 30 Drug Therapy for Heart Failure

CHAPTER 26

Drug Therapy for Hypertension

LEARNING OBJECTIVES

After studying this chapter, you should be able to:

1. Describe how hypertension is classified.
2. Discuss nonpharmacologic measures to control hypertension.
3. Identify the prototype and describe the action, use, contraindications, adverse effects, and nursing implications of the angiotensin-converting enzyme inhibitors.
4. Identify the prototype and describe the action, use, contraindications, adverse effects, and nursing implications of the angiotensin II receptor blockers.
5. Identify the prototype and describe the action, use, contraindications, adverse effects, and nursing implications of the calcium channel blockers.
6. Describe the rationale for using combination drugs in the management of hypertension.
7. Review the recommended use and effects of diuretics, alpha-adrenergic blockers, and beta-adrenergic blockers in the management of hypertension.
8. Implement the nursing process when caring for patients with hypertension.

CLINICAL APPLICATION CASE STUDY

Harold Caudill has a history of primary (essential) hypertension. His medical history includes type 1 diabetes, with early signs of diabetic nephropathy. After having a myocardial infarction (MI) 2 years ago, he has been treated with metoprolol, a beta-adrenergic blocker. In addition, he has been taking the diuretic hydrochlorothiazide to treat the hypertension. His blood pressure today is 138/92 mm Hg, which is consistent with the readings on his last three visits. His physician has added captopril to his treatment regimen.

KEY TERMS

Angioedema: sudden deep swelling or welts under skin, particularly around the eyes and lips

Antiadrenergic: decrease or block the effects of sympathetic nerve stimulation

Autoregulation: ability of body tissues to regulate their own blood flow

Essential hypertension: high blood pressure for which no cause can be found

First-dose phenomenon: orthostatic hypotension with palpitations, dizziness, and perhaps syncope 1 to 3 hours after the first dose of a drug or an increased dose

Secondary hypertension: high blood pressure from an identified cause, such as kidney disease

INTRODUCTION

Antihypertensive drugs are used to treat hypertension, a common, chronic disorder estimated to affect more than 116 million adults and an unknown number of children and adolescents in the United States (CDC, 2021). Hypertension increases risks of myocardial infarction (MI), heart failure, cerebral infarction and hemorrhage, and kidney disease. To understand hypertension and antihypertensive drug therapy, it is necessary first to understand the characteristics of hypertension and the characteristics of antihypertensive drugs.

OVERVIEW OF HYPERTENSION

Regulation of Blood Pressure

Arterial blood pressure reflects the force exerted on arterial walls by blood flow. Blood pressure normally remains constant because of homeostatic mechanisms that adjust blood flow and arterial pressure to supply tissues with needed oxygen and nutrients. The two major determinants of arterial blood pressure are cardiac output (systolic pressure) and peripheral vascular resistance (diastolic pressure).

Cardiac output equals the product of the heart rate and stroke volume (CO = HR × SV). Stroke volume is the amount of blood ejected with each heartbeat (approximately 60 to 90 mL). Thus, cardiac output depends on stroke volume, which is dependent on the force of myocardial contraction, blood volume, and other factors. Peripheral vascular resistance is determined by local blood flow and the degree of constriction or dilation in arterioles and arteries (vascular tone).

Autoregulation of Blood Flow

Autoregulation is the ability of body tissues to regulate their own blood flow. This is a critical homeostatic mechanism of major organs (e.g., heart, brain, kidneys) to preserve oxygenation and function. Local blood flow is regulated primarily by nutritional needs of the tissue, such as lack of oxygen or accumulation of products of cellular metabolism (e.g., carbon dioxide, lactic acid). Local tissues produce vasodilating and vasoconstricting substances to regulate local blood flow. Important chemical mediators affecting vascular flow include histamine, bradykinin, serotonin, and prostaglandins.

Grades and Types of Hypertension

Normal or optimal blood pressure is the level at which minimal vascular damage occurs with sufficient blood flow for tissue oxygenation and waste removal. Hypertension is persistently high blood pressure that exceeds this level and results from abnormalities in blood pressure regulatory mechanisms. It is usually defined as a systolic pressure above 130 mm Hg or a diastolic pressure above 80 mm Hg on multiple blood pressure measurements. The *Eighth Report of the Joint National Committee on Prevention, Detection, Evaluation, and Treatment of High Blood Pressure* (JNC 8), released in 2014, reviewed and updated the current evidence on the detection, evaluation, and treatment of high blood pressure (James et al., 2014). This commentary focused on key thresholds for initiation of pharmacologic treatment of hypertension, including blood pressure targets during treatment and recommendations for antihypertensive therapies. Based on this report and corresponding evidence, the American College of Cardiology (ACC) and American Heart Association (AHA) issued updated guidelines for the categories of hypertension in adults (in mm Hg) (Box 26.1) (Whelton et al., 2018). These recommendations shifted focus from defining threshold levels of hypertension to defining treatment methods for patients with hypertension and establishing outcome measures for treatment effectiveness.

A systolic pressure of 140 mm Hg or greater, with a diastolic pressure of less than 80 mm Hg, is called isolated systolic hypertension and is more common in the elderly. Systolic–diastolic hypertension, which may also occur in older adults, involves elevations of both systolic and diastolic pressures. Both types increase cardiovascular morbidity and mortality, especially heart failure and stroke, and warrant treatment.

A hypertensive emergency, or crisis, is a systolic pressure of 180 mm Hg or more and/or a diastolic pressure of 120 mm Hg or more and significantly increases the risk of acute target organ damage. (A hypertensive urgency is an episode of marked elevation in blood pressure without target organ damage.) The goal of management for hypertensive emergency or crisis is to lower blood pressure within 24 hours.

Although it has frequently been indicated that the causes of primary hypertension, or **essential hypertension** (high blood pressure for which no cause can be found), are not known, this is only partially true. Genetic variations and inherited, behavioral, and environmental factors may increase blood pressure (Unger et al., 2020). These include a body mass index (BMI) higher than 30.0, high alcohol intake, insulin resistance, high salt intake in salt-sensitive people, aging, sedentary lifestyle, and stress. Furthermore, many of these factors are additive, such as BMI higher than 30.0 and alcohol intake. Primary hypertension makes up 90% to 95% of known cases. Appropriate therapy usually controls primary hypertension.

Secondary hypertension (high blood pressure from an identified cause) may result from kidney, endocrine, or central nervous

---

BOX 26.1 Classification of Hypertension (All Values in mm Hg)

- Normal = systolic less than 120 *and* diastolic less than 80
- Elevated = systolic 120 to 129 *and* diastolic less than 80
- Stage 1 hypertension = systolic 130 to 139 *or* diastolic 80 to 89
- Stage 2 hypertension = systolic greater than 140 *or* diastolic 90 or more

Source: Whelton, P. K., Carey, R. M., Aronow, W. S., Casey, D. E., Collins, K. J., Dennison Himmelfarb, C., DePalma, S. M., Gidding, S., Jamerson, K. A., Jones, D. W., MacLaughlin, E. J., Muntner, P., Ovbiagele, B., Smith, S. C. Jr, Spencer, C. C., Stafford, R. S., Taler, S. J., Thomas, R. J., Williams, K. A. Sr,… Wright, J. T. Jr. (2018). 2017 ACC/AHA/AAPA/ABC/ACPM/AGS/APhA/ASH/ASPC/NMA/PCNA guideline for the prevention, detection, evaluation, and management of high blood pressure in adults: A report of the American College of Cardiology/American Heart Association Task Force on Clinical Practice Guidelines. *Circulation, 138*, e484–e594. https://doi.org/10.1161/CIR.0000000000000596

system (CNS) disorders and from drugs that stimulate the sympathetic nervous system (SNS) or cause retention of sodium and water, producing adverse effects. Secondary hypertension can sometimes be cured by managing the underlying condition or cause. Hypertensive emergencies often result from secondary hypertensive conditions such as cerebral hemorrhage, dissecting aortic aneurysm, kidney disease, pheochromocytoma, or eclampsia.

Response to Hypotension

When hypotension (and decreased tissue perfusion) occurs, the SNS is stimulated, the hormones epinephrine and norepinephrine are secreted by the adrenal medulla, angiotensin II and aldosterone are formed, and the kidneys retain fluid. These compensatory mechanisms raise the blood pressure. Specific effects include the following:

- Constriction of arterioles, which increases peripheral vascular resistance
- Constriction of veins and increased venous tone
- Stimulation of cardiac beta-adrenergic receptors, which increases heart rate and force of myocardial contraction
- Activation of the renin–angiotensin–aldosterone mechanism

Chapter 29 contains an additional discussion of the effects and management of hypotension.

Response to Hypertension

When arterial blood pressure is elevated, the following sequence of compensatory events occurs:

- Kidneys excrete more fluid (increase urine output).
- Fluid loss reduces both extracellular fluid volume and blood volume.
- Decreased blood volume reduces venous blood flow to the heart and, therefore, decreases cardiac output.
- Decreased cardiac output reduces arterial blood pressure.
- The vascular endothelium produces vasodilating substances (e.g., nitric oxide (NO) prostacyclin), which reduce blood pressure.

Clinical Manifestations

Initially, and perhaps for years, primary hypertension may produce no symptoms. If symptoms occur, they are usually vague and nonspecific. Hypertension may go undetected, or it may be incidentally discovered when blood pressure measurements are taken as part of a routine physical examination, screening test, or assessment of other disorders.

Symptoms associated with hypertension, if they occur, include headache (may be severe), nausea, vomiting, visual disturbances, neurologic disturbances, weakness, fatigue, disorientation, and decreased level of consciousness (drowsiness, stupor, coma). These symptoms are most frequently associated with significantly elevated blood pressures or hypertensive crisis. Hypertensive emergencies require immediate blood pressure management and reduction with parenteral antihypertensive drugs to limit acute damage to target organs. Over time, the symptoms of hypertension reflect hypertensive-mediated organ damage (HMOD) associated with sustained elevations in blood pressure. Unfortunately, hypertension is often not discovered until after a person experiences angina pectoris, MI, heart failure, stroke, or kidney disease.

Therapy

Goals of Treatment

After the diagnosis of hypertension is established, it is essential that a therapeutic regimen be designed and implemented. Based on guidelines published in 2018 (Whelton et al., 2018), treatment goals vary depending on the population being treated. In patients aged 60 years or older, without diabetes or chronic kidney disease, the treatment goal is a blood pressure of less than 150/90 mm Hg. In patients ages 30 to 59 years who are in general good health and patients 60 years or older with diabetes or chronic kidney disease, the goal of treatment is a blood pressure of less than 140/90 mm Hg. For patients 18 to 30 years of age, the panel recommends a treatment goal of blood pressure less than 140/90 mm Hg, but the evidence supporting the guidelines for this population is more limited.

Lowering blood pressure to any extent is considered beneficial in decreasing the incidence of coronary artery disease (CAD) and stroke. In most instances, it is better to lower blood pressure gradually and to avoid wide fluctuations in blood pressure. However, for patients who have difficulty achieving and maintaining blood pressure in the recommended ranges, referral to a hypertensive specialist is indicated.

Nonpharmacologic Treatment

In their findings, the JNC 8 panel guidelines released recommendations for the management of hypertension (James et al., 2014). Initial interventions include lifestyle modifications (i.e., reduction of weight and sodium intake, regular physical activity, moderate alcohol intake, and no smoking) to achieve and maintain blood pressure below 120/80 mm Hg. Actual blood pressure trends and individual patient risk profiles determine if lifestyle changes with or without drug therapy are the initial treatment option.

Dietary Management

Recent management guidelines distinguish that key behavioral determinants of blood pressure are related to dietary consumption of calories and salt; there is a direct relationship between hypertension and body mass index (Whelton et al., 2018). According to this report, a diet low in sodium and fat along with an increased consumption of fruits, vegetables, and grains may decrease the systolic blood pressure by approximately 11 mm Hg. The Dietary Approaches to Stop Hypertension (DASH) study has demonstrated that people with elevated blood pressure or stage 1 hypertension can reduce their blood pressures by adhering to a diet abundant in fresh fruits and vegetables and low-fat dairy products even without restricting calorie or sodium intake (Moore et al., 2001). The effects of the DASH diet show blood pressure–lowering outcomes that parallel the degree of benefit from drug monotherapy and may include dietary sodium restriction. Effects are evident in people of all ethnicities, particularly African Americans, and in those with significantly higher blood pressures.

Severe restrictions of sodium intake usually are not acceptable to people; however, moderate restrictions (4 to 6 g of salt a day) are beneficial and more easily implemented. Avoiding heavily salted foods (e.g., cured meats, sandwich meats, pretzels, potato chips) and not adding salt to food at the table can achieve this. Research and clinical observations indicate the following:

- Sodium restriction alone reduces blood pressure and is extremely effective when combined with lifestyle modifications.
- Sodium restriction potentiates the antihypertensive actions of diuretics and other antihypertensive drugs. Conversely, excessive sodium intake decreases the antihypertensive actions of all antihypertensive drugs. Patients with unrestricted salt intake who are taking thiazides may lose excessive potassium and become hypokalemic.
- Sodium restriction may decrease dosage requirements of antihypertensive drugs, thereby decreasing the incidence and severity of adverse effects.

Lifestyle Management

Social determinants of health, such as healthcare access and quality, economic stability, educational access and quality, and environmental conditions, contribute to broad health disparities and inequities. Simply promoting lifestyle management will not eliminate health disparities and inequities until there is a focus on improving these social determinants.

Despite the significant racial–ethnic disparities in blood pressure prevalence and management success, recent studies have identified significant heterogeneity in the prevalence of hypertension among specific ethnic–racial groups. A need to disaggregate data to refine high-risk populations and establish targeted interventions is an important step in hypertension management. However, some universal choices have demonstrated success in blood pressure control.

Considerable evidence demonstrates that regular physical activity effectively reduces blood pressure. Research has demonstrated that both aerobic exercise and resistance training have a significant blood pressure–lowering effect (Whelton et al., 2018). However, the direct benefits of exercise on blood pressure control are often difficult to isolate from those of the changes that often accompany exercise, such as improved diet, weight loss, decreased alcohol consumption, and decreased cigarette smoking. The 2017 AHA/ACC Lifestyle Management Guidelines note the importance of regular physical activity as part of a plan of care for adults of all blood pressure levels, including those with hypertension. On average, aerobic physical activity decreases systolic blood pressure by 5 to 8 mm Hg for hypertensive patients. Data suggest that effective results can be expected with aerobic physical activity on interventions of, on average, at least 12 weeks' duration, three to four times per week, lasting on average 40 minutes per session. Besides aerobic activity, the JNC 8 recommendations also included achieving a weight loss goal of at least 10 lb if overweight, limiting alcohol consumption to two drinks or less per day for males and one drink or less per day for females, and ceasing smoking. In summary, it is estimated that each lifestyle change results in a 4 to 5 mm Hg decrease in systolic blood pressure and a 2 to 4 mm Hg decrease in diastolic blood pressure (Whelton et al., 2018).

Drug Management

If lifestyle modifications alone do not produce the target blood pressure (or a systolic blood pressure ≥140 mm Hg or a diastolic blood pressure ≥90 mm Hg), it is important to initiate antihypertensive drug therapy and continue lifestyle modifications. If initial hypertensive diagnosis is stage II Hypertension or there is a high risk of HMOD, it is recommended to initiate antihypertensive drug therapy immediately along with lifestyle modifications (Unger et al., 2020). Drugs used in the management of primary hypertension belong to several different groups, including angiotensin-converting enzyme (ACE) inhibitors; angiotensin II receptor blockers (ARBs), also called angiotensin II receptor antagonists; antiadrenergics; calcium channel blockers (CCBs); diuretics; and direct vasodilators. In general, these drugs act to decrease blood pressure by decreasing cardiac output or peripheral vascular resistance. Evidence indicates that management strategies need to account for race in drug selection for initial therapy. For instance, recommendations for treatment of hypertension in individuals of African American descent, including those with diabetes, includes initial therapy with a CCB and/or thiazide-type diuretic. In non–African American populations, including those with diabetes, there is evidence to support initial drug therapy with an ACE inhibitor, ARB, and/or CCB. This chapter focuses on ACE inhibitors, ARBs, CCBs, and select additional antihypertensive drugs (direct renin inhibitors, alpha$_1$-adrenergic blockers, alpha$_2$ agonists, beta-adrenergic blockers, alpha-/beta-adrenergic blockers, and diuretics); their sites of drug action are identified in Figure 26.1. Various other chapters in this book describe drugs discussed here—for example, chapters related to dysrhythmias (see Chapter 27), angina (see Chapter 28), heart failure (see Chapter 30), and fluid volume excess (see Chapter 34).

Table 26.1 outlines the antihypertensive drugs. Figure 26.2 outlines the International Society of Hypertension's current, evidence-based practice recommendations for the management and treatment of hypertension. Product labeling and current recommendations are the basis for adult dosages. Product labeling and recent clinical research, along with the seminal recommendations from the National High Blood Pressure Education Program Working Group on High Blood Pressure in Children and Adolescents (2004) and Clinical Practice Guideline for Screening and Management of High Blood Pressure in Children and Adolescents (Flynn et al., 2017), are the basis for pediatric dosages.

Current guidelines (Unger et al., 2020; Whelton et al., 2018) suggest that ACE inhibitor, ARB, or CCB be used as first-line therapy, either alone (monotherapy) or with thiazide diuretics (e.g., chlorthalidone, hydrochlorothiazide). Monotherapy is reasonable if the patient has stage 1 hypertension and a BP goal less than 130/80 mm Hg. For African American patients, initial drug therapy guidelines include a combination of thiazide diuretics with an ACE inhibitor, ARB, or CCB (Unger et al., 2020). If the initial drug (and dose) does not produce the desired blood pressure within 1 month of initiating treatment, options for further management include increasing the dose, substituting another drug, or adding a second/additional drug from a different group (Unger et al., 2020). If the patient has a systolic pressure greater than 140 mm Hg or a diastolic blood pressure greater than 90 mm Hg, initial drug therapy with a combination of two antihypertensives is recommended (Whelton et al., 2018). To minimize the impact of medication side effects, two or three medications may be combined at lower doses, rather than increasing doses of monotherapy, to achieve blood pressure

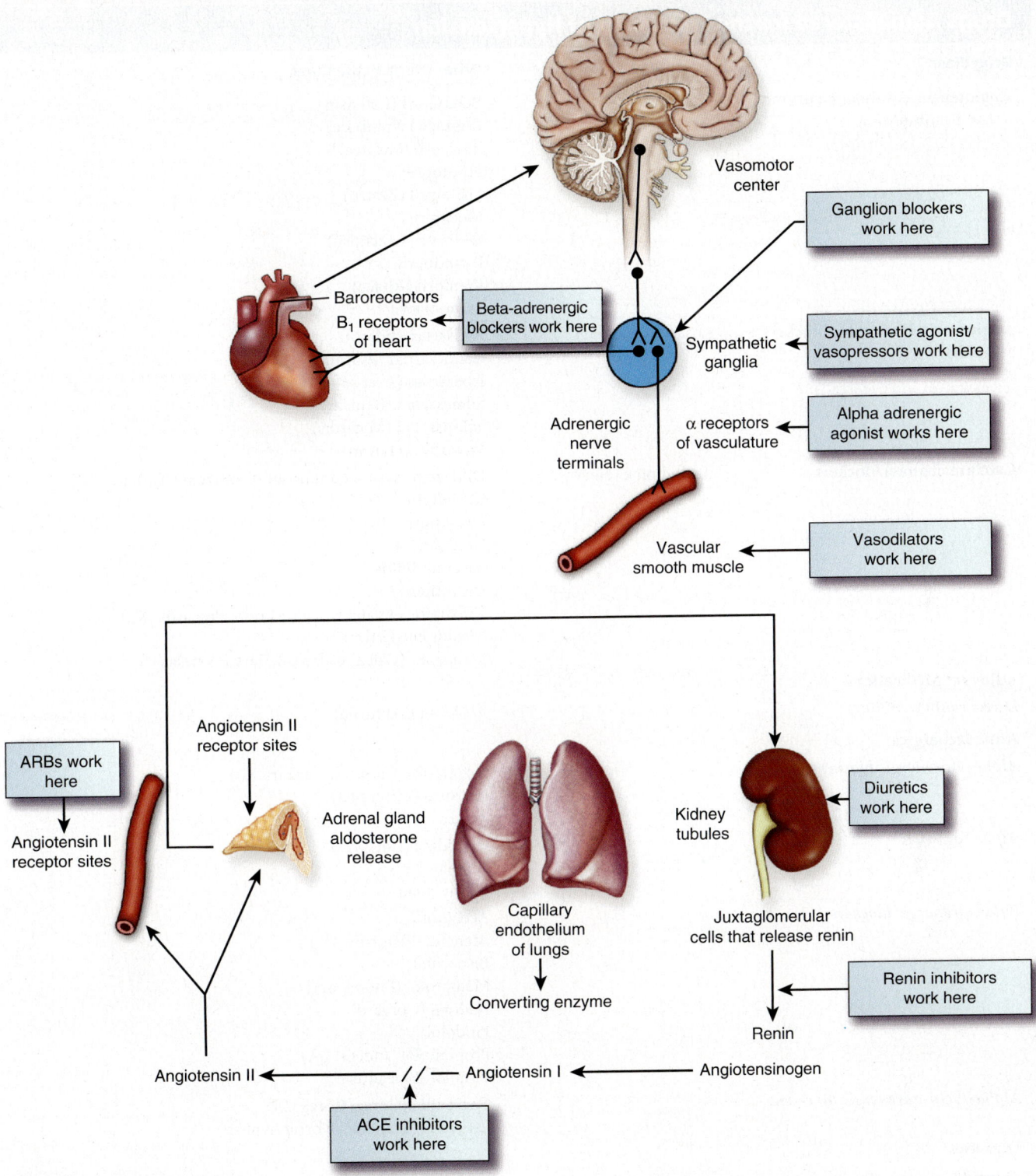

Figure 26.1. Sites of action of antihypertensive drugs. [Reprinted with permission from Karch, A. M. (2020). *Focus on nursing pharmacology* (8th ed., Fig. 43.3, p. 734). Wolters Kluwer.]

treatment goals. If the response is still inadequate, addition of a third drug, including a diuretic if not previously prescribed, is recommended.

When current management is ineffective, it is necessary to reassess the patient's adherence to lifestyle modifications and drug therapy. In addition, it is also important to review other factors that may decrease the therapeutic response, such as the use of over-the-counter appetite suppressants, dietary or herbal supplements, or nasal decongestants, which raise blood pressure. Regardless of the medication selected, the primary determining factor in selecting the appropriate antihypertensive medication(s) and dose(s) is patient response to treatment, with attained blood pressure control being the ultimate outcome measure (Unger et al., 2020; Whelton et al., 2018).

TABLE 26.1

Drugs Administered for the Treatment of Hypertension

Drug Class	Prototype	Other Drugs in the Class
Angiotensin-converting enzyme (ACE) inhibitors	Captopril	Benazepril (Lotensin) Cilazapril (Inhibace) Enalapril (Vasotec) Fosinopril Lisinopril (Zestril) Moexipril Quinapril (Accupril) Perindopril Ramipril (Altace) Trandolapril
Angiotensin II receptor blockers (ARBs)	Losartan (Cozaar)	Azilsartan (Edarbi) Candesartan (Atacand) Irbesartan (Avapro) Olmesartan (Benicar) Telmisartan (Micardis) Valsartan (Diovan)
Calcium channel blockers	Amlodipine (Norvasc)	Diltiazem (sustained release) (Cardizem CD, Cartia XT) Clevidipine Felodipine Isradipine Levamlodipine Nicardipine Nifedipine (Adalat CC, Procardia, Procardia XL) Nisoldipine (Sular) Verapamil (Calan, Calan SR, Tarka, Verelan)
Adjuvant Medications		
Direct renin inhibitors		Aliskiren (Tekturna)
Antiadrenergics		
Alpha₁-adrenergic blockers		Doxazosin (Cardura, Cardura XL) Prazosin (Minipress) Terazosin
Alpha₂ agonists		Clonidine (Catapres) Guanfacine Methyldopa
Beta-adrenergic blockers		Acebutolol Atenolol (Tenormin) Bisoprolol Metoprolol (Lopressor) Nadolol (Corgard) Pindolol Propranolol (Inderal LA) Timolol (Blocadren)
Alpha-/beta-adrenergic blockers		Carvedilol (Coreg, Coreg CR) Labetalol (Trandate, Normodyne)
Diuretics		
Thiazide	Hydrochlorothiazide (Microzide)	Chlorothiazide (Diuril) Chlorthalidone Indapamide Metolazone (Zaroxolyn)
Loop	Furosemide (Lasix)	Bumetanide (Bumex) Torsemide (Demadex)
Potassium sparing	Spironolactone (Aldactone)	Amiloride (Midamor) Triamterene (Dyrenium)
Other vasodilators		Fenoldopam (Corlopam) Hydralazine (Hydra-Zide, BiDil) Minoxidil Sodium nitroprusside (Nitropress)

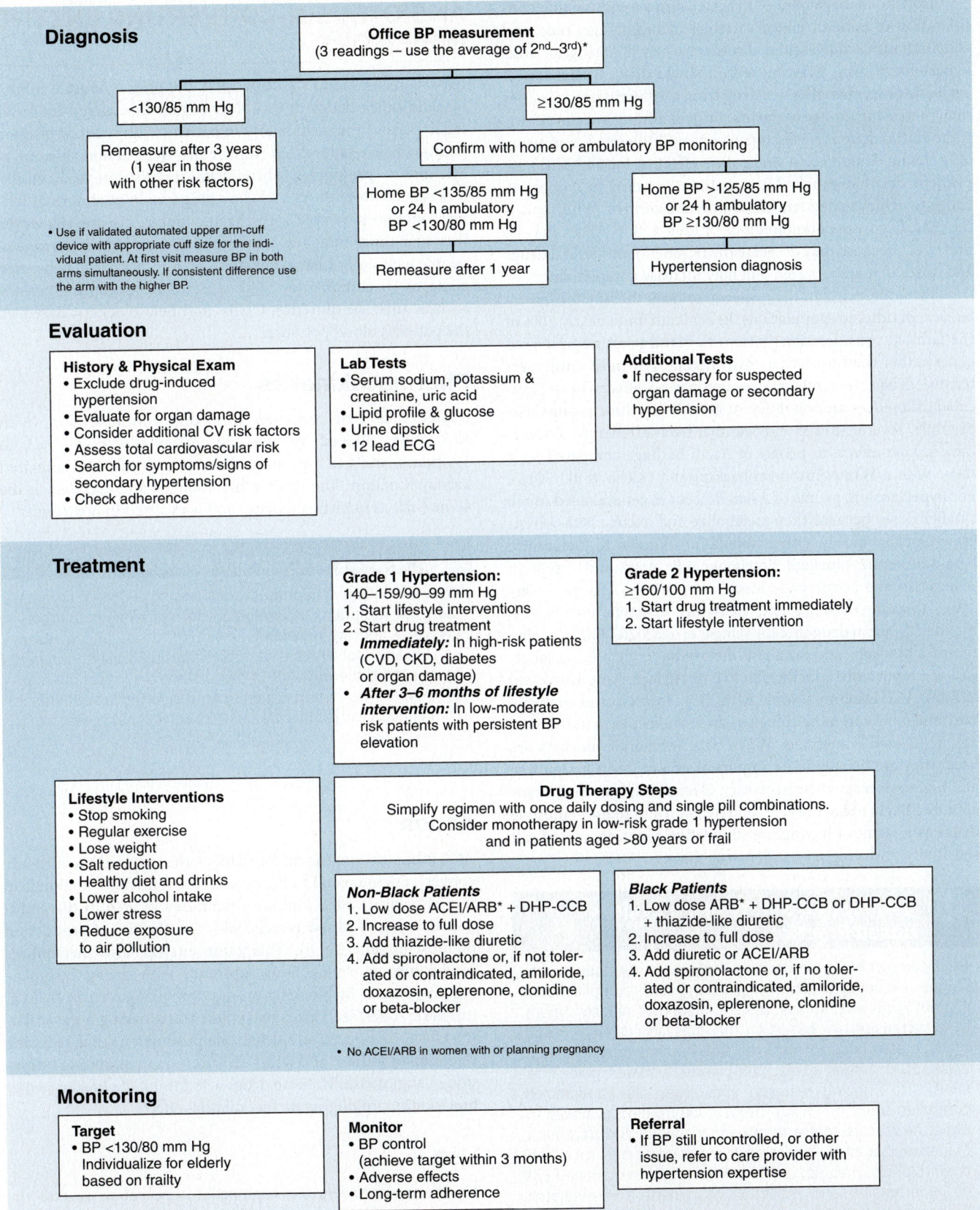

Figure 26.2. The International Society of Hypertension's current, evidence-based practice recommendations for the management and treatment of hypertension. (Unger, T., Borghi, C., Charchar, F., Khan, N., Poulter, N., Prabhakaran, D., Ramirez, A., Schlaich, M., Stergiou, G., Tomaszewski, M., Wainford, R., Williams. B., & Schutte, A. [2020]. 2020 International Society of Hypertension Global Hypertension Practice Guidelines. *Hypertension*, 75, 1334–1357, Figure 6.]

Holistic management of hypertension should include consideration of patient-related variables including age, race, and concomitant cardiovascular disorders when choosing an antihypertensive drug. Starting with a single drug, in the lowest available dose; changing to a drug from a different group, rather than increasing dosage of the first drug or adding a second drug, if the initial drug is ineffective or not well tolerated; and using long-acting drugs (i.e., a single dose effective for 24 hours) are prudent considerations. Many patients require two or more drugs to achieve adequate blood pressure control. When this is the case, fixed-dose combinations or long-acting agents may be preferred, because they decrease the number of individual drugs and doses that are required and may increase compliance.

Variation exists in the response to drug therapy for hypertension in different populations. Experts attribute nearly 70% of the familial considerations related to blood pressure to shared genes rather than to shared environment. For most antihypertensive drugs, research studies comparing effects have indicated differences among different genetic or ethnic groups. For example, several studies indicate that beta-adrenergic blockers have greater effects in people of Asian heritage compared with those with a White European background (Kario et al., 2018). For hypertension, people of Asian descent in general need much smaller doses because they metabolize and excrete beta-adrenergic blockers slowly. Other populations known to metabolize beta-adrenergic blockers slowly include Arab and Egyptian Americans and possibly German Americans. In African Americans, thiazide diuretics and CCBs are effective and recommended as initial drug therapy (Unger et al., 2020). CCBs, alpha$_1$ receptor blockers, and the alpha-/beta-adrenergic blocker labetalol are reportedly equally effective in African Americans and Whites. ACE inhibitors, some ARBs (e.g., losartan and telmisartan), and beta-adrenergic blockers are less effective as monotherapy in African Americans. When beta-adrenergic blockers are used, they are usually one component of a multidrug regimen, and higher doses may be necessary. Overall, African Americans are more likely to have severe hypertension and require multiple drugs as a result of having low circulating renin, increased salt sensitivity, and a higher incidence of obesity.

Quality and Safety Alert: Evidence-Based Practice

Hypertension has wide-ranging implications for patient outcomes, including short-term and long-term complications. Current guidelines for assessment, diagnosis, and treatment of hypertension are based on the latest in evidence-based practice standards for hypertension management [Whelton et al., 2018; Unger, et.al., 2020]. These updated guidelines synthesize ongoing research and large-scale randomized controlled trials, providing the best information available to assist healthcare teams in offering individualized treatment guidelines based on several factors, including age, race, and comorbidities. The updated guidelines reinforce management of hypertension and reduction of hypertensive-mediated organ damage as the ultimate goals. Use of evidence-based data provides specific adjustments based on patient factors aimed at increasing the opportunities for patients to realize those treatment goals. This allows clinicians to treat the patient in a targeted manner based on patient outcomes versus merely treating the condition.

ANGIOTENSIN-CONVERTING ENZYME INHIBITORS

Experts recommend captopril, the prototype ACE inhibitor, and other drugs in this class as first-line agents for treating hypertension, particularly in patients with reduced ejection fraction heart failure, left ventricular dysfunction, history of MI, and/or proteinuric chronic kidney disease. ACE inhibitors reduce proteinuria and slow progression of abnormal kidney function in people with chronic kidney disease. (However, they may cause or aggravate proteinuria and kidney damage in people who do not have diabetes.) ACE inhibitors may be used alone or in combination with other antihypertensive agents, such as thiazide diuretics, CCBs, and beta-blockers, based on the patient's blood pressure.

Pharmacokinetics

Captopril is well absorbed with oral administration (with absorption reduced by food), produces effects within 1 to 1½ hours, and has a prolonged serum half-life with impaired kidney function. The drug is metabolized and excreted in the urine (half as unchanged drug) and is excreted in breast milk.

Quality and Safety Alert: Safety

The metabolism of captopril varies among people of different racial backgrounds. Current guidelines recommend that non–African American individuals, including those with diabetes and chronic kidney disease, receive an ACE inhibitor as part of their drug therapy. ACE inhibitors are only recommended for treatment of hypertension in African American patients in combination with a thiazide diuretic, unless they have chronic kidney disease.

Action

ACE inhibitors such as captopril block the enzyme that normally converts angiotensin I to the potent vasoconstrictor angiotensin II. (ACE [also called kininase] is mainly located in the endothelial lining of blood vessels, which is the site of production of most angiotensin II. This same enzyme also metabolizes bradykinin, an endogenous substance with strong vasodilating properties.) By blocking production of angiotensin II, ACE inhibitors decrease vasoconstriction (thus having a vasodilating effect) and decrease aldosterone production (thus reducing retention of sodium and water). In addition to inhibiting formation of angiotensin II, these drugs also inhibit the breakdown of bradykinin, prolonging its vasodilating effects.

Use

Healthcare providers use captopril to prevent or reverse the remodeling of heart muscle and blood vessel walls that impairs cardiovascular function and exacerbates cardiovascular disease processes. Widely used to treat heart failure and hypertension, the drug may also decrease morbidity and mortality in other cardiovascular disorders. Captopril may be effective as monotherapy in White patients with hypertension or in combination

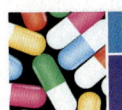

TABLE 26.2
DRUGS AT A GLANCE: Angiotensin-Converting Enzyme Inhibitors

Drug	Routes and Dosage Ranges	
	Adults	**Children 1–17 y of Age (Unless Otherwise Stated)**
Captopril (APO-Capto, PMS-Captopril, TEVA-Captopril)	25 mg PO, 2–3 times daily initially, gradually increased to 50, 100, or 150 mg 2–3 times daily, if necessary; maximum dose 450 mg/d	1.5 mg/kg/d PO in divided doses every 8 h; maximum dose 6 mg/kg/d Neonates, 0.03–0.15 mg/kg/d PO every 8–24 h; maximum dose 2 mg/kg/d
Benazepril	10 mg PO once daily initially, increased to 40 mg daily if necessary, in 1 or 2 doses	0.2 mg/kg PO once daily
Cilazapril (APO-Cilazapril; Inhibace)	2.5 mg once daily; titrate to response; usual dose: 2.5–5 mg once daily (maximum dose: 10 mg/d)	Not labeled for use with pediatrics
Enalapril (Vasotec; ACT-Enalapril, APO-Enalapril, Enalaprilat [Vasotec IV])	5 mg PO once daily, increased to 10–40 mg daily, in 1 or 2 doses, if necessary 1.25 mg/dose IV, given over 5 min every 6 h (Canadian only)	0.08 mg/kg PO; maximum dose 5 mg/d 0.005–0.01 mg/kg/dose every 8–24 h IV (Canadian only)
Fosinopril (APO-Fosinopril, CO Fosinopril)	10 mg PO once daily initially, increased to 40 mg daily if necessary in 1 or 2 doses	>50 kg, 5–10 mg PO once daily
Lisinopril (Zestril; APO-Lisinopril, DOM-Lisinopril)	10 mg PO once daily, increased to 40 mg if necessary	≥6 y, 0.07 mg/kg PO once daily; maximum dose 5 mg/d
Moexipril	Initial dose, 7.5 mg PO (3.75 mg for those who have abnormal kidney function or are taking a diuretic). Maintenance dose, 7.5–30 mg daily, in 1 or 2 doses, adjusted according to blood pressure control	Safety and effectiveness in children have not been established
Perindopril (Coversyl, Auri-Perindopril)	4 mg PO once daily initially; titrate to up to 16 mg/d based on patient response	Safety and effectiveness in children have not been established
Quinapril (Accupril; Accupril, APO-Quinapril)	10 mg PO once daily initially, increased to 20, 40, or 80 mg daily if necessary, in 1 or 2 doses; wait at least 2 wk between dose increments	5–10 mg PO once daily; maximum dose 80 mg once daily
Ramipril (ACT Ramipril, Altace)	2.5 mg PO once daily, increased to 20 mg daily if necessary, in 1 or 2 doses	Safety and effectiveness in children have not been established
Trandolapril (Mavik, Odrik, SANDOZ Trandolapril)	Initial dose, 1 mg PO once daily (0.5 mg for those who have hepatic impairment or abnormal kidney function or are taking a diuretic; 2 mg for African Americans). Maintenance dose, PO 2–4 mg daily, in a single dose, adjusted according to blood pressure control	Safety and effectiveness in children have not been established

with a diuretic in African American patients with hypertension. Clinicians also recommend captopril and other ACE inhibitors for adults with hypertension and diabetes and kidney damage because they slow the progression of albuminuria. In addition, captopril improves post-MI survival when added to the standard therapy of aspirin, a beta-adrenergic blocker, and a thrombolytic.

Table 26.2 presents route and dosage information for captopril and other ACE inhibitors.

Patient-related variables specific to the use of captopril include the following:

- Age:
  - Although limited information is available on the safety and efficacy of captopril in children, neonates and young infants appear to be more sensitive to adverse effects.
  - Captopril has been associated with nephrotoxicity in neonates (Gantenbein et al., 2008).
  - Manufacturer information states that captopril should be used in children only when other measures to control blood pressure have not been successful. Dosing recommendations are to titrate the dose according to the patient's response and use the lowest effective dose.

- Reproduction, pregnancy, and lactation:
  - The U.S. Food and Drug Administration (FDA) has issued a **BOXED WARNING** for use of drugs that directly affect the renin–angiotensin system (such as ACE inhibitors) during pregnancy because their use can cause injury and even death to a developing fetus.
  - ACE inhibitors should be discontinued at the first positive pregnancy test since taking captopril during the first trimester can cause fetal malformation.
- Abnormal kidney function and hepatic impairment:
  - Careful monitoring is required in patients with abnormal kidney function, especially during the first few weeks of therapy, to prevent kidney injury and irreversible kidney failure.
  - Manufacturer recommendations include a reduction in initial dosage and then slow titration over 1- to 2-week intervals to determine the minimum effective dose necessary to achieve desired blood pressure outcome.

Adverse Effects

Captopril is well tolerated and has a low incidence of serious adverse effects (e.g., acute kidney injury, neutropenia, agranulocytosis, thrombocytopenia, proteinuria, glomerulonephritis, **angioedema** [sudden deep swelling or welts under skin, particularly around the eyes and lips]). However, a persistent cough develops in a significant number of patients, especially female patients. Resolution of the cough typically occurs 1 to 4 weeks after discontinuation of captopril but may persist for up to 3 months. Acute hypotension may also occur upon starting captopril, especially in patients with fluid volume deficit. Starting with a low dose taken at bedtime or by stopping diuretics and reducing dosage of other antihypertensive drugs temporarily may prevent this reaction. Hyperkalemia may develop in patients with diabetes or abnormal kidney function or who are taking nonsteroidal anti-inflammatory drugs (NSAIDs), potassium supplements, or potassium-sparing diuretics; these patients should be monitored for this condition.

Contraindications

Contraindications to captopril and other ACE inhibitors include pregnancy, and it is important to discontinue them when pregnancy is detected. Additional contraindications to captopril include known hypersensitivity to the drug or occurrence of angioedema with previous treatment with an ACE inhibitor.

Nursing Implications

Preventing Interactions

Many medications interact with captopril, increasing or decreasing its effects (Box 26.2). Additionally, captopril may increase serum concentrations of digoxin and lithium and increase the risk of adverse reactions and toxicity. ACE inhibitors interact with sacubitril and urapidil, increasing the risk of adverse reactions, especially angioedema.

BOX 26.2 Drug Interactions: Captopril

Drugs That Increase the Effects of Captopril
- Aliskiren
  Increases the risk of hypotension, hyperkalemia, and abnormal kidney function
- Allopurinol
  Increases the risk of severe hypersensitivity reactions, agranulocytosis, neutropenia, and serious infections
- Amiloride, cyclosporine, potassium preparations, spironolactone, tizanidine, triamterene
  Increase the risk of hyperkalemia
- Leflunomide
  Increases the risk of hepatic injury

Drugs That Decrease the Effects of Captopril
- Iron
  Decreases bioavailability, increases risk of adverse/toxic effects of iron
- Lanthanum: *decreases serum concentration of ACEI*

Quality and Safety Alert: Safety

Reportedly, taking captopril and other ACE inhibitors at the same time as potassium-containing salt substitutes (no salt, Morton salt substitute, and others) or large amounts of high-potassium foods (bananas, oranges, and other fruit) increases the risk of hyperkalemia.

Administering the Medication

People should take captopril 1 hour before or 2 hours after meals to enhance absorption. If they have difficulty swallowing, they may crush the tablets. It is necessary to assess blood pressure and pulse on an ongoing basis with initial dosage adjustment and intermittently during therapy.

Assessing for Therapeutic Effects

The nurse monitors response to therapy, looking for a return of blood pressure to target limits without significant adverse effects.

Assessing for Adverse Effects

The nurse monitors for acute hypotension when captopril is started and assesses to make sure the patient does not have a fluid volume deficit that would worsen the likelihood of hypotension. Ongoing nursing assessment would monitor for a persistent cough and regular review of serum potassium levels for indications of hyperkalemia.

Quality and Safety Alert: Safety

It is important to instruct patients who could become pregnant to take measures to prevent pregnancy while taking captopril or other ACE inhibitors because ACE inhibitors are teratogenic.

Patient Teaching

Box 26.3 contains additional patient education guidelines for patients taking antihypertensive drugs.

BOX 26.3 Patient Teaching Guidelines for Antihypertensive Drugs

General Considerations

- Hypertension is a major risk factor for heart attack, stroke, heart failure, and kidney failure. Although it rarely causes symptoms until HMOD occurs, it can be controlled by appropriate management. Learn all you can about the disease process, the factors that cause or aggravate it, and its management.
- Lifestyle changes (i.e., a low-sodium and low-fat diet, regular exercise, and avoiding smoking) may be sufficient to control BP. If drug therapy is prescribed, continue these measures.
- When drug therapy is needed, your prescriber will develop a regimen, including the drug (or drugs), that works best for you. There are numerous antihypertensive drugs, and many can be taken once a day, which makes their use more convenient and less disruptive of daily living. You may need several office visits to find the right drug or drug combination and the right dosage. Changes in drugs or dosages may be needed, especially if you develop other conditions or take other drugs that alter your response to the antihypertensive drugs.
- Antihypertensive drug therapy is usually long term and may produce side effects. Know the brand and generic names of any prescribed drugs and how to take each drug for optimal benefit and minimal adverse effects.
- Antihypertensive drugs must be taken as prescribed for optimal benefits, even if you do not feel well when a medication is started or when dosage is increased. *No antihypertensive drug should be stopped abruptly. If problems develop, they should be discussed with the healthcare prescriber.*
- If treatment is stopped, BP usually increases gradually as the medications are eliminated from the body.
- Sometimes, BP rapidly increases to pretreatment levels or even higher.
- With any of these situations, you are at risk of a heart attack or stroke.
- Stopping one drug of a multidrug regimen may lead to increased adverse effects as well as decreased antihypertensive effectiveness. Thus, antihypertensive drugs should be tapered in dosage and discontinued gradually, as directed by your healthcare provider.
- BP measurements are the only way to tell if your medication is working. Thus, monitor your BP at home, especially when starting drug therapy, changing medications, or changing dosages. Follow manufacturer instructions regarding use, take your BP approximately the same time(s) each day, and keep a record to show to your healthcare provider.
- People sometimes feel dizzy or faint while taking antihypertensive medications. This usually means your BP drops momentarily and is most likely to occur when you start a medication, increase dosage, or stand up suddenly from a sitting or lying position. Prevent or decrease this by moving to a standing position slowly, sleeping with the head of the bed elevated, wearing elastic stockings, exercising legs, avoiding prolonged standing, and avoiding hot baths. If episodes still occur, sit or lie down to avoid a fall and possible injury. Discuss persistent dizziness with your prescriber; this may indicate a need for changing the timing or type of medication.
- It is very important to keep appointments for laboratory testing and follow-up care.
- As with all drugs, keep these medications in the original container, tightly closed, and out of reach of children.

Self- or Caregiver Administration

- Take antihypertensive drugs at prescribed time intervals, about the same time each day. For example, take once-daily drugs as close to every 24 hours as possible; twice-a-day drugs every 12 hours; and if ordered four times daily, take approximately every 6 hours. Taking doses too close together can increase dizziness, weakness, and other adverse effects. Taking doses too far apart may not control BP adequately and may increase risk of heart attack or stroke.
- Take oral captopril on an empty stomach; food decreases drug absorption.
- If you are a sexually active female, use birth control measures when taking angiotensin-converting enzyme (ACE) inhibitors.
- Take most other oral antihypertensive agents with or after food intake to decrease gastric irritation. Candesartan (Atacand), irbesartan (Avapro), losartan (Cozaar), telmisartan (Micardis), and valsartan (Diovan) may be taken with or without food.
- When taking losartan, take the following precautions:
  - Avoid potassium supplements and salt substitutes containing potassium, unless directed by prescriber.
  - Use birth control measures if you are a female and you are sexually active.
  - Contact your healthcare provider immediately if you suspect that you are pregnant.
  - Discuss with your prescriber if you are considering breast-feeding.
- When taking aliskiren, use birth control measures if you are a female and you are sexually active.
- When taking ACE inhibitors, angiotensin II receptor blockers (ARBs), and aliskiren, immediately report hypersensitivity reactions, especially lip or eyelid swelling, throat tightness, and difficulty breathing.
- Avoid taking aliskiren with a high-fat meal because this significantly decreases the amount of available drug.
- With prazosin, doxazosin, or terazosin, take the first dose and the first increased dose at bedtime to prevent dizziness and possible fainting.
- With the clonidine skin patch, apply to a hairless area on the upper arm or torso once every 7 days. Rotate sites.

Other Drugs in the Class

Because of their effectiveness in hypertension and benefits for the heart, blood vessels, and kidneys, the ACE inhibitors are widely used with patients diagnosed with cardiovascular disorders. Drugs in this class also are used in the management of hypertension and heart failure because they decrease peripheral vascular resistance, cardiac workload, and ventricular remodeling. Adverse effects for the class are similar to those outlined with captopril.

Benazepril (Lotensin) is indicated for the treatment of hypertension. Patients may take the drug alone or in combination with thiazide diuretics. Peak plasma concentrations occur within 30 minutes to 1 hour. Once-a-day dosing means that steady-state concentrations of the drug are reached after two or three doses.

Enalapril (Vasotec) is a prodrug used in the treatment of hypertension and heart failure (see Chapter 30). Prescribers may order the drug for use alone or in combination with antihypertensive agents, particularly thiazide diuretics.

> **Quality and Safety Alert: Safety**
>
> Patients started on enalapril who are taking a diuretic occasionally may have symptomatic hypotension following the initial dose of enalapril. The nurse should advocate for the patient's safety and monitor adverse effects.

Fosinopril is indicated for the treatment of hypertension and heart failure. Patients may take the drug alone or in combination with thiazide diuretics. Symptomatic hypotension may occur following the initial dose if the patient has been taking a diuretic. A prodrug, fosinopril, is absorbed very slowly after oral administration and is highly bound to protein. Time to peak concentration is about 3 hours.

Lisinopril (Zestril) is indicated for the treatment of hypertension and heart failure, and the drug is an adjunctive therapy in the management of MI. Prescribers may order it as monotherapy or in combination with thiazide diuretics. Peak serum concentrations of lisinopril occur within about 7 hours. The drug does not undergo metabolism and is excreted unchanged entirely in the urine.

Moexipril, which is administered orally and intravenously, is used in the treatment of hypertension. People may take the drug alone or in combination with thiazide diuretics. Peak serum concentrations occur within about 30 minutes. However, absorption is significantly delayed in the presence of food, and it is important to take the drug in a fasting state. In patients who are currently taking a diuretic, symptomatic hypotension may occasionally occur following the initial dose of moexipril.

Perindopril (Coversyl) is used alone or in combination with other therapies to treat mild to moderate essential hypertension. People should take it at least 1 hour prior to eating. Its peak effect occurs within 1 to 2 hours. Caution is necessary in patients older than 65 years of age; metabolism slows with age, and increased serum plasma levels of the mediation exacerbate fluid retention and hyponatremia.

Quinapril (Accupril) may be used as monotherapy or in combination with thiazide diuretics in the treatment of hypertension or heart failure. Following oral administration, peak concentrations are reached within 1 hour; absorption is decreased with administration with a fatty meal. The drug is highly protein bound and is primarily excreted in the urine.

Ramipril (Altace) is used alone or in combination with other medications, including thiazide diuretics, in the treatment of hypertension. It is also used to reduce the risk of heart attack and stroke in at-risk patients as well as to improve survival in patients with heart failure after a heart attack. After oral administration, peak concentration is reached in 1 hour.

Trandolapril is indicated for the treatment of hypertension alone or in combination with other antihypertensive agents such as hydrochlorothiazide. It is also used post-MI in patients who demonstrate left ventricular systolic dysfunction or in those who are symptomatic from heart failure immediately following an MI.

> **NCLEX Success**
>
> 1. The nurse is reviewing discharge instructions for a patient with a newly initiated order for captopril, an ACE inhibitor. The nurse would indicate that which of the following adverse effects is most common?
>   A. tinnitus
>   B. dry, persistent cough
>   C. muscle weakness
>   D. constipation
>
> 2. The patient with a blood pressure of 154/92 is diagnosed with essential hypertension (stage 2). What would the nurse expect to be potentially included as part of the patient's initial treatment plan along with lifestyle modification? (Select all that apply.)
>   A. ACE inhibitor
>   B. loop diuretic
>   C. angiotensin receptor blocker (ARB)
>   D. calcium channel blocker (CCB)

> **Clinical Application 26.1**
>
> - Mr. Caudill states that he does not understand why he needs an additional medication considering his blood pressure is below 140 mm Hg systolic. How should the nurse respond?

ANGIOTENSIN II RECEPTOR BLOCKERS

Scientists developed ARBs to block the strong blood pressure–raising effects of angiotensin II. ARBs are one of the recommended classes as first-line agents for controlling hypertension, especially with patients initially diagnosed with severe hypertension with left ventricular dysfunction. These drugs resemble ACE inhibitors in their effects on blood pressure and hemodynamics and are as effective in the management of hypertension and possibly heart failure. However, they are less likely to cause hyperkalemia and angioedema than ACE inhibitors, and the occurrence of a persistent cough is rare. The prototype ARB is **Ⓟ losartan** (Cozaar), the first ARB.

Pharmacokinetics

Both losartan and its metabolite are highly bound to plasma albumin, and the drug's active metabolite is 40 times more potent than losartan and largely responsible for the duration of action. The drug undergoes extensive first-pass metabolism, has an onset of 6 hours, and reaches maximum concentrations 1 to 2 hours. Absorption is good. Metabolism is rapid; the cytochrome P450 liver enzymes process losartan to an active metabolite. Excretion is through the kidneys and the liver.

Action

Instead of decreasing production of angiotensin II, like the ACE inhibitors, losartan blocks vasoconstricting and aldosterone-secreting effects of angiotensin II at various receptor sites and prevents angiotensin II from combining at various receptor sites. Losartan may induce a more complete inhibition of the renin–angiotensin system than ACE inhibitors, and they do not affect the response to bradykinin, so losartan is less likely to be associated with non–renin–angiotensin effects (e.g., cough and angioedema). The drug also increases kidney flow and enhances the excretion of chloride, calcium, magnesium, and phosphate.

Although multiple types of receptors have been identified, the angiotensin II receptors, type 1 (AT1) located in brain, kidney, myocardial, vascular, and adrenal tissue, determine most of the effects of angiotensin II on cardiovascular and kidney functions. ARBs block the AT1 receptors and decrease arterial blood pressure by decreasing systemic vascular resistance (see Fig. 26.1).

Use

Prescribers primarily order losartan for use in the treatment of hypertension. Losartan is effective in the treatment of diabetic nephropathy in people with type 2 diabetes who have elevated serum creatinine and proteinuria. After drug therapy begins, maximal effects usually occur within 3 to 6 weeks. It is important to recognize that in African Americans, losartan and other ARBs may be ineffective when used alone. If losartan alone does not control blood pressure, a low dose of a diuretic may be added after 1 to 2 months. A combination product of losartan and hydrochlorothiazide is available.

Table 26.3 presents route and dosage information for losartan and other ARBs.

Patient-related variables specific to the use of losartan and other ARBs include the following:

- Age:
  - Losartan and other ARBs are metabolized by the liver and do not need dose reduction for adults with abnormal kidney function. Use is not recommended in children or adults who have a glomerular filtration rate less than 30 mL/min/1.73 m^2.
- Reproduction, pregnancy, and lactation:
  - The FDA has issued a **BOXED WARNING** ◆ regarding the use of losartan and other ARBs, which directly affect the renin–angiotensin system, because their use can cause injury and even death to a developing fetus.
  - ARBs should be discontinued at the first positive pregnancy test as taking the drug class during the first trimester can cause fetal malformation.
- Abnormal kidney function and hepatic impairment:
  - Caution is warranted for use of all ARBs in biliary tract obstruction or hepatic impairment.
  - A lower starting dose for losartan is recommended because plasma concentrations of the drug and its active metabolite are increased, and clearance is decreased approximately 50% with hepatic dysfunction.
- Specific healthcare environments:
  - In critically ill patients, significant drug–drug interactions and the potential to produce hyperkalemia should be carefully monitored to avoid potentially serious outcomes.

Adverse Effects

Overall, losartan is generally well tolerated, with few side or adverse effects. Adverse effects include dizziness, muscle cramps or weakness, heartburn, diarrhea, and decreased sensitivity to touch. Hyperkalemia may occur, especially for older patients with a history of kidney dysfunction and diabetes, and the serum potassium level should be monitored carefully. While losartan does not directly increase the risk of angioedema, there is an increased risk of angioedema for patients who have a history of angioedema, and the nurse should intervene immediately if this occurs.

Contraindications

Contraindications to losartan include known hypersensitivity to the drug. Pregnancy is a contraindication to use of losartan and other ARBs, and it is essential that the drugs be discontinued as soon as pregnancy is detected to reduce risk of fetal malformation.

Nursing Implications

Preventing Interactions

Many medications interact with losartan, increasing or decreasing its effects (Box 26.4). In addition, several herbs and food alter the effects of losartan. An increased effect occurs with concurrent use of black cohosh, California poppy, celery, garlic, ginger, marshmallow, quinine, and St. John's wort. A decreased effect is observed with grapefruit juice, bayberry, blue cohosh, kola, and licorice.

Administering the Medication

People may take losartan without regard to meals.

Assessing for Therapeutic Effects

The nurse monitors blood pressure to evaluate drug efficacy. Also, the nurse observes for the presence of lifestyle modifications that will improve baseline blood pressure readings (e.g., weight loss, smoking cessation, restricted salt intake).

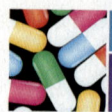

TABLE 26.3
DRUGS AT A GLANCE: Angiotensin II Receptor Blockers

Drug	Routes and Dosage Ranges	
	Adults	**Children 1–17 y of Age (Unless Otherwise Stated)**
Losartan (Cozaar; ACT Losartan, Cozaar)	Initial dose, 50 mg PO once daily initially (25 mg for those who have hepatic impairment or are taking a diuretic). Maintenance dose, PO 35–100 mg daily, in 1 or 2 doses, adjusted according to blood pressure control	≥6 y, 0.7 mg/kg PO once daily; maximum dose 50 mg daily
Azilsartan (Edarbi; Edarbi)	Initial dose 40 mg PO once daily, increase as needed up to 80 mg/d based on patient response	Safety and effectiveness in children have not been established
Candesartan (Atacand; ACH-Candesartan, Atacand)	16 mg PO once daily initially, increased if necessary to a maximum of 32 mg daily, in 1 or 2 doses	1 to <6 y, 0.05–0.4 mg/kg PO per day 6 to <17 y of age <50 kg, 2–16 mg/d PO >50 kg, 4–32 mg/d PO
Irbesartan (Avapro; APO-Irbesartan, Avapro)	150 mg PO once daily initially, increased up to 300 mg, if necessary	6–16 y: 75 mg PO once daily; maximum dose 150 mg
Olmesartan (Benicar; Olmetec, JAMP-Olmesartan)	20 mg PO once daily initially, increased to 40 mg after 2 wk	6–16 y 20 to <35 kg, 10 mg PO once daily; maximum dose 20 mg/d >35 kg, 20 mg PO once daily; maximum dose 40 mg/d
Telmisartan (Micardis; APO-Telmisartan)	40 mg PO once daily initially, increased to maximum of 80 mg daily if necessary	Safety and effectiveness in children have not been established
Valsartan (Diovan; ACT Valsartan, Diovan, DOM-Valsartan)	80 mg PO once daily initially, when used as monotherapy in patients who are not volume depleted; maintenance dose may be increased; however, adding a diuretic is more effective than increasing dose beyond 80 mg	6–16 y, 1.3 mg/kg PO once daily initially up to 40 mg; increase to a maximum of up to 2.7 mg/kg (up to 160 mg) once daily

Assessing for Adverse Effects

The nurse assesses kidney and liver function tests, as well as serum electrolyte levels, particularly potassium. The nurse also observes for the presence of angioedema and other hypersensitivity reactions.

 Quality and Safety Alert: Safety

It is important to instruct patients who could become pregnant to take measures to prevent pregnancy while taking losartan or other ARBs because the drugs are teratogenic.

Patient Teaching

Box 26.3 contains patient education guidelines for the antihypertensive drugs.

Other Drugs in the Class

Azilsartan (Edarbi) may be used as monotherapy or combined with other therapies for hypertension. It has a peak effect within 1½ to 3 hours of administration. Patients should be monitored for the adverse effects of diarrhea, angioedema, hyperkalemia, hypotension, and abnormal kidney function.

Candesartan (Atacand) is used alone or in combination with other drugs to treat hypertension and heart failure. It is available in a fixed combination with hydrochlorothiazide (Avalide). The drug is highly protein bound, crosses the blood–brain barrier poorly, and is excreted in breast milk. After oral administration, the peak serum concentration is reached in about 3 to 4 hours. Food with a high fat content does not affect the bioavailability of candesartan. The adverse effect profile is similar to losartan, and the drug is slightly more effective in reducing blood pressure than losartan.

Irbesartan (Avapro) is used as monotherapy or in combination with other drugs to treat hypertension and is used to treat nephropathy in patients with type 2 diabetes. In patients with volume and salt depletions (e.g., those on hemodialysis), a lower initial dose is recommended. Like candesartan, irbesartan is a bit more effective in reducing blood pressure than losartan. The drug can be administered orally or intravenously. An oral preparation is available in a fixed combination with hydrochlorothiazide

> **BOX 26.4 Drug Interactions: Losartan**
>
> **Drugs That Increase the Effects of Losartan**
> - Alcohol, antihypertensive agents, and diuretics
>   *Increase the risk of hypotension*
> - Aliskiren
>   *Increases the risk of hypotension, hyperkalemia, and abnormal kidney function*
> - Amifostine
>   *Increases the risk of hypotension*
> - Fluconazole
>   *Increases the risk of hypotension through inhibited metabolism*
>
> **Drugs That Decrease the Effects of Losartan**
> - CYP2C9 inducers (e.g., rifampicin, secobarbital), CYP3A4 inducers (e.g., indinavir, clarithromycin) methylphenidate, nonsteroidal anti-inflammatory drugs, peginterferon alfa-2B, and yohimbine
>   *Decrease serum levels*
> - Indomethacin
>   *Decreases antihypertensive effects*
> - Phenobarbital, bromperidol, and rifamycins
>   *Increase metabolism and decrease antihypertensive effects*
>
> CYP, cytochrome P450.

(Avapro HCT). Absorption of oral irbesartan is rapid, and peak concentrations occur within 30 minutes to 2 hours after dosing. Food does not affect the drug's bioavailability.

Olmesartan (Benicar) is used alone or in combination with other drugs to treat hypertension. It is available in a fixed combination with hydrochlorothiazide (Benicar HCT) and with amlodipine (Azor). Absorption is good, and peak concentrations occur within 1 to 2 hours after dosing. The drug is highly protein bound and crosses the blood–brain barrier poorly, but it is excreted in breast milk. Hyperglycemia, dizziness, diarrhea, flulike symptoms, and a spruelike enteropathy are adverse effects. Concomitant use of olmesartan with aliskiren is contraindicated in patients with diabetes.

Telmisartan (Micardis) is used as monotherapy or in combination with other drugs to treat hypertension. It is available in a fixed combination with hydrochlorothiazide (Micardis HCT) and with amlodipine (Twynsta). It is also used in patients 55 years of age or older who are at high risk for developing major cardiovascular events for the risk reduction of death from cardiovascular causes, particularly MI or stroke, and who are unable to take ACE inhibitors. Administration of telmisartan is intravenous or oral. The drug is highly protein bound and is well absorbed, and peak concentrations occur within 30 minutes to 1 hour after dosing. Food slightly reduces bioavailability.

Valsartan (Diovan) is used as monotherapy or in combination with other drugs to treat hypertension. It is available in four fixed combinations: with hydrochlorothiazide (Diovan HCT), with amlodipine (Exforge), with amlodipine and hydrochlorothiazide (Exforge HCT), and with aliskiren (Valturna). The drug is available in oral (tablet and suspension) and intravenous forms. Following oral administration, peak plasma levels occur in 2 to 4 hours. With the tablet, food decreases the bioavailability and the peak plasma level. The suspension has a bioavailability about one and one half times that of the tablet.

CALCIUM CHANNEL BLOCKERS

CCBs are first-line agents for controlling hypertension and may be used as monotherapy or in combination with other drugs. They may be especially useful for people with hypertension who also have angina pectoris, cardiac conduction disorders, other cardiovascular disorders, or pulmonary disorders. Current guidelines recommend that CCBs be used alone or in combination with a thiazide diuretic to treat hypertension. These drugs are especially appropriate as the first-line treatment of hypertension for black patients. They may be used alone or in combination with thiazide-type diuretics. For the purposes of this discussion, **P amlodipine** (Norvasc) serves as the prototype. Note that sustained-release forms of nifedipine, diltiazem, verapamil, and other long-acting drugs (e.g., amlodipine, felodipine) are recommended rather than the short-acting forms because they do not cause precipitous lowering of pressure.

In hypertension, CCBs mainly dilate peripheral arteries and decrease peripheral vascular resistance by relaxing vascular smooth muscle. As a group, the CCBs are well absorbed from the GI tract following oral administration and are highly bound to protein. The drugs are metabolized in the liver and excreted in the urine.

Most of the available CCBs have received FDA approval for use in hypertension. Nifedipine, a short-acting CCB, has been used to treat hypertensive emergencies or urgent hypertensive events.

Note that CCBs (e.g., verapamil) are used for several other cardiovascular disorders. Chapters 27 and 28, respectively, discuss the mechanism of action and use in the management of tachydysrhythmias and angina pectoris.

Pharmacokinetics

Amlodipine is well absorbed with oral administration. Absorption is not reduced by the presence of food. Peak plasma concentration is achieved between 6 and 12 hours after oral administration. Significant initial reductions in blood pressure are achieved with 24 to 48 hours of the initial dose. Therapeutic plasma levels are reached in approximately 7 days with consistent daily dosing. The drug is metabolized in the liver and excreted in the urine.

Action

Amlodipine inhibits the influx of calcium ions across cardiac and smooth muscle during depolarization, resulting in relaxation and vasodilation. This leads to lowered blood pressure.

Use

Healthcare providers use amlodipine to treat hypertension alone or in combination with other antihypertensives. The drug can also be used to treat angina associated with CAD, which is addressed in Chapter 28. Note that no dosage adjustment is necessary in patients with abnormal kidney function.

Table 26.4 provides specific dosage information for amlodipine and other CCBs.

Patient-related variables specific to the use of amlodipine and other CCBs include the following:

- Age:
  - Amlodipine has been shown to be effective in lowering blood pressure in children aged 6 to 17 years.
  - Small sample studies indicate that children younger than 6 years of age may have a weight-adjusted clearance of amlodipine greater than in older children, suggesting that larger than expected doses may be necessary in that age group to obtain the desired response.
  - Older patients have decreased clearance of amlodipine. Therefore, dosing should start with the lowest possible dose and be titrated as necessary.
- Reproduction, pregnancy, and lactation:
  - CCBs are used to treat hypertension during pregnancy; other CCBs are commonly used instead of amlodipine.
  - Amlodipine crosses the placenta and is also present in breast milk, though at typical levels, it does not cause significant risk of adverse effects.
  - The drug's pharmacokinetics may be altered immediately postpartum due to pregnancy-induced pharmacologic changes.
- Abnormal kidney function and hepatic impairment:
  - Amlodipine is metabolized extensively by the liver and the drug may accumulate with hepatic impairment.

TABLE 26.4 DRUGS AT A GLANCE: Calcium Channel Blockers

Drug	Routes and Dosage Ranges — Adults	Children 1–17 y of Age (Unless Otherwise Stated)
Amlodipine (Norvasc; ✦ ACT AmLODIPine, DOM-AmLODIPine)	5–10 mg PO once daily	<6 y, based on weight-based considerations and response
Clevidipine (Cleviprex)	IV: 1–2 mg/h initial infusion, titrate to maintenance dose of 4–6 mg/h (max 21 mg/h)	Safety and effectiveness have not been established
Diltiazem (sustained release) (Cardizem CD, Cartia XT; ✦ ACT Diltiazem CD, APO-Diltiaz CD)	60–120 mg PO twice daily	Safety and effectiveness have not been established
Felodipine (✦ Plendil, SANDOZ Felodipine)	5–10 mg PO once daily	Maximum 10 mg PO daily
Isradipine	2.5–5 mg PO twice daily; may increase to up to 10 mg/d in two divided doses	Immediate release (PO), 0.25–0.2 mg/kg daily in 3–4 doses initially; maximum dose 0.8 mg/kg up to 20 mg daily. Sustained release (PO), 0.15–0.2 mg/kg daily in two divided doses initially; maximum dose 0.8 mg/kg up to 20 mg daily
Levamlodipine (Conjupri)	1.25–2.5 mg PO once daily; titrate to max of 5 mg/d	1.25–2.5 mg PO once daily
Nicardipine	Sustained release (PO), 30–60 mg daily up to 120 mg/d; twice daily IV infusion, 5–15 mg/h	1–3 mcg/kg/min as IV infusion for rapid reduction of blood pressure
Nifedipine (Adalat CC, Procardia, Procardia XL; ✦ Adalat XL, DOM-NIFEdipine)	Sustained release (PO) only, 30–60 mg once daily, increased over 1–2 wk if necessary	Sustained release (PO), 0.25–0.5 mg/kg/d in 1–2 doses; maximum dose 3 mg/kg in 1–2 doses up to 120 mg
Nisoldipine (Sular)	20 mg PO once daily initially, increased by 10 mg/wk or longer intervals to a maximum of 60 mg daily; average maintenance dose, 20–40 mg daily. Adults with liver impairment or >65 y, 10 mg PO once daily initially	Safety and effectiveness have not been established
Verapamil (Calan, Calan SR, Tarka, Verelan; ✦ APO-Verap, Isoptin SR)	Immediate release (PO), 40–120 mg 3 times daily. Sustained release (PO), 180–240 mg once daily. IV, see manufacturer's instructions	IV, see manufacturer's instructions

Adverse Effects

Amlodipine is generally well tolerated. Possible cardiovascular adverse effects occur most frequently and include peripheral edema of the hands, ankles, and feet and pulmonary edema, particularly in patients with heart failure. Other potential adverse effects include symptomatic hypotension, headache, drowsiness, fatigue, dizziness, flushing, palpitations, nausea, and abdominal pain.

Contraindications

Contraindications include hypersensitivity to amlodipine or any of its components.

Nursing Implications
Preventing Interactions

Many medications interact with amlodipine, increasing or decreasing its effects (Box 26.5). Conivaptan, CYP3A4 strong inhibitors (e.g., ketoconazole), may increase plasma concentration levels. Avoid concurrent use. Cyclosporine may decrease the metabolism of CCBs, and the nurse should monitor for hypotension. Dantrolene, a muscle relaxer, can increase the risk of hyperkalemia and enhance amlodipine's reduction of myocardial contractility.

Amlodipine also affects the action of several drugs. Simvastatin serum concentrations may increase when taken concurrently. Concurrent use should be avoided if possible, and due to the increased risk of rhabdomyolysis, the simvastatin dose should be limited to 20 mg/day if patients must take the two drugs concurrently. Foods that affect the action of amlodipine include grapefruit juice (a CYP3A4 inhibitor), which may increase the serum level of the drug. St. John's wort (a CYP3A4 inducer) should be avoided because the herbal supplement may decrease the serum level of the drug.

Administering the Medication

The drug can be given without regard for food.

BOX 26.5 Drug Interactions: Amlodipine

Drugs That Increase the Effects of Amlodipine
- Adenosine
  Increases bradycardia
- Alfuzosin, amifostine, barbiturates, diazoxide, duloxetine, and antihypertensive agents
  Increase hypotensive effects
- Fluconazole and itraconazole
  Inhibit metabolism of amlodipine and increase edema

Drugs That Decrease the Effects of Amlodipine
- Rifampin, rifabutin, bromperidol, carbamazepine, and phenytoin
  Decrease serum level of amlodipine

Assessing for Therapeutic Effects

The nurse monitors blood pressure to evaluate drug efficacy. The nurse also observes for the presence of lifestyle modifications that will improve baseline blood pressure readings (e.g., losing weight, stopping smoking, restricting salt intake).

Assessing for Adverse Effects

The nurse monitors blood pressure and assesses for chest pain and other indications of decreased myocardial oxygen supply frequently on initiation of drug therapy. In patients with severe CAD and/or heart failure, very close monitoring for chest pain, pulmonary edema, and peripheral edema is necessary.

Patient Teaching

Box 26.3 contains patient education guidelines for the antihypertensive drugs, including amlodipine.

Other Drugs in the Class

Diltiazem (Cardizem CD, Cartia XT) is administered for hypertension using the extended-release formulation. As a generic drug is available in once- and twice-daily dosing, it is important to verify that the appropriate extended-release formulation is administered. Diltiazem is also approved as a treatment to improve exercise tolerance for patients who experience angina by decreasing oxygen demand. It is necessary to monitor patients for dysrhythmias, atrioventricular heart block, bradycardia, heart failure, hypotension, headache, and dizziness.

Long-acting dihydropyridines are most commonly used to treat hypertension. If the nondihydropyridine CCBs (diltiazem, verapamil) are prescribed, the extended-release formulations are often used for hypertension; the two drugs can be given for control of angina and for rate control in patients with atrial fibrillation.

Nifedipine is available as Adalat CC, Procardia, and Procardia XL. Nifedipine should not be taken with grapefruit juice. Patients should be monitored for effects of excessive vasodilation, including hypotension, dizziness, and headache. Patient teaching must include that abrupt cessation of taking nifedipine could result in rebound tachycardia. Nifedipine immediate release should be used with caution in elderly patients. Patients taking nifedipine extended release should be monitored for sign and symptoms of GI obstruction.

! Quality and Safety Alert: Safety

Authorities no longer recommend puncturing a nifedipine capsule, because this practice is associated with an increased risk of adverse cardiovascular events precipitated by a rapid and severe decrease in blood pressure.

Verapamil (Calan, Calan SR, Tarka, Verelan) is another CCB used to treat hypertension. It is important not to split or crush extended-release capsules or tablets and not to take the medication with grapefruit juice. The nurse should monitor patients for effects of excessive vasodilation, including hypotension, dizziness, and headache. Felodipine is also used to control hypertension. Patients require monitoring for headache, dizziness, chest pain, and palpitations. Felodipine is available only in extended-release form. Concurrent use with NSAIDs may decrease antihypertensive effects.

Isradipine is used alone or concomitantly with thiazide-type diuretics for treatment of hypertension in adults. As with other CCBs, isradipine is hepatically metabolized via cytochrome P450 isoenzyme CYP3A4, so numerous drug interactions can occur. Grapefruit juice (a CYP3A4 inhibitor) may increase the serum level of the drug, and St. John's wort (a CYP3A4 inducer) may decrease the serum level of the drug.

Unfolding Patient Stories: Junetta Cooper • Part 2

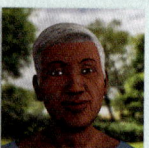

Think back to Junetta Cooper from Chapter 1, a 75-year-old female with coronary artery disease (CAD) and a 20-year history of hypertension controlled with the antihypertensive hydrochlorothiazide. While hospitalized for a cardiac catheterization, her blood pressure is elevated, and the healthcare team is considering the addition of amlodipine. Describe the mechanisms of action in the drug response that are associated with these different antihypertensive medications. How would the nurse explain why hydrochlorothiazide and amlodipine are selected for Junetta? What patient education should the nurse prepare if both medications are ordered for her? Care for Junetta and other patients in a realistic virtual environment: *vSim for Nursing* (thepoint.lww.com/vSimPharm). Practice documenting these patients' care in DocuCare (thepoint.lww.com/DocuCareEHR).

Nicardipine is also a CCB used to manage hypertension. The drug may be taken with or without food but should not be taken with a high-fat meal. It is necessary to monitor for hypotension, chest pain, palpitations, and tachycardia.

Nisoldipine (Sular) is a CCB that may be used to manage hypertension. Patients should take the drug without food. The nurse should monitor for hypotension, chest pain, palpitations, and tachycardia.

Quality and Safety Alert: Safety

Abrupt discontinuation of CCBs may increase frequency and duration of chest pain.

ADDITIONAL MEDICATIONS USED TO TREAT HYPERTENSION

Prescribers may order other drugs for the treatment of hypertension. Additional medications for the management of hypertension are often used in combination with other antihypertensive medications. Table 26.5 lists antihypertensive–diuretic combination products. Table 26.6 presents route and dosage information for additional medications used to treat hypertension.

Diuretics

Diuretics, particularly thiazide diuretics, are often used in combination with other antihypertensive medications to reduce circulating fluid volume and cardiac workload. Thiazide diuretics also contribute to vasodilation and reduced afterload. Current guidelines no longer recommend diuretics as initial monotherapy but do recommend diuretics in combination with first-line drugs such as ARBs, ACE inhibitors, and CCBs (Unger et al., 2020). When diuretic therapy is initiated, blood volume and cardiac output decrease. After long-term administration, cardiac output returns to normal, but there is a persistent decrease in peripheral vascular resistance. Experts have attributed this to a persistent small reduction in extracellular water and plasma volume, decreased receptor sensitivity to vasopressor substances such as angiotensin, direct arteriolar vasodilation, and arteriolar vasodilation secondary to electrolyte depletion in the vessel wall. Current hypertension management guidelines recommend initial drug therapy with two antihypertensive agents for patients with a blood pressure 20/10 mm Hg above goal, and diuretics are frequently part of this combination. Healthcare providers may use diuretics in combination with an ARB, ACE inhibitor, or CCB for initial therapy in all people with hypertension, but diuretics are specifically recommended for any multidrug regimen for African Americans. Diuretics have also demonstrated particularly effectiveness as part of multidrug hypertensive therapy for older adults.

Hydrochlorothiazide is most commonly used, although chlorthalidone has demonstrated a positive effect on the reduction of adverse cardiovascular events. Diazoxide, usually in parenteral form, is indicated for short-term treatment of malignant hypertension. The selective aldosterone blocker, eplerenone, has demonstrated efficacy in African Americans.

Loop diuretics (e.g., furosemide) or potassium-sparing diuretics (e.g., spironolactone) may be useful in some circumstances. Loop diuretics are indicated in people with abnormal kidney function. Potassium-sparing diuretics may precipitate hyperkalemia. Chapter 34 reviews diuretic medications.

Direct Renin Inhibitors

 Aliskiren (Tekturna), the only direct renin inhibitor, decreases plasma renin activity and inhibits the conversion of angiotensinogen to angiotensin I. The drug is used as monotherapy or in combination with other antihypertensive agents for the treatment of hypertension but should never be used in combination with an ACE inhibitor or an ARB. Aliskiren significantly enhances the hypotensive effects of ACE inhibitors and ARBs. A fixed-dose combination with valsartan (Valturna) is available. Aliskiren is poorly absorbed, and steady-state blood levels are reached in about a week. Following oral administration, peak plasma levels are reached in 1 to 3 hours. If taken with a high-fat meal, bioavailability and peak levels are decreased by about 75%. The drug is excreted in the urine. The nurse should monitor for the adverse effects of angioedema, hyperkalemia, symptomatic hypotension, and impaired kidney function. Aliskiren is contraindicated in patients with chronic kidney disease because of the increased risk of abnormal kidney function, hyperkalemia, and hypotension.

TABLE 26.5
DRUGS AT A GLANCE: Oral Antihypertensive Combination Products*

Trade Name	Components						Dosage Ranges
	Angiotensin II Receptor Blocker	Angiotensin-Converting Enzyme Inhibitor	Beta-Adrenergic Blocker	Calcium Channel Blocker	Diuretic	Other	
Accuretic (🍁 Accuretic)		Quinapril 10–20 mg			HCTZ 12.5–25 mg		1–2 tablets once daily
Aldactazide (🍁 Aldactazide 25 or 50, Teva-Spironolactone/HCTZ)					HCTZ 25–50 mg; spironolactone 25–50 mg		1–2 tablets once daily
Atacand HCT (🍁 APO-Candesartan HCTZ, Atacand, DOM-Candesartan)	Candesartan 16 or 32 mg				HCTZ 12.5 or 25 mg		1 tablet daily
Avalide (🍁 Irbesartan-HCT, Avalide)	Irbesartan 150 mg				HCTZ 12.5 mg		1 tablet daily
Azor	Olmesartan 20 or 40 mg			Amlodipine 5 or 10 mg			1 tablet daily
Benicar HCT (🍁 Olmetec, ACT Olmesartan, RIVA-Olmesartan)	Olmesartan 20 or 40 mg				HCTZ 12.5 or 25 mg		1–2 tablets daily
Corzide			Nadolol 40 or 80 mg		Bendroflumethiazide 5 mg		1 tablet daily
Diovan HCT (🍁 Diovan HCT, Valsartan-HCT)	Valsartan 80, 160, or 320 mg				HCTZ 12.5–25 mg		1 tablet daily
Dyazide					HCTZ 25 mg; triamterene 37.5 mg		1 tablet daily
Exforge	Valsartan 160 or 320 mg			Amlodipine 5 or 10 mg			1–2 tablets once daily
Hyzaar (🍁 ACT Losartan/HCT, Hyzaar, ACT Losartan/HCT)	Losartan 100 mg				HCTZ 12.5 mg		1 tablet daily
Lopressor HCT			Metoprolol 25, 50, or 100 mg		HCTZ 12.5 or 25 mg		1–2 tablets daily
Lotrel		Benazepril 10, 20, or mg		Amlodipine 2.5 or 5 mg			1 capsule daily
Maxzide					HCTZ 25–50 mg; triamterene 37.5–75 mg		
Micardis HCT (🍁 Micardis Plus)	Telmisartan 40 or 80 mg				HCTZ 12.5 or 25 mg		1–2 tablets daily

(Continued on page 496)

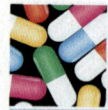

TABLE 26.5
DRUGS AT A GLANCE: Oral Antihypertensive Combination Products* (Continued)

Trade Name	Components						
	Angiotensin II Receptor Blocker	Angiotensin-Converting Enzyme Inhibitor	Beta-Adrenergic Blocker	Calcium Channel Blocker	Diuretic	Other	Dosage Ranges
Tarka (✳ Tarka)		Trandolapril 1, 2, or 4 mg		Verapamil 180 or 240 mg			1 tablet daily
Tenoretic (✳ Tenoretic)			Atenolol 50 or 100 mg		Chlorthalidone 25 mg		1 tablet daily
Twynsta (✳Twynsta)	Telmisartan 40 or 80 mg			Amlodipine 5 or 10 mg			
Vaseretic (✳ TEVA-Enalapril/HCTZ)		Enalapril 5 or 10 mg			HCTZ 12.5 or 25 mg		1–2 tablets daily
Zestoretic (✳ APO-Lisinopril/HCTZ, Zestoretic)		Lisinopril 10 or 20 mg			HCTZ 12.5 or 25 mg		1 tablet daily
Ziac (✳ Ziac)			Bisoprolol 2.5, 5, or 10 mg		HCTZ 6.25 mg		1 tablet daily

*Note that one trade name product may be available in multiple formulations, with variable amounts of antihypertensive, diuretic, or both components.
HCTZ, hydrochlorothiazide.

TABLE 26.6
Additional Medications Used for the Treatment of Hypertension

Drug	Routes and Dosage Ranges	
	Adults	Children 1–17 y of Age (Unless Otherwise Stated)
Direct Renin Inhibitors		
(P) Aliskiren (Tekturna; ✳ Rasilez)	150 mg PO once daily	Safety and effectiveness have not been established
Antiadrenergics		
Alpha₁-Adrenergic Blockers		
Doxazosin (Cardura, Cardura XL; ✳ APO-Doxazosin, DOM-Doxazosin)	1 mg PO once daily initially, increased to 2 mg, then to 4, 8, and 16 mg daily if necessary	Safety and effectiveness have not been established
Prazosin (Minipress; ✳ APO-Prazo, Minipress)	1 mg PO 2–3 times daily initially, increased if necessary to 20 mg in divided doses; average maintenance dose, 6–15 mg daily	Safety and effectiveness have not been established
Terazosin (✳ APO-Terazosin, PMS-Terazosin)	1 mg PO at bedtime initially, may be increased gradually; usual maintenance dose, 1–5 mg once daily	Safety and effectiveness have not been established
Alpha₂ Agonists		
Clonidine (Catapres; ✳ APO-CloNIDine, MINT-CloNIDine)	0.1 mg PO 2 times daily initially, gradually increased up to 2.4 mg daily, if necessary; average maintenance dose, 0.2–0.8 mg daily Transdermal: 0.1 mg/24 h initially, patch applied once every 7 d and increase by 0.1 mg at 1- to 2-wk intervals; usual maintenance dose 0.1–0.3 mg/24 h patch applied once every 7 d	5–25 mcg/kg/d PO, in divided doses, every 6 h; increase at 5- to 7-d intervals, if needed

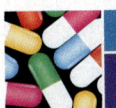

TABLE 26.6 Additional Medications Used for the Treatment of Hypertension (Continued)

Drug	Routes and Dosage Ranges	
	Adults	**Children 1–17 y of Age (Unless Otherwise Stated)**
Guanfacine (✽ Intuniv XR)	1 mg PO daily at bedtime, increased to 2 mg after 3–4 wk and then to 3 mg if necessary	≥12 y, 1 mg daily PO initially: maximum dose 2 mg daily
Methyldopa	250 mg PO 2 or 3 times daily initially, increased gradually until blood pressure is controlled or a daily dose of 3 g is reached	10 mg/kg/d PO in 2–4 divided doses initially, increased or decreased according to response; maximum dose 65 mg/kg/d or 3 g daily, whichever is less
Beta-Adrenergic Blockers		
Acebutolol (✽ APO-Acebutolol)	400 mg PO once daily initially, increased to 800 mg daily if necessary	Safety and effectiveness have not been established
Atenolol (Tenormin; ✽ APO-Atenol), BIO-Atenolol	50 mg PO once daily initially, increased in 1–2 wk to 100 mg once daily, if necessary	0.5–1 mg/kg/d PO in 1 or 2 doses; maximum dose 2 mg/kg up to 100 mg daily in 1 or 2 doses
Bisoprolol (✽ APO-Bisoprolol, RIVA-Bisoprolol)	5 mg PO once daily, increased to a maximum of 20 mg daily if necessary	10 mg PO in a fixed combination with hydrochlorothiazide 6.25 mg daily
Metoprolol (Lopressor; ✽ APO-Metoprolol, APO-Metoprolol SR)	50 mg PO twice daily, gradually increased in weekly or longer intervals if necessary; maximum dose 400 mg daily	Immediate release (PO), 1–2 mg/kg/d in 2 doses; maximum dose 6 mg/kg/d not to exceed 200 mg/d Sustained release (PO), 1 mg/kg once daily not to exceed 50 mg/d; maximum dose not to exceed 200 mg/d
Nadolol (Corgard)	40 mg PO once daily initially, gradually increased if necessary; average dose, 80–320 mg daily	Safety and effectiveness have not been established
Pindolol (✽ APO-Pindol)	5 mg PO 2 or 3 times daily initially, increased by 10 mg/d at 3- to 4-wk intervals to a maximum of 60 mg daily	Safety and effectiveness have not been established
Propranolol (Inderal LA; ✽ APO-Propranolol, Hemangiol)	40 mg PO twice daily initially, gradually increased up to 640 mg daily	1 mg/kg/d PO initially, gradually increased to a maximum of 10 mg/kg/d
Timolol	10 mg PO twice daily initially, increased gradually if necessary; average daily dose, 20–40 mg; maximum daily dose, 60 mg	Safety and effectiveness have not been established
Alpha–Beta-Adrenergic Blockers		
Carvedilol (Coreg, Coreg CR)	6.25 mg PO twice daily for 7–14 d, increase to 12.5 mg twice daily for 7–14 d, and then increase to a maximum dose of 25 mg twice daily if tolerated and needed	Not approved for children <18 y
Labetalol (✽ Trandate, APO-Labetalol)	100 mg PO twice daily, increased by 100 mg twice daily every 2–3 d if necessary; usual maintenance dose, 200–400 mg twice daily; severe hypertension may require 1,200–2,400 mg daily IV injection, 20 mg slowly over 2 min, followed by 40–80 mg every 10 min until the desired blood pressure is achieved or 300 mg has been given IV infusion, mix with IV fluids and infuse at a rate of 2 mg/min	1–3 mg/kg PO daily initially twice daily; increase up to a maximum of 10–12 mg/kg or 1,200 mg daily

(Continued on page 498)

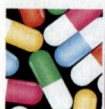

TABLE 26.6

Additional Medications Used for the Treatment of Hypertension (Continued)

Drug	Routes and Dosage Ranges	
	Adults	**Children 1–17 y of Age (Unless Otherwise Stated)**
Diuretics		
Hydrochlorothiazide (Microzide; 🍁 APO-Hydro, TEVA-Hydrochlorothiazide, Urozide)	Hypertension: 12.5–50 mg PO 1 or 2 times daily Elderly: 12.5–25 PO mg/d	2 mg/kg/d PO in 2 divided doses Infants <6 mo, 2–3 mg/kg/d in 2 divided doses
Chlorothiazide (Diuril)	500–2,000 mg/d PO divided in 1–2 times doses Elderly, 500 mg PO once daily or 1 g 3 times/wk 250–1,000 mg IV once or twice daily; maximum dose 1,000 mg	22 mg/kg PO in 2 divided doses Infants <6 mo, 20–40 mg/kg/d in 2 divided doses; maximum dose 375 mg/d IV dosing not well established
Chlorthalidone (🍁 APO-Chlorthalidone)	25–100 mg/d PO Elderly, 12.5–25 mg/d PO or every other day	Not approved in children
Indapamide (🍁 APO-Indapamide, Lozide, MYLAN-Indapamide)	Hypertension: 1.25 mg PO in morning may increase to 5 mg/d	Dosage not established
Furosemide (Lasix; 🍁 APO-Furosemide, Furosemide Special, MINT-Furosemide)	Hypertension: 20–40 mg PO twice daily, gradually increased if necessary Hypertensive crisis: 40–80 mg IV injected over 1–2 min; with kidney failure, much larger doses may be needed PO, IV 5–20 mg once daily	2 mg/kg PO 1 or 2 times daily initially, gradually increased by increments of 1–2 mg/kg per dose if necessary at intervals of 6–8 h; maximum daily dose 6 mg/kg 1 mg/kg IV initially; if diuretic response is not adequate, increase dosage by 1 mg/kg no sooner than 2 h after previous dose; maximum dose 6 mg/kg
Spironolactone (Aldactone, CaroSpir; 🍁 Aldactone, TEVA-Spironolactone)	25–100 mg PO daily	Safety and effectiveness not established
Amiloride (🍁 Midamor)	5–10 mg PO daily	Dosage not established
Triamterene (Dyrenium)	100–300 mg PO daily in divided doses	2–4 mg/kg/d PO in divided doses
Other Vasodilators (Direct Acting)		
Fenoldopam (Corlopam)	Infusion, IV, initial dose based on body weight and then flow rate titrated to achieve desired response; mix with 0.9% sodium chloride or 5% dextrose to a concentration of 40 mcg/mL (e.g., 40 mg of drug [4 mL of concentrate] in 1,000 mL of IV fluid)	Infusion, IV, initial dose based on body weight (0.2 mcg/kg/min) and then flow rate titrated to achieve desired response; may increase dosage every 20–30 min by up to 0.3–0.5 mcg/kg/min; maximum dose 0.8 mcg/kg/min
Hydralazine (Hydra-zide, BiDil; 🍁 APO-HydrALAZINE, Apresoline)	Chronic hypertension: 10 mg PO 4 times daily for 2–4 d, gradually increased up to 300 mg/d, if necessary Hypertensive crisis: 10–20 mg IM, IV, increased to 40 mg if necessary; repeat dose as needed	Chronic hypertension: 0.75 mg/kg/d PO initially in 4 divided doses; gradually increase over 3–4 wk to a maximum dose of 7.5 mg/kg/d if necessary Hypertensive crisis: 0.1–0.2 IM, IV mg/kg every 4–6 h as needed
Minoxidil (🍁 Loniten)	5 mg PO once daily initially, increased gradually until blood pressure is controlled; average daily dose, 10–40 mg; maximum daily dose, 100 mg in single or divided doses	<12 y, 0.2 mg/kg/d PO initially as a single dose, increased gradually until blood pressure is controlled; average daily dose, 0.25–1.0 mg/kg; maximum dose 50 mg/d
Sodium nitroprusside (Nitropress; 🍁 Nipride)	Infusion, IV, 0.5–10 mcg/kg/min; average dose, 3 mcg/kg/min; prepare solution by adding 50 mg of sodium nitroprusside to 250–1,000 mL of 5% dextrose in water and cover promptly to protect from light	Same as adult

> **NCLEX Success**
>
> 3. Orthostatic hypotension is a potential outcome of antihypertensive drugs that places older adults at risk for injury from falls. Instructions given to the patient to decrease this effect include which of the following? (Select all that apply.)
>   A. Take the dose at bedtime.
>   B. Change position slowly when rising from bed or chair.
>   C. Increase fluid intake by 500 mL/day.
>   D. Decrease the dose until symptoms disappear.

Antiadrenergics

Antiadrenergic (sympatholytic) drugs inhibit activity of the SNS. When the SNS is stimulated, the nerve impulse travels from the brain and spinal cord to the ganglia. From the ganglia, the impulse travels along postganglionic fibers to effector organs (e.g., heart, blood vessels). Although SNS stimulation produces widespread effects in the body, the effects relevant to this discussion are the increases in heart rate, force of myocardial contraction, cardiac output, and blood pressure that occur. When the nerve impulse is inhibited or blocked at any location along its pathway, the result is decreased blood pressure.

Alpha$_1$-adrenergic receptor blockers (e.g., prazosin) dilate blood vessels and decrease peripheral vascular resistance. These drugs can be used alone or in multidrug regimens but are not recommended as initial antihypertensive agents. One adverse effect, called the **first-dose phenomenon**, results in orthostatic hypotension, with palpitations, dizziness, and perhaps syncope 1 to 3 hours after the first dose or an increased dose. To prevent this effect, first doses and first increased doses are taken at bedtime. Another effect, associated with long-term use or higher doses, leads to sodium and fluid retention and a need for concurrent diuretic therapy. Centrally acting sympatholytics (e.g., clonidine) stimulate presynaptic alpha$_2$ receptors in the brain and are classified as alpha$_2$ receptor agonists. Taking these drugs leads to the release of less norepinephrine and a reduction of sympathetic outflow from the vasomotor center. Stimulation of presynaptic alpha$_2$ receptors peripherally may also contribute to the decreased sympathetic activity. Reduced sympathetic activity leads to decreased cardiac output, heart rate, peripheral vascular resistance, and blood pressure. Chronic use of clonidine and related drugs may result in sodium and fluid retention, especially with higher doses.

Beta-adrenergic blockers are useful in the treatment of hypertension in patients with ischemic heart disease, especially in those younger than 50 years of age with acute coronary syndrome or recent MI and who have heart failure with reduced ejection fraction. Experts do not recommend beta-blockers as initial monotherapy unless they are specifically indicated; they are most effective when used in combination with ACE inhibitors or ARBs (Unger et al., 2020). Most beta-adrenergic blockers have FDA approval for use in hypertension and are probably equally effective. However, the cardioselective drugs (see Chapter 28) are preferred for people with hypertension who also have asthma, peripheral vascular disease, or diabetes. Research studies demonstrate reduced morbidity and mortality with diuretics and beta-adrenergic blockers used in combination, especially after an MI.

Beta-adrenergic blockers (e.g., propranolol decrease heart rate [chronotropy], force of myocardial contraction [inotropy]), cardiac output, and renin release from the kidneys. The FDA has issued a **BOXED WARNING** for patients with CAD taking oral forms of atenolol, metoprolol, nadolol, propranolol, and timolol; abrupt withdrawal has resulted in exacerbation of angina, the incidence of ventricular dysrhythmias, and the occurrence of MIs. Beta-adrenergic blockers that normally undergo extensive first-pass hepatic metabolism (e.g., acebutolol, metoprolol, propranolol, timolol) may produce excessive blood levels in patients with cirrhosis because the blood containing the drug is shunted around the liver into the systemic circulation. It is necessary to start at a low dose and titrate the dosage carefully. Also, dosage reduction with bisoprolol and pindolol is important in patients with cirrhosis or other hepatic impairment.

Labetalol can be used as monotherapy for initial management of uncomplicated hypertension; however, thiazide diuretics are preferred by JNC 8. Administration is intravenous or oral. Occasionally following intravenous administration, orthostatic hypotension with loss of consciousness reportedly occurs; the hypotension can last for 3 hours or longer.

Other Vasodilators (Direct Acting)

Vasodilator antihypertensive drugs directly relax smooth muscle in blood vessels, resulting in dilation and decreased peripheral vascular resistance. As they reduce afterload, they may be used in management of heart failure. The direct-acting vasodilators are effective in managing a hypertensive emergency.

Nitroprusside (Nitropress) is a potent vasodilator that acts on arterioles and venules. Given by continuous intravenous infusion, the drug has a rapid onset and short duration of action, and it requires continuous blood pressure monitoring. Intra-arterial blood pressure monitoring is recommended during the infusion. Nitroprusside is metabolized to thiocyanate, and it is necessary to measure serum thiocyanate levels if the drug is given longer than 72 hours. If the serum thiocyanate level is more than 12 mg/dL, it is important to stop the infusion after 72 hours. The infusion should last no longer than 48 hours in patients with abnormal kidney function. Hemodialysis reverses the symptoms of thiocyanate toxicity (e.g., nausea, vomiting, muscle twitching or spasm, seizures).

Hydralazine (Hydra-Zide, BiDil) and minoxidil are vasodilators that act mainly on arterioles. These drugs have a limited effect on hypertension when used alone because the vasodilating action that lowers blood pressure also stimulates the SNS and triggers reflexive compensatory mechanisms (vasoconstriction, tachycardia, and increased cardiac output), which raise blood pressure. It is possible to prevent this effect during long-term therapy by also giving a drug that inhibits excessive sympathetic stimulation (e.g., propranolol, an adrenergic blocker). These drugs also cause sodium and water retention, which may be minimized by concomitant diuretic therapy. The FDA has issued a **BOXED WARNING** for minoxidil because the drug can exacerbate angina and precipitate pericardial effusion (which can progress to cardiac tamponade).

Clinical Application 26.2

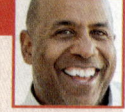

- Discuss the rationale for choosing captopril in Mr. Caudill's case.
- What should the nurse include in teaching Mr. Caudill to minimize adverse effects of the captopril and metoprolol?

NCLEX Success

4. A patient with a history of hypertension comes to the emergency department with double vision and a blood pressure of 240/120 mm Hg. The physician on call orders sodium nitroprusside by continuous infusion, with continual blood pressure monitoring. This drug's immediate action is to lower blood pressure by which of the following mechanisms?

   A. increasing peripheral vascular resistance
   B. increasing cardiac output
   C. dilating venous and arterial vessels
   D. decreasing heart rate

5. A patient in the intensive care unit has been receiving sodium nitroprusside for 2 days. The nurse needs to monitor for which of the following?

   A. thiocyanate toxicity
   B. hyperglycemia
   C. hyperkalemia
   D. metabolic alkalosis

Unfolding Patient Stories: Mary Richards • Part 2

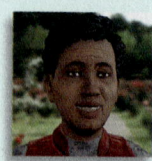

Think back to Chapter 3, where you met Mary Richards, an 82-year-old female who is hospitalized with symptoms of nausea, dizziness, and weakness. She has a history of atrial fibrillation, hypertension, and chronic heart failure managed with furosemide, amlodipine, and digoxin. Upon admission, her current medications are discontinued; they will be replaced with hydrochlorothiazide, bisoprolol, and ramipril once she is stable. What are possible explanations for the medication changes? Why is it important for the nurse to understand the rationale for the adjustment? What nursing assessments verify the safe administration of the new medications and evaluate for potential side effects? What assessment findings would indicate to the nurse an improvement in heart failure and satisfactory medication response versus a need for additional or alternative medications? Care for Mary and other patients in a realistic virtual environment: *vSim for Nursing* (thepoint.lww.com/vSimPharm). Practice documenting these patients' care in DocuCare (thepoint.lww.com/DocuCareEHR).

THE NURSING PROCESS

A concept map outlining the nursing process related to drug therapy considerations in this chapter is found in the map below. Additional nursing implications related to the disease process should also be considered in care decisions.

Assessment
- Assess for conditions and risk factors that may lead to hypertension.
- Assess for the use of oral contraceptives, corticosteroids, appetite suppressants, nasal decongestants, and nonsteroidal anti-inflammatory agents, which may increase blood pressure.
- Assess for signs and symptoms of hypertension.
- Assess blood pressure accurately and repeatedly. As a rule, multiple measurements in which systolic pressure is greater than 130 mm Hg and/or diastolic pressure is greater than 80 mg Hg are necessary to establish a diagnosis of hypertension.

Outcomes of Therapy
The patient will
- Maintain drug regimen as ordered.
- Maintain blood pressure in the recommended range.
- Verbalize or demonstrate knowledge of prescribed drugs and recommended lifestyle changes.
- Recognize signs and symptoms that necessitate professional medical intervention.
- Keep follow-up appointments.

Nursing Interventions
- Implement measures that aid prevention, early detection, and management of hypertension.
- Support the patient with hypertension to adhere to prescribed therapy (see Box 26.3).
- Reinforce the patient's healthy lifestyle changes and supportive interpersonal relationships. Losing weight, stopping smoking, and other changes are most likely to be effective if attempted one at a time.
- Demonstrate and observe return demonstration of recommended techniques for measuring blood pressure. Proper technique is necessary to ensure that antihypertensive drugs and dosages are not changed on the basis of inaccurate blood pressures.

Evaluation
- Observe blood pressure measurement technique and for readings within goal or closer to normal ranges.
- Observe and interview regarding compliance with instructions about drug therapy and lifestyle changes.
- Observe and interview regarding adverse drug effects.

Visit thePoint® at http://thePoint.lww.com/Frandsen13e for answers to NCLEX Success questions (in Appendix A), answers to Clinical Application Case Studies (in Appendix B), additional information on etiology and pathophysiology, and more!

REFERENCES AND RESOURCES

Centers for Disease Control and Prevention (CDC). (2021). *Hypertension Cascade: Hypertension Prevalence, Treatment and Control Estimates Among US Adults Aged 18 Years and Older Applying the Criteria From the American College of Cardiology and American Heart Association's 2017 Hypertension Guideline—NHANES 2015–2018*. US Department of Health and Human Services.

Flynn, J. T., Kaelber, D. C., Baker-Smith, C. M., Blowey, D., Carroll, A. E., Daniels, S. R., de Ferranti, S. D., Dionne, J. M., Falkner, B., Flinn, S. K., Gidding, S. S., Goodwin, C., Leu, M. G., Powers, M. E., Rea, C., Samuels, J., Simasek, M., Thaker, V. V., & Urbina, E. M.; SUBCOMMITTEE ON SCREENING AND MANAGEMENT OF HIGH BLOOD PRESSURE IN CHILDREN. (2017). Clinical Practice Guideline for screening and management of high blood pressure in children and adolescents. *Pediatrics, 140*(3), e20171904.

Gantenbein, M. H., Bauersfeld, U., Baenziger, O., Frey, B., Neuhaus, T., Sennhauser, F., & Bernet, V. (2008). Side effects of angiotensin converting enzyme inhibitor (captopril) in newborns and young infants. *Journal of Perinatology Medicine. 36*(5):448–452.

James, P., Oparil, S., Carter, B., Cushman, W., Dennison-Himmelfarb, C., Handler, J., Lackland, D. T., LeFevre, M. L., MacKenzie, T. D.,

Ogedegbe, O., Smith, S. C. Jr, Svetkey, L. P., Taler, S. J., Townsend, R. R., Wright, J. T. Jr, Narva, A. S., & Ortiz, E. (2014). 2014 evidence-based guideline for the management of high blood pressure in adults report from the panel members appointed to the Eighth Joint National Committee (JNC 8). *Journal of the American Medical Association, 311*(5), 507–520. https://doi.org/10.1001/jama.2013.284427

Kario, K., Chen, C., Park, S., Park, C., Hoshide, S., Cheng, H., Huang, Q., & Wang, J. (2018). Consensus document on improving hypertension management in Asian patients, taking into account Asian characteristics., *Hypertension, 71,* 375–382. https://doi.org/10.1161/HYPERTENSIONAHA.117.10238

Kurtz, T., & Kajiya, T. (2012). Differential pharmacology and benefit/risk of azilsartan compared to other sartans. *Vascular Health Risk Management, 8,* 133–143.

Mann, J. (2022). Choice of drug therapy in primary (essential) hypertension. *Up To Date.*

Moore, T., Conlin, P., Ard, J., Svetkey, L.; for the DASH Collaborative Research Group. (2001). DASH (Dietary Approaches to Stop Hypertension) Diet Is Effective Treatment for Stage 1 Isolated Systolic Hypertension. *Hypertension, 38*:155–158. https://doi.org/10.1161/01.HYP.38.2.155

Norris, T. (2019). *Porth's pathophysiology: Concepts of altered health status* (10th ed.). Wolters Kluwer.

Tucker, R. (2021). *2022 Lippincott's pocket drug guide for nurses.* Wolters Kluwer.

Whelton, P. K., Carey, R. M., Aronow, W. S., Casey, D. E., Collins, K. J., Dennison Himmelfarb, C., DePalma, S. M., Gidding, S., Jamerson, K. A., Jones, D. W., MacLaughlin, E. J., Muntner, P., Ovbiagele, B., Smith, S. C. Jr, Spencer, C. C., Stafford, R. S., Taler, S. J., Thomas, R. J., Williams, K. A. Sr, ... Wright, J. T. Jr. (2018). 2017 ACC/AHA/AAPA/ABC/ACPM/AGS/APhA/ASH/ASPC/NMA/PCNA guideline for the prevention, detection, evaluation, and management of high blood pressure in adults: A report of the American College of Cardiology/American Heart Association Task Force on Clinical Practice Guidelines. *Circulation, 138,* e484–e594. https://doi.org/10.1161/CIR.0000000000000596

Unger, T., Borghi, C., Charchar, F., Khan, N., Poulter, N., Prabhakaran, D., Ramirez, A., Schlaich, M., Stergiou, G., Tomaszewski, M., Wainford, R., Williams, B., & Schutte, A. (2020). 2020 International Society of Hypertension Global Hypertension Practice Guidelines. *Hypertension, 75,* 1334–1357. https://doi.org/10.1161/HYPERTENSIONAHA.120.15026

CHAPTER 27

Drug Therapy for Dysrhythmias

LEARNING OBJECTIVES

After studying this chapter, you should be able to:

1. Describe the principles of therapy in the management of dysrhythmias, including measures that do not involve antidysrhythmic drugs.
2. Identify the prototype and describe the action, use, adverse effects, contraindications, and nursing implications for class I sodium channel blockers.
3. Recognize the prototype and outline the action, use, adverse effects, contraindications, and nursing implications for beta-adrenergic blockers.
4. Identify the prototype and explain the action, use, adverse effects, contraindications, and nursing implications for potassium channel blockers.
5. Identify the prototype and describe the action, use, adverse effects, contraindications, and nursing implications for calcium channel blockers.
6. Classify the drugs used in the management of emergency resuscitation.
7. Implement the nursing process when caring for patients who use selected antidysrhythmic drugs.

CLINICAL APPLICATION CASE STUDY

Marjorie Johnson, a 62-year-old woman with a long-standing history of hypertension, goes to her primary healthcare provider complaining of fatigue, dizziness, and the sensation of her heart beating fast. Her primary care provider transfers her to the emergency department where she is admitted to the hospital with new-onset atrial fibrillation–a rate of 110 to 120 beats/min.

KEY TERMS

Antidysrhythmic: medication used for prevention and treatment of a cardiac dysrhythmia

Automaticity: property of the cardiac cells to generate an electrical impulse

Bradydysrhythmia: dysrhythmia of less than 60 beats/min

Chronotropic: influencing the rate of impulse formation

Conductivity: ability of the cardiac tissue to transmit electrical impulses

Dysrhythmia: abnormality in formation or conduction (or both) of electrical impulse in the heart affecting heart rate and/or rhythm

Ectopic: when an electrical impulse arises from an abnormal focus, anywhere other than the sinoatrial node

Inotropic: influencing the force of myocardial contractility

Paroxysmal supraventricular tachycardia: episodic burst of a rapid heart rate that originates in a part of the heart above the ventricles

Prodysrhythmic effect: tendency of antidysrhythmic drugs to cause the development of new dysrhythmias

Sinus rhythm: electrical activity of the heart initiated by the sinoatrial node

Tachydysrhythmia: dysrhythmia of greater than 100 beats/min

INTRODUCTION

This chapter discusses the **antidysrhythmic** agents, the medications that are used for prevention and treatment of cardiac dysrhythmias. A healthy adult heart normally beats 60 to 100 beats/min. A **dysrhythmia** is an abnormality in formation or conduction (or both) of an electrical impulse in the heart, affecting heart rate and/or rhythm. Dysrhythmias are usually categorized by rate, location, or patterns of conduction. **Tachydysrhythmias** are abnormal heart rhythms with heart rates greater than 100 beats/min. **Bradydysrhythmias** are abnormal heart rhythms with heart rates less than 60 beats/min. A dysrhythmia can become significant if it interferes with cardiac function, thereby altering the ability to adequately pump and causing inadequate perfusion of the body tissues.

OVERVIEW OF DYSRHYTHMIAS

The electrical activity of the heart is initiated by the sinoatrial node (SA) node, often called the natural pacemaker of the heart, and is called **sinus rhythm**. Cardiac dysrhythmias originate in any part of the conduction system or in atrial or ventricular muscle. Any part of the conduction system can spontaneously start an impulse, but the sinoatrial node normally has the fastest ability to generate an impulse. Disturbances in conduction occur from the cardiac cell's ability to generate an electrical impulse (**automaticity**), to transmit electrical impulses (**conductivity**), or both. The inherent characteristic of automaticity allows myocardial cells other than the SA node to depolarize and initiate the electrical impulse that culminates in contraction. This may occur when the SA node fails to initiate an impulse or does so at a slower rate than another conduction focus in the heart. When the electrical impulse arises anywhere other than the SA node, the conduction focus is abnormal or **ectopic**. If the SA node fails to initiate an impulse, automaticity enables other myocardial cells to assume impulse generation. The impulse generation of alternate pacemaker sites with an SA node failure often results in bradydysrhythmias. If the ectopic focus depolarizes at a rate faster than the SA node, the ectopic focus becomes the dominant pacemaker. In many cases, an ectopic pacemaker overriding the SA node results in a tachydysrhythmia. Conditions such as hypoxia, ischemia, or hypokalemia may activate ectopic pacemakers. Ectopic foci indicate myocardial irritability, which can increase responsiveness to stimuli, leading to potentially serious impairment of cardiac function. Atrial fibrillation, the most common sustained dysrhythmia, is the result of disorganized ectopic foci in the atria.

Clinical Considerations

Dysrhythmias may be clinically significant if they interfere with mechanical cardiac function and thus alter the heart's ability to pump sufficient blood to adequately perfuse body tissues. Dysrhythmias affect the rate, rhythm, and strength of contraction, which can have a direct impact on cardiac output. The normal heart can maintain an adequate cardiac output with ventricular rates ranging from 40 to 150 beats/min. The diseased heart, however, may not be able to maintain an adequate cardiac output with heart rates below 60 (i.e., bradydysrhythmias) or above 120 beats/min (i.e., tachydysrhythmias). Atropine, which is used to treat bradydysrhythmias, is discussed in Chapter 48, and digoxin, which is used to treat atrial fibrillation, is discussed in Chapter 30. Box 27.1 describes various types of dysrhythmias.

Clinical Manifestations

Dysrhythmias may be asymptomatic or symptomatic. Mild or infrequent dysrhythmias may be perceived by the patient as palpitations or skipped heartbeats. More severe dysrhythmias may produce the following manifestations, which reflect decreased cardiac output and other hemodynamic changes:

- Hypotension, bradycardia or tachycardia, and irregular rhythm.
- Shortness of breath, dyspnea, and cough from impaired respiration.
- Syncope, dizziness, or mental confusion from reduced cerebral blood flow.
- Chest pain from decreased coronary artery blood flow. Angina pectoris or myocardial infarction may trigger a dysrhythmia or occur as result of a dysrhythmia.
- Anxiety in response to fear of the unknown.
- Oliguria from decreased kidney blood flow.
- Weakness and fatigue from inadequate tissue perfusion.

Nonpharmacologic Management

Management without the use of drugs may be preferable, at least initially, for several dysrhythmias. For example, sinus tachycardia usually results from such disorders as dehydration, fever, infection, or hypotension, and intervention and management should attempt to relieve the underlying cause. For **paroxysmal supraventricular tachycardia** (episodic bursts of a rapid heart rate that originates in a part of the heart above the ventricles) with mild or moderate symptoms, Valsalva maneuver or other measures to increase vagal tone are preferred if the patient is not hypertensive. For unstable, symptomatic patients with atrial tachycardia or ventricular tachycardia with a pulse, immediate synchronized or unsynchronized cardioversion is the initial treatment for emergent rhythm management. For ventricular fibrillation and pulseless ventricular tachycardia, immediate defibrillation is the initial management of choice.

BOX 27.1 Types of Dysrhythmias

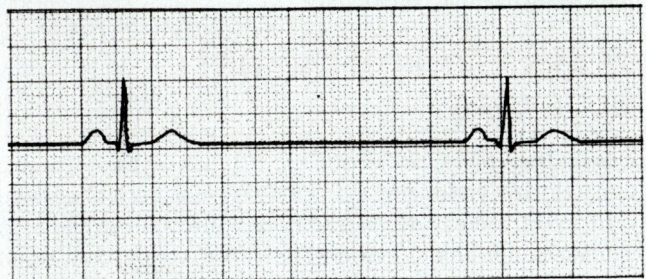
Sinus bradycardia

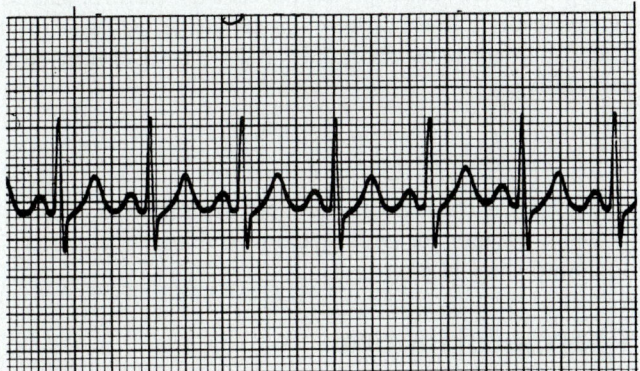
Sinus tachycardia

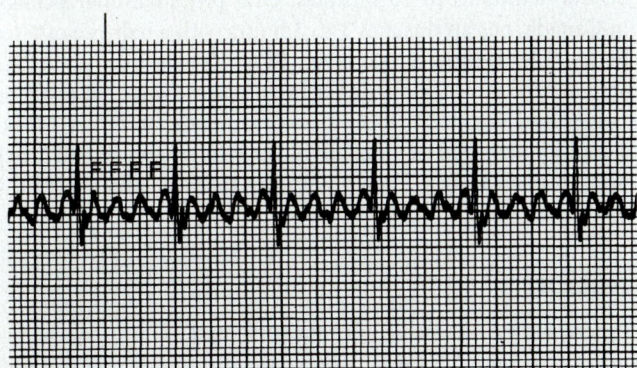
Atrial flutter

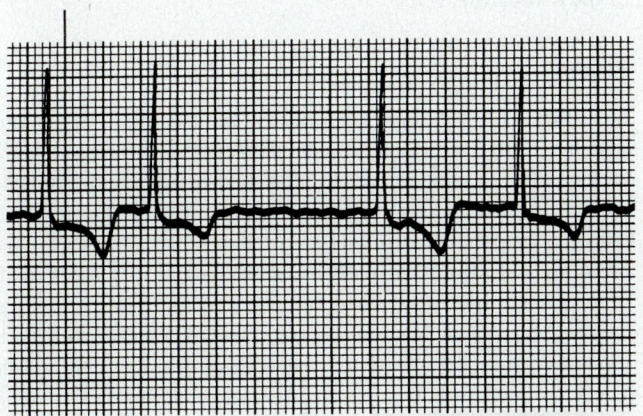
Atrial fibrillation

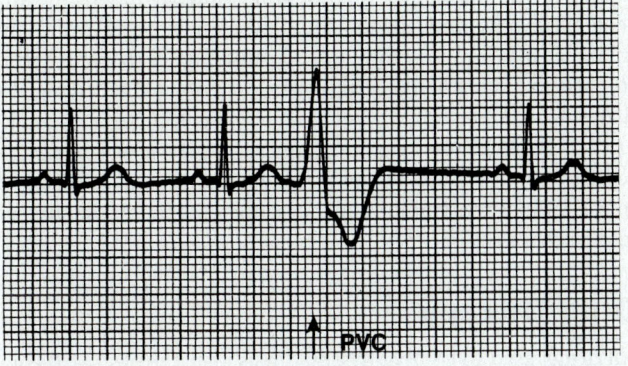
Premature ventricular contraction

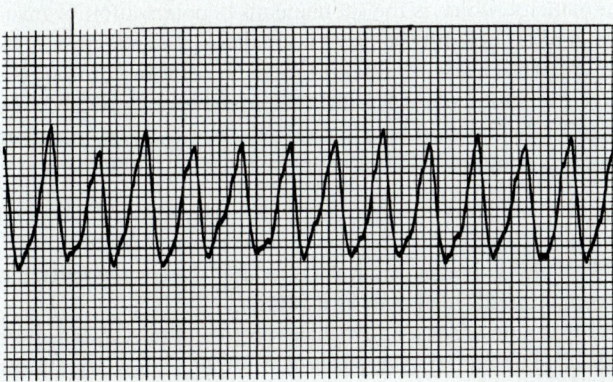
Ventricular tachycardia

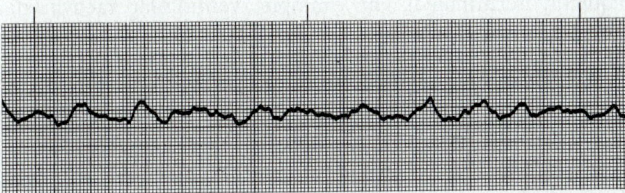
Ventricular fibrillation

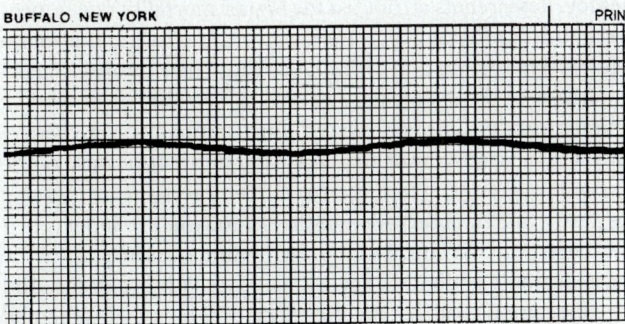
Asystole

In addition to these strategies, use of other nonpharmacologic measures is increasing. The impetus for nonpharmacologic management developed mainly from studies demonstrating that antidysrhythmic drugs could worsen existing dysrhythmias, cause new dysrhythmias, and cause higher mortality rates in patients receiving the drugs than patients not receiving the drugs. Current technology allows clinicians to insert pacemakers and defibrillators (e.g., implantable cardioverter–defibrillators) to control bradydysrhythmias or tachydysrhythmias and to use radio waves (radiofrequency catheter ablation) or surgery to deactivate ectopic foci.

Drug Therapy

All drugs used to combat dysrhythmias alter the electrical conduction system of the heart. The drugs used for the treatment of tachydysrhythmias are the focus of this chapter. They reduce automaticity, which is the spontaneous depolarization of myocardial cells, including ectopic pacemakers. They also slow conduction of electrical impulses through the heart and prolong the refractory period of myocardial cells so they are less likely to be prematurely activated by adjacent cells. Antidysrhythmic drug therapy is commonly indicated in the following conditions:

- Conversion of atrial fibrillation or atrial flutter to normal sinus rhythm.
- Maintaining normal sinus rhythm after electrical conversion from atrial fibrillation or atrial flutter.
- Suppression of a fast or irregular ventricular rate, which alters the cardiac output. Altered cardiac output leads to symptoms of decreased coronary, cerebral, and/or systemic circulation.
- Presence of dangerous dysrhythmias that may be fatal if not quickly terminated. For example, ventricular tachycardia may cause cardiac arrest.

Clinicians use drugs to suppress dysrhythmias, prevent or relieve symptoms, and/or prolong survival. The clinical use of antidysrhythmic drugs for tachydysrhythmias has changed over the years. This change resulted from study outcomes in which patients treated for some dysrhythmias had a higher mortality rate than patients who did not receive antidysrhythmic drug therapy. Researchers attributed the higher mortality rate to **prodysrhythmic effects**, which are effects of antidysrhythmic drugs that worsen existing dysrhythmias or cause new dysrhythmias.

Many of the agents used to treat dysrhythmias do in fact produce prodysrhythmic effects. Thus, rational drug therapy for a cardiac dysrhythmia requires accurate identification of the dysrhythmia, understanding of the basic mechanisms causing the dysrhythmia, observation of the hemodynamic and electrocardiogram (ECG) effects of the dysrhythmia, knowledge of the pharmacologic actions of specific antidysrhythmic drugs, and the expectation that therapeutic effects will outweigh potential adverse effects. Even when these rationale and treatment criteria are met, antidysrhythmic drug therapy is somewhat empiric.

Several different groups of drugs function as antidysrhythmics: class I sodium channel blockers, class II beta-adrenergic blockers, class III potassium channel blockers, and class IV calcium channel blockers (Table 27.1). They are classified according to their mechanisms of action and effects on the conduction system, even though they differ in other respects. Some drugs have characteristics of more than one group and may influence myocardial function beyond just conduction. **Chronotropic** medications affect heart rate. **Inotropic** medications affect the force of myocardial contractility.

CLASS I SODIUM CHANNEL BLOCKERS

Class I drugs block cardiac sodium channels and slow conduction velocity, prolonging refractoriness and decreasing automaticity of sodium-dependent tissue. This inhibits the rapid depolarization phase (Phase 0) of cardiac conduction, resulting in a membrane-stabilizing effect and decreased formation and conduction of electrical impulses. Within the category of class I drugs are subcategories, the class IA, class IB, and class IC medications. The classifications are delineated based on the drugs' mechanism of action and variable rates of channel receptor binding.

CLASS IA

The prototype class IA drug is Ⓟ **procainamide**. Table 27.2 presents dosages for procainamide and the other class IA sodium channel blockers.

Pharmacokinetics

Procainimide has a rapid onset with intravenous (IV) administration. After intramuscular (IM) administration, onset occurs within 15 to 60 minutes. Oral procainamide, available in Canada, has an onset of 1 to 3 hours with a half-life of 6 to 8 hours. Therapeutic serum levels (4 to 10 mcg/mL; Table 27.3) are assessed 6 to 12 hours after IV infusion. Note that reference ranges may vary with laboratory method of analysis used. Toxic symptoms are seen with serum levels greater than 10 to 12 mcg/mL. Procainamide is metabolized by the liver and excreted in the urine.

Action

Procainamide reduces automaticity and slows conduction velocity throughout the cardiac system through direct and indirect anticholinergic effect on cardiac tissue, reducing myocardial contractility. In addition, it prolongs the refractory period of the myocardial cells.

Use

Indications for procainamide include the treatment of (1) ventricular dysrhythmias and (2) paroxysmal supraventricular tachycardia or chronic ventricular tachycardia without heart block. Procainamide is indicated in the treatment of atrial fibrillation when other treatments are ineffective or cannot be used. However, the drug is usually contraindicated in patients with severe, uncompensated heart failure or with second- or third-degree heart block because it depresses myocardial contractility and conduction through the atrioventricular (AV) node. The U.S. Food and Drug Administration (FDA) has issued a **BOXED WARNING ◆** for procainamide and other class 1A drugs (quinidine and disopyramide) because of their known prodysrhythmic properties; the drugs should be reserved for

TABLE 27.1
Drugs Administered for the Treatment of Dysrhythmias

Class of Antidysrhythmic Drug	Prototype	Other Drugs in the Class	Use
Class I Sodium Channel Blockers			
Class IA	Procainamide	Quinidine Disopyramide (Norpace)	Maintenance of normal sinus rhythm after conversion of A-fib or atrial flutter; treatment of symptomatic PVCs, SVT, and VT; prevention of V-fib
Class IB	Lidocaine (Xylocaine)		Treatment of symptomatic PVCs and VT; prevention of V-fib
Class IC		Flecainide Propafenone (Rythmol SR)	Treatment of life-threatening VT or V-fib and SVT unresponsive to other drugs; maintenance of sinus rhythm
Class II Beta-Adrenergic Blockers			
	Propranolol (Inderal LA)	Carvedilol Esmolol Sotalol (Betapace, Sorine, Sotylize)	Treatment of SVT
Class III Potassium Channel Blockers			
	Amiodarone (Nexterone, Pacerone)	Dofetilide (Tikosyn) Dronedarone (Multaq) Ibutilide (Corvert) Sotalol (Betapace, Sorine, Sotylize)	Treatment of VT and V-fib; conversion of atrial flutter or A-fib to sinus rhythm; maintenance of sinus rhythm
Class IV Calcium Channel Blockers			
	Diltiazem (Cardizem, Cardizem CD, Cardizem LA, Tiazac)	Verapamil (Calan, Calan SR, Verelan, Verelan PM)	Treatment of SVT
Unclassified		Adenosine (Adenocard) Magnesium sulfate	Treatment of tachydysrhythmias; SVT Treatment of torsades de pointes

A-fib, atrial fibrillation; PVC, premature ventricular contraction; SVT, supraventricular tachycardia; V-fib, ventricular fibrillation; VT, ventricular tachycardia.

patients with life-threatening ventricular dysrhythmias. In clinical trials, the use of these drugs in individuals with non–life-threatening dysrhythmias has increased mortality, particularly in patients with structural heart disease.

Patient-related variables specific to the use of procainamide and other class 1A drugs include the following:

- Age:
  - Limited data are available about procainamide use in pediatric patients; cardiology consultation is strongly recommended prior to use.
  - For older adults, initial doses of procainamide at the lower end of the dosage range are recommended.
- Abnormal kidney function and hepatic impairment:
  - With abnormal kidney function, reduced dosages of procainamide are necessary based on the creatinine clearance rate, especially in patients with kidney tubular acidosis.
  - Hepatic impairment increases the plasma half-life of several antidysrhythmic drugs, including procainamide; thus, patients with hepatic impairment and hepatic insufficiency are closely monitored and usually receive a reduced dosage less frequently.

Adverse Effects

Adverse effects of procainamide include neuromuscular changes, cardiac dysrhythmias (esp. bradycardia), hypotension, and gastrointestinal (GI) changes, as well as hematologic and hypersensitivity alterations. About 20% to 30% of patients receiving procainamide develop drug-induced lupus erythematosus–like syndrome resulting in multiple neuromuscular and inflammatory changes. Neuromuscular changes include weakness, muscle and joint pain, joint edema, and fatigue. Cardiac dysrhythmias include conduction disturbances, including bradycardia, heart block, and hypotension. GI effects include nausea, vomiting, diarrhea, and liver toxicity. Visual disturbances may also occur.

Contraindications

Procainamide is contraindicated in patients with an allergy to the drug. It is also contraindicated in second- or third-degree heart block, prolonged QT syndrome, myasthenia gravis, pregnancy, and lactation.

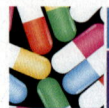

TABLE 27.2
DRUGS AT A GLANCE: Class I Sodium Channel Blockers

Drug	Routes and Dosage Ranges	
	Adults	**Children**
Class IA Procainamide (Apo-Procainamide, Procan SR)	IV loading dose 10–17 mg/kg at 20–50 mg/min or 100 mg every 5 min; maintenance infusion 1–4 mg/min	PO 15–50 mg/kg/d in three to six divided doses every 3–6 h, maximum, 4 g/d IV/IO loading dose 10–15 mg/kg over 30–60 min; maintenance dose of 20–80 mcg/kg/min continuous infusion; max 100 mg/d dose or 2 g/d; or 15 mg/kg given over 30–60 min, followed by maintenance infusion
Quinidine (Apo-Quinidine, Quinate, Novo-Quinidin)	PO 200–600 mg every 6–8 h, or extended-action tablets, 324–648 mg every 8–12 h	PO 30 mg/kg/24 h in four equally divided doses every 6 h; IV (not recommended) 2–10 mg/kg/dose IV every 3–6 h
Disopyramide (Norpace, Norpace CR; Rythmodan)	PO loading dose 200–300 mg (immediate release), maintenance dose 100–300 mg every 6 h depending on patient response; controlled release 200–400 mg every 12 h	>12–18 y: PO 6–15 mg/kg/d in four equal divided doses; max dose 1,600 mg/d >4–12 y: PO 10–15 mg/kg/d in four equal divided doses 1–4 y: PO 10–20 mg/kg/d in four equal divided doses <1 y: PO 10–30 mg/kg/d in four equal divided doses
Class IB Lidocaine (Xylocaine; Xylocaine, Xylocard)	IV (pulseless ventricular fibrillation or ventricular tachycardia) 1–1.5 mg/kg IV bolus; repeat 0.5–0.75 mg/kg every 5–10 min to max dose of 3 mg/kg IV infusion (with return of pulse) 1–4 mg/min (or 20–50 mcg/kg/min)	Safety and efficacy have not been established IV/IO loading dose 1 mg/kg bolus, followed by IV infusion of 20–50 mcg/kg/min with caution
Class IC Flecainide (Apo-Flecainide, Tambocor)	PO 50–100 mg every 12 h initially, increased by 50 mg every 12 h every 4 d until effective or reach maximum dose, 400 mg/d	Safety and efficacy in patients younger than 18 y have not been established
Propafenone (Rythmol SR; Apo-Propafenone, Rythmol)	PO 150 mg every 8 h initially, increase at 3–4 d intervals to 225 mg every 8 h, and then to 300 mg every 8 h; maximum dose of 900 mg/d PO (extended release) 225 mg every 12 h initially may increase at 5-d intervals; maximum 425 mg every 12 h	Safety and efficacy not established

IO, intraosseous.

Nursing Implications

Prior to the start of any new therapy, it is necessary to assess for allergies, second- or third-degree heart block, prolonged QT syndrome, myasthenia gravis, pregnancy, and lactation. Physical assessment includes inspection of the skin for color and the presence of lesions, determination of orientation status, assessment of cranial nerves, determination of bilateral grip strength and reflexes, auscultation of pulse and blood pressure, interpretation of the ECG, checking for edema, and auscultation of bowel sounds. It is also necessary to evaluate hepatic and kidney function as well as to perform a urinalysis and complete blood count. The findings of the physical assessment as well as results of the laboratory work and diagnostic tests help develop the nursing plan of care for the patient who is beginning sodium channel blocker therapy.

TABLE 27.3
Therapeutic Serum Drug Level Ranges of Some Common Antidysrhythmics

Drug	Therapeutic Range (mcg/mL)
Procainamide	4–10
Quinidine	2–6
Disopyramide	2–4
Lidocaine	1.5–5
Flecainide	0.2–1

> **BOX 27.2 Drug Interactions: Procainamide**
>
> **Drugs That Increase the Effects of Procainamide**
> - Ajmaline, citalopram, clarithromycin, domperidone, entrectinib, fexinidazole, fingolimod, flupentixol, gemifloxacin, levofloxacin, moxifloxacin, propafenone, sertindole, thioridazine, QT-prolonging class IA antiarrhythmics, QT-prolonging class III antiarrhythmics
>   *Increase the risk of prolonged QT interval*
> - Cimetidine, erdafitinib, lamotrigine, pacritinib, ranitidine, risdiplam, tafenoquine, trimethoprim
>   *Increase serum concentrations of procainamide*

Preventing Interactions

Preventing drug–drug and drug–food interactions require knowledge of potential effects. Several medications interact with procainamide, increasing or decreasing its effect (Box 27.2). Caution is warranted when using procainamide with concurrent antiarrhythmic medications. With neuromuscular blocking agents, such as succinylcholine, rocuronium, and vecuronium, neuromuscular blocking effects may increase. Grapefruit juice, when given with procainamide, decreases the drug's metabolism and increases the risk of toxic drug effects. Ingesting large amounts of fruit juice or vitamin C may decrease urine pH, which increases the drug's clearance and results in decreased serum concentration.

Administering the Medication

Procainamide is administered intravenously and should be diluted to a maximum concentration of 20 mg/mL in normal saline or 5% dextrose. Serum samples should be drawn 6 to 12 hours after IV infusion has started.

Assessing for Therapeutic Effects

The nurse assesses for improvement in symptoms and for return of an organized cardiac rhythm. Physical assessment includes inspection of the skin for adequate color and perfusion, clear mentation, and pulse and blood pressure within the patient's normal limits. It is also necessary to evaluate the adequacy of hepatic and kidney function through laboratory testing. Therapeutic serum concentrations of procainamide are 4 to 10 mcg/mL; toxic levels are greater than 10 to 12 mcg/mL.

Assessing for Adverse Effects

The nurse assesses patient body systems that are potentially affected by the action of procainamide for adverse effects. Of particular concern are the neuromuscular system, cardiac, GI, and hematologic systems, as well as possible hypersensitivity.

Patient Teaching

The nurse reinforces to the patient that frequent cardiac monitoring and blood tests are important for follow-up; these include regular checks of heart rhythm and blood counts. The additional patient teaching guidelines presented in Box 27.3 are important.

> **BOX 27.3 Patient Teaching Guidelines for Antidysrhythmic Drugs**
>
> - A fast heartbeat normally occurs in response to exercise, fever, and other conditions so that more blood can be pumped and carried to body tissues. An irregular heartbeat occurs occasionally in most people. However, when your healthcare provider prescribes a long-term medication to slow or regularize your heartbeat, this means that you have a potentially serious condition. In addition, the medications can cause potentially serious adverse effects. So, it is extremely important that you take the medications exactly as prescribed. Taking extra doses is dangerous; skipping doses or waiting longer between doses may lead to loss of control of the heart problem.
> - Report dizziness or fainting spells to your healthcare provider. This may mean the medication is decreasing your heart rate or blood pressure too much, which is more likely to occur when starting or increasing the dose of an antidysrhythmic drug. Drug dosages may need to be adjusted.
> - Report any change in vision and complaints of nausea or vomiting, sun sensitivity, tremors, or loss of coordination to your healthcare provider. In addition, report unusual bleeding or bruising, fever, chills, intolerance to heat or cold, shortness of breath, difficulty breathing, cough, swelling of ankles or fingers, palpitation, or difficulty with vision.
> - You may be given a drug classified as an antidysrhythmic or a drug from another group that has antidysrhythmic effects (e.g., a beta-adrenergic blocker such as propranolol, a calcium channel blocker such as diltiazem or verapamil). Follow the instructions for the specific drug ordered.
> - Be sure you know the names (generic and brand) of the medication, why you are receiving it, and what effects you can expect (therapeutic and adverse).
> - You will need continued medical supervision, along with periodic measurements of heart rate and blood pressure, blood tests, and electrocardiograms. Be sure to keep all healthcare appointments.
> - Try to learn the triggers for your irregular heartbeats and avoid them when possible (e.g., excessive caffeinated beverages, strenuous or excessive exercise).
> - Avoid over-the-counter cold and asthma remedies, appetite suppressants, and antisleep preparations, which are all stimulants that can cause or aggravate irregular heartbeats.
> - Take or give medications at evenly spaced intervals to maintain adequate blood levels. Take your medications at the same time each day.
> - Take amiodarone and procainamide with food to decrease gastrointestinal symptoms.
> - Do not crush or chew sustained-release tablets or capsules.
> - Do not drink grapefruit juice if you are taking procainamide because it decreases the metabolism of procainamide and increases the risk of toxic effects.
> - Wear a medical alert tag if recommended stating the health condition you have or the medications you are taking.

Other Drugs in the Class

Quinidine and disopyramide (Norpace), the other class IA medications, also have FDA-issued **BOXED WARNING** ◆ because of their known prodysrhythmic properties that can occur at normal plasma concentrations. As with procainamide, the drugs should be reserved for patients with life-threatening ventricular dysrhythmias because of the lack of evidence of improved survival with their use in patients without life-threatening dysrhythmias.

The use of quinidine and disopyramide (Norpace) has decreased with the availability of newer more effective drugs with less toxicity. Disopyramide increases vascular resistance, which increases the risk to patients with cardiac and vascular comorbidities. In addition, disopyramide is a substrate of CYP3A4, part of the cytochrome P450; therefore, numerous clinically significant drug interactions are known to occur.

CLASS IB

Class IB drugs shorten the repolarization phase. **Lidocaine** (Xylocaine), the prototype class IB drug, is used to treat serious ventricular dysrhythmias associated with acute myocardial infarction, cardiac catheterization, cardiac surgery, and digitalis-induced ventricular dysrhythmias. It decreases myocardial irritability (automaticity) in the ventricles by increasing the electrical stimulation threshold of ventricular myocardial cells. Lidocaine has little effect on atrial tissue and thus is not useful in treating atrial dysrhythmias. The drug differs from procainamide in that it does not decrease AV conduction with usual therapeutic doses. After IV administration of a bolus dose, therapeutic effects occur within 1 to 2 minutes and last approximately 10 to 20 minutes. This characteristic is advantageous in emergency management but limits the use of lidocaine to intensive care settings. Lidocaine is metabolized in the liver; thus, dosage must be reduced in patients with hepatic insufficiency or right-sided heart failure to avoid drug accumulation and toxicity. Serious adverse reactions with lidocaine are uncommon.

Therapeutic serum levels of lidocaine are 1.5 to 5 mcg/mL. Toxic serum levels are greater than 6 mcg/mL. Lidocaine is contraindicated in patients allergic to related local anesthetics (e.g., procaine). Anaphylactic reactions may occur in sensitized persons. Give lidocaine parenterally only as solutions labeled "for cardiac dysrhythmias," and do not use solutions containing epinephrine. Give an IV bolus over 45 to 90 seconds. Table 27.2 provides information about the dosages of lidocaine and related drugs.

> **Quality and Safety Alert: Safety**
>
> Lidocaine solutions that contain epinephrine are for local anesthesia only. It is essential that epinephrine-containing lidocaine solutions never be given intravenously to patients with cardiac dysrhythmias because the epinephrine can cause or aggravate dysrhythmias. Rapid injection of lidocaine (within approximately 30 seconds) produces transient blood levels several times greater than therapeutic range limits. Therefore, there is an increased risk of toxicity without a concomitant increase in therapeutic effectiveness.

CLASS IC

Class IC drugs have no effect on the repolarization phase but primarily block open sodium channels and slow conduction velocity and the refractory period. Flecainide and propafenone (Rythmol SR) are oral agents that greatly decrease conduction in the ventricles. These drugs may cause new dysrhythmias or aggravate preexisting dysrhythmias, sometimes causing sustained ventricular tachycardia or ventricular fibrillation. Thus, it is necessary to begin therapy in a hospital setting in patients with continuous ECG monitoring. The new or aggravated dysrhythmias are more likely to occur with high doses and rapid dose increases. Table 27.2 presents dosage information for these drugs.

Flecainide or propafenone may be used to suppress paroxysmal atrial flutter and fibrillation in patients with minimal or no heart disease. These class IC drugs are recommended for use in life-threatening ventricular dysrhythmias. The FDA has issued two **BOXED WARNING** ◆ for flecainide:

- Drug treatment increases the risk of nonfatal cardiac arrest and death in patients with recent myocardial infarction or chronic atrial fibrillation.
- It is necessary to monitor carefully for a risk of potentially fatal prodysrhythmic effects.

NCLEX Success

1. A nurse is monitoring a patient who has been receiving intravenous procainamide in the critical care unit. The laboratory technician calls to report that the patient's serum procainamide level is 12 mcg/mL. The patient has also developed muscle pain, weakness, drowsiness, fever, and fatigue. The priority action is to

    A. report the findings to the provider immediately
    B. administer the medication as ordered
    C. anticipate that the dosage of the medication will increase
    D. anticipate that the dosage of the medication will decrease

2. A 58-year-old patient is admitted to the coronary care unit for treatment of an acute anterior myocardial infarction. That evening, the patient experiences frequent episodes of ventricular tachycardia with hypotension. The provider tells the nurse to prepare an IV bolus dose of lidocaine. Why is lidocaine administered intravenously at this time—and not orally?

    A. Lidocaine absorption is too erratic when administered orally.
    B. Lidocaine is inactivated by hydrochloric acid.
    C. Most of an absorbed oral dose of lidocaine undergoes first-pass metabolism in the liver.
    D. The onset of action for intravenous lidocaine is 45 to 90 seconds.

CLASS II BETA-ADRENERGIC BLOCKERS

Beta-adrenergic–blocking agents (see Chapter 26) exert antidysrhythmic effects by slowing the stimulation of beta receptors in the heart by the sympathetic nervous system, slowing SA and AV nodal conduction. Blockage of receptors in the SA node and ectopic pacemakers decreases automaticity, and blockage of receptors in the AV node increases the refractory period. Beta-adrenergic blockers are effective for management of dysrhythmias resulting from excessive sympathetic activity. They are most often used to slow the ventricular rate of contraction in atrial flutter and atrial fibrillation.

Class II beta-adrenergic blockers are being used more extensively because of their effectiveness in reducing mortality in patients following myocardial infarction and heart failure. Reduced mortality may result from the ability of the drugs to prevent ventricular fibrillation. Emerging evidence suggests class II beta-adrenergic blockers reduce the development of atrial fibrillation in patients with heart failure. **Propranolol** (Inderal LA), the prototype class II drug, may be given orally for chronic therapy to prevent supraventricular dysrhythmias. It may be administered intravenously for life-threatening dysrhythmias, such as ventricular tachycardia. Table 27.4 presents dosage information for propranolol and the other class II beta-adrenergic blockers.

Pharmacokinetics

For the oral route, the onset of action of propranolol is 1 to 2 hours, with a duration of 6 to 12 hours. For the IV route, the onset of action is less than 5 minutes, with a duration of more than 4 to 6 hours. The drug is metabolized in the liver, and its half-life is 3 to 6 hours (8 to 10 hours with the sustained release form of the medication). The drug is excreted in the urine.

Action

Propranolol competitively blocks beta-adrenergic receptors in the heart and juxtaglomerular apparatus. This action causes a decrease in the influence of the sympathetic nervous system on these tissues and a decrease in the excitability of the heart, cardiac workload, and oxygen consumption. This then causes a release of renin and lowers the blood pressure. In addition, propranolol has a membrane-stabilizing effect that contributes to its antidysrhythmic action.

Use

Propranolol is used in the treatment of cardiac dysrhythmias, especially supraventricular tachycardia. In addition, it has been found to be effective in the treatment of ventricular tachycardia. Other related cardiac indications for propranolol include hypertension, cardiomyopathy, and angina. Propranolol is used in the early treatment of myocardial infarction and has been noted to reduce cardiovascular mortality for patients who survive the acute phase of myocardial infarction. There are no known precautions regarding administration of propranolol in older adults or in those with abnormal kidney function.

TABLE 27.4

DRUGS AT A GLANCE: Class II Beta-Adrenergic Blockers

Drug	Routes and Dosage Ranges	
	Adults	Children
Propranolol (Hemangeol, Inderal LA; Hemangiol, Inderal LA) $Beta_1$ $Beta_2$	PO 10-mg every 8–12 h; titrate to response up to 40 mg every 6–8 h when rate controlled; max dose 320 mg/d IV 1–3 mg slow IVP with careful monitoring, not to exceed 1 mg/min; repeat every 5 min to a total of 5 mg or max dose of 0.1 mg/kg	PO 0.5–1.0 mg/kg/d in divided doses every 6–8 h to maximum daily dose of 16 mg/kg/d or 60 mg/d IV 0.01–0.15 mg/kg slow IVP over 10 min; may give second dose in 6–8 h as needed to maximum age-dependent dose
Acebutolol (Sectral) $Beta_1$	PO 200–400 mg every 12 h, increased gradually to 600–1,200 mg/d in two divided doses	Safety and efficacy not established
Esmolol (Brevibloc) $Beta_1$	IV loading dose 500 mcg/kg/min over 1 min, followed by a maintenance dose of 50 mcg/kg/min over 4 min. If no response in 5 min, repeat the same loading dose, and increase maintenance doses to 100 mcg/kg/min for 4 min. If no response in 5 min, repeat the third (and final) loading dose, and increase maintenance doses to 150 mcg/kg/min. Average maintenance dose 50–200 mcg/kg/min	IV loading dose 100–500 mcg/kg/min over 1 min, followed by a continuous IV infusion of 25–50 mcg/kg/min. Average maintenance dose 50–500 mcg/kg/min
Sotalol (Betapace, Sorine, Sotylize; Rylosol) $Beta_1$ $Beta_2$	PO 80 mg every 12 h initially, titrated to response; average dose, 240–320 mg daily IV 75 mg infused over 5 hours twice daily, after 3 days may increase dose to 112.5 mg twice daily based on patient response	≥2 y with normal kidney function PO 30 mg/m² three times daily can titrate to a maximum of 60 mg/m² in hospital for at least 3 d Infants and children <2 y: see manufacturer's instructions

Patient-related variables specific to the use of propranolol and other class II beta-adrenergic blockers include the following:

- Age:
  - In children, if the drug is administered orally, immediate-release formulations are preferred. The dose should be individualized to the child's weight and therapeutic response.
  - In children, bronchospasm and laryngospasm are the most common serious adverse respiratory effects.
- Reproduction, pregnancy, and lactation:
  - Use of these drugs during the third trimester of pregnancy may increase the risk for bradycardia, hypoglycemia, hypotension, and respiratory depression in the neonate.
  - Newborns should be monitored postpartum for these symptoms and managed accordingly.

Adverse Effects

Some of the known adverse effects to propranolol include allergic reactions, specifically laryngospasm, and central nervous system (CNS) changes, including sleep disorders, agitation, fatigue, and dizziness. Specific cardiovascular effects are bradycardia, heart failure, cardiac dysrhythmias, SA or AV nodal block, peripheral vascular insufficiency, claudication, stroke, pulmonary edema, and hypotension. In addition, dermatologic, GI, genitourinary, musculoskeletal, and respiratory changes occur.

Contraindications

Contraindications to the use of propranolol include allergy to beta-adrenergic–blocking agents, sinus bradycardia, sick sinus syndrome, and second- or third-degree heart block. In addition, other contraindications may include cardiogenic shock, heart failure, bronchial asthma, bronchospasm, and chronic obstructive pulmonary disease,

Nursing Implications

Preventing Interactions

The nurse monitors for important drug–drug interactions when a patient is taking propranolol as well as interference with laboratory tests. Several medications interact with propranolol, increasing or decreasing its effect (Box 27.4). Also, concomitant use of propranolol and glycerin leads to prolonged hypoglycemic effects. Additionally, propranolol interferes with glucose tolerance tests and insulin tolerance tests as well as with glaucoma screening tests.

Administering the Medication

Routes of administration of propranolol (in adults) are oral as well as parenteral. Drug doses significantly differ for oral and parenteral forms; following oral administration, propranolol undergoes first-pass metabolism in the liver and only a portion of the drug reaches systemic circulation. Patients should take the oral form with meals. It is essential that the drug not be discontinued abruptly after long-term therapy; a hypersensitivity to catecholamines may have developed, exacerbating ventricular dysrhythmias. The FDA has issued a **BOXED WARNING** ◆ for propranolol and other beta-adrenergic blockers, stating that abrupt discontinuation of the drug can exacerbate cardiac ischemia, thus increasing the risk of angina pectoris and myocardial infarction. Gradual tapering over a 2-week period, with patient monitoring, is necessary.

Assessing for Therapeutic Effects

After administering propranolol, the nurse monitors the patient until it is determined that the dysrhythmia has resolved. If the patient has received the maximum amount of beta-adrenergic medication and the dysrhythmia persists, use of another pharmacologic agent may be necessary.

Assessing for Adverse Effects

The nurse should monitor for allergic reaction, including laryngospasm, as well as respiratory complications. Cardiovascular effects include bradycardia, heart failure, cardiac dysrhythmias, SA or AV nodal block, peripheral vascular insufficiency, claudication, stroke, pulmonary edema, and hypotension. ECG changes to watch for include heart rates less than 60 beats/min, abnormal heart rhythms, or heart blocks (first-, second-, or third-degree) and/or sinus exit blocks. Other adverse effects relate to the dermatologic, GI, genitourinary, and respiratory systems.

Patient Teaching

The nurse instructs patients to take propranolol with meals. It is important that patients report night cough, swelling of the extremities, slow pulse, confusion, depression, rash, fever, or sore throat to the prescriber. Patients need to realize that they should not stop taking propranolol abruptly because this action can cause the dysrhythmia to worsen. In addition, the nurse should inform patients with diabetes mellitus that propranolol may mask the normal signs of hypoglycemia (e.g., cool, clammy skin; tachycardia); it is necessary to monitor blood or urine glucose carefully. Box 27.3 presents some patient teaching considerations for propranolol and other antidysrhythmics.

Other Drugs in the Class

Acebutolol is a class II beta-adrenergic blocker used in the treatment of ventricular dysrhythmias and hypertension. The onset of beta-blockade action is 1 to 2 hours following oral administration. The drug's duration of action is 12 to 24 hours. Acebutolol undergoes extensive first-pass metabolism and is excreted in the feces and urine.

BOX 27.4 Drug Interactions: Propranolol

Drugs That Increase the Effects of Propranolol
- Verapamil
  Increases the risk of heart block effect

Drugs That Decrease the Effects of Propranolol
- Indomethacin, ibuprofen, piroxicam, sulindac, and barbiturates
  Decrease the effects of blocking the beta-adrenergic receptors in the heart; have less influence on the sympathetic nervous system, excitability of the heart, cardiac workload, and oxygen consumption

Esmolol is a short-acting class II beta-adrenergic blocker with beta$_1$ selectivity approved for the treatment of supraventricular tachycardia and atrial fibrillation/flutter. When given intravenously, the onset of beta-blockade is 2 to 10 minutes. The duration of hemodynamic effect of the drug is 10 to 30 minutes. Esmolol is metabolized and is excreted in the urine.

Sotalol (Betapace, Sorine, Sotylize), which is discussed in detail in the section on potassium channel blockers, has both beta-adrenergic–blocking and potassium channel–blocking activity. At lower doses, class II effects predominate. The drug is used to prevent or treat atrial fibrillation.

CLASS III POTASSIUM CHANNEL BLOCKERS

Although all these drugs share a common mechanism of action, they are very different. The prototype potassium channel blocker **amiodarone** (Nexterone, Pacerone) has electrophysiologic characteristics of sodium channel blockers, beta-adrenergic blockers, and calcium channel blockers. Thus, it has vasodilating effects and decreases systemic vascular resistance, it prolongs conduction in all cardiac tissues and decreases heart rate, and it decreases contractility of the left ventricle. Multiple randomized control trials have demonstrated that amiodarone is the most effective antidysrhythmic agent for preventing atrial fibrillation and maintaining normal sinus rhythm (Al-Khatib et al., 2018). Amiodarone and lidocaine are the drugs of choice for emergent management of life-threatening ventricular dysrhythmias (Panchal et al., 2020). Table 27.5 presents dosage information for amiodarone and the other class III potassium channel blockers.

Pharmacokinetics

The oral form of amiodarone has an onset of 2 days to 3 weeks, with a peak in 3 to 7 hours. The peak effect of the drug is within 1 week to 5 months. Onset of effect may be shorter in pediatric patients and in adult patients who receive an intravenous loading dose. The IV form has an immediate onset, with a peak in 30 to 45 minutes and a duration for as long as the infusion continues. Amiodarone is extensively metabolized in the liver and produces active metabolites. The drug and its metabolites accumulate in the liver, lungs, fat, skin, and other tissues. It has a half-life of 40 to 55 days for oral amiodarone and 9 to 36 days for IV amiodarone. Because of the long serum half-life of amiodarone, loading doses are usually given. These loading doses reduce the time required for therapeutic effects. However, effects may persist for several weeks to months after the drug is discontinued.

Action

Potassium channel blockers such as amiodarone prolong duration of the action potential, slow repolarization, and prolong the refractory period in both the atria and ventricles. To perform these actions, they block cardiac potassium channels.

Use

Amiodarone is used for various types of life-threatening tachydysrhythmias, both ventricular and atrial dysrhythmias. The IV and oral forms of amiodarone differ in their electrophysiologic effects. The oral form is given to treat recurrent ventricular tachycardia or ventricular fibrillation and to maintain a normal sinus rhythm after conversion of atrial fibrillation and

TABLE 27.5
DRUGS AT A GLANCE: Class III Potassium Channel Blockers

Drug	Routes and Dosage Ranges	
	Adults	**Children**
Amiodarone (Nexterone, Pacerone; ✱ Cordarone)	IV loading dose 150 mg over 10 min (15 mg/min), then 1 mg/min over 6 h, then 0.5 mg/min for 18 h PO loading dose 400 mg every 8–24 h (total loading dose of 6–10 g); maintenance dose 100–200 mg/d	IV, IO, loading dose, IV 5 mg/kg over 60 min, max loading dose 300 mg/dose; may repeat initial loading dose to max of 10 mg/kg; maintenance dose varies based on patient response
Dofetilide (Tikosyn)	PO 500 mcg twice daily, reduce dosage based on QT interval response	Not recommended
Dronedarone (Multaq; ✱ Multaq)	PO 400 mg twice daily	Not recommended
Ibutilide (Corvert; ✱ Corvert)	Weight ≥60 kg: IV infusion 1 mg over 10 min Weight <60 kg: IV infusion 0.01 mg/kg over 10 min The dose can be repeated once, if normal sinus rhythm is not restored after 10 min	Not recommended
Sotalol (Betapace, Sorine, Sotylize; ✱ Rylosol) Class II and class III effects	PO 40–80 mg every 12 h initially, adjust gradually every 3 d; max dose 160 mg every 12 h	≥2 y with normal kidney function PO 30 mg/m^2 three times daily can titrate to a maximum of 60 mg/m^2 in hospital for at least 3 d Infants and children <2 y: see manufacturer's instructions

IO, intraosseous.

atrial flutter. The IV form is given mainly for acute suppression of refractory, hemodynamically destabilizing ventricular tachycardia and ventricular fibrillation. The major effect is slowing conduction through the AV node and prolonging the effective refractory period.

The FDA has issued a **BOXED WARNING** for amiodarone, recommending use only in patients with life-threatening dysrhythmias because of the risk of the development of potentially fatal pulmonary toxicity, hepatotoxicity, and worsening dysrhythmias. Low-dose amiodarone may be a pharmacologic choice for preventing recurrent atrial fibrillation after electrical or pharmacologic conversion. The low doses cause fewer adverse effects than the higher ones used for life-threatening ventricular dysrhythmias.

Patient-related variables specific to the use of amiodarone and other class III potassium channel blockers include the following:

- Age:
  - For life-threatening supraventricular tachycardias, pediatric resuscitation guidelines recommend amiodarone to treat ventricular dysrhythmias in pulseless and hemodynamically unstable children.
- Reproduction, pregnancy, and lactation:
  - Amiodarone crosses the placenta and in utero exposure may cause neonatal bradycardia periodic ventricular extrasystoles and QT prolongation.
  - Neonatal elevation of serum T_3 and T_4, hypothyroidism, retardation of fetal growth, and/or premature birth.
  - The manufacturer does not recommend breast-feeding while taking amiodarone; hypothyroidism and bradycardia have developed with exposure through breast-feeding.
- Abnormal kidney function and hepatic impairment:
  - Amiodarone is hepatotoxic so it is necessary to evaluate the liver and monitor liver function tests closely.
- Specific healthcare environments:
  - In the home care setting, close monitoring is needed even with changes in the drug dosage, so careful patient assessment and evaluation are necessary. Continual monitoring of cardiac response to titrate the dosage is essential.

> **Quality and Safety Alert: Evidence-Based Practice**
>
> Over the past two decades, rapid response teams (RRTs) have been put in place with the goal of improving the identification and management of hospitalized patients who are worsening clinically. RRT remains a well-established patient safety strategy that is frequently used. Some form of RRT is present in most hospitals in the United States, although hospitalists are increasingly assuming RRT duties. Despite support from early research and anecdotal reports of the RRTs reducing overall patient death, the benefit has not been supported in multiple systematic reviews. At best, evidence indicates that RRTs slightly decrease unanticipated cardiac arrests but do not alter overall in-hospital mortality.

Adverse Effects

Authorities consider most adverse effects of amiodarone to be dose dependent and reversible. However, maintenance dose selection is difficult because absorption and elimination are variable. With the use of amiodarone, CNS adverse effects, including malaise, fatigue, dizziness, tremors, and ataxia, are the most common. Other common adverse effects include bradycardia, cardiac dysrhythmias (which can be life threatening), hypotension, and heart failure. GI conditions include nausea, vomiting, anorexia, and constipation.

Amiodarone is an iodine-rich drug that has been associated with thyroid dysfunction, with hypothyroidism occurring more frequently than hyperthyroidism. Respiratory adverse effects include serious, potentially fatal pulmonary toxicity (pulmonary fibrosis, pneumonitis, acute respiratory distress syndrome), which may begin with progressive dyspnea and cough with crackles, decreased breath sounds, and pleurisy. Hepatotoxicity may occur and can be life threatening, so liver function tests must be monitored for adverse effects. Corneal microdeposits occur in almost all patients treated for more than 2 months and can lead to blurry vision. Photosensitivity is also an adverse effect and can result in solar dermatitis and blue-gray skin.

Contraindications

Contraindications include hypersensitivity to amiodarone as well as sinus node dysfunction, heart block, cardiogenic shock, severe bradycardia, hypokalemia, and lactation. Allergies to iodine or iodinated contrast agents may not constitute an absolute contraindication to amiodarone but use should be carefully evaluated. Caution is necessary when giving amiodarone to patients who are pregnant or have thyroid or liver dysfunction.

Nursing Implications

> **Quality and Safety Alert: Safety**
>
> The similarity between the names inamrinone and amiodarone has given rise to confusion. Caution is necessary.

Preventing Interactions

When oral amiodarone is used long term, it increases the effects of numerous drugs, worsening existing dysrhythmias or producing new dysrhythmias. Drugs that interact with amiodarone include beta-adrenergic blockers, oral anticoagulants, digoxin, and phenytoin. The effects of interactions with amiodarone may not be apparent until about 7 weeks after the initiation of therapy.

Administering the Medication

Careful patient assessment and evaluation with continual monitoring of cardiac response are necessary for titrating the dosage. Therapy should begin in the hospital with continual monitoring and emergency equipment on standby.

Assessing for Therapeutic Effects

An effect of the medication is to increase the ventricular fibrillation threshold. The nurse assesses the patient's heart rate and the cardiac rhythm; the heart rate and rhythm should be regular, with a rate between 60 and 100 beats/min.

Assessing for Adverse Effects

If the nurse notes any change in heart rate greater than 100 beats/min or less than 60 beats/min or any change in the regularity of the rhythm, increased vigilance in assessing cardiac status is warranted. In addition, the nurse assesses for ectopy and notifies the healthcare provider of any noted rhythm irregularities.

Patient Teaching

Patients should understand that if drug dosages are changed in relation to response of dysrhythmias, they need to be hospitalized during the initiation of amiodarone therapy for continuous cardiac monitoring. Additionally, the nurse should stress the importance of keeping follow-up appointments, including chest x-ray, pulmonary function tests, liver function tests, and ophthalmic examinations. Box 27.3 presents patient teaching information for antidysrhythmic agents.

Other Drugs in the Class

Dofetilide (Tikosyn) is indicated for the maintenance of normal sinus rhythm in symptomatic patients who are in atrial fibrillation for longer than 1 week. Adverse effects increase with decreasing creatinine clearance levels; thus, assessment of kidney function is necessary and initial dosage is dependent on creatinine clearance levels. High dosages in patients with kidney dysfunction result in accumulation of dofetilide and prodysrhythmia (torsades de pointes). The drug has an elimination half-life of approximately 10 hours, with the kidneys being the major route of elimination. It should initially be administered in a setting with personnel and equipment available for emergency use. The FDA has issued a **BOXED WARNING ◆** for dofetilide. It recommends that drug administration initially occur only in a facility that can provide calculations of creatinine clearance, continuous ECG monitoring, and cardiac resuscitation for a minimum of 3 days to minimize the risk of drug-induced dysrhythmia.

Dronedarone (Multaq) is ordered to reduce the risk of hospitalization for atrial fibrillation in patients with a history of persistent or paroxysmal atrial fibrillation. Structurally related to amiodarone, this related drug demonstrates electrophysiologic properties of all four antidysrhythmic classes (sodium channel blockers, potassium channel blockers, beta-adrenergic blockers, and calcium channel blockers). Thus, it inhibits sodium and potassium channels, which prolong the action potential and refractory period in myocardial tissue. The drug also decreases AV node conduction and sinus node function through inhibition of calcium channels and beta receptor blockade. Like amiodarone, the drug inhibits alpha 1 receptor–mediated increases in blood pressure, producing vasodilating effects and decreasing systemic vascular resistance.

The FDA has issued two **BOXED WARNING ◆** for dronedarone because it increases the risk of death, stroke, and heart failure. The drug is contraindicated in the following:

1. Patients with symptomatic heart failure (or New York Heart Association class IV heart failure) because the risk of death doubles in these patients who have had recent decompensation requiring hospitalization.
2. Patients in atrial fibrillation who will not or cannot be cardioverted into normal sinus rhythm. For those with permanent atrial fibrillation, dronedarone doubles the risk of death, stroke, and hospitalization for heart failure.

Ibutilide (Corvert) is indicated for the management of recent onset of atrial fibrillation or atrial flutter, in which the goal is conversion to normal sinus rhythm. The drug enhances the efficacy of cardioversion. It can convert atrial fibrillation to sinus rhythm more rapidly than procainamide or sotalol. Ibutilide is structurally similar to sotalol but lacks clinically significant beta-blocking activity. Studies have demonstrated that ibutilide has no significant advantage compared with amiodarone for the conversion of atrial fibrillation; however, severe hypotension does not occur with ibutilide. Ibutilide is widely distributed and has an elimination half-life of about 6 hours. Most of a dose is metabolized, and the metabolites are excreted in urine and feces. Adverse effects include supraventricular and ventricular dysrhythmias (particularly torsades de pointes) and hypotension. Patients with atrial fibrillation of more than 2 to 3 days' duration must be adequately anticoagulated, generally for at least 2 weeks prior to initiation of ibutilide to prevent adverse effects. The FDA has issued a **BOXED WARNING ◆** recommending that ibutilide be initiated only in a setting of continue ECG monitoring with trained personnel and equipment available for emergency use.

Sotalol (Betapace, Sorine, Sotylize) is approved for prevention or management of ventricular tachycardia and fibrillation. It has also been used, usually in smaller doses, to prevent or treat atrial fibrillation. However, it is less effective than amiodarone in the prophylaxis of atrial fibrillation. As previously mentioned, the drug has both beta-adrenergic–blocking and potassium channel–blocking activities. Class II effects predominate at lower doses, and class III effects predominate at higher doses. Sotalol is well absorbed after oral administration, and peak serum levels are reached in 2 to 4 hours. It has an elimination half-life of approximately 12 hours, and 80% to 90% is excreted unchanged by the kidneys.

Contraindications to the use of sotalol include asthma, sinus bradycardia, heart block, prolonged QT syndrome, cardiogenic shock, heart failure, and previous hypersensitivity to sotalol. The dosage should be individualized, reduced with kidney failure with replacement therapy, and increased slowly (e.g., every 2 to 3 days with normal kidney function or at longer intervals with impaired kidney function). Dysrhythmogenic effects are most likely to occur when therapy is started or when the dosage is increased. Heart failure may occur in patients with markedly depressed left ventricular systolic function. Most adverse effects are attributed to beta-adrenergic blocking activity. Like amiodarone, sotalol may be preferred over a class I agent because it is more effective in reducing recurrent ventricular tachycardia, ventricular fibrillation, and death. The FDA has issued a **BOXED WARNING ◆** for sotalol. This recommends that the drug be initiated only in a facility that can provide cardiac resuscitation and continuous ECG monitoring in the event of life-threatening ventricular tachycardia.

Clinical Application 27.1

- Ms. Johnson begins an IV infusion of amiodarone as well as an anticoagulant. What is the therapeutic goal of the amiodarone infusion? What nursing actions would the nurse implement during the initiation of the infusion?

NCLEX Success

3. The clinical use of class III agents rather than class I agents is preferred for patients with heart disease because the class III agents are associated with
   A. less ventricular fibrillation
   B. increased mortality
   C. more sustained effects
   D. milder adverse effects

4. A 73-year-old patient is about to be discharged from the hospital after treatment for recurrent ventricular fibrillation. To prevent breakthrough ventricular ectopy, the prescriber orders amiodarone, 1,000 mg PO daily as a loading dose for 2 weeks. What patient teaching implications are important regarding this loading dose?
   A. Most of the drug is destroyed in the GI tract and thus a large dose needs to be given.
   B. Older adults require large dosages because of their faster metabolic rate.
   C. A history of ventricular dysrhythmia necessitates a higher dose.
   D. The drug has a long serum half-life.

Clinical Application 27.2

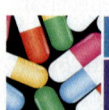

- While Ms. Johnson is receiving the amiodarone infusion, her heart rate decreases to 52 beats/min. The nurse continues to monitor patency of the IV line and the ECG. What other actions should the nurse take?

CLASS IV CALCIUM CHANNEL BLOCKERS

Diltiazem (Cardizem, Cardizem CD, Cardizem LA, Tiazac), the prototype class IV drug, and verapamil are the only calcium channel blockers approved for management of dysrhythmias. Table 27.6 presents dosage information for these drugs. Additional discussion regarding calcium channel blockers is found in Chapters 26 and 28.

Pharmacokinetics

When given intravenously, diltiazem acts within 3 minutes and lasts up to 10 hours. Diltiazem and verapamil are metabolized by the liver, and metabolites are primarily excreted by the kidneys.

Action

Calcium channel blockers obstruct the movement of calcium into conductive and contractile myocardial cells by inhibiting the influx of calcium through its channels, causing a slower conduction through the SA and AV nodes. As antidysrhythmic agents, they act primarily against tachydysrhythmias at SA and AV nodes because the cardiac cells slow channels that depend on calcium influx are found mainly at these sites. Thus, they reduce automaticity of the SA and AV nodes, slow conduction, and prolong the refractory period in the AV node.

Use

Diltiazem, as well as verapamil, is effective only in supraventricular tachycardias. The drug may be given intravenously to terminate acute paroxysmal supraventricular tachycardia, usually within 2 minutes, and in atrial fibrillation and atrial flutter. It is also effective in exercise-related tachycardias. One antidysrhythmic drug may not maintain a normal sinus rhythm, and the use of more than one agent is often necessary.

TABLE 27.6 DRUGS AT A GLANCE: Class IV Calcium Channel Blockers

Drug	Routes and Dosage Ranges	
	Adults	**Children**
Diltiazem (Cardizem, Cardizem CD, Cardizem LA, Tiazac; ✽ Cardizem CD, Diltiazem-CD, Tiazac, Tiazac XC)	IV bolus 0.25 mg/kg over 2 min; repeat 0.35 mg/kg IV over 2 min in 15 min if rate/rhythm unchanged; IV maintenance infusion of 5–15 mg/h based on ventricular response	Safety and efficacy have not been established for use in the treatment of tachydysrhythmias
Verapamil (Calan, Calan SR, Verelan, Verelan PM; ✽ Apo-Verap, Verelan)	PO (immediate release) 120 mg 3 times daily or PO (extended release) 240–480/daily in 1–2 divided doses IV loading dose 5–10 mg over 2 min initially and then additional 10 mg if necessary IV maintenance dose 5 mg/h titrated to goal heart rate	1–15 y: IV injection 0.1–0.3 mg/kg (usual range 2–5 mg for a single dose) over 2 min with continuous ECG monitoring; repeat in 30 min if necessary Verapamil is no longer included in PALS for management of tachydysrhythmias

PALS, pediatric advanced life support.

Patient-related variables specific to the use of diltiazem include the following:

- Age:
  - Safety and efficacy have not been established in pediatric patients.
- Reproduction, pregnancy, and lactation:
  - Calcium channel blockers can be used to treat hypertension in pregnancy although other agents are more commonly prescribed.
  - Patients with existing hypertension continue taking diltiazem during pregnancy unless contraindicated.
  - The risk for serious adverse reactions can be seen in the breast-fed infant; continuing breast-feeding or changing drug therapy in the breast-feeding patient should be considered due to manufacturer recommendations.
- Abnormal kidney function and hepatic impairment:
  - Impaired kidney and hepatic function are contraindications.
- Specific healthcare environments:
  - For patients receiving home care and taking diltiazem, the home care nurse performs a physical assessment, including pulse and blood pressure, with each visit.
  - The home care nurse arranges for follow-up with a 12-lead ECG if alterations in cardiac rhythm occur (e.g., irregular rate or change in baseline heart rate).

Adverse Effects

The most common adverse effect of diltiazem is peripheral edema, which impacts 5% to 15% of all patients taking the medication. Other cardiovascular adverse effects include bradycardia, hypotension, palpitations, and AV block. Adverse effects associated with diltiazem also include CNS symptoms, such as dizziness, sleep/dream disturbances, light-headedness, headache, and weakness. Dermatologic effect includes flushing, photosensitivity, and pruritus. The GI effects most often noted are complaints of nausea and constipation.

Contraindications

Contraindications to the use of diltiazem include allergy to diltiazem, impaired hepatic or kidney function, sick sinus syndrome, second- or third-degree heart block, severe hypertension, cardiogenic shock, acute myocardial infarction with cardiogenic shock, pulmonary congestion, and lactation. Diltiazem, as well as verapamil, is contraindicated in digoxin toxicity because it may worsen heart block. If diltiazem is used with propranolol or digoxin, it is necessary to exercise caution to avoid further impairment of myocardial contractility. Use of IV verapamil with IV propranolol should not take place; it may result in potentially fatal bradycardia and hypotension.

Nursing Implications

Preventing Interactions

Certain drugs increase the effects of diltiazem (Box 27.5). Also, diltiazem increases the serum levels and toxicity of cyclosporine. In addition, there is a decreased metabolism and increased risk of toxic effects if diltiazem is taken with grapefruit juice.

> **BOX 27.5   Drug Interactions: Diltiazem**
>
> **Drugs That Increase the Effects of Diltiazem**
> - Amiodarone
>   *Increases the risk of sinus arrest, decreased myocardial contractility, and hypotension*
> - Atazanavir
>   *Increases the risk of conduction disturbances and atrioventricular block*
> - Beta-adrenergic blockers, flecainide
>   *Cause additive reductions in heart rate, cardiac conduction, and contractility*

Administering the Medication

Careful evaluation to determine the appropriate dosing of calcium channel blockers is warranted. Ensuring that the patient swallows the extended-release or the sustained-release preparations whole rather than cutting, crushing, or chewing is a must.

Assessing for Therapeutic Effects

The nurse monitors the cardiac rate and rhythm for a return to the patient's normal baseline.

Assessing for Adverse Effects

When caring for patients who are receiving diltiazem, the nurse monitors carefully for changes in blood pressure and cardiac rhythm as well as output. (Checking the blood pressure is especially important if the patient is taking nitrates concurrently.) In addition, cardiac rhythm is monitored regularly during dosage stabilization and periodically during long-term therapy. The nurse should also observe for safety issues associated with the development of symptoms such as dizziness and light-headedness.

Patient Teaching

It is important to instruct the patient to report any adverse effects. Box 27.3 outlines patient teaching guidelines.

> **NCLEX Success**
>
> 5. A patient, age 67, is prescribed diltiazem for the treatment of a cardiac rhythm disorder. Which of the following findings would require the nurse to hold the ordered dose of diltiazem and notify the provider for further orders? (Select all that apply)
>   A. Blood pressure of 198/102
>   B. ECG shows 3rd degree atrioventricular block
>   C. ECG shows atrial fibrillation with rapid ventricular response
>   D. Apical heart rate of 42 beats/min

UNCLASSIFIED ANTIDYSRHYTHMIC DRUGS

Adenosine (Adenocard), a naturally occurring component of all body cells, differs chemically from other antidysrhythmic drugs but acts like the calcium channel blockers. It depresses conduction at the AV node and is used to restore normal sinus rhythm in patients with paroxysmal supraventricular tachycardia; it is ineffective in other dysrhythmias. The drug has a very short duration of action (serum half-life of less than 10 seconds) and a high degree of effectiveness. It must be given by a rapid bolus injection, preferably through a central venous line. If given slowly, it is eliminated before it can reach cardiac tissues and exert its action.

Magnesium sulfate is another of the unclassified drugs that may be used intravenously in the management of polymorphic ventricular tachycardia (torsades de pointes). Recent American Heart Association (AHA) practice guidelines do not include routine use of magnesium during the management of cardiac arrest and life-threatening dysrhythmias beyond torsades de pointes. Magnesium assists with regulating the flow of sodium, potassium, and calcium across the cell membrane, which can prevent reinitiation of ventricular tachycardias. Its antidysrhythmic effects may derive from imbalances of magnesium, potassium, and calcium. Hypomagnesemia increases myocardial irritability and is a risk factor for both atrial and ventricular dysrhythmias. Thus, serum magnesium levels should be monitored in patients at risk and replacement therapy instituted when indicated. However, in some instances, magnesium sulfate seems to have antidysrhythmic effects even when serum magnesium levels are normal. Magnesium sulfate to treat torsades de pointes is administered intravenously as a loading dose and then continuous infusion.

> ### Clinical Application 27.3
> Ms. Johnson's atrial fibrillation is converted to normal sinus rhythm pharmacologically. The provider prescribes amiodarone at 200 mg PO daily.
> - Why is she taking amiodarone orally?
> - What patient teaching should be provided to Ms. Johnson regarding the use of amiodarone?

DRUG THERAPY IN EMERGENCY RESUSCITATION OF ADULTS

Drugs are essential for successful resuscitation in emergencies, but initial management of cardiac arrest must also include ensuring adequate ventilation, performing high-quality compressions, restoring circulating volume loss, and identifying the causal event. This section focuses on a brief overview of the best evidence related to the efficacy of drug therapy during resuscitation.

Strengthening systems of care for both out-of-hospital cardiac arrest and in-hospital cardiac arrest is also crucial for improved clinical outcomes. The AHA guidelines provide comprehensive algorithms for basic and advanced life support and post–cardiac arrest care and were comprehensively updated in 2020. Chapter 28 discusses the 2020 AHA recommendations for the evaluation and management of acute coronary syndromes.

Oxygen

Oxygen is one of the most widely used therapeutic agents. The 2020 AHA guidelines strengthened its recommendation for the use of supplemental oxygen to achieve hyperoxia (an abnormally increased concentration of oxygen in tissues and organs) to produce the maximal feasible inspired oxygen during ongoing cardiopulmonary resuscitation or CPR. The use of supplemental oxygen to achieve adequate oxygenation in the early period following resuscitation should be reevaluated in light of the arterial blood gases and potential adverse effects of oxygen toxicity. Experts have cited a dose-dependent association between supernormal oxygen tension postresuscitation and risk of in-hospital death. Titration of oxygen to an oxygen saturation of at least 94% rather than continuing maximum oxygen delivery is emphasized.

Epinephrine

Although no vasopressor medication has ever shown any long-term survival benefit in cardiac arrest, epinephrine is recommended for the treatment of asystole. The 2020 AHA guidelines recommend that epinephrine be administered as early as possible and in regular doses (1 mg IV every 3 to 5 minutes); data do not support improved survival with routine administration of high-dose epinephrine. In addition, because myocardial infarction is often the cause of ventricular fibrillation as the primary rhythm during cardiac arrest, some experts recommend a lower dose of epinephrine with ventricular fibrillation to minimize the vasoconstriction of the coronary arteries caused by epinephrine given at standard doses. Extreme vasoconstriction can produce lactic acidosis at the cellular level and result in metabolic acidosis.

Atropine

The 2020 AHA guidelines recommend atropine (1 mg IV every 3 to 5 minutes with max dose of 3 mg) for bradycardia but no longer recommend the use of atropine for the treatment of asystole because data do not support the use of the drug. Research also does not support the use of atropine for pulseless electrical activity.

Sodium Bicarbonate

Data do not indicate that sodium bicarbonate is generally effective during cardiac arrest, so the drug is not part of routine management. Experts still recommend the drug for use in patients with hyperkalemia and in those with tricyclic antidepressant overdose.

Lidocaine

The 2020 AHA guidelines do not recommend the routine use of lidocaine after return of spontaneous circulation (ROSC). However, experts believe that it may be reasonable to continue lidocaine infusion in the immediate period after ventricular fibrillation or pulseless ventricular tachycardia if lidocaine was given intra-arrest and ROSC was achieved.

Calcium Chloride

Calcium chloride is the first-line therapy for individuals who are hypercalcemic with sudden cardiac death. Calcium chloride is not recommended during cardiac resuscitation in the presence of ventricular fibrillation, in asystole or electromechanical dissociation, or with a risk of existing digitalis toxicity. Untreated hypomagnesemia may make hypocalcemia refractory to drug therapy, so abnormalities in magnesium and calcium should be corrected simultaneously.

MAGNESIUM SULFATE

Magnesium sulfate is recommended during resuscitation only in patients with drug-induced QT prolongation and development of torsades de pointes.

THE NURSING PROCESS

A concept map outlines the nursing process related to drug therapy considerations in this chapter. Additional nursing implications related to the disease process should also be considered in care decisions.

Assessment
- Assess the significance of symptoms in relation to the cardiac dysrhythmias.
- Identify conditions or risk factors that may precipitate the dysrhythmias.
- Observe for adverse drug effects used to manage the dysrhythmias.
- When ECG monitoring is available, assess for type and indications of the dysrhythmias.

Outcomes of Therapy
The patient will
- Receive or take antidysrhythmic drugs accurately.
- Avoid conditions that precipitate dysrhythmias, when feasible.
- Experience improved heart rate, circulation, and activity tolerance.
- Be monitored for therapeutic and adverse drug effects.
- Avoid preventable adverse drug effects.
- Have adverse drug effects promptly recognized and treated if they occur.
- Keep follow-up appointments for monitoring responses to treatment measures.

Nursing Interventions
- Use measures to detect, prevent, and/or minimize dysrhythmias.
- Manage underlying disease processes that contribute to dysrhythmia development. These include cardiovascular (e.g., acute myocardial infarction) and noncardiovascular (e.g., chronic lung disease) disorders.
- Prevent or treat other conditions that predispose to dysrhythmias (e.g., hypoxia, electrolyte imbalance, pain, acid–base imbalance, fluid alterations).
- Encourage the patient to recognize and avoid the negative effects of cigarette smoking, overeating, excessive coffee drinking, and other habits that may cause or aggravate dysrhythmias.
- Implement measures to minimize the incidence and severity of acute dysrhythmias and help the patient comply with drug therapy.
- Monitor heart rate and rhythm and blood pressure every 4 to 6 hours (or as often as clinical condition indicates or is the standard for the care environment where assessing the patient).
- During IV administration of antidysrhythmic drugs, maintain continuous cardiac monitoring and check blood pressure about every 1 to 5 minutes, depending on the onset of action of the drug.
- Check laboratory reports of serum electrolytes and serum drug levels when available. See Table 27.6 for commonly reported serum levels of antidysrhythmic agents. Report and treat abnormal values using established protocols and/or provider's orders.

Evaluation
- Interview and observe for symptom relief and stable vital signs and cardiac rhythm.
- Interview and observe for irregular rhythms, hypotension, and other adverse drug effects.
- Interview and observe for compliance with instructions for taking antidysrhythmic drugs and other aspects of care.

Visit thePoint® *at* **http://thePoint.lww.com/Frandsen13e** *for answers to NCLEX Success questions (in Appendix A), answers to Clinical Application Case Studies (in Appendix B), additional information on etiology and pathophysiology, and more!*

REFERENCES AND RESOURCES

Agency for Healthcare Research and Quality (AHRQ). (2019). *Patient safety primer: Rapid response systems.* https://psnet.ahrq.gov/primers/primer/4/rapid-response-systems

al-Khatib, S. M., Stevenson, W. G., Ackerman, M. J., Bryant, W. J., Callans, D. J., Curtis, A. B., Deal, B. J., Dickfeld, T., Field, M. E., Fonarow, G. C., Gillis, A. M., Granger, C. B., Hammill, S. C., Hlatky, M. A., Joglar, J. A., Kay, G. N., Matlock, D. D., Myerburg, R. J., & Page, R. L. (2018). 2017 AHA/ACC/HRS guideline for management of patients with ventricular arrhythmias and the prevention of sudden cardiac death: A report of the American College of Cardiology Foundation/American Heart Association Task Force on Clinical Practice Guidelines and the Heart Rhythm Society. *Circulation, 138*, e272–e391. https://doi.org/10.1161/CIR.0000000000000549

Berg, K. M., Soar, J., Andersen, L. W., Böttiger, B. W., Cacciola, S., Callaway, C. W., Couper, K., Cronberg, T., D'Arrigo, S., Deakin, C. D., Donnino, M. W., Drennan, I. R., Granfeldt, A., Hoedemaekers, C. W. E., Holmberg, M. J., Hsu, C. H., Kamps, M., Musiol, S., Nation, K. J., ... Nolan J. P. (2020). Adult advanced life support: 2020 international consensus on cardiopulmonary resuscitation and emergency cardiovascular care science with treatment recommendations. *Circulation, 142*(16_suppl 1), S92–S139. https://doi.org/10.1161/CIR.0000000000000893

Brugada, J., Katritsis, D. G., Arbelo, E., Arribas, F., Bax, J. J., Blomström-Lundqvist, C., Calkins, H., Corrado, D., Deftereos, S. G., Diller, G. P., Gomez-Doblas, J. J., Gorenek, B., Grace, A., Ho, S. Y., Kaski, J. C., Kuck, K. H., Lambiase, P. D., Sacher, F., Sarquella-Brugada, G., ... Zaza, A. (2020). 2019 ESC Guidelines for the management of patients with supraventricular tachycardia: The Task Force for the management of patients with supraventricular tachycardia of the European Society of Cardiology (ESC). *European Heart Journal, 41*(5), 655–720. https://doi.org/10.1093/eurheartj/ehz467

Damiani, E., Adrario, E., Girardis, M., Romano, R., Peilaia, P., Singer, M., & Donati, A. (2014). Arterial hyperoxia and mortality in critically ill patients: A systematic review and meta-analysis. *Critical Care, 18*(6), 711.

Gorgels, A. P., van den Dool, A., Hofs, A., Mulleneers, R., Smeets, J. L., Vos, M. A., & Wellens, H. J. (1996). Comparison of procainamide and lidocaine in terminating sustained monomorphic ventricular tachycardia. *The American Journal of Cardiology, 78*, 43–46. https://doi.org/10.1016/s0002-9149(96)00224-x

Hazinski, M. F., Nolan, J. P., & the International Liaison Committee on Resuscitation Editorial Board. (2015). Part 1: Executive summary: 2015 international consensus on cardiopulmonary resuscitation and emergency cardiovascular care science with treatment recommendations. *Circulation, 132*(16), S2–S39.

Karch, A. M. (2023). *2022 Lippincott's pocket drug guide for nurses* (11th ed.). Wolters Kluwer.

Merchant, R. M., Topjain, A. A., Panchal, A. R., Cheng, A., Aziz, K., Berg, K. M., Lavonas, E. J., Magid, D. J., & on behalf of the Adult Basic and Advanced Life Support, Pediatric Basic and Advanced Life Support, Neonatal Life Support, Resuscitation Education Science, and Systems of Care Writing Groups. (2020). Part 1: Executive summary: 2020 American Heart Association guidelines for cardiopulmonary resuscitation and emergency cardiovascular care. *Circulation, 142*(16 Suppl 2), S337–S357. https://doi.org/10.1161/CIR.0000000000000918

Norris, T. (2019). *Porth's pathophysiology: Concepts of altered health status* (10th ed.). Wolters Kluwer.

Panchal, A., Bartos, J., Cabanas, J., Donnino, M., Drennan, I., Hirsch, K., Kudenchuk, P. J., Kurz, M. C., Lavonas, E. J., Morley, P. T., O'Neil, B. J., Peberdy, M. A., Rittenberger, J. C., Rodriguez, A. J., Sawyer, K. N., & Berg, K. M. (2020). Part 3: Adult basic and advanced life support: 2020 American Heart Association guidelines for cardiopulmonary resuscitation and emergency cardiovascular care. *Circulation, 142*, s366–s468. https://doi.org/10.1161/CIR.0000000000000916

Page, R. L., Joglar, J. A., Caldwell, M. A., Calkins, H., Conti, J. B., Deal, B. J., Estes III, N., Field, M. E., Goldberger, Z. D., Hammill, S. C., Indik, J. H., Lindsay, B. D., Olshansky, B., Russo, A. M., Shen, W. K., Tracy, C. M., & Al-Khatib, S. M. (2016). 2015 ACC/AHA/HRS guideline for the management of adult patients with supraventricular tachycardia: A report of the American College of Cardiology/American Heart Association Task Force on Clinical Practice Guidelines and the Heart Rhythm Society. *Journal of the American College of Cardiology, 67*(13), e27–e115. https://doi.org/10.1016/j.jacc.2015.08.856

Zeppenfeld, K., Tfelt-Hansen, J., de Riva, M., Winkel, B. G., Behr, E. R., Blom, N. A., Charron, P., Corrado, D., Dagres, N., de Chillou, C., Eckardt, L., Friede, T., Haugaa, K. H., Hocini, M., Lambiase, P. D., Marijon, E., Merino, J. L., Peichl, P., Priori, S. G., ... Volterrani, M. (2022). 2022 ESC guidelines for the management of patients with ventricular arrhythmias and the prevention of sudden cardiac death: Developed by the task force for the management of patients with ventricular arrhythmias and the prevention of sudden cardiac death of the European Society of Cardiology (ESC) Endorsed by the Association for European Paediatric and Congenital Cardiology (AEPC). *European Heart Journal, 43*(40), 3997–4126. https://doi.org/10.1093/eurheartj/ehac262

CHAPTER 28

Drug Therapy for Coronary Heart Disease

LEARNING OBJECTIVES

After studying this chapter, you should be able to:

1. Examine the nonpharmacologic measures beneficial in controlling or reversing risk factors for cardiovascular disease progression.
2. Identify the prototype and describe the action, use, contraindications, adverse effects, and nursing implications for the organic nitrates in the management of coronary heart disease.
3. Identify the prototype and outline the actions, use, adverse effects, contraindications, and nursing implications for the beta-adrenergic blockers in the management of coronary heart disease.
4. Identify the prototype and describe the actions, use, adverse effects, contraindications, and nursing implications for the calcium channel blockers in the management of coronary heart disease.
5. Evaluate evidence-based considerations in the use of adjuvant drugs administered in the management of patients with acute coronary syndromes.
6. Apply the nursing process in the care of patients with coronary heart disease.

CLINICAL APPLICATION CASE STUDY

Richard Gerald, a 72-year-old patient, has a history of hypertension and coronary artery disease. He stopped smoking and began a regular exercise program after having a non–ST-segment elevation myocardial infarction 2 months ago. He was discharged on nitroglycerin–in a sublingual form and as a transdermal patch (1 in) every 4 hours while awake (off at night)–and on atenolol 50 mg orally daily.

KEY TERMS

Acute coronary syndromes: umbrella term used to describe conditions brought on by sudden, reduced blood flow to the heart in situations where myocardial ischemia is suspected. These include unstable angina, non–ST-segment elevation myocardial infarction, and ST-segment elevation myocardial infarction.

Afterload: amount of vascular resistance that must be overcome to open the aortic valve on the left side of the heart (or pulmonic valve on the right) and eject the blood with systole

Cardioselectivity: ability of a beta-adrenergic blocker to selectively block $beta_1$ receptors

Coronary artery vasospasm: smooth muscle constriction of a coronary artery

Coronary heart disease: stable angina pectoris and acute coronary syndromes, which result from coronary artery disease or spasm

Intima: inner layer of an artery

Media: middle layer of a vessel

Negative chronotropy: causing slowing of the heart rate

Preload: passive stretch of the ventricles just prior to systole

INTRODUCTION

The two broad categories of **coronary heart disease**, chronic coronary artery disease (CAD) and acute coronary syndromes, are on a continuum of disease progression. Stable angina is the classic initial manifestation of chronic CAD. As CAD worsens, the effects of ischemia may lead to **acute coronary syndromes**, an umbrella term used to describe the sequelae of unstable angina and myocardial infarction (MI) with or without elevation in the ST segment.

Coronary artery vasospasm, or smooth muscle constriction of a coronary artery, is another form of angina that can lead to MI, ventricular dysrhythmias, and sudden cardiac death. Termed variant angina (or Prinzmetal or vasospastic angina), this form of angina is not due to an obstructive atherosclerotic lesion but results from the spasm of one or more coronary arteries that reduces blood flow to the myocardium. However, variant angina plays a key role in the development of atherosclerotic lesions.

This chapter introduces the pharmacologic care of the patient experiencing coronary heart disease. Nonpharmacologic treatment measures are also addressed. To understand clinical use of these drugs and nonpharmacologic treatment measures, it is necessary to understand the sequelae of plaque development and rupture as well as the clinical manifestations of CAD.

OVERVIEW OF CORONARY ARTERY DISEASE

Clinical Considerations

In CAD, increased blood levels of low-density lipoprotein (LDL) irritate and damage the **intima** (inner layer) of a portion of a coronary artery, triggering a cycle of protection to the area that sends smooth muscle cells from the **media** (middle layer) of the vessel and stimulating calcium deposition. The effort to protect the damaged area forms a fibrous plaque along the intima, ultimately leading to fixed atherosclerotic plaque. The plaque narrows the lumen of the artery, which restricts the flow of oxygen-carrying blood. When oxygen supply is insufficient, especially during periods of high oxygen demand (e.g., with physical exertion), cardiac ischemia occurs, and the patient may experience stable angina.

Over time, the plaque can harden or rupture, decreasing the diameter of the artery. Inflammation, a key determinant of the vulnerability of plaque, is related to an increase in the activity of macrophages at the site of the plaque; as macrophage activity increases, the vulnerability of the plaque to rupture also increases. With plaque rupture, a thrombus is formed that releases chemical mediators that lead to vasoconstriction. The disrupted plaque and thrombi, together with the vasoconstriction, combine to further narrow the coronary artery and worsen ischemia. At this point, the intraluminal thrombi can occlude an artery outright or detach, move into the circulation, and eventually occlude smaller, distal branches of the artery causing thromboembolism and MI. Catecholamine release along with increased sympathetic tone as seen with tachycardia of any etiology, mental stress, or physical exertion can lead to further cardiac ischemia.

When blood flow is obstructed to all or a portion of a coronary artery, ischemia and ultimately death of the myocardium result. In myocardial cells, in areas of local ischemia failure to maintain the homeostasis of electrolytes leads to electrical instability and dysrhythmias, mechanical dysfunction from reduced contractility and increased diastolic tension, and mitochondrial dysfunction with a shift from aerobic to anaerobic metabolism.

Clinical Manifestations

Stable Angina

When intermittent myocardial oxygen demand surpasses oxygen supply to the heart muscle, the ischemia to the myocardium produces symptoms (Fig. 28.1). Stable angina (also called classic, typical, or exertional angina) is usually precipitated by situations that increase the workload of the heart, such as physical exertion, exposure to cold temperatures, and emotional upset. Recurrent episodes of stable angina usually have the same pattern of onset, duration, and intensity of symptoms.

Although classic anginal pain is typically described as substernal chest pain of a constricting, squeezing, or suffocating nature, patients often report pressure, tightness, heaviness,

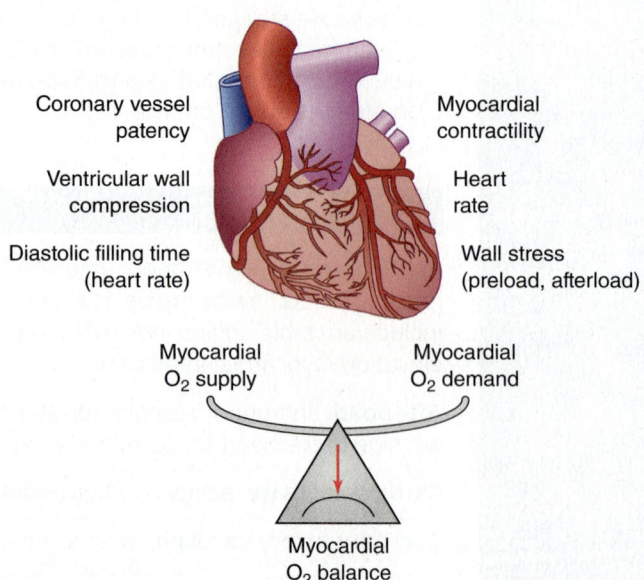

Figure 28.1. Myocardial oxygen supply and demand. (Reprinted with permission from Norris, T. L. (2019). *Porth's pathophysiology: Concepts of altered health states* (10th ed., Fig. 27.4, p. 760). Wolters Kluwer.)

squeezing, or a burning discomfort. They also may report a location other than the chest, including the shoulder, arm, neck, back, upper abdomen, or jaw.

The discomfort is sometimes mistaken for arthritis or for indigestion because it may be associated with nausea, vomiting, dizziness, diaphoresis, shortness of breath, or fear of impending doom. The discomfort is usually brief, typically lasting 5 minutes or less until the balance of oxygen supply and demand is restored. The traditional description of angina derives from studies in males. Females, who report pain other than in the chest, more commonly present with complaints of unusual fatigue, weakness, dizziness, and shortness of breath. Older adults and those with diabetes mellitus may have noncardiac symptoms or may present with silent myocardial ischemia. Note that patients with noncardiac presentations and those with silent ischemia are less likely to be diagnosed accurately and promptly, often placing them outside the therapeutic window of opportunity. They are less likely to receive appropriate treatment (i.e., thrombolytics and interventional therapies), resulting in poorer outcomes.

Variant angina occurs at rest or with minimal exertion, often at night and frequently at the same time each day. Individuals experience cycles of 3- to 6-month clusters of recurring attacks, followed by relatively symptom-free periods.

Quality and Safety Alert: Evidence-Based Practice

Dennis et al. (2021) assessed gender differences in hospitalization incidence, 30-day mortality, and 30-day readmission rates in 2,394 individuals admitted with acute myocardial **infarction (MI)** between January 2013 and June 2019 in one U.S. medical center. The researchers used multivariate logistic regression to estimate gender differences in mortality after adjusting for information found in billing records (e.g., gender, age, principal procedure, insurance status, principal diagnosis, race/ethnicity).

Their findings indicated that males were hospitalized over twice as frequently, yet at around age 65 years, females had greater mortality than men from the MI. On average, female patients were older and somewhat less likely to undergo percutaneous transluminal coronary angioplasty than their male counterparts. Thirty-day readmission rates did not differ by gender.

The study supports other findings that MI symptoms may go underrecognized in females and that additional education is needed to raise awareness of the symptoms of coronary heart disease in females. The inclusion of more females in clinical research trials may help identify treatment strategies that would enhance outcomes in females.

Acute Coronary Syndromes

The symptoms of unstable angina (also called crescendo, rest, or preinfarction angina) are similar to those of stable angina. However, in unstable angina, the acute pain typically occurs at rest and usually lasts longer than 20 minutes. The intensity, timing, and characteristics of the pain show recent increases in severity and frequency, often develop with less exertion than previous episodes of angina and may limit physical activity. Unstable angina differs from non–ST-elevation myocardial infarction (NSTEMI) in that the ischemia is not severe enough to cause sufficient myocardial damage to release detectable quantities of troponins. Because unstable angina often occurs hours or days before acute MI, early recognition and effective management are extremely important in preventing progression to infarction, heart failure, or sudden cardiac death.

In patients with acute coronary syndrome, early risk stratification is performed using a risk assessment system that predicts the risk of further cardiac episodes. Identifying patients at highest risk who may benefit from more aggressive therapeutic management is essential for improved outcomes. Factors that predict severe cardiac events include the presence and extent of ST-segment depression, elevated cardiac biomarkers, evidence of hemodynamic instability, and persistent chest pain despite appropriate medical therapy.

Patients who present without persistent ST-segment elevation may be experiencing an NSTEMI, formerly called a non–Q-wave MI. Their electrocardiogram (ECG) changes may show ST-segment depression or T-wave inversion, other changes, or no changes. An ST-segment elevation MI (STEMI), formerly called a Q-wave MI, is defined by persistent (greater than 20 minutes) ST elevation on ECG, which generally reflects an acute total coronary occlusion. Both NSTEMI and STEMI are characterized by a typical rise and/or fall in biomarkers of myocyte injury. Cardiac troponin I and troponin T are the preferred biomarkers of myocyte injury because they are more specific and sensitive for myocardial tissue than the traditional cardiac isoenzyme creatine kinase (CK)-MB.

Nonpharmacologic Therapy

Nonpharmacologic management of CAD includes risk factor modification, patient education, and revascularization procedures. For patients at any stage of CAD development, irrespective of symptoms of myocardial ischemia, optimal management involves lifestyle changes and drugs to control or reverse risk factors for disease progression. A growing body of evidence corroborates that risk factor management in patients with CAD improves survival, enhances quality of life, reduces recurrent events, and decreases the need for revascularization. Thus, efforts to assist patients in reducing blood pressure, weight, and serum cholesterol levels, when indicated, and developing an exercise program are necessary. For patients with diabetes mellitus, glucose and blood pressure control can reduce the microvascular changes associated with the condition.

In addition, people should avoid circumstances known to precipitate acute attacks, and those who smoke should stop. Smoking is harmful because of the following factors:

- Nicotine increases catecholamines, which, in turn, increase heart rate and blood pressure.
- Carboxyhemoglobin, formed from the inhalation of carbon monoxide in smoke, decreases delivery of blood and oxygen to the heart, decreases myocardial contractility, and increases the risks of life-threatening cardiac dysrhythmias (e.g., ventricular fibrillation) during ischemic episodes.
- Both nicotine and carbon monoxide increase platelet adhesiveness and aggregation, thereby promoting thrombosis.
- Smoking increases the risks of MI, sudden cardiac death, cerebrovascular disease (e.g., stroke), peripheral vascular disease (e.g., arterial insufficiency), and hypertension. It also reduces high-density lipoprotein (HDL) cholesterol.

Additional nonpharmacologic management strategies include surgical revascularization (e.g., coronary artery bypass graft) and interventional procedures that reduce blockages (e.g., primary percutaneous coronary intervention [PCI], intracoronary stent, laser therapy, rotational atherectomy).

Nonpharmacologic management improves patient outcomes. However, most patients still require antianginal and other cardiovascular medications to manage their disease.

Drug Therapy

Upcoming sections discuss the drugs used to treat angina, myocardial ischemia, and infarction. Table 28.1 and the DRUGS AT A GLANCE tables list individual drugs used in the treatment of coronary heart disease, which include the organic nitrates, beta-adrenergic blockers, calcium channel blockers, and adjuvant drugs. These drugs relieve anginal pain by increasing blood supply to the myocardium as well as reducing the oxygen demand of the myocardium. In addition, this chapter includes a brief review of the current evidence related to the indications and effectiveness of additional drugs used in the management of acute MI.

TABLE 28.1
Drugs Administered for the Treatment of Coronary Heart Disease

Drug Class	Prototype	Other Drugs in the Class
Organic nitrates	Nitroglycerin (Nitro-Bid, others)	Isosorbide dinitrate (Isordil) Isosorbide mononitrate
Beta-adrenergic blockers	Atenolol (Tenormin)	Bisoprolol Carvedilol (Coreg) Esmolol (Brevibloc) Metoprolol (Lopressor, Toprol XL) Nadolol (Corgard) Propranolol (Inderal)
Calcium channel blockers	Nifedipine	Amlodipine (Katerzia, Norliqva, Norvasc) Diltiazem (Cardizem) Felodipine Isradipine Nicardipine Verapamil (Calan SR, Verelan)
Adjunct medications	Ranolazine (Ranexa)	Dyslipidemic drugs Antihypertensive drugs Angiotensin-converting enzyme inhibitors Aspirin ADP receptor antagonists Glycoprotein IIb/IIIa receptor antagonists Morphine

ORGANIC NITRATES

The most widely used nitrate is the prototype **nitroglycerin** (Nitro-Bid, Nitro-Dur). Available in multiple forms, it is indicated for the management and prevention of acute chest pain caused by myocardial ischemia.

Pharmacokinetics

Nitroglycerin is 60% bound to protein, undergoes extensive first-pass metabolism in the liver, and has a half-life of 1 to 4 minutes. Excretion occurs in the urine. The onset of action, peak, and duration of action varies with the route of administration:

- Intravenous (IV) drip: onset, immediate; peak, immediate; duration of action, 3 to 5 minutes
- Sublingual (SL): onset, 1 to 3 minutes; peak, 4 to 8 minutes; duration of action, at least 25 minutes
- Translingual spray: onset, 1 to 3 minutes; peak, 4 to 10 minutes; duration of action, at least 25 minutes
- Oral (PO) tablets or capsules (sustained release): onset, about 60 minutes; peak, 2½ to 4 hours; duration of action, 4 to 8 hours
- Topical ointment: onset, 15 to 30 minutes; peak, 60 minutes; duration of action, 7 hours
- Topical transdermal disk: onset, about 30 minutes; peak, 120 minutes; duration of action, 10 to 12 hours

Action

Organic nitrates are converted to nitric oxide, a potent vasodilator, which relaxes smooth muscle in blood vessel walls. The drugs relieve anginal pain by several mechanisms:

- Venous dilation, which reduces venous pressure and decreases venous return to the heart. This decreases blood volume and pressure within the heart (**preload**), which in turn decreases cardiac workload and oxygen demand. This is the main mechanism by which nitroglycerin relieves angina.
- Coronary artery dilation at higher doses, which can increase blood flow to ischemic areas of the myocardium.
- Arteriole dilation, which lowers peripheral vascular resistance (**afterload**). This results in lower systolic blood pressure and, consequently, reduced cardiac workload and balancing supply and demand in the heart.

Use

For relief of sudden-onset angina, fast-acting preparations of nitroglycerin include SL tablets and transmucosal spray. Indications for these preparations include acute-onset chest pain and prophylaxis prior to activities known to provoke angina, such as walking, dancing, or mowing the lawn.

For management of recurrent, chronic angina, long-acting preparations include PO sustained-release tablets and transdermal ointment. With these longer-acting forms, intolerance to their hemodynamic effects may develop, and therefore, the drugs do not relieve chest pain.

> **! Quality and Safety Alert: Safety**
>
> To avoid development of tolerance to nitroglycerin, it is essential to observe a 10- to 12-hour nitrate-free interval.

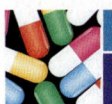

TABLE 28.2
DRUGS AT A GLANCE: Organic Nitrates

Drug	Routes and Dosage Ranges (Adults [Unless Indicated])
ⓟ **Nitroglycerin** (Nitro-Bid, Nitro-Dur, Nitrostat, Nitrolingual, Rectiv; 🍁 Minitran, Nitro-Dur, Nitrostat)	Extended-release tablets or capsules, 2.5 mg PO three or four times/day Sublingual, 0.15–0.6 mg as needed for chest pain Translingual spray, one or two metered doses (0.4 mg/dose) sprayed onto oral mucosa at onset of anginal pain, to a maximum of three doses in 15 min Transmucosal tablet, 1 mg every 3–5 h while awake, placed between upper lip and gum or cheek and gum Topical ointment, 1/2–2 in every 4–8 h; do not rub in Topical transdermal disk, applied once daily IV, 5–10 mcg/min initially, increased in 10–20 mcg/min increments up to 100 mcg/min or more if necessary to relieve pain
Isosorbide dinitrate (Isordil, Dilatrate-SR; 🍁 ISDN)	Sublingual, 5–10 mg as needed or every 2–4 h Regular tablets, 5–80 mg PO two to three times/day Sustained-release capsules, 40 mg PO one to two times daily, maximum 160 mg daily
Isosorbide mononitrate (🍁 Imdur)	5–20 mg PO twice daily, with first dose on arising and the second dose 7 h later Extended-release tablets, 30–60 mg once daily PO in the morning, increased after several days; maximum dose 240 mg once daily

In clinical practice, patients taking nitrates are usually nitrate free during the night, while sleeping, to prevent nitrate tolerance. The oral form of the drug undergoes rapid metabolism in the liver, and relatively small portions ultimately reach the systemic circulation. Thus, the PO form does not relieve acute chest pain but may be useful prophylactically in chronic chest pain. Nitroglycerin ointment is indicated for prevention of chronic angina. This route is convenient to use when the patient can have nothing by mouth (NPO) before surgery and cannot take the usual PO dose.

Angina that is unresponsive to SL, PO, or transdermal preparations calls for IV nitroglycerin. Prescribers may typically order the IV form for management of pain associated with an MI. IV nitroglycerin is useful in the management of angina that is unresponsive to organic nitrates via other routes or to beta-adrenergic blockers. It also may be used to control blood pressure in perioperative or emergency situations and to reduce preload and afterload in severe heart failure. Table 28.2 presents route and dosage information for nitroglycerin and other nitrates.

Concept Mastery Alert

Nitroglycerin is given sublingually, transmucosally, or via IV for immediate relief of anginal pain. Extended-release nitroglycerin, isosorbide dinitrate, and isosorbide mononitrate can be administered orally to prevent anginal pain.

Patient-related variables specific to the use of nitroglycerin and other organic nitrates include the following:
- Age:
  - IV nitroglycerin is the only form of nitroglycerin approved for use in children to treat hypertension and heart failure. Caution and close monitoring are necessary.
  - Older adults may be more vulnerable to hypotension when taking nitroglycerin as a result of volume depletion, concurrent use of other medication, and loss of sympathetic tone.

 Quality and Safety Alert: Safety

Older adults may be at greater risk of falling than younger patients at the therapeutic doses of nitroglycerin because of the risk of hypotension.

- Reproduction, pregnancy, and lactation:
  - Nitroglycerin crosses the placenta.
  - The drug may be used in obstetrical procedures when immediate relaxation of the uterus is necessary.
  - In pregnant patients with preeclampsia, nitroglycerin is used when severe hypertension accompanies pulmonary edema.
  - It is unknown if nitroglycerin is present in breast milk.
- Specific healthcare environments:
  - In the critical care setting, IV nitroglycerin is commonly used given the severity of the patient's clinical condition.
  - Close monitoring of vital signs, along with frequent titration of IV medications, is important in patients who are critically ill.

 Quality and Safety Alert: Safety

The nurse must always check IV compatibility when administering nitroglycerin and other drugs by that route.

Adverse Effects

Most adverse effects of nitroglycerin are related to the hemodynamic changes responsible for preload reduction and vasodilation. The most common adverse effect is a severe headache, which is typically treated with acetaminophen. Other common adverse effects include dizziness, bradycardia, syncope, hypotension, and orthostatic hypotension.

Contraindications

Contraindications to nitroglycerin include hypersensitivity reactions, severe anemia, hypotension, and hypovolemia.

Quality and Safety Alert: Safety

Males taking nitroglycerin or any other nitrate should not use phosphodiesterase enzyme type 5 inhibitors such as sildenafil (Viagra), tadalafil (Cialis), or vardenafil (Levitra) for erectile dysfunction. The combined effect can produce profound, life-threatening hypotension.

Caution is necessary in the following situations:

- In the presence of head injury or cerebral hemorrhage because it may increase intracranial pressure.
- With the use of other antihypertensive agents such as beta-adrenergic blockers. It is essential to observe for extreme episodes of hypotension.
- With abnormal kidney function.

Nursing Implications

Preventing Interactions

Many drugs interact with nitroglycerin, increasing or decreasing its effects (Box 28.1). Several herbs interact with nitroglycerin and can cause profound hypotension, including *N*-acetyl cysteine, arginine, folate, vitamin E, and hawthorn. Vitamin C decrease the effects of nitroglycerin

Administering the Medication

It is important to take a patient's vital signs prior to administration of any form of nitroglycerin. The nurse should withhold the medication with hypotension (systolic blood pressure less than 90 Hg or 30 mm Hg below the patient's normal blood pressure) as well as tachycardia with a heart rate greater than 100 beats/min.

Administration of SL nitroglycerin or translingual spray is essential as soon as chest pain develops. If a patient is hospitalized, it is necessary to call the patient's healthcare provider and obtain a 12-lead ECG at the onset of chest pain. The SL nitroglycerin container should stay in a dry, cool, dark environment, and replacement every 6 months is necessary. Exposure to light deactivates the nitroglycerin tablets. Once opened, the translingual spray has a shelf life of 2 to 3 years.

In acute coronary syndromes, after three SL doses, administered 5 minutes apart, patients outside of the hospital should seek medical attention. While hospitalized, IV dosing should be started and titrated to desired effect. Nitrate tolerance commonly develops within 24 hours in patients on a continuous infusion of nitroglycerin. Extended-release oral nitrate preparations are used post-MI if angina persists after revascularization.

Application of nitroglycerin ointment requires using the dose-measuring application papers supplied with ointment. It is necessary to do the following:

- Squeeze the ointment onto a measuring scale printed on paper; typically, this is 1 or ½ in, depending on the practitioner's order.
- Use the paper to spread ointment onto a nonhairy area of skin (chest, abdomen, thighs; avoid distal extremities) in a thin, even layer, covering a 2- to 3-in area.
- Do not allow the ointment to come in contact with the hand. Do not massage the ointment into the patient's skin because absorption will be increased and interfere with the sustained action.

People should take PO nitrates in the morning after a nitrate-free interval (typically during the night). They should take the tablets or capsules 1 to 2 hours before meals. It is important not to break, crush, or chew sustained-release preparations.

IV nitroglycerin preparations come in glass bottles, polyvinyl chloride (PVC)-free partial-additive bags, and di(2-ethylhexyl) phthalate (DEHP)-free, PVC-free plastic EXCEL containers. Nurses should use these only with special tubing provided by the manufacturer because PVC tubing absorbs 20% to 60% of the nitroglycerin. Inline IV filters that adsorb nitroglycerin should be avoided. In addition, nurses should ensure that IV nitroglycerin is administered via infusion pump and that patients are placed on cardiac monitors. Many hospitals require patients to be in ICUs or step-down units while the nitroglycerin drip is actively being titrated. As previously stated, it is essential to take vital signs frequently with IV administration and recheck them with each titration.

Assessing for Therapeutic Effects

Therapeutic effects of some forms of nitroglycerin may include the relief of acute chest pain as well as a modest decrease in blood pressure. With oral preparations, a decreased frequency of chronic chest pain should occur. Overall, patients should report that they feel better, have no symptoms of cardiac ischemia (i.e., chest pain), and have a higher activity tolerance.

Patient Teaching

Box 28.2 reviews general patient teaching guidelines regarding drugs for the management of coronary heart disease, including nitroglycerin.

Other Drugs in the Class

Isosorbide dinitrate (Isordil) is useful for reducing the frequency and severity of acute anginal episodes, not for acute relief of anginal symptoms. When given sublingually, it acts in about 2 minutes, and its effects last for 2 to 3 hours. When higher doses are given orally, more drug escapes metabolism in the liver and

---

BOX 28.1 Drug Interactions: Nitroglycerin

Drugs That Increase the Effects of Nitroglycerin
- Nifedipine and other calcium channel blockers, alcohol, aripiprazole, benazepril and other angiotensin-converting enzyme inhibitors, codeine and other narcotics, diphenhydramine, tizanidine
  Increase the risk of orthostatic hypotension
- Sildenafil, tadalafil, vardenafil
  Increase the risk of life-threatening hypotension

Drugs That Decrease the Effects of Nitroglycerin
- Acetaminophen, chloral hydrate, dihydroergotamine, sulfonylureas, vasopressin
  Decrease vasodilating effects

BOX 28.2 Patient Teaching Guidelines for Drugs Used for Coronary Heart Disease

General Considerations

- Angina is chest pain that occurs because your heart is not getting enough blood and oxygen. The most common causes are hypertension and atherosclerosis of the coronary arteries. The chest pain usually lasts less than 5 minutes, and episodes can be managed for years without causing permanent heart damage. However, if the pain is severe or prolonged, a heart attack and heart damage may develop. Seek information about your heart condition to prevent or decrease episodes of angina and prevent a heart attack.
- Several types of drugs are used in coronary heart disease, and you may need a combination of drugs for the best effects. Most patients take one or more long-acting drugs to prevent anginal attacks and a fast, short-acting drug (usually nitroglycerin tablets that you dissolve under your tongue or a nitroglycerin solution that you spray into your mouth) to relieve acute attacks. Seek emergency care immediately if rest and three sublingual tablets or oral sprays 5 minutes apart do not relieve chest pain. The long-acting oral medications are not effective in relieving sudden anginal pain.
- As with any medications for serious or potentially serious conditions, it is extremely important to take antianginal medications as prescribed. Do not increase dosage or discontinue the drugs without specific instructions from your healthcare provider.
- Keep sublingual nitroglycerin tablets in the original container; carry them so that they are always within reach but not where they are exposed to body heat. Replace them approximately every 6 months because they become ineffective.
- Record the number and severity of anginal episodes, the number of nitroglycerin tablets required to relieve the attack, and the total number of tablets taken daily. Such a record can help your healthcare provider know when to change your medications or your dosages.
- Headache and dizziness may occur with nitrate antianginal drugs, especially sublingual nitroglycerin. These effects are usually temporary and dissipate with continued therapy. If dizziness occurs, avoid strenuous activity and stand up slowly for approximately an hour after taking the drugs. If headache is severe, you may take aspirin or acetaminophen with the nitrate drug. Do not reduce drug dosage or take the drug less often to avoid headache; loss of effectiveness may occur.
- Keep family members or support people informed about the location and use of medications for heart disease in case help is needed.
- Avoid over-the-counter decongestants, cold remedies, and diet pills, which stimulate the heart and constrict blood vessels and thus may cause angina.
- Avoid alcohol with nitrate drugs. Both the drugs and alcohol dilate blood vessels, and an excessive reduction in blood pressure (with dizziness and fainting) may occur with the combination.
- Avoid concurrent intake of grapefruit juice with a metabolic modulator, as grapefruit juice increases serum drug levels.
- Several calcium channel blockers are available in both immediate-acting and long-acting (sustained-release) forms. It is extremely important that the correct formulation is used consistently.
- Keep all appointments with your healthcare provider.

Self- or Caregiver Administration

- Be aware that specific instructions for administration differ with the type of drug being taken.
- Take or give drugs for heart disease on a regular schedule, at evenly spaced intervals, to increase drug effectiveness in preventing acute attacks of angina. The only exception may be nitroglycerin transdermal paste, which you may be directed not to take at night.
- With nitroglycerin and other nitrate preparations:
  - Use according to instructions for the particular dosage form. The dosage forms were developed for specific routes of administration and are not interchangeable.
  - Take your blood pressure before administering the medication if possible, and anticipate that the drug can decrease blood pressure from the original reading. For sublingual nitroglycerin tablets, place them under the tongue until they dissolve. Take at the first sign of an anginal attack, before severe pain develops. If chest pain is not relieved in 5 minutes, dissolve a second tablet under the tongue. If pain is not relieved within another 5 minutes, dissolve a third tablet. If pain continues or becomes more severe, notify your healthcare provider immediately or report to the nearest hospital emergency room. Sit down when you take the medications. This may help relieve pain and prevent dizziness from the drug.
  - Do not take medications for erectile dysfunction when taking nitroglycerin and other nitrate preparations.
  - For the translingual solution of nitroglycerin, spray onto or under the tongue; do not inhale the spray.
  - Place transmucosal tablets of nitroglycerin under the upper lip or between the cheek and gum and allow them to dissolve slowly over 3 to 5 hours. Do not chew or swallow the tablets.
  - Use the measured paper for accurate nitroglycerin dosage and place the paper with the correct measured dosage of ointment on a nonhairy part of the upper body. Cover the area with plastic wrap or tape, rotate application sites (because the ointment can irritate the skin), and wipe off the previous dose before applying a new dose. Wash hands after applying the ointment.
  - Apply nitroglycerin patches and ointment at the same time each day to clean, dry, hairless areas on the upper body or arms. Note whether the directions require you to remove the patch or ointment at night. Rotate sites to decrease skin irritation. Avoid applying below the knee or elbow or in areas of skin irritation or scar tissue, as the drug is not well absorbed from distal portions of the extremities because of decreased blood flow. Dispose of used patches properly because there is enough residual nitroglycerin to be harmful, especially to children and pets.

(Continued on page 528)

BOX 28.2 Patient Teaching Guidelines for Drugs Used for Coronary Heart Disease (Continued)

- Take oral nitrates on an empty stomach with a glass of water. Oral isosorbide dinitrate is available in regular and sustained-release tablets. Do not crush or chew sustained-release nitrate tablets.
- Place sublingual isosorbide dinitrate tablets under the tongue until they dissolve.
- Stagger administration times if an oral nitrate and topical nitroglycerin are being used concurrently. This minimizes dizziness from low blood pressure and headache, which are common adverse effects of nitrate drugs.
- Report all new dietary supplements to the prescriber because some herbs interact with nitroglycerin.
- With beta-adrenergic blockers:
  - Do not stop taking the drug abruptly because this can cause rebound tachycardia and hypertension. If withdrawal of a beta-adrenergic blocker is planned by your prescriber, a gradual decrease in dose should occur, and you should limit physical activity to a minimum during this period.
  - Move slowly from a sitting to a standing position to avoid orthostatic hypotension.
- Learn how to take your own pulse and blood pressure, report heart rate less than 55 beats/min to your healthcare provider, and withhold medication as instructed. Take your pulse and blood pressure more frequently when the medication is initiated and titrated up or down.
- Be aware of possible adverse effects, including dizziness, wheezing, and low heart rate.
- Take atenolol at the same time each day and avoid drinking large amounts of orange juice.
- If you have diabetes, especially if you are prone to low blood sugar levels, you may need to check your blood sugar levels more frequently and eat consistently because beta-adrenergic blockers mask symptoms of low blood sugar.
- With calcium channel blockers:
  - Increase water and fiber intake as tolerated to decrease constipation.
  - Elevate your feet during the day to avoid ankle swelling.
  - Understand that sustained-release forms are usually taken once daily; do not take more often than prescribed and do not crush or chew.

produces systemic effects in approximately 30 minutes. Therapeutic effects last about 4 hours after PO administration. The effective PO dose is usually determined by increasing the dose until headache occurs, indicating the maximum tolerable dose. Sustained-release capsules also are available.

Isosorbide mononitrate is the metabolite and active component of isosorbide dinitrate. It is well absorbed after PO administration and almost 100% bioavailable. Unlike other PO nitrates, this drug is not subject to first-pass hepatic metabolism. Onset of action occurs within 1 hour, peak effects occur between 1 and 4 hours, and the elimination half-life is approximately 5 hours. It is used only for prophylaxis of angina; it does not act rapidly enough to relieve acute attacks.

Clinical Application 28.1

- Mr. Gerald returns to the clinic for follow-up. His blood pressure is 130/86 mm Hg, and his heart rate is 86 beats/min. He reports that he has been pain free since discharge. He is taking his atenolol as prescribed but reports that he is using the nitroglycerin patch four times a day around the clock because it is easier for his schedule. Given his vital signs, his provider increased the atenolol to 100 mg daily. Mr. Gerald asks the nurse why he needs to take atenolol at all, when he has no pain, and why the dose has been increased. How should the nurse respond? What patient teaching needs to be reinforced?

NCLEX Success

1. A 63-year-old patient continues to complain of chest pain, although the cardiac catheterization showed no significant cardiac disease. The patient notes that the chest pain occurs at the same time each night and typically during the cold weather. What kind of angina is the patient likely experiencing?
   A. stable angina
   B. unstable angina
   C. variant angina
   D. acute coronary syndrome

2. The nurse removes a patient's transdermal nitroglycerin disk at bedtime as ordered to minimize nitrate tolerance. The patient awakens during the night and complains of anginal symptoms. The nurse's action is to do which of the following?
   A. notify the healthcare provider
   B. apply a new transdermal disk
   C. obtain further history of complaints
   D. administer a short-acting nitrate as ordered

3. Concurrent use of nitrates in any form or route of administration with phosphodiesterase enzyme inhibitors produces which of the following?
   A. enhanced erectile potential
   B. significant tachycardia
   C. severe hypotensive effects
   D. mild bronchodilation

BETA-ADRENERGIC BLOCKERS

Beta-adrenergic blockers have become the cornerstone of drug therapy regimens for people with angina, MI, hypertension, heart failure, and dysrhythmias. They inhibit the chronotropic, inotropic, and vasoconstrictor responses to the catecholamines epinephrine and norepinephrine by exerting effects on the three adrenergic receptors (beta$_1$, beta$_2$, and alpha). In the cardiac system, these drugs decrease cardiac workload by slowing heart rate, decreasing blood pressure, and reducing contractility. The drugs are as effective as the organic nitrates in reducing the frequency and severity of anginal symptoms during exercise. People taking the drugs do not develop tolerance during therapy as occurs with the organic nitrates. When started early in patients with acute MI, without signs of heart failure or other hemodynamic instability, beta-adrenergic blocker therapy reduces infarct size and early mortality. Also, with long-term use, these drugs lower the risk of death.

The ability of a drug in this class to selectively block beta$_1$ receptors, principally found in the myocardium, is known as **cardioselectivity**. Therefore, cardioselective beta-adrenergic blockers, such as atenolol, metoprolol, bisoprolol, and esmolol, offer the potential advantage of not interfering with bronchodilation or peripheral vasodilation. In addition to beta$_1$-blockade, noncardioselective beta-adrenergic blockers block beta$_2$ receptors found in smooth muscle in the lungs, blood vessels, and other organs. Examples of noncardioselective beta-adrenergic blockers include propranolol, labetalol, nadolol, carvedilol, and timolol. Labetalol and carvedilol block both beta- and alpha-receptors, thereby decreasing peripheral and coronary vascular resistance. During beta-adrenergic blocker therapy, the beta receptors undergo receptor up-regulation. This means that the number of receptors on the surface of target cells (the beta cells) becomes more sensitive to catecholamines.

Beta-adrenergic blockers are discussed elsewhere in the text in relation to heart failure (see Chapter 30), dysrhythmias (see Chapter 27), hypertension (see Chapter 26), and glaucoma (see Chapter 59). Propranolol (Inderal), the first beta-adrenergic blocker available, is discussed in detail in Chapter 27 and is particularly useful in preventing exercise-induced tachycardia, which can precipitate anginal attacks. This chapter discusses ⓟ **atenolol** (Tenormin) and other beta-adrenergic blockers used to manage angina.

Pharmacokinetics

With PO administration, atenolol undergoes limited first-pass metabolism in the liver. Absorption is rapid and consistent but incomplete. Approximately only 50% of an oral dose is absorbed from the gastrointestinal (GI) tract. The drug is modestly (6% to 16%) bound to plasma, is distributed to the placenta, and is secreted in breast milk. It does not readily cross the blood–brain barrier. Peak blood levels occur between 2 and 4 hours after ingestion. With IV atenolol, onset of action is immediate, duration of action is dose dependent (half-life 6 to 7 hours), and peak blood levels are reached in 5 minutes. The drug is not metabolized and is excreted in the urine and feces.

Action

Atenolol is a cardioselective beta-adrenergic blocker. The cardioselectivity is diminished at higher doses, where it inhibits beta$_2$ receptors in the bronchial and vascular musculature.

Use

Atenolol is useful in the treatment of angina and hypertension as well as for the prophylaxis and treatment of MI. Healthcare providers use atenolol and other beta-adrenergic blockers in long-term management to decrease the frequency and severity of anginal attacks, decrease the need for sublingual nitroglycerin, and increase exercise tolerance. Evidence supports the use of a cardioselective beta-adrenergic blocker, such as atenolol, within the first 24 hours following an acute MI.

> **! Quality and Safety Alert: Safety**
>
> It is important to note that nonselective beta-adrenergic blockers should not be used in patients with variant angina because they are ineffective and may increase the tendency to induce coronary artery vasospasm.

Table 28.3 presents route and dosage information for atenolol and other beta-adrenergic blockers. The U.S. Food and Drug Administration (FDA) has issued a relating to the use of beta-adrenergic blockers in patients with CAD; abrupt withdrawal of oral forms may result in exacerbation of angina, increased incidence of ventricular dysrhythmias, MI, or death. Therefore, it is essential to slowly taper beta-adrenergic blockers before discontinuing them.

Patient-related variables specific to the use of atenolol and other beta-adrenergic blockers include the following:

- Age:
  - Older adults have a higher incidence of multivessel coronary disease, decreased left ventricular function, and comorbid conditions, making beta-adrenergic blockers one of the most frequently prescribed medications in this age group.
  - The incidence of sick sinus syndrome and chronotropic intolerance increases with age and predisposes older adults to bradycardia, syncope, and falls.
- Reproduction, pregnancy, and lactation:
  - Use of atenolol in pregnancy may cause harm to the fetus, including bradycardia, hypoglycemia, and reduced birth weight.
  - If use of a beta-blocker is needed during pregnancy, fetal growth should be monitored; in addition, the newborn should be monitored for 48 hours after delivery for bradycardia, hypoglycemia, and respiratory depression.
- Abnormal kidney function and hepatic impairment:
  - Atenolol is well tolerated in patients with abnormal kidney function, but dosage reduction may be necessary.
  - Beta-adrenergic blockers slow the deterioration of kidney function in chronic kidney disease.

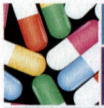

TABLE 28.3
DRUGS AT A GLANCE: Beta-Adrenergic Blockers

Drug	Routes and Dosage Ranges (Adults [Unless Indicated])
ⓟ **Atenolol** (Tenormin; ✺ Tenormin)	50 mg PO once daily, initially, increased to 100 mg daily after 1 wk, if necessary
Bisoprolol (✺ Apo-Bisoprolol, Ava-Bisoprolol)	5 mg PO once daily, initially, increased approximately every 3 d to 10 mg daily, then 20 mg once daily, if necessary
Carvedilol (Coreg, Coreg CR; ✺ Apo-Carvedilol, Auro-Carvedilol)	3.125 mg PO twice a day with food, initially, increased every 2 wk as needed and tolerated to 6.25–25 mg PO twice a day; maximum recommended dose, ≤85 kg: 25 mg twice daily, >85 kg: 50 mg twice daily Extended release, PO 10 mg once daily, initially, increased every 2 wk as needed and tolerated, maximum dose 80 mg/d
Metoprolol (Lopressor, Toprol XL, Kapspargo Sprinkle; ✺ Apo-Metoprolol)	100–450 mg PO daily in two to three divided doses Extended release, 100 mg PO daily in a single dose
Nadolol (Corgard)	40–240 mg PO daily in a single dose
Propranolol (Inderal, Inderal LA, Hemangeol, InnoPran; ✺ Inderal LA, Hemangiol)	80–3,200 mg/d PO in divided doses two to four times/day 0.5–3 mg IV every 4 h until desired response is obtained Extended release, 80 mg PO once daily, maximum dose 320 mg once daily

Adverse Effects

The major cardiac adverse reactions related to beta-adrenergic blockers such as atenolol include heart failure and substantial **negative chronotropy** (causing slowing of the heart rate). A small number of people with chronic heart failure may have an exacerbation of heart failure when they begin taking atenolol or other beta-adrenergic blockers. In these people, sympathetic drive is maintaining cardiac output. The beta-adrenergic blockers decrease this sympathetic drive and therefore cause a low cardiac output state and heart failure. The majority of patients with heart failure do benefit from beta-blockade, and symptoms of heart failure abate.

To manage the negative chronotropy, dosage adjustments may be necessary; the target heart rate should be 55 to 65 beats/min at rest. Use of beta-adrenergic blockers can lead to serious bradydysrhythmias and depression of the atrioventricular node. Noncardiac adverse effects include bronchospasm, especially in patients with chronic obstructive pulmonary disease (COPD) receiving high dosages because of beta$_2$ receptor blockade.

Note that many of the earlier signs of hypoglycemia are adrenergic warning symptoms (e.g., tremors, palpitation, tachycardia). Therefore, the use of beta-adrenergic blockers in patients with diabetes can mask the early warning symptoms of hypoglycemia.

Contraindications

Contraindications to atenolol include known hypersensitivity to the drug, second- or third-degree heart block, and cardiogenic shock, as well as severe bradycardia, heart failure, or hypotension. Caution is warranted with milder bradycardia, heart failure, or hypotension, and asthma.

Nursing Implications

Preventing Interactions

Many medications interact with atenolol, increasing or decreasing its effects (Box 28.3). Additionally, some herbs decrease the effects of atenolol including betel palm, calcium salts, and orange juice.

Administering the Medication

Prior to giving atenolol, the nurse should check the patient's vital signs. It is important to withhold atenolol and notify the prescriber for a resting heart rate of 60 beats/min and/or systolic blood pressure less than 90 mm Hg.

The nurse gives IV beta-adrenergic blockers over 2.5 minutes. Continuous telemetry is necessary for patients receiving an IV bolus or a continuous drip. The effectiveness of beta-adrenergic blockers in relation to relieving angina is dose dependent. It is necessary to titrate the dose of the beta-adrenergic blocker for a target heart rate of 50 to 60 beats/min with normal blood pressure. The nurse monitors the blood pressure every 5 minutes, while the drip is being titrated, and assesses for signs of bronchoconstriction at higher drug dosages where cardioselectivity may be lost.

Assessing for Therapeutic Effects

The nurse evaluates for three main objectives in the patient with chronic angina. One, the patient's frequency and severity of angina are reduced. Two, the patient has improved exercise capacity. Three, there is a reduction or elimination in the use of sublingual nitroglycerin. Ideally, achievement of these goals results in fewer adverse effects.

Assessing for Adverse Effects

The nurse closely monitors the patient's blood pressure and heart rate 2 to 4 hours after the first dose of atenolol. Signs of

> **BOX 28.3** **Drug Interactions: Atenolol**
>
> **Drugs That Increase the Effects of Atenolol**
> - Alcohol
>   Increases the risk of hypotension
> - Atazanavir, dolasetron, saquinavir
>   Increase the risk of heart block
> - Digoxin
>   Increases the risk of bradycardia
> - Diltiazem, verapamil
>   Increase the risk of bradycardia, heart block, and increased left ventricular end-diastolic pressure
> - Reserpine
>   Increases the risk of hypotension and significant bradycardia
> - Sildenafil, tadalafil, vardenafil
>   Increase the risk of life-threatening hypotension
>
> **Drugs That Decrease the Effects of Atenolol**
> - Adrenergic drugs (e.g., epinephrine, isoproterenol)
>   Reverse bradycardia
> - Anticholinergic drugs (e.g., diphenhydramine, ipratropium)
>   Increase heart rate, offsetting slower heart rates of atenolol
> - Indomethacin
>   Decreases the hypotensive effects

hypotension include dizziness and blurred vision; syncope is indicative of bradydysrhythmias. Increased shortness of breath and wheezing are adverse effects seen in patients with COPD who are taking noncardioselective beta-adrenergic blockers or high doses of cardioselective beta-adrenergic blockers. In patients with diabetes prone to hypoglycemia, more frequent assessment of serum glucose levels may be necessary.

Patient Teaching

Box 28.2 includes patient teaching information regarding drugs for the management of coronary heart disease, including atenolol.

Other Drugs in the Class

A variety of other beta-adrenergic blockers are used to treat stable angina.

Metoprolol (Lopressor, Toprol XL) is used alone or in combination with other medications to treat angina and hypertension. Like atenolol, metoprolol is cardioselective and improves survival after an MI. Extended-release tablets are used in the treatment of heart failure. The drug is lipid soluble and almost completely absorbed by the small intestine. Metoprolol has a short half-life, which allows for more rapid dose adjustments based on the patient's blood pressure and heart rate response. It is eliminated by hepatic metabolism and is excreted in the urine. It has a short plasma half-life. Adverse effects include bradycardia, hypotension, dizziness, fatigue, and impotence.

Bisoprolol is used to manage hypertension (see Chapter 26) in patients with stable angina. The drug reduces the workload of the heart and decreases myocardial oxygen demand by decreasing heart rate and the force of myocardial contractions. It is generally well tolerated, and adverse effects are mild and transient; they include nausea, diarrhea, dizziness, fatigue, impotence, bradycardia, and hypotension. At higher doses, the cardioselective properties are diminished, and bisoprolol can cause shortness of breath and wheezing. The drug can mask the early warning symptoms of hypoglycemia, like most of the other beta-adrenergic blockers.

Propranolol (Inderal) is used to reduce the frequency and severity of acute attacks of angina. It is especially useful in preventing exercise-induced tachycardia, which can precipitate anginal attacks. Caution is warranted with hepatic impairment. Nonselective beta-adrenergic blockers such as propranolol can slow down the process of glycogenolysis. Therefore, the occurrence of hypoglycemia increases. Beta-adrenergic blockers also can mask the early symptoms of hypoglycemia such as palpitations and anxiety due to blocked catecholamines. Propranolol is well absorbed after oral administration. It is then metabolized extensively in the liver; a relatively small proportion of an oral dose (approximately 30%) reaches the systemic circulation. For this reason, oral doses of propranolol are much higher than IV doses. Onset of action is 30 minutes after oral administration and 1 to 2 minutes after IV injection. It is important to instruct patients to take the drug at the same time each day, preferably with or immediately following meals, because food may enhance the bioavailability of propranolol. Erectile dysfunction and wheezing are common adverse effects. Also, patients should report shortness of breath, night cough, edema, slow pulse, confusion, depression, rash, fever, or sore throat. In addition, they should understand that propranolol should never be stopped abruptly. Cimetidine may increase beta-adrenergic blocking effects of propranolol by slowing its hepatic clearance and elimination.

Nadolol, which is also noncardioselective, has the same actions, uses, and adverse effects as propranolol, but it has a long half-life and can be given once daily. The drug is excreted by the kidneys, and it is necessary to reduce the dosage in patients with abnormal kidney function.

> **Clinical Application 28.2**
> - While reviewing his medication instructions with Mr. Gerald, the nurse learns that he has a history of erectile dysfunction and has some sildenafil, which was prescribed for him before his MI. What actions should the nurse take?

CALCIUM CHANNEL BLOCKERS

Calcium channel blockers are used to treat an assortment of cardiovascular disorders, including stable angina pectoris and variant angina. Other indications include hypertension, hypertrophic cardiomyopathy, and supraventricular dysrhythmias. There are two main categories of calcium channel blockers: the

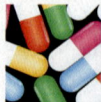

TABLE 28.4
DRUGS AT A GLANCE: Calcium Channel Blockers

Drugs	Routes and Dosage Ranges (Adults [Unless Indicated])
Nifedipine 🍁 Adalat XL, Nifedipine ER)	Angina: immediate release, 10–30 mg PO three times daily; sustained release, 30–60 mg PO once daily, maximum 120 mg/d Hypertension: sustained release only, 30–60 mg once daily, maximum 120 mg/d
Amlodipine (Katerzia, Norliqva, Norvasc; 🍁 Norvasc)	5–10 mg PO once daily
Diltiazem (Cardizem, Cardizem CD, Cartia XT, Matzim LA, Tiazac; 🍁 ACT Diltiazem CD, Apo-Diltiaz SR, Tiazac, Tiazac XC)	Angina or hypertension (immediate release): 30 mg PO four times daily initially, titrate over 1–2 d, usual dose 120–320 mg/d PO in four divided doses Hypertension (sustained release only): 180–240 mg PO once daily
Felodipine (🍁 Plendil, Sandoz-Felodipine)	Hypertension: 5–10 mg PO once daily
Isradipine	Hypertension: 2.5–5 mg PO twice daily
Nicardipine	Angina: immediate release only, 20–40 mg PO three times daily Hypertension: immediate release, same as for angina, above; sustained release, 30–60 mg PO twice daily
Verapamil (Calan SR, Verelan, Verelan PM; 🍁 Covera-HS, Verapamil Hydrochloride Injection, Verelan, Isoptin SR)	Angina: 80–160 mg PO three times daily, maximum dose 480 mg/d Dysrhythmias: 80–120 mg PO three to four times daily; injection, 5–10 mg IV over 2 min or longer, with continuous monitoring of electrocardiogram and blood pressure Hypertension: 120–360 mg/d PO in three divided doses or 240 mg PO (sustained release) once daily

dihydropyridines (nifedipine, amlodipine, nicardipine, nitrendipine) and the nondihydropyridines (verapamil and diltiazem). **Nifedipine** is the prototype.

Pharmacokinetics

Nifedipine is well absorbed after oral administration, with an onset of action of 20 minutes or less. It reaches peak plasma levels within 1 to 2 hours (6 hours or longer for sustained-release forms). Most of the drug is more than 90% protein bound. It undergoes extensive first-pass metabolism in the liver. Excretion occurs in the feces and urine.

Action

Nifedipine inhibits the influx of calcium entering through slow channels, producing vasodilation of the peripheral blood vessels and coronary arteries. However, the drug has a minimal effect on the sinoatrial and atrioventricular nodes. Therefore, it does not affect the heart rate.

Use

Nifedipine has been shown to be effective in the treatment for stable, variant, and unstable angina, mild-to-severe hypertension, and Raynaud phenomenon. Table 28.4 contains route and dosage information for nifedipine and other calcium channel blockers.

Patient-related variables specific to the use of nifedipine and other calcium channel blockers include the following:

- Age:
  - For primary hypertension, nifedipine and other long-acting calcium channel blockers are safe for use in children. They are especially useful in children who have asthma and cannot tolerate beta-adrenergic blockers.
  - Older adults are at higher risk for orthostatic hypotension and for falls while taking calcium channel blockers. Older adults may also have higher plasma concentrations of nifedipine due to decreased hepatic metabolism of the drug, probably because of decreased hepatic blood flow.
- Reproduction, pregnancy, and lactation:
  - An increase in perinatal asphyxia, retardation of intrauterine growth, cesarean delivery, and prematurity have been reported with use during pregnancy.
  - During pregnancy, oral nifedipine is the preferred drug to manage chronic and severe acute-onset hypertension.
  - Nifedipine is considered compatible with breast-feeding, although limited data are available regarding long-term use.
- Abnormal kidney function and hepatic impairment:
  - Dosage adjustment may be necessary with abnormal kidney function and hepatic impairment, and patients must be closely monitored for adverse drug effects.
  - In patients with cirrhosis, bioavailability of oral drugs is greatly increased, and metabolism (of both oral and parenteral drugs) is greatly decreased, causing an increased plasma levels of drug from a given dose (essentially an overdose).
- Specific healthcare environments:
  - In the home care setting, the nurse should check the patient's blood pressure and heart rate at each visit. Also, the nurse should note adverse effects of the drug and suggest measures to minimize fall risk.

Adverse Effects

With nifedipine, cardiac adverse effects due to excessive vasodilation include hypotension, flushing, headache, dizziness, lower limb edema, and reflex tachycardia; these appear to be dose related. Noncardiac adverse effects include constipation, nausea, and gingival hyperplasia.

Contraindications

Contraindications to nifedipine include known hypersensitivity to the drug. It is important not to use nifedipine in the treatment of angina related to overdose with cocaine, amphetamines, or other alpha-adrenergic stimulants. This leads to unopposed stimulation of alpha-adrenergic receptors, causing vasoconstriction and severe, life-threatening hypertension.

Nursing Implications

Preventing Interactions

Many medications interact with nifedipine, increasing or decreasing its effect (Box 28.4). People should not take grapefruit juice with nifedipine because a twofold increase in the effects of the drug may occur. Nifedipine may interact with quinidine, decreasing plasma levels, and digoxin, increasing levels.

Administering the Medication

People may take nifedipine with or without food. It is important not to crush or break sustained-release formulations. It is necessary to take the blood pressure prior to administering nifedipine and withhold the drug for a systolic blood pressure less than 90 mm Hg.

Assessing for Therapeutic Effects

The nurse should note a reduction of angina episodes once the patient has started taking nifedipine. Ideally, in general, the systolic blood pressure should be less than 120 mm Hg.

BOX 28.4   Drug Interactions: Nifedipine

Drugs That Increase the Effects of Nifedipine
- Cisapride, dolasetron, pimozide
  Increase risk of prolongation of QT interval, second- and third-degree heart block, and ventricular dysrhythmias
- Itraconazole
  Increases dose-related negative inotropic effect
- Cimetidine
  Increases peak plasma levels
- Tizanidine
  Increases the risk of hypotension

Drugs That Decrease the Effects of Nifedipine
- Calcium-containing products
  Saturate calcium channels
- Carbamazepine, phenytoin, rifampin
  Induce hepatic enzymes and increase the rate of metabolism

Assessing for Adverse Effects

The nurse should assess for excessive vasodilation. Symptoms include flushing, peripheral edema, and frequent headaches. Hypotension, dizziness, lightheadedness, weakness, peripheral edema, headache, heart failure, pulmonary edema, nausea, and constipation may also occur.

Patient Teaching

 Quality and Safety Alert: Safety

It is essential to teach patients to not stop taking nifedipine abruptly. This may result in rebound tachycardia and hypertension. Patients with coronary heart disease may have exacerbation of angina or acute ischemic events.

Box 28.2 outlines patient teaching guidelines regarding drugs for the management of coronary heart disease, including nifedipine.

Other Drugs in the Class

The other calcium channel blockers vary in clinical indications for use; most are used for stable angina or hypertension, and only diltiazem and verapamil are used to manage supraventricular tachydysrhythmias. In patients with CAD, the drugs are effective as monotherapy but are commonly prescribed in combination with beta-adrenergic blockers. In addition, nimodipine is approved for use only in subarachnoid hemorrhage, in which it decreases spasm in cerebral blood vessels and limits the extent of brain damage.

In variant angina, calcium channel blockers reduce coronary artery vasospasm. In atrial fibrillation or flutter and other supraventricular tachydysrhythmias, diltiazem and verapamil slow the rate of ventricular response. In hypertension, the drugs lower blood pressure primarily by dilating peripheral arteries.

The dihydropyridines used to treat angina besides nifedipine include amlodipine and nicardipine. Amlodipine (Norvasc) is effective in patients with exertional angina, because the drug reduces afterload decreasing myocardial oxygen demand. It is also used for the treatment of coronary spasm in variant angina. The drug is well absorbed by the PO route. Amlodipine has a long elimination half-life (30 to 50 hours) and therefore can be given once daily. Common adverse effects include peripheral edema, fatigue, dizziness, nausea, palpitations, and headache.

Nicardipine (Cardene) is a dihydropyridine calcium channel blocker used for the treatment of chronic stable angina (exertional), hypertension, and Raynaud phenomenon. The drug is available in oral and intravenous forms. The most common side effects are flushing, headaches, dizziness, and peripheral edema. The mechanism of action and clinical effects of nicardipine closely resemble those of nifedipine and the other dihydropyridines, amlodipine and felodipine, except that nicardipine is more selective for cerebral and coronary blood vessels.

Nondihydropyridines, such as diltiazem (Cardizem) and verapamil (Calan SR, Verelan), block the slow calcium channels in the heart. They also decrease the heart rate by slowing conduction through the atrioventricular node and decrease sinoatrial node automaticity. Chapter 27 describes them well.

Whereas nifedipine acts mainly on vascular smooth muscle to produce vasodilation, verapamil and diltiazem have greater effects on the cardiac conduction system. For this reason, these two drugs may also be used for supraventricular tachycardia. They are also effective in the treatment of angina, hypertension, and migraines. Diltiazem is a potent vasodilator of coronary and peripheral vessels, which decreases afterload and decreases workload on the heart. The drug has pharmacologic activity similar to verapamil, although diltiazem and verapamil differ chemically from the dihydropyridines and each other. Adverse effects include hypotension, bradycardia, dizziness, and flushing. Along with other calcium channel blockers, verapamil and diltiazem are known to induce gingival hyperplasia.

ADJUVANT MEDICATIONS

Ranolazine

The anti-ischemic metabolic modulator **ranolazine** (Ranexa) is an approved first-line treatment for chronic angina. However, the drug does not relieve acute angina symptoms and has not shown a benefit in acute coronary syndromes. Conventional antianginal drugs significantly decrease one or more of the determinants of myocardial oxygen demand, such as heart rate, preload, afterload, or myocardial contractility, thus reducing myocardial ischemia. Ranolazine increases the energy production of the heart to preserve cardiac function without decreasing blood pressure or heart rate, but it does not relieve acute anginal attacks and does not have any benefit in treating acute coronary syndromes. Although its mechanism of action is not clearly understood, ranolazine works by preventing both calcium overload and the subsequent increase in diastolic tension. This is all related to inhibition of the late inward sodium channel. Because this sodium channel frequently fails to inactivate in a number of important myocardial disease states such as ischemia and hypertrophy, excess entry of sodium ions leads to activation of the sodium–calcium exchanger, thereby raising calcium concentration. Unlike the other classes of antianginal drugs, ranolazine decreases ischemia but does not possess negative inotropic or chronotropic effects. When compared to placebo in patients with CAD, ranolazine is associated with a decreased frequency of ventricular dysrhythmias, bradycardia, and new-onset atrial fibrillation.

Ranolazine should be reserved for use in two groups of patients: (1) in those who have not had an adequate response to beta-adrenergic blockers or (2) in combination with the blockers for relief of symptoms when initial treatment with the blockers has not been successful. Ranolazine has a dose-dependent ability to prolong the QT interval. Therefore, the drug is contraindicated in patients with preexisting QT-interval prolongation. It is also contraindicated in patients with hepatic disease and in patients taking other drugs that prolong the QT interval. Dose reduction of digoxin and simvastatin may be necessary with concurrent use because ranolazine affects the metabolic pathways of these drugs. Table 28.5 gives route and dosage information for ranolazine.

> **! Quality and Safety Alert: Evidence-Based Practice**
>
> The routine use of oxygen in the setting of acute MIs has been common. However, evidence suggests that its use in patients with acute MI with normal oxygen saturations (≥94% on pulse oximetry) results in no significant difference in mortality when compared to patients breathing room air. Researchers have demonstrated that giving supplemental oxygen to patients without hypoxia does not lead to improved outcomes and has the disadvantages of discomfort of use and additional cost. Abuzaid and colleagues, in a 2018 meta-analysis of seven studies (n = 7,702), confirmed the lack of benefit of routine oxygen therapy in patients with acute MI with normal oxygen saturation levels.
>
> In a secondary analysis of an observational prospective cohort study, Abu-Jaradeh et al. (2019) focused on the safety of oxygen use during emergency transport to the hospital. Of the 2,065 patients enrolled in the parent study, 154 patients had a confirmed acute NSTEMI. The researchers found that in this sample, low flow oxygen at 2 to 6 L/min was not associated with excess risk of major adverse cardiac events in acute ST-elevation MI in the first 30 days, but there was an association with secondary myocardial injury in patients with NSTEMI that the authors suggest needs further investigation.
>
> These findings may result from the fact that hyperoxia has been shown to have a direct vasoconstrictive effect on the coronary arteries, which might occur with the administration of oxygen to patients with normal oxygen saturations.

Dyslipidemic Drugs

Dyslipidemic drugs (i.e., atorvastatin, cholestyramine, niacin) are useful in the management of patients with major risk factors for atherosclerosis and vascular disorders such as CAD, stroke, and peripheral arterial insufficiency when lifestyle changes alone do not reduce blood lipids. These drugs have proven efficacy, and healthcare providers are increasingly using them to reduce morbidity and mortality from coronary heart disease and other atherosclerosis-related cardiovascular disorders. Prescribers order dyslipidemic drugs to decrease blood lipids, prevent or delay the development of atherosclerotic plaque, promote the regression of existing atherosclerotic plaque, and reduce morbidity and mortality from cardiovascular disease. Chapter 10 discusses the dyslipidemic drugs in detail.

Antihypertensive Drugs

Antihypertensive drugs that decrease peripheral vascular resistance are useful in angina. Chapter 26 discusses antihypertensive drugs.

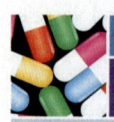

TABLE 28.5

DRUGS AT A GLANCE: Adjuvant Drugs

Drug	Pregnancy Category	Routes and Dosage Ranges (Adults)
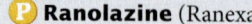 Ranolazine (Ranexa)	C	500 mg PO twice daily, if needed; maximum dose is 1,000 mg twice daily

Angiotensin-Converting Enzyme Inhibitors

Angiotensin-converting enzyme (ACE) inhibitors may be given to most patients routinely unless contraindicated, particularly in those with an anterior infarction, decreased left ventricular function, or heart failure. For those individuals who cannot tolerate an ACE inhibitor, an angiotensin receptor blocker can be given (see Chapter 26).

Aspirin

Aspirin produces an antiplatelet effect by irreversibly acetylating the active site of cyclooxygenase-1 (COX-1), which at lower doses effectively suppress platelet aggregation without affecting important endothelial cell functions. A growing body of evidence supports the use of aspirin in both primary and secondary prevention of cardiovascular events. However, in primary prevention, benefits may be outweighed by the risk of major bleeding. In secondary prevention, aspirin has been shown to substantially reduce mortality when administered during an evolving MI and should be given, unless contraindicated, as soon as possible after the onset of symptoms. The loading dose is 162 to 325 mg of uncoated aspirin; chewing or crushing the tablet establishes a high blood level quickly. Evidence suggests that long-term use of lower doses as opposed to higher dosages does not significantly affect cardiovascular outcomes and causes less risk of bleeding. With NSTEMI and STEMI, enteric-coated aspirin should be avoided initially because the enteric coating delays and reduces drug absorption. Chapter 16 contains additional information regarding aspirin.

Adenosine Diphosphate Receptor Antagonists

Clopidogrel and other adenosine diphosphate (ADP) receptor antagonists, prasugrel and ticagrelor, have antiplatelet effects similar to aspirin and inhibit the ADP (P2Y12) receptor on the surface of platelets. Clopidogrel has three shortcomings: delayed onset of action, irreversible inhibitory effects on platelets with no reversing agent or antidote, and significant individual variability in platelet response. Clopidogrel and ticagrelor are indicated for unstable angina and NSTEMI in patients who are to be treated medically or by planned primary PCI. Administering clopidogrel with aspirin (dual antiplatelet therapy) has been found superior to aspirin alone in decreasing the incidence of cardiovascular death and nonfatal MI—both acutely and for up to 9 to 11 months. Ticagrelor is used to reduce the rate of cardiovascular death, MI, and stroke in patients with a history of MI or acute coronary syndrome. The drug also decreases the rate of stent thrombosis in individuals requiring a stent for the treatment of acute coronary syndromes. Ticagrelor differs from clopidogrel and prasugrel in that receptor blockade is reversible. It is effective and relatively safe when compared to clopidogrel. The most recent data suggest that ticagrelor has broader applicability of use in individuals with acute coronary syndrome as compared to prasugrel. (However, prasugrel seems to be better tolerated.) In addition to aspirin, the ADP antagonists are usually continued for up to 12 months. Further information regarding the ADP receptor antagonists is found in Chapter 9.

Glycoprotein IIb/IIIa Receptor Antagonists

The glycoprotein (GP) IIb/IIIa receptor antagonists eptifibatide and tirofiban inhibit platelet aggregation by preventing activation of GP IIb/IIIa receptors on the platelet surface and the subsequent binding of fibrinogen and von Willebrand factor to platelets. The drugs are used occasionally in combination with heparin or aspirin to prevent clotting before and during invasive heart procedures in patients with NSTEMI. Antiplatelet effects occur during intravenous drug infusion and diminish once the drug is stopped. Additional discussion regarding the GP IIb/IIIa receptors antagonists is found in Chapter 9.

Morphine

Historically, morphine has been useful for relieving pain, reducing anxiety, and decreasing preload and remains a cornerstone in pain management in post-MI patients with unacceptable levels of pain (see Chapter 49). However, findings from the CRUSADE retrospective observational registry (57,039 patients with non–ST-elevation acute coronary syndrome) indicated that treating patients with morphine was associated with decreased survival. Although the exact cause of the negative outcome was not clear, Vaidya et al. (2019) suggested that morphine acts by interfering with the antiplatelet effect of the P2Y12 receptor blockers commonly given to this group of patients.

> **Quality and Safety Alert: Evidence-Based Practice**
>
> Interventions in acute MI are focused on the overall goal of prompt, complete, and sustained reperfusion of the myocardium. Interest in providing evidence-based decisions regarding management strategies that support that goal has given rise to concerns regarding morphine. One study found that the administration of morphine to patients following an NSTEMI increased the risk of death, although another study did not show any increase in adverse events with morphine use. Another study of patients following a STEMI indicated that morphine may interfere with platelet inhibition by disrupting the absorption of the antiplatelet drugs (P2Y12 inhibitors) and other medications. By impeding normal gastric activity, morphine may delay absorption and decrease peak plasma levels of orally administered drugs. Additional research is necessary to determine morphine's ongoing role in pain management following acute MI and whether the drug's effect on delaying the onset of antiplatelet effects could potentially result in early treatment failure in patients receiving antiplatelet drugs.

Thrombolytic Drugs

The purpose of giving thrombolytic agents following a STEMI is to dissolve thrombi and reestablish blood flow as quickly as possible, prevent or limit tissue damage, and maximize functional improvement. These drugs stimulate conversion of plasminogen to plasmin, a proteolytic enzyme that breaks down fibrin, the framework of a thrombus. In coronary circulation, restoration of blood flow reduces morbidity and mortality by limiting MI size. Maximal benefit is achieved when thrombolytic drugs are administered within the first 2 to 3 hours, especially within the first hour. In addition, anticoagulant drugs, such as heparin and warfarin, as well as antiplatelet agents are given following thrombolytic therapy to decrease reformation of a thrombus. Thrombolytic treatment is not recommended as treatment for an NSTEMI.

Alternately, PCI (also called percutaneous transluminal coronary angioplasty) together with certain drugs may be used to reestablish blood flow with a STEMI. Adjunctive therapy with PCI includes antiplatelet and antithrombotic therapy to reduce thrombotic complications. Generally, aspirin, an ADP receptor antagonist, and a GP IIb/IIIa inhibitor are given. Intravenous fractionated heparin is also administered during the PCI to prevent acute coronary closure during the procedure. The goal in both approaches is to minimize total ischemic time and restore blood flow. Therapeutic effects include reversal of symptoms, stabilization of cardiac rhythm, decrease of the ST-segment elevation by 50%, and absence of bleeding complications. Chapter 9 discusses thrombolytic drugs in detail.

NCLEX Success

4. A 72-year-old patient with angina pectoris, who is being discontinued from beta-adrenergic blockers, asks the nurse, "Why can't I just stop taking the drug today if it's not working anyway?" The nurse instructs the patient that failure to taper the drug slowly may lead to which of the following? (Select all that apply)
    A. worsening of her angina symptoms
    B. significant bronchoconstriction
    C. rebound hypertension
    D. acute ischemic event
    E. development of heart failure
    F. drug fever
    G. rebound tachycardia

5. In caring for a patient with chronic angina who has been prescribed the new drug, ranolazine, the nurse is correct in counseling which of the following about this drug?
    A. may be crushed if necessary
    B. must not be taken with beta-adrenergic blockers
    C. must not be taken with meals
    D. should not be taken with grapefruit juice

THE NURSING PROCESS

A concept map outlines the nursing process related to drug therapy considerations in this chapter. Additional nursing implications related to the disease process should also be considered in care decisions.

Assessment
- Assess the length of time and purpose for which patient is taking antianginal drugs (prophylaxis, treatment of acute attacks, or both). If the patient takes nitroglycerin, ask how often it is required, how many tablets are needed for relief of pain, how often the supply is replaced, and where the patient stores or carries the drug.
- Assess the frequency and duration of acute anginal attacks and whether either has increased recently. (An escalation could indicate worsening coronary atherosclerosis and increased risk of acute coronary syndromes.)
- Assess precipitating symptoms during an anginal event, such as chest pain or pressure (e.g., location, quality), shortness of breath, diaphoresis, nausea, and dizziness.
- Assess blood pressure and pulse, ECG reports, serum cholesterol, and cardiac enzymes.
- Assess whether previous invasive procedures were used to diagnose or treat CAD (e.g., cardiac catheterization, PCI, revascularization surgery).

Outcomes of Therapy

The patient will
- Receive or take drugs for coronary heart disease accurately.
- Experience relief of acute chest pain and other anginal symptoms.
- Have fewer episodes of acute chest pain and other anginal symptoms.
- Have increased activity tolerance.
- Identify and manage situations that precipitate anginal attacks.
- Be closely monitored for therapeutic and adverse effects, especially when drug therapy is initiated.
- Avoid preventable adverse effects.
- Verbalize essential information about the disease process, needed dietary and lifestyle changes to improve health status, and drug therapy.
- Identify available resources and support systems and demonstrate appropriate coping strategies.
- Recognize signs and symptoms that necessitate professional medical intervention.
- Keep appointments for follow-up care and monitoring.

Nursing Interventions
- Assist the patient to recognize and avoid precipitating factors (e.g., heavy meals, strenuous exercise) when possible.
- Support the patient while identifying resources, support systems, and effective coping strategies.
- Aid the patient during an acute event to manage symptoms of CAD:
  - Assume that any chest pain may be of cardiac origin.
  - Take a fast-acting nitroglycerin preparation (previously prescribed), up to three SL tablets or three sprays, each 5 minutes apart, as necessary.
  - If chest pain is not relieved with rest and nitroglycerin, assume that an MI has occurred until proven otherwise. In a healthcare setting, keep the patient at rest and notify the patient's prescriber immediately. Outside of a healthcare setting, call 911 for immediate assistance.
- Help the patient develop a more healthful lifestyle in terms of diet and weight control, adequate rest and sleep, regular exercise, and smoking cessation.
- Provide appropriate patient teaching related to drug therapy (see Box 28.2).

Evaluation
- Observe and interview for effective strategies used to relieve acute chest pain and frequency of symptoms.
- Identify CAD lifestyle factors that are being successfully modified or require modification (e.g., diet, weight, activity, smoking cessation).
- Observe effective coping strategies and appropriate use of support system and resources.
- Interview regarding success and adherence with drug therapy.
- Interview and observe for adverse drug effects.

Visit thePoint® at http://thePoint.lww.com/Frandsen13e for answers to NCLEX Success questions (in Appendix A), answers to Clinical Application Case Studies (in Appendix B), additional information on pathophysiology, and more!

REFERENCES AND RESOURCES

Abu-Jaradeh, O., Ahmad, A., Frisch, S. O., Farmand, Z., Landis, P., Mahmoud, A., Callaway, C. W., Martin-Gill, C., & Al-Zaiti, S. S. (2019). Abstract 11501: Supplemental oxygen is associated with larger infarct size but not excess risk of adverse cardiac events in non-ST elevation myocardial infarction. *Circulation (Ovid)*, *140*(Supplement 1), A11501.

Abuzaid, A., Fabrizio, C., Felpel, K., Al Ashry, H. S., Ranjan, P., Elbadawi, A., Mohamed, A. H., Barssoum, K., & Elgendy, I. Y. (2018). Oxygen therapy in patients with acute myocardial infarction: A systematic review and meta-analysis. *American Journal of Medicine*, *131*(6), 693.

Brumström, M., Thompoilos, C., Carlberg, B., Kreutz, R., & Mancia, G. (2021). Methodological aspects of meta-analyses assessing the effect of blood pressure–lowering treatment on clinical outcomes. *Hypertension*, *79*, 491–504.

Dennis, J. A., Zhang, Y., Zhang, F., Kopel, J., Abohelwa, M., & Nugent, K. (2021). Comparison of 30-day mortality and readmission frequency in women versus men with acute myocardial infarction. *Baylor University Medical Center Proceedings*, *34*(6), 668–672. https://doi.org/10.1080/08998280.2021.19453

Elmer, J., & Guyette, F. X. (2022). Early oxygen supplementation after resuscitation from cardiac arrest. *JAMA*, *328*(18), 1811–1813. doi: 10.1001/jama.2022.18620

Gulati, M., Levy, P. D., Mukherjee, D., Amsterdam, E., Bhatt, D., Birtcher, K. K., Blankstein, R., Boyd, J., Bullock-Palmer, R. P., Conejo, T., Diercks, D. B., Gentile, F., Greenwood, J. P., Hess, E. P., Hollenberg, S. M., Jaber, W. A., Jneid, H., Joglar, J. A., Morrow, D. A., ... Shaw, L. J. (2022). 2021 AHA/ACC/ASE/CHEST/SAEM/SCCT/SCMR Guideline for the Evaluation and Diagnosis of Chest Pain: A Report of the American College of Cardiology/American Heart Association Joint Committee on Clinical Practice Guidelines. *Journal of Cardiovascular Computed Tomography*, *16*(1), 54–122. https://doi.org/10.1016/j.jcct.2021.11.009

Lippincott advisor. (2022). http://advisor.lww.com

Rahimi, K., Bidel, Z., Nazarzadeh, M., Copland, E., Canoy, D., Ramakrishnan, R., Pinho-Gomes, A.-C., Woodward, M., Adler, A., Agodoa, L., Algra, A., Asselbergs, F. W., Beckett, N. S., Berge, E., Black, H., Brouwers, F. P. J., Brown, M., Bulpitt, C. J., Cushman, W. C., ... Davis, B. R. (2021). Pharmacological blood pressure lowering for primary and secondary prevention of cardiovascular disease across different levels of blood pressure: An individual participant-level data meta-analysis. *The Lancet*, *397*(10285), 1625–1636.

Stehli, J., Martin, C., Brennan, A., Dinh, D. T., Lefkovits, J., & Zaman, S. (2019). Sex differences persist in time to presentation, revascularization, and mortality in myocardial infarction treated with percutaneous coronary intervention. *Journal of the American Heart Association*, *8*(10), e012161. doi:10.1161/JAHA.119.012161

The Blood Pressure Lowering Treatment Trialists' Collaboration. (2021). Pharmacological blood pressure lowering for primary and secondary prevention of cardiovascular disease across different levels of blood pressure: An individual participant-level data meta-analysis. *Lancet*, *397*(10285), 1625–1636.

Thygesen, K., Alpert, J. S., Jaffe, A. S., Chaitman, B. R., Bax, J. J., Morrow, D. A., White, H. D., & Executive Group on behalf of the Joint European Society of Cardiology (ESC)/American College of Cardiology (ACC)/American Heart Association (AHA)/World Heart Federation (WHF) Task Force for the Universal Definition of Myocardial Infarction. (2018). Fourth universal definition of myocardial infarction. *Journal of the American College of Cardiology*, *72*(18), 2231–2264. doi:10.1016/j.jacc.2018.08.1038

Vaidya, G. N., Khan, A., & Ghafghazi, S. (2019). Effect of morphine use on oral P2Y12 platelet inhibitors in acute myocardial infarction: Meta-analysis. *Indian Heart Journal*, *71*(2), 126–135. https://doi.org/10.1016/j.ihj.2019.03.003

Wyckoff, M. H., Greif, R., Morley, P. T., Ng, K.-C., Olasveengen, T. M., Singletary, E. M., Soar, J., Cheng, A., Drennan, I. R., Liley, H. G., Scholefield, B. R., Smyth, M. A., Welsford, M., Zideman, D. A., Acworth, J., Aickin, R., Andersen, L. W., Atkins, D., Berry, D. C., ... Zelop, C. M. (2022). 2022 International Consensus on Cardiopulmonary Resuscitation and Emergency Cardiovascular Care Science With Treatment Recommendations: Summary From the Basic Life Support; Advanced Life Support; Pediatric Life Support; Neonatal Life Support; Education, Implementation, and Teams; and First Aid Task Forces. *Resuscitation*, *181*, 208–288. https://doi.org/10.1016/j.resuscitation.2022.10.005

CHAPTER 29

Drug Therapy for Shock and Hypotension

LEARNING OBJECTIVES

After studying this chapter, you should be able to:

1. Recognize the effects of cardiac output, preload, and systemic vascular resistance on hemodynamics.
2. Identify the predominant response to and tissue or organ affected by activation of adrenergic receptors and the relationship to patient symptoms.
3. Identify the prototype and describe the action, use, contraindications, adverse effects, and nursing implications of the adrenergic drugs.
4. Describe therapeutic and adverse effects of vasopressor drugs used in the management of hypotension and shock.
5. Implement the nursing process in the care of patients who need drug therapy for acute hypotension and shock.

CLINICAL APPLICATION CASE STUDY

Karsen Sexton, a 78-year-old man, lives alone. His daughter visits him twice a week. Today, she finds her father diaphoretic and disoriented, and she learns that he has had the flu for 3 days and has not been able to keep anything down orally. She calls 911, and Mr. Sexton is transported to the local medical center.

KEY TERMS

Chronotropic effect: causing a change in heart rate

Dromotropic effect: causing a change in speed of electrical conduction in the AV node of the heart

Inotropic effect: causing a change in myocardial contraction

Normotensive: having normal blood pressure

Pressor: effect that increases blood pressure

INTRODUCTION

Blood pressure is important because the various organs adapt to keep blood flowing at certain pressures (autoregulation). Homeostatic mechanisms, including autonomic reflexes, capillary fluid shifts, and variations in neurohormones, normally maintain blood pressure. When hypotension (abnormally low blood pressure) occurs, shock develops if the homeostatic mechanisms are unable to raise blood pressure to the normal range.

Shock is a physiologic continuum initiated by a precipitating event that results from compromised oxygen delivery, oxygen consumption, and/or oxygen utilization. Shock is initially reversible but must be identified and treated immediately to avoid progression to hypoxic injury to vital organs (e.g., brain, heart, kidneys). If untreated, shock causes inadequate flow of nutrients and oxygen to the cells, the inability to meet cellular metabolic needs and oxygen consumption requirements, and resultant cellular and tissue hypoxia and injury. If insufficient tissue perfusion continues, the cell reverts to anaerobic metabolic pathways for energy production, rapidly consuming cellular ATP stores, leading to difficulty regulating intracellular pH.

Acute hypotension is a clinical indicator of shock; therefore, its management will be considered in relation to the underlying cause of shock. This chapter discusses the pharmacologic management of patients who experience shock.

OVERVIEW OF ACUTE HYPOTENSION AND SHOCK

Shock is divided into four potential, although not necessarily exclusive, types based on the underlying cause: hypovolemic, cardiogenic, obstructive, and distributive. In each type, one or more circulatory mechanisms are compromised. Figure 29.1 illustrates how various factors are involved in the development of shock. To understand the role of drug therapy in supporting restoration of balance to these mechanisms, clinical considerations and clinical manifestations of shock must be understood.

Clinical Considerations

Identifying the etiology of shock is important because management varies among the four types and early correction of the underlying cause improves outcomes. In hypovolemic, cardiogenic, and obstructive shock, low cardiac output and inadequate oxygen transport are characteristic. In distributive shock, the main deficit lies in peripheral circulation, with decreased systemic vascular resistance and altered oxygen extraction. Distributive shock can be further divided, depending on cause, into three subtypes.

- Septic shock, the most common cause, is due to massive vasodilation caused by release of mediators of the inflammatory process in response to overwhelming infection. Almost any organism that gains access to the bloodstream can cause septic shock, but most often this kind of shock is associated with Gram-negative and Gram-positive bacteria and fungi.

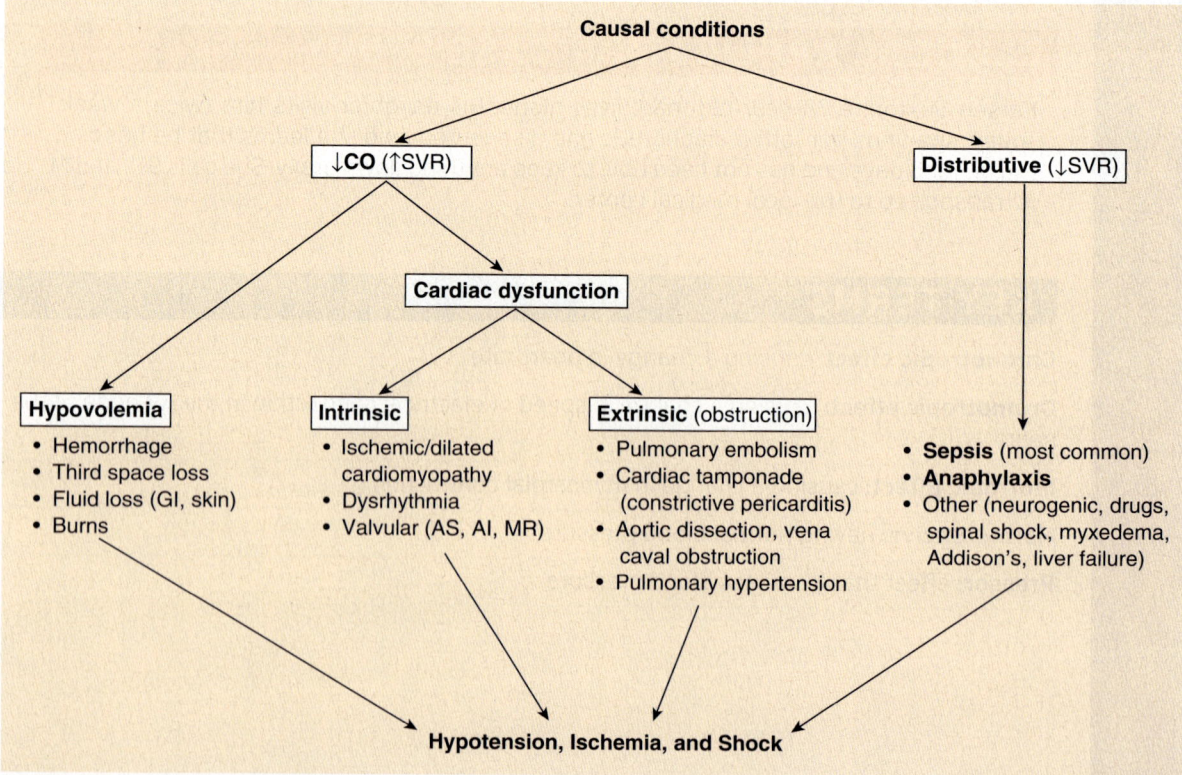

Figure 29.1. Impact of altered cardiac output and systemic vascular resistance on the development of hypotension, ischemia, and shock. AI, aortic insufficiency; AS, aortic stenosis; CO, cardiac output; GI, gastrointestinal; MR, mitral regurgitation; PE, pulmonary embolism; SVR, systemic vascular resistance. (Adapted with permission from Chowdhury, S. H., Cozma, A. I., & Chowdhury, J. H. [2017]. *Essentials for the Canadian medical licensing exam* [2nd ed., Fig. 3.4]. Wolters Kluwer.)

TABLE 29.1
Hemodynamic Profiles of Shock

Type of Shock	Clinical Measurements		
	Preload (Pulmonary Capillary Wedge Pressure, Central Venous Pressure)	Afterload (Systematic Vascular Resistance)	Contractility (Cardiac Output)
Hypovolemic	Decreased	Increased	Decreased
Cardiogenic	Increased	Increased	Decreased
Distributive	Decreased	Decreased	Increased or decreased
Obstructive	Decreased	Increased	Decreased

- Anaphylactic shock is due to massive vasodilation caused by release of histamine in response to a severe allergic reaction.
- Neurogenic shock is a result of massive vasodilation of the peripheral blood vessels from high-level spinal cord injuries.

Clinical Manifestations

Clinical symptoms vary with the stage and type of shock and the degree of impaired perfusion of vital organs. Systemic arterial hypotension is usually present, but the magnitude of the hypotension may appear to be only moderate depending on the patient's baseline blood pressure. In adults with **normotensive** blood pressure, the systolic arterial pressure is less than 90 mm Hg, or the mean arterial pressure is less than 70 mm Hg, with associated tachycardia. In individuals with hemodynamic monitoring in place (e.g., pulmonary artery catheter), a distinct profile emerges based on the type of shock (Table 29.1).

Stages of Shock

The first two stages of shock are more responsive to treatment and are more likely to be reversible. End-stage shock is associated with irreversible end-organ damage and death.

Compensated shock, also known as preshock, is characterized by compensatory responses activated in an attempt to reverse the condition. An increase in heart rate and peripheral vasoconstriction may be sufficient to allow a person to appear asymptomatic and preserve a normal blood pressure. Decreases in oxygen supply cause a short-term transition to anaerobic metabolism, which is unable to sustain ATP production and cellular health for a prolonged period. Symptoms may include tachycardia, change in blood pressure, and potential elevated serum lactate levels (a marker of cellular hypoxia). Prompt recognition and treatment at this stage can completely halt any progression.

Decompensated shock occurs if the condition persists as compensatory mechanisms become overwhelmed, and signs and symptoms of organ dysfunction appear. When cardiac output or blood pressure is too low for prolonged periods, or when cytokine levels are elevated, endothelial damage occurs, and microvascular thrombosis further impairs capillary blood flow. The patient's symptoms reflect that the body is unable to maintain perfusion any longer. Hypotension, symptomatic tachycardia, dyspnea, restlessness, diaphoresis, metabolic acidosis, oliguria, and cool, clammy skin occur. These signs and symptoms of organ dysfunction typically correspond to significant pathophysiologic alterations. With rapid, appropriate treatment, this stage of shock can be reversed.

Irreversible or *end-stage shock* begins to take a permanent toll on the body's organs and tissues and leads to irreversible end-organ damage and multiple organ failure. Overall, organ failure is further accelerated by prior injury or disease. During this stage, the kidneys shut down, and anuria and acute kidney disease develop. Lactic acidosis from anaerobic metabolism further depresses cardiac output and hypotension becomes severe and intractable to treatment. The end point of irreversible shock is death.

MANAGEMENT OF HYPOTENSION AND SHOCK

Initial efforts to reduce the effects of hypotension and shock involve identifying and treating the cause when possible. Management is focused on restoring adequate blood flow to the brain, heart, and kidneys. It may help to place the patient in a recumbent position; give blood transfusions, fluids, and electrolytes; and treat infections. If these measures are ineffective in raising the blood pressure enough to maintain perfusion to vital organs, adrenergic drugs may be used. The usual goal of drug therapy is to maintain tissue perfusion and a mean arterial pressure of at least 80 to 100 mm Hg.

ADRENERGIC DRUGS

Three adrenergic receptors ($beta_1$, $beta_2$, and alpha) are targets of catecholamines, predominately epinephrine and norepinephrine. In order to understand the varying roles adrenergic agonists play in shock, it is necessary to recognize the inherent responses to activation of the adrenergic receptors (Table 29.2). The physiologic sequelae of shock depend on the type(s) of adrenergic receptor activated in response and the number of affected receptors in a particular part of the body.

The usefulness of adrenergic drugs stems mainly from the effects of these drugs on the heart, blood vessels, and bronchi. They are often used as emergency drugs in the treatment of acute cardiovascular and respiratory collapse. In addition, adrenergic drugs are useful in the treatment of allergic reactions. Patients who benefit from these drugs include those in need of restoration of blood pressure in reversing types of hypotensive states.

Adrenergic drugs produce effects similar to those produced by stimulation of the sympathetic nervous system and therefore have widespread effects on body tissues. Some adrenergic drugs, such as norepinephrine, epinephrine, and dopamine, are exogenous formulations of naturally occurring neurotransmitters

TABLE 29.2
Action of Adrenergic Receptors

Adrenergic Receptor	Predominant Effect to Response Activation	Tissue or Organ Affected	Impact
Beta$_1$	Increased force of contraction	Heart	Positive inotropic effect
	Increased heart rate	Heart	Positive chronotropic effect
	Increased speed of electrical conduction	Heart	Positive or negative dromotropic effect
	Increased renin production	Kidneys	Increased blood pressure
Beta$_2$	Bronchodilation	Lungs	
	Vasodilation	Blood vessels	Decreased blood pressure
	Glycogenolysis and gluconeogenesis	Liver	Hyperglycemia for energy
	Decreased insulin secretion	Pancreas	
Beta$_3$	Lipolysis and increased release of free fatty acids into the blood	Adipose tissue	Generates energy
	Relaxation of smooth muscle	Uterus, urinary bladder, and gastrointestinal tract	
Alpha$_1$	Vasoconstriction	Blood vessels	Pressor/vasopressor effect
Alpha$_2$	Inhibition of release of norepinephrine into synapses of sympathetic nervous system	Surface membranes of target tissues and organs (presynaptic)	Antiadrenergic response in body

and hormones. Other adrenergic medications, such as phenylephrine, pseudoephedrine, and isoproterenol, are synthetic chemical relatives of naturally occurring neurotransmitters and hormones. The adrenergic drugs in this chapter are discussed in relation to their use in hypotension and shock. In many cases, a combination of drugs is used, depending on the type of shock and the patient's response to treatment. In an emergency, the drugs may be used to maintain adequate perfusion of vital organs until sufficient fluid volume is replaced and adequate circulation is restored. Additional discussion regarding adrenergic receptors and other adrenergic drugs that produce more localized therapeutic effects are discussed elsewhere (Chapters 31, 33, and 59).

Individual drugs are described in the following section, and indications for use and dosage ranges are listed in Table 29.3. **Norepinephrine** (Levophed) serves as the prototype adrenergic drug in the treatment of hypotension and shock.

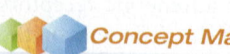
Concept Mastery Alert

Agonists work by activating the receptor to which they bind. Beta$_1$ agonists mimic the action of epinephrine and norepinephrine to raise blood pressure to counteract shock or hypotension.

Pharmacokinetics

Norepinephrine is administered via the intravenous (IV) route. Thus, it has an immediate onset of action with vasopressor duration of 1 to 2 minutes. The drug is metabolized via monoamine oxidase (MAO) and catechol O-methyltransferase, and it is excreted in the urine as inactive metabolites.

Action

Norepinephrine is a pharmaceutical preparation of the naturally occurring catecholamine norepinephrine. It has predominant alpha-receptor agonist effects and results in potent peripheral arterial vasoconstriction. As a result, it increases blood pressure more than it increases heart rate, force of contraction, or cardiac output. The drug is useful in cardiogenic and septic shock; however, the drug's effect in reducing kidney blood flow limits its prolonged use.

Use

Norepinephrine is used to treat severe hypotension and shock that persists after adequate fluid volume replacement. The drug is recommended as the first-choice vasopressor for the management of sepsis and septic shock.

> ### ! Quality and Safety Alert: Evidence-Based Practice
>
> In updated guidelines related to the management of sepsis (Evans et al., 2021), a consensus committee of 60 international experts recommend that initial resuscitation from hypoperfusion from sepsis include IV crystalloids within the first 3 hours of resuscitation and guided fluid resuscitation to maintain a mean arterial pressure of 65 mm Hg or higher. The guidelines recommend that if fluid therapy beyond the initial 30 mL/kg is necessary, small, repeated boluses of fluid should be administered that are guided by stroke volume and/or cardiac output parameters. The guidelines also recommend the use of norepinephrine over dopamine as a first-line drug for septic shock. Norepinephrine is a more potent vasoconstrictor, and in a systematic review and meta-analysis of 11 randomized controlled studies, norepinephrine also resulted in a lower mortality and lower risk of dysrhythmias compared to dopamine.
>
> Since sepsis and septic shock are medical emergencies, early recognition and resuscitation measures to manage the shock are critical to improved outcomes.

TABLE 29.3
DRUGS AT A GLANCE: Drugs Used for Hypotension and Shock

Generic/Trade Name	Adults	Children
Norepinephrine (Levophed; ✦ Levophed)	Hypotension and shock: IV infusion, 8–12 mcg/min initially, titrated to desired response; maintenance dose ranges from 2 to 4 mcg/min Postcardiac arrest: IV infusion, 0.1–0.5 mcg/kg/min initially, titrated to desired response Sepsis and septic shock: IV infusion, 0.01–3 mcg/kg/min	Hypotension and shock: IV infusion, 0.05–0.1 mcg/kg/min; titrated to desired effect; maximum 2 mcg/kg/min
Dobutamine (✦ Dobutrex, Dobutamine Injection, USP)	Cardiac decompensation: IV 0.5–1 mcg/kg/min initially, maintenance dose 2–20 mcg/kg/min, increased to maximum of 40 mcg/kg/min if necessary	Cardiac decompensation: same as adult dosage
Dopamine	Hemodynamic support: IV 5–10 mcg/kg/min initially, maintenance 2–20 mcg/kg/min, gradually increasing to maximum 50 mcg/kg/min Prepare by adding 200 mg of dopamine to 250 mL of IV fluid for a final concentration of 800 mcg/mL or to 500 mL IV fluid for a final concentration of 400 mcg/mL	Hemodynamic support: 2–20 mcg/kg/min, gradually increasing to maximum 50 mcg/kg/min
Epinephrine (Adrenalin, Auvi-Q, EpiPen; ✦ Adrenalin, Allerject, Anapen, EpiPen)	Anaphylaxis: IM (preferred), Sub-Q 0.2–0.5 mg using the 1 mg/mL solution; IV bolus 0.1 mg over 5–10 min using the 0.1 mg/mL solution, continuous infusion 2–15 mcg/min	IV infusion, 0.01 mcg/kg/min
Phenylephrine (Vazculep)	Hypotension and shock IV bolus: 100–180 mcg/dose every 10–15 min as needed not to exceed 500 mcg IV infusion: 100–180 mcg/min or alternatively 0.5 mcg/kg/min	Hypotension and shock IV bolus: 5–20 mcg/kg/dose q10–15 min as needed IV infusion: 0.1–0.5 mcg/kg/min Titrate to effects

Patient-related variables specific to the use of norepinephrine and other adrenergic drugs include the following:

- Age:
  - Norepinephrine is used in children to treat refractory septic shock and persistent pulmonary hypertension.
  - Children are very sensitive to drug effects, including cardiac and central nervous system stimulation, and recommended doses usually should not be exceeded.
  - Norepinephrine must be used with caution in older adults, but its benefit could outweigh any potential risk.
  - Since older adults often have chronic cardiovascular conditions (e.g., angina, dysrhythmias, heart failure, coronary artery disease, hypertension, peripheral vascular disease) that are aggravated by adrenergic drugs, careful monitoring by the nurse is required.
- Reproduction, pregnancy, and lactation:
  - Norepinephrine crosses the placenta.
  - Appropriate administration of norepinephrine and other adrenergic drugs should not be withheld due to concerns of fetal teratogenicity.
  - It is not known if norepinephrine is present in breast milk.
  - Caution is warranted in patients who are breast-feeding.
- Abnormal kidney function and hepatic impairment:
  - Norepinephrine warrants cautious use in patients with kidney failure.
  - The alpha$_1$ activity of norepinephrine causes constriction of renal arteries, thereby diminishing kidney blood flow and urine production.
  - Older adults with kidney disease may not be able to eliminate many adrenergic drugs, causing accumulation of the drug and increased risk of adverse effects.
- Blood flow through the liver is decreased by alpha$_1$ activity of norepinephrine, causing increased hepatic arteriolar and venous resistance, leading to reduced oxygen delivery to the liver.
- Specific healthcare environments:
  - Norepinephrine and other adrenergic drugs are important emergency drugs that may complicate the already complex care of patients who are critically ill.

Adverse Effects

Norepinephrine and other adrenergic drugs can cause significant adverse effects, including the following:

- Possible diminished kidney perfusion and decreased urine output due to vasopressor action

- Possible decreased perfusion to the liver, with subsequent liver damage due to vasopressor action
- Possible irritable cardiac dysrhythmias due to beta$_1$ activity
- Possible increase in myocardial oxygen requirement due to beta$_1$ activity
- Hyperglycemia, hypokalemia, and hypophosphatemia due to beta$_1$ activity
- Severe hypertension and reflex bradycardia
- Limb ischemia due to profound vasoconstriction
- Extravasation at infusion site

> ** Quality and Safety Alert: Safety**
>
> Note that the U.S. Food and Drug Administration (FDA) has issued a **BOXED WARNING** ◆ regarding the potential risk of tissue damage with extravasation of norepinephrine. The drug should be infused into a large vein or central line if possible. The use of leg veins should be avoided in older adults and in those with occlusive disorders. If extravasation occurs, diluted phentolamine should be injected into the area with a small-gauge hypodermic needle as soon as possible to prevent sloughing and necrosis of the tissue.

Contraindications

Contraindications to using norepinephrine include cardiac dysrhythmias, angina pectoris, hypertension, hyperthyroidism, and cerebrovascular disease; stimulation of the sympathetic nervous system worsens these conditions. Narrow-angle glaucoma is a contraindication, because the drugs result in mydriasis, closure of the filtration angle of the eye, and increased intraocular pressure. Hypersensitivity to an adrenergic drug or any component is also a contraindication. For example, the norepinephrine trade preparation Levophed contains sulfites, to which some people may be allergic. However, the generic equivalent does not contain preservatives.

> **NCLEX Success**
>
> 1. When giving a drug with beta$_1$ agonist activity, the nurse knows that which of the following would provide therapeutic benefit? (Select all that apply.)
>   A. vasoconstriction and elevation of the blood pressure
>   B. relaxation of bronchial smooth muscle and bronchodilation
>   C. elevated heart rate and improved force of myocardial contraction
>   D. uterine contraction and induction of labor
>
> 2. The nurse teaches the patient with diabetes who is using adrenergic medications to anticipate which of the following?
>   A. no change in blood glucose levels
>   B. a decrease in blood glucose levels
>   C. an increase in blood glucose levels
>   D. more fluctuation in blood glucose levels
>
> 3. During administration of dopamine, a patient complains of pain at the infusion site. The nurse should recognize which of the following?
>   A. Patient is hypersensitive to the drug, and infusion should be stopped.
>   B. Infusion rate is too fast and should be slowed.
>   C. Medication should be stopped, phentolamine should be infused, and the infusion site should be changed.
>   D. Medication is probably not effective; therefore, patient response should be assessed once all the medication is infused.

Nursing Implications

Preventing Interactions

Remember that norepinephrine reuptake is the major way that sympathetic nerve transmission is terminated. Drugs such as tricyclic antidepressants block norepinephrine reuptake, resulting in stimulation of alpha- and beta-adrenergic receptors. Concurrent use of MAO inhibitors and adrenergic drugs may lead to cardiac dysrhythmias, respiratory depression, and acute hypertensive crisis, with possible intracranial hemorrhage, convulsions, coma, and death. Therefore, MAO inhibitors must not be given with norepinephrine and other adrenergic drugs.

Many other medications interact with norepinephrine, increasing or decreasing its effects (Box 29.1).

Administering the Medication

Administration of norepinephrine should occur through a large vein or on an infusion pump, with titration as ordered to achieve the desired therapeutic response. Close nursing observation and monitoring during drug therapy is essential. Emergency and resuscitative equipment and other drugs should be immediately available to manage any adverse effects.

Assessing for Therapeutic Effects

The nurse should observe signs of adequate tissue perfusion, including a mean arterial pressure of at least 65 mm Hg, heart rate less than 100 beats/min, unlabored breathing, and serum lactate levels and arterial blood gases within normal limits. In addition, urine output should be greater than 30 mL/h. There should be normal mentation; oxygen saturation by pulse oximetry greater than 90%; no dyspnea; and warm, dry skin with no signs of diminished perfusion. Laboratory values (blood urea nitrogen [BUN], creatinine, serum lactate level, aspartate aminotransferase [AST], alanine aminotransferase [ALT], and lactate dehydrogenase [LDH]) should be within normal limits. In addition, with septic shock, the patient should be afebrile with return of the white blood cell count to within normal limits.

Assessing for Adverse Effects

The nurse should assess for signs of complications of vasopressor activity, including diminished kidney perfusion, decreased urine output, decreased liver perfusion, and limb ischemia. The patient should be observed for cardiac dysrhythmias, signs of increased myocardial oxygen requirements, hyperglycemia, hypokalemia, and hypophosphatemia due to beta$_1$ activity.

BOX 29.1 Drug Interactions: Norepinephrine and Other Adrenergic Drugs

Drugs That Increase the Effects of Norepinephrine and Other Adrenergic Drugs

- Anesthetics, general (e.g., propofol), cocaine
  Increase the risk of ventricular irritability, serious cardiac dysrhythmias, or death
- Anticholinergics (e.g., atropine)
  Increase the risk of ventricular dysrhythmias
- Antihistamines, tricyclic antidepressants (e.g., amitriptyline, imipramine), beta-adrenergic blocking agents (e.g., propranolol [Inderal]), doxapram (Dopram), methylphenidate (Ritalin)
  Increase the pressor effect
- Digoxin
  Increases the risk of dysrhythmias
- Ergot alkaloids
  Increase blood pressure and ischemic response
- Monoamine oxidase (MAO) inhibitors (e.g., isocarboxazid [Marplan]); xanthines (in caffeine-containing substances, such as coffee, tea, cola drinks, and theophylline)
  Increase heart rate and blood pressure

Drugs That Decrease the Effects of Norepinephrine and Other Adrenergic Drugs

- Anticholinesterases (e.g., neostigmine, pyridostigmine [Mestinon]) and other cholinergic drugs
  Decrease the effects of norepinephrine
- Antipsychotic drugs (e.g., haloperidol [Haldol]), chlorpromazine
  Paradoxically decrease blood pressure
- Phenothiazines, phentolamine
  Inhibit or reverse the pressor effect

Ongoing assessment of blood pressure and heart rate is critical to avoid severe hypertension and reflex bradycardia. Monitoring the infusion site diligently for infiltration is essential.

Clinical Application 29.1

Mr. Sexton's vital signs are temperature 97°F, pulse 122/min and regular, respirations 28/min, and blood pressure 76/52 mm Hg. His arterial blood gases are pH 7.12, O_2 76 mm Hg, CO_2 30 mm Hg, HCO_3 20 mmol/L, and O_2 saturation 78%. He is in hypovolemic shock, and a physician in the emergency department administers a 1,000-mL normal saline (NS) bolus and starts him on 35% oxygen by face mask.

Within 15 minutes of the start of the fluid bolus, Mr. Sexton is agitated and flushed and complains of palpitations. His vital signs have not improved, and he receives an additional fluid bolus. His blood pressure increases to 80/50 mm Hg, and his heart rate is 118 beats/min after receiving 2,000 mL of NS. His physician then orders an additional 1,000 mL of NS. A nurse gives him IV norepinephrine 8 mcg/min, titrated to a systolic blood pressure greater than 90 mm Hg after receiving the 3 L of IV fluids.

- What are the nursing implications for this patient's reaction to the fluid challenge?
- What assessment is needed relative to the therapeutic and adverse effects of norepinephrine?

Patient Teaching

Patients who are recovering from critical illness will likely have different needs and may require additional services on discharge than they had prior to the shock experience. The nurse should facilitate opportunities to have the patient and family participate in the goal setting and plan of care for discharge as possible.

! Quality and Safety Alert: Teamwork and Collaboration

Before discharge, the interprofessional team should assess the:

- Nature and complexity of posthospital care needs (e.g., patient safety, infection control)
- Impact of the patient's illness on the lifestyle of family or other caregiver and necessary interventions
- Readiness and availability of family or other caregiver to assist with the patient's care needs at home during recovery
- Availability of community or other healthcare resources to assist with care
- Need for special equipment, supplies, or medication

Additional patient teaching guidelines for adrenergic drugs used to manage hypotension and shock, including norepinephrine, are outlined in Box 29.2.

Other Drugs in the Class

Epinephrine (Adrenalin) is a naturally occurring catecholamine produced by the adrenal glands. Epinephrine is an agonist of $alpha_1$, $beta_1$, and $beta_2$ receptors. It can increase the mean arterial pressure by increasing the cardiac index and stroke volume, as well as systemic vascular resistance and heart rate. At low doses, epinephrine stimulates beta receptors, which increases cardiac output by increasing the rate and force of myocardial contractility. It also causes bronchodilation. Larger doses act on alpha receptors to increase blood pressure through vasoconstriction, although its effect of systemic vascular resistance is less than norepinephrine.

In hypotension and shock, epinephrine is administered intravenously. This route has an instant onset, a peak of 20 minutes, and a duration of 20 to 30 minutes. Epinephrine's ability to stimulates $beta_1$ adrenergic receptors in the heart results in positive **inotropic** (increases contractility of the heart), **chronotropic** (increases heart rate), and **dromotropic** (increases speed of conduction through the AV node of the heart) effects. The positive effects produce an increase in blood pressure, tachycardia, hyperglycemia, bronchodilation, and vasoconstriction of arterioles in the skin, mucosa, and most viscera. Most epinephrine is rapidly metabolized in the liver to inactive metabolites, which are then excreted in the urine. The remaining epinephrine is deactivated by reuptake at synaptic receptor sites. Epinephrine

BOX 29.2 Patient Teaching Guidelines for Hypotension and Shock

General Considerations

- Healthcare professionals use adrenergic drugs for short periods in the hospital setting to treat hypotension and shock. Although you will not be discharged on these drugs, patient teaching is aimed at supporting your recovery and preventing the condition from reoccurring.
- If you are receiving IV adrenergic drugs to stimulate your heart or raise your blood pressure, frequent cardiac monitoring and checks of flow rate, blood pressure, and urine output are necessary. These measures increase the safety and benefits of drug therapy. Ask your nurse if you have concerns about your condition or questions about your drug regimen.
- Report adverse reactions such as fast pulse, palpitations, and chest pain so that drug dosage can be reevaluated and therapy changed if needed.

Self-Administration

- Specific considerations for types of shock are addressed below.

For Hypovolemic Shock (Depending on What Caused the Volume Loss)

- Seek help for signs of shock (weak, rapid pulse; cool, clammy skin; faintness, postural dizziness, nausea) if you experience them again.
- Learn how to take your own pulse and blood pressure, and report heart rate greater than 100 beats/min to your healthcare provider. Take your pulse and blood pressure more frequently when you are not feeling well.
- If you have trouble keeping liquids down or have increased diarrhea, notify your healthcare provider.
- If you see blood in your urine or stool, or if you are coughing up blood, contact your healthcare provider.
- Stay hydrated when you are sick or exercising.

For Cardiogenic Shock

- Take care to prevent another heart attack because it is important in avoiding cardiogenic shock.
- Seek prompt medical attention when you experience symptoms of a heart attack.
- Keep family members or support people informed about the location and use of antianginal medications in case you need help.
- Avoid over-the-counter decongestants, cold remedies, and diet pills, which stimulate the heart and constrict blood vessels and thus may cause angina.
- Learn how to take your own pulse and blood pressure, report heart rate less than 55 beats/min to your healthcare provider, and withhold medication as instructed. Take your pulse and blood pressure more frequently when the medication is initiated and titrated up or down.

For Septic Shock

- Avoid contact with people who are sick. Take care to prevent infection (get vaccinated, avoid spread of germs).
- If you are discharged on antibiotics, finish the full course of antibiotics and seek medical attention if adverse effects develop or signs of infection reoccur.

For Anaphylactic Shock

- Learn to self-administer an injection of epinephrine if you have severe allergies. Always carry your injection kit with you. Seek immediate medical care after self-injection of epinephrine.
- If you have a food allergy, always ask about ingredients when eating food prepared by others. At a restaurant, tell your server about your food allergies.
- Wear a medical identification bracelet with the information about your allergy.
- If you have diabetes, monitor your glucose levels carefully because adrenergic medications may elevate them.

---

decreases the splanchnic blood flow and may increase oxygen delivery and consumption. Administration may be associated with an increase in serum lactate levels.

Quality and Safety Alert: Safety

Ratio expressions of epinephrine concentrations are now prohibited on drug labels, and the metric system is now the expected method for expressing the strength of epinephrine.

Epinephrine is the adrenergic drug of choice for relief of anaphylactic shock, the most serious allergic reaction. People susceptible to severe allergic responses should always carry a syringe of epinephrine. EpiPen and EpiPen Jr are prefilled, autoinjection syringes for intramuscular self-administration of epinephrine in emergency situations (see Chapter 33). Epinephrine is also used as treatment of cardiac arrest (see Chapter 27). In addition, epinephrine is used as an additive to local anesthetics for vasoconstrictive effects, which include prolonging the action of the local anesthetic drug, preventing systemic absorption, and minimizing bleeding.

Dopamine, a naturally occurring precursor of norepinephrine and epinephrine, functions as a neurotransmitter. Its action is dose dependent and can stimulate alpha, beta, or dopaminergic receptors, depending on the dose being used. In addition, dopamine acts indirectly by releasing norepinephrine from sympathetic nerve endings and the adrenal glands. At low doses (1 to 5 mcg/kg/min), increased kidney blood flow and urine output occur. At doses greater than 10 mcg/kg/min, stimulation of beta receptors takes place, and there is an increase in heart rate, myocardial contractility, and blood pressure. At the highest doses (20 to 50 mcg/kg/min), beta activity continues, but increasing alpha stimulation (vasoconstriction) may overcome its actions. Undesirable effects at higher doses are tachycardia and increased pulmonary shunting, as well as the potential for decreased splanchnic perfusion and increased pulmonary arterial wedge pressure. If dosages of dopamine exceeding 20 to 30 mcg/kg/min are needed, a more direct-acting vasopressor, such as epinephrine or norepinephrine, may be more beneficial. Dopamine is useful in hypovolemic and cardiogenic shock. Adequate fluid therapy is necessary for maximal **pressor** (increased blood pressure) effect. Acidosis decreases the effectiveness of the drug.

Dobutamine is a sympathomimetic agent and $beta_1$-receptor agonist, although it has some $beta_2$-receptor and minimal alpha-receptor activity. It was developed to provide less vascular activity than dopamine. Dobutamine acts on $beta_1$ receptors in the heart to increase the force of myocardial contraction with a minimal increase in heart rate. In general, at usual doses, it is less likely to cause tachycardia, dysrhythmias, and significant increases in myocardial oxygen consumption than dopamine.

Dobutamine is most useful in cases of shock that require increased cardiac output without the need for blood pressure support. Caution is warranted when administering the drug in patients with moderate or severe hypotension (e.g., systolic blood pressure less than 80 mm Hg), because the peripheral vasodilation may cause a further fall in blood pressure. However, it may increase blood pressure with large doses. In patients with an acute myocardial infarction, dobutamine may increase infarction size because of the potential for increases in myocardial oxygen consumption when oxygen supply is compromised. In addition, it may be useful for short-term management of patients experiencing cardiac decompensation who have not responded to medical therapy while awaiting heart transplant or mechanical circulatory support.

Dobutamine has a short plasma half-life and therefore requires administration by continuous IV infusion. A loading dose is not necessary because the drug has a rapid onset of action and reaches steady state within approximately 10 minutes after the infusion is begun. It is rapidly metabolized to inactive metabolites.

Phenylephrine (Vazculep) is a synthetic adrenergic drug that stimulates alpha-adrenergic receptors to produce vasoconstriction. As a result, it constricts arterioles and raises systolic and diastolic blood pressures. Phenylephrine resembles epinephrine but has fewer cardiac effects and a longer duration of action. Vasoconstriction decreases cardiac output and kidney perfusion and increases peripheral vascular resistance and blood pressure. There is little cardiac stimulation because phenylephrine does not activate $beta_1$ receptors in the heart or $beta_2$ receptors in blood vessels. The drug is excreted primarily in the urine.

Phenylephrine may be given to increase blood pressure in hypotension and shock. Compared with norepinephrine, phenylephrine produces longer-lasting elevation of blood pressure (20 to 50 minutes with injection). When given systemically, phenylephrine produces a reflex bradycardia. This effect may be used therapeutically to relieve paroxysmal atrial tachycardia.

However, other medications such as calcium channel blockers (see Chapters 26 and 27) are more likely to be used for this purpose. As with norepinephrine, reduction of kidney and mesenteric blood flow limits prolonged use. The FDA has issued a **BOXED WARNING** ◆ for parenteral use of Neo-Synephrine that alerts prescribers to be familiar with complete prescribing information before use.

NCLEX Success

4. A patient in cardiogenic shock is started on dobutamine. The healthcare provider's order reads dobutamine 10 mcg/kg/min IV. What effect should the nurse expect after beginning drug therapy?
   A. enhanced cardiac contraction and contractility via stimulation of $alpha_1$, $beta_1$, and $beta_2$ receptors
   B. dilated blood vessels via stimulation of dopamine receptors
   C. increased cardiac output through stimulation of $beta_1$ receptors
   D. constricted blood vessels and increased cardiac output through stimulation of $alpha_1$ receptors

5. A patient receiving norepinephrine for shock has an arterial line in place. The patient's blood pressure has been near 90/42 mm Hg for most of the morning. The blood pressure reading on the continuous monitor suddenly shows a blood pressure of 130/80 mm Hg. The nurse should do which of the following?
   A. decrease the rate of the norepinephrine
   B. call the healthcare provider
   C. stop the norepinephrine infusion
   D. confirm the blood pressure with a manual reading

Clinical Application 29.2

After 1 hour on the norepinephrine IV infusion, Mr. Sexton's blood pressure is 92/52 mm Hg. His urine output is 30 mL/h. His oxygen saturation is 92% on 40% face mask. He is able to appropriately answer questions when aroused and his skin is warm and dry. The patient's heart rate is 96 beats/min and regular. What are the appropriate actions by the nurse?

THE NURSING PROCESS

A concept map outlines the nursing process related to drug therapy considerations in this chapter. Additional nursing implications related to the disease process should also be considered in care decisions.

Assessment

- Assess the patient's condition in relation to hypotension and shock.
- Check blood pressure; heart rate; urine output; skin temperature and color of extremities; level of consciousness; orientation to person, place, and time; and adequacy of respiration. In general, report blood pressure less than 90 mm Hg systolic, mean blood pressure greater than 65 mm Hg, heart rate greater than 100 beats/min, and urine output less than 30 mL/h.
- Assess electrocardiogram and cardiac status for alterations in rhythm or rate.
- Monitor and optimize hemodynamic status, noting and acting on indications of impaired cardiac function. Observe the trend in mixed venous oxygen saturation (SVO_2), stroke index (SI), cardiac index (CI), pulmonary artery occlusive pressure (PAOP), and central venous pressure (CVP) values for effectiveness of treatments and indications for progress of patient toward goals.
- Monitor available laboratory reports for abnormal values. Decreased oxygen saturation levels indicate decreased oxygenation of tissues; abnormal arterial blood gases may indicate metabolic acidosis; an increased hematocrit may indicate hypovolemia; an increased eosinophil count may indicate anaphylaxis; the presence of bacteria in blood cultures may indicate sepsis; and increased serum creatinine and blood urea nitrogen may indicate impending renal failure.

Outcomes of Therapy

The patient will
- Show improvement in tissue perfusion and relief of symptoms.
- Show improved hemodynamic status.
- Guard against recurrence of hypotension and shock, if possible.
- Assess for therapeutic and adverse effects of adrenergic drugs.
- Avoid preventable adverse effects of adrenergic drugs.

Nursing Interventions

- Use measures to prevent or minimize hypotension and shock.
- Recognize impending shock so management can be initiated early.
- Recognize and manage the underlying cause of shock in a particular patient (e.g., replacing fluids; preventing further loss of blood or other body fluids).
- Monitor patients during shock and vasopressor drug therapy.
- Titrate adrenergic drug infusions to maintain blood pressure and tissue perfusion without causing hypertension.
- Check hemodynamic indices (including SVO_2, SI, CI, PAOP, and CVP) every hour and blood pressure and pulse constantly or at least every 5 to 15 minutes during acute shock and titration of vasopressor drug therapy. Intra-arterial monitoring is more reliable than cuff blood pressure measurements in shock conditions.
- Monitor mental status, distal pulses, urine output, and skin temperature and color closely to assess tissue perfusion.
- If possible, administer all vasoactive medications via a central access line. Assess venipuncture sites frequently for signs of infiltration or extravasation. If peripheral sites are used, have phentolamine (Regitine), an alpha-adrenergic blocking agent that reverses vasoconstriction, readily available in any setting where IV adrenergic drugs are used. If infiltration occurs, instill phentolamine through the IV catheter prior to removal. If catheter has been removed, phentolamine may be administered subcutaneously, around the area of extravasation.
- Keep family members informed about patient status and management measures.
- When administering substances known to produce hypersensitivity reactions (penicillin and other antibiotics, allergy extracts, vaccines, local anesthetics), observe the recipient carefully for at least 30 minutes after administration. Have adrenergic and other emergency drugs and equipment readily available in case a reaction occurs.
- Place patient in a recumbent position to improve venous return and blood pressure.
- Provide patient teaching regarding drug therapy (see Box 29.2).

Evaluation

- Observe for improved hemodynamic status, vital signs, color and temperature of skin, urine output, and mental responsiveness.

Visit thePoint® *at* **http://thePoint.lww.com/Frandsen13e** *for answers to NCLEX Success questions (in Appendix A), answers to Clinical Application Case Studies (in Appendix B), additional information on etiology and pathophysiology, and more!*

REFERENCES AND RESOURCES

Ammar, M. A., Ammar, A. A., Wieruszewski, P. M., Bissell, B. D., Long, M. T., Albert, L., Khanna, A. K., & Sacha, G. L. (2022). Timing of vasoactive agents and corticosteroid initiation in septic shock. *Annals of Intensive Care, 12*(1), 1–10.

Evans, L., Rhodes, A., Alhazzani, W., Antonelli, M., Coopersmith, C. M., French, C., Machado, F. R., Mcintyre, L., Ostermann, M., Prescott, H. C., Schorr, C., Simpson, S., Wiersinga, W. J., Alshamsi, F., Angus, D. C., Arabi, Y., Azevedo, L., Beale, R., Beilman, G., … Levy, M. (2021). Surviving Sepsis Campaign: International guidelines for management of sepsis and septic shock 2021. *Critical Care Medicine, 49*(11), e1063–e1143.

Lippincott advisor. (2022). http://advisor.lww.com

Na, S. L., Yang, J. H., Ko, R. E., Chung, C. R., Cho, Y. H., Choi, K. H., Kim, D., Park, T. K., Lee, J. M., Song, Y. B., Choi, J. O., Hahn, J. Y., Choi, S. H., & Gwon, H. C. (2022). Dopamine versus norepinephrine as the first-line vasopressor in the treatment of cardiogenic shock. *PLoS One, 17*(11), e0277087.

Tucker, R. (2022). *2023 Lippincott's pocket drug guide for nurses*. Wolters Kluwer.

UpToDate. (2023). *Drug information*. Lexi-Comp, Inc.

CHAPTER 30

Drug Therapy for Heart Failure

LEARNING OBJECTIVES

After studying this chapter, you should be able to:

1. Describe the differences in heart failure with reduced ejection fraction (HFrEF), or systolic heart failure, and heart failure with preserved ejection fraction (HFpEF), or diastolic heart failure, as they relate to the clinical manifestations of right-sided and left-sided heart failure.
2. Identify the prototype and describe the action, use, adverse effects, contraindications, and nursing implications for the angiotensin receptor–neprilysin inhibitor combination.
3. Identify the prototype and describe the action, use, adverse effects, contraindications, and nursing implications for the sinoatrial node modulator.
4. Recognize the prototype and describe the action, use, adverse effects, contraindications, and nursing implications for the inotropes (cardiac glycosides).
5. Identify the prototype and describe the action, use, adverse effects, contraindications, and nursing implications for the phosphodiesterase inhibitors (cardiotonic–inotropic agents).
6. Identify the prototype and describe the action, use, adverse effects, contraindications, and nursing implications for the human B-type natriuretic peptides.
7. Identify the prototypes and describe the action, use, adverse effects, contraindications, and nursing implications for adjuvant drugs used in the treatment of heart failure.
8. Implement the nursing process in the care of patients undergoing drug therapy for heart failure with left ventricular dysfunction.

CLINICAL APPLICATION CASE STUDY

Dr. Adams is a 59-year-old professor of history at a 4-year college. He tells the nurse practitioner at the campus health center that he has been experiencing increasing shortness of breath and fatigue for the past 6 months. He reports that over the past 2 months he has noticed increased ankle swelling and has gained weight. The nurse practitioner asks Dr. Adams questions to ascertain his past medical history. He states that he has been taking enalapril maleate, 10 mg one time per day for hypertension for many years. He states he was diagnosed with atrial fibrillation 3 years ago and is taking amiodarone 200 mg one time per day. On examination, the nurse practitioner notes that Dr. Adams has pitting edema in his feet and ankles. The nurse practitioner advises Dr. Adams to make an appointment with his cardiologist immediately. The cardiologist diagnoses Dr. Adams with systolic heart failure. The cardiologist increases the dose of enalapril maleate to 20 mg twice a day, prescribes spironolactone (Aldactone), 25 mg every morning, in addition to the amiodarone.

KEY TERMS

Decompensation: the inability of the heart to adequately circulate oxygenated blood to the body's vital organs

Ejection fraction: the percentage of the total amount of blood in the left ventricle that is ejected with each heartbeat

HFpEF: Heart failure with preserved ejection fraction (EF); most commonly associated with diastolic dysfunction that impairs ventricular filling and preload

HFrEF: Heart failure with reduced ejection fraction (EF); most commonly associated with systolic dysfunction that impairs cardiac contractility

Inotropic: related to or influencing the force of myocardial contractility

Phosphene: intermittent enhanced brightness in a limited area of the visual field; appearance of halos or multiple images

Therapeutic index: the margin between effectiveness and toxicity in the blood level of a drug

Ventricular remodeling: dilation and hypertrophy of the ventricles in the initial phases of heart failure, causing the ventricle to assume a spherical shape

INTRODUCTION

Despite significant advances in the management of cardiovascular disease, heart failure remains a leading cause of death in the United States and throughout the world. This chronic, progressive, complex condition occurs when the heart cannot pump enough blood to adequately support perfusion to meet the body tissue's needs for oxygen and nutrients; this is called **decompensation**. Heart failure occurs when cardiac output is reduced due to the heart failing to eject sufficient blood from the ventricle during systole or the ventricles fail to fill adequately during diastole. The pathophysiology of systolic heart failure is complex and impairs cardiac contractility, reduces stroke volume and decreases cardiac output, which is shown in Figure 30.1.

In the United States, heart failure affects 6.2 million patients, is a leading cause of repeated hospitalizations, and accounts for almost $31 billion in health care expenditures annually. As the incidence of heart failure continues to increase, heart failure–associated healthcare costs are expected to reach almost $70 billion annually by 2030 (Patel, 2021). Heart failure has a 50% mortality rate within 5 years of initial diagnosis, and patient outcomes depend on effective management and treatment. This chapter focuses on the management of patients with left ventricular systolic dysfunction, referred to simply as heart failure.

OVERVIEW OF HEART FAILURE

Nurses need to understand the conditions that contribute to the imbalance in supply and demand of oxygen and the clinical manifestations of heart failure to adequately understand the pharmacologic treatment of the problem.

Several clinical conditions can lead to heart failure, including the following:

- Hypertension forces the heart to work harder to overcome increased arterial resistance and maintain cardiac output. Eventually, the heart muscle can no longer accommodate the increased workload and begins to weaken and work less efficiently, ultimately leading to heart failure.
- Coronary artery disease (CAD) reduces blood flow, especially when combined with increased myocardial workload and oxygen demand, leading to myocardial ischemia and myocardial dysfunction. Heart failure results as the myocardium is damaged and unable to function efficiently to support adequate cardiac output.
- Coronary artery endothelial dysfunction contributes to narrowed arterial lumen and decreased blood flow that can trigger the formation of a thrombus that leads to a myocardial infarction. The associated myocardial damage further contributes to the development of heart failure.
- Cardiac dysrhythmias impair the heart's ability to adequately function and pump sufficient blood to meet the demands of homeostasis, resulting in heart failure.
- Heart valve disorders, such as stenosis and regurgitation, disrupt the normal, unidirectional flow of blood through the heart and reduce cardiac output. Heart valve disorders increase myocardial workload, and myocardial compensation for reduced cardiac output frequently results in the development of heart failure.
- Fluid volume overload causes circulatory overload and impairs the pumping ability of the heart, contributing to the development of heart failure. Fluid volume overload can occur in patients with kidney failure. It can also be caused by the excessive administration of intravenous (IV) fluids or blood transfusions or by therapy with certain medications such as corticosteroids, estrogens, and nonsteroidal anti-inflammatory drugs (NSAIDs), which all promote sodium and water retention.
- Hyperthyroidism, a hypermetabolic disorder, and hypothyroidism, a hypometabolic disorder, are contributing factors in the development of heart failure. In hyperthyroidism, thyroid function is increased, which causes a rise in heart rate and myocardial contractility and ultimately cardiac output. The patient is prone to heart failure because of the demands of the increase in cardiac output. In hypothyroidism, the systolic and diastolic functions of the heart are negatively impacted by the lack of adequate metabolic hormones. Additionally, hypothyroidism contributes to the development of cardiac risk factors such as hyperlipidemia, endothelial dysfunction, and obesity.

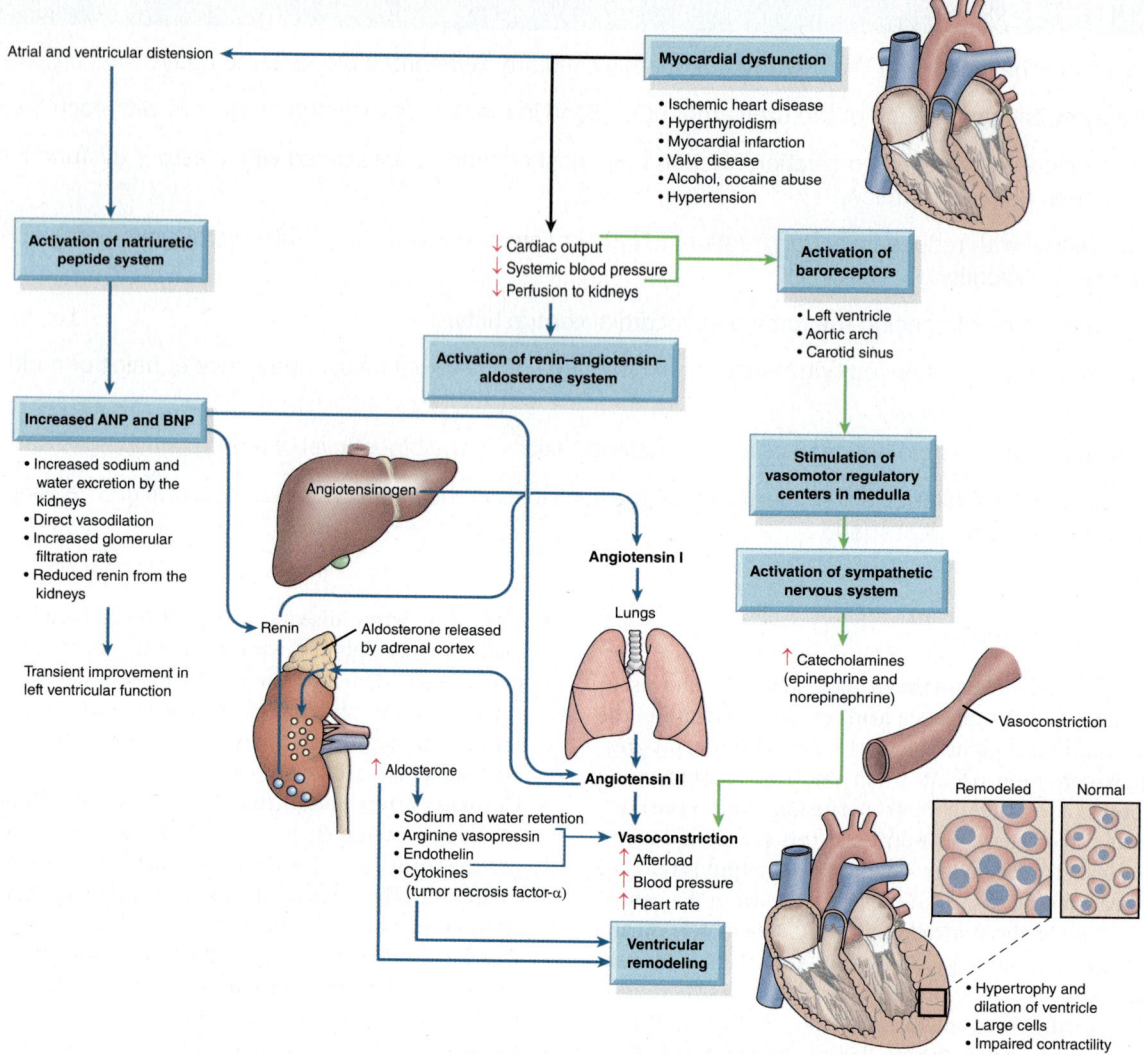

Figure 30.1. The pathophysiology of heart failure. A decrease in cardiac output activates multiple neurohormonal mechanisms that ultimately result in signs and symptoms of heart failure and are targeted with drug therapy. (Adapted from Hinkle, J. L., & Cheever, K. H. [2021]. *Brunner & Suddarth's textbook of medical-surgical nursing* [15th ed.]. Wolters Kluwer Health/Lippincott Williams & Wilkins.)

Types of Heart Failure

Symptoms of heart failure may be classified by the side of the heart that has failed first. While the two types of heart failure impact two different components of cardiac output, their mechanisms and the body's response are intertwined. Over time, left-sided heart failure will cause the right side to fail, producing symptoms associated with both sides of the heart. Clinical manifestations of left- and right-sided heart failure are illustrated in Figure 30.2.

Left-Sided Heart Failure

Left-sided heart failure results in a decrease in cardiac output related to a decrease in stroke volume. There are two types of left-sided heart failure, and drug therapy differs for the two types. Patients with left ventricular dysfunction, called heart failure with reduced ejection fraction (**HFrEF**) or systolic heart failure, have an **ejection fraction** measurement of 40% or less. Ejection fraction is the percentage of the total amount of blood in the left ventricle that is ejected with each heartbeat. This means that as the left ventricle loses its ability to contract normally, only 40% or less of the total amount of blood in the left ventricle is ejected with each heartbeat. In comparison, patients with diastolic heart failure and a preserved left ventricle function (called heart failure with preserved ejection fraction [**HFpEF**]) have an ejection fraction within a normal range, but the left ventricle becomes stiff and loses its ability to relax normally. Because the left ventricle cannot properly fill with blood at rest, an overall decrease in cardiac output occurs due to impaired filling and reduced preload.

Right-Sided Heart Failure

Right-sided heart failure results from an accumulation of blood in the systemic venous system. There are two pumps within the heart. The right-sided pump ejects unoxygenated blood from the systemic circulation into the pulmonary circulation. Failure of the right-sided pump results in an increase in the right atrial, right ventricular, end-diastolic, and systemic venous pressures. The increased pressures impair blood flow from systemic to pulmonary circulation, resulting in systemic fluid volume increases and peripheral edema. The causes of right-sided heart failure are stenosis or regurgitation of the pulmonic or tricuspid valves,

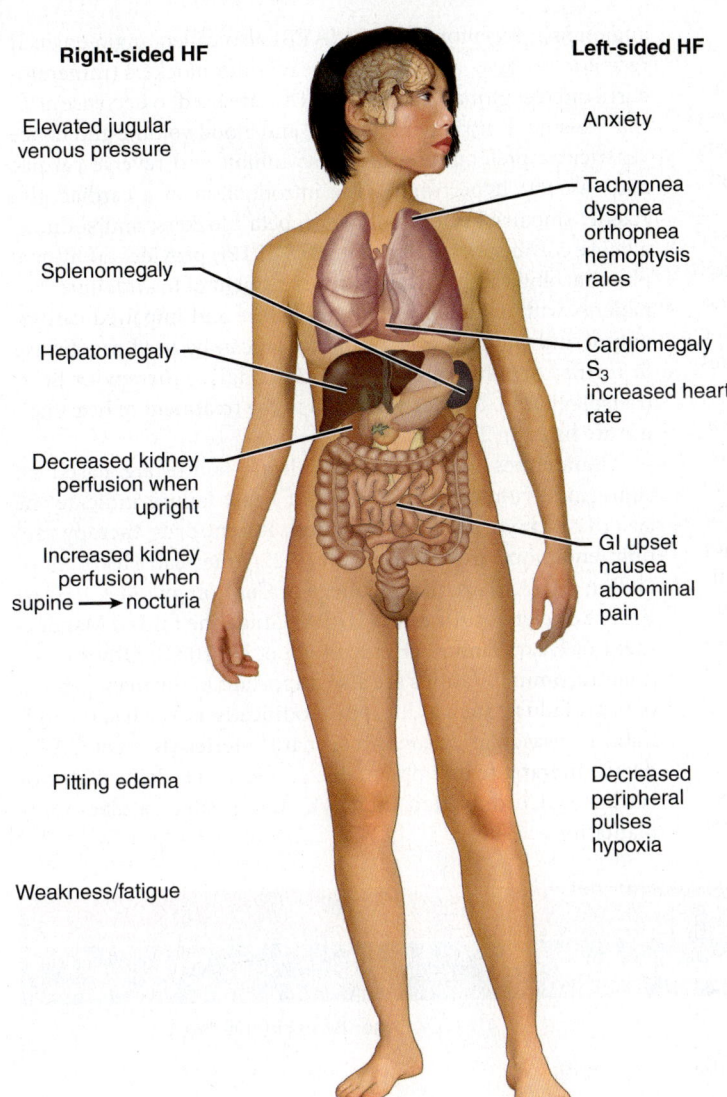

Figure 30.2. Classification of heart failure (HF) and its clinical manifestations. GI, gastrointestinal. (Reprinted with permission from Karch, A. M. (2020). *Focus on nursing pharmacology* (7th ed., Fig. 44.3). Wolters Kluwer.)

right-sided ventricular infarction, cardiomyopathy, or recurrent left-sided heart failure. In some cases, severe pneumonia, pulmonary embolus, or pulmonary hypertension can result in right-sided heart failure.

Clinical Manifestations

Heart failure manifestations are the result of the heart's inability to propel sufficient blood forward to sustain adequate cardiac output and then to pump out adequate amounts of the blood available in the ventricles, resulting in congestion or backward failure. Since systolic and diastolic heart failure involve the left ventricle, the symptoms are very similar and produce inadequate cardiac output. The cardinal manifestations of heart failure are dyspnea, fatigue, weakness, and exercise intolerance. As the congestion backs up to the right side of the heart, jugular vein distention, pulmonary rales, peripheral edema, and weight gain are also seen; these same symptoms are attributed to right-sided heart failure. Orthopnea or pulmonary edema may occur at night while people are supine in bed because the fluid that has shifted from the intravascular space into the interstitial or "third" space during the day when the legs are dependent mobilizes when the legs are elevated. When the third-spaced fluid reenters the circulation, the failing left ventricle cannot pump the blood volume effectively out of the ventricle into the systemic circulation. The pressure in the left atrium increases, resulting in decreased blood flow from the pulmonary vessels. The increase in pulmonary venous pressure forces fluid from the pulmonary capillaries into the alveoli, impairing gas exchange.

Patients with compensated heart failure typically have no symptoms at rest and no edema. In these patients, dyspnea and fatigue occur only with activities that require moderate- to high-level exertion that the heart can no longer accommodate with adequate cardiac output. Patients with symptomatic heart failure have symptoms that occur with minimal exertion or at rest, peripheral edema, and distention of the jugular vein.

Clinical Application 30.1

- Does Dr. Adams have symptoms of right- or left-sided heart failure? Why did his physician prescribe spironolactone?

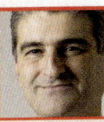

Drug Therapy

Guideline-directed medical therapy (GDMT) includes heart failure clinical evaluation, diagnostic testing, and treatments including pharmacologic therapy and procedural treatments (Heidenreich et al., 2022). The goal of pharmacologic management in heart failure is to slow or reverse the progression of myocardial dysfunction and damage, improve patient symptoms, and reduce morbidity and mortality particularly related to repeated hospitalization risks. Recommendations for the use of individual agents are guided by clinical symptoms and the class and stage of heart failure. Drug therapy that manipulates neurohormonal mechanisms, the renin–angiotensin–aldosterone systems (RAAS), and the natriuretic peptide (NP) system has demonstrated effectiveness in managing heart failure, thereby delaying disease progression and death. Depending on the patient's condition, first-line pharmacologic treatment for symptomatic heart failure could also include diuretics to reduce circulating volume and ventricular preload renin–angiotensin system antagonists to reduce stimulation of the RAAS and decrease myocardial oxygen demand. For example, angiotensin receptor–neprilysin inhibitors (ARNi) are recommended as a first choice for treating symptomatic heart failure and reducing the risk of morbidity and mortality. ARN inhibitors block the harmful effects of the RAAS and sustain the beneficial effects of the NPs while providing direct opposition to increases in angiotensin II. Angiotensin-converting enzyme (ACE) inhibitors, angiotensin receptor blockers (ARB) also called angiotensin II receptor blockers, and aldosterone receptor blockers (mineralocorticoid receptor antagonists [MRA]) are used to decrease arterial pressure, ventricular afterload, and blood volume and hence ventricular preload, and they also inhibit and reverse cardiac and vascular hypertrophy. The introduction of a cardiac glycoside, sinoatrial node modulator, beta-blockers, and sodium-glucose cotransporter 2 inhibitors (SGLT2i) provides additional pharmacologic alternatives in the treatment of heart failure. For patients with acute onset of heart failure and impaired cardiac output, milrinone, a positive inotrope, can be used as a bridge to further definitive treatment such as device therapy or heart transplantation. Medications used in the treatment of heart failure are listed in Table 30.1.

Guidelines for treatment of heart failure are based on signs and symptoms; the stages of heart failure indicate the severity of myocardial dysfunction. Recent drug therapy recommendations are found in the 2022 American Heart Association (AHA)/American College of Cardiology (ACC)/Heart Failure Society of America (HFSA) Guideline for the Management of Heart Failure (Heidenreich et al., 2022). Other treatment recommendations are also important in the management of heart failure, such as lifestyle modifications, cardiac rehabilitation, revascularization of coronary arteries (to treat CAD), device therapy (e.g., implantable cardioverter–defibrillator or cardiac synchronization therapy), and possible cardiac transplantation.

TABLE 30.1

Drugs Administered for the Treatment of Heart Failure

Drug Class	Prototype	Other Drugs in the Class
Angiotensin receptor–neprilysin inhibitors (ARNi)	Sacubitril/valsartan (Entresto)	
Phosphodiesterase inhibitors (cardiotonic–inotropic agents)	Milrinone	
Sinoatrial node modulators	Ivabradine (Corlanor)	
Adjuvant Drugs		
Angiotensin-converting enzyme (ACE) inhibitors	Enalapril maleate (Epaned, Vasotec)	Captopril Fosinopril Lisinopril (Zestril) Perindopril) Quinapril hydrochloride (Accupril) Ramipril (Altace) Trandolapril
Angiotensin receptor blockers (ARB)	Losartan (Cozaar)	Candesartan (Atacand) Valsartan (Diovan)
Aldosterone antagonists	Spironolactone (Aldactone)	Eplerenone (Inspra)
Beta-adrenergic blockers	Metoprolol succinate extended release (Toprol XL)	Bisoprolol Carvedilol (Coreg)
Cardiac glycosides	Digoxin (Lanoxin)	
Loop diuretics	Furosemide (Lasix)	
Sodium-glucose cotransporter-2 inhibitors (SGLT2i)	Dapagliflozin (Farxiga)	Empagliflozin (Jardiance)
Thiazide diuretics	Hydrochlorothiazide (Microzide)	

> ### NCLEX Success
>
> 1. An older adult patient is admitted to the cardiac intensive care unit with acute onset left-sided systolic heart failure with reduced ejection fraction (HFrEF). Which of the following symptoms would the nurse most likely anticipate?
>   A. peripheral edema
>   B. weight gain
>   C. dyspnea
>   D. anxiety

DRUGS THAT INHIBIT THE RENIN–ANGIOTENSIN SYSTEM

Inhibition of the renin–angiotensin system is recommended for patients with HFrEF to reduce morbidity and mortality. Suppressing renin and angiotensin reduces arterial vasoconstriction which reduces resistance, or afterload, and reduces the myocardial workload and improves overall cardiac performance. ACE inhibitors, angiotensin receptor blockers (ARBs), and angiotensin receptor–neprilysin inhibitors (ARNi) are recommended for heart failure. ARNi have demonstrated a significant improvement in heart failure–associated morbidity and mortality and are preferred over ACE inhibitors or ARBs when tolerated (Heidenreich et al., 2022). ACE inhibitors and ARB medications are discussed further in Chapter 26.

ANGIOTENSIN RECEPTOR–NEPRILYSIN INHIBITORS (ARNI)

The heart secretes cardiac NPs in response to changes in cardiac pressure. NPs have a wide range of effects to facilitate cardiac homeostasis related to pressures and volumes. Modulation of the natriuretic system through inhibition of the enzyme neprilysin, which degrades natriuretic (and other vasoactive) peptides, has demonstrated reduced risk of death and hospitalization when added to an ARB in people with chronic heart failure and a reduced ejection fraction. The prototype angiotensin receptor-neprilysin inhibitor (ARNi) **sacubitril/valsartan** (Entresto) blocks the harmful effects of the RAAS and sustains the beneficial effects of the NPs while providing direct opposition to increases in angiotensin II. The drug simultaneously stimulates vasodilation and natriuresis through maintaining increased levels of peptides that would have been degraded by neprilysin and directly blocks vasoconstriction that would have been triggered by angiotensin. The 2022 AHA/ACC/HFSA Guideline for the Management of Heart Failure indicates ARN inhibitors have a significant impact on improving morbidity and mortality for patients with HFrEF when initiated early in symptom management (Desai et al., 2019).

Pharmacokinetics

Sacubitril, the prodrug that inhibits neprilysin, is strongly bound to protein and is converted to an active metabolite by esterases. Following oral administration, peak plasma sacubitril concentrations are reached in approximately 30 minutes. Sacubitril has a half-life of approximately 1½ hours, and the metabolite has a half-life of 11½ hours. The drug and its metabolite are excreted in the urine and feces. Following twice-daily dosing of the drug, steady-state levels of sacubitril and valsartan are reached in 3 days.

Valsartan selectively blocks the binding of angiotensin II to specific tissue receptors found in the vascular smooth muscle and adrenal glands. This, in turn, blocks the vasoconstrictive effect of the RAAS and the release of aldosterone, leading to a decrease in the patient's blood pressure. Chapter 26 contains additional information regarding ARBs and their use in treating hypertension. Valsartan produces direct antagonism of the angiotensin II receptors that produce more efficient blockade of the cardiovascular effects of angiotensin II and less adverse effects than ACE inhibitors. Patients with an allergy to ACE inhibitors may have cross-sensitivity reactions to valsartan and other ARBs.

Action

Sacubitril is a neprilysin inhibitor, and valsartan is an ARB. The beneficial cardiovascular and kidney effects in patients with heart failure appear to result from the increased levels of NPs that are degraded by neprilysin. One method of increasing NP concentrations is to reduce their degradation, which is the action of sacubitril, while simultaneously inhibiting the effects of angiotensin II, which is the action of valsartan. Valsartan also inhibits angiotensin II–dependent aldosterone release.

Use

Sacubitril/valsartan has shown benefits in the management of chronic heart failure with a reduced left ventricular ejection fraction. Dosages for sacubitril/valsartan are given in Table 30.2.

Patient-related variables specific to the use of sacubitril/valsartan include the following:

- Age:
  - Sacubitril/valsartan is indicated for pediatric patients greater than 1 year of age with symptomatic heart failure with left ventricular systolic dysfunction.
  - Dosing is weight-based and oral suspension and tablets are available for administration to pediatric patients.
- Reproduction, pregnancy, and lactation:
  - Drugs that act directly on the RAAS, such as the valsartan, can cause injury and death to the developing fetus if given in the second and third trimester.
  - Sacubitril/valsartan should be discontinued, as soon as possible, once pregnancy is confirmed.
  - Individuals of child-bearing age should be instructed to notify the prescriber if they plan to become pregnant.
  - It is not known if the drug is present in breast milk, so the manufacturer does not recommend breastfeeding.
- Abnormal kidney function and hepatic impairment:
  - In patients who have severe abnormal kidney function, a dose reduction in sacubitril/valsartan is recommended.

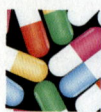

TABLE 30.2
DRUGS AT A GLANCE: Medications to Inhibit Renin–Angiotensin System

Drug	Routes and Dosage Ranges	
	Adults	**Children**
Angiotensin Receptor–Neprilysin Inhibitor		
ⓟ Sacubitril/valsartan (Entresto; ✦ Entresto)	49/51 mg PO twice daily initially; double dose to 97/103 mg twice daily after 2–4 wk as tolerated. If a patient not currently taking an ACE inhibitor or ARB, an initial dose of 24/26 mg twice daily is recommended, double as tolerated every 2 weeks to target dose of 97/103 mg	Children <40 kg: Initial 1.6 mg/kg/dose twice daily, titrate up to 3.1 mg/kg/dose twice daily over 6 weeks Children 40–50 kg: Initial Sacubitril 24 mg/valsartan 26 mg twice daily, titrate up to 72/78 mg twice daily over 6 weeks. Children >50 kg; 49/51 mg twice daily, titrate up to 97/103 mg twice daily over 6 weeks

- In patients who have compromised kidney function, are older adults, or are volume-depleted (including those on diuretic therapy), concomitant use of NSAIDs may result in worsening of kidney function, including possible acute kidney failure. These effects are usually reversible.
- In patients who have moderate hepatic impairment, a dose reduction in sacubitril/valsartan is recommended.
- The drug combination should not be used with patients who have severe hepatic impairment.

Adverse Effects

The most common adverse effects of sacubitril/valsartan are hypotension, hyperkalemia, cough, dizziness, and abnormal kidney function. Angioedema may also occur, and Black patients are at greater risk. Angioedema associated with laryngeal edema may cause airway obstruction and be fatal.

> ❗ **Quality and Safety Alert: Safety**
>
> Blacks are at higher risk of developing angioedema with administration of sacubitril/valsartan.

Contraindications

Sacubitril/valsartan is contraindicated with a hypersensitivity to any component, concomitant use with ACE inhibitors or with aliskiren in patients with diabetes, or a history of angioedema related to previous ACE inhibitor or ARB therapy. The U.S. Food and Drug Administration (FDA) has issued a **BOXED WARNING** ◆ because the drug (valsartan component) can cause fetal harm when administered in pregnancy. The use of drugs that act on the RAAS during the second and third trimesters of pregnancy reduces fetal kidney function and increases fetal and neonatal morbidity and death.

Nursing Implications
Preventing Interactions

Patients taking ACE inhibitors have an adverse/toxic reaction to sacubitril especially related to the occurrence of angioedema. Sacubitril may diminish the effectiveness of hypertension medications such as bromperidol and obinutuzumab. Increases in serum lithium concentrations and lithium toxicity have been reported during concomitant administration of lithium with ARBs. Additional drug interactions that increase or decrease the effect of sacubitril/valsartan are found in Box 30.1. Patients should not take grapefruit juice (a CYP3A4 inhibitor) and St. John's wort (a CYP3A4 inducer) while taking the drug, because adverse effects may occur.

Administering the Medication

Sacubitril/valsartan can be administered without regard to food.

BOX 30.1 Drug Interactions: Sacubitril/Valsartan

Drugs That Increase the Effects of Sacubitril/Valsartan
- Angiotensin-converting enzyme inhibitors
  Increase the risk of angioedema
- Alcohol, antihypertensive agents, and diuretics
  Increase the risk of hypotension
- Aliskiren
  Increases the risk of hypotension, hyperkalemia, and abnormal kidney function
- Eplerenone, drospirenone, and heparin
  Increase the risk of hyperkalemia

Drugs That Decrease the Effects of Sacubitril/Valsartan
- CYP2C9 inducers (e.g., rifampicin, secobarbital), CYP3A4 inducers (e.g., indinavir, clarithromycin), methylphenidate, nonsteroidal anti-inflammatory drugs, peginterferon alfa-2B, and yohimbine
  Decrease serum levels
- Indomethacin
  Decreases antihypertensive effects
- Phenobarbital and rifamycins
  Increase metabolism and decrease antihypertensive effects
- CYP, cytochrome P450.

Assessing for Therapeutic Effects

When switching from an ACE inhibitor or an ARB to sacubitril/valsartan, there should be a "washout" period of 36 hours between administrations of the two drugs to reduce the risk of angioedema.

The nurse should assess for signs of improvement or stabilization of chronic heart failure with patient reports of improved quality of life and decreased hospitalizations. Patients with improved cardiac performance demonstrate increased activity tolerance and alertness, improved appetite, and decreased shortness of breath, cough, nocturia, and irregularity of heart rhythm or rate. Laboratory values (blood urea nitrogen, creatinine, potassium) should remain within acceptable limits.

Assessing for Adverse Effects

The nurse should monitor vital signs and laboratory values and assess the patient for the development of cough or dizziness.

Patient Teaching

Patients of childbearing age should use effective birth control measures while taking sacubitril/valsartan, and they should notify their healthcare provider immediately if they become pregnant. Drugs that act directly on the RAAS can cause injury and death to the developing fetus. Box 30.2 identifies patient teaching guidelines for sacubitril/valsartan.

BOX 30.2 Patient Teaching Guidelines for Sacubitril/Valsartan

- While you are taking this medication, frequent monitoring of your blood pressure will be necessary.
- Do not start, stop, or change the dose of this drug without checking with your provider.
- Talk to your provider (1) if you are taking a salt substitute that contains potassium or a potassium supplement or (2) if you are taking a potassium supplement or a potassium-sparing diuretic.
- Avoid driving and performing other activities that require you to be alert until you see how this drug affects you.
- Get up slowly over a few minutes when sitting or lying down to decrease the chance of feeling dizzy or passing out; use caution and hold the handrail when climbing stairs.
- Have your blood pressure checked often.
- Have blood work checked as you have been told by your healthcare provider. Keep all appointments for laboratory work or provider visits.
- Make sure you drink adequate fluids particularly in hot weather or if you have too much sweating, vomiting or diarrhea. This could lead to low blood pressure.
- Seek medical attention if you have deep swelling or welts under your skin, particularly around your eyes and lips, because this may be a serious reaction called angioedema.
- Notify your provider if you are breast-feeding. You will need to talk about any risks to your baby.

NCLEX Success

2. A 35-year-old female has been prescribed enalapril maleate. What should the nurse teach the patient?
   A. Use effective contraception.
   B. Double the dose if one is missed.
   C. If dizziness occurs, it is not a concern.
   D. There is no change in dose with impaired kidney function.

3. What is the purpose of administering an angiotensin receptor blocker to a patient with heart failure?
   A. It will increase vasoconstriction to increase myocardial contractility.
   B. It will block the influx of calcium across the sinoatrial node.
   C. It will inhibit the enzyme that catalyzes cholesterol synthesis.
   D. It will block the renin–angiotensin II system to increase vasodilation.

Clinical Application 30.2

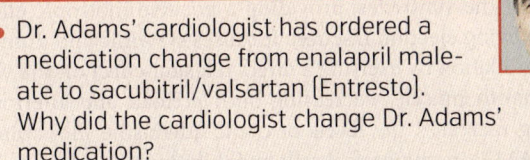

- Dr. Adams' cardiologist has ordered a medication change from enalapril maleate to sacubitril/valsartan (Entresto). Why did the cardiologist change Dr. Adams' medication?
- The cardiologist gives clear instructions to the patient to stop his enalapril maleate for two full days prior to starting the sacubitril/valsartan. Why was that included in the patient's instructions?
- In addition to sacubitril/valsartan, the cardiologist continues the prescribed amiodarone and spironolactone. How will spironolactone assist in decreasing Dr. Adams' symptoms?
- What are the potential interactions between these medications the nurse should be aware of?

PHOSPHODIESTERASE INHIBITORS (CARDIOTONIC–INOTROPIC AGENTS)

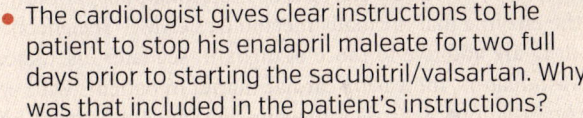 **Milrinone** is the most commonly used phosphodiesterase inhibitor administered for short-term management of acute to severe heart failure to improve myocardial contractility, increase cardiac output, and reduce systemic vascular resistance while awaiting further therapy such as device implantation or cardiac transplant.

Pharmacokinetics

Milrinone is a potent **inotropic** (influences the force of myocardial contractility) agent that is given intravenously by bolus injection followed by continuous infusion. The flow rate of the drug is titrated to maintain adequate circulation. The IV administration of milrinone produces an immediate effect with an

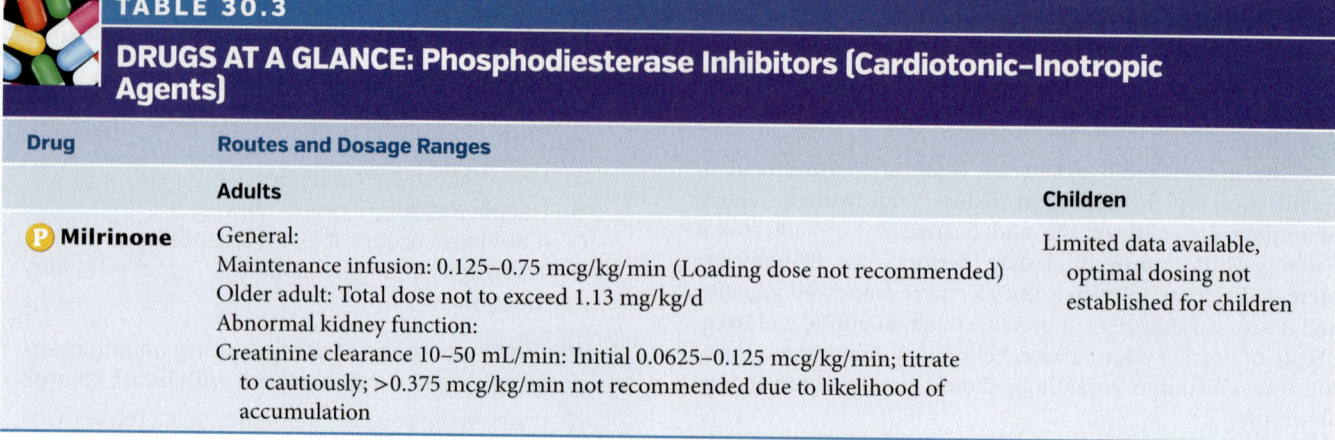

TABLE 30.3
DRUGS AT A GLANCE: Phosphodiesterase Inhibitors (Cardiotonic–Inotropic Agents)

Drug	Routes and Dosage Ranges	
	Adults	**Children**
ⓟ Milrinone	General: Maintenance infusion: 0.125–0.75 mcg/kg/min (Loading dose not recommended) Older adult: Total dose not to exceed 1.13 mg/kg/d Abnormal kidney function: Creatinine clearance 10–50 mL/min: Initial 0.0625–0.125 mcg/kg/min; titrate to cautiously; >0.375 mcg/kg/min not recommended due to likelihood of accumulation	Limited data available, optimal dosing not established for children

onset of action of 5 to 15 minutes. The half-life of this medication is variable and can be as high as 23 hours for patients with severe heart failure, which can lead to accumulation of the medication with prolonged infusions. Dosages for milrinone are given in Table 30.3.

Action

Milrinone's therapeutic action is to increase the force of contraction of the ventricles, providing a positive inotropic effect and improving ejection fraction. It causes systemic and pulmonary vasodilation by exerting a direct relaxant effect on the vascular smooth muscle, decreasing both preload and afterload. The drug increases the levels of cyclic adenosine monophosphate (cAMP) in myocardial cells by inhibiting phosphodiesterase, the enzyme that normally metabolizes cAMP. The effects of this drug are additive to those of digoxin (see later discussion) and vasodilators, increasing cardiac output in patients with systolic heart failure. Because milrinone does not act through beta receptors such as dobutamine, concomitant use of beta-adrenergic blocking drugs does not diminish its effects.

Use

Milrinone is indicated intermediate and long-term as bridge therapy in heart failure. It is useful until a definitive decision is made regarding nonpharmacologic therapy (e.g., coronary revascularization, mechanical circulatory device support, or heart transplantation) to optimize cardiac function and stabilize heart failure patients prior to definitive treatment. Milrinone may also be used as palliative therapy for symptom control in selected patients who are refractory to alternate therapy.

Milrinone (or dobutamine) should be considered for short-term IV administration (1) in patients with acute decompensated heart failure when cardiac output cannot be maintained with diuretics and vasodilators or (2) in patients who are in cardiogenic shock. Routine short-term use of milrinone or dobutamine is not recommended because the drugs are associated with increased mortality in patients with acute decompensated heart failure. Milrinone has limited dosing information available for use with pediatric patients. Because impairment of hepatic function has little effect on milrinone clearance, dosage adjustments are not required for patients with hepatic impairment.

Patient-related variables specific to the use of milrinone include the following:

- Reproduction, pregnancy, and lactation:
  - Milrinone should be administered cautiously in pregnant and lactating patients.
  - It is not known if milrinone is present in breast milk.
- Abnormal kidney function and hepatic impairment:
  - The creatinine clearance level is used to determine the dosage administration for patients with abnormal kidney function (see Table 30.3).
  - Patients with kidney dysfunction may experience prolonged hypotension with milrinone.
- Specific healthcare environments:
  - Milrinone is used mostly in an intensive care unit where the patient's hemodynamic and clinical response to the medication can be monitored.
  - The drug is used in patients with acute heart failure, in weaning patients with pre-existing left ventricular dysfunction from cardiopulmonary bypass, or as a bridging option to support patients with plans to undergo cardiac surgery or transplantation.

Adverse Effects

The most serious adverse effect associated with the administration of milrinone is the development of potentially fatal ventricular dysrhythmias, which reportedly affect 12% to 14% of patients. Hypotension, supraventricular dysrhythmias, chest pain, angina, headache, thrombocytopenia, and hypokalemia may also occur.

Contraindications

The drug is contraindicated in patients who are allergic to milrinone or bisulfites. It is also contraindicated in patients with severe aortic or pulmonic valvular disease.

Nursing Implications

Administering the Medication

Prior to administering milrinone, the nurse assesses the patient for allergy to milrinone or bisulfites. The nurse also obtains an accurate weight and assesses the patient for abnormal kidney function to ensure that an accurate dosage of medication is administered. The patient's cardiac rhythm, blood pressure, and pulse are monitored continuously, and a baseline pulse and blood pressure are recorded. If a marked decline in blood pressure or pulse rate occurs, the rate of administration should be reduced. The nurse assesses for adventitious breath sounds prior to administration and periodically throughout the administration of the drug. A platelet count is drawn prior to administration and at least one time during drug therapy to rule out the adverse effect of thrombocytopenia. Serum electrolyte levels, especially potassium and magnesium, are monitored periodically throughout the administration of the drug. The nurse also monitors and records fluid intake and output.

Milrinone is not compatible with other medications and should not be mixed with any other medications during administration.

> **! Quality and Safety Alert: Safety**
>
> Milrinone and furosemide (Lasix) should not be administered through the same IV line because a precipitate may form.

Patient Teaching

Box 30.3 identifies patient teaching guidelines for milrinone.

> **NCLEX Success**
>
> 4. During the administration of milrinone, the patient's blood pressure decreases from 170/96 to 96/60 mm Hg. What is the first nursing intervention the nurse should perform?
>   A. Call the physician.
>   B. Administer a vasoconstrictor.
>   C. Reduce the infusion rate.
>   D. Reassess the blood pressure.

SINOATRIAL NODE MODULATORS

 Ivabradine (Corlanor), the only drug in its class, is an adjunctive therapy for moderate to severe heart failure when used with drugs with proven morbidity and mortality benefits. Ivabradine is most commonly used with patients who are receiving the maximum tolerated dose of beta-blocker medication with a heartrate >70 bpm (Heidenreich et al., 2022). Ivabradine reduces heart rate, which reduces myocardial demand and adverse outcomes for patients with reduced ejection fraction. Ivabradine is particularly beneficial in reducing hospitalizations for patients with severe heart failure and significantly reduced ejection fraction (Böhm et al., 2015).

Pharmacokinetics

Following oral administration, peak plasma ivabradine concentrations are attained in approximately 1 hour under fasting conditions (about 2 hours with food). The bioavailability of ivabradine is about 40%; the drug undergoes first-pass elimination in the liver and intestines. Metabolism is by CYP3A4-mediated oxidation. Ivabradine has an effective half-life of approximately 6 hours. The drug is excreted in the urine.

Action

Ivabradine produces selective inhibition of the pacemaker ("funny" or f-channels) of the sinoatrial node, with resultant disruption of the current flow. This lengthens diastolic depolarization, resulting in a slower firing of the sinoatrial node and consequently a decrease in heart rate.

Use

Ivabradine is useful for reducing the risk of hospitalization for worsening heart failure in patients with stable, symptomatic chronic heart failure with left ventricular ejection fraction 35% or less; in those who are in sinus rhythm with resting heart rate of 70 beats/min or more; and in those who are either on maximally tolerated doses of beta-adrenergic blockers or in those who have a contraindication to beta-adrenergic blockers. Dosages for ivabradine are given in Table 30.4. Dosage adjustments are based on resting heart rate. Note that no studies have focused on the use of ivabradine in children and that there are no indications that ivabradine dosages in older adults need to be different from those in younger adults.

Patient-related variables specific to the use of ivabradine include the following:

- Reproduction, pregnancy, and lactation:
  - Females of childbearing age should use effective birth control measures while taking ivabradine and should notify the healthcare provider immediately if they become pregnant. In animal studies, ivabradine caused miscarriage, heart and blood vessel problems, and infant death. Whether these effects occur in humans is not known.
  - It is not known if ivabradine passes into breast milk; breast-feeding should be avoided while taking ivabradine.
- Abnormal kidney function and hepatic impairment:
  - Current data do not indicate the need for ivabradine dosage adjustments in patients with impaired kidney function or mild to moderate hepatic dysfunction.
  - No research has studied the effects of ivabradine in patients with severely impaired liver function, and these patients should not take the drug.

> **BOX 30.3 Patient Teaching Guidelines for Milrinone**
>
> - While you are taking this medication, frequent monitoring of your blood pressure, pulse, and heart rhythm will be necessary.
> - You may experience increased urination while you are taking this medication. Because bed rest must be maintained, please call for assistance with toileting.
> - Report pain at the injection site to the nurse.
> - Report any numbness or tingling, shortness of breath, or chest pain.

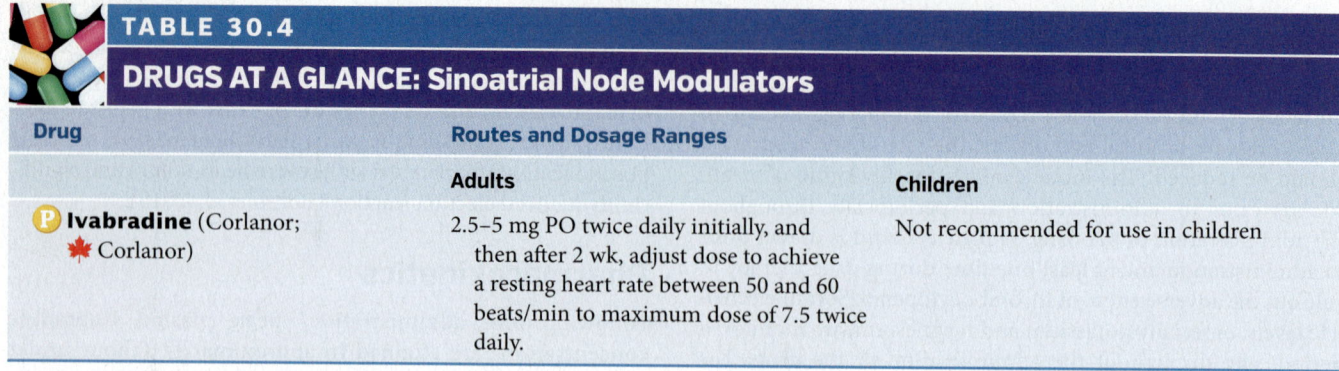

TABLE 30.4

DRUGS AT A GLANCE: Sinoatrial Node Modulators

Drug	Routes and Dosage Ranges	
	Adults	Children
ⓟ Ivabradine (Corlanor; 🍁 Corlanor)	2.5–5 mg PO twice daily initially, and then after 2 wk, adjust dose to achieve a resting heart rate between 50 and 60 beats/min to maximum dose of 7.5 twice daily.	Not recommended for use in children

- Specific healthcare environments:
  - In the critical care setting, administration of ivabradine may be necessary to reduce cardiovascular mortality in the management of patients who are experiencing worsening heart failure.
- Patients who are critically ill may also be receiving additional drugs that are metabolized by CYP3A4 or worsen heart failure.

Adverse Effects

The most common adverse reactions to ivabradine are bradycardia, hypotension, atrial fibrillation, and **phosphene** (intermittent enhanced brightness in a limited area of the visual field, halos, or multiple images).

Contraindications

Ivabradine is contraindicated in acute decompensated heart failure, hypotension, a resting heart rate less than 60 beats/min, sinoatrial block or third-degree AV block, sick sinus syndrome, pacemaker dependence, severe hepatic impairment, and concurrent use with strong CYP3A4 inhibitors, macrolide antibiotics, human immunodeficiency virus (HIV) protease inhibitors, and nefazodone.

Nursing Implications

Preventing Interactions

Ivabradine is primarily metabolized by CYP3A4. Concomitant use of CYP3A4 inhibitors increases ivabradine plasma concentrations, and the use of CYP3A4 inducers decreases them. Increased plasma concentrations may exacerbate bradycardia and conduction disturbances. Additional drugs interact with ivabradine, increasing or decreasing its effect (Box 30.4). Also, patients should not take grapefruit juice (a CYP3A4 inhibitor) or St. John's wort (a CYP3A4 inducer) while taking the drug because adverse effects may occur.

Administering the Medication

Ivabradine should be taken with meals. Food delays absorption by approximately 1 hour and increases plasma exposure by 20% to 40%, extending the action of the drug in the body. As previously stated, patients should avoid drinking grapefruit juice.

Assessing for Therapeutic Effects

Ivabradine causes a dose-dependent reduction in heart rate. The size of the effect is dependent on the baseline heart rate (greater heart rate reduction in patients with higher baseline heart rates). At recommended doses, the heart rate reduction is approximately 10 beats/min at rest and during exercise.

Assessing for Adverse Effects

The nurse should regularly monitor cardiac rhythm, heart rate, and blood pressure. If atrial fibrillation, bradycardia, or hypotension occurs, discontinuation of ivabradine is warranted, and notification of the prescriber is necessary. The nurse should observe for patient reports of phosphenes.

Patient Teaching

The nurse should advise patients to take the medication with meals and to avoid grapefruit juice and St. John's wort. Box 30.5 identifies additional patient teaching guidelines for ivabradine.

ADJUVANT MEDICATIONS USED TO TREAT HEART FAILURE

Adjuvant medications are administered for heart failure to support the treatment and resolution of symptoms. These adjuvant medications are summarized in Table 30.5.

Angiotensin-Converting Enzyme Inhibitors

ACE inhibitors improve morbidity and mortality in patients with heart failure with reduced ejection fractions and have served as the mainstay of heart failure management for over two decades. The prototype ACE inhibitor is ⓟ **enalapril maleate** (Epaned, Vasotec). Enalapril maleate blocks the conversion of angiotensin I to angiotensin II, which is a potent

---

BOX 30.4 *Drug Interactions: Ivabradine*

Drugs That Increase the Effects of Ivabradine

- Moderate CYP3A4 inhibitors (diltiazem, verapamil)
  Increase the risk of bradycardia
- Azole antifungals, macrolide antibiotics, and protease inhibitors
  Increase risk of adverse effects

Drugs That Decrease the Effects of Ivabradine

- CYP3A4 inducers (rifampicin, barbiturates, phenytoin)
  Decrease the effectiveness of ivabradine

> **BOX 30.5** **Patient Teaching Guidelines for Ivabradine (Corlanor)**
>
> - Check your blood pressure, pulse, and heart rhythm as you have been instructed. If your heart rate is less than 50 beats/min, do not take the next dose of medication, and call your provider. Keep all appointments for an electrocardiogram or other tests.
> - Watch for changes in eyesight, including brightness with sudden changes in light. Be cautious while driving, including driving at night.
> - Take your medication with food to maintain consistency in drug effect; avoid grapefruit and grapefruit juice.
> - For patients of childbearing age, use trustworthy birth control while taking this drug, and notify your prescriber if you become pregnant because this drug could harm the baby.

vasoconstrictor. By blocking the production of angiotensin II, enalapril maleate promotes vasodilation (decreasing blood pressure and left ventricular afterload) and decreases aldosterone secretion (increasing serum potassium levels and reducing sodium and water retention). The medication also increases prostaglandin synthesis to decrease blood pressure.

Enalapril maleate is used to treat hypertension, acute and chronic heart failure, and asymptomatic left ventricular dysfunction. Dosages for enalapril maleate in the treatment of HFrEF are provided in Table 30.5 All of the ACE inhibitors have similar effects, but enalapril, captopril, fosinopril, lisinopril (Zestril), quinapril hydrochloride (Accupril), ramipril (Altace), and trandolapril are approved for the treatment of heart failure. Additional information on ACE inhibitors is found in Chapter 26.

The nurse assesses the patient's blood pressure and pulse prior to administration and periodically 4 to 6 hours after administration, because that is the peak of action. The nurse teaches the patient not to stop the medication without the primary health care provider's knowledge and how to recognize adverse effects that need to be reported immediately to the healthcare provider. The nurse instructs females of childbearing age to use contraception while taking the medication because of the risk for fetal abnormalities or death.

Angiotensin Receptor Blockers

Angiotensin receptor blockers (ARBs) oppose the vasoconstricting and aldosterone-secreting effects of angiotensin II at various receptor sites and decrease systemic vascular resistance. Decreased vascular resistance reduces afterload and improves cardiac performance by decreasing myocardial workload and improving blood flow to the myocardium.

The prototype ARB is **losartan** (Cozaar). All of the ARBs have similar effects, but losartan, candesartan (Atacand), and valsartan (Diovan) are approved for the treatment of heart failure and can improve ejection fraction in patients with symptomatic HFrEF, which reduces morbidity and mortality. ARBs can be considered for patients who are not able to use an ARNi or ACE inhibitors due to adverse effects (TRANSCEND Investigators et al., 2008; Wang et al., 2019). Dosages for losartan in the treatment of HFrEF are given in Table 30.5.

The nurse assesses the patient's blood pressure and pulse prior to administration and 6 hours after administration, because that is the peak of action. The nurse teaches the patient not to stop the medication without the primary healthcare provider's knowledge and how to recognize adverse effects, such as angioedema and hypotension, which should be reported immediately to the healthcare provider. The nurse instructs females of childbearing age to use contraception while taking the medication because of the risk for fetal abnormalities or death. Additional information on ARBs is found in Chapter 26.

Diuretics

Strategies aimed at managing the volume overload and pulmonary and/or systemic congestion associated with HFrEF include non-pharmacologic therapy, such as dietary sodium restrictions, and pharmacologic therapy with diuretics. While diuretic medications are effective in managing the congestion in patients with in mild, moderate, and severe heart failure, the impact of diuretics on morbidity and mortality in heart failure is unclear. Therefore, diuretics are recommended to be combined with other GDMT to reduce hospitalizations and prolong survival (Ellison and Felker, 2017). Three drug classes of diuretics are used in heart failure: loop diuretics, thiazide diuretics, and aldosterone antagonists. A further discussion on diuretics is found in Chapter 34.

Loop Diuretics

Loop diuretics are the preferred diuretic agent for most patients with heart failure. **Furosemide** (Lasix), the prototype for the loop diuretics, is administered to patients with moderate to severe heart failure to reduce edema. Loop diuretics cause profound diuresis and, unlike thiazide diuretics, are effective when the glomerular filtration rate is low. Furosemide is also used intravenously to manage symptoms and excess fluid volumes in acute decompensated heart failure. Furosemide is administered with food to prevent gastric upset. When a patient is being treated with furosemide, the nurse weighs the patient daily and reports any increase in weight of greater than 2 lb in 24 hours to the healthcare provider. It is necessary to assess fluid and electrolyte levels frequently to identify extracellular fluid overload or dehydration. The nurse withholds the medication in the event of fluid volume depletion and notifies the healthcare provider. The nurse assesses blood pressure, pulse, and respirations daily. Loop diuretics are potassium wasting; thus, a potassium-rich, low-sodium diet is recommended, and the nurse should instruct the patient on symptoms of hypokalemia such as weakness, fatigue, muscle cramps, and palpitations. Potassium supplements may also be necessary. In patients with diabetes mellitus, the nurse assesses blood glucose levels frequently because furosemide therapy may cause an increase in blood glucose levels.

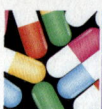

TABLE 30.5

DRUGS AT A GLANCE: Adjuvant Drugs for the Treatment of Heart Failure

Drug	Routes and Dosage Ranges	
	Adults	**Children**
Angiotensin-converting enzyme (ACE) inhibitors		
Ⓟ **Enalapril maleate** (Epaned, Vasotec; 🍁 Taro-Enalapril, Teva-Enalapril, Vasotec)	2.5–20 mg PO daily or BID; Max dose 40 mg/d. Abnormal kidney function: Use smaller initial dose and adjust upward to a maximum of 20 mg/d PO	1 mo to 16 y: initial dose 0.1 mg/kg PO daily or two divided doses. Maximum dose is 0.5 mg/kg/d
Angiotensin-receptor blocker (ARB)		
Ⓟ **Losartan** (Cozaar); 🍁 Cozaar)	25–50 mg PO twice daily initially; doubling dose as tolerated to a target dose of 150 mg/day	Not recommended for use in children with heart failure
Diuretics		
Ⓟ **Furosemide** (Lasix; 🍁 Lasix, Apo-Furosemide, Teva-Furosemide)	20–80 mg PO daily; a second dose can be administered 6–8 h after the initial daily dose. 20–40 mg IV push over 1–2 min; dose can be increased in increments of 20 mg in 2 h. Abnormal kidney function: Up to 4 mg/d has been tolerated. IV bolus injection should not exceed 1 g/d given over 30 min	0.5–2 mg/kg/dose PO every 6–24 h; max dose 6 mg/kg/d. 0.5–2 mg/kg/dose IV or IM every 6–12 h; may increase dosage by 1 mg/kg in 2 h until desired effect is seen or reach max dose of 6 mg/kg/d
Ⓟ **Hydrochlorothiazide** (Microzide; 🍁 Apo-Hydro, Urozide)	25–100 mg PO daily until adequate fluid loss is attained and then 25–100 mg PO daily. Total dose not to exceed 200 mg/d	Infants: 1–3 mg/kg/d PO in 1–2 doses; max dose 37.5 mg/d. Children >2 y: 1–2 mg/kg/d PO in 1–2 doses; max dose 100 mg/d
Ⓟ **Spironolactone** (Aldactone; 🍁 Aldactone, Teva-Spironolactone)	12.5–25 mg once daily PO initially, to 50 mg/d maximum	Not approved for heart failure in children
Beta-Adrenergic Blocking Agents		
Ⓟ **Metoprolol succinate** (Toprol XL; 🍁 Lopressor SR, Metoprolol SR)	12.5–25 mg once daily, to maximum dose of 200 mg	Limited data available, optimal dosing not established for children
Bisoprolol (🍁 Mylan-Bisoprolol, Novo-Bisoprolol, PHL-Bisoprolol)	1.25 mg PO once daily initially to maximum dose of 10 mg once daily	Not recommended for use in children
Carvedilol (Coreg, Coreg CR; 🍁 Auro-Carvedilol, Dom-Carvedilol)	Coreg: 3.125 mg twice daily initially, doubling dose every 2 wk as tolerated; maximum dose based on weight and severity of HF; mild to moderate HF, 85 kg 25 mg twice daily, 85 kg 50 mg twice daily. Severe HF 25 mg twice daily. Coreg CR (extended release): 10 mg once daily initially for 2 wk, doubling dose every 2 wk as tolerated; maximum dose 80 mg once daily	Limited data available, optimal dosing not established for children
Ⓟ **Canagliflozin** (Invokana)	Oral: 100 mg once daily	Not recommended for use in children
Sodium/glucose cotransporter 2 inhibitors (SGLT2i)		
Dapagliflozin (Farxiga)	Oral: 10 mg once daily	Not recommended for use in children
Empagliflozin (Jardiance)	Oral: 10 mg once daily	Not recommended for use in children
Cardiac Glycoside		
Ⓟ **Digoxin** (Lanoxin; 🍁 Apo-Digoxin)	0.125–0.25 mg PO; a loading dose not recommend in heart failure	Children (1–24 mo): 10–15 mcg/kg PO, 10–15 mcg/kg IV in three divided doses per day. Children (2–5 y): 10–15 mcg/kg PO, 8–12 mcg/kg IV in three divided doses per day. Children (5–10 y): 7–12 mcg/kg PO, 5–10 mcg/kg IV in three divided doses per day. Children (older than 10 y): 3–5 mcg/kg PO, 2.5–4 mcg/kg IV in three divided doses per day

Thiazide Diuretics

Thiazide diuretics are the preferred diuretic agent for patients with hypertension and heart failure who have mild fluid congestion. The prototype drug for the thiazide diuretics is P **hydrochlorothiazide** (Microzide). Hydrochlorothiazide (HCTZ) inhibits the reabsorption of sodium and chloride in the distal kidney tubule, moderately increasing the excretion of sodium and water by the kidneys. It is administered primarily for hypertension but is sometimes beneficial in treating edema associated with early or mild heart failure. Decreasing the plasma volume increases cardiac output by decreasing preload and myocardial workload to improve efficiency of myocardial function.

Prior to administering HCTZ, the nurse assesses the patient for allergy to thiazides and sulfonamides. The nurse also assesses the blood pressure and pulse before administering the medication and periodically following administration. HCTZ is also a potassium-wasting diuretic so a potassium-rich, low-sodium diet is recommended, and the nurse should instruct the patient on the symptoms of hypokalemia. In addition, potassium supplements may be necessary. The risk of toxicity and dysrhythmias in the presence of hypokalemia may be a concern, as with the loop diuretics. HCTZ is administered with food to prevent gastric upset. Throughout therapy, the nurse assesses the patient's lungs (for adventitious sounds), heart (for an S_3), and extremities (for peripheral edema), the patient's fluid and electrolyte status, and the patient's weight (daily). Any increase in weight of greater than 2 lb in 24 hours must be reported to the primary healthcare provider.

Aldosterone Antagonists

Increased aldosterone is a major factor in the pathophysiology of systolic dysfunction and heart failure. Aldosterone antagonists, or (mineralocorticoid receptor agonists [MRA]), are an important part of the neurohormonal blockade aimed at blocking the effects of aldosterone. Blocking aldosterone prevents the reabsorption of sodium and increases water loss, reducing fluid volume and preload. For patients with symptomatic heart failure, reducing preload improves myocardial performance by reducing stroke volume and myocardial stretch. Increased aldosterone levels result in interstitial fibrosis, which may decrease systolic function and increase the risk of dysrhythmias. P **Spironolactone** (Aldactone), the prototype drug in this class, is an aldosterone antagonist that reduces aldosterone-induced retention of sodium and water and impaired vascular function by antagonizing the action of aldosterone at mineralocorticoid receptors. In patients with heart failure and inadequate kidney function, spironolactone allows smaller doses of loop diuretics and potassium supplements to be administered as the drug reduces urinary potassium loss. Consequently, aldosterone antagonists are also referred to as potassium-sparing diuretics. Clinical trials have shown that the combination of spironolactone with other drugs improves cardiac function and reduces symptoms, hospitalizations, and mortality in patients with heart failure.

Spironolactone is used to decrease edema in patients with heart failure. A second drug in this class, eplerenone (Inspra), is approved for use in the management of heart failure after myocardial infarction to improve survival.

Clinical Application 30.3

Dr. Adams arrives at the emergency department with dyspnea, fatigue, and weakness and is admitted for treatment of symptomatic heart failure. Dr. Adams' diagnostic testing reveals significantly reduced ejection fraction, and his cardiologist prescribes furosemide IV to treat his symptoms.

- What is the rationale for administering furosemide IV? What would be the expected therapeutic effects?
- What complications from the furosemide IV would the nurse monitor for?
- What dietary modifications are important to reinforce as part of Dr. Adams' care and discharge instructions?

Beta-Adrenergic Blocking Agents

Judicious use of beta-adrenergic blocking agents has been a cornerstone in the treatment of heart failure considering increasing evidence that supports their ability to decrease morbidity and mortality in patients with chronic heart failure. Beta-adrenergic blockers suppress the sympathetic nervous system and the resulting catecholamine excess that eventually damages myocardial cells, reduces myocardial beta receptors, and reduces cardiac output. As a result, over time, **ventricular remodeling** (dilation and hypertrophy of the ventricles) regresses, the heart returns toward a normal shape and function, and cardiac output increases. Although the prototype beta-adrenergic blocking agent is propranolol hydrochloride (Inderal), which is described in detail in Chapter 27, the prototype agent with heart failure is P **metoprolol succinate**.

Class II beta-adrenergic blockers are often administered in patients following myocardial infarction and heart failure because of their effectiveness in improving symptoms, reducing hospitalization, and improving survival. The ability to improve survival may result from the ability of the drug class to prevent ventricular fibrillation. Bisoprolol, carvedilol (Coreg), and sustained-release metoprolol succinate (Toprol XL) are the beta-blockers recommended to reduce mortality and hospitalizations in patients with HFrEF (Heidenreich et al., 2022). These three drugs competitively block the beta-adrenergic receptors in the heart and juxtaglomerular apparatus to decrease the influence of the sympathetic nervous system on these tissues. The resultant diminished excitability of the heart reduces cardiac workload and oxygen consumption. In addition, these three drugs are beneficial in the management of stable, symptomatic heart failure. The drugs reduce the rate of hospitalizations and mortality in patients already receiving ACE inhibitors, diuretics, and/or digoxin.

Prior to the administration of metoprolol, bisoprolol, and carvedilol, the nurse determines if the patient has had any hypersensitivity reactions to beta-adrenergic blockers or conditions that contraindicate use of the medication. The patient should not take the herb betel palm, which blocks the reduction in heart rate produced by beta-adrenergic blocking agents, concurrently. The nurse assesses the patient's weight and cardiopulmonary status and for the presence of dizziness, drowsiness, syncope, or blurred vision. In addition, the nurse instructs the patient to report shortness of breath, night cough, edema, slow pulse, confusion, depression, rash, fever, or sore throat and explains that therapy with a beta-adrenergic blocker should never be stopped abruptly. The FDA has issued a **BOXED WARNING** ◆ for beta-adrenergic blocking agents for patients with coronary artery disease: rapid withdrawal of oral forms of these drugs may result in exacerbation of angina, increased incidence of ventricular dysrhythmias, and the occurrence of myocardial infarctions.

Sodium–Glucose Cotransporter 2 Inhibitors (SGLT2i)

Sodium–glucose cotransporter 2 inhibitors (SGLT2i) have demonstrated decreased mortality when added to the treatment regimen for patients with heart failure with reduced ejection fraction. SGLT2 inhibitors improve glycemic control in patients with type 2 diabetes by blocking reabsorption of glucose in the kidney and promote excretion of excess glucose. This produces a protective effect on the kidney by decreasing protein loss and reducing kidney damage. The clinical outcome benefits for patients with heart failure are thought to be linked to the promotion of natriuresis and diuresis related to the increased urinary glucose excretion (Zhai et al., 2021).

For patients with type 2 diabetes and heart failure, SGLT2 inhibitors treat hyperglycemia, reduce progression of diabetic kidney disease, and reduce heart failure hospitalizations and mortality. Additionally, multiple studies have demonstrated reduced hospitalizations and all-cause mortality for patients with heart failure irrespective of the presence of type 2 diabetes, and the drug is recommended as an adjuvant therapy for symptomatic HFrEF (Packer et al., 2020). The prototype SGLT2 inhibitor is **P canagliflozin** (Invokana). Dapagliflozin (Farxiga), empagliflozin (Jardiance), and canagliflozin have all been demonstrated to improve outcomes in patients with heart failure, but canagliflozin has only been demonstrated to improve outcomes with patients diagnosed with both heart failure and type 2 diabetes. Dapagliflozin and empagliflozin were found to improve clinical outcomes in patients who had heart failure with or without Type 2 diabetes. The nurse should monitor for side and adverse effects related to hypoglycemia and volume depletion and assess for hypotension. The nurse should also monitor the glomerular filtration rate (GFR) and assess for symptoms of declining kidney function and kidney failure with replacement therapy.

Cardiac Glycosides

Cardiac glycosides are rarely used in the first-line management of heart failure because of the availability of other medications with fewer adverse effects. Cardiac glycosides exert positive inotropic effects on the contractility of the heart muscle. **P Digoxin** (Lanoxin), derived from the foxglove plant of the genus *Digitalis*, is the prototype drug of this class. Clinical trials support the use of digoxin in heart failure in patients with left ventricular dysfunction, especially in those with advanced disease, but it is no longer considered a first-line drug. Other drugs, such as ARN inhibitors, ACE inhibitors, ARBs, beta-adrenergic blockers, and diuretics, have demonstrated morbidity and mortality benefits in heart failure and should be maximized first before using digoxin.

Digoxin is the only cardiac glycoside available in the United States. A patient with heart failure experiences decreased contractility of the heart, which impairs the heart's ability to adequately pump blood. Digoxin produces a cardiotonic (positive inotropic) effect that improves the contractility and pumping ability of the heart. Digoxin increases the force of myocardial contractility by inhibiting sodium, potassium, and adenosine triphosphatase (Na, K-ATPase), an enzyme in cardiac cell membranes that decreases the movement of sodium out of myocardial cells after contraction. As a result, calcium enters the cell in exchange for sodium, causing additional calcium to be released from intracellular binding sites and increasing myocardial contractility.

The administration of digoxin requires the nurse to thoroughly assess and monitor the patient's cardiac status. The patient should take digoxin with food or after meals to minimize gastric irritation and the side effects of anorexia, nausea, and vomiting. Digoxin is given with caution to patients with abnormal kidney function, and careful monitoring is required for patients who are critically ill due to the risk of abnormal kidney function. Digoxin use with older adults should consider the potential for abnormal kidney function or hepatic impairment that could lead to accumulation of the drug.

Because of digoxin's narrow **therapeutic index** (the margin between effectiveness and toxicity in the blood level of a drug), the patient is at greater risk for developing digoxin toxicity. Digoxin's adverse effects can cause significant patient harm; the nurse must be extremely cautious with administration and monitoring and be aware of conditions that can increase the risk of digoxin toxicity (Box 30.6). Patients with hypokalemia can develop digoxin toxicity even when the serum digoxin level is not considered to be elevated. Signs of toxicity include potentially life-threatening heart rhythm disturbances, ranging from slow to rapid ventricular rhythm. Premature ventricular contractions (PVCs) occur commonly with digoxin toxicity and are usually perceived as "skipped" heartbeats by patients. However, PVCs have many possible causes and therefore are not specific for digoxin toxicity. Other

---

BOX 30.6 *Factors That Contribute to Digoxin (Lanoxin) Toxicity*

- An accumulation of larger-than-necessary maintenance doses
- Rapid loading or digitalization, whether by one or more large doses or frequent administration of small doses
- Extremes in age (young and old)
- Electrolyte imbalance (hypokalemia, hypomagnesemia, hypercalcemia)
- Fluid imbalance (volume depletion or gastrointestinal losses)
- Hypoxia due to heart or lung disease (hypoxia increases myocardial sensitivity to digoxin)
- Hypothyroidism (slows metabolism of digoxin)
- Concurrent treatment with other drugs affecting the heart, such as quinidine, verapamil (Calan), or nifedipine (Procardia)

adverse effects include dizziness, nausea, vomiting, loss of appetite, abdominal discomfort, vision changes (yellow-green halos and problems with color perception), blurred vision, and mental changes.

Clinical Application 30.4

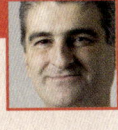

Dr. Adams continues to have symptoms of heart failure with reduced ejection fraction, and so his cardiologist has added dapagliflozin (Farxiga) to his medication therapy.
- Dr. Adams does not have type 2 diabetes. Why is dapagliflozin added to his medication therapy?
- What adverse effects should the nurse observe for while Dr. Adams is taking dapagliflozin?

NCLEX Success

5. A patient is taking furosemide, 40 mg daily, to decrease extracellular fluid related to heart failure. During patient teaching, which of the following points is most important for the nurse to convey?
   A. Sodium intake should be increased due to fluid loss.
   B. Administration of the medication with food will decrease absorption.
   C. The skin should be protected from sun exposure using sunscreen.
   D. Foods that contain potassium should be encouraged to prevent hyperkalemia.

THE NURSING PROCESS

A concept map outlines the nursing process related to drug therapy considerations in this chapter. Additional nursing implications related to the disease process also should be considered in care decisions.

Assessment
- Assess for current or potential heart failure.
  - Identify risk factors for heart failure.
    - Cardiovascular disorders: atherosclerosis, hypertension, coronary artery disease, myocardial infarction, cardiac dysrhythmias, cardiac valvular disease
    - Noncardiovascular disorders: severe infections, hyperthyroidism, pulmonary disease (e.g., cor pulmonale)
    - Other factors: fluid volume overload related to parenteral fluids or blood transfusions, increased age, third spacing
  - Interview and observe for signs and symptoms of chronic heart failure.
    - Mild heart failure: peripheral edema (feet and ankles), dyspnea on exertion, fatigue with ordinary activity
    - Moderate to severe heart failure: more extensive edema, dyspnea at rest, orthopnea, paroxysmal nocturnal dyspnea, cough related to congestion of the respiratory tract with venous blood, confusion from cerebral hypoxia, oliguria from decreased blood flow to the kidneys, anxiety
- Assess baseline vital signs, weight, edema, serum electrolytes (including potassium, magnesium, and calcium), and other laboratory values indicative of cardiovascular function.
- Assess for anticipated therapeutic effects (vital signs and heart rhythm within normal limits, adequate renal function, respiratory congestions and shortness of breath resolved, normal mentation, signs of adequate tissue perfusion, and reports of increased activity tolerance).
- Assess for adverse effects of disease and drug therapy.

Outcomes of Therapy
The patient will
- Take drug therapy safely and accurately.
- Experience improved breathing and less fatigue and edema.
- Verbalize understanding of disease process, recommended lifestyle changes, correct administration and rationale of drug therapy, and when and how to notify the provider.
- Be closely monitored for therapeutic and adverse effects, especially when other drugs are added to or removed from the management regimen.
- Maintain appointments with health care providers to monitor vital signs, serum electrolyte levels (especially potassium level), serum drug levels (such as digoxin), and renal function.

Nursing Interventions
- Implement measures to minimize and prevent heart failure and atrial dysrhythmias.
- Instruct the patient on lifestyle changes:
  - Balanced diet, avoidance of excessive saturated fat and salt, and weight control
  - Smoking cessation
  - Increased levels of regular exercise
  - Limited alcohol intake
- Implement measures to manage hypertension.
- Implement measures to reduce hypoxia.
- Avoid fluid overload, especially in elderly patients.
- Maintain management programs for heart failure, atrial dysrhythmias, and other cardiovascular or noncardiovascular disorders.
- Monitor vital signs, urine output, and serum potassium levels regularly, and compare with baseline values.
- Monitor ECGs when available and compare with baseline or previous ECGs.
- Implement appropriate teaching related to drug therapy.
- Administer oxygen, if needed, to relieve dyspnea, improve oxygen delivery, reduce the work of breathing, and decrease the constriction of pulmonary blood vessels.

Evaluation
- Interview and observe for relief of symptoms (weight loss, increased urine output, decreased peripheral edema, decreased or elimination of shortness of breath, improved activity tolerance, diminished heart rate, increased ability to perform self-care).
- Observe serum drug levels for normal or abnormal values.
- Interview regarding compliance with instructions for the administration of medications.
- Interview and observe for adverse drug effects.
- Observe for achievement of expected outcomes of drug therapy.

Visit thePoint® at http://thePoint.lww.com/Frandsen13e for answers to NCLEX Success questions (in Appendix A), answers to Clinical Application Case Studies (in Appendix B), additional information on the pathophysiology of heart failure, and more!

REFERENCES AND RESOURCES

Böhm, M., Robertson, M., Ford, I., Borer, J. S., Komajda, M., Kindermann, I., Maack, C., Lainscak, M., Swedberg, K., & Tavazzi, L. (2015). Influence of cardiovascular and noncardiovascular comorbidities on outcomes and treatment effect of heart rate reduction with ivabradine in stable heart failure (from the SHIFT trial). *The American Journal of Cardiology*, 116(12), 1890–1897. https://doi.org/10.1016/j.amjcard.2015.09.029

Colucci, W. (2022). Overview of the management of heart failure with reduced ejection fraction in adults. In T. Dardas (Ed.), *UpToDate*. Retrieved May 12, 2022.

Desai, A. S., Solomon, S. D., Shah, A. M., Claggett, B. L., Fang, J. C., Izzo, J., McCague, K., Abbas, C. A., Rocha, R., Mitchell, G. F., & EVALUATE-HF Investigators (2019). Effect of sacubitril-valsartan vs enalapril on aortic stiffness in patients with heart failure and reduced ejection fraction: A randomized clinical trial. *JAMA*, 322(11), 1077–1084. https://doi.org/10.1001/jama.2019.12843

Ellison, D. H., & Felker, G. M. (2017). Diuretic treatment in heart failure. *The New England Journal of Medicine*, 377(20), 1964–1975. https://doi.org/10.1056/NEJMra1703100

Heidenreich, P. A., Bozkurt, B., Aguilar, D., Allen, L. A., Byun, J. J., Colvin, M. M., Deswal, A., Drazner, M. H., Dunlay, S. M., Evers, L. R., Fang, J. C., Fedson, S. E., Fonarow, G. C., Hayek, S. S., Hernandez, A. F., Khazanie, P., Kittleson, M. M., Lee, C. S., Link, M. S., ... Yancy, C. W. (2022). 2022 AHA/ACC/HFSA guideline for the management of heart failure: A report of the American College of Cardiology/American Heart Association Joint Committee on Clinical Practice Guidelines. *Circulation*, 145(18), e895–e1032. https://doi.org/10.1161/CIR.0000000000001063

Hinkle, J. L., Cheever, K. H., & Overbaugh, K. J. (2021). *Brunner and Suddarth's: Textbook of medical-surgical nursing* (15th ed.). Wolters Kluwer.

Jhund, P. S., & McMurray, J. V. (2016). The neprilysin pathway in heart failure: A review and guide on the use of sacubitril/valsartan. *Heart*, 102, 1342–1347.

Lippincott Williams & Wilkins. (2022). *Nursing 2022 Drug Handbook*.

Norris, T. L. (2019). *Porth's Pathophysiology: Concepts of altered health states* (10th ed.). Wolters Kluwer.

Packer, M., Anker, S. D., Butler, J., Filippatos, G., Pocock, S. J., Carson, P., Januzzi, J., Verma, S., Tsutsui, H., Brueckmann, M., Jamal, W., Kimura, K., Schnee, J., Zeller, C., Cotton, D., Bocchi, E., Böhm, M., Choi, D. J., Chopra, V., ... EMPEROR-Reduced Trial Investigators. (2020). Cardiovascular and renal outcomes with empagliflozin in heart failure. *The New England Journal of Medicine*, 383(15), 1413–1424. https://doi.org/10.1056/NEJMoa2022190

Packer, M., Poole-Wilson, P. A., Armstrong, P. W., Cleland, J. G., Horowitz, J. D., Massie, B. M., Rydén, L., Thygesen, K., Uretsky, B. F., & ATLAS Study Group. (1999). Comparative effects of low and high doses of the angiotensin-converting enzyme inhibitor, lisinopril, on morbidity and mortality in chronic heart failure. *Circulation*, 100(23), 2312–2318. https://doi.org/10.1161/01.cir.100.23.2312

Page, R. L., O'Bryant, C. L., Cheng, D., Dow, T. J., Ky, B., Stein, C. M., Spencer, A. P., Trupp, R. J., Lindenfeld, J.; American Heart Association Clinical Pharmacology and Heart Failure and Transplantation Committees of the Council on Clinical Cardiology; Council on Cardiovascular Surgery and Anesthesia; Council on Cardiovascular and Stroke Nursing; & Council on Quality of Care and Outcomes Research. (2016). Drugs that may cause or exacerbate heart failure: A scientific statement from the American Heart Association. *Circulation*, 134(9), e32–e69.

Patel, J. (2021). Heart failure population health considerations. *The American Journal of Managed Care*, 27(9 Suppl), S191–S195. https://doi.org/10.37765/ajmc.2021.88673

Post, T. W. (2019). *Use of beta blockers in heart failure with reduced ejection fraction*. UpToDate.

Solomon, S. D., Zile, M., Pieske, B., Voors, A., Shah, A., Kraigher-Krainer, E., et al. (2012). Prospective comparison of ARNI with ARB on management of heart failure with preserved ejection fraction. *Lancet*, 380(9851), 1387.

Telmisartan Randomised AssessmeNt Study in ACE iNtolerant subjects with cardiovascular Disease (TRANSCEND) Investigators, Yusuf, S., Teo, K., Anderson, C., Pogue, J., Dyal, L., Copland, I., Schumacher, H., Dagenais, G., & Sleight, P. (2008). Effects of the angiotensin-receptor blocker telmisartan on cardiovascular events in high-risk patients intolerant to angiotensin-converting enzyme inhibitors: a randomised controlled trial. *Lancet (London, England)*, 372(9644), 1174–1183. https://doi.org/10.1016/S0140-6736(08)61242-8

Yancy, C. W., Jessup, M., Bozkurt, B., Butler, J., Casey Jr., D. E., Colvin, M. M., Drazner, M. H., Filippatos, G., Fonarow, G. C., Givertz, M. M., Hollenberg, S. M., Lindenfeld, J., Masoudi, F. A., McBride, P. E., Peterson, P. N., Stevenson, L. W., & Westlake, C. (2016). 2016 ACC/AHA/HFSA focused update on new pharmacological therapy for heart failure: An update of the 2013 ACCF/AHA guideline for the management of heart failure. A report of the American College of Cardiology/American Heart Association Task Force on Clinical Practice Guidelines and the Heart Failure Society of America. *Circulation*, 134(13), e282–e293.

Wang, Y., Zhou, R., Lu, C., Chen, Q., Xu, T., & Li, D. (2019). Effects of the angiotensin-receptor neprilysin inhibitor on cardiac reverse remodeling: Meta-analysis. *Journal of the American Heart Association*, 8, e012272.

Zhai, M., Du, X., Liu, C., & Xu, H. (2021). The effects of dapagliflozin in patients with heart failure complicated with type 2 diabetes: A meta-analysis of placebo controlled randomized trials. *Frontiers in Clinical Diabetes and Healthcare*, 2, 703937. https://doi.org/10.3389/fcdhc.2021.703937

Clinical Judgment in Practice: Section 5: Drugs Affecting the Cardiovascular System

A 55-year-old patient is seen by the triage nurse in the emergency department (ED). The patient is 8 weeks post non–ST-elevation myocardial infarction (NSTEMI). The patient also has a 10-year history of hypertension and hyperlipidemia. Upon assessment, the patient complains of shortness of breath, a racing heartbeat, lightheadedness, and slight chest pain. He describes his chest pain as a 4 on a scale of 1 to 10. His vital signs are as follows: T 98.8 orally, RR 28 bpm, HR regular rhythm 136 bpm, BP 92/78 mm Hg, O_2 96% on room air. The patient reports that he waited 6 weeks to resume sexual activity with his wife and has used sildenafil to maintain an erection. He took his sildenafil 50 mg orally 3 hours ago. During sexual intercourse, he began to feel lightheaded and developed chest pain.

He also takes prazosin 1 mg orally three times per day. Prazosin was prescribed due to his resistant hypertension. His blood pressure could not be controlled on combination antihypertensive agents, lisinopril 10 mg with hydrochlorothiazide 12.5 mg.

Step 1: Recognize Cues
Identify the relevant and important information from different sources, such as the medical history or subjective and objective data.

Answer: The patient is 8 weeks post NSTEMI and has a history of hypertension, hyperlipidemia, and erectile dysfunction. The patient complains of shortness of breath, a racing heartbeat, lightheadedness, and slight chest pain. Vital signs are T 98.8 orally, RR 28 bpm, HR regular rhythm 136 bpm, BP 92/78 mm/Hg, O_2 96% on room air. He reports taking sildenafil 50 mg 3 hours ago. He states he became lightheaded and developed chest pain during sexual intercourse.

Step 2: Analyze Cues
Organize and link the recognized cues to the patient's clinical presentation.

Answer: You know that most patients admitted to the ED with a suspected acute coronary syndrome should be questioned about the use of a phosphodiesterase-5 inhibitor. The patient has confirmed he took sildenafil 50 mg 3 hours ago and developed chest pain and lightheadedness. He states that his chest pain is a 4 on a scale of 1 to 10. Normally a patient admitted to the ED with a suspected acute coronary syndrome would be administered nitroglycerin 0.4 mg every 5 minutes for a total of three doses. However, since the patient has taken sildenafil, you know that nitroglycerin is contraindicated due to the fact it will lower blood pressure, and his blood pressure is already low at 92/78 mm Hg. In addition, you know that alpha-1 antihypertensive agents such as prazosin increase the antihypertensive effects when combined with sildenafil.

Step 3: Prioritize Hypotheses
Evaluate hypotheses and rank them according to priority, such as urgency, likelihood, risk, difficulty, and/or time. Cluster your findings to generate a list of problems (actual or potential) you believe the patient is experiencing or may experience and determine the level of urgency. Which problem is of the greatest concern?

Answer: You prioritize the needs of the patient, which include the need to relieve his chest pain, decrease his shortness of breath, and increase his blood pressure and restore his hemodynamic stability.

Step 4: Generate Solutions
Identify expected outcomes and use hypotheses to define a set of interventions for the expected outcomes.

Answer: The ED admission protocol for a suspected acute coronary syndrome requires the administration of oxygen at 2 L per nasal cannula. Since the patient has taken sildenafil in combination with prazosin, the antihypertensive effects are significantly increased. With his blood pressure of 92/78 mm Hg, you anticipate that no treatment to raise the blood pressure will be initiated other than rest and an IV of NS. In addition, the IV access will allow for any further medications to be administered parenterally. You continue to assess the patient's chest pain on a scale of 1 to 10. If the chest pain worsens, you anticipate morphine 10 mg will be administered parenterally. To assess cardiac rhythm, you place the patient on a cardiac monitor and assess the rhythm. You notify the ED provider of the patient's status and anticipate a 12-lead EKG will be ordered. Based on your knowledge of the effect of sildenafil combined with prazosin, you anticipate that with rest and IV fluids, the patient's blood pressure will increase in approximately 4 to 6 hours. The half-life of sildenafil is 4 hours, and the half-life of prazosin is 2 to 3 hours.

Step 5: Take Actions
Implement the solutions that address the highest priorities.

Answer: You start an IV of NS at 125 mL/hour as ordered by the ED provider. You place the patient on a continuous cardiac monitor and monitor his oxygen saturation continuously and his blood pressure every

15 minutes. You place the patient on oxygen 2 L per nasal cannula. The patient is placed on complete bedrest. The patient will require teaching prior to discharge regarding the administration of sildenafil with prazosin.

Step 6: Evaluate Outcomes
Compare observed outcomes against expected outcomes.

Answer: Prior to being discharged, as the ED nurse, you assess the patient's vital signs and cardiopulmonary status. His vital signs are blood pressure 126/78, pulse 76 and regular, and respirations 20 without shortness of breath. He denies chest pain or shortness of breath. He and his wife have been instructed on the increased risk of hypotension when taking sildenafil with prazosin. He agrees to consult with his cardiologist regarding sexual intercourse and the use of sildenafil.

SECTION 6

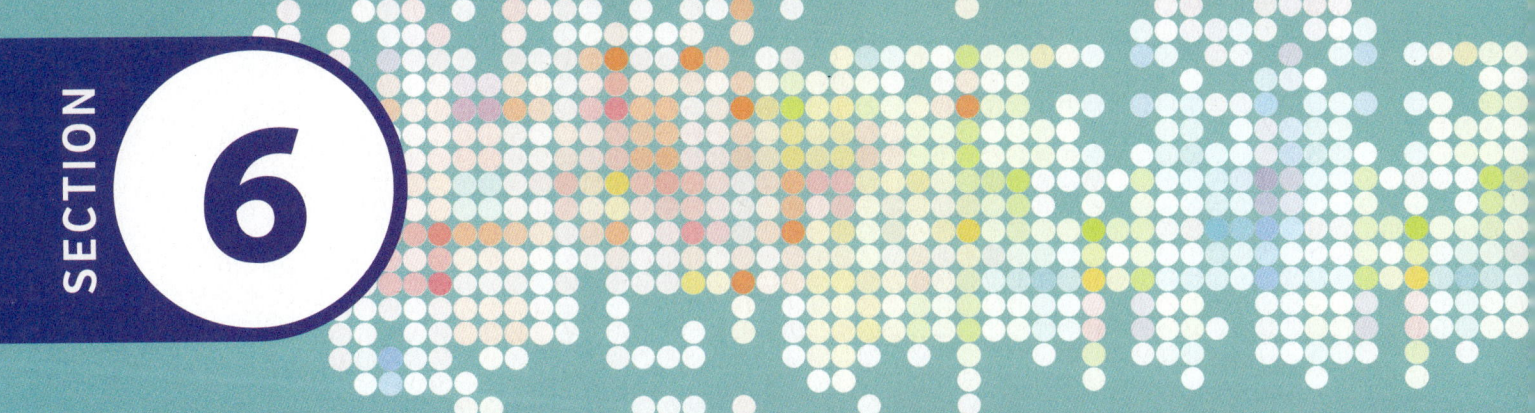

Drugs Affecting the Respiratory System

Chapter 31 Drug Therapy for Nasal Congestion and Cough

Chapter 32 Drug Therapy to Decrease Histamine Effects and Allergic Response

Chapter 33 Drug Therapy for Asthma, Airway Inflammation, and Bronchoconstriction

CHAPTER 31

Drug Therapy for Nasal Congestion and Cough

LEARNING OBJECTIVES

After studying this chapter, you should be able to:

1. Describe characteristics of the common cold and rhinosinusitis.
2. For the nasal decongestants, identify the prototype and describe the action, use, contraindications, adverse effects, and nursing implications.
3. For the antitussive agents, identify the prototype and describe the action, use, contraindications, adverse effects, and nursing implications.
4. For the expectorants, identify the prototype and describe the action, use, contraindications, adverse effects, and nursing implications.
5. For the mucolytics, identify the prototype and describe the action, use, contraindications, adverse effects, and nursing implications.
6. Recognize the concerns of using combination products to treat the common cold.
7. Implement the nursing process with patients receiving nasal decongestants, antitussives, expectorants, and mucolytic agents.

CLINICAL APPLICATION CASE STUDY

Archie Hobbs is a 45-year-old welder at an industrial plant. The occupational nurse at the facility sees a high rate of colds. Mr. Hobbs comes to the health office complaining about his nasal congestion and cough.

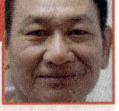

KEY TERMS

Cough: forceful expulsion of air from the lungs

Rhinitis: inflammation of nasal mucosa rhinorrhea

Rhinosinusitis: inflammation of the nasal and paranasal sinus mucosa

Sinusitis: inflammation of the paranasal sinuses (air cells that connect with the nasal cavity and are lined by similar mucosa)

INTRODUCTION

This chapter introduces the pharmacologic care of the patient who is receiving drugs used to treat upper respiratory disorders, such as the common cold and sinusitis, with symptoms such as nasal congestion, cough, and excessive secretions. A more extensive discussion of some of the many drugs used to treat these conditions appears in other chapters; their discussion here relates to their use in upper respiratory conditions.

OVERVIEW OF NASAL CONGESTION AND OTHER RESPIRATORY SYMPTOMS

The common cold, a viral infection of the upper respiratory tract, is the most common respiratory tract infection. Adults usually have 2 to 4 colds per year; schoolchildren may have as many as 10 colds annually. Many types of viruses, most often the rhinovirus, cause colds. Because of the way cold viruses spread, frequent and thorough hand hygiene (by both infected and uninfected people) is the most important protective and preventive measure. The tendency for overmedication and inappropriate use of antibiotics for the common cold is widespread and poses significant risk of complications and drug resistance.

Some of the most common conditions that affect the upper respiratory system are inflammatory responses. **Sinusitis** is the inflammation of the mucous membranes lining the paranasal sinuses. **Rhinitis** is the inflammation of the nasal mucosa. Because sinusitis is almost always accompanied by inflammation of the contiguous paranasal mucosa, the term **rhinosinusitis** is preferred. Sinusitis often results from a viral infection; allergic rhinitis occurs as a response to an allergen. Seasonal rhinitis, or hay fever, occurs in a specific season.

Clinical Manifestations

Nasal Congestion

Nasal congestion occurs when the nasal passages become blocked as membranes lining the nose become swollen due to inflamed blood vessels. The blood vessels in the nasal mucosa become dilated, and the mucous membranes become engorged with blood. Stimulation of the nasal membranes occurs at the same time, resulting in increased mucous secretion.

Cough

Cough (a forceful expulsion of air from the lungs) is a protective reflex response to mechanical, chemical, or inflammatory irritation of the lungs mediated through neurons in the brainstem or cough center. The cough reflex involves central and peripheral mechanisms. A cough helps remove foreign bodies, environmental irritants, or accumulated secretions from the respiratory tract. A cough is productive when secretions are expectorated; it is nonproductive when it is dry, and no sputum is expectorated.

Cough is a prominent symptom of respiratory tract infections (e.g., the common cold, influenza, bronchitis, pharyngitis) as well as chronic obstructive pulmonary diseases (e.g., emphysema, chronic bronchitis). When cough is associated with the common cold, it usually stems from postnasal drainage and throat irritation.

Bronchial Secretions

Bronchial secretions can result from numerous conditions, such as the common cold, where mucus is produced in the chest.

In addition, bronchial secretions can be a symptom of pneumonia, upper respiratory infections, acute and chronic bronchitis, emphysema, and asthma. Postnasal mucus may accumulate in the chest. Alternatively, secretions may be due to nonrespiratory conditions, such as immobility, debilitation, cigarette smoking, or surgery. Surgical procedures involving the chest or abdomen are most likely to be associated with retention of secretions because pain may decrease the patient's ability to cough, breathe deeply, and ambulate.

Excessive secretions may seriously impair respiration by obstructing airways and preventing airflow to and from alveoli, where gas exchange occurs. Secretions also may cause atelectasis (a condition in which part of the lung is airless and collapses) by blocking airflow, and they may cause or aggravate infections by supporting bacterial growth.

Nonpharmacologic Measures

Given the anticipated progression and resolution of a virus, nonpharmacologic measures for symptom relief of a cold can be beneficial. Adequate fluid intake, humidification of the environment, and sucking on hard candy or throat lozenges can help relieve mouth dryness and cough. Additional measures are described in the nursing process concept map.

Drug Therapy

Numerous drugs are available to treat nasal congestion and cough of respiratory disorders. Many are nonprescription drugs that can be obtained alone or in combination with products purchased as over-the-counter (OTC) medications. Available drugs include nasal decongestants, antitussives, expectorants, and mucolytics (Table 31.1). In addition, analgesic agents, such as

TABLE 31.1

Drugs Administered for the Treatment of Nasal Congestion and Cough

Drug Class	Prototype	Other Drugs in the Class
Nasal decongestants	Pseudoephedrine (Sudafed)	Oxymetazoline (Afrin) Phenylephrine (Vazculep)
Antitussives	Dextromethorphan	Benzonatate (Tessalon) codeine Hydrocodone bitartrate (Hysingla ER)
Expectorants	Guaifenesin (glyceryl guaiacolate) (Mucinex, others)	
Mucolytics	Acetylcysteine (Acetadote)	

acetaminophen or ibuprofen (for patients greater than 6 months of age), may provide symptomatic relief. For information on indications and considerations of administering drugs to reduce fever or pain, see Chapter 16.

NASAL DECONGESTANTS

Indications for nasal decongestants are the relief of nasal obstruction and discharge. Adrenergic (sympathomimetic) drugs are most often used for this purpose (see Chapter 29). These agents relieve nasal congestion and swelling by constricting arterioles and reducing blood flow to the nasal mucosa. Oral and topical decongestants are available. **Pseudoephedrine** (Sudafed) is the prototype. In the United States, the OTC sale of cold medicines containing pseudoephedrine is restricted due to the risk of their use in the illicit manufacturing of amphetamine drugs.

Pharmacokinetics

The onset of action of oral pseudoephedrine is approximately 30 minutes and typically peaks in 1 to 2 hours. The drug has a half-life of 4 to 8 hours.

Action

Pseudoephedrine acts directly on adrenergic receptors and acts indirectly by releasing norepinephrine from its storage sites. The drug produces vasoconstriction, which shrinks nasal mucosa membranes, resulting in decreased nasal congestion. It may potentiate the drainage of sinus secretions. In addition, pseudoephedrine may increase irritability of the heart muscle, especially at high doses.

Use

Uses of pseudoephedrine include the temporary relief of symptoms associated with nasal congestion due to the common cold, allergies, and sinuses. Healthcare providers may also use it to reduce local blood flow before nasal surgery and to aid in visualization of the nasal mucosa during diagnostic examinations.

Table 31.2 presents dosage information about various decongestants. It is not necessary to adjust dosages for pseudoephedrine in patients with hepatic impairment. Specific guidelines for adjustment in dosage in the presence of hepatic impairment are not available.

Patient-related variables specific to the use of pseudoephedrine include the following:

- Age:
  - The Food and Drug Administration (FDA, 2023) does not recommend OTC use of pseudoephedrine in infants and children less than 2 years of age due to the risk of serious and life-threatening adverse effects, including seizures, decreased level of consciousness, tachycardia, and death.
  - Research studies in children less than 6 years of age have shown no evidence that the use of pseudoephedrine and other cough and cold preparations are safe and effective.
  - Extended-release tablets should not be administered to children younger than 12 years of age, and children should not be given drugs that are packaged for adults.
  - Older adults are at increased risk of adverse effects from oral nasal decongestants (e.g., hypertension, cardiac dysrhythmias, nervousness, insomnia).

TABLE 31.2
DRUGS AT A GLANCE: Nasal Decongestants

Drug	Routes and Dosage Ranges	
	Adults	**Children**
Pseudoephedrine (Sudafed)	Regular immediate-release tablets, PO 60 mg every 4–6 h Extended-release tablets, PO 120 mg every 12 h or 240 mg every 24 h. Maximum, 240 mg in 24 h	*12 y and older*: same as adults for regular and extended-release tablets *6–12 y*: PO 30 mg every 4–6 h. Maximum, 120 mg/24 h *4 to <6 y*: not recommended, PO 15 mg every 4–6 h. Maximum, 60 mg/24 h *2–4 y*: not recommended *Under 2 y*: not recommended
Oxymetazoline (Afrin) 0.05% spray	Topically, 2–3 sprays in each nostril, every 10–12 h. Maximum, 2 doses/24 h	*6 y and older*: 2–3 sprays in each nostril, every 10–12 h not to exceed 3 days *Under 6 y*: intranasal not recommended
Phenylephrine (❋ Neo-Synephrine)	PO 10 mg every 4 h not to exceed 7 continuous days. Maximum, 60 mg/24 h Intranasal, 2–3 sprays or drops of 0.25%, 0.5%, or 1% solution in each nostril no more often than every 4 h. Maximum, 6 doses/24 h. Not to exceed 3 continuous days	*12 y and older*: same as adults *6 to <12 y*: PO 10 mg every 4 h. Maximum, 60 mg/24 h Intranasal, 1–3 sprays or drops of 0.25% solution in each nostril no more often than every 4 h. Maximum, 6 doses/24 h. Not to exceed 3 continuous days *2 to <6 y*: intranasal, 1 drop of 0.125% solution every 2–4 h. Maximum, 6 doses/24 h. Not to exceed 3 continuous days *<2 y*: not recommended

- Adverse effects from topical agents are less likely in older adults but rebound nasal congestion and systemic effects may occur with overuse.
- Older patients with significant cardiovascular disease should avoid pseudoephedrine.
- Reproduction, pregnancy, and lactation:
  - Due to low or variable benefits to pregnant patients and potential fetal harm, decongestants, including pseudoephedrine, are not the preferred drugs for the treatment of rhinitis during pregnancy.
  - Pseudoephedrine should not be used during the first trimester of pregnancy as the drug may be associated with an increased risk of congenital anomalies.
  - Prolonged use of the drug in later in pregnancy should be avoided.

Quality and Safety Alert: Evidence-Based Practice

In an 8-year surveillance study, Wang et al. (2020) explored the cause of medication errors in children requiring evaluation at a healthcare facility after administration of over-the-counter (OTC) cough and cold medications. The researchers found that medication errors most frequently occurred in children less than 6 years of age who received the wrong amount of a liquid preparation. For common cough and cold preparations, dextromethorphan and diphenhydramine accounted for most medication errors in children in their study.

The risk of errors with administration of OTC cough and cold medications in children can be reduced with further standardization of measuring devices, units of measure, and concentrations of liquid preparations.

Adverse Effects

Notable significant adverse reactions of pseudoephedrine include hypotension, dysrhythmia, impaired coordination, dizziness, excitability, headache, insomnia, restlessness, seizures, vertigo, dysuria, urinary retention, urinary difficulty, and thrombocytopenia. Some people may also experience blurred vision, tinnitus, chest tightness, dry nose, nasal congestion, and wheezing.

Contraindications

Contraindications to pseudoephedrine use include severe hypertension or coronary artery disease because of the drug's cardiac-stimulating and vasoconstricting effects. Another contraindication is narrow-angle glaucoma. Caution is necessary with cardiac dysrhythmias, hyperthyroidism, diabetes mellitus, glaucoma, and prostatic hypertrophy. Patients who take tricyclic or monoamine oxidase inhibitor antidepressants should not receive pseudoephedrine.

Nursing Implications

Preventing Interactions

Many medications interact with pseudoephedrine, increasing its effect (Box 31.1). Caffeine can enhance the adverse effects of pseudoephedrine. The herb coleus may increase the effectiveness of the drug. Tannin-containing herbs such as green or black tea or witch hazel may decrease the absorption and effectiveness of the drug.

BOX 31.1　Drug Interactions: Pseudoephedrine

Drugs That Increase the Effects of Pseudoephedrine
- Cocaine, digoxin, general anesthetics, monoamine oxidase (MAO) inhibitors, other adrenergic drugs, thyroid preparations, and xanthines
  Increase the risk of cardiac dysrhythmias
- Antihistamines, epinephrine, ergot alkaloids, MAO inhibitors, and methylphenidate
  Increase the risk of hypertension due to vasoconstriction

Quality and Safety Alert: Evidence-Based Practice

Drug manufacturers voluntarily label OTC cough and cold products to state: "Do not use in children under 4 years of age." Nurses must emphasize to parents with young children that OTC cough and cold medications lack evidence that they are safe and effective for young children and that these medications pose a risk of potentially life-threatening adverse effects. In patients of any age, in fact, the best available evidence should govern appropriate decisions regarding use of any medication.

Administering the Medication

Patients may take the oral form of pseudoephedrine with or without food. It is important not to crush extended-release preparations.

Quality and Safety Alert: Safety

The FDA encourages drug manufacturers to provide dosing instruments, such as syringes or cups, marked with the correct measurements for administration of liquid medications to children. These alternatives to household spoons for medication measurement contribute to accurate dosing in children.

Assessing for Therapeutic Effects

The nurse assesses for decreased nasal inflammation and congestion after administration of pseudoephedrine. Laboratory monitoring is not necessary.

Assessing for Adverse Effects

The nurse must monitor for cardiac symptoms, particularly in patients with a cardiac history. If anaphylaxis, chest tightness, or throat swelling occurs, it is necessary to discontinue pseudoephedrine immediately.

Patient Teaching

Box 31.2 outlines patient teaching guidelines for nasal decongestants such as pseudoephedrine.

Other Drugs in the Class

Topical preparations (i.e., nasal solutions or sprays) are often preferred for short-term use. They are rapidly effective because they come into direct contact with nasal mucosa. Oxymetazoline (Afrin) is a commonly used nasal spray that acts directly on alpha receptors to produce vasoconstriction of the arterioles in nasal passages. If used longer than the recommended 3 days or in excessive amounts, however, rebound nasal congestion may occur. Topical decongestants are less likely to produce systemic

BOX 31.2 Patient Teaching Guidelines for Nasal Decongestants, Antitussive Medications, Expectorants, and Mucolytics

General Considerations

- These drugs may relieve symptoms but do not cure the disorder causing the symptoms.
- An adequate fluid intake, humidification of the environment, and sucking on hard candy or throat lozenges can help relieve mouth dryness and cough.
- Over-the-counter (OTC) cold remedies should not be used longer than 1 week. Do not use nose drops or sprays more often or longer than recommended. Excessive or prolonged use may damage nasal mucosa and produce chronic nasal congestion.
- Do not increase dosage if symptoms are not relieved by recommended amounts.
- See a healthcare provider if symptoms persist longer than 1 week.
- Inform healthcare providers about any herbal supplements that are being taken.
- Homeopathic preparations are not reviewed or approved by the FDA so have not met the FDA requirements for safety and effectiveness.
- Read the drug fact labels of OTC allergy, cold, and sinus remedies for information about ingredients; many products contain more than the active ingredient. Understand dosages, conditions, or other medications with which the drugs should not be taken and adverse effects.
- Do not combine two drug preparations containing the same or similar active ingredients. For example, pseudoephedrine is the nasal decongestant component of most prescription and OTC sinus and multi-ingredient cold remedies. The recommended dose for immediate-release preparations is usually 30 to 60 mg of pseudoephedrine; doses in extended-release preparations are usually 120 mg. Taking more than one preparation containing pseudoephedrine (or phenylephrine, a similar drug) may increase dosage to toxic levels and cause irregular heartbeats and extreme nervousness.
- Note that many combination products contain acetaminophen or ibuprofen as pain relievers. If you are taking another form of one of these drugs (e.g., Tylenol or Advil), there is a risk of overdosage and adverse effects. Acetaminophen can cause liver damage; ibuprofen is a relative of aspirin that can cause gastrointestinal upset and bleeding. Thus, you need to be sure your total daily dosage is not excessive (with Tylenol, above four doses of 1,000 mg each; with ibuprofen, above 2,400 mg).
- People with diabetes mellitus should read OTC labels for sugar content because many decongestants and cough medicines may contain sucrose, glucose, or corn syrup as a base.

Self-Administration

- Avoid taking excessive amounts of medication or taking recommended amounts too often, as doing so can lead to serious adverse effects.
- Do not chew or crush long-acting tablets or capsules (e.g., those taken once or twice daily). Such actions can cause rapid drug absorption, high blood levels, and serious adverse effects, rather than the slow absorption and prolonged action intended with these products.
- For OTC drugs available in different dosage strengths, start with lower recommended doses rather than "maximum strength" formulations or the highest recommended doses. It is safer to see how the drugs affect you and then increase doses if necessary.
- With topical nasal decongestants:
  - Use only preparations labeled for intranasal use. For example, phenylephrine (Vazculep) is available in both nasal and eye formulations. The two types of solutions cannot be used interchangeably.
  - Phenylephrine preparations may contain different amounts of phenylephrine. Be sure the concentration is appropriate for the person to receive it (e.g., an infant, young child, older adult).
  - Blow the nose gently before instilling nasal solutions or sprays. This clears nasal passages and increases effectiveness of medications.
  - To instill nose drops, lie down or sit with the neck hyperextended and instill medication without touching the dropper to the nostrils (to avoid contamination of the dropper and medication). Rinse the medication dropper after each use.
  - For nasal sprays, sit or stand, squeeze the container once to instill medication, and rinse the spray tip after each use. Most nasal sprays are designed to deliver one dose when used correctly.
  - Report palpitations, dizziness, drowsiness, or rapid pulse. These effects may occur with nasal decongestants and cold remedies and may indicate excessive dosage.
- Take dextromethorphan as directed; increased intake can lead to increased central nervous system impairment.
- Take cough syrups undiluted and avoid eating and drinking for approximately 30 minutes afterward. Part of the beneficial effect of cough syrups stems from soothing effects on the pharyngeal mucosa. Food or fluid removes the medication from the throat.
- If the cough has not improved after 7 days or if symptoms include high fever, skin rash, or persistent headache with cough, seek help from a healthcare provider.
- If you are taking acetylcysteine, understand that increasing fluid intake as directed helps loosen and mobilize secretions. In addition:
- The nebulization may initially cause an unpleasant odor, which soon resolves.
- If the mask leaves a sticky residue on the face, remove it with water.
- Clean the nebulizer equipment after use to minimize infections and prevent buildup of the drug on the equipment.

(Continued on page 578)

BOX 31.2 Patient Teaching Guidelines for Nasal Decongestants, Antitussive Medications, Expectorants, and Mucolytics (Continued)

Administration to Children

- OTC cough and cold medications should not be given to a child under 4 years of age.
- Homeopathic preparations have no known benefits; these should not be given to a child under 4 years of age, as they can cause serious side effects. Imported drugs may be addictive or contain unsafe ingredients.
- Use a dosing instrument, such as a syringe or a cup, marked with the correct measurements to administer liquid medication accurately instead of a household teaspoon.
- Medicines that are packaged and made for adults may overdose your child and should not be given to them.
- Since many medications for children are flavored, reinforce to your toddler or older child that these products are not candy and keep them out of your child's reach.
- Cough drops and lozenges pose a choking risk for young children and should be given cautiously. If swallowed, make sure your child has no problems breathing. If at any point your child has trouble breathing, immediately call 911 for help.

---

effects than oral or parenteral products, but systemic adverse effects may occur; the nurse should watch for them. For patients with cardiovascular disease, topical nasal decongestants are usually preferred. Oral agents are usually contraindicated because of cardiovascular effects (e.g., increased force of myocardial contraction, increased heart rate, increased blood pressure).

NCLEX Success

1. In caring for a patient with nasal congestion, the nurse knows that adrenergic drugs are used as nasal decongestants to relieve symptoms by
   A. constricting arterioles and reducing blood flow to nasal mucosa
   B. stimulating air movement in the lungs
   C. stabilizing mast cells
   D. initiating the cough reflex

2. A patient with nasal congestion is using the OTC decongestant oxymetazoline. The nurse counsels the patient that this medication should be used only for the time recommended on the package and no longer because excessive use may produce
   A. copious lower respiratory tract secretions
   B. ringing in the ears
   C. rebound nasal congestion
   D. a suppressed cough reflex

3. The FDA pediatric safety labeling changes, warning against the use of prescription opioid cough and cold medicines in children younger than 18 years, are based on available data and expert opinion that supports which of the following statements? (Select all that apply.)
   A. A cough should not be suppressed unless it is causing clinical consequences, such as consecutive nights of poor sleep and/or vomiting, rib fractures, or hypoxia.
   B. The safety labeling changes should protect children from unnecessary exposure to opioids.
   C. The risks for prescription opioid cough products typically outweigh the potential benefits in children of all ages.
   D. Addiction or abuse potential is a concern regarding the use of hydrocodone or codeine in children.

ANTITUSSIVES

The goal of antitussive therapy is to suppress nonpurposeful coughing, not productive coughing. Locally acting agents (e.g., throat lozenges, cough drops) may suppress cough by increasing the flow of saliva and by containing demulcents or local anesthetics to decrease irritation of the pharyngeal mucosa. Flavored syrups are often used as vehicles for other drugs.

The nonnarcotic drug **P dextromethorphan** is the antitussive prototype. It is the antitussive drug of choice in most circumstances and the antitussive ingredient in almost all OTC cough remedies (often designated by "DM" on the product label). (Note that some antitussives are narcotics [e.g., codeine, hydrocodone].)

Pharmacokinetics

Following oral administration of dextromethorphan, absorption is rapid. The duration of action is about 3 to 8 hours, with a peak cough-suppressing effect in 15 to 30 minutes. Food decreases the rate and extent of absorption.

Action

Antitussives suppress cough by depressing the cough center in the medulla oblongata or the cough receptors in the throat, trachea, or lungs, effectively elevating the threshold for coughing. Centrally acting antitussives include nonnarcotics and narcotics.

Use

The major clinical indication for use of dextromethorphan is a dry, hacking, nonproductive cough that interferes with rest and sleep. It is not desirable to suppress a productive cough because the secretions need to be removed. There is no information relating to the use of dextromethorphan in older adults (compared with patients of other ages). Table 31.3 gives dosage information for various antitussives.

Evidence supporting the use of dextromethorphan for adults with acute cough due to the common cold is dated, limited, and shows mixed results. Studies show a small improvement at best and the risk of adverse effects may limit the benefit of administration.

Patient-related variables specific to the use of dextromethorphan include the following:

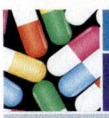

TABLE 31.3
DRUGS AT A GLANCE: Antitussives

Drug	Routes and Dosage Ranges	
	Adults	**Children**
Nonnarcotic ⓿ **Dextromethorphan**	Liquid, lozenges, and syrup, 10–20 mg every 4 h or 20–30 mg every 6–8 h. Maximum, 120 mg/24 h Sustained-action liquid, PO 60 mg every 12 h. Maximum 120 mg/24 h	*12 y and older*: same as adults *6–12 y*: 5–10 mg every 4 h or 15 mg every 6–8 h. Maximum, 60 mg/24 h *2–6 y*: 2.5–7.5 mg every 4–8 h. Maximum, 30 mg/24 h Sustained-action liquid, 6–12 y: 30 mg every 12 h *2–5 y*: 15 mg every 12 h, with caution *Under 2 y*: not recommended
Benzonatate (Tessalon)	PO 100–200 mg three times a day. Maximum, 600 mg/24 h	*10 y and older*: PO 100–200 mg three times a day. Maximum, 600 mg/24 h
Narcotic Codeine (🍁 Codeine Contin, Teva-Codeine)	PO 10–20 mg every 4–6 h. Maximum, 120 mg/24 h	Not recommended for use in children <18 y
Hydrocodone bitartrate (Hysingla ER; 🍁 pdp-Hydrocodone)	PO 1 (5 mg) tablet every 4–6 h up to 30 mg daily	Not recommended for use in children <18 y

- Age:
  - Studies have not demonstrated effectiveness of antitussives, particularly dextromethorphan, in children and adolescents. The American Academy of Pediatrics (Green et al., 2017) advises against the use of antitussives in young people, particularly children less than 2 years of age.
  - Adverse effects of dextromethorphan in children include behavioral disturbances and respiratory depression.
  - Antitussive medications containing opioids should not be used by children under 18 years of age.
- Reproduction, pregnancy, and lactation:
  - Dextromethorphan at standard over-the-counter doses is usually considered acceptable.
  - Products containing alcohol should be avoided during pregnancy and lactation.
  - It is not known if dextromethorphan is present in breast milk.

Adverse Effects

At normal doses, dextromethorphan is known to cause nausea, drowsiness, rash, and difficulty breathing. Doses exceeding recommendations can produce hallucinations and disassociation; dextromethorphan-containing OTC preparations have been used as recreational drugs.

Contraindications

Contraindications to dextromethorphan and other antitussives include known hypersensitivity to the drugs. Concurrent administration of dextromethorphan with an MAO inhibitor or within 2 weeks of discontinuing an MAO inhibitor is contraindicated.

Nursing Implications

Preventing Interactions

Many medications interact with dextromethorphan, increasing its effect (Box 31.3). St. John's wort and tryptophan also interact with the antitussive and increase the risk of serotonin syndrome. No drugs appear to decrease the effect of dextromethorphan.

Administering the Medication

It is necessary to administer dextromethorphan-containing cough syrups undiluted. Appropriate measuring devices should be used to measure liquid medication. The nurse instructs the patient to avoid eating and drinking for approximately 30 minutes afterward. Some caution is warranted with lozenges, which should be dissolved in the mouth to decrease the risk of choking.

Assessing for Therapeutic Effects

The nurse observes for decreased coughing.

Assessing for Adverse Effects

The nurse observes for excessive suppression of the cough reflex (inability to cough effectively when secretions are present) or hallucinations with dosages that exceed recommendations.

Patient Teaching

Box 31.2 outlines patient teaching guidelines for antitussives such as dextromethorphan.

Other Drugs in the Class

Benzonatate (Tessalon), another nonnarcotic antitussive agent, is a peripherally acting drug, unlike dextromethorphan. This antitussive drug acts by anesthetizing stretch receptors in the respiratory passages, thereby decreasing coughing. The nurse advises the patient to swallow the benzonatate capsules whole. Sucking or chewing them may cause numbness of the throat or mouth. Serious adverse effects include a choking feeling, chest pain or numbness, dizziness, confusion, and hallucinations.

The FDA has issued a **BOXED WARNING** ◆ for prescription cough and cold medicines containing codeine or hydrocodone due to the risks of misuse, abuse, addiction, overdose, death, and

BOX 31.3 Drug Interactions: Dextromethorphan

Drugs That Increase the Effects of Dextromethorphan
- Monoamine oxidase inhibitors, serotonin reuptake inhibitors, tricyclic antidepressants, 5-HT1 receptor agonists, ergot alkaloids, lithium, and phenylpiperidine opioids
  Increase the risk of serotonin syndrome
- Alcohol
  Increases central nervous system depression

slowed or difficult breathing. Codeine and hydrocodone, which are both opioid narcotics, have antitussive effects in relatively small doses. Both are centrally acting drugs, like dextromethorphan. In the body, codeine is converted to morphine, and the potential for respiratory depression and death may occur. Other adverse reactions to the narcotic antitussives include nausea, vomiting, constipation, dizziness, drowsiness, pruritus, and drug dependence. Caution is necessary in people, especially children, who have asthma or other chronic breathing problems and who may be more susceptible to respiratory depression. Caution is also necessary in patients with head injuries and increased intracranial pressure, acute abdominal disorders, seizure disorders, abnormal kidney function or hepatic impairment, and prostatic hypertrophy. Additional information about these narcotics is found in Chapter 49.

Clinical Application 31.1

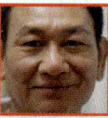

- Mr. Hobbs works in an area with many other people. What should the nurse emphasize to help prevent the further spread of infection throughout the plant?

EXPECTORANTS

Expectorants are agents given orally to liquefy respiratory secretions and allow for their easier removal. The drugs act by moistening the respiratory tract to make the mucus less tenacious. **Ⓟ Guaifenesin** (Mucinex, others) is the prototype expectorant. It is available alone and as an ingredient in many combination cough and cold remedies.

Pharmacokinetics

Guaifenesin is well absorbed following oral administration. The onset of action is 4 to 6 hours, and the duration of action is unknown.

Action

Guaifenesin reduces the viscosity of tenacious secretions by irritating the gastric vagal receptors stimulating respiratory tract fluid. Thus, it increases the volume and decreases the viscosity of respiratory tract secretions.

Use

Used with productive coughs, guaifenesin loosens mucus from the respiratory tract. The drug does not appear to cause unusual adverse effects or problems in older adults. There is no information identifying risk with the use of guaifenesin in older patients compared with younger ones. Table 31.4 presents dosage information for the expectorants.

It is important to note that with excessive respiratory tract secretions, mechanical measures (e.g., coughing, deep breathing, ambulation, chest physiotherapy, forcing fluids) are more likely to be effective than expectorant drug therapy. Research studies do not support the drug's overall effectiveness, and many authorities do not recommend its use.

Patient-related variables specific to the use of guaifenesin include the following:

- Age:
  - Caution is necessary when the drug is used in children younger than 4 years of age.
  - The extended-release tablets should not be used in children younger than 12 years of age.
- Reproduction, pregnancy, and lactation:
  - Taking unnecessary drugs should be avoided during pregnancy, particularly multisymptom formulas with ingredients for a range of symptoms not present in everyone. However, guaifenesin at standard over-the-counter doses is usually considered acceptable.
  - Products containing alcohol should be avoided during pregnancy and lactation.
  - The presence of guaifenesin in breast milk is unknown.

Adverse Effects

Adverse effects of guaifenesin include skin rash, headache, nausea, and vomiting.

Contraindications

Hypersensitivity to guaifenesin is the major contraindication.

TABLE 31.4 DRUGS AT A GLANCE: Expectorants

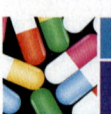

Drug	Routes and Dosage Ranges	
	Adults	**Children**
Ⓟ **Guaifenesin** (glyceryl guaiacolate) (Mucinex, others)	PO 200–400 mg every 4 h. Maximum, 2,400 mg/24 h	*12 y and older*: same as adults *6 to <12 y*: PO 100–200 mg every 4 h. Maximum, 1,200 mg/24 h *4 to <6 y*: PO 50–100 mg every 4 h. Maximum, 600 mg/24 h *2–4 y*: not recommended

Nursing Implications

Administering the Medication

It is necessary to swallow sustained-release capsules or tablets of guaifenesin whole; patients should not break, crush, or chew them. Drinking plenty of water while taking the drug may help loosen mucus in the lungs. People can take it without regard to meals.

Assessing for Therapeutic Effects

The nurse assesses for improvement in cold symptoms, specifically reduction of cough episodes and increased ability to mobilize secretions.

Assessing for Adverse Effects

The nurse assesses for hypersensitivity to the drug and for signs of headache, nausea, and vomiting.

Patient Teaching

Box 31.2 presents patient teaching guidelines for the expectorant guaifenesin.

> **! Quality and Safety Alert: Safety**
>
> It is important to note that guaifenesin liquefies mucus and increases the amount of mucus to be removed. Thus, suction equipment should be available (in the home, if necessary), and the patient and significant others require training in proper use.

> **Clinical Application 31.2**
>
> - Mr. Hobbs has been sick for more than 7 days. He feels that he is getting worse. When the nurse asks him what medication he is taking, he reports that he is using the oxymetazoline (Afrin) that was recommended the last time he was congested. What does the nurse tell him?

MUCOLYTICS

Mucolytics are drugs that are used to liquefy mucus in the respiratory tract by attacking the protein bonds of the mucus. However, no well-designed studies have demonstrated their clinical efficacy. Administration is by inhalation; solutions may be nebulized into a facemask or mouthpiece or instilled directly into the respiratory tract through a tracheostomy. **Acetylcysteine** (Acetadote), the prototype, and sodium chloride solution are the only agents recommended for use as mucolytics. Acetylcysteine has shown small and inconsistent clinical benefits and its limited use may be in patients with refractory symptoms not well controlled by other treatment options.

Pharmacokinetics

Acetylcysteine is rapidly absorbed following inhalation or instillation. The onset of action is 1 minute, the maximum peak effect occurs within 5 to 10 minutes, and the duration of action is 2 to 3 hours.

Action

Acetylcysteine exerts its mucolytic action through its sulfhydryl group, which disrupts the disulfide bonds in the mucoproteins. This reduces the viscosity of mucous secretions. The drug also has antioxidant effects when used at an adequate dose.

> **Concept Mastery Alert**
>
> Expectorants work by increasing production of respiratory secretions, which in turn appears to decrease the viscosity of the mucus. Mucolytics work by breaking down thick and tenacious mucus in the lower portions of the lungs.

Use

Acetylcysteine is used as an adjunctive agent to liquefy viscous mucous secretions. Also, the oral drug is widely used as an antidote in the treatment of acetaminophen overdosage (see Table 2.1 and Chapter 16). Patients should receive an aerosolized bronchodilator 10 to 15 minutes before receiving acetylcysteine.

Table 31.5 presents dosage information for the mucolytics. No studies of acetylcysteine focus specifically on the use of the drug in older adults.

Patient-related variables specific to the use of acetylcysteine include the following:

- Age:
  - Acetylcysteine has no proven benefit in children.
  - The use of acetylcysteine in the management of children with cystic fibrosis has been limited by the development of more effective drugs.

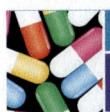

TABLE 31.5
DRUGS AT A GLANCE: Mucolytics

Drug	Routes and Dosage Ranges	
	Adults	**Children**
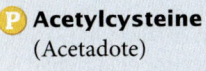 **Acetylcysteine** (Acetadote)	Nebulization, 3–5 mL of a 20% solution or 6–10 mL of a 10% solution every 2–6 h Instillation, 1–2 mL of a 10% or 20% solution every 1–4 h Acetaminophen overdosage, PO 140 mg/kg initially, then 70 mg/kg every 4 h for 17 doses; dilute a 10% or 20% solution to a 5% solution with cola, fruit juice, or water	Not recommended

- Reproduction, pregnancy, and lactation:
  - Acetylcysteine may be used to treat acetaminophen overdose during pregnancy; delay in administration increases the risk of maternal complications.

Adverse Effects

Adverse reactions with inhalation therapy using acetylcysteine include drowsiness, nausea, and vomiting. In some patients, the drug has the potential to cause airway inflammation and bronchospasm and inhibit ciliary function, which has limited its use.

Contraindications

Contraindications include hypersensitivity to acetylcysteine.

Nursing Implications

Administering the Medication

It is necessary to give intermittent aerosol treatments. Typically, these are on arising, before meals, and at bedtime.

Assessing for Therapeutic Effects

The nurse assesses the ability to mobilize secretions and the demonstration of improved respiratory function.

Assessing for Adverse Effects

The nurse assesses for difficulty breathing, inability to expel secretions, bronchospasm, and chest tightness. The nurse also observes for the additional adverse effects of nausea and vomiting.

Patient Teaching

Box 31.2 outlines patient teaching guidelines for the mucolytic acetylcysteine.

HERBAL REMEDIES AND OTHER PREPARATIONS

Herbal remedies and other preparations have been used as cold remedies. However, only herbal preparation and oral zinc preparations have demonstrated ability to reduce the duration and severity of cold symptoms in adults (Box 31.4).

COMBINATION PRODUCTS

Many combination products are available for treating symptoms of the common cold (Table 31.6). Many of the products contain an antihistamine, a nasal decongestant, and an analgesic. Some contain antitussives, expectorants, and other agents as well. Many cold remedies are OTC formulations. Commonly used ingredients include chlorpheniramine (antihistamine), pseudoephedrine (adrenergic nasal decongestant), acetaminophen (analgesic and antipyretic), dextromethorphan (antitussive), and guaifenesin (expectorant). Antihistamines are clearly useful in allergic conditions (e.g., allergic rhinitis; see Chapter 32), but their use to relieve cold symptoms is controversial. First-generation antihistamines (e.g., chlorpheniramine, diphenhydramine) have anticholinergic effects that may reduce sneezing, rhinorrhea, and cough. Also, their sedative effects may aid sleep. Many multi-ingredient cold remedies contain an antihistamine.

The use of OTC products containing pseudoephedrine to manufacture methamphetamine has increased at an alarming rate. Because of this trend, phenylephrine has largely replaced pseudoephedrine in many product formulations in the United States. The Combat Methamphetamine Epidemic Act of 2005 (see Table 1.1) applies to all cough and cold products, including combination products that contain pseudoephedrine.

Quality and Safety Alert: Safety

By law, all pseudoephedrine-containing products, including liquids, gel caps, and pediatric formulas, are stored behind pharmacy counters to restrict purchase limits, control storage, and control sales.

Many products come in several formulations, with different ingredients, and are advertised for different purposes (e.g., allergy, sinus disorders, multisymptom cold, flu remedies). For example, allergy remedies contain an antihistamine; "nondrowsy" or "daytime" formulas contain a nasal decongestant but not an antihistamine; "PM" or "night" formulas contain a sedating antihistamine to promote sleep; pain, fever, and multisymptom formulas usually contain acetaminophen; and "maximum strength" preparations usually refer only to the amount of acetaminophen per dose, usually 1,000 mg for adults. In addition, labels on OTC combination products list ingredients by generic

BOX 31.4 Herbal Remedies and Other Preparations Used as Cold Remedies

Echinacea preparations differ in chemical composition depending on species, parts of the plant, or the season of harvesting. Several well-designed randomized trials and a meta-analysis in adults have concluded that echinacea products are no better than placebo in effectively treating the common cold. In children, a randomized trial found that the incidence of the development of a rash increased without demonstrated clinical efficacy.

Honey and honey-containing products, in a meta-analysis of 14 randomized trials and observational studies [Abuelgasim et al., 2021], demonstrated effectiveness in reducing cough frequency and severity in adults and children with viral upper respiratory infection.

Vitamin C is taken to shorten the duration of colds and alleviate symptoms in adults, although there is no clear consensus that it is effective. However, it appears that vitamin C plays a role in the defense mechanisms of the respiratory system. A recent meta-analysis did not demonstrate the therapeutic benefit of vitamin C in reducing cold duration or severity of symptoms in children.

Zinc sulfate in lozenges and syrup may reduce the duration and severity of cold symptoms in adults. The use of zinc products has not been established in children. However, the U.S. Food and Drug Administration has issued a public health advisory recommending that over-the-counter intranasal zinc-containing products [Zicam] should not be used because of multiple reports of permanent loss of smell.

TABLE 31.6

Representative Multi-Ingredient Nonprescription Cold, Cough, and Sinus Remedies

Trade Name	Ingredients				
	Antihistamine	Nasal Decongestant	Analgesic	Antitussive	Expectorant
Advil Allergy & Congestion Relief	Chlorpheniramine 4 mg	Phenylephrine 10 mg	Ibuprofen 200 mg/tablet		
Advil Cold and Sinus Tablets		Pseudoephedrine 30 mg/tablet	Ibuprofen 200 mg/tablet		
Comtrex Severe Cold & Sinus Tablets		Phenylephrine 5 mg/tablet	Acetaminophen 325 mg/tablet		
Contac Day and Night Cold & Flu Caplets	(Night only) Chlorpheniramine 2 mg/tablet	(Day and night) Phenylephrine 5 mg/tablet	(Day and night) Acetaminophen 500 mg/tablet		
Coricidin D Cold Flu & Sinus	Chlorpheniramine 2 mg/tablet	Phenylephrine 5 mg/tablet	Acetaminophen 325 mg/tablet		
Coricidin HBP Cold & Flu	Chlorpheniramine 2 mg/tablet		Acetaminophen 325 mg/tablet		
Motrin Sinus Headache Tablets		Pseudoephedrine 30 mg/tablet	Ibuprofen 200 mg/tablet		
Robitussin Severe Multisymptom Cough Cold & Flu		Phenylephrine 10 mg/20 mL	Acetaminophen 650 mg/20 mL	Dextromethorphan 20 mg/20 mL	Guaifenesin 400 mg/20 mL
Sinutab Sinus Allergy Maximum Strength Caplets	Chlorpheniramine 2 mg/tablet	Pseudoephedrine 30 mg/tablet	Acetaminophen 500 mg/tablet		
Theraflu Flu, Nighttime Severe Cold & Cough Hot Liquid Powder	Diphenhydramine 25 mg/packet	Phenylephrine 10 mg/packet	Acetaminophen 500 mg/packet		
Vicks NyQuil Severe Cough, Cold & Flu LiquiCaps	Doxylamine 6.25 mg/caplet		Acetaminophen 325 mg/caplet	Dextromethorphan 10 mg/caplet	

name, without identifying the type of drug. This information can be confusing. As a result, consumers, including nurses and other healthcare providers, may not know what medications they are taking or whether some drugs increase or block the effects of other drugs. The FDA recommends that if parents and caregivers use cough and cold products in children older than 4 years of age, it is necessary to read labels carefully, use caution when administering multiple products, and use only measuring devices specifically designed for use with medications.

It is true that single-drug formulations allow flexibility and individualization of dosage, whereas combination products may contain unneeded ingredients and are more expensive. However, many people find combination products more convenient to use.

Clinical Application 31.3

- Mr. Hobbs also complains of a productive cough. He has been taking chlorpheniramine to treat it. What advice should the nurse give to him with regard to the appropriate treatment of a productive cough?

NCLEX Success

4. Cold remedies listed as "nondrowsy" or labeled as "daytime" formulas do not contain
   A. a nasal decongestant
   B. a first-generation antihistamine
   C. a pain reliever
   D. any of the above

5. Which of the following herbal preparations appears to play a role in the defense mechanisms of the respiratory system in adults?
   A. echinacea
   B. vitamin C
   C. zinc gluconate
   D. valerian

THE NURSING PROCESS

A concept map outlines the nursing process related to drug therapy considerations in this chapter. Additional nursing implications related to the disease process should also be considered in care decisions.

Assessment
- Assess the patient's condition in relation to the presence of clinical signs and symptoms for which the drugs are used.
- Assess for the use of treatment measures, including over-the-counter medications, to relieve symptoms and duration of complaints.
- Assess for risk factors (smoking, crowds, contact with people with cold symptoms) that contributed to development of a cold.
- Review history of receiving influenza immunizations.
- Assess for conditions that increase risks of adverse effects or are contraindications to drug therapy.

Outcomes of Therapy
The patient will
- Experience relief of symptoms.
- Take drugs accurately and safely.
- Avoid overuse of decongestants.
- Avoid preventable adverse drug effects.
- Act to avoid recurrence of symptoms.

Nursing Interventions
- Encourage patients to use measures to prevent or minimize the incidence and severity of symptoms. Recommend to patients that they:
  - Avoid smoking cigarettes or breathing secondhand smoke, when possible. Cigarette smoke irritates respiratory tract mucosa, and this irritation causes cough, increased secretions, and decreased effectiveness of cilia in cleaning the respiratory tract.
  - Avoid or limit exposure to crowds, especially during winter when the incidence of colds and influenza is high.
  - Avoid contact with people who have colds or other respiratory infections. This is especially important for patients with chronic lung disease, because upper respiratory infections may precipitate acute attacks of asthma or bronchitis.
  - Maintain a fluid intake of 2,000 to 3,000 mL daily unless contraindicated by cardiovascular or kidney disease.
  - Maintain nutrition, rest, activity, and other general health measures.
  - Practice good hand hygiene techniques.
  - Consider having an annual vaccination for influenza if they are young, older adults, work in high-risk areas, or have chronic respiratory, cardiovascular, or kidney disorders.
- Provide appropriate teaching related to drug therapy (see Box 31.2).

Evaluation
- Interview and observe for relief of symptoms.
- Interview and observe for tachycardia, hypertension, drowsiness, and other adverse drug effects.
- Interview and observe for compliance with instructions about drug use and understanding about need for preventive measures.

Visit thePoint® at **http://thePoint.lww.com/Frandsen13e** *for answers to NCLEX Success questions (in Appendix A), answers to Clinical Application Case Studies (in Appendix B), additional information on pathophysiology, and more!*

REFERENCES AND RESOURCES

Abuelgasim, H., Albury, C., & Lee, J. (2021). Effectiveness of honey for symptomatic relief in upper respiratory tract infections: A systematic review and meta-analysis. *BMJ Evidence-based Medicine*, 26(2), 57–64. https://doi.org/10.1136/bmjebm-2020-111336

FDA Drug Safety Communication. *FDA requires labeling changes for prescription opioid cough and cold medicines to limit their use in adults 18 years and older.* Retrieved February 2023, from www.fda.gov/drugs/drug-safety-and-availability/fda-drug-safety-communication-fda-requires-labeling-changes-prescription-opioid-cough-and-cold

FDA. *Should you give kids medicine for coughs and colds?* Retrieved February 2023, from https://www.fda.gov/consumers/consumer-updates/should-you-give-kids-medicine-coughs-and-colds

Green, J. L., Wang, G. S., Reynolds, K. M., Banner, W., Bond, G. R., Kauffman, R. E., Palmer, R. B., Paul, I. M., & Dart, R. C. (2017). Safety profile of cough and cold medication use in pediatrics. *Pediatrics*, 139(6). https://doi.org/10.1542/peds.2016-3070

Hinkle, J. L., Cheever, K. H., & Overbaugh, K. J. (2021). *Brunner & Suddarth's textbook of medical-surgical nursing* (15th ed.). Wolters Kluwer.

Lam, S., Homme, J., Avarello, J., Heins, A., Pauze, D., Mace, S., Dietrich, A., Stoner, M., Chumpitazi, C. E., & Saidinejad, M. (2021). Use of antitussive medications in acute cough in young children. *Journal of the American College of Emergency Physicians open*, 2(3), e12467. https://doi.org/10.1002/emp2.12467

Lippincott advisor. (2022). http://advisor.lww.com

Nursing2023. (2022). *Drug handbook.* Wolters Kluwer Health/Lippincott Williams & Wilkins.

Schifano, F., Chiappini, S., Miuli, A., Mosca, A., Santovito, M. C., Corkery, J. M., Guirguis, A., Pettorruso, M., Di Giannantonio, M., & Martinotti, G. (2021). Focus on over-the-counter drugs' misuse: A systematic review on antihistamines, cough medicines, and decongestants. *Frontiers in Psychiatry*, 12, 657397–657397. https://doi.org/10.3389/fpsyt.2021.657397

Sloan, V. S., Jones, A., Maduka, C., & Bentz, J. W. G. (2019). A benefit risk review of pediatric use of hydrocodone/chlorpheniramine, a prescription opioid antitussive agent for the treatment of cough. *Drugs—Real World Outcomes*, 6(2), 47–57. https://doi.org/10.1007/s40801-019-0152-6

Tucker, R. (2022). *Lippincott's pocket drug guide for nurses* (10th ed.). Wolters Kluwer.

Wang, G. S., Reynolds, K. M., Banner, W., Bond, G. R., Kauffman, R. E., Palmer, R. B., Paul, I. M., Rapp-Olsson, M., Green, J. L., & Dart, R. C. (2020). Medication errors from over-the-counter cough and cold medications in children. *Academic Pediatrics*, 20(3), 327–332. https://doi.org/10.1016/j.acap.2019.09.006

CHAPTER 32

Drug Therapy to Decrease Histamine Effects and Allergic Response

LEARNING OBJECTIVES

After studying this chapter, you should be able to:

1. Describe the types of hypersensitivity or allergic reactions.
2. Identify the effects of histamine that are blocked by histamine$_1$ (H$_1$) receptor antagonist drugs.
3. Discuss first-generation H$_1$ receptor antagonists in terms of prototype, indications and contraindications, major adverse effects, interactions, and administration.
4. Describe second-generation H$_1$ receptor antagonists in terms of prototype, indications and contraindications, major adverse effects, interactions, and administration.
5. Implement the nursing process in the care of patients receiving antihistamines.

CLINICAL APPLICATION CASE STUDY

Gene Rudolph is a 72-year-old retired mail carrier. His medical history includes hypertension, benign prostatic hypertrophy, and coronary artery disease. He is visiting a medical clinic for a routine blood pressure check. He tells the nurse that he has been having symptoms of nasal congestion, sneezing, and watering of the eyes for the past several weeks and that the symptoms started after he began working in his garden.

KEY TERMS

Anaphylactoid reactions: anaphylaxis-like reaction to a substance without development of immunoglobulin (Ig) E antibody that may occur on first exposure to the causative agent

Anaphylaxis: severe, potentially life-threatening allergic reaction after sensitization to an allergen

Antihistamine: drugs that antagonize the action of histamine, commonly the H$_1$ receptor antagonists

Histamine: first chemical mediator released in immune and inflammatory responses, found mainly in mast cells surrounding blood vessels

Hypersensitivity: allergic reactions that are exaggerated responses by the immune system and that produce tissue injury and may cause serious disease

Serum sickness: type III hypersensitivity response (IgG- or IgM-mediated) characterized by formation of antigen–antibody complexes that induce an acute inflammatory reaction in the tissues

INTRODUCTION

The drugs that antagonize the action of histamine are commonly called **antihistamines**. There are three main types of receptors for histamine, histamine$_1$ (H$_1$), histamine$_2$ (H$_2$), and histamine$_3$ (H$_3$) receptors. This chapter describes the type of allergic reactions and focuses on those drugs that specifically prevent or reduce most of the physiologic effects that histamine normally induces at H$_1$ receptor sites. (http://thePoint.lww.com/Frandsen13e) for additional information related to understanding histamine and its effects on body tissues, the characteristics of allergic reactions, and the selected conditions for which antihistamines are used. Antihistamines that specifically antagonize the H$_2$ receptor sites are found in Chapter 37. Pitolisant, the only H$_3$ receptor antagonist, is discussed in Chapter 57.

OVERVIEW OF HYPERSENSITIVITY (ALLERGIC) REACTIONS

The immune system plays a critical role in protecting the body against microbial invasions. However, this same system can lead to exaggerated immune and inflammatory responses that cause adverse reactions. In predisposed people, harmless environmental antigens that often do not cause a reaction sometimes may trigger an adaptive immune response, immunologic memory, and, on subsequent exposure to the environmental antigen, inflammation responses (see Chapter 16). **Hypersensitivity** involves allergic reactions—exaggerated responses by the immune system that produce tissue injury and may cause serious disease. The mechanisms that eliminate pathogens in adaptive immune responses are essentially identical to those of natural immunity. Allergic reactions may result from specific antibodies, sensitized T lymphocytes, or both, formed during exposure to an antigen.

Traditionally, hypersensitivity reactions are grouped into four types according to the mechanisms by which they are produced (Fig. 32.1). The substances that produce the effect for types I, II, and III hypersensitivity reactions are antibody molecules. The substances responsible for type IV reactions are antigen-specific T cells.

Type I (also called immediate hypersensitivity because it occurs within minutes of exposure to the antigen) is an immunoglobulin E (IgE)-induced response triggered by the interaction of antigen with antigen-specific IgE bound on mast cells, causing mast cell activation. **Histamine**, the first chemical mediator to be released in immune and inflammatory responses, and other mediators are released immediately, and cytokines, chemokines, and leukotrienes are synthesized after activation. Severe **anaphylaxis** (sometimes called anaphylactic shock;

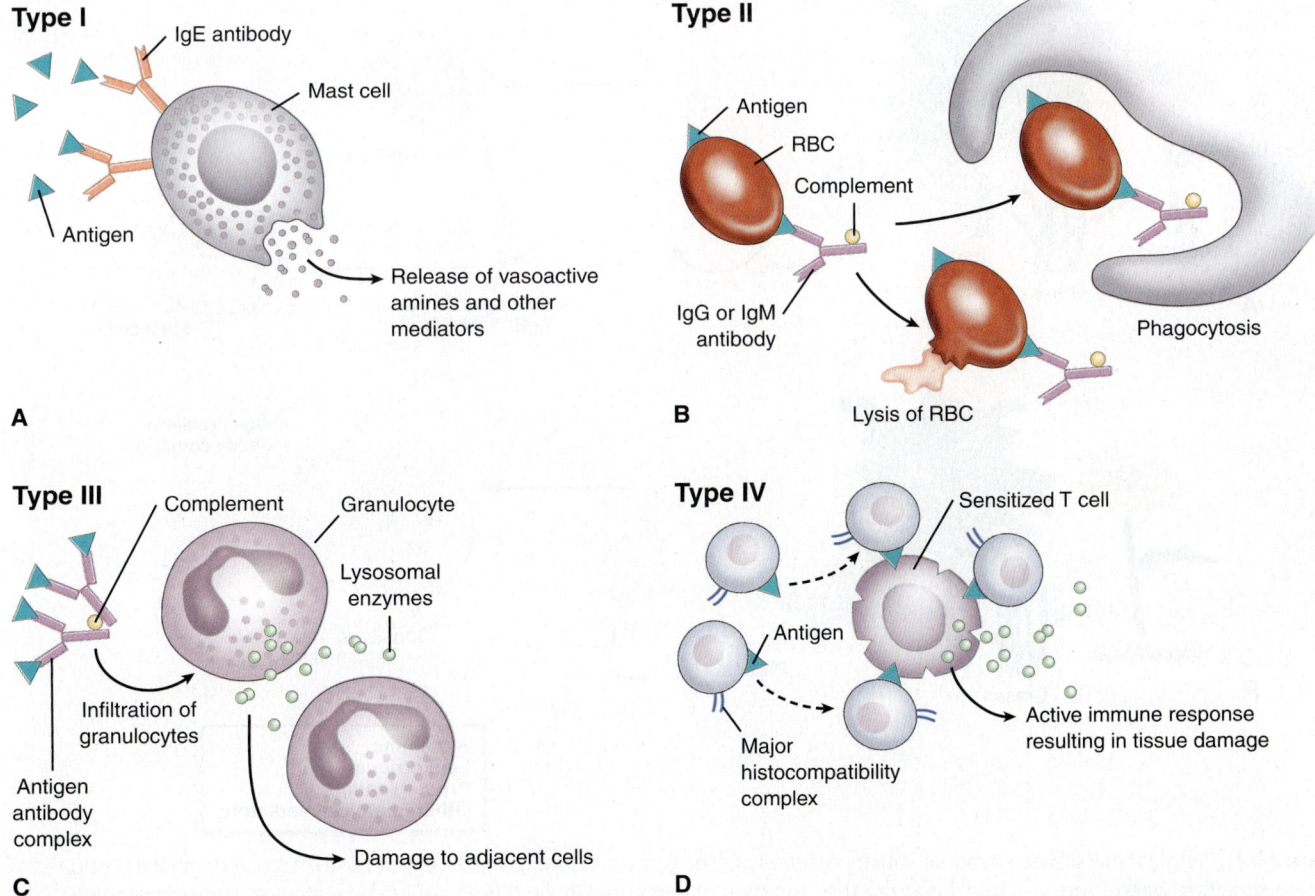

Figure 32.1. Types of hypersensitivity responses: **(A)** type I, atopic or anaphylactic; **(B)** type II, cytotoxic; **(C)** type III, immune complex; and **(D)** type IV, delayed. [Reprinted with permission from Donnelly-Moreno, L. A., & Moseley, B. (2021). *Timby's introductory medical-surgical nursing* (13th ed., Fig. 34.1). Wolters Kluwer.]

see Chapter 29) is a severe, potentially life-threatening allergic reaction after sensitization to an allergen characterized by cardiovascular collapse. Epinephrine, rather than an antihistamine, is the drug of choice for treating severe anaphylaxis.

Type II responses are mediated by IgG or IgM, generating direct damage to the cell surface. These cytotoxic reactions include blood transfusion reactions, hemolytic disease of newborns, autoimmune hemolytic anemia, and some drug reactions. Hemolytic anemia (caused by destruction of erythrocytes) and thrombocytopenia (caused by destruction of platelets), both type II hypersensitivity responses, are adverse effects of certain drugs (e.g., penicillin, methyldopa, heparin).

Type III is an IgG- or IgM-mediated reaction characterized by formation of antigen–antibody complexes that induce an acute inflammatory reaction in the tissues. **Serum sickness**, the prototype of these reactions, occurs when excess antigen combines with antibodies to form immune complexes.

Type IV hypersensitivity (also called delayed hypersensitivity because of the lag time from exposure to antigen until the response is evident) is a cell-mediated response in which sensitized T lymphocytes react with an antigen to cause inflammation mediated by release of lymphokines, direct cytotoxicity, or both. The classic type IV hypersensitivity reaction is the tuberculin test, but similar reactions occur with contact dermatitis and some graft rejection.

Clinical Manifestations

Allergic Rhinitis

Allergic rhinitis is an IgE-mediated inflammatory response of the nasal mucosa caused by a type I hypersensitivity reaction to inhaled allergens (Fig. 32.2). It is a very common disorder characterized by nasal congestion, itching, sneezing, cough, and watery drainage. Itching of the throat, eyes, and ears often occurs as well.

Studies have demonstrated that although antihistamines relieve symptoms of allergic rhinitis, they are not successful in or recommended for treating the common cold. Chapters 17 and 31 describe the drugs besides antihistamines used to manage the condition.

Allergic Contact Dermatitis

Allergic contact dermatitis is a type IV hypersensitivity reaction resulting from direct contact with antigens to which a person has previously become sensitized (e.g., poison ivy or poison oak, cosmetics, hair dyes, metals, drugs applied topically to the skin).

Affected areas of the skin are usually inflamed, warm, edematous, intensely pruritic, and tender to touch. Skin lesions are usually erythematous macules, papules, and vesicles (blisters) that may drain, develop crusts, and become infected. Lesion location may indicate the causative antigen.

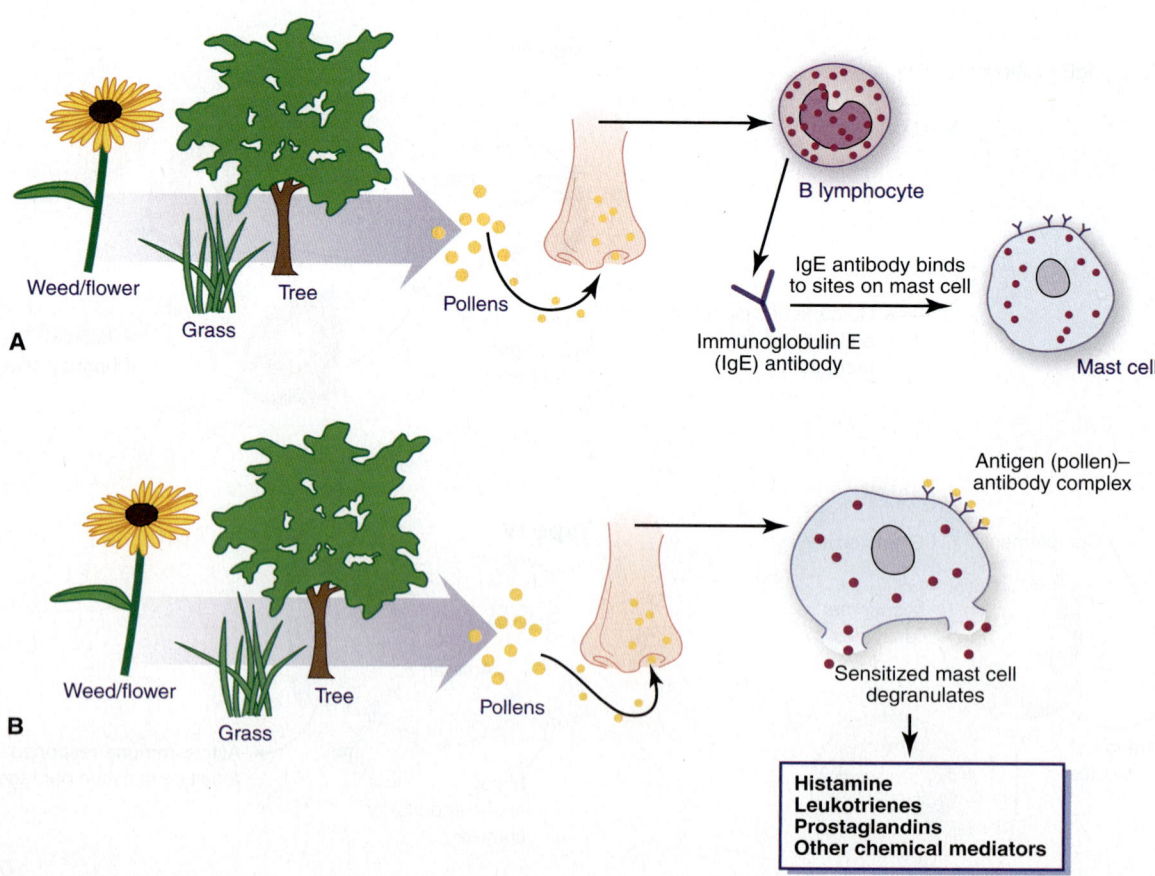

Figure 32.2. Allergic rhinitis: type I hypersensitivity reaction. **A.** The first exposure of mast cells in nasal mucosa to inhaled antigens (e.g., pollens from weeds, grasses, trees) leads to the formation of immunoglobulin E (IgE) antibody molecules. These molecules then bind to the surface membranes of mast cells. This process sensitizes mast cells to the effects of inhaled antigens (allergens). **B.** When sensitized mast cells are reexposed to inhaled pollens or other antigens, they release histamine and other chemical mediators, which then act on nasal mucosa to produce characteristic symptoms of allergic rhinitis.

Allergic Food Reactions

Typically, food allergies are an immune response to the ingestion of a protein. Some food allergens such as shellfish, fish, corn, seeds, bananas, eggs, milk, soy, peanuts, and tree nuts have a higher inherent risk of triggering anaphylaxis than others. However, many other foods have been identified as allergens, including certain fruits and vegetables. There is no known preventive strategy to prevent food allergies except to delay introducing allergy-prone foods to infants until the GI tract has had time to mature. The timing for this varies from food to food and from infant to infant. The most common food allergy among adults is shellfish, often first presenting later in life. Symptoms often occur almost immediately after injection of the food and include the following:

- Itching and tingling around mouth
- Hives
- Swelling of the face, mouth, or throat
- Difficulty swallowing
- Wheezing or shortness of breath
- Dizziness
- Nausea or vomiting

Allergic Drug Reactions

Virtually any drug may induce an immunologic response in susceptible people, and any body tissues may be affected. Allergic drug reactions are complex and diverse and may include any of the types of hypersensitivity described previously. A single drug may induce one or more of these states and multiple symptoms. There are no specific characteristics that identify drug-related reactions, although some reactions commonly attributed to drugs (e.g., skin rashes, drug fever, hematologic reactions, hepatic reactions) rarely occur with plant pollens and other naturally occurring antigens. Usually, however, the body responds to a drug as it does to other foreign materials (antigens).

Allergic drug reactions should be considered when new signs and symptoms develop or when they differ from the usual manifestations of the illness being treated, especially if a reaction:

- Follows ingestion of a drug, especially one known to produce allergic reactions
- Is unpredictable and occurs in only a few patients when many patients receive the suspected drug
- Occurs approximately 7 to 10 days after initial exposure to the suspected drug (to allow antibody production)
- Follows a previous exposure to the same or similar drug (sensitizing exposure)
- Occurs minutes or hours after a second or subsequent exposure
- Occurs after small doses (reduces the likelihood that the reaction is due to dose-related drug toxicity)
- Occurs with other drugs that are chemically or immunologically similar to the suspected drug
- Produces signs and symptoms that differ from the usual pharmacologic actions of the suspected drug
- Produces signs and symptoms usually considered allergic in nature (e.g., anaphylaxis, urticaria, serum sickness)
- Produces similar signs and symptoms to previous allergic reactions to the same or a similar drug
- Increases eosinophils in blood or tissue
- Resolves within a few days of discontinuing the suspected drug

Virtually all drugs have been implicated in anaphylactic reactions. Penicillins and other antimicrobials, radiocontrast media, aspirin and other nonsteroidal anti-inflammatory drugs, and antineoplastics such as L-asparaginase and cisplatin are more common offenders. Less common causes include anesthetics (local and general), opioid analgesics, skeletal muscle relaxants used with general anesthetics, and vaccines. Approximately 10% of severe anaphylactic reactions are fatal. In many cases, it is unknown whether clinical manifestations are immunologic or nonimmunologic in origin.

Serum sickness is a delayed hypersensitivity reaction most often caused by drugs, such as antimicrobials. In addition, many drugs that produce anaphylaxis also produce serum sickness. With initial exposure to the antigen, symptoms usually develop within 7 to 10 days and include urticaria, lymphadenopathy, myalgia, arthralgia, and fever. The reaction usually resolves within a few days but may be severe or even fatal. With repeated exposure to the antigen, after prior sensitization of the host, accelerated serum sickness may develop within 2 to 4 days, with similar but often more severe signs and symptoms.

Systemic lupus erythematosus (SLE) is an autoimmune disorder that may be idiopathic from nondrug causes or induced by hydralazine, procainamide, isoniazid, and other drugs. Clinical manifestations vary greatly, depending on the location and severity of the inflammatory and immune processes, and may include skin lesions, fever, pneumonia, anemia, arthralgia, arthritis, nephritis, and others. Drug-induced lupus produces less kidney and CNS involvement than idiopathic SLE.

Fever often occurs with allergic drug reactions. It may occur alone, with a skin rash and eosinophilia, or with other drug-induced allergic reactions such as serum sickness, SLE, vasculitis, and hepatitis. Dermatologic conditions (e.g., skin rash, urticaria, inflammation) commonly occur with allergic drug reactions and may be the first and most visible manifestations.

Pseudoallergic Drug Reactions

Pseudoallergic drug reactions resemble immune responses (because histamine and other chemical mediators are released), but they do not produce antibodies or sensitized T lymphocytes. **Anaphylactoid reactions** are like anaphylaxis in terms of immediate occurrence, symptoms (rash or hives, difficulty breathing, swelling of body parts), and life-threatening severity. The main difference is that they are not antigen–antibody reactions and, therefore, may occur on first exposure to the causative agent. The drugs bind directly to mast cells, activate the cells, and cause the release of histamine and other vasoactive chemical mediators. Contrast media for radiologic diagnostic tests are often implicated.

Drug Therapy

The H_1 receptor antagonist group contains several classes of antihistamines: alkylamines (e.g., chlorpheniramine), ethanolamines (e.g., clemastine), piperidines (e.g., cyproheptadine), piperazines (e.g., hydroxyzine pamoate), ethylenediamines (tripelennamine), phenothiazines (e.g., promethazine), and a

TABLE 32.1

Drugs Administered to Decrease Histamine Release and the Allergic Response*

Drug Class	Prototype	Other Drugs in the Class
First-generation H_1 receptor antagonists	Diphenhydramine	Chlorpheniramine Clemastine Cyproheptadine Dexchlorpheniramine (Polmon) Hydroxyzine pamoate (Vistaril) Promethazine
Second-generation H_1 receptor antagonists	Cetirizine (Zyrtec Allergy)	Azelastine (Astepro Allergy) Acrivastine and pseudoephedrine (Semprex-D) Loratadine (Claritin) Olopatadine (Patanase)
Third-generation H_1 receptor antagonists	Fexofenadine (Allegra Allergy)	Levocetirizine (Xyzal Allergy 24HR) Desloratadine (Clarinex)

*Table 33.1 lists inhaled drugs used to decrease the histamine response.

miscellaneous group. Choosing an antihistamine is based on the desired effect, duration of action, adverse effects, and other characteristics of available drugs. For most people, a second-generation H_1 receptor antagonist is the first drug of choice. Metabolites of second-generation antihistamines (e.g., fexofenadine, desloratadine, and levocetirizine) are sometimes classed as third-generation antihistamines. These drugs were intended to have increased efficacy with fewer adverse drug reactions than second-generation drugs, although their ability to reduce side effects has not been demonstrated consistently. Table 32.1 lists the drugs given to block the effects of histamine. The H_1 receptor antagonists are categorized into first-, second-, and third-generation drugs. The second- and third-generation drugs are substantially more selective for peripheral histamine H_1 receptors, have decreased ability to cross the blood–brain barrier, and lack anticholinergic effects, thereby providing a better tolerability profile than first-generation agents. The following sections and the DRUGS AT A GLANCE tables describe selected H_1 receptor and H_2 receptor antagonists. (Chapter 33 discusses inhaled drugs used to decrease the histamine response.)

FIRST-GENERATION H_1 RECEPTOR ANTAGONISTS

The oldest H_1 receptor antagonists are relatively inexpensive and widely available. However, they have a limited role in the treatment of most patients because of their numerous adverse effects. They are effective in the relief of allergic symptoms but lack receptor selectivity. Their anticholinergic activity causes poor tolerability of some of these agents, especially compared with the second- and third-generation H_1 receptor antagonists. Patient response and occurrence of adverse drug reactions vary greatly among classes and among drugs within classes.

Ⓟ Diphenhydramine, the prototype first-generation antihistamine, has a high incidence of drowsiness and anticholinergic effects.

Drugs that block the H_1 receptors prevent or reduce most of the physiologic effects that histamine normally induces at H_1 receptor sites. Thus, they

- Inhibit smooth muscle constriction in blood vessels and the respiratory and GI tracts
- Decrease capillary permeability
- Decrease salivation and tear formation

First-generation H_1 antagonists, which are chemically diverse antihistamines (also called nonselective or sedating agents), bind to both central and peripheral H_1 receptors and can cause CNS depression or stimulation. Many of these drugs are currently marketed with or without a prescription, both alone and in combination formulations such as sleep aids.

Pharmacokinetics

Diphenhydramine is well absorbed after oral administration. Immediate-release oral forms act within 15 to 60 minutes and last 4 to 6 hours. Enteric-coated or sustained-release preparations last 8 to 12 hours. For most forms, administration is oral; for a few forms, administration is parenteral. Metabolism is primarily in the liver, and excretion of metabolites and small amounts of unchanged drug occurs in the urine within 24 hours.

Action

Diphenhydramine and the other first-generation H_1 antagonists are structurally related to histamine and occupy the same receptor sites as histamine, which prevents histamine from acting on target tissues. Thus, the drugs are effective in inhibiting vascular permeability, edema formation, bronchoconstriction, and pruritus associated with histamine release. They do not prevent histamine release or reduce the amount released.

Use

Indications for diphenhydramine include hypersensitivity reactions (allergic rhinitis, conjunctivitis, dermatitis), motion sickness, insomnia, and parkinsonism. Table 32.2 gives route and dosage information for some of the first-generation H_1 receptor antagonists.

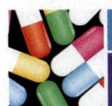

TABLE 32.2
DRUGS AT A GLANCE: First-Generation H₁ Receptor Antagonists

Drug	Routes and Dosage Ranges	
	Adults	**Children**
Diphenhydramine (✦ Diphenhist, PMS-DiphenhydrAMINE)	Hypersensitivity reaction, motion sickness, parkinsonism: PO, 25–50 mg every 4–8 h; IV or deep IM injection 10–50 mg, increased if necessary to a max daily dose of 400 mg Insomnia: PO 50 mg at bedtime Cough (syrup): PO, 25 mg (10 mL) every 4 h, not to exceed 100 mg (40 mL) in 24 h	Weight >10 kg (22 lb), PO 12.5–25 mg every 6–8 h, 5 mg/kg/d, or 150 mg/m²/d; IV 5 mg/kg/d, or 150 mg/m²/d; max oral or parenteral dosage, 300 mg daily Insomnia: ≥12 y, same as adults Cough (syrup) PO 2–6 y, 6.25 mg (2.5 mL) every 4 h, not to exceed 25 mg (10 mL) in 24 h 6–12 y, PO 12.5 mg (5 mL) every 4 h, not to exceed 50 mg (20 mL) in 24 h
Chlorpheniramine (Aller-Chlor, Allergy-Time)	PO, 4 mg PO every 4–6 h; max dose, 24 mg in 24 h Extended-release forms, PO 12 mg every 12 h; max dose, 24 mg in 24 h	2–6 y, PO 1 mg every 4–6 h; max dose, 6 mg in 24 h 6–12 y, PO 2 mg every 4–6 h; max dose, 12 mg in 24 h ≥12 y, same as adults Extended-release forms, ≥12 y, same as adults
Clemastine	Allergic rhinitis: PO 1.34 mg twice daily, increased up to a max of 8.04 mg daily, if necessary Urticaria/angioedema: PO, 2.68 mg 1–3 times daily, increased up to a max of 8.04 mg daily, if necessary	Allergic rhinitis: 6–12 y (syrup only), PO 0.67 mg twice daily, increased up to a max of 4.02 mg daily, if necessary ≥12 y, same as adults Urticaria/angioedema: PO 6 to <12 y (syrup only), PO 1.34 mg twice daily ≥12 y, same as adults
Cyproheptadine	PO, 4 mg every 8 h initially, increase if necessary; max dose 0.5 mg/kg/d	Calculate total daily dosage as 0.25 mg/kg or 8 mg/m² 2–6 y, 2 mg every 8–12 h; max dose, 12 mg/d 7 to <14 y, 4 mg PO every 8–12 h; max dose, 16 mg/d ≥14 y, same as adults
Dexchlorpheniramine (Polmon)	PO, Regular tablets and syrup, 2 mg every 4–6 h	2–5 y, PO 0.5 mg every 4–6 h 6–11 y, PO 1 mg every 4–6 h ≥12 y, same as adults
Hydroxyzine Pamoate (**Vistaril;** ✦ **Atarax, Novo-Hydroxyzin**)	PO, 25 mg every 6–8 h IM, 25–100 mg as needed	<6 y, PO 50 mg daily in divided dose ≥6 y, 50–100 PO mg daily in divided doses
Promethazine	PO, IM, rectally 25 mg, every 4–6 h as needed	≥2 y, 0.5 mg/kg/dose (maximum dose 25 mg) every 12 h as needed

Patient-related variables specific to the use of first-generation H₁ receptor antagonists include the following:

- Age:
  - For safe use in children, close supervision and appropriate dosages are necessary.
  - Young children may experience paradoxical excitement after receiving therapeutic dosages of diphenhydramine and other first-generation H₁ receptor antagonists. After overdose, hallucinations, convulsions, and death may occur.
  - Diphenhydramine is not recommended for use in newborn infants (premature or full term) or children with chickenpox or a flulike infection. When used in young children, doses should be small because of drug effects on the brain and nervous system.
  - Diphenhydramine and other first-generation H₁ receptor antagonists may cause confusion (with impaired thinking, judgment, and memory), dizziness, hypotension, sedation, syncope, unsteady gait, and paradoxical CNS stimulation in older adults. It is possible to misinterpret these effects, especially sedation, as dementia or mental depression.
  - Older males with prostatic hypertrophy may have difficulty voiding while taking these drugs. Some of these adverse reactions derive from anticholinergic effects of the drugs and are likely to be more severe if the patient is also taking other drugs with anticholinergic effects (e.g., tricyclic antidepressants, older antipsychotic drugs, some anti-Parkinson drugs).
  - Despite the increased risk of adverse effects, diphenhydramine is sometimes prescribed as a sleep aid for occasional use in older adults. As with many other drugs, smaller-than-usual dosages are indicated.
- Reproduction, pregnancy, and lactation:
  - Antihistamines may decrease maternal serum prolactin concentrations if taken before breast-feeding is established.

- Diphenhydramine crosses the placenta, but use in pregnancy has not increased the risk for documented congenital anomalies.
- The drug has been shown to have oxytocinlike effects, especially in high dosages.
- Abnormal kidney function and hepatic impairment:
  - In patients with severe abnormal kidney function, it is necessary to give diphenhydramine at a dosing interval of 12 to 18 hours.
- Specific healthcare environments:
  - Patients with critical illness who may be having a blood transfusion or a diagnostic test may receive diphenhydramine, often by injection and usually as a single dose, to prevent allergic reactions.
  - If diphenhydramine is used in the home care setting, the home care nurse needs to assess for drowsiness and safety hazards in the environment (e.g., operating a car or other potentially hazardous machinery).

Concept Mastery Alert

Because many patients self-manage allergy symptoms with over-the-counter (OTC) antihistamines, it is especially important to ask patients with glaucoma, peptic ulcer disease, and urinary retention and those who are pregnant about use of antihistamines, as they may be contraindicated or not recommended for these patients.

Adverse Effects

Diphenhydramine and other first-generation H_1 receptor antagonists usually cause CNS depression (drowsiness, sedation) in therapeutic doses. Some studies have shown that cognitive and performance impairment occurs with the first-generation drugs even when the person does not feel drowsy or impaired. These drugs may cause CNS stimulation (anxiety, agitation) with excessive doses, especially in children. In addition, they have substantial anticholinergic effects (e.g., dry mouth, urinary retention, constipation, blurred vision). In most people, tolerance develops to the sedative effects within a few days if they are not taking other sedative-type drugs or alcoholic beverages.

Contraindications

Contraindication or caution is essential with diphenhydramine in pregnant patients and in patients with hypersensitivity to the drugs, narrow-angle glaucoma, prostatic hypertrophy, stenosing peptic ulcer, and bladder neck obstruction.

Nursing Implications

Preventing Interactions

Several drugs interact with diphenhydramine, increasing its effects (Box 32.1). No drugs reportedly decrease the drug's effects, and no herbs appear to interact with it. Diphenhydramine may reduce the effectiveness of tamoxifen if used concomitantly.

> **BOX 32.1 Drug Interactions: Diphenhydramine**
>
> Drugs that increase the effects of diphenhydramine:
> - Alcohol and other central nervous system depressants (e.g., antianxiety and antipsychotic agents, opioid analgesics, sedative–hypnotics)
>   *Increase central nervous system depression*
> - Monoamine oxidase inhibitors
>   *Decrease metabolism, increase duration of action, and increase sedative and anticholinergic adverse effects*
> - Phenothiazines
>   *Increase risk of dysrhythmias and excessive drowsiness*
> - Pramlintide
>   *Increases risk of constipation*
> - Tricyclic antidepressants
>   *Increase anticholinergic adverse effects*

 Quality and Safety Alert: Safety

It is important not to take diphenhydramine within 14 days of taking a monoamine oxidase inhibitor (isocarboxazid, phenelzine, or tranylcypromine) because of the risk of overstimulation of the sympathetic nervous system.

Administering the Medication

People may take the oral form of diphenhydramine with or without food. Milk may help if stomach upset occurs.

 Quality and Safety Alert: Safety

The nurse should give intramuscular antihistamines deeply into a large muscle mass to decrease tissue irritation. Intravenous (IV) antihistamines are injected slowly, over a few minutes, because severe hypotension may result from rapid IV injection.

To prevent motion sickness, it is necessary to take the drug 30 to 60 minutes before travel.

Assessing for Therapeutic Effects

The nurse observes for a verbal statement of therapeutic effect (relief of symptoms) for the following:

- Decreased nasal congestion when given for hypersensitivity
- Decreased dizziness and nausea when taken for motion sickness
- Drowsiness or sleep when given for insomnia

Assessing for Adverse Effects

The nurse assesses for changes in level of consciousness; dryness of mouth, nose, and throat; blurred vision; urinary retention; and constipation. Gastric effects such as anorexia, nausea, and vomiting are also assessed. In addition, particularly in children, it is necessary to observe for paradoxical excitation (restlessness, insomnia, tremors, nervousness, palpitations).

Patient Teaching

For children with allergies, family members should provide day care staff and school contacts with an emergency plan. Box 32.2

BOX 32.2 Patient Teaching Guidelines for Antihistamines

General Considerations

- People with glaucoma, peptic ulcer, urinary retention, or pregnancy should not take some antihistamines. Inform your physician if you have any of these conditions, or for over-the-counter (OTC) antihistamines, read the label to see if you should avoid a particular drug.
- Antihistamines are most effective before exposure to the stimulus that causes histamine release. For instance, you may want to take these drugs during seasons of high pollen and mold counts.
- Antihistamines may dry and thicken respiratory tract secretions and make them more difficult to remove. Thus, do not take diphenhydramine, which is available OTC, if you have active asthma, bronchitis, or pneumonia.
- First-generation antihistamines cause drowsiness or dizziness and impair mental alertness, judgment, and physical coordination, especially during the first few days. Do not smoke, drive a car, operate machinery, or perform other tasks requiring alertness and physical dexterity until drowsiness has worn off, to avoid injury.
- Avoid using sedating antihistamines with other sedative-type drugs (e.g., alcohol, medications to relieve nervousness or produce sleep), to avoid adverse effects and dangerous drug interactions. Alcohol and other drugs that depress brain function may cause excessive sedation, respiratory depression, and death.
- Do not take more than one antihistamine at a time (e.g., two prescription drugs, two OTC drugs, or a combination of prescription and OTC drugs) because adverse effects are likely. If you do not know whether a particular medication is an antihistamine, consult a healthcare provider. For example, many OTC cold remedies and "nighttime" or "PM" allergy or sinus preparations contain an antihistamine. In addition, the active ingredient in OTC sleep aids is a sedating antihistamine, usually diphenhydramine.
- Avoid prolonged exposure to sunlight and use sunscreens and protective clothing; some antihistamines may increase sensitivity to sunlight and risks of skin damage from sunburn.
- Report adverse effects, such as excessive drowsiness. The healthcare provider may be able to change drugs or dosages to decrease adverse effects.
- If you experience an allergic reaction to a medication, obtain information about the drug thought responsible (including its various names), acceptable alternatives for future drug therapy, and potential sources of the drug. In addition, read the list of ingredients on labels of OTC drug preparations, inform all healthcare providers about the drug reaction before taking any newly prescribed drug, and wear a medical alert device that lists drugs to be avoided. Note that people may be allergic to additives (e.g., dyes, binders, others) rather than the active drug.

Self-Administration

- Take antihistamines only as prescribed or as instructed on packages of OTC preparations to increase beneficial effects and decrease adverse effects. If you miss a dose, do not take a double dose.
- Take most antihistamines with meals to decrease stomach upset. Take loratadine (Claritin) on an empty stomach for better absorption; cetirizine (Zyrtec Allergy) and desloratadine (Clarinex) may be taken with or without food. Do not take fexofenadine with fruit juice as it decreases drug absorption.
- Do not chew or crush sustained-release tablets, and do not open sustained-release capsules. Such actions can cause rapid drug absorption, high blood levels, and serious adverse effects, rather than the slow absorption and prolonged action intended with these products.

---

outlines patient teaching guidelines for diphenhydramine and other antihistamines.

Other Drugs in the Class

Many of the first-generation H_1 receptor antagonists are available alone and in combination with adrenergic nasal decongestants, analgesics, and allergy, cold, and sinus remedies. Most are available as over-the-counter (OTC) drugs, without a prescription.

All other drugs in the class produce a varying degree of drowsiness and can interfere with psychomotor performance, and chronic use should be avoided when possible. Chlorpheniramine and dexchlorpheniramine (Polmon) have similar adverse effects profile as diphenhydramine. Similar interaction patterns exist with other oral H_1 receptor antagonists and diphenhydramine (see Box 32.1).

Hydroxyzine pamoate (Vistaril) or promethazine may be given by injection for nausea and vomiting or to provide sedation but are not usually the first drug of choice for these indications. The U.S. Food and Drug Administration (FDA) has issued a **BOXED WARNING** ◆ for promethazine because of the risk of severe chemical irritation and damage to tissues regardless of the route of administration. Patients younger than 2 years of age should not receive the drug due to the potential for fatal respiratory depression. Although administration may be IV or intramuscular, the oral route should be used as soon as feasible. In addition, cholestatic jaundice has reportedly occurred with promethazine, and use of the drug warrants caution. In children, contraindications to promethazine include hepatic disease, Reye syndrome, history of sleep apnea, and family history of sudden infant death syndrome.

Clinical Application 32.1

- Mr. Rudolph tells the nurse that his wife has a prescription for diphenhydramine, which she takes intermittently at bedtime for insomnia. He says that he knows that diphenhydramine is used to treat allergies and asks if he can use it for his own symptoms. How should the nurse respond?

NCLEX Success

1. The nurse receives an order to administer diphenhydramine. This medication is recommended for use in which of the following?
   A. premature or full-term infants
   B. adults to prevent allergic reactions
   C. children with chickenpox
   D. children with a flulike infection

2. The nurse working in the emergency department anticipates a drug order to treat a severe allergic reaction with anaphylaxis, knowing that the drug of choice for this condition is which of the following?
   A. diphenhydramine
   B. cimetidine
   C. epinephrine
   D. loratadine

3. Because of the action of antihistamines on target tissues, these drugs are effective in producing which of the following actions? (Select all that apply.)
   A. inhibiting vascular permeability
   B. reducing pruritus
   C. minimizing edema formation
   D. preventing histamine release

SECOND-GENERATION H_1 RECEPTOR ANTAGONISTS

Newer-generation H_1 receptor antagonists are much safer than their first-generation counterparts, have a faster onset of action, and have superior potency, selectivity, and efficacy. Unlike the first-generation H_1 receptor antagonists, the second-generation H_1 receptor antagonists do not readily enter the brain from the blood. **Cetirizine** (Zyrtec Allergy), the prototype, and other drugs in this class bind preferentially to peripheral rather than central H_1 receptors. This selectivity significantly reduces the occurrence of adverse drug reactions of the CNS, but drowsiness and CNS depression may occur. The second-generation H_1 receptor antagonists have supplanted the first-generation H_1 receptor antagonists in the symptomatic treatment of allergic rhinitis and in the relief of pruritus in urticaria. In addition, these drugs have a mild beneficial effect in chronic asthma. The drugs are used for treatment of atopic dermatitis or as adjunctive treatment of pruritus and other symptoms in anaphylaxis.

For most agents, onset of action is within 1 hour, and peak serum levels are achieved in 2 to 3 hours. The second-generation agents are also longer acting and require administration once or twice daily. The oral second-generation agents appear to be similarly efficacious to each other. Similar to the older first-generation antihistamines, this generation of agents has less effect on nasal congestion compared with glucocorticoid nasal sprays.

Pharmacokinetics

Cetirizine is rapidly absorbed and reaches peak serum concentrations in 1 hour. The drug is 93% protein bound, and excretion of 50% of the unchanged drug occurs in urine and feces. The drug is present in breast milk.

Action

Cetirizine competes with histamine for binding to histamine receptor sites on effector cells in the GI tract, blood vessels, and respiratory tract, preventing the activation of cells by histamine and thus preventing allergy symptoms. Because the drug does not cross the blood–brain barrier, it does not cause the drowsiness associated with first-generation agents.

Use

Healthcare providers use cetirizine for temporary relief of symptoms of respiratory allergies and urticaria (relief of pruritus). Table 32.3 presents route and dosage information for cetirizine and the other second-generation antihistamines.

> **Quality and Safety Alert: Safety**
>
> If an antihistamine is required during pregnancy, the lowest dose of chlorpheniramine, cetirizine, or loratadine is recommended. However, chlorpheniramine is not recommended during breast-feeding. If a mother takes a second-generation antihistamine while breast-feeding, the infant should be monitored for signs of irritability, jitteriness, or drowsiness.

Patient-related variables specific to the use of second-generation H_1 receptor antagonists include the following:

- Age:
  - Prescription products may be used in children 6 months of age or older for symptoms associated with perennial allergic rhinitis and treatment of uncomplicated skin disorders associated with chronic idiopathic urticaria.
  - OTC products for colds and other respiratory conditions are approved by the FDA in children aged 2 years or older and recommended with caution for use in children younger than 2 years of age. OTC syrup formulations are available for use in younger children.
  - In general, second- and third-generation antihistamines are much safer than first-generation agents for older adults because they are less likely to impair consciousness, thinking, or ability to perform activities of daily living (e.g., driving a car or operating various machines).
  - However, they should be used with caution in older adults as sedation has been reported and normal changes in kidney function may increase adverse effects.
- Reproduction, pregnancy, and lactation:
  - Antihistamines may decrease maternal serum prolactin concentrations if taken before breast-feeding is established.
  - Second-generation antihistamines are less sedating than first-generation drugs, and, if needed to treat rhinitis, the lowest possible dosage is recommended.
  - Cetirizine is present in breast milk, and, if taken by the breast-feeding parent, the drug may cause irritability, jitteriness, or drowsiness in nursing infants.
- Abnormal kidney function and hepatic impairment:
  - Because changes in kidney function related to normal aging have been associated with increased adverse effects

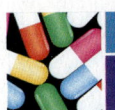

TABLE 32.3
DRUGS AT A GLANCE: Second-Generation H₁ Receptor Antagonists

Drug	Routes and Dosage Ranges	
	Adults	**Children**
Cetirizine (Zyrtec Allergy; APO-Cetirizine, Reactine)	PO, 5–10 mg once daily, to maximum dose of 10 mg daily Abnormal kidney function or hepatic impairment: PO 5 mg once daily	6–12 mo, PO 2.5 mg once daily (syrup available) 12 mo to 2 y, PO 0.5 mg once daily, to a maximum dose of 2.5 mg every 12 h, if needed 2–5 y, PO 2.5 mg (one half tsp) once daily to a maximum dose of 2.5 mg every 12 h or 5 mg once daily, if needed ≥6 y, same as adults
Acrivastine and pseudoephedrine (Semprex-D)	PO, One capsule (acrivastine 8 mg/pseudoephedrine 60 mg) every 4–6 h, to maximum of 4 doses/24 h	≥12, same as adults
Azelastine (Astepro Allergy; Astelin)	Nasal inhalation, (0.1% solution) two sprays per nostrils every 12 h	Nasal inhalation ≥6 mo to ≤5 y, (0.1% solution) one spray per nostrils every 12 h 6 to ≥12 y, (0.1%–0.15% solution) two sprays per nostrils every 12 h 12 y or older, same as adults
Loratadine (Alavert, Claritin)	10 mg PO once daily Abnormal kidney function or hepatic impairment: 10 mg PO every other day	2–5 y, 5 mg PO daily (available in syrup) ≥6 y, same as adults
Olopatadine (Patanase)	Nasal inhalation, two sprays per nostrils every 12 h	Nasal inhalation, 6–11 y, one spray per nostrils every 12 h ≥12 y, same as adults

in those taking the drug, it should be used with caution and the individual's response monitored.
- Because the kidneys play a role in excretion of cetirizine, its use in people with abnormal kidney function warrants caution, and authorities recommend a dosage adjustment.
- Although not specified in manufacturer labeling, dosing adjustments based on glomerular filtration rate are common in those with abnormal kidney function.

Adverse Effects

Adverse effects include drowsiness, headache, dizziness, nausea, vomiting, and fatigue.

Contraindications

Contraindications include known sensitivity to cetirizine or any component of the formulation.

Nursing Implications

Preventing Interactions

Cetirizine does not appear to interact with many drugs, but concomitant use with drugs that also cause the potential for CNS depression may increase the risk of drowsiness and sedation. Theophylline is known to interact with the drug and slightly decrease its clearance. Potentially significant interactions may exist, requiring adjustment in dose or frequency, additional monitoring, or selection of an alternate drug.

Administering the Medication

Administer usually once a day. Food has no effect on the overall absorption of cetirizine but may increase the time it takes to reach peak levels in the blood. It is necessary to shake oral suspensions completely before administration.

Assessing for Therapeutic Effects

The nurse assesses for relief of symptoms, including decreased nasal congestion and cough with seasonal allergic rhinitis. In addition, the nurse assesses for relief of pruritus in urticaria.

Assessing for Adverse Effects

The nurse observes for headache, nausea, vomiting, and fatigue.

Patient Teaching

Box 32.2 summarizes the patient teaching guidelines for antihistamines.

Other Drugs in the Class

Other second-generation H₁ receptor antagonists have similar actions and adverse effect profiles. The level of sedation experienced by patients varies by specific medication and the dose. Acrivastine (Semprex-D) is formulated in combination with pseudoephedrine for symptom relief of seasonal allergic rhinitis. The drug has sedative properties when taken at doses that exceed the recommended dose. Cetirizine, and the intranasal preparations azelastine (Astepro Allergy) and olopatadine

(Patanase), may cause sedation at the recommended dose. Intranasal H_1 receptor antagonists are considered a first-line treatment for allergic rhinitis, although they are generally less effective than intranasal corticosteroids. Intranasal H_1 receptor antagonists are as effective as or superior to oral second-generation antihistamines for treating seasonal allergic rhinitis. Intranasal antihistamines have a clinically significant effect on nasal congestion. The nasal spray leaves an unpleasant taste; however, sniffing gently through the nose after each spray minimizes this taste. When applied to nasal mucosa, the drugs produce peak levels in 2 to 3 hours and last 12 to 24 hours.

Patients should not perform activities that require alertness until they are sure they can engage safely in such activities.

Azelastine nasal spray is available by prescription for adults and children 6 months or older. An OTC preparation (Astepro Allergy) is recommended for adults and children 6 years or older. Olopatadine (Patanase) is only available by prescription as a nasal spray and may be used in children 12 years of age or older.

Loratadine (Claritin) begins to produce effects within 1 to 3 hours, which reach a maximum in 8 to 12 hours and last 24 hours or longer. The drug is metabolized in the liver, and its long duration of action is due, in part, to an active metabolite. The drug should be taken on an empty stomach.

THIRD-GENERATION H_1 RECEPTOR ANTAGONISTS

Like the second-generation H_1 receptor antagonists, third-generation drugs do not readily enter the brain from the blood. Fexofenadine (the metabolite of terfenadine [no longer available]), desloratadine (the metabolite of loratadine), and levocetirizine (a purified isomer of cetirizine) are sometimes classified as third-generation agents. Ⓟ **Fexofenadine** (Allegra Allergy), the prototype, and other drugs in this class bind preferentially to peripheral rather than central H_1 receptors. This selectivity significantly reduces the occurrence of adverse drug reactions, such as drowsiness and sedation, while still providing effective relief of allergic conditions.

Pharmacokinetics

Fexofenadine is rapidly absorbed and reaches peak serum concentrations in about 2.5 hours. It is 60% to 70% protein bound, and excretion of 95% of the unchanged drug occurs in bile and urine. Its effects last for 12 to 24 hours. The drug does not cross the blood–brain barrier, and whether the drug is excreted in breast milk is unknown.

Action

Fexofenadine competes with histamine for binding to histamine receptor sites, preventing the activation of cells by histamine. Competition for the binding sites prevents activation of the H_1 receptors by histamine, thus preventing allergy symptoms from occurring. Because the drug does not cross the blood–brain barrier, it does not cause the drowsiness associated with first-generation agents.

Use

Healthcare providers use fexofenadine for seasonal allergic rhinitis, other minor allergies, and urticaria (relief of pruritus). Table 32.4 presents route and dosage information for fexofenadine and the other third-generation antihistamines. A fexofenadine–pseudoephedrine combination (Allegra-D) is also available for cold and allergy relief, and it is important to review the package literature to ensure appropriate dosing.

Patient-related variables specific to the use of third-generation H_1 receptor antagonists include the following:

- Reproduction, pregnancy, and lactation:
  - Antihistamines may decrease maternal serum prolactin concentrations if taken before breast-feeding is established.

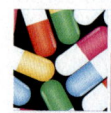

TABLE 32.4

DRUGS AT A GLANCE: Third-Generation H_1 Receptor Antagonists

Drug	Routes and Dosage Ranges	
	Adults	**Children**
Ⓟ Fexofenadine (Allegra Allergy; 🍁 Allegra)	PO, 60 mg twice daily, to maximum of 120 mg/d Abnormal kidney function: 60 mg PO once daily Once-daily formulations: 180 mg once daily (maximum 180 mg/d)	6 mo to 2 y, PO 15 mg twice daily 2–11 y, PO 30 mg twice daily, to maximum of 60 mg/d ≥12, same as adults, to maximum of 120 mg/d (available in syrup)
Desloratadine (Clarinex)	PO, 5 mg once daily	Orally dissolving tablet or liquid: 6–11 mo, PO 1 mg once daily 12 mo to 5 y, 1.25 once daily 6–11 y, 2.5 mg once daily ≥12 y, same as adults
Levocetirizine (Xyzal Allergy 24HR)	PO, 5 mg once daily in evening	6 mo to 5 y, PO 1.25 mg (one half tsp) once daily in evening 6–11 y, PO 2.5 mg (one tsp) once daily in evening ≥12 y, same as adults

- Agents other than fexofenadine are preferred for the treatment of allergic conditions.
- Abnormal kidney function and hepatic impairment:
  - The kidneys play a role in excretion of fexofenadine. Therefore, use of the drug in people with Abnormal kidney function warrants caution, and authorities recommend a dosage adjustment.

Adverse Effects

Adverse effects are usually minor and include headache, nausea, vomiting, dysmenorrhea, and fatigue.

Contraindications

Contraindications include known sensitivity to fexofenadine.

Nursing Implications

Preventing Interactions

Several drugs may interact with fexofenadine, increasing or decreasing its effects (Box 32.3). Some herbs and foods also interact with this drug, including fruit juice (apple, orange, grapefruit), which increases the drug's bioavailability. High-fat meals and chronic use of St. John's wort decrease the bioavailability of fexofenadine.

Administering the Medication

Administration should occur with water only (fruit juice may decrease absorption). It is necessary to shake oral suspensions completely before administration. Oral disintegrating tablets should remain in the blister pack until use.

Quality and Safety Alert: Safety

Patients should take the tablets on an empty stomach. After placement on the tongue, the tablets dissolve in minutes, and swallowing, with or without water, may occur.

BOX 32.3 Drug Interactions: Fexofenadine

Drugs That Increase the Effects of Fexofenadine
- Alcohol, cannabinoids, dimethindene, doxylamine, dronabinol, droperidol, flunitrazepam, and oxycodone
  Increase the potential for sedation
- Azole antifungals (fluconazole, itraconazole, ketoconazole, miconazole) and macrolide antibacterials (azithromycin, clarithromycin, erythromycin)
  Increase the plasma concentration

Drugs That Decrease the Effects of Fexofenadine
- Antacids containing magnesium or aluminum
  Decrease the absorption
- Rifampin
  Decreases the metabolism

Assessing for Therapeutic Effects

The nurse assesses for relief of symptoms, including decreased nasal congestion and cough with seasonal allergic rhinitis. In addition, the nurse assesses for relief of pruritus in urticaria.

Assessing for Adverse Effects

The nurse observes for headache, nausea, vomiting, and fatigue. In females, it is also necessary to assess for dysmenorrhea.

Patient Teaching

Box 32.2 summarizes the patient teaching guidelines for antihistamines.

Other Drugs in the Class

As with second-generation antihistamines, fexofenadine and other third-generation drugs are much safer than the first-generation agents for older adults because they do not impair consciousness, thinking, or ability to perform activities of daily living (e.g., driving a car or operating various machines). The third-generation H_1 receptor antagonists have similar actions and adverse effect profiles.

Levocetirizine (Xyzal Allergy 24HR) is an OTC preparation that has an onset of action of 1 hour, and a single daily dose provides antihistamine activity for 28 hours. The drug can be used with children 6 months or older. Desloratadine (Clarinex) seems to offer no advantage over loratadine as both are two of the least-sedating antihistamines. The drug may be used in children 6 months of age or older.

Quality and Safety Alert: Evidence-Based Practice

A Joint Task Force on Practice Parameters of the American Academy of Allergy, Asthma, and Immunology (Dykewicz et al., 2020) has updated recommendations on the approach to the management of allergic rhinitis. The primary strategy to relieve the symptoms of allergic rhinitis is avoidance of the offending allergen. If avoidance of allergens does not achieve symptom relief in patients with allergic rhinitis, indicated drugs may include the following:

- OTC second-generation antihistamines, such as loratadine, which should provide symptom relief in most situations; first-generation antihistamines not recommended
- Prescription and other OTC drugs
  - Intranasal corticosteroids, such as fluticasone and flunisolide for adults and mometasone (see Chapter 33) for children, when symptoms are moderate to severe
  - Intranasal antihistamines, such as OTC azelastine, if intranasal corticosteroids are not effective or the patient is not a candidate for corticosteroids and as an initial treatment option for patients with seasonal acute rhinitis
- As initial treatment, monotherapy with an intranasal steroid in patients over 12 years of age with symptoms of seasonal acute rhinitis (preferred over a combination of an oral antihistamine and an intranasal steroid)

- For patients older than 15 years of age with moderate-to-severe seasonal allergic rhinitis, an intranasal corticosteroid (recommended over a leukotriene receptor antagonist; see Chapter 33)
- Avoidance of oral decongestants during the first trimester of pregnancy

The use of evidence-based guidelines in the treatment of allergic rhinitis provides effective strategies for symptom relief. Appropriate drug therapy based on best practices maximizes symptom relief and reduces adverse effects. The nurse should educate patients regarding avoidance of the offending allergen and adherence with guidelines for drug use and assess for effective symptom management.

Clinical Application 32.2

- Mr. Rudolph informs the nurse that he thinks he is allergic to the aspirin that he has been taking for his coronary artery disease because he becomes nauseated after taking his daily dose. What questions should the nurse ask Mr. Rudolph to help determine whether he has an allergy to aspirin?

NCLEX Success

4. A patient has asked for an antihistamine to relieve symptoms of an upper respiratory infection. The nurse explains that studies have demonstrated that for treatment of the common cold, which of the following is true of antihistamines?
   A. are effective in relieving cold symptoms
   B. do not relieve symptoms and are not recommended
   C. should be compounded with other products to be effective
   D. relieve nonallergenic symptoms only

5. Which statement by a patient indicates understanding of a nurse's teaching about the adverse effects of diphenhydramine? (Select all that apply)
   A. dry mouth and constipation
   B. drowsiness and sedation
   C. congestion and stuffiness
   D. itching and skin rash
   E. rebound congestion
   F. hypertension
   G. urinary retention
   H. blurred vision

THE NURSING PROCESS

A concept map outlines the nursing process related to drug therapy considerations in this chapter. Additional nursing implications related to the disease process should also be considered in care decisions.

Assessment
- Assess the patient's condition in relation to disorders for which antihistamines are used. For the patient with known allergies, try to determine the factors that precipitate or relieve allergic reactions and specific signs and symptoms experienced during a reaction.
- Assess every patient for a potential hypersensitivity reaction. For example, it is standard practice on first contact to ask a patient if they have any food, drug, or other allergies. The health care provider is likely to get more complete information by asking patients about allergic reactions to specific drugs (e.g., antibiotics such as penicillin, local anesthetics) rather than asking if they are allergic to or cannot take any drugs.
- If a drug allergy is identified, ask about specific signs and symptoms as well as any drugs currently being taken. With previous exposure and sensitization to the same or a similar drug, immediate allergic reactions may occur. With a new drug, antibody formation and allergic reactions usually require a week or longer. Most reactions appear within a month of starting a drug.
- When a suspected allergic reaction occurs (e.g., skin rash, fever, edema, dyspnea), interview the patient or consult medical records about the drug, dose, route, and time of administration. In addition, evaluate all the drugs a patient is taking as a potential cause of the reaction. This assessment may involve searching drug literature to see if the suspected drug is associated with allergic reactions and discussion with physicians and pharmacists.

Outcomes of Therapy
The patient will
- Experience relief of symptoms.
- Take antihistamines accurately.
- Avoid hazardous activities if sedation occurs from antihistamines.
- Avoid preventable adverse drug effects.
- Avoid taking sedative-type antihistamines with alcohol or other sedative drugs.

Nursing Interventions
- For patients with known allergies, assist in identifying and avoiding precipitating factors when possible. If it is a drug allergy, encourage the patient to carry a medical alert device that identifies the drug.
- Monitor the patient closely for excessive drowsiness during the first few days of therapy with antihistamines known to cause sedation.
- Encourage a fluid intake of 2000 to 3000 mL daily, if not contraindicated.
- When indicated, obtain an order and administer an antihistamine before situations known to elicit allergic reactions (e.g., blood transfusions, diagnostic tests that involve contrast media).
- For children with allergies, provide all family members, day care staff, and school personnel with an emergency plan.

Evaluation
- Observe for relief of symptoms.
- Interview and observe for correct drug usage.
- Interview and observe for excessive drowsiness.

Unfolding Patient Stories: Yoa Li • Part 1

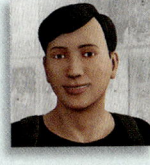

Yoa Li is a 26-year-old male admitted to the hospital for surgical repair of a strangulated groin hernia. He is experiencing symptoms of allergic rhinitis. Recognizing he is NPO pending surgery, what are medication options to relieve nasal congestion and drainage that the nurse can recommend when informing the provider of his symptoms? (Yoa Li's story continues in Chapter 49.)

Care for Yoa and other patients in a realistic virtual environment: **vSim** for Nursing (thepoint.lww.com/vSimPharm). Practice documenting these patients' care in DocuCare (thepoint.lww.com/DocuCareEHR).

Visit **thePoint** at **http://thePoint.lww.com/Frandsen13e** for answers to NCLEX Success questions (in Appendix A), answers to Clinical Application Case Studies (in Appendix B), and more!

REFERENCES AND RESOURCES

Dykewicz, M. S., Wallace, D. V., Amrol, D. J., Baroody, F. M., Bernstein, J. A., Craig, T. J., & Contributors, W. (2020). Rhinitis 2020: A practice parameter update. *The Journal of Allergy and Clinical Immunology, 146*(4), 721–767. https://doi.org/10.1016/j.jaci.2020.07.007

Fein, M. N., Fischer, D. A., O'Keefe, A. W., & Sussman, G. L. (2019). CSACI position statement: Newer generation H1-antihistamines are safer than first-generation H1-antihistamines and should be the first-line antihistamines for the treatment of allergic rhinitis and urticaria. *Allergy, Asthma, and Clinical Immunology: Official Journal of the Canadian Society of Allergy and Clinical Immunology, 15*, 61–61. https://doi.org/10.1186/s13223-019-0375-9

Hall, J. E., & Hall, M. E. (2020). *Guyton and Hall textbook of medical physiology* (14th ed.). Elsevier. ISBN-13: 978-0323597128

Hinkle, J. L., Cheever, K. H., & Overbaugh, K. J. (2021). *Brunner & Suddarth's textbook of medical-surgical nursing* (15th ed.). Wolters Kluwer.

National Guideline Clearinghouse. (2015). *Guideline summary: Clinical practice guideline: Allergic rhinitis.* Retrieved from https://www.guideline.gov

Norris, T. L. (2018). *Porth's pathophysiology: Concepts of altered health states* (10th ed.). Wolters Kluwer.

Nursing2022. (2021). *Drug handbook.* Wolters Kluwer Health/Lippincott Williams & Wilkins.

Xu, H., Zhang, Y., Gu, M., Shan, Y., & Zhang, Q. (2022). A prospective study on the difference of clinical outcomes between elderly and adult patients with allergic rhinitis. *American Journal of Otolaryngology, 43*(4), 103509.

CHAPTER 33

Drug Therapy for Asthma, Airway Inflammation, and Bronchoconstriction

LEARNING OBJECTIVES

After studying this chapter, you should be able to:

1. Describe the clinical manifestations of asthma, airway inflammation, and bronchoconstriction in terms of their pathophysiology.
2. Compare and contrast the short-acting (rescue) and the long-term maintenance inhaled beta$_2$-adrenergic agonists.
3. Identify the prototype drug from each drug class used to treat asthma, airway inflammation, and bronchoconstriction.
4. Recognize drugs used to treat asthma, airway inflammation, and bronchoconstriction in terms of mechanism of action, indications for use, major adverse effects, and nursing implications.
5. Implement the nursing process in the care of patients with asthma, airway inflammation, and bronchoconstriction.

CLINICAL APPLICATION CASE STUDY

Terry Lee, age 38 years, presents to the emergency department in severe respiratory distress, with profound dyspnea, wheezing, and circumoral cyanosis. He received a diagnosis of asthma at age 10. Mr. Lee is admitted to the intensive care unit. His treatment regimen includes albuterol via inhalation every 20 minutes for four doses and intravenous (IV) corticosteroids every 6 hours.

KEY TERMS

Airway hyperresponsiveness: exaggerated bronchoconstrictive response to stimuli

Bronchoconstriction: constriction of the air passages of the lung (as in asthma)

Eosinophilic phenotype: allergic response of individuals with severe asthma who have blood eosinophil counts of 150/μL or greater

Leukotrienes: strong proinflammatory mediators produced by the immune system during trauma, infection, and inflammation that cause bronchoconstriction and inflammation, the major pathologic features of asthma

Maintenance inhalant medications: long-term control beta$_2$-agonists used to achieve and maintain prophylactic control of persistent asthma

Rescue (or reliever) inhalant medications: quick-relief, short-acting beta$_2$-agonists used during periods of acute symptoms and exacerbations

Status asthmaticus: acute, severe asthma

Triggers: factors that initiate asthma symptoms

Work-exacerbated asthma: adverse respiratory outcome resulting from work-related conditions

INTRODUCTION

This chapter describes drugs used to treat asthma and other respiratory disorders characterized by airway inflammation, **bronchoconstriction** (narrowing of the air passages of the lungs), **airway hyperresponsiveness** (exaggerated bronchoconstrictive response to stimuli), and mucosal edema. These signs and symptoms characterize such features as asthma, chronic bronchitis, and emphysema, which are collectively considered the chronic lung diseases. Here, the emphasis is on asthma because of its widespread prevalence, especially in urban populations. To understand the use of drugs in the management of asthma, it is necessary to provide an overview of the condition and its prevalence and clinical manifestations. For further details on the etiology and pathophysiology of asthma, visit thePoint® (http://thePoint.lww.com/Frandsen13e).

OVERVIEW OF ASTHMA

Many people with asthma have sensitivities to certain drugs that can precipitate acute symptoms of asthma. In about 25% of patients with asthma, aspirin and other nonsteroidal anti-inflammatory drugs (NSAIDs) can precipitate an exacerbation. Research has also demonstrated an increased risk of asthma and its exacerbation with the use of acetaminophen.

Some patients are allergic to sulfites and may experience life-threatening asthma attacks if they ingest foods processed with these preservatives (e.g., beer, wine, dried fruit). Patients with severe asthma should be cautioned against ingesting food and drug products that contain sulfites or metabisulfites. The U.S. Food and Drug Administration (FDA) has banned the use of sulfites in foods meant to be served raw, such as salads in salad bars.

Gastroesophageal reflux disease (GERD), a common disorder characterized by heartburn and esophagitis, is also associated with asthma. Asthma that worsens at night may be associated with nighttime acid reflux. Although the precise mechanism of pulmonary symptoms of GERD in asthma is not known, experts suggest that microaspirations or a vagally mediated, reflex type of bronchoconstriction may be involved. Asthma, in turn, may also aggravate GERD, because anti-asthma medications that dilate the airways also relax muscle tone in the gastroesophageal sphincter and may increase acid reflux. The results of randomized trials of acid suppression therapy suggest that gastroesophageal reflux is most likely not a contributor to asthma in patients without esophageal reflux symptoms.

Work-exacerbated asthma (WEA) (i.e., adverse respiratory outcomes resulting from repeated and prolonged work-related conditions) is also a major health problem. People with WEA often have symptoms while in the work environment, with improvement on days off and during vacations. Symptoms sometimes persist after termination of exposure. Different types of agents or conditions at work may exacerbate asthma. Cases of WEA with persistent work-related symptoms can have clinical characteristics (level of severity, medication needs) and adverse socioeconomic outcomes (unemployment, reduction in income) similar to those of cases of occupational asthma. Compared with adults with asthma unrelated to work, people with WEA report more days with symptoms, seek more medical care, and have a lower quality of life.

Management of WEA should focus on reducing work exposures and optimizing standard medical management, with a change in jobs only if these measures are not successful. Additional research is needed (1) to improve the understanding of the risk factors for WEA and its mechanisms and outcomes and (2) to inform and evaluate preventive interventions.

Clinical Manifestations

Asthma is an airway disorder characterized by airway inflammation, bronchoconstriction, and airway hyperresponsiveness to various stimuli. The airway hyperresponsiveness produces an exaggerated contractile response of the airways to stimuli. Resultant symptoms include intermittent dyspnea, wheezing, and cough, with variable expiratory airflow limitations. Wheezing is a high-pitched, whistling sound caused by turbulent airflow through an obstructed airway. Thus, any condition that produces significant airway occlusion can cause wheezing. However, a chronic cough may be the only symptom in some people with asthma. The presence of wheezing or coughing is not a dependable standard for evaluating the severity of an asthma attack.

Patients who use peak expiratory flow rate (PEFR) monitoring can assess the severity of airway constriction through trending of peak flow measurements. In general, a PEFR value 80% or greater of the patient's best PEFR (established when breathing is normal) is considered within a safe range; from 50% to 80% of the PEFR value is a moderate drop; and less than 50% of the patient's best PEFR value is considered a severe reduction in breathing function that requires urgent intervention.

> **Quality and Safety Alert: Safety**
>
> The nurse encourages patients to develop a written asthma action plan with their healthcare provider to identify the correct action for acute episodes of asthma should symptoms worsen or when the PEFR value is less than 50% of the best PEFR.

Quality and Safety Alert: Evidence-Based Practice

Although people with asthma and other allergic diseases are commonly more susceptible to respiratory viruses, which often cause acute exacerbation of asthma, it is unclear whether asthma is a risk factor for severe COVID-19 in children or whether having COVID-19 will negatively affect asthma control.

In a prospective, multicenter study, Vezir et al. (2021) explored the relationship between respiratory and allergic diseases and COVID-19 severity in 75 children and adolescents, ages 5 to 18 years. COVID-19 was asymptomatic/mild in 44 patients and moderate/severe/critical in 31 patients. Patients were evaluated for 1 to 3 months after the COVID-19 infection resolved. Data were collected on complete blood cell count, total immunoglobulin E (IgE) levels, skin prick tests, and spirometry testing results.

Thirty-two patients (42.7%) had an underlying disease. Of these, 10 patients (13%) were identified with asthma, 19 patients (25.3%) with allergic rhinitis, and 3 patients (4%) with atopic rhinitis. There was no difference in COVID-19 symptoms between the patients with or without asthma, nor was there a difference in spirometry parameters. The median total IgE level was significantly higher in the asymptomatic/mild group. The researchers concluded that aeroallergen sensitization and allergic rhinitis in children may be associated with a milder course of COVID-19.

BOX 33.1 Other Bronchoconstrictive Disorders: Chronic Bronchitis and Emphysema

Chronic bronchitis and emphysema, commonly called chronic obstructive pulmonary disease (COPD), usually develop after long-standing exposure to airway irritants such as cigarette smoke. The conditions are also known as chronic obstructive lung disease (COLD), chronic obstructive airway disease (COAD), or chronic airflow limitation (CAL). In both conditions, bronchoconstriction and inflammation are more constant and less reversible than with asthma. Anatomic and physiologic changes occur over several years and lead to increasing dyspnea, activity intolerance, and reduced quality of life. Chronic bronchitis often leads to emphysema.

Chronic Bronchitis

Chronic bronchitis is defined as frequent cough with sputum production for 3 months per year, for two consecutive years. The hallmark of chronic bronchitis is an increase in the number and size of the goblet cells and mucous glands of the airway. This leads to increased mucus in the airways, a factor in narrowing of the airways and causing a cough with sputum. At the cellular level, inflammation infiltrates the airway walls leading to scarring and remodeling that thickens the walls; this further narrows the airways. As chronic bronchitis progresses, there is further thickening and scarring of the wall, limiting airflow.

Emphysema

Emphysema is an enlargement and destruction of the alveoli distal to the terminal bronchioles from long-term lung damage and inflammation. Changes to the alveolar walls decrease the surface area available for gas exchange. Lung elasticity also decreases, leading to loss of supporting structures for the alveoli. Additionally, capillaries feeding the alveoli are destroyed. The small airways that collapse early during expiration cause trapping of carbon dioxide and ultimate reduction of oxygen exchange at the alveoli.

Symptoms vary in incidence and severity from occasional episodes of mild respiratory distress, with normal functioning between exacerbations, to persistent, daily, or continual respiratory distress if not adequately controlled. Inflammation and damaged airway mucosa are chronically present, even when patients appear symptom free. Acute episodes of asthma may last minutes to hours.

Acute, severe asthma that does not respond to the usual use of bronchodilators and is characterized by severe respiratory distress is called **status asthmaticus**. This life-threatening condition requires emergency treatment due to the high probability of respiratory failure. Patients may show signs of acute breathlessness, chest tightness, agitation, confusion, or an inability to concentrate. In status asthmaticus, the lack of wheezing sound or coughing may indicate severe bronchoconstriction, impaired gas exchange in the lungs, and a worsening of the condition.

Other bronchoconstrictive disorders include such conditions as chronic bronchitis and emphysema. Although the characteristics of the diseases are different (Box 33.1), experts increasingly recognize that symptoms previously associated with one disorder may be reported in people with another condition. Importantly, people with mixed symptoms appear to have a poorer quality of life, higher mortality, and greater utilization of healthcare services.

Management

Management of asthma involves prevention of airway inflammation and avoidance of **triggers** (factors that initiate asthma symptoms) for better symptom control. Poor asthma control contributes to unnecessary morbidity and mortality, financial burden, limitations of activities of daily living, and diminishes overall quality of life. Because of asthma's significance as a world health problem, numerous agencies have published asthma guidelines related to the diagnosis, management, and education of asthma. Guidelines emphasize the importance of classifying asthma severity and the assessment of asthma control. Overall guidelines for adults and children with asthma (Box 33.2) center on symptom control and risk reduction. Although the focus of the discussion is on drug therapy, the nurse must consider the nonpharmacologic approaches in the management of the disease.

Nonpharmacologic Approaches

Poor symptom control is a significant predictor of exacerbations of asthma. The nurse should identify any personal or environmental risk factors (e.g., cigarette smoke, mold, dander) that can be treated or modified. Efforts to modify risk factors to decrease the triggers of asthma (e.g., reducing work exposure, avoiding asthma triggers, decreasing stress) could minimize the frequency or severity of asthma episodes.

BOX 33.2 Overall Guidelines for the Treatment of Asthma

Goals of Therapy
- No exacerbations
- Minimal daytime symptoms (less than 3 days/week) or no nighttime symptoms
- No persistent airflow limitations (forced expiratory volume in 1 second [FEV_1] or peak expiratory flow (PEF) at least 90% of personal best
- Maintain normal physical activity levels; for children, no school missed; for adults, no absenteeism from work
- Minimal use of short-acting inhaled beta$_2$-agonist (less than three doses/week)
- Minimal or no adverse effects from medications
- Individual and caregiver ability to act appropriately to manage symptoms, including drug therapy and trigger avoidance measures
- Avoid the risk of asthma-related deaths

General Recommendations
- Establish and teach patients/parents/caregivers about quick-relief measures and long-term control measures. Assist to identify and control environmental factors that aggravate asthma. For acute attacks, gain control as quickly as possible (a short course of systemic corticosteroids may be needed); then step down to the least medication necessary to maintain control.
- Review the treatment regimen every 1 to 6 months. If control is adequate and goals are being met, a gradual stepwise reduction in medication may be possible. If control is inadequate, the treatment regimen may need to be changed. For example, frequent or increasing use of a short-acting beta$_2$-agonist (greater than three times a week with intermittent asthma; daily or increasing use with persistent asthma) may indicate the need to initiate or increase long-term control therapy. However, first reassess the patient's medication techniques (e.g., correct use of inhalers), adherence, and environmental control measures. Maintain a good partnership between person with asthma and caregiver, and healthcare providers. Set mutually agreed to goals for individualized care, create written asthma action plan, and encourage self-management.

Preferred Controller Relief (Adjusted Based on Individual Need and Response to Management)
- **Adults and children older than 5 years:** low-dose inhaled corticosteroid plus short-acting beta$_2$-agonist is preferred. Alternative options include leukotriene antagonist daily. A combination of inhaled steroids and long-acting beta$_2$-agonists leads to faster improvement than inhaled steroid use alone, increases lung function, improves quality of life, and reduces the risk of asthma-related hospitalization or death.
- **Children aged 5 years or younger:** administration of the daily low-dose inhaled corticosteroid by a nebulizer or metered-dose inhaler (MDI) with a holding chamber. Alternatives: a leukotriene modifier or intermittent inhaled corticosteroid.

Rescuer Relief for Acute Exacerbations
- **Adults and children older than 5 years:** increase usual controller-double low-dose inhaled corticosteroid, short-acting, inhaled, beta$_2$-agonist started or increased, as needed.
- **Children aged 5 years or younger:** double low-dose inhaled corticosteroid short-acting beta$_2$-agonist by nebulizer or face mask and spacer or holding chamber.

Low (L), Medium (M), and High (H) Doses of Inhaled Corticosteroids

	Adults (mcg)	Children (6–11 y) (mcg)
Beclomethasone (CFC)	L: 200–500 M: >500–1,000 H: >1,000	L: 100–200 M: >200–400 H: >400
Beclomethasone (HFA)	L: 100–200 M: 200–400 H: >400	L: 50–100 M: >100–200 H: >200
Budesonide (DPI)	L: 200–400 M: 400–800 H: >800	L: 100–200 M: >200–400 H: >400
Budesonide (nebules)	L: n/a M: n/a H: >n/a	L: 250–500 M: >500–1,000 H: >1,000
Ciclesonide (HFA)	L: 80–160 M: >160–320 H: >320	L: 80 M: >80–160 H: >160
Fluticasone furoate (DPI)	L: 100 M: n/a H: >200	L: n/a M: n/a H: >n/a
Fluticasone propionate (DPI)	L: 100–250 M: >250–500 H: >500	L: 100–200 M: 200–400 H: >400
Fluticasone propionate (HFA)	L: 100–250 M: >250–500 H: >500	L: 100–200 M: >200–500 H: >500
Mometasone furoate	L: 110–220 M: >220–440 H: >440	L: 110 M: >220–440 H: >440
Triamcinolone acetonide	L: 400–1,000 M: >1,000–2,000 H: >2,000	L: 400–800 M: >800–1,200 H: >1,200

CFC, chlorofluorocarbon propellant; DPI, dry powder inhaler; HFA, hydrofluoroalkane propellant; n/a, not applicable.

In addition to avoidance of triggers, complementary and alternative medicine (CAM) treatments for asthma may be beneficial. These range from breathing exercises to herbal remedies. However, determining the safety and effectiveness of these therapies is problematic because of a lack of well-designed clinical trials. Overall, a review of asthma studies using a form of CAM therapies found insufficient evidence to support their use as effective asthma treatments; the use of these measures should not supersede or delay management of exacerbations.

Drug Therapy

Bronchodilators and anti-inflammatory drugs are the pharmacologic cornerstones of asthma management. Bronchodilators used to prevent and treat bronchoconstriction include adrenergics, anticholinergics, and xanthines. Anti-inflammatory drugs, such as corticosteroids, leukotriene modifiers, mast cell stabilizers, and immunosuppressant monoclonal antibodies, are used to prevent and treat inflammation of the airways. Reducing inflammation also reduces bronchoconstriction by decreasing mucosal edema and mucous secretions that narrow airways and by decreasing airway hyperresponsiveness to various stimuli. Table 33.1 lists the drugs used for the treatment of asthma.

Overall, the severity of the disease process and a stepwise approach to the patient's response to therapy largely determine the choice of drug and route of administration. An aerosol, which is given by inhalation, acts directly on the airways. Therefore, people with mild asthma can usually take it in smaller doses, and it produces fewer adverse effects than oral or parenteral drugs. A selective, short-acting, inhaled $beta_2$-adrenergic agonist (e.g., albuterol) is the initial drug of choice for acute bronchospasm. Inflammation is a major component of asthma; thus, healthcare providers may give an inhaled corticosteroid early in the disease process, often adding a bronchodilator or mast cell stabilizer. In acute episodes of bronchoconstriction, prescribers often order that a corticosteroid be taken orally or intravenously for several days.

TABLE 33.1

Drugs Administered for the Treatment of Asthma

Drug Class	Prototype	Other Drugs in the Class
Adrenergics	Albuterol (Proventil HFA, Ventolin HFA, ProAir RespiClick)	Epinephrine (Adrenalin) Formoterol (Foradil) Levalbuterol (Xopenex [MDI], Xopenex Concentrate, Xopenex HFA) Metaproterenol (Alupent) Salmeterol (Serevent) Terbutaline
Anticholinergics	Ipratropium bromide (Atrovent)	Tiotropium (Spiriva)
Xanthines	Theophylline (Elixophyllin, Theo-24, Theochron)	
Corticosteroids	Beclomethasone (Qvar RediHaler Beconase AQ, QVAR)	Budesonide (Pulmicort Turbuhaler) Ciclesonide Flunisolide Fluticasone (Flonase) Fluticasone aerosol (Flovent) Fluticasone powder (Flovent Rota disk) Mometasone (Asmanex Twisthaler) Triamcinolone (Azmacort) Hydrocortisone sodium phosphate and sodium succinate Prednisone Methylprednisolone sodium succinate
Leukotriene modifiers	Montelukast (Singulair)	Zafirlukast (Accolate) Zileuton (Zyflo, Zyflo CR)
Immunosuppressant monoclonal antibodies	Omalizumab (Xolair)	Mepolizumab (Nucala) Reslizumab (Cinqair) Benralizumab (Fasenra) Dupilumab (Dupixent) Tezepelumab (Tezspire)
Adjuvant medications		
Mast cell stabilizer		Cromolyn (NasalCrom)

Quality and Safety Alert: Evidence-Based Practice

Evidence indicates that uncontrolled asthma during pregnancy results in problems such as preeclampsia, preterm birth, low birth weight infants, and increased risk of perinatal mortality. Therefore, it is important to maintain optimal control of asthma prior to and during pregnancy. Well-controlled asthma during pregnancy creates little or no increased risk of adverse fetal or maternal complications [Global Initiative for Asthma [GINA], 2022].

Updated guidelines (Global Initiative for Asthma [GINA], 2022) recommend that first-line treatment of acute asthma exacerbation and mild persistent and mild to moderate persistent asthma is a daily inhaled corticosteroid on a regular schedule. Inhaled corticosteroids can decrease the inflammatory symptoms of asthma by reducing airway edema and mucous. Research indicates that use of a daily inhaled corticosteroid was associated with fewer hospitalizations, exacerbations, and death in patients with asthma. For any individual with asthma, long-acting beta$_2$-agonists or long-acting muscarinic antagonists only should be used in combination with inhaled corticosteroids and not as monotherapy.

GINA guidelines no longer recommend inhaled short-acting beta$_2$-agonists, such as albuterol, as initial daily treatment of asthma in adolescents and adults. However, the drug class is still recommended for acute asthma episodes, for those with the first signs of asthma symptoms, and for short-term management of individuals with vigorous exercise-induced asthma.

The use of a combination single maintenance and rescue inhaler containing budesonide and low-dose formoterol is preferred for both maintenance and quick relief in adolescent and adult patients with moderate persistent asthma.

For uncontrolled, persistent asthma, GINA guidelines recommend a long-acting beta$_2$-agonist combined with an inhaled corticosteroid. Both short- and long-acting muscarinic antagonists are no longer recommended for add-on therapy for uncontrolled persistent asthma control.

Management of status asthmaticus entails beta$_2$-agonists in high doses and as often as every 20 minutes for 1 to 2 hours (by metered-dose inhalers [MDIs] with spacer devices or by compressed-air nebulization). However, high doses of nebulized albuterol have been associated with tachycardia, hypokalemia, and hyperglycemia. After symptoms have subsided, dosage reduction usually may occur, with extended dosage intervals. People may take high doses of systemic corticosteroids for several days, intravenously or orally. If the patient can take an oral drug, there is no therapeutic advantage to intravenous (IV) administration.

Quality and Safety Alert: Safety

Because asthma can result in death in a matter of minutes, healthcare providers should counsel patients not to use dietary or herbal supplements in place of prescribed bronchodilating and anti-inflammatory medications. Delays in appropriate treatment can have serious, even fatal, consequences.

ADRENERGICS

Specific effects of adrenergic medications depend mainly on the type of adrenergic receptor activated by the drug. Adrenergic receptors are those responses that are activated by adrenalinelike compounds. The drugs discussed in this chapter are more selective for specific adrenergic receptors or are primarily administered by inhalation to produce more localized therapeutic effects in the management of asthma and bronchoconstriction and thus have fewer systemic adverse effects.

Other adrenergic drugs affect multiple adrenergic receptors and have many clinical uses; other chapters discuss these drugs more extensively (see Chapters 31 and 59).

Administering bronchodilators by inhalation (via nebulizer or MDI) is effective and is recommended for relief of acute asthma episodes. Two general types of inhaled beta$_2$-adrenergic agonists are used for asthma management: **rescue inhalant medications** or reliever medications (quick-relief, short-acting drugs used during periods of acute symptoms and exacerbations) and **maintenance inhalant medications** (long-term control drugs used to achieve and maintain prophylactic control of persistent asthma). Box 33.3 lists the rescue and maintenance medications used in asthma therapy. **Albuterol** (Proventil HFA, Ventolin HFA, ProAir RespiClick), the prototype adrenergic bronchodilator, is a rescue inhalant medication.

Pharmacokinetics

Albuterol is rapidly absorbed following oral administration. With the oral drug, the onset of action is 15 to 30 minutes (extended release, 30 minutes), the peak is 2 to 3 hours, and the duration of action is 8 to 12 hours. With an MDI, the onset of action is 5 to 15 minutes, the peak activity is 1 to 1½ hours, and the duration of action is 3 to 6 hours. The drug quickly undergoes extensive metabolism in the liver.

Action

Albuterol and other drugs in the class stimulate beta$_2$-adrenergic receptors in the smooth muscle of bronchi and bronchioles.

BOX 33.3 Rescue and Maintenance Beta$_2$-Agonist Inhaled Medications

Short-Acting Rescue Medications

- Albuterol
- Metaproterenol
- Levalbuterol
- Albuterol/ipratropium (combines a beta$_2$-agonist and an inhaled anticholinergic bronchodilator)

Long-Acting Maintenance Medications

- Inhaled steroid (beclomethasone, budesonide, ciclesonide, fluticasone, mometasone)
- Salmeterol/fluticasone (combines a beta$_2$-agonist bronchodilator and an inhaled steroid)
- Formoterol/budesonide (combines a beta$_2$-agonist bronchodilator and an inhaled steroid)
- Formoterol/mometasone (combines a beta$_2$-agonist bronchodilator and an inhaled steroid)

The receptors, in turn, stimulate the enzyme adenylyl cyclase to increase production of cyclic AMP. The increased cyclic AMP produces bronchodilation.

Use

Healthcare providers use albuterol to treat bronchospasm in people with asthma and other reversible obstructive airway disease. They also use the drug in those with the first signs of asthma symptoms and short-term management of individuals with vigorous exercise-induced asthma. Table 33.2 gives route and dosage information for albuterol and other adrenergic bronchodilators. In general, children and adolescents may take antiasthmatic medications for the same indications as for adults.

Patient-related variables specific to the use of albuterol and other adrenergic bronchodilators include the following:

- Age:
  - The main risks with adrenergic bronchodilators, particularly in older adults, are excessive cardiac and central nervous system (CNS) stimulation.
  - In all populations, giving the lowest effective dose decreases adverse effects.
- Reproduction, pregnancy, and lactation:
  - Although the drug crosses the placenta, use of albuterol during pregnancy is not associated with an increased risk of fetal malformations (GINA, 2022).
  - Albuterol is the preferred short-acting beta$_2$-adrenergic agonist (SABA) for the management of asthma during pregnancy.
  - Albuterol causes the muscles in the walls of the uterus to relax and may reduce uterine contractility.
  - Although albuterol enters breast milk, it is generally considered compatible with breast-feeding.

Adverse Effects

Administration of albuterol by MDI is associated with fewer systemic effects than administration of higher dosages orally or by nebulizer. Muscle tremor is the most frequent adverse effect. Major adverse effects are excessive cardiac and CNS stimulation. Symptoms of cardiac stimulation include angina, tachycardia, and palpitations. Symptoms of CNS stimulation consist of agitation, anxiety, insomnia, seizures, and tremors. Other reported effects may include serious dysrhythmias and cardiac arrest.

Contraindications

Contraindications to albuterol include known hypersensitivity to the drug, as well as cardiac tachydysrhythmias and severe coronary artery disease. Caution is warranted in hypertension, hyperthyroidism, diabetes, and seizure disorders.

Nursing Implications

Preventing Interactions

Beta-adrenergic blockers inhibit bronchodilation and can induce bronchospasm in patients with asthma who are taking albuterol. Thyroid hormones, theophylline, and some cold products can enhance the stimulatory adverse effects of the drug. Monoamine oxidase inhibitors should be avoided within 14 days of initiating treatment with albuterol to prevent hypertensive crisis. Caffeine-containing products, such as coffee, tea, or cola drinks, can also increase the adverse effects of cardiac and CNS stimulation.

Administering the Medication

Self-administration of albuterol and the other beta$_2$-agonists is usually by MDI. Patients should use an albuterol inhaler before they use any other inhaler. This opens the airways and allows for better absorption of the other drug. The patient should wait 5 minutes or more between using different inhalers, such as one for a corticosteroid. Although most drug references still give a regular dosing schedule (e.g., every 4 to 6 hours) for beta$_2$-agonists, asthma experts recommend that the drugs be used when needed (e.g., to treat acute dyspnea or prevent dyspnea during exercise). With overuse, the drugs lose their bronchodilating effects because the beta$_2$-adrenergic receptors become unresponsive to stimulation. (However, this tolerance does not occur with the long-acting beta$_2$-agonists.)

Assessing for Therapeutic Effects

The nurse observes for decreased dyspnea, wheezing, and respiratory secretions; relief of bronchospasm and wheezing; reduced rate and improved quality of respirations and pulmonary function; and reduced anxiety and restlessness.

Assessing for Adverse Effects

The nurse observes for tachycardia, dysrhythmias, palpitations, restlessness, agitation, and insomnia. These signs and symptoms result from cardiac and CNS stimulation.

Patient Teaching

The nurse helps patients recognize acute asthma attacks and have a plan to treat (or seek help for) exacerbations before respiratory distress becomes severe. Box 33.4 summarizes patient teaching guidelines for antiasthmatic drugs, including albuterol.

> **Quality and Safety Alert: Safety**
> It is essential to ensure that the patient has an adequate supply of albuterol for self-administration.

Other Drugs in the Class

Epinephrine (Adrenalin) is an adrenergic that may be injected subcutaneously in an acute attack of bronchoconstriction, with therapeutic rescue effects in approximately 5 minutes and lasting for approximately 4 hours. However, an inhaled selective beta$_2$-agonist is the drug of choice in this situation. Delivery by aerosol or nebulization of other selective beta$_2$-agonists is effective, even to young children and to patients on mechanical ventilation, and there is seldom a need to give epinephrine or other nonselective adrenergic drugs by injection. Cardiac stimulation is an adverse effect of bronchodilators, and in addition to beta$_2$ receptor stimulation, epinephrine also stimulates beta$_1$-adrenergic receptors in the heart to increase the rate and force of contraction.

Most prescription inhalers use hydrofluoroalkane (HFA) as a propellant.

TABLE 33.2

DRUGS AT A GLANCE: Adrenergic Bronchodilators

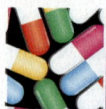

Drug	Routes and Dosage Ranges	
	Adults	**Children**
Albuterol (Proventil HFA, Ventolin HFA, ProAir RespiClick; 🍁 Airomir, Ventolin Discus, Ventolin HFA, Ventolin I.V. Infusion, Ventolin Nebules P.F.)	Inhalation* aerosol (90 mcg/actuation), 2 oral inhalations every 4–6 h; prevention of exercise-induced bronchospasm, 2 inhalations 5 min before exercise Inhalation solution via nebulizer, 2.5 mg 3–4 times daily (in 2.5 mL sterile saline, over 5–15 min) Regular tablets, 2–4 mg PO 3–4 times daily extended-release tablets, 4–8 mg PO every 12 h initially; increase if necessary to a max of 32 mg/d, in divided doses, every 12 h	Inhalation aerosol (90 mcg/actuation); ≥4 y, 4–8 puffs every 20 min for 3 doses then every 1–4 h; adolescents, 4–8 puffs every 20 min for up to 4 h and then every 1–4 h Nebulizer solution, 12 y and older, same as adults; 2–12 y, 1.5 mg/kg (min dose 2.5 mg) every 20 min for 3 doses then 0.15–0.3 mg/kg to max of 10 mg every 1–4 h Immediate-release tablets or syrup, 2–6 y, 0.1–0.2 mg/kg/dose three times daily to max dose of 4 mg; 6–12 y, 2 mg 3–4 times daily; 12 y and older, same as adults; sustained-release tablets, ≥6 y, 0.3–0.6 mg/kg/d divided twice daily to max of 8 mg/d; 12 y and older, same as adults; 6–12 y, 4 mg PO every 12 h initially, increase if necessary to a max of 8 mg/dose twice daily
Epinephrine (Asthmanefrin Refill, S2; 🍁 S2)	Nebulization, racemic (2.25% solution); OTC labeling hand-bulb nebulizer, add 0.5 mL to nebulizer, 1–3 inhalations; dose may be repeated after 3 h, if necessary, for 3 doses to max of 12 inhalations in 24 h	≥4 y, inhalation, same as adults
Formoterol (Perforomist; 🍁 Foradil, Oxeze Turbuhaler)	Nebulizer, 20 mcg/2 mL vial every 12 h	Perforomist not recommended in children
Levalbuterol (Xopenex [MDI], Xopenex Concentrate, Xopenex HFA)	Nebulizer, 0.63–1.25 mg 3 times daily, every 6–8 h to max of 2 inhalations every 4 h MDI, 2 puffs every 4–6 h	≤4 y, 0.31–1.25 mg every 4–6 h as needed 5–11 y, 0.31–0.63 mg every 8 h as needed MDI ≤ 4 y and older, same as adults
Metaproterenol (🍁 Orciprenaline)	PO, 20 mg 3–4 times/d	PO, <6 y 1.3–2.6 mg/kg/d divided every 6–8 h 6–9 y (or <27 kg), 10 mg/dose 3–4 times/d >9 y (or ≥27 kg), same as adults
Salmeterol (Serevent Diskus; 🍁 Serevent Diskhaler Disk, Serevent Diskus)	Inhalation powder, 1 inhalation (50 mcg) every 12 h	Inhalation powder: ≥4 y and older, same as adults
Terbutaline (🍁 Bricanyl Turbohaler)	2.5–5 mg PO every 6–8 h; max dose, 15 mg/d 0.25 mg Sub-Q, repeated every 20 min to 3 h; hold with pulse >120 beats/min	<12 y, PO 0.05 mg/kg/dose 3 times/d to max of 0.15 mg/kg/dose 3–4 times/d or a total of 5 mg/24 h 12–15 y, 2.5 mg PO 3 times/d; max dose, 7.5 mg/d <12 y, Sub-Q 0.005–0.01 mg/kg/dose to max of 0.4 mg/dose every 15–20 min for 3 doses; may repeat every 2–6 h as needed. ≥12 y, same as adults

*Short-acting adrenergic bronchodilators are used mainly by inhalation, as needed, rather than on a regular schedule; MDI, metered-dose inhaler.

BOX 33.4 Patient Teaching Guidelines for Antiasthmatic Drugs

General Considerations

- The symptoms of asthma and other chronic lung diseases frequently overlap and are characterized by constant inflammation of the airways and periodic or persistent labored breathing from constriction or narrowing of the airways. Antiasthmatic drugs are often given in combination to combat these problems. Thus, it is extremely important to know the type and purpose of each drug.
- Except for the short-acting, inhaled bronchodilators (e.g., albuterol), antiasthmatic medications are used long term to control symptoms and prevent acute asthma attacks. This means they must be taken on a regular schedule and continued when symptom free.
- When an asthma attack (i.e., acute bronchospasm with shortness of breath, wheezing respirations, cough) occurs, a fast-acting, inhaled, short-acting bronchodilator (e.g., albuterol) is commonly used to relieve these symptoms. In addition, because most exacerbations are associated with added inflammation, inhaled corticosteroids are frequently increased.
- Try to prevent symptoms and acute asthma attacks by avoiding infections (e.g., use good hand hygiene, avoid people with infections, have annual influenza vaccinations). Also try to avoid or minimize exposure to allergens and other substances that irritate breathing passages (e.g., tobacco smoke, perfume, flowers, hair spray, antiperspirants, cleaning products, and automobile exhaust).

A common cause of acute asthma attacks is not taking medications correctly. Factors that contribute to nonadherence include long-term use, expense, and adverse effects. If you have difficulty taking medications as prescribed, discuss the situation with a healthcare provider. Cheaper medications or lower doses may be effective alternatives. Just stopping the medications may precipitate acute breathing problems.

- If unable to prevent symptoms, early recognition and treatment may help prevent severe distress and hospitalizations. A written asthma action plan can help with decision-making at the onset of acute exacerbation.
- Signs of impending difficulty include increased needs for bronchodilator inhalers, activity limitations, waking at night because of asthma symptoms, and variability in the PEFR, if you use a PEFR meter at home. The first treatment is to use a short-acting, inhaled bronchodilator. If this does not improve breathing, seek emergency care.
- Keep adequate supplies of medications on hand. Missing a few doses of long-term control or "preventive" medications may precipitate an acute asthma attack; not using an inhaled bronchodilator for early breathing difficulty may lead to more severe problems and the need for emergency treatment or hospitalization.
- Use your metered-dose inhalers correctly. Drinking 2 to 3 quarts of fluids, as appropriate, daily helps thin secretions in the throat and lungs and makes them easier to remove.
- Avoid excessive intake of caffeine-containing fluids such as coffee, tea, and cola drinks. These beverages may increase bronchodilation but also may increase heart rate and cause palpitations, nervousness, and insomnia with bronchodilating drugs.
- Obtain an influenza vaccine annually and a pneumococcal vaccine at least once if you have chronic lung disease.
- Inform all healthcare providers about the medications you are taking and do not take over-the-counter drugs or herbal supplements without consulting a healthcare provider. Some drugs can decrease beneficial effects or increase adverse effects of antiasthmatic medications. For example, over-the-counter nasal decongestants, asthma remedies, cold remedies, and antisleep medications can increase the rapid heartbeat, palpitations, and nervousness often associated with bronchodilators. With herbal remedies, none are as effective as standard antiasthmatic medication, and they may cause serious or life-threatening adverse effects.

Self-Administration

- If you need help with metered-dose inhalers, consult a healthcare provider.
- Use short-acting bronchodilator inhalers as needed, not on a regular schedule. If desired effects are not achieved or if symptoms worsen, inform your prescriber. Do not increase dosage or frequency of taking medication. Overuse increases adverse drug effects and decreases drug effectiveness.
- If taking formoterol or salmeterol, which are long-acting, inhaled bronchodilators, do not use more often than every 12 hours. If constricted breathing occurs, use a short-acting bronchodilator inhaler between doses of a long-acting drug. Salmeterol does not relieve acute shortness of breath because it takes approximately 20 minutes to start acting and 1 to 4 hours to achieve maximal bronchodilating effects.
- If taking an oral or inhaled corticosteroid, take on a regular schedule, at approximately the same time each day. The purpose of these drugs is to relieve inflammation in the airways and prevent acute respiratory distress. They are not effective unless taken regularly.
- If taking oral theophylline, take fast-acting preparations before meals with a full glass of water, at regular intervals around the clock. If gastrointestinal upset occurs, take with food. Take long-acting preparations every 8 to 12 hours; do not chew or crush.

(Continued on page 610)

BOX 33.4 — Patient Teaching Guidelines for Antiasthmatic Drugs (Continued)

- Take zafirlukast 1 hour before or 2 hours after a meal; montelukast and immediate-release zileuton may be taken with or without food. Extended-release zileuton should be taken with food. Take montelukast in the evening or at bedtime. This schedule provides maximum beneficial effects during the night and early morning, when asthma symptoms often occur or worsen.
- Use inhalers correctly:
  1. Shake well immediately before each use.
  2. Remove the cap from the mouthpiece.
  3. Exhale to the end of a normal breath.
  4. With the inhaler in the upright position, place the mouthpiece just inside the mouth, and use the lips to form a tight seal or hold the mouthpiece approximately two finger widths from the open mouth.
  5. While pressing down on the inhaler, take a slow, deep breath for 3 to 5 seconds, hold the breath for approximately 10 seconds, and exhale slowly.
  6. Wait 3 to 5 minutes before taking a second inhalation of the drug.
  7. Rinse the mouth with water after each use.
  8. Rinse the mouthpiece and store the inhaler away from heat.
  9. If you have difficulty using an inhaler, ask your provider about a spacer device (a tube attached to the inhaler that makes it easier to use).

Levalbuterol (Xopenex, Xopenex Concentrate, Xopenex [HFA]) is a short-acting $beta_2$-adrenergic agonist used for the prevention and treatment of bronchoconstriction. Formoterol (Foradil) and salmeterol (Serevent) are long-acting $beta_2$-adrenergic agonists used only for prophylaxis of acute bronchoconstriction. They are not effective in acute attacks because they have a slower onset of action than the short-acting drugs (up to 20 minutes for salmeterol). Effects last 12 hours, and the drugs should not be taken more frequently. If additional bronchodilating medication is needed, a short-acting agent (e.g., albuterol) should be used. The FDA has issued a **BOXED WARNING** ◆ indicating that initiating salmeterol in people with significantly worsening or acutely deteriorating asthma may be life-threatening.

Metaproterenol is a relatively selective, intermediate-acting $beta_2$-adrenergic agonist that may be given orally or by MDI. It is used to treat acute bronchospasm and to prevent exercise-induced asthma. In high doses, metaproterenol loses some of its selectivity and may cause cardiac and CNS stimulation.

Terbutaline is a relatively selective $beta_2$-adrenergic agonist and a long-acting bronchodilator. The drug is usually well tolerated, and when symptoms occur, they are minor and require little or no treatment. Common adverse effects include shakiness, drowsiness, and headaches. When given subcutaneously, terbutaline loses its selectivity and has little advantage over epinephrine. The drug is used to treat preterm labor, although it is not approved for this use, has not been shown to be effective, and causes some safety concerns. The nurse should be aware of the FDA's recommendation that oral and injectable terbutaline should not be used for the prevention or treatment of preterm labor.

Clinical Application 33.1

- Mr. Lee may experience adverse effects if albuterol is administered as ordered. For what signs and symptoms should the nurse be alert?
- Mr. Lee's wife is at his bedside. She expresses concern about his treatment with IV corticosteroids, stating that she has heard that many adverse effects are associated with these drugs. Discuss the rationale for the use of IV corticosteroids in this case.

ANTICHOLINERGICS

The anticholinergic bronchodilators are most useful in the long-term management of asthma and other conditions producing bronchoconstriction, such as chronic bronchitis and emphysema. (For additional information about these drugs, see Chapter 48.) The two drugs in the class, the prototype Ⓟ **ipratropium** (Atrovent) and tiotropium, are ineffective in relieving acute bronchospasm by themselves, and they act synergistically with other adrenergic bronchodilators. Prescribers may order them for concomitant use. The drugs improve lung function about 10% to 15% over an inhaled $beta_2$-agonist alone.

Pharmacokinetics

Ipratropium is rapidly absorbed via inhalation with an onset of action within 5 to 15 minutes, a peak effect in 1½ to 2 hours, and a duration of action of 2 to 5 hours. Absorption of the drug is negligible, with excretion in the kidneys and in the feces. Only about 15% of the drug reaches the lower airways.

Action

Ipratropium is chemically related to atropine and blocks the muscarinic acetylcholine receptors in the smooth muscles of the bronchi in the lungs, inhibiting bronchoconstriction and mucus secretion.

Use

Originally, ipratropium was formulated to be taken by inhalation for maintenance therapy of bronchoconstriction associated with asthma, chronic bronchitis, and emphysema. Improved pulmonary function usually occurs in a few minutes. Other uses include treatment of rhinorrhea associated with allergic rhinitis and the common cold. Table 33.3 presents route and dosage information for anticholinergics such as ipratropium.

Patient-related variables specific to the use of ipratropium and other anticholinergics include the following:

- Reproduction, pregnancy, and lactation:
  - Limited data are available about ipratropium in pregnancy, but no adverse effects have been observed in animal reproduction studies.

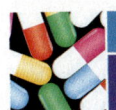

TABLE 33.3
DRUGS AT A GLANCE: Anticholinergics

Drug	Routes and Dosage Ranges	
	Adults	**Children**
P Ipratropium bromide (Atrovent HFA; ❈ Apo-Ipravent Solution, Mylan-Ipratropium, Gen-Ipratropium)	Metered-dose inhaler, 2 inhalations (36 mcg) 4 times/d to max of 12 inhalations in 24 h Nebulizer, 500 mcg every 20 minutes for 3 doses in combination with a short-acting beta-adrenergic agonist, then as needed	Children <5 y, 250 mcg per nebulizer every 20 min if needed for 1 h
Tiotropium (Spiriva HandiHaler, Spiriva Respimat; ❈ Spiriva, Spiriva Respimat)	Spiriva Respimat, 2 inhalations (2.5 mcg) once daily to max of 2 inhalations per 24 h One capsule (18 mcg) in HandiHaler once daily (contents of each capsule should be inhaled twice)	≥12 y, same as adults

- It is not known if nasal ipratropium is excreted in breast milk. The manufacturer recommends using caution when administering nasal ipratropium to patients who are breast-feeding.
- Specific healthcare environments:
  - In patients with critical illness, the drug's use may be limited to synergistic administration with other adrenergic bronchodilators, since ipratropium is ineffective in relieving acute bronchospasm. Administering by nebulization may be necessary.
  - In the home care setting, observation of a patient using an inhalation device can detect errors in the technique and provide opportunity for further education.
  - With inhaled medications, a spacer device may be useful, especially for children and older adults, because less muscle coordination is required to administer a dose and adverse effects may be minimized.

Adverse Effects

Absorption of ipratropium is poor, and it produces few systemic effects. The most common adverse effects are cough, nervousness, nausea, gastrointestinal (GI) upset, headache, and dizziness.

Contraindications

Ipratropium is contraindicated with known hypersensitivity to the drug or to atropine and related substances. Caution is recommended with use in patients with narrow-angle glaucoma, prostatic hypertrophy, and bladder neck obstruction because ipratropium can worsen these conditions.

BOX 33.5 Drug Interactions: Ipratropium

Drugs That Increase the Effects of Ipratropium
- Atropine and other anticholinergic drugs, such as diphenhydramine, dimenhydrinate
  Increase the anticholinergic effects

Drugs That Decrease the Effects of Ipratropium
- Acetylcholinesterase inhibitors
  Decrease in therapeutic effect

Nursing Implications
Preventing Interactions

In general, ipratropium has been shown to have limited drug–drug interactions (Box 33.5) and no herbal interactions. When given as a nasal spray, no interactions reportedly occur.

Administering the Medication

It is appropriate to mix ipratropium bromide inhalation solution in the nebulizer with albuterol or metaproterenol if the mixture is used within 1 hour.

> **! Quality and Safety Alert: Safety**
>
> Administering anticholinergic drugs via the respiratory route instead of the systemic route results in less thickening of respiratory secretions and therefore a reduced incidence of mucus-plugged airways.

Assessing for Therapeutic Effects

The nurse assesses for a reduced rate and improved quality of respirations and pulmonary function. The patient should report that breathing has improved and anxiety is reduced.

Assessing for Adverse Effects

The nurse observes for the presence of a cough, nervousness, nausea, GI upset, headache, and dizziness.

Patient Teaching

Box 33.4 summarizes patient teaching guidelines for antiasthmatic drugs such as ipratropium.

Other Drugs in the Class

Tiotropium (Spiriva) is a long-acting, 24-hour, anticholinergic bronchodilator taken once daily by inhalation for maintenance therapy of bronchoconstriction associated with chronic bronchitis and emphysema. As a muscarinic receptor antagonist, it is closely related to ipratropium but is not used for acute bronchospasm exacerbations. The drug has different pharmacokinetic and pharmacologic properties from ipratropium, and these differences may make it superior to ipratropium as an anticholinergic agent. A patient taking ipratropium should not take tiotropium. The primary adverse effect of tiotropium is dry mouth. Other effects include headache, dizziness, abdominal pain, constipation, diarrhea, flulike symptoms, and chest pain.

When taking tiotropium, the person places a capsule in a piercing chamber (HandiHaler) and then inhales the medication through the mouthpiece. Inhalations are repeated two to three times to ensure that the entire dose is received. When the drug is properly administered, the device makes a distinctive flutter or rattle.

XANTHINES

The xanthines are a group of alkaloids commonly used for their effects as bronchodilators, mainly in treating the symptoms of asthma. However, current clinical practice guidelines do not support or recommend that ⓟ **theophylline** (Elixophyllin, Theo-24, Theochron), the prototype, be used to treat acute asthma attacks. Therefore, this discussion only relates to the oral form of the drug.

Theophylline has a chemical structure similar to that of caffeine. When used, theophylline is usually given orally in an extended-release formulation for chronic disorders, such as chronic obstructive pulmonary disease (COPD).

Pharmacokinetics

Theophylline is rapidly and completely absorbed after oral administration. The onset of action occurs within 15 to 30 minutes by the oral route (extended release, 30 minutes). Peak levels occur in 1 to 2 hours, and the duration of action is 4 to 6 hours (extended release, 12 hours). Metabolism in the liver is extensive. Excretion of metabolites and some unchanged drug involves the kidneys. The drug crosses the placenta, and it enters breast milk.

Action

Theophylline works by relaxing bronchial smooth muscle, promoting bronchodilation. Additionally, the drug suppresses airway responsiveness to stimuli that trigger bronchospasm.

Use

Theophylline was formerly used extensively in the prevention and treatment of bronchoconstriction associated with asthma, bronchitis, and emphysema. Now considered a second-line oral agent, it may be added to a regimen for severe disease that is inadequately controlled by first-line drugs. Most formulations contain anhydrous theophylline (100% theophylline) as the active ingredient, and sustained-action tablets (e.g., Theochron) are more commonly used than other formulations.

To determine theophylline dosage, prescribers should measure serum theophylline levels (therapeutic range is 5 to 15 mcg/mL; toxic levels are 20 mcg/mL or above). It is necessary to draw blood for serum levels 1 to 2 hours after patients have taken immediate-release dosage forms and about 4 hours after they have taken sustained-release forms. In addition, children and cigarette smokers usually need higher doses to maintain therapeutic blood levels because they metabolize theophylline rapidly, and patients with liver disease, congestive heart failure, COPD, or acute viral infections usually need smaller doses because these conditions impair theophylline metabolism. For patients with obesity, prescribers should calculate theophylline dosage on the basis of lean or ideal body weight because theophylline is not highly distributed in fatty tissue. Table 33.4 gives the route and dosage information for oral theophylline.

Patient-related variables specific to the use of theophylline and other xanthine derivatives include the following:

- Age:
  - Use of theophylline preparations is not recommended in children less than 6 months of age, except for preterm infants with apnea.
  - Use of theophylline in children and older adults necessitates close monitoring because dosage needs and rates of metabolism vary widely.
  - Children 6 months to about 16 years of age metabolize theophylline more rapidly than younger or older patients.
  - Children may become hyperactive and disruptive from the CNS-stimulating effects of theophylline; tolerance to these effects usually develops with continued use of the drug.
  - In children younger than 6 months of age, especially premature infants and neonates, drug elimination may be prolonged because of immature liver function.
  - Older adults typically require reduced doses that should be individualized according to serum theophylline levels.

TABLE 33.4

DRUGS AT A GLANCE: Xanthines (Theophylline)

Drug	Routes and Dosage Ranges	
	Adults	**Children**
ⓟ **Immediate-release theophylline** (Elixophyllin, Theo-24, Theochron; Apo-theo LA, Theolair, Uniphyl)	500 mg PO, initially, then 200–300 mg every 6–8 h	7.5 mg/kg PO initially, then 5–6 mg/kg every 6–8 h
Sustained-release theophylline (Theochron, others)	150–300 mg PO every 8–12 h; max dose 13 mg/kg or 900 mg daily, whichever is less	100–200 mg PO every 8–12 h; max dose 24 mg/kg/d

- Reproduction, pregnancy, and lactation:
  - An increased risk of fetal malformations is not associated with use in pregnancy.
  - With use during the third trimester, infants exposed to theophylline should be monitored for adverse events (i.e., irritability, tachycardia, vomiting).
  - Appropriate use of asthma drugs improves pregnancy outcomes (i.e., gestational diabetes, preterm birth).
  - Since theophylline is found in breast milk, breast-feeding the infant just prior to theophylline administration should be considered; the infant needs to be monitored for adverse effects (i.e., irritability, tachycardia, vomiting).
- Abnormal kidney function and hepatic impairment:
  - Patients with Abnormal kidney function can take the usual doses of theophylline, but monitoring of serum drug levels is necessary.
  - Since metabolism of theophylline takes place in the liver, impaired liver function and decreased blood flow to the liver decrease metabolism, requiring a dosage reduction.

Adverse Effects

The therapeutic range of theophylline is narrow, making it and other xanthines second-line asthma treatment. Signs and symptoms of theophylline overdose include anorexia, nausea, vomiting, agitation, nervousness, insomnia, tachycardia and other dysrhythmias, and tonic–clonic convulsions. Ventricular dysrhythmias or convulsions may be the first sign of toxicity. Serious adverse effects frequently occur at serum drug levels above 20 mcg/mL. Overdoses with sustained-release preparations may cause a dramatic increase in serum drug concentrations much later (12 hours or longer) than the immediate-release preparations. Early treatment helps but does not prevent these delayed increases in serum drug levels. Theophylline also increases cardiac output, causes peripheral vasodilation, exerts a mild diuretic effect, and stimulates the CNS.

Contraindications

Contraindications to theophylline include acute gastritis and peptic ulcer disease. Caution is necessary in seizure disorders and cardiovascular disorders that could be aggravated by drug-induced cardiac stimulation.

Nursing Implications

Preventing Interactions

Because theophylline is metabolized by the cytochrome P450 (CYP) enzyme system (CYP1A2), numerous drug–drug interactions using the same enzyme system exist (Box 33.6). Also, the rate of metabolism of theophylline is increased substantially in cigarette smokers (the half-life can be halved). Use of e-cigarettes and nicotine gum appears to have no effect on theophylline metabolism. In addition, caffeine reportedly produces additive cardiac and CNS stimulation. Finally, St. John's wort may decrease the effect of theophylline by increasing its metabolism.

Administering the Medication

To help regulate theophylline dosage and avoid adverse effects, it is necessary to monitor serum drug levels. Patients should take immediate-release oral theophylline before meals with a full glass of water, at regular intervals around the clock. If GI upset occurs, they may take the drug with food to promote dissolution and absorption and decrease the associated nausea and vomiting. They should take sustained-release theophylline every 8 to 12 hours, with instructions not to chew or crush. Doing so causes immediate release of potentially toxic doses.

Assessing for Therapeutic Effects

The nurse observes for therapeutic serum levels of theophylline (5 to 15 mcg/mL). Chronic use of the drug results in improved arterial blood gas levels (normal values on room air: PO_2, 80 to 100 mm Hg; PCO_2, 35 to 45 mm Hg; pH, 7.35 to 7.45), improved exercise tolerance, and decreased incidence and severity of acute attacks of bronchospasm.

Assessing for Adverse Effects

The nurse monitors the serum drug level and observes for tachycardia, dysrhythmias, palpitations, restlessness, agitation, insomnia, nausea, vomiting, and convulsions. Theophylline causes cardiac and CNS stimulation. Toxic serum concentrations (greater than 20 mcg/mL) lead to convulsions, which may occur without preceding symptoms of toxicity and may result in death. IV diazepam (Valium) may control seizures. In patients with seizures, treatment includes securing the airway, giving oxygen, injecting IV diazepam (0.1 to 0.3 mg/kg, up to 10 mg), monitoring vital signs, maintaining blood pressure, providing adequate hydration, and monitoring serum theophylline levels until they are between 15 and 20 mg/mL.

Theophylline also stimulates the chemoreceptor trigger zone in the medulla oblongata, causing nausea and vomiting. In patients without seizures, it may be necessary to induce vomiting, unless the level of consciousness is impaired. In these patients, precautions to prevent aspiration are necessary, especially in children. If overdose is identified within 1 hour of theophylline ingestion, gastric lavage may be helpful if healthcare providers are unable to induce vomiting or vomiting is contraindicated. Experts recommend administration of activated charcoal and a cathartic, especially for overdoses of sustained-release formulations—if the possible benefit exceeds the risk.

In addition, symptomatic treatment of dysrhythmias may be necessary.

BOX 33.6 Drug Interactions: Theophylline

Drugs That Increase the Effects of Theophylline
- Allopurinol, propranolol, quinolones (e.g., ciprofloxacin)
  Decrease metabolism
- Cimetidine, macrolides (e.g., erythromycin, clindamycin)
  Decrease clearance and thereby increase plasma levels

Drugs That Decrease the Effects of Theophylline
- Carbamazepine, phenytoin, rifampicin
  Increase metabolism
- Lithium
  Increases excretion
- Phenobarbital
  Increases metabolism by way of enzyme induction

Patient Teaching

The nurse reinforces the importance of not exceeding the prescribed dose, not crushing long-acting formulations, reporting adverse effects, and keeping appointments for follow-up care. The nurse also instructs patients who smoke to notify their prescriber if they stop smoking, because the dosage of theophylline may need to be reduced. Box 33.4 presents patient teaching guidelines for antiasthmatic drugs.

NCLEX Success

1. A patient begins using an albuterol inhaler and a beclomethasone inhaler for asthma. The patient asks if it matters which inhaler is used first. The best response by the nurse is which of the following?
   A. "You should use the albuterol inhaler first followed in 5 to 10 minutes by the beclomethasone inhaler."
   B. "You should use the beclomethasone inhaler first followed in 5 to 10 minutes by the albuterol inhaler."
   C. "The order in which you use the inhalers does not matter."
   D. "You should not use the inhalers one right after the other."

2. The nurse notes that a patient's serum theophylline level is 25 mcg/mL and that a scheduled dose of the medication is due. The nurse should do which of the following?
   A. Hold the scheduled dose, contact the healthcare provider, and assess the patient for signs of theophylline toxicity.
   B. Administer the dose as scheduled.
   C. Administer only half of the dose and repeat the theophylline level in 4 hours.
   D. Hold the dose until the next meal and administer at that time.

3. A 68-year-old patient, well controlled on theophylline for 2 years, complains of insomnia, nervousness, nausea and vomiting, and tachycardia. The patient, who had smoked one pack of cigarettes per day for 10 years, thought the nervousness was due to recent smoking cessation. After performing an assessment, the nurse practitioner tells the patient that the symptoms are likely due to theophylline toxicity. A serum theophylline level confirms the diagnosis. What is the best explanation for theophylline toxicity in this patient?
   A. Because of their age, the patient is likely having abnormal kidney function.
   B. The patient is not taking the medication as prescribed.
   C. A concurrent medication is altering the metabolism of theophylline.
   D. The metabolism of theophylline has decreased with the recent smoking cessation.

CORTICOSTEROIDS

Chapter 17 describes corticosteroids, which are often ordered for the treatment of many inflammatory conditions. The ability of the corticosteroids to suppress airway inflammation produces beneficial effects, including decreased mucus secretion, decreased edema of airway mucosa, and repair of damaged epithelium, with subsequent reduction of airway reactivity. Corticosteroids are the most consistently effective long-term control medications for asthma. The inhaled drug ⓟ **beclomethasone** (Qvar RediHaler) is the prototype corticosteroid in asthma. Current clinical practice guidelines and GINA recommend the addition of inhaled corticosteroids with administration of a short-acting (rescue) beta$_2$-adrenergic agonist.

Pharmacokinetics

Beclomethasone is rapidly absorbed from the lower respiratory tract or nasal passages. The onset of action is rapid, and the drug peaks in 1 to 2 weeks. Therapeutic effects may not occur until 4 weeks after initial use. Metabolism occurs in the lungs, GI tract, and liver, and excretion predominately occurs in the feces. The drug crosses the placenta. Whether it enters breast milk is unknown.

Action

Corticosteroids suppress the release of inflammatory mediators, block the generation of cytokines, and decrease the recruitment of airway eosinophils (Fig. 33.1). The drugs increase the number and sensitivity of beta$_2$-adrenergic receptors, which restores or increases the effectiveness of beta$_2$-adrenergic bronchodilators. The number of beta$_2$ receptors increases within approximately 4 hours, and improved responsiveness to beta$_2$-agonists occurs within approximately 2 hours.

Use

Beclomethasone is effective in the prophylactic management of asthma. With inhalation, the drug controls asthma that requires corticosteroids as part of the treatment plan. In chronic asthma, patients usually take corticosteroids by inhalation, on a daily schedule. Often, they take them concomitantly with one or more bronchodilators and perhaps another anti-inflammatory drug such as a leukotriene modifier or a mast cell stabilizer. In some instances, the other drugs allow smaller doses of the corticosteroid. For acute flare-ups of symptoms during the treatment of chronic asthma, a systemic corticosteroid may be needed temporarily to regain control. Intranasal administration helps relieve rhinitis that responds poorly to other treatment and minimizes the reoccurrence of nasal polyps after nasal surgery.

In early stages of progressive COPD, patients are unlikely to need corticosteroids. In later stages, however, they usually need periodic short-course therapy for episodes of respiratory distress and a scheduled inhaled corticosteroid for long-term control. When corticosteroids are needed for an acute exacerbation, administration is oral or parenteral.

Table 33.5 provides route and dosage information for beclomethasone and other corticosteroid antiasthmatic drugs.

Patient-related variables specific to the use of beclomethasone and other corticosteroid drugs include the following:

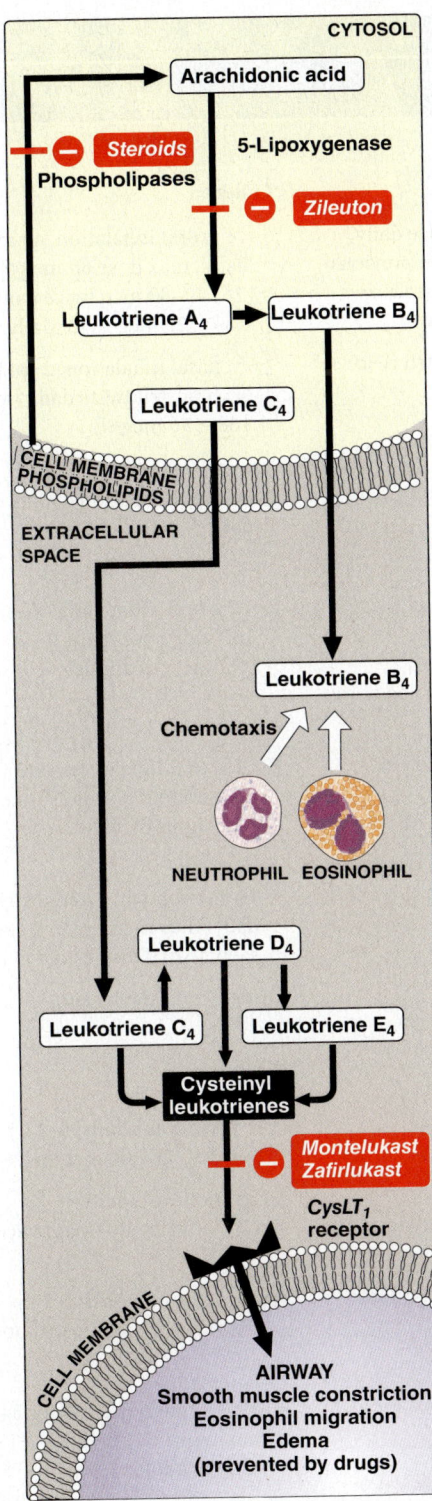

Figure 33.1. Formation of leukotrienes and sites of action of leukotriene-modifying drugs and steroids. CysLT$_1$, cysteinyl leukotriene$_1$. [Reprinted with permission from Whalen, K. (2018). *Lippincott illustrated reviews: Pharmacology* (7th ed., Fig. 39.4). Wolters Kluwer.]

- Age:
  - In general, inhaled corticosteroids are safe and effective in children older than 2 years of age.
  - Major concerns about long-term use in children include decreased adrenal function, growth, and bone mass, with adrenal insufficiency most likely occurring with systemic or high doses of inhaled corticosteroids; monitoring of the effects is necessary.
- Reproduction, pregnancy, and lactation:
  - Available evidence indicates that continuing inhaled corticosteroids, including beclomethasone, in females whose symptoms are adequately controlled is safe during pregnancy.
  - Other agents with more extensive data in pregnant females that cause less systemic absorption may be preferred as an initial therapy in pregnancy (Alhussien, 2018).
- Abnormal kidney function and hepatic impairment:
  - Because elimination of beclomethasone and most corticosteroids is hepatic, dosage reductions may be appropriate.
- Specific healthcare environments:
  - In patients with critical illness, inhaled or nasal beclomethasone with systemic corticosteroids in relatively high doses is necessary when respiratory distress is not relieved by multiple doses of inhaled beta$_2$-agonists.

Adverse Effects

Common adverse effects of beclomethasone include headache, pharyngitis, cough, dry mouth, hoarseness, fungal infection (candidiasis), and nausea. It is possible to decrease local adverse effects of inhaled corticosteroids (oropharyngeal candidiasis, hoarseness) by reducing the dose, administering the drugs less often, rinsing the mouth and throat after use, or using a spacer device. These measures decrease the amount of drug deposited in the oral cavity.

Contraindications

Contraindications to beclomethasone include an allergy to the drug. Recent nasal surgery, injury, or ulcers preclude use of the nasal preparation; the drug can interfere with healing and increase the risk of a nasal infection.

Nursing Implications

Preventing Interactions

Little, if any, of the beclomethasone is absorbed. Therefore, no clinically significant drug–drug or herbal interactions are known to occur.

Administering the Medication

Patients should take inhaled or nasal beclomethasone on a regular schedule. After inhaling, they should rinse the mouth and throat to prevent fungal infection (candidiasis). The drug is not a rescue inhaler, and patients should not take it to resolve an acute asthma event. The recommended inhaled or nasal corticosteroid dose should be the lowest amount of drug required to control symptoms. IV administration offers no therapeutic advantage over oral administration.

Assessing for Therapeutic Effects

The nurse assesses for reversal of asthma symptoms, including reduced airway inflammation, decreased mucus secretion, decreased edema of airway mucosa, and reduced airway

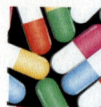

TABLE 33.5
DRUGS AT A GLANCE: Corticosteroids

Drug	Routes and Dosage Ranges	
	Adults	**Children**
ⓟ Beclomethasone (Qvar RediHaler ✦ QVAR)	Oral inhalation, initial 40–80 mcg twice daily; max dose, 320 mcg twice daily; if on previous inhaled corticosteroids, 40–160 mcg twice daily; max dose 320 mcg twice daily	5–11 y, oral inhalation, 40 mcg twice daily; max dose 80 mcg twice daily ≥12 y, 40–80 mcg twice daily; max dose 320 mcg twice daily
ⓟ Beclomethasone (Beconase AQ, Qnasl, Qnasl Children; ✦ Apo-Beclomethasone, Mylan-Beclo AQ, Rivanase AQ)	Nasal inhalation, 2 sprays in each nostril twice daily (total dose 168–336 mcg/d)	≥6 y, nasal inhalation, 2 sprays in each nostril twice daily (total dose 168–336 mcg/d)
Budesonide (Pulmicort Flexhaler; ✦ Pulmicort Nebuamp, Pulmicort Turbuhaler)	Oral inhalation, 200–400 mcg twice daily	≥6 y, oral inhalation 200 mcg twice daily
Ciclesonide (Alvesco ✦ Alvesco)	Oral inhalation, 80 mcg twice daily; max dose 160 mcg twice daily (if receiving bronchodilators alone); max dose 320 mcg twice daily (if receiving inhaled corticosteroids)	2–11 y, oral inhalation, 40, 80, or 160 mcg once daily ≥12 y, same as adults
Flunisolide	Two inhalations twice daily; max dose eight inhalations daily	6–11 y, oral inhalation: one inhalation twice daily; max dose four times daily
Fluticasone (Xhance; ✦ Flonase, Avamys)	4 sprays in each nostril once daily (265 mcg/d)	≥12 y, same as adults 4–11 y: 1 spray in each nostril once daily; may increase to 2 sprays in each nostril for desired effect
Fluticasone aerosol (Flovent Diskus, Arnuity Ellipta, Flovent HFA; ✦ Arnuity Ellipta, Flovent Diskus, Flovent HFA)	Aerosol, 88–220 mcg twice daily	Dosage not established
Fluticasone powder (Flovent Diskus)	Powder, 100–500 mcg twice daily	≥12 y, same as adults; 4–11 y, powder, 50–100 mcg twice daily
Mometasone (Asmanex HFA, Asmanex Twisthaler; ✦ Asmanex Twisthaler)	Aerosol, 100–200 mcg twice daily Inhalation powder (Twisthaler), 110–220 mcg twice daily	≥12 y, same as adults 4–11 y, powder 110 mcg twice daily
Mometasone (Propel Mini; ✦ Apo-Mometasone, Mosaspray, Nasonex)	Nasal inhalation two sprays (50 mcg/spray) in each nostril once daily	≥12 y, same as adults 2–11 y; 1 spray (50 mcg) in each nostril once daily
Prednisone (Prednisone Intensol, Rayos; ✦ Apo-Prednisone, JAA-Prednisone, Teva-Prednisone, Winpred)	Acute asthma: 40–60 mg/d PO for 3–10 d for a short burst	<12 y, 1–2 mg/kg/d PO for 3–10 d; maximum 60 mg daily; ≥12 y, same as adults
Methylprednisolone sodium succinate (Solu-Medrol; ✦ Depo-Medrol, Medrol, Methylprednisolone acetate, Methylprednisolone sodium succinate, Solu-Medrol)	Oral 40–60 mg/d for a short burst; 7.5 mg to 60 mg/d for maintenance of asthma control IV: 40–80 mg/d in divided doses once or twice daily IM (acetate): 240 mg one-time dose in place of a short-course burst	<12 y: 1–2 mg/kg/d PO for 3–10 d; maximum dose: 60 mg daily ≥12 y, same as adults IM (acetate): 7.5 mg/kg up to 240 mg as a one-time dose IV: <12 y, 1–2 mg/kg/d; maximum of 60 mg/d >12 y, same as adults

reactivity. With allergic rhinitis, the nurse assesses for the relief of rhinitis, including clearing of stuffy nose and postnasal drip.

Assessing for Adverse Effects

The nurse observes for the presence of headache, hoarseness, cough, throat irritation, and fungal infection (candidiasis) of mouth and throat. Inhaled corticosteroids are unlikely to produce the serious adverse effects of long-term systemic therapy (see Chapter 17).

Patient Teaching

It is important to instruct patients that oral and nasal inhalations are not interchangeable.

> **Quality and Safety Alert: Safety**
>
> The nurse must remind patients that beclomethasone is not a fast-acting asthma treatment; the drug does not provide immediate relief from asthma-related breathing problems.

Box 33.4 outlines additional patient teaching guidelines.

Other Drugs in the Class

Budesonide (Pulmicort, Pulmicort Flexhaler), ciclesonide, flunisolide, fluticasone (Flonase), and mometasone (Asmanex Twisthaler, Nasonex) are topical corticosteroids for inhalation. Topical administration minimizes systemic absorption and adverse effects; clinical effectiveness of inhaled drugs is due to direct local effects rather than systemic absorption. These preparations may substitute for or allow reduced dosage of systemic corticosteroids.

> **Quality and Safety Alert: Safety**
>
> In people with asthma who are taking an oral corticosteroid, it is necessary to reduce the oral dosage slowly (over weeks to months) when an inhaled corticosteroid is added.

The goal is to use the lowest oral dose necessary to control symptoms. Flunisolide and fluticasone also are available in nasal solutions for the treatment of allergic rhinitis, which may play a role in bronchoconstriction. Because systemic absorption occurs in patients using inhaled corticosteroids (about 20% of a dose), high doses should be reserved for people who otherwise require oral corticosteroids.

Triamcinolone acetonide is not recommended for use in children younger than 2 years of age. Dose-related inhibition of growth has been reported in short and intermediate studies, but long-term studies have found few, if any, decreases in expected adult height. Inhaled corticosteroids have not been associated with significant decreases in bone mass, but more studies of high doses and of drug therapy in adolescents are needed.

Prednisone and methylprednisolone are given to patients who require systemic corticosteroids. Prednisone is given orally and is highlighted as a prototype drug in Chapter 17; methylprednisolone may be given intravenously to patients who are unable to take an oral medication.

LEUKOTRIENE MODIFIERS

Leukotrienes are strong proinflammatory mediators produced by the immune system during trauma, infection, and inflammation. They can cause sustained constriction of bronchioles and immediate hypersensitivity reactions. They also increase mucus secretion and mucosal edema in the respiratory tract. Leukotrienes are formed by the lipoxygenase pathway of arachidonic acid metabolism (see Fig. 33.1) in response to cellular injury. Cysteinyl leukotrienes (cysLTs) are a family of inflammatory lipid mediators of various allergic and hypersensitivity reactions.

Leukotriene modifiers function as either leukotriene-related enzyme inhibitors or leukotriene receptor antagonists to reduce the bronchoconstriction and inflammation caused by leukotrienes. These drugs are effective in a significant portion of patients with asthma. (However, clinical trials that compared leukotriene receptors to inhaled corticosteroids achieved treatment end points more consistently with inhaled corticosteroids.) The prototype leukotriene modifier is **montelukast** (Singulair). The drug antagonizes the cysteinyl leukotriene$_1$ receptor.

Pharmacokinetics

Absorption from the GI tract is rapid. Extensive metabolism takes place in the liver via the CYP3A4, 2C8, and 2C9 enzyme systems, and the drug may interact with other medications metabolized by this system. Excretion of most metabolites occurs in the feces.

Action

Montelukast prevents cysteinyl leukotrienes from binding to its receptors reducing the bronchoconstriction and ultimate inflammation caused by leukotrienes. The drug improves symptoms and pulmonary function tests, decreases nighttime symptoms, and decreases the use of beta$_2$-agonist drugs. The drug is not effective in relieving acute asthma attacks. However, patients may continue taking it concurrently with other drugs during acute episodes.

Use

Healthcare providers use montelukast that is indicated for long-term treatment of asthma in adults and children. It is the only oral tablet approved for management of exercise-induced asthma. In addition, montelukast is the only leukotriene modifier approved for the management of allergic rhinitis or allergies, and it may result in relief of allergic conjunctivitis. The drug can be used with bronchodilators and corticosteroids and elicits a high degree of patient adherence and satisfaction. However, it is less effective than low doses of inhaled corticosteroids. Table 33.6 gives route and dosage information for montelukast and other leukotriene modifiers.

Note that the FDA has issued a **BOXED WARNING** ◆ for montelukast because neuropsychiatric events have been reported in adults, adolescents, and children who take the drug. These symptoms include agitation, aggressive behavior, anxiousness, depression, disorientation, disturbance in attention, dream

TABLE 33.6
DRUGS AT A GLANCE: Leukotriene Modifiers

Drug	Routes and Dosage Ranges	
	Adults	**Children**
ⓟ Montelukast (Singulair; 🍁 Singulair)	10 mg PO once daily in the evening or at bedtime	≥1–2 y, 4 mg (PO granules) once daily in the evening ≥2–6 y, 4 mg (PO granules or chewable tablet) once daily in the evening ≥6–14 y, 5 mg PO chewable tablet once daily in the evening ≥15 y, same as adults
Zafirlukast (Accolate; 🍁 Accolate)	20 mg PO twice daily, 1 h before or 2 h after a meal	5–11 y, 10 mg PO twice daily ≥12 y, same as adults
Zileuton (Zyflo)	Immediate release, 600 mg PO 4 times/d Extended release, 1,200 mg PO twice per day	≥12 y, same as adults

abnormalities, hallucinations, insomnia, irritability, memory impairment, restlessness, suicidal ideation, and tremor.

Patient-related variables specific to the use of montelukast and other leukotriene modifiers include the following:

- Age:
  - Montelukast is approved for use in children 12 months of age and older. Film-coated tablets, chewable tablets, or granules are available.
- Reproduction, pregnancy, and lactation:
  - Based on the best available evidence, montelukast has not shown to increase the risk of teratogenic effects when used in pregnancy (Global Initiative for Asthma [GINA], 2022).
  - Data collection related to the use of montelukast in pregnancy and lactation is ongoing. Manufacturer recommendations indicate that the decision to breast-feed while taking montelukast should consider the risk of infant exposure, the benefits of breast-feeding to the infant, and the benefits of montelukast administration to the mother.
- Abnormal kidney function and hepatic impairment:
  - In patients with hepatic impairment, montelukast produces higher blood levels, and drug elimination is slower. However, no dosage adjustment is necessary for mild to moderate hepatic impairment.

Adverse Effects and Contraindications

Leukotriene modifiers seem relatively devoid of serious toxicity, and adverse effects are typically mild. The most common adverse effects reported are headache, nausea, vomiting, diarrhea, hyperkinesia, psychomotor hyperactivity, and infection.

Contraindications include known hypersensitivity to the drug.

Nursing Implications

Preventing Interactions

Montelukast is metabolized in the liver by the CYP enzyme system, and numerous drug–drug interactions exist, particularly in drugs that utilize the same enzyme system. Box 33.7 summarizes these interactions. St. John's wort may decrease the drug's effect by increasing metabolism of the drug.

Administering the Medication

Oral administration of montelukast is effective. People can take it once or twice a day, in the evening or at bedtime. This schedule provides high drug concentrations during the night and early morning, when asthma symptoms tend to occur or worsen. Food does not significantly affect the drug's bioavailability; people may take it with or without food.

Assessing for Therapeutic Effects

The nurse assesses for stability and improvement of asthma symptoms, relief of allergic rhinitis, or the absence of exercise-induced respiratory symptoms. If the patient's respiratory symptoms are not stable, it is necessary to determine the current frequency and severity of acute attacks as well as factors that precipitate or relieve acute attacks.

Assessing for Adverse Effects

The nurse assesses for headache, nausea, diarrhea, signs of infection, and changes in behavior, including suicidal ideation.

Patient Teaching

The nurse instructs the patient about recognizing signs and symptoms of infection and reporting them to the healthcare provider. Also, the nurse ensures that the patient understands

---

BOX 33.7 *Drug Interactions: Montelukast*

Drugs That Increase the Effects of Montelukast
- Aspirin
  Increases bleeding tendencies

Drugs That Decrease the Effects of Montelukast
- Carbamazepine, erythromycin, phenobarbital, phenytoin, primidone, rifamycin antibiotics, theophylline
  Decrease serum levels

appropriate use of the drug and realizes that the drug should not be used to manage acute asthma symptoms. Box 33.4 outlines additional patient teaching guidelines.

Other Drugs in the Class

Zafirlukast (Accolate) was the first leukotriene modifier, but montelukast is the most widely prescribed and studied worldwide. Like montelukast, zafirlukast antagonizes the cysteinyl leukotriene$_1$ receptor. Well absorbed with oral administration, metabolism of zafirlukast by the CYP enzyme system occurs in the liver, and the drug may interact with other drugs metabolized by the hepatic system. Excretion of most metabolites occurs in the feces. Blood levels of the drug are higher and elimination is slower in older adults than in younger adults. Zafirlukast is approved for use in children older than 5 years of age. The drug enters breast milk, and lactating women should not take it. People should take zafirlukast 1 hour before or 2 hours after a meal; food reduces the bioavailability by approximately 40%. Authorities recommend no dosage adjustments for zafirlukast in patients with Abnormal kidney function.

Zileuton (Zyflo, Zyflo CR), another leukotriene modifier, is a 5-lipoxygenase inhibitor that blocks the first step in leukotriene biosynthesis of the arachidonic acid cascade. Thus, the drug inhibits the formation of leukotrienes B4, C4, D4, and E4 and subsequently the formation of the cysLTs. The most common adverse effect is headache. The extended-release formulation should be taken with food; the immediate-release formulation can be given without regard to food. Monitoring of serum alanine aminotransferase is recommended.

IMMUNOSUPPRESSANT MONOCLONAL ANTIBODIES

Exposure to allergenic material in pollen, dander, and food can cause immune inflammation that leads to allergic asthma. With repeated stimulation of the allergen, IgE antibodies are produced. Monoclonal antibodies specifically bind to target cells or proteins in the hopes of stimulating the patient's immune system to attack those cells. **Omalizumab** (Xolair), a recombinant humanized IgE monoclonal antibody and the prototype, combines with free IgE-blocking receptors on the surfaces of mast cells and basophils so that there is less IgE available to combine with allergens. Omalizumab is the only available anti-IgE therapy approved as adjunctive therapy to inhaled corticosteroids, with the goal of reducing the prevalence of asthma exacerbations and hospitalizations. Chapter 13 further discusses the effects of altering the immune response to an allergen with monoclonal antibodies.

Pharmacokinetics

Absorption is slow following subcutaneous injection. Metabolism occurs in the reticuloendothelial system and the endothelial cells in the liver. Half-life elimination is 26 days. Excretion is primarily through the liver, and intact IgG may be secreted in the bile.

Action

Omalizumab inhibits IgE binding to IgE receptors on mast cells and basophils. This limits the activation and release of mediators in the early and late phases of the allergic response.

Use

Omalizumab is indicated as adjunctive therapy for moderate to severe persistent allergic asthma to a perennial aeroallergen that is not well controlled with a combination of a high-dose inhaled corticosteroid and a long-acting beta$_2$-agonist. Long-term treatment in patients with allergic asthma showed a decrease in asthma exacerbations and corticosteroid use. In addition, the drug is indicated for the treatment of chronic idiopathic urticaria.

Table 33.7 provides route and dosage information for omalizumab and other immunosuppressant monoclonal antibodies.

TABLE 33.7
DRUGS AT A GLANCE: Monoclonal Antibody

Drug	Adults	Children
Omalizumab (Xolair)	150–375 mg every 2–4 weeks Sub-Q, based on body weight and level of total pretreatment serum IgE	≥6–11 y, 75–375 mg every 2–4 weeks Sub-Q, based on body weight and level of total pretreatment serum IgE ≥12 y, same as adults
Mepolizumab (Nucala)	100 mg Sub-Q once every 4 wk	≥12 y, same as adults
Reslizumab (Cinqair)	3 mg/kg IV once every 4 wk	No data available on use in children
Benralizumab (Fasenra; Fasenra)	30 mg Sub-Q every 4 wk for the first 3 doses, then once every 8 wk	≥12 y, same as adults
Dupilumab (Dupixent)	Initial 400 mg (two 200 mg subcutaneous injections) followed by 200 mg given every other week OR an initial dose of 600 mg (two 300 mg injections) followed by 300 mg given every other week	> 6 mo, subcutaneous injection Prefilled pen is only for use ≥ 2 y; Children ≥ 6 y and adolescents ≤ 17 y will need an initial loading dose 5 to <15 kg: Sub-Q: 200 mg every 4 wk 15 to <30 kg: Sub-Q: 300 mg every 4 wk
Tezepelumab (Tezspire)	210 mg Sub-Q every 4 wk	≥12 y, same as adults

Patient-related variables specific to the use of omalizumab and other immunosuppressant monoclonal antibodies include the following:

- Reproduction, pregnancy, and lactation:
  - Information on the use of omalizumab during pregnancy and while breast-feeding is limited.
  - Omalizumab crosses the placenta with fetal exposure highest during the third trimester.
- Specific healthcare environments:
  - Omalizumab is not self-administered at home because of the risk of anaphylaxis; administration occurs in a healthcare facility. However, because anaphylaxis may occur up to 4 days after the drug is administered, the patient and family must be instructed to seek emergency medical treatment for signs of anaphylaxis.

Adverse Effects

The most common adverse effects of omalizumab include local reactions at the injection site, headache, nausea, and fatigue. Anaphylaxis presenting as bronchospasm, hypotension, syncope, urticaria, and/or angioedema of the throat or tongue, cough, flushing, rash, and itching has been reported following administration of the drug. Anaphylaxis has been reported with the first dose and has occurred more than 1 year after initial administration. Because of the risk of anaphylaxis, the FDA has issued a **BOXED WARNING** ◆ for omalizumab.

Contraindications

Contraindications to omalizumab include a known allergy to the drug or a severe hypersensitivity reaction (anaphylaxis) with drug use.

Nursing Implications

Preventing Interactions

No reported drug–drug interactions or herbal interactions occur that decrease or increase the effects of omalizumab.

Administering the Medication

Administration of omalizumab must occur in the healthcare setting because of the risk of life-threatening anaphylaxis with administration. No more than 150 mg (contents of one vial) should be injected at one site. Doses of more than 150 mg should be given at two or more injection sites.

> **Quality and Safety Alert: Safety**
>
> The nurse must take precautions with omalizumab to ensure correct product selection and dose–volume calculations. Prefilled syringes and reconstituted lyophilized powder are available in different concentrations.

Assessing for Therapeutic Effects

The nurse observes for a decrease in the number and severity of asthma exacerbations, better symptom control, and an improvement of airflow limitation. The patient should report a decreased need for rescue medications and oral corticosteroids, as well as an improved reported quality of life.

Assessing for Adverse Effects

The nurse assesses for signs of anaphylaxis, local reactions at the injection sites, headache, nausea, and fatigue.

Patient Teaching

The nurse instructs the patient and family to recognize the signs and symptoms of anaphylaxis and to report them to the healthcare provider. They should understand that the drug must be administered in a healthcare facility and that it may take several months before the patient notices benefits from the drug. Management of local reactions at the site of injection involves the application of local cold compresses or the use of medications such as antihistamines or aspirin. Box 33.4 summarizes additional patient teaching guidelines for antiasthmatic drugs, including omalizumab.

Other Drugs in the Class

Although omalizumab is the only monoclonal antibody that specifically targets IgE, five other monoclonal antibodies target the production of eosinophils in the allergic response of individuals with severe asthma who have blood eosinophil counts of 150/μL or greater (**eosinophilic phenotype**). These include mepolizumab (Nucala) and reslizumab (Cinqair), and benralizumab (Fasenra), an anti–IL-5 receptor alpha antibody. IL-5 is a proeosinophilic cytokine that is a potent mediator of eosinophil hematopoiesis and contributes to eosinophilic inflammation in the airways. Mepolizumab and reslizumab are anti–IL-5 monoclonal antibodies, benralizumab is a monoclonal antibody to IL-5, dupilumab (Dupixent) is a monoclonal antibody that inhibits the activity of both IL-4 and IL-13, and tezepelumab (Tezspire) is a human monoclonal immunoglobulin G2-lambda antibody that binds thymic stromal lymphopoietin (TSLP) reducing blood eosinophils, airway submucosal eosinophils, IgE, fractional exhaled nitric oxide, IL-5, and IL-13. These drugs are considered add-on maintenance for the treatment of severe asthma in adults and children older than or equal to 12 years of age with an eosinophilic phenotype. As with omalizumab, they are not indicated for the relief of acute bronchospasm or status asthmaticus. Table 33.7 contains route and dosage information for the other monoclonal antibodies.

ADJUVANT MEDICATIONS USED TO TREAT ASTHMA

Mast Cell Stabilizers

Mast cell stabilizers are used as an alternative, but not preferred, medication for prophylaxis of acute asthma attacks in patients with mild persistent asthma. They are not effective in acute bronchospasm or status asthmaticus and should not be used in these conditions. Use of one of these drugs may allow reduced dosage of bronchodilators and corticosteroids. Patients may take them prior to exercise or exposure to known allergens. Cromolyn (NasalCrom) stabilizes mast cells and prevents the release of bronchoconstrictive and inflammatory substances when mast cells are confronted with allergens and other stimuli. Administration of mast cell stabilizers is by inhalation. Cromolyn is available in a metered-dose aerosol and a solution for use with a power-operated nebulizer. A nasal solution is also marketed for the prevention and treatment of allergic rhinitis. In patients with impaired kidney or hepatic function, dosage reduction is necessary.

Serious toxicity is relatively absent with mast cell stabilizers. However, the propellants in the aerosols may aggravate coronary artery disease or dysrhythmias. With cromolyn, the nurse assesses for dysrhythmias, hypotension, chest pain, restlessness, dizziness, convulsions, CNS depression, anorexia, and nausea and vomiting. Sedation and coma may occur with overdosage.

Combination Regimens

Combination regimens are commonly used, and one advantage is that smaller doses of each agent can usually be given. This may decrease adverse effects and allow dosages to be increased when exacerbation of symptoms occurs. Table 33.8 summarizes information about available combination inhalation products. Advair, which was developed to treat both inflammation and bronchoconstriction, is more effective than the individual components at the same doses and as effective as concurrent use of the same drugs at the same doses. In addition, the combination reduces the corticosteroid dose by 50% and is more effective than higher doses of fluticasone alone in reducing asthma exacerbations. The combination improves symptoms within 1 week. Additional combination products are likely to be marketed and may improve patient adherence to prescribed drug therapy.

Clinical Application 33.2

- Mr. Lee's symptoms subside, and he is transferred to a medical unit. Mr. Lee tells the nurse that he hopes he does not have another asthma episode of this type again. What efforts does the nurse recommend to reduce the risk of future episodes?

NCLEX Success

4. When teaching a patient about the proper use of metered-dose inhalers, which of the following statements should be included?
    A. "Make sure that you puff out air repeatedly after you inhale the medication."
    B. "After you take a slow, deep breath for 3 to 5 seconds, inhale the medication, hold the breath for approximately 10 seconds and exhale slowly."
    C. "After you inhale the medication once, repeat until you obtain relief."
    D. "Rinse out your mouth before using the inhaler to decrease the development of a mouth infection."

5. A patient using a steroid inhaler complains of anorexia and discomfort when eating. The nurse reports this to the care provider, and the patient receives a diagnosis of oropharyngeal candidiasis. It is possible to decrease this adverse effect by which of the following actions? (Select all that apply.)
    A. reducing the dose
    B. administering the drug more frequently
    C. rinsing the mouth after use
    D. using a spacer device

TABLE 33.8

DRUGS AT A GLANCE: Combination Regimens

Drug	Routes and Dosage Ranges	
	Adults	Children
Fluticasone/salmeterol (Advair Diskus, Advair HFA, AirDuo RespiClick; ✹ Advair, Advair Diskus)	Advair Diskus: oral inhalation, one inhalation, twice daily Advair HFA: oral inhalation, two inhalations, twice daily AirDuo RespiClick: oral inhalation, one inhalation, twice daily	≥12 y, same as adults
Mometasone/formoterol (Dulera; ✹ Zenhale)	Oral inhalation, one inhalation, twice daily	≥12 y, same as adults
Budesonide/formoterol (Symbicort; ✹ Symbicort)	Oral inhalation, two inhalations, twice daily	≥12 y, same as adults
Ipratropium/albuterol (Combivent Respimat; ✹ Apo-Salvent-Ipravent Sterules, Combivent Respimat; Combivent UDV, ratio-Ipra Sal UDV, Teva-Combo Sterinebs)	Aerosol, two inhalations four times daily Nebulizing solution, 1 vial four times daily, increased to six times daily if necessary	Dosage not established

THE NURSING PROCESS

A concept map outlines the nursing process related to drug therapy considerations in this chapter. Additional nursing implications related to the disease process should also be considered in care decisions.

Assessment
- Assess for abnormal breathing patterns (e.g., rate below 12 or above 24 per minute, dyspnea, cough, orthopnea, wheezing, "noisy" respirations) because these may indicate respiratory distress. Severe respiratory distress is characterized by tachypnea, dyspnea, use of accessory muscles of respiration, and hypoxia.
- Assess for early signs of hypoxia, including mental confusion, restlessness, anxiety, and increased blood pressure and pulse rate. Late signs include cyanosis and decreased blood pressure and pulse rate. Hypoxemia is confirmed if arterial blood gas analysis shows decreased PO_2.
- In acute bronchospasm, assess for forceful expiration or wheezing, a characteristic feature of bronchospasm. The absence of wheezing in the presence of increased respiratory effort is an ominous sign.
- In chronic asthma, try to determine the frequency and severity of acute attacks; factors that precipitate or relieve acute attacks; antiasthmatic medications taken occasionally or regularly; allergies; and condition between acute attacks, such as restrictions in activities of daily living due to asthma.
- In chronic bronchitis or emphysema, assess for signs of respiratory distress, hypoxia, cough, amount and character of sputum, exercise tolerance (e.g., dyspnea on exertion, dyspnea at rest), medications, and nondrug treatment measures (e.g., breathing exercises, chest physiotherapy).

Outcomes of Therapy
The patient will
- Self-administer bronchodilating and other drugs accurately.
- Experience relief of symptoms.
- Avoid preventable adverse drug effects.
- Avoid overusing bronchodilating drugs.
- Avoid exposure to stimuli or conditions that cause bronchospasm.

Nursing Interventions
- Use measures to prevent or relieve bronchoconstriction when possible. A specific monitoring plan should be in place, whether peak expiratory flow rate (PEFR) or symptom monitoring. Some measures include coughing, deep breathing, percussion, and postural drainage to mobilize excessive respiratory tract secretions and preventing their retention.
- Help the patient identify and avoid exposure to conditions that precipitate bronchoconstriction.
- Assist patients with asthma to identify early signs of difficulty, including increased need for $beta_2$-adrenergic agonists, activity limitations, and waking at night with asthma symptoms.
- Monitor PEFR as an objective measure of airflow/airway obstruction and to help evaluate the patient's treatment regimen.
- Assist patients in obtaining meters and learning to measure PEFR.
- Assist patients and family in developing an action plan to manage acute attacks of bronchoconstriction, including when to seek emergency care.
- Encourage reduction of anxiety as it may aggravate bronchospasm. Stay with the patient and seek appropriate treatment during an acute asthma attack if feasible.
- Encourage smoking cessation as indicated and provide information, resources, and assistance in doing so.
- Provide appropriate patient teaching related to drug therapy (see Box 33.4).

Evaluation
- Observe for relief of symptoms and improved arterial blood gas values.
- Interview and observe for correct drug administration, including use of inhalers.
- Interview and observe for tachydysrhythmias, nervousness, insomnia, and other adverse drug effects.
- Interview about and observe behaviors to avoid stimuli that cause bronchoconstriction and respiratory infections.

Unfolding Patient Stories: Toua Xiong • Part 1

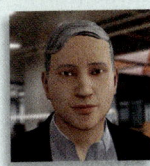

Toua Xiong has a 45-year history of smoking and is diagnosed with emphysema. The provider orders albuterol and ipratropium via metered-dose inhalers. What patient education would the nurse provide on the action and side effects of the medications? How would the nurse explain the use of an inhaler with a spacer and the sequence of medication delivery when the inhalers are ordered for the same time? (Toua Xiong's story continues in Chapter 60.)

Care for Toua and other patients in a realistic virtual environment: **vSim** *for Nursing* (thepoint.lww.com/vSim-Pharm). Practice documenting these patients' care in DocuCare (thepoint.lww.com/DocuCareEHR).

Visit thePoint® *at* http://thePoint.lww.com/Frandsen13e *for answers to NCLEX Success questions (in Appendix A), answers to Clinical Application Case Studies (in Appendix B), additional information on etiology and pathophysiology, and more!*

REFERENCES AND RESOURCES

Alhussien, A. H., Alhedaithy, R. A., & Alsaleh, S. A. (2018). Safety of intranasal corticosteroid sprays during pregnancy: An updated review. *European Archives of Oto-Rhino-Laryngology, 275*(2), 325–333.

Avery, C., Perrin, E. M., & Lang, J. E. (2021). Updates to the pediatrics asthma management guidelines. *JAMA Pediatrics, 175*(9), 966–967. doi:10.1001/jamapediatrics.2021.1494

Brooks, G. D. (2020). Updated evaluation of dupilumab in the treatment of asthma: Patient selection and reported outcomes. *Therapeutics and Clinical Risk Management, 16*, 181–187. https://doi.org/10.2147/TCRM.S192392

Fanta, C. H., & Barrett, N. A. (2022). An overview of asthma management. *UpToDate*. Lexi-comp, Inc.

Galante, C. (2022). Asthma management updates. *Nursing, 52*(2), 25–34. doi:10.1097/01.NURSE.0000806156.52958.3c

Global Initiative for Asthma (GINA). (2022). *Global strategy for asthma management and prevention*. Retrieved June 16, 2022, from http://www.ginasthma.org

Harber, P., Redlich, C. A., Henneberger, P., Lareau, S. C., & Sockrider, M. (2018). Work-exacerbated asthma. *American Journal of Respiratory and Critical Care Medicine, 197*(2), P1–P2.

Hinkle, J. L., Cheever, K. H., & Overbaugh, K. J. (2021). *Brunner & Suddarth's textbook of medical-surgical nursing* (15th ed.). Wolters Kluwer.

King-Biggs, M. B. (2019). Asthma. *Annals of Internal Medicine, 171*(7), ITC49–ITC64. doi:10.7326/AITC201910010

Lippincott. (2022). *Nursing2023 drug handbook* (43rd ed.). Wolters Kluwer.

Norris, T. L. (2019). *Porth's pathophysiology: Concepts of altered health states* (10th ed.). Wolters Kluwer.

Pavord, I. D., Beasley, R., Agusti, A., Anderson, G. P., Bel, E., Brusselle, G., Cullinan, P., Custovic, A., Ducharme, F. M., Fahy, J. V., Frey, U., Gibson, P., Heaney, L. G., Holt, P. G., Humbert, M., Lloyd, C. M., Marks, G., Martinez, F. D., Sly, P. D., … Bush, A. (2018). After asthma: Redefining airways diseases. *The Lancet Commissions, 391*(10118), 350–400. https://doi.org/10.1016/S0140-6736(17)30879-6

Reddel, H. K. (2019). The impact of the Global Initiative for Asthma (GINA): Compass, concepts, controversies and challenges. *Barcelona Respiratory Network Reviews, 5*(1), 4–18.

She, Y., Stephenson, M., Gu, Y., Hu, X., Zhang, M., & Jin, J. (2019). Asthma self-management in children: A best practice implementation project. *JBI Database of Systematic Reviews and Implementation Reports, 17*(5), 985–1002. doi:10.11124/JBISRIR-2017-003775

Vezir, E., Hizal, M., Cura Yayla, B., Aykac, K., Yilmaz, A., Kaya, G., Oygar, P. D., Ozsurekci, Y., & Ceyhan, M. (2021). Does aeroallergen sensitivity and allergic rhinitis in children cause milder COVID-19 infection? *Allergy and Asthma Proceedings, 42*(6), 522–529. https://doi.org/10.2500/aap.2021.42.210087

Clinical Judgment in Practice: Section 6: Drugs Affecting the Respiratory System

A 17-year-old patient is admitted to the emergency department (ED). The patient is on vacation with the family in Florida. The family was eating at a seafood restaurant, and the patient consumed shrimp scampi. Prior to this, the patient had never consumed shrimp as an entrée; the patient had only eaten smaller amounts, such as a shrimp cocktail. Following dinner, the patient began feeling itchy and the lips became swollen. Their vital signs are as follows: T 98.6 orally, P 126 and regular, RR 32 and labored, BP 94/70 mm Hg. The patient has inspiratory and expiratory wheezing per auscultation. The patient states, "It is really hard to breathe, and I itch all over." The tongue and lips are swollen. Currently, the airway is slightly obstructed with an inspiratory stridor.

Step 1: Recognize Cues
Identify the relevant and important information from different sources, such as the medical history or subjective and objective data.

Answer: For dinner the patient ate shrimp. The patient states, "It is really hard to breathe, and I itch all over." The patient's vital signs are as follows: T 98.6 orally, P 126 and regular, RR 32 and labored with an inspiratory stridor, BP 94/70 mm Hg. The tongue and lips are swollen. The patient has inspiratory and expiratory wheezing per auscultation.

Step 2: Analyze Cues
Organize and link the recognized cues to the patient's clinical presentation.

Answer: You are the ED triage nurse. You link the patient's symptoms of itching, swollen lips and tongue, labored respirations with inspiratory stridor, and wheezing following a meal of shrimp scampi as a severe food allergy.

Step 3: Prioritize Hypotheses
Evaluate hypotheses and rank them according to priority, such as urgency, likelihood, risk, difficulty, and/or time. Cluster your findings to generate a list of problems (actual or potential) you believe the patient is experiencing or may experience and determine the level of urgency. Which problem is of the greatest concern?

Answer: You prioritize the needs of the patient, which includes improved respiratory status without an inspiratory stridor, wheezing, and labored respirations. The patient's hemodynamic status will improve with an increased blood pressure without signs and symptoms of allergic shock.

Step 4: Generate Solutions
Identify expected outcomes and use hypotheses to define a set of interventions for the expected outcomes.

Answer: You anticipate the patient will require an IV to provide parenteral fluids to be administered. You also anticipate the administration of parenteral epinephrine and a corticosteroid. You recognize the patient's labored respirations with stridor and place the patient on oxygen at 6 L with a nonrebreather mask. You associate the symptoms of an allergic reaction due to the ingestion of shrimp. You recognize the risk of the patient developing anaphylactic shock. You monitor the patient's BP signs every 5 minutes and cardiac status with continuous cardiac monitoring. As the patient's breathing improves and the signs and symptoms of the severe allergic food reaction begin to resolve, you anticipate the patient will be discharged with an epinephrine autoinjector, oral prednisone, and albuterol inhaler.

Step 5: Take Actions
Implement the solutions that address the highest priorities.

Answer: You start an IV with D_5LR at 125 mL/hour as ordered by the ED provider. The ED provider orders epinephrine IM 0.5 mg using the 1 mg/mL solution to be repeated in 5 to 15 minutes with 0.3 mg epinephrine autoinjector. The ED provider also orders methylprednisolone 125 mg IV. You administer epinephrine IM 0.5 mg and methylprednisolone 125 mg IV. You assess the patient's lung sounds following the administration of epinephrine and methylprednisolone. Fifteen minutes after the epinephrine is administered, a 0.3 mg epinephrine autoinjector is administered. You instruct the patient and family on the medications' actions to improve respiratory rate and ease breathing to reduce air hunger.

Step 6: Evaluate Outcomes
Compare observed outcomes against expected outcomes.

Answer: Following the administration of epinephrine and methylprednisolone, the patient's respiratory rate is 24 and blood pressure 120/80. The inspiratory stridor has resolved. The respirations are unlabored and lung sounds have diminished wheezing in the lower lobes of the lungs. Twelve hours following the administration of one dose of

0.5 mg of epinephrine followed by 0.3 mg of autoinjector epinephrine and methylprednisolone, the patient's breathing is regular and unlabored. The wheezing is completely resolved, and lung sounds are clear per auscultation. Prior to discharge, the patient and family are instructed on the use of the epinephrine autoinjector. The patient and family are also instructed on the action, use, adverse effects, and administration guidelines for albuterol inhaler and oral prednisone. The patient and family are advised that the patient should wear an allergy alert bracelet indicating a seafood allergy. The patient was also instructed that a seafood allergy can result in an allergic reaction to contrast media.

SECTION 7

Drugs Affecting the Kidney and Digestive Systems

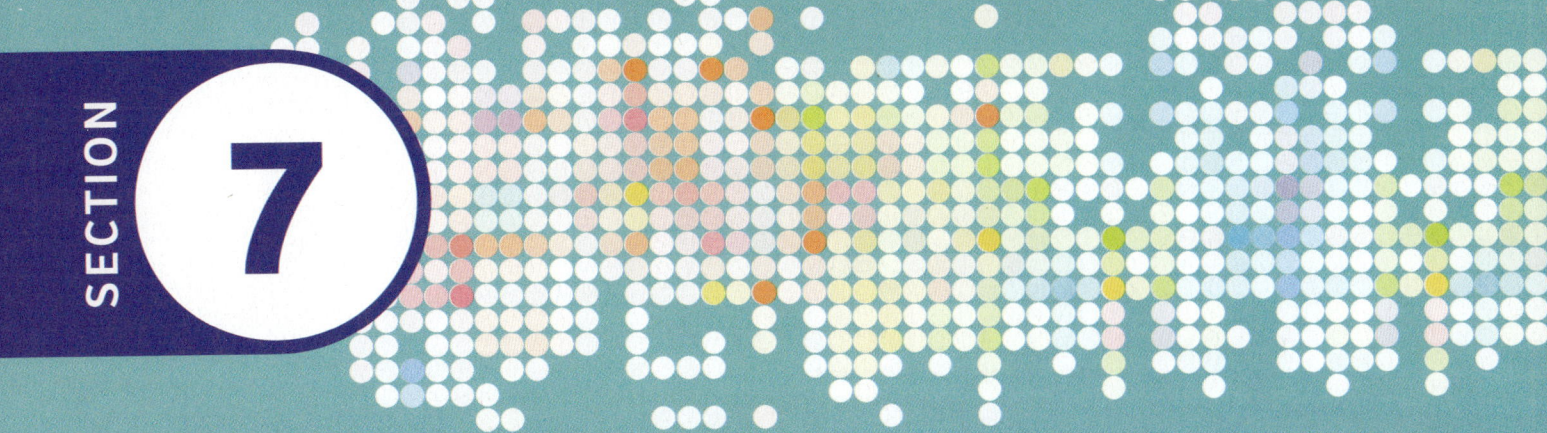

Chapter 34 Drug Therapy for Fluid Volume Excess
Chapter 35 Nutritional Support Products, Vitamins, and Mineral Supplements
Chapter 36 Drug Therapy for Weight Management
Chapter 37 Drug Therapy for Peptic Ulcer Disease and Hyperacidity
Chapter 38 Drug Therapy for Nausea and Vomiting
Chapter 39 Drug Therapy for Constipation and Elimination Problems
Chapter 40 Drug Therapy for Diarrhea

CHAPTER 34

Drug Therapy for Fluid Volume Excess

LEARNING OBJECTIVES

After studying this chapter, you should be able to:

1. Recognize conditions requiring diuretic administration.
2. Identify the loop diuretics in terms of their prototype, mechanism of action, indications for use, major adverse effects, and nursing implications.
3. Describe the thiazide diuretics in terms of their prototype, mechanism of action, indications for use, major adverse effects, and nursing implications.
4. Describe the potassium-sparing diuretics in terms of their prototype, mechanism of action, indications for use, major adverse effects, and nursing implications.
5. Discuss the rationale for using combination products containing a potassium-losing and a potassium-sparing diuretic.
6. Discuss the rationale for concomitant use of a loop diuretic and a thiazide or related diuretic.
7. Implement the nursing process in the care of patients receiving diuretics.

CLINICAL APPLICATION CASE STUDY

Agnes Bass, a 68-year-old woman, presents to the emergency department with acute heart failure complaining of an inability to "catch my breath." Her initial vital signs are temperature 99°F, pulse 108 beats per minute, respirations 28 per minute, and blood pressure 172/90 mm Hg. Her O_2 saturation is 88% on room air. Mrs. Bass has a history of uncontrolled hypertension, and her husband reports that for the past 2 months, they did not have sufficient money to buy her medications.

KEY TERMS

Anasarca: generalized massive edema

Anuria: no urine output

Ascites: accumulation of fluid in the abdominal cavity

Ceiling threshold: near-maximum response of a drug that is yielded by a certain dose

Dependent edema: localized edema occurring in the feet and ankles in people who are ambulatory

Edema: excessive accumulation of fluid in body tissues

INTRODUCTION

Drugs used to treat fluid volume excess, thereby increasing urine formation and output, are referred to as diuretics. These drugs increase kidney excretion of water, sodium, and other electrolytes. They are important therapeutic agents widely used in the management of both edematous (e.g., heart failure, kidney and hepatic disease) and nonedematous (e.g., hypertension, ophthalmic surgery) conditions. Diuretics are also useful in preventing kidney failure by their ability to sustain urine flow.

OVERVIEW OF CONDITIONS REQUIRING DIURETIC AGENTS

To adequately understand the pharmacologic treatment of fluid volume excess, it is important to understand the clinical considerations and manifestations of kidney disorders.

Clinical Considerations

Many clinical conditions alter kidney function. In some conditions, excessive amounts of substances (e.g., sodium, water) are retained; in others, needed substances (e.g., potassium, proteins) are eliminated. Causal conditions include cardiovascular, kidney, hepatic, and other disorders, which may be managed with diuretic drugs. Burns and trauma or allergic and inflammatory reactions may also lead to fluid shifts or loss.

Clinical Manifestations

Clinical manifestations reflect the alterations in fluid and electrolyte balance brought on by the inability of the kidneys to control the volume, composition, and pH of body fluids. **Edema** (excessive accumulation of fluid in body tissues) is a symptom of many disease processes and may occur in any part of the body. Specific manifestations of edema are determined by its location and extent. A common type of localized edema, known as **dependent edema**, occurs in the feet and ankles, especially with prolonged sitting or standing. A less common but more severe type of localized edema in the lungs is pulmonary edema, a life-threatening condition that occurs with circulatory overload (e.g., of intravenous [IV] fluids, blood transfusions) or acute heart failure. Generalized massive edema, or **anasarca**, interferes with the functions of many body organs and tissues.

Drug Therapy

Diuretic drugs act on the kidneys to decrease reabsorption of sodium, chloride, water, and other substances. Major subclasses are the loop diuretics, thiazides and related diuretics, and potassium-sparing diuretics, which act at different sites in the nephron (Fig. 34.1). The choice of diuretic drug depends primarily on the patient's condition.

Major clinical indications for diuretics are edema, heart failure, and hypertension. In edematous states, diuretics mobilize tissue fluids by decreasing plasma volume. In hypertension, the

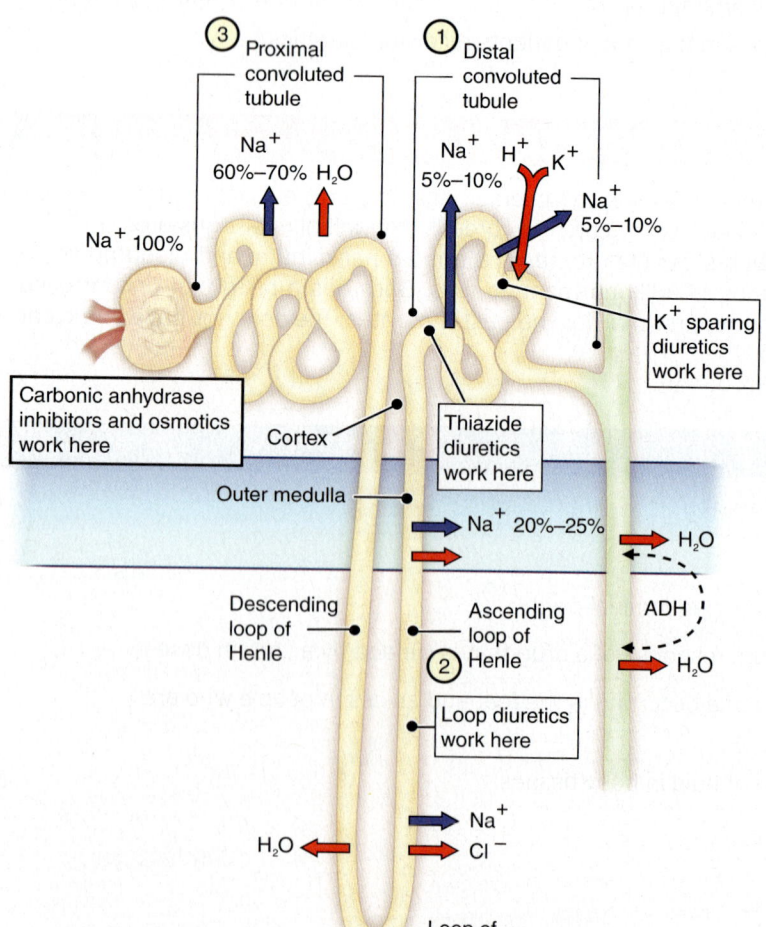

Figure 34.1. Diuretics act at different sites in the nephron to decrease reabsorption of sodium and water and to increase urine output. The main organ of the renal system is the kidney, which houses a tangled mass of nearly 1 million nephrons. The nephron is the structure known for its role in urine production. Different diuretic drugs work in different parts of the nephron: thiazide, thiazide-related in description, and potassium-sparing diuretics work in the distal convoluted tubule [1], loop diuretics in the ascending loop of Henle [2], and carbonic anhydrase inhibitors and osmotic diuretics in the proximal convoluted tubule [3]. Fluid and electrolyte alterations depend on where the specific diuretic works in the kidney. [Reprinted with permission from Aschenbrenner, D. S., & Venable, S. J. [2012]. *Drug therapy in nursing* [4th ed.]. Wolters Kluwer Health/Lippincott Williams & Wilkins.]

TABLE 34.1

Drugs Administered for the Treatment of Fluid Volume Excess

Drug Class	Prototype	Other Drugs in the Class
Loop diuretics	Furosemide (Lasix)	Bumetanide (Bumex) Ethacrynic acid (Edecrin) Torsemide (Soaanz)
Thiazide and thiazide-related diuretics	Hydrochlorothiazide	Chlorothiazide (Diuril) Chlorthalidone (Thalitone) Indapamide Metolazone
Potassium-sparing diuretics	Spironolactone (Aldactone)	Amiloride (Midamor) Eplerenone (Inspra) Triamterene (Dyrenium)
Osmotic diuretics	Mannitol (Osmitrol)	
Combination products		Aldactazide Maxzide (see Table 34.6 for details)

exact mechanism by which diuretics lower blood pressure is unknown, but antihypertensive action is usually attributed to sodium depletion. Initially, diuretics decrease blood volume and cardiac output. With chronic use, cardiac output returns to normal, but there is a persistent decrease in plasma volume and peripheral vascular resistance. Sodium depletion may have a vasodilating effect on arterioles.

Chapters 26 and 30 further discuss the use of diuretic agents in the management of hypertension and heart failure, respectively. The following section describes the types of diuretics, and Table 34.1 lists individual drugs.

LOOP DIURETICS

Loop diuretics are the diuretics of choice when rapid effects are required (e.g., in pulmonary edema) and when kidney function is impaired (creatinine clearance less than 30 mL/min). **Furosemide** (Lasix) is the most used loop diuretic and serves as the prototype for the group. Dosage can be titrated upward as needed to produce greater diuretic effects. Overall, loop diuretics are the most effective and versatile diuretics available for clinical use and, unlike thiazide diuretics, are effective when the glomerular filtration rate (GFR) is low.

Pharmacokinetics

Furosemide is available in oral or IV forms. After oral administration, the diuretic effect of the drug occurs within 30 to 60 minutes, peaks in 1 to 2 hours, and lasts 6 to 8 hours. After IV administration, diuretic effects occur within 5 minutes, peak within 30 minutes, and last about 2 hours. Thus, furosemide produces extensive diuresis for short periods, after which the kidney tubules regain their ability to reabsorb sodium. The kidneys reabsorb more sodium than usual during this postdiuretic phase, so a high dietary intake of sodium can cause sodium retention and reduce or cancel the diuretic-induced sodium loss. Thus, dietary sodium restriction is required to achieve optimum therapeutic benefits. The drug is metabolized and excreted by the kidneys, and drug accumulation does not occur even with repeated doses.

Action

Furosemide and other loop diuretics inhibit sodium and chloride reabsorption in the ascending limb of the loop of Henle, where reabsorption of most filtered sodium occurs. Thus, these potent drugs produce significant diuresis, their sodium-losing effect being up to 10 times greater than that of thiazide diuretics. High doses of furosemide may produce fluid volume depletion and worsen kidney function. Furosemide is often used to manage edema and **ascites** (accumulation of fluid in the abdominal cavity) in patients with hepatic impairment.

Use

Furosemide is useful when given alone or in combination with other antihypertensive agents to treat hypertension. Uses include the management of acute pulmonary edema, heart failure, as well as hepatic and kidney disease. It is feasible to titrate the dosage titrated upward as needed to produce greater diuretic effects. Table 34.2 presents route and dosage information for furosemide and the other loop diuretics.

Patient-related variables specific to the use of furosemide and other loop diuretics include the following:

- Age:
  - Furosemide is the loop diuretic used most often in children.
  - Oral therapy in children is preferred when feasible, and authorities do not recommend doses greater than 6 mg/kg of body weight per day. For maintenance therapy, it is necessary to adjust the dose to the minimum effective level.
  - In preterm infants, furosemide stimulates production of prostaglandin E_2 in the kidneys and may increase the incidence of patent ductus arteriosus and neonatal respiratory distress syndrome.
  - In neonates, furosemide may be given with indomethacin to prevent nonsteroidal anti-inflammatory drug–induced nephrotoxicity (toxic or damaging effects to the kidney) during therapeutic closure of a patent ductus arteriosus.
  - In both preterm and full-term infants, the half-life of furosemide is prolonged but becomes shorter as kidney and hepatic functions develop.

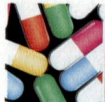

TABLE 34.2
DRUGS AT A GLANCE: Loop Diuretics

Drug	Routes and Dosage Ranges	
	Adults	**Children**
℞ Furosemide (Lasix; ◆APO-Furosemide, Furosemide Special, MINT-Furosemide)	Edema, heart failure: 20–80 mg PO, IM, IV as a single dose initially; if an adequate diuretic response is not obtained, dosage may be gradually increased by 20–40 mg increments at intervals of 6–8 h; for maintenance, dosage range and frequency of administration vary widely and must be individualized; max daily dose, 600 mg orally or 200 mg/dose IM and IV Hypertension: 40 mg PO twice daily, gradually increased if necessary Rapid mobilization of edema: 20–40 mg IV initially, injected slowly; dose may be repeated in 2 h Acute pulmonary edema: initial dose is usually 40 mg IV over 1–2 min, which may be repeated in 60 min at a dose of 80 mg; max dose 200 mg Acute kidney disease: 40 mg IV initially, increased if necessary; max dose, 1–2 g/24 h Hypertensive crisis: 40–80 mg IV injected over 1–2 min; with kidney failure, much larger doses may be needed	Edema, heart failure: 2 mg/kg/dose PO initially; gradually increase by increments of 1–2 mg/kg/dose if necessary at intervals of 6–8 h; max daily dose, 6 mg/kg 1 mg/kg/dose IV initially; if diuretic response is not adequate, increase dosage by 1 mg/kg no sooner than 2 h after previous dose; maintenance dose at intervals of every 6–12 h; max dose, 6 mg/kg
Bumetanide (Bumex; ◆Burinex)	Edema, heart failure: 0.5–2 mg PO per dose 1–2 times daily; may be repeated every 4–5 h to a max dose of 10 mg, if necessary; 0.5–1 mg IV, IM dose repeated in 2–3 h if necessary, may repeat in 2–3 h to a max daily dose of 10 mg; give IV injections over 1–2 min	Edema in infants and children: 0.015–0.1 mg/kg/dose PO, IM, IV every 6–24 h; max dose 10 mg daily
Ethacrynic acid (Edecrin; ◆Edecrin, Sodium Edecrin)	Edema: 50–200 mg PO daily in one to two divided doses; max daily dose, 400 mg; rapid mobilization of edema: 50 mg IV or 0.5–1 mg/kg/dose injected slowly to a max of 100 mg/dose; repeat doses not routinely recommended	1 mg/kg/dose once daily; increase at intervals of 2–3 d as indicated, to max of 3 mg/kg daily
Torsemide (Soaanz)	Heart failure: 10–20 mg PO, IV daily; titrate by doubling the dose to a max of 200 mg daily Hypertension: 5 mg PO daily up to 10 mg for appropriate response Chronic kidney disease: 20 mg daily PO, IV; titrate by doubling the dose to a max of 200 mg daily Hepatic failure: 5–10 mg PO daily up to 40 mg for appropriate response	Heart failure: 10–20 mg PO, IV daily; titrate by doubling the dose to a max of 200 mg daily Hypertension: 5 mg PO daily up to 10 mg for appropriate response Chronic kidney disease: 20 mg daily PO, IV; titrate by doubling the dose to a max of 200 mg daily Hepatic failure: 5–10 mg PO daily up to 40 mg for appropriate response

- In older adults, dose selection requires caution due to potentially decreased cardiac, kidney, or hepatic function and concomitant disease or other drug therapy in this patient population.
- Older adults require monitoring of kidney function because excessive diuresis may cause dehydration, blood volume reduction with circulatory collapse, and the risk of vascular thrombosis and embolism.
- Reproduction, pregnancy, and lactation:
  - Furosemide crosses the placenta.
  - If furosemide is taken during pregnancy, fetal growth must be monitored.
  - Furosemide, or other loop diuretics, can decrease milk volume and suppress lactation; avoid if possible while breast-feeding.
- Abnormal kidney function and hepatic impairment:
  - Furosemide and other loop diuretics are effective in patients with abnormal kidney function.
  - In those with chronic kidney failure, the drugs have lower peak concentrations at their site of action, which decreases diuresis and prolongs kidney elimination.
  - Caution is warranted because diuretic-induced fluid and electrolyte imbalances may precipitate or worsen hepatic encephalopathy and coma.

- Specific healthcare environments:
  - In patients with critical illness, continuous IV infusions of furosemide may be safer, more effective, and less likely to produce adverse effects.

> **Quality and Safety Alert: Evidence-Based Practice**
>
> Use of loop diuretics in managing heart failure has been largely based on expert opinion, dated randomized studies, and a single meta-analysis. Existing evidence indicates that loop diuretics, particularly in high doses, are associated with increased mortality and higher rates of hospitalization from heart failure. Kapelios et al. (2022) conducted a meta-analysis of 159 observational studies involving 96,959 patients to explore whether there is an association between loop diuretics use and dose with outcomes in outpatients with heart failure. Their observational study supported the current evidence. However, without data from large, randomized trials, the strength of the evidence is not robust, and the standard of care is not based on definitive support from the literature. Large, randomized control trials are needed to confirm the best use of loop diuretics in patients with heart failure.

Adverse Effects

Adverse effects of furosemide include fluid and electrolyte imbalances (e.g., hyponatremia, hypokalemia, fluid volume deficit) and ototoxicity. It is usually possible to avoid ototoxicity, which is associated with high plasma drug levels (greater than 50 mcg/mL), by dividing oral doses and by slow injection or continuous infusion of IV doses. Potassium imbalances may occur with diuretic therapy; Box 34.1 offers prevention and management strategies for potassium imbalances.

Contraindications

Contraindications to furosemide include known sensitivity to the drug or **anuria** (no urine output). Patients who are allergic to sulfonamides may also be allergic to furosemide.

> **BOX 34.2 Drug Interactions: Furosemide**
>
> **Drugs That Increase the Effects of Furosemide**
> - Aminoglycosides, cephalosporins
>   *Increase the risk of nephrotoxicity*
> - Corticosteroids, digoxin
>   *Increase the risk of hypokalemia*
>
> **Drugs That Decrease the Effects of Furosemide**
> - Ibuprofen
>   *Inhibits prostaglandins*
> - Phenytoin
>   *Decreases absorption*

Nursing Implications

Preventing Interactions

Several drugs may decrease or increase the effects of furosemide (Box 34.2). Additionally, furosemide may decrease the effects of insulin or oral antidiabetic drugs; blood glucose levels may rise. Several herbs (dandelion, hibiscus, parsley, uva ursi, juniper, buchu, cleavers, horsetail, and gravel root) have a diuretic effect, increasing the effects of furosemide and other diuretics.

Oral aloe can decrease levels of potassium, which may increase potassium losses with the loop diuretics. American ginseng, bayberry, blue cohosh, ginger, kola, and licorice can decrease the effects of diuretics.

Administering the Medication

The nurse gives IV injections of furosemide over 1 to 2 minutes and administers high-dose furosemide continuous IV infusions at a rate of 4 mg/min or less. This decreases or avoids high peak serum levels, which increases the risk of adverse effects, including ototoxicity. If using high doses of furosemide, a volume-controlled IV infusion at a rate of 4 mg or less per minute may be useful. For continuous infusion, it is necessary to mix furosemide with normal saline or

---

> **BOX 34.1 Prevention and Management of Potassium Imbalances**
>
> **Hypokalemia (Serum Potassium Level <3.5 mEq/L)**
>
> Measures to prevent or manage hypokalemia include the following:
>
> - Giving supplemental potassium, usually potassium chloride, in an average dosage range of 20 to 60 mEq daily. Sustained-release tablets are usually better tolerated than liquid preparations.
> - Increasing food intake of potassium. The minimal daily requirement of potassium is unknown; usual recommendations are 40 to 50 mEq daily for the healthy adult. Potassium loss with diuretic drugs may be several times this amount. To provide 50 mEq of potassium daily, estimated amounts of certain foods include 1,000 mL of orange juice, 1,600 mL of apple or grape juice, 1,200 mL of pineapple juice, 4 to 6 bananas, or 30 to 40 prunes.
>   - Some of these foods are high in calories and may be contraindicated, at least in large amounts, for patients with obesity.
>   - The amount of carbohydrate in these foods may be a concern for patients with diabetes.
> - Restricting dietary sodium intake. This reduces potassium loss by decreasing the amount of sodium available for exchange with potassium in kidney tubules.
>
> **Hyperkalemia (Serum Potassium Level >5 mEq/L)**
>
> The following measures help prevent hyperkalemia:
>
> - Avoiding use of potassium-sparing diuretics and potassium supplements in patients with abnormal kidney function
> - Avoiding excessive amounts of potassium chloride supplements
> - Avoiding salt substitutes (half of which are commonly potassium chloride)
> - Maintaining urine output, the major route for eliminating potassium from the body

lactated Ringer solution because 5% dextrose in water, or D_5W, may accelerate degradation of furosemide.

Assessing for Therapeutic Effects

The nurse assesses for decreased or absent edema, increased urine output, and decreased blood pressure. In patients with heart failure or acute pulmonary edema, it is necessary to observe for decreased dyspnea, crackles, cyanosis, and cough.

Assessing for Adverse Effects

Like any effective diuretic, furosemide may cause volume depletion and electrolyte imbalance, especially in patients receiving higher doses and a restricted salt intake. Hypokalemia may develop, especially with rapid diuresis, inadequate oral electrolyte intake, or when cirrhosis is present. Digitalis therapy may exaggerate metabolic effects of hypokalemia, particularly myocardial effects. The nurse should assess the patient for diminished hearing, a sign of ototoxicity. It is necessary to monitor serum electrolytes closely in children because of the frequent changes in kidney function and fluid distribution associated with growth and development.

Patient Teaching

The reason for furosemide use should guide patient teaching. In most instances, it is necessary to initiate measures to limit sodium intake. Key considerations should include not adding salt to food during preparation or at the dinner table, reading food labels carefully to be aware of hidden sources of sodium, and avoiding processed or high-sodium foods. Loop diuretics are potassium wasting; thus, a potassium-rich, low-sodium diet is recommended. The nurse instructs the patient in the use of equipment needed to take routine blood pressure readings. The general teaching guidelines presented in Box 34.3 provide additional patient education information.

BOX 34.3 Patient Teaching Guidelines for Diuretics

General Considerations

- Diuretics increase urine output and are commonly used to manage hypertension, heart failure, and edema (swelling) from heart, kidney, liver, and other disorders.
- While taking a diuretic drug, maintain regular medical supervision so drug effects can be monitored and dosages adjusted when indicated.
- Reducing dietary sodium increases the effectiveness of diuretic drugs and allows smaller doses to be taken, thus reducing the likelihood of adverse effects. Foods to be avoided include excessive table salt and obviously salty foods (e.g., ham, packaged sandwich meats, potato chips, dill pickles, most canned soups), which may aggravate edema or hypertension by causing sodium and water retention.
- Diuretics may cause blood potassium imbalances, and either too little or too much damages heart function. Periodic measurements of blood potassium and other substances are one of the major reasons for regular visits to a healthcare provider.
  - Too little potassium (hypokalemia) may result from the use of potassium-losing diuretics such as hydrochlorothiazide, furosemide (Lasix), and several others. To prevent or treat hypokalemia, your healthcare provider may prescribe a potassium chloride supplement or a combination of a potassium-losing and a potassium-saving diuretic (either separately or as a combined product such as Maxzide or Aldactazide). Your provider may also recommend increased dietary intake of potassium-containing foods (e.g., bananas, orange juice).
  - Too much potassium (hyperkalemia) can result from the use of potassium-saving diuretics, the overuse of potassium supplements, or the use of salt substitutes. Potassium-saving diuretics are not a major cause of hyperkalemia because they are usually given along with a potassium-losing diuretic. Take prescribed potassium supplements as directed. Do *not* use salt substitutes without consulting your primary healthcare provider because they contain potassium chloride instead of sodium chloride. Hyperkalemia is most likely to occur in people with decreased kidney function, which often occurs in older adults and people with diabetes.
- With diuretic therapy, you will have increased urination, which usually lasts only a few days or weeks if you do not have edema. If you do have edema (e.g., in your ankles), you can expect weight loss and decreased swelling as well as increased urination. Check and record your weight two to three times per week (at the same time of day with similar amount of clothing). Rapid weight changes often indicate fluid gain or loss.
- Some commonly used diuretics may increase blood sugar levels and cause or aggravate diabetes. If you have diabetes, you may need larger doses of your antidiabetic medications.
- Diuretics may cause sensitivity to sunlight. Avoid prolonged exposure to sunlight, use sunscreens, and wear protective clothing.
- Do not drink alcoholic beverages or take other medications without the approval of your health care provider.
- If you are taking a diuretic to lower your blood pressure, especially with other antihypertensive drugs, you may feel dizzy or faint when you stand up suddenly. This can be prevented or decreased by changing positions slowly. If dizziness is severe, notify your healthcare provider. Do not drive or operate dangerous machinery until the effects of the drug are known.

Self- or Caregiver Administration

- Take or give a diuretic early in the day, if ordered daily, to decrease nighttime trips to the bathroom. Fewer bathroom trips mean less interference with sleep and less risk of falls. Ask someone to help you to the bathroom if you are older, weak, dizzy, or unsteady in walking (or use a bedside commode).
- Take or give most diuretics with or after food to decrease stomach upset. Torsemide (Soaanz) may be taken without regard to meals.
- If you are taking digoxin, a potassium-losing diuretic, and a potassium supplement, it is crucial that you take these drugs as prescribed to increase beneficial effects and avoid adverse effects. Stopping or changing the dose of one of these medications while continuing the others can lead to serious illness.

Other Drugs in the Class

The pharmacologic characteristics of all loop diuretics are similar; use of another loop diuretic after a lack of response to one loop diuretic at adequate doses is not indicated. Instead, it is necessary to consider combining diuretics with different sites of action if aggressive diuresis is required.

Bumetanide (Bumex) may be used to produce diuresis in some patients who are allergic to or no longer respond to furosemide. It is more potent than furosemide by drug weight, and large doses can be given in small volumes. These drugs differ mainly in potency and produce similar effects at equivalent doses (e.g., furosemide 40 mg = bumetanide 1 mg). Bumetanide should be given by IV injection over 1 to 2 minutes.

Torsemide (Soaanz) is indicated for the treatment of edema associated with heart failure, kidney disease, or hepatic disease. It is also used for the treatment of hypertension alone or in combination with other antihypertensive agents. This drug is highly bioavailable after oral administration. Oral and IV doses are equivalent, and it is possible to switch patients from one route to the other without changing the dosage. To decrease or avoid high peak serum levels, which increase the risk of adverse effects, including ototoxicity, it is necessary to give torsemide intravenously over 2 minutes.

THIAZIDE DIURETICS

Thiazide diuretics are synthetic drugs that are chemically related to the sulfonamides and differ mainly in their duration of action. **Hydrochlorothiazide**, the most used drug in the class, is the prototype. It is not a strong diuretic and works efficiently only when urine flow is adequate. Thiazide diuretics are the drugs of choice for most patients who require diuretic therapy, especially for long-term management of heart failure and hypertension. All drugs in this group have similar effects.

Pharmacokinetics

Hydrochlorothiazide is administered orally and is well absorbed, widely distributed in body fluids, and highly bound to plasma proteins. The drug accumulates only in the kidneys. Diuretic effects usually occur within 2 hours, peak at 4 to 6 hours, and last 6 to 24 hours. Antihypertensive effects usually last long enough to allow use of a single daily dose. Most of the drug is excreted unchanged by the kidneys within 3 to 6 hours.

Action

Hydrochlorothiazide acts to decrease reabsorption of sodium, water, chloride, and bicarbonate in the distal convoluted tubule. Most sodium is reabsorbed before it reaches the distal convoluted tubule, and only a small amount is reabsorbed at this site.

Use

Healthcare providers use hydrochlorothiazide to treat mild to moderate hypertension and the edema associated with heart failure, acute glomerulonephritis, and nephrotic syndrome. However, its effectiveness decreases as the GFR decreases, and it becomes ineffective when the GFR is less than 30 mL/min. Table 34.3 presents route and dosage information for hydrochlorothiazide and the other thiazide diuretics.

Patient-related variables specific to the use of hydrochlorothiazide and other thiazide diuretics include the following:

- Age:
  - Chlorothiazide has more formulations, including a suspension, which may make thiazide preferable to hydrochlorothiazide in young patients. IV hydrochlorothiazide usually is not recommended in children.
  - Thiazides do not commonly cause hyperglycemia, hyperuricemia, or hypercalcemia in children, as they do in adults.
  - Older adults are especially sensitive to adverse drug effects, such as hypotension and electrolyte imbalance. With rapid or excessive diuresis, myocardial infarction, abnormal kidney function, or cerebral thrombosis may occur from fluid volume depletion and hypotension.
  - In older adults, adverse effects may exceed therapeutic benefits at doses greater than 25 mg.
- Reproduction, pregnancy, and lactation:
  - Hydrochlorothiazide crosses the placenta, and maternal use may cause fetal or neonatal thrombocytopenia, jaundice, or other adverse drug effects.
  - When possible, avoid thiazide diuretics in breast-feeding due to the drug's potential to decrease milk volume and suppress lactation.
- Abnormal kidney function and hepatic impairment:
  - The drug may accumulate and increase adverse effects in patients with impaired kidney function. Thus, it is necessary to perform kidney function tests periodically.
  - Patients with severe hepatic impairment are at significant risk for thiazide-induced hypokalemic and hypochloremic alkalosis.
  - Hepatic encephalopathy and death have occurred because of the electrolyte imbalances that accompany diuretic therapy.
  - Blood ammonia levels may become increasingly elevated in people with previously elevated ammonia concentrations.
  - In patients with hepatic impairment, thiazide diuretics should be discontinued promptly if signs of impending hepatic coma (e.g., increased jaundice, tremors, confusion, and asterixis) appear.
- Specific healthcare environments:
  - In patients with critical illness who may require immediate diuresis, hydrochlorothiazide is ineffective because of its slow onset of action; loop diuretics are more likely to be administered in such cases.

> **! Quality and Safety Alert: Safety**
>
> Hydrochlorothiazide should not be given the morning of surgery because it may lead to volume depletion, causing the blood pressure to be labile and undergo frequent changes with general anesthesia.

Adverse Effects

Adverse effects of hydrochlorothiazide include hypersensitivity reactions, hypotension, weakness, dizziness, diarrhea, constipation, electrolyte imbalances (e.g., hyponatremia, hypokalemia, hypochloremia), hyperglycemia, paresthesia, and erectile dysfunction.

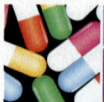

TABLE 34.3
DRUGS AT A GLANCE: Thiazide and Thiazide-Related Diuretics

Drug	Routes and Dosage Ranges	
	Adults	**Children**
ⓟ Hydrochlorothiazide (🍁 APO-Hydro, TEVA-Hydrochlorothiazide, Urozide)	Edema: 25–100 mg daily PO in one to two divided doses; max dose 200 mg/d Hypertension: 12.5–50 mg PO 1 or 2 times daily Older adults, 12.5–25 mg PO	<6 mo, 1–3 mg/kg/d PO in two divided doses; max 37.5 mg daily >6 mo to <2 y, 1–2 mg/kg/d PO on one to two divided doses; max 37.5 mg daily ≥2–12 y, 1–2 mg/kg/d PO on one to two divided doses; max 100 mg daily
Chlorothiazide (Diuril)	Hypertension: 500–2,000 mg/d PO divided in 1–2 times doses Heart failure: 250–500 mg PO once or twice daily; max 1,000 mg/d 500–1,000 mg IV once daily in combination with a loop diuretic	<6 mo, 10–30 mg/kg/d PO in two divided doses; max dose 375 mg daily >6 mo, 10–20 mg/kg/d PO in one to two divided doses; max dose: <2 y, 375 mg daily in children; 2–12 y, 1,000 mg PO daily; >12 y, 2,000 mg PO daily 5–10 mg/kg/d IV in two divided doses up to 20 mg/kg/d; max dose 500 mg
Chlorthalidone (Thalitone; 🍁 APO-Chlorthalidone)	Edema: 50–100 mg PO daily; max 200 mg daily Older adults, 12.5–25 mg/d PO (or every other day) Heart failure: 12.5–25 mg PO once daily; max 100 mg daily	Hypertension: 0.3 mg/kg PO once daily up to 2 mg/kg/d; max 50 mg daily
Indapamide (🍁 APO-Indapamide, Lozide, MYLAN-Indapamide)	Edema: 2.5–5 mg/d PO Hypertension: 1.25 mg PO in morning; may increase to 5 mg/d	Dosage not established
Metolazone (🍁 Zaroxolyn)	Edema: 5–20 mg PO, once daily Hypertension: 2.5 mg once daily; max dose 20 mg daily	Edema, refractory: 0.2–0.4 mg/kg/d in doses every 12–24 h in combination with furosemide

Contraindications

Contraindications to hydrochlorothiazide include known sensitivity to thiazides of sulfonamide-derived agents or kidney decompensation or anuria.

> **❗ Quality and Safety Alert: Safety**
>
> Thiazide diuretics and related drugs must be used cautiously in patients who are allergic to sulfonamide drugs because there is a known cross-sensitivity of some sulfonamide-allergic patients to a sulfonamide nonantibiotic.

Caution is necessary during pregnancy because the drug crosses the placenta and may have adverse effects on the fetus by compromising placental perfusion. It also may increase the risk of congenital anomalies.

Nursing Implications

Preventing Interactions

Several drugs increase or decrease the effects of hydrochlorothiazide (Box 34.4). The thiazide diuretic can increase the effects of angiotensin-converting enzyme inhibitors, other hypertensive agents, allopurinol, calcitriol, and lithium. Several herbs (dandelion, hibiscus, parsley, uva ursi, juniper, buchu, cleavers, horsetail, and gravel root) have a diuretic effect, increasing the effects of hydrochlorothiazide and other diuretics. American ginseng, bayberry, blue cohosh, ginger, kola, and licorice can decrease the effects of diuretics.

Administering the Medication

Hydrochlorothiazide, like all thiazide diuretics, has a **ceiling threshold**, which means that a certain dose yields a near-maximum diuretic response. This dose, known as the ceiling dose, is dependent on the type of diuretic and the extent of a person's disease. As the maximum effect is reached, a subsequent increase in dose does not enhance efficacy. In addition, there is a direct correlation between the dosage increase and the possible onset of adverse effects. When the diuretic dose is less than at ceiling, fluid retention remains following diuresis.

Assessing for Therapeutic Effects

The nurse assesses for the return of blood pressure to acceptable levels and improvement in the edema associated with heart failure and nephrotic syndrome.

BOX 34.4 Drug Interactions: Hydrochlorothiazide

Drugs That Increase the Effects of Hydrochlorothiazide
- Alcohol, barbiturates, monoamine oxidase inhibitors, opioids, phosphodiesterase 5 inhibitors, prostacyclin analogues
  Increase hypotensive effects, possibly contributing to orthostasis
- Beta-adrenergic blockers
  Increase the risk of hyperglycemia, hyperlipidemia, and hyperuricemia
- Carbamazepine
  Increases the risk of hyponatremia
- Chlorpropamide, corticosteroids, digoxin
  Increase the risk of hypokalemia

Drugs That Decrease the Effects of Hydrochlorothiazide
- Cholestyramine
  May significantly decrease absorption
- Methylphenidate, nonsteroidal anti-inflammatory drugs, yohimbine
  Decrease hypotensive effects

Assessing for Adverse Effects

Monitoring for transient or irreversible hearing impairment, tinnitus, or dizziness is important. Ototoxicity is more likely to occur with high serum drug levels (e.g., high doses or in patients with severe abnormal kidney function) or when other ototoxic drugs (e.g., aminoglycoside antibiotics) are being taken concurrently.

Patient Teaching

The nurse instructs the patient regarding the importance of taking the medication as prescribed, keeping follow-up appointments, and watching for signs and symptoms of adverse effects. Box 34.3 presents general patient teaching guidelines.

Other Drugs in the Class

Chlorothiazide (Thalitone) is the only thiazide diuretic that can be given intravenously. Thiazide-related diuretics are nonthiazides whose pharmacologic actions are essentially the same as those of the thiazides; they include chlorthalidone, indapamide, and metolazone. Chlorthalidone has a longer duration of action (48 to 72 hours), which is attributed to slower excretion.

Indapamide, a thiazide-related drug, is the first of a class of diuretics called the indolines. The drug is useful in the treatment of hypertension and can be given with other antihypertensive agents for an additive effect. People can take indapamide without regard to food. Its adverse effect profile is similar to that of hydrochlorothiazide.

Metolazone, another thiazide-related drug, is not generally recommended, but prescribers sometimes use it. Metolazone has some advantages over a thiazide because it is a stronger diuretic, causes less hypokalemia, and can produce diuresis in kidney failure. In children, it is most often used with furosemide, given 30 to 60 minutes before the furosemide dose for greatest effectiveness.

Clinical Application 34.1

After receiving oxygen at 2 L/min on nasal cannula, placement in a high Fowler position, and administration of 40 mg of IV furosemide, Mrs. Bass's vital signs are temperature 99°F, pulse 102 beats per minute, respirations 26 breaths per minute, blood pressure 172/90 mm Hg, and O_2 saturation 89%. Physical assessment findings include crackles on auscultation, productive cough, and bilateral 2+ peripheral edema to the knees. A cardiologist makes a diagnosis of biventricular heart failure.

- What is the rationale for the use of IV furosemide to treat the heart failure?
- What are the clinical manifestations of fluid overload reflected in the assessment findings?

NCLEX Success

1. A patient receives intravenous (IV) furosemide 80 mg for symptoms of severe heart failure. The nurse recognizes that administering the drug slowly by IV push reduces the likelihood of which of the following adverse effects of drug therapy?
   A. hyponatremia
   B. hypokalemia
   C. fluid volume deficit
   D. ototoxicity

2. A patient taking an oral hypoglycemic for management of type 2 diabetes begins taking hydrochlorothiazide. The nurse should monitor for which of the following serum laboratory changes?
   A. hypocalcemia
   B. hypercalcemia
   C. hyperglycemia
   D. hypernatremia

POTASSIUM-SPARING DIURETICS

Potassium-sparing diuretics act by competing for the aldosterone-sensitive Na^+/K^+ channel at the distal tubule of the nephron to decrease sodium and water reabsorption and potassium excretion. **Spironolactone** (Aldactone), the prototype drug in this class, is an aldosterone antagonist that reduces aldosterone-induced retention of sodium and water and impairs vascular function by antagonizing the action of aldosterone at mineralocorticoid receptors.

In patients with heart failure and inadequate kidney function, the addition of spironolactone allows smaller doses of loop diuretics and potassium supplements to be administered as spironolactone reduces urinary potassium loss. Through this action, aldosterone antagonists are also referred to as potassium-sparing diuretics.

Pharmacokinetics

Given orally, the effects of spironolactone are rather slow, requiring several days before full therapeutic effect is achieved; onset, peak, and duration occur between 24 and 48 hours. Absorption is best if the drug is administered with food. The half-life of the drug is 1.3 to 2 hours. Maximal effects may not occur for 6 weeks when the drug is used as an antihypertensive. It is excreted in the feces and urine.

Action

Spironolactone competitively inhibits mineralocorticoid receptors and blocks the effects of aldosterone, a hormone secreted by the adrenal cortex, in the kidney tubules. Spironolactone blocks the sodium-retaining effects of aldosterone, and aldosterone must be present for spironolactone to be effective. This effect promotes retention of sodium and water and excretion of potassium by stimulating the sodium–potassium exchange mechanism in the distal tubule. Independently, the drug is a weak diuretic because urine volume can only be slightly modified in the kidney tubules; it can be combined with other diuretics to increase efficacy.

Use

Primary uses of spironolactone include treatment of heart failure, ascites (in patients with liver disease), hypokalemia, and hypertension, as well as primary and secondary hyperaldosteronism. Also, prescribers often use spironolactone as adjunctive therapy in combination with other drugs to manage chronic heart failure. Clinical trials have shown that the addition of spironolactone improves cardiac function and reduces symptoms, hospitalizations, and mortality in patients with heart failure. Table 34.4 gives route and dosage information for spironolactone and other potassium-sparing diuretics.

Patient-related variables specific to the use of spironolactone and other potassium-sparing diuretics include the following:

- Age:
  - Spironolactone is used to treat hypertension in children. To increase the onset of therapeutic effects, a loading dose of two to three times the daily amount may be administered initially.
  - In infants and children with isolated ventricular septal defects prior to closure, spironolactone may be added to furosemide for more aggressive diuretic therapy if needed to treat moderate heart failure The drug is also used to diagnose primary hyperaldosteronism.

- Reproduction, pregnancy, and lactation:
  - Spironolactone is associated with dose-dependent menstrual irregularities and erectile dysfunction.
  - In utero exposure to spironolactone in animal studies may cause feminization of a male fetus.
  - In late pregnancy, high doses of spironolactone may be connected to restricted intrauterine growth of the fetus.
  - The drug's active metabolite is present in breast milk but is thought to be compatible with breast-feeding.

- Abnormal kidney function and hepatic impairment:
  - Spironolactone accumulates in kidney failure so an extended dosing interval may be ordered.
  - Since spironolactone is primarily metabolized in the liver, it should be avoided in severe hepatic impairment.

- Specific healthcare environments:
  - In patients with critical illness, diuretics that can be administered intravenously are more likely to be used than spironolactone to control the volume, composition, and pH of body fluids.

TABLE 34.4
DRUGS AT A GLANCE: Potassium-Sparing Diuretics

Drug	Routes and Dosage Ranges	
	Adults	Children
Spironolactone (Aldactone, CaroSpir; Aldactone, Teva-Spironolactone)	Edema: 25–200 PO mg daily in one to two divided dosesHeart failure: 12.5–25 mg PO in one to two divided doses once daily; max of 50 mg daily	Edema, hypertension: 1–17 y, 1 mg/kg/d divided every 12–24 h; max does 3.3 mg/kg/d, up to 3.3 mg/kg/d or 100 mg daily, whichever is less
Amiloride (Midamor; Midamor)	Hypertension, heart failure: 5 mg PO once daily, may increase to 10 mg daily as necessary	Hypertension. edema: 0.625 mg/kg/d PO divided every 12–24 h; maximum daily dose: 20 mg/d (limited data available)
Eplerenone (Inspra; Inspra)	Hypertension: 50 mg PO once daily, with increase to 50 mg twice daily if response not adequate; may take 4 wk for full therapeutic response	Safety and effectiveness have not been established
Triamterene (Dyrenium)	Edema: 100–300 mg PO daily in one to two divided doses; max to 300 mg daily	1–2 mg/kg/d PO in two divided doses; max 3–4 mg/kg/d up to 300 mg daily

- Because patients with critical illness can develop abnormal kidney function, the risk of hyperkalemia with spironolactone is potentially harmful in these patients.
- In the home care setting, the nurse should emphasize the need to read the labels of all over-the-counter medications as well as other products, such as salt substitutes, for ingredients, adverse effects, and drug interactions that could complicate the patient's clinical condition.
- The nurse should teach patients and caregivers the signs of hypotension and hyperkalemia and measures to manage these conditions (see Box 34.3).

Adverse Effects

Common adverse effects of spironolactone include dizziness, headache, abdominal cramping, and diarrhea. Because the drug also affects androgen receptors and other steroid receptors, it can cause deepening of the voice, gynecomastia, menstrual irregularities, and testicular atrophy. Its use has been known to cause an increased risk of gastric bleeding, although the mechanism is unknown. Because spironolactone may lead to a dose-related increase in serum potassium levels, assessment of serum potassium levels is important.

The U.S. Food and Drug Administration (FDA) has issued a **BOXED WARNING** ◆ for spironolactone. Investigations have shown that the drug is tumorigenic with chronic toxicity in rats; unnecessary use should be avoided.

Contraindications

Contraindications to spironolactone include known hypersensitivity to the drug. The presence of abnormal kidney function is also a contraindication, as previously discussed, because use of spironolactone may cause hyperkalemia through the inhibition of aldosterone and the subsequent retention of potassium. Spironolactone should be avoided in the first trimester of pregnancy because antiandrogen effects have caused feminization of male fetuses in animal studies.

Nursing Implications

Preventing Interactions

Multiple drugs interact with spironolactone, either increasing or decreasing its effects (Box 34.5). Also, spironolactone increases the half-life of digoxin, which could lead to digitalis toxicity. In addition, spironolactone may reduce kidney clearance of lithium, producing a high risk of lithium toxicity. Several herbs (dandelion, hibiscus, parsley, uva ursi, juniper, buchu, cleavers, horsetail, and gravel root) have a diuretic effect, increasing the effects of spironolactone and other diuretics. American ginseng, bayberry, blue cohosh, ginger, kola, and licorice can decrease the effects of diuretics.

Administering the Medication

It is necessary to administer spironolactone at the same time each day, preferably during the morning, even if the patient feels well. Taking the drug with food increases absorption, and this may decrease gastrointestinal irritation.

BOX 34.5 Drug Interactions: Spironolactone

Drugs That Increase the Effects of Spironolactone
- Angiotensin-converting enzyme inhibitors, angiotensin II receptor blockers, potassium-containing drugs, tacrolimus
  Increase the risk of hyperkalemia
- Beta-adrenergic blockers
  Increase the risk of hyperglycemia and hypertriglyceridemia

Drugs That Decrease the Effects of Spironolactone
- Alcohol, antihypertensive drugs, in particular vasodilators and alpha-blockers
  Increase the risk of hypotension and orthostasis
- Salicylates
  Interfere with the tubular secretion of active metabolite and decrease effectiveness

---

Assessing for Therapeutic Effects

The nurse assesses for decrease or absence of edema, increased urine output, decreased blood pressure, or decreased ascites (in patients with liver disease). Weights are measured and recorded to assist in determining the amount of mobilization of excess fluid. In patients with liver disease, abdominal girth is assessed to determine improvement in ascites.

Assessing for Adverse Effects

The nurse observes for evidence of fluid and electrolyte imbalance, including hyperkalemia, hyponatremia, hypomagnesemia, and hypochloremic alkalosis. Periodic laboratory tests are performed to measure serum electrolytes at appropriate intervals, particularly in older adults and in people with significant abnormal kidney function or hepatic impairment.

Patient Teaching

Routine blood pressure readings are necessary; the nurse instructs the patient about the use of equipment needed for these measurements. The nurse should instruct the patient that the drug may cause dizziness or drowsiness; the patient should curtail activities that require mental alertness (e.g., driving, operating machinery) until the effects of the drug are known. Use in pregnancy is appropriate only when the benefits to the mother outweigh the risks to the fetus. Box 34.3 contains additional patient teaching information.

Other Drugs in the Class

Amiloride (Midamor) and triamterene (Dyrenium) act directly on the distal tubules but do not affect mineralocorticoid receptors. These drugs decrease the exchange of sodium for potassium and have similar diuretic activity. Amiloride enhances kidney prostaglandin production, whereas triamterene decreases prostaglandin production. The drug is also effective in the treatment of lithium-induced nephrogenic diabetes insipidus. The choice of the specific potassium-sparing diuretic drug depends primarily on the patient's condition. Potassium-sparing diuretics are weak diuretics when used alone. Thus, they are usually given in combination with the so-called potassium-losing diuretics to increase diuretic activity and decrease potassium loss. The potassium-sparing diuretics are contraindicated in the presence of abnormal kidney function because their use may cause hyperkalemia through the inhibition of aldosterone and subsequent retention of potassium. Hyperkalemia is the major adverse effect of these drugs.

Eplerenone (Inspra), like spironolactone, competitively inhibits mineralocorticoid receptors. The FDA has approved this drug for use in the management of heart failure after myocardial infarction—to improve survival. Because of the selectivity of eplerenone for aldosterone receptors, people tolerate it better than they do spironolactone; the incidence of endocrine adverse effects, including gynecomastia, menstrual irregularities, and erectile dysfunction, is lower. Hyperkalemia, the most severe adverse effect of spironolactone, also occurs with eplerenone; dosage reduction is recommended with a rise in potassium level. Note that although eplerenone is more selective, with the potential for fewer adverse effects, there is no evidence in clinical trials that its overall efficacy is superior to that of spironolactone, and the cost of treatment may reduce overall use.

> **⚠ Quality and Safety Alert: Safety**
>
> Patients receiving potassium-sparing diuretics must not receive potassium supplements and must not eat foods high in potassium or use salt substitutes. (Salt substitutes contain mostly potassium chloride rather than sodium chloride.)

Box 34.1 presents strategies to manage hyperkalemia.

ADJUVANT MEDICATIONS USED TO TREAT FLUID VOLUME EXCESS

Osmotic Diuretics

Osmotic diuretics produce rapid diuresis by increasing the solute load (osmotic pressure) of the glomerular filtrate. The increased osmotic pressure causes water to be pulled from extravascular sites into the bloodstream, thereby increasing blood volume and decreasing reabsorption of water and electrolytes in the kidney tubules. The drug is freely filterable at the glomerular level, but it is not reabsorbed by the kidney tubules.
 Mannitol (Osmitrol), the prototype, is useful in managing oliguria or anuria, and it may prevent acute kidney injury (AKI) during prolonged surgery, trauma, or infusion of cisplatin, an antineoplastic agent. Mannitol is effective even when kidney circulation and GFR are reduced (e.g., in hypovolemic shock, trauma, dehydration). When administered early in AKI, the drug tends to clear cellular debris and prevent tubular cast formation. Other important clinical uses of hyperosmolar agents include reduction of intracranial pressure before or after neurosurgery, reduction of intraocular pressure before certain types of ophthalmic surgery (see Chapter 59), and urinary excretion of toxic substances.

The onset of diuretic action of mannitol is 1 to 3 hours, and reduction of intracranial pressure occurs in 15 to 30 minutes. Its half-life is approximately 1 to 1.6 hours. Excretion is primarily as unchanged drug in the urine.

Table 34.5 presents route and dosage information for mannitol.

> **Clinical Application 34.2**
>
> - Mrs. Bass has improved, and her vital signs are temperature 98.6°F orally, pulse 84 beats per minute, respirations 18 breaths per minute, blood pressure 132/80 mm Hg, and O_2 saturation 94% on room air. Her physician orders an extra dose of 20 mg of IV furosemide, to be given now. What administration guidelines should the nurse consider?

Combination Products

Thiazide diuretics are available in numerous fixed-dose combinations with nondiuretic antihypertensive agents (see Chapter 26) and with potassium-sparing diuretics. Table 34.6 lists combination diuretic products. Fixed-dose combination products are not indicated for initial therapy of edema or hypertension because therapy should be titrated for the individual patient. However, if the fixed combination represents the dosage so determined, a major benefit of antihypertensive combinations is increased patient convenience and adherence. Additionally, a major purpose of diuretic combinations is prevention of potassium imbalances, typically by combining potassium-sparing and potassium-wasting diuretics.

To prevent or manage hypokalemia and to augment the diuretic effect, people may take a potassium-sparing diuretic concurrently with a potassium-losing diuretic. They may take the two drugs separately or in a fixed-dose combination product.

Alternatively, when an inadequate diuretic response occurs with one of the drugs, people sometimes take two potassium-losing diuretics concurrently. The combination of a loop and a thiazide diuretic has synergistic effects because the drugs act in different segments of the kidney tubule. The synergistic effects

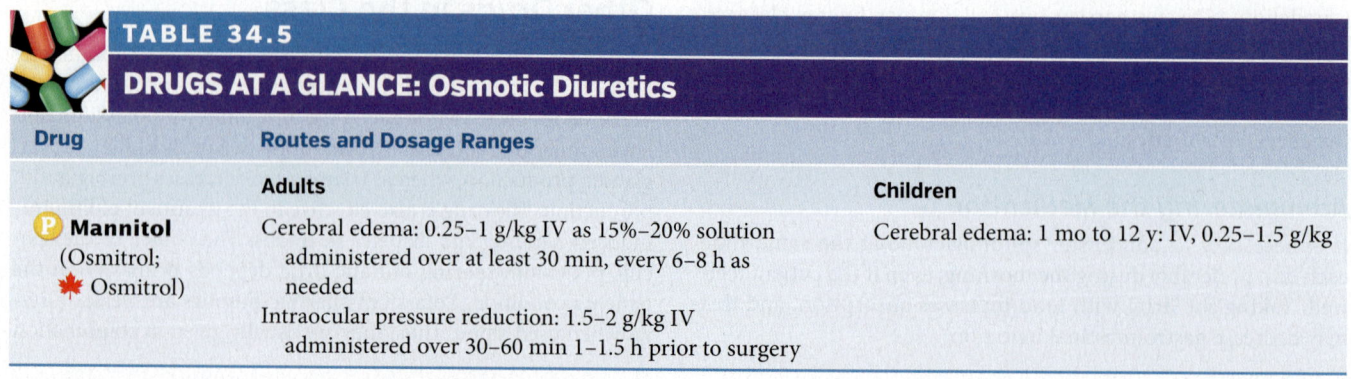

TABLE 34.5
DRUGS AT A GLANCE: Osmotic Diuretics

Drug	Routes and Dosage Ranges	
	Adults	**Children**
Mannitol (Osmitrol; ◆ Osmitrol)	Cerebral edema: 0.25–1 g/kg IV as 15%–20% solution administered over at least 30 min, every 6–8 h as needed Intraocular pressure reduction: 1.5–2 g/kg IV administered over 30–60 min 1–1.5 h prior to surgery	Cerebral edema: 1 mo to 12 y: IV, 0.25–1.5 g/kg

TABLE 34.6

Combination Diuretic Products

Drug Trade Name	Thiazide (Potassium-Losing) Diuretic	Potassium-Sparing Diuretic	Adult Dosage
Aldactazide 25 mg/25 mg (✦ Aldactazide 25)	HCTZ 25 mg	Spironolactone 25 mg	Hypertension, edema: 1–8 tablets PO daily
Aldactazide 50 mg/50 mg (✦ Aldactazide 50)	HCTZ 50 mg	Spironolactone 50 mg	Hypertension, edema: 1–4 tablets PO daily
Maxzide 25 mg/37.5 mg (✦ Apo-Triazide, Pro-Triazide, Teva-Triamterene HCTZ)	HCTZ 25 mg	Triamterene 37.5 mg	Hypertension, edema: 1–2 tablets/capsules PO once daily initially, then adjusted according to response
Maxzide 50 mg/75 mg (✦ Apo-Triazide, Pro-Triazide, Teva-Triamterene HCTZ)	HCTZ 50 mg	Triamterene 75 mg	Hypertension, edema: 1 tablet/capsule PO daily

HCTZ, hydrochlorothiazide.

probably result from the increased delivery of sodium to the distal tubule (where thiazides act) because a loop diuretic blocks sodium reabsorption in the loop of Henle. A commonly used combination is furosemide and hydrochlorothiazide (chlorothiazide can be given intravenously in patients who are unable to take an oral drug). Another combination is furosemide and metolazone. Generally, because a thiazide–loop diuretic combination can induce profound diuresis, with severe sodium, potassium, and volume depletion, only hospitalized patients who can be closely monitored should receive it. Ambulatory patients should take this combination in very low doses or only occasionally to avoid serious adverse events.

NCLEX Success

3. A 53-year-old patient who has had hypertension for 10 years admits to nonadherence with the prescribed antihypertensive therapy. Recently, the patient has begun to experience shortness of breath and ankle swelling. A workup reveals the presence of chronic abnormal kidney function. What classification of diuretic is the first drug of choice for the nurse practitioner to prescribe?
   A. thiazide
   B. loop
   C. osmotic
   D. potassium sparing

4. A nurse is instructing a patient on dietary considerations while taking spironolactone (Aldactone). Which of the following statements made by the patient indicates that teaching has been successful? (Select all that apply.)
   A. "I should not eat foods high in potassium while taking this medication."
   B. "I should use a salt substitute instead of regular salt."
   C. "I should call my nurse practitioner if I have any significant adverse effects from my medications."
   D. "I should not take large amounts of potassium chloride supplements."

5. A patient reports a drug allergy to sulfonamides. Which diuretic drug class should the nurse question if ordered for the patient?
   A. loop diuretics
   B. thiazides
   C. potassium-sparing diuretics
   D. osmotic diuretics

Clinical Application 34.3

- Mrs. Bass says that she enjoys snacks such as potato chips and pretzels. What response should the nurse make?

THE NURSING PROCESS

A concept map outlines the nursing process related to drug therapy considerations in this chapter. Additional nursing implications related to the disease process should also be considered in care decisions.

Assessment

- Useful baseline data include serum electrolytes, creatinine, glucose, BUN, and uric acid, because diuretics may alter these values. Other data are blood pressure readings, weight, amount and appearance of urine output, and measurement of edematous areas such as ankles or abdomen.
- Observe for edema. Visible edema often occurs in the feet and legs of ambulatory patients. Rapid weight gain may indicate fluid retention.
  - With heart failure, numerous signs and symptoms result from edema of various organs and tissues. For example, congestion in the gastrointestinal tract may cause nausea and vomiting; liver congestion may cause abdominal pain and tenderness; and congestion in the lungs (pulmonary edema) causes rapid, labored breathing, hypoxemia, frothy sputum, and other manifestations of severe respiratory distress.
  - Cerebral edema may be manifested by confusion, headache, dizziness, convulsions, unconsciousness, bradycardia, or failure of the pupils to react to light.
  - Ascites, which occurs with hepatic cirrhosis, is an accumulation of fluid in the abdominal cavity. The abdomen appears much enlarged.
- With heart failure, fatigue and dyspnea, in addition to edema, are common symptoms.
- Hypertension (blood pressure greater than 140/90 mm Hg on several measurements) may be the only clinical manifestation present.

Outcomes of Therapy

The patient will
- Take or receive diuretic drugs as prescribed.
- Experience reduced edema and improved control of blood pressure.
- Reduce dietary intake of sodium and increase dietary intake of potassium.
- Avoid preventable adverse drug effects.
- Keep appointments for follow-up monitoring of blood pressure, edema, and serum electrolytes.

Nursing Interventions

- Promote measures to prevent or minimize conditions for which diuretic drugs are used.
  - With edema, helpful measures include the following:
    - Decreasing dietary sodium intake
    - Losing weight, if obese
    - Elevating legs when sitting
    - Avoiding prolonged standing or sitting
    - Wearing support hose or elastic stockings
    - Treating the condition causing edema
- With heart failure and in older adults, it is necessary to administer IV fluids or blood transfusions carefully to avoid fluid overload and pulmonary edema. Fluid overload may occur with rapid administration or excessive amounts of IV fluids.
- With hypertension, helpful measures include decreasing dietary sodium intake, exercising regularly, and losing weight, if obese.
- With edematous patients, interventions to monitor fluid losses include weighing under standardized conditions, measuring urine output, and measuring edematous sites such as the ankles or the abdomen. After the patient reaches "dry weight," these measurements stabilize and can be done less often.
- With patients who are taking digoxin, a potassium-losing diuretic, and a potassium supplement, help them understand that the drugs act together to increase therapeutic effectiveness and avoid adverse effects (e.g., hypokalemia, digoxin toxicity). Thus, stopping or changing dosage of one of these drugs can lead to serious illness.
- Provide patient teaching regarding drug therapy (see Box 34.3).

Evaluation

- Observe for reduced edema and body weight.
- Observe for reduced blood pressure.
- Observe for increased urine output.
- Monitor serum electrolytes for normal values.
- Interview regarding compliance with instructions for diet and drug therapy.
- Monitor compliance with follow-up appointments in outpatients.

Visit thePoint® at http://thePoint.lww.com/Frandsen13e for answers to NCLEX Success questions (in Appendix A), answers to Clinical Application Case Studies (in Appendix B), additional information on pathophysiology, and more!

REFERENCES AND RESOURCES

Ali, S., Navaneethan, S. D., Virani, S. S., & Gregg, L. P. (2022). Revisiting diuretic choice in chronic kidney disease. *Current Opinion in Nephrology and Hypertension*, *31*(5), 406–413.

Girerd, N., & Felker, G. M. (2021). The lower is not always the better: A more comprehensive understanding of loop diuretics in heart failure. *European Journal of Heart Failure*, *23*(7), 1120–1121. https://doi.org/10.1002/ejhf.2182

Hinkle, J. L., Cheever, K. H., & Overbaugh, K. J. (2021). *Brunner and Suddarth's textbook of medical-surgical nursing* (15th ed.). Wolters Kluwer.

Kapelios, C. J., Bonou, M., Malliaras, K., Athanasiadi, E., Vakrou, E., Skouloudi, M., Masoura, C., & Barbetseas, J. (2022). Association of loop diuretics use and dose with outcomes in outpatients with heart failure: A systematic review and meta-analysis of observational studies involving 96,959 patients. *Heart Failure Reviews*, *27*(1), 147–161.

Lippincott advisor. (2022). Retrieved from http://advisor.lww.com.

National Collaborating Centre for Acute and Chronic Conditions (2018). *Chronic heart failure in adults: Diagnosis and management.* National Institute for Health and Clinical Excellence (NICE) (Clinical guideline no. 106). Retrieved January 24, 2020, from https://www.nice.org.uk/guidance/ng106

Norris, T. L. (2019). *Pathophysiology: Concepts of altered health status* (10th ed.). Wolters Kluwer.

Täger, T., Fröhlich, H., Seiz, M., Katus, H. A., & Frankenstein, L. (2019). Ready: Relative efficacy of loop diuretics in patients with chronic systolic heart failure-a systematic review and network meta-analysis of randomised trials. *Heart Failure Reviews*, *24*(4), 461–472. https://doi.org/10.1007/s10741-019-09771-8

Tucker, R. (2021). *2022 Lippincott's pocket drug guide for nurses*. Wolters Kluwer.

Yancy, C. W., Jessup, M., Bozkurt, B., Butler, J., Casey, D. E., Drazner, M. H., Fonarow, G. C., Geraci, S. A., Horwich, T., Januzzi, J. L., Johnson, M. R., Kasper, E. K., Levy, W. C., Masoudi, F. A., McBride, P. E., McMurray, J. J. V., Mitchell, J. E, Peterson, P. N., ... Wilkoff, B. L.; American College of Cardiology Foundation/American Heart Association Task Force on Practice Guidelines, et al. (2013). 2013 ACCF/AHA guideline for the management of heart failure: A report of the American College of Cardiology Foundation/American Heart Association Task Force on practice guidelines. *Circulation*, *128*(16), e240–e327.

CHAPTER 35

Nutritional Support Products, Vitamins, and Mineral Supplements

LEARNING OBJECTIVES

After studying this chapter, you should be able to:

1. Describe the use of vitamins and minerals in specific groups of patients.
2. Identify fat-soluble vitamins used to treat deficiencies, including the nursing implications associated with their administration.
3. Identify water-soluble vitamins used to treat deficiencies, including the nursing implications associated with their administration.
4. Identify minerals used to treat deficiencies, including the nursing implications associated with their administration.
5. Discuss the chelating agents used to remove excess copper, iron, and lead from body tissues.
6. Recognize the benefit of nutritional supplements, including the nursing implications associated with their administration.
7. Apply nursing process skills to prevent, recognize, or treat nutritional imbalances, which may involve monitoring laboratory reports that indicate nutritional status.

CLINICAL APPLICATION CASE STUDY

Jenny Martin, an 86-year-old patient, has lived alone for 10 years since her husband died. She sometimes must limit her food purchases to pay for her medicines and utilities. Thus, her nutritional status is poor. A neighbor, who has not seen Mrs. Martin for a couple of days, finds her lying on the kitchen floor, conscious but with slurred speech. Emergency medical personnel transport her to a hospital emergency department, where she is diagnosed with a left-brain stroke with right hemiparesis, dysarthria, and dysphagia.

Mrs. Martin is unable to swallow foods safely, so the nurses insert a nasogastric tube. A dietician orders a high-calorie commercially prepared formula that contains carbohydrates, protein, fat, vitamins, and minerals.

KEY TERMS

Chelating agents: drugs used to treat metal poisoning (e.g., from iron, lead, or mercury) that bind to the toxic metal, decrease binding of the metal within the body, and promote elimination of the metal

Enteral nutrition: provision of fluid and nutrients to a functional gastrointestinal tract via a feeding tube in a patient who is unable to ingest enough fluid and food

Fat-soluble vitamins: vitamins that are accumulated and stored in the body when taken in excess

Hyperkalemia: greater-than-normal amount of potassium in the blood

Hypokalemia: less-than-normal amount of potassium in the blood

Malabsorption: impaired absorption of nutrients from the gastrointestinal tract

Megaloblastic anemia: anemia characterized by the presence in the blood of megaloblasts (large, abnormal blood cells) associated with vitamin B_{12} deficiency

Megavitamins: large doses of vitamins in excess of the recommended dietary allowance

Parenteral nutrition: intravenous provision of fluid and nutrients to a patient who is unable to ingest enough fluid and food due to a nonfunctional gastrointestinal tract

Water-soluble vitamins: vitamins that are not stored in the body and are rapidly eliminated

INTRODUCTION

Water, carbohydrates, proteins, fats, vitamins, and minerals are required to promote or maintain health, prevent illness, and promote recovery from illness or injury. Water is necessary for cellular metabolism and excretion of metabolic waste products; people need 2,000 to 3,000 mL daily. Carbohydrates and fats mainly provide energy for cellular metabolism. Energy is measured in kilocalories (kcal) per gram of food oxidized in the body. Carbohydrates and proteins supply 4 kcal/g, and fats supply 9 kcal/g. Proteins are structural and functional components of all body tissues; the recommended amount for adults is 50 to 60 g daily.

Vitamins are required for normal body metabolism, growth, and development. They are components of enzyme systems that release energy from ingested carbohydrates, proteins, and fats. They also are necessary for formation of genetic material, red blood cells, hormones, nerve cells, and bone and other tissues. Minerals and electrolytes are essential constituents of cell membranes, many essential enzymes, bone, teeth, and connective tissue. They function to:

- Maintain electrolyte and acid–base balance, osmotic pressure, and nerve and muscle function
- Assist in transfer of compounds across cell membranes
- Influence the growth process

Patients' requirements for these nutrients vary widely, depending on age, sex, size, health or illness status, and other factors. This chapter discusses medications and products to improve nutritional status in patients with deficiency and excess states of selected vitamins, minerals, and electrolytes.

OVERVIEW OF ALTERED NUTRITIONAL STATES

Clinical Considerations

Many patients may be unable to ingest, digest, absorb, or use sufficient nutrients to improve or maintain health. Debilitating illnesses often interfere with appetite and gastrointestinal (GI) function. Drugs often cause anorexia, nausea, vomiting, or diarrhea. The lack of certain vitamins and minerals may impair the function of body organs. Genetic disorders or traumatic injury may also affect nutritional status.

There are two types of vitamins: fat soluble and water soluble. **Fat-soluble vitamins**—vitamins A, D, E, and K—are stored in the body when taken in excess. They are absorbed from the intestine with dietary fat. Absorption requires the presence of bile salts and pancreatic lipase. (Note that vitamin D is discussed in Chapter 44 because of its major role in bone metabolism.) **Water-soluble vitamins**—B complex vitamins and vitamin C—are not stored in the body and are rapidly eliminated.

Historically, the major concern about vitamins concerned whether a person's intake was sufficient to promote health and prevent deficiency diseases. Hence, the Food and Nutrition Board of the National Academy of Sciences established recommendations for daily vitamin intake known as Dietary Reference Intakes (DRIs; Box 35.1).

Many authorities promote vitamin supplements as a means to improve health and prevent or treat illness. However, supplements can be harmful if overused. As a result, DRIs include tolerable upper intake levels (ULs) of some vitamins. Table 35.1 lists the function, recommended daily intake, food sources, and signs and symptoms of deficiency and excess of vitamins.

 Quality and Safety Alert: Safety

No one should take more than the recommended ULs.

Although healthcare providers may order vitamin supplements, people mostly self-prescribe them. Because vitamins are essential nutrients, some people believe that large amounts (megadoses) promote health and provide other beneficial effects. However, excessive intake may cause harmful effects. People should never self-prescribe **megavitamins**, large doses of vitamins in excess of the recommended dietary allowance (RDA).

Minerals maintain acid–base balance and osmotic pressure. They make up part of enzymes, hormones, and vitamins. The body needs minerals for hemoglobin formation, muscle contraction, and skeletal development and maintenance. Minerals present in the body in large amounts (macrominerals) are sodium, potassium, chloride, calcium, magnesium, phosphorus, and sulfur. (Note: Calcium and phosphorus are discussed in Chapter 44 because they play major roles in bone metabolism.) Other minerals are required in small amounts (trace elements). Eight of these (chromium, cobalt, copper, fluoride, iodine, iron, selenium, and zinc) have relatively well-defined roles in human nutrition.

Minerals occur in the body and foods mainly in ionic form. When placed in solution, the components separate into electrolytes. Electrolytes are electrically charged particles found in body fluids and cells (e.g., sodium or potassium ions). At any

BOX 35.1 *Dietary Reference Intakes*

Dietary Reference Intakes (DRIs) are the recommended amounts of vitamins (see Table 35.1) and some minerals (see Table 35.2). The Food and Nutrition Board of the Institute of Medicine revised the current DRIs in 2006; the board intended them to replace the recommended dietary allowances (RDAs) used since 1989. DRIs consist of four subtypes of nutrient recommendations, as follows:

1. **Recommended dietary allowance (RDA)** is the amount estimated to meet the needs of approximately 98% of healthy children and adults in a specific age and gender group. The RDA is used to advise various groups about nutrient intake. It should be noted, however, that RDAs were established to prevent deficiencies and that they were extrapolated from studies of healthy adults. Thus, they may not be appropriate for all groups, such as young children and older adults.
2. **Estimated average requirement (EAR)** is the amount estimated to provide adequate intake in 50% of healthy persons in a specific group. The EAR is a median amount that takes into account the bioavailability of the nutrient and reduction of chronic disease. The EAR is used to determine the RDA.
3. **Adequate intake (AI)** is the amount thought to be sufficient when there is not enough reliable, scientific information to estimate an RDA. The AI is derived from data that show an average intake that appears to maintain health. Although an RDA is expected to meet the needs of all healthy people, an AI does not clearly indicate the percentage of people whose needs will be met.
4. **Tolerable upper intake level (UL)** is the maximum intake considered unlikely to pose a health risk in almost all healthy people in a specified group. The UL is not intended to be a recommended level of intake.
   - **Vitamins.** The ULs for adults (ages 19 to 70 years and older) are D 50 mcg, E 1,000 mg, B_3 (niacin) 35 mg, B_6 (pyridoxine) 100 mg, folate 1,000 mcg, and C 2,000 mg. With vitamin D, pyridoxine, and vitamin C, the UL refers to total intake from food, fortified food, and supplements. With niacin and folate, the UL applies to synthetic forms obtained from supplements, fortified food, or a combination of the two. With vitamin E, the UL applies to any form of supplemental alpha-tocopherol. *These ULs should not be exceeded*. There are inadequate data for establishing ULs for B_1 (thiamine), B_2 (riboflavin), B_5 (pantothenic acid), B_{12} (cyanocobalamin), and biotin. As a result, consuming more than the recommended amounts of these vitamins should generally be avoided.
   - **Minerals.** ULs have been established for magnesium 350 mg, calcium 2.5 g, phosphorus 3 to 4 g, fluoride 10 mg, and selenium 400 mcg. *The UL should not be exceeded for any mineral–electrolyte because all minerals are toxic in overdose*. Except for magnesium, which is set for supplements only and excludes food and water sources, the stated UL amounts include those from both food and supplements.

---

given time, the body must maintain an equal number of positive and negative charges. Therefore, the ions are constantly combining and separating to maintain electrical neutrality or electrolyte balance.

Electrolytes also maintain the acid–base balance of body fluids. Acids are usually anions (e.g., bicarbonate, chloride, phosphate, or sulfate). Bases are usually cations (e.g., sodium, potassium, calcium, and magnesium). Mineral–electrolytes are obtained from foods or supplements. Although most minerals are supplied by a well-balanced diet, studies indicate that most adults and children do not ingest sufficient dietary calcium and that iron deficiency is common in some populations. In addition, some conditions increase requirements (e.g., pregnancy, lactation, and various illnesses), and some drug–drug interactions decrease absorption or use of minerals.

As with vitamins, goals for daily mineral intake have been established as DRIs. Thus far, DRIs and ULs have been established for calcium, fluoride, iron, magnesium, phosphorus, and selenium.

 Quality and Safety Alert: Safety

People should not exceed the UL for any mineral–electrolyte.

Except for the stated amount for magnesium, which excludes food and water sources and considers supplements only, the ULs include those from both foods and supplements. Table 35.2 lists the function, recommended daily intake, and dietary sources of various minerals.

Clinical Manifestations

Tables 35.1 and 35.2 list signs and symptoms associated with deficiency and excess of vitamins and minerals, respectively.

Drug Therapy

Early recognition and treatment of vitamin disorders can prevent a mild deficiency or excess from becoming severe. For deficiency states, oral vitamin preparations are preferred when possible. Multiple deficiencies are common, and a multivitamin preparation used to treat them usually contains more than the recommended daily amount. Use for limited periods is best. When fat-soluble vitamins are given to correct a deficiency, there is a risk of producing excess states. When water-soluble vitamins are given, excesses are less likely but may occur with large doses. For excess states, the usual treatment is to stop administration of the vitamin preparation. There are no specific antidotes or antagonists.

It is important to titrate the amount of mineral supplement closely to the amount needed by the body as there is a risk of producing an excess state. Oral products are preferred for replacement because they are safer, less likely to produce toxicity, more convenient to administer, and less expensive than are parenteral preparations. The U.S. Food and Drug Administration (FDA) regulates the content of supplements for infants and children younger than 4 years of age; however, it does not regulate the content of preparations for older children.

TABLE 35.1

Vitamins

Vitamin/Function	Dietary Reference Intakes	Food Sources	Signs and Symptoms of Deficiency	Signs and Symptoms of Excess
Fat-Soluble Vitamins				
Vitamin A (retinol) Required for normal vision, growth, bone development, skin, and mucous membranes	RDAs Females 14 y and older: 700 mcg Pregnancy, 19 y and older: 770 mcg 14–18 y: 750 mcg Lactation, 19 y and older: 1,300 mcg Lactation, 14–18 y: 1,200 mcg Males 14 y and older: 900 mcg Children 1–3 y: 300 mcg 4–8 y: 400 mcg 9–13 y: 600 mcg Infants (AIs) 1–6 mo, 400 mcg 7–12 mo, 500 mcg	Preformed vitamin A: meat, butter, fortified margarine, egg yolk, whole milk, cheese made from whole milk Carotenoids: turnip and collard greens, carrots, sweet potatoes, squash, apricots, peaches, cantaloupe	Night blindness; xerophthalmia, which may progress to corneal ulceration and blindness; changes in skin and mucous membranes that lead to skin lesions and infections; respiratory tract infections; urinary calculi	Anorexia; vomiting; irritability; skin changes (itching, desquamation, dermatitis); pain in muscles, bones, and joints; gingivitis; enlargement of spleen and liver; increased intracranial pressure; other neurologic signs Congenital abnormalities in newborns whose mothers took excessive vitamin A during pregnancy Acute toxicity, with increased intracranial pressure, bulging fontanelles, and vomiting, may occur in infants who are given vitamin A
Vitamin D (see Chapter 44)				
Vitamin E (antioxidant) Essential in preventing destruction of certain fats, including the lipid portion of cell membranes	RDAs* Adults 15 mg; UL not >1,000 mg Pregnancy ≤18 y: 15 mg; UL not >800 mg 19–50 y: 15 mg; UL not >1,000 mg Lactation 19–50 y: 19 mg; UL not >1,000 mg ≤18 y: 19 mg; UL not > 800 mg Children 1–3 y: 6 mg; UL not >200 mg 4–8 y: 7 mg; UL not >300 mg 9–13 y: 11 mg; UL not above 600 mg 14–18 y: 15 mg; UL not >800 mg Infants (AIs) 1–6 mo: 4 mg 7–12 mo: 5 mg	Cereals, green leafy vegetables, egg yolk, milk fat, butter, meat, vegetable oils	Deficiency is rare	Fatigue, headache, blurred vision, nausea, diarrhea
Vitamin K Essential for normal blood clotting. It activates precursor proteins, found in the liver, into clotting factors II, VII, IX, and X	AIs Males: 120 mcg/d Females: 90 mcg/d (same dose in pregnancy and lactation) AI Children 1–3 y: 30 mcg 4–8 y: 55 mcg 9–13 y: 60 mcg 14–18 y: 75 mcg	Green leafy vegetables (spinach, kale, cabbage, lettuce), cauliflower, tomatoes, wheat bran, cheese, egg yolk, liver	Abnormal bleeding (petechiae, ecchymoses, epistaxis, hematemesis, melena, hematuria, hypovolemic shock)	Clinical manifestations rare; however, when vitamin K is given to someone who is receiving warfarin (Coumadin), the patient can be made "warfarin resistant" for 1 wk or more

(Continued on page 648)

TABLE 35.1

Vitamins (Continued)

Vitamin/Function	Dietary Reference Intakes	Food Sources	Signs and Symptoms of Deficiency	Signs and Symptoms of Excess
Water-Soluble Vitamins				
B Complex Vitamins **Vitamin B$_1$ (thiamine)** A coenzyme in carbohydrate metabolism; essential for energy production	RDAs Females 19 y and older: 1.1 mg Pregnancy: 1.4 mg Lactation: 1.4 mg Males 19 y and older: 1.2 mg Children 1–3 y: 0.5 mg 4–8 y: 0.6 mg 9–13 y: 0.9 mg 14–18 y: females, 1 mg; males, 1.2 mg Infants (AIs) 0–6 mo: 0.2 mg 7–12 mo: 0.3 mg	Meat, poultry, fish, egg yolk, dried beans, whole-grain cereal products, peanuts	Mild deficiency: fatigue, anorexia; retarded growth; mental depression; irritability; apathy, lethargy Severe deficiency (beriberi): peripheral neuritis; personality disturbances; heart failure; edema Wernicke-Korsakoff syndrome in alcoholics	Not established
Vitamin B$_2$ (riboflavin) A coenzyme in metabolism; necessary for growth; may function in production of corticosteroids and red blood cells and in gluconeogenesis	RDAs 19 y and older: 1.1 mg Pregnancy: 1.4 mg Lactation: 1.6 mg Males 19 y and older: 1.3 mg Children 1–3 y: 0.5 mg 4–8 y: 0.6 mg 9–13 y: 0.9 mg 14–18 y: females, 1 mg; males, 1.3 mg Infants (AIs) 1–6 mo: 0.3 mg 7–12 mo: 0.4 mg	Milk, cheddar and cottage cheeses, meat, eggs, green leafy vegetables	Seborrheic dermatitis, glossitis, stomatitis, eye disorders (burning, itching, lacrimation, photophobia, vascularization of the cornea)	Not established
Biotin Part of the vitamin B$_2$ complex; essential in fat and carbohydrate metabolism	AIs Adults 30 mcg/d Children 1–3 y: 8 mcg 4–8 y: 12 mcg 9–13 y: 20 mcg 14–18 y: 25 mcg Infants 1–5 mo: 5 mcg 6–12 mo: 6 mcg	Meat, egg yolk, nuts, cereals, most vegetables	Anorexia, nausea; depression; muscle pain; dermatitis	Not established
Vitamin B$_3$ (niacin) Essential for glycolysis, fat synthesis, and tissue respiration. It functions as a coenzyme in many metabolic processes (after conversion to nicotinamide, the physiologically active form)	RDAs Females 19 y and older: 14 mg Pregnancy (all ages): 18 mg Lactation (all ages): 17 mg Males 19 y and older: 16 mg Children 1–3 y: 6 mg 4–8 y: 8 mg 9–13 y: 12 mg 14–18 y: females, 14 mg; males, 16 mg Infants (AIs) 0–6 mo: 2 mg 7–12 mo: 4 mg	Meat, poultry, fish, peanuts	Pellagra: erythematous skin lesions; GI problems (stomatitis, glossitis, enteritis, diarrhea); CNS problems (headache, dizziness, insomnia, depression, memory loss) Severe deficiency: delusions, hallucinations, impairment of peripheral motor and sensory nerves	Flushing, pruritus, hyperglycemia, increased liver enzymes, uricemia

TABLE 35.1

Vitamins (Continued)

Vitamin/Function	Dietary Reference Intakes	Food Sources	Signs and Symptoms of Deficiency	Signs and Symptoms of Excess
Vitamin B_5 (pantothenic acid) Essential for metabolism of carbohydrate, fat, and protein (e.g., release of energy from carbohydrate; fatty acid metabolism; synthesis of cholesterol, steroid hormones, and phospholipids)	AIs Adults: 5 mg Females 14 y and older: 5 mg Pregnancy: 6 mg Lactation: 7 mg Males 14 y and older: 5 mg Children 1–3 y: 2 mg 4–8 y: 3 mg 9–13 y: 4 mg Infants 1–6 mo: 1.7 mg 7–12 mo: 1.8 mg	Eggs, liver, salmon, yeast, cauliflower, broccoli, lean beef, potatoes, tomatoes	No deficiency state established	Not established
Vitamin B_6 (pyridoxine) A coenzyme in metabolism of carbohydrate, protein, and fat; required for formation of tryptophan and conversion of tryptophan to niacin; helps release glycogen from the liver and muscle tissue; functions in metabolism of the central nervous system; helps maintain cellular immunity	RDAs Females 14–18 y: 1.2 mg 19–50 y: 1.3 mg 51 y and older: 1.5 mg Pregnancy: 1.9 mg Lactation: 2 mg Males 14–50 y: 1.3 mg 51 y and older: 1.7 mg Children 1–3 y: 0.5 mg 4–8 y: 0.6 mg 9–13 y: 1 mg Infants (AIs) 1–6 mo: 0.1 mg 7–12 mo: 0.3 mg	Yeast, wheat germ, liver and other glandular meats, whole-grain cereals, potatoes, legumes	Skin and mucous membrane lesions (seborrheic dermatitis, intertrigo, stomatitis, glossitis), neurologic problems (seizures, peripheral neuritis, mental depression)	Not established
Vitamin B_{12} (cyanocobalamin) Essential for normal metabolism of all body cells, normal red blood cells, normal nerve cells, growth, and metabolism of carbohydrate, protein, and fat	RDAs Females 14 y and older: 2.4 mcg Pregnancy: 2.6 mcg Lactation: 2.8 mcg Males 14 y and older: 2.4 mcg Children 1–3 y: 0.9 mcg 4–8 y: 1.2 mcg 9–13 y: 1.8 mcg Infants (AIs) 0–6 mo: 0.4 mcg 7–12 mo: 0.5 mcg	Meat, eggs, fish, cheese	Pernicious anemia: decreased numbers of RBCs; large, immature RBCs; fatigue; dyspnea Severe deficiency: leukopenia, infection, thrombocytopenia, cardiac dysrhythmias, heart failure Neurologic signs and symptoms: paresthesias in hands and feet, unsteady gait, depressed deep tendon reflexes, loss of memory, confusion, delusions, hallucinations, psychosis Nerve damage may be irreversible	Not established

(Continued on page 650)

TABLE 35.1

Vitamins (Continued)

Vitamin/Function	Dietary Reference Intakes	Food Sources	Signs and Symptoms of Deficiency	Signs and Symptoms of Excess
Folic acid (folate) A B complex vitamin; essential for normal metabolism of all body cells, normal RBCs, and growth	RDAs Females 14 y and older: 400 mcg Pregnancy: 600 mcg Lactation: 500 mcg Males 14 y and older: 400 mcg Older adults (UL): 1,000 mcg Children 1–3 y: 150 mcg 4–8 y: 200 mcg 9–13 y: 300 mcg Infants (AIs) 1–6 mo: 65 mcg 7–12 mo: 80 mcg	Liver, kidney beans, fresh green vegetables (spinach, broccoli, asparagus), fortified grain products (e.g., breads, cereals, rice)	Megaloblastic anemia that cannot be distinguished from the anemia produced by vitamin B_{12} deficiency; impaired growth in children; glossitis; GI problems	Not established
Vitamin C (ascorbic acid) Essential for formation of skin, ligaments, cartilage, bone, and teeth; required for wound healing and tissue repair, metabolism of iron and folic acid, synthesis of fats and proteins, preservation of blood vessel integrity, and resistance to infection	RDAs Females 19 y and older: 75 mg Pregnancy: 19–50 y, 85 mg Lactation: 19–50 y, 120 mg Males 19 y and older: 90 mg Adult smokers: add additional 35 mg/d Children 1–3 y: 15 mg 4–8 y: 25 mg 9–13 y: 45 mg 14–18 y: male, 75 mg; female, 65 mg (pregnancy, 80 mg; lactation, 115 mg) Infants (AIs) 0–6 mo: 40 mg 7–12 mo: 50 mg	Fruits and vegetables, especially citrus fruits and juices	Mild deficiency: irritability, malaise, arthralgia, increased tendency to bleed Severe deficiency: scurvy and adverse effects on most body tissues (gingivitis; bleeding of gums, skin, joints, and other areas; disturbances of bone growth; anemia; and loosening of teeth); if not treated, coma and death may occur	Kidney calculi

*Vitamin E activity is expressed in milligrams of alpha-tocopherol equivalents (alpha-TE).
AI, adequate intake; DRI, Dietary Reference Intake; GI, gastrointestinal; RBC, red blood cell; RDA, recommended dietary allowance; ULs, upper intake levels.

Patient-related variables specific to the use of vitamins and minerals include the following:
- Age:
  - Children need sufficient amounts of vitamins and minerals to support growth and normal body functioning. Dosages should not exceed recommended amounts.
  - For infants (birth to 12 months), the only UL is for vitamin D. For other children, ULs vary according to age. A combined vitamin–mineral supplement every other day may be reasonable, especially for children who eat poorly.
  - There is a risk of overdose in children; this risk is more serious with the fat-soluble vitamins because they are stored long-term within the body. All minerals and electrolytes are toxic in overdose. Because of manufacturers' marketing strategies, many supplements are available in flavors and shapes (e.g., animals, cartoon characters) designed to appeal to children.

> **Quality and Safety Alert: Safety**
>
> Because younger children may think of these supplements as candy and take more than recommended, it is essential that they be stored out of reach and dispensed by an adult.

- Vitamin requirements are the same for older adults as for younger adults, but deficiencies are more common, especially with the fat-soluble vitamins A and D. Assess every older adult regarding vitamin intake (from food and supplements) and use of drugs that interact with dietary nutrients. For most older adults, a daily multivitamin is probably desirable, even for those who seem healthy and able to eat a well-balanced diet.
- In older adults, requirements may be increased during illnesses, especially those affecting GI function. Overdoses,

TABLE 35.2

Minerals and Electrolytes

Mineral/Function	Dietary Reference Intakes	Food Sources	Signs and Symptoms of Deficiency	Signs and Symptoms of Excess
Macrominerals				
Sodium Assists in regulating osmotic pressure, water balance, conduction of electrical impulses in nerves and muscles, and electrolyte and acid–base balance. Influences permeability of cell membranes and assists in movement of substances across cell membranes. Participates in many intracellular chemical reactions. Normal serum sodium = 135–145 mEq/L	Adults (AI) 19–50 y: 1.5 g 51–70 y: 1.3 g 71 y and over: 1.2 g Adults (UL): 2.3 g	Present in most foods; proteins contain large amounts; vegetables and cereals contain small to moderate amounts; fruits contain little or no sodium. Major source in the diet is table salt added to food in processing, cooking, or seasoning. One teaspoon contains 2.3 g of sodium. Water in some areas may contain significant amounts of sodium	Serum sodium <135 mEq/L; anorexia, nausea, and vomiting; ataxia; confusion; delirium; hypotension and tachycardia; muscle tremors; oliguria and increased blood urea nitrogen; seizures; weakness	Serum sodium >145 mEq/L, disorientation, dry skin and mucous membranes, fever, hyperactive reflexes, hypotension, muscle rigidity, tremors and spasms, irritability, cerebral hemorrhage, coma, oliguria, concentrated urine, increased blood urea nitrogen
Potassium Within cells, it helps maintain osmotic pressure, fluid, and electrolyte balance and acid–base balance. In extracellular fluid, it is required for conduction of nerve impulses and contraction of muscle. Helps transport glucose into cells and is required for glycogen formation and storage. Required for synthesis of muscle proteins. Normal serum potassium = 3.5–5 mEq/L	Adults (AI): 4.7 g Adults (UL): not established	Present in most foods, including meat, whole-grain breads or cereals, bananas, citrus fruits, tomatoes, and broccoli	Serum potassium <3.5 mEq/L; dysrhythmias and ECG changes; cardiac arrest; confusion; delirium; hyperglycemia; postural hypotension; muscle weakness; abdominal distension, constipation, paralytic ileus; polyuria; polydipsia, nocturia. Prolonged deficiency may increase blood urea nitrogen and serum creatinine	Serum potassium >5 mEq/L; muscle weakness; cardiotoxicity, with dysrhythmias or cardiac arrest. Cardiac effects are not usually severe until serum levels are 7 mEq/L or above
Chloride Helps maintain osmotic pressure and electrolyte, acid–base, and water balance. Forms hydrochloric acid in gastric mucosal cells. Normal serum chloride = 95–103 mEq/L	Adults (AI) 19–50 y: 2.3 g 51–70 y: 2 g 71 y and over: 1.8 g Adults (UL): 3.6 g	Most dietary chloride is ingested as sodium chloride, and foods high in sodium are also high in chloride	Serum chloride >95 mEq/L; arterial blood pH 7.45; dehydration; hypotension; low respiratory rate and shallow respirations; paresthesias of face and extremities; muscle spasms and tetany, which cannot be distinguished from the tetany produced by hypocalcemia	Serum chloride >103 mEq/L; arterial blood pH < 7.35; increased rate and depth of respirations; lethargy, stupor, disorientation, and coma if acidosis is not treated
Magnesium Required for conduction of nerve impulses and contraction of muscle (especially important in function of cardiac and skeletal muscle). Serves as a component of many enzymes. Essential for metabolism of carbohydrate and protein. Normal serum magnesium = 1.5–2.5 mEq/L	Adults (RDA) Females 19–30 y: 310 mg 31 y and over: 320 mg Males 19–30 y: 400 mg 31 y and over: 420 mg Adults (UL): 350 mg/d from supplements only (does not include intake from food and water)	Present in many foods; diet that is adequate in other respects contains adequate magnesium. Good food sources include nuts, cereal grains, dark green vegetables, and seafood	Serum magnesium <1.5 mEq/L; ataxia; confusion; dizziness; irritability; muscle tremors, carpopedal spasm, nystagmus, and generalized spasticity; seizures; tachycardia, hypotension, premature atrial, and ventricular beats	Serum magnesium >2.5 mEq/L; skeletal muscle weakness; cardiac dysrhythmias, hypotension; respiratory insufficiency; coma

(Continued on page 652)

TABLE 35.2

Minerals and Electrolytes (Continued)

Mineral/Function	Dietary Reference Intakes	Food Sources	Signs and Symptoms of Deficiency	Signs and Symptoms of Excess
Trace Elements				
Chromium — Aids glucose use by increasing effectiveness of insulin and facilitating transport of glucose across cell membranes	Adults (AI) Females 19–50 y: 25 mcg 51 y and over: 20 mcg Males 19–50 y: 35 mcg 51 y and over: 30 mcg Adults (UL): undetermined	Brewer yeast and whole wheat products	Impaired glucose tolerance (hyperglycemia, glucosuria); impaired growth and reproduction; decreased life span	Not established
Cobalt — A component of vitamin B_{12} that is required for normal function of all body cells and for maturation of red blood cells	~1 mg in the form of vitamin B_{12}. There is no established RDA	Animal foods, including liver, muscle meats, and shellfish. Fruits, vegetables, and cereals contain no cobalt as vitamin B_{12}	Deficiency of vitamin B_{12} produces pernicious anemia	Not established
Copper — A component of many enzymes. Essential for correct functioning of the central nervous, cardiovascular, and skeletal systems. Important in formation of red blood cells, apparently by regulating storage and release of iron for hemoglobin	Adults (RDA): 900 mcg Adults (UL): 10,000 mcg	Many foods, including liver, shellfish, nuts, cereals, poultry, and dried fruits	Decreased serum levels; decreased iron absorption; anemia from impaired erythropoiesis; leukopenia. Death can occur. In infants, anemia, chronic malnutrition, and diarrhea or Menkes syndrome (retarded growth and progressive mental deterioration) can occur	Increased serum levels; Wilson disease (a rare genetic disorder characterized by accumulation of copper in the brain, liver, and kidneys). Signs and symptoms vary according to affected organs
Fluoride — A component of tooth enamel. Strengthens the bones. Adequate intake before ages 50–60 y may decrease osteoporosis and fractures during later years	Adults (AI) Females 19–70 y and over: 3 mg Pregnancy and lactation: 3 mg Males 19–70 y and over: 4 mg Children (AIs) 1–3 y: 0.7 mg 4–8 y: 1 mg 9–13 y: 2 mg 14–18 y: 3 mg Infants (AIs) 0–6 mo: 0.01 mg 7–12 mo: 0.5 mg Adults (UL): 10 mg	Beef, canned salmon, eggs. Very little in milk, cereal grains, fruits, and vegetables. Fluoride content of food depends on fluoride content of soil where they are grown	Dental caries and possibly a greater incidence of osteoporosis	Mottling of teeth and osteosclerosis
Iodine — Essential component of thyroid hormones	Adults (RDAs) Females 14 y and over: 150 mcg Pregnancy: 220 mcg Lactation: 290 mcg Males 14 y and over: 150 mcg Children: 1–8 y: 90 mcg; 9–13 y: 120 mcg Infants (AI) 0–6 mo: 110 mcg 7–12 mo: 130 mcg	Iodized salt and seafood are the best sources. In vegetables, iodine content varies with the amount of iodine in soil where they are grown. In milk and eggs, content depends on the amount present in animal feed	Thyroid gland enlargement; possible hypothyroidism	Iodism, with coryza, edema, fever, conjunctivitis, lymphadenopathy, stomatitis, vomiting

TABLE 35.2
Minerals and Electrolytes (Continued)

Mineral/Function	Dietary Reference Intakes	Food Sources	Signs and Symptoms of Deficiency	Signs and Symptoms of Excess
Iron Essential component of hemoglobin, myoglobin, and several enzymes. Hemoglobin is required for transport and use of oxygen by body cells. Myoglobin aids oxygen transport and use by muscle cells. Enzymes are important for cellular metabolism	Adults (RDAs) Females 19–50 y: 18 mg 51 y and over: 8 mg Pregnancy: 27 mg Lactation: 14–18 y: 10 mg 19–50 y: 9 mg Males: 8 mg Children (RDAs) 1–3 y: 7 mg 4–8 y: 10 mg 9–13 y: 8 mg 14–18 y (girls): 15 mg 14–18 y (boys): 11 mg Infants 0–6 mo: 0.27 mg (AI) 7–12 mo: 11 mg RDA Adults (UL): 45 mg	Liver and other organ meats, lean meat, shellfish, dried beans and vegetables, egg yolks, dried fruits, molasses, whole-grain and enriched breads. Milk and milk products contain essentially no iron	Iron deficiency anemia. With gradual development of anemia, minimal symptoms occur. With rapid development or severe anemia, dyspnea, fatigue, tachycardia, malaise, and drowsiness occur	Acute iron intoxication: vomiting, diarrhea, melena, abdominal pain, shock, convulsions, and metabolic acidosis. Death may occur within 24 h if treatment is not prompt Chronic iron overload (hemochromatosis): cardiac dysrhythmias, heart failure, diabetes, bronze pigmentation of the skin, liver enlargement, arthropathy, and others
Selenium Important for function of myocardium and probably other muscles	Adults (RDAs) Females 19–70 y and over: 55 mcg Pregnancy: 60 mcg Lactation: 70 mcg Males 19–70 y and over: 55 mcg Children (RDAs) 1–3 y: 20 mcg 4–8 y: 30 mcg 9–13 y: 40 mcg 14–18 y: 55 mcg Infants (AIs) 0–6 mo: 15 mcg 7–12 mo: 20 mcg Adult UL: 400 mcg	Fish, meat, bread, and cereals	Deficiency most likely with long-term IV therapy. Signs and symptoms include myocardial abnormalities and other muscle discomfort and weakness	Highly toxic in excessive amounts. Signs and symptoms include fatigue, peripheral neuropathy, nausea, diarrhea, and alopecia
Zinc A component of many enzymes that is essential for normal metabolism (e.g., carbonic anhydrase, lactic dehydrogenase, alkaline phosphatase). Necessary for normal cell growth, synthesis of nucleic acids (RNA and DNA), and synthesis of carbohydrates and proteins. May be essential for use of vitamin A	Adults (RDAs) Females 19–70 y and over: 8 mg Pregnancy: 14–18 y: 12 mg 19–50 y: 11 mg Lactation: 14–18 y: 13 mg 19–50 y: 12 mg Males 19–70 y and over: 11 mg Children 1–3 y: 3 mg 4–8 y: 5 mg 9–13 y: 8 mg 14–18 y (girls): 9 mg 14–18 y (boys): 11 mg Infants 0–6 mo (AI): 2 mg 7–12 mo (RDA): 3 mg Adult UL: 40 mg	Animal proteins such as meat, liver, eggs, and seafood. Wheat germ is also a good source	Most evident in growing children and includes impaired growth, hypogonadism in boys, anorexia, and sensory impairment (loss of taste and smell). Also, if the patient has had surgery, wound healing may be delayed	Unlikely with dietary intake but may develop with excessive ingestion or inhalation of zinc. Ingestion may cause nausea, vomiting, and diarrhea; inhalation may cause vomiting, headache, and fever

especially of the fat-soluble vitamins A and D, may cause toxicity; it is necessary to avoid this.
- Abnormal kidney function and hepatic impairment:
  - Patients with acute kidney disease who are unable to eat an adequate diet need a vitamin supplement to meet DRIs. A multivitamin with essential vitamins is recommended for daily use.
  - Decreased Kidney function may promote mineral retention.
  - Vitamin deficiencies commonly occur in patients with chronic liver disease because of poor intake and **malabsorption** (impaired absorption of nutrients from the GI tract).
  - Hepatic failure results in depletion of hepatic stores of vitamin A and other vitamins.

> **Quality and Safety Alert: Patient-Centered Care**
>
> It is important to monitor serum electrolyte levels closely and provide supplements only with great care.

- Specific healthcare environments:
  - Critically ill patients often have organ failure, which alters their ability to ingest and use essential nutrients. They may be undernourished regarding vitamins and minerals.
  - Parenteral multivitamin formulations are available for adults and children.
  - Close monitoring of serum electrolytes is necessary.

Clinical Application 35.1
- Identify findings in the assessment of Mrs. Martin that would put her at risk for vitamin, mineral, and nutritional deficiency.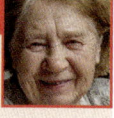

NCLEX Success

1. Which finding in a nursing assessment of a newly admitted patient would be most likely to result in a vitamin deficiency?
   A. a history of liver disease
   B. use of self-prescribed megavitamins
   C. presence of a pressure ulcer
   D. frequent blood transfusions

FAT-SOLUBLE VITAMINS

VITAMIN A

The following discussion concerns vitamin A.

Pharmacokinetics and Use

After oral administration, vitamin A is absorbed from the GI tract along with dietary fat and is primarily stored in the liver. The body can store up to a year's supply of vitamin A in the liver. This vitamin, which is not soluble in the blood, is distributed by attaching to protein carriers in the blood. If a person consumes inadequate amounts of vitamin A, the body uses the vitamin stored in the liver. Vitamin A is metabolized in the liver and eliminated in the feces and urine.

The most important therapeutic use of vitamin A is for replacement in deficiency states. Table 35.3 gives route and dosage information.

Patient-related variables specific to the use of vitamin A include the following:
- Reproduction, pregnancy, and lactation:
  - Doses greater than the RDA are contraindicated in individuals who may become pregnant.

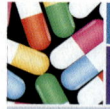

TABLE 35.3
DRUGS AT A GLANCE: Vitamins

Drug	Routes and Dosage Ranges	
	Adults	**Children**
Fat-Soluble Vitamins		
Vitamin A	Deficiency: IM route indicated when oral administration not feasible or absorption insufficient (malabsorption syndrome) 100,000 international units IM daily for 3 d; then 50,000 units PO or IM daily for 2 wk; then 10,000–20,000 units PO daily for another 2 mo; follow with adequate dietary nutrition	Deficiency (severe): Infants 7,500–15,000 units IM daily for 10 d 1–8 y 17,500–35,000 units IM daily for 10 d >8 y and adolescents 100,000 units IM daily for 3 d; then 50,000 units IM daily for 14 d Follow with oral supplementation for 2 mo; infants and children <8 y, 5,000–10,000 units/d; children 8 y or greater and adolescents, 10,000-20,000 units
Vitamin E	Prevention of deficiency: Dose varies by product. Dose range from 100 to 400 units PO daily. (Vitamin E may be ordered in alpha-tocopherol equivalents or ATE)	Deficiency: Infants, children, and adolescents, 25–50 units/kg/d PO

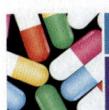

TABLE 35.3
DRUGS AT A GLANCE: Vitamins (Continued)

Drug	Routes and Dosage Ranges	
	Adults	**Children**
Vitamin K or phytonadione (Mephyton; ✳ AquaMEPHYTON, Konakion, Mephyton)	Anti–coagulant-induced prothrombin deficiency: depending on INR and severity of bleeding 2.5–10 mg IV as a single dose over 10–20 min (maximum infusion rate: 1 mg/min) and check INR in 6–12 h with repeat dose if needed; depending on INR 2.5–10 mg. PO as a single dose and check INR in 12–48 h with repeat dose if needed Hypoprothrombinemia due to other causes: 10 mg, once PO, subcutaneous, IV; repeat in 48–72 h if needed; maximum IV infusion rate 1 mg/min	Prevention of hemorrhagic disease: 0.5–1 mg IM within 1 h after birth Treatment of hemorrhagic disease in newborns: 1 mg subcutaneously, IM, or IV daily. Correction in 12–48 h
Water-Soluble Vitamins		
Vitamin B$_1$ (thiamine; ✳ Thiamiject)	Parenteral nutrition supplementation: 6 mg IV daily Deficiency (beriberi): 5–30 mg IM or IV 3 times daily if critically ill; then 5–30 mg/d PO in single or divided doses 3 times daily for 1 mo Alcohol withdrawal syndrome: 100 mg IV daily for several days, followed by 100 mg PO daily or follow institutional protocol Wernicke encephalopathy: 200–500 mg IV (preferred) 3 times daily for 2–7 d; follow with 250 mg once daily for 3–5 d; then decrease to 100 mg daily until no longer at risk	Deficiency (beriberi): Infants: 25–50 mg IV once, followed by 10 mg IM once daily for a week, then 3–5 mg PO for at least 6 wk Children: 10 mg IM or IV once daily for first week then 3–5 mg PO once daily for at least 6 wk (limited data) Adolescents: 100 mg IM or IV up to 7 d, then 10 mg PO once daily (limited data)
Vitamin B$_3$ (niacin, nicotinic acid; ✳ Niaspan, Niaspan FCT, Niodan) Nicotinamide (niacinamide)	Deficiency: up to 100 mg PO daily Pellagra: 50–100 mg oral 3–4 times daily; maximum 500 mg daily Hyperlipidemia: 250 mg PO once daily with evening meal; increase gradually as tolerated to 3 g daily in 2–3 divided doses; alternatively, extended-release tablets 500 mg at bedtime for 4 wk; increase daily dose every 4 wk but not more than 500 mg daily to a maximum of 2 g daily. Adjust to response and tolerance NOTE: Niacin no longer recommended except in specific situations	Pellagra: Children and adolescents 50–300 mg oral 3 times daily for 3–4 wk
Vitamin B$_6$ (pyridoxine)	Deficiency: 10–20 mg IM or IV daily for several 3 wk; then daily PO therapy for several weeks Prevention of vitamin B$_6$ deficiency during isoniazid therapy: 25–50 mg PO daily	Seizures related to vitamin B$_6$ deficiency (infants and children): 100 mg IV; may repeat over 30 min (give in ICU setting due to possible apnea). If IV not feasible: 30 mg/kg/d PO for several days. Maintenance dose: 15–30 mg/kg/d PO not to exceed 500 mg/d
Vitamin B$_{12}$ (cyanocobalamin or hydroxocobalamin) (B$_{12}$ Compliance Injection; Physicians EZ Use B$_{12}$) ✳ Cobex; Cyano Vit B$_{12}$	Deficiency due to inadequate diet or causes other than pernicious anemia: as cyanocobalamin 1,000–2,000 mcg PO daily until deficiency corrected or 1,000 mcg deep subcutaneous or IM 1–3 times/wk or once daily for 1 wk then 1,000 mcg once weekly for 4–8 wk until deficiency corrected; maintenance dose, 1,000–2,000 mcg oral daily or 1,000 mcg deep subcutaneous or IM once monthly Pernicious anemia: initially, cyanocobalamin 1,000 mcg deep subcutaneous or IM once weekly for 4 wk then 1,000 mg once monthly	Deficiency due to inadequate diet or causes other than pernicious anemia: 250–1,000 mcg IM once daily for 1–2 wk followed by weekly dosing Pernicious anemia: Infants, children, and adolescents 100 mcg subcutaneous or IM once daily for 6–7 d; if improved 100 mcg on alternate days for 7 doses, then every 3–4 d for 2–3 wk. Maintenance dose 100 mcg once monthly
Intranasal cyanocobalamin (Nascobal)	Maintenance therapy for remission of pernicious anemia after parenteral vitamin B$_{12}$ therapy: intranasal cyanocobalamin 1 spray (500 mcg) in 1 nostril once weekly. Use alternate route if B$_{12}$ levels low after 1 mo	

(Continued on page 656)

TABLE 35.3
DRUGS AT A GLANCE: Vitamins (Continued)

Drug	Routes and Dosage Ranges	
	Adults	**Children**
Folic acid (FA-8; ✴ JAMP-Folic Acid)	Deficiency, megaloblastic and macrocytic anemia due to folate deficiency: 1–5 mg PO once daily Pregnancy/lactation maintenance dose: 0.8 mg/d	Deficiency, megaloblastic anemia: 0.5–1 mg/d oral, subcutaneous, IM, or IV and then maintenance dose (infant 0.1 mg/d; children 1–3, 0.1–0.3 mg/d; children 4 y and older and adolescents, 0.1–0.4 mg/d)
Vitamin C (ascorbic acid) (Acerola C 500; Asco-Tabs-1,000; Ascocid; many other OTC brand names; ✴ Ascor L 500; Mega-C-Sodium)	Deficiency, depending on severity: 100–1,500 mg PO daily or 70–150 mg subcutaneous/IM/IV daily Burns: 1–2 g subcutaneous/IM/IV daily Wound healing: 300–500 mg subcutaneous/IM/IV daily for 7–10 d pre- and postoperatively	Deficiency: Infants, children, and adolescents 100–300 mg/d PO, IM, or IV in divided doses for 1 wk follow with 100 mg/d for about 1–3 mo

- Excess vitamin A during pregnancy may cause fetal abnormalities. Vitamin A deficiency also causes adverse effects in the fetus.
- Vitamin A requirements increase when breast-feeding.

Adverse Effects and Contraindications

Signs and symptoms of vitamin A toxicity include hair loss, double vision, headaches, vomiting, bone abnormalities, and liver damage. If any signs or symptoms of vitamin A excess appear, it is necessary to stop intake of any known sources of vitamin A.

Contraindications to vitamin A include a history of allergic reaction to the vitamin, hypervitaminosis A, and malabsorption syndrome (oral use only). Caution is warranted in pregnancy. Vitamin A excess during pregnancy can cause fetal defects.

Nursing Implications
Preventing Interactions

Chronic use of mineral oil or bile acid sequestrants may cause vitamin A deficiency by preventing systemic absorption of vitamin A. Mineral oil combines with fat-soluble vitamins and prevents their absorption if both are taken at the same time. Bile salts increase the effects of vitamin A by increasing intestinal absorption of the vitamin. Large doses of vitamin A may increase the anticoagulant effects of warfarin. Antibiotics may cause diarrhea and subsequent malabsorption of vitamin A.

Administering the Medication

People should take vitamin A preparations before meals, on an empty stomach. However, to prevent nausea, it may be necessary to take them after food or meals. (Intramuscular [IM] administration may be necessary.) Also, people should not take oral preparations of vitamin A at the same time as mineral oil; this laxative absorbs the vitamin and thus prevents its systemic absorption.

Assessing for Therapeutic and Adverse Effects

The nurse observes for decreased signs and symptoms of deficiency, such as improved vision, especially in dim light or at night; less dryness in the eyes and conjunctiva (xerophthalmia); and improvement in skin lesions. Night blindness is usually better within a few days. Skin lesions may not disappear for several weeks.

In addition, the nurse observes for signs of hypervitaminosis A, such as anorexia, vomiting, irritability, headache, skin disorders, and pain in muscles, bones, and joints. Serum levels of vitamin A greater than 1,200 IU/dL are toxic. Severity of manifestations depends largely on dose and duration of excess vitamin A intake. Very severe states produce additional clinical signs, including enlargement of the liver and spleen, altered liver function, increased intracranial pressure, and other neurologic manifestations.

Patient Teaching

Box 35.2 identifies patient teaching guidelines for vitamins, including vitamin A.

VITAMIN E

The following discussion concerns vitamin E, or alpha-tocopherol.

Pharmacokinetics and Use

Vitamin E is absorbed from the GI tract if fat absorption is normal. It is primarily stored in adipose tissue. It is metabolized in the liver and eliminated primarily in bile.

The most important therapeutic use of vitamin E is for vitamin E replacement in the narrow, specific circumstances in which vitamin E deficiency occurs. Table 35.3 gives route and dosage information for vitamin E.

Patient-related variables specific to the use of vitamin E include the following:
- Reproduction, pregnancy, and lactation:
  - Vitamin E crosses the placenta. Supplementation is not needed in pregnancy.
  - Vitamin E is found in breast milk. Supplementation is not needed for lactation.

BOX 35.2 Patient Teaching Guidelines for Vitamins

General Considerations
- Certain people may need vitamin supplements. Pregnant people as well as people who smoke, ingest large amounts of alcohol, have impaired immune systems, or are older adults may need to take oral vitamins.
- Avoid taking large doses of vitamins, which do not promote health, strength, or youth.
- Natural vitamins are advertised as being better than synthetic vitamins, but there is no evidence to support this claim. The two types are chemically identical, and the body uses them the same way. Natural vitamins are more expensive.
- Vitamins from supplements exert the same physiologic effects as those obtained from foods.
- Multivitamin preparations often contain minerals as well, usually in smaller amounts than those recommended for daily intake. Large doses of minerals are toxic.
- Supplementary vitamin preparations differ widely in amounts and types of vitamin content.
- When choosing a vitamin supplement, compare ingredients and costs. Store brands are usually effective and less expensive than name brands.

Vitamin A
- Know about dietary sources of vitamin A. Retinol occurs in liver, milk, butter, cheese, cream, egg yolk, fortified milk, margarine, and ready-to-eat cereals. Beta-carotenes occur in spinach, collard greens, kale, mango, broccoli, carrots, peaches, pumpkin, red peppers, sweet potatoes, winter squash, watermelon, apricots, and cantaloupe.
- Understand that excessive amounts of vitamin A are stored in the body and often lead to toxic effects. High doses of vitamin A can result in headaches; diarrhea; nausea; loss of appetite; dry, itching skin; and elevated blood calcium.
- Do not take a supplementary vitamin product that contains more than recommended amounts of vitamin A because of possible adverse effects.
- If you are pregnant or could become pregnant, know that excessive doses of vitamin A during pregnancy may cause birth defects.

Vitamin E
- Know about dietary sources of vitamin E. This vitamin occurs in vegetable oils, margarine, salad dressing, other foods made with vegetable oil, nuts, seeds, wheat germ, dark green vegetables, whole grains, and fortified cereals.
- Be familiar with the signs and symptoms of vitamin E overdose.
- Do not take a supplementary vitamin product that contains more than the recommended amounts of vitamin E.

Vitamin K
- Know about dietary sources of vitamin K. This vitamin occurs in spinach, brussels sprouts, broccoli, cabbage, cauliflower, Swiss chard, lettuce, collard greens, carrots, green beans, asparagus, and eggs.
- Avoid excessive doses of vitamin K. Take this vitamin only as directed by a healthcare provider.
- Keep intake of vitamin K–containing foods constant. Avoid sudden increases or decreases in the amounts of these foods.
- If you are taking warfarin, report any use of vitamin K to your healthcare provider. During warfarin therapy, intake of vitamin K–containing foods should remain constant.

Vitamin B_1, Vitamin B_3, and Vitamin B_6
- Know about dietary sources of vitamins B_1 (thiamine), B_3 (niacin), and B_6 (pyridoxine). Thiamine occurs in whole-grain and enriched breads and cereals, liver, nuts, wheat germ, pork, and dried peas and beans. Niacin occurs in all protein foods and whole-grain and enriched breads and cereals. Pyridoxine occurs in meats, fish, poultry, fruits, green leafy vegetables, whole grains, and dried peas and beans.
- Swallow extended-release products whole; do not break, crush, or chew them. Breaking the product delivers the entire dose at once and may cause adverse effects.
- Take oral niacin preparations, except for timed-release forms, with or after meals or at bedtime to decrease stomach irritation.
- After taking a dose of oral niacin, sit or lie down for approximately 30 minutes after taking a dose. Niacin causes blood vessels to dilate and may cause facial flushing, dizziness, and falls. Facial flushing can be decreased by taking aspirin 325 mg orally, 30 to 60 minutes before a dose of niacin (if aspirin is not contraindicated). Itching, tingling, and headache may occur. These effects usually subside with continued use of niacin.

Vitamin B_{12} and Folic Acid
- Know about dietary sources of vitamin B_{12}. This vitamin occurs in meat, fish, poultry, shellfish, milk, dairy products, eggs, and some fortified foods. Vitamin B_{12} does not occur in plant sources. If you are a strict vegan who consumes no animal products, you are at risk for vitamin B_{12} deficiency unless you take a supplementary source of the vitamin.
- Know about dietary sources of folic acid. This nutrient occurs in liver, okra, spinach, asparagus, dried peas and beans, seeds, and orange juice. Breads, cereals, and other grains are fortified with folic acid.
- Take prescribed vitamins as directed and for the appropriate time. If you have pernicious anemia, you must have vitamin B_{12} injections for the remainder of your life. Any chronic vitamin B_{12} deficiency requires lifelong treatment. If you are pregnant or breast-feeding, requirements may be greater; you usually may need additional vitamin supplements.
- Keep appointments for follow-up visits and obtain the necessary laboratory tests.

Vitamin C
- Know about dietary sources of vitamin C. This vitamin occurs in citrus fruits and juices, red and green peppers, broccoli, cauliflower, brussels sprouts, cantaloupe, kiwi fruit, mustard greens, strawberries, and tomatoes.
- Be aware that vitamin C improves the absorption of iron.
- Understand that vitamin C, which acidifies the urine, may alter the excretion of some drugs.

Adverse Effects and Contraindications

Large amounts of vitamin E are relatively nontoxic but can interfere with vitamin K action (blood clotting) by decreasing platelet aggregation and producing a risk of bleeding. Excessive doses can also cause fatigue, headache, blurred vision, nausea, and diarrhea. If signs or symptoms of vitamin E excess appear, it is essential to stop the intake of any known source of vitamin E.

Contraindications to vitamin E include a history of allergic reaction to vitamin E or hypervitaminosis E. Patients with a history of bleeding disorders or thrombocytopenia should not take vitamin E.

Nursing Implications
Preventing Interactions

Mineral oil and cholestyramine decrease the absorption of vitamin E, which means that vitamin E should not be administered at the same time as these substances. Also, this vitamin may increase the anticoagulant effect of warfarin. Vitamin E may increase the absorption, hepatic storage, and use of vitamin A.

Administering the Medication

People should take oral vitamin E preparations before meals on an empty stomach. However, to prevent nausea, people may also take them after food or meals.

Assessing for Therapeutic and Adverse Effects

The nurse observes for decreased signs and symptoms of vitamin E deficiency. In addition, the nurse checks for signs of hypervitaminosis E, including bleeding, fatigue, headache, blurred vision, nausea, and diarrhea.

Patient Teaching

Box 35.2 identifies patient teaching guidelines for vitamins, including vitamin E.

VITAMIN K

The following discussion concerns vitamin K, or phytonadione.

Pharmacokinetics and Use

After absorption, vitamin K is concentrated in the liver. Minimal amounts of the vitamin are stored. No additional vitamin K is required during pregnancy. It crosses the placental barrier and enters breast milk. Onset of action after an oral dose is 6 to 10 hours and, after an intravenous (IV) dose, 1 to 2 hours. Metabolism occurs rapidly in the liver, and elimination is in the feces and urine.

Vitamin K has two important therapeutic uses: (1) to correct hypoprothrombinemia caused by inadequate levels of vitamin K and (2) to reverse the effects of warfarin (Coumadin) overdose. Table 35.3 gives route and dosage information for vitamin K.

Adverse Effects and Contraindications

No symptoms have been observed from excessive intake of vitamin K. Mild adverse effects of vitamin K intake may include facial flushing, alterations in taste, or redness and pain at the injection site. The FDA has issued a **BOXED WARNING** stating that IV administration of vitamin K may result in an anaphylactic type of reaction with risks of shock, cardiorespiratory arrest, and death, even with drug dilution and slow administration.

Contraindications to vitamin K include a history of allergic reaction as well as a history of allergic reaction to benzyl alcohol or castor oil.

Nursing Implications
Preventing Interactions

Mineral oil as well as cholestyramine and other bile acid sequestrants inhibit the absorption of vitamin K if taken at the same time. Increased vitamin K levels decrease the anticoagulant effect of warfarin. It is necessary to avoid the use of vitamin K as a drug when a patient is receiving warfarin, and significant increases or decreases in dietary vitamin K may necessitate adjustment of the warfarin dose.

Administering the Medication

The oral route for vitamin K administration is preferred when treating nonbleeding patients. The subcutaneous route demonstrates irregular absorption. There is a risk of hematoma formation with the IM route. The IV route is used if there is major bleeding. Both the IM route and the IV route are associated with severe hypersensitivity reactions. For IV administration, dilute dose in minimum of 50 mL of compatible solution; administer slowly using an infusion pump over 10 to 20 minutes depending on dose at rate not to exceed 1 mg/min. Use the IV route only if the oral route is not feasible or there is a greater urgency to reverse anticoagulation. People may take the vitamin without regard to meals. They should avoid taking it at the same time as mineral oil or bile acid sequestrants.

It is necessary to protect all vitamin K preparations from light.

Assessing for Therapeutic and Adverse Effects

The nurse observes for decreased signs and symptoms of vitamin K deficiency. This includes decreased bleeding and more nearly normal blood coagulation tests.

Oral vitamin K rarely produces adverse reactions. Following subcutaneous injection, the nurse observes the injection site for redness and pain. Use of the IM and IV routes requires close observation for anaphylactic reaction as evidenced by chills, fever, diaphoresis, dyspnea, hypotension, bronchospasm, respiratory arrest, cardiac arrest, shock, and death. The means for emergency resuscitation must be immediately available.

Patient Teaching

Box 35.2 identifies patient teaching guidelines for vitamins, including vitamin K.

WATER-SOLUBLE VITAMINS

VITAMIN B COMPLEX: VITAMIN B_1, VITAMIN B_3, AND VITAMIN B_6

Most vitamin B complex deficiencies are multiple, rather than single, and treatment consists of administration of a multivitamin that contains several B complex vitamins. If a single deficiency seems predominant, that vitamin may be given alone or in addition to a multivitamin preparation. Three of the vitamin B complex vitamins are presented together in this section because they have much in common and are prototypical of the B complex vitamins as a whole: vitamin B_1 (thiamine), vitamin B_3 (niacin), and vitamin B_6 (pyridoxine). Vitamin B_{12} (cyanocobalamin) and folic acid are discussed separately below because of their common use in the treatment of anemia.

Pharmacokinetics and Use

Thiamine, niacin, and pyridoxine are absorbed from the GI tract. Pyridoxine is stored in the liver. Niacin and pyridoxine are metabolized in the liver. Thiamine, niacin, and pyridoxine are eliminated by the kidneys in the urine. Table 35.3 gives route and dosage information for the B complex vitamins.

Patient-related variables specific to the use of B complex vitamins include the following:

- Reproduction, pregnancy, and lactation:
  - Water-soluble vitamins cross the placenta. Thiamine requirements increase during pregnancy, and the risk of thiamine deficiency increases with severe nausea and vomiting. Thiamine enters breast milk. Thiamine requirements increase during lactation.
  - The RDA for niacin increases during pregnancy and breast-feeding. Niacin crosses the placenta; discontinue treatment with niacin for hyperlipidemia during pregnancy. Niacin enters breast milk; discontinue breast-feeding if niacin is used to treat hyperlipidemia.
  - Pyridoxine crosses the placenta; it also enters breast milk. Pyridoxine requirements increase with lactation. Pyridoxine use with isoniazid during tuberculosis treatment is continued during pregnancy and lactation.
- Abnormal kidney function and hepatic impairment:
  - Use caution with niacin and pyridoxine in abnormal kidney function.
  - People with liver disease should not take niacin because it may increase liver enzymes and bilirubin causing further liver damage. Long-acting forms may be more hepatotoxic.

Adverse Effects and Contraindications

- Thiamine: history of an allergic reaction to the vitamin
- Niacin: hepatic impairment, active peptic ulcer disease, arterial bleeding, and lactation. Caution is necessary with a history of jaundice, hepatobiliary disease, peptic ulcers, high alcohol consumption, abnormal kidney function, unstable angina, gout, glaucoma, and diabetes. Administration causes vasodilation, which may result in dizziness, hypotension, and injury from falls.
- Pyridoxine (IV form): cardiac disease. Caution is warranted with abnormal kidney function.

Nursing Implications
Preventing Interactions

- Thiamine: no important drug interactions
- Niacin: increases the risk of rhabdomyolysis from the statin dyslipidemics, increases the effectiveness of antihypertensives and vasoactive drugs, and increases the risk of bleeding from anticoagulants. Bile acid sequestrants decrease absorption.
- Pyridoxine: accelerates the peripheral conversion of levodopa into dopamine, thus decreasing the amount of levodopa that is available to cross into the central nervous system (CNS). Isoniazid decreases the effect of pyridoxine.

Administering the Medication

- Thiamine: preferred route of administration is by mouth; people may take it without regard to food. It is necessary to swallow enteric-coated tablets whole, not chewed or crushed. The IM and IV routes are for severe deficiency states only.
- Niacin: people may take oral niacin, except for timed-release forms, with or after meals, which decreases anorexia, nausea, vomiting, diarrhea, and flatulence. They should swallow timed-release forms whole, not chewed or crushed. The nurse should instruct the patient to sit or lie down for about 30 minutes after administration because niacin causes vasodilation and possible dizziness and hypotension.
- Pyridoxine: the general route of administration is oral, and people should swallow sustained-release or enteric forms of pyridoxine whole, not chewed or crushed.

Assessing for Therapeutic Effects

The nurse assesses for decreased signs and symptoms of deficiency. With B complex vitamins, it is necessary to observe for decreased or absent stomatitis, glossitis, seborrheic dermatitis, neurologic problems (neuritis, convulsions, mental deterioration, psychotic symptoms), cardiovascular problems (edema, heart failure), and eye problems (itching, burning, photophobia). Deficiencies of B complex vitamins commonly occur together and produce many similar manifestations.

Assessing for Adverse Effects

Adverse reactions are generally unlikely to occur with B complex multivitamin preparations. They are most likely to develop with large IV doses and rapid administration. The nurse observes for the following:

- Niacin and thiamine (parenteral): hypotension and anaphylactic shock
- Niacin (oral): anorexia, nausea, vomiting, diarrhea, and postural hypotension

Patient Teaching

Box 35.2 identifies patient teaching guidelines for vitamins, including vitamins B_1, B_3, and B_6.

VITAMIN B_{12} (CYANOCOBALAMIN) AND FOLIC ACID

The following discussion concerns vitamin B_{12} (cyanocobalamin) and folic acid.

Pharmacokinetics

- Vitamin B_{12}: requires intrinsic factor, produced by the stomach, for absorption. Normally, vitamin B_{12} is widely distributed and stored principally in the liver (half-life in the liver is 400 days). It is converted into active coenzymes in the tissues and eliminated, very slowly, in the urine.
- Folic acid: absorbed from the proximal small intestine. Folic acid is distributed to all body tissues with high concentrations

in the cerebrospinal fluid. The unused portion is stored in the liver. It is metabolized in the liver to active metabolites. Elimination is in the urine, at a more rapid rate than vitamin B_{12}.

Use

Healthcare providers use vitamin B_{12} to treat vitamin B_{12} deficiency states, whether caused by dietary deficiency, malabsorption, or inadequate secretion of intrinsic factor. They use folic acid as a supplement during infancy, childhood, and pregnancy, as well as to treat folic acid deficiency caused by malabsorption (sprue) or alcoholism. Folate deficiency in alcoholism results from both poor dietary intake and interference with liver processing of folic acid. Deficiency states of both vitamin B_{12} and folic acid present similarly as **megaloblastic anemia** (characterized by abnormally large, immature red blood cells). Proper diagnosis must establish which vitamin is deficient before treatment can begin. If megaloblastic anemia is severe, treatment usually involves both vitamin B_{12} and folic acid.

In pernicious anemia (vitamin B_{12} deficiency caused by the absence of intrinsic factor), vitamin B_{12} must be given by injection because oral forms are not absorbed from the GI tract. The injections must be continued for life. Vitamin B_{12} is also given to prevent pernicious anemia in patients who are strict vegetarians, have had a gastrectomy or bariatric surgery, or have chronic small bowel disease. Although folic acid relieves hematologic disorders of pernicious anemia, giving folic acid alone allows continued neurologic deterioration. Thus, an accurate diagnosis is required.

Patient-related variables specific to the use of vitamin B_{12} and folic acid include the following:
- Reproduction, pregnancy, and lactation:
  - Water-soluble vitamins cross the placenta. Vitamin B_{12} crosses the placenta and enters breast milk. Requirements may increase during pregnancy and lactation.
  - Folic acid supplementation before and during pregnancy decreases the risk of neural tube defects. Anyone planning a pregnancy or who may become pregnant should begin folic acid supplementation.
  - Folic acid crosses the placenta and enters breast milk. Folic acid is used for treatment of anemias due to folate deficiency during pregnancy. Requirements increase during breast-feeding.

Table 35.3 gives route and dosage information for vitamin B_{12} and folic acid.

Adverse Effects

- Vitamin B_{12}: rare. Hypokalemia sometimes results. There is a slight risk of anaphylactic shock and sudden death.
- Folic acid: uncommon. The most serious potential adverse effect is bronchospasm.

Contraindications

- Vitamin B_{12}: history of a sensitivity to vitamin B_{12}, other cobalamins, or cobalt. Vitamin B_{12} should be used with caution when treating folic acid deficiency.
- Folic acid: undiagnosed anemia because the vitamin may mask pernicious anemia. Another contraindication is vitamin B_{12} deficiency (the use of folic acid will improve the patient's megaloblastic anemia while doing nothing to reverse the neurologic problems associated with vitamin B_{12} deficiency).

Nursing Implications
Preventing Interactions

- Vitamin B_{12}: effects decreased by omeprazole and metformin, which decrease absorption of vitamin B_{12} from food.
- Folic acid: effects are decreased by aspirin, chloramphenicol, nonsteroidal anti-inflammatory drugs, sulfa antibiotics, sulfonylureas, triamterene, and trimethoprim. Cholestyramine, oral contraceptives, and sulfasalazine decrease absorption of folic acid. Methotrexate and phenytoin act as antagonists to folic acid. Alcohol alters liver function and leads to poor hepatic storage of folic acid. Folic acid increases phenytoin metabolism, which decreases phenytoin levels.

Administering the Medication

- Vitamin B_{12}: use of the oral form is most convenient, and administration with food increases absorption. Mixing the vitamin with fruit juice is fine, but it is important to consume the mixture quickly because ascorbic acid interferes with the stability of the vitamin.
- Folic acid: oral administration is preferable unless severe malabsorption is present, and people may take the vitamin without regard to food. Folic acid is also available in subcutaneous, IM, or IV forms. It is necessary to protect the parenteral forms from light and heat and store them at room temperature.

> **Quality and Safety Alert: Safety**
>
> Vitamin B_{12} is not safe for IV administration.

Assessing for Therapeutic and Adverse Effects

With vitamin B_{12} and folic acid, the nurse observes for increased appetite, strength, and feeling of well-being; increased reticulocyte counts; and increased number of normal red blood cells, hemoglobin, and hematocrit. Therapeutic effects may be rapid and dramatic.

Patient Teaching

Box 35.2 presents patient teaching guidelines for vitamins, including vitamin B_{12} and folic acid.

VITAMIN C

The following section concerns vitamin C (ascorbic acid).

Pharmacokinetics

Vitamin C is absorbed from the GI tract and is distributed generally. The vitamin is metabolized in the liver and eliminated by the kidneys.

Use

The most important therapeutic use of vitamin C involves the prevention and treatment of scurvy. This vitamin is available alone for oral, IM, or IV administration. It is also an ingredient in most multivitamin preparations. There is no known benefit for taking large amounts of this vitamin, and the nurse should discourage its use. Table 35.3 gives route and dosage information for vitamin C.

Patient-related variables specific to the use of vitamin C include the following:

- Reproduction, pregnancy, and lactation:
  - Because plasma concentrations decrease during pregnancy, some pregnant patients may require supplementation greater than the RDA.
  - Vitamin C is present in breast milk.
- Abnormal kidney function and hepatic impairment:
  - Patients with acute kidney disease who are unable to eat an adequate diet need a vitamin supplement to meet DRIs.
  - It is imperative to avoid large doses of vitamin C because of impaired urinary excretion.
  - Oxalate (a product of vitamin C catabolism) may precipitate in kidney tubules or form calcium oxalate stones, obstruct urine flow, and worsen kidney function.
  - Dialysis removes vitamin C, so patients receiving dialysis require vitamin C replacement.
- Specific healthcare environments:
  - In critically ill patients, conditions that increase the need for vitamin C sometimes warrant larger doses of vitamin C (e.g., extensive burns, delayed fracture or wound healing, delayed postoperative wound healing, or severe febrile or chronic disease states).

Adverse Effects and Contraindications

Usual doses of vitamin C are well tolerated. The most common adverse effects of oral vitamin C (especially megadoses) are abdominal cramps, nausea, vomiting, and diarrhea.

Caution is warranted in patients who are prone to kidney stones, as well as in those with glucose-6-phosphate deficiency or sickle cell anemia.

Nursing Implications
Preventing Interactions

Vitamin C, which acidifies the urine, decreases the elimination of aspirin and other salicylates, which are eliminated more rapidly in alkaline urine.

Administering the Medication

Vitamin C is available in various oral forms. Oral solutions may need mixing with food. Effervescent tablets may need dissolving in water immediately before use. Parenteral forms are also available.

Assessing for Therapeutic and Adverse Effects

Vitamin C deficiency usually begins to resolve rapidly, with improvement seen after only a few days. The nurse assesses for decreased or absent malaise, irritability, and bleeding tendencies (easy bruising of skin, bleeding gums, nosebleeds, and so forth).

Adverse reactions are rare with usual doses and methods of administration.

Patient Teaching

Box 35.2 presents patient teaching guidelines for vitamins, including vitamin C.

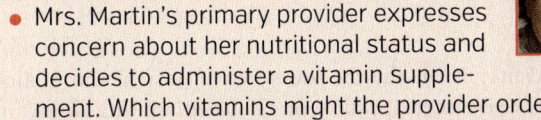

Clinical Application 35.2

- Mrs. Martin's primary provider expresses concern about her nutritional status and decides to administer a vitamin supplement. Which vitamins might the provider order?
- The provider prescribes the anticoagulant warfarin (Coumadin) for Mrs. Martin to aid in preventing another stroke. If she receives an overdose of warfarin, why does the healthcare prescriber order vitamin K? If she is eventually able to eat solid food, what teaching does the nurse provide concerning vitamin K in her diet and warfarin?

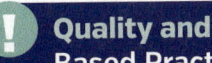

NCLEX Success

2. Which patient taking vitamin A supplements is of most concern to the nurse?
   A. a 21-year-old female who is pregnant
   B. a 32-year-old male with poor night vision
   C. a 55-year-old male with hepatic cirrhosis
   D. a 79-year-old female who is malnourished

3. A nurse is planning to teach a patient about dietary sources of vitamin K. The nurse teaches that foods containing vitamin K include which group?
   A. spinach, brussels sprouts, and broccoli
   B. breads, cereals, and other grains
   C. citrus fruits and juices, as well as strawberries
   D. meat, fish, and poultry

Quality and Safety Alert: Evidence-Based Practice

The FDA-labeled indications for vitamin C are treatment of vitamin C deficiency or for use in conditions requiring increased vitamin C intake (such as burns or wound healing); as a dietary supplement; and for the prevention and treatment of scurvy. An adjunct treatment for sepsis known as a metabolic resuscitation cocktail consists of high-dose vitamin C given intravenously (IV) along with hydrocortisone and vitamin B_1 (thiamine). Recent studies show this treatment less effective than originally thought. In a systematic review and component network meta-analysis, Fujii et al. (2022) found this drug combination did not reduce longer-term mortality. In another systematic review and meta-analysis, Sato et al. (2021) found no reduction in short-term mortality associated with use of high-dose vitamin C given IV; this study did show use of vitamin C associated with shorter duration of vasopressor use and decreased organ failure. Assouline et al. (2021) questioned whether the decline in organ failure was clinically significant and stated that the effect on kidney failure and mortality was unclear. Patients with sepsis have vitamin C and thiamine deficiencies. Experts believe that vitamin C increases synthesis of norepinephrine and vasopressin counteracting septic shock (Assouline et al., 2021). Vitamin C and hydrocortisone act to decrease the effects of the inflammatory cascade. Thiamine reduces kidney stones caused by high-dose vitamin C (Schmidt & Clardy, 2022).

MINERALS

IRON

Iron deficiency is usually the result not of normal elimination but of excessive menstruation or GI bleeding. The following discussion relates to the prototype drug ⓟ **ferrous sulfate (Feosol)**. Ferrous sulfate is often the preparation of choice; it contains 20% elemental iron.

Pharmacokinetics and Use

The fate of iron administered in drug form is the same as that of dietary iron. Only about 10% to 15% of ingested dietary iron is absorbed; although during pregnancy or iron deficiency, this percentage increases. Iron is stored in the small intestine (and in certain other cells) as ferritin as well as in the liver. When needed, iron is released into the bloodstream, bound to transferrin, and transported to the bone marrow for incorporation into hemoglobin.

Iron is not metabolized; the iron in red blood cells is reused. Small amounts of iron are eliminated daily (about 0.5 to 1 mg) in urine, sweat, and sloughing of intestinal mucosal cells. Excess iron is excreted in feces, which turn dark green or black.

The most important therapeutic uses of ferrous sulfate are as a supplement during periods of increased iron use and as treatment for iron deficiency. Table 35.4 gives route and dosage

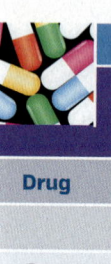

TABLE 35.4

DRUGS AT A GLANCE: Drugs Used in Mineral–Electrolyte and Acid–Base Imbalances

Drug	Indications for Use	Routes and Dosage Ranges	
		Adults	**Children**
Cation Exchange Resin			
Sodium polystyrene sulfonate (Kayexalate; Kionex; 🍁 Kayexalate)	Treatment of hyperkalemia	15–30 g PO once; may repeat up to 4 times per day (maximum daily dose 60 g/d) or 30–50 g rectal every 2–6 h Concomitant administration of sorbitol is not recommended.	1 g/kg/dose PO every 6 h (maximum dose 15 g/dose) or 1 g/kg/dose rectal every 2–6 h (maximum dose 30–50 g/dose). PO route more effective and preferred; in infants and small children, use lower dose by using practical exchange ratio of 1 mEqK⁺/g resin as basis for calculation Pediatric data not available; not for use in children at this time Pediatric data not available; not for use in children at this time
Patiromer (Veltassa; 🍁 Veltassa)	Treatment of hyperkalemia	Initial: 8.4 g PO once daily. Adjust dose by 8.4 g daily at 1-wk intervals (maximum dose 25.2 g/d)	
Sodium zirconium cyclosilicate (SZC) (Lokelma; 🍁 Lokelma)	Treatment of hyperkalemia	Initial: 8.4 g PO once daily. Adjust dose by 8.4 g daily at 1-wk intervals (maximum dose 25.2 g/d) Chronic hyperkalemia: initial 10 g PO 3 times daily for up to 48 h follow with 10 g once daily Severe hyperkalemia (in combination with other acute therapies): 10 g PO 3 times daily for up to 48 h	
Chelating Agents (Metal Antagonists)			
Deferasirox (Exjade; 🍁 APO-Deferasirox; Exjade; Jadenu)	Chronic iron overload	Initially, 20 mg/kg PO daily on empty stomach 30 min before eating; adjust dose every 3–6 mo; should not exceed 40 mg/kg daily	Older than 2 y of age: same as adult; calculate dose to the nearest whole tablet size
Deferoxamine (Desferal; 🍁 Desferal)	Acute iron intoxication Hemochromatosis due to blood transfusions Hemosiderosis due to hemolytic anemia	1 g IV initially and then 500 mg IV every 4 h for two doses, then 500 mg every 4–12 h if needed; maximum dose 6 g/24 h; rate of IV infusion not to exceed 15 mg/kg/h IV route preferred	15 mg/kg/h IV (maximum 80 mg/kg/d, not to exceed 6,000 mg/24 h) IM route not preferred and rarely indicated

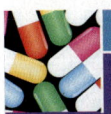

TABLE 35.4
DRUGS AT A GLANCE: Drugs Used in Mineral–Electrolyte and Acid–Base Imbalances (Continued)

Drug	Indications for Use	Routes and Dosage Ranges Adults	Children
Penicillamine (Cuprimine; ❋ Cuprimine) NOTE: Penicillamine should always be administered with a supplement of pyridoxine 25–50 mg PO daily in both adults and children	Wilson disease Cystinuria	Wilson disease: 750–1,500 mg PO daily in divided doses (maximum dose 2,000 mg PO daily; dose based on urinary copper excretion) Cystinuria: 1–4 g/d PO in four divided doses; initiate at 250 mg/d and gradually titrate up to reduce adverse effects; dose titrated based on urinary cystine excretion	Wilson disease: 20 mg/kg/d PO in 2–3 divided doses (round off to the nearest 250 mg dose); dose adjusted based on urinary copper excretion
Succimer (Chemet)	Lead poisoning	10 mg/kg 3 times daily for 5 d followed by 10 mg/kg twice daily for 14 d	10 mg/kg/dose or 350 mg/m²/dose PO every 8 h for 5 d and then every 12 h for 14 d (maximum 500 mg/dose; maximum daily dose 1,500 mg/d); treatment course may be repeated; 2-wk interval between courses recommended; capsule comes only in 100 mg; round the dose to nearest 100 mg; for young children who cannot swallow capsules, capsule contents can be sprinkled on soft food or given with a spoon
Iron Preparations			
Ferrous gluconate (Ferate)	Iron deficiency anemia	Doses in elemental iron (ferrous gluconate contains 12% elemental iron); 27–38 mg every other day or Monday, Wednesday, and Friday	3 mg/kg/d as a single daily dose; up to 60–120 mg once daily
Ⓟ Ferrous sulfate (Fer-In-Sol; Fer-Iron; FeroSul; others; ❋ PMS-Ferrous Sulfate)	Iron deficiency anemia	Doses in elemental iron (ferrous sulfate contains 20% elemental iron); ferrous sulfate doses given 65 mg every other day or on Monday, Wednesday, and Friday	3 mg/kg/d as a single daily dose up to 60–120 mg once daily
Iron dextran injection (INFeD; ❋ DexIron)	Iron deficiency anemia	Dosage is calculated for individual patients according to hemoglobin and weight (see manufacturer's literature); a 25-mg test dose is required before therapeutic doses are given	Same as adults; test dose 10–25 mg
Magnesium Preparations			
Magnesium oxide Magnesium hydroxide Magnesium sulfate	Hypomagnesemia Hypertension or seizures associated with toxemia of pregnancy	Hypomagnesemia: magnesium oxide 800 mg daily with food; magnesium sulfate 1 g IM every 6 h for four doses; magnesium sulfate 1–2 g IV well diluted, over 1–2 h Constipation: magnesium hydroxide (milk of magnesia) 400 mg/5 mL 30–60 mL PO at bedtime Preeclampsia or eclampsia of pregnancy to prevent or control seizures: initially, magnesium sulfate 4–6 g loading dose over 15–30 min at onset of labor; follow with 1–2 g/h continuous infusion for at least 24 h after delivery (maximum infusion rate 3 g/h)	Hypomagnesemia: magnesium oxide PO 10–20 mg/kg/dose up to 4 times per day; magnesium sulfate 25–50 mg/kg/dose IV every 6 h for 2–3 doses; maximum dose 2 g/dose; dilute in appropriate fluid prior to IV infusion; infuse IV solution slowly over 1–4 h

(Continued on page 664)

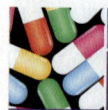

TABLE 35.4
DRUGS AT A GLANCE: Drugs Used in Mineral–Electrolyte and Acid–Base Imbalances (Continued)

Drug	Indications for Use	Routes and Dosage Ranges	
		Adults	**Children**
Potassium Preparation			
ⓟ **Potassium chloride** (K-Tab; Klor-Con; ❋ Apo-K; Micro-K; Slo-Pot 600) NOTE: Give potassium chloride by IV infusion only, *never* IM or IV push; give slowly as a dilute solution; rapid infusion may cause fatal hyperkalemia; always use infusion pump	Prevent or treat hypokalemia	Prevention of hypokalemia: potassium supplement 16–24 mEq PO daily in divided doses; adjust dosage based on serum potassium levels Treatment of hypokalemia: for serum K < 3 mEq: potassium supplement 40 mEq 3–4 times daily PO; for serum K 2.5–3 mEq: IV initial 10–20 mEq/h (maximum infusion rate 20 mEq/h); for serum K < 2.5 mEq: IV central line only, initial 10–40 mEq/h (maximum infusion rate 40 mEq/h) further doses based on serum potassium level and blood pH; give potassium replacement IV only with monitoring of ECG and serum potassium level	Prevention of hypokalemia: potassium supplement 1–2 mEq/kg/d in 1–2 divided doses Treatment of hypokalemia (mild to moderate): Infants, children, and adolescents: potassium supplement 2–5 mEq/kg/d PO in divided doses (not to exceed 1–2 mEq/kg as a single doe or 20 mEq) (whichever is less); treatment of hypokalemia (severe): Infants, children, and adolescents: by intermittent IV infusion 0.5–1 mEq/kg/dose (maximum dose 40 mEq/dose); infuse at rate <0.5 mEq/kg/h
Zinc Preparation			
Zinc sulfate (Orazinc; ❋ Micro-Zn)	Prevent or treat zinc deficiency	Deficiency: zinc sulfate daily dose of 2–3 times zinc RDA	Infants, children, and adolescents: elemental zinc 0.5–2 mg/kg/d once daily
Multiple Mineral–Electrolyte Preparations			
Oral solutions (Pedialyte)	Prevent or treat fluid and electrolyte deficiencies		Amount (PO) individualized according to fluid and electrolyte needs based on estimated fluid loss, age, and weight (see manufacturer's literature)

---

information for ferrous sulfate and other iron preparations. Slow-release or enteric-coated iron products decrease absorption but may cause less gastric irritation.

Patient-related variables specific to the use of iron include the following:

- Reproduction, pregnancy, and lactation:
  - Iron requirements increase during pregnancy. Untreated iron deficiency and iron deficiency anemia may cause adverse events. Treatment is the same as for nonpregnant patients. Ferrous salts are preferred, such as ferrous sulfate.
  - Supplementation is needed for 3 months after Hgb is in the normal range and for at least 6 months postpartum to replenish iron stores.
  - Iron is present in breast milk. Iron requirements increase during breast-feeding. Maternal use of ferrous sulfate increases iron content of breast milk.
  - No adverse events have been observed in breast-feeding infants with maternal use of ferrous sulfate. Ferrous sulfate has been evaluated in multiple studies for treatment of postpartum iron deficiency anemia.

Adverse Effects and Contraindications

The most common adverse effects of ferrous sulfate and other oral iron preparations are GI discomfort, nausea, constipation, diarrhea, and black stools. Liquid forms of iron may temporarily stain the teeth. In iron overload, excess iron is deposited in the heart, liver, and endocrine glands resulting in organ damage and, if untreated, death.

Contraindications to ferrous sulfate include peptic ulceration, ulcerative colitis, regional enteritis, and repeated blood transfusions. Other contraindications are disorders that cause the accumulation of iron stores: hemosiderosis, primary hemochromatosis, and hemolytic anemia (unless iron deficiency anemia is also present).

Nursing Implications
Preventing Interactions

In general, food decreases iron absorption. Examples include cereals, cheese, coffee, eggs, milk, tea, bran and whole-grain breads, and yogurt.

A few drugs increase iron absorption. Most notable is vitamin C, which increases iron absorption by acidifying gastric secretions. Vitamin C, taken at the same time as iron-containing foods or oral iron preparations, increases iron absorption. Taking ferrous sulfate with vitamin C–containing orange juice enhances iron absorption. Some oral iron preparations contain a small amount of vitamin C. Allopurinol may increase the concentration of iron in the liver.

Ferrous sulfate interferes with the absorption of the penicillamine, tetracycline, and fluoroquinolone antibiotics, possibly resulting in decreased antibiotic levels or effect. Ferrous sulfate also decreases the absorption of levodopa, methyldopa, and levothyroxine.

Administering the Medication

People should take iron tablets or capsules before meals, with 8 oz of water or juice, if tolerated. They should not crush or chew sustained-release preparations. Oral iron preparations are better absorbed if taken on an empty stomach. However, because gastric irritation is a common adverse reaction, people more often take iron with or immediately after meals; this may decrease absorption. With liquid preparations, it is necessary to dilute them, take with a straw, and then rinse the mouth afterward to prevent temporary staining of teeth.

Certain interactions affect the timing of iron administration. Ferrous sulfate interferes with the absorption of the penicillamine, tetracycline, and fluoroquinolone antibiotics; therefore, it is necessary to take ferrous sulfate 2 to 4 hours before or after these antibiotics. Because some foods may affect iron absorption, people should take iron at least 2 hours before or after a caffeine-containing beverage or food.

Daily dosing decreases absorption. Current recommendations call for a dose every other day or on Mondays, Wednesdays, and Fridays. IV iron replacement is preferred in many clinical situations (e.g., poor GI absorption, lack of response or poor tolerance of oral iron, and chronic kidney disease).

Assessing for Therapeutic and Adverse Effects

The nurse observes for increased vigor and feeling of well-being, improved appetite, less fatigue, and increased red blood cells, as well as hemoglobin, hematocrit, and reticulocyte count. Therapeutic effects are usually evident within a month unless other problems are also present (e.g., vitamin deficiency, achlorhydria, infection, or malabsorption).

The nurse assesses for GI upset, which may be related to dose. GI symptoms may decrease as therapy progresses. (Enteric-coated products reduce GI upset but also reduce the amount of iron absorbed.) It is also necessary to check for stool color depending on the iron preparation. Oral iron may turn stools black. Although this unabsorbed iron is harmless, it could mask melena.

Patient Teaching

Box 35.3 presents patient teaching guidelines for minerals and electrolytes, including iron.

BOX 35.3 *Patient Teaching Guidelines for Minerals and Electrolytes*

General Considerations

- A well-balanced diet contains all the minerals needed for health in most people. Exceptions are iron and calcium, which are often needed as a dietary supplement in female and children. Note that herbal preparations of chamomile, feverfew, and St. John's wort may inhibit iron absorption. The safest action is to take mineral supplements only on a healthcare provider's advice, in the amounts and for length of time prescribed. All minerals are toxic when taken in excess.
- Keep all mineral or electrolyte substances out of reach of children to prevent accidental overdose. Acute iron intoxication is a common problem among young children and can be fatal. Supervise children about using fluoride supplements (e.g., remind them to spit out oral rinses and gels rather than swallow them).
- Keep appointments with healthcare providers for periodic blood tests and other follow-up procedures when mineral or electrolyte supplements are prescribed (e.g., potassium chloride). This helps prevent ingestion of excessive amounts.
- Minerals are often contained in multivitamin preparations, with percentages of the recommended dietary allowances supplied. These amounts differ in various preparations and should be included in estimations of daily intake.

Iron

- Know about dietary sources of iron. This mineral occurs in beef liver, red meats, fish, poultry, clams, tofu, oysters, lentils, dried peas and beans, fortified cereals, bread, and dried fruits.
- Avoid substituting one iron salt for another, because amounts of elemental iron may vary.
- Take iron preparations with or after meals, with approximately 240 mL of fluid, to prevent stomach upset. Do not take iron with coffee or other caffeine-containing beverages because caffeine decreases absorption. Take iron and caffeine preparations at least 2 hours apart.
- Do not crush or chew slow-release tablets or capsules.
- With liquid preparations, dilute with water, drink through a straw, and rinse the mouth afterward to avoid staining the teeth.
- Expect that stools will be dark green or black. Report constipation or change in color or consistency of stool to the healthcare provider.

Potassium

- Mix oral solutions or effervescent tablets with at least 120 mL of water or juice to improve the taste, dilute the drug, and decrease gastric irritation.
- Do not crush or chew slow-release preparations.
- Take after meals initially to decrease gastric irritation. If no nausea, vomiting, or other problems occur, the drug can be tried before meals because it is better absorbed from an empty stomach.
- Do not stop taking the medication without notifying the healthcare provider who prescribed it, especially if you are also taking diuretics or digoxin.
- Do not use salt substitutes except on the recommendation of a healthcare provider. Salt substitutes contain potassium chloride and may result in excessive intake.
- Serious problems may develop from either high or low levels of potassium in the blood. Know and recognize signs and symptoms of hypokalemia and hyperkalemia.
  - Signs and symptoms of hypokalemia: palpitations, confusion, dizziness, muscle weakness, abdominal distension, frequent voiding of large amounts of urine
  - Signs and symptoms of hyperkalemia: muscle weakness, palpitations, slow pulse, fatigue, shortness of breath

> **Clinical Application 35.3**
>
> Mrs. Martin appears to be anemic and requires iron supplementation.
> - By what route is the iron ordered?
> - How does the nurse determine if this iron therapy is successful?
> - What adverse effects does the nurse observe for?

> **NCLEX Success**
>
> 4. Teaching for a patient who is being started on an iron supplement should include information that the preparation
>   A. may cause diarrhea
>   B. may cause stools to be dark green or black
>   C. should be taken with an antacid
>   D. should not be taken with fruit juice

Other Drugs Used to Treat Iron Deficiency

Iron Dextran

Iron dextran (Dexferrum, INFeD) is a parenteral form of iron useful for treating iron deficiency anemia when oral supplements cannot be used. Indications for use include peptic ulcer or inflammatory bowel disease that may be aggravated by oral iron preparations, the patient's inability or unwillingness to take oral preparations, and a shortage of time for correcting the iron deficiency (e.g., late pregnancy, preoperative status, or excessive blood loss). The FDA has issued a **BOXED WARNING** for iron dextran regarding the risk of anaphylactic reactions and death. Because of this risk, administration should occur only when there is a clear indication. Contraindications include anemias not associated with iron deficiency and hypersensitivity to the drug. Caution is warranted in serious hepatic impairment, rheumatoid arthritis, or other inflammatory diseases as well as a significant history of allergies or asthma. The IV route is preferred to the IM route. It is necessary to give a small test dose before administering a therapeutic dose. The drug has a slow onset of action and peaks in 1 to 2 weeks. Dosage is calculated according to hemoglobin level and weight.

> **Quality and Safety Alert: Patient-Centered Care**
>
> Equipment and drugs for emergency resuscitation must always be available whenever iron dextran IV is administered. Anaphylactic reactions may occur.

Iron Sucrose

Iron sucrose (Venofer) is a parenteral iron supplement given by IV infusion. This supplement is indicated for patients with chronic kidney disease who are not on dialysis and for those who are peritoneal dialysis dependent or hemodialysis dependent. It may be given alone or concurrently with erythropoietin therapy. The major advantage of iron sucrose is a lesser risk of anaphylaxis than with iron dextran; however, hypersensitivity reactions, although rare, can be fatal. Test doses are not necessary. Common adverse effects include headache, heart failure, hypotension, nausea, leg cramps, and sepsis.

POTASSIUM

The following discussion focuses on the prototype **potassium chloride**, or KCl. The oral form of the drug has numerous trade names.

Pharmacokinetics and Use

Potassium is absorbed from the GI tract. The potassium level is normally maintained by the kidneys.

Potassium chloride is usually the drug of choice for preventing or treating **hypokalemia** (less-than-normal amount of potassium in the blood) because deficiencies of potassium and chloride often occur together. Table 35.4 gives route and dosage information for this drug. Healthcare providers may order potassium chloride for patients who are receiving potassium-depleting diuretics (e.g., hydrochlorothiazide, furosemide), those who are receiving digoxin (hypokalemia increases the risk of digoxin toxicity), and those who are receiving IV fluids because of surgical procedures, GI disease, or other conditions. They may also use it to replace chloride in patients with hypochloremic metabolic acidosis.

Patient-related variables specific to the use of potassium include the following:
- Reproduction, pregnancy, and lactation:
  - Potassium requirements are the same in pregnant and nonpregnant patients. No adverse events have been observed following the use of potassium supplements in healthy patients with normal pregnancies. Use with caution if preeclampsia occurs; hyperkalemia is more likely.
  - Potassium is present in breast milk. Concentration is not affected if there is no hyperkalemia from supplementation.

Adverse Effects and Contraindications

Adverse effects of oral potassium are nausea, vomiting, abdominal pain, and diarrhea. Adverse effects of IV potassium include postinfusion phlebitis at the IV site. Overdosage with oral or IV forms or rapid infusion of IV preparations produces **hyperkalemia** (greater-than-normal amount of potassium in the blood), dysrhythmias, heart block, cardiac arrest, respiratory paralysis, and death. Hyperkalemia may occur with the following:

- Concurrent use of potassium chloride with angiotensin-converting enzyme inhibitors or potassium-sparing diuretics
- Salt substitutes that contain potassium instead of sodium if used with potassium supplements
- Penicillin G potassium (potassium salt of penicillin)

Contraindications to potassium supplementation include hyperkalemia, severe abnormal kidney function, acute dehydration, heat cramps, and untreated Addison disease. Caution is necessary in cardiac disease or abnormal kidney function.

Nursing Implications
Administering the Medication

People should take oral preparations with or after meals; this decreases gastric irritation. They should not crush controlled-release or extended-release tablets. It is necessary to mix oral liquids, powders, and effervescent tablets in at least 120 mL of water, juice, or carbonated beverage to disguise the taste.

IV potassium chloride is indicated when a patient cannot take an oral preparation or has severe hypokalemia. The nurse measures the serum potassium level and establishes that urine output is adequate before starting IV potassium therapy. In adults, the maximum concentration for peripheral infusion is 10 mEq/100 mL. The maximum rate of administration for peripheral infusion is 10 mEq/h. With central line administration, higher concentrations and more rapid rates of infusion may be used; concentrations of 20 to 40 mEq/100 mL at a maximum rate of 40 mEq/h have been safely administered (UpToDate, 2022).

> **Quality and Safety Alert: Safety**
>
> It is essential to never give undiluted drug by the IV route or give it by the IV push route.

Well-diluted preparations prevent sudden hyperkalemia, cardiotoxic effects, and phlebitis at the venipuncture site. Careful administration is warranted.

Patient Teaching

Box 35.3 identifies patient teaching guidelines for minerals and electrolytes, including potassium.

> **Clinical Application 35.4**
>
> - Serum electrolytes reveal that Mrs. Martin is hypokalemic. The healthcare provider orders potassium chloride per feeding tube. What steps does the nurse take to administer this medication, and what form of potassium chloride is preferable for administration per feeding tube? What adverse effects does the nurse assess for?
> - Suppose Mrs. Martin is severely hypokalemic and the healthcare provider orders potassium chloride to be given intravenously. What nursing interventions ensure that the ordered potassium supplement is given correctly and safely? What adverse effects may occur if IV administration of this potassium preparation occurs too rapidly?

> **NCLEX Success**
>
> 5. A nurse should question the use of an oral potassium preparation with which one of the following drugs?
>   A. ethacrynic acid
>   B. furosemide
>   C. hydrochlorothiazide
>   D. spironolactone

ADJUVANT MINERALS

Other medications may be necessary in a variety of conditions to support the treatment and resolution of symptoms. Table 35.4 contains information about some of the agents discussed in this section.

Magnesium

Oral magnesium oxide or hydroxide may be useful for mild hypomagnesemia. Parenteral magnesium sulfate may be necessary for moderate to severe hypomagnesemia, convulsions associated with pregnancy, and prevention of hypomagnesemia in total parenteral nutrition. Therapeutic effects in these conditions are attributed to the preparations' depressant effects on the CNS as well as on smooth, skeletal, and cardiac muscles. (Discussion of the use of magnesium products as antacids and cathartics appears in Chapters 37 and 39, respectively.)

Oral magnesium salts may cause diarrhea. Contraindications to magnesium include impaired kidney function or being comatose.

Oral preparations of magnesium oxide or hydroxide act in 3 to 6 hours, are minimally absorbed systemically, and are excreted in the urine. With parenteral magnesium sulfate, IM injections act in 1 hour and last 3 to 4 hours; IV administration produces immediate action that lasts 30 minutes.

Zinc

Zinc sulfate and zinc gluconate are available over the counter in various forms and strengths. Zinc is also an ingredient in several vitamin–mineral combination products. Zinc preparations are given orally as a dietary supplement to prevent or treat zinc deficiency. They have a slow onset of action and a delayed peak. They are metabolized in the liver and excreted in feces. Adverse effects of zinc sulfate are dizziness, restlessness, nausea, vomiting, gastric ulcers, and diarrhea. The FDA recommends that intranasal zinc products not be used because of reports of loss of ability to smell (anosmia) following their use. Zinc-induced anosmia is characterized by rapid onset and stinging and burning.

Multiple Mineral–Electrolyte Preparations

Oral electrolyte solutions (e.g., Pedialyte) contain several electrolytes and a small amount of dextrose. They are used to supply maintenance amounts of fluids and electrolytes when oral intake is restricted. They are especially useful in children for treatment of diarrhea and may prevent severe fluid and electrolyte depletion. The amount given must be carefully calculated, prescribed, and administered to avoid excessive intake. Oral solutions should not be used in severe circumstances in which IV fluid and electrolyte therapy is indicated, and they should not be mixed with other electrolyte-containing fluids, such as milk or fruit juices. In addition, they must be cautiously used in impaired kidney function. There are numerous electrolyte solutions for IV use to maintain or replace electrolytes when the patient is unable to eat and drink.

TREATMENT OF MINERAL EXCESS

Penicillamine

Penicillamine (Cuprimine) is a **chelating agent**, which binds copper, lead, mercury, and zinc to form soluble complexes that are excreted in the urine. Its main use is the removal of excess copper in patients with Wilson disease, a rare condition characterized by accumulation of copper in vital organs. Prophylactic use involves giving the agent to patients in whom this hereditary condition is likely to develop, before clinical manifestations occur. Other uses for penicillamine include cystinuria, a hereditary metabolic disorder characterized by large amounts of cystine in the urine and kidney calculi and lead poisoning.

Succimer

Succimer (or dimercaptosuccinic acid) (Chemet) chelates lead to form water-soluble complexes that are excreted in the urine. Indications include the treatment of lead poisoning in children. After oral administration, peak blood levels are reached in 1 to 2 hours. The drug is metabolized in the liver and excreted in urine and feces, with a half-life of 2 days. The most common adverse effects are anorexia, nausea, vomiting, and diarrhea.

Deferoxamine and Deferasirox

Acute iron overdosage requires treatment with these drugs as soon as possible, even if overdosage is only suspected and the amount taken is unknown. It is unnecessary to wait until the serum iron level is measured.

Deferoxamine (Desferal) is a parenteral drug used to remove excess iron from storage sites (e.g., ferritin, hemosiderin) in the body. It combines with iron to produce a water-soluble compound that can be excreted by the kidneys. IM, IV, and subcutaneous routes may be useful in certain circumstances. The urine becomes reddish brown from the iron content. A common adverse effect is pain or induration at the injection site. The most serious adverse effect is anaphylaxis.

Deferasirox (Exjade) is an iron-chelating agent used to treat chronic iron overload in children and adults who require frequent blood transfusions for severe, chronic anemia. This drug is absorbed with oral administration, with peak plasma levels in 1.5 to 4 hours. It is highly bound to serum albumin, metabolized in the liver, and excreted in bile and feces (with the iron, which binds to the drug). Oral administration should be at the same time each day, before a meal. Patients should not chew or swallow the tablets but dissolve them in water, orange juice, or apple juice. The most common adverse effects are skin rash, fever, headache, and GI problems (e.g., abdominal pain, vomiting, diarrhea, and constipation). The FDA has issued a **BOXED WARNING** ◆ for deferasirox regarding the risk of hepatic impairment and/or abnormal kidney function and GI hemorrhage, all of which can be fatal. It is important to monitor liver and kidney function closely.

Agents Used in the Treatment of Hyperkalemia

The first step in the treatment of hyperkalemia is to eliminate any exogenous sources of potassium. It is essential to treat acidosis, if present, because potassium leaves cells and enters the serum, causing acidosis. Healthcare providers use measures that antagonize the effects of potassium, cause potassium to leave the serum and reenter the cells, and remove potassium from the body. Serum potassium levels and electrocardiographic (ECG) changes are the primary determinants of the treatment regimen.

Sodium Bicarbonate

Sodium bicarbonate is an agent used to control the acidosis associated with hyperkalemia. The dose is 150 mEq in 1 L of 5% dextrose in water over 2 to 4 hours. Experts do not recommend administration of sodium bicarbonate as the only therapy for acute management of hyperkalemia (Mount, 2022).

Calcium Gluconate

Calcium gluconate is a mineral supplement. A 1,000-mg dose (10 mL of a 10% solution) infused over 2 to 3 minutes with constant cardiac monitoring is given to decrease the cardiotoxic effects of hyperkalemia. It may be necessary to repeat the dose after 5 minutes if ECG changes persist or recur. Hypercalcemia potentiates the cardiotoxic effects of digoxin. In patients with hyperkalemia due to digoxin toxicity, administration of digoxin-specific antibody fragments is the preferred therapy (Mount, 2022).

> **Concept Mastery Alert**
>
> Digoxin toxicity is more likely in the presence of hypokalemia, hypomagnesemia, hypercalcemia, and myocardial ischemia.

Glucose and Insulin

IV glucose and insulin are a treatment for hyperkalemia. Infusion causes potassium to move into cells. Glucose, given with insulin, prevents hypoglycemia. Administration of regular insulin 10 units as an IV bolus is followed immediately by 50 mL of 50% dextrose (25 g of glucose). To avoid hypoglycemia, experts recommend administration of IV fluids of 10% dextrose at 50 to 75 mL/h (Mount, 2022). When glucose and insulin are used to lower serum potassium, blood glucose levels should be monitored every hour for 5 to 6 hours.

Gastrointestinal Cation Exchange

With less severe hyperkalemia, sodium polystyrene sulfonate (Kayexalate), a cation exchange resin, administered orally, removes potassium from the body in the stool. However, use of sodium polystyrene sulfonate has the rare but significant risk of intestinal necrosis. Two newer GI cation exchangers are preferred for adults, patiromer and sodium zirconium cyclosilicate (SZC).

> **Quality and Safety Alert: Patient-Centered Care**
>
> Although sorbitol has been given with sodium polystyrene sulfonate orally and as an enema for its laxative effect, recent studies showed an association between the combination and intestinal necrosis. The FDA no longer recommends that sodium polystyrene sulfonate be administered in sorbitol.

NUTRITIONAL PRODUCTS

Various products are available to supplement or substitute for dietary intake. These may consist of vitamins, minerals, liquid enteral formulas, IV fluids and nutrition, and pancreatic enzymes.

Numerous liquid enteral formulas are available for oral or tube feedings, and many are nutritionally complete, except for water, when given in sufficient amounts (e.g., Ensure, Isocal,

Sustacal, Resource). To meet fluid needs, it is necessary to give additional water. Most oral products come in a variety of flavors and contain 1 kcal/mL of formula. Additional products are available formulated for patients with special conditions (e.g., hepatic or kidney failure, malabsorption syndromes) or needs (e.g., high protein, increased calories).

When the GI tract is functional but the patient cannot ingest sufficient food and fluid, the nurse can give high-protein, high-calorie foods (e.g., milkshakes) or nutritionally complete supplements (e.g., Ensure) with meals, between meals, and at bedtime. In patients with a feeding tube, **enteral nutrition** provides fluid and nutrients. When the GI tract is nonfunctional, the nurse often gives IV fluids or **parenteral nutrition**. Most of these solutions are nutritionally incomplete and are used short term to supply fluids, electrolytes, and a few calories; additional nutrition may be necessary.

Use

For short-term use (e.g., 3 to 5 days), the goal is to provide adequate amounts of fluids and electrolytes and enough carbohydrates to minimize oxidation of body protein and fat for energy. The choice of specific solution depends on individual needs, but it should contain at least 5% dextrose. A frequently used solution is 5% dextrose in 0.45% sodium chloride, 2,000 to 3,000 mL per 24 hours (provides approximately 170 kcal/L, water, sodium, and chloride). Vitamins may be added. These solutions are nutritionally inadequate.

For long-term use (weeks to months), the goal is to provide all nutrients required for normal body functioning, including tissue repair. Basic solutions provide water, carbohydrates, proteins, vitamins, and minerals. Patients usually receive fat emulsions (e.g., Intralipid) that are usually given separately to provide additional calories and essential fatty acids (500 mL of 10% emulsion provides 550 kcal).

Patient-related variables specific to the use of nutritional products include the following:

- Age:
  - For children with special needs in relation to nutrients, various enteral formulations are available.
  - Some examples include Lofenalac for children with phenylketonuria; Nursoy and Soyalac, which contain soy protein, for children who are allergic to cow's milk; and Nutramigen and Pregestimil, which contain easily digested nutrients for children with malabsorption or other GI problems. However, parenteral nutrition may be necessary.
- Abnormal kidney function and hepatic impairment:
  - With enteral nutrition, Amin-Aid provides amino acids, carbohydrates, and a few electrolytes for patients with kidney failure. With parenteral nutrition, several amino acid solutions are available for patients with kidney failure (e.g., Aminosyn-RF). Nepro is a formulation for patients receiving dialysis. Suplena, which is lower in protein and some electrolytes than Nepro, is formulated for patients who are not receiving dialysis.
  - For enteral feedings (usually by GI tube) in patients with liver failure, Hepatic-Aid II is available. For parenteral feeding in patients with hepatic failure and hepatic encephalopathy, HepatAmine, a special formula of amino acids, may be useful.
  - Caution is warranted with the use of enteral and parenteral fat preparations in patients with hepatic impairment. Medium-chain triglycerides (e.g., MCT oil), which are used to provide calories in other patients who are malnourished, may lead to coma in patients with advanced cirrhosis. Patients who require parenteral nutrition are at risk for developing high serum triglycerides levels and pancreatitis from administering IV fat emulsions in usual dosages.

Adverse Effects

Adverse reactions, which are usually attributed to the hypertonicity of the preparations, include tachycardia, hypotension, dehydration, nausea, vomiting, diarrhea, and increased urine output. The risk of aspiration of formula is a consideration with tube feeding.

Nursing Implications

Administering the Medication

For oral supplemental feedings, it is necessary to chill liquids or pour them over ice and give them through a straw (unless contraindicated), from a closed container, between meals. This practice may improve formula taste and decrease formula odor. A straw directs the formula toward the back of the throat and decreases contact with taste buds. A closed container also decreases odor.

For tube feedings, the nurse adheres to guidelines for safe administration (positioning, placement of the tube, residual and aseptic management of formula and equipment). When medications are ordered, liquid preparations are preferable. Tablets or powders may stick in the tube lumen, which may mean the full dose of medication does not reach the stomach. Also, the obstruction of the tube is likely. It is important not to mix medications with tube feeding formula; this could interfere with drug absorption.

Assessing for Therapeutic Effects

For patients receiving nutritional formulas, the nurse observes for weight gain and increased serum albumin. For infants and children receiving milk substitutes, the nurse observes for decreased diarrhea and weight gain. Therapeutic effects depend on the reason for use (i.e., prevention or treatment of undernutrition).

Assessing for Adverse Effects

With commercial nutritional formulas (except Osmolite and Isocal), the nurse observes for tachycardia, hypotension, dehydration, nausea, vomiting, diarrhea, and increased urine output. These adverse reactions are usually attributed to the hypertonicity of the preparations. Beginning administration with small amounts of formula, given slowly, may prevent or minimize adverse effects.

Patient Teaching

Box 35.4 presents patient teaching guidelines for nutritional products.

BOX 35.4 Patient Teaching Guidelines for Nutritional Products

- For oral supplements, take or give at the preferred time and temperature, when possible.
- For tube feedings:
  - Use or give with the patient in a sitting position, if possible, to decrease risks of aspirating formula into the lungs.
  - Be sure the tube is placed correctly before each tube feeding. Ask a healthcare provider how to check placement with your type of tube.
  - Be sure the solution is stored at room temperature. Cold formula may cause abdominal cramping.
  - Do not take or give more than 500 mL per feeding, including 60 to 90 mL of water for flushing the tube. This helps to avoid overfilling the stomach and possible vomiting.
  - Take or give slowly, over approximately 30 to 60 minutes. Rapid administration may cause nausea and vomiting.
  - With continuous feedings, change containers and tubing daily. With intermittent feedings, rinse all equipment after each use, and change at least every 24 hours. Most tube feeding formulas are milk based, and infection may occur if formulas become contaminated or equipment is not kept clean.
  - Ask a healthcare provider about the amount of free water. Most people receiving 1,500 to 2,000 mL of tube feeding daily need approximately 1,000 mL or more of free water daily. However, patients' needs vary. Water can be mixed with the tube feeding formula, given after the tube feeding, or given between bolus feedings. Be sure to include the amount of water used for flushing the tube in the total daily intake.
- Caregiver administration for giving medications by tube include the following:
  - Give liquid preparations when available.
  - When liquid preparations are not available, it may be necessary to crush some tablets and empty some capsules and mix them with 15 to 30 mL of water. Ask a healthcare provider which medication can safely be crushed or altered, because some (e.g., long-acting or enteric-coated) can be harmful if crushed.
  - Do not mix medications with the tube feeding formula because some medications may not be absorbed. If the absorption of a drug is affected by the tube feeding formula (e.g., phenytoin), discontinue the tube feeding for the recommended interval prior to drug administration; then, resume feeding at the recommended interval after drug administration.
  - Do not mix medications. Give each one separately.
  - Flush the tube with water before and after each medication to get the medication through the tube and to keep the tube open.
  - For more a more complete discussion of the care of patients with feeding tubes, administration of drugs through feeding tubes, and patient teaching guidelines for home use of feeding tubes, consult a textbook of nursing fundamentals or medical/surgical nursing.

Clinical Application 35.5

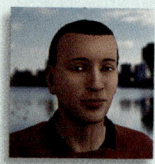

- Mrs. Martin has a percutaneous endoscopic gastrostomy tube. She is to receive a bolus tube feeding of 300 mL at 08:00, 12:00, 17:00, and 21:00 hours, with a flush of free water every 4 hours. What precautions does the nurse take to prevent aspiration of the tube feeding?
- Mrs. Martin receives several medications through the feeding tube. Explain what the nurse does if one of those medications cannot be crushed for administration through the tube. Describe the steps the nurse takes to administer medications through the tube.

Unfolding Patient Stories: Jermaine Jones • Part 1

Jermaine Jones, a 34-year-old patient diagnosed with depression, is assessed by the nurse during a routine clinic visit. The nurse determines that he has lost 8 lb and consumes a beer in place of the evening meal when his wife is working late. What nursing interventions can be implemented to promote good nutrition? What nutritional supplements would the nurse consider for a poor nutritional intake? (Jermaine Jones's story continues in Chapter 55.)

Care for Jermaine and other patients in a realistic virtual environment: *vSim for Nursing* (thepoint.lww.com/vSimPharm). Practice documenting these patients' care in DocuCare (thepoint.lww.com/DocuCareEHR).

THE NURSING PROCESS

A concept map outlines the nursing process related to drug therapy considerations in this chapter. Additional nursing implications related to the disease process should also be considered in care decisions.

Assessment
- Assess dietary intake, nutritional deficiencies, and alcohol intake.
- Assess vitamin intake for deficiencies or megadoses.
- Assess body mass index (BMI).
- Assess deficiencies in B complex vitamins and vitamin C because these are more common.
- Assess for illness, anorexia, nausea, vomiting, and diarrhea.
- Assess for drug interactions and the influence on gains or losses of vitamins, minerals, or electrolytes (e.g., proton pump inhibitors decrease vitamin B_{12}).
- Assess minerals and electrolytes lost with gastric suction, polyuria, diarrhea, or diaphoresis.
- Assess complete blood count and electrolytes: sodium, potassium, chloride, carbon dioxide, and bicarbonate.

Outcomes of Therapy
The patient will
- Demonstrate improvement in nutritional status in relation to body needs.
- Maintain fluid and electrolyte balance as measured by appropriate intake and output and serum electrolyte values.
- Demonstrate appropriate intake of vitamins, minerals, and electrolytes.

Nursing Interventions
- Promote a well-balanced diet for all patients. Five daily servings of fruits and vegetables provide adequate vitamins unless the patient has increased requirements or conditions that interfere with absorption or use of vitamins. A diet that is adequate in protein and calories usually provides adequate minerals and electrolytes. Exceptions are calcium and iron, which are often needed as a dietary supplement in women and children.
- Provide relief for symptoms that are likely to interfere with nutrition, such as pain, nausea, vomiting, or diarrhea.
- Provide palatable supplements at appropriate times for patients who need increased protein–calorie intake and encourage patients to take them.
- Promote exercise and activity. For undernourished patients, this may increase appetite, improve digestion, and aid bowel elimination.
- Minimize the use of sedative-type drugs when appropriate. Although no one should be denied pain relief, strong analgesics and other sedatives may cause drowsiness, decreased desire or ability to eat and drink, constipation, and a feeling of fullness.
- Monitor weight, fluid intake, urine output, vital signs, blood glucose, serum electrolytes, and complete blood count for patients receiving parenteral nutrition. Obtain these values daily, weekly, or as institutional protocols dictate. Adjust monitoring based on patient status whether hospitalized or at home.
- Promote proper use of mineral supplements, which are recommended only for current or potential deficiencies and are toxic in excessive amounts.
- Follow institutional protocols in the care of patients with feeding tubes and in the administration of ordered tube feeding products, and medication administration. Use best practices in relation to assessing correct tube placement, maintaining patency of tubes, positioning of patients, prevention of aspiration, gravity or pump administration of feeding products, and administration of free water and flushes. Avoid the administration of crushed medications to prevent occlusion.
- Provide patient teaching for vitamins (see Box 35.2), minerals and electrolytes (see Box 35.3), and nutritional products (see Box 35.4).

Evaluation
- Observe undernourished patients for quantity and quality of nutrient intake, weight gain, and improvement in laboratory tests of nutritional status (e.g., serum electrolytes, glucose, and proteins).
- Observe children for quantity and quality of food intake and appropriate increases in height and weight.
- Interview and observe for signs and symptoms of complications of enteral and parenteral nutrition.
- When specific vitamins/minerals/electrolytes are being administered, therapeutically observe for improvement in deficiency or excess states as evidenced by improvement in symptoms and absence of adverse effects.

Visit thePoint® *at* **http://thePoint.lww.com/Frandsen13e** *for answers to NCLEX Success questions (in Appendix A), answers to Clinical Application Case Studies (in Appendix B), and more!*

REFERENCES AND RESOURCES

Assouline, B., Faivre, A., Verissimo, T., Sangla, F., Berchtold, L., Giraud, R., Bendjelid, K., Sgardello, S., Elia, N., Pugin, J., de Seigneux, S., & Legouis, D. (2021). Thiamine, ascorbic acid, and hydrocortisone as a metabolic resuscitation cocktail in sepsis: A meta-analysis of randomized controlled trials with trial sequential analysis. *Critical Care Medicine, 49*(12), 2112–2120.

Dudek, S. G. (2021). *Nutrition essentials for nursing practice* (9th ed.). Wolters Kluwer.

Fujii, T., Salanti, G., Bellitti, A., Bellomo, R., Carr, A., Furukawa, T. A., Luethi, N., Luo, Y., Putzu, A., Sartini, C., Tsujimoto, Y., Udy, A. A., Yanase, F., & Young, P. J. (2022). Effect of adjunctive vitamin C, glucocorticoids, and vitamin B1 on longer term mortality in adults with sepsis or septic shock: A systematic review and a component network meta-analysis. *Intensive Care Medicine, 48*, 16–24.

Hinkle, J. H., Cheever, K. H., & Overbaugh, K. J. (2021). *Brunner & Suddarth's textbook of medical-surgical nursing* (15th ed.). Wolters Kluwer.

Hull, R. D., & Garcia, D. A. (2022). Management of warfarin-associated bleeding or supratherapeutic INR. *UpToDate*.

Mount, D. B. (2022). Treatment and prevention of hyperkalemia in adults. *UpToDate*.

National Academy of Science, Institute of Medicine. (2006). In J. J. Otten, J. P. Hellwig & L. D. Meyers (Eds.), *Daily reference intakes: The essential guide to nutrient requirements.* The National Academies Press.

Norris, T. L. (2019). *Porth's pathophysiology: Concepts of altered health states* (10th ed.). Wolters Kluwer.

Nursing 2021 drug handbook. (2021). Wolters Kluwer.

Pazirandeh, S., & Burns, D. L. (2023). Overview of vitamin K. *UpToDate*.

Pazirandeh, S., Burns, D. L., & Griffin, I. J. (2023). Overview of dietary trace elements. *UpToDate*.

Sato, R., Hasagawa, D., Prasitlumkum, N., Ueoka, M., Nishida, K., Takahashi, K., Nasu, M., & Dugar, S. (2021). Effect of IV high-dose vitamin C on mortality in patients with sepsis: A systematic review and meta-analysis of randomized controlled trials. *Critical Care Medicine, 49*(12), 2121–2130.

Schmidt, G. A., & Clardy, P. F. (2022). Investigational and ineffective therapies of sepsis. *UpToDate*.

Sexton, D. J., & McClain, M. T. (2022). The common cold in adults: Treatment and prevention. *UpToDate*.

Taylor, C., Lynn, P., & Bartlett, J. L. (2019). *Fundamentals of nursing: The art and science of person-centered nursing care* (9th ed.). Wolters Kluwer.

UpToDate. (2022). Drug Information. Lexi-Comp Inc.

CHAPTER 36

Drug Therapy for Weight Management

LEARNING OBJECTIVES

After studying this chapter, you should be able to:

1. Describe the clinical manifestations of obesity.
2. Identify the prototype and describe the action, use, adverse effects, contraindications, and nursing implications for the anorexiants.
3. Identify the prototype and describe the action, use, adverse effects, contraindications, and nursing implications for the lipase inhibitors.
4. Identify the prototype and describe the action, use, adverse effects, contraindications, and nursing implications for the glucagonlike peptide-1 receptor agonists.
5. Identify the prototype and describe the action, use, adverse effects, contraindications, and nursing implications for the miscellaneous drugs used for weight management.
6. Implement the nursing process in the care of patients who are overweight or have obesity.

CLINICAL APPLICATION CASE STUDY

Halli Vargas, age 31 years, has had a weight problem all her life. She has been on any number of diets that have a "yo-yo" effect, with weight loss followed by weight gain. She stands 5 ft 5 in tall and weighs 265 lb. Her nurse practitioner starts her on orlistat and prescribes a consultation with a dietitian.

KEY TERMS

Body mass index (BMI): reflection of weight in relation to height; better indicator than weight alone for determining the fitness level of a person

Obesity: BMI of 30 or more kg/m^2

Overweight: BMI of 25 to 29.9 kg/m^2

INTRODUCTION

Obesity, which affects 42.4% of the adult population in the United States, has reached epidemic proportions (Hales et al., 2020). It is associated with multiple chronic diseases, and its negative impact on morbidity, mortality, healthcare costs, and professional and personal quality of life has been well documented. Excess amounts of any of the dietary nutrients are converted to fat and stored in the body, resulting in extra weight and obesity. Although therapeutic lifestyle changes are the cornerstone of population-based interventions to manage obesity, they are often insufficient in achieving recommended treatment targets. Pharmacologic therapy may be necessary. However, once the agents are discontinued, people may regain weight. The importance of a safe and effective use of drugs coupled with therapeutic lifestyle changes has become critical. This chapter discusses obesity and weight management, specifically focusing on drugs to aid weight loss and maintain desired weight.

OVERVIEW OF WEIGHT MANAGEMENT

A better indicator of weight problems than weight alone, **body mass index (BMI)** reflects weight in relation to height. **Overweight** in adults is defined as a BMI of 25 to 29.9 kg/m^2. **Obesity** in adults is defined as a BMI of 30 or more kg/m^2. The desirable range for BMI is 18.5 to 24.9 kg/m^2, with any values below 18.5 indicating underweight and any values of 25 or greater indicating excessive weight. A large waist circumference (greater than 35 in for females, greater than 40 in for males) is another risk factor for overweight and obesity. Using these definitions, it is projected that 68% of adults in America are overweight and 34% have obesity. In children, being overweight is defined as a BMI at or above the 85th and below the 95th sex-specific percentile using the Centers for Disease Control and Prevention (CDC, 2021) BMI-for-age growth charts. Obesity is defined as a BMI at or above the 95th sex-specific percentile. The cause of excessive weight is thought to involve complex and often overlapping interactions among physiologic, genetic, environmental, psychosocial, and other factors.

Physiologic Factors

In general, increased weight is related to an energy imbalance in which energy intake (food/calorie consumption) exceeds energy expenditure. Total energy expenditure represents the energy expended at rest (i.e., the basal or resting metabolic rate), during physical activity, and during food consumption. When a person ingests food, about 10% of the energy content of that food is expended in the digestion, absorption, and metabolism of nutrients. Foods that contain carbohydrates and proteins stimulate energy expenditure; high-fat foods have little stimulatory effect. The energy required to metabolize and to use food reaches a maximum level about 1 hour after the food is ingested. In addition, males tend to expend more energy than do females because they have proportionally more muscle mass. Energy expenditure usually decreases in older adults of all ages because these groups have less muscle tissue and more adipose tissue. Muscle is more metabolically active (i.e., has higher energy needs and burns more calories) than is adipose tissue.

Excessive weight can result from eating more calories, exercising less, or a combination of the two factors. Consuming an extra 500 calories each day for a week result in 3,500 excess calories or 1 lb of fat. Excess calories are converted to triglycerides and stored in fat cells. With continued intake of excessive calories, fat cells increase in both size and number.

The World Health Organization (2020) has advised that lack of physical activity is one of the leading risk factors for increased mortality, stating that individuals who are insufficiently active increase their risk of death by 20% to 30% compared to people who are sufficiently active. Physical activity reduces health risks, including obesity, diabetes, hypertension, depression, and coronary artery disease. Therapeutic lifestyle changes to reduce sedentary behaviors could increase life expectancy in individuals in all age groups.

Genetic Factors

Various studies indicate that a portion of weight variation within a given environment is genetic in origin. For example, identical twins raised in separate environments often have similar body types. Although genomic studies have found over 50 genes related to obesity, most appear to contribute a very small effect. Only rarely can obesity be attributed to a clear inheritance pattern associated linked to a single gene. Most cases of human obesity result mainly from the combination of genetic susceptibility and environmental conditions. Although some people may be genetically predisposed to obesity, it may be possible to counteract a genetic predisposition by making healthy changes in diet, lifestyle, and environment.

Environmental Factors

Environmental factors contributing to the greater number of people who are overweight or have obesity include increased food consumption and decreased physical activity. The ready availability and relatively low cost of a wide variety of foods, in addition to large portion sizes and high-calorie foods, promote overeating. In addition, many social gatherings are associated with eating or overeating.

In relation to physical activity, usual activities of daily living for many people, including work-related activities, require relatively little energy expenditure. In addition, few Americans are thought to exercise in the optimal frequency, intensity, or duration to maintain health and prevent excessive weight gain. For both adults and children, increased time watching television, playing video or computer games, and working on computers contribute to less physical activity and are thought to promote weight gain and obesity. In general, however, it is still unknown whether less physical activity leads to obesity or the physical effects of obesity lead to minimal physical activity.

Psychosocial Factors

Psychosocial disorders may be either a cause or an effect of obesity. Although much is still unknown about the psychological aspects of obesity development, depression and/or abuse may play a role. People with obesity often report symptoms of depression, and some people overeat and gain weight during depressive episodes. It may be that obesity and depression commonly occur together and reinforce each other. A person who is depressed is less likely to take the active measures in diet and exercise that are required to lose weight, even if obesity is a prominent factor in the development of depression.

Other Factors

Diseases are rarely a major cause of the development of obesity. However, numerous disease processes may limit a person's ability to engage in calorie-burning physical activity. In addition, numerous prescription medications reportedly cause weight gain in some or most of the patients who take them (Box 36.1).

BOX 36.1 Effects of Selected Medications on Weight

Antidepressants

Selective serotonin reuptake inhibitors, such as fluoxetine (Prozac, Sarafem) and related drugs, may promote weight loss with short-term use. However, with long-term use, they reportedly may cause as much weight gain as tricyclic antidepressants (TCAs) such as amitriptyline. TCAs have long been associated with excessive appetite and weight gain. Mirtazapine (Remeron) and phenelzine (Nardil) are also associated with weight gain. The effects of bupropion (Wellbutrin and Zyban) on weight are unclear from clinical trials. Gain was reported when bupropion was used as a smoking deterrent, but both gain and loss occurred when it was used as an antidepressant. However, anorexia and weight loss occurred at a higher percentage rate than did increased appetite and weight gain.

Antidiabetic Drugs

Alterations in weight have been reported with diabetic drugs causing either weight gain or weight loss. Weight gain is associated with insulin. Other antidiabetic drugs that are associated with an increase in weight are the sulfonylureas, meglitinides, and the glitazones.

Some antidiabetic drugs are not known to affect weight, including metformin, acarbose, dipeptidyl peptidase-4 inhibitors, and miglitol. Almost all patients with type 2 diabetes eventually require insulin; those who are failing on oral agents generally gain a large amount of body fat when switched to insulin therapy. Although the mechanism of weight gain is unknown, it may be related to the chronic hyperinsulinism induced by long-acting insulins and the sulfonylureas (which increase insulin secretion). Less weight is gained when oral drugs are given during the day and an intermediate- or long-acting insulin is injected at bedtime. This strategy is thought to cause less daytime hyperinsulinemia than the more traditional insulin strategies.

For patients with near-normal weight who have diabetes and who require drug therapy, a sulfonylurea may be given. However, for patients with obesity, metformin is usually the initial drug of choice because it does not promote weight gain. Metformin may also be used to treat children aged 10 to 16 years with obesity and diabetes who require drug therapy.

In the noninterventional CREDIT (Cardiovascular Risk Evaluation in people with type 2 Diabetes on Insulin Therapy) study, weight gain at 1 year was associated with a higher A1C at baseline, a higher insulin dose at baseline and at 1 year, and a lower baseline BMI.

Antiepileptic Drugs

Weight gain commonly occurs with the use of antiepileptic drugs (AEDs). This has been observed for many years with older drugs (e.g., phenytoin, valproic acid, carbamazepine) and with newer-generation AEDs (e.g., gabapentin, lamotrigine, tiagabine). Mechanisms by which the drugs promote weight gain are unclear but may involve stimulation of appetite and/or a slowed metabolic rate. Consequences of weight gain may include increased risks of diabetes, hypertension, and other physical health problems as well as psychological distress over appearance, especially in children and adolescents.

Antihistamines

Histamine$_1$ (H_1) antagonists (e.g., diphenhydramine, loratadine) reportedly increase appetite and cause weight gain.

Antihypertensive Agents

The main antihypertensive drugs reported to cause weight gain are the beta-adrenergic blockers. The drugs can cause fatigue and decrease exercise tolerance and metabolic rate, all of which may contribute to weight gain. Other mechanisms may also be involved. As a result, some clinicians question the use of beta-adrenergic blockers in patients who are overweight or have obesity with uncomplicated hypertension. Alpha-blockers may also cause weight gain but apparently at a low incidence. Angiotensin-converting enzyme (ACE) inhibitors and calcium channel blockers are not reported to promote weight gain.

Antipsychotic Agents

Weight gain is often reported and extensively documented with antipsychotic drugs. Although the exact mechanism is unknown, weight gain has been associated with antihistaminic effects, anticholinergic effects, and blockade of serotonin receptors. In addition, dietary factors and activity levels may also play significant roles.

Clozapine and olanzapine reportedly cause significant weight gain in 40% or more of patients. Compared with clozapine and olanzapine, risperidone causes less weight gain, and quetiapine and ziprasidone cause the least weight gain. Weight gain may lead to nonadherence with drug therapy. In addition to weight gain, clozapine and olanzapine adversely affect glucose regulation and can aggravate preexisting diabetes or cause new-onset diabetes. The extent to which these effects are related to weight gain is unknown. For patients with obesity who have diabetes, or are at risk for developing diabetes, an antipsychotic drug that causes less weight gain would seem the better choice.

Cholesterol-Lowering Agents

Weight gain has been reported with the statin group of drugs; mechanisms and extent are unknown.

Corticosteroids

Systemic corticosteroids may cause increased appetite, weight gain, central obesity, and retention of sodium and fluid. Inhaled and intranasal corticosteroids have little effect on weight.

Gastrointestinal Drugs

Increased appetite and weight gain have been reported with the proton pump inhibitors such as omeprazole and others. The mechanisms and extent are unknown.

Hormonal Contraceptives

The weight gain associated with using hormonal contraceptives may be related more to retention of fluid and sodium than to increased body fat.

Mood-Stabilizing Agent

Weight gain has been reported with long-term use of lithium, with approximately 20% of patients gaining 10 kg (22 lb) or more. This increased weight is attributed to fluid retention, consumption of high-calorie beverages as a result of increased thirst, or a decreased metabolic rate. Weight gain is a common reason for nonadherence with lithium therapy, and weight gain may be more common in females with lithium-induced hypothyroidism and in those who are already overweight.

Age Considerations

Children Who Are Overweight or Have Obesity

In the United States, childhood obesity is reaching epidemic proportions. In 2017–2018, the prevalence of obesity was 19.3% for children and adolescents, aged 2 to 19 years (Fryar et al., 2020). Specifically, the prevalence of obesity was 13.4% among 2- to 5-year-olds, 20.3% among 6- to 11-year-olds, and 21.2% among 12- to 19-year-olds. Childhood obesity is a major public health concern because children with obesity have or are at risk for developing hypertension, dyslipidemias, type 2 diabetes, and other disorders that may lead to reduced quality of life, major disability, and death at younger adult ages than children without obesity. Obesity, type 2 diabetes, and other health problems are mainly attributed to poor eating habits and too little exercise. In addition, the child with obesity after 6 years of age is highly likely to have obesity as an adult and develop obesity-related health problems, especially if a parent has obesity. Obesity in adults that began in childhood tends to be more severe.

Under pressure from parents and advocates to prevent obesity in youth, many school districts have banned soft drinks, candy, and junk foods from school vending machines and cafeterias. The American Beverage Association has agreed to a voluntary ban on the sale of all high-calorie drinks and all beverages in containers larger than 8, 10, and 12 oz in elementary, middle, and high schools, respectively. Several governmental initiatives to combat childhood obesity are available, such as the Supplemental Nutrition Assistance Program (SNAP), the Special Supplemental Nutrition program for Women, Infants, and Children (WIC), and the National School Lunch Program and School Breakfast.

In children, treatment of obesity should focus on healthy eating and increasing physical activity. In general, children should not be put on "diets." For a child who is overweight, the recommended goal is to maintain weight or slow the rate of weight gain so that weight and BMI gradually decline as the child's height increases. If the child has already reached their anticipated adult weight, maintenance of that weight and prevention of additional gain should be the long-term treatment goal. If the child already exceeds their optimal adult weight, the goal of treatment should be a slow weight loss of 10 to 12 lb per year until this weight is reached. As with adults, increased activity is necessary for successful weight loss or management in children. It is possible to implement these measures successfully mainly within a family unit, and family support to assist the child in weight control and a more healthful lifestyle is necessary. In addition, schools should teach children the basic principles of good nutrition and why eating a balanced diet is important to health.

Older Adults Who Are Overweight or Have Obesity

Data from the National Health and Nutrition Examination Survey (NHANES) study for 2017–2018 showed that the age-adjusted prevalence of obesity among older adults aged 60 years and over was 42.8% (Hales et al., 2020). Compared to younger adults, older adults are at greater risk of chronic diseases such as cardiovascular disease, cancer, and osteoporosis; obesity is a major contributor to increased disability and reduced quality of life in later years. In addition, the development of type 2 diabetes remains a risk.

Older adults often enter this life period with excess body weight, less than ideal dietary practices, and less physical activity. Changes in metabolism and absorption of nutrients, age-related loss of bone and muscle mass, and other changes affect nutritional status and the risk of obesity. Excess weight reduces the loss of bone mass, and older adults who are overweight are less likely to suffer hip fractures, a major cause of morbidity and mortality; however, health risks of obesity are greater than any advantages (Box 36.2).

BOX 36.2 Health Risks of Obesity

Obesity is associated with serious health risks. Several disease states and chronic health problems are more prevalent in patients with obesity, as well as increased mortality. Studies indicate that a high body mass index (BMI) is associated with an increased risk of death from all causes, among both males and females, and in all age groups. In addition, a higher death rate occurs in people who gain weight of 10 kg or more after 18 years of age. Some of the major health risks include the disorders listed below. In general, these conditions tend to worsen as the degree of obesity increases and improve with weight loss.

Cancer

Obesity is associated with a higher prevalence of breast, colon, and endometrial cancers. With breast cancer, risks increase in postmenopausal females with increasing body weight. Females who gain more than 20 lb from age 18 to midlife have double the risk of breast cancer compared with those who maintain a stable weight during this period of their life. In addition, central obesity apparently increases the risk of breast cancer independent of overall obesity. In females with central obesity, this additional risk factor may be related to an excess of estrogen (from conversion of androstenedione to estradiol in peripheral fatty tissue) and a deficiency of sex hormone–binding globulin to combine with the estrogen.

Colon cancer seems to be more common in people with obesity. In addition, a high BMI may be a risk factor for a higher mortality rate with colon cancer. Endometrial cancer is clearly more common in females with obesity, with adult weight gain again increasing risk.

Cardiovascular Disorders

Obesity is a major risk factor for cardiovascular disorders and increased mortality from cardiovascular disease. Studies have confirmed the relationship between obesity and increased risk of coronary heart disease (CHD) and stroke in both males and females. In addition, obesity during adolescence is associated with higher rates and greater severity of cardiovascular disease as adults.

Obesity increases risks by aggravating other risk factors such as hypertension, insulin resistance, low high-density lipoprotein (HDL) cholesterol, and hypertriglyceridemia. In addition, obesity seems to be an independent risk factor for cardiovascular disorders, and central obesity may be more important than BMI as a risk factor for death from cardiovascular disease. The increased mortality rate is seen even with modest excess body weight.

BOX 36.2 Health Risks of Obesity (Continued)

Hypertension, dyslipidemia, insulin resistance, and glucose intolerance are known cardiac risk factors that tend to cluster in people with obesity. Hypertension often occurs in people with obesity and is thought to play a major role in the increased incidence of cardiovascular disease and stroke observed in patients with obesity. Metabolic abnormalities that occur with obesity and type 2 diabetes (e.g., insulin resistance and the resultant hyperinsulinemia) aggravate hypertension and increase cardiovascular risks. The combination of obesity and hypertension is associated with cardiac changes (e.g., thickening of the ventricular wall, ischemia, and increased heart volume) that lead to heart failure more rapidly. Weight loss of as little as 4.5 kg (10 lb) can decrease blood pressure and cardiovascular risk in many people with obesity and hypertension.

Diabetes

Obesity is strongly associated with impaired glucose tolerance, insulin resistance, and diabetes. In addition, obesity during adolescence is associated with higher rates of diabetes as adults as well as more severe complications of diabetes at younger ages.

The cellular effects by which obesity causes insulin resistance are unknown. Proposed mechanisms include down-regulation of insulin receptors, abnormal postreceptor signals, and others. Whatever the mechanism, the impaired insulin response stimulates the pancreatic beta cells to increase insulin secretion, resulting in a relative excess of insulin called hyperinsulinemia, and causes impaired lipid metabolism (increased low-density lipoprotein [LDL] cholesterol and triglycerides and decreased HDL cholesterol). These metabolic changes increase hypertension and other risk factors for cardiovascular disease. As with cardiovascular disease and diabetes in general, central obesity seems to increase the likelihood of serious disease. The abdominal fat of central obesity seems to be more insulin resistant than peripheral fat deposited over the buttocks and legs. Intentional weight loss significantly reduces mortality in people with diabetes and obesity.

Dyslipidemias

Obesity strongly contributes to abnormal and undesirable changes in lipid metabolism (e.g., increased triglycerides and LDL cholesterol; decreased HDL cholesterol) that increase risks of cardiovascular disease and other health problems.

Gallstones

Obesity apparently increases the risk of developing gallstones by altering production and metabolism of cholesterol and bile. The risk is higher in females, especially those who have had multiple pregnancies or who are taking oral contraceptives. However, rapid weight loss with very-low-calorie diets is also associated with gallstones.

Metabolic Syndrome

Metabolic syndrome is a group of risk factors and chronic conditions that occur together and greatly increase the risks of diabetes, serious cardiovascular disease, and death. The syndrome is thought to be highly prevalent in the United States. Major characteristics include many of the health problems associated with obesity (e.g., dyslipidemias, hypertension, impaired glucose tolerance, insulin resistance, central obesity). More specifically, metabolic syndrome includes three or more of the following abnormalities:

- Central obesity (waist circumference over 40 in for males and over 35 in for females)
- Serum triglycerides of 150 mg/dL or more or taking medication for high triglycerides
- HDL cholesterol below 40 mg/dL in males and below 50 mg/dL in females or taking medication for low HDL cholesterol
- Blood pressure of 135/85 mm Hg or higher or taking medication for hypertension
- Serum glucose of 110 mg/dL or higher or taking medication for hyperglycemia

Osteoarthritis

Obesity is associated with osteoarthritis (OA) of both weight-bearing joints, such as the hip and knee, and non–weight-bearing joints. Extra weight can stress affected bones and joints, contract muscles that normally stabilize joints, and may alter the metabolism of cartilage, collagen, and bone. In general, people with obesity develop OA of the knees at an earlier age and are more likely than people who maintain a normal weight to require knee replacement surgery.

The important role of obesity in OA is supported by the observation that weight loss delays onset and reduces symptoms and disability. Weight reduction may also decrease infection, wound complications, and blood loss if surgery is required. Despite the benefits of weight loss, however, persons with OA have difficulty losing weight because painful joints limit exercise and activity.

Sleep Apnea

Sleep apnea commonly occurs in persons with obesity. A possible explanation is enlargement of soft tissue in the upper airways that leads to collapse of the upper airways with inspiration during sleep. The obstructed breathing leads to apnea with hypoxemia, hypercarbia, and a stress response. Sleep apnea is associated with increased risks of hypertension, possible right heart failure, and sudden death. Weight loss leads to improvement in sleep apnea.

Miscellaneous Effects

Obesity is associated with numerous difficulties in addition to those described above. These may include the following:

- Nonalcoholic fatty liver disease, which is being increasingly recognized and which may lead to liver failure.
- Poor wound healing.
- Poor antibody response to hepatitis B vaccine.
- A negative perception of people who have obesity that affects their education, socioeconomic, and employment status.
- High costs associated with treatment of the medical conditions caused or aggravated by obesity as well as the costs associated with weight loss efforts.
- In females, obesity is associated with menstrual irregularities, difficulty in becoming pregnant, and increased complications of pregnancy (e.g., gestational diabetes, higher rates of labor induction and cesarean section, and increased risk of neural tube and other congenital defects in offspring of patients with obesity).
- In males, obesity is associated with infertility.
- In children and adolescents, obesity increases risk of bone fractures and muscle and joint pain. Knee pain is commonly reported, and changes in the knee joint make movement and exercise more difficult.

Clinical Manifestations

Common clinical manifestations that characterize overweight and obesity are increased body weight, excess body fat, and a BMI score of 25 kg/m² or greater. Other physical findings include abnormal levels of lipids and lipoproteins, elevated serum levels of insulin, elevated blood pressure, and respiratory difficulties. These metabolic abnormalities place people who are overweight or who have obesity at a significantly higher risk for hypertension, heart disease, diabetes, joint problems, and sleep apnea.

Drug Therapy

The National Heart, Lung, and Blood Institute (NHLBI) of the National Institutes of Health, CDC, and most other organizations generally recommend reserving drug therapy for people with a BMI of 30 or more kg/m² and health problems (e.g., hypertension, dyslipidemia, CHD, type 2 diabetes, sleep apnea) that are likely to improve with weight loss. A loss of 5% to 10% of body weight generally produces a decrease in blood pressure and improved serum lipid concentrations, increased insulin sensitivity, and reduced hyperglycemia, and it may also reduce any related mortality. Drug therapy for obesity should be part of a weight management program that also includes a sensible diet, physical activity, and behavioral modification, and it should be considered only after targeted lifestyle changes fail to achieve therapeutic target weight. A drug may produce adverse effects that can decrease overall benefit. The NHLBI clinical guidelines focus on the identification, evaluation, and treatment of obesity. These guidelines, outlined in Box 36.3, emphasize that drug therapy should be used to decrease medical risk and improve health rather than promote cosmetic weight loss.

Drug therapy for obesity has had a problematic history, mainly because of a series of previous safety-related failures, serious adverse effects, and rapid weight regain when the drugs were stopped. The U.S. Food and Drug Administration

---

BOX 36.3 — **National Heart, Lung, and Blood Institute (NHLBI) Report: Clinical Guidelines on the Identification, Evaluation, and Treatment of Overweight and Obesity in Adults**

- Weight loss reduces health problems. People should decrease blood pressure if they are hypertensive; lower elevated levels of total cholesterol, low-density lipoprotein cholesterol, and triglycerides and raise low levels of high-density lipoprotein cholesterol if they are dyslipidemic; lower elevated blood glucose levels if they have type 2 diabetes.
- Body mass index is used to assess overweight and obesity and to estimate disease risks. Measure waist circumference initially and periodically to assess abdominal fat content. Weigh regularly to monitor body weight.
- The initial goal of weight loss therapy should be to reduce body weight by about 10% from baseline, at a rate of 1 to 2 lb per week for a period of 6 months. Steady weight loss over a longer period reduces fat stores in the body, limits the loss of vital protein tissues, and avoids the sharp decline in metabolic rate that accompanies rapid weight loss. After weight loss, weight maintenance should be the priority goal, because weight regain is a problem with all weight loss programs. In some cases, after a period of weight maintenance, additional losses may be desirable.
- Dietary recommendations include low-calorie diets for weight loss, mainly reducing caloric intake by 500 to 1,000 calories daily. Reducing dietary fat can reduce calories. However, reducing dietary fat without reducing total caloric intake does not produce weight loss. Vitamin and mineral supplements that meet age-related requirements are usually recommended with weight loss programs that provide less than 1,200 kcal for females or 1,800 kcal for males.
- Physical activity recommendations should be part of any weight management program because physical activity contributes to weight loss, may decrease abdominal fat, increases cardiorespiratory fitness, and helps with weight maintenance. Initially, physical activity for 30 to 45 minutes, 3 to 5 days a week, is encouraged. On long term, adults should try to accumulate at least 30 minutes or more of moderate-intensity physical activity on most days of the week.
- In general, weight loss and weight maintenance programs should combine reduced-calorie diets, increased physical activity, and behavior therapy. After weight loss, weight loss maintenance with dietary therapy, physical activity, and behavior therapy should be continued indefinitely. Drug therapy can also be used. However, drug safety and efficacy beyond 1 to 2 years of total treatment have not been established.
- Behavioral modification can be helpful in a weight loss program. The goals are to help patients modify their eating, activity, and thinking habits that predispose to obesity. Techniques include identifying triggers that promote overeating and barriers that keep one from adopting a more healthful lifestyle. One strategy is keeping an accurate record of food/calorie intake and physical activity (most people tend to underestimate food intake and overestimate activity). In addition, stress management, stimulus control, and social support are helpful. Patients who eat more when stressed can learn to manage stress more healthfully. Counseling by a behavioral therapist may be needed. Stimulus control has to do with avoiding or minimizing circumstances that promote overeating (e.g., cooking calorie-dense foods; having high-calorie snacks and "junk food" readily available; eating high-fat, high-calorie foods at fast-food restaurants). Social support involves family, friends, coworkers, and fellow dieters who encourage weight loss efforts rather than sabotage them by urging one to eat high-calorie foods. In general, weight loss regimens that use several of these strategies are more effective.

Reprinted from NHLBI Obesity Education Initiative Expert Panel on the Identification, Evaluation, and Treatment of Obesity in Adults (US). (1998). *Clinical guidelines on the identification, evaluation, and treatment of overweight and obesity in adults: The evidence report.* National Heart, Lung, and Blood Institute.

TABLE 36.1

Drugs Administered for Weight Management

Drug Class	Prototype	Other Drugs in the Class
Noradrenergic sympathomimetic anorexiants	Phentermine hydrochloride	Benzphetamine Diethylpropion Phendimetrazine (Bontril PDM) Phentermine–topiramate (Qsymia)
Lipase inhibitors	Orlistat (Xenical, Alli)	
Glucagonlike peptide-1 receptor agonists	Liraglutide (Saxenda, Victoza)	Semaglutide (Ozempic, Rybelsus)
Miscellaneous agents		Bupropion–naltrexone (Contrave)

(FDA) took or requested manufacturers to remove some drugs (fenfluramine, dexfenfluramine, phenylpropanolamine, sibutramine, and lorcaserin) and some components of many over-the-counter and herbal weight loss products (ephedra and ma huang) off the market because of their adverse effects. Currently, several drugs in various classes have received approval for short- and long-term use in weight the management and treatment of obesity, including the noradrenergic sympathomimetic anorexiants (appetite suppressants), lipase inhibitors, glucagonlike peptide-1 (GLP-1) receptor agonists, and miscellaneous agents (e.g., bupropion–naltrexone). See Table 36.1 for a list of these agents.

NORADRENERGIC SYMPATHOMIMETIC ANOREXIANTS

These adrenergic drugs (see Chapter 29) stimulate the release of norepinephrine and dopamine in the brain; this action in nerve terminals of the hypothalamic feeding center suppresses appetite. FDA approved for short-term use for weight loss, these agents include benzphetamine (Schedule III), diethylpropion (Schedule IV), phendimetrazine (Schedule III), and phentermine (Schedule IV). **Phentermine**, the most frequently prescribed noradrenergic sympathomimetic anorexiant, is the prototype.

Pharmacokinetics

Phentermine is well absorbed orally, metabolized by the liver, and primarily excreted by the kidneys. Time to peak activity is 3 to 4.4 hours, and the half-life elimination is about 20 hours. Under acidic urinary conditions, the half-life is decreased.

Action

Experts believe that phentermine inhibits the reuptake of both serotonin and norepinephrine. The drug causes appetite suppression, which is thought to result from direct stimulation of the satiety center in the hypothalamic and limbic region. As a sympathomimetic amine, the drug has pharmacologic activity similar to the amphetamines.

Use

Phentermine is used to speed weight loss in people who are overweight. The drug is recommended only for short-term use (3 months or less). Combination with a healthy diet and exercise is important. Table 36.2 presents route and dosage information for phentermine and other noradrenergic sympathomimetic anorexiants.

TABLE 36.2

DRUGS AT A GLANCE: Noradrenergic Sympathomimetic Anorexiants (in Adults Unless Specified)

Drug	Route and Dosage Ranges
Phentermine hydrochloride (Adipex-P)	Immediate release: 15–37.5 mg daily or divided twice daily Orally disintegrating tablet: 15–37.5 mg once daily in the morning Adolescents ≥16 y, same as adult dosage
Benzphetamine	Initial: 25 mg once daily; may titrate up to 25–50 mg 1–3 times daily. Maximum dose: 50 mg three times daily
Diethylpropion	Immediate release: 25 mg three times daily before meals Controlled release: 75 mg every morning
Phendimetrazine (Bontril PDM)	Immediate release: 17.5–35 mg 2 or 3 times daily, 1 h before meals. Maximum dose: 70 mg three times daily Sustained release: 105 mg daily in the morning
Phentermine–topiramate (Qsymia)	Initial: 3.75 mg phentermine/23 mg topiramate once daily in the morning for 14 d; then titrate; based on response: 7.5 mg phentermine/46 mg, topiramate daily for 12 wk, then 11.25 mg phentermine/69 mg topiramate daily for 14 d. Maximum dose: 15 mg phentermine/92 mg topiramate daily; reevaluate after 12 wk

Patient-related variables specific to the use of phentermine include the following:

- Age:
  - Phentermine may be useful in adolescents older than 16 years of age who are overweight or who have obesity and may have complications of obesity.
  - Further research into the effectiveness and safety of phentermine in adolescents is needed.
  - Phentermine should not be used in adolescents under 16 years of age.
  - In older adults, anorexiant drugs, including phentermine, should be used very cautiously, if at all.
  - Older adults often have concurrent chronic diseases that increase the risk and seriousness of adverse drug effects.
- Reproduction, pregnancy, and lactation:
  - Drugs for weight loss are not recommended prior to pregnancy due to safety issues and adverse events.
  - Weight loss medications should be discontinued prior to conception.
  - Due to safety concerns, the use of phentermine is contraindicated in breast-feeding patients.
- Abnormal kidney function and hepatic impairment:
  - Clearance of phentermine may be decreased in patients with abnormal kidney function, resulting in an increased risk of toxicity.
  - Limited information is available about the use of phentermine in people with hepatic impairment.

Adverse Effects

The most reported adverse effects with phentermine are nervousness, palpitations, tachycardia, primary pulmonary hypertension, hyperactivity, dry mouth, constipation, and systemic hypertension. Impotence, insomnia, and unpleasant taste may also occur. Tolerance to the drug may occur in as little as 4 to 6 weeks and is an indication for discontinuing the drug. Continued administration or use of large doses does not maintain appetite-suppressant effects. Instead, it increases the incidence of adverse effects.

> **Quality and Safety Alert: Safety**
>
> The nurse should emphasize to patients that phentermine may be habit forming and should be used only as prescribed. There may be an increased risk of drowsiness, so people who take phentermine should not drive a car or operate heavy machinery until they know how the drug affects them.

Contraindications

Contraindications to phentermine use include moderate to severe hypertension, cardiovascular disease, hyperthyroidism, glaucoma, pregnancy, or breast-feeding and a history of drug abuse. Caution is warranted in anxiety or agitation because the drug may have central nervous system (CNS)-stimulating effects. The drug is contraindicated within 14 days of treatment with a monoamine oxidase inhibitor.

Nursing Implications

Preventing Interactions

Several drugs interact with phentermine, increasing or decreasing its effect (Box 36.4). It is important to note that

---

BOX 36.4 Drug Interactions: Phentermine

Drugs That Increase the Effects of Phentermine
- Other tricyclic antidepressants, linezolid
  Increase hypertensive effects
- Other central nervous system stimulants, including alcohol
  Have additive stimulant effects
- Other sympathomimetic drugs (e.g., epinephrine)
  Have additive hypertensive and other cardiovascular effects

Drugs That Decrease the Effects of Phentermine
- Gastrointestinal acidifying agents, methenamine, multivitamins with minerals, urinary acidifying agents
  May decrease serum concentration of phentermine

---

people with diabetes may require increased doses of insulin while taking phentermine because the drug produces effects similar to those caused by stimulating the sympathetic nervous system.

No herbal interactions have been identified.

Administering the Medication

It is necessary to give sustained-release capsules before breakfast or at least 10 to 14 hours before bedtime and instruct patients to swallow the capsule whole and not chew, crush, or open them. Recipients should take immediate-release multiple-dose preparations 30 minutes before meals, with the last dose of the day about 6 hours before going to bed to avoid the possibility of insomnia.

Assessing for Therapeutic Effects

The nurse assesses for the recommended rate of weight loss (1 to 2 lb weekly), minimal adverse effects, and use with a healthy diet and exercise routine.

Assessing for Adverse Effects

The nurse assesses for elevated blood pressure, increased nervousness, hyperactivity, insomnia, or symptoms of dry mouth or constipation.

Patient Teaching

Box 36.5 lists patient teaching guidelines for drugs used in weight management.

NCLEX Success

1. Phentermine aids weight loss by doing which of the following?
    - A. decreasing appetite
    - B. increasing satiety and feelings of fullness
    - C. increasing metabolism
    - D. decreasing absorption of dietary fat

BOX 36.5 Patient Teaching Guidelines for Weight Management and Drugs That Aid Weight Loss

General Considerations

- Because of the extensive health problems associated with overweight and obesity, if your weight is within a normal range, you should try to prevent excessive weight gain by practicing a healthful lifestyle in terms of diet and exercise. You should try to:
  - Manage your weight by balancing calorie intake with physical activity
  - Increase your intake of fruits, vegetables, low-fat and fat-free dairy products, whole grains, and seafood
  - Limit your intake of sodium, saturated and trans fats, cholesterol, refined grains, and foods with added sugars
  - Spread your intake of daily fat, carbohydrate, and protein over three meals
- Further recommendations from the Dietary Guidelines for Americans 2020–2025, published by the U.S. Department of Health and Human Services and the Department of Agriculture in December 2020 (updated every 5 years), are available online at http://www.healthierus.gov/dietaryguidelines.

Self-Administration

- Avoid caffeine.
- Take appetite suppressants in the morning to decrease appetite during the day and avoid interference with sleep at night.
- Do not crush or chew sustained-release products.
- With phentermine, monitor your blood pressure. As body weight decreases, blood pressure usually decreases.
- With liraglutide and semaglutide, allow the drug to warm at room temperature before injecting. Do not use the pen if the drug has changed color, looks cloudy, or has particles in it. Pen-sharing poses a risk for infection.
- With orlistat (Xenical, Alli):
  - Take one capsule with each main meal or up to 1 hour after a meal, up to three capsules daily. If you miss a meal or eat a meal with no fat, you may omit a dose of orlistat.
  - Take a multivitamin containing fat-soluble vitamins (A, D, E, and K) daily, at least 2 hours before or after taking orlistat. Orlistat prevents absorption of fat-soluble vitamins from food or multivitamin preparations if taken at the same time.
- Take the drug with a full glass of water.

---

2. A 42-year-old patient is more than 40 lb overweight and has a 14-year history of type 1 diabetes. The patient is placed on phentermine and has been taking it for the last 8 weeks. The latest serum glycosylated (A1C) hemoglobin levels have risen to 9% even though the patient has maintained a healthy diet and routine exercise program. Phentermine may cause an elevation of A1C levels by doing which of the following?

   A. producing stimulant effects to the sympathetic nervous system
   B. decreasing the level of fat-soluble vitamins
   C. decreasing metabolism to the pancreas
   D. increasing the absorption of dietary fat

Other Drugs in the Class

The FDA has approved a phentermine–topiramate combination (Qsymia), a Schedule IV drug because of the phentermine, for long-term use in weight management. (Topiramate is an AED.) Both drugs affect appetite suppression and satiety enhancement through a combination of mechanisms. In clinical trials, researchers showed that phentermine–topiramate enhanced weight loss in the first year of use compared to a placebo. This combination drug must be used with caution in patients with CHD or hypertension. An increased risk of cleft lip with or without cleft palate has been reported with first trimester exposure to topiramate during pregnancy. In addition, breast-feeding is not recommended due to the potential for adverse effects in the breast-fed infant (e.g., hypertension, tremor, irritability, sleep changes, weight loss).

Other approved noradrenergic sympathomimetic drugs are benzphetamine, diethylpropion, and phendimetrazine. Their mechanisms of action in reducing appetite appear to be secondary to CNS effects, including stimulation of the hypothalamus to release norepinephrine. Diethylpropion is also structurally similar to bupropion. Adverse effects include increases in heart rate, blood pressure, dry mouth, constipation, nervousness, and insomnia. The drugs may counteract the effects of blood pressure medications, so those with hypertension should be observed carefully. As with other weight loss preparations, use during pregnancy is not recommended. In addition, to general concerns, animal reproduction studies suggest that the use of benzphetamine may cause fetal harm. As with phentermine, these drugs are useful on a short-term adjunct in individuals with obesity when diet and exercise have not produced desired results.

LIPASE INHIBITORS

Orlistat (Xenical, Alli), the only FDA-approved weight loss drug available without a prescription, is the prototype lipase inhibitor. A reversible inhibitor of gastric and pancreatic lipases, it slows absorption of dietary fats. Decreased fat absorption leads to decreased caloric intake, resulting in weight loss and improved serum cholesterol values (e.g., decreased total and LDL cholesterol levels). The improvement in cholesterol levels is thought to be independent of weight loss effects.

Pharmacokinetics

Orlistat is not absorbed systemically; it works in the gastrointestinal (GI) tract. Its half-life is 1 to 2 hours. Nearly the entire medication is excreted in feces, 83% as unchanged drug.

Action

Orlistat binds to gastric and pancreatic lipases in the GI tract, and it can prevent the absorption of 30% of ingested fat. Triglycerides, cholesterol, and fat-soluble vitamins from fat-containing foods pass through the intestines unchanged and are not absorbed. Increasing the dose does not increase the percentage.

Use

Orlistat is intended for people identified as clinically obese, not for those who want to lose a few pounds. It is still necessary to decrease consumption of high-fat foods because total caloric intake is a major determinant of weight, and adverse effects (e.g., diarrhea; fatty, malodorous stools) worsen with consumption of a large amount of fat.

The effects of long-term orlistat use are unknown. In addition to weight loss and reduced cholesterol levels, clinical trials found that orlistat results in reduced severity and improved management of other health problems associated with obesity, such as diabetes and hypertension. In general, studies have shown that the addition of orlistat therapy to diet and other lifestyle changes produces greater weight loss than addition of a placebo. In some patients with impaired glucose tolerance, weight loss with orlistat and lifestyle changes prevents or delays the occurrence of diabetes. After the medication is stopped, most patients regain weight.

Table 36.3 presents route and dosage information for orlistat.

Patient-related variables specific to the use of orlistat include the following:

- Age:
  - Although experts do not generally recommend drug therapy for the treatment of childhood obesity, the FDA has approved orlistat for use in children aged 12 years and older and considers the drug to be safe and effective for weight reduction in adolescents who are overweight (see Table 36.3).
  - In adolescents who experience periods of growth spurts, BMI is a better indicator of weight loss because it accounts for weight related to growth.
- Reproduction, pregnancy, and lactation:
  - Obesity increases the risk of infertility.
  - Weight loss medications should be discontinued prior to conception.
  - Although orlistat has minimal systemic absorption, weight loss drugs are not recommended for patients who are breast-feeding due to safety concerns.
- Abnormal kidney function and hepatic impairment:
  - Limited information is available about the use of orlistat in people with abnormal kidney function or hepatic impairment.
  - Manufacturer recommendations advise conservative use and lower dosages, because older adults often have decreased Kidney, cardiac, and hepatic function.

Adverse Effects

The main adverse effects of orlistat are GI symptoms: abdominal pain, oily spotting, fecal urgency and incontinence, flatulence with discharge, fatty stools, and increased defecation. These effects occur in almost all users but usually subside after a few weeks of continued drug usage with moderation of fat intake.

In addition, the drug may cause pancreatitis or, rarely, liver dysfunction, including liver failure.

Contraindications

Contraindications to orlistat include known allergy to the drug and chronic malabsorption syndrome or cholestasis.

Nursing Implications

Preventing Interactions

The body does not absorb orlistat, and no reported drug interactions affecting its action have occurred. However, orlistat may slightly reduce plasma concentrations of amiodarone. By partially inhibiting the absorption of dietary fat, the weight management drug may also decrease the plasma concentration of cyclosporine, which is highly lipid soluble; patients should take orlistat and cyclosporine 2 hours apart. Also, orlistat may decrease the serum concentration of levothyroxine; patients should take levothyroxine and orlistat at least 4 hours apart. In addition, concomitant use of orlistat may increase the lipid-lowering effects of pravastatin.

> **Quality and Safety Alert: Safety**
>
> Orlistat may reduce absorption of fat-soluble vitamins. This has implications for monitoring coagulation parameters if orlistat is used in conjunction with warfarin. The liver uses vitamin K to make blood-clotting proteins; therefore, a decrease in vitamin K increases the international normalized ratio and makes it more difficult to manage warfarin therapy.

Administering the Medication

It is necessary to take orlistat during or up to 1 hour after each main meal containing fat. (People may omit dose if a meal is missed or contains no fat.) Because the drug prevents absorption of the fat-soluble vitamins A, D, E, and K, people who take it should also take a multivitamin daily 2 hours before or after orlistat.

TABLE 36.3

DRUGS AT A GLANCE: Lipase Inhibitors

Drug	Route and Dosage Ranges
Ⓟ Orlistat (Xenical, Alli; Xenical)	Adults and children 12 y of age and older, 120 mg PO three times daily with each main meal containing fat, during or up to 1 h after main meal containing fat Over the counter (Alli), 60 mg PO with each main meal containing fat, up to three capsules daily

Assessing for Therapeutic Effects

The nurse monitors weight loss and BMI. Most weight loss occurs in the first 6 months of therapy, but as patients continue to take orlistat, they can maintain the weight reduction. The metabolic improvements of weight loss are very beneficial for people with obesity-related health problems such as diabetes, dyslipidemia, hypertension, and metabolic syndrome.

Assessing for Adverse Effects

The nurse assesses signs of common adverse GI effects (e.g., diarrhea, flatulence) and reduced concentrations of fat-soluble vitamins. To minimize GI effects, the nurse encourages patients to distribute fat calories over the three main meals and to avoid high-fat meals.

Patient Teaching

Box 36.5 presents patient teaching guidelines for orlistat and other drugs used in weight management.

Clinical Application 36.1

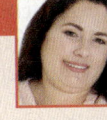

- In addition to proper administration of her medication, what strategies does the nurse review with Ms. Vargas to assist her in being successful with weight loss?
- Ms. Vargas says she needs to lose 140 lb and would like to accomplish this by her next birthday. How does the nurse respond?

GLUCAGONLIKE PEPTIDE-1 RECEPTOR AGONISTS

Some peptides produced in the gut act as key mediators of the gut–brain axis, which is involved in appetite regulation. GLP-1 receptor agonists are a class of drugs that target this pathway and are used in the treatment of type 2 diabetes and obesity. Two GLP-1 receptor agonists have been approved for the treatment of obesity in the United States: **liraglutide** (Victoza, Saxenda), the prototype, and semaglutide (Ozempic). Liraglutide, administered only by subcutaneous injection, is a long-acting analog of endogenous GLP-1 that increases insulin secretion, decreases inappropriate glucagon secretion, increases B-cell growth/replication, and slows gastric emptying. The drug is prescribed for people with type 2 diabetes and is now used under the brand name Saxenda as a treatment for adults who have obesity or are overweight with at least one weight-related comorbid condition. Table 36.4 presents route and dosage information for liraglutide and semaglutide. Additional information related to the role of GLP-1 receptor agonists in the treatment of type 2 diabetes is found in Chapter 41.

Pharmacokinetics

Liraglutide, given subcutaneously, has a bioavailability of about 55% with the time to peak plasma of 8 to 12 hours, with a half-life elimination of about 13 hours. This protracted action enables 24-hour exposure coverage. This action is beneficial for

NCLEX Success

3. Orlistat aids weight loss by doing which of the following?
   A. decreasing appetite
   B. increasing satiety and feelings of fullness
   C. increasing metabolism
   D. decreasing absorption of dietary fat

4. To decrease diarrhea with orlistat, it is important to instruct a patient to do which of the following?
   A. Avoid large amounts of fatty foods.
   B. Drink eight glasses of water daily.
   C. Avoid caffeine-containing beverages.
   D. Increase physical activity.

TABLE 36.4

DRUGS AT A GLANCE: Glucagonlike Peptide-1 Receptor Agonists (in Adults)

Drug	Route and Dosage Ranges
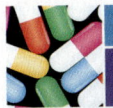Liraglutide (Victoza, Saxenda); 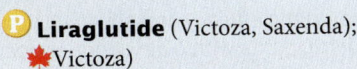Victoza)	Victoza, 0.6 mg subcutaneously daily for 1 wk, increase by 0.6 mg to target of 1.8 mg once daily Initial: Saxenda, 0.6 mg subcutaneously daily for 1 wk, increase by 0.6 mg to target of 3.0 mg once daily
Semaglutide (Ozempic, Rybelsus)	Ozempic initial: 0.25 mg subcutaneously once weekly for 4 wk, then 0.5 mg subcutaneously once weekly for 4 wk, then 1 mg subcutaneously once weekly, 1.7 mg subcutaneously once weekly for 4 wk, then 2.4 mg subcutaneously once weekly starting week 17 and as maintenance dosage Missed doses should be administered as soon as possible within 5 d. If >5 d has lapsed, skip the missed dose, and resume the next scheduled day Rybelsus: 3 mg PO once daily for 30 days and then 7 mg PO once daily, after 14 days dose may be increased to 14 mg PO once daily

glycemic control with once-a-day dosing. Ninety-eight percent of the drug is protein bound. It is excreted as metabolites in the urine and feces.

Action

The drug works in the treatment of obesity by reducing the appetite and feelings of hunger, slowing the release of food from the stomach, and increasing feelings of fullness after eating.

Use

Liraglutide is approved for long-term weight management in adults with BMI of at least 30 or BMI of at least 27 and the presence of weight-related comorbid conditions (i.e., type 2 diabetes, hypertension, high cholesterol, obstructive sleep apnea).

Patient-related variables specific to the use of liraglutide and other GLP-1 receptor agonists include the following:

- Age:
  - In children and adolescents, alternate options for weight loss should be implemented before drug therapy.
  - In children 10 years of age and older, the drug is given for type 2 diabetes.
- Reproduction, pregnancy, and lactation:
  - Liraglutide should not be used for chronic weight loss during pregnancy as the benefits do not justify the potential risk to the fetus.
  - Due to concern for risk to the infant, liraglutide and other GLP-1 receptor agonists are not recommended while breast-feeding.
- Abnormal kidney function and hepatic impairment:
  - Limited data in children with type 2 diabetes show that with mild to severe abnormal kidney function, no dosage adjustment is indicated but the drug should be used with caution.

Adverse Effects

The most common adverse effects associated with liraglutide are diarrhea, nausea, and vomiting. In addition, constipation, abdominal pain, and dyspepsia may also be reported. Acute kidney injury, including acute interstitial nephritis and acute tubular necrosis, has been reported as has gallbladder conditions and hypersensitivity reactions.

Contraindications

Liraglutide should not be used in patients with hypersensitivity to the drug and in those with a history of medullary thyroid cancer or pancreatitis. The FDA has issued a **BOXED WARNING** for use of liraglutide, as the drug has caused thyroid C-cell tumors in rodents, including medullary thyroid carcinoma. Although it is unknown whether the drug causes the development of thyroid C-cell tumors in humans, the drug is contraindicated for patients with a personal or family history of medullary thyroid carcinoma or multiple endocrine neoplasia syndrome type 2.

Nursing Implications

Preventing Interactions

Several drugs interact with liraglutide, increasing or decreasing its effect as an antidiabetic agent. However, no drug or herbal interactions have been identified that affect the drug's effect on weight loss.

Administering the Medication

Liraglutide is administered subcutaneously once daily. If a dose is missed, administer the dose as soon as it is missed. If it is close to the next dose, skip the dose; a double dose should not be administered to make up for a missed one. The safety and effectiveness of liraglutide in combination with other products intended for weight loss have not been established.

Assessing for Therapeutic Effects

The nurse assesses for weight loss, ideally 1 to 2 lb per week, and for healthy lifestyles changes combined with drug therapy to support weight loss goals.

Assessing for Adverse Effects

The nurse assesses for signs of common adverse GI effects (e.g., diarrhea or constipation, nausea, vomiting, dyspepsia). AST and ALT liver enzymes are monitored for elevation of levels above baseline. Persistent severe abdominal pain that may radiate to the back with or without vomiting may be a sign of pancreatitis.

 Quality and Safety Alert: Safety

The FDA identified liraglutide and semaglutide as having the potential to produce drug-induced liver injury; therefore, it is imperative to monitor AST and ALT liver enzyme levels in patients taking these drugs.

Patient Teaching

Box 36.5 presents patient teaching guidelines for liraglutide and semaglutide and other drugs used in weight management.

Other Drugs in the Class

A second drug, semaglutide (Ozempic), shows a similar adverse effect profile as liraglutide and is approved for weight loss in its once-weekly subcutaneous form. The oral form (Rybelsus) is not approved as a weight loss aid but is used to manage blood sugar levels in adults with type 2 diabetes. However, weight loss is an anticipated effect of using Rybelsus.

Quality and Safety Alert: Evidence-Based Practice

Rubino et al. (2022) compared the efficacy and adverse event profiles in two groups of participants with overweight or obesity either receiving once-weekly subcutaneous semaglutide (n = 126) or once-daily subcutaneous liraglutide (n = 127) in addition to counseling for diet and physical activity in the STEP 8 randomized clinical trial. The mean weight change from baseline was −15.8% with semaglutide versus −6.4% with liraglutide at 68 weeks. Gastrointestinal adverse events were reported by 84.1% of participants receiving semaglutide and 82.7% of those receiving liraglutide. Including pharmacologic measures along with counseling regarding lifestyle modifications demonstrated significant weight loss, particularly for those taking semaglutide. Weight reduction can improve risk factors associated with cardiovascular disease.

As with liraglutide, the FDA has issued a BOXED WARNING ◆ for use of semaglutide as the drug has caused thyroid C-cell tumors in rodents, including medullary thyroid carcinoma. Although it is unknown whether semaglutide causes the development of thyroid C-cell tumors in humans, the drug is contraindicated for patients with a personal or family history of medullary thyroid carcinoma or multiple endocrine neoplasia syndrome type 2. Monitoring the drug's effects on pregnancy and infant outcomes is ongoing.

OTHER DRUGS USED FOR WEIGHT MANAGEMENT

Other drugs used for weight management, which have been approved for short-term use, include bupropion–naltrexone (Contrave). Table 36.5 presents route and dosage information for these drugs. Amphetamines were once prescribed, but experts no longer recommend their use. These agents are controlled substances (Schedule II) with a high potential for abuse and dependence (see Chapter 57). Also, they can cause a life-threatening complication in patients who take antidepressants in the form of monoamine oxidase inhibitors (i.e., isocarboxazid, phenelzine).

Bupropion is used for the prevention of weight gain during smoking cessation, as well as for the treatment of depression. It is a relatively weak inhibitor of the neuronal reuptake of dopamine and norepinephrine. Naltrexone is a pure opioid receptor antagonist used to treat alcohol and opioid dependence. Exactly how bupropion–naltrexone leads to weight loss is not fully understood. Effects may result from action on areas of the brain involved in the regulation of food intake, primarily the hypothalamus and the mesolimbic dopamine circuit. The combination is not commonly used as a first-line therapy for weight loss but may be beneficial for an individual with obesity and smokes and desires drug therapy for smoking cessation and obesity.

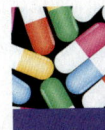

TABLE 36.5

DRUGS AT A GLANCE: Miscellaneous Weight Loss Agents (in Adults Unless Specified)

Drug	Route and Dosage Ranges
Bupropion–naltrexone (Contrave)	Week 1: one tablet (8 mg naltrexone/90 mg bupropion) PO once daily Week 2: one tablet PO twice daily Week 3: two tablets PO in morning and one tablet in evening Week 4: two tablets PO twice daily Maximum daily dose: four tablets (32 mg naltrexone/360 mg bupropion) PO; reevaluate after 12 wk

HERBAL AND DIETARY SUPPLEMENTS USED FOR WEIGHT MANAGEMENT

Many people use herbal or dietary supplements for weight loss, even though reliable evidence of safety and effectiveness is lacking. Some herbal products claim to decrease appetite and increase the rate at which the body burns calories. However, in most cases, there is no scientific evidence that they work at all.

Some supplements for weight loss contain cardiovascular and CNS stimulants that may cause serious, even life-threatening, adverse effects. For example, bitter orange exhibits a non–dose-related increase in heart rate and blood pressure with administration. In general, many consumers often search for an effortless solution without focusing on the benefits of proven weight management techniques (e.g., appropriate diet and exercise) or the potential risks of taking unproven weight loss products. Box 36.6 contains more information about these herbal and dietary supplements.

BOX 36.6 Selected Herbal and Dietary Supplements Used in Weight Management

- Glucomannan expands on contact with body fluids. It is included in weight loss regimens because of its supposed ability to produce feelings of stomach fullness, thereby causing a person to eat less. It also has a laxative effect. There is little evidence to support its use as a weight loss aid. People with diabetes should not use products containing glucomannan; it may cause hypoglycemia alone and increases hypoglycemic effects of antidiabetic medications.
- Guarana, a major source of commercial caffeine, is a component of weight loss products as well as caffeine-containing soft drinks, "energy" drinks, body-building supplements, smoking cessation products, vitamin supplements, candies, and chewing gums. Caffeine is the active ingredient; the amount varies among products, and it is not possible to determine the caffeine content of any product accurately. Advertisers promote guarana as a substance that decreases appetite and increases energy and mental alertness. Dysrhythmias contraindicate its use. The supplement may aggravate gastroesophageal reflux disease and peptic ulcer disease.
- Adverse effects include diuresis, cardiovascular symptoms (premature ventricular contractions, tachycardia), CNS symptoms (agitation, anxiety, insomnia, seizures, tremors), and GI symptoms (nausea, vomiting, diarrhea). Such effects are more likely to occur with higher doses or concomitant use of guarana and other sources of caffeine. Adverse drug–drug interactions include additive CNS and cardiovascular stimulation with beta-adrenergic agonists (e.g., epinephrine, albuterol and related drugs, pseudoephedrine) and theophylline. In addition, concurrent use of cimetidine, fluoroquinolones, or oral contraceptives may increase or prolong serum caffeine levels and subsequent adverse effects.
- Guar gum is a dietary fiber included in weight loss products because it is presumed to be bulk forming and produces feelings of fullness. It may cause esophageal

(Continued on page 686)

BOX 36.6 Selected Herbal and Dietary Supplements Used in Weight Management (Continued)

or intestinal obstruction if not taken with an adequate amount of water and may interfere with the absorption of other drugs if taken at the same time. In a meta-analysis of 20 clinical trials, the fiber was not effective in weight loss. Adverse effects include nausea, diarrhea, flatulence, and abdominal discomfort.

- Hydroxycitric acid, a citric acid derivative extracted from the garcinia cambogia tree, is one of the most highly marketed commercial weight loss supplements. The supplement is purported to suppress appetite in animals, but no reliable studies indicate its effectiveness in humans. In addition, several dozen cases of liver toxicity and even fulminant hepatic failure in people who were taking products containing garcinia cambogia have been reported.
- Although the antioxidants in green tea are reported to improve metabolism aid the effects of some fat-burning hormones, a meta-analysis of clinical trials comparing green tea preparations in adults who are overweight or who have obesity did not demonstrate that green tea significantly influences or helps maintain weight loss. Green tea contains caffeine (20 to 40 mg/cup) that is less than half the amount in coffee.
- Laxative and diuretic herbs (e.g., aloe, rhubarb root, buckthorn, cascara, senna, parsley, juniper, dandelion leaves) are found in several commercial products. These products cause a significant loss of body fluids and electrolytes, not fat. Adverse effects may include low serum potassium levels, with subsequent cardiac dysrhythmias and other heart problems. In addition, long-term use of laxatives may lead to loss of normal bowel function and the necessity for continued use (i.e., laxative dependency).

Clinical Application 36.2

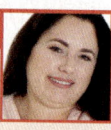

- Ms. Vargas wants to know how orlistat will help her when nothing else in the past has been successful. How does the nurse respond?

Clinical Application 36.3

- Ms. Vargas' prescription is for orlistat three times a day. She takes the drug with breakfast, lunch, and dinner. She often has a meeting that runs through lunch, so she skips lunch but takes her pill on time. At her next clinic appointment, she discusses this with the nurse. How does the nurse respond?

NCLEX Success

5. Drug therapy for weight management may be prescribed for patients with which of the following?

    A. a body mass index (BMI) of 22 kg/m² and a desire to lose 10 lb
    B. a BMI of 24.5 kg/m² and physically fit
    C. a BMI of 30 kg/m² or more with weight-related health problems
    D. a BMI of 25 to 29 kg/m² and healthy

Chapter 36 • Drug Therapy for Weight Management 687

THE NURSING PROCESS

A concept map outlines the nursing process related to drug therapy considerations in this chapter. Additional nursing implications related to the disease process should also be considered in care decisions.

Assessment
- Assess usual drinking and eating patterns, including healthful (e.g., whole-grain breads and cereals, fruits, vegetables, low-fat dairy products) and unhealthful (e.g., sugar-containing beverages and desserts, fried foods, saturated fat, fast foods, high-calorie snack foods) intake. The best way is to ask the patient to keep a food diary for 2 or 3 days. If available, consult a nutritionist to assess a patient's diet and work with the patient to improve health and weight status.
- Assess any patient who is obviously overweight for health problems caused or aggravated by excessive weight (e.g., elevated blood pressure, other cardiovascular problems, diabetes, sleep apnea, osteoarthritis, and other musculoskeletal disorders).
- Calculate the BMI and measure waist circumference.
- Check available reports of laboratory tests. Patients who are overweight may have abnormally high values for total and LDL cholesterol, triglycerides, and blood sugar and low values for HDL cholesterol. If no laboratory reports are available, ask patients if a healthcare provider has ever told them they have high cholesterol or blood sugar.
- List and review all prescription and nonprescription medications the patient is taking and ask about vitamins, herbals, and weight loss supplements.
- Assess motivation for weight loss and usual patterns of physical activity and exercise.

Outcomes of Therapy

The patient will
- Reduce the impact of excessive weight on chronic health problems.
- Modify lifestyle behaviors toward weight loss and weight maintenance at a more healthful level.
- Take weight loss drugs appropriately.
- Avoid unproven weight loss dietary supplements.

Nursing Interventions
- Support programs/efforts to help promote a healthful lifestyle and prevent obesity (e.g., in families and schools).
- Serve as a reliable source of information about weight loss and weight loss drugs and programs.
- For a patient with obesity who reports interest and motivation in losing weight, assist to formulate realistic goals. Losing 5% to 10% of body weight is a reasonable goal and can significantly reduce the medical problems associated with being overweight.
- Assist patients to identify factors that support weight loss efforts (e.g., family and friend encouragement) and factors that sabotage weight loss efforts (e.g., having high-calorie foods readily available, frequently eating at fast-food restaurants).
- Promote exercise and activity. For patients who are overweight or who have obesity, exercise may decrease appetite and distract from eating behaviors as well as increase calorie expenditure.
- Refer patients to a dietitian or nutritionist as indicated.
- Be alert for the psychological consequences of obesity and refer patients for counseling if indicated.
- Instruct patient regarding symptoms of adverse drug effects and effective management of symptoms should they occur.
- Refer children who are overweight or who have obesity to pediatric obesity specialists when possible.
- Provide appropriate teaching related to drug therapy (see Box 36.5).

Evaluation
- Evaluate the safe use of weight loss drugs and the patient's ability to manage any adverse effects.
- Observe patients who are overweight or who have obesity for food intake, weight loss, decreased waist circumference, and appropriate use of exercise.
- Evaluate the patient's perception of level of success in managing weight loss.

Visit **thePoint** at **http://thePoint.lww.com/Frandsen13e** for answers to NCLEX Success questions (in Appendix A), answers to Clinical Application Case Studies (in Appendix B), additional information on etiology and pathophysiology, and more!

REFERENCES AND RESOURCES

Ard, J., Fitch, A., Fruh, S., & Herman, L. (2021). Weight loss and maintenance related to the mechanism of action of glucagon-like peptide 1 receptor agonists. *Advances in Therapy, 38*(6), 2821–2839. https://doi.org/10.1007/s12325-021-01710-0

Centers for Disease Control and Prevention. (2021). *Extended BMI—For age growth charts.* https://www.cdc.gov/growthcharts/Extended-BMI-Charts.html

Centers for Disease Control and Prevention. (2022). *Overweight & obesity.* https://www.cdc.gov/obesity/data/childhood.html

Crescioli, G., Lombardi, N., Bettiol, A., Marconi, E., Risaliti, F., Bertoni, M., Menniti Ippolito, F., Maggini, V., Gallo, E., Firenzuoli, F., & Vannacci, A. (2018). Acute liver injury following Garcinia cambogia weight-loss supplementation: Case series and literature review. *Internal and Emergency Medicine, 13*(6), 857–872. https://doi.org/10.1007/s11739-018-1880-4

Fryar, C. D., Carroll, M. D., & Afful, J. (2020). *Prevalence of overweight, obesity, and severe obesity among children and adolescents aged 2–19 years: United States, 1963–1965 through 2017–2018.* NCHS Health E-Stats.

Hales, C. M., Carroll, M. D., Fryar, C. D., & Ogden, C. L. (2020). *Prevalence of obesity and severe obesity among adults: United States, 2017–2018.* NCHS Data Brief, no 360. National Center for Health Statistics.

Lippincott advisor. (2022). http://advisor.lww.com

Lippincott Williams & Wilkins. (2022). *Nursing 2023 drug handbook* (43rd ed.).

NHLBI Obesity Education Initiative Expert Panel on the Identification, Evaluation, and Treatment of Obesity in Adults (US). (1998). *Clinical guidelines on the identification, evaluation, and treatment of overweight and obesity in adults: The evidence report.* National Heart, Lung, and Blood Institute.

National Heart, Lung, and Blood Institute. (2022). *BMI chart [Measurement instrument].* https://www.nhlbi.nih.gov/health/educational/lose_wt/BMI/bmi_tbl.htm

Perrault, L. (2022). Obesity in adults: Drug therapy. In *UpToDate.* Lexi-Comp, Inc.

Rubino, D. M., Greenway, F. L., Khalid, U., O'Neil, P. M., Rosenstock, J., Sørrig, R., Wadden, T. A., Wizert, A., Garvey, W. T., & STEP 8 Investigators. (2022). Effect of weekly subcutaneous semaglutide vs daily liraglutide on body weight in adults with overweight or obesity without diabetes: The STEP 8 Randomized Clinical Trial. *JAMA, 327*(2), 138.

Sawami, K., Tanaka, A., & Node, K. (2022). Anti-obesity therapy for cardiovascular disease prevention: Potential expected roles of glucagon-like-1 receptor agonists. *Cardiovascular Diabetology, 21*(1), 1–5.

Steirman, B., Afful, J., Carroll, M. D., Chen, T., Davy, O., Fink, S., Fryar, C. D., Gu, Q., Hales, C. M., Hughes, J. P., Ostchega, Y., Storandt, R. J., Akinbami, L. J., & National Center for Health Statistics. (2021). *National Health and Nutrition Examination Survey 2017–March 2020 prepandemic data files development of files and prevalence estimates for selected health outcomes.* NHSR No. 158. http://dx.doi.org/10.15620/cdc:106273

Tucker, R. (2022). *2022 Lippincott pocket drug guide for nurses.* Wolters Kluwer.

U.S. Department of Agriculture and U.S. Department of Health and Human Services. (2020). *Dietary Guidelines for Americans, 2020–2025* (9th ed.). www.DietaryGuidelines.gov

WHO Guidelines on Physical Activity and Sedentary Behaviour. (2020). World Health Organization.

Yanovski, S. Z., & Yanovski, J. A. (2021). Progress in pharmacotherapy for obesity. *JAMA, 326*(2), 129–130. https://doi.org/10.1001/jama.2021.9486

CHAPTER 37

Drug Therapy for Peptic Ulcer Disease and Hyperacidity

LEARNING OBJECTIVES

After studying this chapter, you should be able to:

1. Describe the main characteristics of peptic ulcer disease and gastroesophageal reflux disease.
2. Discuss antacids in terms of the prototype, indications, and contraindications for use, routes of administration, and major adverse effects.
3. Describe histamine$_2$ receptor antagonists in terms of the prototype, indications, and contraindications for use, routes of administration, and major adverse effects.
4. Discuss proton pump inhibitors in terms of the prototype, indications, and contraindications for use, routes of administration, and major adverse effects.
5. Identify the adjuvant medications used to treat peptic ulcer and gastroesophageal reflux disease.
6. Implement the nursing process in the care of patients receiving antacids, proton pump inhibitors, and histamine$_2$ receptor antagonists.

CLINICAL APPLICATION CASE STUDY

Stacy Carpenter, a 54-year-old woman, has been experiencing chronic gastroesophageal reflux disease for several years. Recently, she has been experiencing increasing gastric pain and is concerned that she is also developing a gastric ulcer. Presently, she takes delayed-release omeprazole (Prilosec) 20 mg orally daily, as prescribed. In the past few weeks, she has begun taking three over-the-counter medications: famotidine (Pepcid) 10 mg twice a day as needed to control her heartburn, a combination antacid (Mylanta) 5 mL/dose, and bismuth (Pepto-Bismol) 10 mL. She has had no observable blood in her stools, nor have her stools been discolored. She denies diarrhea or nausea. She does say that the gastric pain feels like someone is "sticking a knife" into her chest. The pain is relieved at times with a change in diet—to what she describes as "bland foods." She has quit drinking milk and limited her intake of other dairy foods because a friend told her these foods were "hard to digest" and made heartburn worse.

KEY TERMS

Achlorhydria: low or absent production of gastric acid in the stomach

Esophagitis: inflammation of the esophagus

Gastritis: acute or chronic inflammation of the gastric mucosa

Helicobacter pylori: gram-negative bacterium found in the gastric mucosa of most patients with chronic gastritis or peptic ulcer disease

Pepsin: proteolytic enzyme that helps digest protein foods

Pyrosis: heartburn

Stress ulcers: gastric mucosal lesions that develop in patients who are critically ill from trauma, shock, hemorrhage, sepsis, burns, acute respiratory distress syndrome, major surgical procedures, or other severe illnesses

INTRODUCTION

Drugs to prevent or treat duodenal and peptic ulcers and acid reflux disorders consist of several groups of agents, most of which alter gastric acid secretion and its effects on the mucosa of the upper gastrointestinal (GI) tract. To aid understanding of drug effects, this chapter presents an overview of both peptic ulcer disease and gastroesophageal reflux disease (GERD) before providing details about specific drugs. For further details on selected upper GI disorders, visit thePoint (http://thePoint.lww.com/Frandsen13e).

OVERVIEW OF PEPTIC ULCER DISEASE AND GERD

Clinical Considerations

Peptic Ulcer Disease

Peptic ulcer disease (PUD) is characterized by ulcer formation in the esophagus, stomach, or duodenum areas of the GI mucosa that are exposed to gastric acid and **pepsin** (proteolytic enzyme that helps digest protein foods). Gastric and duodenal ulcers are more common than esophageal ulcers. Infection with ***Helicobacter pylori*** (gram-negative bacterium found in gastric mucosa) and use of nonsteroidal anti-inflammatory drugs (NSAIDs) account for most cases of PUD.

In addition, stress (e.g., major trauma, severe medical illness) can precipitate ulcer formation. Ulcers are also associated with cigarette smoking. Compared with nonsmokers, smokers are more likely to develop duodenal ulcers, their ulcers heal more slowly with treatment, and the ulcers recur more rapidly.

Cell-protective effects (e.g., secretion of mucus and bicarbonate, dilution of gastric acid by food and secretions, prevention of diffusion of hydrochloric acid from the stomach lumen back into the gastric mucosal lining, the presence of prostaglandin E, alkalinization of gastric secretions by pancreatic juices and bile, perhaps other mechanisms) normally prevent autodigestion of stomach and duodenal tissues and ulcer formation.

Gastroesophageal Reflux Disease

GERD, the most common disorder of the esophagus, is a chronic digestive disease that occurs when stomach acid or, occasionally, bile refluxes into the esophagus. The backwash of acid irritates the lining of the esophagus. The main cause of GERD is thought to be an incompetent lower esophageal sphincter (LES). Several circumstances contribute to impaired contraction of the LES and the resulting reflux, including foods (e.g., fats, chocolate), fluids (e.g., alcohol, caffeinated beverages), medications (e.g., beta-adrenergics, calcium channel blockers, nitrates), gastric distention, cigarette smoking, and recumbent posture.

Clinical Manifestations

Peptic Ulcer Disease

The clinical manifestations of a gastric ulcer are almost opposite to the clinical manifestations of duodenal ulcers; the main differences are the timing and severity of the pain. Gastric ulcers generally cause a dull aching pain, often right after eating. The intake of food does not relieve pain as is the case with a duodenal ulcer. The patient may experience bloating, indigestion, heartburn, or nausea. Gastric ulcers are often manifested by painless bleeding and take longer to heal than do duodenal ulcers. Duodenal ulcers cause heartburn, bloating, severe stomach pain, and a burning sensation at the back of the throat. The symptoms may be worse when the stomach is empty and may flare at night. Typically, the symptoms disappear and then can return.

Gastroesophageal Reflux Disease

Pyrosis (heartburn), which increases with a recumbent position or bending over, is the main symptom of GERD. Effortless regurgitation of acidic fluid into the mouth, especially after a meal and at night, is often indicative. Important protective mechanisms for the esophagus, including gravity, swallowing, and saliva, are effective only when people are upright. At night during sleep in a recumbent position, the effect of gravity is negated, swallowing ceases, and the secretion of saliva is decreased. Consequently, reflux that occurs at night probably results in acid staying in the esophagus longer and causing greater damage. Many people experience both pyrosis and acid reflux from time to time. When they occur regularly, they may be signs of GERD. In addition, there may also be mild-to-severe **esophagitis** (inflammation of the esophagus) or esophageal ulceration. Pain on swallowing usually means erosive or ulcerative esophagitis.

Drug Therapy

Drugs used in the treatment of acid–peptic disorders promote healing of lesions and prevent recurrence of lesions by decreasing cell-destructive effects or increasing cell-protective effects. Several types of drugs are used, alone and in various combinations. Figure 37.1 illustrates the sites of action for drugs used to treat GERD. Antacids neutralize gastric acid and decrease pepsin production, antimicrobials and bismuth can eliminate *H. pylori* infection, histamine$_2$ receptor antagonists (H$_2$RAs) and proton pump inhibitors (PPIs) decrease gastric acid secretion, sucralfate provides a barrier between mucosal erosions or ulcers and gastric secretions, and misoprostol restores prostaglandin activity. The following sections

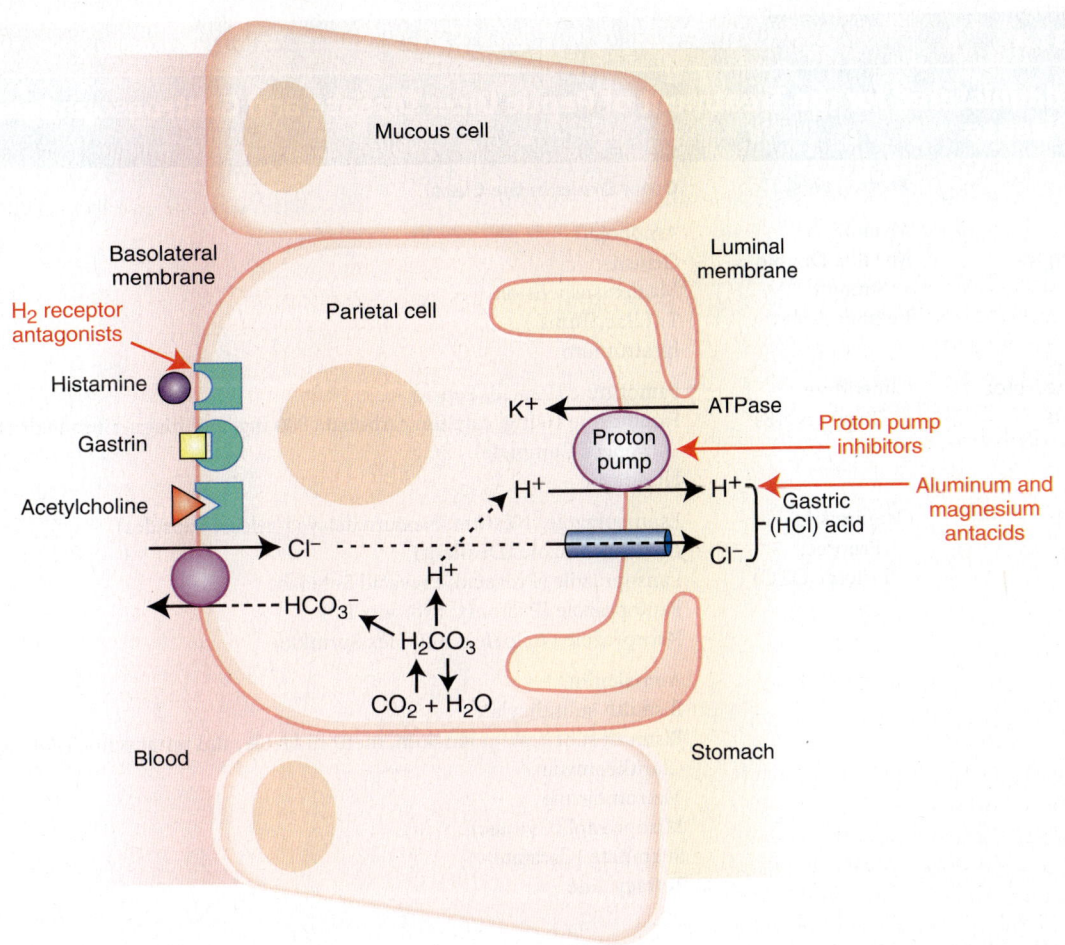

Figure 37.1. Sites of action of drugs for gastroesophageal reflux disease (see *red labels/arrows*). [Adapted with permission from Norris, T. L. (2019). *Porth's pathophysiology: Concepts of altered health states* (10th ed., Fig. 36.10, p. 1066). Wolters Kluwer.]

describe the types of drugs and individual agents. Table 37.1 lists the drugs used for PUD and GERD.

Available drugs are safe and effective.

> **! Quality and Safety Alert: Safety**
>
> Taking some herbal supplements may delay effectiveness of drug therapy and have harmful consequences; therefore, it is important that nurses and other prescribers do not encourage the use of herbs for any acid–peptic disorder and that patients report any concurrent use of supplements.

ANTACIDS

Antacids are oral medicines used to relieve heartburn or acid indigestion by neutralizing excess stomach acid. Although all antacids neutralize gastric acid (50 to 80 mEq of acid is produced hourly), they differ in their ability to neutralize gastric acid, in onset of action, and in adverse effects. Commonly used antacids are mixtures of aluminum, magnesium, and calcium salts and are widely available without a prescription. Antacids may be used to control symptoms and prevent complications of dyspepsia and GERD, but these drugs have been essentially replaced by the effective and cost-effective PPIs and H₂RAs (see later discussion). The magnesium hydroxide–calcium carbonate mixture Ⓟ **Mylanta** is the prototype. In this discussion, the trade name of the drug is used to refer to this antacid. However, since Mylanta does not have a universal formulation, it is important to read the label ingredients as some formulations contain aluminum hydroxide.

Pharmacokinetics and Action

Absorption of Mylanta from the GI tract is minimal. Excretion is in the urine.

As an alkaline substance that neutralizes acids, Mylanta reacts with hydrochloric acid in the stomach to produce neutral, less acidic, or poorly absorbed salts and to raise the pH of gastric secretions. Raising the pH to approximately 3.5 neutralizes more than 90% of gastric acid and inhibits conversion of pepsinogen to pepsin. The antacid has an onset of action of 20 to 60 minutes. In general, aluminum compounds have a low neutralizing capacity (i.e., relatively large doses are required) and a slow onset of action. Magnesium-based antacids have a high neutralizing capacity and a rapid onset of action.

Simethicone, an antiflatulent drug, does not affect gastric acidity. It reportedly decreases gas bubbles, thereby reducing GI distention and abdominal discomfort.

TABLE 37.1

Drugs Administered for the Treatment of Peptic Ulcer Disease and Gastroesophageal Reflux Disease

Drug Class	Prototype(s)	Other Drugs in the Class
Antacids Anticholinergics	Mylanta Mylanta Double Strength Bethanechol	Amphojel Gelusil Maalox suspension Titralac, Tums Ipratropium
Histamine$_2$ receptor antagonists	Cimetidine (Tagamet HB)	Famotidine (Pepcid, Pepcid AC) Famotidine 10 mg, calcium carbonate 800 mg, and magnesium hydroxide 165 mg (Pepcid Complete) Nizatidine
Proton pump inhibitors	Omeprazole (Prilosec, Prilosec OTC)	Esomeprazole (Nexium, Nexium delayed-release capsules) Dexlansoprazole (Dexilant) Lansoprazole (Prevacid, Prevacid SoluTab) Pantoprazole (Protonix, Protonix IV) Rabeprazole (AcipHex, AcipHex Sprinkle)
Adjuvant medications		Amoxicillin Bismuth subsalicylate Bismuth subcitrate potassium, metronidazole, and tetracycline (Pylera) Clarithromycin Metronidazole Misoprostol (Cytotec) Sucralfate (Carafate) Tetracycline

Use

Antacids act primarily in the stomach, and people take them to prevent or treat PUD, GERD, esophagitis, heartburn, **gastritis** (acute or chronic inflammation of the gastric mucosa), GI bleeding, and **stress ulcers**. When pain relief is the goal of treatment, taking antacids on an as-needed basis is usually sufficient. However, it is important not to take them in high doses or for prolonged periods because of potential adverse effects.

Patient-related variables specific to the use of Mylanta and other antacids include the following:

- Age:
  - Ambulatory children may take antacids in doses of 5 to 15 mL every 3 to 6 hours, or after meals, and at bedtime. For prevention of GI bleeding in critically ill children, infants may receive 2 to 5 mL, and children may receive 5 to 15 mL every 1 to 2 hours.
  - Older adults may use all the antiulcer, anti-heartburn drugs. With antacids, smaller doses may be effective because older adults usually secrete less gastric acid than younger adults. Also, with decreased kidney function, older adults are more likely to have adverse effects. Many healthcare providers recommend calcium carbonate antacids (e.g., Tums) as a calcium supplement in older females to prevent or treat osteoporosis.
- Reproduction, pregnancy, and lactation:
  - Antacids are considered first-line therapy for heartburn during pregnancy when lifestyle modifications are inadequate. Most antacids are acceptable during breast-feeding stages; however, those containing sodium bicarbonate are not considered safe due to risks for fluid overload and metabolic alkalosis.
- Abnormal kidney function and hepatic impairment:
  - Patients with kidney failure or with impaired kidney function (creatinine clearance less than 30 mL/min) should not take magnesium-based antacids such as Mylanta because 5% to 10% of the magnesium may be absorbed and accumulate, causing hypermagnesemia. Patients with chronic kidney disease and hyperphosphatemia may take aluminum-based antacids to decrease absorption of phosphates in food. (Aluminum binds with phosphate in the GI tract, preventing phosphate absorption and hyperphosphatemia that commonly occur in kidney failure.) However, aluminum may accumulate in patients with kidney failure, leading to encephalopathy, erythropoietin-resistant anemia, and osteomalacia.
  - Antacids containing calcium carbonate are currently recommended to control phosphate levels in patients with kidney failure with replacement therapy. Antacids with calcium carbonate can cause alkalosis and raise urine pH, and chronic use may cause kidney stones and hypercalcemia.

- Some studies suggest that stomach (gastric) acid suppression alters specific gut bacteria in a way that may promote liver injury and progression of chronic liver disease in at-risk populations.
- Specific healthcare environments:
  - In patients with critical illness, nearly continuous neutralization of gastric acid is desirable to prevent stress ulcers and to treat acute GI bleeding. Dose and frequency of administration must be sufficient to neutralize the gastric acid; a continuous intragastric drip through a nasogastric tube is effective.
  - For patients with a nasogastric tube in place, antacid dosage may be titrated by aspirating stomach contents, determining pH, and then basing the dose on the pH. (Most gastric acid is neutralized, and most pepsin activity is eliminated at a pH above 3.5.)
  - In the home care setting, people commonly take antiulcer, anti-heartburn drugs, usually by self-administration. The home care nurse can assist patients by providing information about taking the drugs correctly and monitoring responses.

Adverse Effects

Calcium compounds may cause hypercalcemia and hypersecretion of gastric acid ("acid rebound") because of stimulation of gastrin release, if large doses are used. Consequently, calcium compounds are rarely used in PUD. Aluminum-containing antacids can cause constipation. Hypophosphatemia and osteomalacia may develop in people who ingest large amounts of aluminum-based antacids over a long period because aluminum combines with phosphates in the GI tract and prevents phosphate absorption. Aluminum compounds are rarely used alone for acid–peptic disorders. Mylanta also contains magnesium. Antacids with magnesium may cause diarrhea and hypermagnesemia. Older adults may experience neuromuscular effects.

Contraindications

People with any signs of appendicitis or inflamed bowel (cramping, soreness, or pain in the lower abdomen) and patients with kidney failure should not take Mylanta.

Nursing Implications

Preventing Interactions

Because antacids are minimally absorbed, few drugs alter their effects. Anticholinergic drugs (e.g., atropine) increase effects by delaying gastric emptying and by decreasing acid secretion themselves. Cholinergic drugs (e.g., pyridostigmine [Mestinon]) decrease effects of antacids by increasing GI motility and rate of gastric emptying. No herbs are known to alter the effects of antacids.

However, antacids may prevent absorption of most drugs taken at the same time, including benzodiazepine antianxiety drugs, corticosteroids, digoxin, H_2RAs (e.g., cimetidine), iron supplements, phenothiazine antipsychotic drugs, phenytoin, fluoroquinolone antibacterials, and tetracyclines. Antacids increase absorption of a few drugs including levodopa, quinidine, and valproic acid. To avoid or minimize these interactions, it is necessary to separate administration times by 1 to 2 hours.

Administering the Medication

Typical prescribing practices with Mylanta and other antacids used to treat active ulcers are to take them 1 and 3 hours after meals and at bedtime for greater acid neutralization. This schedule is effective but inconvenient for many patients.

> **Quality and Safety Alert: Safety**
>
> Liquid antacid preparations must be shaken well before measuring each dose, because these suspensions separate into layers with the medication consolidated at the bottom. Thorough mixing is necessary.

Assessing for Therapeutic Effects

The nurse assesses for decreased epigastric pain in patients with gastric and duodenal ulcers or decreased heartburn in those with GERD. Antacids should relieve pain within a few minutes. Also, it is necessary to assess for decreased GI bleeding (e.g., absence of visible or occult blood in vomitus, gastric secretions, or feces). In addition, the nurse uses pH testing to evaluate the quantity, frequency, and duration of acid reflux episodes, as well as to check the pH of gastric contents. The minimum acceptable pH with antacid therapy is 3.5. Healing usually occurs within 4 to 8 weeks. Finally, the nurse assesses for radiologic or endoscopic reports of ulcer healing.

Assessing for Adverse Effects

With antacids containing magnesium, such as Mylanta, the nurse assesses for diarrhea and hypermagnesemia. The combination of calcium or aluminum may prevent this. Hypermagnesemia may occur in patients with impaired kidney function. With antacids containing only calcium (Titralac, Tums), it is important to observe for constipation. Table 37.2 gives route, dosage, and formulation information for various antacids.

Patient Teaching

Box 37.1 summarizes patient teaching information for antacids.

HISTAMINE$_2$ RECEPTOR ANTAGONISTS

In addition to its other effects, histamine also causes strong stimulation of gastric acid secretion. Vagal stimulation causes release of histamine from cells in the gastric mucosa. The histamine then acts on receptors located on the parietal cells to increase production of hydrochloric acid. These receptors are called the H_2 receptors. Although traditional antihistamines or H_1RAs prevent or reduce other effects of histamine, they do not block histamine effects on gastric acid production.

However, the H_2RAs inhibit both basal secretion of gastric acid and the secretion stimulated by histamine, acetylcholine, and gastrin. **Cimetidine** (Tagamet HB) is the prototype of this class. An over-the-counter (OTC) preparation is available. Prescription forms are also obtainable.

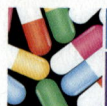

TABLE 37.2 DRUGS AT A GLANCE: Representative Antacid Products

Drug	Components			Route and Dosage Ranges (Adults)
	Magnesium Oxide, Trisilicate or Hydroxide	Aluminum Hydroxide	Other	
ⓟ Mylanta	135 mg/tablet, or 135 mg/5 mL		Calcium carbonate: 400 mg/tablet	5–10 mL or 2–4 chewable tablets PO as needed after meals, at bedtime, or as directed; maximum dose: 10 tablets/day
Mylanta Double Strength	300 mg/tablet		Calcium carbonate: 700 mg/tablet	Chewable tablets: PO 2–4 tablets as needed after meals, at bedtime, or as directed; maximum dose: 8 tablets/day
Gaviscon	14.2 mg/tablet	80 mg/tablet		Chewable tablets: PO 2–4 tablets four times (maximum: 16 tablets in 24 h)
Gelusil	200 mg/tablet or 200 mg/5 mL	200 mg/tablet or 200 mg/5 mL	Simethicone, 25 or 200 mg/5 mL mg/tablet or 20 mg/5 mL	10 or more mL or two or more tablets PO after meals and at bedtime or as directed by physician to a max of 12 tablets or tsp/24 h
Mag-Al	200 mg/5 mL	200 mg/5 mL		10–20 mL PO four times daily, as needed or as directed; max dose, 80 mL/24 h
Titralac, Tums			Calcium carbonate: 750 mg/tablet, 1 g/5 mL (NOTE: one gram of calcium carbonate is equal to 400 mg of elemental calcium	5–10 mL or 1–4 tablets PO after meals as needed or as directed by product labeling or provider to max of 19 tablets or 8 g/24 h as calcium carbonate for up to 2 wk

---

BOX 37.1 — Patient Teaching Guidelines: Drugs Used for Peptic Ulcer Disease and Gastroesophageal Reflux Disease

General Considerations

- These drugs are commonly used to prevent and treat peptic ulcers and heartburn. Peptic ulcers usually form in the stomach or first part of the small bowel (duodenum), where tissues are exposed to stomach acid. Two common causes of peptic ulcer disease are stomach infection with a bacterium called *Helicobacter pylori* and taking nonsteroidal anti-inflammatory drugs (NSAIDs) such as ibuprofen and many others. Heartburn (also called gastroesophageal reflux disease) is caused by stomach acid splashing back onto the esophagus.
- Peptic ulcer disease and heartburn are chronic conditions that are usually managed on an outpatient basis. Complications such as bleeding require hospitalization. Overall, these conditions can range from mild to serious, and it is important to seek information about the disease process, ways to prevent or minimize symptoms, and drug therapy.
- With heartburn, try to minimize acid reflux by elevating the head of the bed; avoiding stomach distention by eating small meals; not lying down for 1 to 2 hours after eating; minimizing intake of fats, chocolate, citric juices, coffee, and alcohol; avoiding smoking (stimulates gastric acid production); and avoiding obesity, constipation, or other conditions that increase intra-abdominal pressure. In addition, take tablets and capsules with 8 oz of water and do not take medications at bedtime unless instructed to do so.
- Most medications for peptic ulcer disease and heartburn decrease stomach acid. An exception is the antibiotics used to treat ulcers caused by *H. pylori* infection. The strongest acid reducers are omeprazole (Prilosec),

BOX 37.1 Patient Teaching Guidelines: Drugs Used for Peptic Ulcer Disease and Gastroesophageal Reflux Disease (Continued)

- dexlansoprazole (Dexilant), esomeprazole (Nexium), lansoprazole (Prevacid), pantoprazole (Protonix), and rabeprazole (AcipHex). Dexlansoprazole, pantoprazole, and rabeprazole are available only by prescription, while the others are approved for nonprescription use. Histamine-blocking drugs such as cimetidine (Tagamet HB), famotidine (Pepcid), and others are available as both prescription and over-the-counter (OTC) preparations. OTC products are indicated for heartburn, and smaller doses are taken than for peptic ulcer disease. These drugs usually should not be taken longer than 2 weeks without the advice of a healthcare provider. (A 2-week treatment with Prilosec OTC can be repeated every 4 months if needed to control heartburn.) The concern is that OTC drugs may delay diagnosis and treatment of potentially serious illness. In addition, cimetidine can increase toxic effects of numerous drugs and should be avoided if you are taking other medications.
- Misoprostol (Cytotec) is given to prevent ulcers from NSAIDs, which are commonly used to relieve pain and inflammation with arthritis and other conditions. This drug should be taken only while taking a traditional NSAID such as ibuprofen. Do not take misoprostol if pregnant and do not become pregnant while taking the drug. If pregnancy occurs during misoprostol therapy, stop the drug and notify your prescriber immediately. Misoprostol can cause abdominal cramps and miscarriage. A related drug, celecoxib (Celebrex), is less likely to cause peptic ulcer disease.
- Numerous antacid preparations are available, but they are not equally safe in all people and should be selected carefully. For example, products that contain magnesium have a laxative effect and may cause diarrhea; those that contain aluminum or calcium may cause constipation (e.g., the antacids Titralac and Tums contain only calcium). Some commonly used antacids (e.g., Gaviscon) are a mixture of magnesium and aluminum preparations, an attempt to avoid both constipation and diarrhea. People with kidney disease should not take products that contain magnesium because magnesium can accumulate in the body and cause serious adverse effects. Thus, it is important to read product labels and, if you have a chronic illness or take other medications, ask your primary provider or pharmacist to help you select an antacid and an appropriate dose.
- All H_2 receptor antagonists (e.g., cimetidine, famotidine) are available by prescription and OTC. When you obtain these drugs with a prescription, avoid concomitant use of OTC versions of the same or similar drugs.

Self- or Caregiver Administration

- Take antiulcer drugs as directed. Underuse decreases therapeutic effectiveness; overuse increases adverse effects. For acute peptic ulcer disease or esophagitis, drugs are given in relatively high doses for 4 to 8 weeks to promote healing. For long-term maintenance therapy, dosage is reduced.
- With omeprazole, rabeprazole sodium, esomeprazole magnesium, and pantoprazole sodium, swallow the capsule whole; do not open, chew, or crush. With Prevacid, the capsule can be opened and the granules sprinkled on applesauce for patients who are unable to swallow capsules. Also, Prevacid granules are available in a packet for preparing a liquid suspension. Follow instructions for mixing the granules exactly. The granules should not be crushed or chewed.
- Take cimetidine with meals or at bedtime. Take famotidine and nizatidine with or without food. Do not take an antacid for 1 hour before or after taking one of these drugs.
- Take sucralfate on an empty stomach at least 1 hour before meals and at bedtime. Also, do not take an antacid for 1 hour before or after taking sucralfate.
- Take misoprostol with food.
- For treatment of peptic ulcer disease, take antacids 1 and 3 hours after meals and at bedtime (4 to 7 doses daily), 1 to 2 hours before or after other medications. Antacids decrease absorption of many medications if taken at the same time. Also, chew chewable tablets thoroughly before swallowing and then drink a glass of water; allow effervescent tablets to dissolve completely and almost stop bubbling before drinking (this increases the surface area of drug available to neutralize gastric acid); and shake liquids well before measuring the dose. A high-fiber diet, adequate fluid intake (2,000 to 3,000 mL daily), and exercise may help prevent constipation if it occurs with Mylanta therapy.
- With Pepcid AC orally disintegrating tablets, open the blister package with dry hands immediately before use, place the tablet on the tongue, and allow the tablet to dissolve with saliva. Taking it with liquids is not necessary.

Pharmacokinetics

After oral administration, absorption is good. Cimetidine is distributed in almost all body tissues. Onset varies. After a single dose, peak blood level is reached in all routes in 1 to 1.5 hours, the half-life is 2 hours, and an effective concentration is maintained for about 6 hours. Onset of the drug after intravenous (IV) and intramuscular (IM) administration is rapid. Metabolism takes place in the liver. Excretion of the unchanged oral dose occurs unchanged in the urine within 24 hours; some excretion takes place in the bile, with elimination in the feces.

Action

Cimetidine inhibits the action of histamine at the H_2 receptors of the stomach, decreasing the amount, acidity, and pepsin content of gastric juices. A single dose can inhibit acid secretion for 6 to 12 hours, and a continuous IV infusion can inhibit secretion for prolonged periods.

Prescribers often advise taking antacids concurrently with H_2RAs such as cimetidine to relieve pain. The pain relief usually occurs after 1 week. Patients should not take the antacid and the H_2RA at the same time (except for Pepcid Complete) because the antacid reduces absorption of the H_2RA.

Use

Indications for use of cimetidine include prevention and treatment of PUD, GERD, esophagitis, GI bleeding due to acute stress ulcers, and Zollinger–Ellison syndrome. With gastric or duodenal ulcers, healing occurs within 6 to 8 weeks; with esophagitis, healing occurs in about 12 weeks. The U.S. Food and Drug Administration (FDA) has approved the OTC preparations for the treatment of heartburn.

Table 37.3 gives route and dosage information for cimetidine and other H_2RAs.

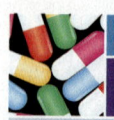

TABLE 37.3
DRUGS AT A GLANCE: Histamine$_2$ Receptor Antagonists

Drug	Routes and Dosage Ranges	
	Adults	**Children**
P Cimetidine (Tagamet HB; ✱ Apo-Cimetidine)	Duodenal or gastric ulcer: PO 800 mg once daily at bedtime or 300 mg four times daily or 400 mg twice daily Maintenance: 400 mg PO at bedtime IV injection, 300 mg diluted in 20 mL of 0.9% NaCl solution every 6–8 h IV intermittent infusion: 300 mg diluted in 50 mL of dextrose or saline solution every 6 h Impaired kidney function (creatinine clearance <30 mL/min): 25 mg/h IV for prevention of GI bleeding; 300 mg PO or IV every 12 h, may increase to every 8 h if tolerated 300 mg IM every 6–8 h GERD: 800 mg PO twice daily or 400 mg four times daily Prevention of upper GI bleeding: 50 mg/h continuous IV infusion Heartburn: 200 mg PO once or twice daily as needed Impaired kidney function: 300 mg PO or IV every 8–12 h	Limited data available Treatment and Maintenance duodenal or gastric ulcer: ≥5 y–<16 y, PO 2 to 40 mg/kg/d in 3–4 divided doses for 4 to 8 wk, followed by 5 to 8 mg/kg/dose once daily at bedtime GERD: <16 y, PO 20 to 40 mg/kg/d ≥16 y, PO 300 mg four times daily or 800 mg at bedtime or 400 mg twice daily for up to 8 wk Zollinger–Ellison syndrome: ≥16 y, PO 300 mg four times daily; adjusted to patient response; maximum daily dose 2,400 mg/d
Famotidine (Pepcid, Pepcid AC; ✱ Apo-famotidine; Teva-famotidine) Famotidine 10 mg, calcium 800 mg, and magnesium hydroxide 165 mg (Pepcid Complete)	Duodenal or gastric ulcer: 40 mg PO or IV once daily at bedtime or 20 mg twice daily for 4–8 wk; maintenance, 20 mg PO or IV once daily at bedtime Zollinger–Ellison syndrome: 20 mg PO every 6 h, increased if necessary IV injection: 20 mg every 12 h, diluted to 5 or 10 mL with 5% dextrose or 0.9% sodium chloride IV infusion: 20 mg every 12 h, diluted with 100 mL of 5% dextrose or 0.9% sodium chloride Impaired kidney function (creatinine clearance <50 mL/min): 20 mg PO or IV every 24–48 h GERD: 20 mg PO twice daily for 6–12 wk Heartburn (Pepcid Complete): 1–2 tablets PO chewed, daily as needed	GERD: <3 mo, 0.5 mg/kg/dose PO daily for 8 wk 3 mo ≤1 y: PO 0.5 mg/kg/dose twice daily, IV famotidine not adequately studied in patients <1 y with GERD Peptic ulcer: 1–16 y, 0.5 mg/kg/d PO at bedtime or divided twice daily up to 40 mg/d GERD with or without esophagitis: 1.0 mg/kg/d PO divided twice daily up to 40 mg twice daily
Nizatidine ✱ Axid, Dom-Nizatidine)	Duodenal or gastric ulcer: 300 mg PO once daily at bedtime or 150 mg PO twice daily; maintenance, 150 mg PO once daily at bedtime GERD: 150 mg PO twice daily Heartburn: 75 mg PO 30–60 min before meals Impaired kidney function (creatinine clearance [CrCl] 20–50 mL/min), 150 mg PO daily; CrCl <20 mL/min, 150 mg PO every 72 h	Limited data available GERD: ≤11 y, 5 mg/kg/dose twice daily; maximum daily dose 300 mg daily ≥12, 150 mg twice daily; maximum daily dose 300 mg daily Esophagitis: ≥6 mo to ≤11 y, 5 mg/kg/dose twice daily ≥12 y, 150 mg twice daily; maximum daily dose: 300 mg daily

GERD, gastroesophageal reflux disease, including erosive esophagitis; GI, gastrointestinal.

Patient-related variables specific to the use of cimetidine and other H₂RAs include the following:

- Age:
  - With cimetidine, older adults are more likely to experience adverse effects, especially confusion, agitation, and disorientation.
- Reproduction, pregnancy, and lactation:
  - Cimetidine is effective and approved for use during pregnancy and lactation.
  - Famotidine and nizatidine are contraindicated during pregnancy due to the risk for congenital anomalies.
  - Of the H₂RAs, cimetidine has the greatest excretion in breast milk.
- Abnormal kidney function and hepatic impairment:
  - Use of cimetidine and other H₂RAs in patients with impaired kidney function requires caution and dosage reduction. Cimetidine may cause mental confusion in patients with abnormal kidney function.
  - The drug also blocks secretion of creatinine in kidney tubules, thereby decreasing creatinine clearance and increasing serum creatinine level.
  - Partial metabolism of cimetidine and other H₂RAs occurs in the liver, increasing drug level higher than anticipated in patients with impaired liver function.
  - Cimetidine inhibits the hepatic metabolism of many other drugs; this is a major concern.
  - For patients on hemodialysis, cimetidine administration should occur at the end of dialysis.
- Specific healthcare environments:
  - In patients who are critically ill, H₂RAs have a longer half-life and lower clearance rate than in people who are healthy due to decreased perfusion rates and delayed kidney excretion.
  - It is unclear if the benefit of such prophylactic practice achieves the desired outcome through all population groups.
  - In the home care setting, the nurse must assess for potential drug–drug interactions and adverse effects in patients taking cimetidine.

Adverse Effects

Common adverse effects of cimetidine include diarrhea, dizziness, drowsiness, headache, confusion, and gynecomastia. They occur infrequently following the usual doses and standard duration of treatment. Adverse effects are more likely with prolonged use of high doses, with increasing age, and with impaired kidney or hepatic function.

Contraindications

Contraindications include known hypersensitivity to cimetidine. Caution is warranted in people with abnormal kidney function and hepatic impairment.

Nursing Implications

Preventing Interactions

Antacids decrease absorption of cimetidine, so the drugs should not be given at the same time. No drugs are known to increase or decrease the effects of cimetidine. Additionally, no herbs increase or decrease the effects of cimetidine.

Quality and Safety Alert: Safety

Cimetidine contributes to multiple-drug interactions. As a known inhibitor of many isozymes of the cytochrome P450 (CYP450) drug-metabolizing system in the liver, it interferes with the hepatic metabolism of other drugs. Consequently, the clearance of affected drugs from the body is slower, and the increased serum levels are more likely to cause adverse effects and toxicity unless dosage is reduced.

Drugs that are affected by cimetidine include antidysrhythmics (e.g., lidocaine, propafenone, quinidine), the anticoagulant warfarin, anticonvulsants (e.g., carbamazepine, phenytoin), benzodiazepine antianxiety or hypnotic agents (e.g., alprazolam, diazepam, flurazepam, triazolam), beta-adrenergic blockers (e.g., labetalol, metoprolol, propranolol), the bronchodilator theophylline, calcium channel blocking agents (e.g., verapamil), tricyclic antidepressants (e.g., amitriptyline), and sulfonylurea antidiabetic drugs. In addition, cimetidine may increase serum levels (e.g., fluorouracil, procainamide and its active metabolite) and pharmacologic effects of other drugs (e.g., respiratory depression with opioid analgesics) by unidentified mechanisms. Cimetidine also may decrease effects of several drugs, including drugs that require an acidic environment for absorption (e.g., iron salts, indomethacin, fluconazole, tetracyclines) and miscellaneous drugs (e.g., digoxin, tocainide) by unknown mechanisms. The accumulation of the antihistamines, terfenadine, and astemizole, may result in a prolongation of the QT interval and could lead to the development of ventricular dysrhythmias such as torsades de pointes. Cimetidine also may decrease the effects of drugs that require an acidic environment for absorption (e.g., iron salts, indomethacin, fluconazole, tetracyclines) and miscellaneous drugs (e.g., digoxin, tocainide) by unknown mechanisms.

Administering the Medication

H₂RAs are available in a wide array of products, and it is essential to take precautions to ensure that the formulation, dosage strength, and method of administration are appropriate for the intended use.

Oral administration of a single oral dose occurs at bedtime, and administration of multiple oral doses of cimetidine occurs with meals and at bedtime.

Quality and Safety Alert: Safety

With any oral solution, it is important to measure the liquid with a marked measuring spoon or medicine cup, not with a tablespoon.

- IV administration requires dilution and administration over at least 2 minutes. For intermittent infusion, it is necessary to dilute and infuse over 15 to 20 minutes.
- IM administration does not require dilution. Injection is given deep into a large muscle group.

Assessing for Therapeutic Effects

The nurse assesses for decreased epigastric pain with gastric and duodenal ulcers or decreased heartburn with GERD.

Assessing for Adverse Effects

With H$_2$RAs, the nurse assesses for diarrhea or constipation, headache, dizziness, muscle aches, fatigue, skin rashes, mental confusion, delirium, coma, depression, and fever. Adverse effects are uncommon and usually mild with recommended doses. The nurse assesses for central nervous system effects, which have been associated with high doses in older adult patients or in those with impaired kidney function. With long-term administration of cimetidine, other observed adverse effects include decreased sperm count and gynecomastia in men and galactorrhea in women.

Patient Teaching

Box 37.1 summarizes patient teaching guidelines that apply to the H$_2$RAs.

Other Drugs in the Class

Unlike cimetidine, famotidine (Pepcid, Pepcid AC) and nizatidine do not affect the cytochrome P450 drug–metabolizing system in the liver and therefore do not interfere with the metabolism of other drugs. Use of these other drugs may be preferable in patients who are critically ill because they often require numerous other drugs with which cimetidine may interact.

Famotidine and nizatidine pharmacokinetics are similar to cimetidine. Nizatidine is not available in a parenteral formulation. Compared with cimetidine, the other drugs cause similar effects except they are less likely to cause mental confusion and gynecomastia (antiandrogenic effects). Moderate-to-severe abnormal kidney function decreases clearance and prolongs half-life of famotidine and nizatidine. Nizatidine increases serum salicylate levels in people taking high doses of aspirin.

> ### Clinical Application 37.1
> - Ms. Carpenter visits her primary care physician, who orders an esophagogastric duodenoscopy. This confirms the presence of a gastric ulcer in the antrum of her stomach. Omeprazole is increased to 40 mg once daily, and she continues to take the antacids plus sucralfate as prescribed.

NCLEX Success

1. When taking a patient's history, the nurse notes that the patient is taking warfarin and cimetidine concurrently. The nurse should anticipate which of the following?
   A. Warfarin effects would be increased.
   B. Cimetidine effects would be increased.
   C. Warfarin effects would be decreased.
   D. Cimetidine effects would be decreased.

2. A 69-year-old patient seen in the GI clinic for heartburn is prescribed famotidine. Which of the following statements by the patient indicates an understanding of the patient teaching received related to minimizing acid reflux? (Select all that apply.)
   A. Take the medication with no more than 2 oz of water
   B. Elevate the head of the bed
   C. Avoid smoking
   D. Minimize intake of fats, chocolate, citric juices, coffee, and alcohol
   E. Avoid lying down for 1 to 2 hours after eating
   F. Avoid constipation

PROTON PUMP INHIBITORS

PPIs are the most potent inhibitors of gastric acid secretion available. PPIs are like the H$_2$RAs in terms of effects but have a different mode of action. Compared with H$_2$RAs, PPIs suppress gastric acid more strongly, for a longer period. This effect provides faster symptom relief and faster healing in acid-related diseases. Rates of ulcer recurrence are similar. Because PPIs are more effective than H$_2$RAs, certainly in the short term, PPIs are more popular. **Omeprazole** (Prilosec), the first drug in the class to be developed, is still widely used and serves as the prototype.

> ### ! Quality and Safety Alert: Safety
> The PPIs have been identified as having pharmacogenomic interactions, especially as drugs in this class are known inhibitors of the CYP2C19 isoenzyme.

Pharmacokinetics

Omeprazole is well absorbed after oral administration and highly bound to plasma proteins (about 95%). Metabolism occurs in the liver, and excretion takes place in the urine (about 75%) and bile or feces. The half-life of the drug is 1 to 1.5 hours. Acid-inhibiting effects occur within 2 hours and last 72 hours or longer. When the drug is discontinued, effects persist for 48 to 72 hours or longer, until the gastric parietal cells can synthesize additional H$^+$, K$^+$-ATPase.

Action

Omeprazole binds irreversibly to the gastric proton pump (e.g., the enzyme H$^+$, K$^+$-ATPase) to prevent the "pumping" or release of gastric acid from parietal cells into the stomach lumen, thereby blocking the final step of acid production. Inhibition of the proton pump suppresses gastric acid secretion in response to all primary stimuli, histamine, gastrin, and acetylcholine. Thus, omeprazole and other drugs in the class inhibit both daytime (including meal-stimulated) and nocturnal (unstimulated) acid secretion.

Use

Omeprazole and other PPIs are usually the drug class of choice for treatment of PUD, including duodenal and gastric ulcers;

GERD with erosive esophagitis; and Zollinger–Ellison syndrome. With duodenal and gastric ulcers, healing may occur after 2 weeks compared with 4 weeks using H$_2$RAs. With GERD, PPIs usually eliminate symptoms within 1 to 2 weeks and heal esophagitis within 8 weeks. Lower doses can prevent recurrence of esophagitis, maintain symptom relief, and heal esophagitis. Higher doses or longer therapy may be needed for severe GERD.

In patients with *H. pylori*–associated ulcers, eradication of the bacterium with antimicrobial drugs is preferable to long-term maintenance therapy with antisecretory drugs. Therapy with bismuth, a PPI, and two or three antimicrobial drugs is the most effective regimen (see Medications Used to Treat *H. pylori*). Table 37.4 presents route and dosage information for omeprazole and other PPIs.

TABLE 37.4
DRUGS AT A GLANCE: Proton Pump Inhibitors

Drug	Routes and Dosage Ranges	
	Adults	**Children**
Omeprazole (Prilosec, Prilosec OTC; Losec, Olex)	Gastric ulcer: 40 mg PO once daily for 4–8 wk Duodenal ulcer: 20 mg PO once daily for 4–8 wk GERD, with erosive esophagitis: 20 mg PO once daily Zollinger–Ellison syndrome: 60 mg PO once daily Heartburn: 20 mg PO for 14 d; may repeat treatment every 4 mo if needed *H. pylori* infection: 40 mg PO daily for 14 d, then 20 mg daily for 14 d, with clarithromycin	1–16 y GERD: 5–10 kg, 5 mg 10–20 kg, 10 mg ≥20 kg, 20 mg PO
Dexlansoprazole (Dexilant; Dexilant)	GERD: 30 mg PO once daily for 4 wk	≥12 y: 30 mg PO once daily for 4 wk
Esomeprazole (Nexium, Nexium IV, Nexium Delayed-Release Capsules; Nexium)	GERD: 20–40 mg PO once daily for 4–8 wk; maintenance, 20 mg PO once daily, 20–40 mg IV daily up to 10 d	1 mo to <1 y, 0.5 mg/kg IV infused over 10–30 min 1–11 y, GERD, 30 mg PO once daily for up to 12 wk; >30 kg, 15 mg PO once daily for up to 12 wk 12–17 y, GERD, 10 mg PO once daily for up to 8 wk, <55 kg 10 mg IV; ≥55 kg 20 mg IV infused over 10–30 min Healing erosive esophagitis: <20 kg 10 mg PO once daily for up to 8 wk; ≥20 kg 10 or 20 mg PO once daily for up to 8 wk
Lansoprazole (Prevacid, Prevacid SoluTab; Prevacid, Prevacid FasTab)	Duodenal ulcer: 15 mg PO daily for healing and maintenance Gastric ulcer: 30 mg PO once daily, up to 8 wk Erosive esophagitis: 30 mg PO daily up to 8 wk; maintenance, 15 mg PO daily *H. pylori* infection: 30 mg PO (with amoxicillin and clarithromycin) three times daily for 10–14 d Hypersecretory conditions: 60–90 mg PO daily	1–11 y, GERD: ≤30 kg, 30 mg PO once daily for up to 12 wk; >30 kg, 15 mg PO once daily for up to 12 wk 12–17 y GERD: 30 mg PO once daily for up to 8 wk Nonerosive GERD: 15 mg PO once daily for up to 8 wk Healing erosive esophagitis: 15 mg PO once daily Hypersecretory conditions: 60 mg PO once daily
Rabeprazole (AcipHex; AcipHex Sprinkle; Pariet)	Duodenal ulcer: 20 mg PO once daily up to 4 wk GERD: 20 mg PO once daily for healing and maintenance Zollinger–Ellison syndrome: 60 mg PO once or twice daily	12 y and more, GERD 20 mg PO once daily for up to 8 wk

GERD, gastroesophageal reflux disease, including erosive esophagitis; GI, gastrointestinal; *H. pylori, Helicobacter pylori.*

Patient-related variables specific to the use of omeprazole and other PPIs include the following:

- Age:
  - In infants and children, omeprazole and the other PPIs have gained widespread popularity for the management of peptic ulcers and GERD as well as the eradication of *H. pylori*. These drugs are acid-labile, and oral formulations consist of capsules that contain enteric-coated granules. A chewable form of omeprazole exists, and a pharmacist can prepare a liquid formulation.
  - Older adults tolerate PPIs well. PPIs are probably the drug of choice for treating symptomatic GERD because evidence suggests that patients 60 years of age and older require stronger antisecretory effects than younger adults. However, long-term use (greater than 1 year) is associated with increased risk of hip fractures in people older than 50 years of age; the risk of fractures increases the longer the medications are taken and is greater in people who take higher dosages of PPIs. The increased risk of fractures may be due to decreased calcium absorption due to **achlorhydria** (low or absent production of gastric acid in the stomach) from PPI therapy. It is important to consider appropriate dose and duration of therapy when treating GERD in older adults. An increased risk of dementia risk has also been associated with the use of PPIs in certain individuals.
- Reproduction, pregnancy, and lactation:
  - Omeprazole is contraindicated during pregnancy as some research has indicated that congenital anomalies include cardiac defects. Lansoprazole, pantoprazole, and rabeprazole can safely be used during pregnancy.
  - Although studies suggest that PPIs are excreted in the breast milk, they are used in breast-feeding in the neonate population with success and few negative effects.
- Abnormal kidney function and hepatic impairment:
  - With omeprazole, bioavailability is increased because of decreased first-pass metabolism, and plasma half-life is increased. Metabolism of PPIs occurs in the liver, and use of these drugs may cause transient elevations in liver function tests. However, dosage adjustments are not recommended.
- Specific healthcare environments:
  - In patients with critical illness, PPIs are the strongest gastric acid suppressants used prophylactically. The drugs are usually well tolerated. IV administration, if necessary, is an option.

Adverse Effects

Adverse effects are reported with both short- and long-term use. Nausea, diarrhea, and headache are the most frequently reported adverse effects. Use of high-dose PPIs or long-term use of the drugs carries a possible increased risk of bone fractures due to hypocalcemia. In addition, long-term use of PPIs can affect absorption of dietary vitamin B_{12} and magnesium leading to subsequent deficiencies.

Contraindications

Contraindications include known hypersensitivity to omeprazole.

Nursing Implications

Preventing Interactions

Drug interactions with the PPIs are relatively few. Omeprazole increases blood levels of some benzodiazepines (diazepam, flurazepam, triazolam), phenytoin, and warfarin, probably by inhibiting hepatic metabolism. Coadministration of clopidogrel with PPIs may reduce the cardioprotective effects of clopidogrel. Clarithromycin increases effects of omeprazole and may increase blood levels. No herbs have been reported to increase or decrease the effects of omeprazole.

Administering the Medication

Omeprazole must be administered before food intake. Two 20-mg oral capsules or suspension packets are not equivalent to one 40-mg dose. The 20- and 40-mg dosages contain the same amount of sodium bicarbonate; substituting two 20-mg doses for one 40-mg dose results in the administration of too much sodium bicarbonate. The patient should swallow the tablets or capsules whole, without crushing or chewing, because the drug formulations are delayed-release and long-acting. Crushing or chewing destroys these effects.

Assessing for Therapeutic Effects

The nurse assesses for decreased epigastric pain with gastric and duodenal ulcers and for decreased heartburn with GERDs.

Assessing for Adverse Effects

The nurse observes for the presence of headache, diarrhea, abdominal pain, nausea, and vomiting. With long-term use, the nurse should assess for signs of malabsorption of magnesium (i.e., seizures, hyperreflexia, muscle cramps), calcium (i.e., Chvostek and Trousseau signs), and vitamin B_{12} (i.e., muscle weakness, fatigue, dizziness).

Patient Teaching

Box 37.1 lists general teaching guidelines that apply to PPIs.

Other Drugs in the Class

The actions and pharmacokinetics of the other PPIs, including dexlansoprazole (Dexilant), esomeprazole (Nexium), lansoprazole (Prevacid), pantoprazole (Protonix), and rabeprazole (AcipHex), are similar to those of omeprazole. However, differences in their metabolism may lead to specific drug interactions. The PPIs are metabolized by the CYP450 system, with CPY2C19 having the predominant role in all PPIs but rabeprazole, which is metabolized primarily by CYP3A4.

Dexlansoprazole capsules should be swallowed whole and not chewed. However, the capsules may be opened and sprinkled on a tablespoon of applesauce if a person is not able to swallow the capsule. Capsules may also be opened and administered via a nasal gastric tube. Doses greater than 30 mg do not provide additional benefit during the maintenance phase. Note that two 30-mg orally disintegrating tablets are not interchangeable with one 60-mg delayed-release capsule.

Esomeprazole capsules can be opened, mixed with 50 mL of water, and swallowed or administered via nasogastric tube. Flush tube with water after administration. IV esomeprazole can be injected over no less than 3 minutes or infused over 10 to 30 minutes into a dedicated IV line. Flush the IV line with 5%

dextrose or lactated Ringer solution before and after esomeprazole administration.

Lansoprazole and rabeprazole should be used cautiously, and dosage should be reduced in patients with severe liver impairment. Patients with phenylketonuria should be advised that orally disintegrating tablets of lansoprazole may contain aspartame. Lansoprazole may cause drowsiness or dizziness. For patients who are unable to swallow capsules, lansoprazole (and esomeprazole) capsules can be opened and the granules mixed with applesauce or other acidic substances; this preserves the coating of the granules, allowing them to remain intact until they reach the small intestine. Chewing or crushing destroys the coating. For a liquid suspension, it is possible to mix the lansoprazole granules with 30 mL of water (use no other liquids), stir well, and swallow it immediately, without chewing the granules.

The nurse ensures that oral pantoprazole is taken with or without food as per the manufacturer's recommendations. The nurse may administer IV pantoprazole over 15 minutes, injecting the drug into a dedicated line or the Y-site of an IV infusion. Specific directions for pantoprazole administration include the following:

- Use the in-line filter provided; if injecting in a Y-site, place the filter below the Y-site closest to the patient.
- Flush the IV line with 5% dextrose, 0.9% NaCl, or lactated Ringer solution before and after administration.

Omeprazole and esomeprazole have the greatest potential for drug interactions. Esomeprazole appears to interfere with the metabolism of other drugs to a lesser degree than omeprazole. The metabolism of pantoprazole undergoes the same metabolism but is followed rapidly by sulfate conjugation. Because of this, pantoprazole has the lowest potential for drug interactions with other agents metabolized by the CYP450 system. Rabeprazole is metabolized by CYP2C19 but shows a strong affinity for CYP3A4 and is associated with very few known drug interactions. Although dexlansoprazole and lansoprazole are potent inhibitors of CYP2C19 and other CYP450 isoforms, these drugs are metabolized primarily by CYP3A4. Interactions with theophylline have been reported, increasing serum theophylline levels.

Clinical Application 37.2

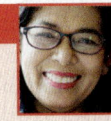

The patient education includes instructions for Ms. Carpenter about how to take her medication properly and measures to avoid gastric irritation.
- What content should the teaching plan include?
- What foods are included or excluded in her nutritional intake?

ADJUVANT MEDICATIONS USED TO TREAT PUD AND GERD

Administration of adjuvant medications may support the treatment and resolution of symptoms of acid peptic disorders. Table 37.5 summarizes these adjuvant medications.

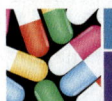

TABLE 37.5

DRUGS AT A GLANCE: Adjuvant Medications Used to Treat Peptic Ulcer Disease and Gastroesophageal Reflux Disease

Drug	Route and Dosage Ranges	
	Adults	**Children**
Misoprostol (Cytotec)	100–200 mg PO four times daily with meals and at bedtime	Safety and effectiveness not established
Sucralfate (Carafate; 🍁 Sucralfate-1, Sulcrate, Sulcrate Suspension Plus)	Active ulcer: 1 g PO four times daily before meals and at bedtime; maintenance, 1 g PO two times daily	Safety and effectiveness not established
Amoxicillin (Moxatag 🍁 Pro-Amox, Novamoxin)	500 mg–1 g two to three times daily, Moxatag 775 mg ER	Dosing not established with *H. pylori* infection
Clarithromycin (🍁 ACCEL-Clarithromycin, ACT-Clarithromycin, APO-Clarithromycin, Biaxin)	500 mg PO three times daily	Dosing not established with *H. pylori* infection
Metronidazole (🍁 Flagyl)	250 mg PO four times daily	Dosing not established with *H. pylori* infection
Tetracycline (🍁 APO-Tetra, Nu-Tetra)	500 mg PO four times daily	Dosing not established with *H. pylori* infection; tetracycline can discolor teeth in children 8 y of age or less
Bismuth subsalicylate	525 mg PO (2 tablets or 30 mL) four times daily	<3 y, consult physician 3–6 y, 1/3 tablet or 5 mL PO 6–9 y, 2/3 tablet or 10 mL PO 9–12 y, 1 tablet or 15 mL PO Dosage may be repeated every 30–60 min, if needed, up to 8 doses in 24 h

H. pylori, *Helicobacter pylori*.

Miscellaneous Medications

Prostaglandin: Misoprostol

Naturally occurring prostaglandin E, which is produced in mucosal cells of the stomach and duodenum, inhibits gastric acid secretion and increases mucus and bicarbonate secretion, mucosal blood flow, and perhaps mucosal repair. It also inhibits the mucosal damage produced by gastric acid, aspirin, and NSAIDs. When synthesis of prostaglandin E is inhibited, erosion and ulceration of gastric mucosa may occur. This is the mechanism by which aspirin and other NSAIDs are thought to cause gastric and duodenal ulcers (see Chapter 16).

Misoprostol (Cytotec) (see Table 37.5) is a synthetic form of prostaglandin E approved for concurrent use with NSAIDs to protect gastric mucosa from NSAID-induced erosion and ulceration. It is indicated for patients at high risk for GI ulceration and bleeding, such as those taking high doses of NSAIDs for arthritis and older adults. The FDA has issued a **BOXED WARNING** to alert healthcare professionals that misoprostol is contraindicated in females of childbearing potential, unless effective contraceptive methods are being used, and during pregnancy, because it may induce abortion, premature birth, or congenital anomalies. In fact, misoprostol is one of the drugs used for medical abortions in lieu of surgical evacuation.

The most common adverse effects are diarrhea (occurs in 10% to 40% of recipients), which may be severe enough to lead to dosage reduction or stopping the drug, and abdominal cramping. Other adverse effects include nausea, vomiting, headache, uterine cramping, and vaginal bleeding. Older adults often take large doses of NSAIDs for arthritis and therefore are at risk for development of acute gastric ulcers and GI bleeding. Thus, they may be candidates for treatment with misoprostol. However, they may be unable to tolerate the misoprostol-induced diarrhea and abdominal discomfort. Dosage reduction to prevent severe diarrhea and abdominal cramping may be necessary.

Sucralfate

Sucralfate (Carafate) is a preparation of sulfated sucrose and aluminum hydroxide that binds to normal and ulcerated mucosa. Prescribers use it to prevent and treat PUD. For ulcer treatment, it requires use for 4 to 8 weeks unless healing is confirmed by radiologic or endoscopic examination. When used in the long term to prevent ulcer recurrence, dosage reduction is necessary.

Sucralfate is effective even though it does not inhibit secretion of gastric acid or pepsin, and it has little neutralizing effect on gastric acid. Its mechanism of action is unclear, but it is thought to act locally on the gastric and duodenal mucosa. Possible mechanisms include binding to ulcer and forming a protective barrier between the mucosa and gastric acid, pepsin, and bile salts; neutralizing pepsin; stimulating prostaglandin synthesis in the mucosa; and exerting healing effects through the aluminum component. Sucralfate is effective in healing duodenal ulcers and in maintenance therapy to prevent ulcer recurrence. In general, the rates of ulcer healing with sucralfate are similar to the rates with H_2RAs.

Adverse effects are low in incidence and severity because sucralfate is not absorbed systemically. Constipation and dry mouth are most often reported. Older adults tolerate sucralfate well. The main disadvantages of using sucralfate are that the tablet is large; it must be given at least twice daily; it requires an acid pH for activation and should not be given with an antacid, H_2RA, or PPI; and it may bind to other drugs and prevent their absorption. Sucralfate decreases absorption of ciprofloxacin and other fluoroquinolones, digoxin, phenytoin, warfarin, as well as the PPI lansoprazole. If a person takes both sucralfate and any of these drugs, to avoid or minimize this interaction, they should do the following:

- Take lansoprazole about 30 minutes before sucralfate.
- Take ciprofloxacin and other fluoroquinolones, digoxin, phenytoin, warfarin, or other drugs 2 hours before sucralfate, if it is possible.

In addition, antacids decrease the effects of sucralfate, and people should not take these within 30 minutes before or after administration of sucralfate.

Medications Used to Treat *H. pylori*

Combination Therapy With Antibiotics

The choice of the initial antibiotic regimen to treat *H. pylori* should be guided by treatment history. For instance, taking an antibiotic within the past few years may lead to resistance to the drug. Also, drug therapy using an antibiotic with a known allergy must be avoided. Few regimens have consistently achieved high eradication rates, so several treatment regimens have been used. For example, combination drug therapy including at least two antibiotics and an acid reducer (e.g., clarithromycin-based triple therapy with clarithromycin, amoxicillin, and a PPI, or clarithromycin-based triple therapy with clarithromycin, metronidazole, and a PPI) may be used. Alternatively, bismuth subsalicylate (bismuth quadruple therapy with bismuth, metronidazole, tetracycline, and a PPI) is recommended for patients with PUD who are known to be infected with *H. pylori*.

Effectiveness of *H. pylori* eradication after antibiotic treatment can be confirmed by a urea breath test, stool antigen test, or upper endoscopy-based testing. A positive result on one of these tests is indicative of a tenacious *H. pylori* infection, suggesting that the bacteria have become resistant to the action of one of the selected antibiotics. In situations where therapy is ineffective, alternate *H. pylori* therapy, including levofloxacin triple therapy (levofloxacin, amoxicillin/metronidazole, and a PPI); high-dose dual therapy consisting of amoxicillin and a PPI; and rifabutin triple therapy (rifabutin, amoxicillin, and a PPI) have been used with success.

In addition, alternate treatment approaches to *H. pylori* have demonstrated some success by splitting up the antibiotics rather than taking them all at once. Sequential therapy may be more effective than standard triple therapy considering the increasing frequency of resistant strains of *H. pylori*; however, the complexity of therapy may make adherence difficult. Furthermore, some North American clinical practice guidelines recommend against using sequential therapy as a first-line regimen given the lack of data from North American trials.

Table 37.5 presents examples of drug combinations used to treat *H. pylori*. For convenience, some of the recommended drug combinations are packaged together. The treatment regimen that is selected must consider local antibiotic resistance patterns (if known), previous exposure and allergies to specific antibiotics, cost, side effects, and ease of administration. Section 4 of this book contains additional information about antibiotic therapy.

> **Quality and Safety Alert: Safety**
>
> As noted previously, metronidazole, a nitroimidazole antibiotic, antiprotozoal medication, is sometimes included as part of a multidrug regimen to treat *H. pylori* (see Chapter 21).
>
> Consuming alcohol while using metronidazole can cause a disulfiramlike reaction with effects that can include flushing, tachycardia, diaphoresis, nausea, vomiting, or headache. Patients must be informed that even a very small amount of alcohol can produce the reaction; the risk persists for up to 48 hours after completion of treatment.

> **Quality and Safety Alert: Evidence-Based Practice**
>
> Roszczenko-Jasiriska et al. (2020) summarized the treatment of *H. pylori* in what they termed the post-antibiotic era. Antibiotic therapy remains a part of the treatment plan with the use of quadruple therapy with a PPI, bismuth, metronidazole (MTZ), and tetracycline (TC) or levofloxacin (LVF).
>
> The use of probiotics in combination with antibiotic therapy appears to be more effective, in both children and adults, compared with a standard therapy alone. In addition, probiotics in combination with antibiotic therapy have been found to produce beneficial effects to barrier protection of the gastrointestinal environment, enhance the immune system, and cause inhibitory effects on pathogens, including *H. pylori*. Probiotics can also decrease the side effects of nausea and vomiting, diarrhea, and taste disturbance. Phytomedicine, use of plant extracts, is also gaining ground as an aspect of treatment. Natural Chinese medicine has long been used as complementary and collaborative therapy. One Chinese drug (Jinghua Weikang Capsule) with the components of *Chenopodium ambrosioides* and *Adina pilulifera* is commonly used as an additive to *H. pylori* therapy in China.

Bismuth Subsalicylate

Prescribers use bismuth subsalicylate to coat ulcers, protecting them from stomach acid to treat *H. pylori*. Other uses include treatment of diarrhea and nausea. Commonly known as pink bismuth, it is the active ingredient in OTC medications such as Pepto-Bismol and Kaopectate. Bismuth subsalicylate is also used in combinations with other drugs to treat *H. pylori*. However, as a salicylate, this drug can cause serious bleeding problems when used alone in patients with ulcers.

> **Quality and Safety Alert: Safety**
>
> People with an allergy to aspirin or other salicylates should not take bismuth subsalicylate.

People who are taking chewable tablets should chew them and then swallow them. If they are taking the liquid form of this medication, they should shake the bottle well and use a measuring device or cup. Adverse effects of bismuth subsalicylate include ringing in the ears or hearing loss. A darkening of the stools or tongue may occur, which is a harmless effect that disappears once the drug is stopped. If ear-related problems occur, it is necessary to discontinue the drug and have a prescriber evaluate the patient.

NCLEX Success

3. Which fact regarding administration should the nurse include in patient teaching about the drug sucralfate?
   A. Take sucralfate concurrently with an antacid.
   B. Take sucralfate after meals.
   C. Take sucralfate before meals.
   D. Take sucralfate 2 hours before meals.

4. The nurse would question the use of misoprostol in which population?
   A. children under 5 years of age
   B. adults with concurrent use of antacid
   C. pregnant people at all stages of pregnancy
   D. older adults with concurrent use of cimetidine

5. Adverse effects of cimetidine include which of the following? (Select all that apply.)
   A. headache
   B. constipation
   C. gynecomastia
   D. diarrhea
   E. confusion

Clinical Application 37.3

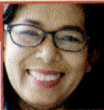

- What measures could Ms. Carpenter take to prevent or minimize GERD?
- What additional patient teaching regarding antacid therapy would the nurse provide Ms. Carpenter?

THE NURSING PROCESS

A concept map outlines the nursing process related to drug therapy considerations in this chapter. Additional nursing implications related to the disease process should also be considered in care decisions.

Assessment
- Assess all patients for signs and symptoms of increased gastric acid secretion evidenced by heartburn, reflux, belching, abdominal pain, nausea, and any signs of hematemesis or blood in stools.
- Assess for history of aspirin, acetaminophen, ibuprofen, or other NSAID intake.
- Assess for times of pain occurrence (e.g., ask: does pain lessen after eating?, do certain foods exacerbate pain and discomfort?).
- Assess patients for smoking or alcohol intake.
- Assess patient for psychological stress.
- Assess patient for OTC "ulcer therapy."

Outcomes of Therapy

The patient will
- Take medications at specific times ordered.
- Decrease or eliminate smoking and alcohol intake.
- Remain upright after eating.
- Eat frequent small meals.
- Avoid foods high in fat and acidity.
- Maintain adequate levels of nutrition and fluids, rest and sleep, and exercise.
- Cope with anxiety and stress.
- Keep appointments for follow-up care.
- Prevent or recognize and promptly treat adverse drug effects.
- Avoid pregnancy.
- Maintain family and other emotional/social support systems.
- Receive optimal instructions and information about nutritional intake and avoidance of NSAIDs.

Nursing Interventions
- Instruct patients to verify times for medication therapy and the rationale for dosing intervals.
- Instruct patients about positioning after eating and while sleeping.
- Instruct patients about adverse effects of medications.
- Inform patients about additional diagnostic test results, changes in therapeutic regimen, and evidence of progress.
- Consult other healthcare team members (e.g., physician, dietitian, social worker) on the patient's behalf when indicated.
- Assist patients in learning strategies to manage day-to-day activities and stress relief measures.

Evaluation
- Interview and observe for accurate drug administration.
- Interview and observe for therapeutic and adverse drug effects with each patient contact.
- Interview regarding knowledge and attitude toward the drug therapy regimen, including follow-up care and symptoms to report to healthcare providers.
- Interview regarding a 24-hour dietary recall for diet compliance.
- Observe and assess outpatients regarding ability to comply with follow-up care.

Unfolding Patient Stories: Suzanne Morris • Part 1

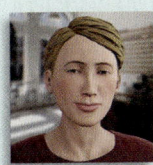

Suzanne Morris, age 43, is diagnosed with peptic ulcer disease. She is prescribed triple combination therapy with amoxicillin, clarithromycin, and pantoprazole for *H. pylori*. What patient education would the nurse provide for each medication? (Suzanne Morris's story continues in Chapter 44.)

Care for Suzanne and other patients in a realistic virtual environment: **vSim** for Nursing. Practice documenting these patients' care in DocuCare (thepoint.lww.com/DocuCareEHR).

Visit thePoint® at http://thePoint.lww.com/Frandsen13e for answers to NCLEX Success questions (in Appendix A), answers to Clinical Application Case Studies (in Appendix B), and more!

REFERENCES AND RESOURCES

Amorim, D. C., Travassos, M. P. P., Dias, I. T., Gurgel, H. Q., et al. (2021). Adverse reactions of proton pump inhibitors: A literature review. *Journal of Young Pharmacists, 13*(1), 25–27.

Brun, M. M., Deijkers, R. L. M., Bazuin, R., Elzakker, E., & Pijls, B. B. (2021). Proton-pump inhibitors are associated with increased risk of prosthetic join infection in patients with total hip arthroplasty: A case-cohort study. *Acta Orthopaedica, 92*(4), 431–435.

Guevara, B., & Cogdill, A. G. (2020). *Helicobacter pylori*: A review of current diagnostic and management strategies. *Digestive Diseases and Sciences, 64*, 1917–1931.

Hamzah, A. B., & Fauzi, A. (2021). Comprehensive management of *Helicobacter pylori* infection. *The Indonesian Journal of Gastroenterology Hepatology and Digestive Endoscopy, 22*(2).

Ji, J., & Yang, H. (2020). Using probiotics as supplementation for *Helicobacter pylori* antibiotic therapy. *International Journal of Molecular Sciences, 21*(1136), 1–15.

Keikha, M., & Karbalaei, M. (2021). Probiotics as the live microscopic fighters against Helicobacter pylori gastric infections. *BMC Gastroenterology*. https://doi.org/10.1186/s12876-021-01977-1

Lafferty, L. (2020). Drug-induced nutrient deficiencies and proton pump inhibitors. *Nutritional Perspectives: Journal of the Council on Nutrition of the American Chiropractic Association, 13–21*(238), 1–18.

Lin, J., Xiong, Z., Geng, X., & Cui, M. (2020). Rebamipide with proton pump inhibitors (PPIs) versus PPIs alone for the treatment of endoscopic submucosal dissection-induced ulcers: A meta-analysis. *BioMed Research International*, 1–10.

Mounsey, A., Barzin, A., & Rietz, A. (2020). Functional dyspepsia: Evaluation and management. *American Family Physician, 101*(2), 85–88.

Nyssen, O. P., Perez-Aisa, A., Tepes, B., Rodrigo-Saez, L., Romero, P. M., et al. (2020). Helicobacter pylori first-line and rescue treatment in patient allergic to penicillin; Experience from the European Registry on *H. pylori* management (HP-EuReg). *Helicobacter, 25*, e12686, 1–11.

Patel, T. A., Patel, M., Rajagopalan, K., Patel, R., Shaika, A. S., et al. (2021). Safety and efficacy of almagate and simethicone combination in symptomatic management of GERD: Post-marketing observational TRIALMA study. *Journal of Clinical and Diagnostic Research, 14*(3).

Roszczenko-Jasiriska, P., Wojtys, M. I., & Jagusztyn-Krynicka, E. K. (2020). *Helicobacter pylori* treatment in the post-antibiotic era—Searching for new drug targets. *Applied Microbiology and Biotechnology, 104*, 9891–9905.

Seo, J., Bortolin, K., & Jones, N. L. (2020). Review: Helicobacter pylori infection in children. *Helicobacter, 25*(Suppl 11), e12742.

Simon, M., Levy, E. I., & Vandenplas, Y. (2021). Safety considerations when managing gastro-esophageal reflux disease in infants. *Expert Opinion on Drug Safety, 20*(1), 37–49.

Singeap, A., Huiban, L., Chiriac, S., Cuciureanu, T., & Trifan, A. (2020). The role of alginate-based therapy in gastroesophageal reflux disease. *Romanian Journal of Medical Practice, 15*(3), 285–291.

Sloan, J. A., & Katz, P. O. (2021). Proton pump inhibitors in 2021: Pros, cons, and everything in between. *Foregut, 2*, 145–151.

Song, M. J., Kim, S., Boo, D., Park, C., Yoo, S., Yoon, H., & Cho, Y. (2021). Comparison of proton pump inhibitor and histamine 2 receptor antagonists for stress ulcer prophylaxis in the intensive care unit. *Scientific Reports, 11*, 18467. https://doi.org/10.1038/s41598-021-98069-7

Teng, G., Liu, Y., Ting, W., Wang, W., Wang, H., & Hu, F. (2020). Efficacy of sucralfate-combined quadruple therapy on gastric mucosal injury induced by *Helicobacter pylori* and its effect on gastrointestinal flora. *BioMed Research International, 20*, 1–14.

Thelin, C. S., & Richter, J. E. (2020). Review article: The management of heartburn during pregnancy and lactation. *Alimentary Pharmacology and Therapeutics, 51*(4), 421–434.

Young, A., Kumar, M. A., & Thots, P. N. (2020). GERD: A practical approach. *Cleveland Clinic Journal of Medicine, 87*(4), 223–230.

Zhang, Y., Liang, M., Sun, C., Sone, J., Cheng, C., Shi, T., Min, M., & Sun, Y. (2020). Proton pump inhibitors use and dementia risk a meta-analysis of cohort studies. *European Journal of Clinical Pharmacology, 76*(2), 139–147.

CHAPTER 38

Drug Therapy for Nausea and Vomiting

LEARNING OBJECTIVES

After studying this chapter, you should be able to:

1. Discuss the phenothiazines in terms of indications and contraindications for use, routes of administration, and major adverse effects.
2. Describe selected antihistamines used to control nausea and vomiting in terms of indications and contraindications for use, routes of administration, and major adverse effects.
3. Discuss the 5-hydroxytryptamine$_3$ receptor antagonists in terms of indications and contraindications for use, routes of administration, and major adverse effects.
4. Describe the substance P/neurokinin 1 antagonist aprepitant in terms of indications and contraindications for use, routes of administration, and major adverse effects.
5. Identify the prototype drug for each drug class.
6. Identify nonpharmacologic measures to reduce nausea and vomiting.
7. Implement the nursing process in the care of patients receiving drugs for the management of nausea and vomiting.

CLINICAL APPLICATION CASE STUDY

Nellie Snyder is a 38-year-old woman with breast cancer who is receiving radiation and chemotherapy. She is experiencing significant nausea and vomiting.

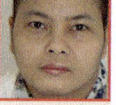

KEY TERMS

Anticipatory nausea and vomiting: conditioned response prior to chemotherapy that is triggered by fears of recurrence of significant nausea and vomiting

Cannabinoid: derivative of marijuana

Emesis: stomach contents produced with vomiting

Emetogenic: having the ability to cause vomiting

Motion sickness: action in which rapid changes in body motion stimulate receptors in the inner ear (vestibular branch of the auditory nerve, which is concerned with equilibrium) and nerve impulses are transmitted to the vomiting center

Nausea: an unpleasant sensation of abdominal discomfort accompanied by an urge to vomit

Rescue antiemetic: antiemetic use after a prophylactic antiemetic drug regimen was unsuccessful in preventing emesis

Vomiting: expulsion of stomach contents up through the esophagus and out of the mouth

INTRODUCTION

Nausea and vomiting are common symptoms experienced by virtually everyone at some time. **Nausea**, an unpleasant sensation of abdominal discomfort accompanied by an urge to vomit, may occur without vomiting, and **vomiting**, the expulsion of stomach contents up through the esophagus and out of the mouth and occasionally nose, may occur without prior nausea, but the two symptoms often occur together. Antiemetic drugs are used to prevent or treat nausea and vomiting. They are usually contraindicated if their use may prevent or delay diagnosis or may mask signs and symptoms of drug toxicity.

OVERVIEW OF NAUSEA AND VOMITING

Symptoms of nausea and vomiting may accompany almost any illness or stress situation. A drug or condition that causes nausea or vomiting is said to be **emetogenic**. Some common causes of nausea and vomiting include the following:

- Gastrointestinal (GI) disorders
- Cardiovascular, infectious, neurologic, or metabolic disorders
- Adverse effects of drug therapy or radiation therapy
- Pain and other noxious stimuli, such as unpleasant sights and odors, and motion sickness
- Emotional disturbances and physical or mental stress
- Postoperative status, which may include pain, impaired GI motility, and various medications
- Pregnancy
- Migraines

Clinical Manifestations

As mentioned, nausea is an unpleasant abdominal sensation that is often, but not always, accompanied by vomiting. Nausea and vomiting can be triggered by diverse stimuli and are mediated by the interaction between the brain and the gastrointestinal tract. **Anticipatory nausea and vomiting** triggered by memories and fear of nausea and vomiting are mediated by afferent signals from the higher centers of the cerebral cortex to the vomiting center. Noxious stimuli, such as unpleasant odors or sights, as well as pain, are transmitted by afferent pathways from the sensory organs to the vomiting center. In **motion sickness**, rapid changes in body motion stimulate receptors in the inner ear (vestibular branch of the auditory nerve, which is concerned with equilibrium), and nerve impulses are transmitted to the vomiting center. When vomiting occurs, **emesis** is the stomach contents produced.

Drug Therapy

Antiemetic drugs are indicated to prevent and treat nausea and vomiting associated with surgery, pain, motion sickness, cancer chemotherapy, radiation therapy, pregnancy, and other causes. Several classes of these drugs are available, which antagonize the neurotransmitter receptors that play a role in the physiology of nausea and vomiting by acting on the vomiting center, the chemoreceptor trigger zone (CTZ) (one of the central sites that relay stimuli to the vomiting center), cerebral cortex, vestibular apparatus, or a combination of these. The antiemetic drugs in this chapter are classified according to their primary action. However, some agents affect multiple receptors.

In general, the antiemetic drugs are more effective in prophylaxis than treatment and most are available in oral, parenteral, and rectal dosage forms. Generally, oral forms are preferred for prophylactic use, and rectal or parenteral forms are preferred for therapeutic use. Prompt treatment of short-term vomiting is more effective than managing long-term vomiting.

Nurses should be aware that pregnant patients should not take any medication without the guidance of their healthcare provider. Some antiemetics are dangerous during pregnancy and can cause damage to the fetus. However, when the nausea and vomiting associated with pregnancy are not controlled with lifestyle measures, some pharmacologic interventions may be appropriate. Interventions used depend on the severity of the disorder and are focused on improving the symptoms while minimizing risks to patient and fetus. See Chapter 6 for additional information on antiemetics used during pregnancy.

With all antiemetics, there is risk of adverse effects such as dizziness, drowsiness, mood changes, and other mind-altering effects, and patients should avoid hazardous activities and using alcohol while taking the medication.

> **Quality and Safety Alert: Evidence-Based Practice**
>
> Hesketh et al. (2020), on behalf of the American Society of Clinical Oncology (ASCO), completed a systematic review of literature to update the society's clinical practice guidelines related to management of nausea and vomiting during chemotherapy. The systematic review reinforced the importance of ongoing symptom monitoring throughout therapy. The researchers maintained the classified chemotherapy regimens based on emetogenicity and evaluated additional drugs in terms of their emetogenic potential. The four accepted categories based on the risk of emesis in the absence of antiemetic prophylaxis were as follows:
>
> - Highly emetogenic: greater than 90% risk of emesis
> - Moderately emetogenic: greater than 30% to 90% risk of emesis
> - Low emetogenic: 10% to 30% risk of emesis
> - Minimally emetogenic: less than 10% risk of emesis
>
> Emetogenic risk and other characteristics guide the drug regimens used to prevent chemotherapy-induced vomiting. The recommendations serve as a framework for clinical decision-making and are used along with consideration of individual variations among those receiving chemotherapy.

Table 38.1 and the following sections describe major antiemetic drugs.

PHENOTHIAZINES

Phenothiazines are first-generation (typical) antipsychotic drugs that depress the central nervous system (CNS). They are the first group of drugs to exhibit extensive activity in the prevention of chemotherapy-induced emesis; they are also used to treat schizophrenia or psychosis (see Chapter 56). These drugs act primarily by antagonizing D_2-dopamine receptors in the area postrema of the midbrain, therefore, decreasing the effect of dopamine in the brain. They also possess M_1-muscarinic and H_1-histamine blocking effects, activity associated with significant adverse effect profiles. The Beers Criteria identifies this class of drugs as

TABLE 38.1

Drugs Administered for the Treatment of Nausea and Vomiting

Drug Class	Prototype	Other Drugs in the Class
Phenothiazines	Prochlorperazine (Compro)	Chlorpromazine Perphenazine
Antihistamines	Hydroxyzine (Vistaril)	Diphenhydramine Dimenhydrinate (Dramamine) Doxylamine succinate with pyridoxine hydrochloride (Diclegis, Bonjesta) Meclizine (Antivert, Dramamine Less Drowsy)
5-HT_3 (serotonin) receptor antagonists	Ondansetron (Zofran, Zuplenz)	Dolasetron Granisetron (Sancuso, Sustol) Palonosetron (Aloxi)
Substance P/neurokinin 1 receptor antagonists	Aprepitant (Cinvanti, Emend)	Netupitant/palonosetron (Akynzeo) Rolapitant (Varubi)
Miscellaneous agents		Olanzapine (Zyprexa) Dronabinol (Marinol, Syndros) Nabilone (Cesamet) Fructose, dextrose, and orthophosphoric acid (Emetrol) Scopolamine (Transderm Scop)

potentially inappropriate for older individuals and, when used in pediatric patients less than 18 years of age, dopamine antagonists, such as prochlorperazine, are identified on the Key Potentially Inappropriate Drugs in Pediatrics (KIDs) list.

Dosage and route of administration depend primarily on the reason for use. Doses of phenothiazines are much smaller for antiemetic effects than for antipsychotic effects; not all phenothiazines are effective antiemetics. In this discussion, Ⓟ **prochlorperazine** (Compro), the most commonly used antiemetic drug in this class, serves as the prototype.

Pharmacokinetics

Prochlorperazine has low and variable absorption following oral administration and undergoes extensive first-pass metabolism in the liver. Clinical effects are apparent within 30 minutes after oral, 10 minutes after intramuscular, and about 60 minutes after rectal administration. Peak antiemetic effect with intravenous administration is 30 to 60 minutes after administration. The effects last 3 to 4 hours with oral and intramuscular administration and 3 to 12 hours with rectal. Metabolism primarily occurs in the liver, with excretion mainly in the feces.

Action

Prochlorperazine and other phenothiazines have widespread effects on the body. The therapeutic effects in nausea and vomiting are attributed to their ability to block dopamine from receptor sites in the brain and CTZ.

Use

Prochlorperazine is moderately effective for nausea caused by various GI disorders and mild to moderate emetogenic chemotherapy. The drug is used for the prevention and treatment of nausea and vomiting associated with surgery, anesthesia, migraines, chemotherapy, and motion sickness. Table 38.2 presents specific information about the use of prochlorperazine and other phenothiazines in the treatment of nausea and vomiting, including dosages for adults and children.

Patient-related variables specific to the use of prochlorperazine and other phenothiazines include the following:

- Age:
  - Prochlorperazine should not be used in children with hepatic disease, Reye syndrome, a history of sleep apnea, or a family history of sudden infant death syndrome.
  - Increased risk for sedation and extrapyramidal symptoms (EPS) occurs in children.
  - Newer agents (e.g., ondansetron and aprepitant) are recommended for management of postoperative nausea and vomiting in pediatric patients.
  - Older adults may have increased concerns with the adverse anticholinergic effects (e.g., dizziness, acute confusion, delirium, dry mouth, tachycardia, blurred vision, urinary retention, constipation).
- Reproduction, pregnancy, and lactation:
  - Use of prochlorperazine may interfere with pregnancy tests, causing false-positive results.
  - Antipsychotic use during the third trimester of pregnancy has a risk for abnormal muscle movements (EPS) and withdrawal symptoms in newborns following delivery. Symptoms in the newborn may include agitation, feeding disorder, hypertonia, hypotonia, respiratory distress, somnolence, and tremor.
  - It is unknown if prochlorperazine is present in breast milk. However, other phenothiazines are excreted in breast milk.
- Abnormal kidney function and hepatic impairment:
  - Use cautiously in children and adults with abnormal kidney function and hepatic impairment to avoid adverse effects, toxicity, or increased sensitivity to phenothiazines.
  - The U.S. Food and Drug Administration (FDA) has issued a ◆ BOXED WARNING ◆ for use in older adults with dementia-related psychosis due to an increased risk of death.

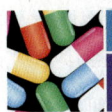

TABLE 38.2
DRUGS AT A GLANCE: Phenothiazines

Drug	Routes and Dosage Ranges	
	Adults	**Children**
Prochlorperazine (Compro; ❋ PMS-Prochlorperazine, Prochlorazine)	PO 10–25 mg 3 or 4 times daily (sustained-release capsule, 10 mg twice daily) IM 5–10 mg every 3–4 h to a maximum of 40 mg daily IV 2.5–10 mg every 3–4 h Rectal suppository 25 mg twice daily	>10 kg: PO 0.4 mg/kg/d, in 3 or 4 divided doses IM 0.2 mg/kg as a single dose Rectal suppository dosage form no longer available in the United States
Chlorpromazine (❋ Teva-Chlorpromazine)	PO 10–25 mg every 4–6 h IM, IV 25–50 mg every 4–6 h IV (during surgery) 2 mg at 2-min intervals to not exceed 25 mg	>6 mo and ≤45.5 kg: PO, IM, IV 0.55 mg/kg/dose every 6–8 h as needed. Max for children <5 y or weighing <22.7 kg is 40 mg/d; max for children ≥5 y or weighing 22.7–45.5 kg is 75 mg/d >6 mo and >45.5 kg: PO 10–25 mg every 4–6 h as needed IM, IV 25 mg; if no hypotension, then 25–50 mg every 4–6 h as needed
Perphenazine (❋ PMS-Perphenazine)	PO 8–16 mg daily in divided doses Max daily dose 24 mg if necessary	>12 y: PO 8 mg daily in divided doses. Early dose reduction is desirable

Adverse Effects

Adverse effects with phenothiazines include orthostatic hypotension, exacerbation of asthma, cholestatic jaundice, extrapyramidal reactions, anticholinergic effects (i.e., blurred vision, urinary retention, dry mouth, constipation, drowsiness, confusion), and Q wave and T wave alterations on the electrocardiogram.

Contraindications

Contraindications to the use of prochlorperazine include known hypersensitivity to the drug. Cautious use is necessary in people with glaucoma because the drug possesses antimuscarinic activity increasing the potential to precipitate acute angle closure glaucoma.

Nursing Implications

Preventing Interactions

Several medications interact with prochlorperazine, increasing its effects (Box 38.1). Herbal interactions with prochlorperazine have been reported with kava kava, St. John's wort, and valerian; an increased risk of CNS depression is a possibility. No herbs or foods that decrease the effects of prochlorperazine have been identified.

Administering the Medication

Parenteral administration of prochlorperazine is by the deep intramuscular route. Skin contact with the solution may cause contact dermatitis. If intravenous administration is necessary, patients should remain flat following administration and be observed for at least 20 minutes to decrease the risk of hypotension.

Assessing for Therapeutic Effects

The nurse observes for prevention or resolution of nausea and vomiting.

Assessing for Adverse Effects

The nurse assesses for associated adverse anticholinergic effects (dry mouth, blurred vision, urinary retention, constipation, acute confusion). The nurse must be aware that hallucinations, convulsions, and sudden death may occur with excessive doses. The nurse also assesses tissue integrity with intramuscular injection as the drug may cause severe tissue injury; burning and pain at the IV site justify immediate discontinuation of the drug.

Patient Teaching

The nurse teaches patients taking prochlorperazine to use the lowest effective dosage to prevent the development of EPS and other adverse effects.

Box 38.2 presents additional patient teaching guidelines.

BOX 38.1 Drug Interactions: Prochlorperazine

Drugs That Increase the Effects of Prochlorperazine

- Escitalopram, flunitrazepam, gabapentin, and zolpidem
  Have additive respiratory depressant effects
- Ethanol
  Increases the risk of central nervous system depression and psychomotor impairment
- Amisulpride
  Increases the risk of neuroleptic malignant syndrome
- Amiodarone, fluconazole, itraconazole, nortriptyline
  Increases the risk of abnormal heart rhythms

BOX 38.2 Patient Teaching Guidelines for Antiemetic Drugs

General Considerations

- Try to identify and avoid the circumstances that cause or aggravate nausea and vomiting.
- Take antiemetics before the causative event when possible, for greater preventative effects.
- Do not eat, drink, or take oral medications during acute vomiting episodes, to avoid aggravating the stomach upset.
- Lie down to help nausea and vomiting subside; activity tends to increase stomach upset.
- After your stomach has settled down, try to take enough fluids to prevent dehydration and potentially serious problems. Tea, broth, and gelatins are usually tolerated.
- If drowsy from antiemetic drugs, do not drive, operate dangerous machinery, or perform hazardous tasks requiring alertness, coordination, or physical dexterity, to avoid injury.
- If you take antiemetic drugs regularly, do not drink alcohol or take other drugs without consulting a healthcare provider. Several drugs interact with antiemetic agents, increasing adverse effects.

Self- or Caregiver Administration

- Do not increase dosage, take more often, or take when drowsy, dizzy, or unsteady on your feet. Several of the drugs cause sedation and other adverse effects, which are more severe if too much is taken.
- To prevent motion sickness, take medication 30 minutes before travel and then every 4 to 6 hours, if necessary, to avoid or minimize adverse effects.
- Take or give antiemetic drugs 30 to 60 minutes before a nausea-producing event, when possible. This includes cancer chemotherapy, radiation therapy, changing of painful dressings, or other treatments.
- Take dronabinol only when you can be supervised by a responsible adult because of its sedative and mind-altering effects.

Other Drugs in the Class

Phenothiazines are effective antiemetic agents. However, because of their adverse effects (e.g., sedation, cognitive impairment, extrapyramidal reactions), they are mainly indicated if vomiting is severe and cannot be controlled by other measures or only when a few doses are needed.

Chlorpromazine is used less often than prochlorperazine for nausea and vomiting but is more commonly used in the treatment of psychosis and psychotic symptoms in other disorders (see Chapter 56). It is also used with intractable hiccups and treatment of nausea and vomiting associated with anesthesia. Perphenazine has a side effect profile similar to that of prochlorperazine and is used to manage severe nausea and vomiting and in the treatment of schizophrenia (see Chapter 56). However, the FDA has issued a **BOXED WARNING** for perphenazine because older patients with dementia-related psychosis treated with perphenazine and other antipsychotic drugs have an increased risk of death. It is important to reduce the dose as soon as possible to minimize significant adverse effects, including bradycardia, cardiac arrest, hypotension, catatoniclike states, EPS, and a blue-gray discoloration of the skin.

ANTIHISTAMINES

Antihistamines are used primarily to prevent histamine from exerting its widespread effects on body tissues (see Chapter 32). The antihistamines used as antiemetic agents are the "classic" antihistamines or H_1 receptor blocking agents (as differentiated from cimetidine and related drugs, which are H_2 receptor blocking agents). Not all antihistamines are effective as antiemetic agents. **Hydroxyzine** (Vistaril) is the prototype of the class.

Pharmacokinetics

When administered orally, hydroxyzine is rapidly absorbed from the GI tract, with its effect noticeable within 30 minutes. The drug is metabolized in the liver, and the main metabolite is cetirizine. The half-life of hydroxyzine is, on average, 14 hours for adults, but it can be as short as 5 hours for small children and as long as 30 hours for older adults. Hydroxyzine is excreted into the urine in the form of its metabolites.

Action

Hydroxyzine and other antihistamines are thought to relieve nausea and vomiting by blocking the action of acetylcholine in the brain.

Use

Hydroxyzine may be effective in treating nausea and vomiting and preventing and treating motion sickness. Hydroxyzine is also used as a sedative to treat anxiety. Additionally, the drug is given in combination with other medications during anesthesia. Table 38.3 presents dosage information for the antihistamines.

Patient-related variables specific to the use of hydroxyzine include the following:

- Age:
  - In children, the recommended dosage of hydroxyzine is based on age and weight.
  - Dosage reduction may be appropriate with older adults due to an increased sedative potential.
  - According to the Beers Criteria, hydroxyzine is considered potentially inappropriate for use in older adults.
- Reproduction, pregnancy, and lactation:
  - Hydroxyzine crosses the placenta and potential withdrawal symptoms have been observed in neonates following chronic maternal use during pregnancy.
  - Use in early pregnancy is contraindicated by the manufacturer.
  - It is unknown if hydroxyzine is present in breast milk although sedation has been found in exposed breast-fed infants.

TABLE 38.3

DRUGS AT A GLANCE: Antihistamines

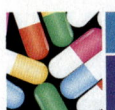

Drug	Routes and Dosage Ranges	
	Adults	**Children**
ⓟ **Hydroxyzine** (Vistaril; 🍁 NOVO-Hydroxyzine, Atarax, PMS-Hydroxyzine HCl)	PO IM 25–100 mg every 4–6 h as needed	IM 1.1 mg/kg in 4 divided doses (max 100 mg)
Dimenhydrinate (Dramamine) (🍁 Gravol)	PO 50–100 mg every 4–6 h as needed (max 400 mg in 24 h) IM 50 mg as needed IV 50 mg in 10 mL of sodium chloride injection, over 2 min (max 100 mg every 4 h)	6–12 y: PO 25–50 mg every 4–6 h (max 150 mg in 24 h) IM 1.25 mg/kg four times daily (max 300 mg in 24 h)
Doxylamine succinate with pyridoxine hydrochloride (Diclegis, Bonjesta; 🍁 Diclectin)	Nausea and vomiting of pregnancy: Doxylamine 10 mg/pyridoxine 10 mg/tablet (Diclegis): 2 tablets at bedtime on day 1 and 2; if symptoms continue, 1 tablet in morning and 2 tablets at bedtime on day 3; if symptoms continue, increase to 1 tablet in morning, 1 tablet in midafternoon, and 2 tablets at bedtime on day 4 (to max of doxylamine 40 mg/pyridoxine 40 mg [4 tablets] per day) Doxylamine 20 mg/pyridoxine 20 mg (Bonjesta): initial: one tablet at bedtime on day 1; if symptoms persist on day 2, increase to 1 tablet in morning and 1 tablet at bedtime (maximum: doxylamine 40 mg/pyridoxine 40 mg [2 tablets] per day)	Not indicated for use in children
Meclizine (Antivert, Dramamine Less Drowsy)	Motion sickness: PO 25–50 mg 1 h before travel Vertigo: PO 25–100 mg daily in divided doses	Motion sickness, >12 y: PO 25–50 mg/d divided into 2 or 3 doses

- Abnormal kidney function and hepatic impairment:
  - Because hydroxyzine is excreted in the urine, dosage adjustments and more intensive monitoring of adverse effects may be required in people with abnormal kidney function.
  - Likewise, because hydroxyzine is metabolized in the liver, dosage adjustments and more intensive monitoring of adverse effects may be required in people with hepatic impairment.
- Specific healthcare environments:
  - In the home setting, antiemetics are usually given orally or by rectal suppository. The home care nurse may need to assess patients for possible causes of nausea and vomiting and assist patients and caregivers with appropriate use of the drugs and other interventions to prevent fluid and electrolyte depletion.

Adverse Effects

With hydroxyzine, adverse anticholinergic effects include drowsiness, dizziness, confusion, dry mouth, thickened respiratory secretions, blurred vision, urinary retention, and tachycardia. In addition, hydroxyzine is associated with a possible risk of prolonged QT interval on ECG, and torsade de pointes.

Contraindications

Contraindications to hydroxyzine include known sensitivity to the drug. Patients in early pregnancy or individuals with a prolonged QT interval on ECG should not receive the drug.

Nursing Implications

Preventing Interactions

Many medications interact with hydroxyzine, increasing its effects (Box 38.3). Several medications that can cause CNS depression, such as sedatives, tranquilizers, muscle relaxants, and antidepressants, can have an increased sedative effect with the concomitant use of hydroxyzine. Kava kava, kratom, and valerian may enhance the adverse effect of CNS depressants. No herbs or foods appear to decrease or increase the effects of hydroxyzine.

Administering the Medication

Oral administration of hydroxyzine is often unsuccessful with nausea and vomiting. It is important to give the medication intramuscularly deep into a large muscle, not subcutaneously. IV administration can result in a sterile abscess with damage to tissue. Excessive sedation may occur with usual doses of antiemetics and is more likely with high doses. This may be minimized by avoiding high doses and assessing the patient's level of consciousness before each dose. Teaching safety precautions with sedating drugs may also be needed.

Assessing for Therapeutic Effects

The nurse assesses for the absence of nausea and vomiting.

Assessing for Adverse Effects

The nurse assesses for the presence of anticholinergic effects, including blurred vision, urinary retention, constipation, thick

BOX 38.3 Drug Interactions: Hydroxyzine

Drugs That Increase the Effects of Hydroxyzine
- Alcohol, gabapentin, levetiracetam, and lamotrigine
  Increase the risk of respiratory depression
- Seroquel
  Increases the risk of severe extrapyramidal reactions

secretions, and blurred vision. Patients with narrow-angle glaucoma, prostatic hyperplasia, and asthma are at greater risk for adverse effects.

Patient Teaching

Box 38.2 outlines patient teaching guidelines.

Other Drugs in the Class

Diphenhydramine, dimenhydrinate (Dramamine), and meclizine (Antivert, Dramamine Less Drowsy) are also used to prevent nausea, vomiting, dizziness, and vertigo associated with motion sickness. Diphenhydramine is more commonly used for symptomatic relief of allergic symptoms caused by histamine release, including nasal allergies and allergic dermatosis, as an adjunct to epinephrine in the treatment of anaphylaxis, and short-term insomnia, and prevention or treatment of motion sickness. Although diphenhydramine is often used for insomnia, the American Academy of Sleep Medicine guidelines do not recommend the drug for the treatment of chronic insomnia due to the absence of evidence for clinically significant improvement (Sateia et al., 2017). Meclizine is also given to manage vertigo associated with disease affecting the vestibular system. Dimenhydrinate and meclizine are available over-the-counter and are sold under the name Dramamine. Meclizine is dispensed by prescription. For vestibular diseases, meclizine should be taken at the onset of symptoms. Dimenhydrinate typically takes a minimum of 4 hours to take full effect. Meclizine becomes effective in about 1 hour.

A combination of doxylamine succinate, an antihistamine, and pyridoxine, a form of vitamin B6 (Diclegis, Bonjesta), is specifically approved for the treatment of nausea and vomiting during pregnancy for patients who do not respond to conservative management. The drug is taken daily on a routine basis and not PRN. Systematic reviews of clinical trials have shown that pyridoxine alone improves mild to moderate nausea in pregnancy but does not significantly reduce vomiting; however, the combination is effective in controlling nausea and vomiting.

Both Diclegis and Bonjesta exert delayed-release properties. However, Bonjesta has an immediate rapid release phase followed by a delayed release phase providing faster symptom relief than Diclegis.

Of note, another combination of doxylamine and pyridoxine, Bendectin, was voluntarily withdrawn from the market in 1983 because of lawsuits alleging teratogenicity. However, there was no proven association between its use and congenital anomalies. This erroneous concern contributed to a 30-year setback in prescription treatment for nausea and vomiting during pregnancy, until Diclegis was approved in 2013. Currently, strong scientific evidence, including a meta-analysis of controlled studies on outcome of pregnancies in patients taking the drug combination, have established the efficacy and fetal safety of the combination.

> **Quality and Safety Alert: Evidence-Based Practice**
>
> Mares et al. (2022) designed a questionnaire to explore subjective effectiveness of the diverse management approaches to treat hyperemesis gravidarum, the most severe form of nausea and vomiting of pregnancy. Available therapies have remained virtually unchanged over the last few decades, and affected patients commonly have partial relief to the antiemetics currently recommended. There were 786 pregnant participants who responded to a survey distributed online to hyperemesis gravidarum support groups, personal social media, and institutional email. Of those respondents, 66.6% were diagnosed formally with hyperemesis gravidarum. Results of the study indicated that most participants tried at least three medications without success or with adverse effects. Sixty-eight percent of those taking medications experienced adverse effects (e.g., fatigue, constipation, headache, anxiety, depression). Although a variety of antiemetic drugs were reported used, ondansetron was the most commonly used drug reported. The results of the study can inform the development of guidelines that can successfully manage the symptoms of hyperemesis gravidarum.

NCLEX Success

1. The nurse knows that antiemetics are most effective when administered
   A. before an emetogenic event occurs
   B. during an episode of nausea but before vomiting has occurred
   C. after the patient has experienced nausea and vomiting
   D. any time; timing of administration has no impact on drug effectiveness

2. The nurse would question an order for which of the following antiemetics for treatment of motion sickness–induced nausea?
   A. prochlorperazine
   B. dimenhydrinate
   C. meclizine
   D. scopolamine

5-HYDROXYTRYPTAMINE$_3$ (5-HT$_3$) OR SEROTONIN RECEPTOR ANTAGONISTS

The 5-HT$_3$ receptor antagonists approved for use in the United States are the cornerstones of therapy for the control of acute emesis caused by chemotherapy agents with moderate to high emetogenic potential. In addition, the class is usually considered drugs of first choice for postoperative nausea and vomiting. **Ondansetron** (Zofran, Zuplenz) is the prototype of the 5-HT$_3$ receptor antagonists.

Pharmacokinetics

Oral ondansetron is well absorbed from the GI tract and undergoes some first-pass metabolism. The drug's half-life is 3 to 5.5 hours in most patients and 9 to 20 hours in patients with moderate or severe liver impairment. With the oral forms (disintegrating tablet or soluble film), action begins in 30 to 60 minutes and peaks in about 2 hours. With the IV form, onset and peak of drug action are immediate. The bioavailability is slightly increased by the presence of food but is unaffected by antacids.

Action

Ondansetron and the other 5-HT_3 receptor antagonists antagonize serotonin receptors, preventing their activation by the effects of emetogenic drugs and toxins.

Use

Ondansetron is used to prevent or treat moderate to severe nausea and vomiting associated with cancer chemotherapy, radiation therapy, and postoperative status. Table 38.4 presents dosage information for the 5-HT_3 receptor antagonists.

Patient-related variables specific to the use of ondansetron and other 5-HT_3 receptor antagonist include the following:

- Age:
  - The ASCO recommends the use of a 5-HT_3 receptor antagonist plus a corticosteroid before administering high-dose chemotherapy or chemotherapy with high to moderate emetic risk to pediatric oncology patients.
- Reproduction, pregnancy, and lactation:
  - Ondansetron may be considered for the treatment of severe or refractory nausea and vomiting during the first 10 weeks of pregnancy.
  - Ondansetron can be used as a multidrug regimen to prevent nausea and vomiting associated with cesarean delivery.
  - It is unknown whether ondansetron is present in breast milk.
- Abnormal kidney function and hepatic impairment:
  - The drug's half-life is significantly increased in patients with moderate to severe hepatic impairment, which increases the risk of adverse effects.
- Specific healthcare environments:
  - In the home setting, the nurse must assist patients and caregivers with appropriate use of the drugs and other interventions to prevent fluid and electrolyte depletion.

Adverse Effects

Adverse effects include diarrhea, headache, dizziness, constipation, fatigue, transient elevation of liver enzymes, and pain at the injection site.

Contraindications

Contraindications to ondansetron include known hypersensitivity to the drug. Ondansetron and other drugs in the class may prolong QT interval on the electrocardiogram and should be avoided in patients taking class I and class III antidysrhythmic agents because of concerns about the development of torsade de pointes.

Nursing Implications

Preventing Interactions

Phenytoin, carbamazepine, rifampin, and other inducers of the cytochrome 450 (CYP) 3A4 enzymes increase the clearance of ondansetron and decrease serum concentrations. No dosage adjustment of ondansetron appears necessary for people taking these drugs based on available data. The use of ondansetron with apomorphine is contraindicated due to the potential of a significant drop of blood pressure or loss of consciousness with concurrent use. St. John's wort may decrease ondansetron levels.

Administering the Medication

It is important to leave the disintegrating tablet in the blister pack until administration. Gentle removal is essential; it is necessary to peel back the blister backing and not push the tablet through the foil. The oral film dissolves rapidly on the tongue, without the need for water.

Assessing for Therapeutic Effects

The nurse assesses for verbal reports of decreased nausea and the absence of vomiting.

Assessing for Adverse Effects

Because headache and diarrhea are the most common adverse effects, the nurse gives special attention when assessing for these effects. It is also necessary to evaluate for stamina and balance. The nurse should note that the use of ondansetron may mask a progressive ileus and gastric distension following abdominal surgery or in patients with chemotherapy-induced nausea and vomiting.

Patient Teaching

The nurse teaches patients with phenylketonuria that the oral disintegrating tablets contain phenylalanine. Box 38.2 presents other patient teaching guidelines.

Other Drugs in the Class

The other 5-HT_3 receptor antagonist drugs (granisetron, dolasetron, and palonosetron) may be more beneficial in the prevention of chemotherapy-induced nausea and vomiting than as rescue drugs.

Clinical Application 38.1

- Ms. Snyder's oncologist orders ondansetron 32 mg IV to be administered 30 minutes prior to her chemotherapy and 8 to 16 mg PO every 8 hours as needed. She also receives metoclopramide 10 mg PO four times a day (30 minutes before meals and at bedtime). For what adverse effects of ondansetron does the nurse assess?

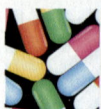

TABLE 38.4

DRUGS AT A GLANCE: 5-Hydroxytryptamine$_3$ (5-HT$_3$ or Serotonin) Receptor Antagonists

Drug	Routes and Dosage Ranges	
	Adults	**Children**
Ondansetron (Zofran, Zuplenz; ❋ ACT Ondansetron, APO-Ondansetron, Zofran ODT)	Chemotherapy-induced nausea and vomiting (highly emetogenic chemotherapy): PO, 8 mg, given day chemotherapy is administered, IV 8 mg or 0.15 mg/kg given as a single dose on the day of chemotherapy; IV doses >16 mg not recommended by manufacturer due to the potential for prolongation of QT internal on electrocardiogram; given in regimen that includes dexamethasone and aprepitant or fosaprepitant Chemotherapy-induced nausea and vomiting (moderately emetogenic chemotherapy): PO, 16 mg, given as 8 mg twice daily on day chemotherapy is administered, IV 8 mg or 0.15 mg/kg given as a single dose on day of chemotherapy; IV doses >16 mg not recommended due to the potential for prolongation of QT internal on electrocardiogram; given in regimen that includes dexamethasone and aprepitant or fosaprepitant Prevention of radiation therapy–induced nausea and vomiting: PO 8 mg 1–2 h before irradiation then 8 mg every 8 h after first dose for 102 d after completion of radiation Postoperative nausea and vomiting prevention: IV, IM 4 mg 1/2 h before end of anesthesia, IV 4 mg given over 2–5 min, PO 8 mg as an oral disintegrating tablet or soluble film ½–1 h before surgery; PO can be repeated in high-risk patients at discharge and on days 1 and 2	Chemotherapy-induced nausea and vomiting: >6 mo: IV 0.15 mg/kg for 3 doses, given ½ h before chemotherapy, repeat in 4 and 8 h. Infuse over 15 min 4–11 y: PO 4 mg given for 3 doses ½ h before chemotherapy, repeat in 8 and 16 h for 1–2 d after chemotherapy completed ≥12 y: PO 8 mg ½ h before chemotherapy, repeat Postoperative nausea and vomiting, prevention ≥5 mo to 12 y: ≤40 kg to IV 0.1 mg/kg, max 4 mg/dose >40 kg: IV 4 mg Given over 2–5 min; PO may be administered, if indicated
Dolasetron	Chemotherapy-induced nausea and vomiting: PO, 100 mg, given up to 1 h prior to chemotherapy Postoperative nausea and vomiting: IV 12.5 mg 15 min before reversal of anesthesia, PO 100 mg within 2 h prior to surgery	Chemotherapy-induced nausea and vomiting (>2 y): PO 1.8 mg/kg (max 100 mg) given up to 1 h prior to chemotherapy Postoperative nausea and vomiting (>2 y): IV 0.35 mg/kg (max 12.5 mg) 15 min before the reversal of anesthesia or with nausea or vomiting PO 1.2 mg/kg (max 100 mg) within 2 h prior to surgery
Granisetron (Sancuso, Sustol; ❋ APO-Granisetron, NAT-Granisetron)	Chemotherapy-induced nausea and vomiting: IV, 10 mcg/kg over 5 min, beginning ½ h prior to chemotherapy PO, 2 mg, given up to 1 h prior to chemotherapy, or 1 mg given up to 1 h prior to chemotherapy and repeated in 12 h PO, 2 mg, given up to 1 h prior to chemotherapy Transdermal patch: apply one patch at least 24 h prior to chemotherapy for prophylaxis; remove patch 24 h after chemotherapy completion. Patch may be worn up to 7 d Postoperative nausea and vomiting: IV 1 mg undiluted immediately before induction or reversal or after surgery	Chemotherapy-induced nausea and vomiting (2–16 y): IV 10 mcg/kg beginning ½ h prior to chemotherapy
Palonosetron (Aloxi; ❋ Aloxi)	Prevention of chemotherapy-induced nausea and vomiting: IV 0.25 mg about 30 min prior to chemotherapy Prevention of postoperative nausea and vomiting: IV 0.075 mg as a single dose immediately prior to induction of anesthesia	Prevention of chemotherapy-induced nausea and vomiting (≥1 mo): IV 20 mcg/kg (max 1.5 mg) ≥17 y: see adult dosage

SUBSTANCE P/NEUROKININ 1 ANTAGONISTS

Substance P is a peptide neurotransmitter in the neurokinin family. It plays a role in mediating acute chemotherapy-induced nausea and vomiting (along with serotonin) and is believed to be the primary mediator of delayed nausea and vomiting associated with chemotherapy. The drug ⓟ **aprepitant** (Emend, Cinvanti) and its prodrug fosaprepitant (Emend IV) are the prototype of the substance P/neurokinin 1 antagonists. As a prodrug, fosaprepitant is rapidly converted in the body to aprepitant with parenteral administration. Cinvanti is the IV form of aprepitant. Aprepitant and other substance P/neurokinin 1 antagonists are typically used in combination with a 5-HT$_3$ receptor and/or a glucocorticoid for patients receiving highly emetic chemotherapy.

Pharmacokinetics

Aprepitant is orally absorbed, reaching peak levels 4 hours after administration. It is highly protein bound. The drug is metabolized in the liver and is excreted in urine and feces. Because aprepitant undergoes extensive hepatic metabolism by CYP450 enzyme systems, it has the potential for multiple drug interactions. After administration, the prodrug form, fosaprepitant, is converted in the body to aprepitant within 30 minutes.

Action

Aprepitant exerts its antiemetic effect by blocking the activity of substance P at NK1 receptors in the brain, inhibiting the signal to the brain that causes nausea. The drug has little or no effect on serotonin, dopamine, or corticosteroid receptors.

Use

The antiemetic guidelines of the ASCO recommend the use of aprepitant in combination with a serotonin receptor antagonist and dexamethasone with chemotherapeutic drugs with high emetic risk. Prescribers often order aprepitant as part of combination therapy along with a 5-HT$_3$ receptor antagonist and corticosteroids to treat both acute and delayed nausea and vomiting associated with chemotherapy. Other indications include prevention of postoperative nausea and vomiting. The drug is also recommended as part of a chemotherapy regimen in protocols including anthracycline, cyclophosphamide, and other chemotherapeutic agents known to cause moderate emetic risk.

The FDA has stipulated that the IV prodrug of the oral formulation (fosaprepitant) should no longer be used to prevent nausea and vomiting associated with cancer chemotherapy in pediatric and adult patients because of the risk of abnormal heart rhythm.

Table 38.5 contains dosage information for aprepitant.

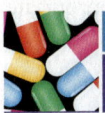

TABLE 38.5
DRUGS AT A GLANCE: Substance P/Neurokinin 1 Receptor Antagonists

Drug	Routes and Dosage Ranges	
	Adults	**Children**
ⓟ **Aprepitant** (Emend, Cinvanti; ✳ Emend, Emend Tri-Pack)	Prevention of nausea and vomiting associated with highly emetic and moderately emetic chemotherapy (administered as part of a four-drug treatment that also includes a 5-HT$_3$ receptor antagonist, olanzapine, and dexamethasone): Day 1: PO 125 mg 1 h before chemotherapy or IV 130 mg ½ h over 15 min before chemotherapy Days 2 and 3: PO 80 mg in the morning	≥6 mo to <12 y (6–<30 kg) day 1: PO suspension 3 mg/kg 1 h before chemotherapy and then 2 mg/kg on days 2 and 3 (regimen also includes a 5-HT$_3$ receptor antagonist, olanzapine, and dexamethasone, as indicated) ≥12 y: PO 125 mg prior to chemotherapy on day 1, followed by 80 mg once daily on days 2 and 3 (regimen also includes a 5-HT$_3$ antagonist, olanzapine, and dexamethasone, as indicated)
Netupitant/palonosetron (Akynzeo)	Day 1: PO one capsule (netupitant 300 mg/palonosetron 0.5 mg) about 1 h before prior chemotherapy (regimen also includes dexamethasone)	Safety and efficacy in children not established
Rolapitant (Varubi)	Day 1: PO one capsule about 1 h before prior chemotherapy (regimen also includes dexamethasone) Highly emetogenic: Day 1: PO 180 mg 1–2 h prior to chemotherapy (in combination with dexamethasone given on days 1, 2, 3, and 4 and a 5-HT$_3$ receptor antagonist) Moderately emetogenic: Day 1: PO 180 mg 1–2 h prior to chemotherapy (in combination with dexamethasone given on day 1 and a 5-HT$_3$ receptor antagonist and olanzapine, given as indicated)	Safety and efficacy in children not established

Patient-related variables specific to the use of aprepitant include the following:

- Age:
  - Limited evidence suggests that aprepitant is well tolerated in children receiving the drug in combination with standard antiemetics for chemotherapy-induced nausea and vomiting.
- Reproduction, pregnancy, and lactation:
  - The efficacy of hormonal contraceptives may be reduced during administration of and for 28 days following the last dose of aprepitant. An alternate method of contraception is needed during this time.
- Abnormal kidney function and hepatic impairment:
  - No dosage adjustment is required in patients with kidney disease, including those with kidney failure with replacement therapy receiving dialysis.
  - No adjustment is required in dosage for patients with mild to moderate hepatic impairment. However, no data are available regarding its use in people with severe hepatic impairment, and caution is warranted.

Adverse Effects

Aprepitant is well tolerated, with the most common adverse effects being fatigue, weakness, dizziness, abnormal heart rhythm, headache, and hiccups. Infusion site pain has been reported with IV administration.

Contraindications

Contraindications to aprepitant include known hypersensitivity to the drug or use in combination with ranolazine, pimozide, or cisapride.

Nursing Implications
Preventing Interactions

Aprepitant is extensively metabolized by the CYP3A4 enzyme, which is particularly important in drug metabolism. Certain drugs may increase or decrease the effects of aprepitant and are affected by aprepitant's inhibitory effects (Box 38.4). It is essential to reduce oral doses of dexamethasone or methylprednisolone by 50% and the IV dose of methylprednisolone by 25% when coadministered with aprepitant because of CYP3A4 inhibition.

Aprepitant also produces significant interactions that alter the effectiveness of other medications. The drug reduces the effectiveness of oral contraceptives for up to 28 days after administration; therefore, alternate contraceptive methods are recommended during treatment and for 1 month following administration of aprepitant.

Quality and Safety Alert: Safety

Aprepitant induces the metabolism of warfarin. It is necessary to monitor the international normalized ratio (INR) for 2 weeks after treatment is initiated, especially for the first 7 to 10 days, because a clinically significant drop in INR may occur.

BOX 38.4 Drug Interactions: Aprepitant

Drugs That Increase the Effects of Aprepitant
- CYP3A4 inhibitors, such as macrolide antibiotics, protease inhibitors, azole antifungal agents, nefazodone, cyclosporine, danazol, diltiazem, and verapamil
  Alter metabolism, increasing serum levels

Drugs That Decrease the Effects of Aprepitant
- CYP3A4 inducers, such as carbamazepine, phenytoin, rifampin, phenobarbital, and nevirapine
  Alter metabolism, decreasing serum levels

Foods and herbs are also known to affect aprepitant concentrations. Grapefruit juice decreases the metabolism of aprepitant. Because this effect can last up to 24 hours, repeated juice consumption can result in a cumulative increase in the serum level of aprepitant. In contrast, St. John's wort is known to cause a decrease in serum levels.

Administering the Medication

Patients should take aprepitant by mouth as directed with a full glass of water, with or without food. Typically, the first dose is taken 1 hour before chemotherapy and then daily in the morning for the next 2 days after the chemotherapy treatment. The approved IV form, fosaprepitant, a prodrug, in a dose of 150 mg, is bioequivalent to aprepitant, 125 mg, and it is appropriate to use these forms interchangeably.

Assessing for Therapeutic Effects

The nurse assesses for the absence of nausea and vomiting after chemotherapy or during the postoperative period.

Assessing for Adverse Effects

The nurse observes for the presence of adverse effects, such as fatigue, weakness, dizziness, headache, or hiccups. In addition, it is necessary to assess for a normal heart rhythm.

Patient Teaching

The nurse instructs patients to take the medication before the onset of nausea and vomiting. Alternate antiemetic medication (**rescue antiemetic**) may be necessary for who already have nausea and vomiting. Box 38.2 presents additional patient teaching guidelines.

Other Drugs in the Class

Netupitant is available in an oral fixed combination tablet with palonosetron (Akynzeo). The combination of a selective 5-HT_3 receptor antagonist and a substance P/neurokinin 1 receptor antagonist is used for the prevention of acute and delayed nausea and vomiting associated with initial and repeat courses of cancer chemotherapy, including, but not limited to, highly emetogenic chemotherapy. Netupitant prevents nausea and vomiting during both the acute and delayed phases, and palonosetron prevents nausea and vomiting during the acute phase and after cancer chemotherapy.

> **! Quality and Safety Alert: Evidence-Based Practice**
>
> Navari et al. (2021) evaluated the pooled efficacy from three cisplatin registration trials (total n = 1,197), each with arms containing a netupitant/palonosetron combination and an aprepitant regimen. The analysis revealed that the netupitant/palonosetron combination was more effective in preventing nausea and vomiting in days 3 to 5 following chemotherapy than the aprepitant regimen. Simultaneously targeting two critical antiemetic pathways with a single-dose combination preparation decreased the frequency of medications and the amount of additional rescue medications required to control nausea and vomiting symptoms. In addition, protecting patients from chemotherapy-induced nausea and vomiting can positively impact a patient's quality of life.

Rolapitant (Varubi) has a longer plasma half-life (~7 days) than either aprepitant or fosaprepitant, but unlike these drugs, which are moderate inhibitors of CYP3A4, rolapitant does not inhibit this metabolic pathway. Therefore, no adjustment of dexamethasone is required. Rolapitant does inhibit the CYP2D6 enzyme, which is responsible for metabolizing certain drugs, such as thioridazine; the use of both drugs together is contraindicated. Adverse effects include headache, lack of energy and strength, dyspepsia, constipation, and erythema.

MISCELLANEOUS ANTIEMETICS

Several miscellaneous agents are used individually or in multidrug regimens in the treatment of nausea and vomiting. Table 38.6 presents the dosage information for the miscellaneous agents.

Although corticosteroids are used mainly as antiallergic, anti-inflammatory, and antistress agents (see Chapter 17), they have antiemetic effects as well. Dexamethasone and methylprednisolone are commonly used in the management of chemotherapy-induced emesis and postoperative nausea and vomiting, either alone or in combination regimens with $5\text{-}HT_3$ receptor antagonists and/or substance P/neurokinin 1 receptor antagonists. With short-term use, adverse effects associated with corticosteroids are mild (e.g., euphoria, insomnia, mild fluid retention).

Benzodiazepine antianxiety drugs (see Chapter 54) are not antiemetics, but they are often used in multidrug regimens to prevent nausea and vomiting associated with cancer chemotherapy. The drugs produce relaxation, relieve anxiety, and inhibit cerebral cortex input to the vomiting center. They are often prescribed for patients who experience anticipatory nausea and vomiting before administration of anticancer drugs. Lorazepam (Ativan) is commonly used for this purpose but is not recommended as a single-agent antiemetic.

Olanzapine (Zyprexa) is a second-generation (atypical) antipsychotic often used in the treatment of bipolar disorder and schizophrenia. Current practice guidelines by ASCO (Hesketh et al., 2020) recommend adding olanzapine to antiemetic prophylaxis to reduce the likelihood of nausea among adults who are treated with high emetic risk antineoplastic agents. In adults who did not receive olanzapine and who experience nausea or vomiting despite optimal prophylaxis, the drug should be considered in addition to continuing the standard antiemetic regimen. As antiemetic prophylaxis postoperatively in adults and children, the IV or oral formulations can be administered, as indicated.

TABLE 38.6
DRUGS AT A GLANCE: Miscellaneous Agents

Drug	Routes and Dosage Ranges	
	Adults	**Children**
Olanzapine (Zyprexa; ❋ ACT Olanzapine OPT, TEVA-Olanzapine)	PO 10 mg on day 1 followed by 10 mg once daily, days 2–4 (in combination with dexamethasone and palonosetron on day 1 only)	Use in children not recommended for treatment of chemotherapy-induced nausea and vomiting
Dronabinol (Marinol, Syndros)	PO 5 mg/m² (square meter of body surface area) 1–3 h before chemotherapy and then every 2–4 h for a total of 4–6 doses daily. Dosage can be increased by 2.5 mg/m² increments to a maximal dose of 15 mg/m² if necessary	Same as adults for treatment of chemotherapy-induced nausea and vomiting
Nabilone (Cesamet; ❋ ACT-nabilone, Cesamet, PMS-nabilone)	PO initially, 1–2 mg twice daily; first dose 1–3 h before chemotherapy; may be administered 2–3 doses daily for course of chemotherapy continued to 48 h after the last dose	Limited data in select situations; first dose administered 1–3 h before chemotherapy <18 kg: PO 0.5 mg twice daily 19–30 kg: PO 1 mg twice daily >30 kg: 1 mg 3 times daily
Fructose, dextrose, and orthophosphoric acid (Emetrol)	PO 15–30 mL repeated at 15-min intervals until vomiting ceases not to exceed 5 doses over 1 h	≥2 y: PO 5–10 mL repeated at 15-min intervals until vomiting ceases not to exceed 5 doses over 1 h ≥12 y: refer to adult dosing
Scopolamine (Transderm Scop; ❋ Buscopan, Transderm-V)	Motion sickness: PO, IM, subcutaneous, 0.6–1.0 mg as a single dose Transdermal disc (1.5 mg scopolamine): placed behind the ear every 3 d if needed	Motion sickness: PO, subcutaneous, 0.006 mg as a single dose to max of 0.3 mg/dose; may be repeated every 6–8 h

Marijuana (*Cannabis*) is a schedule I drug, and 37 U.S. states, the District of Columbia, Guam, Puerto Rico, and the U.S. Virgin Islands allow the use of medical marijuana with a prescription (or signed medical statement) for registered qualifying patients who would likely benefit from marijuana. Patients have used it to treat chemotherapy-induced nausea and vomiting. Although marijuana has been used for centuries in treating nausea and vomiting and has been found to be an effective antiemetic agent, marijuana's potential in the treatment of cancer is still largely unknown. There remains insufficient evidence for a recommendation regarding its use in the most recent practice guidelines for management of chemotherapy- and radiation-induced nausea and vomiting (Hesketh et al., 2020). Dronabinol (Marinol, Syndros) and nabilone (Cesamet) are synthetic **cannabinoids** (derivatives of marijuana) that have demonstrated antiemetic activity and are FDA approved for the treatment of nausea and vomiting caused by chemotherapy. However, concern about their abuse potential and their rather unfavorable adverse effect profiles, especially in older adults, may limit their clinical utility. Both cannabinoids are approved in patients who have failed to respond adequately to conventional antiemetic treatments, and national clinical practice guidelines propose that this agent be considered as a rescue antiemetic for refractory nausea and vomiting. Synthetic cannabinoids have the same adverse effects as marijuana, including psychiatric symptoms (euphoria, tachycardia, abnormality in thinking, paranoia, drowsiness), and a high potential for abuse. Dronabinol can cause dizziness, drowsiness, mood changes, and other mind-altering effects. Use caution when increasing the dose of dronabinol and nabilone because there is an increased frequency of dose-related adverse reactions at higher dosages. In addition, the drugs may cause a withdrawal syndrome when abruptly discontinued. Withdrawal symptoms (e.g., insomnia, irritability, restlessness) in as little as 12 hours are most likely to occur with high doses or prolonged use, and around 24 hours postdronabinol discontinuation, withdrawal symptoms may intensify to include hot flashes, sweating, hiccoughs, rhinorrhea, loose stools, and anorexia. Sleep disturbances may persist for several weeks.

Quality and Safety Alert: Safety

Drugs with abuse potential are labeled in the Controlled Substance Act (see Chapter 1) on a schedule from I to V, from most to least risk of abuse, respectively. Marijuana is labeled schedule I as any cannabinoid found in the plant is automatically controlled in schedule I. Synthetic preparations nabilone, under the trade name Cesamet, and a liquid version of dronabinol, under the trade name Syndros, are schedule II drugs. Dronabinol as an oral capsule, under the trade name Marinol, is a schedule III drug under federal narcotic laws. The difference in schedule classification of the trade name drugs of dronabinol may be the result of the date of approval, the research findings regarding abuse potential, and other factors. Assess individuals taking these drugs for adverse effects and withdrawal symptoms.

Fructose, dextrose, and orthophosphoric acid (Emetrol) is a hyperosmolar solution with phosphoric acid. This drug is thought to reduce smooth muscle contraction in the GI tract and is available as an over-the-counter medication in syrup form. Because this solution contains fructose, patients with diabetes mellitus should consult their healthcare provider before using it.

Scopolamine (Transderm Scop), an M1 muscarinic receptor antagonist, is a major anticholinergic drug (see Chapter 48) effective in relieving nausea and vomiting associated with motion sickness and radiation therapy. It is predominantly used as a transdermal patch to prevent motion sickness.

NCLEX Success

3. When administering 5-HT$_3$ receptor antagonists before cancer chemotherapy, the nurse should also be prepared to administer which of the following adjunctive medications?
   A. prochlorperazine
   B. dexamethasone
   C. dronabinol
   D. hydroxyzine

4. A woman sends her partner to the store to purchase an over-the-counter product to resolve the vomiting she has experienced during a migraine. She has a history of diabetes and hypertension. She has an appointment with her healthcare provider in the morning. Which of the following drugs would be the best for the partner to purchase?
   A. prochlorperazine
   B. fructose, dextrose, and orthophosphoric acid
   C. meclizine
   D. dimenhydrinate

5. A 30-year-old patient has been ordered dronabinol. Which of the following statements are true for dronabinol? (Select all that apply.)
   A. The drug is most effective when given every 2 hours.
   B. It is approved for nausea and vomiting related to chemotherapy in people with cancer.
   C. Adverse effects include drowsiness or euphoria.
   D. Insufficient research is available to support its use as a treatment for nausea and vomiting.
   E. It is approved as an appetite stimulant for anorexia in people with AIDS.
   F. The drug is used as a first-line treatment in women with hyperemesis gravidarum associated with pregnancy.

Clinical Application 38.2

- Ms. Snyder is concerned about the amount of medication she is receiving. She asks the nurse to withhold her antiemetics until she actually vomits. What is the best way to respond to Ms. Snyder?

NONPHARMACOLOGIC MANAGEMENT

Nonpharmacologic techniques have become an acceptable adjunct to antiemetic drug therapy. The use of herbal supplements has also received support.

Acupuncture and Acupressure

Practitioners use acupuncture and acupressure to stimulate the pericardium 6 site, which is generally thought to be effective in the management of chemotherapy-induced nausea and vomiting and motion sickness. Acupuncture is one of the most well studied of all the nonpharmacologic techniques, but interpretation of the results of randomized trials is hampered by a high risk of bias in most studies and a lack of standardization of treatment methods and comparison groups. Acupressure wristbands may also be useful in the treatment of nausea and vomiting associated with motion sickness.

Herbal Supplements

The use of ginger in traditional Chinese and Indian medicine has a long history. The herb's components are thought to interact with 5-HT_3 receptors, which may account for the antiemetic activity. Clinical trials suggest that the herb can effectively reduce nausea and vomiting associated with motion sickness, pregnancy, and surgery. However, evidence of the herb's success against chemotherapy-induced nausea and vomiting is mixed. ASCO guidelines (2020) state that insufficient evidence exists to recommend for or against the use of ginger to prevent chemotherapy-induced nausea and vomiting. However, ASCO endorsed the Society for Integrative Oncology's evidence-based guideline for the use of integrative therapies after breast cancer treatment, stating that ginger could be considered as an addition to antiemetic drugs to control nausea and vomiting during chemotherapy (Lyman et al., 2018).

Additional high-quality studies are needed to establish the clinical efficacy of ginger as a complementary therapy in the treatment of nausea and vomiting.

Clinical Application 38.3

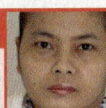

- What nursing measures, in addition to the administration of antiemetic medication, should the nurse suggest to Ms. Snyder to reduce her nausea and vomiting?

THE NURSING PROCESS

A concept map outlines the nursing process related to drug therapy considerations in this chapter. Additional nursing implications related to the disease process should also be considered in care decisions.

Assessment
- Identify risk factors for nausea and vomiting and frequency, duration, and precipitating causes.
- Interview for any measures, including antiemetic drugs, that successfully relieve nausea and vomiting.
- When possible, observe and measure the vomitus.

Outcomes of Therapy

The patient will
- Receive antiemetic drugs at appropriate times, by indicated routes.
- Take antiemetic drugs as prescribed for outpatient use.
- Obtain relief of nausea and vomiting.
- Eat and retain food and fluids.
- Report increased comfort.
- Maintain body weight.

Nursing Interventions
- Use measures to prevent or minimize nausea and vomiting.
- Assist patient to identify situations and avoid stimuli that cause or aggravate nausea and vomiting.
- Administer analgesics before painful diagnostic tests and dressing changes or other therapeutic measures, as pain may cause nausea and vomiting.
- Administer antiemetic drugs 30 to 60 minutes before a nausea-producing event, when possible (e.g., radiation therapy, cancer chemotherapy, travel).
- Adjust the timing of any oral drugs that cause gastric irritation, nausea, and vomiting by taking with or just after food if food does not alter the beneficial effects of drug.
- Assess the patient's condition and report to the health care provider reoccurring nausea and vomiting. In some instances, a drug (e.g., digoxin, an antibiotic) may need to be discontinued or reduced in dosage. In other instances (e.g., paralytic ileus, GI obstruction), preferred treatment is restriction of oral intake and nasogastric intubation.
- Suggest that a woman eat dry crackers before rising in the morning and ingest small, frequent protein meals to help prevent nausea and vomiting associated with pregnancy.
- Avoid administering oral intake of food, fluids, and drugs during acute episodes of nausea and vomiting. Oral intake may increase vomiting and risks of fluid and electrolyte imbalances.
- Give replacement fluids and electrolytes. Offer small amounts of food and fluids orally when tolerated and according to patient preference.
- Record vital signs, intake and output, and body weight at regular intervals if nausea or vomiting occurs frequently.
- Decrease environmental stimuli when possible (e.g., noise, odors). Allow the patient to lie quietly in bed when nauseated. Decreasing motion and activity may decrease stimulation of the vomiting center in the brain.
- Help the patient rinse his or her mouth after vomiting. Rinsing decreases the bad taste and corrosion of tooth enamel caused by gastric acid.
- Provide requested nonpharmacologic remedies when possible (e.g., a cool, wet washcloth to the face and neck).
- Provide appropriate education for any drug therapy (see Box 38.2).

Evaluation
- Observe and interview for decreased nausea and vomiting.
- Observe and interview regarding ability to maintain adequate intake of food and fluids and baseline weight.
- Observe and interview regarding appropriate use of antiemetic drugs.

Visit thePoint® *at* **http://thePoint.lww.com/Frandsen13e** *for answers to NCLEX Success questions (in Appendix A), answers to Clinical Application Case Studies (in Appendix B), additional material on etiology and pathophysiology, and more!*

REFERENCES AND RESOURCES

American College of Obstetricians and Gynecologists. (2018). ACOG Practice Bulletin #189. Nausea and vomiting of pregnancy. *Obstetrics and Gynecology*, *131*, e15–e30.

Elvir-Lazo, O. L., White, P. F., Yumul, R., & Cruz Eng, H. (2020). Management strategies for the treatment and prevention of postoperative/post discharge nausea and vomiting: an updated review. *F1000Research*, *9*. F1000 Faculty Rev-983. https://doi.org/10.12688/f1000research.21832.1

Estoup, A. C., Moise-Campbell, C., Varma, M., & Stewart, D. G. (2016). The impact of marijuana legalization on adolescent use, consequences, and perceived risk. *Substance Use & Misuse*, *51*(14), 1881–1887.

Fiaschi, L., Nelson-Piercy, C., Deb, S., King, R., & Tata, L. J. (2019). Clinical management of nausea and vomiting in pregnancy and hyperemesis gravidarum across primary and secondary care: A population-based study. *BJOG: An International Journal of Obstetrics & Gynaecology*, *126*, 1201–1211. doi: 10.1111/1471-0528.15662

Gan, T. J., & Habib, A. S. (2016). *Postoperative nausea and vomiting: A practical guide*. Cambridge University Press.

Garnock-Jones, K. P. (2016). Fosaprepitant Dimeglumine: A review in the prevention of nausea and vomiting associated with chemotherapy. *Drugs*, *76*(14), 1365–1372. https://doi.org/10.1007/s40265-016-0627-7

Hesketh, P. J. (2022). Prevention and treatment of chemotherapy-induced nausea and vomiting in adults. In *UpToDate*. Lexi-Comp, Inc.

Hesketh, P. J., Kris, M. G., Basch, E., Bohlke, K., Barbour, S. Y., Clark-Snow, R. A., Danso, M. A., Dennis, K., Dupuis, L. L., Dusetzina, S. B., Eng, C., Feyer, P. C., Jordan, K., Noonan, K., Sparacio, D., & Lyman, G. H. (2020). Antiemetics: American Society of Clinical Oncology Clinical Practice guideline update. *Journal of Clinical Oncology*, *38*(24), 2782–2797.

Hinkle, J. H., Cheever, K. H., & Overbaugh, K. (2021). *Brunner & Suddarth's textbook of medical-surgical nursing* (15th ed.). Wolters Kluwer.

Kovac, A. L. (2021). Postoperative nausea and vomiting in pediatric patients. *Paediatric Drugs*, *23*(1), 11–37. https://doi.org/10.1007/s40272-020-00424-0

Longstreth, G. F., & Hesketh, P. J. (2022). Characteristics of antiemetic drugs. In *UpToDate*. Lexi-Comp, Inc.

Lyman, G. H., Greenlee, H., Bohlke, K., Bao, T., De Michele, A. M., Deng, G. E., & Cohen, L. (2018). Integrative therapies during and after breast cancer treatment: ASCO endorsement of the SIO clinical practice guideline. *Journal of Clinical Oncology*, *36*(25), 2647–2655. https://doi.org/10.1200/JCO.2018.79.2721

Mares, R., Morrow, A., Shumway, H., Zapata, I., Forstein, D., & Brooks, B. (2022). Assessment of management approaches for hyperemesis gravidarum and nausea and vomiting of pregnancy: A retrospective questionnaire analysis. *BMC Pregnancy and Childbirth*, *22*(1), 1–8.

Navari, R. M., Biner, G., Bonizzoni, E., Clark-Snow, R., Olivaris, S., & Roeland, E. J. (2021). Single-dose netupitant/palonosetron versus 3-day aprepitant for preventing chemotherapy induced nausea and vomiting: A pooled analysis. *Future Oncology*, *17*(23), 3027–3035. https://doi.org/10.2217/fon-2021-0023

Norris, T. L. (2018). *Porth's pathophysiology: Concepts of altered health states*. Wolters Kluwer.

Razvi, Y., Chan, S., McFarlane, T., McKenzie, E., Zaki, P., DeAngelis, C., Pidduck, W., Bushehri, A., Chow, E., et al. (2019). ASCO, NCCN, MASCC/ESMO: A comparison of antiemetic guidelines for the treatment of chemotherapy-induced nausea and vomiting in adult patients. *Supportive Care in Cancer*, *27*(1), 87–95. https://doi.org/10.1007/s00520-018-4464-y

Sateia, M. J., Buysse, D. J., Krystal, A. D., Neubauer, D. N., & Heald, J. L. (2017). Clinical practice guideline for the pharmacologic treatment of chronic insomnia in adults: An American Academy of Sleep Medicine Clinical Practice Guideline. *Journal of Clinical Sleep Medicine*, *13*(2). https://doi.org/10.5664/jcsm.6470

CHAPTER 39

Drug Therapy for Constipation and Elimination Problems

LEARNING OBJECTIVES

After studying this chapter, you should be able to:

1. Educate patients about nonpharmacologic measures to prevent or treat constipation.
2. Identify the prototype and describe the action, use, contraindications, adverse effects, and nursing implications of the laxatives.
3. Identify the prototype and describe the action, use, contraindications, adverse effects, and nursing implications of the cathartics.
4. Identify the prototype and describe the action, use, contraindications, adverse effects, and nursing implications of guanylate cyclase-C (GC-C) agonists.
5. Identify the prototype, indications, dosages, and routes for the miscellaneous agents used to treat constipation and other conditions.
6. Implement the nursing process in the care of patients with constipation.

CLINICAL APPLICATION CASE STUDY

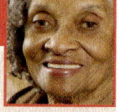

Doris Campbell, an 84-year-old woman, is complaining about being constipated. Her past health history includes arthritis, osteoporosis, hemorrhoids, and peptic ulcer disease. As a home care nurse, you frequently see patients who complain of constipation.

KEY TERMS

Constipation: infrequent and painful expulsion of hard, dry stools

Defecation: bowel elimination that is normally stimulated by movements and reflexes in the gastrointestinal tract

Fecal impaction: mass of hard, dry stool in the rectum; caused by chronic constipation

Flatulence: expulsion of gas through the rectum

INTRODUCTION

Constipation is the infrequent and painful expulsion of hard, dry stools. Drug therapy for constipation and elimination problems includes laxatives and cathartics, which are used to promote bowel elimination (defecation). The term *laxative* implies mild effects, with elimination of soft, formed stool. The term *cathartic* implies strong effects, with elimination of liquid or semiliquid stool. Although different effects may depend more on the dose than on the particular drug used, the names laxatives and cathartics are used in this chapter to specify the harshness of the level of response expected at normal doses of the drugs.

OVERVIEW OF CONSTIPATION

Generally, constipation is difficult to define clearly because normal frequency of stools varies as a symptom and differs from person to person. Constipation is a symptom, not a disease.

Several factors can cause or contribute to constipation, although in most people, no single cause can be found. Constipation may be associated with normal or slow bowel transit, defecatory dysfunction, or both. Several risk factors are associated with the development of constipation, including age, diet and lifestyle (particularly decreased levels of physical activity), and certain drugs and disease processes.

Clinical Manifestations

Constipation involves infrequent **defecation**, bowel elimination that is stimulated by movements and reflexes in the gastrointestinal (GI) tract. Because of variations in diet and other factors, there is no "normal" number of stools, but the traditional medical definition of functional constipation in adults includes three or fewer bowel movements per week. In adults, the use of a multisymptom criterion-based checklist (Rome III criteria for functional constipation) requires two or more of six symptoms during at least one fourth of the bowel movements. Along with fewer than three stools per week, symptoms include straining, a sensation of incomplete evacuation, a sensation of anorectal blockage, hard stools, and use of manual evacuation. Normal bowel elimination should produce a soft, formed stool without pain.

In children, the criteria that define constipation are slightly different. In those younger than 4 years of age, the Rome III criteria for functional constipation include two of the following symptoms: fewer than two stools per week, at least one episode of incontinence per week after the acquisition of toileting skills, stool retention, painful bowel movements, large mass of stool in the rectum, and large-diameter stools that may obstruct the toilet. In those aged 4 years and older, the criteria include two defecations in the toilet per week, stool retention, painful bowel movements, large mass of stool in the rectum, large-diameter stools that may obstruct the toilet, and a history of retentive posturing or excessive volitional stool retention.

Physicians may measure the bowel transit time to find the cause of constipation or locate whether a specific part of the intestine is slowing down movement more than another. Because different people have different transit times, experts disagree on the usefulness of the test. Some providers do not recommend bowel transit time testing or do so only when lifestyle changes have not produced desired results.

Lifestyle Changes

Nonpharmacologic treatment of people with constipation has included the use of fiber, fluid supplementation, prebiotics, probiotics, and behavioral therapy. There is some evidence that fiber supplements and adequate fluid intake improve the frequency and consistency of stools. Children with constipation should eat a balanced diet, containing juices that contain sorbitol, such as prune, pear, and apple juice (for infants), and whole grains, fruits, and vegetables (for children). Bowel transit time depends on what types of food eaten and the quantity of fluid ingested; research indicates that people who eat increased fruits, vegetables, and whole grains tend to have shorter transit times than do people who eat mostly sugars and starches. In addition, people should be advised to try to defecate after meals, thereby taking advantage of normal postprandial increases in colonic motility.

Behavioral interventions, such as biofeedback therapy, have been successful in improving symptoms of constipation.

> **Quality and Safety Alert: Teamwork and Collaboration**
>
> Factors that improve the chance of successfully resolving constipation with biofeedback are the motivation of the patient and therapist; the intensity and frequency of the retraining program; and a team approach that includes a broad scope of participants, such as the patient and their significant others, behavioral psychologist, and dietitian. The role of significant others is especially important in children.

> ### Clinical Application 39.1
>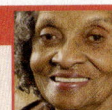
> - Given Mrs. Campbell's complaint of constipation, what does the nurse assess regarding the patient's bowel pattern and risk of constipation?

Drug Therapy

Laxatives and cathartics are given to prevent or treat constipation and are somewhat arbitrarily classified as:

- Laxatives: bulk-forming, lubricant or emollient, and surfactant agents (stool softeners)
- Cathartics: saline and stimulant agents
- Miscellaneous agents

Table 39.1 lists the specific drugs used for the treatment of constipation by class.

Clinically, the choice of a laxative or cathartic often depends on the reason for use and the patient's condition, as shown in Table 39.2. There are several indications for use:

- To relieve constipation in pregnant patients, older adult patients whose abdominal and perineal muscles have become weak and atrophied, children with megacolon, and patients receiving drugs that decrease intestinal motility (e.g., opioid analgesics, drugs with anticholinergic effects)

TABLE 39.1

Drugs Administered for the Treatment of Constipation

Drug Class	Prototype(s)	Other Drugs in the Class
Laxatives		
Bulk-forming	Psyllium preparations (Metamucil, Konsyl, Natural Fiber, Reguloid)	Methylcellulose (Citrucel, Soluble Fiber Therapy) Polycarbophil (FiberCon, FiberGen, Fiber-Lax)
Lubricant laxative		Mineral oil (GoodSense Mineral Oil, Fleet Oil, Fleet Mineral Oil Enema)
Stool softeners		Docusate calcium Docusate sodium (Colace, Docusil, Docuprene)
Cathartics		
Stimulant	Bisacodyl (Dulcolax)	Castor oil Glycerin (Glycerin, Pedia-Lax, Sani-Supp Pediatric) Senna preparations (Ex-Lax Maximum Strength, Senokot)
Saline		Magnesium citrate solution (Citroma, GoodSense Magnesium Citrate) Magnesium hydroxide (Milk of Magnesia, Pedia-Lax, Phillips) Polyethylene glycol (PEG) solution (GaviLAX, GlycoLax, HealthyLax, MiraLAX, PEGyLAX) Polyethylene glycol–electrolyte solution (PEG-ES) (Colyte, GaviLyte-N, GoLYTELY, NuLYTELY, TriLyte)
Guanylate Cyclase-C Agonists	Linaclotide (Linzess)	Plecanatide (Trulance)
Miscellaneous		Lactulose (Constulose, Kristalose) Lubiprostone (Amitiza) Sorbitol Prucalopride (*Motegrity*) Tegaserod (Zelnorm)

- To prevent straining at stool in patients with coronary artery disease (e.g., post–myocardial infarction), hypertension, cerebrovascular disease, and hemorrhoids and other rectal conditions
- To empty the bowel in preparation for bowel surgery or diagnostic procedures (e.g., colonoscopy, barium enema)
- To accelerate elimination of potentially toxic substances from the GI tract (e.g., orally ingested drugs or toxic compounds)
- To prevent absorption of intestinal ammonia in patients with hepatic encephalopathy
- To obtain a stool specimen for parasitologic examination
- To accelerate excretion of parasites after anthelmintic drugs have been administered
- To reduce serum cholesterol levels (psyllium products)

In addition, safety, clinical response, cost, and convenience all influence the choice of the initial treatment selected.

LAXATIVES

Bulk-forming laxatives are soluble fibers that are largely unabsorbed by the intestine. When water is added, these substances swell and become gel-like. Bulk-forming laxatives are the most physiologic laxatives because their effect is similar to that of increased intake of dietary fiber. Generally, bulk-forming laxatives are preferred for long-term use. The bulk-forming laxative **psyllium** (Metamucil; others) is the prototype laxative.

Pharmacokinetics

Psyllium usually acts within 12 to 24 hours, although it may take as long as 2 to 3 days to exert its full effects. Excretion is in the stool.

Action

Psyllium is essentially unabsorbed by the body. It works by mechanical action to absorb excess water while stimulating normal bowel elimination. The drug adds bulk and size to the fecal mass that stimulates peristalsis and defecation. It also may act by pulling water into the intestinal lumen.

Use

Uses of psyllium include treatment of occasional constipation or bowel irregularity. The drug may also help lower cholesterol when combined with a diet low in cholesterol and saturated fat. It may also be useful in the treatment of diarrhea. It should be noted that because psyllium, like most laxatives, is not absorbed or metabolized extensively, it can usually be used without difficulty in patients with hepatic impairment. Table 39.3 presents route and dosage information for the psyllium and other bulk-forming laxatives as well as surfactant and lubricant laxatives.

Patient-related variables specific to the use of psyllium include the following:

TABLE 39.2

Use of Laxatives and Cathartics for Specific Conditions

Indication	Preferred Drug Regimen
For patients in whom straining is potentially harmful or painful such as those with coronary artery disease (e.g., post–myocardial infarction), hypertension, cerebrovascular disease, anal fissures, or hemorrhoids	Stool softeners (e.g., docusate sodium) are the agents of choice.
For children For occasional use to cleanse the bowel for endoscopic or radiologic examinations	Saline or stimulant cathartics are acceptable (e.g., magnesium citrate, polyethylene glycol–electrolyte solution, bisacodyl). These drugs should not be used more than once per week. Frequent use is likely to produce laxative abuse.
For long-term use of laxatives or cathartics in patients who are debilitated, older, or unable or unwilling to eat an adequate diet	Bulk-forming laxatives (e.g., Metamucil) usually are preferred. However, because obstruction may occur, these agents should not be given to patients with difficulty in swallowing or adhesions or strictures in the GI tract or to those who are unable or unwilling to drink adequate fluids.
To accelerate elimination of potentially toxic substances from the GI tract (e.g., orally ingested drugs or toxic compounds)	Sorbitol may be given with activated charcoal to remove toxic substances.
To prevent absorption of intestinal ammonia in patients with hepatic encephalopathy	Lactulose acidifies the stool and traps ammonia and eliminates it with other fecal material.
For fecal impaction	In adults, a rectal suppository (e.g., bisacodyl) or an enema (e.g., oil retention or Fleet Enema) is preferred. Oral laxatives are contraindicated when fecal impaction is present but may be given after the rectal mass is removed. In children, polyethylene glycol with or without electrolytes and mineral oil have been shown to be effective for initial disimpaction. After the impaction is relieved, measures should be taken to prevent recurrence. If dietary and other nonpharmacologic measures are ineffective or contraindicated, use of a bulk-forming agent daily or another laxative once or twice weekly may be necessary.
For adults with irritable bowel syndrome with constipation For children with functional constipation	If a trial of soluble fiber and polyethylene glycol is unsuccessful, lubiprostone, linaclotide, or plecanatide may be administered to adults. In women under 65 y of age, tegaserod may be considered. Insufficient evidence exists to support the use of probiotics in children with FC. To date, PEG is the laxative of the first choice for both disimpaction (high dose 1–1.5 g/kg/d) and maintenance treatment (0.2–0.8 g/kg/d) lactulose, lactitol, and magnesium hydroxide are available, but studies have shown a lower efficacy than PEG for all of these agents. Stimulant laxatives, such as diphenylmethanes (e.g., bisacodyl) and anthraquinones (e.g., senna) are often used for short periods of time and are associated with more side effects, such as abdominal pain.

- Age:
  - Although psyllium-containing products are available without a prescription, children should take them only under the supervision of a healthcare provider.
  - Psyllium is one of the many laxatives that is often used or overused in older adults, thus nondrug measures to prevent constipation are much preferred. If a regular laxative is required, a bulk-forming psyllium compound (e.g., Metamucil) is best because it is most physiologic in its action.
- Reproduction, pregnancy, and lactation:
  - Since psyllium is not absorbed systemically, the drug is safe in pregnancy when administered with oral adequate fluids.

Adverse Effects

Psyllium or any fiber product may result in severe **flatulence** (expulsion of gas through the rectum) and bloating. In addition, there have been reports of abdominal cramping and esophageal or bowel obstruction.

Contraindications

Contraindications to the use of psyllium include the presence of undiagnosed abdominal pain. The danger is that the drugs may cause an inflamed organ (e.g., the appendix) to rupture and spill GI contents into the abdominal cavity with subsequent peritonitis, a life-threatening condition. Other contraindications are known allergy to the drug and intestinal obstruction and **fecal impaction**, a mass of hard, dry stool in the rectum.

Quality and Safety Alert: Safety

People who have difficulty swallowing, including those with esophageal stricture or other narrowing or obstruction of the GI tract, should not take psyllium.

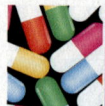

TABLE 39.3 DRUGS AT A GLANCE: Laxatives

Drug	Routes and Dosage Ranges	
	Adults	Children
Bulk-Forming		
Psyllium preparations (Metamucil, Natural Vegetable Fiber, Reguloid; Metamucil)	PO 2.5–30 g daily in divided doses, stirred in at least 8 oz water or other liquid	6–11 y: PO 1.25–15 g daily in divided doses in 8 oz water 12 y and older: PO same dosage as adults
Methylcellulose (Citrucel, Good Sense Fiber, Soluble Fiber Therapy)	PO powder 2 g up to three times daily with water (8 oz or more) PO caplets two up to six times daily	6–11 y: PO 1 g in 8 oz water up to three times daily; 1 caplet up six times daily 12 y and older: PO same dosage as adults
Polycarbophil (FiberCon, Fiber-Lax)	PO 1250 mg 1–4 times daily or PRN with 8 oz of fluid; maximum dose 4 g/24 h	6–12 y: PO 625 mg 1–4 times daily or PRN; maximum dose 2 g/24 h 12 y and older: PO same dosage as adults
Stool Softeners		
Docusate sodium (Colace, Docusil, Colace, Dosolax, Soflax, Taro-Docusate)	PO 50–360 mg once daily or in divided doses Rectal 283 mg/5 mL in one enema 1–3 times daily	2–6 y: products vary, consult labels 6–11 y: PO 100 mg daily 12 y and older: PO same dosage as adults
Lubricants		
Mineral oil (GoodSense Mineral Oil, Fleet Oil, Fleet Mineral Oil Enema)	PO 15–45 mL at bedtime or in divided doses, maximum 45 mL/d Rectal enema, 118 mL as single dose	Older than 6 y: PO 5–15 mL at bedtime; rectal enema, 30–60 mL

Nursing Implications

Preventing Interactions

With psyllium, no known drug or herbal interactions exist. However, the laxative may reduce or delay the absorption of certain medications, including carbamazepine, digoxin, lithium, tricyclic antidepressants, and warfarin. People should take psyllium at least 1 hour before or 2 to 4 hours after taking other medications. There is also a potential risk of psyllium interfering with nutrient absorption, but clear evidence is not available.

Administering the Medication

It is important to take the drug with at least 8 oz of water or another liquid. With the psyllium-containing preparation Metamucil, there have been reports of obstruction in the GI tract when the compound was taken with insufficient fluid. People should take capsules one at a time with ample fluids.

Assessing for Therapeutic Effects

The nurse assesses for relief from constipation within 12 to 72 hours.

Assessing for Adverse Effects

The nurse assesses for choking or trouble swallowing, severe stomach pain or cramping, nausea or vomiting, rectal bleeding, or constipation lasting longer than 7 days.

Patient Teaching

Patients should take the medication as directed with a full glass of liquid, as soon as it is mixed. Maintaining adequate overall intake of fluids also helps improve bowel regularity. Box 39.1 lists patient teaching guidelines for the laxatives and cathartics.

> **Quality and Safety Alert: Safety**
>
> Psyllium products may contain sugar, sodium, potassium, or artificial sweeteners. This may be of concern to patients who have diabetes, high blood pressure, kidney disease, or phenylketonuria. It is important to teach patients to check the product label if they have these conditions.

Other Drugs in the Class

Other laxative products facilitate relief of constipation through different physiologic mechanisms. Lubricant and surfactant laxatives are briefly discussed in this section.

Lubricant Laxative

Mineral oil is the only lubricant laxative used clinically. It lubricates the fecal mass and slows colonic absorption of water from the fecal mass, but its exact mechanism of action is unknown. Effects usually occur in 6 to 8 hours. Oral mineral oil may cause several adverse effects and is not recommended for long-term use. Mineral oil is probably most useful as a retention enema to soften hard, dry feces and aid in their removal. Oral use of mineral oil may cause potentially serious adverse effects (decreased absorption of fat-soluble vitamins and some drugs; lipid pneumonia if aspirated into the lungs). Thus, mineral oil is not an oral laxative of choice in any condition, although occasional use in the alert patient is unlikely to be harmful. It should not be used regularly. With mineral oil, lipid pneumonia and decreased absorption of vitamins A, D, E, and K can occur.

BOX 39.1 Patient Teaching Guidelines for Laxatives and Cathartics

General Considerations

- Eat foods high in dietary fiber daily. Fiber is the portion of plant food that is not digested. It is contained in fruits, vegetables, and whole-grain cereals and breads. Bran, the outer coating of cereal grains such as wheat or oats, is an excellent source of dietary fiber and is available in numerous cereal products.
- If one is having chronic constipation and is unable or unwilling to eat enough fiber-containing foods in the diet, the next best action is regular use of a bulk-forming laxative (e.g., Metamucil) as a dietary supplement. When taken daily, these can prevent constipation. However, these laxatives may take 2 to 3 days to work and are not effective in relieving acute constipation.
- Drink at least 6 to 10 glasses (8 oz each) of fluid daily if not contraindicated.
- Exercise regularly. Walking and other activities aid movement of feces through the bowel.
- Establish a regular time and place for bowel elimination. The defecation urge is usually strongest after eating, and the defecation reflex is weakened or lost if repeatedly ignored.
- *Never* take laxatives and cathartics when acute abdominal pain, nausea, or vomiting is present. Doing so may cause a ruptured appendix or other serious complication.
- Laxative and cathartics use should be temporary and not regular. Regular use may prevent normal bowel function, cause adverse drug reactions, and delay treatment for conditions that cause constipation.
- After taking a strong laxative or cathartic, it takes 2 to 3 days of normal eating to produce enough feces in the bowel for a bowel movement. Frequent use of a strong laxative promotes loss of normal bowel function, loss of fluids and electrolytes that your body needs, and laxative dependence.
- Urine may be discolored if one takes a laxative containing senna (e.g., Senokot). The color change is not harmful.
- The use of strong laxatives for weight control is inappropriate and dangerous because it can lead to life-threatening fluid and electrolyte imbalances, including dehydration and cardiovascular problems.

Self- or Caregiver Administration

General Use

- With bulk-forming laxatives, mix in 8 oz of fluid immediately before taking, and follow with additional fluid, if able. *Never* take the drug dry. Adequate fluid intake is essential.
- With bisacodyl tablets, swallow whole (do not crush or chew), and do not take within 1 hour of an antacid or milk. This helps prevent stomach irritation, abdominal cramping, and possible vomiting.
- Take magnesium citrate or milk of magnesia on an empty stomach with 8 oz of fluid to increase effectiveness.
- Refrigerate magnesium citrate before taking to improve taste and retain effectiveness.
- Mix lactulose with fruit juice, water, or milk, if desired, to improve taste.
- Take lubiprostone (Amitiza) with food.
- Notify your healthcare provider if severe diarrhea develops while taking lubiprostone.

Use in Children

- Keep a diary or log to record bowel movements; the use of medication; and episodes of fecal incontinence, abdominal pain, and other symptoms.
- Plan, encourage, and observe a program of regular toilet sitting. A child should sit on the toilet shortly after a meal, for 5 to 10 minutes, two to three times per day. Toilet-sitting episodes should occur at the same time each day and be timed with a timer.
- Structure a reward system tailored to the appropriate developmental period of the child. This system should provide rewards (stickers, reading a book, special toys used only during toilet sitting, handheld game) for effort (i.e., toilet sitting) rather than success (i.e., having a bowel movement in the toilet).
- Do not make negative comments about incontinence of stool. Do not scold or otherwise punish a child for soiling episodes or lack of success in having a bowel movement.
- Should aversion to using a school bathroom create constipation issues with school-age children, seek the aid of the school and teacher; the child may benefit from use of a private bathroom.

Quality and Safety Alert: Safety

Lipid pneumonia can be prevented by not giving mineral oil to patients with dysphagia or impaired consciousness. Decreased absorption of fat-soluble vitamins can be prevented by not giving mineral oil with or shortly after meals or for longer than 2 weeks.

Surfactant Laxatives (Stool Softeners)

Surfactant laxatives (e.g., docusate sodium) decrease the surface tension of the fecal mass to allow water to penetrate the stool. They also act as a detergent to facilitate admixing of fat and water in the stool. As a result, stools are softer and easier to expel. These agents have little, if any, laxative effect. Their main value is to prevent straining while expelling stool. They usually act within 1 to 3 days and should be taken daily.

Clinical Application 39.2

- Based on Mrs. Campbell's past health history, what is the most likely drug of choice to relieve her constipation?

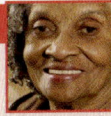

NCLEX Success

1. Which of the following points should be included when teaching patients about measures to promote healthy bowel function? (Select all that apply.)
    A. increasing activity
    B. eating a low-residue diet
    C. maintaining adequate fluid intake
    D. establishing regular bowel habits

2. Which of the following oral medications is safe to use in a 60-year-old patient with dysphagia who is constipated?
    A. methylcellulose
    B. psyllium
    C. mineral oil
    D. docusate sodium

3. A laxative is contraindicated in a patient
    A. with cancer taking daily narcotics for pain control
    B. complaining of abdominal pain and distention
    C. scheduled for a colonoscopy
    D. with limited mobility due to Parkinson disease

CATHARTICS

The stimulant cathartics are the strongest and most abused laxative products. Two types of cathartics exist: stimulant and saline. **Bisacodyl** (Dulcolax), a stimulant cathartic, is the prototype cathartic.

Pharmacokinetics

Bisacodyl is very poorly absorbed in the small intestine following oral administration or in the large intestine following rectal administration. It has a half-life of 16 hours. The drug is metabolized in the liver. Bisacodyl is primarily excreted in the feces, and any systemically absorbed portion of the drug is excreted in the urine.

Action

Bisacodyl and other stimulant cathartics act by irritating the GI mucosa and pulling water into the bowel lumen. As a result, feces move through the bowel too rapidly to allow colonic absorption of fecal water, so there is elimination of a watery stool.

Use

Bisacodyl is prescribed for the relief of constipation and as part of bowel preparation before medical examinations and surgery. The drug is also used in the management of neurogenic bowel dysfunction. The use of bisacodyl is not restricted in patients with abnormal kidney function or hepatic impairment. Table 39.4 provides route and dosage information for bisacodyl as well as other stimulant and saline cathartics.

Patient-related variables specific to the use of bisacodyl and other stimulant laxatives include the following:

- Age:
  - Stimulant laxatives are generally avoided in children younger than 6 years of age for occasional constipation, unless otherwise directed by a clinician. Bisacodyl can be used short term as rescue therapy or cautiously in children with difficult-to-treat constipation.
  - Cathartics are often used or overused in older adults; measures such as maintaining adequate fluids, a high-fiber diet, and exercise are much preferred.
- Reproduction, pregnancy, and lactation:
  - Use of bisacodyl should be limited during pregnancy due to an increased risk of adverse events, such as electrolyte abnormalities.
  - Some dosage forms contain a benzyl alcohol derivative, which has been associated with a potentially fatal toxicity ("gasping syndrome") in neonates. The dosage form should be avoided or used with caution.

Adverse Effects

Common adverse effects of bisacodyl include abdominal pain and cramping, nausea, diarrhea, and weakness.

Contraindications

Contraindications to bisacodyl include known allergy to the drug. Additionally, the presence of undiagnosed abdominal pain or intestinal obstruction or fecal impaction precludes its use.

Nursing Implications

Preventing Interactions

Medications interact with bisacodyl to decrease its effect (Box 39.2). Bisacodyl should not be taken within an hour after ingesting milk, because milk increases gastric pH and may reduce the resistance of the enteric coating of the tablet, resulting in earlier release of the drug.

Administering the Medication

It is necessary to take bisacodyl on an empty stomach or at bedtime. Patients should swallow the drug whole.

> **! Quality and Safety Alert: Safety**
>
> People should not use bisacodyl frequently or for longer than 1 week because it may produce serum electrolyte and acid-base imbalances (e.g., hypocalcemia, hypokalemia, metabolic acidosis, or alkalosis).

The nurse inserts bisacodyl rectal suppositories to the length of the index finger, next to the rectal mucosa.

Assessing for Therapeutic Effects

Oral formulations produce laxative effects in 6 to 12 hours, and a single bedtime dose of bisacodyl usually produces a morning bowel movement. Rectal forms of bisacodyl typically produce a bowel movement within 15 minutes to 1 hour.

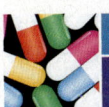

TABLE 39.4
DRUGS AT A GLANCE: Cathartics

Drug	Routes and Dosage Ranges	
	Adults	**Children**
Stimulants		
ⓟ Bisacodyl (Dulcolax, Correct, Gentle Laxative)	PO 10–15 mg Rectal suppository, 10 mg	6 y and older: PO 5 mg; rectal suppository, 5 mg
Castor oil (GoodSense Castor Oil)	PO 15–60 mL as a single dose	2–11 y: PO 5–15 mL as single dose ≥12 y: PO refer to adult dosing
Glycerin (Fleet Liquid Glycerin Supp, Pedia-Lax)	Rectal suppository, 1 adult suppository once daily as needed or directed	2–6 y: rectal pediatric suppository once daily as directed
Senna preparations (Ex-Lax, Geri-kot, Senna-Tabs, Senokot)	Granules, PO 1 level tsp once or twice daily Syrup, PO 10–15 mL once or twice daily Tablets, PO 2 tablets once or twice daily For geriatric, obstetric, or gynecologic patients, reduce all dosages by half	2–6 y: PO syrup 2.5–3.75 mL at bedtime, not to exceed 3.75 mL twice daily 6–12 y: PO 5–7.5 mL at bedtime not to exceed 7.5 mL twice daily ≥12 y: 10–15 mL at bedtime not to exceed 15 mL twice daily Tablets PO 2–6 y: PO ½ tablet (4.3 mg) at bedtime, not to exceed 1 tablet twice daily 6–12 y: PO 5–7.5 mL at bedtime, not to exceed 7.5 mL twice daily ≥12 y: 10–15 mL at bedtime, not to exceed 15 mL twice daily
Saline		
Magnesium citrate solution (Citroma, GoodSense Magnesium Citrate)	PO 195–300 mL given once or in divided doses	2–6 y: PO 60–90 mL given once or in divided doses 6–11 y: PO 90–210 mL given once or in divided doses 12 y and older: PO same dosage as adults
Magnesium hydroxide (Milk of Magnesia, Pedia-Lax, Phillips Milk of Magnesia)	Tablet, chewable 311 mg/tablet: 8 tablets/d once daily at bedtime or in divided doses Liquid: PO 2,400–4,800 once daily at bedtime or in divided doses	Liquid: 2–5 y: PO 400–1200 mg once daily at bedtime or in divided doses 6–11 y: PO 1,200–2,400 mg once daily at bedtime or in divided doses 12 y and older: PO same dosage as adults Concentrated liquid: 2–5 y: PO 2.5–7.5 mL at bedtime 6–11 y: PO 7.5–15 mL at bedtime 12 y and older: PO same dosage as adults
Polyethylene glycol (PEG) solution (GaviLAX, GlycoLAX, HealthyLax, MiraLAX, PEGyLAX; ✸ Lax-A-Day, Pegalax, Relaxa)	PO 17 g in 4–8 oz water or beverage or as ordered for bowel preparation before colonoscopy	Off-label: limited data available Disimpaction: PO 1–1.5 g/kg/d by mouth for up to 6 days Maintenance: PO 0.2–0.8 g/kg/d daily in 60 mL of noncarbonated beverage
Polyethylene glycol–electrolyte solution (PEG-ES) (Colyte, GaviLyte-N, GoLYTELY; ✸ Colyte, Klean-Prep, PegLyte)	For bowel cleansing before GI examination: PO 240 mL every 10 min until 4 L is consumed or until rectal fluid clear	Disimpaction ≥6 mo: PO 25 mL/kg/h until rectal fluid clear to maximum of 1 L/h for 4 h/d for 2 d

Assessing for Adverse Effects

The nurse monitors for bowel elimination patterns and the presence of diarrhea. In addition, the nurse should monitor for the existence of abdominal pain and cramping, nausea, or weakness.

Patient Teaching

With bisacodyl tablets, it is important to instruct the patient to swallow the tablets without chewing and not to take them within an hour after ingesting milk or gastric antacids or while receiving H_2 receptor blocker therapy. This prevents abdominal

> **BOX 39.2 Drug Interactions: Bisacodyl**
>
> **Drugs That Decrease the Effects of Bisacodyl**
> - Anticholinergic drugs (e.g., atropine)
>   *Slow intestinal motility, increasing constipation*
> - H_2 receptor blockers (e.g., ranitidine)
>   *Decrease stomach acid, resulting in premature tablet dissolution and gastric irritation*
> - Proton pump inhibitors (e.g., omeprazole)
>   *Decrease stomach acid, resulting in premature tablet dissolution and gastric irritation*

cramping and vomiting associated with premature tablet dissolution and gastric irritation.

Box 39.1 presents additional patient teaching guidelines for the laxatives and cathartics.

Other Drugs in the Class

Stimulant Cathartics

Besides bisacodyl, other stimulant cathartics, such as glycerin, given as a rectal suppository, and oral castor oil and senna preparations, are available. In addition to its irritant, stimulant effects, glycerin exerts hyperosmotic effects in the colon, acting within 30 minutes. Other oral laxative preparations causing less adverse effects (i.e., electrolyte imbalances) are recommended over castor oil and senna preparations. However, their over-the-counter availability increases their use. Ingestion of castor oil may be associated with induction of labor so it should be avoided as a laxative during pregnancy.

Saline Cathartics

Saline cathartics (e.g., magnesium citrate, milk of magnesia) are not well absorbed from the intestine. Consequently, the drugs increase osmotic pressure in the intestinal lumen and cause water retention. Distention of the bowel leads to increased peristalsis and decreased intestinal transit time for the fecal mass. The resultant stool is semifluid. These cathartics are used when rapid bowel evacuation is needed. With oral magnesium preparations, effects occur within ½ to 6 hours.

Saline cathartics are generally useful and safe for short-term treatment of constipation, cleansing the bowel before endoscopic examinations, and treating fecal impaction. However, they are not safe for frequent or prolonged use or for certain patients because they may produce fluid and electrolyte imbalances. For example, patients with impaired kidney function are at risk for hypermagnesemia with magnesium-containing laxatives because some of the magnesium is absorbed systemically. Patients with congestive heart failure are at risk for fluid retention and edema with sodium-containing cathartics. Saline cathartics containing phosphate, sodium, magnesium, or potassium salts are usually contraindicated or must be used cautiously in the presence of impaired kidney function and in people who follow a sodium-restricted diet for hypertension. Ten percent or more of the magnesium in magnesium salts may be absorbed and cause hypermagnesemia, and potassium salts may cause hyperkalemia. Polyethylene glycol–electrolyte solution (PEG-ES) (e.g., NuLYTELY) is formulated for rapid and effective bowel cleansing without significant changes in water or electrolyte balance. The drug is a nonabsorbable oral solution that induces diarrhea within 30 to 60 minutes and rapidly evacuates the bowel, usually within 4 hours. The drug has little effect on abdominal pain. The adverse effects of bloating and abdominal discomfort may limit the use of PEG-ES. It is a prescription drug used for bowel cleansing before GI examination (e.g., colonoscopy) and is contraindicated in patients with GI obstruction, gastric retention, colitis, or bowel perforation. Combination products, available by prescription, such as HalfLytely combine polyethylene glycol with a stimulant cathartic, bisacodyl, to evacuate the colon in preparation for a colonoscopy. Polyethylene glycol solution (MiraLAX) is an oral laxative that may be used to treat occasional constipation. Effects may require 2 to 4 days. It is an over-the-counter drug, and people should not take it for longer than 2 weeks.

> **NCLEX Success**
>
> 4. A nurse is caring for a patient preparing to undergo a colonoscopy. Which of the following drugs are commonly used to enhance bowel cleansing? (Select all that apply.)
>   A. polyethylene glycol–electrolyte solution
>   B. bisacodyl
>   C. psyllium
>   D. docusate sodium
>
> 5. Which of the following mechanisms of action is shown by over-the-counter drug magnesium hydroxide (milk of magnesia)?
>   A. increased gastric secretions
>   B. increased osmotic pressure in the intestinal lumen
>   C. binding to diarrhea-causing bacteria for excretion
>   D. decreased gastrointestinal motility

GUANYLATE CYCLASE-C AGONISTS

Guanylate cyclase-C (GC-C) agonists are not laxatives but work to proactively manage symptoms of chronic idiopathic constipation and irritable bowel syndrome with constipation. Routine use supports more frequent and complete bowel movements and helps to relieve overall abdominal symptoms (i.e., pain, discomfort, bloating) associated with IBS-C. **Linaclotide** (Linzess) was the first approved treatment in this class of drugs and serves as the prototype. This class of drugs is discussed below, and Table 39.5 gives dosage information.

Pharmacokinetics

Linaclotide is minimally available systemically, and minimal tissue distribution is detected at recommended doses. The drug is metabolized within the GI tract to an active metabolite, and both the metabolite and the parent drug undergo degradation in the intestinal lumen. Excretion is mainly in the feces.

TABLE 39.5

DRUGS AT A GLANCE: Guanylate Cyclase-C Agonists Administered for the Treatment of Constipation

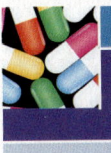

Drug	Routes and Dosage Ranges	
	Adults	**Children**
ⓟ Linaclotide (Linzess; 🍁 Constella)	For chronic idiopathic constipation: PO 145 mcg once daily For irritable bowel syndrome with constipation: PO 290 mcg once daily	≤2 y: contraindicated 2–17 y: safety and efficacy not established
Plecanatide (Trulance)	For chronic idiopathic constipation: PO 3 mg once daily	≤6 y: contraindicated 7–16 y: safety and efficacy not established

Action

Linaclotide (Linzess) increases the secretion of chloride and water in the intestines by binding to GC-C on the surface of intestinal epithelium. This local action in the intestine softens stools, accelerates bowel movements, and calms pain-sensing nerves.

Use

Linaclotide is used to treat adults with chronic idiopathic constipation and irritable bowel syndrome with constipation.

Patient-related variables specific to the use of linaclotide include age. The FDA has issued a **BOXED WARNING** for use of linaclotide in children. The warning states that the drug is contraindicated in children younger than 2 years of age; death from dehydration has been reported in nonclinical studies from administration of a single, adult oral dose. In addition, the drug should be avoided in children and adolescents 2 through 17 years of age.

Adverse Effects

The most common adverse effects include diarrhea, abdominal discomfort, and headache.

Contraindications

Contraindications to linaclotide include administration to children less than 2 years of age, known or suspected mechanical gastrointestinal obstruction, or known allergy to the drug.

Nursing Implications

Preventing Interactions

Since linaclotide metabolism occurs within the gastrointestinal tract and plasma concentrations are not measurable following administration of a recommended dosage, no significant drug interactions are known. No herbal interactions that increase or decrease the drug's effects of have been identified.

Administering the Medication

The drug should be given on an empty stomach at least 30 minutes before the first meal of the day. A high-fat breakfast may increase stool frequency and loose stools with administration of linaclotide.

Assessing for Therapeutic Effects

The nurse monitors for improvement of symptoms, such as improved spontaneous bowel movement and frequency, decrease in abdominal pain, and decrease straining during bowel movements.

> **! Quality and Safety Alert: Evidence-Based Practice**
>
> In a randomized, double-blind, controlled trial, Schoenfeld et al. (2018) explored the efficacy and safety of low-dose linaclotide for chronic irritable bowel syndrome with constipation in 1,223 patients (mean age = 46 years, White = 71%, female = 77%). Inclusion criteria included less than three spontaneous bowel movements per week without the use of laxative, suppository, or enema during the preceding 24 hours and at least one of the following symptoms during 25% or more of bowel movements for at least 12 weeks within the preceding 6 months: straining, lumpy or hard stools, and a sensation of incomplete evacuation. Findings demonstrated that once-daily linaclotide (72 mcg) significantly improved symptoms in male and female patients in 12 weeks and the need to discontinue the drug due to diarrhea was low.

Assessing for Adverse Effects

The nurse monitors for bowel elimination patterns and the presence of ongoing constipation or diarrhea. In addition, the nurse should monitor for the existence of abdominal pain and cramping, nausea, or weakness.

Patient Teaching

Patient education should stress the importance of taking the medication on a regular basis at breakfast and not PRN. The medication needs to be kept in the original container and tightly closed to protect the medication from moisture. General patient teaching guidelines are listed in Box 39.1.

Other Drugs in the Class

Plecanatide (Trulance) is indicated in adults for the treatment of chronic idiopathic constipation and irritable bowel syndrome with constipation in adults. The efficacy and adverse effects of plecanatide are similar to linaclotide. The drug is contraindicated with suspected or known mechanical gastrointestinal obstruction and in children younger than 6 years of age. The FDA has issued a **BOXED WARNING** for use of plecanatide due to the risk of serious dehydration in children. Death from dehydration has been reported in nonclinical studies following administration of a single, adult oral dose.

MISCELLANEOUS AGENTS FOR CONSTIPATION

Several miscellaneous agents are used in the treatment of constipation. These drugs are discussed briefly below, and Table 39.6 gives dosage information.

Lactulose (Constulose, Kristalose) is a disaccharide that is not absorbed from the GI tract. It exerts laxative effects by pulling water into the intestinal lumen. It is used to treat constipation but is commonly given for hepatic encephalopathy, a condition that usually results from alcoholic liver disease in which ammonia accumulates and causes stupor or coma. Lactulose decreases production of ammonia in the intestine. The goal of treatment is usually to maintain two to three soft stools daily; effects usually occur within 24 to 48 hours. It is important to use the drug cautiously because it may produce electrolyte imbalances and dehydration.

> **Concept Mastery Alert**
>
> Lactulose treats constipation by producing lactic and acetic acids in the colon, which lower the colonic pH; the reduced pH favors the formation of the nonabsorbable NH_4^+ from NH_3 (ammonia), trapping NH_4^+ in the colon and thus reducing plasma ammonia concentrations. In addition, the cathartic effects of a hyperosmolar load in the colon improve gastrointestinal transit, allowing less time for ammonia absorption.

Lubiprostone (Amitiza) is a chloride channel activator indicated for the treatment of chronic idiopathic constipation in adults, opioid-induced constipation in adults, and irritable bowel syndrome with constipation only in female patients greater than 18 years of age. At the time of approval, the efficacy of lubiprostone in males was not conclusively demonstrated. The drug acts locally in the apical membrane of the GI tract, producing increased intestinal fluid secretion and improved fecal transit. This mode of action is particularly beneficial in individuals with opioid-induced constipation as the effect bypasses the antisecretory effects of opiates, suppressing secretomotor neuron excitability.

Lubiprostone exerts its effect locally by activating chloride channels in the GI tract to increase the secretion of chloride-rich fluids into the intestine. Increased intestinal fluid secretion stimulates intestinal motility, improving the passage of stool. It

TABLE 39.6

DRUGS AT A GLANCE: Miscellaneous Drugs Administered for the Treatment of Constipation

Drug	Routes and Dosage Ranges	
	Adults	**Children**
Lactulose (Constulose, Enulose, Kristalose)	For constipation: PO 10–20 g (15–30 mL) daily; maximum dose 60 mL daily Portal systemic encephalopathy: PO 20–30 g (30–45 mL) 3 or 4 times daily, adjusted to produce two or three soft stools daily Rectally as retention enema, 300 mL with 700 mL water or normal saline, retained 30–60 min, every 4–6 h	Infants: PO 2.5–10 mL daily in divided doses Older children: PO 40–90 mL daily in divided doses
Lubiprostone (Amitiza)	For chronic idiopathic constipation: PO 24 mcg twice daily with food For irritable bowel syndrome with constipation: females ≥18 y, 8 mcg twice daily Opioid-induced constipation: PO 24 mcg twice daily	Safety and efficacy in children have not been established
Sorbitol	As hyperosmolar laxative, PO 30–150 mL (as 70% solution) Rectal enema, 120 mL as 25%–30% solution	2–11 y: PO 2 mg/kg (as 70% solution); rectal enema, 30–60 mL as 25%–30% solution 12 y and older: same as adult dose
Prucalopride (Motegrity; ✱Resotran)	For chronic idiopathic constipation: PO 2 mg once daily	Not approved for use in children
Tegaserod (Zelnorm)	For irritable bowel syndrome with constipation in women: PO 6 mg two times daily before meals	Not approved for use in children

is metabolized by enzymes in the stomach and excreted in the urine and feces.

Adverse effects of lubiprostone include nausea, particularly in older adults, and severe diarrhea. Taking the drug with food may decrease nausea. Acute-onset dyspnea that resolves within a few hours has been observed following the first and subsequent doses of lubiprostone. Syncope and hypotension may also occur and generally resolve prior to the next dose or following discontinuation. Hypotension may require hospitalization, particularly in patients who are also taking drugs that produce a hypotensive effect. In addition, methadone may decrease the therapeutic effect of the agent.

Sorbitol is a monosaccharide that pulls water into the intestinal lumen and has laxative effects. It is often given with sodium polystyrene sulfonate (Kayexalate), a potassium-removing resin used to treat hyperkalemia, prevent constipation, and aid expulsion of the potassium–resin complex. It can also be given with activated charcoal to eliminate toxins in the body. Maternal use during pregnancy is not expected to result in fetal exposure to the drug.

Tegaserod (Zelnorm) is used as a short-term treatment of irritable bowel syndrome with constipation in female patients less than 65 years of age. Efficacy and safety have not been established in males. The drug is contraindicated with moderate to severe kidney or liver disease and in females over the age of 65 years. The drug is also contraindicated in patients with a history of myocardial infarction, angina, stroke, or transient ischemic attack. Common adverse effects include headache and abdominal pain. The drug should be taken 30 minutes before meals as food decreases the drug's bioavailability and prolongs maximum effectiveness for 1 to 2 hours following a meal.

Prucalopride (Motegrity) is a serotonin 5-HT_4 receptor agonist used to treat chronic idiopathic constipation in adults. The drug enhances normal GI motility. The drug is contraindicated in adults with intestinal perforation or obstruction due to structural or functional disorder of the gut wall, obstructive ileus, and severe inflammatory conditions of the GI tract such as ulcerative colitis and Crohn disease. Caution should be used with administration in people with abnormal kidney function. Common adverse effects include headache, abdominal pain, nausea, and diarrhea. Diarrhea may be severe, particularly during the first week of treatment, and usually resolves within a few days. Dizziness has been reported, so patients should be instructed to avoid operating machinery and other tasks that require mental alertness. Suicide ideations have been reported, and patients should be monitored for worsening of depression or development of suicidal thoughts and behaviors.

Clinical Application 39.3

- Mrs. Campbell is concerned about not having a bowel movement. She takes a psyllium preparation at 8 a.m. She does not have a result by noon, so she takes milk of magnesia. She has not had a stool by supper, so she takes a glycerin suppository. She has diarrhea throughout the night. What patient education is appropriate?

THE NURSING PROCESS

A concept map outlines the nursing process related to drug therapy considerations in this chapter. Additional nursing implications related to the disease process should also be considered in care decisions.

Assessment
- Assess patients for current or potential constipation.
- Signs and symptoms include the following:
  - Decreased number and frequency of stools (fewer than two to three stools per week, depending on age)
  - Passage of dry, hard stool
  - Abdominal distention and discomfort
  - Flatulence
  - Sensation of incomplete evacuation
  - History of retentive posturing or excessive volitional stool retention
  - Large mass of stool in rectum
- Presence of risk factors
  - Diet with minimal fiber (e.g., small amounts of fruits, vegetables, and whole-grain products)
  - Low fluid intake (e.g., less than 2000 mL daily)
  - Immobility or limited activity
  - Use of drugs that reduce intestinal function and motility (e.g., opioid analgesics, antacids containing aluminum or calcium, anticholinergics, calcium channel blockers, clozapine, diuretics, iron, phenothiazines, cholestyramine, colestipol, sucralfate, tricyclic antidepressants, vincristine)
  - Overuse of antidiarrheal agents, which may also cause constipation
  - Conditions that may reduce intestinal function and motility (e.g., depression, eating disorders such as anorexia nervosa, hypothyroidism, hypercalcemia, multiple sclerosis, Parkinson's disease, spinal lesions)
  - Hemorrhoids, anal fissures, or other conditions characterized by painful bowel elimination
  - Elderly or debilitated status

Outcomes of Therapy
The patient will
- Take drugs appropriately to promote normal bowel function and prevent constipation.
- Use nondrug measures to promote normal bowel function and prevent constipation.
- Regain normal patterns of bowel elimination.
- Avoid excessive losses of fluids and electrolytes from laxative use.
- Be protected from excessive fluid loss, hypotension, and other adverse drug effects, when possible.
- Be assisted to avoid constipation when at risk (e.g., has illness or injury that prevents activity and food and fluid intake; takes medications that decrease GI function).

Nursing Interventions
- Assist patients with constipation and caregivers to
  - Understand the importance of diet, exercise, and fluid intake in promoting normal bowel function and preventing constipation.
  - Increase activity and exercise.
  - Increase intake of dietary fiber (e.g., vegetables, fruits, cereal grains).
  - Drink at least 2000 mL of fluid daily, if not contraindicated.
  - Establish and maintain a routine for bowel elimination (e.g., going to the bathroom immediately after breakfast).
  - Recognize importance of and comply with drug therapy (see Box 39.1).
- Monitor patient responses.
  - Record number, amount, and type of bowel movements.
  - Record vital signs. Hypotension and weak pulse may indicate deficient fluid volume.

Evaluation
- Observe and interview for improved patterns of bowel elimination.
- Observe for use of nondrug measures to promote bowel function.
- Observe for appropriate use of laxatives.
- Observe and interview regarding adverse effects of laxatives.

Visit thePoint® *at* **http://thePoint.lww.com/Frandsen13e** *for answers to NCLEX Success questions (in Appendix A), answers to Clinical Application Case Studies (in Appendix B), additional material on etiology and pathophysiology, and more!*

REFERENCES AND RESOURCES

DeMicco, M., Barrow, L., Hickey, B., Shailubhai, K., & Griffin, P. (2017). Randomized clinical trial: Efficacy and safety of plecanatide in the treatment of chronic idiopathic constipation. *Therapeutic Advances in Gastroenterology, 10*, 837–851

DiPiro, J. T., Talbert, R. L., Yee, G. C., Wells, B. G., Posey, L. M., & Matzke, G. R. (2020). *Pharmacotherapy: A pathophysiologic approach* (11th ed Kindle ed.). McGraw-Hill Education

Hinkle, J. H., Cheever, K. H., & Overbaugh, K. J. (2022). *Brunner & Suddarth's textbook of medical-surgical nursing* (15th ed.). Wolters Kluwer

Karch, A. M. (2019). *Focus on Nursing Pharmacology* (8th ed.). Wolters Kluwer

Lippincott advisor. (2022). Retrieved from http://advisor.lww.com

Lippincott Williams & Wilkins. (2022). *Nursing 2023 drug handbook* (43rd ed.).

Norris, T. L. (2019). *Pathophysiology: Concepts of altered health status* (10th ed.). Wolters Kluwer.

Paquette, I. M., Varma, M., Ternent, C., Melton-Meaux, G., Rafferty, J. F., Feingold, D., et al. (2016). The American Society of Colon and Rectal Surgeons' Clinical Practice Guideline for the Evaluation and Management of Constipation. *Diseases of the Colon & Rectum, 59*(6), 479–492. 10.1097/DCR.0000000000000599

Philichi, L. (2018). Management of childhood functional constipation. *Journal of Pediatric Health Care, 32*(1), 103–111

Schoenfeld, P., Lacy, B. E., Chey, W. D., Lembo, A. J., Kurtz, C. B., Reasner, D. S., et al. (2018). Low-dose linaclotide (72 μg) for chronic idiopathic constipation: A 12-week, randomized, double-blind, placebo-controlled trial. *American Journal of Gastroenterology, 113*(1), 105–114. 10.1038/ajg.2017.230

Shah, E. D., Kim, H. M., & Schoenfeld, P. (2018). Efficacy and tolerability of guanylate cyclase c agonists for irritable bowel syndrome with constipation and chronic idiopathic constipation: systematic review and meta-analysis. *The American Journal of Gastroenterology, 113*(3), 329–338 https://doi.org/10.1038/ajg.2017.495

Tabbers, M. M., DiLorenzo, C., Berger, M. Y., Faure, C., Langendam, M. W., Nurko, S., et al. (2014). Evaluation and treatment of functional constipation in infants and children: Evidence based recommendations from ESPGHAN and NASPGHAN. *Journal of Pediatric Gastroenterology and Nutrition, 58*(2), 258–274

Wald, A. (2023). Treatment of irritable bowel syndrome in adults). UpToDate. Lexi-Comp, Inc

CHAPTER 40

Drug Therapy for Diarrhea

LEARNING OBJECTIVES

After studying this chapter, you should be able to:

1. Identify patients at risk for development of diarrhea.
2. Describe opioid-related antidiarrheal agents in terms of the prototype, indications and contraindications for use, routes of administration, and major adverse effects.
3. Identify adjuvant drugs used to manage diarrhea.
4. Apply the nursing process in the care of patients receiving drug therapy for diarrhea.

CLINICAL APPLICATION CASE STUDY

Joseph Mendoza is a 47-year-old salesman who travels extensively as part of his job. He returned from a trip to Asia 2 days ago, and since his return, he has had abdominal cramping and bloating and an average of four watery bowel movements per day. Mr. Mendoza comes to the clinic seeking advice about how to manage his symptoms. He denies nausea and vomiting. His vital signs are temperature 99.4°F, pulse 82 beats/min, respirations 22 breaths/min, and blood pressure 124/72 mm Hg lying and 120/72 mm Hg standing.

KEY TERMS

Diarrhea: increase in the liquidity of stool or frequency of defecation to more than three stools per day

Inflammatory bowel disorders: disorders in which inflamed mucous membranes secrete large amounts of fluids into the intestinal lumen, along with mucus, proteins, and blood; characterized by impaired absorption of water and electrolytes

Irritable bowel syndrome: functional disorder of intestinal motility with no evidence of inflammation or tissue changes

Traveler's diarrhea: form of diarrhea caused by the enterotoxigenic strain of *Escherichia coli*, typically from fecal contamination of food or water

INTRODUCTION

The focus of this chapter is the description of drugs used to relieve the symptoms of diarrhea, specifically the opioid-related agents. Topics of discussion include the general characteristics of these drugs, their mechanisms of action, indications for and contraindications to their use, and their nursing implications. The section on adjuvant medications briefly addresses specific drugs, including antibacterial agents, used to manage underlying disease processes that cause diarrhea.

OVERVIEW OF DIARRHEA

Clinical Considerations

Diarrhea, an increase in the liquidity of stool or frequency of defecation to more than three stools per day, is a common condition experienced by virtually everyone. It is a symptom of numerous conditions and not a disease. Diarrhea is a manifestation of basic mechanisms that increase bowel motility, cause secretion or retention of fluids in the intestinal lumen (lactose intolerance or toxins such as cholera or laxatives and other drugs), or cause inflammation or irritation of the gastrointestinal (GI) tract (*Escherichia coli, Salmonella*, rotaviruses, *Giardia*). It is common for more than one of the mechanisms to be involved in the pathogenesis of a given situation. As a result, bowel contents are rapidly propelled toward the rectum, and absorption of fluids and electrolytes is limited.

Clinical Manifestations

Diarrhea may be acute or chronic and mild or severe. Most episodes of acute diarrhea are defensive mechanisms by which the body tries to rid itself of irritants, toxins, and infectious agents. These episodes of frequent liquid or semiliquid stools are usually self-limiting and subside within 24 to 48 hours without serious consequences. If severe or prolonged, acute diarrhea may lead to serious fluid and electrolyte depletion, especially in young children and older adults. Chronic diarrhea may cause malnutrition and anemia and is often characterized by remissions and exacerbations.

Fever, vomiting, and bloody stools are associated with acute diarrhea, and the presence of these symptoms may help determine the cause. Fever is common and often linked with invasive pathogens. Vomiting is frequently found in illness caused by ingestion of bacterial toxins or viruses. Invasive and cytotoxin-releasing pathogens are known to cause bloody stools, and enterotoxigenic strain *E. coli* O157:H7 infection is suspected in the absence of fecal leukocytes. Bloody stools are not associated with viral agents and enterotoxins that release bacteria.

Some causes of diarrhea include the following:

- *Excessive use or abuse of laxatives*
- *Undigested, coarse, or highly spiced food in the GI tract*
- *Lack of digestive enzymes*
- *Intestinal infections with viruses, bacteria, or protozoa*
- *Inflammatory bowel disorders* (disorders in which inflamed mucous membranes secrete large amounts of fluids into the intestinal lumen, along with mucus, proteins, and blood; characterized by impaired absorption of water and electrolytes)
- *Irritable bowel syndrome (IBS)* (functional disorder of intestinal motility with no evidence of inflammation or tissue changes)
- *Drugs*
- *Intestinal neoplasms*
- *Functional disorders*
- *Hyperthyroidism*
- *Surgical excision of portions of the intestine, especially the small intestine*
- *Human immunodeficiency virus (HIV) infection/acquired immunodeficiency syndrome (AIDS)*.

For further details on the etiology of diarrhea, visit **thePoint** http://thePoint.lww.com/Frandsen13e.

Nonpharmacologic Therapy

In most cases of acute, nonspecific diarrhea in adults, fluid losses are not severe, and patients need only simple replacement of fluids and electrolytes to replace those lost in the stool. Acceptable replacement fluids during the first 24 hours include clear liquids (e.g., flat ginger ale, decaffeinated cola drinks or tea, broth, gelatin)—2 to 3 L. Also, a diet consisting of bland foods (e.g., rice, soup, bread, salted crackers, cooked cereals, baked potatoes, eggs, applesauce) is best. People may resume their regular diet after 2 or 3 days.

Drug Therapy

Antidiarrheal drugs include a variety of agents, most of which are discussed in other chapters. When used for treatment of diarrhea, these drugs may be prescribed to relieve the symptom or the underlying cause of the symptom. Overall, opiates and opiate derivatives (see Chapter 49) are the most effective agents for symptomatic treatment of diarrhea. Although morphine, codeine, and related drugs are effective in relieving diarrhea, they are rarely used for this purpose because of their adverse effects. The synthetic drugs diphenoxylate and loperamide have replaced these drugs. Uses include only treatment of diarrhea; they do not cause morphinelike adverse effects in recommended doses. Table 40.1 summarizes drugs used to manage diarrhea.

OPIATE-RELATED ANTIDIARRHEAL AGENTS

The oral opioid **diphenoxylate with atropine** (Lomotil) is the prototype used to treat moderate-to-severe diarrhea. A Schedule V controlled substance, diphenoxylate requires a prescription.

Pharmacokinetics

Diphenoxylate with atropine is well absorbed by the oral route with an onset of action of 45 to 60 minutes. The duration of action is 3 to 4 hours. The drug is metabolized in the liver to active metabolites and is excreted in the bile and feces.

Action

Diphenoxylate with atropine slows peristalsis by acting on the smooth muscles in the intestine.

TABLE 40.1
Drug Therapy for Diarrhea

Drug Class	Prototype	Other Drugs in the Class
Opiate-related antidiarrheals	Diphenoxylate with atropine sulfate (Lomotil)	Loperamide (Imodium A-D) Paregoric
Adjuvant antidiarrheal medications		Alosetron (Lotronex) Bismuth subsalicylate (Pepto-Bismol) Cholestyramine (Prevalite) Colestipol (Colestid) Nitazoxanide (Alinia) Octreotide (Sandostatin) Polycarbophil preparations (FiberCon) Rifaximin (Xifaxan)

Use

Prescribers order diphenoxylate with atropine to treat diarrhea. Table 40.2 provides dosage information for diphenoxylate with atropine and other opiate-related drugs.

Patient-related variables specific to the use of diphenoxylate include the following:

- Age:
  - In children, signs of atropine overdose may occur with usual doses of diphenoxylate, which contains atropine.
  - Children younger than 2 years of age should not take the drug, and those from age 2 to less than 13 years should take the liquid preparation to enhance the accuracy of proper dosage administration.
  - If children show no improvement in symptoms in 48 hours, treatment with diphenoxylate with atropine is likely to be ineffective.
  - In children, large doses of anticholinergics, such as diphenoxylate with atropine, may produce a paradoxical reaction characterized by hyperexcitability. The oral solution may contain 15% alcohol.
  - In older adults, diarrhea may occur from laxative abuse and bowel-cleansing procedures before GI surgery or diagnostic tests.
  - Fluid volume deficits may rapidly develop in older adults with diarrhea. General principles of fluid and electrolyte replacement, measures to decrease GI irritants, and drug therapy apply as for younger adults.
  - Older people may safely take most antidiarrheal drugs, but cautious use is indicated to avoid inducing constipation.
- Reproduction, pregnancy, and lactation:
  - Limited data are available to inform use of the drug in pregnancy.
  - The drug is present in breast milk so caution should be exercised with use in lactation.

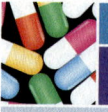

TABLE 40.2
DRUGS AT A GLANCE: Opiate-Related Antidiarrheal Agents

Drug	Routes and Dosage Ranges	
	Adults	**Children**
P Diphenoxylate with atropine sulfate (Lomotil; ❋ Lomotil)	5 mg (2 tablets or 10 mL of liquid) PO three or four times daily; max daily dose 20 mg	Liquid preparation (2.5-mg diphenoxylate and 0.025-mg atropine per 5 mL); contraindicated in children <2 y of age 2 y, 1.5–3 mL: PO four times daily 3 y, 2–3 mL: PO four times daily 4 y, 2–4 mL: PO four times daily 5 y, 2.5–4.5 mL: PO four times daily 6–8 y, 2.5–5 mL: PO four times daily 9–12 y, 3.5–5 mL: PO four times daily
Paregoric	5–10 mL PO 1–4 times daily (max of 4 doses) until diarrhea is controlled	PO 0.25–0.5 mL/kg 1–4 times daily (maximum of 4 doses) until diarrhea is controlled
Loperamide (Imodium A-D; ❋ Apo-Loperamide, Diarr-Eze)	4 mg PO initially, then 2 mg after each loose stool to a maximal daily dose of 16 mg. For chronic diarrhea, dosage should be reduced to the lowest effective amount (average 4–8 mg daily)	Contraindicated in children <2 y of age 2–5 y, 13–20 kg: 1 mg three times daily 6–8 y, 20–30 kg: PO 2 mg twice daily 8–12 y, >30 kg: PO 2 mg three times daily

- Abnormal kidney function and hepatic impairment:
  - Use of diphenoxylate with atropine warrants extreme caution in patients with severe hepatorenal disease because hepatic coma may be precipitated. Care is also necessary in patients with abnormal results of liver function tests.
- Specific healthcare environments:
  - In patients with critical illness, administration of antibacterial drugs may cause diarrhea by altering the normal bacterial flora in the intestine.
  - In the critical care unit and the home environment, it is important to observe for fluid and electrolyte imbalance and assess the cause of diarrhea before treating the condition.

Adverse Effects

Adverse effects of diphenoxylate with atropine include tachycardia, dizziness, headache, flushing, nausea and vomiting, dry skin and mucous membranes, and urinary retention. Hypotension and respiratory depression have occurred, particularly with doses greater than ordered.

Contraindications

Contraindications to the use of diphenoxylate with atropine include diarrhea caused by toxic materials, microorganisms that penetrate intestinal mucosa (e.g., pathogenic *E. coli*, *Salmonella*, *Shigella*), and antibiotic-associated colitis. In these circumstances, antidiarrheal drugs that slow peristalsis may aggravate and prolong diarrhea.

Nursing Implications

Preventing Interactions

Increased levels of diphenoxylate with atropine may result with the use of methotrimeprazine and pramlintide. Decreased drug levels may result from concurrent use of acetylcholinesterase inhibitors. Use of alcohol may increase central nervous system (CNS) depression. There are no known herbal interactions with diphenoxylate.

Administering the Medication

Administration is oral.

> **Quality and Safety Alert: Safety**
>
> With liquid diphenoxylate and atropine, it is necessary to use only the calibrated dropper furnished by the manufacturer for measuring doses accurately.

Assessing for Therapeutic Effects

After drug administration, the nurse monitors the number and consistency of stools and fluid and electrolyte balance. The nurse also assesses for the return of normal pattern of bowel movements and signs of normal fluid and electrolyte balance (adequate hydration, urine output, and skin turgor). In addition, it is important to assess for resumption of usual activities of daily living.

Assessing for Adverse Effects

The nurse assesses for hypotension and respiratory depression due to the effects of diphenoxylate. The nurse observes for signs of the effects of atropine, including tachycardia, thirst, flushing, urinary retention, and dry skin and mucous membranes.

Patient Teaching

Once the diarrhea is under control, it is important that diphenoxylate with atropine be discontinued. The nurse ensures that patients who take this drug understand how to use it. Box 40.1 outlines patient teaching guidelines for antidiarrheal drugs.

Other Drugs in the Class

The choice of antidiarrheal agent depends largely on the cause, severity, and duration of diarrhea. Loperamide (Imodium A-D) is a synthetic derivative of meperidine that decreases GI motility by its effect on intestinal muscles and is an unscheduled, nonprescription drug. Because loperamide does not penetrate the CNS well, it does not cause the CNS effects associated with opioid use and lacks potential for abuse. Although adverse effects are generally few and mild, loperamide can cause abdominal pain, constipation, dizziness, drowsiness, fatigue, nausea, and vomiting. For nonprescription use, dosages for adults should not exceed 8 mg per day; with supervision by a health care provider, maximum daily dosage is 16 mg per day. In general, it is necessary to discontinue loperamide after 48 hours if clinical improvement has not occurred. The Food and Drug Administration (FDA) has issued a **BOXED WARNING** because torsades de pointes, cardiac arrest, and death have been reported in people using higher than recommended dosages of loperamide. With loperamide, the nurse monitors patients with hepatic impairment for signs of CNS toxicity. The drug normally undergoes extensive first-pass metabolism, which may be lessened by liver disease. As a result, a larger portion of a dose reaches the systemic circulation and may cause adverse effects. Treatment of overdose may involve naloxone, gastric lavage, and administration of activated charcoal. A dosage adjustment may be necessary.

Paregoric is a schedule III drug alone and a schedule V in the small amounts combined with other drugs; it contains 0.4 mg/mL of morphine. The main effects of paregoric are to increase the muscular tone of the intestine, to inhibit normal peristalsis, and to suppress coughing. Practitioners use it as an antidiarrheal and as an antitussive. In recommended doses over the short term, paregoric does not produce euphoria, analgesia, or dependence.

> **Quality and Safety Alert: Safety**
>
> Confusing paregoric (camphorated tincture of opium) with the much more potent drug opium tincture is a common and potentially fatal drug error. Opium tincture is much more concentrated than is paregoric and contains 10 mg/mL of morphine. Labels on opium tincture packaging should identify it as a poison, giving the strength of morphine as 10 mg/mL and containing the statement, "Warning! Do not use opium tincture in place of paregoric."

Clinical Application 40.1

- What recommendations for management of the diarrhea does the nurse practitioner most likely make?

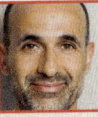

BOX 40.1 Patient Teaching Guidelines for Antidiarrheals

General Considerations

- Taking a medication to stop diarrhea is not always needed or desirable because diarrhea may mean the body is trying to rid itself of irritants or bacteria. Treatment is indicated if diarrhea is severe, is prolonged, or occurs in young children or older adults, who are highly susceptible to excessive losses of body fluids and electrolytes.
- Try to drink 2 to 3 quarts of fluid daily. This helps prevent dehydration from fluid loss in stools. Water, clear broths, and noncarbonated, caffeine-free beverages are recommended because they are unlikely to cause further diarrhea.
- Avoid highly spiced or "laxative" foods, such as fresh fruits and vegetables, until diarrhea is controlled.
- Frequent and thorough hand washing and careful food storage and preparation can help prevent diarrhea.
- Consult a healthcare provider if diarrhea is accompanied by severe abdominal pain or fever or lasts longer than 3 days or if stools contain blood or mucus. These signs and symptoms may indicate more serious disorders for which other treatment measures are needed.
- Stop antidiarrheal drugs when diarrhea is controlled to avoid adverse effects such as constipation.
- Bismuth subsalicylate (Pepto-Bismol) and loperamide (Imodium A-D) are available over the counter; diphenoxylate (Lomotil) is a prescription drug.
- Diphenoxylate and loperamide may cause dizziness or drowsiness and should be used with caution if driving or performing other tasks requiring alertness, coordination, or physical dexterity. In addition, alcohol and other drugs that cause drowsiness should be avoided.
- Pepto-Bismol may temporarily discolor bowel movements a grayish-black.
- Keep antidiarrheal drugs out of reach of children.

Self- or Caregiver Administration

- Do not administer Pepto-Bismol to children due to the risk of Reye syndrome.

- Take or give antidiarrheal drugs only as prescribed or directed on nonprescription drug labels.
- Do not exceed maximal daily doses of diphenoxylate (Lomotil), loperamide, or paregoric.
- With liquid diphenoxylate, use only the calibrated dropper furnished by the manufacturer for accurate measurement of dosages.
- Use caution driving or operating heavy machinery with diphenoxylate and atropine, which may cause drowsiness or dizziness, until the effects of the medication are known.
- Be aware that diphenoxylate can cause dry mouth; sucking on hard candy or chewing gum may alleviate it.
- With Pepto-Bismol liquid, shake the bottle well before measuring the dose; with tablets, chew them well or allow them to dissolve in the mouth.
- Add at least 30 mL of water to each dose of paregoric to help the drug dose reach the stomach. The mixture appears milky.
- Take cholestyramine or colestipol with at least 4 oz of water. These drugs should never be taken without fluids because they may block the gastrointestinal tract. Also, do not take within 4 hours of other drugs because they may combine with and inactivate other drugs.
- Take rifaximin with or without food for 3 days. Notify your healthcare prescriber if your condition worsens or does not improve after 1 to 2 days.
- Use caution driving or operating machinery if experiencing dizziness while using rifaximin.
- With Alinia, if you have diabetes, be aware that the oral suspension contains 1.48 g of sucrose per 5 mL.
- With Lotronex, if you become constipated, notice blood in your bowel movements, or experience a new worse or different pain in your stomach or abdomen, *stop* taking the drug and notify your healthcare prescriber.

NCLEX Success

1. An appropriate nursing measure when treating a 5-year-old child with a 1-day onset of mild diarrhea involves encouraging which of the following?
   A. regular diet
   B. intake of clear liquids
   C. intake of milk products
   D. no fluids for 24 hours

2. A 28-year-old patient is hospitalized on antibiotic therapy. The patient is experiencing fever, abdominal pain, and diarrhea containing mucus, pus, and blood. The best nursing intervention in this situation is to do which of the following?
   A. Continue the antibiotic because the patient has signs of a gastrointestinal infection.
   B. Monitor the patient's vital signs and notify the provider if there is further deterioration.
   C. Withhold the antibiotic and notify the provider of the patient's condition.
   D. Encourage fluid intake because fever is a sign of dehydration.

3. A 68-year-old patient has been taking nonprescription loperamide for diarrhea. Which of the following symptoms should the nurse explain are signs of adverse effects? [Select all that apply.]
   A. abdominal pain
   B. dizziness
   C. bloody diarrhea
   D. fatigue
   E. torsades de pointes

ADJUVANT MEDICATIONS USED TO TREAT DIARRHEA

Specific drug therapy for diarrhea depends on the cause of the symptoms and may include the use of hormones, bulk-forming products, enzymatic replacement therapy, bile salt–binding drugs, antibacterial agents, and 5-HT$_3$ serotonin receptor antagonists. Table 40.3 presents route and dosage information for these drugs.

Bismuth Salts

Bismuth salts have antibacterial and antiviral activity. Bismuth subsalicylate (Pepto-Bismol), a commonly used over-the-counter (OTC) drug, also has antisecretory and possibly anti-inflammatory effects because of its salicylate component.

> **Quality and Safety Alert: Safety**
>
> People with an allergy to aspirin and aspirin products should not take bismuth subsalicylate as the drug is a salicylate.

This salt causes a temporary and harmless darkening of the tongue or stool.

Octreotide

Octreotide acetate (Sandostatin) is a synthetic form of somatostatin, a hormone produced in the anterior pituitary gland and

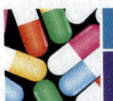

TABLE 40.3

DRUGS AT A GLANCE: Adjuvant Antidiarrheal Medications

Drug	Routes and Dosage Ranges	
	Adults	**Children**
Alosetron (Lotronex)	0.5 mg PO twice a day; may increase to 1 mg after 4 wk if needed	Not recommended
Bismuth subsalicylate (Pepto-Bismol)	2 tablets or 30 mL PO every 30–60 min, if needed, up to 8 doses in 24 h	Under 3 y, consult pediatrician 3–6 y, 1/3 tablet or 5 mL PO every 30–60 min as needed 6–9 y, 2/3 tablet or 10 mL PO every 30–60 min as needed 9–12 y, 1 tablet or 15 mL PO every 30–60 min as needed
Cholestyramine (Prevalite; Novo-Cholamine) Binds and inactivates bile salts in the intestine (see Chapter 10)	16–32 g/d in 120–180 mL of water PO, in 2–4 divided doses before or during meals and at bedtime	Based on limited data: Children and adolescents, 240 mg/kg/day PO, in 2–3 divided doses; suggested maximum daily dose: 8 g/day
Colestipol (Colestid; Colestid) Binds and inactivates bile salts in the intestine (see Chapter 10)	15–30 g/d in 120–180 mL of water PO, in 2–4 divided doses before or during meals and at bedtime	Drug not used to manage diarrhea in children
Nitazoxanide (Alinia) Inhibits growth of certain protozoa	500 mg (tablet or suspension) PO every 12 h for 3 d	12–47 mo, 5 mL (100 mg) PO every 12 h for 3 d 4–11 y, 10 mL (200 mg) PO every 12 h for 3 d ≥12 y, see adult dose
Octreotide (Sandostatin; Sandostatin) Decreases secretions and motility in GI tract (see Chapter 24)	100–150 mcg every 8 h SC, 50–100 mcg every 8 h IV divided over 2–4 doses; start at 200–300 mcg/d divided over 2–4 doses for 2 wk and then individualize dose to response	1–10 mcg/kg every 12 h SC, IV
Polycarbophil preparations (FiberCon, Care One Fiber; Equalactin) Absorbs water and toxins and decreases fluidity of stools (see Chapter 39)	1 g PO, 1–4 times daily; do not exceed 4 g in 24 h; for severe diarrhea, repeat dose every 30 min but do not exceed max dose	Under 6 y, products vary, so consult labels; for severe diarrhea, repeat dose every 30 min but do not exceed max dose 6–12 y, 500 mg PO 1–4 times daily; do not exceed 2 g in 24 h
Rifaximin (Xifaxan; Zaxine) Affects *E. coli* in the GI tract	550 mg PO 3 times a day for 14 d	≥12 y, see adult dosing

in the pancreas. The drug may be effective in diarrhea because it decreases GI secretion and motility. Uses include diarrhea associated with carcinoid syndrome, intestinal tumors, HIV/AIDS, and diarrhea that does not respond to other antidiarrheal drugs. Commonly reported adverse effects are diarrhea, headache, cardiac dysrhythmias, and injection site pain.

Polycarbophil

Polycarbophil (e.g., FiberCon) and psyllium are most often used as bulk-forming laxatives. They are occasionally used in diarrhea to adsorb toxins and water, decreasing the fluidity of stools. Polycarbophil is the only adsorbent drug evaluated to be effective by the FDA OTC review panel. Polycarbophil absorbs large amounts of water and produces stools of gelatin-like consistency. It may cause abdominal discomfort and bloating and may reduce the absorption of coadministered medications.

Bile-Binding Drugs

Cholestyramine (Prevalite) and colestipol (Colestid) are useful in treating diarrhea due to bile salt accumulation in conditions such as Crohn disease or surgical excision of the ileum. Although limited data are available in children, the drug is used to manage diarrhea secondary to intestinal failure or short bowel syndrome.

Antibacterial Drugs

Practitioners recommend antibacterial drugs for bacterial enteritis when diarrhea lasts longer than 48 hours, when the patient passes six or more loose stools in 24 hours, when diarrhea is associated with fever, or when blood or pus is present in the stools. In bacterial gastroenteritis or diarrhea, the choice of antibacterial drug depends on the causative microorganism and susceptibility tests. Antibacterial drugs are effective in preventing **traveler's diarrhea** (caused by the enterotoxigenic strain of *Escherichia coli*, typically from fecal contamination of food or water), but authorities usually do not recommend them because their use may promote the emergence of drug-resistant microorganisms. Although effective in reducing diarrhea due to *Salmonella* and *E. coli* intestinal infections, antibiotics may induce a prolonged carrier state during which the infection can be transmitted to other people.

Rifaximin (Xifaxan) is a structural analog of the antimycobacterial drug rifampin. This nonsystemic antibiotic remains in the gut and is not absorbed into the bloodstream. Researchers developed it specifically to treat traveler's diarrhea due to noninvasive strains of *E. coli* in patients older than 12 years of age. Use for diarrhea in the presence of fever or bloody stools or due to pathogens other than *E. coli* is not warranted. As with the use of other broad-spectrum antibiotics, superinfections may occur, requiring termination of the rifaximin. Adverse effects of rifaximin may include flatulence, headache, stomach pain, urgent bowel movements, nausea, constipation, fever, vomiting, and dizziness.

> ### ! Quality and Safety Alert: Evidence-Based Practice
>
> The 2016 American College of Gastroenterology (ACG) guideline provides the organization's most current recommendations for the diagnosis, management, and prevention of acute diarrheal infections in adults in US-based and travel settings. The ACG (Riddle et al., 2016) provided the treatment recommendations based on systematic review of the related literature.
>
> Recommendations regarding treatment of US-based acute diarrheal infections include the use of balanced electrolyte rehydration, probiotics or prebiotics, and administration of bismuth subsalicylates to control the frequency of stools. The group did not recommend the use of antibiotics for community-acquired diarrhea because the infection is typically viral in nature, and its duration is not shortened using antibiotics. Further, there is not enough evidence that empiric antimicrobial treatment for routine acute diarrheal infection should be used except in cases where the likelihood of a bacterial basis is sufficient to justify the potential adverse effects of antibiotic administration.
>
> The guidelines reinforced that prevention strategies for acute diarrheal illness in travel settings include the use of bismuth for travelers who can adhere to the frequent dosing requirements and do not have contraindications to use. In addition, administration of antibiotic prophylaxis has demonstrated moderate-to-good effectiveness and may be considered in high-risk groups for short-term use. However, the use of probiotics and prebiotics for prevention of traveler's diarrhea is not consistently strong and is currently not recommended.

Nitazoxanide (Alinia) is an antiprotozoal agent used specifically for treating diarrhea resulting from infection with *Giardia lamblia* or *Cryptosporidium parvum* (see Chapter 25). Caution is necessary when administering nitazoxanide concurrently with highly plasma protein–bound medications such as warfarin because the active metabolite of nitazoxanide is highly plasma protein–bound, and such concurrent use may result in competitive drug interactions.

Selective 5-HT$_3$ Receptor Antagonist

Alosetron (Lotronex) is a selective 5-HT$_3$ receptor antagonist indicated for treating females with chronic severe diarrhea–predominant IBS that has not responded to conventional therapy. Clinical studies have not demonstrated safety and efficacy of alosetron in males. Alosetron is rapidly absorbed orally with a bioavailability of 50% to 60%. It is moderately plasma protein–bound (82%). Extensively metabolized by the cytochrome 450 enzyme system (CYP2C9, CYP3A4, and CYP1A2), its multiple metabolites produced are excreted primarily in the urine. Caution is essential with concurrent administration with CYP1A2 and CYP3A4 inhibitors. Contraindications include concurrent administration with fluvoxamine, and severe hepatic impairment is also a contraindication. Reduced dosages to prevent drug accumulation and toxicity may be necessary in some females older than 65 years of age.

An FDA-issued **BOXED WARNING** ◆ alerts nurses to the serious GI adverse effects of alosetron. Severe constipation, with possible obstruction, perforation, and hemorrhage, is the most common problem. Ischemic colitis (reduced blood flow to the intestinal tract resulting in tissue damage [symptoms of abdominal pain, blood in stool, a feeling of urgency to move bowels]) has also occurred. These serious conditions have resulted in hospitalizations, blood loss necessitating transfusion, surgery, and death in severe cases. It is important not to give alosetron to patients with a history of GI disorders, including chronic or severe constipation or sequelae of constipation, intestinal obstruction, stricture, toxic megacolon, GI perforation and/or adhesions, ischemic colitis, impaired intestinal circulation, thrombophlebitis or hypercoagulable state, Crohn disease or ulcerative colitis, and diverticulitis.

To ensure safe and appropriate use of alosetron, the drug manufacturer has established a prescribing program, and only qualified healthcare providers enrolled in the program can prescribe this medication. Pharmacists must provide patients with a medication guide developed by the manufacturer at the time the medication is dispensed that includes the risks of taking alosetron and the situations under which the drug should be immediately discontinued. Each patient must sign a patient–physician agreement indicating that they (1) understand the risks of taking alosetron and agree to take the medication; (2) will discontinue taking alosetron if constipation occurs; (3) will immediately notify the physician if constipation or signs of ischemic colitis occur; and (4) will stop taking alosetron and contact the physician after 4 weeks of therapy with alosetron if the symptoms of IBS are not controlled.

NCLEX Success

4. A patient with diarrhea begins complaining of eye pain after administration of diphenoxylate with atropine. The nurse should do which of the following?

   A. Offer an over-the-counter analgesic such as acetaminophen.
   B. Discontinue the diphenoxylate with atropine and notify the provider.
   C. Tell the patient that this is a common side effect and will soon pass.
   D. Apply a cool compress to the eyes for relief of the discomfort.

5. A 28-year-old female with chronic severe diarrhea–predominant irritable bowel syndrome (IBS) has been given a new prescription for alosetron, and the nurse is providing education about this medication. Which of the following if said by the patient indicates that the patient teaching has been successful? (Select all that apply.)

   A. "I will stop taking the medication if constipation occurs."
   B. "I will notify my health care provider if constipation occurs."
   C. "I understand the risk of taking alosetron and agree to take the medication as prescribed."
   D. "I will stop taking alosetron and contact my healthcare provider after 4 weeks of therapy with alosetron if the symptoms of my IBS are not controlled."
   E. "If I run out of medications on a weekend, I should go to the closest urgent care center for a new prescription."
   F. "I will stop taking alosetron and contact my health care provider if I get belly pain, blood in my stool, or a feeling of urgency to move my bowels."

Clinical Application 40.2

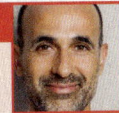

- Mr. Mendoza's culture report identifies an enterotoxigenic strain of *E. coli* (ETEC). What is the most likely drug of choice for him?

THE NURSING PROCESS

A concept map outlines the nursing process related to drug therapy considerations in this chapter. Additional nursing implications related to the disease process should also be considered in care decisions.

Assessment

- Try to determine the duration of diarrhea; number of stools per day; amount, consistency, color, odor, and presence of abnormal components (e.g., undigested food, blood, pus, mucus) in each stool; precipitating factors; accompanying signs and symptoms (i.e., nausea, vomiting, fever, abdominal pain, or cramping); and measures used to relieve diarrhea. When possible, look at stool specimens for possible clues to causation. Blood may indicate inflammation, infection, or neoplastic disease; pus or mucus may indicate inflammation or infection. Infections caused by *Shigella* organisms produce blood-tinged mucus. Infections caused by *Salmonella* or *E. coli* usually produce green, liquid or semiliquid stools. Inflammatory bowel disorders often produce nonbloody mucus.
- Try to determine the cause of the diarrhea. This includes questioning about such causes as chronic inflammatory diseases of the bowel, food intake, possible exposure to contaminated food, living or traveling in areas of poor sanitation, and use of laxatives or other drugs that may cause diarrhea. When available, check laboratory reports on stool specimens (e.g., culture reports).
- With severe or prolonged diarrhea, especially in young children and older adults, assess for dehydration, hypokalemia, and other fluid and electrolyte disorders.

Outcomes of Therapy

The patient will
- Take antidiarrheal drugs appropriately.
- Obtain relief from acute diarrhea (reduced number of liquid stools, reduced abdominal discomfort).
- Maintain fluid and electrolyte balance.
- Maintain adequate nutritional intake.
- Avoid adverse effects of antidiarrheal medications.
- Reestablish normal bowel patterns after an episode of acute diarrhea.
- Have fewer liquid stools with chronic diarrhea.

Nursing Interventions

- Provide instruction about the use of measures to prevent diarrhea.
- Prepare and store food properly and avoid improperly stored foods and those prepared under unsanitary conditions. Dairy products, cream pies, and other foods may cause diarrhea (food poisoning) if not refrigerated.
- Wash hands before handling any foods, after handling raw poultry or meat, and always before eating.
- Chew food well.
- Do not overuse laxatives (i.e., amount per dose or frequency of use). Many OTC products contain senna or other strong stimulant laxatives.
- Provide education about drug therapy (see Box 40.1).
- Provide supportive care, which is necessary regardless of whether antidiarrheal drugs are used.
- Replace fluids and electrolytes (2–3 quarts daily). Fluids such as weak tea; water; bouillon; clear soup; noncarbonated, caffeine-free beverages; and gelatin are usually tolerated and helpful. If the patient cannot tolerate adequate amounts of oral liquids or if diarrhea is severe or prolonged, intravenous fluids may be needed (i.e., solutions containing dextrose, sodium chloride, and potassium chloride).
- Avoid foods and fluids that may further irritate GI mucosa (e.g., highly spiced foods; "laxative" foods, such as raw fruits and vegetables).
- Increase frequency and length of rest periods, and decrease activity. Exercise and activity stimulate peristalsis.
- If perianal irritation occurs because of frequent liquid stools, cleanse the area with mild soap and water after each bowel movement, then apply an emollient, such as white petrolatum (Vaseline).

Evaluation

- Observe and interview for decreased number of liquid or loose stools.
- Observe for signs of adequate food and fluid intake (e.g., good skin turgor and urine output, stable weight).
- Observe for appropriate use of antidiarrheal drugs.
- Observe and interview for return of prediarrheal patterns of bowel elimination.
- Interview regarding knowledge and use of measures to prevent or minimize diarrhea.

Visit thePoint® at http://thePoint.lww.com/Frandsen13e for answers to NCLEX Success questions (in Appendix A), answers to Clinical Application Case Studies (in Appendix B), additional information on etiology, and more!

REFERENCES AND RESOURCES

Centers for Disease Control and Prevention. (2022). *Travelers' diarrhea*. Retrieved April 18, 2022, from https://wwwnc.cdc.gov/travel/page/travelers-diarrhea

Fernandes, H. V. J., Houle, S. K. D., Johal, A., & Riddle, M. S. (2019). Travelers' diarrhea: Clinical practice guidelines for pharmacists. *Canadian Pharmacists Journal, 152*(4), 241–250. https://doi.org/10.1177/1715163519853308

Hinkle, J. L., Cheever, K. H., & Overbaugh, K. J. (2021). *Brunner & Suddarth's textbook of medical-surgical nursing* (15th ed.). Wolters Kluwer.

Karch, A. M. (2023). *Focus on nursing pharmacology* (9th ed.). Wolters Kluwer.

LaRocque, P., & Harris, J. B. (2022). Approach to the adult with acute diarrhea in resource-rich settings. In *UpToDate*. Lexi-Comp, Inc.

Lippincott advisor. (2022). Retrieved from http://advisor.lww.com

Riddle, M. S., DuPont, H. L., & Connor, B. A. (2016). ACG clinical guideline: Diagnosis, treatment, and prevention of acute diarrheal infections in adults. *American Journal of Gastroenterology, 111*(5), 602–622.

Schnadower, D., O'Connell, K. J., Van Buren, J. M., Vance, C., Tarr, P. I., Schuh, S., Hurley, K., Rogers, A. J., Poonai, N., Roskind, C. G., Bhatt, S. R., Gouin, S., Mahajan, P., Olsen, C. S., Powell, E. C., Farion, K., Sapien, R. E., Chun, T. H., Freedman, S. B., & on Behalf of the Pediatric Emergency Care Applied Research Network and Pediatric Emergency Research Canada. (2021). Association between diarrhea duration and severity and probiotic efficacy in children with acute gastroenteritis. *The American Journal of Gastroenterology, 116*(7), 1523–1532. doi:10.14309/ajg.0000000000001295

Shane, A. L., Mody, R. K., Crump, J. A., Tarr, P. I., Steiner, T. S., Kotloff, K., Langley, J. M., Wanke, C., Warren, C. A., Cheng, A. C., Cantey, J., & Pickering, L. K. (2017). 2017 Infectious Diseases Society of America clinical practice guidelines for the diagnosis and management of infectious diarrhea. *Clinical Infectious Diseases: An Official Publication of the Infectious Diseases Society of America, 65*(12), 80. https://doi.org/10.1093/cid/cix669. https://doi.org/10.1093/cid/cix669

Clinical Judgment in Practice: Section 7: Drugs Affecting the Kidney and Digestive Systems

A 62-year-old patient is admitted to the hospital for a total hip replacement. The admitting nurse is gathering the patient's medical history. During the admission interview, the patient states they have experienced severe nausea and vomiting with general anesthesia. The patient states, "Ten years ago I had a hysterectomy and I vomited for 12 hours after surgery. The anesthetist told me to make sure I told anesthesia if I ever had another surgery."

Step 1: Recognize Cues
Identify the relevant and important information from different sources, such as the medical history or subjective and objective data.

Answer: The patient states, "Ten years ago I had a hysterectomy and I vomited for 12 hours after surgery. The anesthetist told me to make sure I told anesthesia if I ever had another surgery."

Step 2: Analyze Cues
Organize and link the recognized cues to the patient's clinical presentation.

Answer: The patient has a past medical history of nausea and vomiting following the administration of general anesthesia.

Step 3: Prioritize Hypotheses
Evaluate hypotheses and rank them according to priority, such as urgency, likelihood, risk, difficulty, and/or time. Cluster your findings to generate a list of problems (actual or potential) you believe the patient is experiencing or may experience and determine the level of urgency. Which problem is of the greatest concern?

Answer: You identify the priority preoperative care is the prevention of nausea and vomiting in the postoperative phase of the patient's care.

Step 4: Generate Solutions
Identify expected outcomes and use hypotheses to define a set of interventions for the expected outcomes.

Answer: Since the patient has a past medical history of nausea and vomiting in the postoperative phase following the administration of general anesthesia, you anticipate that the patient will require a scopolamine patch, dexamethasone, and ondansetron. You also anticipate that the scopolamine patch will be administered in the preoperative phase, dexamethasone will be administered following the induction of anesthesia, and ondansetron will be administered at the end of surgery. The patient will require the insertion of an IV for the administration of preoperative, intraoperative, and postoperative medications.

Step 5: Take Actions
Implement the solutions that address the highest priorities.

Answer: You start an IV with LR ordered by the orthopedic surgeon. You apply a scopolamine patch behind the right ear. Prior to the induction of anesthesia, dexamethasone 4 mg IV will be administered. In addition, at the end of surgery, ondansetron 4 mg will be administered IV. You instruct the patient on the action and use of scopolamine, dexamethasone, and ondansetron on the prevention of postoperative nausea and vomiting.

Step 6: Evaluate Outcomes
Compare observed outcomes against expected outcomes.

Answer: In the postanesthesia care unit, the patient does not experience postoperative nausea and vomiting.

SECTION 8

Drugs Affecting the Endocrine System

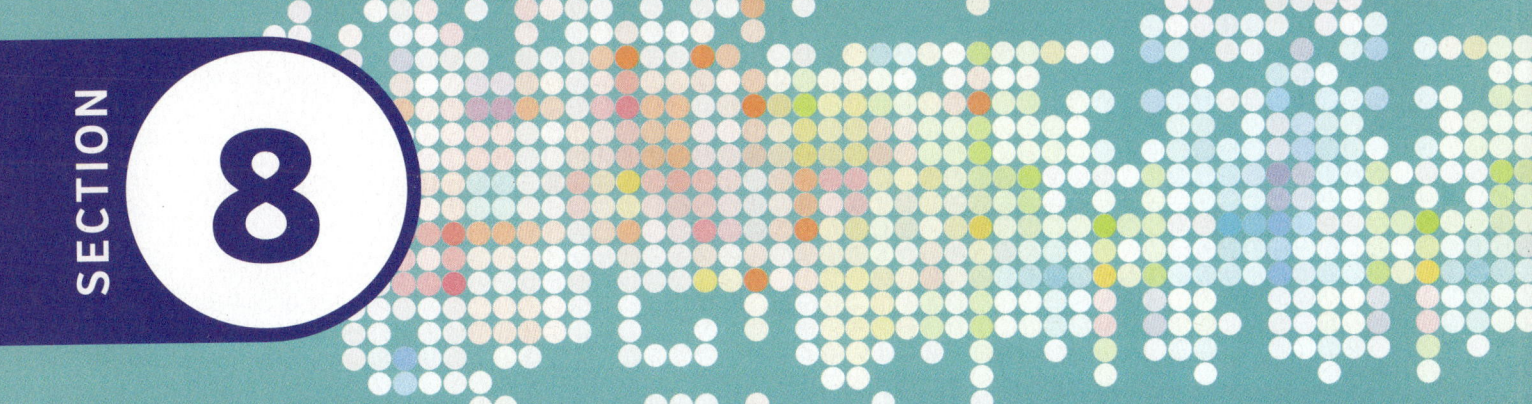

Chapter 41 Drug Therapy for Diabetes Mellitus

Chapter 42 Drug Therapy for Hyperthyroidism and Hypothyroidism

Chapter 43 Drug Therapy for Pituitary and Hypothalamic Dysfunction

Chapter 44 Drug Therapy to Regulate Calcium and Bone Metabolism

Chapter 45 Drug Therapy for Adrenal Cortex Disorders

CHAPTER 41

Drug Therapy for Diabetes Mellitus

LEARNING OBJECTIVES

After studying this chapter, you should be able to:

1. Differentiate between type 1 and type 2 diabetes mellitus.
2. Identify the clinical manifestations of type 1 and type 2 diabetes mellitus.
3. Identify the prototype and describe the action, use, adverse effects, contraindications, and nursing implications for the insulins.
4. Discuss characteristics of the various types of insulins and insulin analogs.
5. Identify the various prototypes, and describe the actions, uses, adverse effects, contraindications, and nursing implications for the oral antidiabetic drugs.
6. Identify the different prototypes and describe the actions, uses, adverse effects, contraindications, and nursing implications for the sulfonylureas, alpha-glucosidase inhibitors, biguanide, thiazolidinediones, meglitinides, dipeptidyl peptidase 4 (DPP-4) inhibitors, amylin analogs, incretin mimetics, and sodium–glucose cotransporter 2 inhibitors.
7. Apply the pharmacokinetics, pharmacodynamics, and pharmacotherapeutics of the angiotensin-converting enzyme inhibitors, angiotensin II receptor blockers, and the statins in the care of the diabetic patient.
8. Implement the nursing process in the care of patients receiving medications for the treatment of diabetes mellitus, including explaining the benefits of maintaining glycemic control in preventing complications, assisting patients or caregivers in learning how to manage diabetes care and to administer medications, and assessing and monitoring patients' adherence to prescribed management strategies.

CLINICAL APPLICATION CASE STUDY

Alfred Smith, a 56-year-old librarian, visits his physician because he has been feeling more tired and weak than usual for the past 2 months. On questioning, the physician learns that Mr. Smith often gets up in the middle of the night to urinate and drinks a glass of water. He also has numbness and tingling in his hands and feet, as well as blurred vision, which affects his job. Laboratory results show an impaired fasting glucose of 160 mg/dL and urinalysis of 4+ glucose. His lipid panel also shows total cholesterol of 240 mg/dL, high-density lipoprotein cholesterol of 22 mg/dL, and triglycerides of 400 mg/dL. Mr. Smith receives a diagnosis of type 2 diabetes, and his physician places him on metformin (Glucophage XR) 500 mg by mouth once daily. He also receives information about a diet and exercise routine to help control his diabetes.

KEY TERMS

Blood glucose level: blood sugar level in the body

Blood glucose meter: device that measures how much glucose is in the blood

Diabetes mellitus: chronic disease characterized by disordered metabolism of carbohydrates, fats, and protein, and hyperglycemia, due to a deficiency in the amount on action of insulin; the three main forms of diabetes are type 1, type 2, and gestational diabetes

Glucagon: pancreatic hormone that raises blood glucose levels by stimulating the liver to convert glycogen into glucose; it opposes insulin

Gluconeogenesis: formation of glucose from noncarbohydrate sources such as fats and amino acids

Glucose: sugar in the blood; major stimulus of insulin secretion

Impaired fasting glucose: fasting blood glucose level between 100 and 125 mg/dL; also referred to as prediabetes

Insulin: protein hormone secreted by beta cells in the pancreas; facilitates glucose utilization by cells. Absence of insulin results in diabetes mellitus

Insulin pump: wearable delivery system for continuous subcutaneous insulin infusion; the insulin dosage is programmed into the pump, and the appropriate amount of insulin is injected through a needle into the adipose tissue

Ketoacidosis: metabolic acidosis due to accumulation of ketone bodies formed by the breakdown of fatty acids and amino acids for energy in the absence of insulin

INTRODUCTION

Diabetes mellitus is characterized by disordered metabolism of carbohydrates, fats, and proteins, and hyperglycemia, due to a deficiency in the amount on action of insulin. **Insulin** is a protein hormone secreted by beta cells in the pancreas that facilitates **glucose** (blood sugar) utilization. Insulin plays a major role in metabolism of carbohydrate, fat, and protein. **Glucagon** is a hormone that raises blood glucose levels by stimulating the liver to convert glycogen into glucose. Glucagon secretion complements the effects of insulin on blood glucose. The effects of insulin are presented in detail in Box 41.1.

The three main forms of diabetes are type 1, type 2, and gestational diabetes. Treatment of diabetes mellitus includes drugs to maintain **blood glucose levels** (blood sugar levels in the body) within the normal range and prevent complications. Insulin and oral antidiabetic agents are two of the several types of medications used to lower blood glucose in diabetes mellitus. New drug therapies include amylin analogs, incretin mimetics, and dipeptidyl peptidase 4 (DPP-4) inhibitors. It is important that nurses understand the characteristic of diabetes mellitus and the clinical use of insulin, oral hypoglycemic medications, and the newer drugs. They also need to be familiar with the effects of dietary herbal supplements on blood glucose levels.

OVERVIEW OF DIABETES

Metabolic problems occur early in people with diabetes mellitus and are related to changes in the metabolism of carbohydrate, fat, and protein. A major clinical manifestation of disordered metabolism is hyperglycemia or fasting blood glucose levels exceeding 126 mg/dL. A person with a fasting blood glucose level between 100 and 125 mg/dL is said to have **impaired fasting glucose** (IFG) or prediabetes. Fasting plasma glucose, a 75-g glucose tolerance test, and hemoglobin A1C are used to test for prediabetes and type 2 diabetes. Plasma blood glucose is used to diagnose the acute onset of type 1 diabetes in individuals with symptoms of hyperglycemia.

Vascular problems include atherosclerosis throughout the body. Macrovascular (moderate and large vessels) clinical manifestations include hypertension, myocardial infarction, stroke, and peripheral vascular disease. Changes in small blood vessels (microvasculature) especially affect the retina and kidney, resulting in retinopathy and chronic kidney disease.

Type 1 Diabetes

Type 1 diabetes, a common chronic disorder of childhood, results from an autoimmune disorder that destroys pancreatic beta cells. Although it may occur at any age, it usually appears after 4 years of age and peaks in incidence at 10 to 12 years for females and 12 to 14 years for males. A subtype of type 1 diabetes, latent autoimmune diabetes of the adult, begins in adulthood. Symptoms of traditional type 1 diabetes usually develop when 10% to 20% of functioning beta cells remain, but they may occur at any time if acute illness or stress increases the body's demand for insulin beyond the capacity of the remaining beta cells to secrete it. Eventually, destruction of all beta cells occurs, resulting in no insulin production.

Type 2 Diabetes

Type 2 diabetes is characterized by hyperglycemia and insulin resistance. The hyperglycemia results from increased

> **BOX 41.1** *Effects of Insulin on Metabolism*
>
> **Carbohydrate Metabolism**
> - Insulin increases glucose transport into the liver, skeletal muscle, adipose tissue, the heart, and some smooth muscle organs (such as the uterus); it must be present for muscle and fat tissues to use glucose for energy.
> - Insulin regulates glucose metabolism to produce energy for cellular functions. If excess glucose is present after this need is met, it is converted to glycogen and stored for future energy needs or converted to fat and stored. The excess glucose transported to liver cells is converted to fat only after glycogen stores are saturated. When insulin is absent or blood glucose levels are low, these stored forms of glucose can be reconverted. The liver is especially important in restoring blood sugar levels by breaking down glycogen or by forming new glucose.
>
> **Fat Metabolism**
> - Insulin promotes transport of glucose into fat cells, where it is broken down. One of the breakdown products is alpha-glycerophosphate, which combines with fatty acids to form triglycerides. This is the mechanism by which insulin promotes fat storage.
> - When insulin is lacking, fat is released into the bloodstream as free fatty acids. Blood concentrations of triglycerides, cholesterol, and phospholipids are also increased. The high blood lipid concentration probably accounts for the atherosclerosis that tends to develop early and progress more rapidly in people with diabetes mellitus. Also, when more fatty acids are released than the body can use as fuel, some fatty acids are converted into ketones. Excessive amounts of ketones produce acidosis and coma.
>
> **Protein Metabolism**
> - Insulin increases the total amount of body protein by increasing transport of amino acids into cells and synthesis of protein within the cells. The basic mechanism of these effects is unknown.
> - Insulin potentiates the effects of growth hormone.
> - Lack of insulin causes protein breakdown into amino acids, which are released into the bloodstream and transported to the liver for energy or gluconeogenesis. The lost proteins are not replaced by synthesis of new proteins, and protein wasting causes abnormal functioning of many body organs, severe weakness, and weight loss.

production of glucose by the liver and decreased uptake of glucose in liver, muscle, and fat cells. Insulin resistance means that higher-than-usual concentrations of insulin are required. Thus, insulin is present but unable to work effectively (i.e., inhibits hepatic production of glucose and causes glucose to move from the bloodstream into liver, muscle, and fat cells). Most insulin resistance is attributed to impaired insulin action at the cellular level, possibly related to postreceptor, intracellular mechanisms.

Historically, the onset of type 2 diabetes typically occurred after 40 years of age. More recently, however, type 2 diabetes is increasingly prevalent among children and adolescents. Type 2 is a heterogeneous disease and probably involves both genetic predisposition and environmental factors. Obesity is a major cause; with obesity and chronic ingestion of excess calories, along with a sedentary lifestyle, more insulin is required. Another risk factor for the development of type 2 diabetes is the presence of metabolic syndrome, which is characterized by abdominal obesity (excessive fat tissue in and around the abdomen), hypertriglyceridemia, low high-density lipoprotein (HDL) cholesterol, hypertension, and/or IFG. Metabolic syndrome has become increasingly common in the United States.

Compared with type 1, type 2 usually has a gradual (insidious) onset, produces less severe symptoms initially, is easier to control, and causes less diabetic **ketoacidosis** (DKA) (metabolic acidosis due to accumulation of ketone bodies formed by the breakdown of fatty acids and amino acids for energy in the absence of insulin) and less kidney failure but more myocardial infarctions and strokes. However, it does not necessarily require exogenous insulin because endogenous insulin is still produced. About 90% of people with diabetes have type 2 disease; 20% to 30% of them require exogenous insulin at some point in their lives. Metformin is most commonly prescribed for the initial management of type 2 diabetes. The addition of insulin may be indicated if the patient presents with catabolic symptoms, including polyuria, polydipsia, and weight loss.

Clinical Manifestations

Most signs and symptoms stem from a lack of effective insulin and the subsequent metabolic abnormalities. The incidence and severity depend on the amount of effective insulin, and conditions such as infection, rapid growth, pregnancy, or other factors may increase demand for insulin. Most early symptoms result from disordered carbohydrate metabolism, which causes excess glucose to accumulate in the blood (hyperglycemia). Hyperglycemia produces glucosuria, which, in turn, produces polydipsia, polyuria, dehydration, and polyphagia.

Glucosuria usually appears when the blood glucose level is approximately twice the normal value and the kidneys receive more glucose than can be reabsorbed. However, kidney threshold varies, and the amount of glucose lost in the urine does not accurately reflect blood glucose. In children, glucose tends to appear in urine at much lower or even normal blood glucose levels. In older people, the kidneys may be less able to excrete excess glucose from the blood. As a result, blood glucose levels may be high with little or no glucose in the urine.

When large amounts of glucose are present, water is pulled into the kidney tubule. This results in a greatly increased urine output (polyuria). The excessive loss of fluid in urine leads to increased thirst (polydipsia) and, if fluid intake is inadequate, to dehydration. Dehydration also occurs because high blood glucose levels increase osmotic pressure in the bloodstream and fluid is pulled out of the cells in the body's attempt to regain homeostasis. Polyphagia (increased appetite) occurs because the body cannot use ingested foods. People with uncontrolled diabetes lose weight because of abnormal metabolism.

Complications of diabetes mellitus are common and potentially disabling or life threatening. Diabetes is a leading cause of myocardial infarction, stroke, blindness, leg amputation, and kidney failure. These complications result from hyperglycemia and other metabolic abnormalities that accompany a lack of effective insulin. The metabolic abnormalities associated with hyperglycemia can cause early, acute complications, such as DKA or hyperosmolar hyperglycemic nonketotic coma (HHNC; see Box 41.2). Eventually, metabolic abnormalities lead to damage in blood vessels and other body tissues. For example, atherosclerosis develops earlier, progresses more rapidly, and becomes more severe in people with diabetes. Microvascular changes lead to nephropathy, retinopathy, and peripheral neuropathy. Other complications include musculoskeletal disorders, increased numbers and severity of infections, and complications of pregnancy.

 Quality and Safety Alert: Evidence-Based Practice

Jonas et al. (2021) conducted a review of data from PubMed/MEDLINE, Cochrane Library, and trial registries through 2019 to 2021 on the evidence on screening prediabetes and diabetes to inform the U.S. Preventive Services Task Force. The main outcomes and measures included information on mortality, cardiovascular morbidity, diabetes-related morbidity, diabetes development, quality of life, and any noted harm from the disease. Two articles under review revealed no difference between the screening and control groups for specific or all causes of mortality at 10 years. The United Kingdom Prospective Diabetes Study revealed improved health outcomes with intense glucose control utilizing sulfonylureas and insulin. Overweight persons had intensive glucose control with metformin and possessed improved health outcomes at 10 years. Changes in lifestyle to promote health reduced the incidence of prediabetes. In addition, metformin showed a significant reduction in diabetes incidence and an overall reduction in weight and body mass index.

BOX 41.2 Acute Complications of Diabetes Mellitus

Diabetic Ketoacidosis

This life-threatening complication occurs with severe insulin deficiency. In the absence of insulin, glucose cannot be used by body cells for energy, and fat is mobilized from adipose tissue to furnish a fuel source. The mobilized fat circulates in the bloodstream, from which it is extracted by the liver and broken down into glycerol and fatty acids. The fatty acids are further changed in the liver to ketones (e.g., acetoacetic acid, acetone), which then enter the bloodstream and are circulated to body cells for metabolic conversion to energy, carbon dioxide, and water.

The ketones are produced more rapidly than body cells can use them, and their accumulation produces acidemia (a drop in blood pH and an increase in blood hydrogen ions). The body attempts to buffer the acidic hydrogen ions by exchanging them for intracellular potassium ions. Hydrogen ions enter body cells, and potassium ions leave the cells to be excreted in the urine. Another attempt to remove excess acid involves the lungs. Deep, labored respirations, called *Kussmaul respirations*, eliminate more carbon dioxide and prevent formation of carbonic acid. A third attempt to regain homeostasis involves the kidneys, which excrete some of the ketones, thereby producing acetone in the urine.

Two major causes of diabetic ketoacidosis (DKA) are omission of insulin and illnesses such as infection, trauma, myocardial infarction, or stroke. DKA worsens as the compensatory mechanisms fail. Clinical signs and symptoms become progressively more severe. Early ones include blurred vision, anorexia, nausea and vomiting, thirst, and polyuria. Later ones include drowsiness, which progresses to stupor and coma; Kussmaul respirations; dehydration and other signs of fluid and electrolyte imbalances; and decreased blood pressure, increased pulse, and other signs of shock.

Insulin therapy is a major part of any treatment for DKA. Patients with DKA have a deficiency in the total amount of insulin in the body and a resistance to the action of the insulin that is available, probably due to acidosis, hyperosmolality, infection, and other factors. To be effective, insulin therapy must be individualized according to frequent measurements of blood glucose. Low doses, given by continuous intravenous (IV) infusion, are preferred in most circumstances so that the brain has time to equilibrate and account for fluid shifts.

Additional measures include identification and treatment of conditions that precipitate DKA, administration of IV fluids to correct hyperosmolality and dehydration, administration of potassium supplements to restore and maintain normal serum potassium levels, and administration of sodium bicarbonate to correct metabolic acidosis. Infection is one of the most common causes of DKA. If no obvious source of infection is identified, cultures of blood, urine, and throat swabs are recommended. When infection is identified, antimicrobial drug therapy may be indicated.

Hyperosmolar Hyperglycemic Nonketotic Coma

Hyperosmolar hyperglycemic nonketotic coma (HHNC) is another type of diabetic coma that is potentially life threatening. It is relatively rare and carries a high mortality rate. The term *hyperosmolar* refers to an excessive amount of glucose, electrolytes, and other solutes in the blood in relation to the amount of water.

Like DKA, HHNC is characterized by hyperglycemia, which leads to osmotic diuresis and resultant thirst, polyuria, dehydration, and electrolyte losses, as well as neurologic signs ranging from drowsiness to stupor to coma. Additional clinical problems may include hypovolemic shock, thrombosis, kidney problems, or stroke. In contrast with DKA, hyperosmolar coma occurs in people with previously unknown or mild diabetes, usually after an illness; occurs in hyperglycemic conditions other than diabetes (e.g., severe burns, corticosteroid drug therapy); and does not cause ketosis.

Treatment of HHNC is similar to that of DKA in that insulin, IV fluids, and potassium supplements are major components. Regular insulin is given by continuous IV infusion, and dosage is individualized according to frequent measurements of blood glucose levels. IV fluids are given to correct the profound dehydration and hyperosmolality, and potassium is given IV to replace the large amounts lost in urine during a hyperglycemic state.

Drug Therapy

Medications used in the treatment of diabetes mellitus depend on the type of diabetes and degree of glycemic control. Healthcare providers use many medications to control diabetes (Table 41.1). Insulin is the prototype drug for treatment of type 1 diabetes. Several different classes of other drugs are also available for the treatment of type 2 diabetes (Fig. 41.1). Patients with diabetes may be using herbal supplements, and nurses should be aware that some of these substances affect blood glucose levels. Alfalfa, aloe bilberry, bitter melon, burdock, celery, coriander, damiana, dandelion root, garcinia, garlic, ginseng, gymnema, juniper, marshmallow, and stinging nettle increase the risk of hypoglycemia when combined with antidiabetic agents.

> **Clinical Application 41.1**
> - What additional condition does Mr. Smith have?
> - What are the complications related to this diagnosis?

INSULINS

Insulin in its various forms is the only effective drug treatment for type 1 diabetes, where pancreatic beta cells are unable to secrete endogenous insulin and metabolism is severely impaired. **Regular insulin** (HumuLIN R U-500, HumuLIN R U-500 KwikPen) is the prototype. Over-the-counter (OTC) preparations include HumuLIN R, Novolin R, and Novolin R ReliOn. Insulin is also necessary in patients with type 2 diabetes who cannot control their disease with diet, weight control, and oral agents. Any person with diabetes may need insulin during times of stress, such as illness, infection, or surgery. Other uses of insulin include control of diabetes induced by chronic pancreatitis, surgical excision of pancreatic tissue, hormones and other drugs, and pregnancy (gestational diabetes). In patients who do not have diabetes, healthcare providers use insulin to prevent or treat hyperglycemia induced by IV parenteral nutrition and to treat hyperkalemia. In hyperkalemia, an IV infusion of insulin and dextrose solution causes potassium to move from the blood into the cells; it does not eliminate potassium from the body.

All insulin in the United States is human insulin. Pork and bovine insulins, which were more antigenic, are no longer manufactured in the United States. The name human insulin means that the synthetic product is identical to endogenous insulin (i.e., has the same number and sequence of amino acids).

Types of Insulin

Insulins differ in onset and duration of action. They are usually categorized as rapid, short, intermediate, or long acting. The synthesis of insulin analogs, which are structurally similar chemicals, involves altering the type or sequence of amino acids in insulin molecules.

Rapid-Acting Insulin

Rapid-acting insulins have a rapid onset (15 minutes or less) and have a short duration of action (4 to 8 hours). All rapid-acting insulins are approved for use in external **insulin pumps** that administer a continuous subcutaneous infusion. Rapid-acting products include insulin lispro (Humalog, Admelog, Humalog KwikPen), insulin aspart (NovoLog, Fiasp, NovoLog FlexPen), and insulin glulisine (Apidra, Apidra SoloStar). Lispro, the first insulin analog to be marketed, is identical to human insulin except for the reversal of two amino acids (lysine and proline). It is absorbed more rapidly and has a shorter half-life after subcutaneous injection than regular (short-acting) human insulin. As a result, lispro is similar to physiologic insulin secretion after a meal, more effective at decreasing postprandial hyperglycemia, and less likely to cause hypoglycemia before the next meal. Injection just before a meal produces hypoglycemic effects similar to those of an injection of conventional regular insulin given 30 minutes before a meal. Aspart has an even more rapid onset and shorter duration of action. Glulisine has the shortest onset of action (5 to 10 minutes).

Afrezza is an inhaled regular insulin analog. The FDA has issued a **BOXED WARNING** 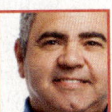 for this insulin, stating that patients with diabetes and chronic lung disease who take it are at risk for acute bronchospasm. Acute bronchospasm has been reported in patients with asthma and chronic obstructive pulmonary disease, and Afrezza is contraindicated in these patients who need insulin. The Institute for Safe Medication Practices also lists Afrezza as a drug with heightened risk for significant patient harm. Before ordering Afrezza, prescribers should collect a detailed medical history, perform a physical examination, and evaluate the patient's spirometry. The insulin requirements can vary with the use of Afrezza; thus, careful blood glucose monitoring is necessary. Afrezza is administered at the beginning of every meal. The cartridges should be stored at room temperature. Afrezza is not recommended for treatment of DKA. The most common adverse effect of inhaled insulin is hypoglycemia. Inhaled insulin must be used in combination with long-acting insulin in patients with type 1 diabetes.

Intermediate-Acting and Long-Acting Insulin

Intermediate-acting insulin preparations such as isophane (NPH) suspension possess zinc insulin crystals that have been modified by protamine in a neural buffer. The addition of zinc assists in slowing the absorption and thus prolongs the duration of action.

Long-acting insulin preparations include insulin glargine and insulin detemir. Healthcare providers use them to provide a basal amount of insulin through 24 hours, similar to normal, endogenous insulin secretion.

Several mixtures of an intermediate- and a short-acting insulin are available and in common use. U-100, the main insulin concentration in the United States, contains 100 units of insulin per milliliter of solution. Accurate measurement requires an orange-tipped syringe designed for use only with U-100 insulin.

Absorption

After subcutaneous injection, insulin is absorbed most rapidly from the abdomen, followed by the upper arm, thigh, and buttocks. Absorption is delayed or decreased by injection into subcutaneous tissue with lipodystrophy or other lesions, by circulatory problems such as edema or hypotension, by insulin-binding antibodies (which develop after 2 or 3 months of insulin administration), and by injecting cold (i.e., refrigerated) insulin.

TABLE 41.1

Drugs Administered for the Treatment of Diabetes Mellitus

Drug Class	Prototype	Other Drugs in the Class
Insulins	Insulin (HumuLIN R U-500, HumuLIN R U-500 KwikPen, *over-the-counter* HumuLIN R, Novolin R, Novolin R ReliOn)	Rapid-acting insulins or analogs: Insulin lispro (HumuLIN N KwikPen, HumuLIN N, Novolin N ReliOn, Novolin N) Insulin aspart (NovoLog, Fiasp, NovoLog FlexPen) Insulin glulisine (Apidra, Apidra SoloStar). Intermediate-acting insulin: Isophane insulin suspension (NPH Humulin N, Novolin N) Long-acting insulins: Insulin glargine (Lantus) Insulin detemir (Levemir)
Sulfonylureas	Glyburide (Glynase)	Glimepiride (Amaryl) Glipizide (Glucotrol, Glucotrol XL, GlipiZIDE) Chlorpropamide Tolazamide Tolbutamide
Biguanide	Metformin (Glumetza, Riomet)	
Alpha-glucosidase inhibitors	Acarbose (Precose)	Miglitol
Thiazolidinediones	Rosiglitazone (Avandia)	Pioglitazone (Actos)
Meglitinides	Repaglinide (Prandin)	Nateglinide (Starlix)
Dipeptidyl peptidase 4 (DPP-4) inhibitor	Sitagliptin (Januvia)	Alogliptin (Nesina) Linagliptin (Tradjenta) Saxagliptin (Onglyza)
Glucagonlike peptide 1 receptor agonist (incretin mimetics)	Exenatide (Bydureon BCise, Byetta)	Albiglutide (Tanzeum) Dulaglutide (Trulicity) Liraglutide (Saxenda, Victoza) Lixisenatide (Adlyxin, Adlyxin Starter Kit) Semaglutide (Ozempic, Rybelsus)
Amylin analogs	Pramlintide (SymlinPen 120, SymlinPen 60)	
Angiotensin-converting enzyme inhibitors	Enalapril maleate (Vasotec)	Benazepril hydrochloride (Lotensin) Captopril (Capoten) Fosinopril (Monopril) Lisinopril (Prinivil, Zestril) Moexipril hydrochloride (Univasc) Perindopril erbumine (Aceon, Coversyl) Quinapril hydrochloride (Accupril) Ramipril (Altace) Trandolapril (Mavik, Gopten)
Angiotensin II receptor antagonists	Losartan (Cozaar)	Azilsartan medoxomil (Edarbi) Candesartan cilexetil (Atacand) Eprosartan mesylate (Teveten) Irbesartan (Avapro) Olmesartan medoxomil (Benicar)
Thiazidelike diuretics	Hydrochlorothiazide (HCTZ)	Hydrochlorothiazide (HydroDiuril)
Antiplatelet	Acetylsalicylic acid (Aspirin)	Acetylsalicylic acid/methocarbamol (Robaxisal)
HMG-CoA reductase inhibitors	Simvastatin (Zocor)	Atorvastatin calcium (Lipitor) Fluvastatin (Lescol, Lescol SL) Lovastatin (Altoprev, Mevacor) Pitavastatin calcium (Livalo) Pravastatin (Pravachol) Rosuvastatin (Crestor)

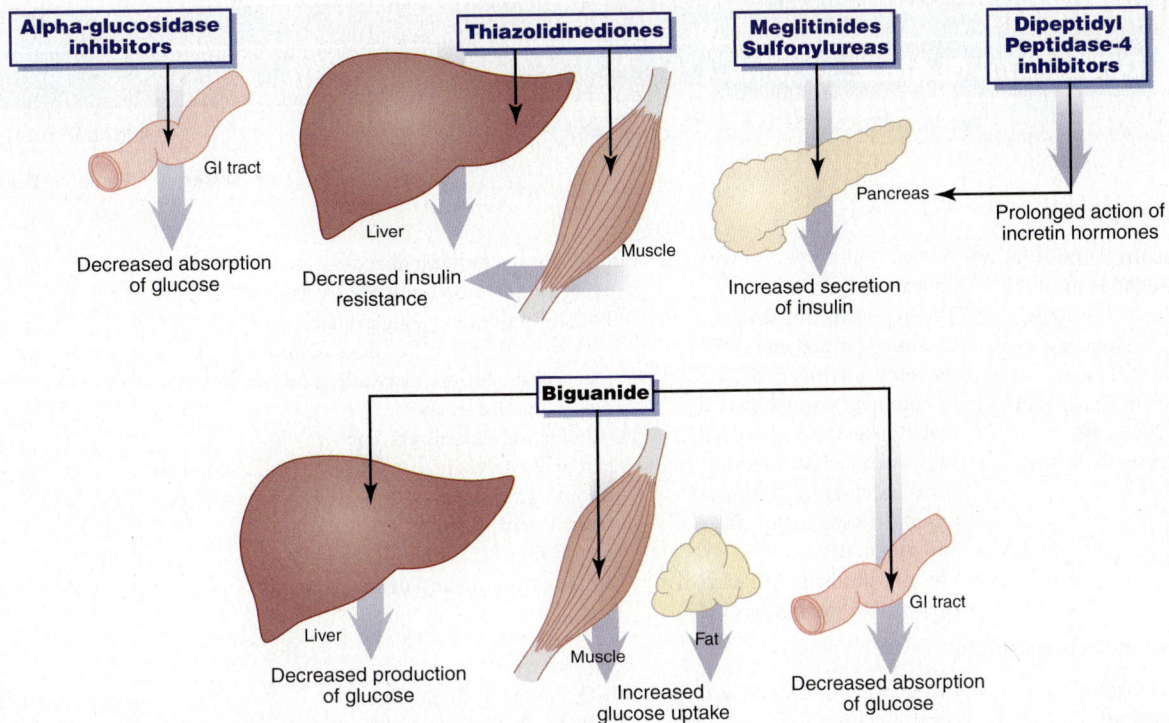

Figure 41.1. Actions of oral antidiabetic drugs. The drugs lower blood sugar by decreasing absorption or production of glucose, by increasing secretion of insulin, or by increasing the effectiveness of available insulin (decreasing insulin resistance).

Absorption may also be increased when administered in an extremity before the patient engages in a sport that requires use of the specific extremity (i.e., swimming, tennis, or jogging).

Table 41.2 gives information about insulins, including routes and dosages.

Choice of Insulin

When insulin therapy is indicated, the physician may choose from several preparations that vary in composition, onset, duration of action, and other characteristics. Some factors to be considered include the following:

- Regular insulin (insulin injection) has a rapid onset of action when administered IV; therefore, it is the insulin of choice during acute situations, such as DKA, severe infection or other illness, and surgical procedures.
- Isophane insulin (NPH) is often used for long-term insulin therapy. For many patients, a combination of NPH and short-acting insulin provides more consistent control of blood glucose levels. Although several regimens are used, a common one is a mixture of regular and NPH insulins administered before the morning and evening meals. A commercial mixture is more convenient and probably more accurate than a mixture prepared by a patient or caregiver, if the proportions of insulins are appropriate for the patient.
- Insulin lispro, aspart, or glulisine may be used instead of regular subcutaneous insulin in most situations, but safe use requires both healthcare providers and patients to be aware of differences.
- Insulin glargine or insulin detemir may be used to provide a basal amount of insulin over 24 hours, with a short-acting or rapid-acting insulin at meal times. Short-acting insulin, such as regular, will act in 15 to 30 minutes, whereas rapid-acting insulin begins to act immediately upon administration.

Pharmacokinetics

Regular insulin is rapidly absorbed after IV, intramuscular (IM), and subcutaneous administration. All of these forms of regular insulin are considered to be of short duration with a slow action. It is primarily metabolized in the liver, and a small amount is metabolized in the kidneys. Less than 2% of the drug is excreted in the urine.

Action

Insulin and its analogs replace endogenous insulin, and this exogenous insulin has the same effects as the pancreatic hormone. The insulins lower blood glucose levels by increasing glucose uptake by body cells, especially skeletal muscle and fat cells, and by decreasing glucose production in the liver.

Use

Insulin is used to lower blood glucose, and the dosage must be individualized according to blood glucose levels. **Blood glucose meters** are devices that measure how much glucose is in the blood. A specially coated test strip containing a fresh sample of blood (obtained by pricking the skin, usually the finger or forearm, with a lancet) is inserted in the meter, which then measures the amount of glucose in the blood. The FreeStyle Libre 2 System and Dexcom G6 Glucose Monitoring System have afforded greater ease in monitoring blood glucose levels. These systems

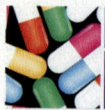

TABLE 41.2
DRUGS AT A GLANCE: Insulins

Drug	Characteristics	Routes and Dosage Ranges	Action (Hours) Onset	Peak	Duration
Short-acting insulin					
Insulin (HumuLIN R U-500, HumuLIN R U-500 KwikPen, *over-the-counter* HumuLIN R, Novolin R, Novolin R ReliOn; ✸ Entuzity KwikPen)	• A clear liquid solution with the appearance of water • The hypoglycemic drug of choice for patients with diabetes in/with acute or emergency situations, diabetic ketoacidosis (DKA), hyperosmolar nonketotic coma, severe infections or other illnesses, major surgery, and pregnancy • The only insulin preparation that can be given intravenously (IV)	Sub-Q, dosage individualized according to blood glucose levels. For sliding-scale dosing available as a high, medium, or low dose before meals and bedtime, depending on blood glucose levels IV, dosage individualized. For ketoacidosis, regular insulin may be given by direct injection, intermittent infusion, or continuous infusion and is based on hourly blood and urine glucose levels	1/2–1	2–3	5–7
Intermediate-acting insulins					
Isophane insulin suspension (HumuLIN N KwikPen, HumuLIN N, Novolin N ReliOn, Novolin N)	• Commonly used for long-term administration • Modified by addition of protamine (a protein) and zinc • A suspension with a cloudy appearance when correctly mixed in the drug vial • Given *only* sub-Q • Hypoglycemic reactions are more likely to occur during mid to late afternoon • Not recommended for use in acute situations	Sub-Q, dosage individualized. Initially, 7–26 units may be given once or twice daily	1–1½	8–12	18–24
Insulin mixtures					
NPH 70%, regular 30% (Humulin 70/30, Novolin 70/30; ✸ Humulin 70/30, Novolin ge 30/70, Novolin ge 40/60, Novolin ge 50/50) NPH 50%, regular 50% (Humulin 50/50)	• Controls postprandial hyperglycemia • Not recommended for DKA or hyperosmolar hyperglycemic reaction				
Insulin analogs					
Insulin lispro (Humalog, Admelog, Humalog KwikPen; ✸ Humalog, Humalog KwikPen)	• A synthetic insulin of recombinant DNA origin, created by reversing two amino acids • Has a faster onset and a shorter duration of action than human regular insulin • Intended for use with a longer-acting insulin	Sub-Q, dosage individualized, 15 min before meals. May also be given in external insulin pumps	1/4	1–1½	6–8
Insulin aspart (NovoLog, Fiasp, NovoLog FlexPen; ✸ NovoRapid)	Similar to lispro	Sub-Q, dosage individualized	1/4	1–3	3–5

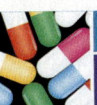

TABLE 41.2
DRUGS AT A GLANCE: Insulins (Continued)

Drug	Characteristics	Routes and Dosage Ranges*	Onset	Peak	Duration
Insulin glargine (SoloStar; ✹ SoloStar)	• Long-acting • Provides basal amount of insulin • Must *not* be diluted or mixed with any other insulin or solutions	Sub-Q, dosage individualized, once daily at bedtime	1.1	None	24
Insulin glulisine (Apidra; ✹ Apidra SoloStar; Apidra)	• Clear, colorless solution • More rapid onset of action and shorter duration of action than regular human insulin • Should be used in regimens that include a longer-acting insulin or basal insulin analog • May be mixed with NPH insulin for injection only. Draw up Apidra first and then NPH insulin. Do NOT mix Apidra with other insulins in sub-Q infusion pumps	Sub-Q by injection or continuous infusion pump, dosage individualized When used as a mealtime insulin, give up to 15 min before or within 20 min of beginning the meal	1/12–1/6 (5–10 min)	1	4
Insulin detemir (Levemir, Levemir FlexTouch; ✹ Levemir)	• Long-acting • Provides basal amount of insulin • Must not be diluted or mixed with other insulins	Sub-Q once or twice daily, dosage individualized	1	None	6–23
Analog mixtures					
Insulin lispro protamine (Humalog Mix, Humalog Mix 50/50, Humalog Mix 50/50 KwikPen, Humalog Mix 75/25, Humalog Mix 75/25 KwikPen; ✹ Humalog Mix 25, Humalog Mix 50) Insulin lispro 25% (Humalog Mix 75/25)	• Same onset, peak, and duration as individual components	Sub-Q, dosage individualized			
Insulin, recombinant (Afrezza)		Initial dose: insulin-naive patients, 4 units at each meal Patients previously on sub-Q mealtime (prandial) insulin: ≤4 units injected dose per meal: 4 units inhalation dose per meal 5–8 units injected dose per meal: 8 units inhalation per meal 9–12 units injected dose per meal: 12 units inhalation dose per meal 13–16 units injected dose per meal: 16 units inhalation per meal 17–20 units injected dose per meal: 20 units inhalation dose per meal	12–15 min		160–180 min

*When mixing insulins, always draw up the clear insulin first and then add the cloudy insulin.

allow the patient to insert a sensor in the arm or abdomen and read glucose levels on a monitor or smartphone. The patient's blood sugar levels are recorded and stored in the monitoring device or smartphone. The sensors are changed every 2 weeks.

The outcome of care is to administer enough insulin to alleviate symptoms of hyperglycemia and to reestablish metabolic balance without causing hypoglycemia (Box 41.3). An initial dose of 0.4 to 1 units/kg/d may be started and then adjusted to maintain blood glucose levels (tested before meals and at bedtime) of 80 to 130 mg/dL in adults. For children and adolescents, insulin is used to maintain glucose levels (tested before meals and at bedtime) of 90 to 150 mg/dL. However, many factors influence blood glucose response to exogenous insulin and therefore influence insulin requirements.

Factors That Influence Insulin Requirements

Factors that increase insulin requirements include weight gain, increased caloric intake, pregnancy, decreased activity, acute infections, hyperadrenocorticism (Cushing disease), primary hyperparathyroidism, acromegaly, hypokalemia, and drugs such as corticosteroids, epinephrine, levothyroxine, and thiazide diuretics. Patients with a body mass index (BMI) or 30.0 or higher may require 2 units/kg/d because of resistance to insulin in peripheral tissues.

BOX 41.3 Hypoglycemia: Characteristics and Management

Hypoglycemia may occur with insulin, meglitinides, oral sulfonylureas, amylin analogs (pramlintide [Symlin]), and incretin mimetics (exenatide [Byetta]). When hypoglycemia is suspected, the blood glucose level should be measured if possible, although signs and symptoms and the plasma glucose level at which they occur vary from person to person. Hypoglycemia is blood glucose below 60 to 70 mg/dL and is especially dangerous at approximately 40 mg/dL or below. Central nervous system effects may lead to accidental injury or permanent brain damage; cardiovascular effects may lead to cardiac dysrhythmias or myocardial infarction. Causes of hypoglycemia include the following:

- Intensive insulin therapy (i.e., continuous subcutaneous [sub-Q] infusion or three or more injections daily)
- Omitting or delaying meals
- An excessive or incorrect dose of insulin or an oral agent that causes hypoglycemia
- Altered sensitivity to insulin
- Decreased clearance of insulin or an oral agent (e.g., with abnormal kidney function)
- Decreased glucose intake
- Decreased production of glucose in the liver
- Giving an insulin injection via the intramuscular (IM) rather than the sub-Q route
- Drug interactions that decrease blood glucose levels
- Increased physical exertion
- Ethanol ingestion

Hormones That Raise Blood Sugar

Normally, when hypoglycemia occurs, several hormones (glucagon, epinephrine, growth hormone, and cortisol) work to restore and maintain blood glucose levels. Glucagon and epinephrine, the dominant counterregulatory hormones, act rapidly because they are activated as soon as blood glucose levels start declining. Growth hormone and cortisol act more slowly, about 2 hours after hypoglycemia occurs.

People with diabetes who develop hypoglycemia may have impaired secretion of these hormones, especially those patients with type 1 diabetes. Decreased secretion of glucagon is often evident in patients who have had diabetes for 5 years or longer. Decreased secretion of epinephrine also occurs in people who have been treated with insulin for several years. Decreased epinephrine decreases tachycardia, a common sign of hypoglycemia, and may delay recognition and treatment.

The Conscious Patient

Treatment of hypoglycemic reactions consists of immediate administration of a rapidly absorbed carbohydrate. For the conscious patient who is able to swallow, the carbohydrate is given orally. Foods and fluids that provide approximately 15 g of carbohydrate include the following:

- Liquids or fruit juices.
- Teaspoons of sugar.
- Commercial glucose products (e.g., Glutose, B-D Glucose). These products must be swallowed to be effective.
- Symptoms usually subside within 15 to 20 minutes. If they do not subside, the patient should take another 10 to 15 g of oral carbohydrate.
- *If acarbose or miglitol has been taken with insulin or a sulfonylurea and a hypoglycemic reaction occurs, glucose (oral or intravenous [IV]) or glucagon must be given for treatment.* Sucrose (table sugar) and other oral carbohydrates do not relieve hypoglycemia because the presence of acarbose or miglitol prevents their digestion and absorption from the gastrointestinal tract.

The Unconscious Patient

Carbohydrates cannot be given orally. Therefore, the choices are parenteral glucose or glucagon.

- In the healthcare facility, administer 25% to 50% dextrose solution.
- In home or elsewhere, give sub-Q or IM glucagon 0.5 to 1 mg if available, and there is someone to inject it.
- Glucagon is a pancreatic hormone that increases blood sugar by converting liver glycogen to glucose. It is effective only when liver glycogen is present. Some patients cannot respond to glucagon because glycogen stores are depleted by conditions such as starvation, adrenal insufficiency, or chronic hypoglycemia. The hyperglycemic effect of glucagon occurs more slowly than that of IV glucose and is of relatively brief duration. If the patient does not respond to one or two doses of glucagon within 20 minutes, IV glucose is indicated.

Avoid Overtreatment

Caution is necessary in the treatment of hypoglycemia. Although the main goal of treatment is to relieve hypoglycemia and restore the brain's supply of glucose, a secondary goal is to avoid overtreatment and excessive hyperglycemia.

Factors that decrease insulin requirements include weight reduction; decreased caloric intake; increased physical activity; development of abnormal kidney function; stopping administration of corticosteroids, epinephrine, levothyroxine, and diuretics; hypothyroidism; hypopituitarism; recovery from hyperthyroidism; recovery from acute infections; and the "honeymoon period," which may occur with type 1 diabetes.

People who need less than 0.5 units/kg/d may produce some endogenous insulin, or their tissues may be more responsive to insulin because of exercise and good physical conditioning.

In acute situations, dosage of regular insulin needs frequent adjustments based on measurements of blood glucose. When insulin is given intravenously in a continuous infusion, 20% to 30% binds to the IV fluid container and the infusion tubing.

Dosage of insulin for long-term therapy is determined by blood glucose levels at various times of the day and is adjusted when indicated (e.g., because of illness or changes in physical activity). Titrating insulin dosage may be difficult and time consuming; it requires cooperation and collaboration between patients and healthcare providers.

Insulin has been used successfully with all currently available types of oral agents (alpha-glucosidase inhibitors, biguanide, thiazolidinediones, meglitinides, and sulfonylureas).

Patient-Related Variables

Patient-related variables specific to the use of insulin include the following:

- Age:
  - Type 1 diabetes requires insulin injections in children.
  - Infants who experience prolonged episodes of hypoglycemia and persistent hyperglycemia are at risk for diminished brain development that effects learning (Levitsky & Misra, 2022).
  - Rotation of injection sites in infants and young children with type 1 diabetes is important to prevent lipodystrophy.
  - Type 2 diabetes is on the rise in children and can be managed with oral diabetic agents and/or insulin. Weight management is recommended.
  - It is essential to synchronize children's insulin injections with three meals and three snacks per day at regularly scheduled times. Though difficult to maintain, this schedule is extremely important in promoting child growth and development.
  - Children with type 1 diabetes receive either multiple daily insulin injections or continuous subcutaneous administration through an insulin pump.
  - Children with type 1 diabetes should partake in 60 minutes of moderate- to vigorous-intensity aerobic activity daily. The child and family members should be taught to check blood glucose levels before, during, and after exercise.
  - A preexercise glucose of 90 to 250 mg/dL is optimal, and carbohydrate snacks should be available to the child during exercise in the event their blood sugar decreases. The child and caregivers should be taught about the effects of hypoglycemia after exercise and overnight.
  - Strategies to reduce the postexercise hypoglycemia include reducing mealtime dosing preceding the exercise, increasing carbohydrate intake preceding exercise, eating bedtime snacks, using continuous glucose monitoring, and/or reducing basal insulin doses.
  - During illness, children are highly susceptible to dehydration. If blood glucose levels fall below 250 mg/dL, the child should be administered sugar-containing gelatins, juices, or other beverages.
  - Adolescents and young adults may resist adhering to treatment by delaying, omitting, or decreasing dosage to fit in socially (e.g., by eating more, "sleeping in," drinking alcohol) or to control their weight, which may lead to repeated episodes of ketoacidosis. Also, adolescent females may be more at risk for developing eating disorders.
  - Older adults require close monitoring of blood glucose levels and control of cardiovascular risk factors.
  - Older adults may also have impaired vision, poor manual dexterity, or other problems that decrease their ability to administer insulin, monitor glucose levels, manage diet, and exercise.
- Reproduction, pregnancy, and lactation:
  - Poorly controlled diabetes during pregnancy can be associated with increased risk of adverse outcomes for both patient and baby.
  - There can be an increased risk of DKA, preeclampsia, preterm delivery, abortion, and still birth.
  - Insulin is the preferred treatment for type 1 and type 2 diabetes with pregnancy.
  - During lactation, glycemic control is recommended.
- Abnormal kidney function and hepatic impairment:
  - Blood glucose levels in patients with abnormal kidney function and/or hepatic impairment should be monitored frequently to determine the need for dosage adjustments. In such patients, dosage is difficult to predict because less insulin is degraded by the kidneys (normally about 25%), which may lead to higher blood levels of insulin if dosage is not reduced.
  - Vigilance is required to prevent dangerous hypoglycemia, especially in patients with unstable or worsening kidney function.
  - Muscles and other tissues are less sensitive to insulin, and this resistance may result in an increased blood glucose level if dosage is not increased.
- Specific healthcare environments:
  - Insulin rather than oral agents is more likely used in critical illness and surgery. (See Box 41.4 for information about perioperative insulin therapy.)
  - Critically ill patients, with and without diabetes, often experience hyperglycemia associated with insulin resistance.
  - Hyperglycemia may complicate the progress of critically ill patients, resulting in complications such as postoperative infections, poor recovery, and increased mortality.
  - Tight glycemic control is required to prevent complications and improve mortality with critical illness.
  - The home care nurse teaches patients how to use the drug effectively; how to recognize medication responses that should be reported to the healthcare provider, such as symptoms of hypoglycemia; and, when a patient is receiving a combination of insulins, their different types, onsets, and therapeutic ranges.

Contraindications

The only clear-cut contraindication to the use of insulin is hypoglycemia, because of the risk of brain damage (see Box 41.3).

> ### BOX 41.4 Perioperative Insulin Therapy
>
> Patients with diabetes who undergo major surgery have increased risks of both surgical and diabetic complications. Risks associated with surgery and anesthesia are greater if diabetes is not well controlled and complications of diabetes (e.g., hypertension, diabetic kidney disease, vascular damage) are already evident. Hyperglycemia and poor metabolic control are associated with increased susceptibility to infection, poor wound healing, and fluid and electrolyte imbalances. Risks of diabetic complications are increased because the stress of surgery increases insulin requirements and may precipitate diabetic ketoacidosis. Metabolic responses to stress include increased secretion of catecholamines, cortisol, glucagon, and growth hormone, all of which increase blood glucose levels. In addition to hyperglycemia, protein breakdown, lipolysis, ketogenesis, and insulin resistance occur. The risk of hypoglycemia is also increased.
>
> The goals of treatment are to avoid hypoglycemia, severe hyperglycemia, ketoacidosis, and fluid and electrolyte imbalances. Maintenance of blood glucose levels between 80 and 180 mg/dL during the perioperative period is desirable. Because surgery is a stressful event that increases blood glucose levels and the body's need for insulin, insulin therapy is usually required. A 25% reduction of the insulin dose in the evening before surgery is likely to achieve perioperative blood glucose in the target range with decreased risk for hypoglycemia. Oral hypoglycemic agents such as metformin are withheld the day of the surgery. If NPH is used, give half of the NPH dose or 60% to 80% of a long-acting analog or pump basal insulin. Blood glucose is monitored every 4 to 6 hours while the patient is NPO, and prescribers should dose with short-acting insulin as needed.
>
> The goal of insulin therapy is to avoid ketosis from inadequate insulin and hypoglycemia from excessive insulin. Specific actions depend largely on the severity of diabetes and the type of surgical procedure. Diabetes should be well controlled before any type of surgery. Minor procedures usually require little change in the usual treatment program; major operations usually require a different medication regimen.

Nursing Implications

Preventing Interactions

Patients who take insulin may have other diseases that require therapeutic drugs. Certain medications can interfere with insulin, increasing or decreasing the effects, thus causing hypoglycemia or hyperglycemia (Box 41.5).

Administering the Medication

Oral administration of insulins is not effective because the proteins are destroyed by proteolytic enzymes in the GI tract. Sub-Q administration is preferred, and for regular insulin, the IV route may be appropriate. However, one important consideration with IV insulin therapy is that 30% or more of a dose may adsorb into containers of IV fluid or infusion sets.

Young children usually adjust to injections and blood glucose monitoring better when the parents express less anxiety about these vital procedures. Parents should be taught to monitor blood glucose of infants and young children more frequently than children ages 3 years and older.

Administration of insulin for infants and toddlers who weigh less than 10 kg or require less than 5 units of insulin per day can be difficult because small doses are difficult to measure in a U-100 syringe. Use of diluted insulin allows more accurate administration. The most common dilution strength is U-10 (10 units/mL), and a diluent is available from insulin manufacturers for this purpose. It is necessary to clearly label vials of diluted insulin and discard them after 1 month.

> ### BOX 41.5 Drug Interactions: Insulin
>
> **Drugs That Increase the Effects of Insulin**
>
> - Angiotensin-converting enzyme inhibitors (e.g., captopril)
>   Increase the risk of hypoglycemia
> - Alcohol
>   May promote increased hypoglycemia; inhibits gluconeogenesis (in people with or without diabetes)
> - Antidiabetic drugs, oral
>   May alter blood glucose levels; increasingly being used with insulin in the treatment of type 2 diabetes (The risks of hypoglycemia are greater with the combination.)
> - Antimicrobials (sulfonamides, tetracyclines)
>   Increase the risk of hypoglycemia
> - Beta-adrenergic blocking agents (e.g., propranolol)
>   Increase hypoglycemia by inhibiting the effects of catecholamines on gluconeogenesis and glycogenolysis (effects that normally raise blood glucose levels in response to hypoglycemia); may also mask signs and symptoms of hypoglycemia (e.g., tachycardia, tremors) that normally occur with a hypoglycemia-induced activation of the sympathetic nervous system
>
> **Drugs That Decrease the Effects of Insulin**
>
> - Adrenergics (e.g., albuterol, epinephrine)
>   Increase insulin requirements
> - Anabolic corticosteroids (e.g., prednisone)
>   Increase insulin requirements
> - Estrogens and oral contraceptives
>   Increase insulin requirements
> - Glucagon
>   Raises blood glucose by converting liver glycogen to glucose
> - Levothyroxine
>   Increases insulin requirements due to hyperglycemia
> - Phenytoin
>   Raises blood sugar by inhibiting insulin secretion
> - Thiazide diuretics (e.g., hydrochlorothiazide)
>   Increase risk of hyperglycemia due to change in glucose control

> **Quality and Safety Alert: Safety**
>
> Before administering insulin, patient safety requires that two nurses always check the dosage.

Timing

Patients with type 1 diabetes administer rapid-acting or short-acting insulin prior to meals. Patients with type 2 diabetes may take at least two insulin injections daily, with one half to two thirds of the total daily dose in the morning before breakfast and the remaining one half or one third before the evening meal or at bedtime. With regular insulin before meals, it is very important that the medication be injected 30 to 45 minutes before meals so that the insulin is available when blood sugar increases after meals. With insulin lispro, aspart, or glulisine before meals, it is important to inject the medication about 15 minutes before eating. Insulin glargine or detemir is most commonly given at bedtime. However, it may be administered in the morning or in split doses as needed.

It is important for patients who use external insulin pumps to understand the pharmacokinetics of the insulin used in the pump. The healthcare provider overseeing the patient's insulin pump sets the basal insulin settings that provide the continuous insulin needed throughout the day. However, the patient needs to have an understanding of how much and when to administer the insulin for meals. Figure 41.2 presents information concerning the insulin pump.

Selection of Subcutaneous Sites for Injections and Pumps

Several factors affect insulin absorption from injection sites, including the site location, environmental temperature, and exercise or massage. Studies indicate that insulin is absorbed fastest from the abdomen, followed by the deltoid, thigh, and hip.

Because of these differences, many clinicians recommend rotating injection sites within areas. This technique decreases rotations between areas and promotes more consistent blood glucose levels. With regard to temperature, insulin is absorbed more rapidly in warmer sites and environments. In relation to exercise, people who exercise should avoid injecting insulin into subcutaneous tissue near the muscles to be used. The increased blood flow that accompanies exercise promotes rapid absorption and may lead to hypoglycemia.

For the patient with an insulin pump, the most commonly recommended sites are the abdomen and lower back so that absorption rates remain consistent (see Fig. 41.2). It is extremely important that the patient rotate sites and avoid placing a site into scar tissue, which also affects insulin absorption.

Timing of Food Intake

Patients receiving insulin need food at the peak action time of the insulin and at bedtime. They usually take the food as a between-meal and a bedtime snack. These snacks help prevent hypoglycemic reactions between meals and at night. When hypoglycemia occurs during sleep, there may be a delay in recognition and treatment, which may allow the reaction to become more severe.

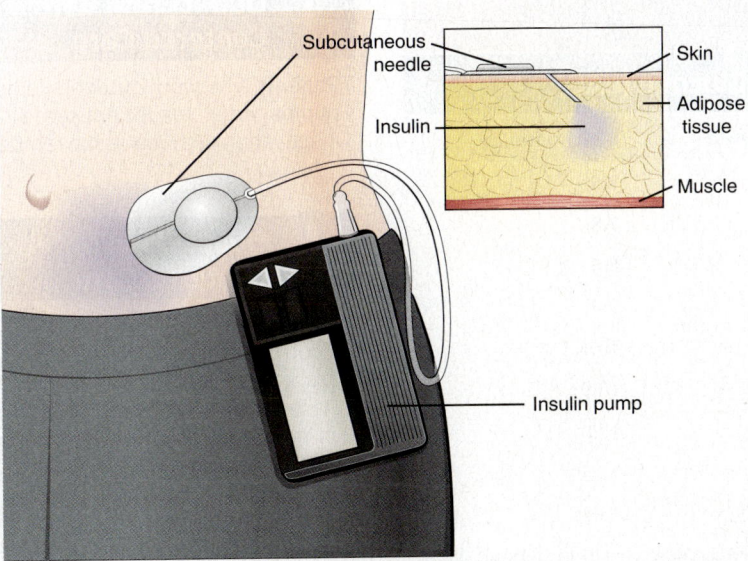

Figure 41.2. Continuous subcutaneous (sub-Q) insulin infusion pump. The insulin dosage is programmed into the pump's computer, and the appropriate amount of insulin is injected into the adipose tissue through a needle inserted into the sub-Q area. Insulin pumps are being increasingly used, especially by adolescents and young adults who want flexibility in diet and exercise. These devices allow continuous subcutaneous administration of regular insulin, insulin aspart, or insulin glulisine. A basal amount of insulin is injected (e.g., 1 unit per hour or a calculated fraction of the dose used previously) continuously, with bolus injections before meals. This method of insulin administration maintains more normal blood glucose levels and avoids wide fluctuations. Candidates for insulin pumps include patients with diabetes that is poorly controlled with other methods and those who are able and willing to care for the devices properly. The MiniMed Paradigm Real-Time System (Medtronic), the world's first integrated insulin pump and continuous glucose monitoring system, is now available in the United States. The Guardian RT System is an insulin pump and displays glucose readings every 5 minutes. It sounds an alarm when glucose levels reach high or low glucose limits preset by the clinical professional. The study completed on the RT System demonstrated that patients using the RT continuous glucose monitoring technology had better control of their blood glucose than did patients using fingersticks only.

Assessing for Therapeutic Effects

Patients with type 1 diabetes self-monitor their blood glucose by testing 6 to 10 times daily. Patients with type 2 diabetes and using basal insulin may test their blood glucose up to four times a day. In patients with type 2 diabetes not using insulin, routine glucose monitoring has limited clinical benefit. The more often the patient can check blood glucose levels, the greater possibility of tighter glucose control.

Healthcare providers also look at the glycosylated hemoglobin (hemoglobin A1C) levels to assess the effectiveness of treatment. Because glucose stays attached to hemoglobin for the life of the red blood cell, which is about 120 days, the hemoglobin A1C level reflects the average blood glucose level over the past 3 months. The normal hemoglobin A1C level is less than 7%. The American Diabetes Association has provided healthcare professionals with the estimated average glucose (eAG). This is a new term in diabetes management, which allows healthcare professionals to report A1C results to patients using the same units (mg/dL or mmol/L). Thus, the patient can see routinely the blood glucose measurements. Table 41.3 describes the relationship between A1C and eAG. This information assists healthcare providers in educating patients on glucose control.

Assessing for Adverse Effects

Assessing for signs and symptoms of hypoglycemia is essential (see Box 41.3). It is necessary to assess for tachycardia, palpitations, nervousness, weakness, confusion, hunger, and sweating. A decrease in blood glucose activates the sympathetic nervous system to produce a stress response. The nurse also assesses for such CNS effects as mental confusion, incoherent speech, visual changes, convulsions, and coma. In addition, the nurse assesses the skin and subcutaneous fat for dimpling, atrophy, or hypertrophy of the injection sites. These effects are indicative of lipodystrophy that prevents proper absorption of insulin.

Avoiding hypoglycemia is a major goal in infants and young children because of potentially damaging effects on growth and development. There may be a delay in recognition of hypoglycemia because signs and symptoms are vague, and children may be unable to communicate them to parents or caregivers. Most pediatric endocrinologists recommend maintaining blood glucose levels between 100 and 200 mg/dL to prevent hypoglycemia. It is important never to skip the bedtime snack and blood glucose measurement.

Signs and symptoms of hypoglycemia in older children are similar to those in adults (e.g., hunger, sweating, and tachycardia). In young children, hypoglycemia may be manifested by changes in behavior, including severe hunger, irritability, and lethargy. In addition, mental functioning may be impaired in all age groups, even with mild hypoglycemia. Any time hypoglycemia is suspected, it is essential that blood glucose be tested.

Infants are at the highest risk of severe hypoglycemia, which can be difficult to detect due to the infant's inability to communicate the symptoms. In addition, the clinical signs are less specific than those experienced by an older child. Infants may present with poor feeding, lethargy, hypotonia, or jitteriness (Levitsky & Misra, 2022).

TABLE 41.3

Estimated Average Glucose (eAG)

A1C (%)	eAG (mg/dL)	eAG (mmol/L)
6	126	7.0
6.5	140	7.8
7	154	8.6
7.5	169	9.4
8	183	10.1
8.5	197	10.9
9	212	11.8
9.5	226	12.6
10	240	13.4

The relationship between A1C and eAG is described by the formula $28.7 \times A1C - 46.7 = eAG$.

Flyer describing the relationship between A1C and eAG (link is external).
Questions and answers regarding estimated average glucose (eAG).
Use of eAG in Patient Care Powerpoint presentation.
Translating the hemoglobin A1C assay into estimated average glucose values (link is external). David M. Nathan, Judith Kuenen, Rikke Borg, Hui Zheng, David Schoenfeld, and Robert J. Heine, for the A1C-Derived Average Glucose (ADAG) Study Group. Diabetes Care 2008.
Translating the hemoglobin A1C assay (link is external) Editorial. Richard Kahn and Vivian Fonseca. Diabetes Care 2008
A statement (link is external) from the American Association for Clinical Chemistry regarding the reporting of eAG.
Managing diabetes. Retrieved from: https://www.cdc.gov/diabetes/managing/managing-blood-sugar/a1c.html

Quality and Safety Alert: Patient-Centered Care

Patients who work outdoors in hot weather and have insulin pumps are at risk for not receiving the insulin because of its inactivation with increased temperatures.

Quality and Safety Alert: Patient-Centered Care

Infections and other illnesses may cause wide fluctuations in blood glucose levels and interfere with metabolic control. For example, viral infections cause hypoglycemia; others, especially chronic infections, may cause hyperglycemia and insulin resistance and may precipitate ketoacidosis. As a result, insulin requirements may vary widely during illness episodes and should be based on blood glucose and urine ketone levels. Hypoglycemia often develops in young children, partly because of anorexia and smaller glycogen reserves.

During illness, children are highly susceptible to dehydration, and an adequate fluid intake is very important. Many clinicians recommend sugar-containing liquids (e.g., regular sodas, clear juices, and regular gelatin desserts) if blood glucose values are lower than 250 mg/dL. When blood glucose values are above 250 mg/dL, children should receive diet soda, unsweetened tea, and other fluids without sugar.

Patient Teaching

It is important to teach the patient and family about all aspects of diabetes care (Box 41.6). It is also essential to teach them about the insulins and their administration (Box 41.7).

BOX 41.6 Patient Teaching Guidelines for Antidiabetic Drugs (General)

- Wear or carry diabetic identification (e.g., a MedicAlert necklace or bracelet) at all times.
- Stay informed about how to control the disease, minimize complications, and achieve optimal quality of life. Although much information is available from healthcare providers, an additional major resource is the American Diabetes Association (http://www.diabetes.org)
- A consistent schedule of diet, exercise, and medication generally results in the best control of blood sugar levels and the least risk of complications.
- Maintaining healthy weight and avoiding excessive caloric intake decrease the need for medication and the workload of the pancreas. Exercise helps body tissues use insulin better, which promotes more normal blood glucose levels and decreases long-term complications.
- Notify a healthcare provider if you are unable to take a medication. If you take insulin, know what type(s) you are taking, how to obtain more, and how to store it.
- Regular and isophane (NPH) insulins and mixtures (e.g., Humulin) are available over the counter; lispro (Humalog), aspart (NovoLog), glargine (Lantus), glulisine (Apidra), and detemir (Levemir) require a prescription.
- Unopened vials of insulin should be refrigerated. An opened vial may be stored at room temperature for 28 days. DO NOT freeze insulin.
- Keep several days' supply of insulin and syringes on hand to allow for weather or other conditions that might prevent replacement of insulin or other supplies.
- If you take exenatide, store it in the original package in the refrigerator and discard unused portion after 30 days. Alert your healthcare provider if you experience acute abdominal discomfort.
- If you take pramlintide, opened vials can be kept in the refrigerator or at room temperature for up to 28 days.
- Know the signs and symptoms of high blood sugar (hyperglycemia): increased blood glucose and excessive thirst, hunger, and urine output. Persistent hyperglycemia may indicate a need to change some aspect of the treatment program, such as diet or medication.
- Know the symptoms of low blood sugar (hypoglycemia): sweating, nervousness, hunger, weakness, tremors, and mental confusion. Hypoglycemia may indicate too much medication or exercise or too little food. Treatment is a rapidly absorbed source of sugar, which usually reverses symptoms within 10 to 20 minutes. If alert and able to swallow, take 4 oz of fruit juice; 4 to 6 oz of a sugar-containing soft drink; a piece of fruit or 1/3 cup of raisins; two to three glucose tablets (5 g each); a tube of glucose gel; 1 cup of skim milk, tea, or coffee with two teaspoons of sugar; or eight Life Savers candies. Avoid taking so much sugar that hyperglycemia occurs.
- If you take acarbose (Precose) or miglitol (Glyset) along with insulin, glimepiride (Amaryl), glipizide (Glucotrol), or glyburide (DiaBeta, Glynase) and a hypoglycemic reaction occurs, you must take some form of glucose (or glucagon) for treatment. Sucrose (table sugar) and other oral carbohydrates do not relieve hypoglycemia because the presence of acarbose or miglitol prevents their digestion and absorption from the gastrointestinal (GI) tract.
- Have a family member or another person who is able to recognize and manage hypoglycemia in case you are unable to obtain or swallow a source of glucose. If you take insulin, glucagon should be available in the home, and a caregiver should know how to give it.
- Make regular visits to healthcare providers, preferably a team of specialists in diabetes care; regular vision, retinal eye examination, and glaucoma testing; and special foot care. In addition, if you have hypertension or elevated lipid levels, treatment can help prevent heart attacks and strokes.
- Avoid other prescriptions and over-the-counter drugs unless these are discussed with the physician treating the diabetes because adverse reactions and interactions may occur.
- If you wish to take any kind of herbal or dietary supplement, discuss this with your healthcare provider. There has been little study of these preparations in relation to diabetes; many can increase or decrease blood sugar and alter diabetes control. If you start a supplement, check your blood sugar frequently to see how it affects your blood glucose level.
- Test blood regularly for glucose according to your individualized needs. Test more often when medication dosages are changed or when you are ill. A blood sample can be obtained from a fingertip or other location such as the forearm. Glucose concentrations measured at different sites may vary; the fingertips are the most accurate site and are preferred if hypoglycemia is suspected.
- Reduce insulin dosage or eat extra food if you expect to exercise more than usual. Recommendations should be individualized and worked out with healthcare providers in relation to the type of exercise.
- Ask for written instructions about managing "sick days," and call your physician if unsure about what you need to do. Although each person needs individualized instructions, some general guidelines include the following:
  - Continue your antidiabetic medications unless instructed otherwise. Additional insulin also may be needed, especially if ketosis develops. Ketones (acetone) in the urine indicate insulin deficiency or insulin resistance.
  - Check blood glucose levels before meals and at least four times daily; test urine for ketones when the blood glucose level exceeds 250 mg/dL or with each urination. If unable to test urine, have someone else do it.
  - Rest, keep warm, do not exercise, and keep someone with you if possible.
  - If unable to eat solid food, take easily digested liquids or semiliquid foods. About 15 g of carbohydrate every 1 to 2 hours is usually enough and can be provided by half cup of apple juice, applesauce, cola, cranberry juice, eggnog, cream of wheat cereal, custard, vanilla ice cream, regular gelatin, or frozen yogurt.
  - Drink 2 to 3 quarts of fluids daily, especially if you have a fever. Water, tea, broths, clear soups, diet soda, or carbohydrate-containing fluids are acceptable.
  - Record the amount of fluid intake as well as the number of times you urinate, vomit, or have loose stools.
  - Seek medical attention if a premeal blood glucose level is more than 250 mg/dL, if urine acetone is

(Continued on page 764)

BOX 41.6 Patient Teaching Guidelines for Antidiabetic Drugs (General) (Continued)

present, if you have fever above 100°F, if you have several episodes of vomiting or diarrhea, or if you have difficulty in breathing, chest pain, severe abdominal pain, or severe dehydration.
- Know that illness is a stress response and can increase or decrease your blood glucose. The body will have increased secretions of glucagon, epinephrine, growth hormone, cortisol, and hormones that raise blood glucose levels, and this will require an increase in medication to lower blood sugar. If you are unable to eat, hypoglycemia will result. Illnesses that lower blood sugar include viral infections, nausea, and vomiting. These conditions can result in dehydration and changes in fluids and electrolytes, leading to diabetic ketoacidosis.

BOX 41.7 Patient Teaching Guidelines for Insulin

- Follow instructions for times of administration as nearly as possible. Accurate timing (e.g., in relation to meals) can increase benefits and decrease risks of hypoglycemic reactions.
- Wash hands; wash injection site, if needed.
- Draw up insulin in a good light, being very careful to draw up the correct dose. If you have trouble seeing the syringe markers, get a magnifier or ask someone else to draw up the insulin. Prefilled syringes or cartridges for pen devices are also available.
- Instructions may vary about cleaning the top of the insulin vial and the injection site with an alcohol swab and about pulling back on the plunger after injection to see if any blood enters the syringe. Follow your healthcare provider's orders.
- Inject straight into the fat layer under the skin, at a 90-degree angle. If very thin, pinch up a skinfold and inject at a 45-degree angle.
- Rotate injection sites. Your healthcare provider may suggest a rotation plan. Many people rotate between the abdomen and the thighs. Do not inject insulin within 2 inches of the "belly button" or into any skin lesions.
- If it is necessary to mix two insulin preparations, ask for specific instructions about the technique and then follow it consistently. There is a risk of inaccurate dosage of both insulins unless measured very carefully. Commercial mixtures are also available for some combinations.
- Carry sugar, candy, or a commercial glucose preparation for immediate use if a hypoglycemic reaction occurs.

Clinical Application 41.2

Mr. Smith comes back 6 months later after an increase in metformin extended release 500 mg four times per day because of poor glycemic control and failure to adhere to a diet and exercise regimen. His physician orders 6 units of Humulin 70/30 once daily in the morning.
- At what time does the nurse tell Mr. Smith to expect hypoglycemia to occur?
- What teaching does the nurse provide to Mr. Smith about preparing and injecting the insulin?

NCLEX Success

1. A patient with newly diagnosed type 1 diabetes is beginning daily insulin injections. The nurse is preparing to teach the patient about insulin injections. What should the nurse include in the teaching plan?
   A. Understand that ketones in the urine indicate the need for a decrease in the number of units of insulin.
   B. Administer the insulin at the same time every day regardless of meals.
   C. Rotate the insulin injection sites.
   D. Increase the insulin dosage just prior to exercise.

2. Which of the following insulins cannot be administered in a continuous subcutaneous insulin infusion pump?
   A. insulin lispro
   B. insulin aspart
   C. insulin glulisine
   D. insulin glargine

Unfolding Patient Stories: Juan Carlos • Part 2

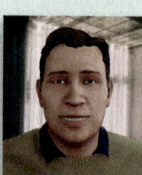

Recall Juan Carlos, a 52-year-old male with diabetes mellitus type 2, hypertension, and hyperlipidemia, whom you first met in Chapter 12. He is hospitalized for antibiotic treatment and surgical debridement of a diabetic foot ulcer. He is to receive his maintenance insulin detemir (Levemir) 5 units SC and a sliding-scale insulin aspart (NovoLog) 4 units SC for a fingerstick glucose of 225. What factors may be causing an increase in Juan's insulin requirement? How would the nurse explain the characteristics of each insulin? What patient education would the nurse provide when Juan asks the nurse to combine the insulins for one injection and why he needs frequent fingersticks?

Care for Juan and other patients in a realistic virtual environment: *vSim for Nursing* (thepoint.lww.com/vSim-Pharm). Practice documenting these patients' care in DocuCare (thepoint.lww.com/DocuCareEHR).

SULFONYLUREAS

The sulfonylureas are the oldest and largest group of oral agents used in patients with type 2 diabetes. They are not commonly prescribed due to the increased risk of hypoglycemia. The sulfonylureas stimulate insulin secretions in patients who still have some beta cell production in the pancreas. Second-generation sulfonylureas have replaced the first-generation sulfonylureas (e.g., chlorpropamide, tolazamide, tolbutamide). Glyburide (Glynase) is the prototype of the second-generation sulfonylurea class (Table 41.4). The sulfonylurea medications are chemically similar to sulfonamide antibacterial drugs. When these drug classes are administered concurrently, the patient's blood glucose levels should be assessed routinely throughout the day.

BIGUANIDE

The only drug available in this class is the prototype **metformin** (Glumetza, Riomet). Experts prefer to call it an antihyperglycemic rather than a hypoglycemic because it does not cause hypoglycemia, even in large doses, when used alone.

Pharmacokinetics

Absorption of metformin occurs in the small intestine, and it circulates without binding to plasma proteins. The drug has a serum half-life of 1.3 to 4.5 hours. It is not metabolized in the liver and is excreted unchanged in the urine.

Action

Metformin reduces the production of glucose by the liver. It also decreases the intestinal absorption of glucose to increase insulin sensitivity. This action increases the uptake of glucose, thus enhancing its utilization to produce energy.

Use

People may take metformin alone or in combination with insulin or other oral agents. Prescribers widely order it as the initial drug in newly diagnosed type 2 diabetes, mainly because it does not cause the weight gain associated with most other oral agents. Authorities consider metformin to be weight neutral and ideal for overweight people with type 2 diabetes, who have been known to lose weight on this medication, further improving insulin sensitivity. Table 41.5 presents dosage information about metformin.

TABLE 41.4

DRUGS AT A GLANCE: Sulfonylureas

Drug	Routes and Dosage Ranges	
	Adults	**Children**
Glyburide (Glynase; APO-GlyBURIDE, DiaBeta, DOM-GlyBURIDE, SANDOZ-GlyBURIDE, TEVA-GlyBURIDE)	Initial dose, 2.5–5 mg PO with breakfast Maintenance dose, 1.25–20 mg/d PO given as single or divided doses; increase in increments of no more than 2.5 mg at weekly intervals based on patient's blood glucose Older adult initial: 1.25 mg/d PO	Not recommended
Chlorpropamide (APO-ChlorproPAMIDE)	PO 250 mg daily; may be increased or decreased by 50–125 mg at 3- to 5-d intervals; titrate after 5–7 d Maintenance: 100–250 mg daily Severe diabetes: 500 mg daily avoid doses >750 mg daily	Not recommended
Glimepiride (Amaryl; Amaryl, Apo-Glimepiride; Novo-Glimepiride, PMS-Glimepiride, ratio-Glimepiride, Sandoz-Glimepiride)	Initial dose, 1–2 mg PO once daily, with breakfast or first main meal; maximum starting dose, 2 mg or less Maintenance dose, 1–4 mg once daily; after a dose of 2 mg is reached, increase dose in increments of 2 mg or less at 1- to 2-wk intervals, based on blood glucose levels; maximum recommended dose, 8 mg once daily When administered with insulin, administer glimepiride 8 mg PO once daily with insulin at the breakfast or the first main meal of the day	Safety and efficacy not established
Glipizide (GlipiZIDE XL Glucotrol; Glucotrol XL)	Initial dose, 5 mg PO daily in a single dose, 30 min before breakfast; maximum dose, 40 mg daily In elderly, may start with 2.5 mg daily Extended-release, once daily with breakfast	Safety and efficacy not established
Tolazamide	PO 100–250 mg/d; 500 mg in 2 divided doses	Safety and efficacy not established
Tolbutamide	PO 1–2 g/d as a single dose in the morning or in divided doses throughout the day; maintenance dose, 0.25 mg to 3 g/d Geriatric: Initial dose: 250 mg one to three times per day	Safety and efficacy not established

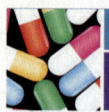

TABLE 41.5
DRUGS AT A GLANCE: Metformin (Biguanide)

Drug	Routes and Dosage Ranges	
	Adults	**Children**
ⓟ **Metformin** (Glumetza, Riomet; ✹ ACT MetFORMIN, APO-MetFORMIN ER, Glumetza, Glycon, JAMP-MetFORMIN)	500 mg BID or 850 mg once daily PO; maximum dosage: 2,550 mg/d in divided doses 500–1,000 mg once daily; dosage may be increased by 500 mg at 1–2 wk; maximum daily dose, 2,000 mg/d Glumetza: 500–1,000 mg once daily; increase by 500 mg weekly; maximum daily dose, 2,000 mg/d	>10 y, 500 mg BID PO with meals; maximum dosage, 2,000 mg/d in divided doses; oral suspension is administered in the evening 17 y and older, see adult dose

Patient-related variables specific to the use of metformin include the following:

- Age:
  - Children ≥10 years of age may be administered an oral suspension. The recommended dosage of the oral suspension of 500 mg/5 mL in the evening may be titrated at 500-mg increments each week, to a maximum dose of 2,000 mg/day. The dosage of the tablet form of 500 to 1,000 mg daily with the evening meal can be increased by 500 to 1,000 mg every 7 to 14 days. A gradual increase in dose will allow better glycemic control and assist in decreasing the GI symptoms that occur.
  - Dosage titration to the maximum amount recommended for younger adults is not appropriate for older adults. Contraindications in older adults often include cardiovascular disorders that increase risks of fluid retention and congestive heart failure. A **BOXED WARNING** for metformin states that patients 80 years of age or older should not take the drug because of the risk of lactic acidosis.

- Reproduction, pregnancy, and lactation:
  - Metformin may increase ovulation in premenopausal patients.
  - Metformin crosses the placenta; however, the risk of congenital anomalies or negative fetal outcome has not been reported for patients taking metformin for gestational or type 2 diabetes.
  - Dosage may need to be increased in the third trimester.
  - Metformin is present in breast milk. Breast-feeding is acceptable if the relative infant dose is <10. Do not breast-feed at the metformin serum peak (immediate release: 2 to 3 hours; extended release: 7 hours; extended-release suspension: 4.5 hours).

- Abnormal kidney function and hepatic impairment:
  - Assess kidney function before starting the drug and at least annually during long-term therapy. Discontinue metformin if abnormal kidney function occurs or serum lactate increases.
  - Parenteral radiographic contrast media containing iodine (e.g., Cholografin, Hypaque) may cause kidney failure and have been associated with lactic acidosis in patients receiving metformin. Discontinue metformin at least 48 hours before such diagnostic tests and resume the drug at least 48 hours after, once tests indicate that kidney function is normal.
  - Avoid use in patients with clinical or laboratory evidence of hepatic impairment because of increased risk of lactic acidosis.

> **❗ Quality and Safety Alert: Patient-Centered Care**
>
> Patients admitted for minor surgery should discontinue metformin the day of surgery. The blood glucose level should be monitored closely and a rapid-acting subcutaneous insulin may be required. Metformin should be held for 48 hours following surgery and until normal kidney function is established. Patients admitted for surgery greater than 2 hours should be instructed to discontinue metformin 24 hours prior to surgery. The blood glucose level should be monitored closely. The patient may require an IV infusion of regular insulin due to hyperglycemia. Metformin is resumed in 48 hours following surgery and once normal kidney function resumes.

Adverse Effects

The primary adverse effect of metformin is lactic acidosis. Other adverse effects include hypersensitivity reactions, dizziness, nausea, vomiting, abdominal discomfort or cramping, malabsorption of amino acids, and diarrhea.

Contraindications

Contraindications to metformin include diabetes complicated by fever, severe infections, severe trauma, major surgery, acidosis, or pregnancy (insulin is indicated in these conditions). Patients with serious hepatic impairment or abnormal kidney function, cardiac or respiratory insufficiency, hypoxia, or a history of lactic acidosis should not take the drug because these conditions may increase production of lactate and the risk of potentially fatal lactic acidosis (see note above about **BOXED WARNING** ◆).

Nursing Implications

Preventing Interactions

Some drugs increase the effects of metformin (Box 41.8). Use with sulfonylureas, furosemide, cationic drugs such as digoxin, and vancomycin increases the risk of hypoglycemia.

> **BOX 41.8 Drug Interactions: Metformin**
>
> **Drugs That Decrease the Effects of Metformin**
> - Corticosteroids (systemic and inhaled)
>   *Result in hyperglycemia*
> - Luteinizing hormone, somatotropin, and thiazide diuretics
>   *Increase risk of hyperglycemia*
>
> **Drugs That Increase the Effects of Metformin**
> - Alcohol
>   *Increases risk of hypoglycemia and lactic acidosis*
> - Cephalexin, cimetidine, dalfampridine, and glycopyrrolate
>   *Interferes with metabolism and increases blood levels*
> - Corticosteroids (oral and inhaled)
>   *May suppress the hypothalamic–pituitary–adrenal axis, leading to adrenal crisis, leading to hypoglycemia*
> - Furosemide
>   *Increases blood levels*
> - Pegvisomant
>   *Increases risk of hypoglycemia*
> - Sulfonylurea hypoglycemic agents
>   *Increases risk of hypoglycemia*

Administering the Medication

The nurse should assess kidney function before starting metformin and at least annually during long-term therapy. Patients should take metformin with meals to decrease GI distress. They should swallow the extended-release formulation whole and take it with the evening meal. Patients should discontinue the drug immediately if they are diagnosed with a myocardial infarction.

Assessing for Therapeutic Effects

The nurse assesses fasting, preprandial, and postprandial blood glucose for normal or near-normal levels. Also, the nurse assesses for improvement in hemoglobin A1C levels.

Assessing for Adverse Effects

The nurse assesses the skin for eczema, pruritus, erythema, and urticaria, which are all indicative of a hypersensitivity reaction. It is also necessary to assess the GI response to the medication. In addition, the nurse assesses for abdominal pain, nausea, vomiting, and diarrhea. It is essential to check the liver function to determine the onset of lactic acidosis. Blood lactate levels are above 5 mmol/L, and blood pH is below 7.35. Symptoms and signs of lactic acidosis may include drowsiness, malaise, respiratory distress, bradycardia, and hypotension.

Patient Teaching

Box 41.6 presents general patient teaching guidelines for the antidiabetic drugs. Box 41.9 presents patient teaching guidelines for the oral antidiabetic drugs.

> **BOX 41.9 Patient Teaching Guidelines for Oral or Injectable Antidiabetic Drugs**
>
> - Take glipizide or glyburide (DiaBeta) approximately 30 minutes before meals; take glimepiride with breakfast or the first main meal. Take Glucotrol XL with breakfast.
> - Take acarbose or miglitol (Glyset) with the first bite of each main meal. The drugs need to be taken with food because they act by decreasing sugar absorption. Starting with a small dose and increasing it gradually helps to prevent bloating, "gas pains," and diarrhea.
> - Take metformin (Glucophage) with meals to decrease stomach upset.
> - Take Glucophage XR with the evening meal.
> - Stop metformin 48 hours before any diagnostic test requiring a contrast media with iodine, and do not begin taking it again until 48 hours after.
> - Take repaglinide (Prandin) or nateglinide (Starlix) about 15 to 30 minutes before meals (two to four times daily). Doses may vary from 0.5 to 4.0 mg, depending on fasting blood glucose levels. Dosage changes should be at least 1 week apart. If you skip a meal, skip that dose; if you eat an extra meal, take an extra dose.
> - Know the signs and symptoms of hypoglycemia with repaglinide and how to treat the condition immediately.
> - Keep candy or simple sugars available to treat mild hypoglycemia.
> - Take pioglitazone (Actos), rosiglitazone (Avandia), and sitagliptin (Januvia) without regard to meals. If you take rosiglitazone or pioglitazone, report shortness of breath, chest pain, swelling, and fatigue.
> - If you take glimepiride, glipizide, glyburide, repaglinide, or nateglinide alone or in combination with other antidiabetic drugs, be prepared for hypoglycemic reactions (as with insulin; see Box 41.7). Acarbose, miglitol, metformin, pioglitazone, and rosiglitazone do not cause hypoglycemia when taken alone. Do not skip meals and snacks; this increases the risk of hypoglycemic reactions.
> - If you exercise vigorously, you may need to decrease your dosage or eat more. Ask for and follow the specific instructions ordered by the healthcare provider related to the type and frequency of exercise.

ALPHA-GLUCOSIDASE INHIBITORS

Alpha-glucosidase inhibitors inhibit alpha-glucosidase enzymes (e.g., sucrase, maltase, amylase) in the GI tract, thereby delaying digestion of complex carbohydrates into glucose and other simple sugars. **Acarbose** (Precose), the prototype alpha-glucosidase inhibitor, is known best for improving glycosylated hemoglobin levels. The drug is obtained through the fermentation process of microorganisms. Because acarbose does not enhance insulin, it works best when given with a sulfonylurea to control blood glucose levels.

Pharmacokinetics

Acarbose has a rapid onset of action and peaks in 1 hour. The drug is metabolized by the digestive enzymes and intestinal bacteria in the GI tract. It is minimally distributed and excreted in the urine and feces.

Action and Use

Acarbose works to delay the digestion of carbohydrates to diminish the increase in blood glucose after meals.

It may be necessary to combine acarbose with insulin or an oral agent, usually a sulfonylurea. Low initial doses and gradual increases decrease GI upset (e.g., bloating, diarrhea) and promote patient adherence. Patients taking acarbose should continue their diet, exercise, and blood glucose testing routines. Acarbose does not alter insulin secretion or cause hypoglycemia. Table 41.6 presents dosage information for acarbose and other alpha-glucosidase inhibitors.

Patient-related variables specific to the use of alpha glucosidase inhibitors include the following:

- Age:
  - Infants >4 months and young children who have experienced gastroesophageal reflux and have had Nissen fundoplication surgery may develop dumping syndrome (reactive hypoglycemia). It is recommended acarbose 12.5 to 25 mg is administered before each bolus feeding of complex carbohydrate formula.
  - Acarbose can decrease levels of digoxin (often prescribed for older adults). Patients who take both drugs need close monitoring.
  - Aging adults may have fat loss, resulting in weight reduction. In adults who weigh less than 60 kg, it is necessary to decrease the maximum dosage.
- Reproduction, pregnancy, and lactation:
  - Agents other than acarbose and miglitol are recommended for pregnant individuals with type 2 diabetes.
  - Acarbose and miglitol is not recommended with lactation.
- Abnormal kidney function and hepatic impairment:
  - Alpha-glucosidase inhibitors accumulate in patients with abnormal kidney function. However, dosage reduction is not helpful because the drugs act locally, within the GI tract.
- These drugs are contraindicated with cirrhosis.
- Specific healthcare environments:
  - Post gastric bypass surgery, patients are at risk for postprandial hyperinsulinemic hypoglycemia. It is recommended that acarbose is administered 25 to 100 mg three times daily at the start of each meal. If the patient eats more frequently, administer 25 to 50 mg up to six times per day.

Adverse Effects

There are no serious adverse effects of acarbose. However, acarbose can cause gastric upset because the drug is metabolized in the GI tract. It also has the potential to produce leukopenia, thrombocytopenia, and anemia. In addition, elevated serum transaminase levels may occur with the administration of acarbose. In the event of an increase in the AST and/or ALT levels, acarbose should be discontinued (McIver & Tripp, 2021).

Contraindications

Contraindications to acarbose include hypersensitivity, DKA, hepatic cirrhosis, inflammatory or malabsorptive intestinal disorders, and severe abnormal kidney function.

Nursing Implications

Preventing Interactions

As mentioned previously, acarbose can decrease digoxin levels, and patients taking digoxin require close monitoring. Certain drugs may increase or decrease the effects of acarbose (Box 41.10).

Administering the Medication

People should take acarbose at the beginning of each meal so that it is present in the GI tract with food and able to delay digestion of carbohydrates. Never administer acarbose with cola products. The combination will result in a worsening of abdominal symptoms such as abdominal pain and bloating.

TABLE 41.6

DRUGS AT A GLANCE: Alpha-Glucosidase Inhibitors

Drug	Routes and Dosage Ranges	
	Adults	Children
ⓟ **Acarbose** (Precose; Glucobay; MAR-Acarbose)	Monotherapy: initially 25 mg PO three times per day with first bite of each meal; may start with 25 mg/d and gradually increase if gastrointestinal (GI) side effects are a problem Patients weighing 60 kg or less, maximum dosage 50–100 mg three times per day PO Patients weighing more than 60 kg, maximum dosage 100 mg three times per day PO	Diabetes type 2: Children 10 years and older: PO 25 mg three times per day with the first bite of the main meal Dumping Syndrome after Nissen Fundoplication: Infants 4 months or older who have failed nutritional manipulations: PO 12.5–25 mg before each bolus feeding
Miglitol	Monotherapy: initial dose 25 mg PO three times per day at the first bite of each meal; may start at 25 mg PO daily if severe GI effects are seen Maintenance: 100 mg PO three times per day	Safety and efficacy not established

BOX 41.10 Drug Interactions: Acarbose

Drugs That Decrease the Effects of Acarbose
- Corticosteroids (systemic and inhaled)
  Result in hyperglycemia
- Luteinizing hormone, somatotropin, and thiazide diuretics
  Increase risk of hyperglycemia

Drugs That Increase the Effects of Acarbose
- Corticosteroids (inhaled)
  May suppress the hypothalamic–pituitary–adrenal axis, leading to adrenal crisis, leading to hypoglycemia
- Pegvisomant
  Increased risk of hypoglycemia

Assessing for Therapeutic Effects

After acarbose administration, the increase in blood glucose levels after a meal is smaller. The nurse assesses the patient's response to the medication by checking for diminished blood glucose levels without signs and symptoms of hypoglycemia.

Assessing for Adverse Effects

The nurse assesses for GI effects such as diarrhea, abdominal pain, and flatulence. The nurse also assesses the complete blood (cell) count for leukopenia, thrombocytopenia, and anemia.

Patient Teaching

Box 41.6 presents general patient teaching guidelines for the antidiabetic drugs. Box 41.9 presents patient teaching guidelines for the oral antidiabetic drugs.

Other Drugs in the Class

Miglitol has the same action, use, adverse effects, and contraindications as acarbose.

THIAZOLIDINEDIONES

Thiazolidinediones are sometimes called "glitazones" and are also referred to as insulin sensitizers. These drugs decrease insulin resistance, a major factor in the pathophysiology of type 2 diabetes. **Rosiglitazone maleate** (Avandia) is the prototype for the thiazolidinediones (Table 41.7). At the present time, it is rarely prescribed due to the risk of heart failure and atherosclerotic cardiovascular events. The same is true of pioglitazone. In some cases, pioglitazone may be administered as a second- or third-line therapy when other oral agent combination is not providing adequate glycemic control.

MEGLITINIDES

Meglitinides are nonsulfonylureas that lower blood sugar by stimulating pancreatic secretion of insulin. **Repaglinide** is the prototype meglitinide drug. The ability of repaglinide to work effectively depends on the existence of functioning beta cells left in the pancreas. Administration in combination with metformin or insulin results in a greater reduction in a patient's hemoglobin A1C than when either medication is administered alone.

Pharmacokinetics

Absorption of repaglinide from the GI tract is good, and peak plasma level occurs within 1 hour. The drug has a plasma half-life of 1 to 1.5 hours and is highly bound (greater than 98%) to plasma proteins. Metabolism occurs in the liver. Excretion of metabolites is in urine and feces. Metabolism and removal of repaglinide from the bloodstream occurs within 3 to 4 hours after a dose. This decreases the workload of pancreatic beta cells (i.e., decreases duration of beta cell stimulation), allows serum insulin levels to return to normal before the next meal, and decreases risks of hypoglycemic episodes.

TABLE 41.7 DRUGS AT A GLANCE: Thiazolidinediones

Drug	Routes and Dosage Ranges	
	Adults	Children
Rosiglitazone (Avandia; Avandia)	4 mg as a single oral dose or divided into two doses; if adequate response not seen in 8–12 wk, may be increased to 8 mg PO daily	Not recommended
Pioglitazone (Actos; ACCEL Pioglitazone, ACH-Pioglitazone, ACT Pioglitazone, JAMP-Pioglitazone)	PO 15–30 mg once daily; maximum dosage 45 mg Combination therapy with sulfonylurea or metformin: 15–30 mg daily PO added to the established dose of the other agent; if hypoglycemia occurs, reduce the dose of the other agent Combination therapy with insulin: decrease insulin does by 10%–25%; individualize based on glycemic response	Safety and efficacy not established

Action

Repaglinide works by closing potassium channels in pancreatic beta cells, which causes calcium channels to open and release insulin. The ability to lower blood glucose is dependent on the amount of functioning beta cells in the pancreas.

Use

Repaglinide can be used as monotherapy with diet and exercise or in combination with metformin or thiazolidinediones. Dosage is flexible, depending on food intake, but patients should eat within a few minutes after taking a dose to avoid hypoglycemia. Table 41.8 presents dosage information for the meglitinides, including repaglinide.

Patient-related variables specific to the use of meglitinides include the following:

- Reproduction, pregnancy, and lactation:
  - Repaglinide and nateglinide are not recommended with pregnancy or lactation.
- Abnormal kidney function and hepatic impairment:
- Assess kidney function before initiating therapy.
  - Decrease the initial dosage for patients with kidney disease.
  - Make incremental dosage changes very slowly in both abnormal kidney function and hepatic impairment, as higher serum drug levels are noted for a longer period.

Adverse Effects

Hypoglycemia is the most common adverse effect of repaglinide. Other adverse effects are upper respiratory congestion and gastric upset.

Contraindications

Repaglinide is contraindicated in patients with hypersensitivity, type 1 diabetes, or DKA. It is contraindicated with the administration of gemfibrozil.

Nursing Implications

Preventing Interactions

The risk of severe hypoglycemia is associated with the use of repaglinide with gemfibrozil and itraconazole. Therefore, such drug combinations should be avoided (Box 41.11).

Administering the Medication

Patients should take repaglinide just before or up to 30 minutes before meals. If a meal is skipped, the drug dose should be skipped; if a meal is added, a drug dose should be added.

Assessing for Therapeutic Effects

The nurse assesses fasting, preprandial, and postprandial blood glucose for normal or near-normal levels. It is also important to assess for improvement in hemoglobin A1C levels.

Assessing for Adverse Effects

The nurse assesses for dizziness, weakness, and hunger. In addition, the nurse assesses for gastric upset and respiratory congestion.

Patient Teaching

Box 41.6 presents general patient teaching guidelines for the antidiabetic drugs. Box 41.9 presents patient teaching guidelines for the oral antidiabetic drugs, including repaglinide.

Other Drugs in the Class

Nateglinide is a nonsulfonylurea, known as a meglitinide analog, that blocks the ATP-dependent potassium channels to depolarize the membrane and facilitate calcium to reenter the calcium channels. The increase in intracellular calcium then stimulates the release of insulin from pancreatic beta cells. The drug is rapidly absorbed, reaching a peak of action in 1 hour. It is 98% protein bound to albumin and metabolized in the liver by hydroxylation. The drug then undergoes glucuronide conjugation by CYP2C9 and CYP3A4. When combined with metformin or insulin, repaglinide is more effective than nateglinide in lowering hemoglobin A1C.

TABLE 41.8 DRUGS AT A GLANCE: Meglitinides

Drug	Routes and Dosage Ranges	
	Adults	Children
P Repaglinide (✱ ACT Repaglinide, APO-Repaglinide, Auro-Repaglinide)	0.5–4 mg PO taken three or four times a day 15–30 min before meals; maximum dosage 16 mg/d PO; wait 1 wk before making dose adjustment Severe abnormal kidney function: starting dose 0.5 mg PO	Not recommended
Nateglinide	120 mg PO three times daily, 1–30 min before meals; omit dose if skipped a meal 60 mg PO three times per day may be tried if patient is near HbA1c goal	Safety and efficacy not established

> **BOX 41.11** **Drug Interactions: Repaglinide**
>
> **Drugs That Increase the Effects of Repaglinide**
> - Cimetidine, erythromycin, ketoconazole, and miconazole
>   *Increase serum concentrations of repaglinide, leading to hypoglycemia*
> - Corticosteroids (oral or inhaled)
>   *May suppress the hypothalamic–pituitary–adrenal axis, leading to adrenal crisis, leading to hypoglycemia*
> - Nonsteroidal anti-inflammatory drugs and other agents that are highly bound to plasma proteins
>   *May displace drug from binding sites, increasing blood levels*
> - Pegvisomant
>   *Increases the risk of hypoglycemia*
> - Sulfonamides
>   *May inhibit hepatic metabolism, increasing blood levels*
>
> **Drugs That Decrease the Effects of Repaglinide**
> - Adrenergics, corticosteroids, estrogens, niacin, oral contraceptives, and thiazide diuretics
>   *Increase the risk of hyperglycemia*
> - Corticosteroids (systemic and inhaled)
>   *Diminish the effect of acarbose, resulting in hyperglycemia*
> - Luteinizing hormone, somatotropin, and thiazide diuretics
>   *Increase the risk of hyperglycemia*
> - Carbamazepine and rifampin
>   *Induce drug-metabolizing enzymes in the liver, which leads to faster inactivation*

NCLEX Success

3. The nurse is assessing a patient who has just begun taking glyburide. Which of the following is a therapeutic outcome for this patient? (Select all that apply.)
   A. a glycosylated hemoglobin (hemoglobin A1C) of 10%
   B. a decrease in polyuria
   C. a decrease in polyphagia
   D. a fasting blood glucose of 108 mg/dL

4. A patient with type 2 diabetes is scheduled to have a cardiac catheterization in 1 week, and the nurse makes a preprocedure phone call. The nurse instructs the patient to stop taking which medication 2 days before the procedure?
   A. sitagliptin
   B. insulin
   C. glyburide
   D. metformin

DIPEPTIDYL PEPTIDASE 4 INHIBITORS

Glucagonlike peptide 1 (GLP-1) has been known for some time to have a hypoglycemic action via its ability to stimulate insulin secretion. Recent advances have overcome the problems associated with short half-life and inactivation of the incretin hormone. The DPP-4 enzyme inhibitor Ⓟ **sitagliptin** (Januvia) is a medication that solves these problems.

Pharmacokinetics

Sitagliptin is rapidly absorbed and distributed with 3% protein bound. The drug is metabolized minimally by CYP3A4 and CYP2C8, resulting in a 12-hour circulating half-life for GLP-1. The peak of action is 1 to 4 hours. Eighty-seven percent of the medication is excreted in the urine with 79% unchanged. Approximately 13% is excreted in the feces.

Action

Sitagliptin minimizes the rate of inactivation of the incretin hormones to increase hormone levels and prolong their activity. Incretin hormones stimulate insulin release in response to a meal to normalize glucose levels. This action increases and lengthens the release of insulin and decreases hepatic glucose production to promote glycemic control.

Use

Patients with type 2 diabetes mellitus take sitagliptin in addition to following an exercise and diet regimen. They may also take it in combination with metformin and/or thiazolidinediones. Table 41.9 presents dosage information for sitagliptin and other DPP-4 enzyme inhibitors.

Patient-related variables specific to the use of DPP 4 inhibitors include the following:

- Reproduction, pregnancy, and lactation:
  - Dipeptidyl peptidase 4 inhibitors are not recommended during pregnancy for patients with type 2 diabetes. Patients should use effective contraception during therapy.
  - Agents other than the DPP-4 inhibitors are recommended in pregnancy and lactation.
- Abnormal kidney function and hepatic impairment:
  - No dosage adjustments are recommended with DPP-4 inhibitors.
  - Patients with an elevated creatinine clearance require decreased dosages initially.
  - Dosage adjustments are also necessary in the early stage of chronic kidney disease.

Adverse Effects

Common adverse effects of sitagliptin are upper respiratory tract infection, stuffy or runny nose, sore throat, and headache.

Contraindications

Contraindications to sitagliptin use include type 1 diabetes mellitus, insulin use, or the common production of ketones in the urine. Another contraindication is kidney failure with replacement therapy. Strict avoidance of other medications known to cause hypoglycemia, such as sulfonylureas, is warranted.

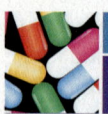

TABLE 41.9
DRUGS AT A GLANCE: Dipeptidyl Peptidase 4 (DPP-4) Inhibitors

Drug	Routes and Dosage Ranges	
	Adults	**Children**
ⓟ Sitagliptin (Januvia; ✦ Januvia)	100 mg/d PO as monotherapy or combined with metformin, pioglitazone, rosiglitazone, or other oral drugs Abnormal kidney function: creatinine clearance of 30–50 mL/min, 50 mg/d PO; creatinine clearance <30 mL/min, 25 mg/d PO	Not recommended
Alogliptin (Nesina; ✦ Nesina)	25 mg PO once daily	Not recommended
Linagliptin (Tradjenta; ✦ Tradjenta)	5 mg PO once daily	Safety and efficacy not established
Saxagliptin (Onglyza; ✦ Onglyza; APO-Saxagliptin; Sandoz Saxagliptin)	2.5–5 mg PO daily Limit dose to 2.5 mg when used with a strong CYP3A4/5 inhibitor or with abnormal kidney function	Safety and efficacy not established

The FDA has identified a risk of heart failure associated with DPP-4 inhibitors. This risk is more pronounced in patients with kidney and heart disease.

Nursing Implications

Administering the Medication

Patients should take sitagliptin once daily with or without food. If they forget to take a dose, they should take it as soon as possible. However, if a dose is skipped, patients should take only one dose per day.

Assessing for Therapeutic Effects

The nurse assesses fasting, preprandial, and postprandial blood glucose for normal or near-normal levels. It is also important to assess for improvement in hemoglobin A1C levels.

Assessing for Adverse Effects

The nurse assesses the patient for signs and symptoms of upper respiratory infection.

> **❗ Quality and Safety Alert: Safety**
> In 2015, the FDA issued a warning that the DPP-4 inhibitors may cause joint pain that can be severe or cause disability. Patients should be instructed not to stop the medication and consult with the prescriber.

Patient Teaching

Box 41.6 presents general patient teaching guidelines for the antidiabetic drugs. Box 41.12 gives some patient teaching guidelines for the newer antidiabetic drugs, including sitagliptin.

Other Drugs in the Class

Alogliptin (Nesina), linagliptin (Tradjenta), and saxagliptin (Onglyza) inhibit DPP-4 to prolong the incretin levels. The incretin hormones and glucose-dependent insulinotropic polypeptide regulate the glucose homeostasis. The synthesis of insulin increases, allowing the release of insulin from beta cells. In addition, glucagon secretion from the alpha cells decreases. This decrease also reduces production of hepatic glucose. It is important to note that alogliptin and saxagliptin have the potential to increase the risk of heart failure when administered to patients with heart or kidney disease.

 NCLEX Success

5. A patient with type 2 diabetes begins taking sitagliptin for the management of blood glucose levels. Which statement by the patient indicates an understanding of this medication?
   A. "I will take two doses in the morning if my blood sugar is high."
   B. "By taking this medication, I am able to eat more."
   C. "Now that I am taking this medication, I don't have to exercise anymore."
   D. "I will take this medicine once a day."

BOX 41.12 Patient Teaching Guidelines for the Newer Antidiabetic Drugs

- Use correct technique for injecting amylin analogs and incretin mimetics:
  - Inject pramlintide (Symlin) subcutaneously into the abdomen or thighs before meals. Do not mix in same syringe with insulin. Insulin dosages may be reduced by 50% when taking pramlintide.
  - Inject exenatide (Byetta) subcutaneously into the abdomen, thigh, or upper arm within 60 minutes before morning and evening meal.
  - Rotate the injection site of pramlintide and do not give in the same site where insulin is administered.

AMYLIN ANALOGS

Some people with type 1 or type 2 diabetes cannot achieve optimal glucose control with insulin therapy alone. **Pramlintide acetate** (SymlinPen 120, SymlinPen 60) is a drug used as an adjunctive treatment with mealtime insulin that is important in the regulation of glucose control during the postprandial period. A synthetic analog of amylin, pramlintide is a peptide hormone secreted with insulin by the beta cells of the pancreas.

Pharmacokinetics

Pramlintide has a rapid onset of action, reaching its peak in 20 minutes, with a 3-hour duration of action. Sixty percent of the drug is protein bound. It is metabolized primarily in the kidney system and excreted in the urine.

Action

Pramlintide slows gastric emptying, which helps regulate the postprandial rise in blood glucose. The drug also suppresses postprandial glucagon secretion, thus helping to maintain better blood glucose control. It also increases the sense of satiety, possibly reducing food intake and promoting weight loss.

Use

Taken immediately before meals, pramlintide mimics the body's natural processes. Oral hypoglycemic drugs and insulin dosages are usually up to 50% lower as well, depending on the patient's response to the drug. Patients with type 2 disease may combine pramlintide and insulin therapy with metformin or sulfonylureas. Table 41.10 gives dosage information for pramlintide.

Patient-related variables specific to the use of amylin analogs include reproduction, pregnancy, and lactation. Pramlintide has a low potential to cross the placenta. It is not known if pramlintide is present in breast milk. The manufacturer states that the decision to breast-feed during therapy should consider the risk and benefit to the infant as well as the benefit to the patient.

Adverse Effects

Adverse effects include anorexia, nausea, vomiting, and headache. Nausea tends to decrease with time. Careful titration of the dosage to the therapeutic level may reduce it. A **BOXED WARNING** alerts nurses to the danger of severe insulin-induced hypoglycemia with pramlintide therapy, especially in type 1 diabetes.

Contraindications

The only contraindications to pramlintide are hypersensitivity and gastroparesis.

Nursing Implications

Preventing Interactions

Some drugs may increase the effects of pramlintide (Box 41.13). Pramlintide also can cause increased effects of gastric emptying if combined with anticholinergic drugs or drugs that slow gastric absorption of nutrients. It is essential to avoid pramlintide with such drugs.

Administering the Medication

Subcutaneous injection of pramlintide before meals is necessary. The patient should not use pramlintide if a meal is skipped or if a dose is forgotten. It is necessary to inject pramlintide into a site (thigh or abdomen) that is at least 2 inches away from the insulin site injection. Opened vials of pramlintide may be stored in a refrigerator or at room temperature for up to 28 days.

It is essential not to mix pramlintide in the same injection with mealtime insulin. Patients with type 2 diabetes should take oral hypoglycemic drugs at least 1 hour before or 2 hours after injecting pramlintide.

Assessing for Therapeutic Effects

The nurse assesses fasting, preprandial, and postprandial blood glucose for normal or near-normal levels. It is also important to assess for improvement in the hemoglobin A1C levels.

Assessing for Adverse Effects

The nurse assesses for signs and symptoms of hypoglycemia, the only serious adverse effect.

Patient Teaching

Box 41.6 presents general patient teaching guidelines for the antidiabetic drugs. Box 41.12 gives some patient teaching guidelines for the newer antidiabetic drugs, including pramlintide.

TABLE 41.10

DRUGS AT A GLANCE: Amylin Analog (Pramlintide)

Drug	Routes and Dosage Ranges	
	Adults	Children
Pramlintide (Symlin, Symlin Pen; SymlinPen 60, SymlinPen 120)	Type 2 diabetes: initially 60 mcg sub-Q injection immediately prior to major meals. Dose can be increased to 120 mcg if needed Type 1 diabetes: initially 15 mcg sub-Q injection immediately prior to major meals; titrate 15-mcg increments to maintenance dose of 30 or 60 mcg as tolerated	Not recommended

| BOX 41.13 | Drug Interactions: Pramlintide |

Drugs That Increase the Effects of Pramlintide
- Anticholinergics
  May further slow gastrointestinal motility and intestinal absorption of drug
- Alpha-glucosidase inhibitors
  Increase risk of hypoglycemia

GLUCAGONLIKE PEPTIDE 1 RECEPTOR AGONISTS (INCRETIN MIMETICS)

Before starting a patient with type 2 diabetes on insulin, the provider should consider a new option for treatment of diabetes. The glucagonlike peptide 1 receptor agonist is also known as the incretin mimetic ⓟ **exenatide** (Bydureon BCise, Byetta 10 MCG Pen, Byetta 5 MCG Pen), a synthetic GLP-1 analog; it is possible to improve glycemic control in patients with type 2 diabetes who are already taking an oral hypoglycemic medication but having difficulty in achieving glycemic control.

Pharmacokinetics

Exenatide has a rapid onset, and the peak effect occurs in 2 hours. The drug is metabolized minimally and has proteolytic degradation following glomerular filtration. It remains in the body for 8 to 10 hours, which means that dosages must be 6 hours apart. It has a 2.4-hour half-life and is excreted in the urine.

Action

Exenatide acts as a natural helper hormone by stimulating the pancreas to secrete the right amount of insulin based on the food that was just eaten. This helps reduce the problem of high blood glucose after meals. The drug also halts **gluconeogenesis** (formation of glucose from noncarbohydrate sources such as fats and amino acids) by the liver, keeping it from making too much glucose after a meal. Exenatide slows gastric emptying, which serves to reduce the sudden rise of blood glucose after a meal, and it also quickly stimulates a feeling of satiety when eating. This fosters a sense of fullness, which causes the patient to eat less and potentially lose weight.

Use

When oral medications, diet, and exercise together have not assisted in reaching the target hemoglobin A1C goal, prescribers may now order exenatide. The FDA has approved its use with oral medications such as sulfonylureas, metformin, and/or thiazolidinediones. Major advantages of exenatide over insulin are increased satiety and weight loss. Exenatide is also now being used as monotherapy in combination with diet and exercise for newly diagnosed adults with type 2 diabetes. Table 41.11 provides route and dosage information for exenatide and other incretin mimetics.

Patient-related variables specific to the use of glucagonlike peptide 1 receptor agonists (incretin mimetics) include the following:

- Age:
  - Children *>10 years* and adolescents with type 2 diabetes should be prescribed Bydureon BCise 2 mg subcutaneously once weekly, without regard to meals.
- Reproduction, pregnancy, and lactation:
  - Glucagonlike peptide 1 receptor agonists are not recommended for patients with type 2 diabetes who are planning to become pregnant.
  - Agents other than GLP-1 receptor agonists should be used to treat type 2 diabetes during pregnancy and with lactation.
- Abnormal kidney function and hepatic impairment:
  - No dosage adjustments are required with hepatic impairment.
  - In abnormal kidney function, refer to the manufacturer's recommendations for dosage adjustments. GLP-1 receptor agonists should not be administered to patients with kidney failure with replacement therapy.

Adverse Effects

Major adverse effects of exenatide are hypoglycemia, GI distress, and nausea. Many patients experience nausea at first, and healthcare providers should encourage them to continue the medication if at all possible because the nausea usually subsides and becomes a feeling of fullness. A rare but serious side effect is the development of acute pancreatitis.

Contraindications

Contraindications to exenatide include a known hypersensitivity to the drug. Patients with liver disease or elevated liver enzymes should not receive it with HMG-CoA reductase inhibitors. Lactation is also a contraindication.

The FDA has issued a **BOXED WARNING** ◆ for exenatide; C-cell thyroid cancer has developed in studies of animals that were given the drug. Patients should be monitored routinely for thyroid nodules, and the drug is contraindicated in patients with a family history of endocrine neoplasia syndrome type 2.

Nursing Implications

Preventing Interactions

Like pramlintide, exenatide may reduce the absorption of concurrently administered oral medications due to slow gastric emptying (see Box 41.13).

Administering the Medication

Patients administer exenatide subcutaneously twice a day within 60 minutes of the morning and evening meal (at least 6 or more hours apart). No dosage adjustment is necessary based on blood glucose levels or the amount of food a patient is able to consume. If patients forget a dose, they should not inject exenatide after a meal. Injection sites include the subcutaneous tissue of the upper arm or leg and the abdomen areas.

TABLE 41.11

DRUGS AT A GLANCE: Glucagon-Like Peptide-1 Receptor Agonist (Incretin Mimetics)

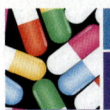

Drug	Routes and Dosage Ranges	
	Adults	**Children**
ⓟ **Exenatide** (Bydureon BCise, Byetta 10 MCG Pen, Byetta 5; 🍁 Bydureon, Byetta 10 MCG PEN, Byetta 5 MCG PEN)	5 mcg by subcutaneous injection within 60 min before morning and evening meals or two main meals of day ~6 h apart; may be increased to 10 mcg twice a day after 1 mo of therapy if needed	BCise: Subq: 2 mg once weekly without regard to meals
Dulaglutide (Trulicity; 🍁 Trulicity)	0.75 mg by subcutaneous injection once weekly; may increase to 1.5 mg once weekly if adequate glycemic response; maximum 1.5 mg once weekly	Not recommended for use in children
Liraglutide (Saxenda, Victoza; 🍁 Saxenda, Victoza)	Initially 0.6 mg sub-Q once daily for 1 wk; then increase dose to 1.2–1.8 mg once daily to achieve glycemic control	>10 years old and adolescents: 0.6 mg subcutaneous once daily for at least 1 wk; may increase by 0.6 mg/d increments at weekly intervals to achieve glycemic control. Maximum daily dose: 1.8 mg/d
Lixisenatide (Adlyxin, Adlyxin Starter Pack; 🍁 Adlyxin)	10 mcg subcutaneous once daily for 14 d; on day 15, increase to 20 mcg once daily; maintenance dose: 20 mcg once daily	Not recommended for use in children
Semaglutide (Ozempic; 🍁 Ozempic) Semaglutide (Rybelsus 🍁Rybelsus)	0.25 mg subcutaneous once weekly for 4 wk then increase to 0.5 mg once weekly for at least 4 wk. Maximum dose is 1 mg once weekly Missed doses should be administered as soon as possible within 5 d. If >5 d has lapsed, skip the missed dose, and resume the next scheduled day PO 3, 7, 14 mg on an empty stomach >30 min before the first food, beverage of the day with <4 *ounces* of plain water only	Not recommended for use in children

It is essential that exenatide be stored at all times in the original packaging in a refrigerator at 36°F to 46°F, protected from light, kept dry, and discarded once opened after 30 days.

Assessing for Therapeutic Effects

The nurse assesses fasting, preprandial, and postprandial blood glucose for normal or near-normal levels. It is also important to assess for improvement in hemoglobin A1C levels.

Assessing for Adverse Effects

It is important that patients and their caregivers recognize the signs and symptoms of hypoglycemia, a possible adverse effect of exenatide, and be prepared to treat hypoglycemia with fast-acting sugar or glucagon. If patients are unable to eat or plan to skip a meal, they should not take the drug. Patients taking exenatide should report any unusual abdominal discomfort to their healthcare providers because acute pancreatitis is a possible adverse effect of the medication.

Patient Teaching

Box 41.6 presents general patient teaching guidelines for the antidiabetic drugs. Box 41.12 gives some patient teaching guidelines for the newer antidiabetic drugs.

Other Drugs in the Class

Dulaglutide (Trulicity) is injected subcutaneously. They are agonists of human GLP-1 receptor to enhance glucose-dependent insulin secretion and slow gastric emptying. As with exenatide, all drugs in the class possess a **BOXED WARNING** ◆; C-cell thyroid cancer has developed in studies of animals that were given the drug. Routine monitoring for thyroid nodules is warranted, and a family history of endocrine neoplasia syndrome type 2 is a contraindication. Dulaglutide has an increased risk for the development of pancreatitis. Instruct the patient to notify the prescriber of persistent severe abdominal pain.

Liraglutide is administered subcutaneously. Liraglutide is used in children aged 12 years and older for weight management. It is also used in children aged 10 years and older for treatment of type 2 diabetes.

Lixisenatide is administered as a stand-alone therapy or in combination with insulin or other oral agents. It is contraindicated in patients who have an increased serum or urinary ketone level.

Semaglutide is administered orally or subcutaneously. The oral form is Rybelsus. The subcutaneous form is Ozempic.

Semaglutide should be discontinued at least 2 months prior to a planned pregnancy; adverse events with congenital anomalies were noted in animal reproduction studies.

> **! Quality and Safety Alert: Patient Safety**
>
> In March 2021, the FDA identified the following medications as having the potential to produce the serious side effect of drug-induced liver injury: lixisenatide, exenatide, semaglutide, liraglutide, and dulaglutide, and the drug combinations insulin glargine and lixisenatide, as well as insulin degludec and liraglutide. It is imperative that the AST and ALT liver enzyme levels be monitored.

SODIUM–GLUCOSE COTRANSPORTER 2 (SGLT2) INHIBITORS

In 2013, the FDA approved the first the sodium–glucose cotransporter 2 (SGLT2) inhibitors. The prototype of this class is **canagliflozin** (Invokana). The drug inhibits kidney SGLT2, thus blocking reabsorption of glucose in the kidney. In addition, it promotes the excretion of excess glucose in the urine. All the SGLT2 inhibitors provide kidney protection by decreasing the protein loss and reducing the damage caused by hyperfiltration.

Pharmacokinetics

Canagliflozin is 99% bound to albumin. The peak of action is 1 to 2 hours. For a 100-mg dose, the half-life of the drug is 10.6 hours, and for a 300-mg dose, it is 13.1 hours. The drug is metabolized by glucuronidation. The elimination of the drug is 30% in the urine and 52% in the feces.

Action

The proximal kidney tubule is the site where the majority of filtered glucose is reabsorbed, and in this tubule, canagliflozin inhibits SGLT2. This action provides the patient with type 2 diabetes greater excretion of glucose by the kidney.

Use

Prescribers order canagliflozin in combination with other antidiabetic agents to promote improvement in glycemic control in patients with type 2 diabetes. Table 41.12 gives route and dosage information for canagliflozin and other SGLT2 inhibitors.

Patient-related variables specific to the use of sodium–glucose cotransporter 2 (SGLT2) inhibitors include the following:

- Age:
  - Patients aged 65 years and older may have an increased risk of hypotension, dizziness, syncope, and dehydration. Also, hemoglobin A1C reductions are less than in younger patients.
- Reproduction, pregnancy, and lactation:
  - SGLT2 inhibitors are not recommended for patients with type 2 diabetes who are planning to become pregnant.
  - SGLT2 inhibitors are not recommended during pregnancy or lactation.
- Abnormal kidney function and hepatic impairment:
  - Patients with severe hepatic impairment should not take canagliflozin.
  - In patients with an estimated glomerular filtration rate of 45 to 59 mL/min, the dosage of canagliflozin should not exceed 100 mg daily. It is not recommended that patients with an estimated glomerular filtration rate less than 45 mL/min take canagliflozin.

Adverse Effects

The loss of body fluids leads to dehydration, hypotension, syncope, and dehydration. The metabolic adverse effects include increased low-density lipoprotein, hyperphosphatemia, hyperkalemia, hypermagnesemia, and increased creatinine. Because of increases in urine glucose, patients are prone to genital mycotic infections. Approximately 12% of females develop vulvovaginal candidiasis. Four percent of males develop inflammation of the glans penis; this includes balanitis/balanoposthitis, balanitis candida, and fungal genital infection. A rare adverse effect of canagliflozin is necrotizing fasciitis of the perineum. The administration of potassium-sparing diuretics with SGLT2 inhibitors causes hyperkalemia.

In addition, in June 2016, the FDA identified the risk of acute kidney injury with canagliflozin. Health Canada found evidence of a link between bone-related adverse effects, including demineralization of the bone and risk of bone fractures. In May 2017, an FDA alert was issued. There is a twofold increased risk of lower limb amputations in patients taking canagliflozin.

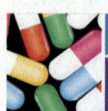

TABLE 41.12

DRUGS AT A GLANCE: Sodium–Glucose Cotransporter 2 (SGLT2) Inhibitors

Drug	Routes and Dosage Ranges	
	Adults	**Children**
Canagliflozin (Invokana; 🍁 Invokana)	PO 100 mg once daily prior to the first meal of the day; may increase to 300 mg once daily to patients with eGFR > 60 mL/m²	Not recommended for use in children
Dapagliflozin (Farxiga; 🍁 Farxiga)	PO 5 mg once daily; may increase to 10 mg daily	Not recommended for use in children
Empagliflozin (Jardiance; 🍁 Jardiance)	PO 10 mg once daily; may increase to 25 mg once daily	Not recommended for use in children

Contraindications

Severe abnormal kidney function and hypersensitivity reactions contraindicate the administration of canagliflozin.

Nursing Implications

Preventing Interactions

SGLT2 inhibitors combined with angiotensin-converting enzyme (ACE) inhibitors, angiotensin II receptor blockers (ARBs), and loop diuretics that have hypotensive effects will lead to symptoms of syncope, hypotension, and hyperkalemia. In addition, hyperkalemia will result with potassium-sparing diuretics. St. John's wort will decrease the serum concentration of the SGLT2 inhibitors, leading to hyperglycemia. Certain drugs may interact with canagliflozin (Box 41.14).

Administering the Drug

Prior to administering SGLT2 inhibitors, patients should be well hydrated. The initial dose should be low. Patients should take the drugs with the first meal of the day. Box 41.15 gives patient teaching guidelines for canagliflozin and the other SGLT2 inhibitors.

Assessing for Therapeutic Effects

The nurse assesses fasting, preprandial, and postprandial blood glucose for normal or near-normal levels. It is also important to assess for improvement in hemoglobin A1C levels.

Assessing for Adverse Effects

It is imperative to assess the patient's hydration level and blood pressure for signs and symptoms of syncope and hypotension. The nurse should assess the potassium level and alert the prescriber of hyperkalemia. In the event of hyperkalemia, it is important to check the patient's cardiac rhythm for dysrhythmia.

Other Drugs in the Class

Following the development of canagliflozin, dapagliflozin (Farxiga) and empagliflozin (Jardiance) became available. These two drugs have the same action, use, adverse effects, and contraindications as canagliflozin.

BOX 41.14 Drug Interactions: Canagliflozin

Drugs That Increase the Effects of Canagliflozin
- Alpha-lipoic acid, androgens, insulin, or antidiabetic agents (oral or subcutaneous, monoamine oxidase inhibitors, pegvisomant, quinolone antibiotics, salicylates, selective serotonin reuptake inhibitors)
  Increase hypoglycemic effects

Drugs That Decrease the Effects of Canagliflozin
- Carbamazepine, efavirenz, fosphenytoin, phenobarbital, phenytoin, primidone, and ritonavir
  Decreases the serum concentration of canagliflozin

BOX 41.15 Patient Teaching Guidelines for the Sodium–Glucose Cotransporter 2 (SGLT2) Inhibitors

- Administer without regard to food with the first meal of the day.
- For patients with stable glycemic control, hemoglobin A1C should be monitored every 6 months.
- Maintain adequate hydration of 2,000 to 3,000 mL/d.
- Instruct on hypotension and syncope.
- Do not consume salt substitutes.

COMBINATION DRUG THERAPY FOR TYPE 2 DIABETES

Combination drug therapy is an increasing trend in type 2 diabetes that is not controlled by diet, exercise, and single-drug therapy. Useful combinations include drugs with different mechanisms of action, and several rational combinations are currently available. Most studies have involved combinations of two drugs; some three-drug combinations are also being used. All combination therapy should be monitored with periodic measurements of fasting plasma glucose and glycosylated hemoglobin levels. If adequate glycemic control is not achieved, oral drugs may need to be discontinued and insulin therapy started. A list of some two-drug combinations are as follows:

- **Insulin plus a sulfonylurea.** Advantages include lower fasting blood glucose levels, decreased glycosylated hemoglobin levels, increased secretion of endogenous insulin, smaller daily doses of insulin, and no significant change in body weight. The role of insulin analogs in combination therapy is not clear. One regimen, called BIDS, uses bedtime insulin, usually NPH, with a daytime sulfonylurea, usually glyburide.
- **Insulin plus a glitazone.** Thiazolidinediones increase the effectiveness of insulin, whether endogenous or exogenous.
- **Sulfonylurea plus acarbose or miglitol.** This combination is approved by the FDA for patients who do not achieve adequate glycemic control with one of the drugs alone.
- **Sulfonylurea plus metformin.** Glimepiride is approved by the FDA for this combination.
- **Sulfonylurea plus a thiazolidinedione.** The sulfonylurea increases insulin, and the thiazolidinedione increases insulin effectiveness.
- **Metformin plus a meglitinide.** If one of the drugs alone does not produce adequate glycemic control, the other one may be added. Dosage of each drug should be titrated to the minimal dose required to achieve the desired effects.
- **Metformin plus a thiazolidinedione.** If metformin alone does not produce adequate glycemic control, a thiazolidinedione may be added. Pioglitazone is approved by the FDA for this combination.
- **Metformin or thiazolidinedione plus sitagliptin.** Sitagliptin may be added as adjunctive therapy with metformin or a thiazolidinedione to achieve desired glycemic control.
- **Metformin or sulfonylurea plus exenatide.** Exenatide may be added as adjunctive therapy with metformin or a sulfonylurea to achieve desired glycemic control.

- **Mealtime insulin plus metformin, thiazolidinedione, and/or sulfonylurea plus pramlintide.** Pramlintide may be given with mealtime insulin in people with type 2 diabetes to achieve better postprandial glucose control.
- **Dapagliflozin and saxagliptin (Qtern).** This drug combination is an adjunct to diet and exercise to improve glycemic control in patient with type 2 diabetes. It is designed to treat increase glucose levels for patients not controlled on dapagliflozin alone or currently taking dapagliflozin and saxagliptin.
- **Dapagliflozin, saxagliptin, and metformin (Qternmet XR).** The administration of this combination is intended for patients who are already taking metformin. If the patient has not been taking dapagliflozin, then the therapy is started with dapagliflozin 5 mg, saxagliptin 5 mg, and metformin 1 g daily.

ADJUVANT MEDICATIONS USED TO TREAT DIABETES

For most patients, the goals of treatment are to maintain blood glucose at normal or near-normal levels; promote normal metabolism of carbohydrate, fat, and protein; prevent acute and long-term complications; and prevent hypoglycemic episodes. There is strong evidence that strict control of blood sugar delays the onset and slows progression of complications of diabetes. In addition to glycemic control, other measures can be used to help prevent complications of diabetes. Table 41.13 summarizes these adjuvant medications.

Angiotensin-Converting Enzyme Inhibitors

The prototype ACE inhibitor is ⓟ **enalapril maleate** (Vasotec). Enalapril maleate blocks the conversion of angiotensin I to angiotensin II, thereby decreasing blood pressure. Enalapril maleate has protective effects on the kidneys in both type 1 and type 2 diabetes and in both normotensive and hypertensive people. Although ACE inhibitors are also used in the treatment of hypertension, their ability to delay nephropathy seems to be independent of antihypertensive effects. Additional measures to preserve kidney function include effective treatment of hypertension, limited intake of dietary protein, prompt treatment of urinary tract infections, and avoidance of nephrotoxic drugs when possible. Serum potassium levels and creatinine levels should be monitored.

Angiotensin II Receptor Blockers

ⓟ **Losartan** (Cozaar) is the prototype ARB. In kidney studies of patients with diabetes and nephropathy, losartan reduced the incidence of kidney failure with replacement therapy in 28% of the patients. ARBs do not prevent nephropathy but reduce the rate of progression. Serum potassium levels and creatinine levels should be monitored.

Thiazidelike Diuretics

ⓟ **Hydrochlorothiazide** (HCTZ) is the prototype thiazide-like diuretics. Thiazidelike diuretics have been shown to reduce

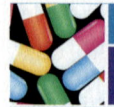

TABLE 41.13
DRUGS AT A GLANCE: Adjuvant Drugs for the Treatment of Diabetes Mellitus

Drug	Routes and Dosage Ranges	
	Adults	**Children**
ⓟ **Enalapril maleate** (Epaned, Vasotec; ✤ ACT Epaned, APO Epaned, JAMP Epaned, NOVO Vasotec)	2.5 mg PO daily or twice daily; maintenance daily dosage is 2.5–20 mg daily Abnormal kidney function: use smaller initial dose, and adjust upward to a maximum of 40 mg/d PO	1 mo to 16 y: initial dose 0.08 mg/kg PO once daily Maximum dose: 5 mg
ⓟ **Losartan** (Cozaar; ✤ ACT Losartan, AG-Losartan, SANDOZ Losartan, TEVA Losartan)	50 mg PO once daily; can be increased to 100 mg once daily based on blood pressure response Diabetic nephropathy: 50 mg PO once daily; can be increased to 100 mg once daily based on blood pressure response	≥6 y to ≤16 y: 0.7 mg/kg once daily Maximum initial dose: 50 mg/d
ⓟ **Hydrochlorothiazide** (✤ APO Hydro, BIO Hydrochlorothiazide)	25 mg/d in morning; may not need more than 50 mg with other ACES and ARBS	2–12 y: 1–2 mg/kg/d (0.5–1 mg/lb) orally daily as a single dose or in 2 divided doses Maximum dose: 100 mg/d
ⓟ **Acetylsalicylic acid (ASA)** (Aspirin; ✤ Novasen, Asaphen)	75–162 mg/d	Not recommended
ⓟ **Simvastatin** (Zocor, Zocor, FloLipid; ✤ ACT Simvastatin, AG Simvastatin, Auro Simvastatin)	20–40 mg PO once daily in the evening Abnormal kidney function: starting dose 5 mg/d PO and increase slowly	10–17 y: 10 mg/d PO in evening

cardiovascular events in diabetes. Serum potassium levels and creatinine levels should be monitored.

Antiplatelet Agent

Aspirin therapy is considered a primary prevention strategy in patients with diabetes who are at increased cardiovascular risk.

HMG-CoA Reductase Inhibitors

The prototype HMG-CoA reductase inhibitor is **simvastatin** (Zocor). Simvastatin inhibits HMG-CoA reductase, the enzyme that catalyzes the first step in cholesterol synthesis, which ultimately reduces serum cholesterol. Current research suggests that a number of treatment strategies may be beneficial in reducing the cardiovascular disease risk associated with type 2 diabetes mellitus. Some clinicians are recommending the routine use of statins such as simvastatin to reduce the risk of occlusive arterial disease in all patients with diabetes, regardless of cholesterol level.

Clinical Application 41.3

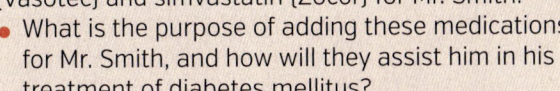

In addition to the addition of insulin to Mr. Smith's medication regimen, the physician also prescribes enalapril maleate (Vasotec) and simvastatin (Zocor) for Mr. Smith.
- What is the purpose of adding these medications for Mr. Smith, and how will they assist him in his treatment of diabetes mellitus?

Clinical Application 41.4

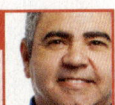

The goal of care for Mr. Smith is to increase his ability to achieve good glycemic control and prevent complications related to diabetes mellitus.
- In addition to his primary physician, what other types of healthcare providers should be involved in his care to allow him to achieve this goal?
- What additional teaching could the nurse provide to Mr. Smith to help prevent physical and emotional complications?

THE NURSING PROCESS

A concept map outlines the nursing process related to drug therapy considerations in this chapter. Additional nursing implications related to the disease process should also be considered in care decisions.

Assessment

- Assess the patient's history, including age at onset of diabetes, prescribed control measures and their effectiveness, the ease or difficulty of adhering to the prescribed treatment, occurrence of complications such as ketoacidosis, and whether other disease processes have interfered with diabetes control.
- Assess the patient's:
  - **Diet.** Ask about the prescribed nutritional plan and use of herbal or dietary.
  - **Activity.** Ask the patient to describe usual activities of daily living, and exercise.
  - **Medication.** Assess the type or insulin or anti-diabetic agent. Assess hypoglycemic reactions due to the medication administered.
  - **Monitoring methods.** Testing the blood for glucose and the urine for ketones (e.g., when blood sugar is elevated, when ill and unable to eat) are the two main methods of self-monitoring glycemic control.
  - **Skin and mucous membranes.** Inspect for signs of infection and other lesions. Women with diabetes are susceptible to monilial vaginitis and infections under the breasts. Check the sites of insulin injection for atrophy (dimpling or indentation), hypertrophy (nodules or lumps), and fibrosis (hardened areas). Inspect the feet for calluses, ulcers, and signs of infection. Check pedal pulses, color, and temperature in both feet to evaluate arterial blood flow.
  - **Eyes.** Ask about difficulties with vision and if eyes are examined regularly. Cardiovascular system. Assess blood pressure and ask about chest pain and pain in the legs with exercise (intermittent claudication).
  - **Genitourinary system.** Assess for signs of urinary tract infection, polyuria, and impotence in men.
  - **Blood glucose levels.** Assess blood sugar reports for abnormal levels. Two or more fasting blood glucose levels greater than 126 mg/dL or two random levels greater than 200 mg/dL are diagnostic of diabetes. Decreased blood sugar levels are especially dangerous at 40 mg/dL or below.
  - **Glycosylated hemoglobin level.** Assess the glycosylated hemoglobin (also called glycated hemoglobin and HbA1c) level when available.

Outcomes of Therapy

The patient will
- Learn self-care activities.
- Manage drug therapy to prevent or minimize hypoglycemia and other adverse effects.
- Develop a consistent pattern of diet and exercise.
- Use available resources to learn about the disease process and how to manage it.
- Take diabetes medications accurately.
- Self-monitor blood glucose and urine ketones appropriately.
- Keep appointments for follow-up and monitoring procedures by a healthcare provider.

Nursing Interventions

- Instruct the patient and family about diet, exercise, and the use of insulin or antidiabetic agents.
- Self-monitoring of blood glucose levels allows the patients to see the effects of diet, exercise, and hypoglycemic medications on blood glucose levels and may promote compliance.
- Test urine for ketones when the patient is sick, when blood glucose levels are greater than 200 mg/dL, and when episodes of nocturnal hypoglycemia are suspected. Instruct patients and family to test urine when indicated.
- Promote early recognition and treatment of problems by observing for signs and symptoms of urinary tract infection, peripheral vascular disease, vision changes, ketoacidosis, hypoglycemia, and others.
- Discuss the importance of regular visits to healthcare facilities for blood sugar measurements, weights, blood pressure measurements, and eye examinations.
- Perform and teach correct foot care. Also, teach the patient to report any lesions on the feet to the physician.
- Provide appropriate patient teaching for any drug therapy and combination drug therapy for patients with type 2 diabetes mellitus (Boxes 41.6, 41.7, 41.9, 41.12 and 41.15).

Evaluation

- Check blood sugar reports regularly for normal or abnormal values.
- Check glycosylated hemoglobin reports when available.
- Interview and observe for therapeutic and adverse responses to diabetic drugs.
- Interview and observe for compliance with prescribed treatment.
- Interview patients and family members about the frequency and length of hospitalizations for diabetes mellitus.

Visit thePoint® at http://thePoint.lww.com/Frandsen13e for answers to NCLEX Success questions (in Appendix A), answers to Clinical Application Case Studies (in Appendix B), additional information about pathophysiology and etiology, and more!

REFERENCES AND RESOURCES

American Diabetes Association. (2022a). *eAG/A1C conversion calculator*. Retrieved March 19, 2022, from https://eAG/A1C Conversion Calculator | American Diabetes Association

American Diabetes Association. (2022b). *Understanding A1C: Diagnosis*. Retrieved February 3, 2022, from https://www.diabetes.org/a1c/diagnosis

Centers for Disease Control. (2019). *Prevalence of Diagnosed Diabetes*. Retrieved February 4, 2022, from https://www.cdc.gov/diabetes/data/statistics-report/diagnosed-diabetes.html

Hinkle, J. L., Cheever, K. H., & Overbaugh, K. (2022). *Brunner & Suddarth's textbook of medical-surgical nursing* (15th ed.). Wolters Kluwer.

Inzucchi, S. E., & Lupsa, B. (2022). Thiazolidinediones in the treatment of type 2 diabetes mellitus). *UpToDate*. Lexi-Comp, Inc.

Jonas, D. E., Crotty, K., Yun, J., Middleton, J. C., Feltner, C., Taylor-Phillips, S., Barclay, C., Dotson, A., Baker, C., Balio, C. P., Voisin, C. E., & Harris, R. (2021). Screening for prediabetes and type 2 diabetes updated evidence report and systematic review for the US Preventive Services Task Force. *Journal of the American Medical Association*, 326(8), 744–760.

Laffel, L., & Svoren, B. (2022). Epidemiology, presentation, and diagnosis of type 2 diabetes mellitus in children and adolescents. *UpToDate*. Lexi-Comp, Inc.

Levitsky, L., & Misra, M. (2022). Management of type 1 diabetes mellitus in children and adolescents. *UpToDate*. Lexi-Comp, Inc.

Lippincott Advisor. (2022). *Drug information*. Wolters Kluwer Inc.

McIver, L. A., & Tripp, J. (2021). Acarbose. In *Stat Pearls*. Retrieved March 17, 2022, https://www.ncbi.nlm.nih.gov/books/NBK493214/

Norris, T. L. (2019). *Porth's Pathophysiology: Concepts of altered health states* (10th ed.). Wolters Kluwer.

UpToDate. (2022). *Drug Information*. Lexi-Comp, Inc.

U.S. Food and Drug Administration. (2015). *FDA drug safety communication: FDA warns that DPP-4 inhibitors for type 2 diabetes may cause severe joint pain*. Retrieved March 19, 2022, from https://www.fda.gov/drugs/drug-safety-and-availability/fda-drug-safety-communication-fda-warns-dpp-4-inhibitors-type-2-diabetes-may-cause-severe-joint-pain

U.S. Food and Drug Administration. (2021). *January-March 2021 Potential signals of serious risk/new safety information identified by the FDA Adverse Event Reporting System*. Retrieved March, from 19, 2022 https://www.fda.gov/drugs/questions-and-answers-fdas-adverse-event-reporting-system-faers/january-march-2021-potential-signals-serious-risksnew-safety-information-identified-fda-adverse

Wexler, D. J. (2022). Overview of general medical care in nonpregnant adults with diabetes mellitus). *UpToDate*. Lexi-Comp, Inc.

CHAPTER 42

Drug Therapy for Hyperthyroidism and Hypothyroidism

LEARNING OBJECTIVES

After studying this chapter, you should be able to:

1. Understand the physiologic effects of thyroid hormone.
2. Describe the clinical considerations and manifestations of hyperthyroidism.
3. Describe the clinical considerations and manifestations of hypothyroidism.
4. Identify the prototype and describe the action, use, adverse effects, contraindications, and nursing implications of the drugs administered for the treatment of hyperthyroidism.
5. Identify the prototype and describe the action, use, adverse effects, contraindications, and nursing implications of the drugs administered for the treatment of hypothyroidism.
6. Understand the use of immunosuppressive drug therapy for the treatment of thyroid eye disease.
7. Implement the nursing process in the care of patients receiving medications for the treatment of hyperthyroidism or hypothyroidism.

CLINICAL APPLICATION CASE STUDY

Brenda Zalewski, a 45-year-old woman, had a goiter as a child and a thyroidectomy at age 12. She has been taking a synthetic thyroid preparation since that time. Ms. Zalewski takes a maintenance dose of levothyroxine (Synthroid) 0.1 mg orally daily. She is 5 ft 8 in tall and weighs 215 lb.

KEY TERMS

Euthyroid: normal thyroid gland function

Goiter: enlarged thyroid gland

Graves disease: an autoimmune disorder in which thyrotropin receptor antibodies stimulate the thyroid-stimulating hormone (TSH) receptors, increasing thyroid hormone production and release.

Hyperthyroidism: excessive synthesis and secretion of thyroid hormone; usually involves an enlarged thyroid gland known as a goiter

Hypothyroidism: diminished secretion of thyroid hormone

Myxedema: hypothyroidism that occurs after early childhood may be caused when inflammatory disease of the thyroid or another acquired defect destroys parts of the gland

Myxedema coma: severe, life-threatening hypothyroidism

Primary hypothyroidism: occurs when disease or destruction of thyroid gland tissue causes inadequate production of thyroid hormones

Thyroid storm: rare but severe complication characterized by extreme symptoms of hyperthyroidism; most likely to occur in patients with hyperthyroidism that has been inadequately treated, especially when stressful situations occur; also known as thyrotoxic crisis

Thyroiditis: an autoimmune disorder characterized by inflammation of the thyroid gland

INTRODUCTION

This chapter introduces the pharmacologic care of the patient experiencing increased or decreased function of the thyroid gland. To fully appreciate the management of hyperthyroidism and hypothyroidism, the two types of thyroid disorders requiring drug therapy, it is necessary to understand the characteristics, clinical manifestations, and pathophysiology of the thyroid gland.

OVERVIEW OF THE THYROID GLAND

Physiology

Normal serum levels of thyroid hormones and a **euthyroid** physiologic state (normal thyroid gland function) require a functioning thyroid gland and feedback mechanism. The thyroid gland produces three hormones: thyroxine, triiodothyronine, and calcitonin. Thyroxine (also called T_4) contains four atoms of iodine, and triiodothyronine (also called T_3) contains three atoms of iodine. Chapter 44 discusses calcitonin functions in calcium metabolism.

Production of T_3 and T_4 depends on the presence of iodine and tyrosine in the thyroid gland. In a series of chemical reactions, iodine atoms become attached to tyrosine, an amino acid derived from dietary protein, to form the thyroid hormones T_3 and T_4. After they are formed, the hormones are stored within the chemically inactive thyroglobulin molecule. Tyrosine forms the basic structure of thyroglobulin. Thyroid hormones are released into the circulation when the thyroid gland is stimulated by thyroid-stimulating hormone (TSH or thyrotropin) from the anterior pituitary gland (Fig. 42.1) through a negative feedback mechanism. The hormones become largely bound to plasma proteins, with only the small unbound ones remaining biologically active. T_3, the most active thyroid hormone, mediates the cellular actions of the other thyroid hormone. T_3 is more potent than T_4 and has a more rapid onset but a shorter duration of action. T_3 binds to two receptors that regulate the expression of many genes. The bound thyroid hormones are released to tissue cells very slowly. In tissue cells, the hormones combine with intracellular proteins so they are again stored. They are released slowly within the cell, and as they are used over days or weeks, they release iodine atoms. Most of the iodine is reabsorbed and used to produce new thyroid hormones; the remainder is excreted in the urine.

Thyroid hormones profoundly affect major physiologic processes, such as metabolism, growth, and development. By controlling the rate of cellular metabolism, these hormones influence the functioning of virtually every cell in the body. The heart, skeletal muscle, liver, and kidneys are especially responsive to the hormones' stimulating effects. The brain, spleen, and gonads are less responsive. Normal levels of thyroid hormones are essential for normal growth and development, especially fetal and neonatal brain and skeletal development

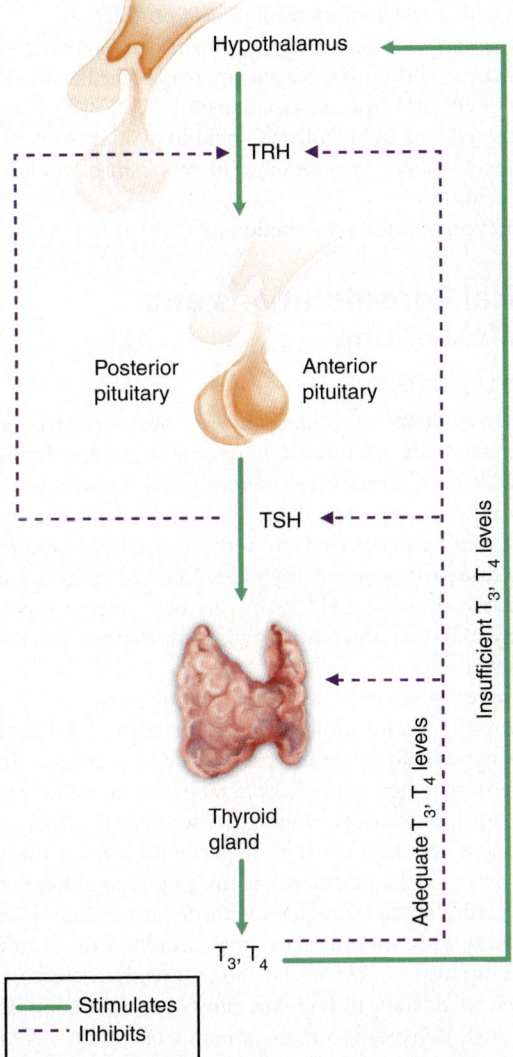

Figure 42.1. Thyroid-releasing hormone (TRH) from the hypothalamus stimulates the anterior pituitary to release thyroid-stimulating hormone (TSH). It also inhibits the hypothalamus from releasing TRH. TSH stimulates the thyroid gland to release T_3 and T_4. It also inhibits the hypothalamus from releasing TRH and the anterior pituitary from releasing more TSH. The release of T_3 and T_4 from the thyroid gland inhibits TRH release from the hypothalamus, TSH release from the pituitary, and further T_3 and T_4 release from the thyroid gland. Falling T_3 and T_4 levels stimulate the hypothalamus to release TRH, and the process repeatedly continues to maintain effective hormone levels. ACTH, adrenocorticotropic hormone; CRH, corticotropin-releasing hormone; FSH, follicle-stimulating hormone; GH, growth hormone; GHRH, growth hormone–releasing hormone; GnRH, gonadotropin-releasing hormone; LH, luteinizing hormone; PIF, prolactin-inhibiting factor; PRL, prolactin; PRF, prolactin-releasing factor; SRIF, somatotropin release–inhibiting factor.

and maturation. Thyroid hormone deficiency is not compatible with human health.

Thyroid hormones also influence linear growth; brain function, including intelligence and memory; neural development; dentition; and bone development. These hormones are thought to act mainly by controlling intracellular protein synthesis. Some specific physiologic effects include:

- Increased rate of cellular metabolism and oxygen consumption with a resultant increase in heat production
- Increased heart rate, force of contraction, systemic vascular resistance, and cardiac output (increased cardiac workload)
- Increased carbohydrate metabolism
- Increased fat metabolism, including increased lipolytic effects of other hormones and metabolism of cholesterol to bile acids
- Inhibition of pituitary secretion of TSH

Clinical Considerations and Manifestations

Hyperthyroidism

Hyperthyroidism is characterized by excessive synthesis and secretion of thyroid hormone(s) by the thyroid and usually involves an enlarged thyroid gland, known as a **goiter**. The enlarged thyroid gland has an increased number of cells. Endogenous hyperthyroidism most commonly results from Graves disease or nodular thyroid goiter. Other causes include thyroiditis, overtreatment with thyroid drugs, functioning thyroid carcinoma, and pituitary adenoma that secretes excessive amounts of TSH.

Graves disease is an autoimmune disorder in which thyrotropin receptor antibodies stimulate the TSH receptors, increasing thyroid hormone production and release. In nodular thyroid goiter, growth of established nodules and new nodule formation trigger the hyperthyroidism. Graves disease is the most common cause of hyperthyroidism in the United States; however, the prevalence of toxic nodular goiter increases in older adults and in regions with dietary iodine deficiency. The hyperplastic thyroid gland may secrete 5 to 15 times the normal amount of thyroid hormone, greatly increasing body metabolism. Specific physiologic effects vary (see Clinical Manifestations), depending on the amount of circulating thyroid hormone, and they usually increase in incidence and severity over time if hyperthyroidism is not treated.

Subclinical hyperthyroidism is defined as a reduced TSH (less than 0.1 microunit/L) and normal T_3 and T_4 levels. The most common cause is excess thyroid hormone therapy. Subclinical hyperthyroidism is a risk factor for osteoporosis in postmenopausal females who do not take estrogen replacement therapy, because it leads to reduced bone mineral density. It also greatly increases the risk of atrial fibrillation in patients older than 60 years of age.

Hypothyroidism

Hypothyroidism is characterized by diminished secretion of thyroid hormone. **Primary hypothyroidism** occurs when disease or destruction of thyroid gland tissue causes inadequate production of thyroid hormones. Common causes of primary hypothyroidism include chronic (Hashimoto's) **thyroiditis**, an autoimmune disorder characterized by inflammation of the thyroid gland, and treatment of hyperthyroidism with antithyroid drugs, radiation therapy, or surgery. Other causes include previous radiation to the thyroid area of the neck and treatment with amiodarone, lithium, or iodine preparations. Secondary hypothyroidism occurs when there is decreased TSH from the anterior pituitary gland or decreased thyrotropin-releasing hormone (TRH) secreted from the hypothalamus, which disrupts the negative feedback mechanism.

Clinical Manifestations

Several signs and symptoms of altered thyroid function are characteristic. Table 42.1 lists the specific effects of hyperthyroidism and hypothyroidism.

Hyperthyroidism

Thyroid storm or thyrotoxic crisis is a rare but severe complication characterized by extreme symptoms of hyperthyroidism, such as severe tachycardia, fever, dehydration, heart failure, and coma. It is most likely to occur in patients with inadequately treated hyperthyroidism, especially when stressful situations occur (e.g., trauma, infection, surgery, emotional upset).

It should be noted that iodine is present in foods (especially seafood and kelp) and in radiographic contrast dyes. Instances of iodine-induced hyperthyroidism have been reported after ingestion of dietary sources of iodine.

Hypothyroidism

Hypothyroidism is the result from a congenital or acquired defect that results in thyroid hormone deficiency. Congenital hypothyroidism is a type of hypothyroidism that occurs when a child is born with a poorly functioning or absent thyroid gland. Now uncommon in the United States, congenital hypothyroidism once occurred because of a lack of iodine in the mother's diet; however, salt with iodine supplements has virtually eliminated frank iodine deficiency. Symptoms are rarely present at birth but develop gradually during infancy and early childhood, and they include poor growth and development, lethargy and inactivity, feeding problems, slow pulse, subnormal temperature, and constipation. If congenital hypothyroidism is untreated until the child is several months old, irreversible intellectual deficits are likely to result.

Hypothyroidism occurring after early childhood, or **myxedema**, may be caused when inflammatory diseases of the thyroid or another acquired defect destroys parts of the gland. The condition occurs much more often in females than in males. Myxedema may be classed subclinical or clinical. Subclinical hypothyroidism, the most common thyroid disorder, involves a mildly elevated serum TSH and normal serum thyroxine levels. It is usually asymptomatic. If the thyroid gland cannot secrete enough hormones despite excessive release of TSH, hypothyroidism occurs, and a goiter may occur from the overstimulation. Clinical hypothyroidism produces variable signs and symptoms, depending on the amount of circulating thyroid hormone. Initially, manifestations (see Table 42.1) are mild and vague. They usually increase in incidence and severity over time as the thyroid gland gradually atrophies and functioning glandular tissue is replaced by nonfunctioning fibrous connective tissue.

TABLE 42.1

Thyroid Disorders and Their Effects on Body Systems

Hypothyroidism	Hyperthyroidism
Cardiovascular Effects	
Increased capillary fragility	
Decreased cardiac output	Increased cardiac output
Decreased blood pressure	Increased systolic blood pressure Decreased diastolic blood pressure
Decreased heart rate	Tachycardia
Cardiac enlargement	Cardiac dysrhythmias
Heart failure	Heart failure
Anemia	
More rapid development of atherosclerosis and its complications (e.g., coronary artery and peripheral vascular disease)	
	Increased blood volume
Central Nervous System Effects	
Apathy and lethargy	Nervousness
Emotional dullness	Emotional instability
Slow speech, perhaps slurring and hoarseness as well	Restlessness
Hypoactive reflexes	Hyperactive reflexes
Forgetfulness and mental sluggishness	Anxiety
Excessive drowsiness and sleeping	Insomnia
Metabolic Effects	
Intolerance of cold	Intolerance of heat
Subnormal temperature	Low-grade fever
Increased serum cholesterol	
Weight gain	Weight loss despite increased appetite
Gastrointestinal Effects	
Decreased appetite	Increased appetite
Constipation	Abdominal cramps Diarrhea Nausea and vomiting
Muscular Effects	
Weakness	Weakness
Fatigue	Fatigue
Vague aches and pains	Muscle atrophy Tremors
Integumentary Effects	
Dry, coarse, and thickened skin	Moist, warm, flushed skin due to vasodilation and increased sweating
Puffy appearance of the face and eyelids	Localized edema around the eyeballs, which produces characteristic eye changes, including exophthalmos
Dry and thinned hair Thick and hard nails	Hair and nails soft

TABLE 42.1

Thyroid Disorders and Their Effects on Body Systems (Continued)

Hypothyroidism	Hyperthyroidism
Reproductive Effects	
Prolonged menstrual periods Infertility or sterility Decreased libido	Amenorrhea or oligomenorrhea
Miscellaneous Effects	
Increased susceptibility to infection	Increased susceptibility to infection
Increased sensitivity to narcotics, barbiturates, and anesthetics due to slowed metabolism of these drugs	
	Dyspnea Hoarse, rapid speech Polyuria Excessive perspiration

Myxedema coma is a severe, life-threatening hypothyroidism characterized by coma, hypothermia, cardiovascular collapse, hypoventilation, and severe metabolic disorders such as hyponatremia, hypoglycemia, and lactic acidosis. Predisposing factors include exposure to cold, infection, trauma, respiratory disease, and administration of central nervous system (CNS) depressants (e.g., anesthetics, analgesics, sedatives).

> **! Quality and Safety Alert: Safety**
>
> A person with severe hypothyroidism cannot metabolize and excrete the CNS depressants. It is necessary to assess the patient for signs of adverse drug effects.

NCLEX Success

1. A patient has been treated for ventricular dysrhythmias with amiodarone. What is the patient at risk for developing?
   - A. Graves disease
   - B. thyroiditis
   - C. thyroid storm
   - D. congenital hypothyroidism

Drug Therapy

The goal of treatment is to restore the euthyroid state and normal metabolism. In hyperthyroidism, the goals are to reduce thyroid hormone production to relieve symptoms, return serum TSH and thyroid hormone levels to normal, and avoid complete destruction of the thyroid gland. Antithyroid drugs act by decreasing the production or release of thyroid hormones. The thioamide drugs inhibit the synthesis of thyroid hormones. Iodine preparations inhibit the release of thyroid hormones and cause them to be stored within the thyroid gland. Radioactive iodine emits rays that destroy the thyroid gland tissue.

In hypothyroidism, the goal of thyroid replacement therapy is to administer a dosage in sufficient amounts to compensate for the thyroid deficit to resolve symptoms and restore serum TSH and thyroid hormone to normal. TSH is the most reliable marker of adequacy of replacement therapy, and a serum value within the reference range is often considered the therapeutic target. Table 42.2 summarizes the drugs administered for thyroid disease.

ANTITHYROID DRUGS

 Propylthiouracil is the prototype of the thioamide antithyroid drugs. The drug has been the cornerstone of pharmacologic management for hyperthyroidism in adults for over half a century.

Pharmacokinetics

Propylthiouracil is well absorbed with oral administration, and peak plasma levels occur within 30 minutes. The drug's plasma half-life is 1 to 2 hours. However, its duration of action depends on the half-life within the thyroid gland rather than the plasma half-life. Because this time is relatively short, the drug must be given every 8 hours. It is metabolized in the liver and excreted in urine.

Action

Propylthiouracil acts by inhibiting production of thyroid hormones and peripheral conversion of T_4 to the more active T_3. The drug does not interfere with release of thyroid hormones previously produced and stored. Thus, therapeutic effects do not occur for several days or weeks until the stored hormones have been used.

Use

Healthcare providers may use propylthiouracil alone to treat hyperthyroidism, as part of the preoperative preparation for thyroidectomy, before or after radioactive iodine therapy, and in the treatment of thyroid storm. Treatment of hyperthyroidism changes the rate of body metabolism, including

TABLE 42.2
Drugs Administered for the Treatment of Hyperthyroidism and Hypothyroidism

Drug Class	Prototype	Other Drugs in the Class
Antithyroid drug	Propylthiouracil	Methimazole (Tapazole) Strong iodine solution (Lugol solution) Saturated solution of potassium iodide (SSKI; ThyroShield) Sodium iodide ^{131}I (Hicon)
Beta-adrenergic–blocking agent	Propranolol hydrochloride (Inderal, Inderal LA, Innopran XL l)	
Thyroid drug	Levothyroxine (Ermeza, Euthyrox, Synthroid, Levoxyl)	

the rate of metabolism of many drugs. In the hyperthyroid state, drug metabolism may be very rapid, and higher doses of most drugs may be necessary to achieve therapeutic results. When the patient becomes euthyroid, the rate of drug metabolism decreases. Consequently, it is necessary to evaluate and likely reduce doses of all medications to avoid severe adverse effects. Table 42.3 contains the standard route and dosage information for propylthiouracil and other antithyroid drugs.

Patient-related variables specific to the use of propylthiouracil include the following:

- Age:
  - Propylthiouracil is not recommended for use in pediatric patients due to reports of severe liver toxicity. Use in children should be limited to patients who have developed minor toxic reactions to methimazole and who are not candidates for surgery. If propylthiouracil is

TABLE 42.3
DRUGS AT A GLANCE: Drugs for Hyperthyroidism (Antithyroid Drugs)

Drug	Routes and Dosage Ranges	
	Adults	**Children**
ⓟ **Propylthiouracil** (✳ Halycil)	300–400 mg/d PO in divided doses every 8 h, until the patient is euthyroid; then 100–150 mg/d in three divided doses, for maintenance	6–10 y: PO 50–150 mg/m²/d divided every 8 h >10 y: PO 150–300 mg/d divided every 8 h
Methimazole (✳ Tapazole, APO-Methimazole, JAMP Methimazole, Mar-Methimazole)	Hyperthyroidism associated with Graves Disease: Free T_4 levels 1–1.5 times UNL: 5–10 mg PO once daily Free T_4 levels >1.5–2 times UNL: 10–20 mg PO once daily Free T_4 levels >2 times UNL: 20–40 mg PO once daily	0.4 mg/kg/d PO initially, in three divided doses every 8 h; maintenance dose, one half initial dose
Potassium iodide and iodine (Lugol solution)	Thyroidectomy preparation: 5–7 drops PO three times per day for 10 d before surgery Thyrotoxic crisis: 4–8 drops every 6–8 h; initial dose ≥1 h following the initial dose of either propylthiouracil or methimazole	Thyroidectomy preparation: 3–5 drops PO three times per day for 10 d before surgery Thyrotoxic crisis: 4–8 drops every 6 h; initial dose 2 h following the initial dose of either propylthiouracil or methimazole
Potassium iodide saturated solution of potassium iodide (iOSAT, ThyroSafe, ThyroShield, Pima, SSKI)	Thyroidectomy preparation: 50–100 mg PO three times per day for 10 d before surgery	Thyroidectomy preparation: 150–350 mg PO three times per day for 10 d before surgery
Sodium iodide I^{131} (Iodotope, i3odine Max, Hicon)	Dosage (PO, IV) as calculated by a radiologist trained in nuclear medicine	Dosage (PO, IV) as calculated by a radiologist trained in nuclear medicine

prescribed, a short course of therapy of limited duration should be used. Aspartate aminotransferase (AST) and alanine aminotransferase (ALT) levels should be monitored. If the levels rise two to three times the upper normal limits and do not lower within a week, therapy should be discontinued.
- For pediatric patients, administer in three equally divided doses at approximately 8-hour intervals.
- In older adults, propylthiouracil (or methimazole) may be useful, but radioactive iodine is often preferable because it is associated with fewer adverse effects than other antithyroid drugs or surgery. Older patients must be monitored closely for hypothyroidism, which usually develops within 1 year after receiving treatment for hyperthyroidism.
- Reproduction, pregnancy, and lactation:
  - Patients taking propylthiouracil should use effective contraception and postpone pregnancy until stable euthyroid state is achieved.
  - Propylthiouracil crosses the placenta, and adverse events have been noted during pregnancy including maternal and fetal liver damage and hypothyroidism in the fetus/neonate.
  - Propylthiouracil is present in breast milk. The infant should be assessed for adequate growth and development. Propylthiouracil should be administered 3 to 4 hours before breast-feeding.
- Abnormal kidney function and hepatic impairment:
  - The FDA has issued a **BOXED WARNING** ◆ for propylthiouracil stating that severe liver injury resulting in death or acute liver failure may occur within 6 months of treatment. Routine liver function testing to assess for liver failure is important.

Adverse Effects

Administration of propylthiouracil may have several adverse effects, including the following:

- Signs and symptoms of hypothyroidism: bradycardia, heart failure, anemia, coronary artery disease, peripheral vascular disease, slow speech and body movements, emotional and mental dullness, excessive sleeping, increased weight, constipation, and skin changes
- Hematologic effects: leukopenia, agranulocytosis (puts patient at risk for sepsis, rare but severe, earliest symptoms likely to be sore throat and fever), and hypoprothrombinemia
- Dermatologic effects: rash, pruritus, and alopecia
- CNS effects: headache, dizziness, loss of taste, drowsiness, and paresthesias
- Gastrointestinal (GI) effects: nausea, vomiting, abdominal discomfort, gastric irritation, and cholestatic hepatitis
- Other reported effects: lymphadenopathy, edema, joint pain, and drug fever

Contraindications

The only contraindication to propylthiouracil is a known hypersensitivity reaction to the medication.

Nursing Implications

Preventing Interactions

Propylthiouracil may increase the effect of anticoagulants, which may put patients at risk for bleeding. Use with amiodarone, potassium iodide, and sodium iodide reverses thyroid hormone efficacy. Lithium acts synergistically with propylthiouracil to produce hypothyroidism.

Administering the Drug

Patients should take propylthiouracil around the clock in evenly divided doses. If they choose to take one dose of the medication without food, they should take all doses without food. (The same is true if they take it with food.)

Assessing for Therapeutic Effects

The nurse assesses for a slower pulse rate, slow speech, normal level of activity without the signs of hyperactivity, decreased nervousness and tremors, increased sleep patterns, and weight gain. The therapeutic effects should be apparent in 1 to 2 weeks, but a euthyroid state may not occur for 6 to 8 weeks.

Assessing for Adverse Effects

The nurse assesses the patient's heart rate and peripheral pulses for increases, the lung sounds for crackles, and the heart sounds for an audible S_3; these are all indicative of heart failure. The patient is also assessed for slow speech and emotional status (dullness). In addition, the nurse checks for increased periods of rest, increased weight, constipation, and skin changes. Finally, the nurse assesses for CNS depression and gastric irritation, as well as for fever or sore throat, the first signs of agranulocytosis. It is important to assess the white blood count for leukopenia.

Patient Teaching

All patients should receive instructions about the signs and symptoms of acute liver failure and seek immediate medical treatment should those symptoms occur. Box 42.1 identifies additional patient teaching guidelines for propylthiouracil.

Other Drugs in the Class

Methimazole (Tapazole) is similar to propylthiouracil in terms of action, use, and adverse effects. It is also well absorbed with oral administration and rapidly reaches peak plasma levels.

> **Quality and Safety Alert: Safety**
>
> Because of the risk of fetal abnormalities associated with methimazole, patients who are able to become pregnant should have a pregnancy test before beginning the drug. Methimazole should be avoided during the first trimester; it is safe to use in the second and third trimesters.

Strong iodine solution (Lugol solution) and saturated solution of potassium iodide (SSKI) are iodine preparations sometimes used in short-term treatment of hyperthyroidism. These drugs inhibit release of thyroid hormones, causing them to

> **BOX 42.1** **Patient Teaching Guidelines for Propylthiouracil**
>
> - To decrease the production of thyroid hormone by an overactive thyroid gland, it is necessary to take antithyroid drugs for 1 year or longer to return thyroid hormone levels to normal.
> - Have periodic tests of thyroid function. Dosage adjustments may be necessary.
> - Have periodic tests of liver function tests during the first 6 months of treatment.
> - Ask the prescriber if it is necessary to avoid or restrict amounts of seafood or iodized salt during antithyroid drug therapy.
> - Take this drug at regular intervals around the clock, usually every 8 hours.
> - Report fever, sore throat, unusual bleeding or bruising, headache, skin rash, yellowing of the skin, or vomiting to the prescriber. If these adverse effects occur, the drug dosage may be reduced or the drug may be discontinued.
> - Consult a healthcare provider before taking over-the-counter (OTC) drugs. Some OTC drugs (e.g., cough syrups, asthma medications, multivitamins) may contain iodide, which can increase the likelihood of goiter and the risk of adverse effects from excessive doses of iodide.
> - Take your pulse daily and report rates above 100 and below 60 beats/min to the prescriber.
> - Check your weight two to three times per week, and if it increases suddenly, call your healthcare provider.
> - Consult a healthcare provider if signs or symptoms of a rash occur.

accumulate in the thyroid gland. Lugol solution is usually used to treat thyrotoxic crisis and to decrease the size and vascularity of the thyroid gland before thyroidectomy. SSKI is more often used as an expectorant but may be given as preparation for thyroidectomy. Iodine preparations should not be followed by propylthiouracil, methimazole, or radioactive iodine because the latter drugs cause release of stored thyroid hormone and may precipitate acute hyperthyroidism.

Sodium iodide ^{131}I (Hicon) is a radioactive isotope of iodine. The thyroid gland cannot differentiate between regular iodide and radioactive iodide, so it picks up the radioactive iodide from the circulating blood. As a result, small amounts of radioactive iodide can be used as a diagnostic test of thyroid function, and larger doses are used therapeutically to treat hyperthyroidism. Therapeutic doses act by emitting beta and gamma rays, which destroy thyroid tissue and thereby decrease production of thyroid hormones. The drug is also used to treat thyroid cancer. It is safe, effective, inexpensive, and convenient. One disadvantage is hypothyroidism, which usually develops within a few months and requires lifelong thyroid hormone replacement therapy. Another disadvantage is the delay in therapeutic benefits. Results may not be apparent for 3 months or longer, during which time it is necessary to bring severe hyperthyroidism under control with one of the thioamide antithyroid drugs. Note that after radioactive iodine therapy, patients should not expectorate or cough freely because their saliva will be radioactive for 24 hours.

ADJUVANT MEDICATION USED TO TREAT HYPERTHYROIDISM

The drug **propranolol** (Inderal, Inderal LA, Innopran XL) is a beta-adrenergic-blocking agent that is recommended in all patients with symptomatic hyperthyroidism. It is particularly useful in older adults who have resting heart rates greater than 90 beats/min or have a history of cardiovascular conditions, such as dysrhythmias, angina pectoris, and hypertension. When given to patients with hyperthyroidism, propranolol blocks beta-adrenergic receptors in various organs and thereby controls symptoms of hyperthyroidism resulting from excessive stimulation of the sympathetic nervous system. These symptoms include tachycardia, palpitations, excessive sweating, tremors, and nervousness. Propranolol is useful for controlling symptoms during the delayed response to thioamide drugs and radioactive iodine, before thyroidectomy, and in treating thyrotoxic crisis. When patients become euthyroid and definitive treatment has controlled hyperthyroid symptoms, it is necessary to taper propranolol and discontinue it. Table 42.4 gives route and dosage information for propranolol.

TABLE 42.4

DRUGS AT A GLANCE: Adjuvant Drugs for the Treatment of Hyperthyroidism (Propranolol)

Drug	Routes and Dosage Ranges	
	Adults	**Children**
Propranolol hydrochloride (Inderal, Inderal LA, Innopran XL; ✤ Inderal, Inderal LA, Hemangeol, InnoPran XL)	Thyrotoxicosis: 30–160 mg/d in 1–4 divided doses PO	Thyrotoxicosis: Infants and Children: PO 0.5–2 mg/kg/d divided every 8 h: maximum dose: 40 mg/dose Adolescents: PO 10–40 mg every 6–8 h

THYROID EYE DISEASE MEDICATIONS

Thyroid eye disease (TED) is known as Graves orbitopathy. It is an autoimmune disorder of the retro-orbital tissues. The condition is exacerbated by stress, pregnancy, and radioactive iodine therapy.

The clinical presentation varies from a unilateral dry-eye disease to bilateral sight-threatening complications. Treatment for TED includes reversal of hyperthyroidism, smoking cessation, administration of IV methylprednisolone (Chapter 17), and IV infusion of teprotumumab. The secondary therapy for TED is tocilizumab or rituximab (Chapter 13) (Davis & Burch, 2023).

Glucocorticoids

IV methylprednisolone is administered with a 500 mg dose once weekly for weeks 1 to 6, then 250 mg once weekly for weeks 7 to 12 with a cumulative dose of 4.5 to 5 g over 12 weeks. TED usually improves within 4 weeks. Approximately one half of patients have a good response within 6 months. Patients on long-term glucocorticoid therapy will require skeletal assessments to determine the increased risk of fracture.

Immunosuppressants

Teprotumumab is administered every 3 weeks IV 10 mg/kg as an initial dose, then 20 mg/kg for a total of eight infusions. Adverse effects of the teprotumumab infusions include nausea, muscle spasms, hyperglycemia, and hearing impairment. Patients with type 2 diabetes may have impaired glycemic control.

Tocilizumab targets IL-6. It is administered to patients who do not respond to glucocorticoid therapy. Rituximab is an anti-B-cell antibody that produces a decrease in thyrotropin receptor antibody and depletion of B cells in the retro-orbital tissues. High doses of the antibody are associated with severe immunosuppression. However, when used for TED, lower dosages are administered, thus decreasing the severe immunosuppression.

NCLEX Success

2. How does propranolol control symptoms of hyperthyroidism?
   A. Propranolol blocks the alpha-adrenergic receptor sites.
   B. Propranolol stimulates the thyroid gland to decrease thyroid production.
   C. Propranolol impedes the beta-adrenergic receptors in various organs.
   D. Propranolol lowers blood pressure to decrease metabolism.

3. A patient taking propylthiouracil develops a sore throat and fever. What does the nurse suspect is wrong with this patient?
   A. The patient has developed a goiter.
   B. The patient has an elevated liver function.
   C. The patient has developed a hypersensitivity reaction.
   D. The patient has agranulocytosis.

THYROID DRUGS

Levothyroxine (Ermeza, Euthyrox, Synthroid, Levoxyl), a synthetic preparation of thyroxine, serves as the prototype thyroid drug and is considered the standard of care for long-term treatment of hypothyroidism. This potent form of T_4 contains a uniform amount of hormone and can be administered orally and parenterally.

Pharmacokinetics

Absorption of levothyroxine varies after oral administration from 48% to 79%. Taking the drug on an empty stomach increases absorption. In malabsorption syndromes, this results in excessive loss of the drug in the feces. Most (99%) of the circulating drug is bound to serum proteins, including thyroid-binding globulin as well as thyroid-binding prealbumin and albumin. Levothyroxine has a long half-life, about 6 to 7 days in a euthyroid state, but it is prolonged to 9 to 10 days in hypothyroidism and shortened to 3 to 4 days in hyperthyroidism. The drug is metabolized in the liver and excreted in the urine.

Action

Levothyroxine increases the metabolic rate in the body's tissues, increasing oxygen consumption, respiratory rate, and heart rate. It also increases the metabolism of fats, carbohydrates, and proteins and enhances the growth process.

Use

Healthcare providers use levothyroxine as replacement therapy for people with hypothyroidism. Other uses include the following:

- Treatment and prevention of euthyroid goiters in patients with pituitary suppression of TSH
- Management of thyroid cancer
- Prevention of goitrogenesis, hypothyroidism, and thyrotoxicosis during pregnancy (in combination with antithyroid medications)
- Treatment of myxedema coma

Table 42.5 provides route and dosage information for levothyroxine. The FDA has issued a **BOXED WARNING** cautioning prescribers not to order thyroid hormones, either alone or with other therapeutic agents, for the treatment of obesity or for weight loss. Significant and serious complications may develop in euthyroid people who take thyroid hormones.

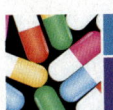

TABLE 42.5
DRUGS AT A GLANCE: Levothyroxine

Drug	Routes and Dosage Ranges	
	Adults	**Children**
P Levothyroxine (Ermeza, Euthyrox, Synthroid, Levoxyl; ❋ Synthroid, Levoxyl, Tirosint, Levothroid)	Primary hypothyroidism: Adjust initial dose by 12–25 mcg/day every 3–6 wk based on clinical response and serum TSH. Patients ≤60 y without evidence of coronary heart disease: PO 1.6 mcg/kg/d Patients >60 y without evidence of coronary heart disease: PO 25–50 mcg once daily Patients with coronary heart disease: PO 12.5–50 mcg once daily; monitor for onset of cardiac symptoms Myxedema coma: IV initial loading dose IV 200–400 mcg as a slow bolus; followed by a daily replacement dose of 50–100 mcg until patient improved clinically and can transition to oral therapy Thyroid-stimulating hormone (TSH) suppression in well-differentiated thyroid cancer, 1.6–2 mcg/kg/d PO may be needed; highly individualized	Congenital hypothyroidism, PO 1–3 mo, 10–15 mcg/kg/d 3–6 mo, 8–10 mcg/kg/d 6–12 mo, 6–8 mcg/kg/d 1–5 y, 5–6 mcg/kg/d 6–12 y, 4–5 mcg/kg/d >12 y, 2–3 mcg/kg/d Growth and puberty complete, 1.7 mcg/kg/d, same as adults

Patient-related variables specific to the use of levothyroxine include the following:

- Age:
  - In children, replacement therapy with thyroid hormone is essential for normal growth and development. The dosage of levothyroxine must be adjusted according to growth. Determination of the maintenance dosage requires periodic radioimmunoassay of serum thyroxine levels and periodic radiographs to follow bone development. To monitor drug effects on growth in children, height and weight are recorded and compared with growth charts at regular intervals. Close monitoring for adverse drug effects is necessary.
  - In older adults, thyroid hormone replacement with levothyroxine increases the heart's workload and may cause serious adverse effects, especially in those with cardiovascular disease. In such patients, cautious treatment is necessary. Thus, use of smaller initial dosages and smaller drug increments at longer intervals than prescribed for younger adults is essential. Periodic measurements of serum TSH levels are necessary to monitor drug therapy and to adjust doses when indicated. Also, regular monitoring of blood pressure and pulse is essential. In general, levothyroxine should not be given if the resting heart rate is more than 100 beats/min.
- Reproduction, pregnancy, and lactation:
  - Hypothyroidism increases the risk of irregular menses and infertility. Treatment with levothyroxine is recommended to normalize thyroid function in infertile patients.
  - Levothyroxine has not been shown to increase the risk of congenital abnormalities or miscarriage. Normal levels of maternal thyroid hormones are required for fetal development.
  - Levothyroxine is present in breast milk. The decision to breast-feed must consider the risk of infant exposure. The World Health Organization (WHO) considers levothyroxine to be compatible with breast-feeding.
- Abnormal kidney function and hepatic impairment:
  - Hepatic metabolism of levothyroxine in patients with hypothyroidism is slow, so drug metabolism may be delayed. Many drugs given to these patients have a prolonged effect. It is therefore important to assess drug reactions in patients with hepatic impairment.
- Specific healthcare environments:
  - In the critical care unit, management of patients in thyroid storm or thyrotoxic crisis is common. Increased rate of cellular metabolism and oxygen consumption occurs with a resultant increase in heat production. The hypermetabolic state increases the metabolism of medications, so increased or more frequent dosing may be necessary.

Adverse Effects

Adverse effects of levothyroxine include signs and symptoms of hyperthyroidism. Other more serious adverse effects are tachycardia, cardiac dysrhythmias, angina pectoris, myocardial infarction, and heart failure. Nervousness, hyperactivity, insomnia, diarrhea, abdominal cramps, nausea, vomiting, weight loss, fever, and an intolerance to heat have also been reported.

Most adverse reactions stem from excessive doses, and signs and symptoms produced are the same as those occurring with hyperthyroidism. Excessive thyroid hormones make the heart work very hard and fast in attempting to meet tissue demands for oxygenated blood and nutrients. Symptoms of myocardial ischemia occur when the increased cardiac workload is prolonged. Cardiovascular problems are more likely to occur in older adult patients or in those who already have heart disease.

Contraindications

Contraindications to levothyroxine include a known hypersensitivity to active or extraneous constituents of the drug, thyrotoxicosis, and acute myocardial infarction related to hypothyroidism.

Caution is warranted in Addison disease. Affected patients require corticosteroids prior to administration of levothyroxine. Thyroid hormones increase tissue metabolism and tissue demands for adrenocortical hormones. If adrenal insufficiency is not treated first, administration of thyroid hormone may cause acute adrenocortical insufficiency, a life-threatening condition. Also, caution is necessary during lactation and with coronary artery disease or angina.

Nursing Implications

Preventing Interactions

Many medications interact with levothyroxine, increasing and decreasing its effects (Box 42.2).

Administering the Medication

Several factors affect the dosage of levothyroxine: the choice of drug, age and general condition, severity and duration of hypothyroidism, and clinical response to drug therapy. It is essential to individualize the dosage to approximate the amount of thyroid hormone needed to make up the deficit in endogenous hormone production. As a rule, the initial dosage is relatively small, and gradual increases at approximately 2-week intervals are appropriate until symptoms are relieved and a normal serum TSH level (0.5 to 4.2 microunits/L) is reestablished. Determination of the maintenance dosage for long-term therapy depends on the patient's clinical status and periodic measurement of serum TSH.

People should take levothyroxine in the morning on an empty stomach. If the pulse rate prior to administering the drug is more than 100 beats/min, it is important to notify the prescriber.

When giving levothyroxine to an infant or young child, it may be necessary to crush the tablet and add a small amount of formula or water. The child should take the solution with the medication soon after it is mixed; avoid storing the liquid for long periods. The crushed tablet may also be sprinkled on a small amount of food and then administered. Because the bioavailability of levothyroxine is reduced when administered with enteral tube feedings, a dosage increase may be required. Also, frequent thyroid function tests (every 1 to 3 weeks) are required with prolonged administration by enteral feedings.

Assessing for Therapeutic Effects

In hypothyroidism, thyroid replacement therapy is life-long. Medical supervision is necessary frequently during early treatment and at least annually after the patient's condition has stabilized, and maintenance dosage has been determined. The brand of medication should be consistent; patients should not change brands. The nurse assesses for the following conditions:

- Increasing energy and diminished sleep
- Level of alertness and interest in the environment and surroundings
- Increased pulse rate and blood pressure
- Bowel regularity and decreased symptoms of constipation
- Reversal of coarseness of the skin and hair
- Laboratory values (should decrease as the thyroid hormone is replaced): serum cholesterol, creatinine phosphokinase, lactate dehydrogenase, and aspartate aminotransferase

In patients with congenital hypothyroidism, the nurse records the patient's height periodically to determine an increase in linear growth.

In patients with myxedema, the nurse assesses for decreased edema and loss of weight.

> **Quality and Safety Alert: Evidence-Based Practice**
>
> Karatas and Hacioglu (2022) conducted a study to determine the factors that cause hypothyroidism and the effectiveness of treatment. One hundred and eighty participants, each diagnosed with hypothyroidism, were enrolled in the study. Participants were recruited in an endocrine outpatient clinic and were grouped according to treatment effectiveness. The groups were compared in terms of age, gender, medication adherence, thyroid antibodies, antithyroglobulin, and thyroid heterogenicity. Of those, age, thyroid antibodies, and treatment adherence were found to be the factors that influenced the success of hypothyroidism treatment. The study revealed that patients with low treatment adherence to levothyroxine therapy experienced a higher rate of treatment failure. These findings demonstrate that high treatment failure, and levothyroxine treatment adherence, is an important subjective factor to determine treatment efficacy.

Assessing for Adverse Effects

The nurse assesses for tachycardia and any cardiac dysrhythmias. Excessive thyroid hormones make the heart work very hard and fast to meet the tissue demands for oxygenated blood and nutrients. It is necessary to assess for chest pain, edema, and signs of heart failure. Symptoms of myocardial infarction occur when the myocardium does not have an adequate supply of oxygenated blood. Symptoms of heart failure occur when the increased cardiac workload is prolonged.

Patient Teaching

Box 42.3 provides patient teaching guidelines for levothyroxine.

> **BOX 42.2** **Drug Interactions: Levothyroxine**
>
> **Drugs That Increase the Effects of Levothyroxine**
> - Activating antidepressants (bupropion, venlafaxine), adrenergic asthmatic agents (albuterol, epinephrine), nasal decongestants
>   *Increase the effects of thyroid hormones*
>
> **Drugs That Decrease the Effects of Levothyroxine**
> - Antacids, cholestyramine, iron, sucralfate
>   *Decrease the absorption of levothyroxine*
> - Antihypertensives, propranolol
>   *Decrease cardiac-stimulating effects*
> - Estrogens, oral contraceptives
>   *Increase thyroxine-binding globulin, thereby increasing the amount of bound, inactive levothyroxine in patients with hypothyroidism*
> - Phenytoin, rifampin
>   *Induce enzymes, leading to more rapid metabolism*

BOX 42.3 Patient Teaching Guidelines for Levothyroxine

- Understand that thyroid hormone is required for normal body functioning and for life. When your thyroid gland is unable to produce enough thyroid hormone, levothyroxine is used as a synthetic substitute. Thus, levothyroxine therapy for hypothyroidism is life-long; stopping it may lead to a life-threatening illness.
- Have periodic tests of thyroid function.
- Understand that dosage adjustments may occur according to clinical response and results of thyroid function tests.
- Do not switch from one drug brand to another; effects may be different.
- Consult a healthcare provider before taking over-the-counter drugs that stimulate the heart or cause nervousness (e.g., asthma remedies, cold remedies, decongestants). Levothyroxine stimulates the central nervous system and the heart; excessive stimulation may occur if it is taken with other stimulating drugs. In addition, you should probably limit your intake of caffeine-containing beverages to two to three servings daily.
- Take the drug every morning, on an empty stomach, for best absorption. Also, do not take the drug with an antacid (e.g., Tums, Maalox), an iron preparation, or sucralfate (Carafate). These drugs decrease absorption of levothyroxine. If it is necessary to take one of these drugs, take levothyroxine 2 hours before or 4 to 6 hours after the other drug.
- Take the drug at about the same time each day for more consistent blood levels and more normal body metabolism.
- Report chest pain, heart palpitations, nervousness, or insomnia to the prescriber. These adverse effects result from excessive stimulation and may indicate that drug dosage or intake of other stimulants needs to be reduced.

Clinical Application 42.1

While Ms. Zalewski is in the hospital, the nurse is administering her medications. Hospital routine is to administer all once-daily medications at 9:00 a.m. When reviewing the medication administration orders, the nurse notes that Ms. Zalewski is to receive levothyroxine (Synthroid) at 9:00 a.m. Patients usually receive their breakfast trays between 8:00 and 8:30 a.m.
- What action should the nurse take with regard to the administration of levothyroxine?

Clinical Application 42.2

Ms. Zalewski has been discharged from the hospital and is being seen by the home care nurse. During the visit, the nurse reviews all of Ms. Zalewski's medications. Ms. Zalewski states she is taking aluminum hydroxide gel (Amphojel) every morning when she arises to prevent gastric distress after breakfast.
- How will the administration of Amphojel affect her levothyroxine?
- What patient teaching should the home care nurse provide to Ms. Zalewski?

NCLEX Success

4. The home care nurse is visiting a patient who has a diagnosis of hypothyroidism. The patient is being treated with levothyroxine. The assessment of the patient reveals the following findings: an audible S_3, crackles in the lower lobes, edema of the lower extremities, and a heart rate of 120 beats/min. What does the nurse suspect the patient has developed?
   A. myocardial infarction
   B. thrombophlebitis
   C. pulmonary embolism
   D. heart failure

5. A 21-year-old female is taking levothyroxine for hypothyroidism. She has recently become sexually active and would like to take an oral contraceptive. Which of the following aspects of patient teaching is most accurate?
   A. A low-dose oral contraceptive agent is permissible with levothyroxine.
   B. Oral contraceptive agents increase the amount of thyroid hormone.
   C. For protection from pregnancy, it is necessary to use an oral contraceptive and an alternative form of birth control.
   D. Oral contraceptive agents result in diminished levothyroxine levels due to inactivation.

THE NURSING PROCESS

A concept map outlines the nursing process related to drug therapy considerations in this chapter. Additional nursing implications related to the disease process should also be considered in care decisions.

Assessment
- Assess for signs and symptoms of thyroid disorders (see Table 42.1). During the course of treatment with thyroid or antithyroid drugs, the patient should be monitored for indicators of hypothyroidism, euthyroidism, and hyperthyroidism, which can indicate therapeutic and adverse drug effects.
- Check laboratory reports for serum TSH (normal = 0.5–4.2 microunits/mL) when available. An elevated serum TSH is the first indication of primary hypothyroidism and commonly occurs in middle-aged women, even in the absence of other signs and symptoms. Serum TSH is used to monitor response to drugs that alter thyroid function.

Outcomes of Therapy
The patient will
- Achieve normal blood levels of thyroid hormone.
- Receive or take drugs accurately.
- Experience relief of symptoms of hypothyroidism or hyperthyroidism.
- Be assisted to cope with symptoms until therapy becomes effective.
- Avoid preventable adverse drug effects.
- Maintain the therapeutic and avoid the adverse effects of drug therapy.

Nursing Interventions
- Use nondrug measures to control symptoms, increase effectiveness of drug therapy, and decrease adverse reactions. Some areas for intervention include the following:
- Patients with hypothyroidism are very intolerant of cold, due to their slow metabolism rate. Chilling and shivering should be prevented because of added strain on the heart. Provide blankets and warm clothes as needed. Patients with hyperthyroidism are very intolerant of heat and perspire excessively, due to their rapid metabolism rate. Provide cooling baths and lightweight clothing as needed.
- Hypothyroid patients are often overweight because of a slow metabolism rate. Thus, a low-calorie, weight-reduction diet may be indicated. In addition, an increased intake of high-fiber foods is usually needed to prevent constipation as a result of decreased GI secretions and motility. Hyperthyroid patients are often underweight because of a rapid metabolism rate. They often need extra calories and nutrients to prevent tissue breakdown. With hypothyroidism, patients need an adequate intake of low-calorie fluids to prevent constipation. With hyperthyroidism, patients need large amounts of fluids (3000–4000 mL/d) unless contraindicated by cardiac or renal disease. With hypothyroidism, encourage activity to maintain cardiovascular, respiratory, GI, and musculoskeletal function. With hyperthyroidism, encourage rest and quiet, nonstrenuous activity. Because patients differ in what they find restful, this must be determined with each patient.
- Hypothyroid patients are likely to have edema and dry skin. When edema is present, inspect pressure points, turn often, and avoid trauma when possible. Edema increases risks of skin breakdown and decubitus ulcer formation. Also, increased capillary fragility increases the likelihood of bruising from seemingly minor trauma. When skin is dry, use soap sparingly and lotions and other lubricants freely.
- Hyperthyroid patients may have exophthalmos. In mild cases, use measures to protect the eye. For example, dark glasses, local lubricants, and patching of the eyes at night may be needed. If the eyelids cannot close, they are sometimes taped shut to avoid corneal abrasion. In severe exophthalmos, corticosteroids and diuretics are usually given.

Evaluation
- Interview and observe for compliance with instructions for taking medications.
- Observe for relief of symptoms.
- Check laboratory reports for normal blood levels of TSH or thyroid hormones.
- Interview and observe for adverse drug effects.
- Check appointment records for compliance with follow-up procedures.

Visit thePoint® at http://thePoint.lww.com/Frandsen13e for answers to NCLEX Success questions (in Appendix A), answers to Clinical Application Case Studies (in Appendix B), and more!

REFERENCES AND RESOURCES

Davies, T. F., & Burch, H. B. (2023). Treatment of thyroid eye disease. *UpToDate*. Lexi-Comp, Inc.

Hinkle, J. H., Cheever, K. H., & Overbaugh, K. J. (2021). *Brunner & Suddarth's textbook of medical-surgical nursing* (15th ed.). Wolters Kluwer.

Karatas, S., & Hciogu, Y. (2022). Determinants of levothyroxine treatment in patient with hypothyroidism. *Cyprus Journal of Science*, 7(5), 593–596. doi:10.4274/cjms.2022.2022-8

Norris, T. L. (2019). *Porth's pathophysiology concepts of altered health states* (10th ed.). Wolters Kluwer.

Ross, D. S. (2022). Graves' hyperthyroidism in nonpregnant adults: Overview of treatment. *UpToDate*. Lexi-Comp, Inc.

Shah, S. S., & Patel, B. C. (2023). Thyroid eye disease. [Updated 2022 May 26]. In *StatPearls [Internet]*. StatPearls Publishing. Available from https://www.ncbi.nlm.nih.gov/books/NBK582134

UpToDate. (2023). *Drug Information*. Lexi-Comp, Inc.

CHAPTER 43

Drug Therapy for Pituitary and Hypothalamic Dysfunction

LEARNING OBJECTIVES

After studying this chapter, you should be able to:

1. Identify clinical considerations and manifestations of growth deficiency in children, diabetes insipidus, central precocious puberty, and acromegaly.
2. Identify the prototype and describe the action, use, adverse effects, contraindications, and nursing implications of the anterior pituitary hormone used to treat growth hormone deficiency in children.
3. Identify the prototype and describe the action, use, adverse effects, contraindications, and nursing implications of the posterior pituitary hormone used to treat diabetes insipidus.
4. Identify the prototype and describe the action, use, adverse effects, contraindications, and nursing implications of the hypothalamic hormone drugs used to treat precocious puberty.
5. Identify the prototype and describe the action, use, adverse effects, contraindications, and nursing implications of the hypothalamic hormone drugs used to treat acromegaly.
6. Implement the nursing process in the care of the patient receiving specific pituitary and hypothalamic hormones.

CLINICAL APPLICATION CASE STUDY

Jose Rojas is a 24-year-old man who has suffered a head injury while riding his motorcycle without a helmet. He has been admitted for observation, with multiple abrasions and a blow to the head. He begins to produce massive amounts of clear, pale-yellow urine. The healthcare provider diagnoses diabetes insipidus and orders desmopressin 0.2 mL intranasally in two divided doses.

KEY TERMS

Acromegaly: a chronic disease, resulting from excessive secretion of growth hormone (GH); characterized by an abnormal pattern of bone and connective tissue growth associated with an increased incidence of diabetes mellitus and hypertension

Diabetes insipidus: a condition that results from a dysfunction in the posterior pituitary lobe with excretion of large quantities of dilute urine due to deficient production of antidiuretic hormone (ADH).

Precocious puberty: the onset of pubertal development that is 2 to 2.5 standard deviations earlier than population norms. Children diagnosed with precocious puberty develop secondary sexual characteristics prior to the age of 9 (males) and 8 (females).

INTRODUCTION

This chapter introduces the pharmacologic care of the patient experiencing increased or decreased function of the hormones secreted by the hypothalamus and pituitary gland. It focuses on drug therapy for growth hormone (GH) deficiency in children, diabetes insipidus, central precocious puberty, and acromegaly.

The hypothalamus of the brain and the pituitary gland interact to control most metabolic functions of the body and to maintain homeostasis (Fig. 43.1). They are anatomically connected by a funnel-shaped hypophyseal stalk. The hypothalamus controls secretions of the pituitary gland. The pituitary gland, in turn, regulates secretions or functions of other body tissues called target tissues. The pituitary gland is two glands, each with different structures and functions. The anterior pituitary is composed of different types of glandular cells that synthesize and secrete different hormones. The posterior pituitary is anatomically an extension of the hypothalamus and is composed mainly of nerve fibers. Although it does not manufacture any hormones itself, it stores and releases hormones synthesized in the hypothalamus. Hormones are chemical messengers with specific regulatory effect on the cells that control various bodily functions. For further details on the physiology of pituitary hormones, visit thePoint http://thePoint.lww.com/Frandsen13e.

OVERVIEW OF PITUITARY AND HYPOTHALAMIC DYSFUNCTION

Clinical Considerations and Manifestations of Growth Hormone Deficiency, Diabetes Insipidus, Precocious Puberty, and Acromegaly

Growth Hormone Deficiency in Children

The definition of growth deficiency in children is growth below the third percentile of the established normal values. There are several causes of GH deficiency. Mutation of a transcription factor (POUF1; also known as PIT-1) leads to variable recessive peptide hormone deficiencies that may be associated with anterior pituitary hypoplasia. Also, mutation of a transcription factor (PROP1), which causes a failure to activate POUF1/PIT-1 gene expression, results in pituitary hypoplasia and/or familial multiple pituitary hormone deficiency.

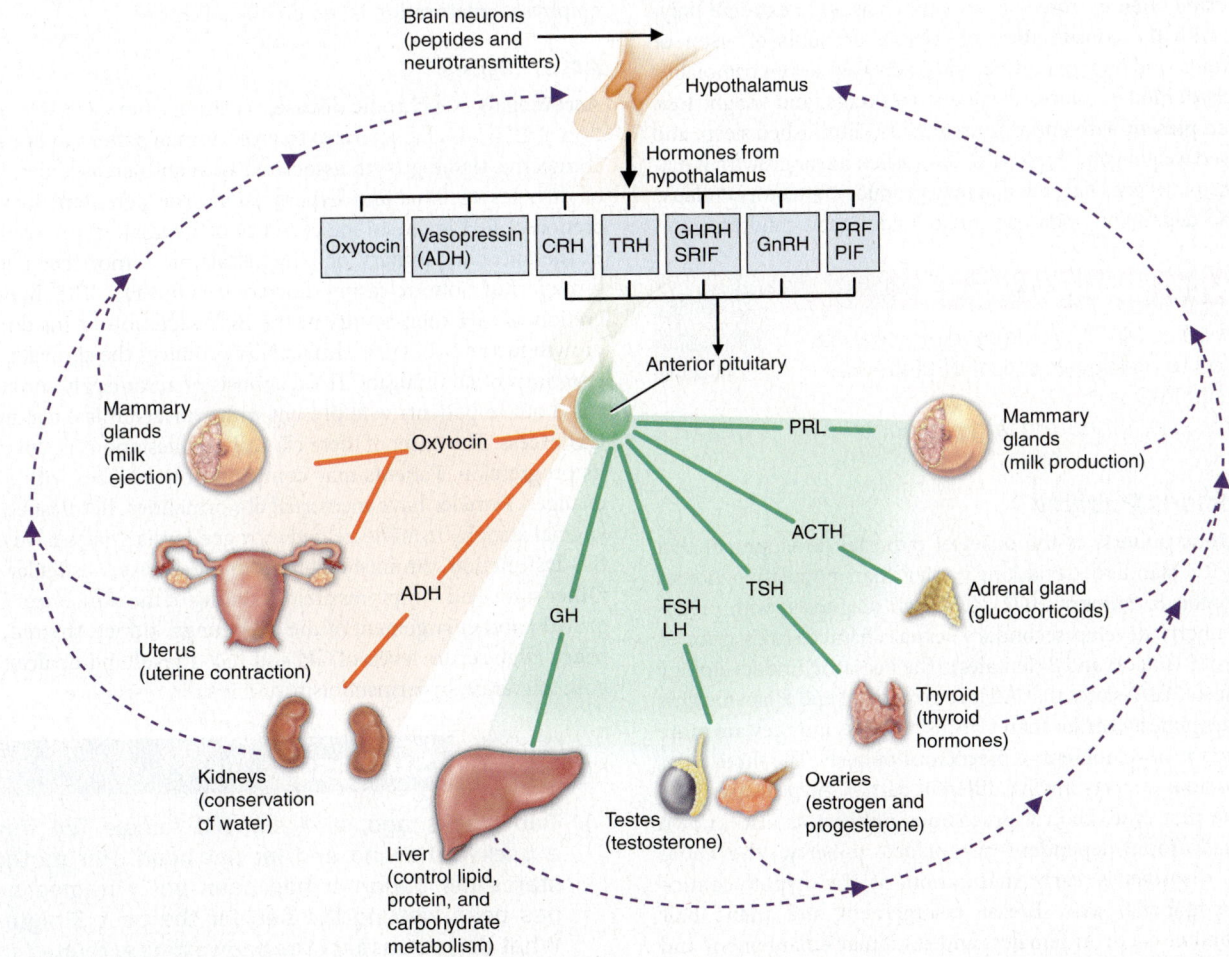

Figure 43.1. Hypothalamic and pituitary hormones and their target organs. The hypothalamus produces hormones that act on the anterior pituitary or are stored in the posterior pituitary. The anterior pituitary produces hormones that act on various body tissues and stimulate production of other hormones. ACTH, adrenocorticotropic hormone; ADH, antidiuretic hormone; CRH, corticotropin-releasing hormone or factor; FSH, follicle-stimulating hormone; GH, growth hormone; GnRH, gonadotropin-releasing hormone; LH, luteinizing hormone; PIF, prolactin-inhibiting factor; T_3, triiodothyronine; T_4, thyroxine; TRH, thyrotropin-releasing hormone; TSH, thyroid-stimulating hormone.

In addition, mutations in the anterior pituitary cells are sources of GH deficiency.

Idiopathic short stature is present when a child's stature falls below two standard deviations of the mean for age. The child has no endocrine, metabolic, or other condition to account for the GH deficiency.

Diabetes Insipidus

Diabetes insipidus is a condition that results from a dysfunction in the posterior pituitary lobe with excretion of large quantities of dilute urine due to deficient production of antidiuretic hormone (ADH). With the absence of ADH, the kidneys filter the water but do not reabsorb it. When this occurs, the circulating fluid volume decreases, producing increased thirst and large amounts of urine production.

Diabetes insipidus may be idiopathic, hereditary, or acquired. Causes include lesions in the posterior pituitary, hypothalamus, or infundibular stem that interfere with ADH synthesis, transport, and release. These lesions in the central nervous system (CNS) can be the result of a tumor, aneurysm, or thrombus. Other causes are the removal of the pituitary gland, immunologic disorders, or infections.

Characteristic features include polyuria, with excretion of dilute urine ranging from 4 L to as much as 30 L; extreme polydipsia, with the consumption of copious amounts of water or other fluids; and hypernatremia, with increased serum osmolality. The dehydration produces dizziness, weakness, and weight loss. Children present with enuresis, irritability, diminished sleep, and decreased weight gain along with diminished linear growth. If diabetes insipidus goes untreated, it may produce circulatory collapse and CNS depression or damage in both adults and children.

> **Clinical Application 43.1**
> - How has Mr. Rojas' head injury contributed to the development of diabetes insipidus?
> - Why is he producing large amounts of dilute urine?

Precocious Puberty

Precocious puberty is the onset of pubertal development that is 2 to 2.5 standard deviations earlier than population norms (Harrington & Palmert, 2022). Children diagnosed with precocious puberty develop secondary sexual characteristics prior to the age of 9 (males) and 8 (females). The Pediatric Endocrinology Fact Sheet (2020) states that African American and Hispanic girls may start puberty earlier than Caucasian girls, and they are more prone to the development of precocious puberty. The three types of precocious puberty involve different pathologic processes.

The first type, central precocious puberty, is also known as gonadotropin-dependent precocious puberty. The cause of this disorder is early maturation of the hypothalamic–pituitary–gonadal axis. Breast enlargement and pubic hair development occur in females, and testicular enlargement and pubic hair development occur in males. Other signs of this disorder include accelerated linear bone growth, increased bone age, and pubertal levels of some gonadal hormones such as follicle-stimulating hormone (FSH) and luteinizing hormone (LH) in females and testosterone in males. Idiopathic central precocious puberty is often due to the presence of genetic variants that are associated with early puberty. The most common lesion that results in central precocious puberty is hamartomas. These are benign tumors of the tuber cinereum. CNS irradiation rarely results in the development of central precocious puberty, but it can result in GH deficiency.

The second type, peripheral precocity, also known as gonadotropin-independent precocious puberty, is a result of excess secretion of the estrogen and androgen sex hormones from the gonads or adrenal glands. In females, pituitary tumors are rare but do cause this type of precocious puberty. Exposure to estrogen creams used by menopausal care providers of females may also lead to precocious puberty. A follicular cyst of the ovaries is the most common cause of peripheral precocity. Ovarian tumors may also cause peripheral precocity. In preadolescent males, Leydig cell tumors may be the cause. These tumors, which result in an asymmetric enlargement of the testes, are benign; surgical removal is appropriate.

The third type, benign or nonprogressive pubertal variants (previously called incomplete precocious puberty), is isolated breast development in preadolescent females or hormone-mediated characteristics (e.g., acne or axillary or pubic hair) in males. It is necessary to confirm the diagnosis using radiographic examination of the bone age—determining when the epiphyseal maturation is marginally advanced.

Acromegaly

Acromegaly is a chronic disease, resulting from excessive secretion of GH. It is characterized by an abnormal pattern of bone and connective tissue growth associated with an increased incidence of diabetes mellitus and hypertension. The persistent hypersecretion of GH is due to the presence of a somatotroph adenoma of the anterior pituitary or a hypothalamic tumor that releases growth hormone-releasing hormone (GHRH). The hypersecretion of GH then results in the liver secretion of insulin-like growth factor 1 (IGF-1). This activity produces the clinical manifestations of acromegaly. The diagnosis of acromegaly should be ruled out in patients who present with typical clinical features of GH excess. The onset of these clinical manifestations is slow, as is its progression. Patients may complain of headaches with visual changes. Females have menstrual abnormalities, hot flashes, and vaginal atrophy from decreased estrogen levels. Males have erectile dysfunction, diminished libido, and decreased testicular size. Other signs and symptoms are thickening of the skin, linear bone growth, and enlargement of the liver, lungs, kidney, thyroid, and heart. High serum levels of GH and IGF-1 result in impaired glucose tolerance, hyperinsulinism, and insulin resistance.

NCLEX Success

1. Two weeks ago, a 4-year-old female fell from a backyard swing and hit her head. Her mother states her daughter had been potty trained but has been wetting the bed for the past 3 nights. What do you suspect the bedwetting is related to?
    A. regression in development due to changes in the home
    B. drinking juices prior to bedtime
    C. a urinary tract infection
    D. possible diabetes insipidus

TABLE 43.1

Drugs Administered for the Treatment of Hypothalamic Hormonal Changes

Drug Class	Prototypes	Other Drugs in the Class
Hypothalamic hormones	Leuprolide acetate (Lupron) Octreotide acetate (Sandostatin, Sandostatin LAR Depot)	Goserelin (Zoladex) Histrelin (Vantas, Supprelin LA) Lanreotide (Somatuline Depot) Nafarelin (Synarel) Pasireotide (Signifor, Signifor LAR) Triptorelin (Trelstar Mixject)

synthesized more drug formulations. Tables 43.1 and 43.2 list the exogenous hormones used in the treatment of hormonal dysfunction.

ANTERIOR PITUITARY HORMONE DRUGS FOR GROWTH DEFICIENCY IN CHILDREN

The prototype anterior pituitary hormone is GH. Administered therapeutically, GH is not natural but rather synthesized from bacteria using recombinant DNA technology. ⓟ **Somatropin** (Genotropin, Humatrope; others) is therapeutically equivalent to endogenous GH produced by the anterior pituitary gland.

Pharmacokinetics

Somatropin is well absorbed. Most of the drug is metabolized in the liver and kidneys. A small amount is excreted unchanged by the kidneys.

Drug Therapy

Although pituitary and hypothalamic hormones have few therapeutic uses, they have important functions when used in certain circumstances. Hypothalamic hormones are synthesized into drug formulations that are administered to treat endometriosis, metastatic breast cancer, advanced prostate cancer, uterine fibroid tumors, vasoactive intestinal tumors, and diarrhea, as well as central precocious puberty. Manufacturers have

Action

Somatropin has the same sequence of amino acids as endogenous GH; it stimulates skeletal, linear, muscle, and organ growth. Stimulation of cartilage growth at the epiphyseal plate promotes linear growth. Lean body mass and bone mass increase, and fat mass decreases. Stimulation of erythropoietin results in an increase of red blood cells. The drug increases protein synthesis and hepatic glucose output. Absorption of nutrients from the GI tract improves.

TABLE 43.2

Drugs Administered for the Treatment of Pituitary Hormonal Changes

Hormone	Hormonal Action
Anterior Pituitary Hormones	
Corticotropin (Acthrel, HP Acthar Gel)	Stimulates the synthesis of hormones by the adrenal cortex
Cosyntropin (Cortrosyn)	Stimulates the adrenal cortex to synthesize and secrete adrenocortical hormones
Follitropin alfa/beta (Follistim AQ, Gonal-F, Gonal-F RFF Redi-Ject)	Stimulates ovulation
Human chorionic gonadotropin (Pregnyl)	Induces ovulation
Menotropins (Menopur)	Induces ovulation
Pegvisomant (Somavert)	GH receptor antagonist
Recombinant chorionic gonadotropin alpha (Ovidrel)	Induces ovulation
Somatropin (Genotropin, Humatrope, Norditropin, Nutropin, Serostim)	Stimulates skeletal, linear, muscle, and organ growth
Thyrotropin alfa (Thyrogen)	Stimulates the secretion of thyroglobulin
Posterior Pituitary Hormones	
Desmopressin (DDAVP, Stimate)	Increases the permeability of kidney tubular epithelium to cAMP leading to concentrated urine
Vasopressin (Vasostrict)	Increases cAMP
Oxytocin (Pitocin)	Increases uterine contractility

Use

The main clinical use of somatropin is for children whose growth is impaired by a deficiency of endogenous GH. The drug is ineffective when impaired growth results from other causes or after puberty, when epiphyses of the long bones have closed. Also, it is useful in the treatment of growth failure associated with chronic kidney disease as well as short stature associated with Turner syndrome, being born small for gestational age, Prader-Willi syndrome, idiopathic short stature, certain genetic mutations, and Noonan syndrome. In addition, somatropin is useful in adults with GH deficiency. Table 43.3 gives route and dosage information for somatropin and other anterior pituitary hormone drugs.

TABLE 43.3
DRUGS AT A GLANCE: Anterior Pituitary Hormone Drugs

Drug	Routes and Dosage Ranges	
	Adults	**Children**
Somatropin (Genotropin, Genotropin MiniQuick, Humatrope, Norditropin FlexPro, Nutropin AQ NuSpin 10, Serostim; Omnitrope, Genotropin GoQuick, Genotropin MiniQuick, Humatrope, Norditropin, NordiFlex, Norditropin Simplex, Nutropin AQ NuSpin, Nutropin AQ pen, Saizen, Serostim)	Initial for patients <60 years of age without diabetes mellitus, glucose intolerance, or obesity: 0.2–0.4 mg/d subcutaneous; in patients transitioning from pediatric treatment, higher doses (e.g., 50% of the dose used in childhood may be needed). Patients >60 years of age with diabetes mellitus, glucose intolerance, or obesity: 0.1–0.2 mg/d subcutaneous FOR SPECIFIC BRAND NAME DOSING REVIEW DRUG INSERT	0.16–0.24 mg/kg/wk subcutaneously divided equally and given 6–7 d/wk
Lonapegsomatropin (Skytrofa)		Children and adolescents weighing >11.5 kg; initial dose 0.24 mg/kg/dose once weekly; round dose to the newest prefilled cartridge as follows: 11.5–<14 kg: 3 mg once weekly 14–<16.5 kg: 3.6 mg once weekly 16.5–<20 kg: 4.3 mg once weekly 20–<24 kg: 5.2 mg once weekly 24–<29 kg: 6.3 mg once weekly 29–<35 kg: 7.6 mg once weekly 35–<42 kg: 9.1 mg once weekly 42–<51 kg: 11 mg once weekly 51–<60.5 kg: 13.3 once weekly 60.5–70 kg: 15.2 once weekly 70–<85 kg: 18.2 mg once weekly 85–100 kg: 22 mg once weekly
Corticotropin (Acthar)	Diagnostic use, up to 80 units IM, subcutaneous as a single injection HP Acthar Gel, 40–80 units IM, subcutaneous every 24–72 h 80–120 units IM daily for 2–3 wk	Infants and children <2 y: 75 units/m²/dose twice daily IM for 2 wk; followed by a gradual taper over a 2-wk period
Cosyntropin (Cortrosyn; Cortrosyn, Synacthen Depot)	0.25 mg IM, IV (equivalent to 25 units ACTH)	Older than 2 y, same as adult dose Younger than 2 y, 0.125 mg IM, IV
Human chorionic gonadotropin (hCG) (Novarel, Pregnyl; Pregnyl)	Ovulation induction: IM: 5,000–10,000 units 1 d following last dose of menotropin Cryptorchidism and male hypogonadism: 500–4,000 units IM 2–3 times per week for several weeks	Preadolescent males, cryptorchidism and hypogonadism: see adult dose
Recombinant chorionic gonadotropin alpha (Ovidrel; Ovidrel)	250 mcg subcutaneous in 1 dose, 1 d after treatment with menotropins	

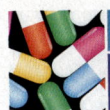

TABLE 43.3
DRUGS AT A GLANCE: Anterior Pituitary Hormone Drugs (Continued)

Drug	Routes and Dosage Ranges	
	Adults	**Children**
Follitropin alfa/beta (Gonal-t, Gonal-F RFF Redi-Ject; 🍁 Gonal-F, Gonal-F Pen)	75 IU subcutaneous of FSH to maximum daily dose of 300 units Prefilled pen, 300–900 IU IV of FSH as individualized dosage	
Menotropins (Menopur; 🍁 Menopur)	Initially 225 units subcutaneously; can be increased to maximum daily dose of 450 units for a maximum of 20 d to be followed by hCG to induce ovulation	
Pegvisomant (Somavert; 🍁 Somavert)	Load, 40 mg subcutaneous Maintenance, 10 mg daily subcutaneous, titrate by 5 mg increments or decrements every 4–6 wk according to IGF-1 levels to maximum of 30 mg/d	
Thyrotropin alfa (Thyrogen; 🍁 Thyrogen)	0.9 mg IM every 24 h for 2 doses or every 72 h for 3 doses	Younger than 16 y, dosage not established

Patient-related variables specific to the use of somatropin include the following:

- Age:
  - Pediatric patients diagnosed with Prader-Willi syndrome who have severe obesity or severe respiratory impairment should not be administered somatropin.
  - Failure to increase the growth rate during the first year of therapy is indicative of the need to assess adherence to treatment and evaluation of the growth failure, such as hypothyroidism, undernutrition, advanced bone age, and antibodies to recombinant human growth hormone.
  - In older adults, reduced dosages may be necessary to minimize adverse effects. Patients who are 65 years of age or older may be more sensitive to the action of GH. Clinicians should avoid using GH in the older adults except as hormone replacement following pituitary gland removal. Treatment should begin at the low end of the dosage range.
- Reproduction, pregnancy, and lactation:
  - Adequate somatropin use prior to conception may improve fertility with hypopituitarism.
  - The Pediatric Endocrine Society guidelines suggest discontinuation of somatropin during pregnancy (Fleserium et al., 2016).
  - Adverse events have not been reported in infants who are breast-fed following maternal use.
- Abnormal kidney function and hepatic impairment:
  - Although chronic abnormal kidney function or severe hepatic disease decreases kidney or hepatic metabolism, respectively, there are no recommended dosing changes in patients with kidney or hepatic dysfunction.
  - Patients on dialysis should take somatropin before bedtime or 3 to 4 hours after the procedure.
  - Children receiving the drug for chronic abnormal kidney function should take it until kidney transplantation.
- Specific healthcare environments:
  - Somatropin should not be initiated in patients with acute critical illness because of complications following open heart or abdominal surgery, trauma, or acute respiratory failure. Increased mortality may occur.

Adverse Effects

Adverse effects are not common and are fewer in children than in adults. Mild edema, headache, localized muscle pain, weakness, and hyperglycemia may occur. Patients with diabetes are more likely to develop hyperglycemia; they require close monitoring, and diabetic medications may require adjustment. Antibodies to the drug may develop, but this does not interfere with its growth-stimulating effects. Otitis media may occur in children. Hypersensitivity reactions are possible.

Patients with chronic kidney failure, Turner syndrome, and Prader–Willi syndrome are at increased risk for intracranial hypertension; symptoms include headache, papilledema, visual changes, nausea, and vomiting. When intracranial hypertension occurs, it is important to stop treatment, but it is appropriate to start the drugs again after symptoms resolve.

A special set of warnings accompanies the use of somatropin in treating short stature in patients with Prader–Willi syndrome. Fatalities have been reported following the use of somatropin in these patients. Risk factors associated with these fatalities are severe obesity, sleep apnea, respiratory impairment, respiratory infection, and male sex. It is essential to discontinue use of somatropin if any signs of upper airway obstruction occur or if snoring develops or increases.

Contraindications

Contraindications to somatropin include closed epiphyses, preproliferative or severe nonproliferative diabetic retinopathy, active malignancy, acute critical illness (as described previously), or active underlying intracranial lesions. Patients with Prader-Willi syndrome who have severe obesity or severe respiratory impairment should not take the drug.

Caution is necessary in hypothyroidism, GH deficiency caused by intracranial lesions, and diabetes.

Nursing Implications

Preventing Interactions

Long-term use of corticotropin or corticosteroids inhibits the growth response to somatropin. Patients require monitoring to determine this lack of effect. Somatropin decreases insulin sensitivity, resulting in hyperglycemia. Patients most at risk for increased insulin sensitivity are those with obesity, Turner syndrome, or a family history of diabetes mellitus. Antihyperglycemic drugs may require dosage adjustments.

Administering the Medication

Administration may be subcutaneous or intramuscular (IM). The subcutaneous route is preferred; here are guidelines for its use:

- To prepare the solution, inject the supplied diluent into the vial containing the drug by aiming the stream of liquid against the glass wall of the vial.
- Swirl the vial gently. Do not shake it.
- After reconstitution, make sure the solution is clear. Do not inject a cloudy solution.
- Rotate injection sites.
- Store the reconstituted drug in the refrigerator; use within the time period recommended by the manufacturer.
- If the patient develops sensitivity to the diluent, reconstitute the drug with sterile water for injection. When administering the drug to infants, use only sterile water as the diluent. With sterile water, administer only one dose per vial and use the reconstituted drug within 24 hours; discard any unused portion.
- There is a preservative-free form of somatropin. Not all forms are approved for IM injection.
- Administer the correct dosage daily.

For patients on hemodialysis, give the drug before bedtime or 3 to 4 hours after dialysis. For long-term cycling peritoneal dialysis, give the drug in the morning after completion of dialysis. For long-term ambulatory dialysis, give the drug in the evening at the time of the overnight exchange.

Quality and Safety Alert: Safety

When administering somatropin, it is essential that after one nurse calculates the dosage, another nurse rechecks the calculation.

Assessing for Therapeutic Effects

The nurse observes for increased skeletal growth and development. Appropriate increases in height and weight should occur. It is necessary to measure the child's height frequently. The child should take somatropin until a satisfactory height has been achieved, epiphyseal closure occurs, or until no further stimulation of growth occurs. Periodic tests of growth curve and bone age are also important.

BOX 43.1 Patient Teaching Guidelines for Somatropin

Parent or Caregiver Information

- Keep appointments for all follow-up visits and diagnostic tests.
- Report any lack of growth to the healthcare practitioner.
- Report any new-onset limping or hip or knee pain.
- Monitor the glucose level as ordered by the healthcare practitioner.
- Administer the medication subcutaneously or intramuscularly and rotate sites to prevent tissue damage.

Assessing for Adverse Effects

It is important to have periodic tests of serum glucose levels and thyroid function as well as frequent eye examinations. Monitoring of serum and urine calcium should occur. Hypercalciuria may develop within 2 to 3 months after the start of therapy. Assess the patient for flank pain and colic. Patients who fail to respond to somatropin should receive testing for GH antibodies. Children who have GH deficiency may develop slipped capital femoral epiphyses more frequently, and those with scoliosis may see a progression of the condition. The nurse assesses the patient for severe hip or knee pain or the development of a limp.

The nurse carefully assesses patients with malignancies or GH deficiency secondary to an intracranial lesion to ensure that enlargement or recurrence of the lesion is not occurring. Reportedly, there is an increased risk of a second neoplasm in adults who had cancer as children and who have been treated with somatropin. It is necessary to monitor patients with Prader–Willi syndrome carefully for signs of respiratory infection.

Patient Teaching

Box 43.1 presents patient teaching information for somatropin.

Other Drugs in the Class

Lonapegsomatropin (Skytrofa) is a long-acting pegylated prodrug of a human growth hormone. It assists in linear bone, skeletal muscle, and organ growth through the stimulation of chondrocyte proliferation and differentiation, lipolysis, protein synthesis, and hepatic glucose output stimulating erythropoietin to increase red blood cell mass. It exerts both insulin-like and diabetogenic effects, thus producing an elevation in blood-glucose concentration.

Other Anterior Pituitary Hormone Drugs

Corticotropin (HP Acthar Gel), which is obtained from animal pituitary glands, is mainly of historical interest. Corticotropin (ACTH) is effective in treating infantile seizures in patients 2 months to 2 years of age. For therapeutic purposes, adrenal corticosteroids have replaced it. It may be used occasionally as a diagnostic test to differentiate primary adrenal insufficiency (Addison disease, which is associated with atrophy of the adrenal gland) from secondary adrenal insufficiency caused by inadequate pituitary secretion of corticotropin. However, cosyntropin (Cortrosyn), a synthetic formulation, is more commonly used to test for suspected adrenal insufficiency (see Chapter 45).

> **Quality and Safety Alert: Patient-Centered Care**
>
> Acute relapses of multiple sclerosis with new or worsening neurologic symptoms that persist for greater than 24 hours and are not attributable to heat overexertion or infection can be treated with repository corticotropin injection. This treatment is particularly beneficial in patients who are allergic to corticosteroid therapy. The exact mechanism of action of the drug is unknown, but it has been attributed to its ability to stimulate the adrenal corticosteroids, leading to an indirect modulation of multiple inflammatory processes.

Human chorionic gonadotropin (hCG) produces physiologic effects similar to those of naturally occurring LH. In males, it is used to evaluate the ability of Leydig cells to produce testosterone, to treat hypogonadism caused by pituitary deficiency, and to treat cryptorchidism (undescended testicle) in preadolescent males. In females, recombinant hCG choriogonadotropin alpha (Ovidrel) is used in combination with menotropins to induce ovulation in the treatment of infertility. Excessive doses or prolonged administration can lead to sexual precocity, edema, and breast enlargement caused by oversecretion of testosterone and estrogen (see Chapter 6).

Menotropins (Menopur) are available in a gonadotropin preparation obtained from the urine of postmenopausal women that contains both FSH and LH. The drug is usually combined with hCG to induce ovulation in the treatment of infertility caused by lack of pituitary gonadotropins (see Chapter 6).

Pegvisomant (Somavert) is a GH receptor antagonist used in the treatment of acromegaly in adults who are unable to tolerate or are resistant to other management strategies. The drug selectively binds to GH receptors, blocking the binding of endogenous GH. In general, it is necessary to individualize the dosage according to response. Dosage reduction of hypoglycemic agents may be required because the drug may increase glucose tolerance. Increased dosages of pegvisomant may be necessary when administered with narcotics. Caution is warranted in older adults and in kidney or hepatic disease. At the initiation of therapy, baseline liver function tests should be assessed. Liver function should be assessed monthly for the first 6 months, quarterly for the next 6 months, and biannually the following year.

Thyrotropin alfa (Thyrogen) is a synthetic formulation of TSH used as a diagnostic adjunct for serum thyroglobulin testing in people with well-differentiated thyroid cancer who have previously undergone a thyroidectomy. The test may or may not involve radioiodine imaging, because there is a risk of missing the diagnosis of thyroid cancer. Thyroid hormone withdrawal thyroglobulin testing radioactive imaging is the standard test for evaluating the presence, extent, and location of thyroid cancer. Thyrotropin alfa requires caution in patients with coronary artery disease and with a large amount of residual thyroid tissue; the drug produces a temporary rise of thyroid hormone concentration in the blood.

Follitropin alfa and beta (Gonal-F) are drug preparations of FSH. The purpose of these drugs is to stimulate ovarian function in the treatment of infertility, and females may take them sequentially with hCG. Follitropin alfa and follitropin beta are recombinant products that appear to be well tolerated and have similar efficacy. A new liquid formulation of follitropin alfa/beta (Gonal-F RFF Redi-ject) is available in a prefilled and ready-to-use multidose FSH injection (see Chapter 6).

> **NCLEX Success**
>
> 2. A male child with type 1 diabetes mellitus receives a prescription for somatropin. How will this medication affect the child's insulin needs?
>   A. His insulin needs will decrease.
>   B. He will need a sulfonylurea added to his insulin.
>   C. His insulin needs will remain the same.
>   D. His insulin needs will increase.
>
> 3. A female child is taking somatropin. Her mother asks the nurse when her daughter will no longer need the medication. Which of the following is the nurse's best response?
>   A. It will be stopped if she develops obesity.
>   B. It will be stopped when she has stopped growing.
>   C. It will be stopped when she no longer wants to take the medication.
>   D. It will be stopped if she has a test showing that the epiphysis of the bone is open.

POSTERIOR PITUITARY HORMONE DRUGS FOR DIABETES INSIPIDUS

Desmopressin acetate (DDAVP, Stimate) is the prototype posterior pituitary hormone medication. It is a synthetic analog of ADH. It reduces urine volume and serum osmolality in patients with diabetes insipidus. It increases the reabsorption of water by the kidney.

Pharmacokinetics

For the intranasal form, the onset of action is 15 to 30 minutes, and the peak of action is 60 to 90 minutes. For the intravenous (IV) form, the onset of action is 30 minutes, and peak of action is 1.5 to 2 hours. For the oral form, the onset of action is 60 minutes, and the peak of action is 60 to 90 minutes. For the subcutaneous form, the onset of action, peak of action, and duration of action are unknown. For all forms, the duration of action is approximately 6 to 14 hours. The half-life of the intranasal, IV and subcutaneous, and oral preparations is approximately 3.5, 3, and 2 to 3 hours, respectively. Elimination of all forms of the medication takes place in the urine.

Action

Desmopressin increases cyclic adenosine monophosphate (cAMP) in the cells of the kidney tubule to increase the water permeability, decreasing urine volume and increasing its osmolality. The drug increases the plasma level of von Willebrand factor, clotting factor VIII, and tissue plasminogen activator (a protein involved in the breakdown of blood clots) to shorten the activated partial thromboplastin and bleeding times.

Use

The main clinical use for desmopressin is for the treatment of neurogenic diabetes insipidus. However, synthetic hormones are useful for other purposes. Table 43.4 contains route and dosage information for desmopressin and other posterior pituitary hormones.

TABLE 43.4

DRUGS AT A GLANCE: Posterior Pituitary Hormone Drugs

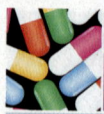

Drug	Routes and Dosage Ranges	
	Adults	**Children**
ⓟ **Desmopressin** (DDAVP, Stimate; 🍁 DDAVP, Apo-Desmopressin)	Diabetes insipidus: intranasally 0.1–0.4 mL/d, in 1–3 doses, or, give 0.5–1 mL, IV or subcutaneously daily in two divided doses. For PO administration to adults and children over 4 y of age: Initially, 0.05 mg, orally twice daily Hemophilia A, von Willebrand disease: IV 0.3 mcg/kg in 50 mL sterile saline, infused over 15–30 min (if used preoperatively give 30 min prior to procedure)	Diabetes insipidus: 3 mo to 12 y, 0.05–0.3 mL/d in 1–2 doses intranasally Hemophilia A, von Willebrand disease: Weight more than 10 kg, same as adult dosage Weight 10 kg or less, 0.3 mcg/kg IV in 10 mL of sterile saline
Vasopressin (Vasostrict)	0.25–0.5 mL (5–10 units) IM, subcutaneously, intranasally on cotton pledgets 2–3 times daily	0.125–0.5 mL (2.5–10 units) IM, subcutaneously, intranasally on cotton pledgets 3–4 times daily
Oxytocin (Pitocin; 🍁 Oxytocic Agent)	Induction of labor: initially, 10 units in 1,000 mL of D_5W, lactated Ringer's, or normal saline infused IV at 0.5–2 mU/min titrated every 30–60 min until 9–10 mU/min or normal contraction pattern has been achieved Postpartum hemorrhage: 10–40 units in 1,000 mL of D_5W, lactated Ringer's, or normal saline, IV, infused at rate to control bleeding, not to exceed 40 mU/min	

Patient-related variables specific to the use of desmopressin include the following:

- Age:
  - When administering intranasal desmopressin in children, ensure that the nasal passages are intact, clean, and free of obstruction prior to administration.
- Reproduction, pregnancy, and lactation:
  - Pregnant patients being treated with desmopressin for diabetes insipidus should continue treatment.
  - Desmopressin is present in breast milk. The decision to breast-feed during therapy should consider the risk of infant exposure. Desmopressin is considered acceptable for use during breast-feeding.
- Abnormal kidney function and hepatic impairment:
  - A creatinine clearance less than 50 mL/minutes contraindicates the use of desmopressin.

Adverse Effects and Contraindications

Adverse effects of desmopressin reportedly occur in less than 5% of cases. The most common effects are erythema, swelling, and burning of the parenteral injection site. Other adverse effects include drowsiness, headache, dizziness, lethargy, shortness of breath, gastric irritation with heartburn, abdominal cramping, vulval pain, nasal congestion, and nasal irritation. The U.S. Food and Drug Administration (FDA) has issued a **BOXED WARNING** stating that severe hyponatremia may develop as a result of the medication, leading to seizures and death. Another **BOXED WARNING** stipulates that changes in fluid volume status may result in cardiac arrest in patients with known cardiovascular disease.

Contraindications include hypersensitivity to the drug or any component of its formulation. A creatinine clearance less than 50 mL/minutes contraindicates the use of desmopressin

Nursing Implications

Preventing Interactions

Several medications interact with desmopressin, increasing or decreasing its effects (Box 43.2).

Administering the Medication

Guidelines for administration are as follows:

- Use the IM, IV, and subcutaneous preparations for central diabetes insipidus. Withdraw the dosage from the ampule and administer it using a small gage needle and syringe (e.g., an insulin syringe).
- For hemophilia A, von Willebrand disease (type 1), and prevention of surgical bleeding in patients with uremia, dilute in normal saline solution and infuse over 15 to 30 minutes.
- For intranasal administration, ensure that nasal passages are intact, clean, and free of obstruction before giving intranasally. The nasal spray pump delivers only doses of 10 mcg DDAVP. If doses other than these are necessary, use the nasal tube delivery system as directed below.

BOX 43.2 Drug Interactions: Desmopressin

Drugs That Increase the Effects of Desmopressin
- Carbamazepine and chlorpropamide
  Increase the risk of antidiuretic effects
- Selective serotonin reuptake inhibitors and tricyclic antidepressants
  Increase the risk of hyponatremia

Drugs That Decrease the Effects of Desmopressin
- Alcohol
  Decreases the diuretic effect

- Insert the top of the dropper into the tube in a downward position. Then squeeze the dropper until the solution reaches the desired calibrated dose and disconnect the dropper.
- Hold the tube 3/4 in. from the end and insert one end into the nostril until the fingertips reach the nostril. Place the opposite end into the patient's mouth while the patient holds their breath.
- Have the patient tilt the head back and blow into the tube, and into the nostril, with a strong, short puff. (In children, the nurse or an adult needs to blow into the tube.)

Assessing for Therapeutic Effects

The desired therapeutic effects are decreased urine output, increased urine specific gravity, decreased signs of dehydration, and decreased thirst. It is important to assess the serum electrolytes, particularly the sodium and potassium levels. The sodium level should be 135 to 145 mEq/L. The nurse assesses serum osmolality; it should be in the normal range of 285 to 295 mOsm/kg H_2O. It is necessary to interview the patient to determine if they are thirsty. The nurse assesses skin turgor, mucous membranes, and production of tears for signs of rehydration. In patients with von Willebrand disease, it is important to determine the factor VIII coagulant effect; the normal factor VIII is 55% to 145%.

Assessing for Adverse Effects

The nurse assesses for hyponatremia, which can lead to diminished mental status and seizures. Serum osmolality may be less than 285 mOsm/kg H_2O. It is also necessary to assess fluid volume status for signs of dehydration, as well as urine output and urine specific gravity. Also, the nurse assesses the parenteral injection site for rash or erythema.

Patient Teaching

Box 43.3 presents patient teaching information for desmopressin.

Clinical Application 43.2

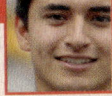

When providing patient teaching to Mr. Rojas:
- What are the signs and symptoms of diabetes insipidus?
- What is the action of desmopressin?
- What is the therapeutic effect of desmopressin?
- How does the nurse administer desmopressin intranasally using a nasal tube?

Other Posterior Pituitary Hormone Drugs

Vasopressin (Vasostrict) had been used off-label for the treatment of central diabetes insipidus, although it has since been discontinued. However, the Vasostrict formulation is used to increase blood pressure in patients experiencing septic or postcardiotomy syndrome. Patients with postcardiotomy syndrome have a febrile illness with inflammation of the pleura or pericardium. This condition can also occur following a myocardial infarction with the placement of a pacemaker. Therapeutically, vasopressin replaces ADH; the drug increases tubular reabsorption of water. It stimulates the arginine vasopressin, oxytocin, and purinergic receptors. The stimulation of these receptors yields an increase in systemic vascular resistance and mean arterial blood pressure to decrease the heart rate. In addition, the stimulation of the receptors causes an increase in cAMP, which in turn increases water permeability, decreasing urine output.

Oxytocin (Pitocin) is a synthetic drug that exerts the same physiologic effects as the posterior pituitary hormone. Thus, it promotes uterine contractility and is used clinically to induce labor and in the postpartum period to control bleeding. It is essential that oxytocin be used only when clearly indicated and when the patient can be supervised by well-trained personnel, as in a hospital (see Chapter 6).

BOX 43.3 Patient Teaching Guidelines for Desmopressin

- Report drowsiness, headache, dizziness, lethargy, shortness of breath, gastric irritation with heartburn, abdominal cramping, vulval pain, nasal congestion, and nasal irritation to the health care provider.
- When using the DDAVP nasal spray pump, insert the top of the dropper into the tube in a downward position. Squeeze the dropper until the solution reaches the desired calibrated dose and disconnect the dropper. Then hold the tube 3/4 in. from the end and insert it into the nostril until the fingertips reach the nostril. Place the opposite end of the tube in the mouth while holding your breath. Tilt the head back and blow into the tube with a strong, short puff into the nostril.
- When administering subcutaneously, rotate injection sites.

NCLEX Success

4. A patient has just received desmopressin. Which electrolyte is most important to assess?
   A. sodium
   B. chloride
   C. potassium
   D. calcium

HYPOTHALAMIC HORMONE DRUGS

DRUGS FOR CENTRAL PRECOCIOUS PUBERTY

Leuprolide acetate (Eligard, Lupron) is equivalent to gonadotropin-releasing hormone (GnRH). The drug is more potent than the natural hormone.

Pharmacokinetics

Leuprolide has a transient onset of action. The drug is 43% to 49% protein-bound. It is metabolized to pentapeptide in the hypothalamus and anterior pituitary and is excreted in the urine.

Action

An LH-releasing hormone agonist, leuprolide acts as a potent inhibitor of gonadotropin secretion, thus suppressing production of ovarian and testicular steroids. This action decreases LH and FSH to decrease testosterone in males and estrogen in females. (Testosterone levels are below levels required for reproduction.)

Use

Leuprolide is useful for the treatment of central precocious puberty in children. Experts recommended that the drug be administered to females until age 11 and males until age 12. Other uses include treatment of advanced prostate cancer, endometriosis, and uterine fibroids. Table 43.5 gives the route and dosage information for the hypothalamic hormones.

Patient-related variables specific to the use of leuprolide include the following:

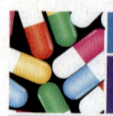

TABLE 43.5
DRUGS AT A GLANCE: Hypothalamic Hormones

Drug	Routes and Dosage Ranges	
	Adults	**Children**
ⓟ **Leuprolide acetate** (Camcevi, Eligard, Lupron Depot, Fensolvi; ✹ Eligard, Lupron, Lupron Depot)	Advanced prostate cancer: 1 mg subcutaneously daily Endometriosis: 3.75 mg IM depot injection once monthly for up to 6 mo or 11.25 mg IM every 3 mo for up to 6 mo Uterine fibroids: 3.75 mg IM depot injection once monthly for up to 3 consecutive mo or 11.25 mg IM depot injection for 1 dose	Central precocious puberty: Dosing regimens and route of administration may vary; carefully review drug inserts Lupron Depot: <25 kg: Initial: IM 7.5 mg every 4 wk; titrate dose in 3.75 mg increments every 4 wk until clinical or laboratory tests indicate adequate suppression >25–37.5 kg: Initial: IM 11.25 mg every 4 wk; titrate dose in 3.75 mg increments every 4 wk until clinical or laboratory tests indicate adequate suppression >37.5 kg: Initial: IM 15 mg every 4 wk; titrate dose in 3.75 mg increments every 4 wk until clinical or laboratory tests indicate suppression Long-acting formulation: Fensolvi: subcutaneous: 45 mg every 6 mo
ⓟ **Octreotide acetate** (SandoSTATIN, SandoSTATIN LAR; ✹ Sandostatin LAR)	Acromegaly: 50–100 mcg subcutaneous or IV 3 times daily; long-acting, give 20 mg, IM (intragluteally), at 4-wk intervals for 3 mo	Hypothalamic obesity: Children >8 years-adolescents: 5 mcg/kg/d in 3 divided doses may be increased bimonthly at 5 mcg/kg/d: Maximum dose: 15 mcg/kg/d in 3 divided doses daily
Goserelin (Zoladex; ✹ Zoladex, Zoladex LA)	Advanced prostate cancer: Implant into upper abdominal wall, Advanced breast cancer: 3.6 mg subcutaneously every 28 d or 10.8 mg SC every 3 mo	
Histrelin (Vantas, Supprelin LA)	Prostate cancer: 50 mg subcutaneous implant inserted every 12 mo	Central precocious puberty: Children >2 years: 50 mg subcutaneous implant every 12 mo; discontinue at the appropriate time for the onset of puberty
Lanreotide (Somatuline Depot; ✹ Somatuline Autogel)	Subcutaneous: initial dose 90 mg once every 4 wk for 3 mo; after initial 90 d of therapy, adjust dose based on clinical response	≥16 y: refer to adult dosing
Nafarelin (Synarel; ✹ Synarel)	Endometriosis: 1 spray (200 mcg) in one nostril in the morning and 1 spray in the other nostril in the evening (400 mcg/d), starting between the 2nd and 4th day of the menstrual cycle If regular menstruation persists after 2 mo, may increase dose to 2 sprays in the morning and evening; total duration of therapy not to exceed 6 mo	Central precocious puberty: 2 sprays (400 mcg) in each nostril morning and evening (1,600 mcg/d), until resumption of puberty is desired
Pasireotide (Signifor LAR; ✹ Signifor LAR)	Initial 40 mg IM once every 28 d for patients who have not normalized IGF-1 levels after 3 mo; increase to a maximum dose of 60 mg	Dosage not established
Triptorelin (Trelstar Mixject, Triptodur; ✹ Trelstar, Decapeptyl)	Advanced prostate carcinoma: 3.75 mg once every 4 wk, 11.25 mg once every 12 wk, or 22.5 mg once every 24 wk IM Controlled ovarian hyperstimulation for assisted reproductive technologies: 0.1 mg subcutaneously once daily initiated on day 2 or 3 or days 21–23 of menstrual cycle	Central precocious puberty: Children >2 years: Triptodur IM 22.5 mg once every 24 wk; discontinue therapy at appropriate age of onset of puberty

- Age:
  - In pediatric and adult patients, do not use a fractional dose of the 3-, 4-, or 6-month depot formulation, or a combination of doses of the monthly depot formulation or any depot formulation due to different release characteristics. Do not use a combination of syringes to achieve a particular dose. Do not administer IV.
- Reproduction, pregnancy, and lactation:
  - Treatment with leuprolide usually inhibits ovulation and stops menstruation; however, contraception is not ensured. Non-hormonal contraception is recommended.
  - Evaluate pregnancy status prior to use and throughout treatment in patients who could become pregnant.
  - Leuprolide will cause fetal harm.
  - It is not known if leuprolide enters breast milk.
- Abnormal kidney function and hepatic impairment:
  - No dosage adjustments are needed with abnormal kidney function or hepatic impairment.

Adverse Effects and Contraindications

The most common adverse effect of leuprolide is pain at the injection site. Less than 2% of the people who receive the drug have reported vasodilation, labile emotions, rash, acne, and allergic reaction. In the postmarketing phase of leuprolide use, seizures have been reported with the use of long-acting leuprolide. Patients aged 65 and older are prone to drug-related QT prolongation. Decreased bone density has been confirmed in adults taking leuprolide. There are conflicting data regarding bone density in children.

Contraindications include known hypersensitivity to the medication's formulation, GnRH, or GnRH antagonists.

Nursing Implications

Preventing Interactions

Leuprolide may decrease the therapeutic effect of antidiabetic drugs, resulting in hyperglycemia.

Administering the Medication

Administration of Lupron Depot should occur as a single injection. The depot suspension is stable for 24 hours after reconstitution. It is important to rotate the injection sites and not to use areas of the body that are compressed or rubbed.

Assessing for Therapeutic Effects

The nurse assesses for a decrease in mature sexual characteristics. Gonadotropins (testosterone in males; estrogen in females) should decrease to prepubertal levels. These effects occur within 2 to 4 weeks after therapy has begun.

Assessing for Adverse Effects

The nurse assesses for pain at the injection sites. It is also necessary to assess for signs of a hypersensitivity reaction to the medication, such as a rash or erythema.

Patient Teaching

Box 43.4 presents patient teaching information for leuprolide.

> **BOX 43.4 Patient Teaching Guidelines for Leuprolide**
>
> - Administer the medication subcutaneously or intramuscularly.
> - Use a calendar to mark the dates of future injections.
> - Report any pain, burning, itching, or tingling of the injection site to the healthcare provider.
> - Patients prescribed leuprolide who are sexually active should use a nonhormonal form of birth control.

Other Hypothalamic Hormone Drugs

Goserelin (Zoladex), histrelin (Vantas), nafarelin (Synarel), and triptorelin (Trelstar Mixject) are equivalent to GnRH. After initial stimulation of LH and FSH secretion, chronic administration of therapeutic doses inhibits gonadotropin secretion. This action results in decreased production of testosterone and estrogen, which is reversible when administration is stopped. In children with central precocious puberty, gonadotropins decline to prepubertal levels. As with leuprolide, these effects occur within 2 to 4 weeks of beginning drug treatment.

Oral administration of these GnRH equivalents is ineffective, because enzymes in the GI tract destroy the medication. Administration of most of these drugs is by injection; they are available in depot preparations that nurses can give once a month (or less often). Adverse effects are basically those of testosterone or estrogen deficiency. The drugs may also cause or aggravate depression.

DRUGS FOR ACROMEGALY

Octreotide acetate (Sandostatin, Sandostatin LAR Depot) has pharmacologic actions similar to the anterior pituitary hormone somatostatin. Scientists first synthesized this somatostatin analog in 1979.

Pharmacokinetics

Octreotide is rapidly and completely absorbed when given IV and subcutaneously with a rapid onset and a peak in 30 minutes. It is released slowly in the microsphere of the muscle; therefore, when given intramuscularly, the onset and duration are unknown, but the peak occurs in 1 to 2 weeks. Its half-life is 1.5 hours. Octreotide is metabolized in the liver and excreted by the kidneys.

Action

Octreotide mimics the natural hormone somatostatin by inhibiting serotonin release. The drug also inhibits gastrin, vasoactive intestinal peptide, insulin, glucagon, secretin, motilin, and pancreatic polypeptide. In acromegaly, it suppresses GH and IGF-1. In fact, octreotide inhibits GH, glucagon, and insulin more than endogenous somatostatin. The drug also suppresses LH response to GnRH and the secretion of thyroid-stimulating hormone (TSH).

Use

Prescribers order octreotide for patients with acromegaly to reduce levels of GH. In addition, they use it to (1) treat secretory diarrhea and GI bleeding and (2) inhibit tumor GH and solid tumors. Table 43.5 presents route and dosage information for this drug.

Patient-related variables specific to the use of octreotide acetate include the following:

- Age:
  - All pediatric dosing is based on the immediate release non-long-acting injection solution.
  - Serious and fatal adverse effects have been reported in pediatric patients. IV doses have resulted in bradycardia. Most severe events or death occurred in neonates, infants, and children under the age of 2.
  - In older adults, the LAR depot suspension and injection solution has an increased half-life by 46% and clearance is decreased by 26%. Dosing should be at the lowest end of the dosage range.
- Reproduction, pregnancy, and lactation:
  - Octreotide may be used in patients with acromegaly who are trying to conceive. It should be discontinued once pregnancy is confirmed.
  - If control of acromegaly symptoms is required during pregnancy, the short-acting octreotide is recommended.
  - Octreotide is present in breast milk.
- Abnormal kidney function and hepatic impairment:
  - Patients on kidney dialysis require a reduced dosage of the drug by 50%.
  - For those with cirrhosis of the liver, the initial dosage should be 10 mg intramuscularly over 4 weeks. The dosage is titrated weekly based on the patient's response.

Adverse Effects

Octreotide may cause CNS effects such as headache, dizziness, light-headedness, and fatigue. Cardiac effects such as bradycardia and heart failure may also occur. Other effects include hyperglycemia, pruritus, abdominal pain, loose stools, nausea, and cholelithiasis. Reportedly, approximately 20% of patients report back pain, myalgia, upper respiratory infections, and shortness of breath.

Contraindications

Contraindications to octreotide include a known hypersensitivity to the drug or any component of the formulation. It is important to use the drug cautiously in patients with pancreatitis, gallbladder or bile disorders, cardiac abnormalities, diabetes, or nutritional disorders; the medication may cause or exacerbate these conditions.

Nursing Implications
Preventing Interactions

The combination of octreotide with alfuzosin, artemether, chloroquine, ciprofloxacin, dronedarone, indacaterol, levofloxacin, lumefantrine, pimozide, propafenone, quetiapine, quinine, tetrabenazine, thioridazine, toremifene, vandetanib, vemurafenib, and ziprasidone results in a prolonged QTc with an increased risk of ventricular dysrhythmia and cardiac arrest. The combination of octreotide and codeine increases the metabolism of codeine, and the combination of cyclosporine and octreotide decreases the serum concentration of cyclosporine. The administration of octreotide with food may alter the absorption of dietary fats. The following herbs and foods increase the effects of octreotide: alfalfa, aloe, bilberry, bitter melon, burdack, celery, damiana, fenugreek, garcinia, garlic, ginger, ginseng, gymnema, marshmallow, and stinging nettle.

Administering the Medication

Administration is by injection. It is important to administer the medication between meals to prevent fat malabsorption. Storage of the ampules requires refrigeration. For IV administration, dilute in 50 to 200 mL 5% dextrose in water or normal saline and infuse over 15 to 30 minutes. It may be given by IV push over 3 minutes.

With a depot injection, administration should occur immediately after the medication is mixed. The nurse administers the depot injections intramuscularly, deep in the intragluteal site—never in the deltoid. With an IM or subcutaneous injection, the sites of administration are rotated.

It is necessary to withdraw the drug for 4 weeks once per year.

Assessing for Therapeutic Effects

The nurse assesses for diminished bone growth. The patient is interviewed to determine if headaches and visual changes have subsided. Also, it is necessary to assess females for a decrease in hot flashes and regulation of the menstrual cycle.

Assessing for Adverse Effects

The nurse assesses for alertness (e.g., Is there any fatigue?) and interviews the patient about headache or light-headedness. The nurse checks the blood glucose for glucose tolerance. Approximately 2% to 27% of patients develop hyperglycemia. Also, the nurse assesses the heart rate for bradycardia and an audible S_3, indicating the onset of heart failure. In addition, the patient is assessed for abdominal pain, nausea, or pain between the shoulder blades, indicating the onset of cholelithiasis. Finally, it is important to check for musculoskeletal pain, fever, cough, and congestion, including the respiratory rate and effort that indicates the onset of shortness of breath.

Patient Teaching

Box 43.5 presents patient teaching information for octreotide.

Other Drugs in the Class

Lanreotide (Somatuline Depot) is administered subcutaneously for the treatment of acromegaly and gastroenteropancreatic neuroendocrine tumor. It is important to assess for GI symptoms. It was reported that 20% of patients experience gallbladder-related symptoms and cholelithiasis.

Pasireotide (Signifor, Signifor LAR) is administered deep intramuscularly for acromegaly and Cushing disease. The nurse

BOX 43.5 Patient Teaching Guidelines for Octreotide

- Administer the medication subcutaneously or intramuscularly.
- Contact the healthcare provider to determine the time for withdrawal of the medication. It should be withdrawn for 4 weeks one time per year.
- Have follow-up diagnostic tests and keep the schedule of those tests.
- Monitor blood glucose.
- Notify the healthcare provider if abdominal pain or pain between the shoulder blades develops.
- Have follow-up gallbladder ultrasounds to detect cholelithiasis.

assesses for elevation of aspartate aminotransferase and alanine aminotransferase as well as for bradycardia and QT prolongation. Hazardous drug handling protocols must be in place to administer this medication. When doing the receipt of the drug, unpacking the drug, and storing it, gloves must be worn.

Quality and Safety Alert: Evidence Based-Practice

Sahin et al. (2022) conducted a study of 150 patients diagnosed with acromegaly being treated with somatostatin receptor ligand. The study revealed patients suffered from vitamin B_{12} deficiency. Thus, it is important to monitor and assess patients treated with somatostatin receptor ligand for vitamin B_{12} deficiency.

NCLEX Success

5. A patient with acromegaly is planning a trip to South Africa. The patient is taking chloroquine to prevent malaria and octreotide for acromegaly. What is the patient at risk for developing?
   A. diarrhea
   B. ventricular dysrhythmia
   C. hepatotoxicity
   D. urinary retention

THE NURSING PROCESS

A concept map outlines the nursing process related to drug therapy considerations in this chapter. Additional nursing implications related to the disease process should also be considered in care decisions.

Assessment
- Assess for disorders for which hypothalamic and pituitary hormones are given.
- Assess for the following:
  - For children with impaired growth, assess height and weight (actual and compared with growth charts) and diagnostic radiographic reports of bone age.
  - For patients with diabetes insipidus, assess baseline blood pressure, weight, ratio of fluid intake to urine output, urine specific gravity, and laboratory reports of serum electrolytes.

Outcomes of Therapy

The patient will
- Experience relief of symptoms without serious adverse effects.
- Take or receive the drug accurately.
- Adhere to procedures for monitoring and follow-up.

Nursing Interventions
- For children receiving GH, help the family set reasonable goals for increased height and weight and comply with accurate drug administration and follow-up procedures (e.g., periodic radiographs to determine bone growth and progress toward epiphyseal closure; recording height and weight at least weekly).
- For patients with diabetes insipidus, help them develop a daily routine to monitor their response to drug therapy (e.g., weigh themselves; monitor fluid intake and urine output for approximately equal amounts; check urine specific gravity [should be at least 1.015] and replace fluids accordingly).

Evaluation
- Interview and observe for adherence to instructions for taking the drug(s).
- Observe for relief of symptoms for which pituitary hormones were prescribed.
- Observe for effective coping with the underlying condition and the effects of treatment.

Visit thePoint® at http://thePoint.lww.com/Frandsen13e for answers to NCLEX Success questions (in Appendix A), answers to Clinical Application Case Studies (in Appendix B), physiology of anterior pituitary hormones, posterior pituitary hormones, and hypothalamic hormones, and more!

REFERENCES AND RESOURCES

Bichet, D. G. (2021). Urine output in diabetes insipidus. *UpToDate*. Lexi-Comp, Inc.

Fleseriu, M., Hashim, I. A., Karavitakie, N., et al. (2016). Hormonal replaced in hypopituitarism in adults: An Endocrine Society Clinical Practice Guideline. *Journal of Clinical Endocrinal Metabolism. 101*(11), 3888–3921. https://doi.org/10.1210/jc.2016-2118.

Hashim, I. A., Karavitaki, N., Melmed, S., Murad, M. H., Salvatori, R., & Samuels, M. H. (2016). Hormonal replacement in hypopituitarism in adults: An Endocrine Society clinical practice guideline. *Journal of Clinical Endocrinology Metabolism, 9*(1), 64–76.

Harrington, J., & Palmert, M. R. (2022). Definition, etiology, and evaluation of precocious puberty. In *UpToDate*. Lexi-Comp, Inc.

Hinkle, J. H., Cheever, K. H., & Overbaugh, K. J. (2021). *Brunner & Suddarth's textbook of medical-surgical nursing* (15th ed.). Wolters Kluwer.

Liddle, R. A. (2021). Physiology of somatostatin and its analogues. In *UpToDate*. Lexi-Comp, Inc.

Melmed, S., & Katzneson, L. (2021). Diagnosis of acromegaly. In *UpToDate*. Lexi-Comp, Inc.

Norris, T. L. (2019). *Porth's pathophysiology concepts of altered health states* (10th ed.). Wolters Kluwer.

Pediatric Endocrinology Fact Sheet. (2020). Precocious puberty: A guide to families. *Pediatric Endocrine Society*. Retrieved February 25, 2023. https://pedsendo.org/wp-content/uploads/2020/06/E-Precocious-Puberty.pdf

Sahin, S., Eskazan, T., Cicek, E., Ozogul, Y. Y., Durcan, E., Sulu, C., Ozkaya, H. M., Hatemi, A. I., & Kadioglu, P. (2022). The association between somatostatin receptor ligand and vitamin B_{12} in patients with acromegaly. *Turkish Journal of Endocrinology and Metabolism, 26*(2), 67–72. https://doi.org/10.5152/tjem.2022.22030

Takacs, D. S., & Katyayan, A. (2022). *Infantile spasms: Management and prognosis. UpToDate*. Lexi-Comp, Inc.

UpToDate (2023). *Drug information*. Lexi-Comp, Inc.

CHAPTER 44

Drug Therapy to Regulate Calcium and Bone Metabolism

LEARNING OBJECTIVES

After studying this chapter, you should be able to:

1. Examine the roles of parathyroid hormone, calcitonin, and vitamin D in regulating calcium metabolism.
2. Evaluate the use of calcium and vitamin D supplements, as well as calcitonin, in the treatment of osteoporosis.
3. Identify the prototype and describe the action, use, adverse effects, contraindications, and nursing implications of the bisphosphonates used in the treatment of osteoporosis.
4. Outline appropriate management strategies of hypercalcemia as a medical emergency.
5. Implement the nursing process in the care of the patient receiving drug therapy to regulate calcium and bone metabolism.

CLINICAL APPLICATION CASE STUDY

Carolyn Taylor, a 68-year-old retired teacher, has chronic venous insufficiency and osteoporosis. She has suffered two fractures from falls in recent years. Mrs. Taylor has been menopausal for 16 years and has not been on estrogen replacement therapy due to her vascular disease. Her healthcare provider prescribes alendronate once weekly.

KEY TERMS

Bisphosphonates: class of drugs that binds to bone and inhibits calcium resorption from bone

Calcitonin: hormone from the thyroid gland whose secretion is controlled by the concentration of ionized calcium in the blood flowing through the thyroid gland; its function is to lower serum calcium in the presence of hypercalcemia

Hypercalcemia: abnormally high blood calcium level (greater than 10.5 mg/dL)

Hyperparathyroidism: excessive production of parathyroid hormone (PTH)

Hypocalcemia: abnormally low blood calcium level (less than 8.5 mg/dL)

Hypoparathyroidism: insufficient production of PTH

Osteoporosis: decreased bone density and weak, fragile bones that often lead to fractures, pain, and disability

Paget disease: inflammatory skeletal disease that affects older people

Parathyroid hormone (PTH): hormone secreted by the parathyroid gland; secretion is stimulated by low serum calcium levels and inhibited by normal or high levels

Tetany: neuromuscular irritability characterized by numbness and tingling of the lips, fingers, and toes, twitching of facial muscle, spasms of skeletal muscle, carpopedal spasm, laryngospasm, and convulsions

Vitamin D (calciferol): fat-soluble vitamin that includes both ergocalciferol (obtained from foods) and cholecalciferol (formed by exposure of skin to sunlight); it functions as a hormone and plays an important role in calcium and bone metabolism

INTRODUCTION

Three hormones regulate calcium and bone metabolism—parathyroid hormone (PTH), calcitonin, and vitamin D—and act to maintain normal serum levels of calcium. When serum calcium levels are decreased, hormonal mechanisms raise them; when they are elevated, hormonal mechanisms lower them (Fig. 44.1). Overall, the hormones alter absorption of dietary calcium from the gastrointestinal (GI) tract, movement of calcium from bone to serum, and excretion of calcium through the kidneys.

Disorders of calcium and bone metabolism include hypocalcemia, hypercalcemia, osteoporosis, Paget disease, and bone breakdown associated with breast cancer and multiple myeloma. Drugs used to treat these disorders mainly alter serum calcium levels or strengthen bone. This chapter describes the characteristics of the hormones, calcium, phosphorus, and some associated disorders.

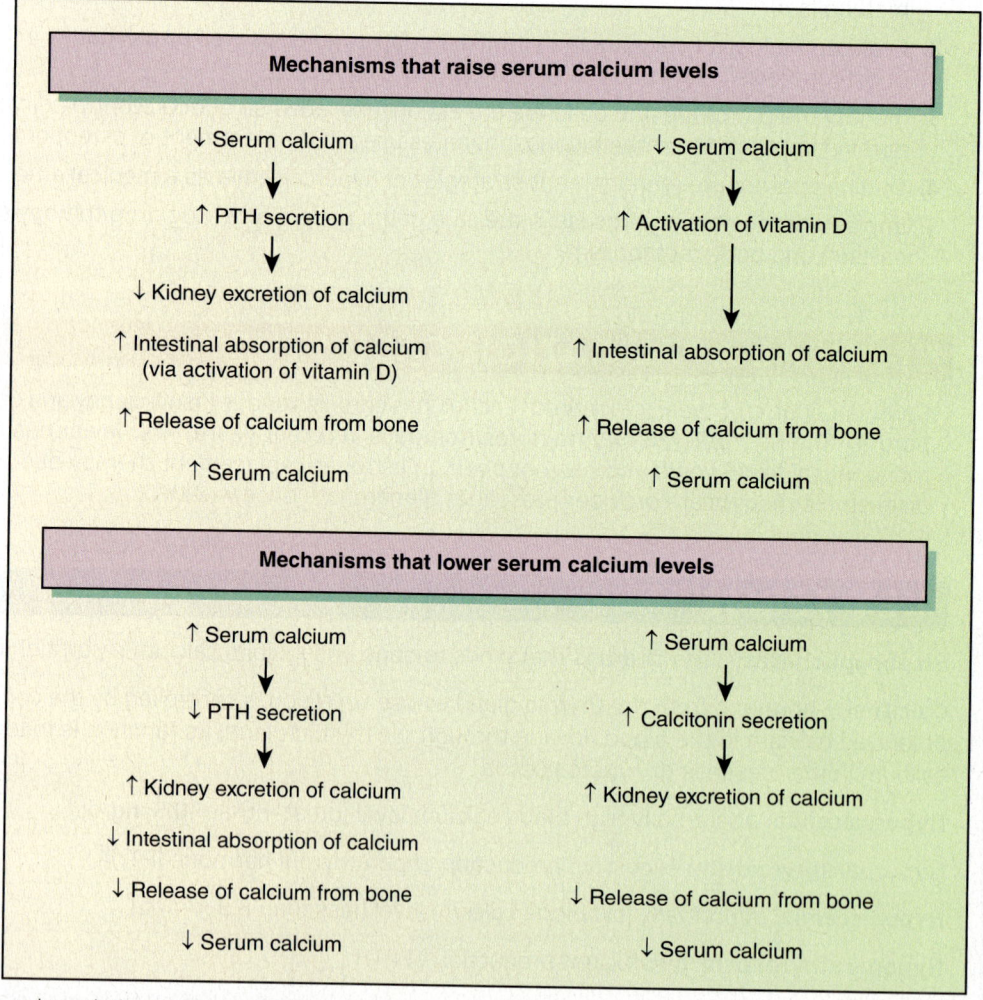

Figure 44.1. Hormonal regulation of serum calcium levels. When serum calcium levels are low (hypocalcemia), there is increased secretion of parathyroid hormone (PTH) and increased activation of vitamin D. These mechanisms lead to decreased loss of calcium in the urine, increased absorption of calcium from the intestine, and increased resorption of calcium from bone. These mechanisms work together to raise calcium levels to normal. When serum calcium levels are high (hypercalcemia), there is decreased secretion of PTH and increased secretion of calcitonin. These mechanisms lead to increased loss of calcium from the intestine and decreased resorption of calcium from bone. These mechanisms lower serum calcium levels to normal.

OVERVIEW OF CALCIUM AND BONE METABOLISM

Hypocalcemia, an abnormally low serum calcium level (less than 8.5 mg/dL), stimulates **parathyroid hormone (PTH)** secretion. PTH secretion is inhibited by normal or high levels of calcium. **Hypercalcemia** is an abnormally high serum calcium level (greater than 10.5 mg/dL). The inhibition of PTH with hypercalcemia is a negative feedback system. Because phosphate is closely related to calcium in body functions, PTH also regulates phosphate metabolism. In general, when serum calcium levels increase, serum phosphate levels decrease, and vice versa. Thus, an inverse relationship exists between calcium and phosphate.

When the serum calcium level falls below the normal range, PTH raises the level by acting on bone, intestines, and kidneys. In bone, breakdown is increased, so that calcium moves from bone into the serum. In the intestines, there is increased absorption of calcium ingested in food (PTH activates vitamin D, which increases intestinal absorption). In the kidneys, there is increased reabsorption of calcium in the kidney tubules and less urinary excretion. The opposite effects occur with phosphate (PTH decreases serum phosphate and increases urinary phosphate excretion).

Calcium and phosphorus are discussed together because they are closely related physiologically. These mineral nutrients occur in many of the same foods, from which they are absorbed together. Calcium and phosphorus both play critical roles in cellular structure and function and, as calcium phosphate, in formation and maintenance of bones and teeth. The characteristics and functions of calcium and phosphorus can be found on thePoint.

Disorders of parathyroid function are related to **hypoparathyroidism** (insufficient production of PTH) or **hyperparathyroidism** (excessive production of PTH). Most often, the cause of hypoparathyroidism is removal of or damage to the parathyroid glands during neck surgery. Most often, the cause of hyperparathyroidism is a tumor or hyperplasia of a parathyroid gland. It also may result from ectopic secretion of PTH by malignant tumors (carcinomas of the lung, pancreas, kidney, ovary, prostate gland, or bladder). Clinical manifestations and treatment of hypoparathyroidism are the same as those of hypocalcemia. Clinical manifestations and treatment of hyperparathyroidism are the same as those of hypercalcemia.

Calcitonin is a hormone from the thyroid gland whose secretion is controlled by the concentration of ionized calcium in the blood flowing through the thyroid gland. When the serum level of ionized calcium increases, secretion of calcitonin

---

BOX 44.1 Calcium and Bone Disorders

Hypocalcemia

Hypocalcemia is an abnormally low blood calcium level (i.e., less than 8.5 mg/dL). Causes may include inadequate intake of calcium and vitamin D, numerous disorders (e.g., diarrhea or malabsorption syndromes that cause inadequate absorption of calcium and vitamin D, hypoparathyroidism, kidney failure, severe hypomagnesemia, hypermagnesemia, acute pancreatitis, rhabdomyolysis, tumor lysis syndrome, vitamin D deficiency), and several drugs (e.g., cisplatin, cytosine arabinoside, foscarnet, ketoconazole, pentamidine, agents used to treat hypercalcemia). Calcium deficits caused by inadequate dietary intake affect bone tissue rather than serum calcium levels. Two mechanisms result in hypocalcemia associated with kidney failure. First, inability to excrete phosphate in urine leads to accumulation of phosphate in the blood (hyperphosphatemia). Because phosphate levels are inversely related to calcium levels, hyperphosphatemia induces hypocalcemia. Second, when kidney function is impaired, vitamin D conversion to its active metabolite is impaired. This results in decreased intestinal absorption of calcium.

Clinical manifestations are characterized by increased neuromuscular irritability, which may progress to tetany. In young children, hypocalcemia may be manifested by convulsions rather than tetany and erroneously diagnosed as epilepsy. This may be a serious error because anticonvulsant drugs used for epilepsy may further decrease serum calcium levels. Severe hypocalcemia may cause lethargy or confusion.

Hypercalcemia

Hypercalcemia is an abnormally high blood calcium level (i.e., greater than 10.5 mg/dL). It may be caused by hyperparathyroidism, hyperthyroidism, malignant neoplasms, vitamin D or vitamin A intoxication, aluminum intoxication, prolonged immobilization, adrenocortical insufficiency, and ingestion of thiazide diuretics, estrogens, and lithium. Cancer is a common cause, especially carcinomas (of the breast, lung, head and neck, or kidney) and multiple myeloma. Cancer stimulates bone breakdown, which increases serum calcium levels. Increased urine output leads to fluid volume deficit. This leads, in turn, to increased reabsorption of calcium in kidney tubules and decreased kidney excretion of calcium. Decreased kidney excretion potentiates hypercalcemia. Patients at risk for hypercalcemia should be monitored for early signs and symptoms, so treatment can be started before severe hypercalcemia develops.

Clinical manifestations are caused by the decreased ability of nerves to respond to stimuli and the decreased ability of muscles to contract and relax. Hypercalcemia has a depressant effect on nerve and muscle function. Gastrointestinal (GI) problems with hypercalcemia include anorexia, nausea, vomiting, constipation, and abdominal pain. Central nervous system problems include apathy, depression, poor memory, headache, and drowsiness. Severe hypercalcemia may produce lethargy, syncope, disorientation, hallucinations, coma, and death. Other signs and symptoms include weakness and decreased tone in skeletal and smooth muscle, dysphagia, polyuria, polyphagia, and cardiac dysrhythmias. In addition, calcium may be deposited in various tissues, such as the conjunctiva, cornea, and kidneys. Calcium deposits in the kidneys (renal calculi) may lead to irreversible damage and impairment of function.

Osteoporosis

Osteoporosis is characterized by decreased bone density (osteopenia) and weak, fragile bones that often lead to fractures, pain, and disability. Although any bones may be affected, common fracture sites are the vertebrae of the

BOX 44.1 Calcium and Bone Disorders (Continued)

lower dorsal and lumbar spines, wrists, and hips. Risk factors include female sex, advanced age, small stature, lean body mass, White or Asian race, positive family history, low calcium intake, menopause, sedentary lifestyle, nulliparity, smoking, excessive ingestion of alcohol or caffeine, high protein intake, high phosphate intake, hyperthyroidism, and chronic use of certain medications (e.g., corticosteroids, phenytoin). Postmenopausal women are at high risk because of estrogen deficiency, age-related bone loss, and a low peak bone mass. Osteoporosis occurs in men but less often than in women. Both men and women who take high doses of corticosteroids are at high risk because the drugs demineralize bone. In addition, kidney transplant recipients can acquire osteoporosis from corticosteroid therapy, decreased kidney function, increased PTH secretion, and cyclosporine immunosuppressant therapy.

Osteopenia or early osteoporosis may be present and undetected unless radiography or a bone density measurement is done. If detected, treatment is needed to slow bone loss. If undetected or untreated, clinical manifestations of osteoporosis include shortened stature (a measurable loss of height), back pain, spinal deformity, or a fracture. Fractures often occur with common bending or lifting movements or falling.

Paget Disease

Paget disease is an inflammatory skeletal disease that affects older people. Its etiology is unknown. It is characterized by a high rate of bone turnover and results in bone deformity and pain. It is treated with nonnarcotic analgesics and drugs that decrease bone resorption (e.g., bisphosphonates, calcitonin).

---

increases. The function of calcitonin is to lower serum calcium in the presence of hypercalcemia, which it does by decreasing movement of calcium from bone to serum and increasing urinary excretion of calcium. The action of calcitonin is rapid but of short duration. Thus, this hormone has little effect on long-term calcium metabolism.

Vitamin D (calciferol) is a fat-soluble vitamin that includes both ergocalciferol (obtained from foods) and cholecalciferol (formed by exposure of the skin to sunlight). It functions as a hormone and plays an important role in calcium and bone metabolism. The main action of vitamin D is to raise serum calcium levels by increasing intestinal absorption of calcium and mobilizing calcium from bone. It also promotes bone formation by providing adequate serum concentrations of minerals. Vitamin D is not physiologically active in the body. It must be converted to an intermediate metabolite in the liver and then to an active metabolite (1,25-dihydroxyvitamin D or calcitriol) in the kidneys. PTH and adequate hepatic and kidney function are required to produce the active metabolite.

Deficiency of vitamin D causes inadequate absorption of calcium and phosphorus. This, in turn, leads to low levels of serum calcium and stimulation of PTH secretion. In children, this sequence of events produces inadequate mineralization of bone (rickets), a rare condition in the United States. In adults, vitamin D deficiency causes osteomalacia, a condition characterized by decreased bone density and strength.

Bone is a mineralized connective tissue that functions as structural support and a reservoir for calcium, phosphorus, magnesium, sodium, and carbonate. The role of bone in maintaining serum calcium levels takes precedence over its structural function (bone may be weakened or destroyed as calcium leaves bone and enters serum). Bone tissue is constantly being formed and broken down in a process called remodeling. Bone tissue removal is referred to as resorption. During childhood, adolescence, and early adulthood, formation usually exceeds breakdown (resorption) as the person attains adult height and peak bone mass. After approximately 35 years of age, resorption is greater than formation. **Osteoporosis** occurs when bone strength (bone density and bone quality) is impaired, leading to increased porousness and vulnerability to fracture. Hormonal deficiencies, some diseases, and some medications (e.g., glucocorticoids) can also increase resorption, resulting in loss of bone mass and osteoporosis. Table 44.1 presents an overview of the prevention and treatment of osteoporosis.

Clinical Manifestations

The calcium disorders are hypocalcemia and hypercalcemia, either of which can be life threatening. Hypocalcemic emergencies, for example, may result in **tetany** (neuromuscular irritability). Tetany is characterized by numbness and tingling of the lips, fingers, and toes; twitching of facial muscles; spasms of skeletal muscle; carpopedal spasm; laryngospasm; and convulsions. The bone disorders discussed in this chapter are those characterized by increased resorption of calcium and loss of bone mass. These disorders weaken the bone, possibly leading to osteoporosis, with fractures, pain, and disability. Box 44.1 describes the selected calcium and bone disorders.

Drug Therapy

Healthcare providers use a variety of drugs to regulate calcium and bone metabolism:

- Treatment of hypocalcemia and prevention and treatment of osteoporosis: calcium and vitamin D supplements
- Treatment of hypercalcemia: bisphosphonates, calcitonin, corticosteroids, 0.9% sodium chloride intravenous (IV) infusion, and other agents
- Treatment of osteoporosis: bisphosphonates, calcitonin, estrogens, and antiestrogens

Clinical Application 44.1

- Mrs. Taylor, who has osteoporosis, should take preventive measures in addition to taking her prescribed medication. One important measure is to increase the intake of foods that contain high levels of calcium. What dietary recommendations should the nurse make?

TABLE 44.1
Prevention and Treatment of Osteoporosis

Prevention/Treatment	Rationale
Adequate dietary intake of calcium at all ages Calcium supplementation if needed	Promotes normal bone development and maintenance Promotes peak bone mass Allows for more bone loss before osteoporosis develops
Adequate dietary intake of vitamin D Vitamin D supplementation if at risk (older adults and patients on chronic corticosteroid therapy)	Ensures adequate stores of vitamin D to maintain normal serum and bony calcium
Lifestyle changes Adequate exercise Smoking cessation	Vigorous, weight-bearing exercise promotes and maintains strong bone Smoking decreases the amount of active estrogen that accelerates bone loss
Use of bisphosphonates (e.g., alendronate)	Used for prevention and treatment Reduces bone resorption and increases bone mass and strength
Preventive measures for patients on chronic corticosteroid therapy (prednisone >7.5 mg daily) Calcium and vitamin D supplements Lifestyle changes Use of bisphosphonates Use of low doses of corticosteroids or nonsystemic route, if possible	Corticosteroids decrease calcium absorption, increasing risk of osteoporosis. Lower doses or nonsystemic routes decrease corticosteroid effect on calcium absorption
Preventive measures for patients taking phenytoin Calcium and vitamin D supplements Drug treatment if bone density is low	Phenytoin increases hepatic metabolism of vitamin D
Treatment in women (if actual bone loss is present) Calcium/vitamin D supplements Alendronate 10 mg daily or 70 mg weekly OR Risedronate 5 mg daily or 35 mg weekly or 150 mg monthly Dose reduction if on corticosteroids	Bisphosphonates decrease the rate of bone breakdown, slow the rate of bone loss, increase bone mineral density, reduce the risk of vertebral fractures, and slow the progression of vertebral deformities and loss of height
Treatment in men Calcium/vitamin D supplements Use of bisphosphonates Testosterone supplements Dose reduction if on corticosteroids	Low testosterone levels may contribute to osteoporosis in men

CALCIUM PREPARATIONS

Calcium is available in many different forms. These preparations differ mainly in the amounts of calcium they contain and their routes of administration. It is important to note that even if people have normal serum levels of calcium, their diets may not contain enough calcium; they may need calcium supplements. Experts believe that the diets of most people of all ages, but especially of young women and older adults, are deficient in calcium.

Pharmacokinetics and Action

Absorption of calcium occurs in the small intestine, where approximately one third of the amount consumed is absorbed. PTH and vitamin D increase the absorption of calcium. Excretion primarily occurs in the feces, with the remainder excreted by the kidneys. PTH decreases kidney excretion of calcium.

Oral and IV calcium preparations replace lost calcium and help maintain normal calcium levels.

Use

Oral calcium (e.g., calcium carbonate or calcium citrate) provides supplemental calcium when diet alone is insufficient to meet body requirements. Also, it is useful for the treatment of chronic, nonemergent hypocalcemia, regardless of the cause. In addition, it provides relief from symptoms of acid indigestion and heartburn. Finally, it can decrease bone loss and fractures, especially in women. Calcium citrate is reportedly better absorbed than calcium carbonate.

IV calcium is essential for the treatment of acute, severe hypocalcemia, which is a medical emergency. It may be necessary to give repeated doses, to give a continuous infusion, or to use oral supplements to avoid symptoms of hypocalcemia and maintain normal serum calcium levels (measured every 4 to 6 hours). In calcium blocker overdose, calcium gluconate is given by IV infusion to help reverse the vasodilation and decreased myocardial contractility caused by the calcium channel blocker.

Table 44.2 gives route and dosage information for several calcium supplements.

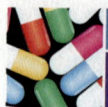

TABLE 44.2
DRUGS AT A GLANCE: Calcium and Vitamin D Preparations

Drug	Routes and Dosage Ranges	
	Adults	**Children**
Oral Calcium Products		
Calcium acetate (Calphron; ✹ PhosLo) 25% calcium	1,334 mg PO with each meal; increase gradually to 2,001–2,668 mg with each meal	Limited data available. Individualize dose; initial dose 667–1,000 mg with each meal; titrate to response
Calcium carbonate precipitated (Os-Cal, Tums; ✹ Apo-Cal, Os-Cal, Tums) 40% calcium	500–4,000 mg daily in 1–3 divided doses	Infants, children, and adolescents. As elemental calcium 30–75 mg/kg/d PO in 4–5 divided doses
Calcium citrate (Cal-Citrate; ✹ Osteocit) 21% calcium	200 mg to 1 g/d as elemental calcium in single dose or divided doses	Limited data available. Infants, children, and adolescents. As elemental calcium 30–75 mg/kg/d in 4–5 divided doses
Calcium gluconate (Cal-Glu) 9% calcium (✹ Calcium Sandoz)	19–50 y: 1,000 mg/d Females 51 y and older: 1,200 mg/d Males 51–70 y: 1,000 mg/d	Same as above for calcium citrate
Parenteral Calcium Products		
Calcium chloride 10 mL of 10% solution contains 273 mg (13.6 mEq) of calcium; ✹ (Calciject)	Hypocalcemia: 200–1,000 mg IV every 1–3 d	Hypocalcemia: 2.7–5 mg/kg/dose IV every 4–6 h (maximum dose 1,000 mg)
Calcium gluconate 10 mL of 10% solution contains 93 mg (4.65 mEq) of calcium; calcium gluconate preferred over calcium chloride	Hypocalcemia (IV) Mild: 1,000–2,000 mg over 2 h Moderate to severe: 4,000 mg over 4 h Severe (with seizures): 1,000–2,000 mg over 10 min; repeat every 60 minutes until symptoms resolve	Hypocalcemia (infants, children, adolescents <17 years): 29–60 mg/kg/dose IV every 6 hours or 8–13 mg/kg/h IV continuously (adolescents 17 years or older) 1,000–2,000 mg/dose IV every 6 hours or 5.4–21.5 mg/kg/h IV continuously Symptomatic (with seizures): 100–200 mg/kg/dose over 5–10 min IV or intraosseous (maximum dose 1,000–2,000 mg/dose; repeat as needed or follow with continuous IV infusion of 8–32 mg/kg/h
Vitamin D Preparations		
Calcitriol (Rocaltrol; ✹ Rocaltrol)	0.25 mcg PO daily initially and then adjusted according to serum calcium levels (usual daily maintenance dose 0.5–1 mcg)	1–5 y: 0.25–0.75 mcg PO daily 6 y or older: refer to adult dose
Cholecalciferol (vitamin D3) (Delta-D; D-Vi-Sol; ✹ D-Tabs; EURO-D)	DRI (19–70 y): 600 IU PO daily	DRI Birth to 12 mo: AI, 400 PO IU/d 1–18 y: RDA, 600 PO IU/d
Ergocalciferol (vitamin D2) (Calciferol, Drisdol; ✹ D-Forte, SANDOZ D-Forte)	19–70 y: 600 IU/d PO	Same as cholecalciferol
Paricalcitol (Zemplar; ✹ Zemplar)	Secondary hyperparathyroidism associated with chronic kidney disease: 0.04–0.1 mcg/kg IV every other day initially; increase by 2–4 mcg at 2- to 4-wk intervals if necessary; reduce dosage or stop therapy if hypercalcemia occurs	Secondary hyperparathyroidism associated with chronic kidney disease 5 y and older: same as adults (small studies only)

AI, adequate intake; DRI, dietary reference intake; RDA, recommended dietary allowance.

Patient-related variables specific to the use of calcium include the following:

- Age:
  - In older adults, calcium deficiency commonly occurs because of long-term dietary deficiencies of calcium and impaired absorption of calcium from the intestine.
- Reproduction, pregnancy, and lactation:
  - Calcium crosses the placenta.
  - Calcium is required for fetal growth. Intestinal absorption and urinary excretion of calcium increase during pregnancy.
  - The amount of calcium reaching the fetus is determined by physiologic changes in the pregnant patient, which are generally not influenced by patient diet or supplementation.
  - Calcium is present in breast milk. Calcium is required for milk production. The amount of calcium in breast milk is not altered by calcium intake in the breast-feeding patient.
- Abnormal kidney function and hepatic impairment:
  - In abnormal kidney function, calcium dosage adjustments may be necessary depending on serum calcium levels.
  - Kidney disease produces impairment in calcium metabolism.
  - Calcium acetate is used to treat hyperphosphatemia. It reduces serum phosphate by reducing absorption from food; it binds with dietary phosphate to produce insoluble calcium phosphate, which is excreted in the feces.
  - In hepatic impairment, dosage adjustments are not required.

Adverse Effects

GI effects of hypercalcemia include anorexia, nausea, vomiting, abdominal pain, and constipation. Central nervous system effects are apathy, poor memory, depression, drowsiness, and disorientation. Cardiac effects include dysrhythmias, and an electrocardiogram (ECG) shows a prolonged QT interval and an inverted T wave. Weakness and decreased tone in skeletal and smooth muscles, dysphagia, polyuria, and polydipsia may also occur.

Contraindications

Contraindications to calcium preparations include cancer with bone metastases, as well as ventricular fibrillation, hypercalcemia, hypophosphatemia, and kidney stone.

Nursing Implications

Preventing Interactions

Bran, rhubarb, spinach, and whole grain cereals decrease the effectiveness of calcium preparations. Several medications interact with calcium supplements, increasing or decreasing their effects (Box 44.2).

Also, it is important to note that oral calcium preparations interfere with the absorption of numerous drugs, including atenolol and fluoroquinolones, when the calcium is taken at the same time. In the case of oral tetracyclines, the calcium combines with the antibiotic, preventing its absorption.

In addition, calcium preparations and digoxin have similar effects on the myocardium. Therefore, if a patient taking digoxin receives calcium, the risks of digoxin toxicity and cardiac dysrhythmias increase. It is essential to use this combination very cautiously. Use of calcium with phenytoin decreases absorption of both drugs. IV calcium antagonizes the effects of verapamil.

> **BOX 44.2** **Drug Interactions: Calcium Preparations**
>
> **Drugs That Increase the Effects of Calcium**
> - Thiazide diuretics
>   *Reduce calcium losses in the urine*
> - Vitamin D
>   *Increases absorption of calcium*
>
> **Drugs That Decrease the Effects of Calcium**
> - Calcitonin
>   *Interferes with absorption of calcium*
> - Corticosteroids (prednisone and others)
>   *Lower calcium levels by various mechanisms*
> - Phosphates
>   *Lower calcium levels by various mechanisms*

Administering the Medication

Calcium is available in many different forms; the nurse ensures that the form being given is the correct one. The nurse also makes sure to:

- Administer oral preparations with or after meals to increase absorption. If used as an antacid, administer after a meal.
- Administer oral preparations separately from atenolol and fluoroquinolones and more than 2 to 3 hours before or after giving oral tetracycline.
- Dilute IV preparations in a compatible fluid and administer slowly as a continuous infusion or in divided doses; check pulse and blood pressure closely; monitor the ECG if possible. IV solutions may cause dysrhythmias and hypotension if administered too rapidly.
- Carefully observe the IV site during administration because IV calcium is irritating to tissues.
- Do not administer parenteral forms intramuscularly.

Assessing for Therapeutic Effects

The nurse observes for relief of symptoms of neuromuscular irritability and tetany, such as decreased muscle spasms, decreased paresthesias, absence of Chvostek sign, and absence of Trousseau sign. The nurse also assesses laboratory results for return of serum calcium levels to the normal range of 8.5 to 10.5 mg/dL.

Once the hypocalcemia is stabilized, the aim of treatment is management of the underlying cause or prevention of recurrence. If diarrhea or malabsorption is the cause, treatment of the underlying condition decreases loss of calcium from the body and increases absorption. It is also necessary to measure serum magnesium levels; treatment of hypomagnesemia is essential before treatment of hypocalcemia can be effective.

Assessing for Adverse Effects

The nurse assesses for increased thirst, inability to eat, and increased urination, as well as for constipation and abdominal pain. It is necessary to assess for diminished memory, disorientation, and drowsiness. The nurse checks the ECG for a prolonged QT interval and inverted T wave that results from hypercalcemia.

BOX 44.3 Patient Teaching Guidelines for Calcium Preparations

- Consult with your healthcare provider before taking calcium supplements.
- If you need a calcium supplement, your healthcare provider may recommend calcium carbonate 500 mg twice daily. This calcium supplement contains the most elemental calcium by weight (40%). It is inexpensive and available in a nonprescription form as the antacid Tums, which contains 500 mg of calcium per tablet.
- Consume good sources of dietary calcium that include milk, yogurt, hard natural cheese, bok choy, broccoli, Chinese/Napa cabbage, collards, kale, okra, turnip greens, fortified breakfast cereals, fortified orange juice, and dried peas and beans.
- Do not take a calcium supplement with an iron preparation, tetracycline, ciprofloxacin, or phenytoin. Instead, take the drugs at least 2 hours apart to avoid calcium interference with drug absorption.
- Avoid rhubarb, spinach, bran, and whole-grain cereals in the meal before taking calcium because these foods interfere with calcium absorption.
- Take oral calcium 1 to 1.5 hours after meals if gastrointestinal upset occurs.
- Take oral calcium with a full glass of water.
- Report anorexia, nausea, vomiting, abdominal pain, dry mouth, thirst, or polyuria.

Patient Teaching

Box 44.3 presents patient teaching guidelines for calcium preparations.

Clinical Application 44.2

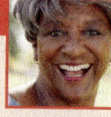

- What instructions should the nurse give Mrs. Taylor about taking oral calcium supplements?

NCLEX Success

1. The nurse must administer a tetracycline antibiotic to a patient who takes an oral calcium supplement with each meal. When should the nurse administer the tetracycline?
   A. 2 hours before meals
   B. 30 minutes before meals
   C. with meals
   D. 1 hour after meals

2. The nurse is administering a continuous IV infusion of calcium properly diluted in a compatible IV fluid. Which one of the following would it be most important for the nurse to monitor?
   A. cardiac rhythm
   B. urine output
   C. hearing changes
   D. musculoskeletal pain

VITAMIN D

Vitamin D is a fat-soluble vitamin used in chronic hypocalcemia if calcium supplements alone cannot maintain serum calcium levels within a normal range. It is also used to prevent deficiency states and treat hypoparathyroidism and osteoporosis. Although authorities agree that dietary intake is better than supplements, some suggest a vitamin D supplement for people who ingest less than the recommended amount. The recommended dietary allowance, or RDA, for vitamin D is 15 mcg/day for individuals 1 to 70 years of age and 20 mcg/day for adults aged 71 years and older to prevent and treat osteoporosis. Adequate intake for infants 0 to 12 months is 10 mcg/day.

Pharmacokinetics and Action

As a drug, vitamin D is absorbed from the GI tract. It is stored in the liver, skin, and other tissues for months. It is metabolized into its active form in the liver and kidneys. Half of an oral dose is eliminated in the bile.

Vitamin D increases calcium and phosphorus absorption from the GI tract. It also promotes movement of calcium and phosphorus from the bones to maintain normal serum calcium levels. In the kidneys, vitamin D decreases elimination of calcium and phosphorus.

Use

Vitamin D is useful for the treatment of rickets, other vitamin D deficiency diseases, and hypoparathyroidism. It is important to take vitamin D supplements cautiously and not overuse them; excessive amounts can cause serious problems, including hypercalcemia. Table 44.2 gives route and dosage information for some vitamin D preparations.

Vitamin D is also useful if a calcium preparation alone cannot maintain serum calcium levels within a normal range. When vitamin D is given to treat hypocalcemia, frequent measurements of serum calcium levels determine dosage. Usually, people take higher doses initially, and lower doses are appropriate for maintenance therapy. Calcium salts and vitamin D are available over the counter in many combined preparations promoted as dietary supplements (Table 44.3). These mixtures are not indicated for maintenance therapy in chronic hypocalcemia.

Patient-related variables specific to the use of vitamin D include the following:

- Age:
  - A vitamin D supplement is recommended for infants who are partially or completely breast-fed because breast milk contains only small quantities of vitamin D.
- Reproduction, pregnancy, and lactation:
  - A vitamin D supplement is recommended for pregnant patients with the dose in a standard prenatal vitamin.
  - For routine vitamin D supplementation, the 2010 IOM recommend 600 IU daily for all reproductive age patients during pregnancy and lactation (Dawson-Hughes, 2023).
  - Vitamin D is present in breast milk following normal maternal exposure to sunlight and adequate dietary sources.

TABLE 44.3

Selected Calcium/Vitamin D Combination Products*

Drug	Calcium (mg of Elemental Calcium)/ Tablet or Capsule	Vitamin D International Units/Tablet
Caltrate 600 + D3	600	800
Citracal Maximum	315	250
Citracal + D Slow Release	600	500
Citracal Calcium Gummies	250	500
Os-Cal Calcium + D3	500	200
Os-Cal Extra + D3	500	600
Os-Cal Chewable	500	600

*In general, the upper intake level for vitamin D is 100 mcg/d.

- Abnormal kidney function and hepatic impairment:
  - Kidney disease interferes with metabolism of vitamin D precursors to the active form of vitamin D in the kidneys. If vitamin D therapy is necessary for treating osteomalacia in abnormal kidney function, calcitriol is preferable as it is the active form of vitamin D and undergoes no metabolism.
  - Hepatic impairment requires no vitamin D dosage adjustments.

Adverse Effects

The principal adverse effects of excessive vitamin D use are hypervitaminosis D and hypercalcemia. This is most likely to occur with chronic ingestion of high doses daily. In children, accidental ingestion may lead to acute toxicity. Of particular significance with vitamin D excess are kidney stones, irreversible kidney damage, and muscle and bone weakness. Box 44.1 discusses symptoms of hypercalcemia, such as tetany.

Contraindications

Contraindications to vitamin D include hypercalcemia and vitamin D toxicity. It is necessary to withhold all preparations containing vitamin D.

Nursing Implications

Preventing Interactions

Several medications interact with vitamin D, increasing or decreasing its effects (Box 44.4).

Administering the Medication

People may take vitamin D without regard to food. It is important not to take both the vitamin and magnesium-containing antacids or mineral oil.

BOX 44.4 Drug Interactions: Vitamin D

Drugs That Increase the Effects of Vitamin D
- Thiazide diuretics
  Inhibit kidney excretion

Drugs That Decrease the Effects of Vitamin D
- Cholestyramine resin
  Decreases the intestinal absorption of vitamin D
- Mineral oil
  Prevents the absorption of vitamin D
- Phenytoin
  Accelerates vitamin D metabolism in the liver

Assessing for Therapeutic Effects

The nurse observes for a decrease in symptoms of hypocalcemia and symptoms of rickets or osteomalacia. It is necessary to check that the following laboratory results are normal: serum calcium level, blood urea nitrogen and serum creatinine, and serum phosphate. Improved bone health, as documented by radiograph, should be evident.

Assessing for Adverse Effects

Serum calcium must be monitored; if hypercalcemia occurs, the nurse must stop the drug and notify the healthcare provider. It is necessary to observe for signs and symptoms of vitamin D excess, including headache, somnolence, weakness, irritability, hypertension, cardiac dysrhythmias, kidney stones, polydipsia, polyuria, and bone and muscle pain.

Patient Teaching

Box 44.5 presents patient teaching guidelines for vitamin D.

BOX 44.5 Patient Teaching Guidelines for Vitamin D

- Take vitamin D supplements only if recommended by your primary healthcare provider.
- Avoid over-the-counter drugs and magnesium-containing antacids unless recommended by the healthcare provider.
- Immediately report early symptoms of vitamin D intoxication: weakness, nausea, vomiting, dry mouth, constipation, muscle or bone pain, and metallic taste.
- Be aware that certain drugs interact with vitamin D, such as thiazide diuretics, phenytoin, cholestyramine resin, and mineral oil, and increase or decrease the effects of the vitamin.
- Learn about good dietary sources of vitamin D. Food sources of vitamin D include cod liver oil, oysters, mackerel, most fish, egg yolks, fortified milk, some ready-to-eat cereals, and margarine.
- Understand that a source of vitamin D besides diet is sunlight on the skin. Adequate sun exposure allows the body to produce enough vitamin D to meet daily requirements. Factors that limit vitamin D production through sun exposure include lack of exposure, geographic location, season, use of sunblock, and darker skin pigmentation.

Clinical Application 44.3

- Mrs. Taylor has developed kidney failure with replacement therapy and receives hemodialysis three times per week. She requires a vitamin D supplement. Why would she receive the active form of vitamin D, calcitriol (Rocaltrol)?

BISPHOSPHONATES

Bisphosphonates are drugs that bind to bone and inhibit calcium resorption from bone. Although indications vary, the drugs are used mainly in the treatment of hypercalcemia and osteoporosis. **Alendronate** (Fosamax) is the prototype bisphosphonate.

Pharmacokinetics and Action

Alendronate is poorly absorbed from the intestinal tract. It is not metabolized. The drug bound to bone is slowly released into the bloodstream. Most of the drug that is not bound to bone is excreted in the urine.

Alendronate suppresses osteoclast activity on newly formed resorption surfaces, which reduces bone turnover. This means that bone formation exceeds resorption at remodeling sites, leading to progressive gains in bone mass.

Use

Although the main use of alendronate is to prevent and treat osteoporosis in postmenopausal women, it is also used to treat osteoporosis in men. Other uses include the treatment of **Paget disease**, an inflammatory bone disease that affects older people, and glucocorticoid-induced osteoporosis in both sexes. Table 44.4 gives route and dosage information for alendronate and other bisphosphonates.

Patient-related variables specific to the use of alendronate include the following:

- Age:
  - In children, alendronate is used for disorders characterized by bone fragility and poor bone calcification (such as osteogenesis imperfecta) and in osteopenia associated with cystic fibrosis; it is also used for osteopenia in nonambulatory patients (e.g., cerebral palsy or muscular dystrophy).
- Reproduction, pregnancy, and lactation:
  - Effective contraception is recommended if alendronate is used in patients who are sexually active and able to become pregnant. Discontinue use as early as possible prior to a planned pregnancy.
  - It is unknown if alendronate crosses the placenta but due to its lower molecular weight, fetal exposure is expected. Available data have not shown exposure to alendronate during pregnancy significantly increases the risk of adverse fetal events. Monitor exposed infants for hypocalcemia after birth.
  - It is unknown if alendronate is present in breast milk. The decision to breast-feed considers risk of infant exposure, benefits of breast-feeding, and benefits of alendronate treatment to the breast-feeding patient.
- Abnormal kidney function and hepatic impairment:
  - Alendronate is not recommended in severe abnormal kidney function (creatinine clearance less than 35 mL/min).
  - In hepatic impairment, no dosage adjustment is necessary.

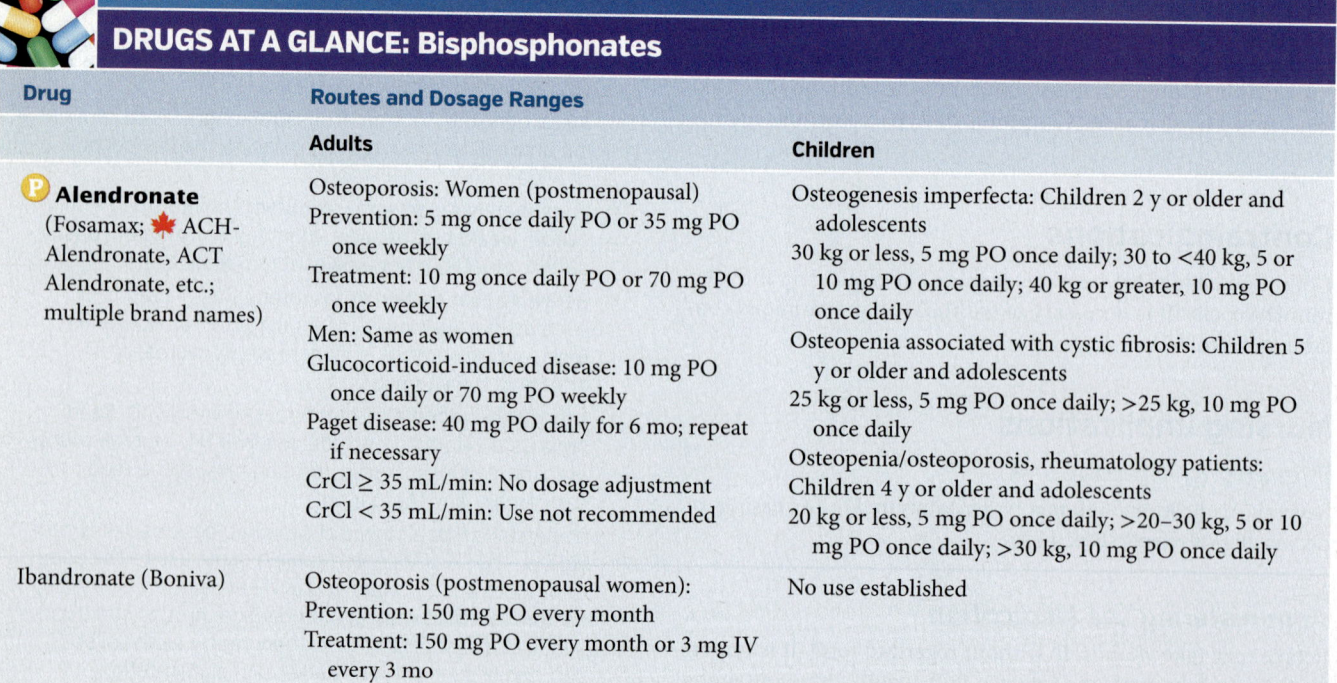

TABLE 44.4
DRUGS AT A GLANCE: Bisphosphonates

Drug	Routes and Dosage Ranges	
	Adults	**Children**
Alendronate (Fosamax; ACH-Alendronate, ACT Alendronate, etc.; multiple brand names)	Osteoporosis: Women (postmenopausal) Prevention: 5 mg once daily PO or 35 mg PO once weekly Treatment: 10 mg once daily PO or 70 mg PO once weekly Men: Same as women Glucocorticoid-induced disease: 10 mg PO once daily or 70 mg PO weekly Paget disease: 40 mg PO daily for 6 mo; repeat if necessary CrCl ≥ 35 mL/min: No dosage adjustment CrCl < 35 mL/min: Use not recommended	Osteogenesis imperfecta: Children 2 y or older and adolescents 30 kg or less, 5 mg PO once daily; 30 to <40 kg, 5 or 10 mg PO once daily; 40 kg or greater, 10 mg PO once daily Osteopenia associated with cystic fibrosis: Children 5 y or older and adolescents 25 kg or less, 5 mg PO once daily; >25 kg, 10 mg PO once daily Osteopenia/osteoporosis, rheumatology patients: Children 4 y or older and adolescents 20 kg or less, 5 mg PO once daily; >20–30 kg, 5 or 10 mg PO once daily; >30 kg, 10 mg PO once daily
Ibandronate (Boniva)	Osteoporosis (postmenopausal women): Prevention: 150 mg PO every month Treatment: 150 mg PO every month or 3 mg IV every 3 mo	No use established

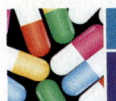

TABLE 44.4
DRUGS AT A GLANCE: Bisphosphonates (Continued)

Drug	Routes and Dosage Ranges	
	Adults	**Children**
Pamidronate (PMS-Pamidronate; Pamidronate Disodium Omega)	Hypercalcemia of malignancy: 60–90 mg IV as a single dose over 2–24 h (maximum 90 mg/dose) Breast cancer: 90 mg IV over 2 h every 3–4 wk (maximum 90 mg/dose) Multiple myeloma: 90 mg IV over 4 h once monthly Paget disease: 30 mg IV over 4 h once daily for 3 consecutive days (total dose 90 mg)	Hypercalcemia: Initial treatment 0.5–1 mg/kg IV (maximum dose 90 mg); repeat if needed at interval of 24 h or more Osteogenesis imperfecta: Infants/children <2 y: First cycle 0.25 mg/kg IV day 1 and then 0.5 mg/kg/dose IV days 2 and 3; subsequent cycles 0.5 mg/kg/dose once daily for 3 d; repeat cycles every 2 mo for total 9 mg/kg yearly Children 2–3 y: First cycle 0.38 mg/kg IV day 1 and then 0.75 mg/kg/dose IV days 2 and 3; subsequent cycles 0.75 mg/kg/dose once daily for 3 d; repeat cycles every 3 mo for total 9 mg/kg yearly Children >3 y and adolescents: First cycle 0.5 mg/kg IV day 1 and then 1 mg/kg/dose days 2 and 3; subsequent cycles 1 mg/kg/dose once daily for 3 d; repeat cycles every 4 mo for total 9 mg/kg yearly
Risedronate (Actonel; Actonel, Actonel DR)	Osteoporosis (postmenopausal women) Prevention/treatment: 5 mg PO once daily or 35 mg PO once weekly or 150 mg PO once monthly. If glucocorticoid induced, 5 mg PO once daily Paget disease: 30 mg PO (immediate release) once daily for 2 mo	No use established
Zoledronic acid (Reclast, Zometa; Aclasta, TARO-Zoledronic Acid)	Osteoporosis: 5 mg IV once per year Hypercalcemia of malignancy: 4 mg IV max given as a single dose. May repeat after 7 d	Osteoporosis (primary or secondary). Limited data available. Children <2 y first dose 0.0125 mg/kg/dose IV; maintenance 3 mo after first dose 0.025 mg/kg/dose every 3 mo. Children 2 y or older and adolescents first dose 0.0125 mg/kg/dose IV; second dose 3 mo after first dose 0.025 mg/kg/dose IV; maintenance begin 6 mo after first dose 0.05 mg/kg/dose every 6 mo (maximum dose 4 mg/dose). Doses adjusted based on lumbar spine BMD. Administer acetaminophen or ibuprofen 30 min prior to infusion and 6 h following infusion

CrCl, creatinine clearance; BMD, bone mineral density.

Adverse Effects

Adverse effects of alendronate are usually minor if the doses taken for prevention or treatment of osteoporosis are used and the drug is taken as directed. Patients who do not follow the dosing instructions are at greater risk for esophagitis, dysphagia, and esophageal ulcers/erosions. Other effects include headache, musculoskeletal pain (sometimes severe), and decreased serum calcium. More severe effects may occur with the higher doses taken for Paget disease.

Rare adverse effects include atypical femur fracture and osteonecrosis of the jaw. Patients on long-term therapy are at greater risk for femur fracture. Greater risk of osteonecrosis of the jaw occurs with higher drug potency, higher cumulative dose, and parenteral route of administration. Experts recommend a drug holiday after 5 years of alendronate therapy if there is a low risk of fracture. Alendronate is restarted if there is a decrease in bone mineral density or a new osteoporotic fracture (Rosen, 2021).

Quality and Safety Alert: Evidence-Based Practice

Bauer and Abrahamsen (2021), after reviewing multiple studies, recommend that patients with osteoporosis without previous hip, vertebral, or multiple nonspine fractures who are successfully treated with oral bisphosphonates for 5 years or with IV bisphosphonates for 3 years receive a 3- to 5-year drug holiday. A drug holiday reduces the risk of the serious adverse effect of atypical femur fracture.

Contraindications

Contraindications to alendronate include hypersensitivity to the drug, abnormalities of the esophagus that delay esophageal emptying, and inability to stand or sit upright for at least 30 minutes. People with hypocalcemia require correction of the low serum calcium levels before beginning therapy with alendronate.

Caution is warranted with active upper GI conditions.

BOX 44.6 Drug Interactions: Alendronate

Drugs That Increase the Effects of Alendronate
- Aspirin and nonsteroidal anti-inflammatory drugs
  Increase the risk of gastrointestinal effects when combined with alendronate

Drugs That Decrease the Effects of Alendronate
- Antacids and calcium supplements
  Interfere with alendronate absorption if they are taken within 2 hours of the drug

Nursing Implications

Preventing Interactions

Several medications interact with alendronate, increasing or decreasing its effects (Box 44.6). Any food interferes with absorption of alendronate.

Administering the Medication

Alendronate must always be taken with a full glass of water, not juice or coffee, at least 30 minutes before breakfast and before taking other drugs. The person must remain upright (with the head elevated 90 degrees if in the bed, sitting upright in a chair, or standing) for at least 30 minutes after administration. These interventions promote absorption and decrease esophageal and gastric irritation.

Assessing for Therapeutic and Adverse Effects

The nurse observes for improved bone density and absence of fractures. Early osteopenia and osteoporosis are asymptomatic. Measurement of bone density is the only way to quantify bone loss.

It is also necessary to observe for GI adverse effects, including abdominal distention, acid regurgitation, dysphagia, esophagitis, and flatulence.

Patient Teaching

Box 44.7 gives patient teaching guidelines for alendronate.

BOX 44.7 Patient Teaching Guidelines for Alendronate

- Take tablets on waking only with 6 to 8 oz of water or more at least 30 minutes before eating or drinking anything else, including food, beverages, or other drugs. Waiting longer than 30 minutes improves absorption.
- Do not lie down for at least 30 minutes after taking alendronate to reduce the risk of esophageal irritation and aid movement of the drug to the stomach.
- Report adverse effects to the healthcare provider immediately, especially esophageal pain, irritation, or burning; heartburn; dyspepsia, nausea, or vomiting; or difficulty swallowing.

Other Drugs in the Class

Other bisphosphonates include ibandronate (Boniva), pamidronate (Aredia), risedronate (Actonel), and zoledronic acid (Reclast, Zometa). Ibandronate, risedronate, and zoledronic acid (Reclast), like alendronate, are used to prevent and treat osteoporosis. Both ibandronate and risedronate are available in oral preparations to be taken once monthly. Zoledronic acid, as Reclast, is administered IV once a year. Pamidronate is not approved by the U.S. Food and Drug Administration (FDA) for osteoporosis but may be useful for various bone-related conditions such as Paget disease and bone lesions.

Common adverse effects of bisphosphonates include nausea and vomiting. Serious adverse effects may include anemia, jaw osteonecrosis, neutropenia, infections, and kidney damage.

Clinical Application 44.4

- The nurse is giving instructions to Mrs. Taylor on the proper administration method for taking alendronate. What important instructions must the nurse include?

NCLEX Success

3. A patient has a serum calcium level of 6.8 mg/dL. The healthcare provider orders a vitamin D supplement. Which one of the following laboratory values for serum calcium indicates that the vitamin D is effective?
   A. 5.5 mg/dL
   B. 6.8 mg/dL
   C. 7.5 mg/dL
   D. 8.5 mg/dL

4. The nurse is caring for a patient who takes alendronate. Which adverse effects should the nurse observe for?
   A. numbness and tingling of the extremities
   B. irregular pulse rate and angina
   C. acid reflux and difficulty swallowing
   D. rash and skin lesions

5. The healthcare provider has prescribed alendronate for the patient. Which one of the following should the nurse include in discharge teaching?
   A. "Take alendronate first thing in the morning with orange juice."
   B. "Take alendronate at bedtime with a glass of milk."
   C. "Take alendronate first thing in the morning with water."
   D. "Take alendronate on a full stomach after breakfast."

OTHER MEDICATIONS USED TO TREAT BONE DISORDERS AND HYPERCALCEMIA

Other drugs are used to treat bone disorders and hypercalcemia. Table 44.5 presents route and dosage information for these drugs.

Calcitonin (Miacalcin) is used in the treatment of hypercalcemia, Paget disease, and postmenopausal osteoporosis. In hypercalcemia, calcitonin lowers serum calcium levels by inhibiting bone resorption. Calcitonin is most likely to be effective in hypercalcemia caused by hyperparathyroidism, prolonged immobilization, or certain malignant neoplasms. In acute hypercalcemia, healthcare providers may use calcitonin along with other measures to lower serum calcium rapidly. A single injection of calcitonin decreases serum calcium levels in approximately 2 hours, and its effects last approximately 6 to 8 hours. In Paget disease, calcitonin slows the rate of bone turnover, improves bone lesions on radiologic examination, and relieves bone pain. In osteoporosis, calcitonin prevents further bone loss in the presence of adequate calcium and vitamin D. Calcitonin does not cross the placenta; weigh risks and benefits to the patient if breast-feeding.

Denosumab (Prolia, Xgeva) is an antiresorptive drug. Prolia is used to treat osteoporosis in postmenopausal women at high risk for fracture. Xgeva is used to prevent skeletal-related events in bone metastases from solid tumors. Denosumab decreases bone resorption and increases bone mass and strength. The drug is administered subcutaneously at 6-month intervals. Adverse effects include fatigue, weakness, back pain, extremity pain, hypocalcemia, hypophosphatemia, nausea, diarrhea, peripheral edema, hypertension, headache, skin rash, and dermatitis. Significant adverse effects include fractures (femur or vertebrae), infection, and osteonecrosis of the jaw. Patients of reproductive potential require contraception during denosumab therapy and for 5 months after the last dose. During pregnancy, exposure to the drug may cause fetal harm. Weigh risks and benefits of breast-feeding.

Phosphate salts (Neutra-Phos) inhibit intestinal absorption of calcium and increase deposition of calcium in bone. (Neutra-Phos is an oral combination of sodium phosphate and potassium phosphate.) Oral salts are effective in the treatment of hypercalcemia due to any cause. A potential adverse effect of phosphates is calcification of soft tissues due to deposition of calcium phosphate, which can lead to severe impairment of function in the kidneys and other organs. It is important to give phosphates only when hypercalcemia is accompanied by hypophosphatemia (serum phosphate less than 3 mg/dL) and kidney function is normal to minimize the risk of soft tissue calcification. Frequent monitoring of serum calcium, phosphate, and creatinine levels is necessary, and the dose reduction should

TABLE 44.5

DRUGS AT A GLANCE: Drugs Used to Treat Other Bone Disorders and Hypercalcemia

Drug	Routes and Dosage Ranges	
	Adults	**Children**
Calcitonin (Miacalcin; Calcimar)	Hypercalcemia: 4 units/kg subcutaneously or IM every 12 h; can be increased after 1–2 d to 8 units/kg every 12 h; limit total duration of therapy to 24–48 h Paget disease: 100 units/d subcutaneously or IM Postmenopausal osteoporosis: nasal spray, 200 units daily (1 spray in 1 nostril daily); subcutaneously or IM, 100 units daily	Osteogenesis imperfecta: Infants >6 mo, children, and adolescents: 2 units/kg/dose subcutaneously or IM three times/wk
Denosumab (Prolia, Xgeva; Prolia, Xgeva)	Osteoporosis, bone loss, breast cancer and prostate cancer treatment (Prolia): 60 mg subcutaneously every 6 mo Prevention of skeletal-related events with solid tumor bone metastases (Xgeva): 120 mg subcutaneously every 4 wk	Treatment of giant cell tumor of the bone (Xgeva): Skeletally mature adolescents weighing 45 kg or more, 120 mg subcutaneously once every 4 wk (during the first month, give additional 120 mg on days 8 and 15)
Potassium phosphate; sodium phosphate	Hypercalcemia: elemental phosphorus 250–500 mg PO four times per day	Hypercalcemia: 4 y of age or older, elemental phosphorus 250 mg PO four times per day
Raloxifene (Evista; ACT Raloxifene, APO-Raloxifene, Evista)	Postmenopausal osteoporosis: prevention/treatment: 60 mg PO once daily	No use established
Teriparatide (Forteo; Forteo)	Postmenopausal osteoporosis, osteoporosis in men, glucocorticoid-induced osteoporosis: 20 mcg subcutaneous daily for up to 2 y (first dose, sitting, or lying down)	No use established

occur if serum phosphate exceeds 4.5 mg/dL or the product of serum calcium and phosphate exceeds 60 mg/dL. Use with caution in preeclampsia and during breast-feeding.

Raloxifene (Evista) is a selective estrogen receptor modulator that is used to prevent or treat postmenopausal osteoporosis. It acts like estrogen in some body tissues and prevents the action of estrogen in other body tissues. It has estrogenic effects in bone tissue, thereby decreasing bone breakdown and increasing bone mass density. It has antiestrogen effects in breast and uterine tissue. Raloxifene increases the risk of deep vein thrombosis or pulmonary emboli; the risk of death due to stroke may be increased in women with coronary heart disease or in women at risk for coronary events. Raloxifene is not indicated for patients of reproductive potential; it is contraindicated during pregnancy.

Teriparatide (Forteo) is a recombinant DNA version of PTH that is approved for the treatment of osteoporosis in women. This drug increases bone formation by increasing the number of bone-building cells (osteoblasts). It also increases serum levels of calcium and the active form of vitamin D. In clinical trials, teriparatide increased vertebral bone mineral density and decreased vertebral fractures. Experts recommend the drug for use in patients with severe osteoporosis or those who have not responded adequately to other treatments. Patients with an increased risk of osteosarcoma, such as those with Paget disease, prior radiation, unexplained elevation of alkaline phosphatase, and open epiphyses, should avoid using teriparatide. Adverse effects include nausea, headache, back pain, dizziness, syncope, and leg cramps. It is necessary to administer the drug with the patient sitting or lying down to prevent orthostatic hypotension.

Teriparatide is rapidly and well absorbed after subcutaneous injection. Bioavailability is 95%, and peak serum levels occur in 30 minutes. The drug is metabolized and excreted through the liver, kidneys, and bone. It is not expected to accumulate in bone or other tissues, to interact significantly with other drugs, or to require dosage adjustment with abnormal kidney function or hepatic impairment. Discontinue the drug in pregnancy; avoid use if breast-feeding.

Emergency Treatment of Hypercalcemia

Acute hypercalcemia (severe symptoms or a serum calcium level greater than 14 mg/dL) is a medical emergency, and rehydration is a priority. It is essential to administer an IV saline solution (0.9% sodium chloride) at an initial rate of 200 to 300 mL/h and then adjust it to maintain a urine output of 100 to 150 mL/h. Authorities no longer recommend the routine use of loop diuretics, such as furosemide, in the absence of heart failure or abnormal kidney function. Because sodium, potassium, and water are also lost in the urine, replacement with IV fluids is necessary.

In addition, patients who are symptomatic should receive calcitonin subcutaneously. Long-term control of hypercalcemia requires addition of a bisphosphonate; zoledronic acid and pamidronate are preferred agents. These two bisphosphonates are given intravenously and reach their maximum effect in 2 to 4 days (Shane & Berenson, 2022).

THE NURSING PROCESS

A concept map outlines the nursing process related to drug therapy considerations in this chapter. Additional nursing implications related to the disease process should also be considered in care decisions.

Assessment
- Assess for risk factors and manifestations of hypocalcemia and calcium deficiency:
  - Assess dietary intake of dairy products, other calcium-containing foods, and vitamin D.
  - Assess serum calcium. The normal total serum calcium level is approximately 8.5 to 10.5 mg/dL (SI units 2.2–2.6 mmol/L). Approximately half of the total serum calcium (4–5 mg/dL) should be free ionized calcium, the physiologically active form. To interpret serum calcium levels accurately, serum albumin levels and acid–base status must be considered. Low serum albumin decreases the total serum level of calcium by decreasing the amount of calcium that is bound to protein; however, the ionized concentration is unaffected by serum albumin levels. Metabolic and respiratory alkalosis increase the binding of calcium to serum proteins, thereby maintaining normal serum calcium but decreasing the ionized values. Conversely, metabolic and respiratory acidosis decrease binding and therefore increase the concentration of ionized calcium.
  - Assess Chvostek and Trousseau signs.
- Assess for conditions in which hypercalcemia is likely to occur: cancer, prolonged immobilization, or vitamin D overdose.
- Assess ECG changes indicative of hypercalcemia, which include a shortened QT interval and an inverted T wave.
- Assess for risk factors and manifestations of osteoporosis, especially in postmenopausal women and in men and women on chronic corticosteroid therapy.
- If Paget disease is suspected, assess for an elevated serum alkaline phosphatase level and abnormal bone scan reports.

Outcomes of Therapy

The patient will
- Achieve and maintain normal serum levels of calcium.
- Increase dietary intake of calcium-containing foods to prevent or treat osteoporosis.
- Use calcium or vitamin D supplements in recommended amounts.
- Adhere to instructions for safe drug use and follow-up treatment of hypocalcemia, hypercalcemia, or osteoporosis.
- Be monitored closely for therapeutic and adverse effects of drugs used to treat hypercalcemia.

Nursing Interventions
- Assist all patients in meeting the recommended daily requirements of calcium and vitamin D. Instruct the patient that the best dietary source is milk and other dairy products, including yogurt.
- Recommend that adults drink at least two 8 oz glasses of milk daily (unless contraindicated by the patient's condition). This supplies half of the daily recommended amount of calcium.
- Instruct parents that children need approximately four glasses of milk or an equivalent amount of calcium in milk and other foods to support normal growth and development.
- Teach pregnant and lactating women to consume four glasses of milk or the equivalent to meet increased needs, in addition to prescribed vitamin and mineral supplements.
- Instruct postmenopausal women who take estrogens to consume at least 1,000 mg of calcium daily. Those who do not take estrogen need at least 1,500 mg.
- Instruct patients on calorie restrictions to consume low-calorie sources such as skim milk and low-fat yogurt.
- Educate patients about additional sources of vitamin D. Sun exposure is also needed to supply adequate amounts of vitamin D.
- Instruct patients who have an inadequate intake of calcium to take a calcium supplement to prevent osteoporosis.
- Instruct patients with hypercalcemia to drink 3,000 to 4,000 mL of fluid daily to prevent kidney stone.

Evaluation
- Check laboratory reports of serum calcium levels for normal values.
- Interview and observe for relief of symptoms of hypocalcemia, hypercalcemia, or osteoporosis.
- Interview and observe intake of calcium-containing foods.
- Question about normal calcium requirements and how to meet them.
- Interview and observe for accurate drug usage and adherence to follow-up procedures.
- Interview and observe for therapeutic and adverse drug effects.

Unfolding Patient Stories: Suzanne Morris • Part 2

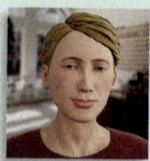

Think back to Suzanne Morris, the 43-year-old female from Chapter 37 who is treated for peptic ulcer disease (PUD) with amoxicillin, clarithromycin, and pantoprazole. During the clinic visit, she expresses concern about a family history of osteoporosis. What patient education should the nurse provide on factors that can influence the development of osteoporosis? If Suzanne's diet is insufficient, what oral supplements would the nurse consider for osteoporosis prevention? What are the nursing implications when administering oral supplements for osteoporosis prevention with her current medications for PUD?

Care for Suzanne and other patients in a realistic virtual environment: *vSim for Nursing* (thepoint.lww.com/vSimPharm). Practice documenting these patients' care in DocuCare (thepoint.lww.com/DocuCareEHR).

Visit thePoint at http://thePoint.lww.com/Frandsen13e for answers to NCLEX Success questions (in Appendix A), answers to Clinical Application Case Studies (in Appendix B), and more!

REFERENCES AND RESOURCES

Bauer, D. C., & Abrahamsen, B. (2021). Bisphosphonate drug holidays in primary care: When and what to do next? *Current Osteoporosis Reports, 19*, 182–188.

Dawson-Hughes, B. (2023). Vitamin D deficiency in adults: Definition, clinical manifestations, and treatment. In *UpToDate*. Lexi-Comp, Inc.

Hinkle, J. L., Cheever, K. H., & Overbaugh, K. J. (2022). *Brunner & Suddarth's textbook of medical-surgical nursing* (15th ed.). Wolters Kluwer.

Nursing 2022 Drug handbook. Wolters Kluwer.

Rosen, H. N. (2021). *Pharmacology of bisphosphonates*. In *UpToDate*. Retrieved June 21, 2022.

Shane, E., & Berenson, J. R. (2022). *Treatment of hypercalcemia*. In *UpToDate*. Retrieved July 5, 2022.

UpToDate. (2022). *Drug information*. Lexi-Comp, Inc.

CHAPTER 45

Drug Therapy for Adrenal Cortex Disorders

LEARNING OBJECTIVES

After studying this chapter, you should be able to:

1. Understand the clinical considerations and manifestations of Addison disease.
2. Understand the clinical considerations and manifestations of Cushing disease.
3. Explain how corticotropin (ACTH) is used in the diagnosis of adrenocortical insufficiency.
4. Explain how cosyntropin (Cortrosyn) is used in the diagnosis of adrenocortical insufficiency.
5. Identify the prototypes and describe the action, use, adverse effects, contraindications, and nursing implications for the drugs used in the treatment of Addison disease.
6. Identify the prototypes and describe the action, use, adverse effects, contraindications, and nursing implications for the drugs used in the treatment of Cushing disease.
7. Implement the nursing process in the care of the patient with Addison disease or Cushing disease.

CLINICAL APPLICATION CASE STUDY

Rosa James is a 68-year-old woman who is being seen by her nurse practitioner with symptoms of muscle weakness and fatigue. She states that she has felt depressed. Physical assessment reveals dark pigmentation of the mucous membranes and skin on the knuckles, knees, and elbows. She appears dehydrated with poor skin turgor. Her blood pressure is 84/50 mm Hg. Blood chemistry reveals sodium level of 132 mEq/L and a potassium level of 5.5 mEq/L. Mrs. James is admitted to the hospital with suspected Addison disease, and an endocrine consult is ordered.

KEY TERMS

Acute adrenal crisis (or Addisonian crisis): acute adrenocortical insufficiency

Adrenocortical excess: increase in adrenocortical function

Adrenocortical insufficiency: decrease in adrenocortical function

INTRODUCTION

This chapter introduces the pharmacologic care of the patient with adrenocortical insufficiency and the patient with adrenocortical excess. The adrenal glands are attached to the upper portion of each kidney. The adrenal cortex of each adrenal gland secretes steroid hormones. The hypothalamic–pituitary–adrenal (HPA) axis regulates hormone secretion. The hypothalamus secretes corticotropin-releasing hormone (CRH), which in turn stimulates the pituitary gland to secrete adrenocorticotropic hormone (ACTH) (Fig. 45.1). The ACTH then stimulates the adrenal cortex to secrete glucocorticoid hormone (cortisol). As the levels of adrenal or steroid hormones increase, the levels of CRH and ACTH decrease through a negative feedback mechanism. For discussion of corticosteroids, see Chapter 17, and for discussion about the types of hormones secreted by the hypothalamus, including CRH, see Chapter 43.

OVERVIEW OF ADDISON DISEASE

Clinical Considerations and Manifestations

Adrenocortical insufficiency is a decrease in adrenocortical function. There are two forms of adrenocortical insufficiency. Primary adrenal insufficiency, or Addison disease, occurs when adrenal cortical hormones are deficient. ACTH levels are elevated because the feedback mechanism is not working. Secondary adrenal insufficiency occurs when there is a disorder in the HPA system.

Primary adrenal insufficiency most commonly results from an autoimmune disorder that has destroyed the layers of the adrenal cortex. Other causes of adrenal cortex destruction include metastatic carcinoma, fungal infections such as histoplasmosis, cytomegalovirus, amyloid disease, and hemochromatosis. Hemorrhage of the adrenal cortex related to anticoagulant therapy, coronary artery bypass graft surgery, giving birth, or trauma also leads to primary adrenal insufficiency.

Secondary adrenal cortical insufficiency results from hypopituitarism or surgical removal of pituitary gland. The abrupt withdrawal of oral glucocorticoids also causes secondary adrenal insufficiency. Patients who have endogenous steroid production from a nonendocrine tumor have adrenocortical insufficiency.

Primary adrenocortical insufficiency is associated with the destruction of the adrenal cortex. The resulting deficiency in the mineralocorticoids causes an increase in the loss of urinary sodium, chloride, and water. The patient becomes hyponatremic, and the cardiac output decreases. This progression of the disease is known as **acute adrenal (or Addisonian) crisis**, which is acute adrenocortical insufficiency. The loss of sodium leads to retention of potassium, resulting in symptoms of hyperkalemia.

The clinical manifestations of adrenocortical insufficiency are evident when approximately 90% of the adrenal cortex has been destroyed. These signs and symptoms reflect loss of sodium, water, and chloride. Findings include decreased cardiac output, dehydration, weakness, and fatigue. Excessive sodium loss results in cardiovascular collapse and shock. Other symptoms include lethargy, weakness, fever, anorexia, nausea, vomiting, and weight loss. Hyperkalemia and hypoglycemia are present. (Any patient with unexplained severe hypoglycemia requires assessment for adrenal insufficiency.) Hyperpigmentation of the gums and mucous membranes is also present;

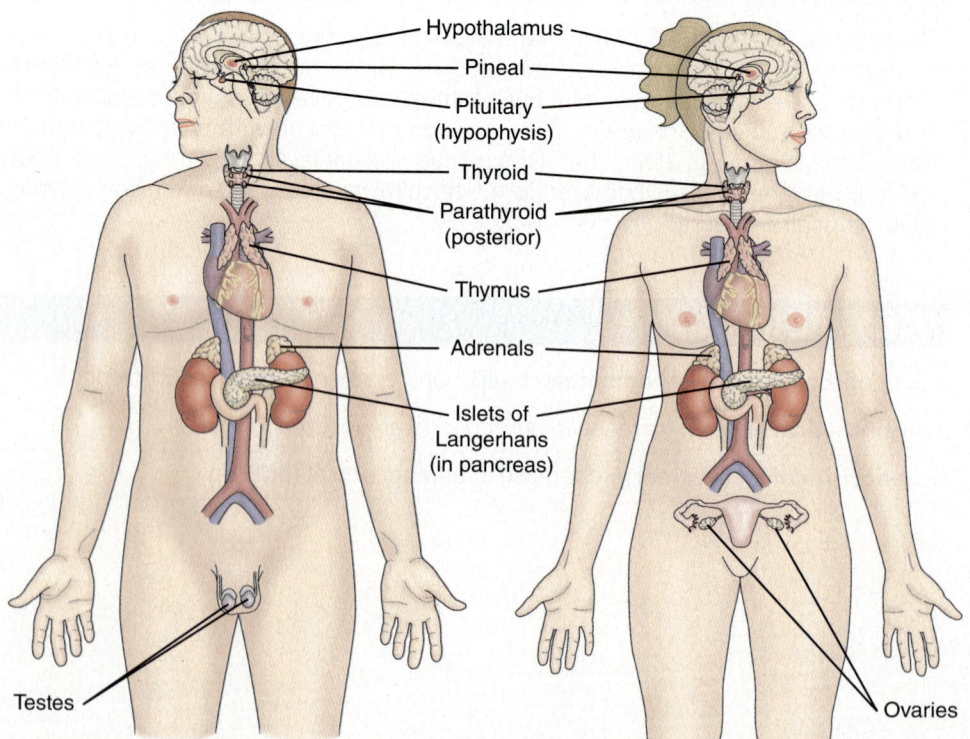

Figure 45.1. The adrenal glands are located on the top of each kidney. Adrenocorticotropic hormone is secreted by the pituitary gland.

they may be bluish black. Females have diminished axillary and pubic hair, but males have few effects from the lack of androgens due to the production of hormones by the testes.

Acute adrenal crisis, or Addisonian crisis, is a life-threatening condition that occurs when Addison disease is the underlying problem and the patient is exposed to minor illness or increased stress. Nausea, vomiting, hypotension, muscle weakness, and vascular collapse are present. There may be a craving for salt.

Clinical Application 45.1

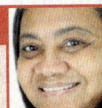

- Mrs. James is hyponatremic. When assessing her cardiac status, what findings would the nurse expect?
- On the second day of Mrs. James' hospital admission, her sodium level is 125 mEq/L. What condition does the nurse suspect?

Quality and Safety Alert: Evidence-Based Practice

Bala et al. (2022) conducted a retrospective study collecting clinical and laboratory data from adrenal insufficiency due to autoimmune adrenalitis in pediatric patients from 2015 to 2020. Primary adrenal insufficiency is rare in children and potentially life-threatening. Pediatric patients present with non-specific symptoms, and it is imperative to establish a diagnosis of adrenal insufficiency. The eight patients identified in the study presented with chronic fatigue, weight loss, altered mental status, and seizures. The median duration of symptoms was 4.5 months. The diagnosis of adrenal insufficiency was confirmed with the serum cortisol and plasma ACTH measurement. The researchers also concluded that appropriate treatment should be instituted and that signs and symptoms of other autoimmune diseases should be investigated.

Diagnosis

Patients commonly present to their primary healthcare provider with vague symptoms of adrenocortical insufficiency. However, as the adrenocortical insufficiency progresses, acute hypotension results and acute adrenal crisis may develop. Making the diagnosis of adrenocortical insufficiency involves laboratory work. This includes early morning serum cortisol and plasma ACTH levels. A serum cortisol level less than 3 mcg/dL, or 80 nmol/L, is indicative of adrenocortical insufficiency. (The normal morning level of serum cortisol is greater—10 to 20 mcg/dL, or 275 to 555 nmol/L.) An ACTH level greater than 22.0 nmol/L is indicative of (primary) adrenocortical insufficiency. (The normal morning level of ACTH is less than 18 nmol/L.)

Confirming the diagnosis of adrenocortical insufficiency requires a short plasma corticotropin stimulation test. The examiner administers corticotropin in the morning, and a subnormal blood cortisol level in the morning and afternoon confirms the diagnosis. A higher cortisol level in the morning is a sign that a person does not have adrenal insufficiency. In a patient with adrenal insufficiency, the response to the corticotropin, or ACTH, is the same both morning and afternoon.

Another test that confirms the diagnosis of adrenocortical insufficiency is the standard high-dose test. It is a three-step process:

1. Measurement of baseline serum cortisol
2. Intravenous (IV) administration of 250 mcg of ACTH 30 minutes later
3. Measurement of serum cortisol 30 to 60 minutes later

An increase of *at least* 18 to 20 mcg/dL is considered normal. No increase in serum cortisol indicates the presence of adrenocortical insufficiency.

Diagnosis of secondary adrenocortical insufficiency in its early stages requires the low-dose test. It is also used for the diagnosis of chronic partial pituitary ACTH deficiency. This test involves the administration of 1 mcg of cosyntropin (Cortrosyn) as an IV bolus. Normally, an increase in cortisol occurs in 20 minutes. In patients with adrenocortical insufficiency, there is no increase in the serum cortisol level.

OVERVIEW OF CUSHING DISEASE

Clinical Considerations and Manifestations

Adrenocortical excess, an increase in adrenocortical function, is the cause of Cushing disease. In most patients, increased adrenocortical function results from excessive corticotropin, leading to hyperplasia of the adrenal cortex. In a smaller percentage of patients, adrenocortical excess is the result of a cortisol-secreting adrenal tumor, whether from too much corticotropin (ACTH) or a primary tumor of the adrenal gland. A malignant tumor of the adrenal gland can produce many corticosteroids, whereas the benign adrenal tumor only produces one corticosteroid that is secreted by the adrenal gland. Other, much less common causes are hyperplasia of the adrenal gland or ectopic production of ACTH by malignancies such as bronchogenic carcinoma. Long-term treatment with pharmacologic glucocorticoids leads to iatrogenic Cushing syndrome.

Patients with Cushing disease often present with classic signs and symptoms. These include obesity, with a heavy trunk and thin extremities, a fatty "buffalo hump" at the neck and supraclavicular region, and a moon-faced appearance. The skin becomes fragile and tears easily, and broad purple striae and bruises may develop. Wound healing may be impaired. The hair is thin. Females have virilization with the appearance of masculine traits such as increased facial hair, breast atrophy, enlarged clitoris, disrupted menses, and voice deepening. Libido is diminished or absent in males and females. Depression, weakness, and lassitude may also occur.

The excessive secretion of corticotropin leads to osteoporosis and fractures, which are caused by the increase in calcium reabsorption from the bone. Blood glucose levels are also increased, and glucose intolerance may occur as a result of increased hepatic gluconeogenesis and resistance to insulin. Peptic ulcers may develop because of increased secretion of gastric acid and pepsin.

Diagnosis

The diagnosis of Cushing disease requires an overnight dexamethasone suppression test. The patient takes dexamethasone,

TABLE 45.1

Drugs Administered for Addison Disease

Drug Class	Prototypes	Other Drugs in the Class
Adrenocorticoid/mineralocorticoids	Hydrocortisone (Alkindi Sprinkle, Cortef, Solu-CORTEF)	None
Mineralocorticoids	Fludrocortisone	None

a synthetic glucocorticoid, 1 mg orally at 11 p.m. A serum cortisol level is drawn at 8 a.m. A cortisol level of less than 5 mcg/dL indicates that the HPA axis is functioning normally. Cortisol levels are higher in patients with adrenal or ectopic tumors.

DRUGS USED TO TREAT ADDISON DISEASE

The goal of treatment for Addison disease is to replace the adrenocorticoids to correct adrenal insufficiency. It is important to replace both the mineralocorticoid and adrenocorticoid. Lifetime hormone replacement is necessary. Table 45.1 summarizes the adrenocorticoid and mineralocorticoids Administered for the treatment of adrenocortical insufficiency.

ADRENOCORTICOIDS/MINERALOCORTICOIDS

The prototype **hydrocortisone** (Alkindi Sprinkle, Cortef, Solu-CORTEF), a combination of a mineralocorticoid and adrenocorticoid, is useful in acute and chronic adrenal insufficiency.

Pharmacokinetics

The oral preparation of hydrocortisone has a 1- to 2-hour onset of action, a peak of action in 1 to 2 hours, and a duration of action of 1 to 1.5 days. The parenteral preparation of the drug has an immediate onset of action, an unknown peak of action, and a duration of action of 1 to 1.5 days. Metabolism occurs in the liver. Excretion is in the kidneys.

Action

Hydrocortisone enters the cells and binds to the receptors in the cytoplasm to decrease inflammation; it suppresses the migration of polymorphonuclear lymphocytes and decreases capillary permeability. The mineralocorticoid in the drug increases the retention of sodium.

Use

Healthcare providers use hydrocortisone to replace adrenocorticoids and mineralocorticoids in patients with Addison disease. The drug is also useful in congenital adrenal hyperplasia. Table 45.2 gives route and dosage information for adrenocorticoids and mineralocorticoids.

Patient-related variables specific to the use of hydrocortisone include the following:

- Age:
  - In infants and children, the dose is individualized depending on the severity of the adrenal insufficiency and the response to the medication. Because the drug may affect growth velocity, it is important to carefully assess growth and development. Also, the neonate's respiratory status is assessed closely after administration of parenteral hydrocortisone. Some preparations contain benzyl alcohol, which may cause gasping syndrome in neonates.
  - In premature neonates, the use of high-dose dexamethasone for the treatment of bronchopulmonary dysplasia

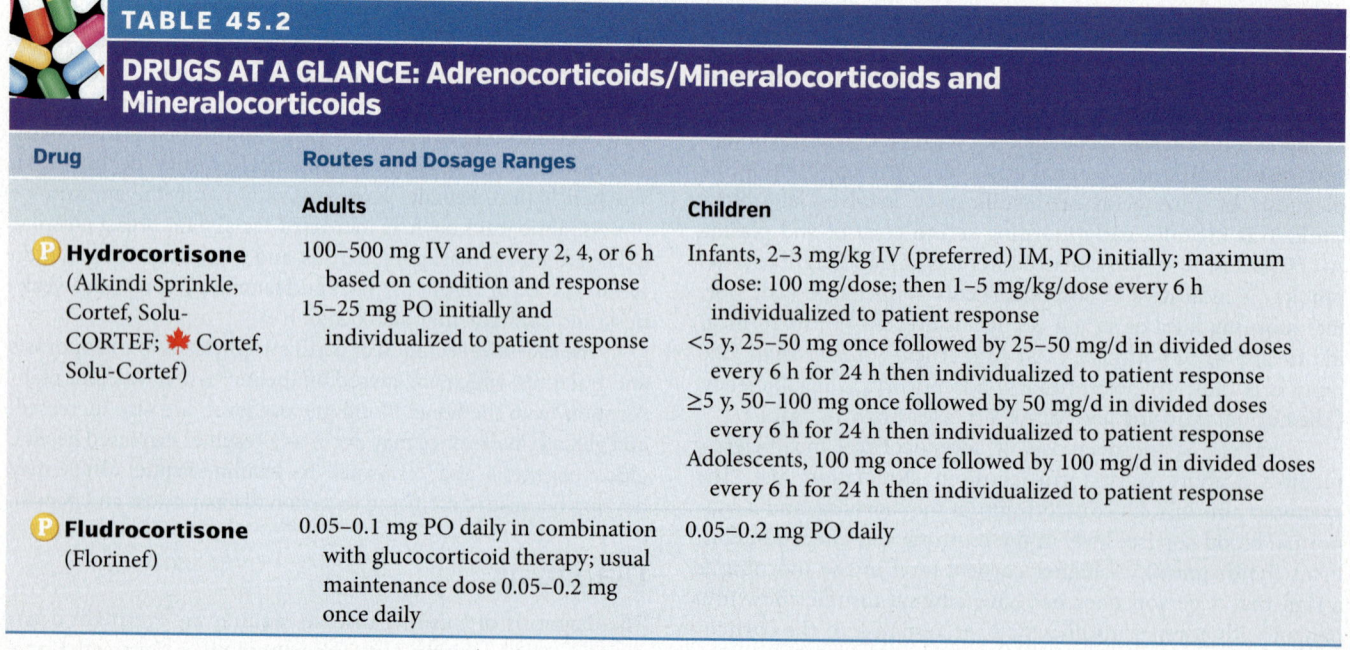

TABLE 45.2

DRUGS AT A GLANCE: Adrenocorticoids/Mineralocorticoids and Mineralocorticoids

Drug	Routes and Dosage Ranges	
	Adults	**Children**
Hydrocortisone (Alkindi Sprinkle, Cortef, Solu-CORTEF; ✦ Cortef, Solu-Cortef)	100–500 mg IV and every 2, 4, or 6 h based on condition and response 15–25 mg PO initially and individualized to patient response	Infants, 2–3 mg/kg IV (preferred) IM, PO initially; maximum dose: 100 mg/dose; then 1–5 mg/kg/dose every 6 h individualized to patient response <5 y, 25–50 mg once followed by 25–50 mg/d in divided doses every 6 h for 24 h then individualized to patient response ≥5 y, 50–100 mg once followed by 50 mg/d in divided doses every 6 h for 24 h then individualized to patient response Adolescents, 100 mg once followed by 100 mg/d in divided doses every 6 h for 24 h then individualized to patient response
Fludrocortisone (Florinef)	0.05–0.1 mg PO daily in combination with glucocorticoid therapy; usual maintenance dose 0.05–0.2 mg once daily	0.05–0.2 mg PO daily

(approximately >0.5 mg/kg/day) has been associated with adverse neurodevelopmental outcomes.
- Use caution in older adults due to the increased risk of adverse effects with systemic corticosteroids. It is imperative to use the smallest possible effective dose for the shortest duration of time.
- Reproduction, pregnancy, and lactation:
  - The development of oral clefts or decreased birth weight has been associated with first trimester systemic corticosteroid use.
  - For treatment of adrenal insufficiency in pregnant patients, hydrocortisone is the preferred corticosteroid.
  - Pregnant patients with adrenal insufficiency should be monitored at least once per trimester.
  - Corticosteroids are present in breast milk and are generally considered acceptable in breast-feeding patients.
- Abnormal kidney function and hepatic impairment:
  - No dosage adjustments are necessary with abnormal kidney function or hepatic impairment.

Adverse Effects

Hydrocortisone has significant adverse effects, including the following:

- Cardiac effects: fluctuations in blood pressure, shock, dysrhythmias, myocardial infarction, embolism, circulatory collapse, heart failure, and cardiac arrest
- Central nervous system (CNS) effects: vertigo, headache, and depression
- Dermatologic effects: fragile skin that tears easily, petechiae, ecchymoses
- Gastrointestinal (GI) effects: peptic or esophageal ulcers, pancreatitis, increased appetite, and weight gain
- Hematologic effects: sodium and fluid retention
- Metabolic effects: hyperglycemia and Cushing syndrome
- Musculoskeletal effects: osteoporosis and spontaneous fractures (long-term administration)
- Reproductive (female) effects: amenorrhea and irregular menses
- Other effects: immunosuppression, muscle weakness, impaired wound healing, and anaphylaxis

Contraindications

Contraindications to hydrocortisone include a known hypersensitivity to the drug or any component of the formulation as well as a serious infection. The U.S. Food and Drug Administration (FDA) has issued a **BOXED WARNING** stating that patients who are being treated with hydrocortisone should not receive live virus vaccines.

Nursing Implications

Preventing Interactions

Several medications interact with hydrocortisone, increasing or decreasing its effects (Box 45.1). Echinacea may increase the

---

BOX 45.1 Drug Interactions: Hydrocortisone

Drugs That Increase the Effects of Hydrocortisone
- Estrogen, hormonal contraceptives, ketoconazole, troleandomycin
  Increase steroid blood levels

Drugs That Decrease the Effects of Hydrocortisone
- Cholestyramine, phenobarbital, phenytoin, rifampin
  Decrease steroid blood levels

---

effects of hydrocortisone, whereas St. John's wort may decrease the drug's effects. Hydrocortisone has numerous other interactions. Combination of hydrocortisone with certain drugs may result in the following effects:

- Salicylates: increased serum salicylate levels
- Acetylcholinesterase drugs: diminished therapeutic effect
- Anticoagulants: increased bleeding; it is necessary to monitor the prothrombin time and the international normalized ratio closely
- Food: interference with calcium absorption
- Alcohol: increased risk of gastric mucosal irritation and development of gastric ulcers

Administering the Medication

People should take the oral preparation with food to decrease gastric irritation.

> **Quality and Safety Alert: Safety**
> Administration of hydrocortisone should take place every morning before 9 a.m. This minimizes HPA suppression.

It is necessary to dilute hydrocortisone sodium succinate to 50 mg/mL and administer the drug as an IV bolus over 30 seconds or over 10 minutes for doses ≥500 mg. For intermittent IV infusion, dilution to 1 mg/mL and administration over 20 to 30 minutes are appropriate.

Assessing for Therapeutic Effects

The nurse assesses the patient's blood pressure, pulse, and respirations for improved cardiac function. The sodium level and fluid volume status are assessed for return to normal range with retention of sodium and water. It is important to assess for increased strength and energy as well as for improved mood and ability to cope with stress.

Assessing for Adverse Effects

The nurse assesses for hypertension, heart failure, or alterations in cardiac output. It is important to assess for normal menses and diminished virilization in females. Also, the nurse checks the patient's ability to fight infection (e.g., normal white blood cell count). In addition, serum blood sugar is assessed to rule out hypoglycemia or hyperglycemia.

> **BOX 45.2 Patient Teaching Guidelines for Hydrocortisone**
>
> - Take the oral preparation of hydrocortisone every day at 9:00 a.m.
> - Space other doses of hydrocortisone evenly throughout the day.
> - Do not stop the medication abruptly or without notifying the prescriber.
> - Inform the healthcare provider of increased stress, as the medication dosage may need to be increased.
> - Increase calcium intake if hydrocortisone is administered for a prolonged period.
> - Administer antacids between doses of hydrocortisone to prevent gastric irritation.
> - Monitor blood sugar daily.
> - Wear a medic alert bracelet.
> - Report swelling, weight gain, muscle weakness, tarry stools, moon face, fever, infection, inability of wounds to heal, and fatigue.

Patient Teaching

Box 45.2 presents patient teaching guidelines for hydrocortisone.

> **Clinical Application 45.2**
>
> - Mrs. James' endocrinologist orders hydrocortisone 200 mg intravenously every 4 hours. How does the nurse dilute the drug, and over what period does the nurse administer it?
> - One hour following the administration of the medication, the endocrinologist orders blood glucose testing. What is the rationale for blood glucose testing?
> - What is the action of hydrocortisone?

MINERALOCORTICOIDS

If a patient with Addison disease requires additional mineralocorticoid supplementation, then (P) **fludrocortisone**, a synthetic steroid, is useful. A patient usually takes it in combination with a glucocorticoid. It is important to note that fludrocortisone has also proved effective for the treatment of orthostatic hypotension in older adults.

Pharmacokinetics and Action

Fludrocortisone is absorbed rapidly and completely and is 42% protein-bound. The drug reaches a peak serum level in approximately 1.7 hours, and it has a 3.5-hour serum half-life. Metabolism occurs in the liver. The site of excretion is unknown.

Fludrocortisone has strong mineralocorticoid action. This drug produces sodium retention and potassium excretion to increase blood pressure.

Use

Healthcare providers use fludrocortisone for partial replacement of mineralocorticoids in the treatment of primary and secondary adrenocortical insufficiency resulting from Addison disease.

Patient-related variables specific to the use of fludrocortisone include the following:

- Age:
  - In young children who have taken high doses of fludrocortisone for long periods, the drug may cause hypercortisolism suppression of the HPA axis. This suppression can lead to adrenal crisis.
  - Because fludrocortisone may affect growth velocity, pediatric patients require routine assessment of growth and development.
  - In older adults, the lowest dose possible for the shortest duration is used to prevent the risk of adverse effects.
- Reproduction, pregnancy, and lactation:
  - Use of systemic corticosteroids during pregnancy requires administration of the lowest possible dosage.
  - It is not known if fludrocortisone enters breast milk. The manufacturer recommends cautious use of fludrocortisone during breast-feeding.
- Abnormal kidney function and hepatic impairment:
  - No dosage adjustments are recommended with abnormal kidney function or hepatic impairment.
  - Patients with hepatic impairment or cirrhosis who take fludrocortisone for long periods require close monitoring for fluid retention.

Adverse Effects and Contraindications

The endocrine and metabolic effects of fludrocortisone are HPA axis suppression, growth suppression, hyperglycemia, and hypokalemia alkalosis. The most commonly reported cardiopulmonary adverse effects include heart failure, edema, and hypertension. Other adverse effects include peptic ulcer, acne, bruising, rash, cataracts, muscle weakness, and diaphoresis.

Contraindications include known hypersensitivity to the medication or any component of its formulation as well as a systemic fungal infection.

Nursing Implications

Preventing Interactions

Many medications interact with fludrocortisone, increasing or decreasing its effects (Box 45.3). Amphotericin B, indacaterol, loop diuretics, and thiazide diuretics in combination with fludrocortisone enhance the hypokalemic effect of fludrocortisone. Warfarin in combination with fludrocortisone enhances the anticoagulant effect, placing the patient at risk for hemorrhage.

Administering the Medication

People should take fludrocortisone concomitantly with a glucocorticoid to enhance effectiveness and produce a more normal adrenal response. It is necessary to store the drug in an airtight, light-protected container at a temperature of 59°F to 86°F.

Assessing for Therapeutic Effects

The nurse assesses sodium levels for increased values and potassium levels for decreased values. It is also important to assess

> **BOX 45.3** **Drug Interactions: Fludrocortisone**
>
> **Drugs That Decrease the Effects of Fludrocortisone**
> - Acetylcholinesterase inhibitors, neuromuscular agents
>   *Increase muscle weakness*
> - Aminoglutethimide
>   *Increases metabolism of fludrocortisone*
> - Antacids
>   *Decrease bioavailability of fludrocortisone*
> - Barbiturates, primidone
>   *Decrease serum concentration of fludrocortisone*
>
> **Drugs That Increase the Effects of Fludrocortisone**
> - Antifungal agents, calcium channel blockers, macrolide antibiotics
>   *Decrease the metabolism of corticosteroids*
> - Aprepitant, estrogens, fosaprepitant, mifepristone, mitotane, telaprevir
>   *Increase serum concentration of fludrocortisone*

intake, output, and blood pressure. The nurse monitors the patient's weight and assesses fluid volume status. If the weight increases by 5 lb in 1 week, it is necessary to notify the prescriber.

Assessing for Adverse Effects

In children, it is essential to assess growth patterns. In all patients, the nurse assesses the patient's fluid and electrolyte status for hypokalemia and alkalosis. Patients are assessed for pedal edema, hypertension, crackles in the lungs, and an audible S_3 that is indicative of heart failure. It is important to assess the GI system for burning, epigastric pain, and bleeding, which are signs of peptic ulcer disease. The nurse assesses the skin for bruising and rash. Muscle weakness is also assessed.

> **BOX 45.4** **Patient Teaching Guidelines for Fludrocortisone**
>
> - Eat foods high in potassium such as bananas, potatoes, and orange juice.
> - Consume foods high in calcium and vitamins A and D such as dairy products.
> - Take supplements containing vitamins B_6 and C, folate, zinc, and phosphorous.
> - Decrease sodium in the diet and limit salt intake.
> - Report muscle weakness, numbness, fatigue, depression, increased urination, changes in heart rhythm, epigastric pain, and tarry stools.
> - Monitor weight and report an increase of 5 lb to the primary healthcare provider.
> - See an ophthalmologist every 6 months to determine if cataracts have formed.
> - Have periodic laboratory tests as ordered by the prescriber.
> - Report swelling of feet, hands, and shortness of breath to the primary healthcare provider.
> - Report any infections or injuries to the primary healthcare provider.
> - Wear medical alert identification.

Patient Teaching

Box 45.4 contains patient teaching guidelines for fludrocortisone.

> **NCLEX Success**
>
> 1. A patient is taking fludrocortisone acetate for adrenal insufficiency. Which of the following symptoms indicates that the patient is hypokalemic?
>   A. tetany
>   B. irregular pulse rate
>   C. decreased pulse rate
>   D. muscle weakness
>
> 2. The administration of fludrocortisone is necessary in which of the following conditions?
>   A. hypoglycemia
>   B. hypernatremia
>   C. hypercalcemia
>   D. hyperphosphatemia
>
> 3. A patient receives a prescription of hydrocortisone for adrenal insufficiency. It is necessary to report which of the following conditions to the primary healthcare provider?
>   A. fever
>   B. headache
>   C. insomnia
>   D. neuropathic pain

DRUGS USED TO TREAT CUSHING DISEASE

The treatment of Cushing disease depends on the cause of the medical condition. The most common treatment of hypercortisolism is transsphenoidal surgery. Drug therapy is indicated in several situations: when surgery is contraindicated, in preparation for surgery, in occult ectopic ACTH syndrome, with a recurrence of hypercortisolism following surgery, and with treatment using radiation therapy to the pituitary.

GLUCOCORTICOID RECEPTOR ANTAGONISTS

Glucocorticoid receptor antagonists are administered when surgery to treat corticotroph tumors is delayed or contraindicated. The two medications used to normalize the 24-hour urinary cortisol are cabergoline and pasireotide. Cabergoline is an ergot derivative. Its off-label use is to normalize urinary free cortisol levels in the treatment of Cushing syndrome. Pasireotide is a somatostatin analog to maximize the reduction of urinary free cortisol. The maximum reduction of cortisol is usually noted in approximately 2 months.

Cabergoline is a long-acting dopamine receptor agonist. It has a high affinity for D_2 receptors in the anterior pituitary. It inhibits lactation and hyperprolactinemia. Cabergoline is administered orally with food. Cabergoline is extensively distributed to the pituitary gland. It is 40% to 42% protein-bound, with a half-life of 63 to 69 hours. Metabolism of the drug takes place in the liver by hydrolysis. The peak of action is 2 to 3 hours, with 60% excretion in the feces and approximately 20% in the urine. Patients with impaired liver function will see an increase in cabergoline levels. Hot flashes, edema, and orthostatic hypotension are the most commonly reported adverse effects. Patients who have a history of cardiac valvular disease should not be administered cabergoline. It is also contraindicated in patients with a known ergot hypersensitivity.

Pasireotide (Signifor, Signifor LAR) binds to somatostatin receptor with high affinity for sst_1, sst_2, sst_3, and sst_5. It inhibits ACTH secretion and causes decreased cortisol secretion. Patients with severe hepatic impairment should avoid this medication. If symptoms of hepatic impairment develop, the medication should be discontinued. Gloves should be worn when unpacking, administering, or disposing of pasireotide. Assess the patient for peripheral edema, hyperglycemia, diarrhea, and prolonged partial thromboplastin time. Assess the serum alanine aminotransferase and serum aspartate aminotransferase; if there is an elevation of ALT and AST, the medication dosage should be reduced or discontinued. In addition, assess the blood glucose for elevation.

11-DEOXYCORTISOL INHIBITORS

In Cushing disease, the goal of drug therapy is to inhibit one or more enzymes contained in cortisol synthesis. The antifungal drug (see Chapter 24) **ketoconazole** can inhibit these enzymes. It also prevents the conversion of 11-deoxycortisol to cortisol. Table 45.3 identifies the drugs administered for the treatment of Cushing disease.

Pharmacokinetics and Action

Ketoconazole is absorbed rapidly in the GI tract. The drug is protein-bound. It is metabolized in the liver and excreted by the kidneys.

TABLE 45.3
Drugs Administered for Cushing Disease

Drug Class	Prototype	Other Drugs in the Class
Glucocorticoid receptor antagonists	N/A	Ergot derivative: Cabergoline Somatostatin analog: Pasireotide (Signifor, Signifor LAR)
11-Deoxycortisol inhibitors	Ketoconazole	Metyrapone (Metopirone) Etomidate (Amidate)
Antineoplastics	Mitotane (Lysodren)	None

Ketoconazole acts by inhibiting the first step in cortisol biosynthesis and the conversion of deoxycortisol to cortisol.

Use

Healthcare providers use ketoconazole to control cortisol secretion in Cushing disease. Table 45.4 presents route and dosage information for the drugs used in Cushing disease.

Patient-related variables specific to the use of ketoconazole include the following:

- Age:
  - There are no specific variables based on age.
- Reproduction, pregnancy, and lactation:
  - Patients treated with ketoconazole may experience a decrease in ovulatory disturbances and should be informed of the potential return of fertility.
  - Ketoconazole may cause fetal harm.
  - Ketoconazole is present in breast milk.
- Abnormal kidney function and hepatic impairment:
  - No dosage adjustments are necessary with abnormal kidney function.
  - Use of ketoconazole is contraindicated in acute or chronic liver disease.

Adverse Effects and Contraindications

The most commonly reported adverse effects associated with ketoconazole include pruritus, headache, sedation, nausea, vomiting, and abdominal pain. Gynecomastia, impotence, and decreased libido may occur and are related to the decrease in testosterone production. The FDA has issued a **BOXED WARNING** ◆ stating that ketoconazole can cause hepatotoxicity. Therefore, it is contraindicated in acute or chronic liver disease.

Contraindications include a known hypersensitivity to the medication.

Nursing Implications

Preventing Interactions

Some medications interact with ketoconazole, decreasing its effects (Box 45.5). Ketoconazole combined with echinacea puts the patient at risk for hepatotoxicity. In addition, a **BOXED WARNING** ◆ alerts that ketoconazole increases the plasma concentration of methadone, pimozide, cisapride, disopyramide, dronedarone, and ranolazine, and it may prolong QT intervals on an electrocardiogram. Coadministration increases the risk of life-threatening ventricular dysrhythmias, such as torsades de pointes.

Administering the Medication

People should take ketoconazole with water, coffee, tea, or fruit juice. The presence of stomach acid enhances absorption.

Assessing for Therapeutic Effects and Adverse Effects

The nurse assesses for a decrease in blood pressure and checks the blood glucose for normal levels. It is also important to assess

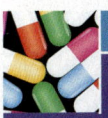

TABLE 45.4
DRUGS AT A GLANCE: Glucocorticoid Receptor Antagonists, 11-Deoxycortisol Inhibitors, and Antineoplastics

Drug	Routes and Dosage Ranges	
	Adults	Children
Glucocorticoid Receptor Antagonists		
Cabergoline	0.5 mg PO daily	Not administered to children
Pasireotide (Signifor, Signifor LAR)	0.6 or 0.9 mg subcutaneous two times per day Signifor LAR: Initial: 10 mg once every 28 d; may increase dose to a maximum of 40 mg once every 28 d	Not administered to children
11-Deoxycortisol Inhibitors		
ⓟ Ketoconazole (Apo-Ketoconazole, Teva-Ketoconazole)	200–400 mg PO 2–3 times per day	Cushing syndrome: second line therapy: Children >12 y and adolescents: Initial PO 400–600 mg/d in 2–3 divided doses; doses can be increased by 200 mg/d every 7–28 d based on patient response. Peripheral precocious puberty: Children > 2 y and adolescents: PO 10–20 mg/kg/d in 3 divided doses
Metyrapone (Metopirone)	250 mg PO four times daily (max dose 6,000 mg) Diagnostic test for hypothalamic–pituitary adrenocorticotropic hormone (ACTH) function: single dose, 30 mg/kg (max 3 g) at midnight; multiple dose, 750 mg/kg every 4 h for 6 doses	Diagnostic test for ACTH function: single dose, 30 mg/kg (min 250 mg; max 750 mg) at midnight; multiple dose, 15 mg/kg every 4 h for 6 doses
Etomidate (Amidate)	0.04–0.05 mg/kg IV per hour titrated to serum cortisol level	Same as adults
Antineoplastics		
ⓟ Mitotane (Lysodren; ✹ Lysodren)	Adrenocortical carcinoma: 2–6 g/d in 3–4 divided doses and then increase incrementally to 9–10 g/d in 3–4 divided doses; max tolerated range is 2–16 g/d, usually 9–10 g/d; max studied dose is 18–19 g/d Cushing syndrome: 500 mg PO three times per day; max dose 4,000–8,000 mg in three divided doses per day	Safety and efficacy not established

for increased muscle strength and cardiopulmonary status without edema or crackles in the lower lobes and audible S_3.

Assessing for adverse effects is also necessary. The nurse assesses for skin irritation and pruritus; nausea, vomiting, and headache; and diminished libido, gynecomastia, and impotence.

Patient Teaching

Box 45.6 presents patient teaching guidelines for ketoconazole.

> **Quality and Safety Alert: Patient-Centered Care**
>
> Stomach acid increases the absorption of some medications, like ketoconazole. Coffee, tea, and fruit juice increase the acidity in the stomach, enhancing the absorption of these medications.

BOX 45.5 Drug Interactions: Ketoconazole

Drugs That Decrease the Effects of Ketoconazole
- Antacids, anticholinergics
  Decrease absorption, thus decreasing serum levels
- Isoniazid, rifampin
  Increase metabolism

BOX 45.6 Patient Teaching Guidelines for Ketoconazole

- Take the medication with water, coffee, tea, or fruit juice. Acidic drinks enhance absorption.
- Take the drug with food to prevent gastrointestinal upset.
- Do not take antacids.
- Maintain serum liver enzyme laboratory tests as ordered by the prescriber.
- Report clay-colored stools, extreme thirst, and yellowing of skin or eyes. These signs and symptoms indicate elevated liver enzymes.

Other Drugs in the Class

Metyrapone and etomidate are also administered for their inhibition of 11-deoxycortisol. Metyrapone (Metopirone) blocks the final step in cortisol biosynthesis and increases adrenal androgen production. The drug also decreases cortisol production. It is administered as an adjunctive agent to prevent further release of ACTH in patients with mild Cushing disease or following radiation therapy of the pituitary gland.

Etomidate (Amidate) also blocks the production of cortisol. Normally administered to produce sedation, it is a local anesthetic and is discussed in Chapter 50. Prescribers order it for patients with ectopic secretion of ACTH (Cushing disease).

> **Quality and Safety Alert: Safety**
>
> Etomidate has not demonstrated sedation at recommended doses for Cushing disease. However, patients should be managed in an intensive care unit with sedation scoring every 2 hours for the first 24 hours, then every 12 hours, to assess for sedation.

Etomidate lowers serum cortisol to normal in approximately 10 hours. Cortisol levels should be measured every 4 to 6 hours.

ANTINEOPLASTICS

Healthcare providers use the antineoplastic drug **mitotane** (Lysodren) for the treatment of adrenocortical carcinoma. The drug may also be useful for therapy of Cushing disease caused by such carcinoma.

Pharmacokinetics and Action

Mitotane is absorbed rapidly, with approximately 40% of the drug absorbed in the GI tract. The onset of action is 2 to 4 weeks. The half-life of mitotane is 18 to 159 days. The drug is metabolized in the liver and deposited in the adipose tissues. It is eliminated in the urine and feces.

Mitotane is an adrenolytic agent that causes the adrenal cortex to atrophy. The drug affects the mitochondrial adrenal cortical cells, resulting in decreased production of cortisol. It also alters the peripheral metabolism of steroids.

Use

Mitotane is used for the treatment of an inoperable adrenocortical carcinoma. Its unlabeled use is for treatment of Cushing syndrome. Table 45.4 gives route and dosing information for mitotane.

Patient-related variables specific to the use of mitotane include the following:

- Age:
  - Mitotane is associated with moderate emetic potential, so antiemetic use is recommended with pediatric patients.
- Reproduction, pregnancy, and lactation:
  - Use of effective birth control is recommended in patients receiving mitotane.
  - Mitotane crosses the placenta and has the potential to cause fetal harm.
  - Mitotane is present in breast milk, and breast-feeding should be discontinued with its use.
- Abnormal kidney function and hepatic impairment:
  - No dosage adjustments are recommended in patients with abnormal kidney function or mild-to-moderate hepatic impairment.
  - Mitotane is not recommended in severe hepatic impairment.

Adverse Effects and Contraindications

The CNS effects of mitotane include depression, lethargy, and dizziness. GI effects are anorexia, nausea, vomiting, and diarrhea. Neuromuscular effects include weakness and muscle tremors.

Contraindications include known hypersensitivity to the drug.

Nursing Implications

Preventing Interactions

Mitotane increases the metabolism of phenytoin, phenobarbital, and warfarin. The antineoplastic drug decreases the effect of potassium-sparing diuretics. Alcohol increases the CNS depression associated with mitotane.

Administering the Medication

The FDA has issued a stating that it is necessary to withhold mitotane in the event the patient develops shock or with trauma, because the primary action of the drug is adrenal suppression, and adrenal crisis can occur. The onset of shock or trauma should lead to a temporary discontinuation of mitotane followed by the administration of steroids.

> **Quality and Safety Alert: Safety**
>
> The Institute for Safe Medication Practices considers mitotane to be a drug that has a heightened risk of causing significant patient harm when used in error.

Assessing for Therapeutic Effects

The nurse assesses for a decrease in blood pressure. It is necessary to check the blood glucose for normal levels. The nurse also assesses for increased muscle strength and cardiopulmonary status without edema or crackles in the lower lobes and audible S_3.

Assessing for Adverse Effects

The nurse assesses for CNS depression, which may place the patient at risk for injury. It is also important to assess the gait for safety with walking. The nurse assesses for decreased weight related to anorexia or fluid and electrolyte balance related to nausea and vomiting, as well as for muscle weakness and tremors.

Patient Teaching

Box 45.7 presents patient teaching guidelines for mitotane.

NCLEX Success

4. A patient has received a diagnosis of Cushing disease and is taking ketoconazole. Which of the following conditions affects the treatment plan?
   A. hypertension with administration of hydrochlorothiazide
   B. type 2 diabetes with the administration of metformin
   C. migraine headaches with the administration of ergotamine
   D. heart failure with the administration of digoxin

5. A patient receiving mitotane for an inoperable adrenocortical carcinoma is admitted to the emergency department following an automobile accident. The patient is diaphoretic and unresponsive. The patient's blood pressure is 80/30 mm Hg. What medication should the nurse anticipate administering?
   A. a steroid
   B. an anticoagulant
   C. a beta-adrenergic blocker
   D. a sulfonylurea

BOX 45.7 Patient Teaching Guidelines for Mitotane

- Understand that this drug will decrease the tumor mass but will not cure the disease.
- Report signs and symptoms of adrenal insufficiency, including weakness, fatigue, orthostatic hypotension, nausea, anorexia, vomiting, increase skin pigmentation, and weight loss.
- Do not operate machinery due to diminished alertness and central nervous system depression.

THE NURSING PROCESS

A concept map outlines the nursing process related to drug therapy considerations in this chapter. Additional nursing implications related to the disease process should also be considered in care decisions.

Assessment
- For the patient with Addison's disease, the major focus of the assessment should be on the severity of symptoms and the effectiveness of drug therapy for the treatment of the disease. Assess for dehydration, hypovolemia, hypoglycemia, hyperkalemia, weight loss, hyperpigmentation of gums and mucous membranes, and depression.
- For the patient with Cushing's disease, the major focus of the assessment should be on the severity of symptoms, body image, and drug therapy of the treatment of the disease. Assess for glucose intolerance, fragile skin tissues, truncal obesity, peripheral edema, osteoporosis, moon face, buffalo hump, irritability, and decreased wound healing.

Outcomes of Therapy

The patient will
- Take the drug correctly.
- Practice measures to decrease the need for corticosteroids and minimize adverse effects.
- Be monitored regularly for adverse drug effects.
- Keep appointments for follow-up care.
- Be assisted to cope with body image changes.
- Verbalize or demonstrate essential drug information.

Nursing Interventions
- For the patient taking long-term, systemic mineralocorticoid/glucocorticoid therapy, use supplementary drugs as ordered and nondrug measures to decrease dosage and adverse effects of corticosteroid drugs. Specific measures include the following:
  - Help set reasonable goals of drug therapy. For example, partial relief of symptoms may be better than complete relief if the latter requires larger doses or longer periods of treatment with systemic drugs.
  - Dietary changes may be beneficial. Salt restriction may help prevent hypernatremia, fluid retention, and edema. Foods high in potassium may help prevent hypokalemia. A diet high in protein, calcium, and vitamin D may help prevent osteoporosis. Increased intake of vitamin C may help decrease bleeding in the skin and soft tissues.
  - Avoid exposing the patient to potential sources of infection by washing hands frequently, using aseptic technique when changing dressings, keeping healthcare personnel and visitors with colds or other infections away from the patient, and following other appropriate measures.
  - Handle tissues very gently during any procedures (e.g., bathing, assisting out of bed, venipunctures).

Evaluation
- Interview and observe for relief of symptoms for which mineralocorticoids, adrenocorticoids, cortisol, 11-deoxycortisol inhibitors, and antineoplastic agents have been prescribed.
- Interview and observe for accurate drug administration.
- Interview and observe for use of nondrug measures indicated for the condition being treated.
- Interview and observe for adverse drug effects on a regular basis.
- Interview regarding drug knowledge and effects to be reported to healthcare providers.

Visit thePoint® at http://thePoint.lww.com/Frandsen13e for answers to NCLEX Success questions (in Appendix A), answers to Clinical Application Case Studies (in Appendix B), and more!

REFERENCES AND RESOURCES

Bala, N. M., Goncalves, R. S., Caetano, R. S., Cardoso, R., Dinis, I., & Mirante, A. (2022). Autoimmune primary adrenal insufficiency in children. *Journal of Clinical Research in Pediatric Endocrinology*, 14(3), 308–312. https://doi.org/10.4274/jcrpe.galenos.2022.2021-11-9

Hinkle, J. L., Cheever, K. H., & Overbaugh, K. J. (2021). *Brunner & Suddarth's textbook of medical-surgical nursing* (15th ed.). Wolters Kluwer.

Nieman, L. K. (2022a). Clinical manifestations of adrenal insufficiency in adults. In *UpToDate*. Lexi-Comp, Inc.

Nieman, L. K. (2022b). Medical therapy of hypercortisolism (Cushing's syndrome). In *UpToDate*. Lexi-Comp, Inc.

Nieman, L. K. (2022c). Overview of the treatment of Cushing's syndrome. In *UpToDate*. Lexi-Comp, Inc.

Nieman, L. K. (2022d). Treatment of adrenal insufficiency in adults. In *UpToDate*. Lexi-Comp, Inc.

UpToDate. (2023). *Drug information*. Lexi-Comp, Inc.

Clinical Judgment in Practice: Section 8: Drugs Affecting the Endocrine System

A 15-year-old patient is seen by the pediatric nurse practitioner (PNP) for the required school physical. The patient's body mass index is greater than 30. The abdominal area is noted with excessive fat tissue in and around the abdomen. The PNP notes that the patient has developed metabolic syndrome. Metabolic syndrome is a clustering of risk factors for type 2 diabetes. The patient has hyperglycemia, dyslipidemia, and hypertension. The patient's hemoglobin A1C is 7.0%. The low-density lipoprotein is 225 mg/dL. The patient's blood pressure is 140/88. The patient's mother reports that the patient plays video games approximately 2 hours per day. The patient has good grades, but with virtual learning, the patient's computer use has increased significantly.

At the initial visit, the PNP prescribes metformin 500 mg extended release with the evening meal. The patient is placed on a calorie reduction diet. The patient and the patient's mother are referred to the dietician and certified diabetic educator. After 3 months on metformin, the patient has only lost 7 lb. The hemoglobin A1C is 6.8%.

Step 1: Recognize Cues
Identify the relevant and important information from different sources, such as the medical history or subjective and objective data.

Answer: At the initial visit, the patient's body mass index is greater than 30, the hemoglobin A1C is 7.0%, the low-density lipoprotein is 225 mg/dL, and the blood pressure is 140/88. The patient's mother reports the patient has a sedentary lifestyle with the increased use of virtual learning and playing video games. After 3 months on metformin, the patient has only lost 7 lb and the hemoglobin A1C is 6.8%.

Step 2: Analyze Cues
Organize and link the recognized cues to the patient's clinical presentation.

Answer: As the PNP, you link the patient's loss of 7 lb and the patient's hemoglobin A1C of 6.8%, a slight improvement from the initial visit. You determine that an improvement in the patient's weight loss and improvement of hemoglobin A1C will be enhanced with the addition of semaglutide as follows:

- Weeks 1 to 4: 0.25 mg once weekly
- Weeks 5 to 8: 0.5 mg once weekly
- Weeks 9 to 12: 1 mg once weekly
- Weeks 13 to 16: 1.7 mg once weekly
- ≥Week 17: Maintenance dose 2.4 mg once weekly

Step 3: Prioritize Hypotheses
Evaluate hypotheses and rank them according to priority, such as urgency, likelihood, risk, difficulty, and/or time. Cluster your findings to generate a list of problems (actual or potential) you believe the patient is experiencing or may experience and determine the level of urgency. Which problem is of the greatest concern?

Answer: You prioritize the needs of the patient, which include the need to lose weight and to decrease the hemoglobin A1C. The patient and family are instructed on the action, use, administration, adverse effects, and therapeutic effects of semaglutide. The patient will engage in a support group for adolescents diagnosed with type 2 diabetes. The school nurse meets with the patient weekly to review the patient's diet and exercise.

Step 4: Generate Solutions
Identify expected outcomes and use hypotheses to define a set of interventions for the expected outcomes.

Answer: The patient will have a decrease in hemoglobin A1C with the administration of semaglutide and metformin. The patient will reduce carbohydrate intake to aid in weight loss and decrease hemoglobin A1C. The patient will increase physical activity.

Step 5: Take Actions
Implement the solutions that address the highest priorities.

Answer: You arrange for the patient to attend biweekly support group meetings for adolescents diagnosed with type 2 diabetes. You instruct the patient and family on a diet with an increased intake of fruits and vegetables. You also instruct the patient on the need to reduce carbohydrate intake, and you and the patient set goals to reduce the intake of fast food. In addition, you and the patient set the goal for them to swim 3 times per week for 30 minutes.

Step 6: Evaluate Outcomes
Compare observed outcomes against expected outcomes.

Answer: By week 9 of semaglutide administration, the patient has lost 14 lb and the hemoglobin A1C is 5.8%. In addition, the patient's blood pressure is 126/74. The patient's low-density lipoprotein is 150.

SECTION 9

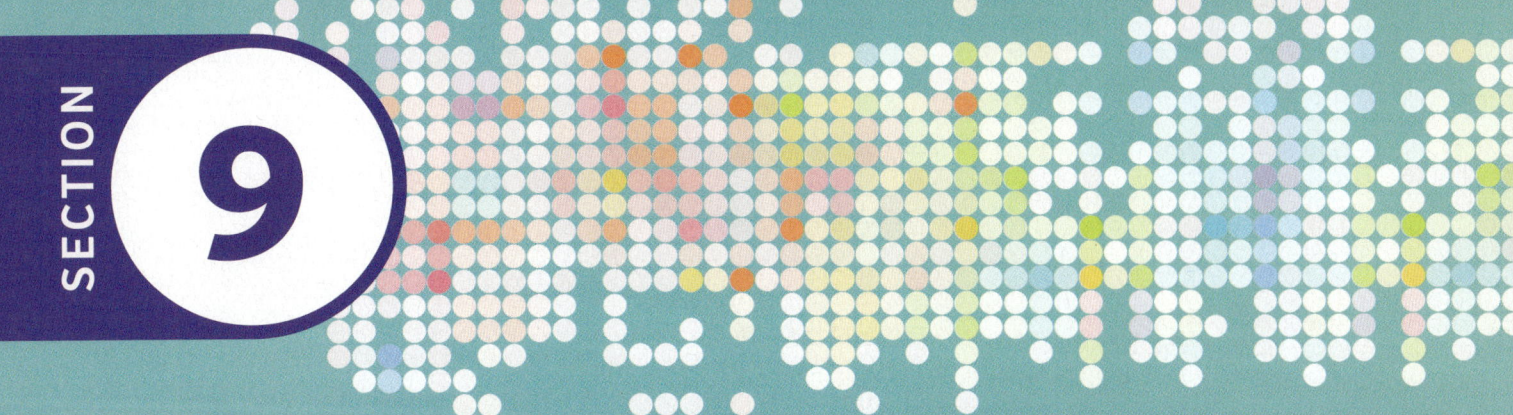

Drugs Affecting the Autonomic and Central Nervous Systems

Chapter 46 Physiology of the Autonomic and Central Nervous Systems and Indications for the Use of Drug Therapy

Chapter 47 Drug Therapy for Myasthenia Gravis, Alzheimer Disease, and Other Conditions Treated With Cholinergic Agents

Chapter 48 Drug Therapy for Parkinson Disease, Urinary Spasticity, and Disorders Requiring Anticholinergic Drug Therapy

Chapter 49 Drug Therapy With Opioids

Chapter 50 Drug Therapy With Local Anesthetics

Chapter 51 Drug Therapy With General Anesthetics

Chapter 52 Drug Therapy for Migraines and Other Headaches

Chapter 53 Drug Therapy for Seizure Disorders and Skeletal Muscle Disorders

Chapter 54 Drug Therapy for Anxiety and Insomnia

Chapter 55 Drug Therapy for Depression and Mood Disorders

Chapter 56 Drug Therapy for Psychotic Disorders

Chapter 57 Drug Therapy for Attention Deficit Hyperactivity Disorder and Narcolepsy

Chapter 58 Drug Therapy for Substance Use Disorders

CHAPTER 46

Physiology of the Autonomic and Central Nervous Systems and Indications for the Use of Drug Therapy

LEARNING OBJECTIVES

After studying this chapter, you should be able to:

1. Identify the physiologic effects of the sympathetic nervous system.
2. Differentiate the subtypes and functions of sympathetic nervous system receptors.
3. Identify the physiologic effects of the parasympathetic nervous system.
4. Differentiate the subtypes and functions of parasympathetic nervous system receptors.
5. Describe signal transduction and the intracellular events that occur when receptors of the autonomic nervous system are stimulated.
6. Recognize the terminology and general characteristics of drugs affecting the autonomic nervous system.

CLINICAL APPLICATION CASE STUDY

Jennifer Johnson, age 35 years, runs 5 miles daily before work. One morning while running, she encounters a bear on the jogging trail. She begins to hyperventilate and can feel her heart racing. She also begins to sweat profusely, and her pupils begin to dilate. The bear runs into the woods when a car approaches.

KEY TERMS

Affinity: rate of binding of ligands that demonstrates a tendency or strength of the effect

Agonist: a ligand that can bind to a receptor, alter the function of the receptor, and trigger a physiologic response for that receptor

Antagonist: a ligand that binds to a receptor but fails to activate the physiologic response for that receptor

Down-regulation: a process by which a cell decreases the quantity of a cellular component in response to an external variable; also called desensitization

First messenger: extracellular ligand that binds to a cell surface receptor and initiates intracellular activity

Ligands: substances such as neurotransmitters (e.g., acetylcholine and norepinephrine) medications, and hormones that bind to receptors in the autonomic nervous system

Second messenger: the second messenger is the molecule inside the cell that acts to transmit signals from a receptor to the target. The second messenger is the link between events that are occurring outside the cell

Signal transduction: when receptors located on target tissues are stimulated by a ligand, a cascade of intracellular events is initiated

Up-regulation: a process by which a cell increases the quantity of a cellular component in response to an external variable; also called hypersensitization

INTRODUCTION

The nervous system has two main divisions: the central nervous system (CNS) and the peripheral nervous system (PNS) (Fig. 46.1). The CNS includes the brain and spinal cord. It receives and processes incoming sensory information and responds by sending out signals that initiate or modify body processes. The PNS includes all the neurons and ganglia found outside the CNS. Afferent neurons carry sensory input from the periphery to the CNS and modify motor output through the action of reflex arcs. Efferent neurons carry motor signals from the CNS to the peripheral areas of the body. Ganglia are nerve cell clusters that house the cell bodies of the afferent nerves.

The efferent portion of the PNS has two subdivisions: the somatic nervous system and the autonomic nervous system (ANS). The somatic nervous system innervates skeletal muscles and controls voluntary movement. The ANS, without conscious thought or effort, controls involuntary activities in smooth muscle, in secretory glands, and in the visceral organs of the body such as the heart.

STRUCTURE AND FUNCTION OF THE AUTONOMIC NERVOUS SYSTEM

Structural centers in the CNS, including the hypothalamus, brainstem, and spinal cord, regulate the ANS. There are two parts of the ANS: the sympathetic nervous system (SNS) and the parasympathetic nervous system. The functions of the ANS can be broadly described as activities designed to maintain a constant internal environment (homeostasis), to respond to stress or emergencies, and to repair body tissues.

Nerve impulses are generated and transmitted to body tissues in the SNS and the parasympathetic nervous system, as they are in the CNS. Preganglionic nerve impulses travel from the CNS along the presynaptic nerves to ganglia. Ganglia are bundles of nerve tissue composed of the terminal end of the presynaptic neuron and clusters of postsynaptic neuron cell bodies. A neurotransmitter is released from the terminal end of the presynaptic neuron, allowing the nervous impulse to bridge the synapse between the presynaptic and postsynaptic nerves. The postganglionic impulses travel from the ganglia to target

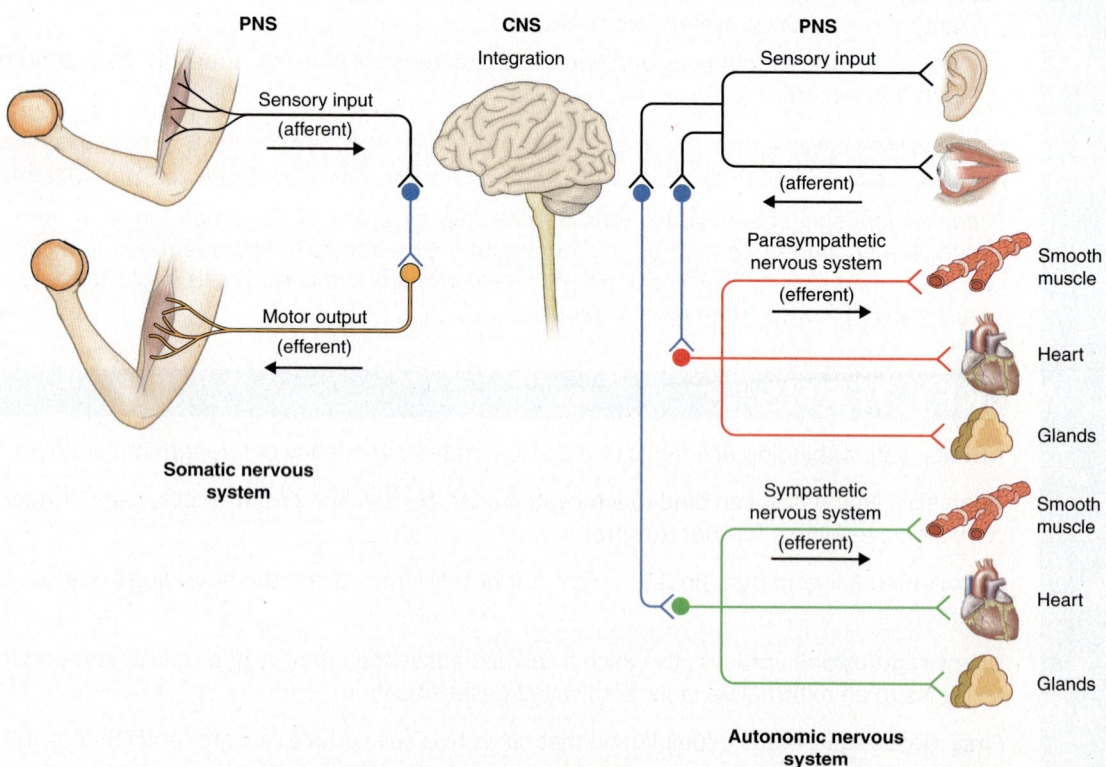

Figure 46.1. Divisions of the human nervous system. The nervous system can be divided anatomically into the central (brain and spinal cord) nervous system (CNS) and the peripheral (sensory organs and nerves) nervous system (PNS). The nervous system can be functionally divided into the somatic nervous system and the autonomic nervous system (ANS). The somatic nervous system leads to contraction of muscle fibers through efferent (motor) neurons. The autonomic nervous system controls the heart, glands, and hollow organs and is essential in maintaining homeostasis. (Reprinted with permission from Plowman, S. A., & Smith, D. L. (2017). *Exercise physiology for health, fitness, and performance* (5th ed.) Philadelphia, PA: Wolters Kluwer.)

or effector tissues of the heart, blood vessels, glands, other visceral organs, and smooth muscle. A neurotransmitter is released from the terminal end of the postsynaptic neuron, allowing the impulse to reach the effector tissue, stimulate a receptor, and bring about a response (Fig. 46.2).

The primary neurotransmitters of the ANS are acetylcholine and norepinephrine. Acetylcholine is synthesized from acetyl-coenzyme A and choline. It is released at preganglionic fibers of both the SNS and parasympathetic nervous system and at postganglionic fibers of the parasympathetic nervous system. Acetylcholine is also released from postganglionic sympathetic neurons that innervate the sweat glands and from motor neurons of the somatic nervous system that innervate the skeletal muscles. The nerve fibers that secrete acetylcholine are called cholinergic fibers. Acetylcholine acts on receptors in body organs and tissues to cause parasympathetic effects.

Norepinephrine is synthesized from the amino acid tyrosine by a series of enzymatic conversions that also produce dopamine and epinephrine (i.e., tyrosine → dopamine → norepinephrine → epinephrine). Except in the adrenal medulla, where most of the norepinephrine is converted to epinephrine, the chemical reaction stops with norepinephrine. This neurotransmitter is released at most postganglionic fibers of the SNS. Norepinephrine-secreting nerve fibers are called adrenergic fibers. Norepinephrine acts on receptors in body organs and tissues to cause sympathetic effects.

Ligands are substances such as neurotransmitters (e.g., acetylcholine and norepinephrine), medications, and hormones that can bind to receptors in the ANS. **Affinity** is the rate of binding of ligands that demonstrates a tendency or strength of the effect. A ligand that can bind to a receptor, alter the function of the receptor, and trigger a physiologic response for that receptor is called an **agonist**. Ligands that bind to a receptor but fail to activate the physiologic response to that receptor are **antagonists**. When receptors located on target tissues are stimulated by a ligand, a cascade of intracellular events known as **signal transduction** is initiated.

The extracellular ligand that binds to the cell surface receptor to initiate the intracellular activity is the **first messenger**. In most cases, this ligand–receptor interaction activates a cell membrane–bound G protein and an effector enzyme, which then activate a molecule inside the cell called a **second messenger**. The second messenger is the molecule inside the cell that acts to transmit signals from a receptor to the target. The second messenger is the link between events that are occurring outside the cell (i.e., receptor activation by the ligand) and resulting events that will occur inside the cell, such as opening ion channels, stimulating other enzymes, and increasing intracellular calcium levels. These intracellular events ultimately produce the physiologic responses to neurotransmitter and hormone release or drug administration. Figure 46.3 illustrates the intracellular events of signal transduction that

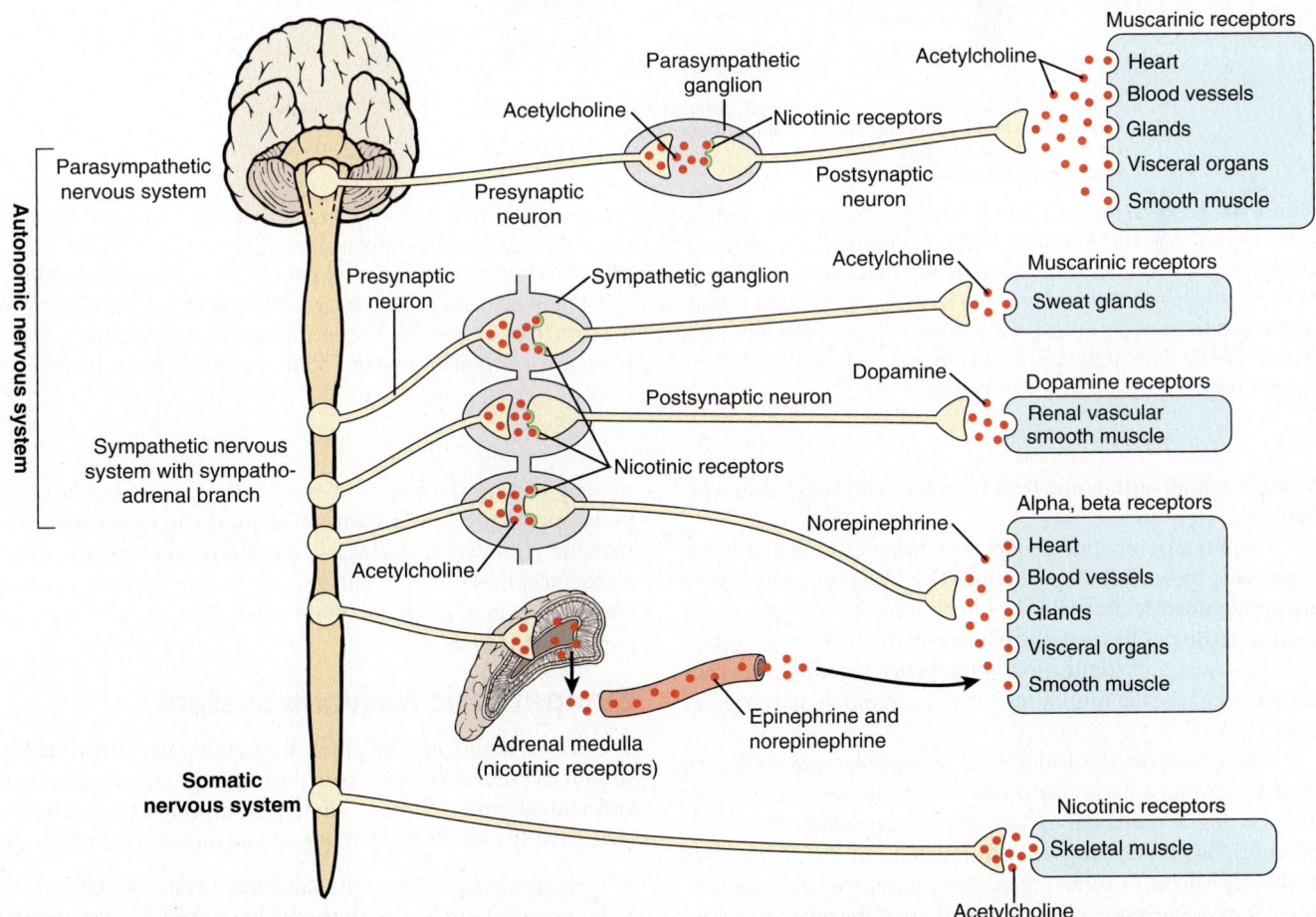

Figure 46.2. Organization of the autonomic and somatic nervous systems. [Reprinted with permission from Brophy, K., Scarlett-Ferguson, H., Webber, K. S., Abrams, A. C., Pennington, S. S., & Lammon, C. B. (2011). *Clinical drug therapy for Canadian practice* (2nd ed.) Philadelphia, PA: Wolters Kluwer Health | Lippincott Williams & Wilkins.]

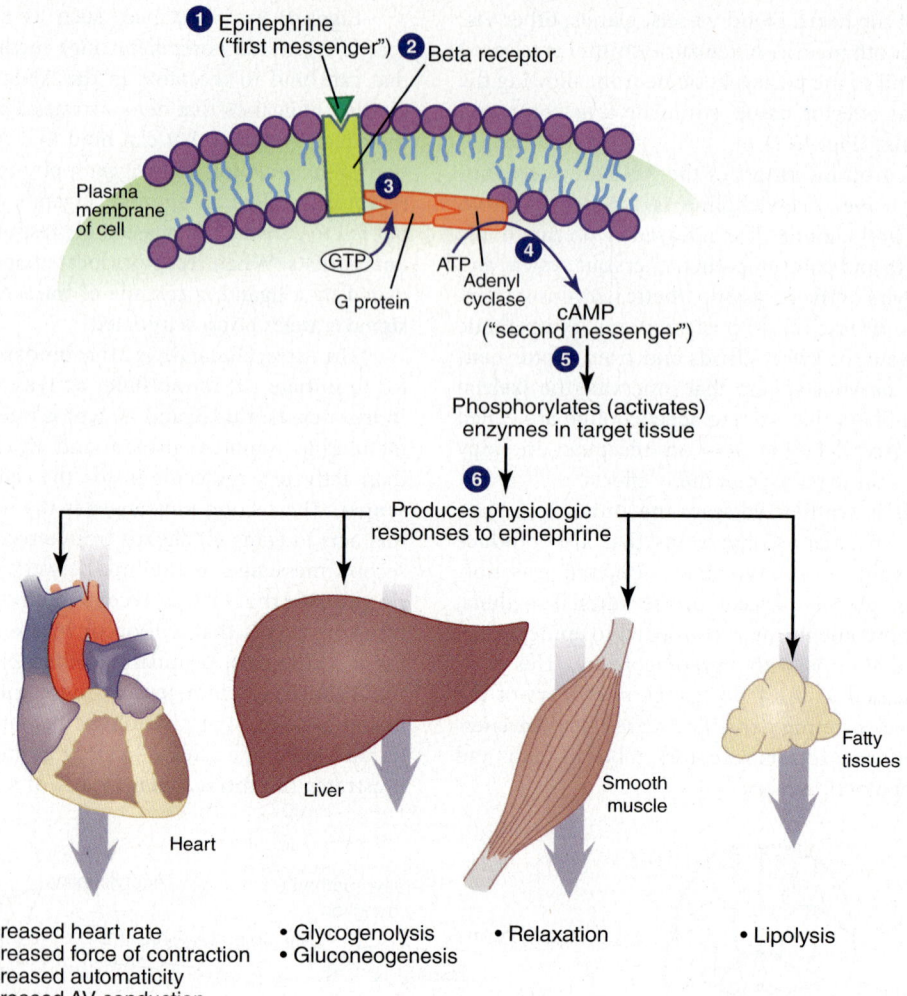

Figure 46.3. Signal transduction mechanism for an adrenergic beta receptor. Epinephrine (*1*), the "first messenger," interacts with a beta receptor (*2*). This hormone–receptor complex activates a G protein, which reacts with a guanosine triphosphate (GTP) (*3*). The activated G protein then activates the enzyme adenyl cyclase, which (*4*) catalyzes the conversion of adenosine triphosphate (ATP) to cyclic adenosine monophosphate (cAMP), the "second messenger" (*5*). cAMP activates enzymes, which bring about the biologic responses to epinephrine (*6*). AV, atrioventricular. (Reprinted with permission from Brophy, K., Scarlett-Ferguson, H., Webber, K. S., Abrams, A. C., Pennington, S. S., & Lammon, C. B. (2011). *Clinical drug therapy for Canadian practice* (2nd ed.) Philadelphia, PA: Wolters Kluwer Health | Lippincott Williams & Wilkins.)

occur when an adrenergic beta receptor is stimulated by epinephrine.

Involuntary muscles in organs and tissues in the body are innervated by both divisions of the ANS. However, most organs are predominantly controlled by one system. For example, in the gastrointestinal (GI) tract, the parasympathetic nervous system predominates, and stimulation of the parasympathetic nervous system regulates the routine activities of digestion and elimination.

The two divisions of the ANS are usually antagonistic in their actions on a particular organ. When the sympathetic system excites a particular organ, the parasympathetic system often inhibits it and vice versa. Stimulation of the ANS causes excitatory effects in some organs but inhibitory effects in others. For example, sympathetic stimulation of the heart causes an increased rate and force of myocardial contraction, and parasympathetic stimulation decreases rate and force of contraction, thereby resting the heart. In the GI tract, stimulation of the parasympathetic nervous system promotes digestion, and sympathetic stimulation decreases blood flow and impairs digestion. Exceptions to this antagonistic action include sweating and regulation of arteriolar blood vessel diameter, which is controlled by the SNS.

Sympathetic Nervous System

The SNS is stimulated by physical or emotional stress, such as strenuous exercise or work, pain, hemorrhage, intense emotions, and temperature extremes. The reaction produced by the SNS is essentially a whole-body response and includes the following:

- Increased arterial blood pressure and cardiac output
- Increased blood flow to the brain, heart, and skeletal muscles; decreased blood flow to the viscera, skin, and other organs not needed for "fight or flight" (whether real or imaginary)

- Increased rate of cellular metabolism, with increased oxygen consumption and carbon dioxide production
- Increased breakdown of muscle glycogen for energy
- Increased blood glucose
- Increased mental activity and ability to think clearly
- Increased muscle strength
- Increased rate of blood coagulation
- Increased rate and depth of respiration
- Pupil dilation to aid vision
- Increased sweating (Note that acetylcholine is the neurotransmitter for this sympathetic response—not the normal postganglionic neurotransmitter, which is norepinephrine.)

These responses are protective mechanisms designed to help the person cope with the stress or escape from it. The intensity and duration of the sympathetic response depend on the existing amounts of the neurotransmitters norepinephrine and epinephrine.

Neurotransmitters

Norepinephrine is synthesized in adrenergic nerve endings and released into the synapse when adrenergic nerve endings are stimulated. It exerts intense but brief effects on presynaptic and postsynaptic adrenergic receptors. The effects of norepinephrine are terminated by reuptake of most of the neurotransmitter back into the nerve endings, where it is packaged into vesicles for reuse as a neurotransmitter. This reuptake and termination process can be inhibited by cocaine and tricyclic antidepressant medications and is responsible for the activation of the SNS seen with these drugs. The remainder of the norepinephrine, which was not taken back into the nerve endings, diffuses into surrounding tissue fluids and blood or is metabolized by monoamine oxidase (MAO) or catechol-O-methyltransferase (COMT).

Norepinephrine also functions as a circulating neurohormone, along with epinephrine. In response to adrenergic nerve stimulation, norepinephrine and epinephrine are secreted into the bloodstream by the adrenal medullae and transported to all body tissues. They are continually present in arterial blood in amounts that vary according to the degree of stress present and the ability of the adrenal medullae to respond to stimuli. The larger proportion of the circulating hormones (approximately 80%) is epinephrine.

Norepinephrine and epinephrine exert the same effects on target tissues as those caused by direct stimulation of the SNS. However, the effects last longer because the hormones are removed from the blood more slowly. The enzymes MAO and COMT metabolize these hormones, mainly in the liver. Box 46.1 outlines the strength and type of response to activation of alpha and beta receptors.

Dopamine is also an adrenergic neurotransmitter and a catecholamine. In the brain, dopamine is essential for normal function. In peripheral tissues, its main effects are on the heart and blood vessels of the kidney system and viscera, where it produces vasodilation.

BOX 46.1 Response to Activation of Alpha and Beta Receptors

Activation of $alpha_1$ and $beta_1$ receptors causes stimulatory responses:
- When activating $alpha_1$ receptors, norepinephrine causes a greater response than does epinephrine.
- When activating $beta_1$ receptors, epinephrine and norepinephrine cause equal responses.

Activation of $alpha_2$, $beta_2$, and $beta_3$ receptors causes inhibitory responses:
- When activating $alpha_2$ receptors, epinephrine causes a greater or equal response than does norepinephrine.
- When activating $beta_2$ receptors, epinephrine causes a significantly greater response than does norepinephrine.

Clinical Application 46.1

- When Mrs. Johnson returns home, she tells her husband about the experience and states "I have never been so scared in my whole life." She tells her husband that even though she was afraid, she remembers being able to think clearly and feeling physically stronger after she spotted the bear.
- Explain Mrs. Johnson's physiologic response to the experience. What additional symptoms does this physiologic response trigger?

Adrenergic Receptors

When norepinephrine and epinephrine act on body cells that respond to sympathetic nerve or catecholamine stimulation, they interact with two distinct adrenergic receptors, alpha and beta. Norepinephrine acts mainly on alpha receptors, and epinephrine acts on both alpha and beta receptors. These receptors have been further subdivided into $alpha_1$, $alpha_2$, $beta_1$, $beta_2$, and $beta_3$ receptors.

Quality and Safety Alert: Evidence-Based Practice

Chawla et al. [2019] published a commentary article in *Critical Care*, promoting the use of broad-spectrum vasopressors for the management of septic shock. Septic shock impairs the sympathetic modulation of the heart and the vasculature. The first-line vasopressor for septic shock is norepinephrine with fluid resuscitation. The authors conclude that using broad-spectrum vasopressors with different mechanisms of action will improve outcomes of shock. Teboul et al. [2018] suggest that patients in severe septic shock require high doses of norepinephrine to achieve targeted mean arterial pressure, due to the downward regulation of the *alpha*₁-adrenergic receptors. High-dose norepinephrine can injure the myocardial cells, so the use of vasopressin can be administered as adjunctive medication to reduce the dosage of norepinephrine. Vasopressin will elevate blood pressure and restore vascular tone. Other vasopressors that can also improve outcomes are selepressin or terlipressin. The oral vasopressin midodrine has had positive outcomes in the recovery phase of septic shock and has shortened the patient's stay in the intensive care unit.

Quality and Safety Alert: Evidence-Based Practice

Patients who are critically ill with the diagnosis of sepsis require large quantities of IV fluids, which cause a significant positive fluid balance to meet the needs of cardiac output, systemic blood pressure, and perfusion to the kidneys. Akbar et al. (2021) conducted a randomized, nonblind clinical trial on adult patients with septic shock admitted to the intensive and emergency care units. The study had two treatment groups: the norepinephrine group and the fluid resuscitation group. The researchers conducted a test on the urinary albumin to creatinine ratio, increase of serum creatinine values, ratio of arterial oxygen partial pressure to fractional inspired oxygen, and intra-abdominal pressure at the time of the septic shock diagnosis, then at 3 hours and at 24 hours after the treatment was given. Based on the analysis, a significant difference in all study variables was identified in the fluid resuscitation group compared to the norepinephrine group. The fluid resuscitation group was at higher risk of fluid overload than the norepinephrine group. Thus, early norepinephrine administration can reduce fluid administration and prevent overload in the resuscitation of patients with septic shock.

When dopamine acts on body cells that respond to adrenergic stimulation, it can activate $alpha_1$ and $beta_1$ receptors as well as dopaminergic receptors. Only dopamine can activate dopaminergic receptors. Dopamine receptors are located in the brain, in blood vessels of the kidneys and other viscera, and probably in presynaptic sympathetic nerve terminals. Activation (agonism) of these receptors may result in stimulation or inhibition of cellular function. Like alpha and beta receptors, dopamine receptors are divided into several subtypes (D_1–D_5), and specific effects depend on which subtype of receptor is activated. Additional discussion about the adrenergic receptors is found in Table 29.2, which describes the locations of adrenergic receptors in the body and the response that occurs when each receptor is stimulated.

The intracellular events resulting from signal transduction after stimulation of adrenergic receptors are thought to include the following mechanisms:

- *$Alpha_1$ receptors*: Activation of $alpha_1$ receptors in smooth muscle cells is thought to open ion channels, allow calcium ions to move into the cell, and produce muscle contraction (e.g., vasoconstriction, gastrointestinal and bladder sphincter contraction).
- *$Alpha_2$ receptors*: In the brain, some of the norepinephrine released into the synaptic cleft between neurons returns to the nerve endings from which it was released and stimulates presynaptic $alpha_2$ receptors. This negative feedback prevents calcium-mediated release of norepinephrine from storage vesicles into the synapse, resulting in decreased sympathetic outflow and an antiadrenergic effect. In addition, $alpha_2$ receptors cause a decrease in cyclic adenosine monophosphate (cAMP), resulting in smooth muscle contraction.
- *$Beta_1$, $beta_2$, and $beta_3$ receptors*: Activation of these receptors stimulates activity of adenyl cyclase (an enzyme in cell membranes), which increases intracellular cAMP activity. cAMP serves as a second messenger and can initiate several different intracellular actions, such as cardiac contraction, smooth muscle relaxation, and glycogenolysis. An enzyme called phosphodiesterase rapidly degrades cAMP to 5′-adenosine monophosphate. Drugs such as theophylline inhibit phosphodiesterase and increase cAMP concentrations, resulting in bronchodilation (see Chapter 33).
- *Dopaminergic receptors D_1 and D_5*: Activation of these receptors is thought to stimulate the production of cAMP, as does activation of $beta_1$ and $beta_2$ receptors.
- *Dopaminergic receptors D_2, D_3, and D_4*: Activation of this receptor is thought to inhibit formation of cAMP and to alter calcium and potassium ion currents. D_3 and D_4 receptors are grouped with D_2 receptors, but the effects of their activation have not been clearly delineated.

The number of receptors and the binding activity of receptors to target organs and tissues are dynamic and may be altered. These phenomena are most clearly understood with beta receptors. For example, when chronically exposed to high concentrations of substances that stimulate their function, the beta receptors decrease in number and become less efficient in stimulating adenyl cyclase. **Down-regulation**, also called desensitization, is a process by which a cell decreases the quantity of a cellular component in response to an external variable. Conversely, when chronically exposed to substances that block their function, the receptors may increase in number and become more efficient in stimulating adenyl cyclase. **Up-regulation**, also called hypersensitization, is a process by which a cell increases the quantity of a cellular component in response to an external variable. The resulting increase in beta-adrenergic responsiveness may lead to an exaggerated response when the blocking substance is withdrawn.

NCLEX Success

1. Activation of the sympathetic nervous system will result in which of the following? (Select all that apply.)
    A. increased rate and depth of respiration
    B. pupil dilation to aid vision
    C. increased blood pressure and heart rate
    D. increased urine output

2. A drug that has the same effects on the human body as stimulation of the sympathetic nervous system is called which of the following? (Select all that apply.)
    A. sympathomimetic agent
    B. adrenergic drug
    C. beta-adrenergic agonist drug
    D. alpha-adrenergic blocking agent

3. When the body is exposed to high concentrations of substances that stimulate their function, the resulting decrease in beta-adrenergic responsiveness is called which of the following? (Select all that apply.)
    A. desensitization
    B. down-regulation
    C. fight or flight
    D. norepinephrine reuptake

Parasympathetic Nervous System

Experts often describe processes stimulated by the parasympathetic nervous system as "rest and digest" because of their resting, reparative, or vegetative functions. They include digestion, excretion, cardiac deceleration, anabolism, and near vision.

Approximately 75% of all parasympathetic nerve fibers are in the vagus nerves. These nerves supply the thoracic and abdominal organs; their branches go to the heart, lungs, esophagus, stomach, small intestine, proximal half of colon, the liver, gallbladder, pancreas, and upper portions of the ureters. Other parasympathetic fibers supply pupillary sphincters and circular muscles of the eye; lacrimal, nasal, submaxillary, and parotid glands; descending colon and rectum; lower portions of the ureters and bladder; and genitalia.

Specific body responses to parasympathetic stimulation include the following:

- Dilation of blood vessels in the skin
- Decreased heart rate, possibly bradycardia
- Increased secretion of digestive enzymes and motility of the GI tract
- Constriction of smooth muscle of bronchi
- Increased secretions from glands in the lungs, stomach, intestines, and skin (sweat glands)
- Constricted pupils (from contraction of the circular muscle of the iris) and accommodation to near vision (from contraction of the ciliary muscle of the eye)
- Contraction of smooth muscle in the urinary bladder
- Contraction of skeletal muscle
- Release of nitrous oxide from the endothelium of blood vessels, resulting in decreased platelet aggregation, decreased inflammation, relaxation of vascular smooth muscle, and dilation of blood vessels

Neurotransmitters

Parasympathetic responses are regulated by acetylcholine, a neurotransmitter in the brain, ANS, and neuromuscular junctions. Acetylcholine is formed in cholinergic nerve endings from choline and acetyl-coenzyme A, in a chemical reaction catalyzed by choline acetyltransferase. After its release from the nerve ending, the effect of acetylcholine on receptors of the parasympathetic nervous system is brief and measured in milliseconds. The action of acetylcholine on receptors is terminated because of rapid metabolism by acetylcholinesterase, an enzyme present in the nerve ending and on the surface of the receptor organ. Acetylcholinesterase splits the active acetylcholine into inactive acetate and choline. The choline is taken up again by the presynaptic nerve terminal and reused to form more acetylcholine. Acetylcholine exerts excitatory effects at nerve synapses and neuromuscular junctions and inhibitory effects at some peripheral sites such as the heart.

Cholinergic Receptors

When acetylcholine acts on body cells that respond to parasympathetic nerve stimulation, it interacts with two types of *cholinergic* receptors: *nicotinic* and *muscarinic*. Nicotinic receptors are located in motor nerves and skeletal muscles. When they are activated by acetylcholine, the cell membrane depolarizes and produces muscle contraction. Muscarinic receptors are located in most internal organs, including the cardiovascular, respiratory, GI, and genitourinary systems. When muscarinic receptors are activated by acetylcholine, the affected cells may be excited or inhibited in their functions.

Nicotinic and muscarinic receptors have been further subdivided; two types of nicotinic and five types of muscarinic receptors have been identified. Although the subtypes of cholinergic receptors have not been as well characterized as those of the adrenergic receptors, the intracellular events resulting from signal transduction after receptor stimulation are thought to include the following mechanisms:

- *Muscarinic$_1$ receptors*: Muscarinic$_1$ receptors are expressed primarily in the CNS, autonomic ganglia, and the gastric and salivary glands. Activation of these receptors results in a series of processes during which phospholipids in the cell membrane and inside the cell are broken down. One of the products of phospholipid metabolism is inositol phosphate. Inositol phosphate acts as a second messenger to increase the intracellular concentration of calcium. Calcium also acts as a second messenger and functions to activate several intracellular enzymes, initiate contraction of smooth muscle cells, increase secretions of exocrine glands, increase cognitive function, and decrease dopamine release.
- *Muscarinic$_2$ receptors*: Receptor activation results in inhibition of adenyl cyclase in the heart, smooth muscle, and brain. As a result, less cAMP is formed to act as a second messenger and stimulate intracellular activity. Receptor stimulation also results in activation of potassium channels in cell membranes of the heart. The overall consequences of M$_2$ activation are inhibition of cardiac function, increased contraction of smooth muscle, and inhibition of neuronal transmission.
- *Muscarinic$_3$ receptors*: Muscarinic$_3$ receptors are expressed primarily in the CNS, smooth muscle, glands, and heart. Activation apparently causes the same cascade of intracellular processes as with activation of the M$_1$ receptors, resulting in decreased dopamine release, increased smooth muscle contraction, and increased glandular secretion. In addition, nitrous oxide is generated from vascular endothelial cells, resulting in dilation of vessels.
- *Muscarinic$_4$ receptors*: Activation of these receptors in the CNS results in a molecular response similar to M$_2$ receptor activation. Muscarinic$_4$ activation results in inhibition of acetylcholine release in the striatum, a subcortical portion of the forebrain. These receptors have a regulatory effect on dopaminergic neurotransmission, and activation facilitates dopamine release. Alterations in M$_4$ receptors may contribute to disorders such as Parkinson disease.
- *Muscarinic$_5$ receptors*: Receptor activation results in a molecular response similar to M$_1$ receptor activation. The receptor has been identified in CNS tissues (especially the substantia nigra); its activation results in dilation of cerebral arteries and arterioles and facilitation of dopamine release. In addition, stimulation of M$_5$ receptors decreases cAMP levels.

Quality and Safety Alert: Safety

Muscarinic$_5$ activation also plays a role in augmentation of drug-seeking behavior and reward.

Although five muscarinic receptor subtypes have been identified, currently available drug therapies do not selectively differentiate among the various receptor subtypes:

- *Nicotinic$_n$ receptors*: These receptors are located on autonomic ganglia and the adrenal medulla. Activation results in enhanced transmission of nerve impulses at all parasympathetic and sympathetic ganglia and release of epinephrine from the adrenal medullae.
- *Nicotinic$_m$ receptors*: These are located at neuromuscular junctions in skeletal muscle. Their activation causes muscle contraction.
- *Nicotinic$_{CNS}$ receptors*: These receptors are located on presynaptic nerve fibers in the brain and spinal cord. Their activation promotes the release of acetylcholine in the cerebral cortex.

Nicotinic receptors are composed of five different protein subunits. The protein subunits that make up a nicotinic$_n$ receptor vary from those that make up a nicotinic$_m$ receptor, thus allowing the development of medications that are more selective in their actions.

Quality and Safety Alert: Safety

Neuromuscular-blocking medications such as pancuronium, which act selectively at nicotinic$_m$ receptors, can paralyze skeletal muscles in patients when limiting movement is therapeutic (such as in patients who are ventilated or during surgery), without adversely affecting other functions of the ANS.

CHARACTERISTICS OF AUTONOMIC DRUGS

Many drugs are used clinically because of their ability to stimulate or block activity of the SNS or parasympathetic nervous system. Drugs that stimulate an activity act like endogenous neurotransmitter substances; drugs that block an activity prevent the actions of both endogenous substances and stimulating drugs. Specific drugs that either stimulate or block the SNS are well described in the cardiac section of this text. Chapters 47 and 48 discuss the influence of drugs on the PNS.

Because ANS receptors are widespread throughout the body, drugs that act on the ANS usually affect the entire body rather than certain organs and tissues. Drug effects depend on which branch of the ANS is involved and whether it is stimulated or inhibited by drug therapy. Thus, knowledge of the physiology of the ANS is required if drug effects are to be understood and predicted. In addition, it is becoming increasingly important to understand receptor activity and the consequences of stimulation or inhibition. More drugs are being developed to stimulate or inhibit particular subtypes of receptors. This is part of the continuing effort to design drugs that act more selectively on particular body tissues and decrease adverse effects on other body tissues. For example, drugs such as terbutaline (see Chapter 33) have been developed to stimulate beta$_2$ receptors in the respiratory tract and produce bronchodilation (a desired effect) with decreased stimulation of beta$_1$ receptors in the heart (an adverse effect).

The terminology used to describe autonomic drugs is often confusing because different terms are used to refer to the same phenomenon. Thus, sympathomimetic, adrenergic, and alpha- and beta-adrenergic agonists are used to describe a drug that has the same effects on the human body as stimulation of the SNS. Parasympathomimetic, cholinomimetic, and cholinergic are used to describe a drug that has the same effects on the body as stimulation of the parasympathetic nervous system. There are also drugs that oppose or block stimulation of these systems. Sympatholytic, antiadrenergic, and alpha- and beta-adrenergic blocking drugs inhibit sympathetic stimulation. Parasympatholytic, anticholinergic, and cholinergic blocking drugs inhibit parasympathetic stimulation. This text uses the terms adrenergic, antiadrenergic, cholinergic, and anticholinergic when describing medications.

NCLEX Success

4. A drug that has the same effects on the body as stimulation of the parasympathetic nervous system is described as
   A. cholinergic
   B. sympatholytic
   C. antiadrenergic
   D. parasympatholytic

5. Activation of the parasympathetic system will result in which of the following? (Select all that apply.)
   A. dilation of blood vessels in the skin
   B. decreased heart rate
   C. increased motility of the gastrointestinal tract
   D. constriction of smooth muscle of bronchi

THE NURSING PROCESS

A concept map outlines the nursing process related to drug therapy considerations in this chapter. Additional nursing implications related to the disease process should also be considered in care decisions.

Assessment
- Assess for potential contraindications to the use of adrenergic medications: angina, hypertension, and tachydysrhythmias.
- Throughout treatment, monitor vital signs, level of consciousness, and gas exchange.
- Assess for the therapeutic effects of adrenergic drug therapy.
- Assess for the adverse effects of adrenergic drug therapy.
- Assess for patient's understanding about drug therapy and use of over-the-counter medications.

Outcomes of Therapy
The patient will
- Receive or take drugs that affect the sympathetic and parasympathetic nervous systems accurately.
- Recognize that many of these drugs should not be stopped abruptly.
- Have fewer episodes of symptoms.
- Be closely monitored for therapeutic and adverse effects, especially when drug therapy is started.
- Avoid preventable adverse effects.
- Verbalize essential information about the drug therapy.
- Demonstrate appropriate coping strategies.
- Recognize signs and symptoms that necessitate professional medical intervention.
- Keep appointments for follow-up care and monitoring.

Nursing Interventions
- Use appropriate measures to prevent symptoms.
- Provide appropriate patient teaching related to drug therapy.

Evaluation
- Observe and interview for relief of symptoms.
- Observe effective coping strategies and appropriate use of support system and resources.
- Interview regarding success and adherence with drug therapy.
- Interview and observe for adverse drug effects.

Visit thePoint® at http://thePoint.lww.com/Frandsen13e for answers to NCLEX Success questions (in Appendix A), answers to Clinical Application Case Studies (in Appendix B), and more!

REFERENCES AND RESOURCES

Akbar, R., George, Y., Madjid, A. S., Sedano, R., & Tantri, A. (2021). Early administration of norepinephrine prevents the occurrence of fluid overload in the resuscitation of septic shock patients. *Critical Care & Shock, 24*(5), 257–268. 152665705

Chawla, L. S., Ostermann, M., Forni, L., & Tidmarsh, G. F. (2019). Broad spectrum vasopressors: A new approach to the initial managements of septic shock. *Critical Care, 23*(124), 1–3. doi: 10.1186/s13054-019-2420-y

Lippincott Advisor. (2022). *Drug information*. Wolters Kluwer.

Manaker, S. (2022). Use of vasopressors and inotropes. *UpToDate*. Lexi-Comp, Inc.

Norris, T. L. (2019). *Porth's pathophysiology: Concepts of altered health states* (10th ed.). Wolters Kluwer Health/Lippincott Williams & Wilkins.

Teboul, J. L., Duranteau, J., & Russel, J. A. (2018). Intensive care medicine in 2050: Vasopressors in sepsis. *Intensive Care Medicine, 44*, 1130–1132. doi: 10.1007/s00134-017-4909-7

UpToDate. (2022). *Drug information*. Lexi-Comp, Inc.

CHAPTER 47

Drug Therapy for Myasthenia Gravis, Alzheimer Disease, and Other Conditions Treated With Cholinergic Agents

LEARNING OBJECTIVES

After studying this chapter, you should be able to:

1. Understand the characteristics and major manifestations of myasthenia gravis.
2. Identify the prototype and describe the action, use, adverse effects, contraindications, and nursing implications for acetylcholinesterase inhibitors used in myasthenia gravis.
3. Understand the characteristics and major manifestations of Alzheimer disease.
4. Identify the prototype and describe the action, use, adverse effects, contraindications, and nursing implications for reversible cholinesterase inhibitors used in Alzheimer disease.
5. Identify the prototype and describe the action, use, adverse effects, contraindications, and nursing implications for antiamyloid monoclonal antibody medication used in Alzheimer disease.
6. Identify the prototype and describe the action, use, adverse effects, contraindications, and nursing implications for cholinergic agonist drugs.
7. Describe the pharmacologic care of the patient with toxicity of acetylcholinesterase agents.
8. Implement the nursing process in the care of patients undergoing drug therapy for myasthenia gravis, Alzheimer disease, and urinary retention.

CLINICAL APPLICATION CASE STUDY

Mary Collins, a 35-year-old woman, is diagnosed with myasthenia gravis. She has generalized fatigue and tiredness. She also has ptosis that develops in the evening and difficulty chewing at dinner time. She has been prescribed pyridostigmine.

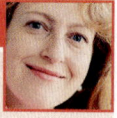

KEY TERMS

Acetylcholine: neurotransmitter in the cholinergic system located in many areas of the brain, with high concentrations in the motor cortex and basal ganglia (also a neurotransmitter in the autonomic nervous system and at peripheral neuromuscular junctions); exerts excitatory effects at synapses and at the nerve–muscle junction and inhibitory effects at some peripheral sites, such as organs supplied by the vagus nerve

Acetylcholinesterase: enzyme that acts on the neurotransmitter acetylcholine, breaking it into choline and an acetate group; found mainly at neuromuscular junctions, its activity serves to terminate synaptic transmission

Alzheimer disease (AD): most common type of dementia; characterized by a significant loss of neurons in addition to shrinkage of large cortical neurons, with plaques and neurofibrillary tangles

Cholinergic drugs: agents that stimulate the parasympathetic nervous system in the same manner as acetylcholine

Myasthenia gravis (MG): chronic autoimmune neuromuscular disease characterized by varying degrees of weakness of the skeletal (voluntary) muscles of the body

INTRODUCTION

The neuromuscular conditions myasthenia gravis (MG) and Alzheimer disease (AD) are characterized by disruptions in neurologic and autoimmune processes. This chapter discusses the acetylcholinesterase inhibitor medications used for the treatment of MG as well as the medications used to improve memory related to AD. It also covers selected drugs used to treat atony of the gastrointestinal (GI) and urinary smooth muscle, which may result in paralytic ileus and urinary retention.

OVERVIEW OF MYASTHENIA GRAVIS

Myasthenia gravis (MG) is a chronic autoimmune neuromuscular disease characterized by varying degrees of painless weakness of the skeletal (voluntary) muscles of the body. Normally, when nerve impulses travel down the nerve, the nerve endings release a neurotransmitter called **acetylcholine**. This neurotransmitter is in the cholinergic system located in many areas of the brain with high concentrations in the motor cortex and basal ganglia. Acetylcholine travels from the neuromuscular junction and binds to acetylcholine receptors, which are activated and generate a muscle contraction. MG results from a defect in the transmission of nerve impulses to muscles.

The hallmark of the disorder is muscle weakness that increases during periods of activity and improves after periods of rest. The term *myasthenia gravis*, which is Latin and Greek in origin, literally means "grave muscle weakness." With the therapies currently available, however, most cases of MG are not as "grave" as the name implies. In fact, most people who have MG have an average life expectancy.

MG occurs in all ethnic groups and sexes. It most commonly affects young adult females (younger than 40 years of age) and older males (older than 60 years of age).

Clinical Manifestations

The clinical manifestations of MG may affect any voluntary muscle, but muscles that control eye and eyelid movement, facial expression, and swallowing are most frequently affected. The onset of the disorder may be sudden, and symptoms often are not immediately recognized as MG. In most cases, the first noticeable symptom is weakness of the eye muscles. In others, difficulty in swallowing and slurred speech may be the first signs. The degree of muscle weakness involved in MG varies greatly among people, ranging from a localized form limited to eye muscles (ocular myasthenia) to a severe or generalized form in which many muscles—sometimes including those that control breathing—are affected.

Symptoms, which vary in type and severity, may include a drooping of one or both eyelids (ptosis), blurred or double vision (diplopia) due to weakness of the muscles that control eye movements, unstable or waddling gait, a change in facial expression, difficulty in chewing and swallowing, shortness of breath, impaired speech (dysarthria), and weakness in the arms, hands, fingers, legs, and neck.

Diagnosis

Diagnosis of MG with edrophonium is no longer recommended. However, edrophonium is administered during neuromuscular blockade reversal with atropine. Immunologic assays to detect acetylcholine receptor antibodies are now used. AChR-Ab is the first laboratory test for MG confirmation; further immunoassays include MuSK and LRP4 antibodies. Almost all patients with MG (approximately 85%) are seropositive for these antibodies (Bird, 2022a).

Myasthenia Crisis

Myasthenia crisis is characterized by respiratory insufficiency, worsening of tongue and swallowing muscle weakness, and in rare cases, respiratory failure. It can be precipitated by infection, surgery, pregnancy, or a spontaneous response of MG. Current management and treatment include plasma exchange, intravenous immune globulin (IVIG), high-dose glucocorticoids, and monitoring and assessment of respiratory muscle strength (Bird & Levine, 2022).

Drug Therapy

Cholinergic drugs stimulate the parasympathetic nervous system in the same manner as acetylcholine. These drugs act directly to stimulate the cholinergic receptors. Figure 47.1 shows the mechanism of action by interacting with the postsynaptic cholinergic receptor. **Acetylcholinesterase** is an enzyme that acts on the neurotransmitter acetylcholine, breaking it into choline and an acetate group. It is found mainly at neuromuscular junctions and its activity serves to terminate synaptic transmission. The acetylcholinesterase inhibitor drugs are cholinergic drugs that inhibit the enzyme acetylcholinesterase, thereby slowing acetylcholine metabolism at autonomic nerve synapses. The acetylcholinesterase inhibitor drugs are also known as indirect-acting cholinergics. Other cholinergic drugs act directly to stimulate cholinergic receptors (Fig. 47.2).

Acetylcholinesterase inhibitor drugs are classified as either reversible or irreversible inhibitors of acetylcholinesterase. The reversible inhibitors exhibit a moderate duration of action and have several therapeutic uses—in MG and, as described later in this chapter, in AD. Table 47.1 lists medications used to treat MG.

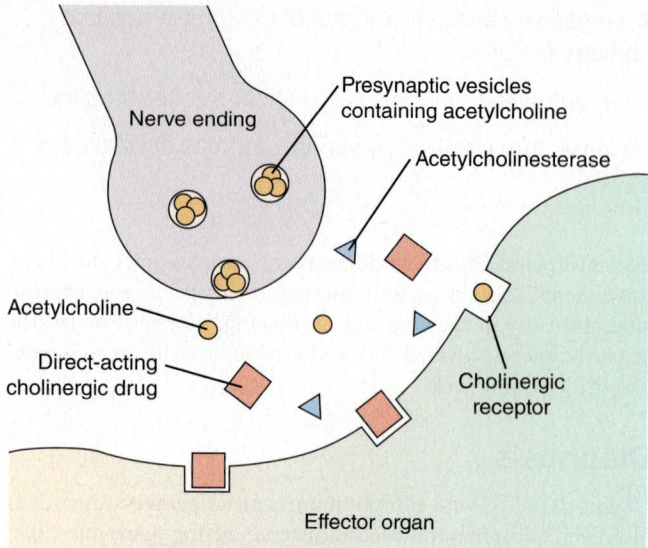

Figure 47.1. Mechanism of drug action. Direct-acting cholinergic drugs interact with postsynaptic cholinergic receptors on target effector organs, activating the organ in a similar fashion as the neurotransmitter acetylcholine.

ACETYLCHOLINESTERASE INHIBITORS (INDIRECT-ACTING CHOLINERGICS)

The initial therapy for mild to moderate MG is an oral acetylcholinesterase inhibitor (Bird, 2022b). P Pyridostigmine (Mestinon, Regonol) is the **prototype drug** of the class. Neostigmine was the prototype of the class but is no longer used. Healthcare providers use pyridostigmine for the long-term treatment of MG and as an antidote for tubocurarine and other nondepolarizing skeletal muscle relaxants used in surgery.

Pharmacokinetics

In the United States, pyridostigmine is available in an oral preparation for MG and IV use for the reversal of nondepolarizing neuromuscular blocking agents. Oral pyridostigmine's onset of action is 30 minutes with a 3- to 4-hour duration of action. The oral half-life is 1 to 2 hours. The parenteral administration has a 2- to 5-minute onset of action with a 1.5-hour half-life and a 2- to 3-hour duration of action. The oral and parenteral forms are excreted by the kidneys.

Action

Pyridostigmine inhibits the destruction of acetylcholine by acetylcholinesterase, facilitating the transmission of impulses across the neuromuscular junction. The drug increases tone and contractibility of smooth muscle (see Figs. 47.1 and 47.2).

Use

The major use of pyridostigmine is the treatment of MG. In addition, it reverses the action of nondepolarizing neuromuscular blocking agents such as muscle relaxants or tubocurarine, which is used in surgery.

Table 47.2 presents dosage information for pyridostigmine.

Patient-related variables specific to the use of pyridostigmine include the following:

- Age:
  - The oral preparation for children must be swallowed, not crushed or chewed.
  - Neonates of myasthenic birthing parents may have transient difficulties with swallowing, sucking, and breathing.
  - Older adults are more likely to experience adverse drug reactions due to age-related physiologic changes.
- Reproduction, pregnancy, and lactation:
  - Oral pyridostigmine is the agent of choice with MG during pregnancy.
  - Exacerbation of MG symptoms may occur with breast-feeding related to patient fatigue. Pyridostigmine is acceptable in lactation.
- Abnormal kidney function and hepatic impairment:
  - When administering to patients with impaired kidney function, begin with the lowest possible dose and monitor kidney function.
  - There are no dosage adjustments in hepatic impairment.

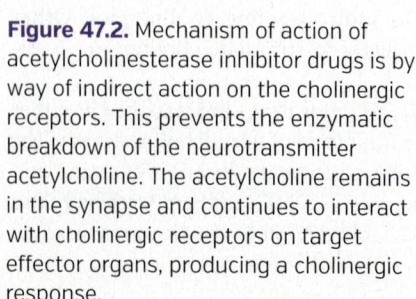

Figure 47.2. Mechanism of action of acetylcholinesterase inhibitor drugs is by way of indirect action on the cholinergic receptors. This prevents the enzymatic breakdown of the neurotransmitter acetylcholine. The acetylcholine remains in the synapse and continues to interact with cholinergic receptors on target effector organs, producing a cholinergic response.

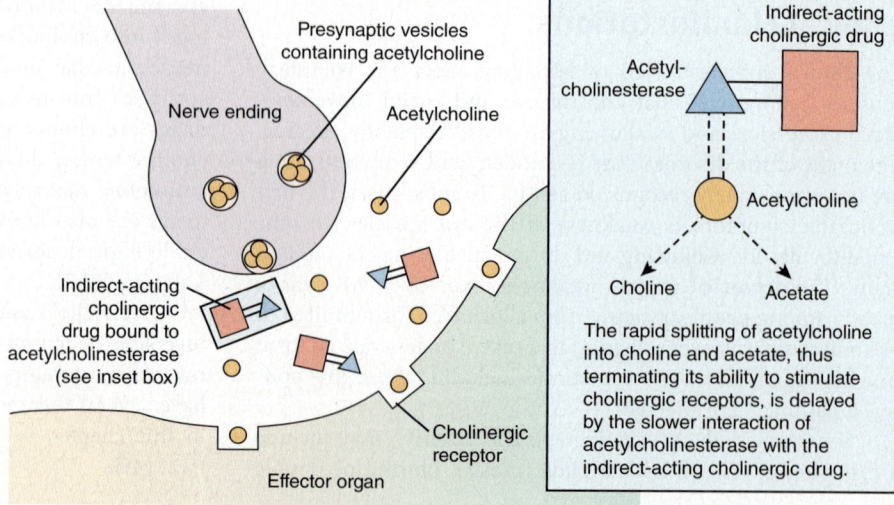

TABLE 47.1

Drugs Administered for the Treatment of Myasthenia Gravis (MG), Alzheimer Disease (AD), and Urinary Retention

Drug Class	Prototype	Other Drugs in the Class
Acetylcholinesterase inhibitors	Pyridostigmine (Mestinon, Regonol)	Physostigmine
Cholinesterase inhibitors	Donepezil (Aricept)	Galantamine (Razadyne, Razadyne ER) Rivastigmine (Exelon, Exelon Patch)
NMDA receptor antagonist	Memantine (Namenda, Namenda XR)	
Cholinesterase–NMDA receptor antagonist	Donepezil–memantine (Namzaric)	
Antiamyloid monoclonal antibody	Aducanumab (Aduhelm)	
Cholinergic agonist	Bethanechol (Urecholine)	

- Specific healthcare environments:
  - Use cautiously in patients with bromide sensitivity.
  - In critically ill patients, if there is inadequate reversal of nondepolarizing neuromuscular blocking agents, mechanical ventilation may be required until adequate recovery is attained. Also, atropine may be required in the event of cholinergic crisis.

Clinical Application 47.1

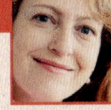

Following the administration of pyridostigmine, Ms. Collins is able to swallow and breathe more effectively.
- Why is pyridostigmine administered?
- What is the action of pyridostigmine?
- Why has Ms. Collins' breathing improved, and why is she now able to swallow?

Adverse Effects

Pyridostigmine's adverse effects of abdominal cramping, diarrhea, increased salivation and bronchial secretions, nausea, sweating, and bradycardia can be controlled with the administration of glycopyrrolate, propantheline, and hyoscyamine. The diarrhea can be controlled by loperamide or diphenoxylate.

Pyridostigmine and other acetylcholinesterase inhibitors can have toxic effects. Cholinergic crisis is a drug-induced overstimulation of the parasympathetic nervous system, requiring discontinuation of any anticholinesterase drug that the patient has been receiving. Atropine sulfate should be readily available whenever cholinergic drugs are given. It is important to note that atropine reverses only the muscarinic effects of cholinergic drugs, primarily in the heart, smooth muscle, and glands. Atropine does not interact with nicotinic receptors and, therefore, cannot reverse the nicotinic effects of skeletal muscle weakness due to overdose of indirect anticholinergic drugs.

Atropine sulfate is also administered for the management of mushroom poisoning. Muscarine, an alkaloid found in small quantities in the *Amanita muscaria* mushroom, is the source of the name for the muscarinic receptors in the parasympathetic nervous system; muscarine can stimulate these receptors. Some mushrooms found in North America, such as *Clitocybe* and *Inocybe* mushrooms, however, contain much larger quantities of muscarine. Accidental or intentional ingestion of these mushrooms results in cholinergic crisis and is potentially fatal.

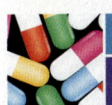

TABLE 47.2

DRUGS AT A GLANCE: Acetylcholinesterase Inhibitors

Drug	Routes and Dosage Ranges	
	Adults	**Children**
ⓟ Pyridostigmine (Mestinon, Regonol; ✦ Mestinon, Mestinon-SR)	MG Initially, PO 60–1,500 mg/d; usually 600 mg/d divided into 5–6 doses. Individualize dose to control symptoms. IM, IV slowly: 1/30th the oral dose; sustained release 180–360 mg PO at HS	MG Neonates of birthing parents with MG who have difficulty with sucking/breathing/swallowing: 0.05–0.15 mg/kg IM. Change to syrup as soon as possible Children: 7 mg/kg (200 mg/m²)/d in 5–6 divided doses
Physostigmine	Initially, IM, IV 0.5–2 mg. Give IV slowly, no faster than 1 mg/min to avoid adverse effects of bradycardia, respiratory distress, and seizures. May repeat every 10–30 min until response occurs	Infants, children, and adolescents: IM and IV Initial: 0.02 mg/kg; maximum: 0.5 mg per dose; may repeat every 5–10 min until response occurs (maximum total dose, 2 mg)

BOX 47.1 Drug Interactions: Pyridostigmine

Drugs That Increase the Effects of Pyridostigmine
- Succinylcholine, dipyridamole
  Increase neuromuscular blocking

Drugs That Decrease the Effects of Pyridostigmine
- Atropine
  Decreases the effects of pyridostigmine by unknown mechanism
- Corticosteroids
  May result in muscular depression

Contraindications

Contraindications to pyridostigmine include known hypersensitivity and any allergic reaction to anticholinergic muscle stimulants.

Nursing Implications

Preventing Interactions

Several drugs interact with pyridostigmine (Box 47.1), increasing or decreasing its effects.

Administering the Medication

It is important to administer IV pyridostigmine slowly and have atropine available as an antidote in the event of a cholinergic crisis or hypersensitivity to pyridostigmine. The availability of a sustained-release form is an advantage. When this form is taken at bedtime, the patient does not have to take other medications during the night and does not awaken too weak to swallow. In some cases, it may be necessary for immediate-release and sustained-release to be used concurrently.

Clinical Application 47.2

Ms. Collins forgot if she had taken her pyridostigmine. Since she assumed she had not taken it, she immediately administered a dose. Thirty minutes after the administration of pyridostigmine, Ms. Collins develops copious salivary secretions and respiratory depression.
- What do these symptoms indicate?
- What patient education should Ms. Collins have been taught related to cholinergic crisis?
- What emergency medication will be administered?

! Quality and Safety Alert: Patient-Centered Care

Patients with MG will experience more serious symptoms of muscle weakness if they get the flu or pneumonia. It is important that they receive flu vaccine annually and pneumonia vaccine as appropriate for the patient's age and comorbid states. COVID-19 vaccines and boosters are also important.

Assessing for Therapeutic Effects

When pyridostigmine is given to patients with MG, it is necessary to observe for increased muscle strength; decreased difficulty with chewing, swallowing, and speech; and decreased or absent ptosis of eyelids. When administered to reverse the effects of nondepolarizing neuromuscular blocking agents, the nurse observes for increased skeletal muscle strength.

Assessing for Adverse Effects

The nurse assesses for increased central nervous system (CNS) effects, such as twitching or hyperesthesia, as well as for increased secretions, acute bronchitis, or exacerbation of asthma. It is necessary to assess for nausea and vomiting, which are common GI effects. To prevent these GI side effects, glycopyrrolate, propantheline, or hyoscyamine sulfate may be administered. These anticholinergic agents have little or no effect on the nicotinic receptors. In addition, the nurse observes neonates of birthing parents with MG who have received pyridostigmine for difficulty breathing, swallowing, or sucking.

Quality and Safety Alert: Safety

It is important to avoid the following drugs in patients with MG. They may exacerbate the symptoms of the disease.
- Fluoroquinolones
- Aminoglycosides
- Neuromuscular blocking agents
- Lidocaine and procaine
- Magnesium sulfate
- Penicillamine
- Beta-blockers
- Anticonvulsants
- Statins
- Glucocorticoids
- Live attenuated vaccines

Patient Teaching

Box 47.2 identifies patient teaching guidelines for pyridostigmine.

BOX 47.2 Patient Teaching Guidelines for Acetylcholinesterase Inhibitors: Pyridostigmine

- Wear a medical alert identification device if you are taking long-term cholinergic drug therapy for MG.
- Record symptoms of MG and effects of drug therapy, especially when drug therapy is initiated and medication doses are being titrated. The amount of medication required to control symptoms of MG varies greatly, and the physician needs this information to adjust the dosage correctly.
- Do not overexert yourself if you have MG. Rest between activities. Although the dose of medication may be increased during periods of increased activity, it is desirable to space activities to obtain optimal benefit from the drug, at the lowest possible dose, with the fewest adverse effects.
- Report increased muscle weakness, difficulty breathing, or recurrent of myasthenic symptoms to your physician. These are signs of drug underdosage (myasthenic crisis) and indicate a need to increase or change drug therapy.
- Report adverse reactions, including abdominal cramps, diarrhea, excessive oral secretions, difficulty in breathing, and muscle weakness. These are signs of drug overdosage (cholinergic crisis) and require immediate discontinuation of drugs and treatment by a physician. Respiratory failure can result if this condition is not recognized and treated properly. Atropine may be administered for overdose of cholinergic drugs.

Other Drugs in the Class

Physostigmine is the only other acetylcholinesterase inhibitor. It is a carbamate that prolongs both central and peripheral effects of acetylcholine. It can cross the blood–brain barrier. Unlike other drugs in this group, physostigmine is not a quaternary amine and does not carry a positive charge; therefore, it is more lipid soluble. It is sometimes used as an antidote for overdose of anticholinergic drugs, including atropine, antihistamines, tricyclic antidepressants, and phenothiazine antipsychotics. However, its potential for causing serious adverse effects limits its usefulness. It should be administered intravenously no faster than 0.5 mg/minute to prevent bradycardia, seizures, and respiratory depression.

NCLEX Success

1. What is the therapeutic effect for the administration of pyridostigmine extended-release at bedtime?
   A. increases urinary frequency
   B. allows for increased swallowing
   C. decreases heart rate
   D. prevents hallucinations

2. A patient is admitted to the emergency department with muscle weakness. Their family states the patient was recently diagnosed with myasthenia gravis. The patient took their morning dose without an improvement in symptoms. The physician orders an additional dose of pyridostigmine. What medication should be available in the event of a cholinergic crisis?
   A. pralidoxime
   B. diphenhydramine
   C. atropine
   D. travoprost

IMMUNOSUPPRESSIVE THERAPY FOR MYASTHENIA GRAVIS

Patients who do not achieve control of symptoms on pyridostigmine may require immunosuppressive therapy to treat underlying immune dysregulation. Prescribers may use glucocorticoids initially and later add a nonsteroidal immunosuppressive agent such as azathioprine or mycophenolate. These drugs reduce the long-term use of glucocorticoids (Bird, 2022b).

Azathioprine

Prescribers use azathioprine on an off-label basis for the treatment of MG. The drug blocks the purine pathway and inhibits RNA, DNA, and protein synthesis. Azathioprine is well absorbed orally and is 30% protein bound. The metabolism of the drug is by 6-mercaptopurine via glutathione S-transferase reduction. The initial dose administered is 50 mg orally per day, with the dose increased every 1 to 2 weeks to a target of 2.5 to 3 mg/kg/d. The drug may be administered as monotherapy or in combination with pyridostigmine and/or glucocorticoids.

The dose increase in the medication should be 25 mg/day with a gradual increase to 25 to 50 mg/day every 2 weeks up to 150 mg/day if flulike symptoms develop. Adverse effects include malaise, hepatotoxicity, increased risk of infection, and myalgia.

Mycophenolate

Mycophenolate (CellCept), another drug used on an off-label basis for MG, may be appropriate for patients who remain significantly asymptomatic on pyridostigmine. Mycophenolate inhibits inosine monophosphate dehydrogenase, which then inhibits de novo guanosine nucleotide synthesis. The drug exhibits a cytotoxic effect on T and B lymphocytes, which are dependent on these pathways for proliferation. Mycophenolate is rapidly and extensively absorbed. It must be administered on an empty stomach. The initial therapy is 500 mg orally twice daily, with an increase to a maintenance dose of 1 to 1.5 g.

The U.S. Food and Drug Administration (FDA) has issued a **BOXED WARNING** ◆ for mycophenolate. It states that patients who can become pregnant must be instructed about the increased risk of congenital malformations and first trimester pregnancy loss. Prior to beginning therapy, a negative pregnancy test is required. Two types of birth control are recommended.

Efgartigimod Alfa

Efgartigimod alfa (Vyvgart) is recommended for patients with MG who are antiacetylcholine receptor antibody positive. Efgartigimod alfa is a neonatal Fc receptor antagonist. It is a human IgG1 antibody fragment. The binding of this fragment to the neonatal Fc receptor reduces the circulating IgG. The drug is administered by IV injection for MG. The IV fluid bag should be at room temperature. The dosage is 10 mg/kg with a maximum dose of 1.2 g every 4 weeks. Following the IV administration, the patient should be monitored for an infusion reaction.

Efgartigimod alfa is metabolized by degrading the proteolytic enzymes into small peptides and amino acids. The half-life is 3 to 5 days and excreted in the urine. Patients with MG who are pregnant should use other forms of treatment for the disease. Sexually active male patients should use effective contraception during treatment and for 90 days after the last dose. Given the immunosuppressive action of the drug, combining it with other immunomodulator medications will increase immunosuppression. The patient should be monitored for infection.

OVERVIEW OF ALZHEIMER DISEASE

Alzheimer disease (AD) is the most common form of dementia. It is characterized by a significant loss in neurons in addition to shrinkage of large cortical neurons, with plaques and neurofibrillary tangles. The most common early symptom of AD is difficulty remembering newly learned information because the neurologic changes typically begin in the part of the brain that affects learning. As AD advances through the brain, it leads to increasingly severe symptoms, including disorientation and mood and behavior changes; deepening confusion about events, time, and place; unfounded suspicions about family, friends, and professional caregivers; more serious memory loss and behavior changes; and difficulty speaking, swallowing, and walking.

The goal of drug therapy for AD is to slow the loss of memory and cognition, thus preserving the independence of the individual person for as long as possible. Studies have shown that vitamin E, estrogen, and anti-inflammatory agents lower the risk of AD. Practice guidelines developed by the Alzheimer's Association (2018) recommend early diagnosis and treatment of AD with cholinesterase inhibitors for all patients with mild to moderate symptoms. Although these drugs do not cure the disease, they do delay the onset of the disease somewhat and bring about a slight improvement in cognition and function. Improvement in cognitive function is seen in approximately 12 weeks with continuous therapy. The reversible cholinesterase inhibitors are also known as indirect-acting cholinergic drugs that improve memory by elevating acetylcholine in the cerebral cortex of the brain.

> **Quality and Safety Alert: Evidence-Based Practice**
>
> Liu et al. (2022) conducted a study on the efficacy of donepezil for the treatment of Alzheimer disease. The research revealed strong evidence that treatment with donepezil delays the progression of Alzheimer disease. The medication targets key proteins and essential pathways associated with enhanced memory.

CHOLINESTERASE INHIBITORS: REVERSIBLE INDIRECT-ACTING CHOLINERGICS

This class of drugs for the treatment of AD or dementia interferes with the enzyme that allows for the production of acetylcholinesterase to increase acetylcholine and improve memory.

 Donepezil (Adlarity, Aricept) is the prototype drug in this class. Treatment of mild, moderate, or severe AD is the primary use for this centrally acting reversible cholinesterase inhibitor. Table 47.1 lists the cholinesterase inhibitors used in the management of AD.

Pharmacokinetics

Absorption of donepezil after oral administration is good, and it is unaffected by food. The drug is highly bound (96%) to plasma proteins. The peak of action occurs in 3 to 8 hours. Metabolism takes place in the liver, producing several metabolites, some of which are pharmacologically active. Excretion of these metabolites and some unchanged drug occurs mainly in urine.

Action

Donepezil increases acetylcholine in the brain by inhibiting its metabolism, leading to elevated acetylcholine levels in the cortex. This slows the neuronal degradation that occurs in AD.

Use

Long-term studies have shown that donepezil delays the progression of AD for up to 55 weeks. Other uses include enhancing memory in other neurologic conditions such as multiple sclerosis, treating MG, or treating overdoses of atropine and centrally acting anticholinergic drugs (e.g., those used for parkinsonism). Table 47.3 presents dosage information for donepezil and related drugs.

Patient-related variables specific to the use of donepezil include the following:

- Age:
  - Older adults are more likely to experience adverse drug effects because of age-related physiologic changes and superimposed pathologic conditions.
- Reproduction, pregnancy, and lactation:
  - Animal studies have revealed adverse effects on the fetus.
  - It is unknown if donepezil is present in breast milk.
- Abnormal kidney function and hepatic impairment:
  - No dosage adjustment with abnormal kidney function.
  - Liver disease may impair the drug's hepatic metabolism, resulting in increased adverse effects. Monitor a patient's liver function and clinical response to the medication carefully.
- Specific healthcare environments:
  - Donepezil is used in critically ill patients who may have delirium (a form of acute cognitive dysfunction that manifests as a fluctuating change in mental status, with inattention and altered level of consciousness).
  - In the home care setting, the nurse must work with responsible family members to ensure accurate drug administration.

Adverse Effects

The most common adverse effects of donepezil are headache, dizziness, depression, vertigo, and insomnia. Possible drug-related GI conditions include nausea, vomiting, diarrhea, abdominal muscle cramps, anorexia, and GI bleeding. The most serious adverse effects are breathing problems (e.g., asthma, chronic obstructive pulmonary disease), fainting, and heart disease (e.g., sick sinus syndrome, other heart conduction disorders). Dyspnea has been reported and is more common in patients who have previous lung disease. In addition, fatigue and anorexia may occur. Other adverse effects include seizures and trouble urinating.

Contraindications

Contraindications to donepezil include known hypersensitivity to the drug. Patients with lung disease or heart disease such as sick sinus syndrome should not take this medication.

Nursing Implications

Preventing Interactions

Many medications interact with donepezil, increasing or decreasing its effects (Box 47.3).

Administering the Medication

Before administering donepezil, the nurse assesses the patient for allergy, orientation, and contraindications. Administration should occur at bedtime each day. If the patient is taking an oral disintegrating tablet, the nurse ensures that the medication is dissolved on the tongue.

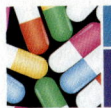

TABLE 47.3
DRUGS AT A GLANCE: Drugs Used for the Treatment of Alzheimer Disease

Drug	Routes and Dosage Ranges	
	Adults	**Children**
Cholinesterase Inhibitors		
ⓟ Donepezil (Adlarity, Aricept; 🍁 Aricept, Aricept RDT	5 mg PO daily at bedtime for 4–6 wk, then increase to 10 mg daily if needed	Dosage not established
Galantamine (Razadyne ER; 🍁 Auro-Galantamine ER, Mylan-Galantamine ER)	8 mg PO daily initially, with food; increase to 16 mg/d after 4 wk if needed. May continue to increase every 4 wk up to max dose of 24 mg/d	Dosage not established
Rivastigmine (Exelon; 🍁 Exelon, Rivastigmine Patch 5, 10, or 15, SANDOZ Rivastigmine)	1.5 mg PO twice daily with food initially. May titrate to higher doses at 1.5 mg intervals every 2 wk to a maximum dose of 6 mg twice daily TDS initially 4.6 mg/24 h patch. Increase to 9.5 mg/24 h patch after 4 wk. Max dose 13.3 mg/24 h patch	Dosage not established
NMDA Receptor Antagonist		
ⓟ Memantine (Namenda, Namenda Titration Pak, Namenda XR, Namenda XR Titration Pak; 🍁 Ebixa)	5 mg PO daily, increase dose by 5 mg/wk to a target dose of 20 mg daily; doses >5 mg should be given twice/day. Severe abnormal kidney function: 5 mg PO 2 times/d	Dosage not established
Acetylcholinesterase–NMDA Receptor Antagonist		
Donepezil–memantine (Namzaric)	Recommended starting dose is 7 mg/10 mg daily, with a maximum dose of 28/10 mg daily; administer in evening without regard to meals	Dosage not established
Antiamyloid Monoclonal Antibody		
Aducanumab (Aduhelm)	IV 1 mg/kg once every 4 weeks for 1 and 2 infusions; 3 mg/kg every 4 weeks for 3 and 4 infusions; 6 mg/kg every 4 weeks for 5 and 6 infusions	Dosage not established

TDS, transdermal delivery system.

> **! Quality and Safety Alert: Safety**
>
> The brand names for donepezil (Aricept) and rabeprazole (AcipHex) are a source of confusion. It is essential to use caution when administering either of these drugs.

Assessing for Therapeutic Effects

The nurse assesses for improved memory and reduction of dementia. This involves assessing daily for memory changes, forgetfulness, and mood.

BOX 47.3 Drug Interactions: Donepezil

Drugs That Increase the Effects of Donepezil
- Theophylline
  Increases the risk of toxicity
- Cholinesterase inhibitors
  Increase the risk of toxicity

Drugs That Decrease the Effects of Donepezil
- Anticholinergics
  Decrease the efficacy
- Nonsteroidal anti-inflammatory drugs
  Increase the risk of gastrointestinal bleeding

Assessing for Adverse Effects

The nurse assesses for signs and symptoms of GI upset such as nausea, diarrhea, and vomiting. If GI bleeding is suspected, it is important to obtain an order for laboratory tests such as complete blood count and bleeding time. The nurse should also assess the patient for sleep disturbances due to the risk of insomnia.

Patient Teaching

Box 47.4 identifies patient teaching guidelines for donepezil.

Other Drugs in the Class

Galantamine hydrobromide (Razadyne ER) slows the degradation of acetylcholine by increasing it in the cerebral cortex. Rivastigmine (Exelon, Exelon Patch) increases acetylcholine in the CNS. Each medication is used to slow the symptoms of mild to moderate dementia. In addition, rivastigmine is administered for Parkinson disease. The oral preparations of both medications should be administered with food to reduce gastric distress. Galantamine is contraindicated with severe hepatic or abnormal kidney function. Rivastigmine is contraindicated with carbamate derivatives. The most common adverse effects of galantamine are insomnia, tremor, dizziness, somnolence, headache, bradycardia, and syncope.

> **BOX 47.4** **Patient Teaching Guidelines for Cholinesterase Inhibitors: Donepezil**
>
> - Take this drug at bedtime.
> - Place orally disintegrating tablet on your tongue; allow it to dissolve and then drink water.
> - Know that this drug does not cure the disease but is thought to slow down the degeneration associated with the disease.
> - Continue taking this drug if no change in symptoms is noted.
> - Arrange for regular blood tests and follow-up visits while adjusting to this drug.
> - Note that the following side effects may occur: nausea, vomiting (eat frequent small meals), insomnia, fatigue, and confusion (use caution if driving or performing tasks that require alertness).
> - Report severe nausea, vomiting, changes in stool or urine color, diarrhea, changes in neurologic functioning, and yellowing of the eyes or skin to your healthcare provider.

Oral rivastigmine lasts 12 hours, making twice-a-day dosing possible. Rivastigmine transdermal is applied as a patch once a day. The site of the transdermal application should be rotated. The site used should not be used again for a period of 14 days. Metabolism occurs in the liver, and excretion takes place in the feces. The side effect profile of rivastigmine is similar to that of donepezil.

NCLEX Success

3. A nurse is teaching family members how to administer donepezil for Alzheimer disease. The instructions should include which of the following?

    A. Take the medication with food.
    B. Take the medication on an empty stomach.
    C. Take the medication at bedtime.
    D. Take the medication at the start of each day.

N-METHYL-D-ASPARTATE RECEPTOR ANTAGONIST

Memantine (Namenda, Namenda Titration Pak) is the prototype *N*-methyl-D-aspartate (NMDA) receptor antagonist. The drug is administered to patients with moderate to severe AD. Its neuroprotective action is different from that of the cholinesterase inhibitors.

Pharmacokinetics

Memantine is well absorbed orally, with 100% absorption in the GI tract. It is easily distributed and easily transported across the blood–brain barrier. The drug is 45% protein bound. Its peak of action occurs in 3 to 7 hours with the immediate-release formulation and in 9 to 12 hours with the extended-release formulation. It is partially metabolized by the liver, independent of the cytochrome P450 enzyme system. The terminal elimination half-life is 60 to 80 hours.

Action

Glutamate is an excitatory amino acid in the CNS and is known to contribute to origin and development of AD. In patients with Alzheimer's, overstimulation of the glutamate receptors occurs, leading to cell death. NMDA is a glutamate receptor in which memantine induces an antagonistic effect. When the NMDA receptors are overstimulated, magnesium is prevented from reentering and blocking the channel from closing. Thus, an influx of calcium results, and neuronal cell death subsequently occurs. Memantine can bind to the magnesium site to block the excitatory function by slowing intracellular calcium accumulation. This action prevents nerve damage but does not affect glutamate.

Use

Memantine is used to slow the progression of moderate to severe AD.

Patient-related variables specific to the use of memantine include reproduction and pregnancy and lactation status. Adverse events in animal studies have been observed. It is not known if memantine is present in breast milk.

Contraindications

Contraindications include any hypersensitivity reaction to memantine. Also, patients with kidney failure should not take the drug.

Nursing Implications

Preventing Interactions

Memantine interacts with carbonic anhydrase and alkalinizing agents, resulting in increased serum concentration of memantine. Also, trimethoprim may lead to memantine toxicity.

Administering the Medication

Memantine should be administered without regard to meals. The extended-release capsule should be swallowed whole; it should not be chewed. The capsule can be opened and sprinkled on applesauce, which must be consumed immediately. The liquid formulation should be squirted in the corner of the patient's mouth and should not be mixed with any other liquid.

Assessing for Therapeutic Effects

The nurse assesses for improved memory and reduction in dementia. The nurse also assesses for changes in memory and mood.

Assessing for Adverse Effects

The nurse should assess the patient for changes in blood pressure. Hypertension occurs in 4% of patients who take memantine, and hypotension may result with the extended-release formulation. The nurse should assess for CNS adverse effects such as dizziness, confusion, anxiety, fatigue, and hallucinations. In addition, the patient is assessed for diarrhea, constipation, vomiting, abdominal pain, urinary incontinence, back pain, and cough. Finally, the nurse assesses for signs and symptoms of a hypersensitivity reaction.

Patient Teaching

Instruct the patient's caregiver about the administration of memantine. Because of the CNS effects, the patient should be protected from falls related to dizziness. In the event the patient develops GI symptoms, urinary incontinence, back pain, or cough, the prescriber should be notified. In addition, the caregiver should be instructed about hypersensitivity reactions, including skin rash, dyspnea, or bronchospasm.

> **NCLEX Success**
>
> 4. A patient diagnosed with Alzheimer disease has used donepezil for 4 years. Their daughter notices the patient's memory is worsening. Which of the following medications might be more successful for enhancing the patient's memory?
>   A. tacrine
>   B. rivastigmine
>   C. memantine
>   D. galantamine

CHOLINESTERASE INHIBITOR–N-METHYL-D-ASPARTATE RECEPTOR ANTAGONIST

Donepezil and memantine are available as a combination of a cholinesterase inhibitor and an NMDA—as Namzaric. For the actions of this combination drug, see previous discussions. Donepezil–memantine is administered to patients with moderate to severe dementia. This oral agent is for patients who are stabilized on 10 mg donepezil once daily but are not taking memantine. Initial dose of memantine extended-release of 7 mg combined with donepezil 10 mg once daily. The dosage can be increased weekly with a maintenance dose of memantine extended-release of 28 mg and donepezil 10 mg daily.

The nurse must assess for cardiovascular adverse effects. The donepezil may cause bradycardia and heart block. Patients should be protected from falls; there is a risk of syncopal episodes. Diarrhea, nausea, and vomiting may develop and commonly resolve in 1 to 3 weeks. As with other medications administered for AD, it is important to monitor the patient's mental status and ability to perform activities of daily living.

ANTIAMYLOID MONOCLONAL ANTIBODY

Aducanumab (Aduhelm) is a monoclonal antibody approved by the FDA for patients with AD with beta-amyloid plaques. It is the first immunomodulator medication used to treat the biology of the disease.

Pharmacokinetics

Aducanumab is a monoclonal IgG1 antibody that binds to amyloid-β. It is metabolized by degrading the catabolic pathways into small peptides and amino acids. It has a long duration of action with a half-life elimination of 24.8 days.

Action

The action of aducanumab is the reduction of amyloid plaques.

Use

Aducanumab is used for mild cognitive impairment or mild dementia in patients with a confirmed diagnosis of amyloid plaques.

Patient-related variables specific to the use of aducanumab include reproduction and pregnancy and lactation status. Adverse pregnancy events were inconclusive in animal studies. It is unknown if aducanumab is present in breast milk.

Adverse Effects

The reported adverse effects include microhemorrhages, brain edema, and diarrhea. The patient will be prone to headaches and falls with drug toxicity.

Contraindications

There are no reported contraindications.

Nursing Implications

Preventing Interactions

Efgartigimod alfa's therapeutic effect will be diminished if combined with aducanumab.

Administering the Drug

Aducanumab is diluted prior to intravenous administration. The infusion bags are refrigerated when stored and should be warmed prior to administration. Administer by IV infusion over 60 minutes in a sterile, low protein binding 0.2 or 0.22 micron in-line filter. The infusions should be at least 21 days apart.

Assessing for Therapeutic and Adverse Effects

Amyloid-related imagery with magnetic resonance imaging (MRI) should be conducted to assess for resolution of symptoms. If the imagery reveals symptoms of toxicity, the dosage is adjusted or discontinued by the prescriber. In addition,

MRI results indicating an intracerebral bleed will require discontinuation of the medication.

Patient Teaching

According to Press and Buss (2022), the approval of aducanumab was controversial. It has been primarily administered in research settings. For patients receiving treatment with aducanumab, the patient and family should be taught to report any signs of headache, increased confusion, or visual field changes. The patient should be protected from falls. MRI monitoring is essential with drug therapy.

CHOLINERGIC AGONIST

(P) Bethanechol is the prototype cholinergic agonist. Cholinergic agonists are frequently used in the treatment of urinary retention (see Table 47.1). The patient may describe a sensation of bladder fullness or incomplete bladder emptying; a neurogenic bladder results in urinary retention or leakage.

Pharmacokinetics

Bethanechol is well absorbed in the GI tract. The onset of action is 30 minutes, and the medication reaches its peak in 60 to 90 minutes. The duration of action is 1 to 6 hours. The site of metabolism and elimination is not known. The drug does not cross the blood–brain barrier but does cross the placenta, and it enters breast milk.

Action

Bethanechol is a parasympathomimetic agent that acts at the cholinergic receptors in the urinary and GI tracts to increase muscle tone. The increased tone of the detrusor muscle in the urinary bladder allows for bladder emptying.

Use

Bethanechol is administered during the acute postoperative and postpartum periods for the treatment of nonobstructed urinary retention and neurogenic atony of the bladder muscle. Table 47.4 gives dosage information for this drug.

Patient-related variables specific to bethanechol include reproduction and pregnancy and lactation status. Animal reproduction studies have not been conducted. It is unknown if bethanechol enters the breast milk.

Adverse Effects

Cardiovascular adverse effects to bethanechol include transient heart block, orthostatic hypotension with large doses, and cardiac arrest. Reported GI adverse effects are abdominal discomfort, increased salivation, nausea, vomiting, and fecal incontinence. Genitourinary effects include urinary urgency. Other adverse effects are flushing, sweating, malaise, and dyspnea.

Contraindications

Contraindications to bethanechol include known hypersensitivity to the drug or other cholinergic agent as well as hyperthyroidism, peptic ulcer disease, intestinal obstruction, asthma, bradycardia, coronary artery disease, epilepsy, and parkinsonism. Patients should not take bethanechol in the postoperative phase of bladder neck or GI surgery.

Nursing Implications

Preventing Interactions

Several drugs, including cholinergic agents, atropine, procainamide, epinephrine, and ganglionic blockers, increase the effects of bethanechol. This causes a significant drop in blood pressure.

Administering the Medication

Administration of bethanechol should occur 1 hour before meals or 2 hours after meals to prevent nausea and vomiting. Therapy should begin using the lowest possible dosage, which is then increased as tolerated.

Assessing for Therapeutic Effects

The nurse assesses the patient's ability to void 1 hour following the administration of the medication. The nurse also interviews the patient regarding the relief of symptoms of bladder fullness.

Assessing for Adverse Effects

The nurse assesses the patient's blood pressure lying, sitting, and standing. It is also necessary to assess an electrocardiogram for signs of heart block or impending cardiac arrest. In addition, the nurse assesses for cholinergic crisis with sweating and flushing. Finally, the nurse assesses for GI effects such as abdominal pain, nausea, and vomiting.

TABLE 47.4

DRUGS AT A GLANCE: Cholinergic Agonist Used for the Treatment of Urinary Retention

Drug	Routes and Dosage Ranges	
	Adults	Children
(P) Bethanechol	10–50 mg PO 3–4 times/d; initial dose of 5–10 mg with gradual increases hourly until desired effect is seen; or until 50 mg is given	Safety and efficacy not established

> **BOX 47.5 Patient Teaching Guidelines for Bethanechol**
>
> - Take the medication on an empty stomach.
> - Report difficulty urinating to your healthcare provider.
> - Report diarrhea, headache, belching, substernal pressure, or pain to your healthcare provider.

Patient Teaching

Box 47.5 identifies patient teaching guidelines for bethanechol.

> **NCLEX Success**
>
> 5. A 40-year-old patient is taking bethanechol for urinary retention. The physician increases the dosage from 30 to 40 mg. For which of the following adverse effects should the nurse assess?
>   A. pulmonary edema
>   B. bronchospasm
>   C. orthostatic hypotension
>   D. pulse deficit

IRREVERSIBLE ANTICHOLINESTERASE TOXICITY

Most irreversible anticholinesterase agents are highly lipid soluble and can enter the body by a variety of routes, including the eye, skin, respiratory system, and GI tract. Because they readily cross the blood–brain barrier, their effects are seen peripherally as well as centrally.

Some of the agents used by terrorists are irreversible anticholinesterases. In 1995, a terrorist group released sarin gas on a number of subway trains in Tokyo, Japan. Sarin is a toxic nerve gas that produces a cholinergic crisis characterized by excessive cholinergic (muscarinic) stimulation and neuromuscular blockade. This cholinergic crisis occurs because the irreversible anticholinesterase poison binds to the enzyme anticholinesterase and inactivates it. Consequently, acetylcholine remains in cholinergic synapses and causes excessive stimulation of muscarinic and nicotinic receptors. Other nerve gases that produce these effects include tabun and soman. In addition, the organophosphate insecticides malathion and parathion have the same cholinergic effects.

Emergency treatment includes decontamination procedures such as removing contaminated clothing, flushing the poison from skin and eyes, and using activated charcoal and lavage to remove ingested poison from the GI tract. Pharmacologic treatment includes administering atropine to counteract the muscarinic effects of the poison (e.g., salivation, urination, defecation, bronchial secretions, laryngospasm, bronchospasm). Atropine acts by blocking the acetylcholine at the parasympathetic sites of the smooth muscle, salivary glands, and the CNS to dry secretions and increase cardiac output. The severity of the poisoning dictates the dosage of atropine. The U.S. Department of Defense uses atropine in the form of AtroPen for the initial treatment of muscarinic symptoms.

In addition, a second drug is necessary to relieve the neuromuscular blockade produced by nicotinic effects of the poison. This drug, pralidoxime (Protopam), a cholinesterase reactivator, is a specific antidote for overdose with irreversible anticholinesterase agents. (Other indications for pralidoxime include control of overdose by anticholinesterase drugs used to treat MG.) It treats toxicity by causing the anticholinesterase poison to release the enzyme acetylcholinesterase. The reactivated acetylcholinesterase can then degrade excess acetylcholine at the cholinergic synapses, including the neuromuscular junction. It is important to note that pralidoxime cannot cross the blood–brain barrier; thus, it is effective only in the peripheral areas of the body. It is essential that pralidoxime is given as soon after the poisoning as possible. If too much time passes, the bond between the irreversible anticholinesterase agent and acetylcholinesterase becomes stronger, and pralidoxime is unable to release the enzyme from the poison.

Because pralidoxime is excreted in the urine, dosage reduction is necessary in the presence of abnormal kidney function. During the administration of the medication, continuous monitoring of the patient is essential due to the risk of tachycardia and cardiac arrest. The peak onset of action is 5 to 15 minutes. The half-life is 74 to 77 minutes. Excretion of unchanged drug occurs in the urine.

Treatment of anticholinesterase overdose may also require diazepam or lorazepam to control seizures. The mechanism of action of diazepam is not understood, but the drug is thought to act in the limbic system. It potentiates gamma-aminobutyric acid, an inhibitory neurotransmitter. Close monitoring of the patient's electrocardiogram during drug administration is necessary. Mechanical ventilation may be necessary to treat respiratory paralysis.

Table 47.5 summarizes the miscellaneous medications used for the treatment of irreversible anticholinesterase toxicity.

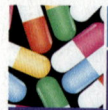

TABLE 47.5

DRUGS AT A GLANCE: Miscellaneous Drugs Used for Treatment of Irreversible Anticholinesterase Toxicity

Drug	Routes and Dosage Ranges	
	Adults	**Children**
Atropine sulfate (AtroPen)	Neuromuscular blockade reversal: IV 15–30 mcg/kg administered with pyridostigmine or 5–7 mcg/kg administered with edrophonium Muscarine-containing mushroom poisoning: IV 1–2 mg; titrate and repeat as needed Organophosphate or carbamate insecticide or nerve agent poisoning: AtroPen: mild symptoms: IM 2 mg at initial exposure If severe symptoms develop after first dose, rapidly give two additional doses within 10 min; do not exceed three doses	Mushroom poisoning (muscarine): IV 0.02 mg/kg/dose; minimum dose 0.1 mg; titrate and repeat as needed AtroPen: IM <7 kg: 0.25 mg/dose (yellow pen) 6.8–18 kg: 0.5 mg/dose (blue pen) 18–41 kg: 1 mg/dose (dark red pen) >41 kg: 2 mg/dose (green pen) Administer the weight-based dose as soon as exposure is known or suspected: 2 additional doses should be repeated in rapid succession 10 min after the first dose; do not administer more than 3 doses
Pralidoxime (Protopam)	Use in conjunction with atropine 1–2 g IV or IM; repeat in 1–2 h if muscle weakness has not been relieved, then at 10- to 12-h intervals if cholinergic signs recur Organophosphate poisoning: loading dose 1,000–2,000 mg IV, repeat bolus of 1,000–2,000 mg after 1 h and repeat 10–12 h thereafter Mild symptoms: 600 mg IM, repeat every 15 min (maximum dose 1,800 mg) Severe symptoms: 600 mg; repeat twice in rapid succession to deliver a total of 1,800 mg Persistent symptoms: repeat entire series beginning 1 h after last injection	Use in conjunction with atropine 20–50 mg/kg/dose; repeat in 1–2 h if muscle weakness is not improved, then 10- to 12-h intervals if cholinergic signs recur Organophosphate poisoning (<16 y): 20–50 mg/kg IV (max dose 2,000 mg/dose); repeat after 1 h and every 10- to 12-h if muscle weakness persists Mild symptoms: 15 mg/kg repeat every 15 min for persistent symptoms (max dose: 45 mg/kg; may administer in rapid succession) Severe symptoms: 15 mg/kg; repeat twice in rapid succession 45 mg/kg total dose Persistent symptoms: may repeat entire series (45 mg/kg) beginning 1 h after last dose
Diazepam (Valium; Diastat AcuDial, Diastat Pediatric, Diazepam Intensol) (✺ Apo-Diazepam, BIO-Diazepam, Diazemuls, Diastat, Valium)	5–10 mg IV slowly; may repeat in 10–15 min; max dose: 30 mg	Infants, children, adolescents; IV 0.15–0.2 mg/kg (max dose: 10 mg); may repeat once

Chapter 47 • Drug Therapy for Myasthenia Gravis, Alzheimer Disease, and Other Conditions Treated With Cholinergic Agents

THE NURSING PROCESS

A concept map outlines the nursing process related to drug therapy considerations in this chapter. Additional nursing implications related to the disease process should also be considered in care decisions.

Assessment
- Myasthenia gravis
  - Assess for muscle weakness in mild to moderate disease: ptosis (drooping) of the upper eyelid and diplopia (double vision) caused by weakness of the eye muscles.
  - In severe disease, assess for difficulty in chewing, swallowing, and speaking; accumulation of oral secretions, which the patient may be unable to expectorate or swallow; decreased skeletal muscle activity, including impaired chest expansion; and eventual respiratory failure.
- Alzheimer disease
  - Assess for abilities and limitations in relation to memory, cognitive functioning, and self-care activities.
  - Assess for preexisting conditions that may be aggravated by a cholinergic drug.
- Urinary retention
  - Assess for bladder distention.
  - Assess for time and amount of previous urination and fluid intake.

Outcomes of Therapy
The patient will
- Verbalize or demonstrate correct drug administration.
- Improve in self-care abilities.
- Regain usual patterns of urinary and bowel elimination.
- Maintain effective oxygenation of tissues.
- Report adverse drug effects.
- For patients with myasthenia gravis, at least one family member will verbalize or demonstrate correct drug administration, symptoms of too much or too little drug, and emergency care procedures.
- For patients with dementia, a caregiver will verbalize or demonstrate correct drug administration and knowledge of adverse effects to be reported to a health care provider.

Nursing Interventions
- Use measures to prevent or decrease the need for cholinergic drugs. Ambulation, adequate fluid intake, and judicious use of opioid analgesics or other sedative-type drugs help prevent postoperative urinary retention.
- In myasthenia gravis:
  - Schedule activities to avoid excessive fatigue and to allow adequate rest periods. This may be beneficial, because muscle weakness is aggravated by exercise and improved by rest.
  - Recommend that one or more family members be trained in cardiopulmonary resuscitation.
- In Alzheimer disease, assist and teach caregivers to
  - Maintain a quiet, stable environment and daily routines to decrease confusion (e.g., verbal or written reminders, simple directions, adequate lighting, calendars, personal objects within view and reach).
  - Avoid altering dosage or stopping the drug without consulting the prescribing physician.
  - Be sure that the patient keeps appointments for supervision and blood tests.
- With long-term drug use, assist patients and families to establish a schedule of drug administration that best meets the patient's needs.
- Do not give cholinergic drugs for bladder atony and urinary retention or for paralytic ileus in the presence of an obstruction.

Evaluation
- Observe and interview about the adequacy of urinary elimination.
- Observe abilities and limitations in self-care.
- Question the patient and at least one family member of the patient with myasthenia gravis about correct drug usage, symptoms of underdosage and overdosage, and emergency care procedures.
- Question caregivers of patients with dementia about the patient's level of functioning and response to medication.

Visit **thePoint**® *at* **http://thePoint.lww.com/Frandsen13e** *for answers to NCLEX Success questions (in Appendix A), answers to Clinical Application Case Studies (in Appendix B), additional material on etiology and pathophysiology, and more!*

REFERENCES AND RESOURCES

Alzheimer's Association. (2018) *Dementia care practice recommendations*. Retrieved: May 3, 2023 https://www.alz.org/media/Documents/alzheimers-dementia-care-practice-recommendations.pdf

Alzheimer's Association. (2019). *What is Alzheimer's disease?* Retrieved June 30, 2022, from https://www.alz.org/alzheimers-dementia/what-is-alzheimers

Alzheimer's Association. (2022). *Aducanumab approved for treatment of Alzheimer's disease*. Retrieved June 30, 2022, from https://www.alz.org/alzheimers-dementia/treatments/aducanumab

Bird, S. J. (2022a). Diagnosis of MG. In *UpToDate*. Lexi-Comp, Inc.

Bird, S. J., & Levine, J. M. (2022). Myasthenic crisis. In *UpToDate*. Lexi-Comp, Inc.

Bird, S. (2022b). Overview of the treatment of MG. In *UpToDate*. Lexi-Comp, Inc.

Hinkle, J. H., Cheever, K. H., & Overbaugh, K. J. (2022). *Brunner & Suddarth's textbook of medical-surgical nursing* (15th ed.). Wolters Kluwer.

Liu, L., Zhu, Y., Fu, P., & Yang, J. (2022). Research on the mechanism of donepezil in treating Alzheimer's disease. *Frontiers in Aging Neuroscience., 14* 10.3389/fnagi.2022.822480

National Institutes of Health. (2022). *Alzheimer's disease fact sheet*. Retrieved June 29, 2022, from https://www.nia.nih.gov/health/alzheimers-disease-fact-sheet

Norris, T. (2019). *Porth's pathophysiology concepts of altered health states* (10th ed.). Wolters Kluwer.

Press, D., & Buss, S. (2022). Treatment of dementia. In *UptoDate*. Lexi-Comp, Inc.

UpToDate. (2022). *Drug information*. Lexi-Comp, Inc.

Wright, C. (2022). Treatment and prevention of vascular cognitive impairment and dementia. In *UpToDate*. Lexi-Comp, Inc.

CHAPTER 48

Drug Therapy for Parkinson Disease, Urinary Spasticity, and Disorders Requiring Anticholinergic Drug Therapy

LEARNING OBJECTIVES

After studying this chapter, you should be able to:

1. Describe the major characteristics and manifestations of Parkinson disease.
2. Understand the pathophysiology of Parkinson disease.
3. Describe the types of commonly used anti-Parkinson drugs.
4. Identify the prototype and describe the action, use, adverse effects, contraindications, and nursing implications for the dopamine receptor agonists.
5. Identify the prototype and describe the action, use, adverse effects, contraindications, and nursing implications for the catechol-*O*-methyltransferase (COMT) inhibitors.
6. Identify the prototype and describe the action, use, adverse effects, contraindications, and nursing implications for a COMT inhibitor and decarboxylase inhibitor/dopamine precursor.
7. Implement the nursing process in the care of patients undergoing drug therapy for Parkinson disease.
8. Describe the general characteristics of anticholinergic drugs.
9. Identify the prototype and describe the action, use, adverse effects, contraindications, and nursing implications for belladonna alkaloids and derivatives.
10. Identify the prototype and describe the action, use, adverse effects, contraindications, and nursing implications for centrally acting anticholinergic drugs.
11. Identify the prototype and describe the action, use, adverse effects, contraindications, and nursing implications for anticholinergic medications used for gastrointestinal and urinary disorders.
12. Implement the nursing process in the administration of anticholinergic agents.

CLINICAL APPLICATION CASE STUDY

Lee Stokes, age 61, visits his primary healthcare provider. He is experiencing pill-rolling movement of the right hand and fingers; slow, stooped movement; a shuffling gait with the absence of arm movement; and excessive salivation. His physician diagnosed Mr. Stokes with Parkinson disease and started him on levodopa–carbidopa (Sinemet) 25-mg carbidopa–100-mg levodopa four times a day and benztropine mesylate at bedtime.

KEY TERMS

Akinesia: rigid limbs

Anticholinergic drug: drug that inhibits the actions of acetylcholine in the brain

Antimuscarinic drug: drug that interacts with muscarinic cholinergic receptors in the brain, secretory glands, heart, and smooth muscle to produce an anticholinergic response

Basal ganglia: area in the midbrain that controls smooth voluntary movement

Bradykinesia: inability to move

Catechol-O-methyltransferase (COMT) inhibitor: medication that inhibits the metabolism of levodopa in the periphery

Cycloplegia: paralysis in the ciliary muscle of the eye

Dopamine receptor agonist: drug that corrects the neurotransmitter imbalance by increasing levels of dopamine

Hypertensive crisis: severe increase in blood pressure that can lead to a stroke

Muscarinic receptors: located in most internal organs, including the cardiovascular, respiratory, gastrointestinal (GI), and genitourinary systems; when activated by acetylcholine, the affected cells may be excited or inhibited in their functions

Mydriasis: pupil dilation

Nicotinic receptors: located in motor nerves and skeletal muscles; when activated by acetylcholine, the cell membrane depolarizes and produces muscle contraction

Parkinson disease: the most common form of parkinsonism, which is a chronic, progressive, degenerative disorder of the central nervous system (CNS) characterized by resting tremor, bradykinesia, rigidity, and postural instability

Parkinsonism: a general term for a group of neurologic disorders that cause problems with movement

Quaternary amines: anticholinergic drugs that carry a positive charge and are lipid insoluble; they do not readily cross the cell membranes, are poorly absorbed from the GI tract, and do not cross the blood–brain barrier

Substantia nigra: region of the midbrain with dopamine cells

Tertiary amines: anticholinergic drugs that are unchanged lipid-soluble molecules, are able to cross cell membranes readily, and are well absorbed from the GI tract and conjunctiva, and they cross the blood–brain barrier

Wearing off: periods of the day when the medication is not working well, causing worsening of parkinsonian symptoms

INTRODUCTION

The first part of this chapter discusses Parkinson disease and the medications administered to decrease the symptoms of the disease. The second part discusses anticholinergic drugs administered to decrease secretions and prevent urinary urgency.

OVERVIEW OF PARKINSON DISEASE

Parkinsonism is a general term for a group of neurologic disorders that cause problems with movement. **Parkinson disease** is the most common form of parkinsonism, which is a chronic, progressive, degenerative disorder of the central nervous system (CNS) characterized by resting tremor, bradykinesia, rigidity, and postural instability. Manifestations of Parkinson disease also may occur with other CNS diseases, brain tumors, and head injuries. Drugs that deplete dopamine stores or block dopamine receptors, including the older antipsychotic drugs (phenothiazines and haloperidol), reserpine, and metoclopramide, can produce movement disorders such as secondary parkinsonism (which also involves extrapyramidal reactions; see Chapter 56). Treatment can be pharmacologic, nonpharmacologic, and/or surgical.

Idiopathic parkinsonism results from progressive destruction of or degenerative changes in dopamine-producing nerve cells in the **substantia nigra** in the **basal ganglia**, the area in the midbrain that controls smooth voluntary movement. The basal ganglia in the brain normally contain substantial amounts of the neurotransmitters dopamine and acetylcholine. The correct balance of dopamine and acetylcholine is important in regulating posture, muscle tone, and voluntary movement. People with Parkinson disease have an imbalance in these neurotransmitters, resulting in a decrease in inhibitory brain dopamine and a relative increase in excitatory acetylcholine.

Clinical Manifestations

The first symptom of Parkinson disease is often a resting tremor that begins in the fingers and thumb of one hand ("pill-rolling" movements), eventually spreading over one side of the body and progressing to the contralateral limbs. Other common symptoms include inability to move (**bradykinesia**), rigid

TABLE 48.1

Drugs Administered for the Treatment of Parkinson Disease

Drug Class	Prototype	Other Drugs in the Class
Dopamine receptor agonist	Levodopa–carbidopa	Amantadine (Gocovri, Osmolex ER) Apomorphine hydrochloride (Apokyn) Bromocriptine mesylate (Parlodel, Cycloset) Pramipexole dihydrochloride (Mirapex, Mirapex ER) Rasagiline (Azilect) Ropinirole Rotigotine transdermal (Neupro) Safinamide (Xadago) Selegiline hydrochloride (Emsam, Zelapar)
Catechol-*O*-methyltransferase (COMT) inhibitors	Tolcapone (Tasmar)	Entacapone (Comtan)
COMT inhibitor and decarboxylase inhibitor/dopamine precursor	Levodopa, carbidopa, and entacapone (Stalevo)	

limbs (**akinesia**), shuffling gait, stooped posture, masklike facial expression, and a soft speaking voice. Less common manifestations may include depression, personality changes, loss of appetite, sleep disturbances, speech impairment, or sexual difficulty. Approximately 15% to 20% of people with Parkinson disease develop dementia. The severity of disease manifestations usually worsen over time. However, disease progression is often quite gradual, and patients may retain near-normal functional abilities for several years.

Drug Therapy

Drugs used in Parkinson disease include **dopamine receptor agonists**, which help correct the neurotransmitter imbalance by increasing levels of dopamine, and **catechol-*O*-methyltransferase (COMT) inhibitors**, which inhibit the metabolism of levodopa in the periphery. See Table 48.1. (The older belladonna alkaloids and the newer centrally acting anticholinergic agents inhibit the actions of acetylcholine in the brain. As previously stated, these medications are discussed later in this chapter.)

DOPAMINE RECEPTOR AGONISTS

Levodopa (L-dopa), the original prototype dopamine receptor agonist, was developed in the 1960s. It is routinely administered with the drug carbidopa; therefore, the combination medication is discussed as the prototype. **Ⓟ Levodopa–carbidopa** (Sinemet, Dhivy, Duopa, Rytary) is well established as the most effective drug for the symptomatic treatment of idiopathic Parkinson disease. (Carbidopa is used only in conjunction with levodopa.) The combination is particularly effective for the management of akinetic symptoms.

Clinical Application 48.1

- A nurse is providing patient teaching to Mr. Stokes and his family. The family inquires about the progression of Parkinson disease. What does the nurse tell the patient and the family with regard to disease progression?

Pharmacokinetics

In peripheral tissues (e.g., gastrointestinal [GI] tract, liver), levodopa is metabolized extensively by the enzyme aromatic amino acid decarboxylase (AADC) and to a lesser extent by COMT. Because most levodopa is metabolized in peripheral tissues, large doses are required to obtain therapeutic levels of dopamine in the brain. These large amounts increase adverse drug effects. To reduce levodopa dosage and decrease adverse effects, carbidopa, an AADC inhibitor, is given to decrease the peripheral metabolism of levodopa. The combination of levodopa and carbidopa greatly increases the amount of available levodopa, so that levodopa dosage can be reduced by approximately 70%. When carbidopa inhibits the decarboxylase pathway of levodopa metabolism, the COMT pathway becomes more important (see COMT Inhibitors for a discussion of entacapone and tolcapone).

Levodopa is well absorbed from the small intestine after oral administration, reaches peak serum levels within 30 to 90 minutes, and has a short serum half-life (1 to 3 hours). Absorption is decreased by delayed gastric emptying, hyperacidity of gastric secretions, and competition with amino acids (from digestion of protein foods) for sites of absorption in the small intestine. Pyridoxine (vitamin B_6) promotes the breakdown of levodopa, reducing its effectiveness. Levodopa is metabolized to 30 or more metabolites, some of which are pharmacologically active and probably contribute to drug toxicity; the metabolites are excreted primarily in the urine, usually within 24 hours.

Action

Dopaminergic drugs increase the amount of dopamine in the brain by various mechanisms (Fig. 48.1). If levodopa is administered alone, large doses must be taken to produce therapeutic effects. Carbidopa combined with levodopa prevents the decarboxylation of the levodopa, which makes levodopa more available for transportation to the brain. Levodopa is the metabolic precursor of dopamine, and after levodopa crosses the blood–brain barrier, it converts to dopamine in the brain. This is thought to be the mechanism

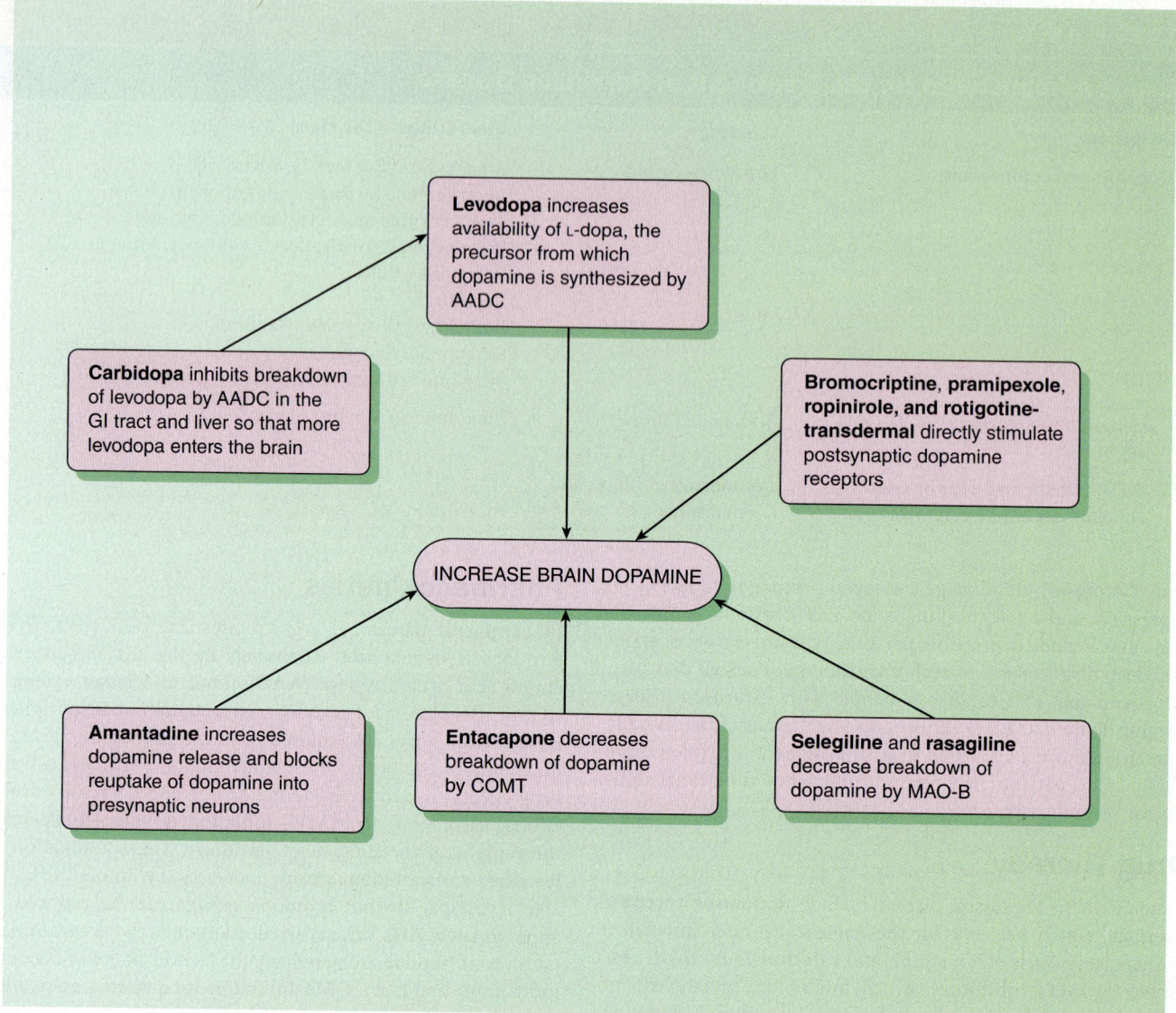

Figure 48.1. Mechanisms by which dopaminergic drugs increase dopamine in the brain. AADC, amino acid decarboxylase; COMT, catechol-O-methyltransferase; MAO-B, monoamine oxidase B.

whereby the drug relieves symptoms of Parkinson disease. Carbidopa does not cross the blood–brain barrier and does not affect levodopa metabolism.

Use

Levodopa–carbidopa is a treatment of idiopathic Parkinson disease, postencephalitic and arteriosclerotic parkinsonism, and parkinsonism related to carbon dioxide and manganese intoxication. Prescribers may also order levodopa to reduce the symptoms of restless legs syndrome (RLS). People with RLS experience paresthesias of the muscles, particularly in the calf and thighs, creating the urge to move. Movement relieves the paresthesia, which returns when the person is at rest or trying to sleep. The disorder may result in insomnia, mental distress, and, in some cases, suicide.

Levodopa and carbidopa are usually given together in a fixed-dose formulation called Sinemet. Table 48.2 gives the doses of this combination and other dopamine receptor agonists used to treat Parkinson disease.

Patient-related variables specific to the use of levodopa–carbidopa include the following:

- Age:
  - Safe and effective use in children has not been established for most anti-Parkinson drugs including levodopa–carbidopa.
  - Anti-Parkinson drugs are most likely to be used in children for other purposes, such as to stimulate growth hormone in children with Down syndrome.
  - In older adults, it may be necessary to reduce dosages of levodopa–carbidopa because of an age-related decrease in peripheral AADC, the enzyme that carbidopa inhibits. Older patients who take dopamine agonist drugs have a greater risk of hallucinations; they may also experience dementia and drowsiness.
- Reproduction, pregnancy, and lactation:
  - Carbidopa can be detected in the umbilical cord, but fetal absorption is minimal.
  - Levodopa in present in breast milk. The decision to breastfeed should be determined by the prescriber.

TABLE 48.2
DRUGS AT A GLANCE: Dopamine Receptor Agonists

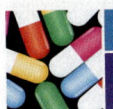

Drug	Routes and Dosage Ranges	
	Adults	**Children**
ⓟ Levodopa–carbidopa (Dhivy, Duopa, Rytary, Sinemet; 🍁 APO-Levocarb, APO-Levocarb CR, TEVA-Levocarbidopa)	One tablet containing 10-mg carbidopa and 100-mg levodopa or 25-mg carbidopa and 100-mg levodopa PO 3 times per day; increased by 1 tablet daily or every other day up to 6 tablets/d Patients who are switched from levodopa alone to levodopa–carbidopa: if <1,500 mg/d; one tablet containing 25-mg carbidopa and 100-mg levodopa PO 3–4 times per day; if >1,500 mg/d; one tablet containing 25-mg carbidopa and 250-mg levodopa PO 3–4 times per day; the dosage is adjusted by 1/2–1 tablet/d (initial dose should be 25% of initial dose of levodopa) CR form: carbidopa 50 mg–levodopa 200 mg 2 times daily at intervals not <6 h Inhaled levodopa 42 mg per inhalation for OFF episodes of parkinsonism	Safety and efficacy not established
Amantadine hydrochloride (Gocovri, Osmolex ER; 🍁 PDP-Amantadine)	*Anti-Parkinson*: 100 mg PO 2 times per day (maximum dosage 400 mg/d) *Antiviral*: 200 mg/d or 100 mg 2 times per day PO. Start within 24–48 h of exposure and continue 24–48 h after symptoms resolved. Treatment commonly 5 d	Safety and efficacy have not been established in children under the age of 1 y 1–9 y: 4.4–8.8 mg/kg/d PO in one or two divided doses not to exceed 150 mg/d >10 y and <40 kg: 5 mg/kg/d in two divided doses >10 y and >40 kg, 100 mg twice daily
Apomorphine hydrochloride (Apokyn, Kynmobi, Kynmobi Titration Kit; 🍁 Kynmobi, Movapo)	Parkinson disease off time episode: monitor blood pressure with administration: administer test dose 2 mg subcutaneous; if there is response, administer 2 mg and may increase dose by 1 mg every few days with max dose of 6 mg; if no response, administer the second test dose of 4 mg; if well tolerated, administer 3 mg; may increase by 1 mg every few days with max dose of 6 mg; if no response, give the third test dose 3 mg; if well tolerated, administer 2 mg for off time episodes; may increase to 3 mg after a few days	Safety and efficacy not established
Bromocriptine mesylate (Parlodel, Cycloset)	1.25 mg PO twice daily; increase by 2.5 mg daily in 2- to 4-wk intervals as needed (max dosage: 100 mg/d)	>16 years same as adult Limited data on children <11 years
Pramipexole dihydrochloride (Mirapex, Mirapex ER; 🍁 ACT-Pramipexole, APO-Pramipexole, Mirapex)	0.125 mg PO 3 times per day gradually increase every 5–7 d to a max dose of 0.5–1.5 mg 3 times per day Extended release: 0.375 mg PO daily, may increase to 0.75 mg per dose after 5–7 d up to a max dose of 4.5 mg/d RLS: 0.125 mg taken 2–3 h before bed, dose can be increased every 4–7 d Abnormal kidney function: CrCl 30–50 mL/min: 0.125 mg 2 times per day (max dose, 0.75 mg 3 times per day); CrCl 15–29 mL/min, 0.125 mg/d (max dosage 1.5 mg/d)	Safety and efficacy not established
Rasagiline (Azilect; 🍁 APO-Rasagiline, Azilect, TEVA-Rasagiline)	1 mg PO daily as monotherapy; (max dose: 1 mg/d); PO; with levodopa: 0.5 mg/d with max dose of 1 mg/d based on tolerance Hepatic impairment: 0.5 mg PO daily	Safety and efficacy not established

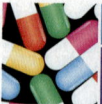

TABLE 48.2
DRUGS AT A GLANCE: Dopamine Receptor Agonists (Continued)

Drug	Routes and Dosage Ranges	
	Adults	**Children**
Ropinirole hydrochloride (✦ ACT-Ropinirole, JAMP-Ropinirole, PMS-Ropinirole)	0.25 mg PO 3 times per day; titrate up by 0.25 mg/dose 3 times per day every week to a target dose of 1 mg 3 times per day; may be increased by 1.5 mg/d every week (max dosage: 9 mg/d) and then 3 mg/d weekly to a max dosage of 24 mg/d Extended release: 2 mg/d for 1–2 wk and then increase by 2 mg/d at 1-wk intervals; max dosage 24 mg/d RLS: 0.25 mg/d 1–3 h before bedtime for 2 d, may increase to 0.5 mg for the 1st week and then increase to 1 mg/d to a max dose of 3 mg during week 6 and to a max dosage of 4 mg starting at 7 wk	Safety and efficacy not established
Rotigotine (Neupro; ✦ Neupro)	2 mg/24-h transdermal patch; may increase by 2 mg weekly based on clinical response	Safety and efficacy not established
Safinamide (Xadago)	50 mg PO once daily; after 2 wk may increase to 100 mg once daily	Safety and efficacy not established
Selegiline hydrochloride (Eldepryl, Emsam, Zelapar; ✦ APO Selegiline, DOM Selegiline, MYLAN Selegiline, PMS Selegiline, TEVA Selegiline)	5 mg PO 2 times per day with breakfast and lunch; dosages >10 mg/d are associated with increased risk of toxicity due to MAO inhibition Geriatric dosage: start with 5 mg in the morning ODT: 1.25 mg/d with levodopa-carbidopa therapy for 6 wk; may increase to 2.5 mg/d based on tolerance (max 2.5 mg/d); transdermal, start with 6 mg/d; may titrate by 3 mg/d every 2 wk (max 12 mg/d)	Depression: adolescents >17 y, transdermal; refer to adult dosing

- Abnormal kidney function and hepatic impairment:
  - Caution is necessary with the use of levodopa–carbidopa in patients with kidney failure. Dosage adjustments are required.
  - With levodopa, cautious use in patients with hepatic impairment is warranted, and dosage reduction may be necessary.
  - Reduced dosages are indicated with severe hepatic impairment. It is important to monitor liver transaminase enzymes frequently to assess for liver impairment. At the earliest sign of hepatotoxicity, drug withdrawal is essential, and there should be no reinstatement.
- Specific healthcare environments:
  - In critically ill patients, caution is necessary with the use of levodopa in those with severe neurologic, cardiac, or hepatic injuries. Dosage adjustment to the lowest level required for therapeutic effects is essential.
  - In the home care setting, the nurse can help patients and caregivers understand that the purpose of drug therapy is to control symptoms and that noticeable improvement may not occur for several weeks.
  - Caregivers may need to be informed that most activities (e.g., eating, dressing) take longer and require considerable effort by patients with parkinsonism.

Adverse Effects

Because of the adverse effects and recurrence of parkinsonism symptoms after a few years of levodopa therapy, levodopa is usually reserved for patients with significant symptoms and functional disabilities. The adverse effects addressed here are related to levodopa–carbidopa. The most common CNS adverse effects are headache and anxiety. The most severe adverse effect is depression with suicidal tendencies.

Cardiovascular adverse effects include ectopic beats, tachycardia, anginal pain, palpitations, hypotension, vasoconstriction, dyspnea, bradycardia, and a widened QRS. The medication can also cause orthostatic hypotension during the first few weeks but usually subsides. Concurrent administration of nonselective monoamine oxidase (MAO) inhibitors used in the treatment of depression and levodopa can result in extreme elevations in blood pressure or **hypertensive crisis**. (MAO exists in two types, MAO-A and MAO-B, both of which are found in the CNS and peripheral tissues.)

In addition, some patients report anorexia, bruxism, and nausea and vomiting. Other less common adverse effects are piloerection, azotemia, and gangrene with prolonged use. Dermatologic effects such as hypersensitivity, anaphylaxis, and urticaria occur less frequently.

Contraindications

Contraindications to the use of levodopa–carbidopa include a known hypersensitivity to the drug. The drug can dilate pupils and raise intraocular pressure; thus, narrow-angle glaucoma is also a contraindication. Levodopa may activate malignant melanoma; people with suspicious skin lesions or a history of melanoma should not take it. To avoid the severe hypertension that may occur with concurrent use of some MAO inhibitors and levodopa, it is essential that MAO inhibitors be discontinued

14 days prior to beginning levodopa therapy. In addition, use of levodopa warrants caution in patients with severe cardiovascular, pulmonary, kidney, hepatic, or endocrine disorders; depression; and peptic ulcer disease.

Nursing Implications

Preventing Interactions

The administration of levodopa–carbidopa with an MAO inhibitor can precipitate a hypertensive crisis. Postural hypotension occurs with the administration of tricyclic antidepressants and levodopa–carbidopa. Methyldopa combined with levodopa increases CNS effects. Dysrhythmic effects are increased when combined with halogenated general anesthetics. Several drugs interact with levodopa–carbidopa, increasing or decreasing its effects (Box 48.1). A high-protein meal increases the effects of levodopa–carbidopa and kava decreases its effects.

Administering the Medication

The nurse ensures that

- Levodopa–carbidopa is administered with or just after food or following a meal to reduce nausea and vomiting.
- Sinemet CR is not crushed.
- Levodopa is not given with iron preparations or multivitamin–mineral preparations that contain iron.
- Levodopa–carbidopa is not administered with a high-protein diet. Adequate hydration is also necessary.

In addition, the nurse should ensure a temperature-controlled environment to prevent hyperpyrexia.

> **Quality and Safety Alert: Patient-Centered Care**
>
> When administering levodopa, carbidopa, and other medications for Parkinson disease, it is critical to give medications to the patient on time for optimal therapeutic effect.

BOX 48.1 Drug Interactions: Levodopa–Carbidopa

Drugs That Increase the Effects of Levodopa–Carbidopa
- Monoamine oxidase inhibitors
  Increase the risk of hypertensive crisis

Drugs That Decrease the Effect of Levodopa–Carbidopa
- Anticholinergics
  Increase anticholinergic effects by delaying gastric emptying
- Pyridoxine (vitamin B$_6$)
  Stimulates decarboxylase, the enzyme that converts levodopa to dopamine, causing metabolism in the peripheral tissues and decreasing medication distribution to the central nervous system
- Phenytoin, papaverine, tricyclic antidepressants, and benzodiazepines
  Decrease drug efficacy

Assessing for Therapeutic Effects

With levodopa and other dopaminergic agents, the nurse observes for improvement in mobility, balance, posture, gait, speech, handwriting, and self-care ability. Elimination of drooling and seborrhea may occur. Mood elevation may result. After 2 to 5 years, the medication may lose its overall effectiveness, and the dosage may need to be increased. The nurse needs to be aware of symptoms such as ataxic gait, tremors of the hands and fingers, drooling, and masklike facial expressions.

Assessing for Adverse Effects

The nurse assesses for anorexia, nausea, and vomiting. These symptoms usually disappear after a few months of levodopa–carbidopa therapy. As previously stated, giving the drug with food minimizes these effects. The nurse also assesses the patient's blood pressure in the sitting and standing positions to identify signs of orthostatic hypotension. This effect, too, commonly dissipates a few weeks after beginning therapy. Levodopa and its metabolites stimulate beta-adrenergic receptors in the heart. Patients with preexisting coronary artery disease may take propranolol (Inderal) to counteract cardiac dysrhythmia effects. It is necessary to assess the patient for dyskinesia. The involuntary movements of the tongue, mouth, and face are common adverse effects. Decreasing the dose of the medication decreases dyskinesia.

Patient Teaching

Box 48.2 identifies patient teaching guidelines for levodopa–carbidopa.

Other Drugs in the Class

Amantadine hydrochloride is an anti-Parkinson and antiviral agent (see Chapter 23). It increases the dopamine release in the nigrostriatal pathway of patients with Parkinson disease. It is absorbed in the GI tract with an onset of action of

---

BOX 48.2 Patient Teaching Guidelines for Levodopa–Carbidopa

- Do not crush the sustained-release preparation.
- Do not take multivitamin preparations containing pyridoxine.
- Understand that there are adverse effects of medication such as drowsiness, dizziness, and orthostatic hypotension.
- Change positions slowly to prevent drop in blood pressure.
- Avoid alcohol.
- Take the medication with food to prevent nausea and vomiting.
- Do not take the medication with a high-protein meal.
- Report fainting, light-headedness, irregular heart rate, uncontrolled facial movements, urinary retention, nausea, and vomiting to the prescriber.
- Notify the prescriber of any increase in symptoms such as static gait, altered mobility, and "pill-rolling."

36 to 48 hours, a peak of action of 1.5 to 8 hours, and a half-life of 10 to 25 hours. It crosses the placenta and enters the breast milk. It is excreted unchanged in the urine. The most common adverse effects of amantadine are dizziness, light-headedness, and insomnia. The nurse instructs the patient to report swelling of the fingers or ankles, difficulty walking, urinary retention, tremors, slurred speech, or thoughts of suicide to the healthcare provider. It is important not to discontinue this drug abruptly.

Apomorphine hydrochloride (Apokyn, Kynmobi, Kynmobi Titration Kit) is an anti-Parkinson agent administered to patients with advanced Parkinson disease for "off time," or "off" episodes (when the medication is not adequately controlling the patient's symptoms) to assist in diminishing the symptoms of hypomobility. It is administered subcutaneously. Doses are incremental, generally ranging from 20 to 40 mg. The most common dosage is 30 mg, or 0.3 mL, and the maximum dosage is 60 mg. The patient's blood pressure must be monitored for hypertensive crisis during the administration. When apomorphine is administered to patients with a known cardiac history, periodic electrocardiogram results should be monitored as well as serum electrolytes.

Bromocriptine mesylate (Parlodel, Cycloset) is an ergot derivative that directly stimulates dopamine receptors in the brain. It is used in the treatment of idiopathic Parkinson disease, with levodopa–carbidopa, to prolong effectiveness and to allow reduced dosage of levodopa. Administration to patients with a history of myocardial infarction with residual dysrhythmia requires caution.

Inbrija is an orally inhaled levodopa inhalation powder and a dopamine precursor. Inbrija is administered for the intermittent treatment of **wearing off** (which is noted when levodopa's effect wears off before the next dose) in patients with Parkinson disease already treated with levodopa–carbidopa. Inbrija must be used concurrently with levodopa–carbidopa. Unpredictable off periods occur in Parkinson disease without an obvious relationship between the time of levodopa administration and the appearance of off episodes. It may be related to the fact that the GI system may become delayed in the absorption of levodopa, and levels will be altered. The advantage of Inbrija is the systemic pulmonary route, which enables its effect to control parkinsonism to be more consistent than that of levodopa. Clinical trials revealed a 10-minute onset of action with an 84-mg dose of Inbrija and improvement in motor function within 30 minutes. The drug comes in a capsule form, to be administered only through the Inbrija inhaler, which comes with the medication. Each capsule dose is 42 mg; the inhaler holds one capsule at a time. The approved daily dose is 84 mg up to five times daily as needed for OFF period symptoms in Parkinson disease. The maximum daily dose is 420 mg. Adverse reactions include cough, low blood pressure, chest discomfort, headache, hallucinations, nausea/vomiting, decreased red blood cell count, and sputum discoloration. Concerns related to adverse effects include hallucinations, thinking/behavioral changes, CNS depression, dyskinesias, and neuroleptic malignant syndrome.

Pramipexole (Mirapex, Mirapex ER) and ropinirole (Requip, Requip XL) stimulate dopamine receptors in the brain. It is administered for early and late stages of Parkinson disease. In early stages, one of these drugs can be used alone to improve motor performance, improve ability to participate in usual activities of daily living, and delay levodopa therapy. In advanced stages, one of these drugs can be used with levodopa and perhaps other anti-Parkinson drugs to provide more consistent relief of symptoms between doses of levodopa and allow reduced dosage of levodopa. These drugs, which are not ergot derivatives, may not cause some adverse effects associated with bromocriptine (e.g., pulmonary and peritoneal fibrosis, constriction of coronary arteries). It is unknown if fetal development is affected with these medications or if these medications are present in breast milk. Ropinirole is administered for RLS.

Pramipexole is rapidly absorbed with oral administration. Peak serum levels are reached in 1 to 3 hours after a dose and steady-state concentrations in about 2 days. The drug is less than 20% bound to plasma proteins and has an elimination half-life of 8 to 12 hours. Most of the drug is excreted unchanged in the urine; only 10% is metabolized. As a result, kidney failure may cause higher-than-usual plasma levels and possible toxicity. However, hepatic disease is unlikely to alter drug effects.

Rasagiline (Azilect) is an irreversible MAO inhibitor. It is indicated for initial treatment for idiopathic parkinsonism and as an adjunct therapy with levodopa to reduce "off time" when movements are poorly controlled. In addition, rasagiline has the potential to increase serotonin neurotransmission. When given with other drugs that enhance stimulation of serotonergic receptors (e.g., antidepressants, St. John's wort, dextromethorphan, and meperidine), serotonin syndrome, a potentially fatal CNS toxicity reaction characterized by hyperpyrexia and death, can occur. Rasagiline should be discontinued at least 14 days before beginning treatment with most antidepressants or other MAO inhibitors. Fluoxetine should be discontinued at least 5 weeks before initiating rasagiline, due to its long half-life. Rasagiline is well absorbed orally, metabolized in the liver, and excreted primarily by the kidney. Because it has not been determined to be selective for MAO-B in humans, it is contraindicated with foods containing tyramine or sympathomimetic amine–containing medications (e.g., nonprescription cold preparations and anesthetics), because of the risk of hypertensive crisis, and with antidepressants (e.g., tricyclic antidepressants, selective serotonin reuptake inhibitors, serotonin–norepinephrine reuptake inhibitors, mirtazapine), meperidine, and dextromethorphan because of the potential for inducing serotonin syndrome. Evidence of fetal harm has been observed in animal studies. It is unknown if rasagiline is present in breast milk.

Ropinirole is also well absorbed with oral administration. It reaches peak serum levels in 1 to 2 hours and steady-state concentrations within 2 days. It is 40% bound to plasma proteins and has an elimination half-life of 6 hours. It is metabolized by the cytochrome P450 enzymes in the liver to inactive metabolites, which are excreted through the kidneys. Less than 10% of ropinirole is excreted unchanged in the urine. Thus, hepatic failure may decrease metabolism, allow drug accumulation, and increase adverse effects. Kidney failure does not appear to alter drug effects. Ropinirole is prescribed for RLS. It is unknown the effects on fetal development or presence in breast milk.

Rotigotine (Neupro) is an anti-Parkinson agent that is a dopamine agonist. It is a transdermal patch in which the mechanism of action is unknown. When starting the medication, the patient should be aware that decreases in blood pressure can place the patient at risk for falls. Instruct the patient to cautiously change positions due to orthostatic hypotension. It is unknown the effects on fetal development or presence in breast milk.

Safinamide (Xadago) is a monoamine type B inhibitor that blocks the catabolism of dopamine, to increase the dopamine level and dopaminergic activity in the brain. It is administered as an adjunctive therapy with levodopa to increase motor function. It is important to monitor blood pressure with the administration of safinamide. The administration of dosages ≤ 100 mg will interact with tyramine-containing foods. Evidence of fetal harm has been observed in animal studies. It is unknown if safinamide is present in breast milk.

Selegiline (Emsam, Zelapar) inhibits the metabolism of dopamine by MAO, which exists in two types (as previously stated). These types are differentiated by their relative specificities for individual catecholamines. MAO-A acts more specifically on tyramine, norepinephrine, epinephrine, and serotonin. This enzyme is the main subtype in GI mucosa and in the liver and is responsible for metabolizing dietary tyramine. If MAO-A is inhibited in the intestine, tyramine in various foods is absorbed systemically rather than deactivated. As a result, there is excessive stimulation of the sympathetic nervous system, and severe hypertension and stroke can occur. This life-threatening reaction can also occur with some medications (e.g., sympathomimetics) that are normally metabolized by MAO. MAO-B metabolizes dopamine; in the brain, most MAO activity is due to type B. At oral dosages of 10 mg/day or less, selegiline inhibits MAO-B *selectively* and is unlikely to cause severe hypertension and stroke. However, at dosages greater than 10 mg/day, selectivity is lost and metabolism of both MAO-A and MAO-B is inhibited. Dosages greater than 10 mg/day should be avoided in patients with Parkinson disease. Selegiline inhibition of MAO-B is irreversible, and drug effects persist until more MAO is synthesized in the brain, which may take several months.

In early Parkinson disease, selegiline may be effective as monotherapy (level A). In advanced disease, prescribers order the drug to enhance the effects of levodopa. Its addition aids symptom control and allows the dosage of levodopa–carbidopa to be reduced. Once proposed to have neuroprotective properties, authorities now believe that there is insufficient evidence to recommend the use of selegiline to confer neuroprotection in patients with Parkinson disease (level U). Selegiline can be administered for depression. In the event of pregnancy, other antidepressants should be considered. It is unknown if selegiline enters breast milk.

Quality and Safety Alert: Evidence-Based Practice

Binde et al. (2020) compared the effectiveness of dopamine agonist and monoamine oxidase type-B inhibitors for the treatment of Parkinson disease. The researchers performed a systematic review of the literature of randomized controlled trials investigating four dopamine agonists and three MAO-B inhibitors. In 79 publications, they found that the investigated drugs were effective compared to placebo. Dopamine agonists were effective in treating Parkinson symptoms both in monotherapy and in combination with levodopa. Selegiline was the best option in combination with levodopa.

NCLEX Success

1. A 65-year-old patient has been taking levodopa for several weeks for symptoms of Parkinson disease. Which of the following symptoms indicates that they are not receiving an adequate dose for the treatment of their symptoms?
   A. edema of the feet and ankles
   B. widened QRS complex
   C. static gait
   D. increased intraocular pressure

2. A 56-year-old patient is taking levodopa–carbidopa for Parkinson disease. During therapy, the patient becomes light headed and dizzy. Which of the following is a potentially serious adverse effect of the drug treatment?
   A. orthostatic hypotension
   B. diminished fluid volume
   C. hematuria
   D. jaundice

Clinical Application 48.2

- Mr. Stokes has been having "off time" symptom development. His neurologist orders rasagiline (Azilect). He develops an upper respiratory viral infection with a cough. He begins to take dextromethorphan hydrobromide (Robitussin) every 4 hours. What is Mr. Stokes at risk for developing?
- What symptom does the nurse assess Mr. Stokes for when combining rasagiline and dextromethorphan hydrobromide?

CATECHOL-*O*-METHYLTRANSFERASE INHIBITORS

Tolcapone (Tasmar) is the prototype COMT inhibitor. COMT plays a role in brain metabolism of dopamine and metabolizes approximately 10% of peripheral levodopa. By inhibiting COMT, tolcapone increases levels of dopamine in the brain and relieves symptoms more effectively and consistently.

Pharmacokinetics

Tolcapone is absorbed rapidly and is highly protein bound. It is metabolized in the liver and possesses a 2- to 3-hour half-life. It crosses the placenta and enters the breast milk. It is excreted in the feces and urine.

Action

The main mechanism of action of tolcapone seems to be inhibiting the metabolism of levodopa in the bloodstream, thus increasing the plasma concentration and duration of action of the drug. It may also inhibit COMT in the brain and prolong the activity of dopamine at the synapse.

TABLE 48.3

DRUGS AT A GLANCE: Catechol-O-Methyltransferase Inhibitors

Drug	Routes and Dosage Ranges	
	Adults	**Children**
℗ **Tolcapone** (Tasmar)	100 mg PO 3 times per day with levodopa-carbidopa (max dose: 200 mg 3 times per day); doses of levodopa >600 mg may need reduced Because of the risk of potentially fatal acute fulminant liver failure, tolcapone should ordinarily be used in patients with Parkinson disease on L-dopa/carbidopa who are experiencing symptom fluctuations and are not responding satisfactorily to or are not appropriate candidates for other adjunctive therapies	Safety and efficacy not established
Entacapone (Comtan; 🍁 Comtan, Mylan-Entacapone)	200 mg PO administered with each dose of levodopa/carbidopa up to 8 times per day (max dose: 1,600 mg daily)	Safety and efficacy not established

Use

Tolcapone is useful for the treatment of signs and symptoms of idiopathic Parkinson disease. Administration is only in conjunction with levodopa–carbidopa, and a reduction in levodopa dosage is required. If a patient does not show a clinical benefit within 3 weeks of starting treatment, discontinuation of tolcapone is necessary.

Table 48.3 presents the dosage information for tolcapone and other drugs in its class.

Patient-related variables specific to the use of tolcapone include the following:

- Age:
  - In older patients, dosage is reduced and adjusted slowly to prevent adverse effects.
- Reproduction, pregnancy, and lactation:
  - Adverse fetal effects in animal studies have been observed.
  - It is not known if tolcapone is present in breast milk.
- Abnormal kidney function and hepatic impairment:
  - Caution is warranted in the administration of tolcapone to patients with abnormal kidney function because it is excreted in the urine.
  - If liver values are greater than two times the upper limit of normal, tolcapone is discontinued.
  - Patients with moderate to severe hepatic impairment should not take tolcapone at doses exceeding 100 mg three times per day. The FDA has issued a **BOXED WARNING** ◆ stating that patients who take tolcapone risk potentially fatal acute fulminant liver failure. Liver function tests must be monitored before therapy begins and every 2 weeks thereafter.

Adverse Effects

Tolcapone produces adverse effects in several major body systems, including the CNS, cardiovascular system, dermatologic system, GI system, and respiratory system. The most severe adverse effect is fulminant liver failure, which may be fatal. CNS adverse effects include disorientation, confusion, hallucinations, and psychosis. Dry mouth, dizziness, and orthostatic hypotension may also occur.

Contraindications

Contraindications to tolcapone include a hypersensitivity to the drug. Other contraindications are liver disease, nontraumatic rhabdomyolysis, hyperpyrexia, and confusion. Caution is warranted with hypertension, hypotension, and abnormal kidney function.

Nursing Implications

Preventing Interactions

Tolcapone and other COMT medications must not be administered with MAO inhibitors due to the risk of hypertensive crisis.

Administering the Medication

It is necessary to administer tolcapone in conjunction with levodopa–carbidopa and to monitor the patient's response to the medication. The addition of the drug may require a decrease in the levodopa dosage. Abrupt withdrawal of tolcapone can lead to serious complications. Tapering over 2 weeks is necessary to prevent adverse effects.

Assessing for Therapeutic Effects

The decrease or absence of symptoms of Parkinson disease such as improved gait and mobility, diminished tremors, and rigidity is indicative of tolcapone's therapeutic effectiveness.

Assessing for Adverse Effects

The nurse assesses for disorientation and confusion, light-headedness, and orthostatic hypotension. It is necessary to take blood pressure lying down, sitting, and standing up. Frequent monitoring of liver enzymes is essential.

Patient Teaching

Box 48.3 presents patient teaching guidelines for tolcapone.

Other Drugs in the Class

Entacapone (Comtan) is well tolerated and safer than tolcapone, and thus, more commonly prescribed. This COMT inhibitor is well absorbed after oral administration and reaches a peak plasma level in 1 hour. It is highly protein bound (98%), has a half-life of

BOX 48.3 Patient Teaching Guidelines for Tolcapone

- Do not stop the medication abruptly; taper it over 2 weeks.
- Take the medication in conjunction with levodopa–carbidopa.
- Use barrier contraceptives while using this medication.
- Do not breast-feed while taking the medication.
- Use caution when operating machinery due to central nervous system (CNS) depression.
- Use hard candy to decrease dry mouth.
- Have liver function tests as scheduled.
- Avoid concurrent use of alcohol or other CNS depressants.

about 2.5 hours, and is metabolized in the liver to an inactive metabolite. The dosage must be reduced by 50% in the presence of impaired liver function. The parent drug and metabolite are 90% excreted through the biliary tract and feces, and 10% of excretion occurs in the urine. Adverse effects include confusion, dizziness, drowsiness, hallucinations, nausea, and vomiting, which can be reduced by lowering the dose of either levodopa or entacapone. Although clinical trials report few instances of liver enzyme elevation or hemoglobin decreases, it is recommended that liver enzymes and red blood cell counts be measured periodically.

NCLEX Success

3. A 35-year-old patient has begun to take tolcapone in addition to levodopa–carbidopa for Parkinson disease. Which of the following is the priority nursing intervention?

    A. Arrange to assess the patient for hypertension early in the morning.
    B. Evaluate the patient's ability care for themselves.
    C. Have the patient take levodopa–carbidopa 2 hours after tolcapone.
    D. Instruct the patient to report tea-colored urine to the prescriber.

CATECHOL-*O*-METHYLTRANSFERASE INHIBITOR AND DECARBOXYLASE INHIBITOR/DOPAMINE PRECURSOR

One anti-Parkinson drug is a combination of **levodopa**, **carbidopa**, and **entacapone** (Stalevo). This chapter discusses this medication in a separate class because it combines medications from two separate classes. Administration of Stalevo allows for greater convenience and improved Parkinson symptom management. Use of the drug combination provides the patient with the convenience of one medication.

Pharmacokinetics

The combination drug Stalevo has the same pharmacokinetics as those of levodopa–carbidopa and entacapone.

Action

Levodopa is the metabolic precursor of dopamine. Depleted in Parkinson disease, levodopa is circulated in the plasma and crosses the blood–brain barrier, where it is converted to dopamine by the striatal enzymes. Carbidopa inhibits the peripheral plasma breakdown of levodopa by inhibiting decarboxylation, thus increasing levodopa. Entacapone is a reversible and selective inhibitor of COMT. It alters the pharmacokinetics of levodopa, allowing for more sustained levodopa serum levels and increased concentrations for absorption across the blood–brain barrier.

Use

Stalevo is used for the treatment of idiopathic Parkinson disease. Table 48.4 presents the dosage information for Stalevo.

Patient-related variables specific to use of the combination drug Stalevo include the following:

- Reproduction, pregnancy, and lactation:
    - Carbidopa can be detected in the umbilical cord, but fetal absorption is minimal.
    - Levodopa is present in breast milk. The decision to breast-feed should be determined by the prescriber.
    - The effects of entacapone on fetal development or its presence in breast milk are unknown.

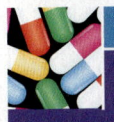

TABLE 48.4

DRUGS AT A GLANCE: Catechol-*O*-Methyltransferase Inhibitor and Decarboxylase Inhibitor/Dopamine Precursor

Drug	Routes and Dosage Range	
	Adults	Children
Levodopa–carbidopa–entacapone (Stalevo; 🍁 Stalevo)	Dosing forms: Levodopa 50 mg–carbidopa 12.5 mg–entacapone 200 mg PO daily Levodopa 75 mg–carbidopa 18.75 mg–entacapone 200 mg Levodopa 100 mg–carbidopa 25 mg–entacapone 200 mg Levodopa 125 mg–carbidopa 31.25 mg–entacapone 200 mg Levodopa 150 mg–carbidopa 37.5 mg–entacapone 200 mg Levodopa 200 mg–carbidopa 50 mg–entacapone 200 mg	Safety and efficacy not established

- Abnormal kidney function and hepatic impairment:
  - Cautious administration of Stalevo is necessary in patients with severe abnormal kidney function. Dosage reduction to prevent further abnormal kidney function may be warranted.
  - Cautious administration is also necessary in patients with hepatic impairment because the medication is metabolized in the liver.

Adverse Effects

Stalevo may affect the GI, dermatologic, respiratory, and cardiovascular systems. GI adverse effects include diarrhea as well as nausea, vomiting, bruxism, dry mouth, and excess salivation. The development of diarrhea is indicative of drug-induced colitis, and it is necessary to discontinue Stalevo if diarrhea occurs. Somnolence has been reported in which patients fall asleep without warning. This adverse effect is linked to entacapone. Also, the risk of melanoma may increase. If dyskinesia occurs, it may be necessary to reduce the dose. As with other anti-Parkinson medications, hypotension is a risk, along with heart attack, stroke, and cardiovascular death. Also, there is an increased risk of cardiovascular events in patients who received Stalevo versus those who received Sinemet. However, studies show that the risk of cardiovascular events is not statistically significant, but research is continuing. In addition, postmarketing studies report that impulsivity and compulsive behaviors may occur.

Contraindications

Contraindications to the use of Stalevo include a known sensitivity to the levodopa, carbidopa, or entacapone. The concurrent use of MAO inhibitors, or use within 14 days, is also a contraindication. Levodopa may trigger melanoma; therefore, patients with a history of melanoma should not receive Stalevo. Also, it is important to note that ergot-derived dopamine agonists administered with Stalevo have been associated with fibrotic complications such as pleural effusion, pleural thickening, and pulmonary infiltrates.

Nursing Implications

Preventing Interactions

The administration of catecholamines such as epinephrine, dopamine, and methyldopa enhances the action of entacapone, one of the components of Stalevo.

Administering the Medication

Patients whose medication regimen is being changed to Stalevo should be administered levodopa and the adjunctive entacapone. The levodopa dose should be adjusted prior to the conversion to Stalevo therapy. The dose should be individualized based on the therapeutic response. The presence of dyskinesia necessitates a dosage adjustment, such as by changing the strength or adjusting the dosing intervals. Fractionated doses are not recommended, and only one tablet should be administered at each dosing interval. The maximum daily dose is eight 50-, 75-, 100-, 125-, and 150-mg tablets and only six 200-mg tablets. (Patients who take more than 600 mg/day of levodopa should not switch directly to Stalevo.) Patients should swallow the tablets whole—not crushed, broken, or chewed. Stalevo can be administered without regard to meals. To prevent fluctuation in levodopa absorption, it is necessary to distribute protein intake throughout the day. People should take iron, iron supplements, and multivitamins that contain minerals separately from Stalevo.

Assessing for Therapeutic Effects

The decrease or absence of Parkinson symptoms such as muscle rigidity, excessive salivation, "pill-rolling," and tremors is indicative of Stalevo's therapeutic effectiveness.

Assessing for Adverse Effects

The nurse assesses the patient's cardiovascular status, including heart rate and blood pressure, to determine alterations in cardiovascular symptoms. It is also necessary to assess for chest pain, confusion, and weakness of extremities related to cerebrovascular accident or myocardial infarction. In addition, the nurse assesses the patient's skin for unusual skin lesions and checks the patient's fecal elimination for drug-induced colitis. It is important to teach the family to report any statements that indicate suicidal ideations. The nurse assesses for abnormal compulsive urges.

Patient Teaching

Patient education for Stalevo is the same as the patient education for the drug's individual components: levodopa, carbidopa, and entacapone (see Box 48.2). With entacapone, the nurse instructs the patient to report hallucinations and diarrhea. It is also necessary to tell the patient that urine may become brownish orange; this reaction is normal and not harmful. In addition, the nurse tells the patient to protect against falls due to orthostatic hypotension; patients can stand up slowly.

NCLEX Success

4. A 76-year-old patient is taking levodopa–carbidopa–entacapone. Which of the following is the priority nursing intervention?
   A. administering with a high-protein meal
   B. administering with meals only
   C. assessing for diarrhea
   D. assessing for constipation

Clinical Application 48.3

- Mr. Stokes' prescriber switches him from levodopa–carbidopa to levodopa–carbidopa–entacapone. He asks his nurse what the difference is between the medication he once took and what he is now taking. What patient education does the nurse provide?

OVERVIEW OF ANTICHOLINERGIC DRUGS

Anticholinergic drugs inhibit the actions of acetylcholine in the brain and affect the parasympathetic nervous system. Most anticholinergic drugs interact with muscarinic cholinergic receptors in the brain, secretory glands, heart, and smooth

TABLE 48.5
Common Tertiary Amine and Quaternary Amine Anticholinergic Drugs

Tertiary Amines	Quaternary Amines
Atropine	Glycopyrrolate (Robinul, Cuvposa)
Benztropine mesylate	Ipratropium bromide (Atrovent HFA)
Darifenacin hydrobromide	Methscopolamine bromide (Pamine)
Dicyclomine hydrochloride (Bentyl)	Tiotropium bromide (Spiriva)
Flavoxate hydrochloride	Trospium chloride
Oxybutynin chloride (Ditropan XL, Gelnique, Gelnique Pump)	
Scopolamine hydrobromide (Transderm Scop)	
Solifenacin succinate (Vesicare)	
Tolterodine tartrate (Detrol, Detrol LA)	
Trihexyphenidyl hydrochloride	

muscle and are sometimes called **antimuscarinic drugs**. **Nicotinic receptors** are located in motor nerves and skeletal muscles; when activated by acetylcholine, the cell membrane depolarizes and produces muscle contraction. When given at high doses, a few anticholinergic drugs are able to block nicotinic receptors in autonomic ganglia and skeletal muscles. Glycopyrrolate (Robinul) is an example of such a medication. This drug class includes belladonna alkaloids and their derivatives, such as atropine, and many synthetic substitutes.

Most anticholinergic medications are either **tertiary amines** or **quaternary amines** (Table 48.5). Tertiary amines are uncharged lipid-soluble molecules. Atropine and scopolamine are tertiary amines and, therefore, are able to cross cell membranes readily. They are well absorbed from the GI tract and conjunctiva, and they cross the blood–brain barrier. Tertiary amines are excreted in the urine.

Quaternary amines carry a positive charge and are lipid insoluble. Some belladonna derivatives and synthetic anticholinergics are quaternary amines. Consequently, they do not readily cross cell membranes. They are poorly absorbed from the GI tract and do not cross the blood–brain barrier. Quaternary amines are excreted largely in the feces.

Clinical Use

The widespread effects of anticholinergic drugs limit their clinical usefulness. Consequently, several synthetic drugs have been developed in an effort to increase the selectivity of action on particular body tissues, especially to retain the antispasmodic and antisecretory effects of atropine while eliminating its adverse effects. This effort has been less than successful—all the synthetic drugs produce atropinelike adverse effects when doses are sufficient.

Some synthetic drugs are used for antispasmodic effects in GI disorders and overactive urinary bladder. Another group of synthetic drugs includes centrally active anticholinergics used in the treatment of Parkinson disease; these drugs balance the relative cholinergic dominance that causes the movement disorders associated with parkinsonism. Specific body systems and conditions in which anticholinergic medications are administered are listed in Table 48.6.

Drug Therapy

Anticholinergic drugs act by occupying receptor sites on target organs innervated by the parasympathetic nervous system, thereby leaving fewer receptor sites free to respond to acetylcholine (Fig. 48.2). Parasympathetic response is absent or decreased,

TABLE 48.6
Body System and Indication of Anticholinergic Use

Body System	Indication for Anticholinergic Use
Cardiac	Bradycardia, heart block with hypotension and shock: increases heart rate and prevent vagal stimulation
Gastrointestinal	Peptic ulcer disease, gastritis, pylorospasm, and diverticulitis: relieves pain and relaxes gastrointestinal smooth muscle Irritable bowel, colitis: reduces frequent bowel movements and abdominal discomfort
Genitourinary	Urinary incontinence and frequency: reduces urinary muscle spasm Cystitis, urethritis, and prostatitis: decreases pain and frequency Enuresis, paraplegia, and neurogenic bladder: increases bladder capacity
Otolaryngology	Head and neck surgery and bronchoscopy: reduces respiratory tract secretions
Ophthalmology	Mydriatic and cycloplegic effects: dilate pupils
Respiratory	Asthma, chronic bronchitis: produces bronchodilation
Metabolic	Mushroom poisoning and organophosphate pesticide poisoning: reduces cholinergic stimulation; salivation, urination, defecation, bronchial secretions, laryngospasm, and bronchospasm

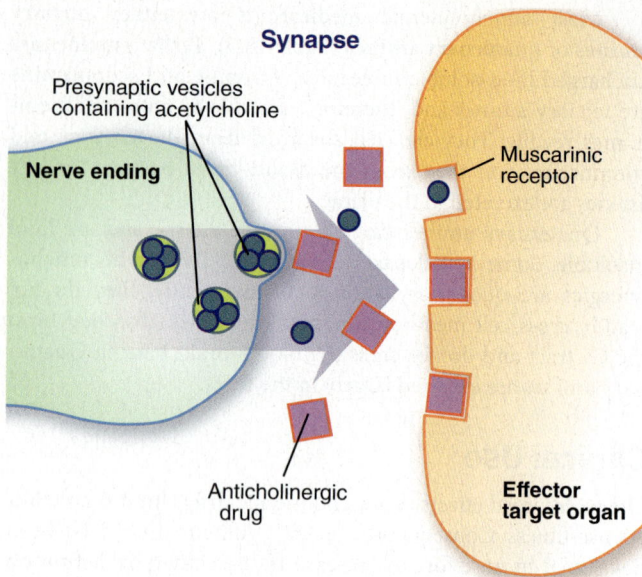

Figure 48.2. Mechanism of action of anticholinergic drugs. Anticholinergic (antimuscarinic) drugs prevent acetylcholine from interacting with muscarinic receptors on target effector organs, thus blocking or decreasing a parasympathetic response in these organs.

depending on the number of receptors blocked by anticholinergic drugs and the underlying degree of parasympathetic activity. **Muscarinic receptors** are located in the most internal organs, including the cardiovascular, respiratory, GI, and genitourinary systems; when activated by acetylcholine, the affected cells may be excited or inhibited in their functions. Because cholinergic muscarinic receptors are widely distributed in the body, anticholinergic drugs produce effects in a variety of locations, including the CNS, heart, smooth muscle, glands, and the eye.

Specific effects on body tissues and organs include the following:

- CNS stimulation followed by depression, which may result in coma and death. This is most likely to occur with large doses of anticholinergic drugs that cross the blood–brain barrier (atropine, scopolamine, and anti-Parkinson agents).
- Decreased cardiovascular response to parasympathetic (vagal) stimulation that slows heart rate. Atropine is the anticholinergic drug most often used for its cardiovascular effects.
- Bronchodilation and decreased respiratory tract secretions. Anticholinergics block the action of acetylcholine in bronchial smooth muscle when given by inhalation. This action reduces intracellular guanosine monophosphate (GMP), a bronchoconstrictive substance. When anticholinergic drugs are given systemically, respiratory secretions decrease and may become viscous, resulting in mucous plugging of small respiratory passages. Administering the medications by inhalation decreases this effect while preserving the beneficial bronchodilation effect.
- Antispasmodic effects in the GI tract due to decreased muscle tone and motility. The drugs have little inhibitory effect on gastric acid secretion with usual doses and insignificant effects on pancreatic and intestinal secretions.
- **Mydriasis** (pupil dilation) and **cycloplegia** (paralysis in the ciliary muscle) in the eye. Normally, anticholinergics do not change intraocular pressure, but with narrow-angle glaucoma, they may increase intraocular pressure and precipitate an episode of acute glaucoma. When the pupil is fully dilated, photophobia may be uncomfortable, and reflexes to light and accommodation may disappear.
- Miscellaneous effects. These include decreased secretions from salivary and sweat glands; relaxation of ureters, urinary bladder, and the detrusor muscle; and relaxation of smooth muscle in the gallbladder and bile ducts.

Table 48.7 lists the various anticholinergic medications.

BELLADONNA ALKALOID AND DERIVATIVES

Atropine sulfate, the prototype of the anticholinergic drugs, is a naturally occurring belladonna alkaloid that can be extracted from the belladonna plant or prepared synthetically. It is usually prepared as atropine sulfate, a salt that is very soluble in water. Atropine sulfate is also classified as a muscarinic antagonist.

Pharmacokinetics

Atropine is well absorbed after all forms of administration. The peak effect occurs in 0.7 to 4 minutes with intravenous (IV) preparations, 30 minutes with intramuscular (IM) preparations, 1 to 2 hours with subcutaneous preparations, and 1.5 to 4 hours with inhalation preparation. The pharmacologic effects last for about 4 hours, except for ocular effects, which last for up to 2 weeks in normal eyes. The drug is absorbed systemically when applied locally to mucous membranes. Atropine crosses the blood–brain barrier and enters the CNS, where large doses produce stimulant effects and toxic doses produce depressant effects. It is metabolized in the liver and rapidly excreted in the urine. Atropine crosses the placenta and enters the breast milk.

Action

Atropine competitively blocks the effects of acetylcholine at muscarinic cholinergic receptors that mediate the effects of parasympathetic postganglionic impulses. It also prevents the action of acetylcholine in the CNS. Atropine depresses the salivary and bronchial secretions, dilates the bronchi, and increases cardiac output. Large doses can decrease motility of the GI and GU tracts. In addition, it relaxes the pupil of the eye and prevents the accommodation for near vision.

Use

In the past, atropine was used to control the symptoms of Parkinson disease—to relieve tremors and decrease rigidity. The development of the centrally acting anticholinergic agents has replaced the use of atropine for Parkinson disease.

The most common use of atropine is the restoration of cardiac rate and arterial pressure during anesthesia when vagal stimulation produced by intra-abdominal traction causes a decrease in pulse rate, lessening the degree of atrioventricular

TABLE 48.7

Anticholinergic Medications

Drug Class	Prototype	Other Drugs in the Class
Belladonna alkaloids and derivatives	Atropine sulfate (Atropen)	Homatropine bromide Ipratropium bromide (Atrovent HFA) Scopolamine hydrobromide Tiotropium bromide (Spiriva HandiHaler)
Centrally acting anticholinergic agents	Benztropine mesylate	Trihexyphenidyl hydrochloride
Gastrointestinal antisecretory/antispasmodic	Dicyclomine hydrochloride (Bentyl)	Glycopyrrolate (Robinul)
Urinary antispasmodic	Oxybutynin chloride (Ditropan XL, Gelnique, Oxytrol, Oxytrol for women)	Darifenacin hydrobromide Flavoxate hydrochloride Solifenacin succinate (Vesicare) Tolterodine tartrate (Detrol and Detrol LA) Trospium chloride

block when increased vagal tone is a factor. Atropine also relieves bradycardia and syncope due to hyperactive carotid sinus reflex. It also serves as an antidote for cardiac collapse with an overdose of parasympathomimetic drugs also known as cholinergic agents and cholinesterase inhibitors such as physostigmine.

Also, practitioners administer atropine in the preanesthesia stage to reduce respiratory tract secretions.

In addition, atropine is an antidote for mushroom poisoning (*Amanita muscaria*). Symptoms of muscarinic poisoning include salivation, lacrimation, visual disturbances, bronchospasm, diarrhea, bradycardia, and hypotension. Atropine prevents the poison from interacting with muscarinic receptors, thus reversing the toxic effects. Muscarinic poisoning can also occur from cholinergic agonist drugs, cholinesterase inhibitor drugs, and insecticides that contain organophosphates.

Table 48.8 presents the dosage information for atropine sulfate and the other belladonna alkaloids.

Patient-related variables specific to the use of atropine sulfate include the following:

- Age:
  - Systemic anticholinergics, including atropine, have essentially the same indications and adverse effects in children of all ages as in adults. However, the effects may be more severe in children, who are especially sensitive to these drugs.
  - Children may experience facial flushing and skin rashes, as well as hyperpyrexia or atropine fever.
  - It is necessary to administer atropine cautiously in older adults, for whom CNS reactions are more likely to occur.
- Specific healthcare environments:
  - In critically ill patients, when atropine is administered for cardiovascular symptoms, the patient's cardiac status is monitored with an electrocardiogram.

Adverse Effects

Atropine sulfate may adversely affect several body systems. Cardiovascular adverse effects include bradycardia (low doses) and tachycardia (high doses). CNS adverse effects include blurred vision, mydriasis, cycloplegia, photophobia, and increased intraocular pressure. In older adults, nervousness, weakness, confusion, and excitement are common. The most severe GI adverse effect is paralytic ileus. Genitourinary effects are urinary hesitancy and retention. The patient may also complain of decreased sweating, which leads to heat prostration.

Overdose of atropine or other anticholinergic drugs produces the usual pharmacologic effect such as decreased secretions, increased heart rate, relaxation of the bronchial smooth muscle, and decreased GI and genitourinary tone in severe and exaggerated forms. The anticholinergic overdose syndrome is characterized by hyperthermia; hot, dry, flushed skin; dry mouth; mydriasis; delirium; tachycardia; paralytic ileus; and urinary retention. Myoclonic movements and choreoathetosis may be evident. Seizures, coma, and respiratory arrest may also occur. Treatment involves the use of activated charcoal to absorb the ingested drug. Hemodialysis, hemoperfusion, peritoneal dialysis, and repeated doses of charcoal are not effective.

Physostigmine salicylate (see Chapter 47), an acetylcholinesterase inhibitor, is a specific antidote for overdose of anticholinergics. It is usually given intravenously at a slow rate of 1 mg/min because rapid administration may cause bradycardia, hypersalivation (with subsequent respiratory distress), and seizures. The IM/IV adult dose is 0.5 to 2 mg, IM or IV, and may be repeated every 10 to 30 minutes until a response is achieved. Additional doses may be required for life-threatening anticholinergic effects. For infants, children, and adolescents, give IM or IV at an initial dose of 0.02 mg/kg, with a maximum dose of 2 mg. The drug should be administered IV no faster than 0.5 mg/min to prevent bradycardia, respiratory distress, and seizures. The pediatric dose is warranted only for life-threatening cases. For infants, children, and adolescents, give IM or IV at an initial dose of 0.02 mg/kg, with a maximum dose of 2 mg. Administer IV no faster than 0.5 mg/min to prevent bradycardia, respiratory distress, and seizures. Repeated doses may be given every 5 to 10 minutes if life-threatening dysrhythmias, convulsions, or coma occurs with anticholinergic overdose. However, the benefit of repeat dosing must be balanced against the risk of physostigmine overdose. Excessive administration of physostigmine can precipitate a cholinergic crisis, leading to seizures and dysrhythmias. Atropine is the antidote for physostigmine overdose.

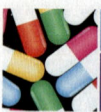

TABLE 48.8
DRUGS AT A GLANCE: Belladonna Alkaloids and Derivatives

Drug	Routes and Dosage Ranges	
	Adults	**Children**
ⓟ **Atropine sulfate** (Atropen) **Ophthalmic atropine** (Isopto Atropine; 🍁 Dioptics Atropine Solution, Isopto Atropine)	IM, SC, or IV 0.4–1 mg preoperatively; may repeat every 4–6 h (max dose 3 mg) Amblyopia and mydriasis: instill a drop in the conjunctiva 40 min maximal dilation time; may repeat up to 2 times daily	IM, IV: neonatal; 0.02 mg/kg/dose; IM, SC, IV: infant, children <12 y; 0.02 mg/kg/dose; give 30–60 min prior to the procedure, may repeat every 4–6 h (max dose 1 mg/procedure); children >12 y; 0.02 mg/kg/dose; give 30–60 min prior to procedure, may repeat every 4–6 h (max dose 2 mg/procedure) Mydriasis: infants >3 mo and children <3 y, instill one drop 1% solution 40 min prior to dilation time. Max dose of one drop per eye/d. Children >3 y and adolescents: instill 1 drop 1% solution 40 min prior to dilation time
Homatropine bromide (Homatropine; 🍁 Isopto Homatropine)	For refraction: instill 1–2 drops of 2% or 5% solution into the affected eye before the procedure. May repeat in 5–10 min as needed For uveitis: instill one or two drops of 2% or 5% solution into the affected eye every 3–4 h	Refraction/uveitis: infants >3 mo, children, and adolescents, instill 1–2 drops of 5% solution into the affected eye up to every 3–4 h
Hyoscyamine sulfate (Anaspaz, Ed-Spaz, Hyosyne, Levsin; 🍁 Levsin)	PO, 0.125–0.25 every 4 h PRN daily before meals and at bedtime (max dose 1.5 mg/d) PO (timed-release formula): 0.375–0.75 mg every 12 h (max dose 1.5 mg/d); IM, IV, SC: 0.25–0.5 mg up to 4 times daily every 4 h	Children <2 y: oral drops 0.125 mg/mL based on age and wt repeat dose every 4 h PRN. 3.4–<5 kg, 4 drops with maximum 24 drops/daily; 5 to <7 kg, 5 drops with max 30 drops/daily; 7 to <10 kg, 6 drops with max 36 drops/daily; >10 kg: 8 drops with max 48 drops/daily. Children 2–12 y: tablets—0.0625–0.125 mg every 4 h PRN with max 0.75 mg/daily. Oral drops: 0.125 mg/mL; 0.03125–0.125 mg every 4 h PRN with max 0.75 mg/daily
Ipratropium bromide (Atrovent HFA; 🍁 Apo-Ipravent Solution, Apo-Ipravent Sterules, Atrovent HFA)	COPD, oral inhalation; nebulizer, 500 mcg every 6–8 h; MDI, 2 inhalations 4 times/daily with max dose 12 inhalations/daily Acute asthma exacerbation (off-label): for oral inhalation, give with short-acting beta-adrenergic agonist. Nebulizer: 500 mcg every 20 min for 3 doses and then PRN. MDI: 8 inhalations every 20 min PRN up to 3 h. Rhinorrhea: two sprays/nostril of 0.06% spray 4 times daily	COPD: <12 y—see adult dosing Acute asthma (off-label) <5 y; nebulizer 250 mcg every 20 min PRN for 1 h; ≤12 y; nebulizer 250–500 mcg every 20 min every 3 h and then PRN: MDI, <5 y; 2 inhalations every 20 min if needed for 1 h; ≤12 y; 4–8 inhalations every 20 min PRN up to 3 h Rhinorrhea: children 5–11 y, 0.06%—two sprays in each nostril 3 times/daily. Children ≥12 y and adults: 0.06%—two sprays in each nostril 4 times/daily
Scopolamine (Transderm Scop; 🍁 Buscopan)	PO 0.4–0.8 mg daily every 8–12 h PRN Transdermal: apply disk 4 h before antiemetic effect is needed. Replace every 3 d For refraction: instill one or two drops into the eye 1 h before refracting For iridocyclitis: instill one or two drops into eye(s) up to 4 times daily	Apply one transdermal disk behind the ear at least 4 h prior to exposure every 3 d as needed For refraction: instill one drop of 0.25% to the eye twice daily for 2 d before the procedure For iridocyclitis: instill one drop of 0.25% to the eye up to 3 times daily
Tiotropium bromide (Spiriva HandiHaler, Spiriva Respimat; 🍁 Spiriva, Spiriva Respimat)	Asthma: oral inhalation with Spiriva Respimat (1.25 mcg), two inhalations 2.5 mcg once daily with max two inhalations/24 h COPD: oral inhalation with HandiHaler, inhale each capsule twice to ensure drug delivery; Spiriva Respimat (2.5 mcg) two inhalations (5 mcg) once daily with max 2 inhalations/24 h	Children >6 y and adolescent: oral inhalation Spiriva Respimat—see adult dosing

Diazepam or a similar drug may be given for excessive CNS stimulation (e.g., delirium, excitement) that accompanies anticholinergic toxicity. Ice bags, cooling blankets, and tepid sponge baths may help reduce fever. Artificial ventilation and cardiopulmonary resuscitative measures are used if excessive depression of the CNS causes coma and respiratory failure. Infants, children, and the older adults are especially susceptible to the toxic effects of anticholinergic drugs.

Contraindications

Contraindications to the use of atropine include a known hypersensitivity to anticholinergic agents. It is also contraindicated with the herbal supplements aloe, senna, and cascara, which increase atropine's effects. Other contraindications include glaucoma, stenosing peptic ulcer, pyloroduodenal obstruction, bronchial asthma, and bladder neck obstruction, as well as hepatic or kidney disease.

Nursing Implications

Preventing Interactions

Drugs that increase the anticholinergic effects of atropine include amantadine, antihistamines, tricyclic antidepressants, quinidine, disopyramide, and procainamide.

Administering the Medication

Prior to administering atropine, the nurse assesses for hypersensitivity to anticholinergic agents, glaucoma, stenosing peptic ulcer, paralytic ileus, bronchial asthma, bladder neck obstruction, and cardiac dysrhythmias. The patient should be well hydrated and the environment should be cool to protect from hyperpyrexia. If the patient has a history of urinary retention, the patient should void before administration of the drug.

Assessing for Therapeutic Effects

The nurse assesses the heart rate if atropine is administered for bradycardia. In preoperative patients, the nurse assesses for diminished secretions, particularly when the drug is administered for head and neck surgery. Patients with Parkinson disease or Parkinson-like syndromes require assessment for decreased spasticity and tremors.

Assessing for Adverse Effects

The nurse assesses for the following conditions, which may indicate a severe anticholinergic reaction:

- Changes in rate, quality, and rhythm of the heart that indicates ventricular tachycardia.
- Urinary retention.
- Bowel sounds for signs of paralytic ileus.
- Photophobia, mydriasis, blurred vision, and increased intraocular pressure.
- Dry mouth.
- Increased temperature. Older adults and children are prone to hyperpyrexia due to suppression of perspiration and heat loss.

Patient Teaching

Box 48.4 identifies patient teaching guidelines for atropine sulfate.

> **BOX 48.4** *Patient Teaching Guidelines for Atropine Sulfate*
>
> - Avoid excessive high temperatures.
> - Drink water frequently.
> - Rinse the mouth frequently.
> - Maintain good dental hygiene.
> - Use hard candy to decrease dry mouth.
> - Void before taking the medication.
> - Visit the ophthalmologist regularly.
> - Notify your prescriber if fluid intake is greater or less than urine output.
> - Notify your prescriber if you develop a fever.
> - Notify your prescriber if weakness becomes severe.
> - Avoid the use of machinery if visual acuity or alertness is impaired.

Other Drugs in the Class

Homatropine, ipratropium (Atrovent HFA), tiotropium bromide (Spiriva HandiHaler, Spiriva Respimat), and scopolamine are all similar to atropine and produce anticholinergic effects. Homatropine is an eye drop that produces mydriasis (Chapter 59). Ipratropium is an inhaled nasal spray for the treatment of rhinorrhea. The aerosol form of ipratropium lessens the respiratory secretions and reduces mucus-plugged airways. Tiotropium bromide is administered for chronic obstructive pulmonary disease (COPD). It is a long-acting muscarinic, anticholinergic, quaternary ammonium compound that inhibits M_3 receptors in smooth muscle, resulting in bronchodilation. Tiotropium is indicated for daily maintenance treatment of bronchospasm associated with COPD. It is not indicated for acute episodes of bronchospasm (i.e., rescue therapy). Tiotropium is eliminated via the kidney system, and patients with moderate to severe kidney dysfunction should be carefully monitored for drug toxicity. Scopolamine is administered orally, parenterally, and by transdermal adhesive disk behind the ear. The transdermal disk is routinely used to relieve motion sickness. Scopolamine can produce amnesia, euphoria, relaxation, and sleep. It crosses the placenta and should be avoided with preeclampsia and eclampsia.

NCLEX Success

5. A 62-year-old patient is admitted to the cardiac intensive care unit. They are in sinus bradycardia with a rate of 48 beats/min. What is the drug of choice for sinus bradycardia?

   A. atropine sulfate
   B. epinephrine
   C. isoproterenol
   D. dopamine

CENTRALLY ACTING ANTICHOLINERGICS

Older anticholinergic drugs such as atropine are rarely used to treat Parkinson disease because of their undesirable peripheral effects (e.g., dry mouth, blurred vision, photophobia, constipation, urinary retention, tachycardia). Newer, centrally acting synthetic anticholinergic drugs are more selective for muscarinic receptors in the CNS and are designed to produce fewer adverse effects. The prototype centrally acting anticholinergic agent is P **benztropine mesylate**.

Pharmacokinetics

Benztropine is administered orally and parenterally. The oral form has an onset of action of 60 minutes and a 6- to 10-hour duration of action, with a peak effect of 7 hours. The parenteral form has an onset of action within a few minutes and a similar duration of action. The drug is absorbed from the GI tract and metabolized in the liver. It crosses the blood–brain barrier and the placenta. It is unknown how the drug is excreted.

Action

The anticholinergic activity of benztropine takes place in the CNS. Experts believe that the drug helps normalize the imbalance of cholinergic and dopaminergic neurotransmission in the basal ganglia of the brain to reduce rigidity, akinesia, and tremor. It suppresses the secondary symptoms of parkinsonism such as excessive salivary secretions and drooling.

Use

Benztropine mesylate is used for adjunctive therapy of all forms of parkinsonism: arteriosclerotic, idiopathic, and postencephalitic. It is also administered to control extrapyramidal disorders such as tardive dyskinesia due to neuroleptic drugs (phenothiazines). In addition, it is commonly used as a supplement with trihexyphenidyl, carbidopa, or levodopa. Table 48.9 lists the dosages of the centrally acting anticholinergic agents.

Patient-related variables specific to the use of centrally acting anticholinergics include the following:

- Age:
  - In older adults, cautious administration and strict adherence to dosing regulations are necessary. Patients older than 60 years of age can develop increased sensitivity to the CNS effects of all anticholinergic medications.
- Reproduction, pregnancy, and lactation:
  - Paralytic ileus has been reported in newborns if benztropine and chlorpromazine were prescribed during the second or third trimesters.
  - It is not known if benztropine enters the breast milk.

Adverse Effects

CNS adverse effects of benztropine include disorientation, confusion, hallucinations, memory loss, psychoses, agitation, euphoria, light-headedness, depression, giddiness, and heaviness of the limbs. With the administration of high doses, an inability to move certain muscle groups may occur. Peripheral anticholinergic effects include tachycardia, palpitation, hypotension, orthostatic hypotension, blurred vision, dry mouth, urinary retention, decreased sweating, and elevated temperature.

Contraindications

There are several contraindications to the use of benztropine mesylate. Glaucoma is a problem because the drug can increase intraocular pressure. GI obstruction, prostatic hypertrophy, and urinary bladder neck obstruction are other complications because of the drug's effect on smooth muscle and sphincter tone. Also, myasthenia gravis is a contraindication, because blockade of acetylcholine receptor sites at neuromuscular synapses exacerbates muscle weakness.

Caution is necessary in patients with cardiovascular disorders (e.g., tachycardia, dysrhythmias, and hypertension) because parasympathetic blockade may allow a harmful increase in sympathetic dominance. Also, caution is warranted in older adult patients with preexisting cognitive impairments because acetylcholine is an important neurotransmitter in memory function.

Nursing Implications

Preventing Interactions

Benztropine has the same interactions as atropine. Phenothiazines and tricyclic antidepressants combined with benztropine mesylate can cause confusion, hallucinations, and paralytic ileus.

TABLE 48.9
DRUGS AT A GLANCE: Centrally Acting Anticholinergics

Drug	Routes and Dosages	
	Adults	**Children**
P **Benztropine mesylate** (🍁 Benztropine Omega, PMS-Benztropine)	0.5–1 mg PO, IM, IV at bedtime; may increase up to 6 mg given at bedtime or in 2–4 divided doses For acute dystonia: PO, IM, IV 1–2 mg (orally) 1–2 times/daily up to 7–28 d to prevent recurrence; IM/IV is preferred over oral route for severe acute dystonic reactions	Safety and efficacy have not been established
Trihexyphenidyl	1 mg/daily PO; increase by 2-mg increments at 3- to 5-d intervals until a total of 6–10 mg is given daily in divided doses 3–4 times daily at mealtimes and bedtimes PO 1 mg initially. Increase as needed to control symptoms	Safety and efficacy have not been established

Administering the Medication

If the patient is experiencing GI upset, it is necessary to administer benztropine with food. The drug may be taken before meals in the presence of a dry mouth and after meals if drooling or nausea occurs. Ice chips or lozenges may counteract symptoms of dry mouth. The patient should void prior to the administration of the medication. Dosage reduction during the summer months may be necessary.

Assessing for Therapeutic Effects

The nurse assesses for decreased rigidity and tremor as well as for a decrease in oral secretions and an absence of drooling.

Assessing for Adverse Effects

The nurse monitors the patient's intake and output. If difficulty with urination results, a dosage reduction may be necessary. The nurse assesses for signs and symptoms of paralytic ileus such as intermittent constipation, abdominal pain, diminished bowel sounds on auscultation, and distention. It is also necessary to assess the heart rate for tachycardia. In addition, the nurse assesses the inability to move certain muscle groups. Checking the patient's ambulation for signs of muscle weakness and unsteady gait helps.

Patient Teaching

Box 48.5 identifies patient teaching guidelines for benztropine.

Other Drugs in the Class

Trihexyphenidyl is used in the treatment of parkinsonism and extrapyramidal reactions caused by some antipsychotic drugs. This drug relieves smooth muscle spasm by a direct action on the muscle and by inhibiting the parasympathetic nervous system. It supposedly has fewer adverse effects than atropine, but approximately half of the recipients report mouth dryness, blurring of vision, and other adverse effects common to anticholinergic drugs. Trihexyphenidyl requires the same precautions as other anticholinergic drugs and is contraindicated in glaucoma. Administration of trihexyphenidyl during pregnancy has not shown any adverse effects. It is not known if it enters the breast milk.

> **Clinical Application 48.4**
>
> Mr. Stokes has been prescribed benztropine mesylate 3 mg PO at bedtime. He resides in Wisconsin and lives there for much of the year, but he spends the winter months in Corpus Christi, Texas:
> - The nurse should educate Mr. Stokes regarding the administration of benztropine mesylate. What specific guidelines are important to mention?
> - What adverse effect is Mr. Stokes at risk for during the time he spends in Corpus Christi?

GASTROINTESTINAL ANTICHOLINERGICS (ANTISECRETORY/ANTISPASMODIC)

Dicyclomine hydrochloride (Bentyl) and glycopyrrolate (Robinul) are older medications previously administered for the treatment of peptic ulcer disease. The use of these medications has declined with the advent of the proton pump inhibitors. However, they are still prescribed for irritable bowel syndrome. **Dicyclomine hydrochloride** (Bentyl) is the prototype GI anticholinergic medication.

Pharmacokinetics

Dicyclomine is available for oral and parenteral administration. Its onset of action is 1 to 2 hours, and its duration of action is 4 hours. It is metabolized in the liver and excreted by the kidneys. The drug crosses the placenta and enters the breast milk.

Action

Dicyclomine is a GI smooth muscle relaxant. It competitively blocks the effects of acetylcholine at muscarinic cholinergic receptors that mediate the effects of the parasympathetic postganglionic impulses.

Use

Prescribers order dicyclomine for the treatment of irritable bowel syndrome. Table 48.10 gives the dosage information for this drug and related agents.

Patient-related variables specific to the use of dicyclomine hydrochloride include the following:

- Age:
  - Children have experienced serious respiratory and/or CNS reactions leading to death, particularly in infants.
  - In older adults, onset of adverse effects is increased; use of dicyclomine requires caution.

BOX 48.5 Patient Teaching Guidelines for Benztropine Mesylate

- Avoid excessive high temperatures.
- Avoid alcohol, sedatives, and over-the-counter medications, including cough and cold remedies.
- Drink water frequently.
- Rinse the mouth frequently.
- Maintain good dental/oral hygiene.
- Use hard candy to decrease dry mouth.
- Void before taking the medication.
- Visit the ophthalmologist regularly.
- Notify your prescriber if fluid intake is greater or less than urine output.
- Notify your prescriber if you develop a fever.
- Notify your prescriber if weakness becomes severe.
- Avoid the use of machinery if visual acuity or alertness is impaired.

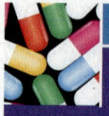

TABLE 48.10
DRUGS AT A GLANCE: Gastrointestinal Anticholinergics (Antisecretory/Antispasmodic)

Drug	Routes and Dosage Ranges	
	Adults	**Children**
ⓟ **Dicyclomine hydrochloride** (Bentyl; 🍁 JAMP Dicyclomine, Protylol, RIVA-Dicyclomine)	20 mg PO 4 times daily/7 d; increase to 40 mg 4 times/daily after 1 wk; if no efficacy in 2 wk or if adverse effects require a dose of <80 mg/d, discontinue therapy. Safety is not established for doses >80 mg/daily that exceed 2 wk. IM 10–20 mg 4 times/daily for 1–2 d and then to oral therapy as soon as possible	Safety and efficacy have not been established
Glycopyrrolate (Robinul, Cuvposa, Glycate; 🍁 Cuvposa)	Preoperatively to reduce secretions: 4 mcg/kg IM 30–60 min prior to anesthesia Reversal of bradycardia/vagal reflexes intraoperatively: IV, 0.1 mg single dose, may repeat PRN at 2- to 3-min intervals Reversal muscarinic effects of cholinergic agents: 0.2 mg IV for each 1 mg of neostigmine or 5-mg pyridostigmine administered	Preoperatively to reduce secretions: <2 y, 4–9 mcg/kg IM 30–60 min prior to anesthesia Reversal of bradycardia/vagal reflexes intraoperatively (all ages): 4 mcg/kg/dose IV (max dose, 0.1 mg); may repeat PRN at 2- to 3-min intervals Reversal muscarinic effects of cholinergic agents (all ages): See adult dosing

- Reproduction, pregnancy, and lactation:
  - Antispasmodic agents are often administered during pregnancy. Dicyclomine should be avoided during pregnancy and is contraindicated during lactation.

Adverse Effects

Adverse effects of dicyclomine are blurred vision, dry mouth, altered taste perception, nausea, vomiting, dysphagia, urinary hesitancy, urinary retention, and irritation at the injection site.

Contraindications

Dicyclomine possesses the same contraindications as the belladonna derivatives and the centrally acting anticholinergics. Contraindications to the belladonna derivatives include hypersensitivity, glaucoma, some ulcers, bronchial asthma, urinary bladder neck obstruction, and hepatic or kidney disease. Contraindications to the use of centrally acting anticholinergics also include glaucoma, GI obstruction, and urinary bladder neck obstruction, as well as prostatic hypertrophy and myasthenia gravis.

Nursing Implications
Preventing Interactions

Dicyclomine has interactions similar to those of the previous anticholinergics. The combination of antipsychotic agents with dicyclomine results in decreased effectiveness of the antipsychotic medications. Tricyclic antidepressants and amantadine combined with dicyclomine produces increased anticholinergic effects. If dicyclomine is administered with digoxin or atenolol, there is a greater reduction in the heart rate or blood pressure than if the medications are administered alone.

Administering the Medication

As with the other anticholinergic medications, it is necessary to have the patient void before taking dicyclomine. Patients receiving the IM preparation should be switched to the oral form as soon as possible because of the increased anticholinergic effects of the parenteral formulation.

Assessing for Therapeutic Effects

If dicyclomine is working, the patient reports a decrease in abdominal pain.

Assessing for Adverse Effects

The nurse assesses for altered taste perception, dry mouth, nausea, and vomiting, as well as for urinary retention. Administering the parenteral preparation requires assessment for injection site irritation.

Patient Teaching

Patient teaching for dicyclomine is the same as for atropine and benztropine (see Boxes 48.5 and 48.6).

URINARY ANTISPASMODICS

Anticholinergic drugs are the drugs of choice for their antispasmodic effects on smooth muscle to relieve the symptoms of urinary incontinence and frequency that accompany an overactive bladder. In infections, such as cystitis, urethritis, and prostatitis, the drugs decrease the frequency and pain of urination. The drugs are also given to increase bladder capacity in enuresis, paraplegia, and neurogenic bladder. ⓟ **Oxybutynin** (Ditropan XL, Gelnique, Oxytrol), the prototype, is a urinary antispasmodic that is available in oral and transdermal forms.

Pharmacokinetics

The oral preparation of oxybutynin has an onset of action 30 to 60 minutes, a peak of 3 to 6 hours, and a duration of 6 to 10 hours. The transdermal preparation has an onset of action of 24 to 48 hours, a variable peak, and a duration of action of 96 hours. The medication is metabolized in the liver and is excreted in the urine. It crosses the placenta and may enter the breast milk.

Action

Oxybutynin acts directly to relax the smooth muscle and inhibits the effects of acetylcholine at muscarinic receptors. A less potent anticholinergic than atropine, oxybutynin is more potent as an antispasmodic and devoid of antinicotinic activity at the skeletal neuromuscular junctions or autonomic ganglia.

Use

Oxybutynin is administered for the relief of bladder instability associated with voiding in patients with uninhibited neurogenic and reflex neurogenic bladder. The extended-release tablets decrease the symptoms of overactive bladder, incontinence, urgency, and frequency. Table 48.11 gives the dosage information for oxybutynin and other urinary antispasmodics.

Patient-related variables specific to the use of oxybutynin include the following:

- Age:
  - In children 6 years and older, the extended-release formulation of oxybutynin can be used for the treatment of symptoms of detrusor muscle overactivity associated with neurologic conditions such as spina bifida.
  - In older adults, dosage should not exceed 2.5 mg PO two to three times per day.
- Reproduction, pregnancy, and lactation:
  - There is no report of adverse fetal events in animal studies.
  - It is not known if oxybutynin enters the breast milk.
- Abnormal kidney function and hepatic impairment:
  - The use of oxybutynin in abnormal kidney function requires caution because of its elimination in the urine.
  - The use of oxybutynin in hepatic impairment requires caution because it is metabolized by the liver.

Adverse Effects

The adverse effects of oxybutynin are consistent with the previous anticholinergic agents discussed in this chapter. The most commonly reported CNS adverse effects include drowsiness, dizziness, and blurred vision. Other adverse effects are dry mouth, nausea, urinary hesitancy, and decreased sweating.

TABLE 48.11 DRUGS AT A GLANCE: Urinary Antispasmodics

Drug	Routes and Dosages	
	Adults	**Children**
Oxybutynin (Ditropan XL, Gelnique, Oxytrol, Oxytrol for women; APO-Oxybutynin, Ditropan XL, DOM-Oxybutynin, Gelnique, MYLAN-Oxybutynin)	PO: 5 mg 2 or 3 times daily; max dose 5 mg 4 times daily. Extended release: 5 mg increments at intervals weekly; max 30 mg/daily. Gel 10%: use contents of one sachet (100 mg/g) once/d TDS: apply one 3.9 mg/d twice weekly every 3–4 d Geriatrics: IR, start with 2.5 mg 2–3 times daily/ increase with caution	PO: infants, ≤5 y 0.1–0.2 mg/kg 2–3 times per day (max 5 mg/dose) Children >5 y and adolescents: 5 mg PO twice daily (max dosage 5 mg 3 times per day) Extended release: >6 y and adolescents, 5 mg daily; dosage may be adjusted in 5 mg increments at weekly intervals up to a max dose of 20 mg/daily
Darifenacin hydrobromide (APO-Darifenacin, Enablex, JAMP-Darifenacin)	7.5 mg PO once daily. May increase to 15 mg once daily if needed to control symptoms	Safety and efficacy have not been established
Flavoxate hydrochloride	100–200 mg PO 3 or 4 times daily. Reduce when symptoms improve	Children >12 y: see adult dosing
Solifenacin succinate (Vesicare; ACT-Solifenacin, APO-Solifenacin, JAMP-Solifenacin, Vesicare)	5 mg once PO daily. May increase to 10 mg once daily if needed to control symptoms	Safety and efficacy have not been established
Tolterodine tartrate (Detrol, Detrol LA; Detrol, Detrol LA, APO-Tolterodine, MINT-Tolterodine, MYLAN-Tolterodine)	IR: 2 mg PO twice daily. May decrease to 1 mg when symptoms improve. Reduce doses to 1 mg PO twice daily in the presence of hepatic impairment ER: 4 mg/daily; dose may be lowered to 2 mg/daily based on response	Safety and efficacy have not been established
Trospium chloride (Sanctura XR, Trosec)	IR: 20 mg PO twice daily at least 1 h before meals or on an empty stomach ER: 60 mg/daily in morning	Safety and efficacy have not been established

Contraindications

Contraindications to oxybutynin are hypersensitivity to the medication, pyloric or duodenal ulcer, obstructive intestinal lesions, intestinal atony, megacolon, colitis, obstructive uropathies, glaucoma, myasthenia gravis, cardiovascular instability, and urinary retention.

Nursing Implications

Preventing Interactions

Use of oxybutynin in combination with phenothiazines results in increased anticholinergic effects. The phenothiazines inhibit the cytochrome 450 enzyme CYP3A4 in the liver. This enzyme is required in the metabolism of oxybutynin. The inhibition of the enzyme results in a greater amount of oxybutynin that has not undergone first-pass metabolism contributing to oxybutynin toxicity. This same effect occurs if haloperidol is administered with oxybutynin. Also, use of oxybutynin together with haloperidol reduces the effect of the haloperidol and results in the development of tardive dyskinesia. Administration of oxybutynin with amantadine or nitrofurantoin leads to increased toxicity of oxybutynin.

Administering the Medication

It is important that the extended-release medication is not cut, crushed, or chewed.

Assessing for Therapeutic Effects

The nurse assesses for patient reports of decreased urinary incontinence, urgency, and frequency.

Assessing for Adverse Effects

The nurse assesses for CNS depression. The nurse also assesses for urinary hesitancy and retention as well as for impotence. In addition, it is necessary to assess for allergic reactions to the medication such as urticarial reactions.

Patient Teaching

Box 48.6 identifies the patient teaching guidelines for oxybutynin.

BOX 48.6 Patient Teaching Guidelines for Oxybutynin Chloride

- Do not cut, crush, or chew extended-release tablets.
- Apply the transdermal patch to dry intact skin over the abdomen, hip, or buttock every 3 to 4 days (twice weekly). Do not put on waistline. Remove the old system before applying a new one. Select a new site when applying a new system.
- Have periodic bladder examinations to evaluate the therapeutic response.
- Drink water frequently.
- Rinse the mouth frequently.
- Maintain good dental/oral hygiene.
- Use hard candy to decrease dry mouth.
- Avoid excessive high temperatures.
- Notify your prescriber if fluid intake is greater or less than urine output.
- Notify your prescriber if you develop a fever.

Other Drugs in the Class

Darifenacin, flavoxate, solifenacin (Vesicare), tolterodine (Detrol, Detrol LA), and trospium chloride are antimuscarinic, anticholinergic agents, which inhibit bladder contractions and reduce urinary urgency. Dosages are reduced in abnormal kidney function and hepatic insufficiency. They should be used cautiously in older adults. Darifenacin also has local anesthetic and analgesic effects. Solifenacin may prolong QT intervals, especially at higher dosages, potentially resulting in dysrhythmias. Trospium chloride should be taken on an empty stomach. When taken with food, absorption is delayed. Trospium has the potential for interaction with other drugs that are eliminated by active tubular secretion (e.g., digoxin, procainamide, pancuronium, morphine, vancomycin, metformin, tenofovir), resulting in increased serum concentration of either trospium or the coadministered drug because of competition for the urinary tubular pump.

Chapter 48 • Drug Therapy for Parkinson Disease, Urinary Spasticity, and Disorders Requiring Anticholinergic Drug Therapy

THE NURSING PROCESS

A concept map outlines the nursing process related to drug therapy considerations in this chapter. Additional nursing implications related to the disease process should also be considered in care decisions.

Assessment
- Assess for signs and symptoms of Parkinson disease and drug-induced extrapyramidal reactions, such as the following, depending on the severity and stage of progression:
  - Slow movements (bradykinesia) and difficulty in changing positions, assuming an upright position, eating, dressing, and other self-care activities
  - Stooped posture
  - Accelerating gait with short steps
  - Tremor at rest (e.g., "pill-rolling" movements of fingers)
  - Rigidity of arms, legs, and neck
  - Masklike, immobile facial expression
  - Speech problems (e.g., low volume, monotonous tone, rapid, difficult to understand)
  - Excessive salivation and drooling
  - Dysphagia
  - Excessive sweating
  - Constipation from decreased intestinal motility
  - Mental depression from self-consciousness and embarrassment over physical appearance and activity limitations. The intellect is usually intact until the late stages of the disease process.

Outcomes of Therapy
The patient will
- Experience relief of excessive salivation, muscle rigidity, spasticity, and tremors.
- Experience improved motor function, mobility, and self-care abilities.
- Increase knowledge of the disease process and drug therapy.
- Take medications as instructed.
- Avoid falls and other injuries from the disease process or drug therapy.

Nursing Interventions
- Use measures to assist the patient and family in coping with symptoms and maintaining function. These include the following:
  - Arrange for physical therapy for heel-to-toe gait training, widening stance to increase balance and base of support, and other exercises.
  - Encourage ambulation and frequent changes of position, assisted if necessary.
  - Help with active and passive range-of-motion exercises.
  - Encourage self-care as much as possible.
- It may help to cut meat; open cartons; give frequent, small meals; and allow privacy during mealtime.
- If the patient has difficulty chewing or swallowing, chopped or soft foods may be necessary.
- Hook-and-loop-type fasteners or zippers are easier to handle than buttons.
- Slip-on shoes are easier to manage than laced ones.
- Spend time with the patient and encourage socialization with other people. Victims of Parkinson disease tend to become withdrawn, isolated, and depressed.
- Schedule rest periods. Tremor and rigidity are aggravated by fatigue and emotional stress.
- Provide facial tissues if drooling is a problem.
- Provide appropriate patient teaching related to drug therapy (see Boxes 48.2, 48.3, 48.4, 48.5, and 48.6).

Evaluation
- Interview and observe for relief of symptoms.
- Interview and observe for increased mobility and participation in activities of daily living.
- Interview and observe regarding correct usage of medications.

Visit thePoint® *at* **http://thePoint.lww.com/Frandsen13e** *for answers to NCLEX Success questions (in Appendix A), answers to Clinical Application Case Studies (in Appendix B), and more!*

REFERENCES AND RESOURCES

Binde, C. D., Tvete, I. F., Gasemyr, J. I., Natvig, B., & Klemp, M. (2020). Comparative effectiveness of dopamine agonists and monoamine oxidase type-B inhibitors for Parkinson' disease: A multiple treatment comparison analysis. *European Journal of Clinical Pharmacology, 76*, 1731–1743. https://doi.10.1007/s00228-020-02961-6

Hinkle, J. H., Cheever, K. H., & Overbaugh, K. J. (2022). *Brunner & Suddarth's textbook of medical-surgical nursing* (15th ed.). Wolters Kluwer.

Lippincott Advisor. (2022). *Drug information.* Wolters Kluwer.

Norris, T. (2019). *Porth's pathophysiology: Concepts of altered health states* (10th ed.). Wolters Kluwer.

Parkinson Disease Foundation. (2022). *Statistics on Parkinson's.* Retrieved July 2, 2022, from https://www.parkinson.org/Understanding-Parkinsons/Statistics

Spindler, M. A., & Tarsy, D. (2022). Initial pharmacological treatment of Parkinson disease. In *UpToDate*.

UpToDate. (2022). *Drug information.* Lexi-Comp, Inc.

CHAPTER 49

Drug Therapy With Opioids

LEARNING OBJECTIVES

After studying this chapter, you should be able to:

1. Recognize the usefulness as well as public health concerns related to opioid drug therapy for acute and chronic pain.
2. Recognize the impact of the opioid epidemic on individuals and society and the national strategies to reduce opioid-associated deaths.
3. Identify the prototype and describe the action, use, adverse effects, contraindications, and nursing implications for the opioid agonists.
4. Identify the prototype and describe the action, use, adverse effects, contraindications, and nursing implications for the opioid antagonists.
5. Implement the nursing process in the care of the patient receiving opioid medications for pain.

CLINICAL APPLICATION CASE STUDY

Darlene Hoffman, a 50-year-old woman, is receiving treatment for ovarian cancer. After surgery, she arrives on the unit from the postanesthesia care unit (PACU) complaining of lower back pain of 2 out of 10 on a 10-point pain scale. She received a total of 10 mg of morphine sulfate in the PACU. Her vital signs are temperature 98.2°F, pulse 82 beats/min, respirations 22 breaths/min, and blood pressure 124/72 mm Hg, with an O_2 saturation of 94% on 2 L/min nasal cannula.

KEY TERMS

Abuse-deterrent formulations: preparations designed to decrease the ability to crush or dissolve opioids to reduce the risk of misuse

Agonist substitution treatment: a process for treating addiction and the associated withdrawal by using a substance (such as buprenorphine or methadone) to substitute for a stronger full agonist opioid (such as heroin) and slowly tapering it off

Breakthrough pain: episodic bursts of intense pain that "breaks through" the pain control of the medication regime

Ceiling effect: a phenomenon of certain drugs that limits the ability to produce a further effect above a particular dosage level

Drug diversion: the illegal distribution or misuse of prescription drugs for purposes not intended as prescribed

Neonatal abstinence syndrome: neonatal withdrawal from substances exposed to in utero

Opioid-naive: patients who do not meet opioid-tolerant criteria and have not had at least 60 mg of morphine or an equianalgesic dose of another opioid for a week or longer

Opioid-tolerant: patients who have been taking at least 60 mg of morphine or an equianalgesic dose of another opioid for a week or longer

Patient-controlled analgesia: any method used by patients to administer their own pain medication, typically used to indicate administration through a controlled intravenous pump

Risk evaluation and mitigation strategy (REMS): A requirement by the U.S. Food and Drug Administration (FDA) that manufacturers of approved opioid analgesic products have drug-compliant education programs available to prescribers

Tolerance: decreased effect from initial response to an opioid that requires a higher dose of the drug to achieve the same level of response reached initially

INTRODUCTION

Pain is an unpleasant sensory and emotional experience associated with or resembling that associated with actual or potential tissue injury (IASP, 2020). The perception of pain is part of the clinical presentation in many acute and chronic disorders and is one of the most difficult sensations for patients to cope with across the course of a disease. It impels a person to remove the cause of the damage or seek relief from the pain. This chapter aids in the understanding of pain-relieving opioid drugs used to treat acute and chronic pain. In addition, this chapter provides an overview of opioid misuse (Box 49.1), identifying it as a major global public health issue, and discusses the association of opioids with unintentional overdoses and drug-related deaths.

OVERVIEW OF PAIN

Pain is the most common symptom prompting people to seek healthcare. When not managed effectively, pain may greatly impair quality of life and ability to perform activities of daily living. Opioid analgesics are drugs that provide pain relief by affecting people's perception and tolerance of moderate-to-severe pain.

Defining the multidimensional concept of pain presents challenges, as pain has various pathologic mechanisms and implications and differs broadly in quality, intensity, and duration. Pain occurs when tissue damage (e.g., nerve damage, actual tissue injury, cancer, surgery) from pain-producing substances activates pain receptors, increases the sensitivity of pain receptors, or stimulates the release of inflammatory substances. Pain may be classified according to its origin in body structures (e.g., somatic, visceral, neuropathic), duration (e.g., acute, chronic), or cause (e.g., cancer). Pain also can negatively impact a person's level of functioning, mental health, work productivity, and quality of life. For further details on the etiology and pathophysiology of pain, and types of pain, visit thePoint® http://thePoint.lww.com/Frandsen13e.

Clinical Manifestations

Pain is a subjective experience, and a patient's self-reporting of pain is considered the gold standard of pain assessment measurements because it is a personal experience that offers the most valid measurement of pain. However, numerous factors, including mood, sleep disturbances, fatigue, and medications, may influence self-reporting. Cultural, gender, age, and other

---

BOX 49.1 *Overview of Opioid Misuse*

The United States continues to experience an opioid epidemic, made worse by a surge in fentanyl-related overdose deaths over the last decade. Much of the early use and misuse of opioids resulted from the mistaken belief that they were not addictive. Roughly 143 million opioid prescriptions were dispensed from US pharmacies in 2020 (CDC, 2020). While that represents a 40% decrease in opioid prescriptions from its peak in 2010, opioid-related deaths have continued to increase. With increased scrutiny on prescription use, individuals misusing opioids progressed to cheaper and more easily available heroin. As deaths increased, users turned to synthetic opioids (mostly fentanyl). The number of deaths from accidental overdose of opioids–both prescription and nonprescription–has eclipsed that of every other drug *combined* and is now the leading cause of accidental death in the United States. Data from the Centers for Disease Control and Prevention (CDC, 2021) indicated that in 2021, the leading cause of death in the age group of those 18 to 45 years was unintentional injuries. Illicitly manufactured fentanyl or fentanyl analogs comprise approximately 90% of the synthetic opioids category, making fentanyl the major cause of fatal drug overdose. That number exceeded COVID-19 as the second highest leading cause of death that year. Furthermore, the CDC reported that total opioid-related deaths in 2021 were 106,699; for a 12-month period ending in October 2022, the total deaths from opioid were reported at 101,750, primarily the result of synthetic opioids, such as fentanyl. It is anticipated that the FDA's recent approval of naloxone availability over the counter will reduce fatal opioid overdoses with easier lay access to the drug.

> **BOX 49.1** *Overview of Opioid Misuse* (Continued)
>
> Accidental death from opioids also occurs when certain drugs are mixed and marketed as other drugs to make drugs such as heroin or fentanyl more potent and cheaper to produce. The drug isotonitazene or "ISO" is a synthetic opioid sourced from China that was never approved for medical use in the United States. The drug is more potent than fentanyl and was first reported in 2019 after entering the illicit drug market. In 2023, the U.S. Drug Enforcement Administration published a warning regarding an outbreak of deaths resulting from ingestion of isotonitazene. The drug structurally differs from fentanyl and is not detected by hospital-based rapid drug screens for opioids. Symptoms of toxicity of isotonitazene are similar to other opioids, and naloxone reverses the effects. With no approved medical use, numerous overdose deaths associated with poisoning from isotonitazene highlight the importance of an individual taking prescription drugs only as ordered for them by a provider and dispensed by a licensed pharmacist.
>
> Opioids taken during pregnancy expose the fetus in utero to these substances, producing neonatal withdrawal from opioids. **Neonatal abstinence syndrome** is the term used to describe neonatal withdrawal. Clinical signs vary for each infant based on the type and amount of drug exposure, the time of last maternal drug use, and the drug's half-life. Typically, symptoms begin within 48 to 72 hours of birth and include neurologic (irritability, myoclonus, tremors, hyperreflexia, seizures, high-pitched cry, decreased sleeping, yawning), autonomic (sweating, low-grade fever), and gastrointestinal (excessive sucking, poor feeding, excessive weight loss, vomiting, diarrhea) symptoms.
>
> Since 2017, the U.S. Department of Health and Human Services (HHS) has declared opioid overdose as a public health emergency and has introduced a strategy to combat the opioid crisis, focusing on better addiction prevention, treatment, and recovery services; collecting better data on the epidemic; targeting better evidence-based methods of pain management; better utilization of opioid-reversing drugs; and better research on pain and addiction. In 2023, the Secretary of HHS renewed the opioid public health emergency with interventions to further deemphasize the approach of criminalizing addiction to one of recognizing and treating addiction appropriately as a disease and emphasizing harm reduction strategies. President Biden's National Drug Strategy focused on the major drivers of the opioid epidemic: untreated addiction and drug trafficking actions. The government's strategy also included expanding access to high-impact harm reduction tools such as naloxone, preventing substance misuse among school-aged children and young adults, and supporting community-led coalitions implementing evidence-based prevention strategies across the country. Despite this national agenda, more than 250 Americans die each day from an overdose (CDC, 2021).

psychosocial factors can play a role in manifestations of pain. Individuals learn the concept of pain through their life experiences.

A variety of pain measurement tools exists, including visual analog scales, verbal or numerical rating scales, or picture scales. The pain measurement tool chosen should be appropriate to the individual patient, considering developmental, cognitive, emotional, language, and cultural factors. A mnemonic device (SOCRATES) can be used to assess the clinical manifestations of pain. Its meaning appears below:

- Site
- Onset
- Character
- Radiation
- Associations with other symptoms
- Time course (pattern)
- Exacerbating/relieving factors
- Severity

Nurses can use observational tools for patients who cannot communicate their pain for various reasons (e.g., unconsciousness, language barrier, cognitive impairment). These tools involve several behaviors, including facial expressions, limb movements, vocalization, restlessness, and guarding as indicators of pain. In patients with pain, vital signs may demonstrate tachycardia, tachypnea, and hypertension.

Drug Therapy

Opioid analgesics relieve moderate-to-severe pain by inhibiting adenylate cyclase, which coordinates the transmission of pain signals from peripheral tissues to the brain, reducing the perception of pain sensation in the brain, producing sedation, and decreasing the emotional upsets often associated with pain. The drugs also inhibit the production of pain and inflammation by prostaglandins and leukotrienes in peripheral tissues. With repeated opioid use, adenylate cyclase adapts, reducing the ability of the opioids to inhibit pain signals. Thus, patients no longer respond to an opioid as they originally did and so require a higher dose of the drug to achieve the same level of response reached initially. This response is the cause of opioid **tolerance**.

Opioid drugs are commonly used to treat moderate-to-severe pain, although evidence is not definitive regarding their short- and long-term benefits, particularly in lieu of the risks. Some opioids are also be used to treat coughing (Chapter 32) and diarrhea (Chapter 40). Most of the opioids are Schedule II drugs under federal narcotics laws and may lead to drug misuse and dependence (see Chapter 1). The U.S. Food and Drug Administration (FDA) has issued **BOXED WARNING ◆** warnings for all opioid analgesics because of the potentially fatal adverse effects of respiratory depression, coma, and death, as well as the dependence, abuse, and misuse liability of the opioids as a drug class. The FDA requires drug companies with approved opioid analgesic products to have an opioid **risk evaluation and mitigation strategy (REMS)** to provide drug-compliant education programs to prescribers. Because of wide-spread opioid misuse, the FDA has approved **abuse-deterrent formulations** that reduce the ability to crush the tablets for three opioids—oxycodone (Xtampza ER), morphine (Mitigo, MorphaBond [ER]), and hydrocodone (Hysingla)—in an attempt to reduce the risk of misuse. These formulations target the known or anticipated

TABLE 49.1

Drugs (Opioids) Administered for the Treatment of Pain

Drug Class	Prototype	Other Drugs in the Class
Agonists	Morphine sulfate (Duramorph, Infumorph, Kadian, MS Contin, Mitigo)	Codeine Fentanyl (Actiq) Hydrocodone (Hysingla) Hydromorphone (Dilaudid) Meperidine (Demerol) Methadone (Methadose) Oxycodone (OxyContin, Xtampza ER) Oxymorphone Tramadol (Ultram, ConZip)
Agonists/antagonists	Butorphanol	Buprenorphine (Subutex) Nalbuphine Pentazocine
Antagonists	Naloxone Narcan, Zimhi	Naltrexone (Vivitrol)

routes of misuse for a specific opioid, such as crushing to snort or dissolving to inject.

In 2022, the CDC released its *Clinical Practice Guideline for Prescribing Opioids for Pain* that provides pain management recommendations for adults seen in outpatient settings for acute (<1-month duration), subacute (1–3-month duration), and chronic (>3-month duration) pain, excluding adults receiving palliative or end-of-life care and those with sickle cell disease. The guideline further emphasizes that policies should allow for providers making clinical decisions that account for each patient's unique circumstances. The guideline does not support stopping opioid use abruptly. Table 49.1 outlines the subgroups of opioid analgesics: the opioid agonists, agonists/antagonists, and antagonists. The larger group of agonists includes morphine and morphine-like drugs. These agents have activity at mu and kappa receptors and thus produce prototypical effects. As their name indicates, the agonists/antagonists have both agonist and antagonist activities. Antagonists are antidote drugs that reverse the effects of agonists. In addition, numerous combinations of opioid and nonopioid analgesics (see Chapter 16) are available and commonly used in most healthcare settings.

Healthcare providers are now able to take advantage of several approaches to perioperative pain management using medications from different drug classes to suppress pain by blocking multiple pain pathways. Many approaches are considered opioid sparing, which allows a clinically significant reduction in the dose of opioids given. This reduces opioid adverse effects without sacrificing pain control. In addition, properly managed pain reduces healthcare costs and improves postoperative outcomes.

> **! Quality and Safety Alert: Safety**
>
> Respiratory depression is a possible adverse effect for patients taking opioids, but the concern can be minimized by (1) avoiding concomitant use of other drugs such as alcohol and benzodiazepines, which depress the central nervous system (CNS), and (2) careful monitoring of the response to the drug and the dosage. It is important to use additional caution when administering narcotics to patients with underlying respiratory disorders, such as chronic pulmonary disease or sleep apnea.

Despite that, the use of long-term opioid therapy for chronic pain has escalated concerns about addiction, tolerance, and diversion, which often leads to suboptimal pain management that results in decreased quality of life. Providers must balance the possibility of addiction against the benefits of the therapy. Lack of understanding of addiction and mislabeling of patients as addicts may result in unnecessary withholding of opioid medications. The management of pain in patients with a history of addiction or a coexisting psychiatric disorder requires special consideration by a pain management specialist.

It was previously thought that the ability to use opioids effectively on a long-term basis for pain management was limited because of the risk of tolerance. However, data have shown that tolerance is not a major drawback to long-term opioid use. In patients with cancer, what initially appears to be tolerance is usually progression of the disease. In patients who do not have cancer, the failure to respond to increasing doses of opioids may result from several factors, including tolerance, disease progression, and opioid-induced sensitivity to noxious stimuli.

Drug diversion, the illegal distribution or misuse of prescription drugs for purposes not intended as prescribed, is a major concern. The ability of the healthcare team, including the patient, to provide ongoing communication during each transition in care can reduce the risk of diversion. Activities that may help rule out diversion include urine and/or blood drug screening, pill counts, and regular patient follow-up to review treatment efficacy. State prescription monitoring program databases, where available, are useful in monitoring compliance and enhance communication. In addition, legislation and regulatory policies should not deter the use of opioids where medically indicated for moderate-to-severe pain, and the treatment plan is reasonably designed to mitigate the risk of addiction and misuse.

OPIOID AGONISTS

Morphine sulfate (Duramorph, Infumorph, Kadian, MS Contin, Mitigo), the prototype, is an opium alkaloid used mainly to relieve moderate-to-severe pain. A Schedule II–controlled drug, administration is most often oral or parenteral. Patient response depends on route of administration and dosage.

Pharmacokinetics

Morphine is well absorbed after oral (PO), intramuscular (IM), subcutaneous, and intravenous (IV) administration. However, PO formulations undergo significant first-pass metabolism in the liver, which means that PO doses must be larger than injected doses to have equivalent therapeutic effects. After PO administration of fast-acting (e.g., immediate release) formulations, peak activity occurs in about 60 minutes. After IV injection, maximal analgesia and respiratory depression usually occur within 10 to 20 minutes. After IM injection, these effects occur in about 30 minutes. After subcutaneous injection, morphine effects may be delayed up to 60 to 90 minutes. The duration of action is 5 to 7 hours.

Action

Morphine relieves pain by binding to receptors in the brain, spinal cord, and peripheral tissues. When bound to the drug, receptors function like gates that close and thereby block or decrease transmission of pain impulses from one nerve cell to the next. The receptors also activate the endogenous analgesia system. The major types of receptors are mu, kappa, and delta. Most of the effects of morphine (analgesia; CNS depression, with respiratory depression and sedation; euphoria; decreased gastrointestinal [GI] motility; and physical dependence) are attributed to activation of the mu receptors. Analgesia, sedation, and decreased GI motility occur with activation of kappa receptors. The endogenous analgesia system involves the delta receptors, which may not bind with opioid drugs.

Use

The main indication for morphine is to prevent or relieve moderate-to-severe acute or chronic pain. Specific conditions for morphine include acute myocardial infarction, biliary colic, kidney colic, burns and other traumatic injuries, and postoperative states. Healthcare providers usually give morphine for chronic pain, such as that associated with terminal cancer, only when other measures and milder drugs are ineffective. Other clinical uses of morphine include the following:

- Before and during surgery to promote sedation, decrease anxiety, facilitate induction of anesthesia, and decrease the amount of anesthesia required
- During labor and delivery (obstetric analgesia; note that morphine crosses the placenta)
- Treatment of GI disorders, such as abdominal cramping and diarrhea
- Treatment of acute pulmonary edema
- Treatment of severe, unproductive cough (codeine may be used)
- Unlabeled use: relief of dyspnea associated with acute left ventricular failure and pulmonary edema.

Table 49.2 gives dosages of morphine sulfate and other opioid agonists.

Patient-related variables specific to the use of morphine sulfate and other opioid agonists include the following:

- Age:
  - Oral solutions are of multiple strengths, so precautions should be taken to avoid confusion between the different concentrations when administering morphine to children. All prescriptions should have the concentration stated and the dose designated in milligrams of morphine, not by volume in milliliters.
  - Children may be unable to communicate their discomfort, or they may fear injections and so may be undertreated or their pain may be overlooked.
  - Monitory for respiratory depression in children, particularly neonates.
  - In older adults, the duration of morphine's action may be longer, increasing the risk of adverse effects.
  - Older adults are especially sensitive to respiratory depression, excessive sedation, confusion, and other adverse effects of morphine. However, they should receive adequate analgesia, along with vigilant monitoring.
  - With morphine use in older adults, observe voiding and urine output since acute urinary retention is more likely to occur.
- Reproduction, pregnancy, and lactation:
  - Long-term use of opioids may cause infertility or sexual dysfunction in females and males from secondary hypogonadism.
  - Morphine crosses the placenta and maternal use of opioids may be associated with poor fetal growth, stillbirth, preterm delivery, and congenital anomalies (i.e., neural tube defects, congenital heart defects, gastroschisis).
  - Opioid use during pregnancy, including as part of obstetric analgesia/anesthesia during labor and delivery, can cause a decrease in fetal heart rate.
  - The FDA has issued a **BOXED WARNING** advising that prolonged use of morphine during pregnancy can result in neonatal abstinence syndrome.
  - If morphine use is necessary, it may be safer to wait 4 to 6 hours after opioid administration to nurse an infant.
- Abnormal kidney function and hepatic impairment:
  - Patients with abnormal kidney function or hepatic impairment should take minimal doses of morphine for the shortest effective time because usual doses may produce profound sedation and a prolonged duration of action.
  - Morphine produces an active metabolite that may accumulate in patients with abnormal kidney function.
  - Since morphine is extensively metabolized by the liver, it may accumulate and cause increased adverse effects in the presence of hepatic impairment if the dosage is not reduced, especially with chronic use.
- Specific healthcare environments:
  - Patients with critical illness are commonly in pain or at high risk for development of pain. Morphine is usually given by IV bolus injection or continuous infusion.

> **Quality and Safety Alert: Safety**
>
> When children's doses are calculated based on adult doses, fractions and decimals often result, which greatly increases the risk of a dosage error. It is advisable to have two people do the calculations independently and compare results.

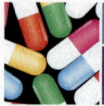

TABLE 49.2
DRUGS AT A GLANCE: Opioid Agonists

Drug	Routes and Dosage Ranges	
	Adults	**Children**
ⓟ **Morphine** (Duramorph, Infumorph, Kadian, MS Contin, Mitigo; ✦ M.O.S.-S.R, MS Contin SRT, Statex, Teva-Morphine SR)	PO immediate release, 5–30 mg every 4 h PRN PO controlled release, 30 mg or more every 8–12 h IM, subcutaneously 5–20 mg/70 kg every 4 h PRN IV injection, 2–10 mg/70 kg, diluted in 5 mL water for injection and injected slowly, over 5 min IV continuous infusion, 0.1–1 mg/mL in 5% dextrose in water solution, by controlled infusion pump Epidurally, 2–5 mg/24 h; intrathecally, 0.2–1 mg/24 h Rectal, 10–20 mg every 4 h PCA dosing based on institutional protocols; standard parameters: 2-mg bolus, 1-mg dose, lockout interval 10 min, 4-h maximum limit 30 mg, basal rate not recommended for starting PCA Older adult, PCA dosing per institutional protocols typically 25% of adult dose and requires more intense monitoring and dose individualization	<1 y: PO, 80–200 mcg/kg every 4 h 1–2 y: PO, 200–400 mcg/kg every 4 h 2–12 y: PO, 200–500 mcg/kg every 4 h; max oral starting dose is 5 mg. subcutaneous, 0.05–0.2 mg/kg (up to 15 mg) every 4 h neonate: subcutaneous, 25–50 mcg/kg every 6 h 1–6 mo: subcutaneous, 100 mcg/kg every 6 h 6 mo–2 y: subcutaneous, 100 mcg/kg every 4 h 2–12 y: subcutaneous, 100–200 mcg/kg every 4 h, max starting dose 2.5 mg
Buprenorphine (Subutex; ✦ BuTrans, Sublocade)	Withdrawal- sublingual: 2-day induction, adjust dose in increments of 2–4 mg to target dose of 16 mg once daily; max, 24 mg once daily	Neonatal abstinence syndrome: Full-term infant, sublingual solution (0.075 mg/mL) Initial: 5.3 mcg/kg/dose every 8 h Ages 2–12 y, 2–6 mcg/kg IM or slow IV injection every 4–6 h ≥13 y, same as adult dosage
Codeine (✦ Codeine Contin, PMS-Codeine, Ratio-Codeine)	Pain: PO, subcutaneous, IM 15–60 mg every 4–6 h PRN; usual dose 30 mg; max, 360 mg/24 h Cough: PO 10–20 mg every 4 h PRN; max, 120 mg/24 h	1 y or older, pain: PO, subcutaneous, IM 0.5 mg/kg every 4–6 h PRN 2–6 y, cough: PO 2.5–5 mg every 4–6 h; max, 30 mg/24 h 6–12 y, cough: PO 5–10 mg every 4–6 h; max, 60 mg/24 h
Fentanyl (Actiq, ✦ Abstral, Fentora, Matrix Patch, PMS-Fentanyl MTX)*	Preanesthetic sedation: IM 0.05–0.1 mg 30–60 min before surgery Analgesic adjunct to general anesthesia: IV total dose of 0.002–0.05 mg/kg, depending on surgical procedure Adjunct to regional anesthesia: IM or slow IV (over 1–2 min) 0.05–0.1 mg PRN Postoperative analgesia: IM 0.05–0.1 mg, repeat in 1–2 h if needed General anesthesia: IV 0.05–0.1 mg/kg with oxygen and a muscle relaxant (max dose 0.15 mg/kg with open heart surgery, other major surgeries, and complicated neurologic or orthopedic procedures) Chronic pain (Duragesic transdermal system): 2.5–10 mg every 72 h	Children weighing at least 10 kg: conscious sedation or preanesthetic sedation, 5–15 mcg/kg of body weight (100–400 mcg), depending on weight, type of procedure, and other factors; max dose, 400 mcg, regardless of age and weight. 2–12 y: general anesthesia induction and maintenance, IV 2–3 mcg/kg
Hydrocodone (Hysingla ER) Hydrocodone (with acetaminophen: Paracetamol, Lortab, Vicodin HP) (with ibuprofen: Ibudone, Reprexain, Vicoprofen, Xylon; ✦ Vicoprofen)	Hysingla ER: 20 mg once daily and then increase 10–20 mg every 3–5 d PRN With acetaminophen: 1–2 tablets every 4–6 h as needed for pain, not to exceed 4 g of acetaminophen daily With ibuprofen: 1 tablet (hydrocodone 2.5–0 mg/ibuprofen 200 mg) every 4–6 h as needed for pain, not to exceed five tablets daily; consider reducing dosing in older adults	2–13 y or <50 kg: hydrocodone 0.1–0.2 mg/kg/dose, not to exceed 6 doses a day or the max recommended dose of acetaminophen. ≥16 y: refer to adult dosing for hydrocodone with ibuprofen. Extended-release products containing hydrocodone should not be given to children younger than 6 y and should be used with caution in children 6–12 y

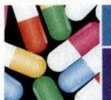

TABLE 49.2

DRUGS AT A GLANCE: Opioid Agonists (Continued)

Drug	Routes and Dosage Ranges	
	Adults	**Children**
Hydromorphone (Dilaudid; ❋ Hydromorph Contin, Jurnista)	PO 2–4 mg every 4–6 h PRN IM, subcutaneous, IV 1–2 mg every 4–6 h PRN (may be increased to 4 mg for severe pain) Rectal suppository 3 mg every 6–8 h	Safety and effectiveness not established in children
Meperidine (Demerol; ❋ Demerol)	PO, IM, IV, subcutaneous, PO 50–150 mg every 3–4 h Obstetric analgesia: IM, subcutaneous 50–100 mg when pain becomes regular; may repeat at 1- to 3-h intervals	<18 y: Use with caution due to risk of respiratory depression >1 y: PO, IM, subcutaneous 1.1–1.8 mg/kg/dose, up to adult dose, every 3–4 h as needed
Methadone (Methadose ❋ Metadol, Metadol-D)	PO (opioid naive) initial 2.5 mg every 8–12 h IV, IM, subcutaneous, initial 2.5–10 mg every 8- to 12-h titrate slowly to effect	Neonatal abstinence syndrome: Initial: 0.05–0.1 mg/kg/dose PO, IV every 6 h or 0.05–0.1 mg/kg/dose PO, IV every 4 h Pain: following pain management with opioids, methadone dose selection, dose reduction, and duration of oral weaning limited
Oxycodone (OxyContin, Xtampza ER; ❋ Oxy IR, OxyNEO, PMS-Oxycodone CR, Supeudol)	PO, immediate release, 5 mg every 6 h PRN; 10–30 mg every 4 h PRN for other formulations PO, controlled release, 10 mg every 12 h, increased if necessary	Safety and effectiveness not established in young children >12 y: PO, 0.2 to 0.9 mg/kg/day (0.05–0.15 mg/kg/dose q4–6h).
Oxymorphone	PO (opioid naive), 5–10 mg every 4–6 h; conversion from stable parenteral dose 10 times the total parenteral requirement in divided doses every 4–6 h PO, extended release (opioid naive), 5 mg every 12 h, increased by 5–10 mg every 12 h every 3–7 d until pain relieved; conversion from stable parenteral dose 10 times the total parenteral requirement in two divided doses IM, subcutaneous 1–1.5 mg every 4–6 h PRN IV 0.5 mg every 4–6 h PRN Labor analgesia: IM 0.5–1 mg	Safety and effectiveness not established in children
Tramadol (Ultram, ConZip; ❋ Durela, Tridural, Ultram, Zytram XL)	PO 50–100 mg every 4–6 h PRN (max dose, 400 mg/d) Abnormal kidney function (CrCl < 30 mL/min): PO 50–100 mg every 12 h (max dose, 200 mg/d) Hepatic impairment (cirrhosis): PO 50 mg every 12 h Older adults (65–75 y): same as adults, unless they also have abnormal kidney function or hepatic impairment Older adults (>75 y): <300 mg daily, in divided doses	Not approved for children <17 y ≥17 y, PO 1 mg/kg every 4–6 h (max dose 2 mg/kg or 100 mg)

*Actiq, Fentora are special preparations for specific uses. (Check manufacturers' instructions for dosage and administration instructions.)

Morphine is commonly used to manage pain associated with disease processes and invasive diagnostic and therapeutic procedures. In intensive care units, morphine and other opioid agonists are also used concurrently with sedatives and neuromuscular blocking agents, which increase the risks of adverse drug reactions and interactions. In general, morphine should be given continuously or on a regular schedule of intermittent doses, with supplemental or bolus doses when needed for **breakthrough pain**, episodic bursts of intense pain that "break through" the pain control provided by the pain medication.

One effective method of pain management is **patient-controlled analgesia** (PCA), which allows a person in pain to administer their own pain relief. Commonly, an IV device regulated by programmable settings delivers morphine at a preset bolus dosage when the patient presses a button. It is possible to program a lockout period into the pump so that the frequency

BOX 49.2 Assessment for Appropriateness of Patient-Controlled Analgesia

- Preprocedure cognitive assessment (patient must be cognitively competent to actively participate in pain management)
  - Assess mental status, level of consciousness, and developmental status.
  - Assess patient's (and family's) ability to comprehend teaching regarding the patient's role in managing pain, specific information on pump operation, safety measures, and when to alert a nurse.
- Is the patient opioid-tolerant or opioid-naive?
  - Opioid-tolerant: patients who have been taking at least 60 mg of morphine or an equianalgesic dose of another opioid for a week or longer.
  - Opioid naive: patients who do not meet opioid-tolerant criteria and have not had narcotics in the amounts given above for a week or more.
- Pain assessment: use a consistent standard pain assessment tool, such as the 0 to 10 pain scale or the 0 to 10 Faces Pain Scale for children.
- Sedation assessment
  - Assess sedation using a consistent tool (e.g., Ramsay Sedation Scale [RAS], Riker Sedation-Agitation Scale [SAS] or Richmond Agitation and Sedation Scale [RASS]).
  - This is a critical component; sedation precedes respiratory depression because less opioid is required to produce it.
- Respiratory assessment
  - Assess rate, quality, and sounds of respirations.
  - Assess oxygen saturation using pulse oximetry.

---

of administration is controlled, as well as the basal amount of drug to be delivered. When starting a continuous IV infusion of pain medication, a healthcare professional gives a loading dose to attain therapeutic blood levels quickly. The nurse assesses pain scores after initiation, after any change in pump setting, and periodically using a standardized pain rating scale to assess pain relief response to the PCA medication based on hospital protocol. Box 49.2 outlines specific assessment considerations prior to and throughout the administration of opioids using PCA.

With some types of chronic pain, such as those occurring with low back pain or osteoarthritis, morphine is not indicated for long-term use. Treatment involves nonopioid medications, physical therapy, and other measures. The home care nurse may need to explain the reasons for not using opioids on a long-term basis and help patients and caregivers learn alternative methods of relieving discomfort. The nurse should also assess for the effectiveness of the opioid in relieving pain as well as any signs that might indicate addiction, diversion, or tolerance.

With cancer pain, the goal of treatment is to prevent or relieve pain and keep patients comfortable. Thus, the home care nurse must assist patients and caregivers in understanding the appropriate use of morphine in cancer care, including administration on a regular schedule, storing the drugs to avoid use by people other than the patient, and avoiding theft and diversion to street use. The nurse also must be proficient in using and teaching various routes of drug administration and in arranging regimens with potentially very large doses and various combinations of drugs. In addition, the nurse must make an active effort to prevent or manage adverse effects, such as a bowel program to prevent constipation.

Additional guidelines include the following:

- Morphine should be given on a regular schedule, around the clock. Patients should be awakened, if necessary, to prevent pain recurrence.
- PO, rectal, and transdermal routes of administration are generally preferred over injections.
- When long-acting forms of morphine are given on a regular schedule, fast-acting forms also need to be available for breakthrough pain. If supplemental or "rescue" doses are needed frequently, the baseline dose of long-acting medication may need to be increased.
- In addition to morphine, other drugs may be used to increase patient comfort (see Other Drugs in the Class). In addition, multimodal anesthesia, including the use of select antidepressants and anticonvulsants to decrease neuropathic pain, may enhance the efficacy of pain management.

Adverse Effects

Morphine has widespread pharmacologic effects, especially in the CNS and the GI system. These effects occur with usual doses and may be therapeutic or adverse, depending on the reason for use. CNS effects include analgesia; CNS depression, ranging from drowsiness to sleep to unconsciousness; decreased mental and physical activity; respiratory depression; nausea and vomiting; and pupil constriction. Sedation and respiratory depression are major adverse effects and potentially life-threatening. In the GI tract, morphine slows motility, and it may cause constipation and smooth muscle spasms in the bowel and biliary tract.

Contraindications

Contraindications include hypersensitivity to morphine, significant respiratory depression, acute or chronic lung disease (if in unmonitored setting or if resuscitative equipment unavailable), upper airway obstruction, concurrent use of monoamine oxidase inhibitors (MAOIs) or use in the last 14 days and GI obstruction. The drug should be used with caution with hypotension, thyroid dysfunction, liver or kidney disease, increased intracranial pressure and head injury, seizure disorders, severe alcoholism, concurrent use of benzodiazepines or other CNS depressants.

Nursing Implications
Preventing Interactions

Drugs that increase the effects of morphine are found in Box 49.3. Naloxone is known to reverse the effects of morphine. Herbs such as kava, valerian, and St. John's wort may

| BOX 49.3 | **Drug Interactions: Morphine Sulfate** |

Drugs That Increase the Effects of Morphine Sulfate

- Alcohol, antidepressants, antipsychotics, barbiturates, benzodiazepines, and sedatives
  Increase the risk of drowsiness, confusion, memory loss, or respiratory distress
- Antihistamines
  Increase sedation and the risk of constipation and urinary retention
- Monoamine oxidase (MAO) inhibitors
  Increase the risk of hypotension, respiratory depression, or coma; patients should not take morphine and an MAO inhibitor within 14 days of each other.
- Other narcotics or opiates
  Increase the risk of hypotension, respiratory depression, or coma

increase the sedative effect of morphine. The FDA has issued a BOXED WARNING for the combined use of morphine and other opioid analgesics with the benzodiazepines and other drugs that depress the CNS. The risk of serious adverse reactions, including slowed or difficult breathing and death, has been reported.

Administering the Medication

Although the dose of morphine can be titrated upward for adequate analgesia, unacceptable adverse effects (e.g., excessive sedation, respiratory depression, nausea, and vomiting) may limit the dose. With PO administration, patients may take the drug without regard to food. However, if GI upset occurs, food is acceptable. It is essential that PO forms are not broken or crushed. The nurse dilutes and administers IV doses slowly to minimize the likelihood of adverse effects.

It is necessary to monitor respiration closely in neonates. The antagonist naloxone should be readily available (see "Opioid Antagonists"). Other guidelines for morphine administration include:

- Assess for pain on a regular schedule around the clock (e.g., every 1 to 2 hours). It is important to use a consistent method for assessing severity, such as a visual analog or numeric scale. If the patient can communicate, the nurse asks about the location, severity, and so forth. If the patient is unable to communicate needs for pain relief, as is often the case during critical illnesses, the nurse must evaluate posture, body language, risk factors, and other possible indicators of pain.
- In patients with trauma and other critical illnesses, administer morphine by IV infusion over a prolonged period. Healthcare providers may also give the drug by transdermal patch or by epidural infusion, depending on the patient's condition. For information about the use of PCA, see Box 49.2.
- As previously stated, the nurse administers morphine by the recommended routes (e.g., PO, IV, epidural) rather than IM injections, because IM injections are painful and frightening for children. For any child receiving parenteral medications, it is essential to assess vital signs and level of consciousness regularly.

 Quality and Safety Alert: Safety

The reversal effects of naloxone with IM or subcutaneous administration may be delayed or erratic in pediatric patients, patients who are hypotensive, or patients with peripheral vasoconstriction or hypoperfusion due to inconsistent or delayed drug absorption.

Assessing for Therapeutic Effects

The nurse assesses for decreased pain (patient reports) and general feeling of well-being. The nurse ensures that the patient is free from adverse effects. Tolerance (the initial dose of a substance loses its effectiveness over time) occurs with morphine and other opioids (see Chapter 2).

Assessing for Adverse Effects

The nurse should assess for increases in respiratory distress, cardiac rhythm disturbances, and increasing somnolence. The FDA has issued BOXED WARNING for all opioid analgesics because of the potentially fatal adverse effects of respiratory depression, coma, and death, as well as the risks of drug misuse and dependence. Assessing for pruritus and urticaria, which may indicate an allergic reaction, is also important. Sweating may be a sign of tolerance and dependence in some patients taking morphine. Box 49.4 presents measures to recognize and manage toxicity with opioid use. Additionally, Box 49.5 identifies measures to recognize and manage withdrawal from opioids.

Patient Teaching

Box 49.6 presents patient teaching guidelines for morphine sulfate and other opioids.

| BOX 49.4 | **Recognition and Management of Toxicity With Opioid Use** |

- Acute toxicity or overdose can occur from therapeutic use or from misuse by people who are drug-dependent.
- Overdose may produce severe respiratory depression and coma.
- The main goal of treatment is to restore and maintain adequate respiratory function.
- Managed by inserting an endotracheal tube and starting mechanical ventilation or by giving an antagonist, such as naloxone.
- Emergency supplies should be readily available in any setting where opioids are used.

BOX 49.5 Prevention and Management of Withdrawal With Opioid Use

- Abstinence from opioids after chronic use produces a withdrawal syndrome characterized by anxiety; restlessness; insomnia; perspiration; pupil dilation; piloerection (goose bumps); anorexia, nausea, and vomiting; diarrhea; elevation of body temperature, respiratory rate, and systolic blood pressure; muscle cramps; and dehydration.
- Signs and symptoms in neonates include tremor, restlessness, increased muscle tone, screaming, fever, sweating, tachycardia, vomiting, diarrhea, respiratory distress, and possibly seizures.
- Although all opioids produce similar withdrawal syndromes, the onset, severity, and duration vary.
  - With morphine, symptoms begin within a few hours of the last dose, reach peak intensity in 36 to 72 hours, and subside over 8 to 10 days.
  - With methadone, symptoms begin in 1 to 2 days, peak in about 3 days, and subside over several weeks.
- Heroin, meperidine, methadone, morphine, oxycodone, and oxymorphone are associated with more severe withdrawal symptoms than other opioids.
- If an antagonist such as naloxone (Narcan) is given, withdrawal symptoms occur rapidly and are more intense but of shorter duration.
- Recognition and treatment of early, mild symptoms of withdrawal can prevent progression to severe symptoms.
  - One technique is to give the opioid from which the person is withdrawing, which immediately reverses the signs and symptoms of withdrawal. Then, dosage is gradually reduced over several days.
  - Another technique is to substitute a long-acting opioid (e.g., methadone) for a short-acting opioid. Methadone is usually given in an adequate dose to control symptoms, once or twice daily, and then is gradually tapered over 5 to 10 days.
  - In neonates undergoing withdrawal, methadone or buprenorphine may be used.

Clinical Application 49.1

- Mrs. Hoffman complains of pain in her lower back with an intensity of 7 out of 10. Her vital signs remain stable. To manage her pain, her prescriber has ordered morphine 4 to 8 mg intravenously, every 2 to 4 hours as needed, to be given over 5 minutes, as well as oxycodone 5 mg with acetaminophen 500 mg orally (after 24 hours), every 4 to 6 hours, as needed, not to exceed six doses in 24 hours. When assessing pain in Mrs. Hoffman, what are the major considerations?
- Mrs. Hoffman tells the nurse that she does not want to take morphine because she is afraid that she will become addicted. What is the best response regarding addiction to narcotics?
- What major adverse effects of analgesics should the nurse observe for in Mrs. Hoffman once the morphine is administered?

Unfolding Patient Stories: Yoa Li • Part 2

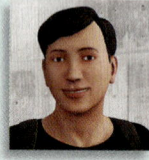

Recall Yoa Li, a 26-year-old male with a strangulated groin hernia from Chapter 32. He arrived on the medical-surgical unit following surgical repair of the hernia. What are the desired outcomes for postoperative pain management? What assessments should the nurse perform when administering morphine intravenously and evaluating Yoa's response?

Care for Yoa and other patients in a realistic virtual environment: *vSim for Nursing* (thepoint.lww.com/vSim-Pharm). Practice documenting these patients' care in DocuCare (thepoint.lww.com/DocuCareEHR).

Other Drugs in the Class

Several other opioid agonists are available and are described below and in Table 49.2. Factors such as patient variability, the type of pain (i.e., acute vs. chronic), length of administration of the previous drug, and drug tolerance may influence drug

! Quality and Safety Alert: Evidence-Based Practice

Schieber et al. (2019) explored trends and patterns of geographic variation in opioid prescribing practices in the United States by state from 2006 to 2017 and found considerable variation occurring with prescribing patterns among states. The researchers found that during this time, the number of opioids prescribed decreased, but long-term prescriptions increased. One of the six measures described is the milligrams of a prescribed opioid weighted to national and state populations for each study year. This measure, expressed as MME, is based on the opioid's analgesic potency relative to morphine. The authors used an administrative database to provide these weighted estimates of the number of retail opioid prescriptions dispensed in the United States. The study reported that each year between 2006 and 2017, an estimated 233.7 million opioid prescriptions (211.0 billion MME) met the study's inclusion criteria and were filled in retail pharmacies in the United States. In 2017, pharmacies filled enough opioid prescriptions to theoretically provide every individual living in the United States with 5 mg of hydrocodone bitartrate every 4 hours around the clock for 3 weeks. States with the greatest MME per person in 2017 were Tennessee, Oklahoma, Delaware, and Alabama. Updated information from the CDC from 2020 indicates that the five states with the greatest number of opioid prescriptions are Alabama, Arkansas, Tennessee, Louisiana, and Kentucky (https://wonder.cdc.gov/).

Trend information in state prescribing patterns may be useful when designing state-specific intervention programs. In addition, analysis of interventions used in states with the lowest MME per person may help promote a decline in trends and patterns.

BOX 49.6 Patient Teaching Guidelines for Opioid Analgesics

General Considerations

- For acute episodes of pain that occur at irregular intervals, most opioids may be taken as needed; for acute pain that occurs daily and for chronic pain, the drugs should be taken on a regular schedule, around the clock.
- When a choice of pain-relieving medication is available, use the least amount of the mildest drug that is likely to be effective in a particular situation.
- If desired effects are not achieved, report to your healthcare provider. Do not increase the dose and do not take medication more often than prescribed. Although these principles apply to all medications, they are especially important with opioid analgesics because of potentially serious adverse effects and because analgesics may mask pain for which medical attention is needed.
- Do not drink alcohol or take other drugs that cause drowsiness (e.g., some antihistamines, sedative-type drugs for nervousness or anxiety, sleeping pills) while taking opioids for pain. Combining drugs with similar effects may lead to excessive sedation and difficulty in breathing.
- Do not smoke, cook, drive a car, or operate machinery when drowsy or dizzy or when vision is blurred from medication.
- Sit or lie down at least 30 to 60 minutes after receiving an opioid by injection. Injected drugs may cause dizziness, drowsiness, and falls when walking around. If it is necessary to stand up, ask someone for assistance.
- If hospitalized, ask a healthcare provider about methods of pain management. For example, if anticipating surgery, ask how postoperative pain will be managed, how you need to report pain and request pain medication, and so on. It is better to take adequate medication and be able to cough, deep breathe, and walk around than to avoid or minimize pain medication and be unable to perform activities that promote recovery and healing. Do not object to having bed rails up or asking for assistance when receiving a strong narcotic analgesic. These are safety measures to prevent falls or other injuries because these drugs may cause drowsiness, weakness, unsteady gait, and blurred vision.
- Avoid constipation, a common adverse effect of opioid analgesics. It may be prevented or managed by eating high-fiber foods, such as whole-grain cereals, fruits, and vegetables; drinking 2 to 3 quarts of fluid daily; and being as active as tolerated. If you take these medicines for more than a few days, or if you are the caregiver for someone who takes them, ask a healthcare provider about a bowel program to prevent constipation. A possible regimen is a daily stool softener (e.g., docusate) and a daily or every other day laxative (e.g., bisacodyl), preferably started at the same time as the narcotic. Docusate and bisacodyl are available over the counter.

Self-Administration

- Take oral opioid analgesics with 6 to 8 ounces of water, with or after food to reduce nausea.
- Do not crush or chew long-acting tablets (e.g., MS Contin, OxyContin). The tablets are formulated to release the active drug slowly, over several hours. Crushing or chewing causes immediate release of the drug, with a high risk of overdose and adverse effects, and shortens the duration of pain-relieving effects.
- You may experience these side effects: nausea, loss of appetite (take the drug with food and lie quietly), constipation (notify your healthcare provider if this is severe; a laxative may help), dizziness, sedation, drowsiness, and impaired visual acuity (avoid driving or performing other tasks requiring alertness, visual acuity).
- Omit one or more doses if severe adverse effects occur, and report to a healthcare provider. Also, report a skin rash.
- Take these drugs exactly as prescribed. Avoid alcohol, antihistamines, sedatives, tranquilizers, and over-the-counter drugs.
- Do not take any leftover medication for other disorders, and do not let anyone else take your prescription medications.

---

selection. To calculate the dose of a specific opioid agonist, a prescriber may consult an equianalgesic chart, a conversion table that lists equivalent doses of these pain-relieving drugs. Table 49.3 outlines the approximate equivalent doses and equianalgesic dose ratios of common opioids.

Codeine is an opium alkaloid used for analgesic and antitussive effects. This Schedule II drug has weaker analgesic and antitussive effects and milder adverse effects than morphine. Compared with other opioid analgesics, codeine is more effective when given orally and is less likely to lead to misuse and dependence. The injected drug is more effective than the oral drug in relieving pain, but onset (15 to 30 minutes), peak (30 to 60 minutes), and duration of action (4 to 6 hours) are about the same. Half-life is about 3 hours. Larger doses are required for analgesic than for antitussive effects. Codeine is often given with acetaminophen for additive analgesic effects. The cytochrome P450 2D6 (CYP2D6) family of enzymes metabolizes the opioid to morphine in the liver, which is responsible for codeine's analgesic effects.

Quality and Safety Alert: Safety

The CYP2D6 enzyme is inherited as an autosomal recessive trait. As many as 10% of Whites, 7% of Blacks, and 5% of Asians have inadequate amounts or activity of the CYP2D6 enzymes and are classified as poor metabolizers (see Chapter 2). These individuals may therefore receive less pain relief with the usual therapeutic doses of codeine and other opioids metabolized by CYP2D6. In addition, 21% of Asians, 5% of Whites, and 5% of Blacks are classified as ultrarapid metabolizers of the CYP2D6 enzymes and quickly metabolize codeine to its morphine, its active metabolite. This increases the risk of adverse effects, including respiratory depression and CNS depression.

TABLE 49.3

Approximate Equivalent Doses and Equianalgesic Dose Ratios of Common Opioids

Drug	Approximate equivalent doses (oral immediate-release preparations)	Approximate equianalgesic dose ratio (morphine sulfate: alternate opioid)
Morphine	30 mg	1:1 (reference standard)
Codeine*	200 mg	1:7
Oxycodone	20 mg	1.5:1
Oxymorphone	10 mg	3:1
Fentanyl patch (Duragesic)	No oral equivalent	—
Hydrocodone	30 mg	1:1
Hydromorphone	7.5 mg	1:4
Tramadol	300 mg	0.1:1

*Generally not recommended with codeine due to high variability in response.

Data from *Calculating total daily dose of opioids for safer dosage*. US Centers for Disease Control and Prevention. Retrieved February 21, 2023, from https://www.cdc.gov/drugoverdose/pdf/calculating_total_daily_dose-a.pdf (Accessed on February 21, 2023).

The FDA has issued a **BOXED WARNING** regarding the cautious use of codeine in children, particularly for pain management following surgery, after reports of the death of children taking codeine who are ultrarapid metabolizers of the drug.

Prescribers sometimes order codeine for moderate pain, often with a nonopioid analgesic. The multimodal combination of opioid and nonopioid drugs produces additive analgesic effects and may allow smaller doses of opioids.

Fentanyl (Duragesic, Sublimaze, others) is a potent opioid agonist and Schedule II–controlled substance that is widely used for preanesthetic medication, postoperative analgesia, and chronic pain that requires an opioid analgesic. It has become one of the most abused opioids. Because of the high risk of respiratory depression, the drug is contraindicated in the use of acute pain, including management of headaches or migraines, or for postoperative pain outside the hospital setting. It should not be administered in patients who are **opioid-naive** (those who have not had at least 60 mg of morphine or an equianalgesic dose of another opioid for a week or longer); the FDA has issued a **BOXED WARNING** for fentanyl, reporting that fatal respiratory depression has occurred following use in opioid-intolerant patients and with improper dosing. In addition, the substitution of buccal fentanyl for any other fentanyl product may result in fatal overdose because the pharmacokinetic profiles are significantly different. There are numerous routes of administration, including IV and IM injection, transdermal application, sublingual tablets and spray, lozenges, and nasal spray. These formulations are not interchangeable on a microgram-per-microgram basis, and current dosages must be exchanged appropriately using a conversion table. The United States and Canadian guidelines differ, so it is necessary to consult the appropriate conversion table.

Duragesic is available as a transdermal formulation of fentanyl. Duragesic is for treatment of chronic and severe malignant pain. After deposition of active drug in the skin, systemic absorption slowly occurs. Duragesic has a slow onset of action (12 to 24 hours), but it lasts about 72 hours. When a Duragesic patch is removed, the drug continues to be absorbed from the skin deposits for 24 hours or longer.

With a transdermal formulation, a fast-acting formulation should be available for acute pain. An oral lozenge on a stick (Actiq) and a buccal tablet (Fentora) are approved to treat acute (breakthrough) pain in people who have been receiving opioids and have become opioid-tolerant. Because of a risk of respiratory depression, recommended dosages must not be exceeded with any formulation.

Hydrocodone (Hysingla), a Schedule III drug, is similar to codeine in its analgesic and antitussive effects. It is available only in oral combination products for cough and with acetaminophen or ibuprofen for pain. Its half-life is about 4 hours, and its duration of action is 4 to 6 hours. Hydrocodone is metabolized to hydromorphone by the CYP2D6 enzymes.

Hydromorphone (Dilaudid) is a Schedule II, semisynthetic derivative of morphine that has the same actions, uses, contraindications, and adverse effects as morphine. It is more potent on a milligram-to-milligram basis and more effective orally than morphine. Effects occur in 15 to 30 minutes, peak in 30 to 90 minutes, and last 4 to 5 hours. Hydromorphone is metabolized in the liver to inactive metabolites that are excreted through the kidneys.

Meperidine (Demerol) is a synthetic drug similar to morphine in action and adverse effects. After injection, analgesia occurs in 10 to 20 minutes, peaks in 1 hour, and lasts 2 to 4 hours. After an oral dose, about half is metabolized in the liver and never reaches the systemic circulation. Prescribers order meperidine infrequently for therapeutic purposes, mainly because it produces a neurotoxic metabolite (normeperidine). Normeperidine accumulates with chronic use, large doses, or kidney failure and produces CNS stimulation characterized by agitation, hallucinations, and seizures. The half-life of normeperidine is 15 to 30 hours, depending on kidney function, and the effects of normeperidine are not reversible with opioid antagonist drugs. Meperidine is not recommended for cancer pain management or for use in older adults.

Methadone (Methadose) is a Schedule II synthetic opioid agonist similar to morphine but with a longer duration of action. It is usually given orally, and onset and peak of action occur in 30 to 60 minutes. Effects last 4 to 6 hours initially and longer with repeated use. The usual half-life is 15 to 30 hours, and this also lengthens with repeated use. Prescribers order methadone for severe pain and in **agonist substitution treatment** in the detoxification and maintenance treatment of opiate dependence. Agonist substitution treatment is a process to treat opioid use syndrome by using a substance (such as methadone) to substitute for a strong full agonist (such as heroin) that has been abused. The FDA has issued a **BOXED WARNING** advising about serious adverse effects (e.g., death, overdose, and serious cardiac dysrhythmias) reported in patients taking methadone.

Oxycodone (OxyContin, Xtampza ER) is a derivative of codeine used to relieve moderate pain; its pharmacologic actions are similar to those of other opioid analgesics. It is a Schedule II drug of misuse. With oral administration, action starts in 15 to 30 minutes, peaks in 60 minutes, and lasts 4 to 6 hours. Its half-life is unknown. It is metabolized by the CYP2D6 enzymes and excreted through the kidneys.

An agonist narcotic, oxycodone is used, alone or in combination with acetaminophen, for the treatment of moderate-to-severe pain. The drug is available in tablets, capsules, and solutions. Immediate-release products are intended for patients who are narcotic naive. Extended-release products are intended only for patients who are opioid-tolerant. When giving extended-release products every 12 hours, the goal is to relieve pain around the clock. Thus, these effects are most useful for patients with terminal cancer or other chronic pain conditions.

Unfortunately, OxyContin is a popular drug of misuse and is associated with many deaths and much criminal activity. Most deaths have resulted from inappropriate use through diversion either (1) by chewing, crushing, and snorting through the nose or (2) crushing and injecting the drug. Chewing or crushing destroys the long-acting feature and constitutes an overdose. As a result, the FDA has issued a **BOXED WARNING** ◆ for the extended-release tablets and capsules because of serious, life-threatening, or fatal respiratory depression. Crushing, chewing, or dissolving can cause rapid release and a potentially fatal dose. As previously discussed, the FDA has approved an abuse-deterrent formulation that is designed to prevent the tablets from being chewed or crushed.

Oxymorphone, a Schedule II drug, is a derivative of morphine with actions, uses, and adverse effects similar to those of morphine. Used for acute and chronic pain and for analgesia during labor, administration can be administered IV, IM, and PO. Oral tablets are available in immediate-release and extended-release formulations. The FDA has issued **BOXED WARNING** ◆ cautioning that accidental ingestion of even one dose of extended-release oxymorphone, particularly in children, can result in a fatal overdose. Also, when taken with a high-fat meal, peak concentration is increased up to 50%; both formulations should be taken 1 hour before or 2 hours after eating.

Tramadol (Ultram, ConZip) is an oral, synthetic, Schedule IV opioid that acts at the central opioid receptors for moderate-to-severe pain. It is effective and well tolerated in older adults and in people with acute or chronic pain, back pain, fibromyalgia, osteoarthritis, and neuropathic pain. Because it has a low potential for producing tolerance and misuse, it may be used in long term for the management of chronic pain. It is not chemically related to opioids and is not a controlled drug. Its mechanism of action includes binding to mu opioid receptors and inhibiting reuptake of norepinephrine and serotonin in the brain, actions that interfere with transmission of pain signals. Analgesia occurs within 1 hour of administration and peaks in 2 to 3 hours with immediate-release tablets. Tramadol is associated with less risk of respiratory depression and constipation than morphine but carries a risk of serotonin syndrome, especially when combined with other serotonergic agents, such as the selective serotonin reuptake inhibitors, serotonin norepinephrine reuptake inhibitors, tricyclic antidepressants, and monoamine oxidase (MAO) inhibitors.

Tramadol is available in oral immediate-release tablets alone and in combination with acetaminophen as well as an extended-release tablet that can be given once daily. The drug is well absorbed after oral administration, even if taken with food. The CYP3A4 and CYP2D6 enzymes metabolize the drug, and it forms an active metabolite. Dosage reduction in people with abnormal kidney function or hepatic impairment is necessary.

NCLEX Success

1. When caring for a patient who is receiving morphine, it is most important that the nurse regularly assess for which of the following?
    A. respiratory depression
    B. hyperactive bowel sounds
    C. frequent urination
    D. insomnia

2. A patient has an order for morphine sulfate 2 mg intravenously every 2 hours following a cholecystectomy. The patient has a history of IV drug misuse. The patient reports that their pain is 7 out of 10 (with 10 being the worst) and requests the morphine every hour. What is the nurse's appropriate response?
    A. to instruct the patient about possible adverse effects
    B. to tell the patient that you can administer the drug only every 2 hours
    C. to use distraction techniques to help the patient forget the pain
    D. to notify the surgeon of the patient's request

3. The nurse is taking care of a newborn who was exposed to opioids throughout the pregnancy. Which of the following assessment findings in the newborn are associated with neonatal abstinence syndrome? (Select all that apply.)
    A. Rectal temperature of 100.6 degrees
    B. High-pitched cry
    C. Vomiting
    D. Flaccid reflexes
    E. Seizures
    F. Poor feeding
    G. Excessive weight loss.

OPIOID AGONISTS/ANTAGONISTS

Opioid agonists/antagonists act on the same pain receptors in the CNS as morphine and other opiates, resulting in interference with pain transmission and/or pain sensation. These agents have agonist activity at some receptors and antagonist activity at others. Because of their agonist activity, they are potent analgesics with a lower misuse potential than pure agonists. However, they are considered second-line drugs for treatment of moderate-to-severe pain. Because of their antagonist activity, they should not be given to people who have been receiving analgesics, and they may produce withdrawal symptoms in people with dependence. Pentazocine was the original prototype, but its use is marginal. **Butorphanol** will serve as the prototype in this discussion. Butorphanol is a synthetic, Schedule IV agonist similar to morphine in analgesic effects and ability to cause respiratory depression. Prescribers order it for moderate-to-severe pain. Administration may be parenteral; after IM or IV use, analgesia peaks in 30 to 60 minutes. Alternatively, administration may be topical to nasal mucosa by a metered spray; after nasal application, analgesia peaks within 1 to 2 hours.

Pharmacokinetics

Butorphanol is rapidly and well absorbed following IV, IM, and nasal administration. Onset of action occurs within a few minutes with IV administration and within 15 minutes with the other routes. Time to peak concentration is 20 to 40 minutes (IM) and 30 to 60 minutes (nasal), and the duration of action is usually 3 to 4 hours with IV and IM routes and 4 to 5 hours with nasal administration. The drug crosses the placenta, and it also enters breast milk.

Action

Butorphanol is an agonist of kappa opiate receptors and a partial agonist of mu opiate receptors in the CNS, causing inhibition of ascending pain pathways. The drug alters the perception of pain and produces analgesia. Like morphine, it has a sedative effect. The FDA has issued a **BOXED WARNING** with concerns that butorphanol subjects users to the risks of opioid addiction, abuse, and misuse, which can lead to overdose and death.

Use

Butorphanol is used to treat moderate-to-severe pain that has not been adequately managed with alternative treatments. The drug is also used as a preoperative medication and as a supplement to multimodal anesthesia. Table 49.4 presents dosage information for butorphanol and the other opioid agonists/antagonists.

Patient-related variables specific to the use of butorphanol include the following:

- Age:
  - The safety of butorphanol has not been established in children younger than 18 years of age.
  - In older adults, an increased frequency of adverse effects has been reported, particularly with the intranasal route; begin with a low dose at least 6 hours apart.

TABLE 49.4
DRUGS AT A GLANCE: Opioid Agonists/Antagonists

Drug	Routes and Dosage Ranges	
	Adults	**Children**
Butorphanol (Butorphanol)	IM, IV 1–4 mg every 3–4 h PRN Nasal spray 1 mg (one spray in one nostril) every 3–4 h PRN Older adults: IM 1–2 mg every 6–8 h PRN Abnormal kidney function or hepatic impairment: IM 1–2 mg every 6–8 h	Not recommended for children younger than 18 y
Buprenorphine (Butrans, Sublocade, Belbuca, Buprenex)	Heroin withdrawal IV, 0.3 to 0.9 (diluted in 50–100 mL of NS) over 20–30 min every 6–12 h with gradual tapering once symptoms resolve	Not recommended for children
Buprenorphine/naloxone (Suboxone, Bunavail, Zubsolv; Mylan-Buprenorphine/Naloxone, Suboxone)	Short-acting opioid dependency: Suboxone film, day 1, initial buprenorphine 2–4 mg/naloxone 0.5–1.0 mg film sublingually approximately every 2 h to control acute withdrawal symptoms up to total dose of buprenorphine 8 mg/naloxone 2 mg; day 2 up to buprenorphine 16 mg/naloxone 4 mg Zubsolv, day 1, initial sublingual tablet, buprenorphine 1.4 mg/naloxone 0.36 mg and to control withdrawal symptoms increase in those increments every 1.5–2 h to a total day 1 dose up to buprenorphine 5.7 mg/naloxone 1.4 mg; day 2, up to buprenorphine 4.2 mg/naloxone 2.9 mg once daily Maintenance: Bunavail, buccal film, buprenorphine 8.4 mg/naloxone 1.4 mg	≥16 y, same as adult dosage
Nalbuphine (Nubain)	IM, IV, subcutaneous 10 mg/70 kg every 3–6 h PRN; max dose in non–opioid-dependent patients: 20 mg as a single dose, max daily dose 160 mg Surgical anesthesia supplement: induction IV 0.3–3 mg/kg to 5 mg/kg over 10–15 min, maintenance doses of 0.25–0.5 mg/kg as required	≥1 y IM, IV, subcutaneous 0.1–0.2 mg/kg every 3–4 h as needed; 20 mg max as a single dose, max daily dose 160 mg
Pentazocine (Talwin)	IV, 30 mg (do not exceed) every 3–4 h (max dose 360 mg) IM, subcutaneous, 30–60 mg every 3–4 h (max dose 360 mg) Labor analgesia: IM, 30 mg once IV, 20 mg every 2–3 h PRN (max dose 60 mg)	5–8 y: IM 15 mg 9–14 y: IM 30 mg 1–16 y: preoperative/preanesthetic, IM 0.5 mg/kg

- Reproduction, pregnancy, and lactation:
  - Butorphanol injection is approved for the management of pain during labor with a fetus greater than 37 weeks of gestation and in no signs of respiratory distress; a temporary decrease in fetal heart rate is anticipated as is a risk of apnea or respiratory distress in the newborn.
  - The FDA has issued a **BOXED WARNING** ◆ regarding the risk of neonatal abstinence syndrome in newborns that may occur with prolonged maternal use of butorphanol and other opioids during pregnancy.
- Abnormal kidney function and hepatic impairment:
  - Butorphanol should be used with caution and administered at least 6 hours between doses in patients with abnormal kidney function.
  - Patients with extensive liver impairment, with decreased metabolism, may have accentuated adverse effects; administer doses at least 6 hours apart.

Adverse Effects

The adverse effects of butorphanol include headache, dizziness, drowsiness, vertigo, constipation, nausea and/or vomiting, dizziness, and euphoria. Reported effects with the nasal spray include nasal congestion, cough, dyspnea, and rhinitis. With both injection and intranasal routes, the type and incidence of adverse effects are similar to those of morphine, but butorphanol may be more likely to cause hallucinations. Also, some drugs of the opioid class, including butorphanol, produce dose-related symptoms, including delusions and/or delirium, which mimic psychosis.

Unlike morphine, the respiratory depressant action of butorphanol is subject to a **ceiling effect**; there is no further effect (in this case, respiratory depression) above a particular dosage level. The **BOXED WARNING** ◆ issued for morphine also applies to butorphanol because of its potentially fatal adverse effects of respiratory depression, coma, and death, as well as risks of drug misuse and dependence.

Contraindications

Caution is necessary when administering butorphanol to patients with acute asthma who are unmonitored or if resuscitative equipment is not available or with patients with significant respiratory depression.

Nursing Implications

Preventing Interactions

The FDA has issued a **BOXED WARNING** ◆ regarding concomitant use of intranasal butorphanol with CYP3A4 inhibitors because of the risk of increased or prolonged adverse effects, including potentially fatal respiratory depression. In addition, discontinuing a CYP3A4 inducer while taking butorphanol may result in an increased butorphanol plasma level. The nurse should be aware that alcohol and other CNS depressants add to the sedative effect of butorphanol. Concomitant use with the phenothiazines or benzodiazepines increases the risk of respiratory depression, hypotension, profound sedation, or coma.

Administering the Medication

Administration of butorphanol is by IM and IV injection or intranasal spray. Before giving IV butorphanol and other drugs together in a syringe or at a tubing Y-site, a pharmacist needs to confirm that combination is compatible.

Assessing for Therapeutic Effects

The nurse assesses for pain relief. However, tolerance can be a problem, and it may be necessary to adjust the dosage of butorphanol.

Assessing for Adverse Effects

The nurse assesses for respiratory depression, CNS depression, and possible signs of withdrawal in patients who are **opioid-tolerant** (those who have been taking at least 60 mg of morphine or an equianalgesic dose of another opioid for a week or longer). The signs of withdrawal from butorphanol include tremors and anxiety. In patients taking the nasal spray, the nurse assesses for nasal congestion cough, dyspnea, and rhinitis. When used for pain relief during labor, the nurse monitors the drug effect on the heart rate of the fetus and for the presence of apnea or respiratory distress in the newborn.

Patient Teaching

The nurse ensures that patients are instructed to notify the prescriber if the pain does not disappear, becomes worse, or changes in location or type. Patients should not stop taking butorphanol abruptly, and they should take care when changing positions quickly or operating equipment that requires mental alertness. Box 49.6 outlines additional patient teaching guidelines.

Other Drugs in the Class

Buprenorphine (Belbuca, Buprenex, Butrans, Subutex), a synthetic opioid, is approved for the treatment of acute pain, chronic pain, and opioid dependence. As a Schedule III drug, it has potential for low-or-moderate physical dependence or high psychological dependence, with a high affinity to mu-opioid receptors, providing relative resistance to the effective reversal by naloxone. It is the first drug for opioid use disorder that can be prescribed in a provider's office, significantly increasing access to treatment.

Buprenorphine is used in agonist substitution treatment. By tapering down the substitute, the patient's withdrawal symptoms and cravings are suppressed, and the effects of other opioids are blocked, thereby reducing use. This may help the patient to better engage in the recovery process to produce better outcomes.

The FDA has issued numerous **BOXED WARNING** ◆ recognizing the risk of fatal overdose from accidental exposure to buccal film and transdermal patches, especially in children. In addition, the FDA has concerns that the drug has addiction, abuse, and misuse concerns, which can lead to overdose and death and concerns about the drug's respiratory depression, and neonatal abstinence syndrome. The FDA requires an REMS for buprenorphine.

Buprenorphine also comes compounded with naltrexone to prevent injection diversion. It is dosed daily, has a long half-life, and prevents withdrawal in patients who are opioid-dependent. It can be in tablet, sublingual film, or injectable formulations. Dosages vary by the formulation of buprenorphine/naloxone. For instance, 8 mg/2 mg sublingual film is equivalent to buprenorphine/naloxone 4.2 mg/0.7 mg buccal film is equivalent to buprenorphine/naloxone 5.7 mg/1.4 mg sublingual tablet. There is a ceiling effect in which further increase above

24 mg in dosage does not increase the effects on respiratory or cardiovascular function.

Nalbuphine is a synthetic analgesic used for moderate-to-severe pain. It is not a controlled drug. Administration is IV, IM, or subcutaneous. After IV injection, action starts in 2 to 3 minutes, peaks in 15 to 20 minutes, and lasts for 3 to 6 hours. After IM or subcutaneous injection, action begins in less than 15 minutes, peaks in 30 to 60 minutes, and lasts for 3 to 6 hours. The most common adverse effect is sedation; at recommended doses, other effects are minimal.

> ### Clinical Application 49.2
> - Twenty-four hours after surgery, Mrs. Hoffman is started on oxycodone 5 mg with acetaminophen 500 mg orally, with her pain level at 3 out of 10. She can ambulate independently and is eating and voiding without difficulty. In planning for discharge, what instruction does the nurse provide to Mrs. Hoffman regarding the adverse effects of oxycodone with acetaminophen?

OPIOID ANTAGONISTS

An antagonist (antidote) reverses analgesia and the CNS and respiratory depression caused by agonists. However, an opioid antagonist does not relieve the depressant effects of other drugs, such as sedative–hypnotic, antianxiety, and antipsychotic agents. The chief clinical use of an antagonist is to relieve opioid-induced CNS and respiratory depression. The prototype of this class is **naloxone** (Narcan, Zimhi). It is essential that this drug be readily available in all healthcare settings in which opioids are given. In addition, inhaled naloxone is now available either (1) with a prescription in all states or (2) without a prescription to patients and their caregivers using narcotics for pain in many states. Some states have approved peace officers (first responders) to carry naloxone when on duty. In 2023, the FDA approved the over-the-counter availability of naloxone 4 mg nasal spray. Other formulations and dosages of naloxone remain available by prescription only.

Pharmacokinetics

Therapeutic effects occur within minutes after injection (IV [about 2 minutes], IM [2 to 5 minutes], or subcutaneous [2 to 5 minutes]) or intranasal administration (8 to 13 minutes); they last 1 to 2 hours. Naloxone has a shorter duration of action than opioids, and repeated injections are usually necessary. To combat the effects of a long-acting drug such as methadone, patients may need injections for 2 to 3 days.

Action

Naloxone (antidote) reverses analgesia and the CNS and respiratory depression caused by agonists. It is a competitive mu-opioid receptor antagonist that competes with opioids for mu-receptor sites in the brain and thereby prevents binding with receptors or displaces opioids already occupying receptor sites. When opioids cannot bind to receptor sites, they are "neutralized" and cannot exert their effects on body cells.

> ### ! Quality and Safety Alert: Evidence-Based Practice
> In a study of eight first-responders providing data on 261 attempted overdose reversals using naloxone nasal spray (4 mg dose per device), Avetian et al. (2018) found that the drug was successful in reversing opioid overdose in 98.8% (242/245) of cases, with 73.5% (125/170) having a response within 5 minutes of naloxone administration. Survival was reported in 92% (245/261 cases). The findings from these case reports support the importance of early intervention with naloxone in the reversal of opioid overdose.

Use

Naloxone has long been the drug of choice to treat respiratory depression caused by opioid overdose. Given intravenously, naloxone begins to reverse CNS and respiratory depression induced by opioids in minutes. If the IV route is unavailable, the nasal spray should be immediately administered. Table 49.5 gives dosage information for naloxone.

Patient-related variables specific to the use of naloxone include the following:

- Age:
  - Recommended route in children and adults is IV to control absorption. The endotracheal route is preferred if IV or the intraosseous route (in children) is not available. Outside the healthcare environment, intranasal spray should be used as soon as possible.
  - Cautious use is required in neonates and children with smaller kilogram-based weight dosing.
- Reproduction, pregnancy, and lactation:
  - Naloxone should not be withheld when needed in cases of maternal opioid overdose; it may precipitate fetal and/or maternal opioid withdrawal.
  - The benefits of breast-feeding to the infant and the benefits of treatment to the breast-feeding parent should be greater that the risk of infant exposure.
- Abnormal kidney function and hepatic impairment:
  - In children, kidney and hepatic function may affect the response to the medication.
  - Use of naloxone in abnormal kidney function and hepatic impairment requires caution.
  - Impaired kidney function leads to slower drug excretion.
  - Impaired abnormal kidney function and hepatic impairment increases risk of accumulation and toxicity.
- Specific healthcare environments:
  - Patients with critical illness with increased intracranial pressure, seizure disorders, head trauma, or respiratory depression should not receive naloxone.
  - Patients with coma of unknown origin may receive the drug to determine if the cause of the mental status change could result from opioids.

Adverse Effects

Adverse effects of naloxone include tremors, drowsiness, sweating, decreased respirations, hypertension, and nausea and vomiting. Naloxone itself has minimal toxicity.

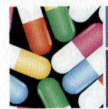

TABLE 49.5
DRUGS AT A GLANCE: Opioid Antagonists

Drug	Routes and Dosage Ranges	
	Adults	**Children**
ⓟ Naloxone (Narcan, Zimhi; ✣ Naloxone hydrochloride injection)	Overdose: IV 0.4–2 mg, repeat every 2–3 min if needed. Give IM or subcutaneously (contents of 1 autoinjector [0.4 mg]) if unable to give IV; also may give 2½ times initial IV dose via endotracheal tube Narcan nasal spray: 4 or 8 mg (contents of 1 nasal spray) as single dose; may repeat every 2–3 min in alternating nostrils until medical assistance available Postoperative reversal: IV 0.1–0.2 mg every 2–3 min until desired level of reversal is attained	Overdose: IV (preferred), intraosseous: Birth to 5 y or weight <20 kg: 0.1 mg/kg; may repeat every 2–3 min if needed ≥5 y or weight ≥20 kg: 2 mg/dose; may repeat every 2–3 min if needed
Nalmefene	Overdose: Non-opioid-dependent IV (preferred), IM, subcutaneous 0.5 mg, if no evidence of withdrawal, 1 mg 2–5 min later Opioid-dependent IV (preferred), IM, subcutaneous 0.1 mg, if no evidence of withdrawal, 0.5 mg. May repeat 1 mg 2–5 min later	Not approved for use in children
Naltrexone (Vivitrol; ✣ APO-Naltrexone, ReVia)	PO initial 25 mg, if no signs of withdrawal, 50 mg every 24 h; alternate dosing can be used with supervised administration IM, 380 mg once every 4 wk	Not approved for use in children

Contraindications

Contraindications to naloxone include known hypersensitivity to the drug and presence of narcotic misuse. The drug may precipitate withdrawal, producing tachycardia, hypertension, and violent behavior.

Nursing Implications

Assessing for Therapeutic Effects

The nurse assesses for reversal of opioid effects, including improved respiratory function and decreased sedation.

Assessing for Adverse Effects

The nurse assesses for decreased respirations and elevated blood pressure. With the use of naloxone, the nurse is prepared to repeat the dose. The return of pain is a factor to be considered.

Other Drugs in the Class

Naltrexone (Vivitrol) is an opiate antagonist that acts in the brain to prevent opiate effects (e.g., pain relief, feelings of well-being), making it effective in decreasing the desire to take opiates and in treating alcohol dependence. Professionals commonly use naltrexone as part of a complete treatment program for substance misuse (e.g., compliance monitoring, counseling, support, behavioral contract, lifestyle modification); healthcare providers administer the medication. The drug decreases the desire to drink alcohol, and the dose is based on the patient's medical condition and response to treatment.

Contraindications to naltrexone include concurrent use of opiates, including methadone. Such use can cause sudden withdrawal symptoms (see Box 49.5). After discontinuing opiates, at least 7 days should pass before a person starts taking naltrexone. To confirm the absence of opioids, healthcare providers should verify self-reporting of opioid abstinence in patients with addiction using urine analysis. If results for opioids are positive or there are signs of opiate withdrawal, a naloxone challenge test (administering small doses of naltrexone and observing for signs of withdrawal) is typically necessary. It is important to assess liver function in patients taking naltrexone because liver problems may occur.

NCLEX Success

4. A patient is difficult to arouse after IV administration of morphine sulfate. The patient has a respiratory rate of 7 breaths/min. Which of the following (with appropriate prescriber orders) are priority nursing actions? (Select all that apply.)
   A. Administer oxygen.
   B. Administer naloxone.
   C. Insert a urinary catheter.
   D. Increase the IV fluid rate.
   E. Place the patient in semi-Fowler position.

5. For an overdose of morphine sulfate, which drug should the nurse have on hand to counteract an overdose?
   A. phenytoin
   B. tramadol
   C. naloxone
   D. atropine sulfate

THE NURSING PROCESS

A concept map outlines the nursing process related to drug therapy considerations in this chapter. Additional nursing implications related to the disease process should also be considered in care decisions.

Assessment

- Assess the patient with regard to pain, initially to determine appropriate interventions to be implemented. Assess the patient after interventions are implemented. Increase data collection by interviewing family members about the patient's pain. Specific assessment data include:
  - Location. Determine the location of the pain and whether it radiates. Intensity or severity. Have the patient rate their pain utilizing an accepted scale. Assess pain in relation to time, activities, and other signs and symptoms.
  - Assess for pain on a regular schedule around the clock (e.g., every 1–2 hours). If the patient is unable to communicate needs for pain relief, as is often the case during critical illnesses, evaluate posture, body language, risk factors, and other possible indicators of pain.
- Administer analgesics before painful procedures, when indicated. Provide nursing care that does not promote tissue or muscle damage.
- For uncontrolled or unexpected pain, reassess and consider alternative causes for the pain.

Outcomes of Therapy

The patient will
- Understand the use of nonpharmacological and pharmacological therapies for pain relief.
- Maintain safety with the administration of pharmacological agents to relieve pain.
- Avoid or be relieved of pain.
- Use opioid analgesics appropriately.
- Avoid preventable adverse effects.
- Be monitored for excessive sedation and respiratory depression.
- Be able to communicate and perform other activities of daily living when feasible.

The patient and caregivers will
- Verbalize expected adverse effects of pain management medications.
- Verbalize effective management of adverse effects of pain management medications.

Nursing Interventions

- Use measures to prevent, relieve, or decrease pain when possible. General measures include those that promote optimal body functioning and those that prevent trauma, inflammation, infection, and other sources of painful stimuli. Specific interventions include the following:
- Use sterile technique when caring for wounds, urinary catheters, or IV lines.
- Use exercises, ambulation, and position changes to promote circulation and musculoskeletal function.
- Rub or massage the painful area to stimulate other nerve fibers that block the nerve fibers carrying pain signals from entering the spinal cord.
- Handle any injured tissue gently, to avoid further trauma.
- Prevent bowel or bladder distention.
- Apply heat or cold, as indicated.
- Use relaxation or distraction techniques.
- When caring for children in pain:
  - Recognize that expressions of pain may differ according to age and developmental level. Infants may cry and have muscular rigidity and thrashing behavior. Preschoolers may behave aggressively or complain verbally of discomfort. Young school-aged children may express pain verbally or behaviorally, often with regression to behaviors used at younger ages.
  - Adolescents may be reluctant to admit they are uncomfortable or need help. With chronic pain, children of all ages tend to withdraw and regress to an earlier stage of development.
- Adults and children are better able to cope with pain when they are informed about what is happening to them and are assisted in developing coping strategies.

Evaluation

- Ask patients about their levels of comfort or relief from pain.
- Observe behaviors that indicate the presence or absence of pain, including ability to complete activities of daily living.
- Observe for presence or absence of sedation and respiratory depression.
- Observe signs of drug-seeking behavior (possibly indicating dependence).

Visit **thePoint** at **http://thePoint.lww.com/Frandsen13e** for answers to NCLEX Success questions (in Appendix A), answers to Clinical Application Case Studies (in Appendix B), additional information on etiology and pathophysiology, and more!

REFERENCES AND RESOURCES

Avetian, G. K., Fiuty, P., Mazzella, S., Koppa, D., Heye, V., & Hebbar, P. (2018). Use of naloxone nasal spray 4 mg in the community setting: A survey of use by community organizations. *Current Medical Research and Opinion, 34*(4), 573–576.

CDC. (2021). *Wide-ranging online data for epidemiologic research (WONDER).* National Center for Health Statistics. http://wonder. http://wonder.cdc.gov

Cohen, S. P., & Hooten, W. M. (2019). Balancing the risks and benefits of opioid therapy: The pill and the pendulum. *Mayo Clinic Proceedings, 94*(12), 2385–2389. Elsevier.

Dowell, D., Haegerich, T., & Chou, R. (2019). No shortcuts to safer opioid prescribing. *New England Journal of Medicine, 380,* 2285–2287.

Dowell, D., Ragan, K. R., Jones, C. M., Baldwin, G. T., & Chou, R. (2022). Prescribing opioids for pain—The new CDC Clinical Practice Guideline. *New England Journal of Medicine, 387,* 2011–2013. 10.1056/NEJMp2211040

Han, Y., Yan, W., Zheng, Y., Khan, M. Z., Yuan, K., & Lu, L. (2019). The rising crisis of illicit fentanyl use, overdose, and potential therapeutic strategies. *Translational Psychiatry, 9*(1), 282. https://doi.org/10.1038/s41398-019-0625-0

International Association for the Study of Pain (IASP). (2020). https://www.iasp-pain.org/publications/iasp-news/iasp-announces-revised-definition-of-pain/

Lippincott Advisor. (2023). http://advisor.lww.com

Lyden, J., & Binswanger, I. A. (2019). The United States opioid epidemic. *Seminars in Perinatology, 43*(3), 123–131. https://doi.org/10.1053/j.semperi.2019.01.001

Portenoy, R. K., Mehta, Z., & Ahmed, E. (2023). *Cancer pain management with opioids: Optimizing analgesia.* UpToDate. Lexi-Comp, Inc.

Raja, S. N., Carr, D. B., Cohen, M., Finnerup, N. B., Flor, H., Gibson, S., Keefe, F. J., Mogil, J. S., Ringkamp, M., Sluka, K. A., Song, X.-J., Stevens, B., Sullivan, M. D., Tutelman, P. R., Ushida, T., & Vader, K. (2020). The revised International Association for the study of pain definition of pain: Concepts, challenges, and compromises. *Pain, 161*(9), 1976–1982. https://doi.org/10.1097/j.pain.0000000000001939

Rosenquist, R. (2023). *Abuse-deterrent opioids.* UpToDate. Lexi-Comp, Inc.

Schieber, L. Z., Guy, P. G., Seth, P., Young, R., Mattson, C. L., Mikosz, C. A., & Schieber, R. A. (2019). Trends and patterns of geographic variation in opioid prescribing practices by state, United States, 2006-2017. *JAMA Network Open, 2*(3), e190665. https://doi.org/10.1001/jamanetworkopen.2019.0665

Shafi, A., Berry, A. J., Sumnall, H., Wood, D. M., & Tracy, D. K. (2022). Synthetic opioids: A review and clinical update. *Therapeutic Advances in Psychopharmacology, 12,* 20451253221139616. https://doi.org/10.1177/20451253221139616

Shah, M. & Huecker, M. R. (2022 January) [Updated 2022 Sep 9]. Opioid withdrawal. In: *StatPearls* [Internet]. StatPearls Publishing. https://www.ncbi.nlm.nih.gov/books/NBK526012/

Smith, L. A., Burns, E., & Cuthbert, A. (2018). Parenteral opioids for maternal pain management in labour. *Cochrane Database of Systematic Reviews, 6,* CD007396. https://doi.org/10.1002/14651858.CD007396.pub3

Strain, E. (2023). Approach to treating opioid use disorders. *UpToDate.* Lexi-Comp, Inc.

Tucker, R. (2023). *2023 Lippincott's pocket drug guide for nurses* (11th, North America edition). Wolters Kluwer.

Yeo, Y., Johnson, R., & Heng, C. (2022). The public health approach to the worsening opioid crisis in the United States calls for harm reduction strategies to mitigate the harm from opioid addiction and overdose deaths. *Military Medicine, 187*(9–10), 244–247. https://doi.org/10.1093/milmed/usab485. https://doi.org/10.1093/milmed/usab485

CHAPTER 50

Drug Therapy With Local Anesthetics

LEARNING OBJECTIVES

After studying this chapter, you should be able to:

1. Identify the various methods of administering local anesthetic agents.
2. Recognize the symptoms of local anesthetic systemic toxicity and strategies used to manage the condition.
3. Identify the prototype, and describe the action, use, adverse effects, contraindications, and nursing implications for amide local anesthetics.
4. Identify the prototype, and describe the action, use, adverse effects, contraindications, and nursing implications for ester local anesthetics.
5. Implement the nursing process in the care of patients receiving local anesthetics.

CLINICAL APPLICATION CASE STUDY

Lexi Scruggs, a 7-year-old girl, was swinging from the monkey bars on the school playground. She lost her grip and fell, cutting her left knee on a piece of glass. At the emergency department, she requires 10 sutures to close the jagged cut. She receives lidocaine (Xylocaine) prior to cleaning and suturing the wound.

KEY TERMS

Bier block anesthesia: regional limb anesthesia provided by local anesthesia and an extremity tourniquet

Epidural anesthesia: injection of local anesthetic into the epidural space, either in the lumbar or in the thoracic spine area

Field block anesthesia: subcutaneous injection of local anesthetic around the margin of the surgical or procedural site

Local anesthetic systemic toxicity (LAST): systemic absorption of a local anesthetic agent that results in excitation of the central nervous system

Peripheral nerve block anesthesia: blocking a nerve or group of nerves, called a plexus or ganglion, to a specific area of the body

Spinal anesthesia: injection of anesthetic into the subarachnoid space of the spinal canal in the lumbar area

Topical anesthesia: application of a local anesthetic on the skin or mucous membranes

INTRODUCTION

This chapter serves two primary purposes: (1) introduce the fundamentals of local anesthesia and (2) discuss the implementation of safe perioperative nursing care during the administration of local anesthesia.

The local anesthetic agents are classified as amides and esters. The molecular structure of amide local anesthetics includes an amide linkage, while ester local anesthetics contain an ester linkage. The amide group is more commonly used in clinical practice.

OVERVIEW OF LOCAL ANESTHESIA

Local anesthetics, given to produce loss of sensation and motor activity, are injected into localized areas of the body. These agents decrease the permeability of the nerve cell membrane to ions, especially sodium. They stop the nerve from depolarizing, preventing the sodium ions from entering the nerve, which means that the nerve impulses can no longer be initiated or conducted by the anesthetized nerves. Thus, local anesthetics prevent the nerve cells from transmitting pain impulses and sensory stimulation and sending signals for skeletal muscle movement. This loss of function occurs in the following sequence: temperature, touch, proprioception, and skeletal muscle tone. These effects diminish as the drug molecules diffuse out of the neurons into the bloodstream. The drugs are then transported to the liver for metabolism to inactive metabolites and eventual excretion in the urine.

To better understand the care required for patients receiving local anesthesia, it is important to identify the types of local anesthesia. **Topical anesthesia** involves the application of a local anesthetic on the skin or mucous membrane. **Bier block anesthesia** is a regional limb anesthesia that involves a local anesthesia and the application of a tourniquet. **Peripheral nerve block anesthesia** involves blocking a nerve or group of nerves, called a plexus or ganglion, to a specific area of the body. **Field block anesthesia** is the subcutaneous injection of a local anesthetic around the margin of the surgical or procedural site. **Epidural anesthesia** is the injection of local anesthetic into the epidural space, either in the lumbar or in the thoracic spine area. Finally, **spinal anesthesia** is an anesthetic injection into the subarachnoid space of the spinal canal in the lumbar area.

Methods of Administration

There are several different methods to administer local anesthesia.

- Topical anesthesia involves the application of ointment, lotion, cream, lotion, or drop of local anesthetic to the skin or mucous membranes in the eyes, nose, throat, mouth, urethra, anus, or rectum. These preparations are used to relieve pain and itching of dermatoses, sunburn, minor skin wounds, hemorrhoids, sore throat, and other conditions.
- Bier block anesthesia involves the use of a tourniquet on an extremity; this form of anesthesia is utilized for short procedures on the hand and forearm.
- Peripheral nerve block anesthesia involves blocking a nerve or group of nerves, called a plexus or ganglion, through the injection of an anesthetic into a specific area of the body.
- Field block anesthesia involves using an anesthetic agent to block nerves en masse, not individually, to form a barrier proximal to the surgical site. This method is often used for tooth extraction.
- Neuraxial anesthesia is performed by placing a needle between vertebrae and injecting medication into the epidural space. Neuraxial blocks include epidural, spinal, and caudal blocks.

Age-Related Considerations

Local anesthetics are used in children and older adults in much the same way as they are used in adults. Nursing care should include support and reassurance, assessing for skin breakdown related to immobility and safety precautions.

Infants are at particular risk for systemic absorption and toxicity from topically applied local anesthetics. Tight diapers and occlusive dressings can increase systemic absorption.

Older adults are more at risk for adverse effects, including neurologic, cardiovascular, and dermatologic effects. They are also more prone to developing toxicity because of possible hepatic and abnormal kidney function and polypharmacy. Longer monitoring and regular reorientation and reassurance are important.

Local Anesthetic Systemic Toxicity

Although the use of local anesthetics is usually safe, they have the potential to cause toxic systemic or local reactions when administered improperly and, in some cases, may cause unintended effects even when administered appropriately. **Local anesthetic systemic toxicity (LAST)** is the most severe and life-threatening effect associated with the use of any local anesthetic. The incidence of LAST is a rare but well-recognized complication that may occur with a large overdose, particularly involving inadvertent intravascular injection. The consequences may be severe, potentially resulting in death. LAST occurs when the local anesthetic is absorbed systemically, resulting in extreme central nervous system (CNS) excitation followed by cardiovascular excitation and cardiovascular collapse. Manifestations usually occur 1 to 5 minutes after the injection but may be delayed for as long as 1 hour. Initial symptoms may include analgesia, circumoral numbness, metallic taste, tinnitus or auditory changes, and agitation. These may progress to seizure activity and then lead to symptoms of CNS depression, including coma, respiratory arrest, ventricular dysrhythmias, and cardiovascular collapse.

Treatment of LAST consists of stopping the injection of the local anesthetic immediately and attending to airway management, seizure suppression, and management of dysrhythmias, hypotension, and subsequent cardiac arrest. The use of lipid emulsion therapy with 20% lipid emulsion (lipid rescue therapy) is an effective antidote and should be started early in resuscitation process. Lipid emulsion should be available in any area where neuraxial or peripheral nerve blocks are performed, such as pre- and postanesthesia units, operating rooms, and labor and delivery suites.

> **Quality and Safety Alert: Safety**
>
> Although propofol is prepared in a lipid emulsion, it should not be substituted for a 20% lipid solution for the management of LAST because the vasodilation and cardiac depression associated with a large dose of propofol may counteract resuscitation efforts.

Table 50.1 lists the common drugs administered for local anesthesia. The use of topical anesthetics is especially important in children, who are administered local anesthesia before suturing, insertion of an intravenous (IV) line, or vaccination administration. Box 50.1 summarizes the use of topical anesthesia in children.

TABLE 50.1

Drugs Administered for Local Anesthesia

Drug Class	Prototype	Other Drugs in the Class
Amides	Lidocaine (Lidomark 1/5, Lidomark 2/5, Xylocaine, Xylocaine MPF)	Bupivacaine (Bupivacaine Fisiopharma, Bupivacaine Spinal, Marcaine Preservative Free, Marcaine Spinal, Sensorcaine, Saracoll)
		Mepivacaine (Carbocaine, Carbocaine Preservative Free, Polocaine, Polocaine Dental, Polocaine-MPF, Scandonest 3% Plain)
		Ropivacaine (Naropin)
Esters	Chloroprocaine (Clorotekal, Nesacaine, Nesacaine-MPF)	Benzocaine (Allevacaine, Anacaine, Anbesol Cold Sore Therapy, Baby Anbesol, Benz-O-Sthetic, Blistex, Cepacol INSTAMAX, GoodSense Oral Pain Relief, HurriCaine One, Hurricaine, Hurricane Snap-n-Go, HurriPak Starter Kit, Instant Oral Pain Relief Max, Ivy-Rid, Dentapaine, LolliCaine, Ora-film, Zilactin Baby)
		Tetracaine (Altacaine, Ametop)

BOX 50.1 Topical Anesthesia Used in Children

Common drugs used for topical anesthesia include the following:

- Eutectic mixture of local anesthetics (EMLA): This cream-based mixture of lidocaine and prilocaine is applied to intact skin. The cream penetrates intact skin to provide local anesthesia and decrease pain of vaccinations and venipuncture. The cream is applied at the injection site with an occlusive dressing at least 60 minutes before the vaccination or venipuncture. EMLA should never be applied to abraded skin or mucous membranes.
- Lidocaine, epinephrine, and tetracaine (LET): This combination of lidocaine (4%), epinephrine (0.1%), and tetracaine (0.5%) is an aqueous solution or gel that blocks the sensory and motor nerves. It inhibits axonal sodium channels, thus blocking conduction of action potential. Epinephrine causes local vasoconstriction, whereas lidocaine and tetracaine produce numbness and weakness. It is used for laceration repair.
- Needle-free lidocaine delivery: Lidocaine is administered by compressed gas. It reduces pain at the site of venipunctures or intravenous line insertion.
- Liposomal lidocaine (LMX 4 or LMX 5): This solution contains lidocaine encapsulated in liposomes. It is applied to intact skin with the use of an occlusive dressing.

Quality and Safety Alert: Evidence-Based Practice

Local anesthetic agents are commonly administered during labor and delivery. The most common local anesthetics used are epidural, spinal, and pudendal nerve blocks. Subcutaneous infiltration is administered before perineal tear repair. Routine use of local anesthetics may result in local anesthetic systemic toxicity (LAST). LAST is a potential complication and nurses must be aware of the signs and symptoms of toxicity. Bowsher et al. (2018) stated that the knowledge in assessing patients for adverse effects has been overlooked. Nurses need to be aware of safe maximum doses, signs and symptoms of toxicity, the immediate management of symptoms, and both the type and location of the antidote. Anesthesia providers need to inform the nurse of the maximum dose administered. Clinical features of LAST include perioral paresthesia, metallic taste in the mouth, tinnitus, dizziness, headache, muscle twitching, palpitations, seizures, confusion, cardiac arrhythmias, hypotension, shock, bradycardia, tachycardia, respiratory depression, respiratory arrest, and cardiac arrest. Anesthesia practitioners in this study were asked to name three clinical features. Overall, only 9% could name three symptoms. In conclusion, nurses caring for these patients in the postpartum phase should be able to assess and identify patients who are at risk for LAST and report to the patient's healthcare provider.

NCLEX Success

1. A 50-year-old patient is 1-day postoperative following abdominal surgery for resection of colon cancer. Which of the following pain control devices is most effective in treating their pain?
   A. lidocaine using IV regional anesthesia
   B. bupivacaine by the epidural route
   C. benzocaine by the transdermal route
   D. fentanyl citrate by patient-controlled analgesia

2. Local anesthetics reduce the excitability neuronal cell membranes by decreasing permeability to which ion?
   A. sodium
   B. potassium
   C. chloride
   D. magnesium

AMIDES

Lidocaine (Lidomark 1/5, Lidomark 2/5, Xylocaine, Xylocaine-MFP) is the prototype amide local anesthetic agent. The drug has a rapid effect, and when combined with epinephrine, this effect is prolonged. An additional discussion of lidocaine as a treatment for ventricular dysrhythmias is found in Chapter 27.

Pharmacokinetics and Action

The pharmacokinetics of lidocaine depends on the route of administration. The onset of action may be almost immediate, with a peak of 2 to 5 minutes and a duration of 30 to 120 minutes. Lidocaine has an elimination half-life of 96 minutes, and therefore, a single dose should not be repeated during this period. The drug is metabolized in the liver into two active metabolites, and most is excreted in the urine.

Lidocaine diminishes pain by blocking nerve conduction. It decreases the neuronal membrane's permeability to sodium ions. This action then inhibits the depolarization and blocks nerve conduction.

Use

Clinicians use lidocaine in its various forms to obtain local anesthesia. Specific uses include the following:

- Topical preparation: used to relieve pain associated with postherpetic neuralgia.
- Injectable solution: used for infiltration of the skin or subcutaneous administration prior to the insertion of an IV or central venous catheter, spinal, epidural, or a minor emergency procedure such as suturing or a minor surgical procedure.
  - 1% to 2% solution: administered intravenously preceding administration of a painful IV medication such as propofol (Diprivan) in the surgical arena. Lidocaine 1% to 2% is also used in conjunction with other local anesthetics to achieve epidural anesthesia, appropriate for surgical procedures, treatment of postoperative pain, or management of labor pain. In addition, it can be administered as surface anesthesia for a diagnostic procedure of the upper respiratory tract, such as a medical bronchoscopy.
  - 0.5% to 2% solution: administered for IV regional anesthesia. Bier block anesthesia, or IV regional anesthesia, is regional limb anesthesia produced by a local anesthetic such as lidocaine and a pneumatic extremity tourniquet. The tourniquet prevents lidocaine from entering the general circulation and provides a bloodless surgical field.
  - 4% solution: administered through a nebulizer and inhaled into the lungs to produce anesthesia for a diagnostic procedure, such as a bronchoscopy.
  - 2% and 4% viscous solution: administered for topical oropharyngeal anesthesia (gargle or swish, and spit for oral anesthesia, swallow for pharyngeal anesthesia), awake fiberoptic intubation and bronchoscopy, and upper endoscopy.

Patient-related variables specific to the use of lidocaine include the following:

- Age:
  - Children and adolescents should be administered lidocaine 1% or 2% preservative-free solution.
- Reproduction, pregnancy, and lactation:
  - Lidocaine injection is approved for obstetric analgesia.

Table 50.2 gives route and dosage information for lidocaine and other amide local anesthetics.

TABLE 50.2
DRUGS AT A GLANCE: Amides

Drug	Routes and Dosage Ranges	
	Adults	**Children**
Lidocaine (Lidomark 1/5, Lidomark 2/5, Xylocaine, Xylocaine-MPF, ✶ Xylocaine, Xylocaine Plain, Xylocard)	Cutaneous infiltration, maximum: 4.5 mg/kg not to exceed 300 mg, with epinephrine 500 mg; do not repeat within 2 h Infiltration, 0.5% or 1% Peripheral nerve block, 1% or 2%, 3–40 mL Epidural, 1%, 1.5%, or 2%, 20–30 mL in 3–5 mL increments, allowing time to detect toxic manifestations Topical, 1.8%–5% jelly, gel, cream, ointment, solution, patch, spray	Anesthesia, local injectable, 5 mg/kg/dose not to exceed adult maximum dose of 300 mg/dose; do not repeat within 2 h; administer lowest concentrations to allow for larger volumes
Bupivacaine (Bupivacaine Fisiopharma, Bupivacaine Spinal, Marcaine Preservative Free, Marcaine Spinal, Sensorcaine, Saracoll; ✶ Marcaine, Marcaine Spinal, Sensorcaine)	Cutaneous infiltration, maximum single dose 175 mg, with epinephrine 200 mg Local anesthesia, 0.25% Spinal, 0.75% in 8.25% dextrose, 1–2 mL Epidural, 0.25% or 0.5%, 20–30 mL in 3–5 mL increments, allowing time to detect toxic manifestations Caudal, 0.25% or 0.5%, 15–30 mL Peripheral nerve block, 0.25% or 0.5%, 3–40 mL, maximum 400 mg/d	≥12 y, same as adults Caudal, 0.25%, 0.5–1.3 mL/kg, maximum drug volume 20 mL, not to exceed 2 mg/kg or 3 mg/kg with epinephrine
Mepivacaine (Carbocaine, Carbocaine Preservative-Free, Polocaine, Polocaine Dental, Scandonest 3% Plain; ✶ Carbocaine, Polocaine)	Maximum single dose, 300 mg, with epinephrine 500 mg Maximum dose per 24 h, 1,000 mg Infiltration, 0.5% or 1%, up to 40 mL of 1%, up to 50 mL with epinephrine Therapeutic block pain management, 1–5 mL of 1% (maximum 50 mg) or 1–5 mL of 2% (maximum: 100 mg) Caudal and epidural block, 15–30 mL of 1% (max 200 mg) or 10–25 mL (max 375 mg) or 10–20 mL of 2% (max 400 mg)	Local or regional anesthesia: max single or total dose 5–6 mg/kg (to adult max); only concentration <2% should be used in children <3 y or <14 kg
Ropivacaine (Naropin; ✶ Naropin)	Maximum single dose, 200 mg, with epinephrine 250 mg Infiltration, 0.2% or 0.5% Epidural, 0.5%, 0.75%, or 1%, 15–30 mL Peripheral nerve block, 0.5% or 0.75%, 10–40 mL	Caudal, 0.2%, 0.5–1.25 mL/kg, not to exceed 2 mg/kg Epidural, 0.2%, 0.7 mL/kg (wait 45 min for repeat dosing, reduce dose by 1/3–1/2)

Adverse Effects

Adverse effects of lidocaine are often dose related and vary with the route of administration. They include allergic reactions (e.g., skin rash; itching; hives; swelling of the face, lips, or tongue), swelling, burning and pain at application site, headache, shivering, and nausea and vomiting.

Contraindications

A known hypersensitivity or allergic reaction to an amide local anesthetic rules out the use of lidocaine in any form. Any patient may experience hypersensitivity reactions to any local anesthetic. If lidocaine is combined with sulfites, the patient may develop a laryngospasm. Other contraindications include severe trauma, sepsis, blood dyscrasias, and cardiac abnormalities, including heart block.

Nursing Implications

Preventing Interactions

Medications that increase the effects of lidocaine are found in Box 50.2. St. John's wort decreases the serum concentration of the anesthetic.

Administering the Medication

The nurse ensures that the appropriate preparation of lidocaine is administered properly. For topical anesthesia, it is necessary to

- Apply the gel formulation to the skin of the affected area, approximately 1/8 in thick. The area becomes numb in 20 to 60 minutes.
- Swish the oral solution in the mouth and then spit it out. When pharyngeal anesthesia is needed, the patient gargles and then swallows the medication.
- Apply Lidoderm to the most painful area of the skin. Patients should not expose this preparation to an external heat source such as a heating pad.
- Apply the lido patch (lidocaine and menthol) to the most painful area of the skin after removing the protective film. First, remove the old patch and cleanse the skin.
- Use a nebulizer following dilution in normal saline or sterile water.

Quality and Safety Alert: Safety

Although lidocaine is administered intravenously for specific conditions (e.g., to mitigate venous irritation with propofol administration and for ventricular dysrhythmias), only a qualified provider should administer the injectable form of lidocaine for a neuraxial or peripheral nerve block. When administering lidocaine for a peripheral nerve block, the practitioner will aspirate prior to starting the injection and then every 5 mL thereafter (for larger injection volumes) to prevent accidental intravenous injection.

Assessing for Therapeutic Effects

The therapeutic effect of lidocaine is dependent on the route of administration, concentration of the medication, vascularization of the site, and the patient's physical condition. The nurse

BOX 50.2 Drug Interactions: Lidocaine

Drugs That Increase the Effects of Lidocaine
- Antidysrhythmic drugs (amiodarone, dronedarone, beta-adrenergic blockers mexiletine), barbiturates, conivaptan, and darunavir
  Increase serum concentration
- Procainamide
  Increases the neurologic and cardiac effects

assesses the patient's sense of touch at 2 to 5 minutes after the application of lidocaine to determine if the patient is experiencing numbness at the site. It is also important to ask the patient if they sense any pain, pressure, or discomfort. The nurse should ask the patient questions throughout the procedure to determine if sensation is returning to the site.

Assessing for Adverse Effects

The nurse assesses the skin for redness, hives, or rash, indicating a hypersensitivity reaction. It is necessary to assess the respiratory status and lung sounds for signs of bronchospasm related to hypersensitivity. (Respiratory adverse effects are more common when lidocaine is administered by nebulizer.) The nurse observes for CNS symptoms (i.e., altered taste, anxiety, agitation, paresthesia), which typically occur before seizure activity. Also, the nurse assesses the cardiovascular status for tachycardia and hypertension, leading to cardiovascular collapse. Ongoing patient monitoring should occur after administration of the drug for at least 12 hours because cardiovascular depression due to local anesthetics can persist or recur.

Quality and Safety Alert: Safety

Facilities that commonly administer local anesthetics in doses sufficient to produce LAST are more prepared to correct this medical emergency if they have an established and regularly reviewed plan for management of LAST as well as a readily available local anesthetic toxicity kit and instructions for its use. This kit includes 20% Intralipid (20% IV fat emulsion). Any site where regional anesthesia is administered should have this available.

Patient Teaching

Box 50.3 identifies patient teaching guidelines for lidocaine.

BOX 50.3 Patient Teaching Guidelines for Lidocaine

- Report pain.
- Report tachycardia and anxiety.
- Do not drink fluids or eat after gargling with viscous lidocaine for at least 60 minutes due to risk of aspiration.
- Prior to applying lido patch, remove the old patch, cleanse the skin, and apply the new patch to the most painful site.
- When numbness dissipates following epidural or spinal anesthesia, do not ambulate without assistance until instructed to do so.

Other Drugs in the Class

Bupivacaine (Bupivacaine Fisiopharma, Bupivacaine Spinal, Marcaine Preservative free, Marcaine Spinal, Sensorcaine, Saracoll) is used for local, regional, epidural, and spinal anesthesia for diagnostic and therapeutic procedures. The drug is more potent and has a longer duration of action than lidocaine, procaine, or mepivacaine. Consequently, if systemically absorbed, the drug has a higher risk of toxicity than most other local anesthetics, and patients often have seizures as the first manifestation of toxicity. It is important to administer a test dose before the full dosage and ensure that resuscitative equipment is available. Bupivacaine is contraindicated for local infiltration in pregnancy. The FDA has issued a **BOXED WARNING** alerting providers to the risk in obstetrical patients of cardiac arrest with difficult resuscitation or death with the use of 0.75% concentration of bupivacaine for epidural anesthesia. Caution should be used with the drug in older, debilitated, and acutely ill patients. The 0.75% concentration is used for spinal anesthesia, typically for surgical procedures where a high degree of muscle relaxation and prolonged effects are necessary, including when prolonged postprocedure pain control is preferred.

Mepivacaine (Carbocaine, Polocaine) is used to produce local or regional analgesia. It is also used for local infiltration, peripheral neural, and central neural with epidural and caudal anesthesia. Adverse effects include hypersensitivity and LAST.

> **Quality and Safety Alert: Safety**
>
> Bupivacaine is highly cardiotoxic and should never be administered intravenously or for Bier block anesthesia.

NCLEX Success

3. Which of the following medications prolongs the effect of local anesthetics?
   A. propofol
   B. epinephrine
   C. calcium
   D. labetalol

4. A patient has been administered lidocaine via an epidural. Which of the following symptoms indicate the patient is having an adverse reaction to the anesthesia? (Select all that apply.)
   A. blood pressure of 130/86 mm Hg
   B. metallic taste in mouth
   C. pulse rate of 76 beats/min
   D. crackles in the right lower lobe of the lung
   E. circumoral numbness
   F. anxiety

Clinical Application 50.1

- How does lidocaine produce numbness in Lexi's knee?
- What assessments does the nurse make to determine whether Lexi is anesthetized so that the wound can be cleaned?

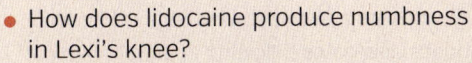
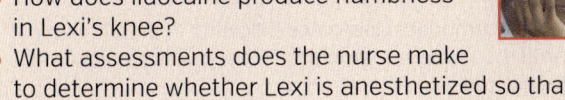

ESTERS

Chloroprocaine hydrochloride (Clorotekal, Nesacaine, Nesacaine-MPF) serves as the prototype ester local anesthetic. While allergic reactions to local anesthetics are rare, the decreasing use of the esters has further reduced their frequency, as most are due to para-aminobenzoic acid, a common metabolite of esters. Ester local anesthetics are metabolized in the blood by plasma cholinesterase (pseudocholinesterase).

Pharmacokinetics

Chloroprocaine is absorbed rapidly at the injection site. The onset of action is 6 to 12 minutes, with a duration of 1 hour. The serum half-life varies with the age of the patient. In adults, the half-life elimination is 20 to 25 seconds; in neonates, half-life elimination is about 43 seconds. The drug is rapidly metabolized in the liver into two active metabolites, and most is excreted in the urine unchanged. Chloroprocaine exhibits rapid onset, which can be further enhanced by increasing the concentration (3% preparation compared to 2%). As a result of rapid metabolism, it has a short duration of action.

Action

The action of chloroprocaine is similar to that of lidocaine. Chloroprocaine reversibly decreases the influx of sodium into the nerve cell and depresses depolarization to prevent conduction of the nerve impulse.

Use

Chloroprocaine is used to produce local anesthesia by nerve block, infiltration, or neuraxial blocks. The utility of chloroprocaine is generally limited to epidural anesthesia where a very rapid onset is desired (emergent cesarean section). Chloroprocaine's short duration of action limits its use otherwise, though a preservative-free preparation has seen increased use in spinal anesthesia for short outpatient procedures.

> **Quality and Safety Alert: Safety**
>
> Chloroprocaine is available with and without preservatives. Chloroprocaine with preservatives should not be used for neuraxial anesthesia.

Patient-related variables specific to the use of chloroprocaine include the following:

- Age:
  - In children and older adults, reduce dosage consistent with age and physical status.
- Reproduction, pregnancy, and lactation:
  - Chloroprocaine crosses the placenta, but exposure to the fetus is limited due to the short maternal half-life. It may cause varying degrees of maternal, fetal, or neonatal toxicity involving the CNS, peripheral vascular tone, and cardiac function.
  - It is unknown if chloroprocaine is present in breast milk.

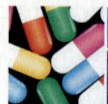

TABLE 50.3

DRUGS AT A GLANCE: Esters

Drug	Routes and Dosage Ranges	
	Adults	Children
ⓟ **Chloroprocaine** (Clorotekal, Nesacaine, Nesacaine-MPF)	Max single dose, 800 mg, with epinephrine 1,000 mg Infiltration, 1% or 2% Spinal, 1%, 20-60 mg Epidural or caudal, 2% or 3%, 15–25 mL Peripheral nerve block, 1% or 2%, 0.5–10 mL	Max dose (without epinephrine), 11 mg/kg Infiltration, 0.5% or 1% Peripheral nerve block, 1%–1.5%
Benzocaine (Allevacaine, Anacaine, Anbesol Cold Sore Therapy, Baby Anbesol, Benz-O-Sthetic, Blistex, Cepacol INSTAMAX, GoodSense Oral Pain Relief, HurriCaine One, Hurricaine, Hurricane Snap-n-Go, HurriPak Starter Kit, Instant Oral Pain Relief Max, Ivy-Rid, Dentapaine, LolliCaine, Ora-film, Zilactin Baby)	Topical anesthesia, oral: gel or spray 20%: apply a small amount to mucosa to achieve topical anesthesia Topical, external: ointment 5%, spray 5% and 20%: apply to affected area or use 1 spray up to 3–4 times daily as needed	Check product insert for pediatric dosage
Tetracaine (Altecaine; 🍁 Ametop)	Topical anesthesia, ocular: 1–2 drops of 0.5%, can repeat every 5–10 min up to 5 doses Spinal anesthesia, 2–15 mg; dosage varies with anesthetic procedure	Check product insert for pediatric dosage

Table 50.3 gives route and dosage information for chloroprocaine and other ester local anesthetics.

Adverse Effects

The most severe adverse effects of chloroprocaine, as with lidocaine, include LAST and hypersensitivity reactions.

Contraindications

Contraindications include known hypersensitivity to chloroprocaine or similar drugs that contain para-aminobenzoic acid. Patients with pseudocholinesterase deficiency may exhibit a longer duration of action.

Nursing Implications

Preventing Interactions

Sulfonamides and antihypertensive drugs may cause hypotension. In addition, St. John's wort decreases the serum concentration of chloroprocaine.

Assessing for Therapeutic Effects

Assessing the effects of chloroprocaine is the same as for lidocaine. The therapeutic effect of chloroprocaine is dependent on the route of administration, concentration of the medication, vascularization of the site, and the patient's physical condition. It is necessary to assess the sense of touch and to ask the patient if they sense any pain, pressure, or discomfort.

Assessing for Adverse Effects

The nurse assesses the skin for redness, hives, or rash, indicating a hypersensitivity reaction. It is necessary to assess the respiratory status and lung sounds for signs of bronchospasm related to hypersensitivity. The nurse assesses the CNS for excitability and the cardiovascular status for tachycardia and hypertension, leading to cardiovascular collapse.

Do not use solutions if crystals, cloudiness, or discoloration is present.

Patient Teaching

Box 50.4 identifies patient teaching guidelines for chloroprocaine.

Other Drugs in the Class

Benzocaine (Anacaine, Anbesol, Benz-O-Sthetic, Blistex, Cepacol, Dentapaine, Topex Topical Anesthetic) is a topical ester local anesthetic in many over-the-counter (OTC) products applied for skin irritation related to minor burns, sunburns, and insect bites. There are several other trade names for benzocaine; those listed are most common. Application of the 5% to 20% topical solution relieves hemorrhoid pain. The use of oral solutions relieves mouth and gum irritation, such as teething pain in infants greater than or equal to 2 years of age.

BOX 50.4 Patient Teaching Guidelines for Chloroprocaine

- Following dental procedures, do not eat or drink until numbness disappears and swallowing reflex is intact.
- When numbness dissipates following epidural or spinal anesthesia, do not ambulate without assistance until instructed to do so.
- Report anxiety, rash, hives, or redness.

> **! Quality and Safety Alert: Safety**
>
> Benzocaine has an FDA warning against use of OTC oral preparations in infants and children less than 2 years of age due to the potential for development of methemoglobinemia, a condition where the oxygen carrying capacity of hemoglobin is greatly diminished.

NCLEX Success

5. A child returns to school after a dental procedure requiring anesthesia. He visits the school nurse's office to take his pain medication. The most important assessment the nurse should make before administering the pain medication is to assess the
   A. prescription for an expiration date
   B. child's blood pressure and pulse
   C. child's mouth for bleeding
   D. child's mouth for numbness

Tetracaine is a topical, ophthalmic, and spinal anesthetic that is metabolized in the liver and excreted in the urine. The topical preparation can be applied to the skin prior to IV catheter placement or venipuncture. While the topical form should not be applied to the eyes, ears, mucous membranes, or broken skin, ophthalmic drops are instilled in the eye for ocular procedures. When administering the drops, ensure that the applicator does not touch the eye. Spinal anesthesia is accomplished by the injection of tetracaine in the subarachnoid space. The patient is at risk for cardiac arrest if the medication is administered too rapidly. As with any neuraxial or regional nerve block, it is important to have resuscitation equipment available.

Clinical Application 50.2

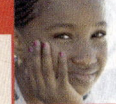

- What does the nurse teach Lexi's mother about the anesthetic?

THE NURSING PROCESS

A concept map outlines the nursing process related to drug therapy considerations in this chapter. Additional nursing implications related to the disease process should also be considered in care decisions.

Assessment
- Assess the patient's status in relation to the application and response of the local anesthetic.
- Assess his or her understanding of the administration of the topical, spinal, and epidural anesthesia.
- Interview him or her regarding any past experience with anesthesia, particularly the development of LAST.
- Identify what medications, both prescription and over-the-counter or complementary and alternative therapies, he or she is taking.
- Assess his or her skin integrity.
- If the patient is to receive local anesthesia for treatment of an injury, assess his or her psychosocial response to the injury and administration of local anesthesia.
- If the patient is to receive local anesthesia for a procedure, assess his or her vital signs preprocedure, immediately following the administration of the local anesthetic, throughout the procedure, and postprocedure.

Outcomes of Therapy
The patient will
- Experience a reduced level of anxiety in the preprocedure and postprocedure phases.
- Understand the benefits and risks of local anesthesia.
- Have no adverse effects from local anesthesia.
- Understand the expected outcome or limitations of local anesthesia, including the following:
  - Postprocedure pain
  - Limited mobility
  - Recovery

Nursing Interventions
- Instruct the patient to report symptoms of redness, hives, or rash.
- Instruct the patient to report anxiety.
- Provide accurate information to the patient regarding surgery, emergency care, the diagnostic procedure, or during the obstetrical delivery.
- Assess the patient's psychosocial status.
- Monitor vital signs before, during, and after the local anesthetic has been administered.
- Instruct the patient about postanesthesia care.

Evaluation
- Be familiar with your institution's practice guidelines and benchmark goals to help direct therapy and evaluate recovery from anesthesia.
- Observe that patient planning/goals are met.
- Assess the effectiveness of perioperative nursing interventions and medication therapy.

Visit thePoint® *at* **http://thePoint.lww.com/Frandsen13e** *for answers to NCLEX Success questions (in Appendix A), answers to Clinical Application Case Studies (in Appendix B), and more!*

REFERENCES AND RESOURCES

AORN. (2023). Strategies to prevent local anesthetic system toxicity. *AORN Journal*, 117(1), 1–10. doi:10.1002/aorn13860

Baldor, R., & Mathes, B. M. (2022). Digital nerve block. In M. Ganetsky (Ed.), *UpToDate*. Wolters Kluwer.

Bowsher, G. M., Deepak, S., & Edwards, A. (2018). Multidisciplinary knowledge of local anaesthetic system toxicity in maternity care: A pilot study. *British Journal of Midwifery*, 26(2), 103–108.

Butterworth, J. F., & Lahaye, L. (2022). Clinical use of local anesthetics in anesthesia. In M. Crowley (Ed.), *UpToDate*. Wolters Kluwer.

Flood, P., & Rathmell, J. P. (2021). *Stoelting's pharmacology & physiology in anesthetic practice* (6th ed.). Wolters Kluwer.

Gabriel, R. A., Swisher, M. W., Sztain, J. F., Furnish, T. J., Ilfeld, B. M., & Said, E. T. (2019). State of the art opioid-sparing strategies for postoperative pain in adult surgical patients. *Expert Opinion on Pharmacotherapy*, 20(8), 949–961.

Gropper, M., Cohen, N. H., Eridsson, L. I., Fleisher, L. A., Wiener-Kronish, J. P., & Young, W. L. (2019). *Miller's anesthesia* (9th ed.). Elsevier Saunders.

Hoffman, J. M., McLaren, A. C., Glass, C. M., & Overstreet, D. J. (2023). Extended release of bupivacaine from temperature-responsive hydrogels provides multi-day analgesia for postoperative pain. *Pain Medicine*, 24(2), 113–121. doi:10.1093/pm/pnac119

Hsu, D. C. (2022a). Subcutaneous infiltration of local anesthetics. In M. Ganetsky (Ed.), *UpToDate*. Wolters Kluwer.

Hsu, D. C. (2022b). Clinical use of topical anesthetics in children. In J. F. Wiley (Ed.), *UpToDate*. Wolters Kluwer.

Iseki, T., Tsukada, S., Wakui, M., Kurosaka, K., & Yoshiya, S. (2019). Percutaneous periarticular multi-drug injection at one day after arthroplasty as a component of multimodal pain management: A randomized control trial. *BioMed Central*. 20, 61. https://doi.org/10.1186/s12891-019-2451-1

Jiang, J., & Tang, T. (2022). Allergy to local anesthetics is a rarity: Review of diagnostics and strategies for clinical management. *Clinical Reviews in Allergy & Immunology*. https://doi.org/10.1007/s12016-022-08937-x

Lippincott Advisor. (2022). *Drug information*. Wolters Kluwer Publishing.

Neal, J. M., Neal, E. J., & Wienberg, G. L. (2021). American Society of Regional Anesthesia and Pain Medicine Local Anesthetic Systemic Toxicity checklist: 2020 version. *Regional Anesthesia and Pain Medicine*, 43, 150–153.

Norris, T. L. (2019). *Porth's Pathophysiology: Concepts of altered health status* (10th ed.). Wolters Kluwer.

Patacsil, J. A., McAuliffe, M. S., Feyh, L. S., & Sigmon, L. L. (2016). Local anesthetic adjuvants providing the longest duration of analgesia for single-injection peripheral nerve blocks in orthopedic surgery: A literature review. *AANA Journal*, 84(2), 95–103.

Schatz, M. (2020). Allergic reactions to local anesthetics. In A. M. Fedweg (Ed.), *UpToDate*. Wolters Kluwer.

Suresh, S., Ecoffey, C., & Bosenberg, A. (2018). The European society of regional anaesthesia and pain therapy/American society of regional anesthesia and pain medicine recommendations on local anesthetics and adjuvants dosage in pediatric regional anesthesia. *Regional Anesthesia and Pain Medicine*, 43(2), 211–216.

Tayeb, B. O., Eidelman, A., Eidelman, C. L., McNicol, E. D., & Carr, D. B. (2017). Topical anaesthetics for pain control during repair of dermal laceration. *Cochrane Database of Systematic Reviews*, 2, CD005364. doi:10.1002/14651858.CD005364.pub3

UpToDate. (2022). *Drug information*. Lexi-Comp, Inc.

Wick, E. D., Grant, J. C., & Wu, C. L. (2017). Postoperative multimodal analgesia pain management with nonopioid analgesics and techniques: A review. *JAMA Surgery*, 152(7), 691–697.

CHAPTER 51

Drug Therapy With General Anesthetics

LEARNING OBJECTIVES

After studying this chapter, you should be able to:

1. Define general anesthesia.
2. Describe the three phases of general anesthesia.
3. Identify the fundamental principles of balanced anesthesia.
4. Describe how inhalation anesthetics are delivered, and describe how this process is different from intravenous anesthetics.
5. Identify the prototype and describe the action, use, adverse effects, contraindications, and nursing implications for the inhalation and intravenous general anesthetic agents.
6. Identify the prototype and describe the action, use, adverse effects, contraindications, and nursing implications for the neuromuscular blocking agents.
7. Identify the prototype and describe the action, use, adverse effects, contraindications, and nursing implications for the adjuvant medications administered to patients receiving general anesthesia.
8. Implement the nursing process in the care of patients receiving general anesthesia.

CLINICAL APPLICATION CASE STUDY

Harriet Wilberson, 60-year-old woman with a body mass index (BMI) greater than 30, has chronic cholecystitis and a history of allergic asthma. Despite dietary modification, she continues to have right abdomen pain, nausea, and bloating sensation. Ms. Wilberson believes that her numerous food allergies are the cause of these symptoms. She is scheduled for a laparoscopic cholecystectomy in an ambulatory surgical facility. Because Ms. Wilberson has an anaphylactic penicillin allergy, the surgeon has ordered preoperative intravenous gentamicin and clindamycin. The anesthesia practitioner has completed a preanesthetic evaluation and plans to administer a general endotracheal anesthetic. You are the nurse assigned to her care.

KEY TERMS

Amnesia: memory loss (of limited duration in anesthesia)

Analgesia: reduction or absence of pain

Balanced anesthesia: four elements of general anesthesia (amnesia, analgesia, hypnosis, and muscle relaxation) achieved by a combination of medications to produce a state of physiologic and pharmacologic equilibrium

Emergence: return to consciousness from general anesthesia

Fasciculation: transitory muscle contractions that occur after the administration of a depolarizing muscle relaxant

General anesthesia: medication-induced reversible unconsciousness with loss of protective reflexes

Hypnosis: unconsciousness

Induction: rendering the patient unconscious by using inhalation anesthetics, intravenous anesthetics, or both

Maintenance anesthesia: administering a continuous level of inhalation and/or intravenous anesthetic to sustain general anesthesia until the procedure is complete

Malignant hyperthermia: potentially fatal hypermetabolic response after exposure to volatile inhalation anesthetics or the drug succinylcholine

Minimum alveolar concentration: quantitative measure of the potency of inhalation anesthetics

Monitored anesthesia care: sedation administered by an anesthesia practitioner

Rapid sequence induction: intubation procedure that uses cricoid pressure and omits face mask ventilation to reduce the risk of aspiration

Residual neuromuscular blockade: inadequate reversal or no reversal from the effects of nondepolarizing neuromuscular blocking agents (formerly known as recurarization)

Total intravenous anesthesia (TIVA): a method of general anesthesia that replaces the inhalation agent with an intravenous anesthetic for the induction and maintenance of anesthesia

INTRODUCTION

This chapter introduces the fundamentals of general anesthesia and the implementation of nursing care during the administration of general anesthesia. The administration of general anesthesia is a complex task that requires the expertise of a certified registered nurse anesthetist (CRNA), anesthesiologist (physician), or both. The CRNA and anesthesiologist may practice independently or as a team. They are physically present and actively providing care during the entire anesthetic process.

In some circumstances, complications from anesthesia can be immediately life threatening. To promote patient safety, the operating room and postanesthesia care unit (PACU) must be controlled environments. With knowledge of anesthesia drug classes and their actions, the nurse can recognize adverse consequences and intervene to avoid detrimental outcomes. The nurse must have an organized differential approach to clinical problems. It is necessary to provide lifesaving interventions and then seek the cause of the difficulty. Airway, breathing, circulation, and supplemental oxygen is an important approach to all clinical problems. Fortunately, present-day anesthetic medications are generally safe with rapid onset and recovery.

The goal of this chapter is to learn the basic aspects of anesthesia and anesthetic medications. Because this chapter is not about medication therapy for a disease process, the content focuses on understanding the medications, adverse effects (or after effects), and nursing care.

OVERVIEW OF GENERAL ANESTHESIA

General anesthesia is defined as a medication-induced reversible unconsciousness with loss of protective reflexes. There is the misconception that general anesthesia is a deep sleep. It is much deeper and more like a drug-induced coma. Arousal, even to painful stimuli, cannot occur. Therefore, it is possible to perform surgery or other unpleasant therapeutic or diagnostic procedures such as endoscopy or interventional radiology that would be unreasonable or impossible to accomplish in a conscious person.

Clinical Manifestations

The concept of using several drugs to achieve a state of physiologic and pharmacologic equilibrium under general anesthesia is called **balanced anesthesia**. Balanced anesthesia refers to the following four elements of general anesthesia, which are designed to work collectively to produce a state of physiologic and pharmacologic equilibrium and superior outcome of each:

1. **Amnesia** or memory loss (of limited duration in anesthesia)
2. **Analgesia** or a reduction or absence of pain
3. **Hypnosis** or unconsciousness
4. Muscle relaxation or immobility

Suppression of the sympathetic nervous system in response to noxious stimuli is also desired. Depending on the procedure, the anesthesia practitioner combines one or more of these elements by selecting appropriate medications. Generally, a major surgical procedure that requires tracheal intubation requires all of these elements to some degree.

Drug Therapy

Selection of anesthesia and adjuvant medications depends on a variety of conditions, including the requirements of the procedure; the patient's age, health status, medical conditions, weight, drug allergies, and results of laboratory or diagnostic tests; and the patient's and/or surgeon's preferences (if relevant). Using this information, the anesthesia practitioner develops a plan of care that maintains the patients' health and physiologic homeostasis.

The administration of a general anesthetic can be divided into three phases. The first phase is **induction**, or rendering the patient unconscious by using inhalation anesthetics, intravenous anesthetics, or both. Adult patients usually receive a rapid-acting intravenous anesthetic medication. Pediatric patients more often breathe an inhalation anesthetic through a face mask. Called a mask induction, this allows an anesthesia practitioner or a nurse to perform the venipuncture for intravenous solutions after the patient is under general anesthesia. Before induction, the patient, whether adult or child, may receive a benzodiazepine that provides rapid anxiolytic and amnestic effects. The induction phase also includes securing and maintaining a patent airway.

The next phase is maintenance or **maintenance anesthesia**, which is administering a continuous level of inhalation and/or intravenous anesthetics until the procedure is complete. Adjunctive medications may be used at this time, such as antiemetics (see Chapter 38), opioids (see Chapter 49), nonopioid analgesics, local anesthetics, and neuromuscular blocking agents.

The concluding phase is **emergence**. As the procedure ends, the general anesthetic medications are stopped, and the patient is permitted to wake up and return to a state of consciousness. As the patient emerges from the anesthetic, the anesthesia practitioner may use medications to reverse the effects of neuromuscular blocking agents. The patient is then transported to the PACU or perhaps the intensive care unit (ICU) for close observation, monitoring of vital signs and neurologic status, and additional nursing or medical care.

Five drug classes are used to achieve balanced anesthesia: benzodiazepines, analgesics, inhalation anesthetics, intravenous anesthetics, and neuromuscular blocking agents. Benzodiazepines or inhalation anesthetics are used to achieve amnesia. Opioid or nonopioid medications are used to achieve analgesia. Inhalation or intravenous anesthetics are used to achieve hypnosis. Neuromuscular blocking agents and, to some extent, inhalation anesthetics are used to achieve muscle relaxation. Within each class, every medication has unique properties that determine onset, duration, elimination, and other characteristics. The anesthesia practitioner can select from several medications in each class to achieve balanced anesthesia. Knowledge of the synergistic, additive, or antagonistic effects of anesthetic medications helps inform the appropriate dose and combination.

Nurses should be aware that the U.S. Food and Drug Administration (FDA) warns that lengthy or repeated use of general anesthetic and sedation drugs during surgeries or procedures in pediatric patients younger than 3 years or in pregnant patients during their third trimester may affect the fetus or child's neurologic development.

Table 51.1 lists the general anesthetics and neuromuscular blocking agents discussed in this chapter.

INHALATION ANESTHETICS

Inhalation anesthetics are volatile organic liquids administered by inhalation for induction and maintenance of general anesthesia. Volatile means having the ability to evaporate readily and release a gas. Today's volatile inhalation anesthetics are halogenated ethers, which contain fluorine. The stability of the fluorine carbon bond helps reduce solubility, decreasing metabolism and organ toxicity. **Isoflurane** (Forane), an extremely physically stable methyl ethyl ether, is the prototype inhalation anesthetic. Although not the first inhalation anesthetic introduced for clinical use, it is the oldest of three remaining volatile inhaled anesthetics used in the United States. After isoflurane's introduction in 1981, it quickly replaced competitors due to its improved potency, low tissue solubility and metabolism, and chemical responses. Currently, it is the most potent inhalation anesthetic available. Isoflurane has a mild pungent or ethereal odor and can irritate the airways when concentration increases. Therefore, it does not lend itself to inhalation mask inductions. However, it makes an excellent maintenance anesthetic after using an intravenous induction medication.

Pharmacokinetics

Inhalation of isoflurane results in its delivery as a gas to the lungs. From there, it diffuses rapidly into the arterial vascular system, travels throughout the vascular system, and crosses the blood–brain barrier. As the inhaled concentration of the anesthetic increases or decreases, the depth of anesthesia also changes. Several factors determine the speed of onset, but the desired level of anesthesia can be obtained in just a few minutes. The characteristics of intermediate solubility and high potency of isoflurane allow for easy regulation of the depth of anesthesia, and it is possible to sustain its effect on the brain for an extended period of time.

Metabolism of isoflurane principally occurs in the liver, although some metabolism takes place in the kidney. Approximately 0.2% of the anesthetic undergoes complete metabolism. Therefore, absorption (uptake) and elimination are primarily through the alveoli and involve ventilation of the lungs. At the conclusion of the anesthesia, the patient receives 100% oxygen. This creates a reverse gradient, and the lungs eliminate the anesthetic. Awakening usually takes place within 10 minutes, and the patient is coherent within 15 to 30 minutes.

TABLE 51.1
General Anesthetics and Neuromuscular Blocking Agents

Drug Class	Prototype	Other Drugs in the Class
Inhalation anesthetics	Isoflurane (Forane)	Desflurane (Suprane) Nitrous oxide Sevoflurane (SoJourn, Ultane)
Intravenous anesthetics	Propofol (Diprivan, Fresenius Propoven; Propofol-Lipuro)	Etomidate (Amidate) Ketamine (Ketalar) Methohexital (Brevital Sodium)
Neuromuscular blocking agents	Vecuronium	Atracurium Cisatracurium (Nimbex) Mivacurium Pancuronium Rocuronium Succinylcholine (Anectine, Quelicin)
Adjuvant drugs		Dexmedetomidine (Precedex) Fentanyl (Sublimaze, Actiq, Fentora, Lazanda, Subsys) Midazolam (Nayzilam)

Action

Isoflurane produces amnesia, skeletal muscle relaxation, and hypnosis. It, therefore, blocks the perception of pain. Its ability to provide analgesia is unclear. The exact mechanism of action of inhalation anesthetics has not been established. However, the drug may amplify the effect of inhibitory neurotransmitter targets such as the gamma-aminobutyric acid (GABA) and glycine receptors. Activation of brain GABA receptors results in a loss of consciousness and amnesia, and the spinal cord glycine receptors cause immobility or absence of response to noxious stimuli. The action of inhalation anesthetics also involves the antagonism of excitatory N-methyl-D-aspartate (NMDA) receptors and possibly other unidentified molecular sites.

Isoflurane produces a dose-dependent change in several organ systems. As the isoflurane concentration increases, blood pressure decreases and heart rate may increase.

The respiratory rate increases, but the tidal volume diminishes, resulting in an overall decrease in minute ventilation. Isoflurane produces moderate bronchodilation. Once the patient emerges from general anesthesia, the depressant effects normally resolve within 30 minutes. Therefore, residual effects may be observed in the PACU. In addition, as concentration increases, there is progressive skeletal muscle relaxation likely due to the effect on spinal cord glycine receptors. This enhances the action of neuromuscular blocking agents.

Use

Isoflurane is indicated for the induction and maintenance of general anesthesia in people of all ages, in those who are healthy, and in those who are critically ill. It can be used alone to maintain general anesthesia or more commonly in combination with other agents to produce balanced anesthesia. Table 51.2 summarizes the use of the inhalation anesthetic agents.

Patient-related variables specific to the use of isoflurane include the following:

- Age:
  - In adults, coughing, breath holding, and bronchospasm may occur during induction. The use of an ultra-short-acting barbiturate may avoid these symptoms.
  - In patients less than 3 years, repeated exposure to isoflurane may have detrimental effects on the child's brain development.
- Abnormal kidney function and hepatic impairment:
  - Isoflurane reduces kidney blood flow and urine output.
  - Adequate hydration during the perioperative period maintains normal kidney function, so the drug is considered safe in patients with abnormal kidney function.
  - Isoflurane is associated with very mild and brief postoperative hepatic dysfunction, but the incidence of hepatotoxicity is rare.
- Reproduction, pregnancy, and lactation:
  - In the third trimester of fetal development, repeated exposure to isoflurane may have detrimental effects on the fetal brain development.
  - Based on pharmacokinetic properties, the use of isoflurane while breast-feeding may be considered acceptable.

Adverse Effects

Inhalation anesthetics such as isoflurane are associated with cardiovascular and respiratory depression. They can also cause airway irritation and progress to coughing, laryngospasm, or bronchospasm in susceptible patients such as smokers or asthmatics. In addition, inhalation anesthetics are known to cause postoperative nausea and vomiting (PONV), especially after 2 or more hours of exposure.

There is also a very rare possibility of immune-mediated hepatotoxicity that can result in death. In the obstetrical patient, all volatile inhalation anesthetics, including isoflurane, decrease the tone of uterine smooth muscle, increasing the risk of bleeding during surgery such as cesarean section. Additionally, an alteration in the thermoregulatory system with or without hypothermia may cause shivering after emergence.

Malignant hyperthermia, a genetic disorder, is a potentially fatal hypermetabolic response after exposure to volatile inhalation anesthetics or to the depolarizing neuromuscular blocking agent succinylcholine. Several myopathies such as muscular dystrophy have a predisposition to malignant hyperthermia. The symptoms and their timing vary and include hypercapnia, tachycardia, elevated temperature, body rigidity, mixed metabolic and respiratory acidosis, mottling and sweating,

TABLE 51.2
DRUGS AT A GLANCE: Inhalation Anesthetics

Drug	Routes and Dosage Ranges	
	Adults	**Children**
ⓟ Isoflurane (Forane)	MAC in 100% O_2, 40 yo: 1.17%	MAC values are generally lower in newborns but higher in infants and then progressively decrease with age
Desflurane (Suprane)	MAC in 100% O_2, 40 yo: 6.6%	MAC in 100% O_2, 9 mo old, 10%; 3 y old, 8.9% (range 5.2%–10%); dosage must be individualized based on response
Nitrous oxide	MAC in 100% O_2, 40 yo: 104% (range up to 70%)	Refer to adult dosing; dosage must be individualized based on response
Sevoflurane (Ultane)	MAC in 100% O_2, 40 yo: 1.8%	MAC in 100% O_2, 1–6 mo, 3%; 6 mo to ≤1 y, 2.8%; 1 to ≤3 y, 2.8%; 3–12 y, 2.5% (0.5%–3%)

MAC, minimum alveolar concentration.

masseter spasm (rigid jaw), hyperkalemia, elevated creatine kinase (CK), myoglobinuria, and kidney failure. Prompt treatment with intravenous dantrolene sodium (Dantrium, Revonto, Ryanodex) (see Chapter 53), oxygenation and hyperventilation, hydration, and body cooling improves outcomes. Additional medications are necessary to treat the acidosis, hyperkalemia, and dysrhythmias and to prevent kidney failure.

Contraindications

Factors that rule out the use of volatile anesthetics include a family history of malignant hyperthermia, a history of hepatic dysfunction after halogenated inhalation anesthetics, or any risk of a sensitivity reaction. In patients who have a history of severe PONV, the anesthetist may substitute the inhalation anesthetic with a technique called **total intravenous anesthesia (TIVA)**. TIVA is a method of general anesthesia that replaces the inhalation agent with an intravenous anesthetic for induction and maintenance of anesthesia, thus producing fewer emetic and nonmalignant hyperthermia symptoms.

Quality and Safety Alert: Safety

With the exception of cesarean section, surgery while pregnant would be performed only under urgent or emergent circumstances. The benefits of surgery must outweigh the risks. Therefore, a preoperative pregnancy test is routinely ordered before elective procedures in patients who can bear children. Should a pregnant patient require surgery, the anesthesia practitioner designs effective strategies and tailors the anesthetic to avoid the possibility of patient harm, fetal teratogenicity, and premature labor.

The more advanced the pregnancy, the smaller the chance that the medications and inhalation anesthetics affect the unborn child. Authorities generally agree that anesthesia and surgery after the first trimester can be conducted in a safe manner and that the risk of fetal teratogenicity is minimal to nonexistent. Both the nurse and anesthesia practitioner serve as an advocate and minimize the possibility of harm to the patient and unborn child.

Nursing Implications

Preventing Interactions

Isoflurane combined with dopamine, ephedrine, epinephrine, isoproterenol, or norepinephrine may be capable of producing cardiac dysrhythmias. Alcohol, kava, St. John's wort, and valerian increase the effects of isoflurane.

Administering the Medication

Anesthesia practitioners use inhalation anesthetics widely in their daily practice. The choice of inhalation anesthetic is based on several factors such as the pharmacokinetic profile, preexisting medical conditions, and history of previous reactions.

The administration of inhalation anesthetics requires the use of an anesthesia machine. These devices vary in features and sophistication. It only takes a very small amount of isoflurane (1% to 3%) to produce general anesthesia. The inhalation anesthetic, along with oxygen, air, and sometimes nitrous oxide, is delivered to the patient's lungs through a plastic breathing circuit that connects to a mask, endotracheal tube, or supraglottic airway device such as the laryngeal mask airway.

The term **minimum alveolar concentration** (MAC) is a quantitative measure of the potency of inhalation anesthetics. It is the concentration of anesthetic necessary to suppress a response to pain in 50% of patients who receive a noxious stimulus such as a surgical incision. MAC values vary with the age of the patient. Furthermore, MAC values are additive. With the addition of other medications such as benzodiazepines, opioids, intravenous anesthetics, or nitrous oxide, MAC values decrease. For example, the MAC of isoflurane is 1.15% in adults when it is administered alone. However, when in combination with 70% nitrous oxide, the MAC of isoflurane decreases to 0.5%.

Assessing for Therapeutic Effects

Assessing the patient for the therapeutic effects of inhalation anesthetics is the responsibility of the anesthesia practitioner.

Assessing for Adverse Effects

Because inhalation anesthetics may lead to low blood pressure and respiratory depression, it is prudent to provide oxygen and frequently assess the blood pressure and quality of breathing or ventilation early in the postoperative period. Monitoring oxygen saturation as measured by pulse oximetry helps guide therapy. The nurse may treat postoperative shivering with warm blankets or forced-air warming devices. Nausea and vomiting may occur after surgery using isoflurane. Treatment involves antiemetics (see Chapter 38). If symptoms possibly indicate malignant hyperthermia, it is imperative that the nurse notify the anesthesia practitioner immediately.

Quality and Safety Alert: Evidence-Based Practice

Zengin and Ergun (2022) conducted a retrospective assessment of the association between inhalation anesthesia and postoperative complications in patients with a BMI higher than 40 undergoing bariatric surgery compared to those receiving TIVA. The study reviewed similar demographics of 213 women and 65 men. The comparison of the clinical characteristics of the study showed that the rate of admission to the intensive care unit and complications were higher in the TIVA group rather than the inhalation anesthesia group. Morbid obesity contributes to higher rates of anesthesia and surgery-related complications.

Patient Teaching

Box 51.1 identifies patient teaching guidelines for the inhalation anesthetics, including isoflurane.

Other Drugs in the Class

Several other inhaled anesthetic agents are available. These inhalation anesthetics further reduce body tissue solubility and allow rapid induction and emergence from anesthesia, making them valuable adjuncts in ambulatory surgery.

Desflurane (Suprane) is a completely fluorinated methyl ethyl ether. Of the currently available inhalation anesthetics, it is the least soluble and least potent, with negligible metabolism. These characteristics favor rapid induction, emergence, and return of protective airway reflexes. Patients benefit from faster recovery and return of normal cognition. However, desflurane

| BOX 51.1 | **Patient Teaching Guidelines for General Anesthetics** |

- Ask your healthcare practitioner for information about the administration and effects of the general anesthetic agent(s) you may receive. Feel free to ask questions. Learn about the postoperative/postprocedural recovery phase.
- If you will be receiving an intravenous anesthetic such as propofol, be aware that there may be pain, burning, or stinging when the medication is injected into the intravenous catheter and flows into the vein. (Preinduction opioids and simultaneous administration of intravenous lidocaine also help relieve the discomfort.)
- Refrain from smoking prior to surgery.
- Discontinue complementary and alternative medicine products, including herbal supplements, for 2 weeks prior to surgery.
- Do not ingest alcohol for 24 hours prior to the scheduled surgery or procedure.
- Ask your healthcare practitioner about diagnostic testing to screen for malignant hyperthermia or atypical plasma cholinesterase if you have a family history.

is very pungent, making mask inhalation induction impractical. Moreover, desflurane produces airway irritation and increases the incidence of coughing, breath holding, or laryngospasm. Unlike other inhalation anesthetics, desflurane may cause mild bronchoconstriction.

Sevoflurane (Ultane) is a completely fluorinated methyl isopropyl ether that has about half the potency of isoflurane. Its solubility is extremely low. Therefore, induction, emergence, and recovery are fast. In addition, sevoflurane is nonpungent and results in the least amount of airway irritation. It provides a pleasant inhalation mask induction in both adults and children without the need of an initial intravenous anesthetic. Furthermore, it produces bronchodilation similar or perhaps greater than isoflurane. These properties make sevoflurane a popular choice for patients with reactive airway disease or chronic obstructive pulmonary disease. In young children, sevoflurane is associated with emergence or postoperative agitation but does not seem to have long-term implications.

In addition to the volatile anesthetics, the inorganic inhalation agent nitrous oxide can be used in combination with other anesthetic medications. Also known as laughing gas, it is not a volatile agent like isoflurane because it is a gas at room temperature. Unfortunately, the potency of nitrous oxide is low, and it cannot produce general anesthesia by itself. However, its additive effect will permit a lower concentration or dose of the volatile or intravenous anesthetics. Nitrous oxide produces amnesia, analgesia, and euphoria. Because it has a greater solubility in blood than nitrogen, it diffuses into closed body cavities and expands. This can place undue pressure in the bowels, middle ear, and other spaces created by surgery or disease. As a result, it is contraindicated in many types of surgeries and preexisting medical conditions.

NCLEX Success

1. The nurse is circulating in the operating room when the anesthesia practitioner declares a malignant hyperthermia emergency. Which of the following symptoms are indicative of malignant hyperthermia? (Select all that apply.)
   A. muscle rigidity
   B. bradycardia
   C. rash
   D. hypercapnia
   E. increased serum creatinine
   F. hyperkalemia

2. A 32-year-old patient with a history of reactive airway disease is admitted to the hospital for an appendectomy. Which of the following inhalation anesthetic agents, if any, is contraindicated?
   A. isoflurane
   B. sevoflurane
   C. desflurane
   D. nitrous oxide

Clinical Application 51.1

- The anesthesia practitioner has decided to use sevoflurane, an inhalation anesthetic, for Ms. Wilberson's cholecystectomy. Why is this anesthetic an appropriate choice?

INTRAVENOUS GENERAL ANESTHETICS

Intravenous general anesthetics render a patient unconscious in a fast and safe manner. Introduced in 1934, the fast-acting barbiturates revolutionized the often slow and difficult procedure of inducing the surgical patient using only the inhalation anesthetics available at that time. 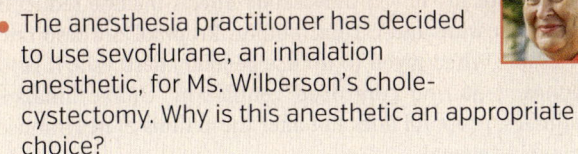 **Propofol** (Diprivan, Fresenius Propoven, Propofol-Lipuro) is the prototype intravenous anesthetic with wide acceptance and extensive use for surgical, therapeutic, and diagnostic procedures. Unlike barbiturates, awakening from propofol is associated with negligible aftereffects such as lingering sedation, confusion, and nausea. Fortunately, no intravenous general anesthetic triggers malignant hyperthermia.

Quality and Safety Alert: Patient-Centered Care

In March 2021, during the COVID-19 pandemic, the FDA issued an emergency use authorization of Propofol-Lipuro 1% emulsion for infusion in the intensive care unit setting. It is used to maintain sedation administered as a continuous infusion for patients older than 16 years who require mechanical ventilation. The Fact Sheet for Healthcare Providers can be accessed at: https://www.fda.gov/media/146682/download.

Pharmacokinetics

Following intravenous administration, propofol provides smooth hypnosis in less than 1 minute. Chiefly metabolized in the liver to water-soluble inactive metabolites, the drug is excreted by the kidneys. Elimination of the anesthetic is not altered by chronic hepatic impairment or abnormal kidney function. Propofol, which is very lipid soluble, easily crosses the blood–brain barrier. The cessation of the effect of propofol is dependent on its redistribution away from the central nervous system (CNS). Therefore, because of both extensive redistribution and high metabolic clearance, recovery from anesthesia is rapid, usually within 10 minutes. However, very long administration times, with large dosages, can result in delayed emergence from anesthesia.

Action

Propofol produces amnesia and hypnosis. It, therefore, blocks the perception of pain. It does not provide analgesia. Propofol causes depression of the CNS by amplifying the inhibitory neurotransmitter GABA. The action of propofol may also involve modulation of excitatory NMDA receptors, glycine receptors, and the endocannabinoid system. Furthermore, propofol has anticonvulsant properties.

Propofol produces a dose-dependent change in several organ systems. This effect is exacerbated in hypovolemia and significant cardiac disease or in older adult patients or those who are critically ill. Cardiovascular effects include reductions in blood pressure and cardiac output. Propofol is a respiratory depressant. When given to induce general anesthesia, it results in apnea, requiring controlled ventilation. Unlike inhalation anesthetics, propofol does not alter the actions of neuromuscular blocking agents.

Use

Propofol is indicated for the induction and maintenance of general anesthesia. It can be used alone to maintain general anesthesia (TIVA) or more commonly combined with other medications to produce a balanced anesthesia. Because of propofol's antiemetic properties, it is frequently used for the induction and maintenance of general anesthesia with patients at high risk for PONV. Propofol can produce bronchodilation, which is therapeutic for patients with asthma and chronic obstructive pulmonary disease. Moreover, propofol suppresses laryngeal reflexes, making it a suitable choice when inserting a supraglottic airway device.

Propofol can be titrated and used in lesser amounts to provide light, moderate, or deep sedation, in addition to its use as a general anesthetic. When an anesthesia practitioner administers propofol or similar medications for sedation, it is called **monitored anesthesia care**. During conscious or moderate sedation, the patient can be aroused with stimulation and maintains protective airway reflexes. However, anesthesia practitioners may provide deep sedation in particularly uncomfortable procedures or minor surgery. Deeply sedated patients are not easily aroused and may partially or entirely lose protective airway reflexes. Airway obstruction can be corrected with repositioning or use of an oral or nasal airway. Decreases in tidal volume and respiratory rate may necessitate assisted ventilation. The level of deep sedation can rapidly change into general anesthesia, necessitating a clinician educated in airway management and the recognition and treatment of anesthetic-related complications.

Table 51.3 summarizes the use of the intravenous anesthetics.

TABLE 51.3

DRUGS AT A GLANCE: Intravenous Anesthetics

Drug	Routes and Dosage Ranges	
	Adults	**Children**
Propofol (Diprivan, Fresenius Propoven; Propofol-Lipuro; Diprivan, TEVA-Propofol)	Induction: Healthy: 2–2.5 mg/kg IV or 40 mg every 10 s until hypnosis Older adults or debilitated: 1–1.5 mg/kg IV or 20 mg every 10 s until hypnosis Maintenance: 100–200 mcg/kg/min IV Sedation: 10–20 mg IV PRN titrated to effect or 25–75 mcg/kg/min IV	Induction: Healthy: 2.5–3.5 mg/kg over 20–30 s Debilitated: lower dose Maintenance: 125–300 mcg/kg/min IV
Etomidate (Amidate)	Induction: 0.2–0.6 mg/kg IV, average dose 0.3 mg/kg IV	Induction: 0.2–0.4 mg/kg IV (>10 y of age)
Ketamine (Ketalar; Ketalar)	Induction: 0.5–2 mg/kg IV or, if IV access not available, 4–6 mg/kg IM Maintenance infusion: up to 1 mg/kg/h Sedation and analgesia: 1–2 mg/kg IV, repeat 0.5–1 mg/kg every 5–10 min	Induction: <16 yo, 1–3 mg/kg IV; 5–10 mg/kg IM, adolescents >16 yo 1–4.5 mg/kg IV; 6.5–13 mg/kg IM Sedation and analgesia: 1–2 mg/kg IV, repeat 0.5–1 mg/kg every 5–15 min
Methohexital (Brevital Sodium)	Induction: 1–1.5 mg/kg IV Sedation: 0.75–1 mg/kg, repeat 0.5 mg/kg every 2–5 min	Induction: 1–2.5 mg/kg IV

Patient-related variables specific to the use of propofol include the following:

- Age:
  - In pediatric patients less than 3 years of age, repeated exposure to propofol may have detrimental effects on the child's brain development.
  - Propofol is identified as a Key Potentially Inappropriate Drug in Pediatrics.
- Reproduction, pregnancy, and lactation:
  - Propofol is not recommended for obstetrical use, including cesarean section deliveries.
  - Propofol crosses the placenta and may be associated with neonatal CNS and respiratory depression.
  - Breast-feeding is not recommended with the use of propofol.
- Specific healthcare environments:
  - In the ICU, propofol is used to sedate patients on mechanical ventilation. Propofol infusion syndrome affects children and adults and is characterized by metabolic acidosis, rhabdomyolysis, dysrhythmias, and multiorgan failure. Monitor for elevation in lactic acidosis, CK levels, and triglyceride levels.

Adverse Effects

The rapid intravenous administration of propofol can be unpleasant because of the emulsion formula. On injection, pain, burning, or stinging at the intravenous site may occur. Occasionally, hiccups and myoclonic movements are observed during induction with propofol.

Contraindications

The anesthesia practitioner exercises caution in patients with disorders of lipid metabolism and pancreatitis. Patients who are allergic to soybean or soy products, or eggs or egg products, should not receive propofol. Generic formulations of propofol are preservative free, whereas the trade preparation Diprivan contains disodium edetate (EDTA or metabisulfite). Metabisulfite can cause bronchoconstriction and wheezing in susceptible patients. Therefore, the anesthetic practitioner must exercise discretion in the choice of propofol formulation in patients with a history of reactive airway disease or an allergy to sulfites.

Nursing Implications

Preventing Interactions

Alcohol, kava, St. John's wort, and valerian increase the effects of propofol.

Administering the Medication

Similar to inhalation anesthetics, propofol is widely used in daily practice. The choice of propofol is based on several factors such as the pharmacokinetic profile, preexisting medical conditions, and allergies.

Propofol is either injected manually or attached to an electronic pump to provide a precise dose for continuous infusion. Electronic pumps are especially useful for maintenance anesthesia or sedation.

The administration of propofol should be individualized according to concomitant anesthetic medications and comorbidities. It should be titrated to the desired effect while maintaining cardiovascular stability. Age-appropriate doses are necessary. The handling of propofol requires aseptic technique because the emulsion-based formulation favors the growth of pathogens.

Propofol may be administered in the ICU, where the nurse managing the patient must be skilled in the care of critically ill patients and educated in advanced life support, including airway management.

Assessing for Therapeutic Effects

Assessing the patient for the therapeutic effects of intravenous anesthetics is the responsibility of the anesthesia practitioner.

Assessing for Adverse Effects

When caring for a patient who received propofol, the hypnosis or sedation dissipates quickly. Adverse effects are few.

Patient Teaching

Box 51.1 identifies patient teaching guidelines for intravenous anesthetics, including propofol.

Other Drugs in the Class

Other intravenous anesthetics with differing profiles are available for use. Etomidate (Amidate) is a short-acting anesthetic that appears to promote cardiovascular stability, even in critically ill patients. As an imidazole-containing compound, it is structurally dissimilar to the other intravenous anesthetics. Like propofol, etomidate amplifies the inhibitory neurotransmitter GABA and results in quick patient recovery because of its redistribution to other tissues. However, etomidate suppresses steroid synthesis, leading to short-term adrenocortical suppression. Symptoms may include weakness and hypotension. There is some evidence that the use of etomidate in critically ill patients results in increased mortality. The risks versus benefits of using etomidate in this patient population should be carefully considered. In addition, when compared with other intravenous anesthetics, etomidate causes more PONV.

Ketamine (Ketalar) is a dissociative anesthetic, which means that it produces a trancelike state or detached feeling. It causes hypnosis, amnesia, and potent analgesia. A noncompetitive NMDA receptor antagonist that blocks glutamate, it is opioid-sparing and does not rely on opioid receptors. Because of these unique properties, ketamine can be used as a sedative or total anesthetic. Ketamine has sympathomimetic effects and is commonly used in the care of critically ill patients because it maintains blood pressure and heart rate as long as catecholamine reserves are present. The anesthetic has a versatile profile, and administration may be intravenous, intramuscular, oral, or nasal. When carefully titrated, ketamine preserves airway reflexes and adequate ventilation. It is also an excellent bronchodilator. Because ketamine increases salivation, prior administration of glycopyrrolate is recommended.

The FDA has issued a **BOXED WARNING ◆** for ketamine. A phencyclidine derivative, it can produce emergence delirium, hallucinations, and unpleasant dreams. Symptoms of this effect may include confusion, agitation, and nystagmus.

Psychological effects can last up to 24 hours. Reducing adverse effects involves using the lowest necessary doses and premedicating with benzodiazepines. With the exception of required nursing care and vital signs, the nurse minimizes stimulation and permits the patient to recover in a calm, quiet environment with gentle reorientation. Monitoring to ensure a complete recovery from anesthesia is essential. The anesthesia practitioner may have to treat severe reactions. A responsible adult should accompany the patient home. Esketamine (Spravato), the pure S-enantiomer of ketamine, is currently available as a nasal spray for the treatment of depression. Esketamine demonstrates better analgesic and anesthetic effects with less psychomimetic properties compared to ketamine; thus, there is interest in using this drug for analgesia, sedation, and anesthesia once an IV preparation becomes available.

Methohexital sodium (Brevital) is an ultrashort-acting barbiturate with a fast recovery period. Although it was predominantly used to induce anesthesia before the introduction of propofol, it may be used to induce rapid anesthesia, which is then maintained with an inhaled anesthetic. The anesthetic depresses the cardiovascular and respiratory system. Patients with porphyria should not receive barbiturates, which are highly alkaline and cause venous irritation. Venous infiltration results in local tissue damage. Incompatibility with other medications results in precipitation, so it is necessary to flush the intravenous line before and after injecting barbiturates. Methohexital does not raise the seizure threshold. Therefore, it is the drug of choice when providing short-term anesthesia prior to electroconvulsive therapy.

The FDA has issued a **BOXED WARNING** ◆ for methohexital. Appropriately educated clinicians should be available to continuously monitor the patient and provide age-specific resuscitative measures if necessary. The use of deep sedation requires that clinicians be dedicated to patient monitoring and care and not be participating in the surgery or procedure.

Clinical Application 51.2

- Ms. Wilberson stated in the nursing interview that she has a history of food allergies. Before administration of the anesthetic, the nurse and anesthesia practitioner need to assess for which food allergies?

NCLEX Success

3. A seriously ill pediatric patient has been admitted to the ICU. The patient is intubated, and propofol is used for long-term sedation so the patient does not "fight" the ventilator. Which of the following laboratory values should be monitored? (Select all that apply.)
   A. complete blood count
   B. triglycerides
   C. alkaline phosphatase
   D. lactate
   E. creatine kinase
   F. luteinizing hormone

NEUROMUSCULAR BLOCKING AGENTS

Modern neuromuscular blocking agents, or muscle relaxants, are divided into two classes: nondepolarizing and depolarizing. **Vecuronium**, an intermediate acting, nondepolarizing aminosteroid compound, is the prototype. There are several nondepolarizing muscle relaxants. Succinylcholine is the only depolarizing agent used in the United States. Each agent has unique characteristics (see Other Drugs in the Class), and the anesthesia practitioner makes the appropriate choice based on the health history of the patient as well as the length and type of procedure.

Pharmacokinetics

Maximum neuromuscular blockade with vecuronium occurs within 3 to 5 minutes, and the duration of action to 95% recovery is 45 to 65 minutes. The onset and duration are dose dependent. For example, larger doses result in faster onset and longer duration. The cessation of effect is dependent on the redistribution of the medication away from the neuromuscular junction. Vecuronium has an extensive hepatic uptake and metabolism, which accounts for a rapid decline in plasma concentration. Because of its lipid solubility, about 40% of the vecuronium is excreted in the bile. Hepatic metabolites and unchanged vecuronium are excreted in the urine. Because of the distribution to peripheral compartments, large and repeated dosing can result in accumulation of vecuronium and active metabolites.

Action

Vecuronium acts by temporarily blocking nerve impulses at the neuromuscular junction. It can be titrated to produce weakness through complete paralysis. The inhibition of nerve transmission occurs at the postsynaptic nicotinic acetylcholine (ACh) receptors. Because vecuronium is structurally similar to ACh, it binds to the receptors on the muscle and prevents normal function of ACh, producing skeletal muscle paralysis. As vecuronium redistributes and metabolizes, ACh effectively takes over, and normal functioning of skeletal muscle resumes. Vecuronium has no abnormal effects on the cardiovascular system.

Use

The use of vecuronium and other neuromuscular blocking agents is often necessary because inhalation or intravenous anesthetics alone may not produce the skeletal muscle relaxation a surgeon needs when performing an operation. Muscles may need to be relaxed so that proper exposure occurs. Also, it is essential for absolutely no movement to occur with delicate repairs. In addition, neuromuscular blocking agents facilitate easy tracheal intubation and mechanical ventilation by relaxing the vocal cords, jaw, and associated respiratory muscles.

Table 51.4 summarizes the use of the neuromuscular blocking agents.

Patient-related variables specific to the use of vecuronium include the following:

- Age:
  - Infants between the age of 7 weeks and 1 year are more sensitive to vecuronium and take longer to recover.
  - Children younger than 10 years may require higher initial doses and more frequent supplementation to maintain sedation.
  - Cautious use of vecuronium is necessary in older adult patients. Age-related reduction in organ clearance prolongs the effect of the anesthetic.
- Abnormal kidney function and hepatic impairment:
  - When larger doses of vecuronium are administered and the patient has significant kidney dysfunction, the clearance is inhibited, resulting in drug accumulation and prolonged muscle paralysis.
  - Patients with significant hepatic impairment such as cirrhosis or cholestasis can experience slow elimination and prolonged muscle paralysis.
- Reproduction, pregnancy, and lactation:
  - The pharmacokinetics of vecuronium are altered in pregnancy. The use of vecuronium in cesarean section has shown that umbilical venous concentrations were 11% of maternal values at delivery.
  - It is not known if vecuronium is present in breast milk.
- Specific healthcare environments:
  - Vecuronium or other nondepolarizing neuromuscular blocking agents are administered in critical care situations to enhance the therapeutic effects of mechanical ventilation.

Clinical Application 51.3

- During laparoscopic procedures such as Ms. Wilberson's cholecystectomy, the surgeon has long metal instruments inside the body, perhaps next to major blood vessels. The anesthesia practitioner administers vecuronium during the procedure, in addition to the sevoflurane. What is the purpose of using vecuronium?

Adverse Effects

Nondepolarizing neuromuscular blocking agents can result in allergic reactions during anesthesia such as anaphylaxis or mild dermatologic conditions such as urticaria or erythema.

Contraindications

In the case of a patient who reports a known hypersensitivity or allergy to vecuronium or nondepolarizing neuromuscular blocking agents, the anesthesia practitioner modifies the anesthetic plan.

Nursing Implications

The maintenance of the patient's airway and respiratory function following the administration of neuromuscular blocking agents such as vecuronium is the most important nursing implication. The anesthetist ensures respiratory function during the period of anesthesia.

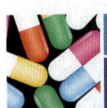

TABLE 51.4

DRUGS AT A GLANCE: Neuromuscular Blocking Agents

Drug	Routes and Dosage Ranges	
	Adults	**Children**
P Vecuronium	Intubation: 0.08–0.1 mg/kg IV Maintenance: 0.01–0.015 mg/kg IV PRN or 0.8–1.2 mcg/kg/min	Intubation: 0.08–0.1 mg/kg IV Maintenance: infants, 0.8–1,7 mcg/kg/min, children and adolescents, 0.8–2.5 mcg/kg/min
Atracurium	Intubation: 0.4–0.5 mg/kg IV Maintenance: 0.08–0.1 mg/kg IV PRN or 2–15 mcg/kg/min	Intubation: 0.3–0.4 mg/kg IV Maintenance: <2 yo, 6–14 mcg/kg/min, >2 yo, 2–15 mcg/kg/min
Cisatracurium (Nimbex; ✹ Cisatracurium Omega)	Intubation: 0.15–0.2 mg/kg IV Maintenance: 0.03 mg/kg IV PRN or 1–3 mcg/kg/min	Intubation: 0.1–0.15 mg/kg IV Maintenance: 1–4 mcg/kg/min
Pancuronium	Intubation: 0.04–0.1 mg/kg IV Maintenance: 0.01 mg/kg IV PRN	Intubation: 0.05–0.15 mg/kg IV Maintenance: 0.05–0.15 mg/kg IV PRN
Rocuronium	Intubation: 0.45–0.6 mg/kg IV Rapid sequence induction: 0.6–1.2 mg/kg IV Maintenance: 0.1–0.3 mg/kg IV PRN or 4–16 mcg/kg/min	Intubation: 0.45–0.6 mg/kg IV Rapid sequence induction: 0.6–1.2 mg/kg IV Maintenance: 0.075–0.15 mg/kg IV PRN or 7–12 mcg/kg/min
Succinylcholine (Anectine, Quelicin; ✹ Quelicin Chloride)	Intubation: 0.3–1.1 mg/kg IV, 3–4 mg/kg IM (150 mg max) Rapid sequence induction: 1–1.5 mg/kg IV	Intubation: Infants <6 mo 2–3 mg/kg IV Infant >6 mo and children 1–2 mg/kg IV Adolescents 1–1.5 mg/kg IV

> **BOX 51.2 Drug Interactions: Vecuronium**
>
> **Drugs That Increase the Effects of Vecuronium**
> - Abobotulinumtoxin A, aminoglycosides, calcium channel blockers, cyclosporine, inhalation anesthetics, lincosamide antibiotics, lithium, local anesthetics, magnesium salts, polymyxins, quinidine, spironolactone, tetracyclines, and vancomycin
>   *Act in a complex way*
>
> **Drugs That Decrease the Effects of Vecuronium**
> - Acetylcholinesterase inhibitors; calcium; chronic use of carbamazepine, fosphenytoin, or phenytoin
>   *Act in a complex way*
>
> **Drugs That May Increase or Decrease the Effects of Vecuronium Depending on Dose and Comorbidities**
> - Corticosteroids, loop diuretics
>   *Act in a complex way*

Preventing Interactions

Numerous medications interact with vecuronium (Box 51.2).

Administering the Medication

Neuromuscular blocking agents are intravenous drugs that may be injected manually. Or, like propofol, they may be attached to an electronic pump to provide a controlled continuous infusion. Vecuronium is the only muscle relaxant supplied in powder form, and it must be reconstituted with sterile normal saline prior to use.

After administration of vecuronium is complete, it may be necessary for the anesthetist to reverse its effects so that the patient can regain baseline skeletal muscle function. The anesthetist uses an anticholinesterase, such as neostigmine, edrophonium, or pyridostigmine, which inhibits acetylcholinesterase, the enzyme responsible for degrading ACh. This allows an increase in synaptic ACh, which displaces the neuromuscular blocking agent, thus resulting in the return of muscle movement. Anticholinesterases must always be given with an anticholinergic, such as glycopyrrolate or atropine, to prevent adverse effects at other cholinergic receptor sites in the body, particularly the heart (bradycardia, asystole) and lungs (bronchoconstriction).

Sugammadex (Bridion) is a newer reversal agent without cholinergic effects. It can be used to reverse only the steroidal nondepolarizing neuromuscular blockers vecuronium and rocuronium. Sugammadex has been shown to reverse neuromuscular blockade more quickly and completely than neostigmine. Research suggests that the use of suggamadex reduces postoperative pulmonary complications. Its use is sometimes restricted to patients at high risk due to its cost.

Assessing for Therapeutic Effects

Most often, anesthesia practitioners use a device called a peripheral nerve stimulator to monitor the level of neuromuscular blockade, which allows them to better select the correct dosing regimen for maintenance and reversal of muscle relaxation. When administered in the ICU, the nurse may be responsible for monitoring the level of paralysis. Because nondepolarizing neuromuscular blocking agents have no anesthetic or analgesic properties, medication-induced hypnosis and amnesia must be provided to ensure patient comfort.

Assessing for Adverse Effects

The actions of nondepolarizing neuromuscular blocking agents such as vecuronium may persist after emergence from anesthesia and manifest as **residual neuromuscular blockade**, formerly known as recurarization, in the PACU. This may occur after inadequate reversal or no reversal from the effects of nondepolarizing neuromuscular blocking agents. Patients at risk include those with liver and kidney disease, acid–base or electrolyte imbalance, hypothermia, critical illness, myopathic disorders, and neuromuscular diseases such as myasthenia gravis or myasthenic (Eaton-Lambert) syndrome. In addition, older patients or those taking medications that may intensify or prolong the actions of neuromuscular blocking agents are at risk. Residual neuromuscular blockade can elevate the risk of upper airway obstruction, aspiration, and hypoventilation with respiratory acidosis and hypoxia. Therefore, it is essential to assess airway, breathing, and circulation. The nurse assesses the quality of respirations by observing the rate and depth. Subtle signs such as difficulty swallowing or double vision may be present, and patients may have a weak and ineffective cough. Difficulties with vocalization and taking a deep breath are possible. The nurse assesses the patient's ability to sustain a head lift for 5 seconds and assesses the strength of the patient's hand grip. If the patient shows any signs or symptoms of respiratory distress, the nurse immediately begins supplemental high-flow oxygen by mask and notifies the anesthesia practitioner. Reversal medications and supported ventilation are necessary.

Patient Teaching

Box 51.1 identifies patient teaching guidelines for vecuronium.

> **Clinical Application 51.4**
> - On admission to the PACU, Ms. Wilberson complains of difficulty breathing in a weak voice. She has trouble lifting her head. What would be the initial nursing actions?
> - What aspect of Ms. Wilberson's care and anesthetic provide clues as to the cause of her symptoms?

Other Drugs in the Class

Nondepolarizing Neuromuscular Blocking Agents

Other aminosteroids in addition to vecuronium include the long-acting (greater than 60 minutes) pancuronium and the intermediate-acting (less than 60 minutes) rocuronium. Pancuronium is useful when prolonged paralysis is indicated. In addition, it has the ability to stimulate the vagus nerve and accelerate the heart rate. However, patients with hepatic insufficiency and abnormal kidney function or significant disease may experience prolonged paralysis. Pancuronium is rarely used due to the risk of residual neuromuscular blockade. Rocuronium has a rapid onset in high doses and is the drug of choice when succinylcholine is contraindicated. While it is categorized with vecuronium as an intermediate-acting muscle relaxant, it has a slightly quicker onset with standard dosing.

The benzylisoquinolinium nondepolarizing neuromuscular blocking agents are mivacurium, atracurium, and cisatracurium. Mivacurium is short acting and was originally developed as a nondepolarizing alternative to succinylcholine. Its low potency and propensity for histamine release limits its use (histamine can produce hypotension, bronchospasm, tachycardia, and skin flushing). It is more commonly used in pediatrics. Cisatracurium, an isomer of atracurium, is three times as potent. Both drugs are useful when anesthetizing patients with compromised kidney or hepatic function, because elimination is not dependent on enzymatic, liver, or kidney pathways. Cisatracurium has a longer duration than atracurium. At higher doses, atracurium releases histamine, whereas cisatracurium does not.

Depolarizing Neuromuscular Blocking Agent

Succinylcholine (Anectine, Quelicin) is a rapid-onset and short-duration depolarizing muscle relaxant administered by intravenous or intramuscular injection. The structure of succinylcholine is two acetylcholine molecules connected by a methyl group. Succinylcholine attaches to postsynaptic nicotinic ACh receptors and activates them. The depolarization caused by succinylcholine results in momentary contractions of the muscles called **fasciculation**; the patient's entire body may twitch and move for about 5 to 10 seconds. After fasciculation, succinylcholine remains attached to the receptor, and there is flaccid muscle paralysis for approximately 5 to 10 minutes. Succinylcholine is metabolized in the blood by plasma cholinesterase. There are no reversal medications for succinylcholine.

The primary use for succinylcholine is paralysis for tracheal intubation, especially when it is necessary to quickly protect the airway. **Rapid sequence induction** is a tracheal intubation procedure that uses cricoid pressure to occlude the esophagus and omits face mask ventilation to reduce the risk of aspiration. This type of induction is indicated in patients at increased risk for pulmonary aspiration, such as for emergency procedures when an empty stomach cannot be guaranteed. Succinylcholine is also used to relax the vocal cords and terminate a laryngospasm.

The adverse effects of succinylcholine include bradycardia, hyperkalemia, and postoperative myalgia. Because there is a risk of abrupt hyperkalemia and cardiac arrest, it is important to avoid using succinylcholine in patients with preexisting hyperkalemia, major burns or extensive tissue damage, denervation conditions such as paraplegia, prolonged illness with immobility, stroke, or motor neuron disease. In patients at risk, serum electrolytes with potassium levels help guide therapy. Malignant hyperthermia is also possible with succinylcholine, so it is contraindicated with confirmed or suspicious history of this condition. In addition, it is avoided in disease processes associated with malignant hyperthermia. Finally, two scenarios cause prolonged paralysis after administration of succinylcholine. The first is decreased plasma cholinesterase, which can result from severe illness that may include liver disease and interactions with other medications. The prolonged effect is usually small. The other scenario is the genetic condition called atypical plasma cholinesterase. Paralysis can last from approximately 30 minutes to many hours. Patients remain intubated and are observed in the ICU until the paralysis spontaneously resolves. During this time, they receive a drug to induce hypnosis.

The FDA has issued a **BOXED WARNING** ◆ for succinylcholine because of the risk of sudden cardiac arrest from rapid onset rhabdomyolysis and hyperkalemia. (This condition most likely occurs in males younger than 8 years of age with Duchenne muscular dystrophy.) Because of the possibility of undiagnosed myopathy in children, the use of succinylcholine in this population is reserved for emergency airway control and intubation to prevent aspiration.

> **NCLEX Success**
>
> 4. An anesthesia practitioner administers succinylcholine. What is the expected effect of this drug? (Select all that apply.)
>   - A. decrease in anxiety
>   - B. fasciculations
>   - C. muscle relaxation
>   - D. apnea
>   - E. analgesia
>
> 5. A patient is admitted to the postanesthesia care unit following surgery, where they received vecuronium. The patient is unable to raise their head and develops shortness of breath. What are the priority nursing interventions? (Select all that apply.)
>   - A. Draw an arterial blood gas.
>   - B. Notify the anesthesia practitioner.
>   - C. Administer furosemide.
>   - D. Apply high-flow oxygen.
>   - E. Intubate the patient.

ADJUVANT MEDICATIONS USED IN GENERAL ANESTHESIA

The adjuvant medications are administered during the preoperative, intraoperative, and postoperative phase in support of balanced anesthesia. Table 51.5 summarizes the chief adjuvant medications administered to support balanced anesthesia.

Benzodiazepines

Benzodiazepines are a valuable adjunct to all types of anesthesia. This includes sedation, regional techniques such peripheral nerve blocks, spinal anesthetics, epidural anesthetics, and general anesthesia. Benzodiazepines produce amnesia, anxiolysis, and sedation and have anticonvulsant properties (see Chapter 54). At high doses, benzodiazepines can induce hypnosis.
Ⓟ **Midazolam** (Nayzilam), the prototype drug in this class, is a short-acting intravenous medication. Midazolam is the most common medication administered prior to surgical, diagnostic, or therapeutic procedures. Furthermore, when given for procedures that only require sedation, midazolam can be continuously administered to maintain sedation. Because midazolam also can be administered in flavored syrup orally, as an

TABLE 51.5

DRUGS AT A GLANCE: Adjuvant Drugs Used in General Anesthesia

Drug	Routes and Dosage Ranges	
	Adults	**Children**
P Midazolam (Nayzilam)	0.5–2 mg IV in 0.5–1-mg increments	0.25–0.5 mg/kg PO (20 mg max) 0.1–0.15 mg/kg IM Children >6 to <6 yo 0.05–0.1 mg/kg IV, (6 mg max) Children >6 yo 0.025–0.05 IV, (10 mg max) Adolescents 1–2.5 mg IV PRN, (10 mg max)
P Fentanyl (Sublimaze, Abstral, Fentora, Ionsys; ❋ Abstral, Duragesic, Fentora)	Balanced anesthesia adjunct: 25–100 mcg IV, 1–2 mcg/kg/h Sedation/analgesia: 0.5–1 mcg/kg IV PRN titrated to effect, reduce dose if used with other sedatives	Balanced anesthesia adjunct: 0.5–3 mcg/kg IV PRN, 1–2 mcg/kg/min 4–10 mcg/kg higher range for complex surgeries
P Dexmedetomidine (Precedex; ❋ Precedex)	Loading dose: 0.5–1 mcg/kg over 10 min Maintenance: 0.2–1 mcg/kg/h	Loading dose: 0.5–2 mcg/kg over 10 min Maintenance: 0.5–1 mcg/kg/h

intranasal spray, or intramuscularly, it is a valuable adjunct in pediatric anesthesia.

Remimazolam (Byfavo) is an ultrashort-acting benzodiazepine introduced in 2020. Remimazolam has a very short duration of action due to its organ-independent metabolism by ester hydrolysis in the blood. It can be used safely in patients with liver or kidney disease without exhibiting a longer duration of action.

The FDA has issued a **BOXED WARNING** ◆ for midazolam and remimazolam because of profound respiratory depression that may result in hypoxia, brain damage, or death. Rapid intravenous administration to neonates has resulted in hypotension and seizures. It is essential to titrate both drugs carefully according to age and medical conditions. Following administration, continuous monitoring for respiratory depression is required, and if necessary, age-specific resuscitative measures should be implemented. Flumazenil is a benzodiazepine antagonist that reverses the effects of midazolam and remimazolam.

Opioid Analgesics

When pain is anticipated, opioid analgesics are a component of the anesthetic technique. Opioids (see Chapter 49) bind to several classes of opioid receptors in the nervous system and tissues. The prototype intravenous opioid analgesic is **P** fentanyl (Sublimaze, Actiq, Fentora, Lazanda, Subsys). A synthetic opioid that is about 100 times more potent than morphine sulfate, fentanyl can be used to supplement sedation, regional techniques, and general anesthesia. Common adverse effects of all opioids are respiratory depression, nausea and vomiting, altered mentation, urinary retention, and itching. Other commonly used opioids in anesthesia practice include remifentanil (Ultiva), sufentanil (Dsuvia), alfentanil (Alfenta), and hydromorphone (Dilaudid). Naloxone (Narcan) (see Chapter 49) is an antagonist that reverses the effects of opioids.

Alpha-2 Adrenergic Agonist

P Dexmedetomidine (Precedex) is an alpha-2 receptor agonist that acts on the brain and spinal cord, resulting in sedation, analgesia, and anxiolysis without respiratory depression. Dexmedetomidine is used to provide sedation for surgical, therapeutic, and diagnostic procedures and also as an adjunct to general anesthesia. Hypotension and bradycardia can occur, particularly when dexmedetomidine is used with medications that have similar effects (propofol). Dexmedetomidine is administered as a continuous infusion using an electronic pump for precise dosing. The length of the infusion will influence the time to complete recovery.

THE NURSING PROCESS

A concept map outlines the nursing process related to drug therapy considerations in this chapter. Additional nursing implications related to the disease process should also be considered in care decisions.

Assessment

A systematic preoperative interview is conducted prior to the surgery or diagnostic procedure to determine the physical and psychological preparation of the patient. This helps predict the possible implications or interactions with anesthesia. Although the anesthesia provider is responsible for the assessment and treatment of the patient, the care of the patient is a team process.
- **Assess the patient's status in relation to the anesthesia administration and his or her surgical experience preoperatively.**
  - Assess the patient's understanding of the perioperative process.
  - Assess the patient's health and surgical history, including allergies to medications, eggs or soy products, latex, or anesthesia-related products.
  - Interview the patient about the surgical experience and administration of anesthetics, including a family or patient history of malignant hyperthermia or atypical plasma cholinesterase.
  - Assess medications, both prescription and over-the-counter or complementary and alternative therapies, taken in the past 2 weeks, and the day of surgery.
- **Implement preoperative assessments.**
  - Assess blood count, chemistry panel, coagulation profile, fasting blood sugar, HbA1c, ECG, chest radiation, and pregnancy test.
  - Assess baseline vital signs, level of consciousness, and orientation.
- **Assess the patient's response to general anesthesia.**
  - Assess vital signs continuously.
  - Assess physiologic response to anesthesia.
- **Implement postanesthesia/postoperative assessment.**
  - Assess airway, vital signs, level of consciousness, pain.
  - Assess for postoperative nausea and vomiting.

Outcomes of Therapy

The patient will
- Understand the expected outcome or limitations of the anesthesia, including the following:
  - Level of pain
  - Postoperative nausea and vomiting
  - Expectations during the surgery or procedure and recovery period
- Adhere to preoperative instructions (a coherent patient may be necessary for selected surgical or diagnostic procedures):
  - Cessation of alcohol, complementary and alternative therapies, and smoking
  - Essential medications day of surgery
- Experience partial or complete amnesia while in the surgical suite:
- Experience control of pain to acceptable level.
- Experience control of PONV so as not to cause excessive pain, dehydration, or disrupt the surgical repair.
- Have no adverse effects from the anesthesia.

Nursing Interventions

- Provide accurate information to the patient about the surgical or diagnostic procedure, the planned anesthetic, and the expected outcomes.
- Instruct the patient to report symptoms such as pain, nausea, difficult breathing, weakness, lightheadedness, itching, and chest pain.
- Assess the patient's preoperative psychological status.
- Be available to assist the anesthesia provider during tracheal intubation and extubation.
- Monitor vital signs, fluid intake or output, or perform other responsibilities in coordination with the anesthesia provider.
- Do not move or reposition an intubated patient without prior coordination with the anesthesia provider.
- Know the location of emergency equipment such as a difficult airway cart, malignant hyperthermia cart, or code cart.
- Refrain from inappropriate discussion during surgery. Even during general anesthesia or sedation, a patient may have recall of conversation or events.
- Be cognizant that anesthetics have the potential for rapid and profound changes in physiologic stability and that the nurse may be required to assist the anesthesia provider at any time.
- Assist the anesthesia provider with the transport from the operating room to the PACU or ICU.
  - Continue to evaluate airway patency, breathing, and circulation during transport and on arrival to the PACU or ICU. Supplemental oxygen may be necessary, especially for pediatric and elderly patients.
  - Information includes the anesthetic technique and medications used, time of last narcotic, intake and output, pertinent events during the surgery or procedure, length of anesthetic, stability during procedure, and whether neuromuscular blocking agents were reversed and at what time.
  - Develop a customized plan of patient care with the anesthesia provider.
- When the patient is transferred from the PACU to the division or outpatient suite, maintain and assess:
  - Pulse oximetry oxygen saturation
  - Airway, circulation, Level of consciousness and motor function
  - Temperature, pain, PONV, emotional comfort and intake and output

Evaluation

- Be familiar with your institution's practice guidelines and benchmark goals to help direct therapy and evaluate recovery from anesthesia.
- Observe that patient planning/goals are met.
- Assess the effectiveness of perioperative nursing interventions and medication therapy.

Visit thePoint® at **http://thePoint.lww.com/Frandsen13e** for answers to NCLEX Success questions (in Appendix A), answers to Clinical Application Case Studies (in Appendix B), and more!

REFERENCES AND RESOURCES

Bittner, E. A. (2022). Neuromuscular blocking agents in critically ill patients: Use, agent selection, administration, and adverse effects. In P. E. Parson, G. Finlay & M. Crowley (Eds.), *UpToDate*. Wolters Kluwer.

Falk, S. A., & Fleisher, L. E. (2022). Overview of anesthesia. In S. B. Jones, N. A. Nussmeier & W. Chen (Eds.), *UpToDate*. Wolters Kluwer.

Feinleib, J., Kwan, L. H., & Yamani, A. (2022). Postoperative nausea and vomiting. In N. F. Holt, A. Davidson & M. Crowley (Eds.), *UpToDate*. Wolters Kluwer.

Flood, P., & Rathmell, J. P. (2021). *Stoelting's pharmacology and physiology in anesthesia practice* (6th ed.). Wolters Kluwer.

Gan, T. J., Belani, K. G., Bergese, S., Chung, F., Diemunsch, P., Habib, A. S., Jin, Z., Kovac, A. L., Meyer, T. A., Urman, R. D., Apfel, C. C., Ayad, S., Beagley, L., Candiotti, K., Englesakis, M., Hedrick, T. L., Kranke, P., Lee, S., Lipman, D., et al. (2020). Fourth Consensus Guidelines for the Management of Postoperative Nausea and Vomiting. *Anesthesia & Analgesia*, 131(2), 411–448.

Khorsand, S. M. (2022). Maintenance of general anesthesia: Overview. In G. P. Joshi & N. A. Nussmeier (Eds.), *UpToDate*. Wolters Kluwer.

Nettina, S. M. (Ed.) (2019). *Lippincott manual of nursing practice* (11th ed.). Wolters Kluwer.

Renew, J. R. (2022). Clinical use of neuromuscular blocking agents in anesthesia. In G. P. Joshi & M. Crowley (Eds.), *UpToDate*. Wolters Kluwer.

Rosero, E. B. (2022). Monitored anesthesia care in adults. In G. P. Joshi & M. Crowley (Eds.), *UpToDate*. Wolters Kluwer.

UpToDate. (2022). *Drug Information*. Lexi-Comp, Inc.

Zengin, S. U., & Ergun, M. O. (2022). Retrospective assessment of the association between inhalation anesthesia and post-operative complication in morbidly obese patients undergoing bariatric surgery. *Journal of Surgical Medicine*, 6(3), 258–262. doi: 10.28982/josam.1083644

CHAPTER 52

Drug Therapy for Migraines and Other Headaches

LEARNING OBJECTIVES

After studying this chapter, you should be able to:

1. Identify the major manifestations of cluster headaches, migraine headaches, tension-type headaches, and menstrual migraine headaches.
2. Identify the prototype and describe the action, use, adverse effects, contraindications, and nursing implications for nonsteroidal anti-inflammatory drugs administered as abortive therapy for migraines.
3. Describe the action, use, adverse effects, contraindications, and nursing implications for acetaminophen–aspirin–caffeine combinations administered as abortive therapy for headaches.
4. Identify the prototype and describe the action, use, adverse effects, contraindications, and nursing implications for ergot alkaloids administered as abortive therapy.
5. Identify the prototype and describe the action, adverse effects, contraindications, and nursing implications for triptans administered as abortive therapy.
6. Identify the prototype and describe the action, adverse effects, contraindications, and nursing implications for calcitonin gene–related peptide antagonists administered as abortive therapy.
7. Identify the prototype and describe the action, use, adverse effects, contraindications, and nursing implications for estrogen administered for menstrual migraines.
8. Identify the medications used for the prevention of migraine headaches.
9. Describe the action, use, adverse effects, contraindications, and nursing implications for antiemetic drugs used in the treatment of migraine headaches.
10. Implement the nursing process in the care of patients who suffer from migraine headaches.

CLINICAL APPLICATION CASE STUDY

Tanya Van Art, who is 18 years of age, has experienced headaches since she was 13. In the past year, the headaches have been increasing in severity. While at work this past week, she developed a severe headache with nausea and vomiting and was admitted to the emergency department (ED). On admission, her blood pressure was 180/90 mm Hg and her pain was 10 on a 10-point scale. She denied having any aura preceding the onset of the headache or any vision changes at onset or now. In the ED, she received sumatriptan 6 mg subcutaneous injection, ketorolac 30 mg IV, and dihydroergotamine 1 mg combined with metoclopramide 10 mg.

The diagnosis was acute migraine headache.

KEY TERMS

Abortive therapy: medications administered to treat the symptoms of migraine headache

Aura: subjective sensation that immediately precedes a migraine headache, consisting of a breeze, odor, or light

Cluster headache: recurrent, severe, unilateral orbitotemporal headache

Menstrual migraine headache: migraine headache associated with a drop in circulating estrogen that occurs 2 to 3 days prior to the onset of menses; also called estrogen-associated headaches

Migraine headache: unilateral pain in the head that may or may not be accompanied by an aura; may be associated with vertigo, nausea, vomiting, and photophobia

Preventive therapy: administration of medications to prevent the onset of migraine headaches

Tension-type headache: headache associated with nervous tension or anxiety

Vascular constriction: narrowing of the blood vessels

INTRODUCTION

Headaches are among the most common disorders, yet the focus on their importance as a public health concern was limited until 30 years ago. Although headache disorders can be debilitating for a relatively large minority of the population, most individuals experience a headache from time to time, the disorder is not fatal, and it does not result in permanent disability. These factors have delayed the focus on headache disorders.

This chapter discusses the various types of headaches, including cluster, migraine, and tension-type, all of which produce pain. However, the pain experienced by patients and the physiology involved varies with each type of headache. To aid understanding of drug therapy for cluster, migraine, and tension-type headaches, this chapter presents clinical manifestations of the different types of headaches. This chapter also considers the pharmacologic treatment for each of these headaches. For further details on the pathophysiology of headaches, visit thePoint® http://thePoint.lww.com/Frandsen13e.

OVERVIEW OF HEADACHES

Cluster headache belongs to a group of headache conditions, called the trigeminal autonomic cephalalgias, all of which involve unilateral, often severe headache symptoms. Cluster headache is the most common syndrome and presents with recurrent and severe orbitotemporal headache. Evidence suggests that the syndrome demonstrates a familial pattern and is four times more prevalent in females than in males.

Migraine headache is a severe and disabling neurologic disorder resulting from an inherited tendency for the brain to lose control of its inputs. Annually, this condition affects approximately 12% to 15% of the general population, with 17% of females and 6% of males. It occurs most commonly in persons between 30 and 39 years of age, although children may have migraine headaches. Migraine is associated with a huge socioeconomic impact when symptoms are episodic and chronic in nature. The headache involves unilateral pain in the head that may or may not be accompanied by an **aura**. An aura is a subjective sensation that immediately precedes the migraine headache consisting of a breeze, odor, or light. Migraine headaches may also be associated with vertigo, nausea, vomiting, and photophobia.

Migraine predominately affects females more often than does males. In part, the increased incidence in females may be the result of circulating estrogen. Menstruation may be the most common and potent trigger of a migraine attack. **Menstrual migraine headaches**, also called estrogen-associated headaches, are most commonly brought on with a drop in circulating estrogen 2 to 3 days prior to the onset of menses. Nearly one in four U.S. households includes a person who experiences migraine.

Tension-type headache, previously described as tension or stress headache, muscle contraction headache, and psychogenic headache, is the most common headache in the general population. The tension-type headache is associated with nervous tension or anxiety. Many individuals do not seek help for the condition, because the headache is intermittent, mild, and often indistinctive. This type of headache is the least studied of all the primary headache disorders despite having a high socioeconomic impact. A tension-type headache was once thought to be the result of chronic contraction of the scalp muscles, but that concept is no longer considered valid.

Clinical Manifestations

Cluster Headache

A cluster headache typically occurs up to eight times per day with pain commonly lasting 15 to 180 minutes. In the episodic form, the attacks typically occur daily for a period of 6 to 12 weeks followed by a period of remission that can last for up to a year or longer. In the chronic form, remission is not part of the cluster attack.

Cluster symptoms are indicative of both parasympathetic hyperactivity and sympathetic impairment. A person with cluster headache presents with severe orbital, supraorbital, or temporal pain accompanied by ipsilateral autonomic symptoms such as ptosis, miosis, lacrimation, conjunctival injection, rhinorrhea, and nasal congestion. Sweating and cutaneous blood flow also increase on the side of the pain, particularly in areas of sympathetic deficit. The symptoms typically resolve with the headache, but mitosis and ptosis, signs of sympathetic paralysis, can persist but intensify during attacks. In addition, patterns of circadian rhythmicity are a hallmark of the syndrome.

Migraine Headache

A migraine headache with an aura has four phases: prodrome, aura, headache, and recovery. The prodrome phase occurs hours or days before the onset of a migraine headache. Symptoms include depression, irritability, feeling cold, cravings, loss of appetite, alterations in activity, polyuria, diarrhea, and constipation. The aura phase, which occurs only in some patients, involves an aura lasting 1 hour with focal neurologic symptoms, visual disturbances, or vision in only half of the visual field.

The headache phase is characterized by vasodilation and a decline in serotonin levels. A throbbing headache becomes more intense, lasting for several hours. The headache can become incapacitating, with photophobia, nausea, and vomiting. The recovery phase involves slow subsiding of the pain. There may be muscle contractions in the neck and scalp, with localized tenderness, tiredness, and alterations in mood. The patient may sleep for hours after the recovery phase.

Symptoms in females with a menstrual headache may vary from this pattern. These headaches are not commonly associated with an aura, although females may experience an aura during periods of nonmenstrual attacks. In addition, menstrual migraines tend to be more severe, last longer, and be less responsive to abortive treatment.

Chronic migraine is diagnosed by the presence of a migraine headache without an aura for 8 days or more per month for 3 months. The headache is unilateral, pulsating with moderate to severe intensity, and aggravated by activity.

Tension-Type Headache

A wide variation exists in the experiences of people who suffer from a tension-type headache. Characteristic signs and symptoms include bilateral, nonthrobbing head pain of mild to moderate intensity. Patients may describe pressure, head fullness, or a bandlike sensation around the head, or they may report a feeling like a heavyweight is on their head or shoulders without other associated features. Tension-type headaches are classified into three subtypes based on the frequency of headache episodes:

- Infrequent: headache less than 1 day per month
- Frequent: headache 1 to 14 days per month
- Chronic: headache 15 or more days per month

Management of the condition varies based on the subtype. Infrequent or low-frequency episodic subtype patterns are managed with acute symptomatic treatment; prophylactic treatments are added for high-frequency and chronic headaches. In addition, impact on the quality of life increases with the headache frequency of the subtype.

Drug Therapy
Cluster Headache

Drug therapy to prevent cluster headaches should begin with the onset of a cluster episode. Verapamil is recommended as initial preventive therapy. Topiramate can be administered in combination with verapamil. Glucocorticoids are administered for patients who have infrequent cluster headaches and last less than 2 months. Treatment of a cluster headache involves subcutaneous sumatriptan and high-flow (100%) oxygen. Because the adverse effects of oxygen use are less than those of sumatriptan, high-flow oxygen may be administered for 15 minutes to determine effectiveness. Although oxygen may be effective in some patients, resuming the use of high-flow oxygen within a short period of time following relief of the headache should be avoided, because evidence shows that the frequency of cluster headaches may increase in some patients with overuse of high-flow oxygen. Ergot derivatives, lidocaine, and octreotide are also effective in the treatment of acute cluster headaches. Cluster headaches often are not treated as effectively as migraines. New guidelines have suggested that sumatriptan, administered subcutaneously, and zolmitriptan nasal spray, augmented by high-flow oxygen, may be effective. Steroid injections as well as calcium channel blockers may offer an option. Nonpharmacologic options include occipital and vagal nerve stimulation.

Migraine Headaches

Drug therapy to manage a migraine is guided mainly by several factors: (1) the severity of the attacks; (2) the presence of associated symptoms, such as nausea and vomiting; (3) the type of treatment setting (outpatient or inpatient); and (4) patient-specific factors, such as the patient's medication preference and the presence of vascular risk factors. There are two specific courses of treatment for migraine headaches: abortive and preventive therapy. **Abortive therapy** is the administration of medications to treat the symptoms of migraine headache. **Preventive therapy** is the administration of medications to prevent the development of a migraine headache. The emergency management of severe migraine attacks includes the following medications:

- Sumatriptan 6 mg subcutaneous injection
- Antiemetics: dopamine receptor blockers as prescribed
  - Prochlorperazine 10 mg IV or IM
  - Metoclopramide 10 mg IV
  - Chlorpromazine 0.1 mg/kg (or 12.5 mg) single dose as a slow IV infusion (1 mg/min) maximum dosage: 25 mg
- Dihydroergotamine 1 mg combined with metoclopramide 10 mg IV
- Ketorolac 30 mg IV or 60 mg IM (15 mg IV or 30 mg IM for patients older than 65 years, less than 50 kg, or abnormal kidney function)

Medications used in the treatment of migraine headaches are listed in Table 52.1.

The abortive agents administered for the treatment of migraine headaches include nonsteroidal anti-inflammatory agents, acetaminophen–aspirin with caffeine medication, the ergot alkaloids, the triptans (serotonin receptor [5-HT_{1B} and 5-HT_{1D}] agonists), and the calcitonin gene–related receptor antagonists (gepants). Although it can produce nervousness and dizziness, caffeine was found to be an effective analgesic adjuvant in the acute treatment of migraine headache. The pharmacologic and nonpharmacologic treatment of long-term migraine is to reduce the frequency, severity, and disability. The initial pharmacotherapy for acute treatment of migraine is the administration of triptans subcutaneously. In addition, intravenous metoclopramide and prochlorperazine are also used in eligible adults who present to an ED with acute migraine. Metoclopramide has been shown to be highly effective in relieving migraine-associated symptoms. In children, ketorolac, administered intramuscularly or intravenously, is highly effective, relieving migraine pain within 60 minutes.

Initial abortive therapy for females who experience acute menstrual migraines is the same as that for migraine occurring at any other time. People who suffer from migraines take preventive medications, which are discussed later in this chapter.

> **Quality and Safety Alert: Evidence-Based Practice**
>
> Hartford et al. (2022) analyzed the treatment patterns and outcomes for acute migraines in pediatric patients. The authors examined retrospective data on treatment, length of stay, and emergency department (ED) charges. The data also included ethnicity and language preference. The researchers examined whether the patients received oral, intranasal, or intravenous (IV) administration of medications to treat migraine pain. A total of 833 patients with a median age of 14.8 years with 67% female, 51% non-Hispanic White, 23% Hispanic, 8.3% Black or African American, and 4.3% Asian were included. Of the study participants, 287 received oral or intranasal and 546 received IV medications. The study revealed that patients who were Asian, Black or African American, and Hispanic or had a language preference other than English had a significantly lower chance of receiving IV treatment despite similar pain scores as those treated with IV medications. Patients in the group receiving IV treatment had longer lengths of stay and higher ED charges. The results of this study confirm the need to improve equity for all patients receiving ED care.

Clinical Application 52.1

- What are the recommended medications for acute migraine treatment in the ED?
- What does the nurse discuss about auras and migraine-associated vision changes?

Tension-Type Headaches

Acute therapy for tension-type headaches entails the use of nonpharmacologic methods such as rest, relaxation techniques, or stress reduction strategies as well as medication. Pharmacologic treatment of tension-type headaches includes acetaminophen, aspirin, and nonsteroidal anti-inflammatory drugs (NSAIDs) (see Chapter 16). Studies have shown that tricyclic drugs can reverse the central sensitization and chronicity of these headaches. In addition, a meta-analysis of eight placebo-controlled clinical trials found that botulinum toxin type A led to a small decrease in number of headaches per month, although the result was not statistically significant.

NONSTEROIDAL ANTI-INFLAMMATORY DRUGS (NSAIDS)

Ibuprofen is the traditional prototype of the NSAIDs (see Chapter 16). However, naproxen sodium is more commonly prescribed for the treatment of migraine headaches because it is more rapidly absorbed and produces more rapid analgesia. Thus, 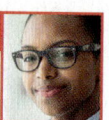 **naproxen** (Naprosyn) or **naproxen sodium** (Aleve) serves as the prototype described in detail in this chapter.

Pharmacokinetics

There are two types of naproxen: naproxen and naproxen sodium. Naproxen has an onset of action of 1 hour, a peak of action of 2 to 4 hours, and duration of action of 7 hours or less. Naproxen sodium has an onset of action of 1 hour, a peak of action of 1 to 2 hours, and the same duration of action as naproxen. Metabolism of both agents occurs in the liver, and they have a half-life of 12 to 15 hours. Excretion is in the urine. Naproxen and naproxen sodium cross the placental barrier and enter the breast milk.

Action

Naproxen is a nonselective inhibitor of cyclooxygenase resulting in the inhibition of prostaglandin synthesis of COX-1 and

TABLE 52.1

Drugs Administered for the Treatment of Migraine Headache

Drug Class	Prototype	Other Drugs in the Class
Nonsteroidal anti-inflammatory drugs	Naproxen (Aleve, Anaprox DS, Naprosyn, Naprosyn EC, Goodsense Naproxen Sodium, Naprelan)	Ketorolac tromethamine
Analgesic	Aspirin–acetaminophen–caffeine (Excedrin)	
Ergot alkaloids	Ergotamine tartrate (Ergomar)	Dihydroergotamine (Migranal, Trudhesa)
Triptans	Sumatriptan (Imitrex, Onzetra Xsail, others)	Almotriptan Eletriptan (Relpax) Frovatriptan (Frova) Naratriptan Rizatriptan (Maxalt, Maxalt-MLT) Zolmitriptan (Zomig)
Estrogen	Estradiol	
Calcitonin gene–related peptide receptor antagonist	Ubrogepant (Ubrelvy)	Atogepant (Qulipta) Rimegepant (Nurtec)
Antiemetic	Chlorpromazine hydrochloride	Metoclopramide (Reglan) Prochlorperazine (Compro)

COX-2. Naproxen sodium improves the solubility of naproxen through faster absorption and rapid onset of action.

Use

Prescribers order naproxen sodium to reduce the pain resulting from an acute migraine headache. Table 52.2 presents dosage information for naproxen and related drugs.

Patient-related variables specific to the use of naproxen and naproxen sodium include the following:

- Age:
  - Older people should not take more than 200 mg of naproxen sodium every 12 hours.
  - In pediatric patients who are 12 years of age or older, improved efficacy has been shown when using a fixed dose combination of naproxen with sumatriptan.
- Reproduction, pregnancy, and lactation:
  - NSAIDs may delay or prevent rupture of ovarian follicles. This may be associated with infertility that is reversible upon discontinuation of the medication. Consider discontinuation of the medication in patients having difficulty conceiving.
  - The use of NSAIDs close to conception may be associated with miscarriage due to the inhibition of cyclooxygenase 2 with implantation.
  - Avoid maternal use of NSAIDs beginning at 20 weeks' gestation. If it is necessary to administer NSAIDs at 20 to 30 weeks, use the lowest possible dose.
  - Naproxen is present in the breast milk. Consideration must be given to the risk versus benefit of breast-feeding.
- Abnormal kidney function and hepatic impairment:
  - In patients with kidney disease, caution is necessary with the administration of naproxen sodium because the kidney system excretes the drug. It should be avoided in patients with advanced kidney disease.
  - In patients with hepatic impairment, caution is warranted with the administration of naproxen sodium because the site of metabolism is the liver.

Adverse Effects

The most severe adverse effects of naproxen sodium include bronchospasm and anaphylaxis. Gastrointestinal (GI) adverse effects include GI bleeding, nausea, dyspepsia, and GI pain. The U.S. Food and Drug Administration (FDA) has issued a **BOXED WARNING** ◆ stating that naproxen sodium may put patients at increased risk for cardiovascular events and GI bleeding.

Contraindications

Contraindications to naproxen or naproxen sodium include a known allergy to aspirin or other NSAIDs as well as pregnancy and lactation. It is important to administer the medication cautiously to patients with asthma, cardiovascular dysfunction, hypertension, GI bleeding, and peptic ulcer.

Nursing Implications

Administering the Medication

Administer naproxen with food, milk, or antacids to decrease adverse GI effects. Patients should swallow the extended-release tablet whole. The drug suspension must be shaken well before administration.

Preventing Interactions

The administration of naproxen sodium with lithium results in increased lithium levels and the risk of lithium toxicity.

Assessing for Therapeutic Effects

Following the administration of naproxen or naproxen sodium, the patient should exhibit diminished pain. The nurse assesses the patient's pain level using a pain scale.

Assessing for Adverse Effects

The nurse assesses the patient for GI upset, dyspepsia, or bleeding. Pulmonary function and lung sounds are assessed for bronchospasm or anaphylactic reaction.

TABLE 52.2

DRUGS AT A GLANCE: Nonsteroidal Anti-inflammatory Drugs*

Drug	Routes and Dosages	
	Adults	**Children**
ⓟ **Naproxen** (Naprosyn)	375–500 mg PO two times per day	10 mg/kg PO in two divided doses
ⓟ **Naproxen** (Aleve, Anaprox DS, Naprosyn, Naprosyn EC, Goodsense Naproxen Sodium, Naprelan; 🍁 Aleve, Maxidol, Naproxen, others)	Prevention, 250–500 mg PO two times per day Treatment, 750 mg PO initially, an additional 250–500 mg may be given if needed 25 8 (max 1,200 mg/24 h)	>6 y and adolescents: 5–7 mg/kg/dose PO every 8–12 h; maximum dose: 1,000 mg/d
Ketorolac tromethamine (🍁, ALTI-Ketorolac, APO-Ketorolac, Toradol)	15–30 mg IV every 6 h to a maximum of 120 mg/d; 30–60 mg IM	>2–16 y: 0.5 mg/kg IV up to a maximum of 15 mg

*Drugs used in headache treatment.

> **BOX 52.1 Patient Teaching Guidelines for Naproxen Sodium**
>
> - Take the medication with meals to prevent gastrointestinal upset.
> - Do not cut, crush, or chew tablets.
> - Do not operate machinery if dizziness or drowsiness occurs.
> - Report sore throat, fever, rash, itching, edema, visual changes, and black, tarry stools to your healthcare provider.

Patient Teaching

Box 52.1 identifies patient teaching guidelines for naproxen sodium.

Other Drugs in the Class

People with migraine headaches often seek treatment in the ED when the more commonly used abortive therapies are ineffective. In the emergency setting, ketorolac tromethamine is the most frequently administered intravenous drug.

> **Clinical Application 52.2**
> - What is the rationale for administering ketorolac and prochlorperazine to Ms. Van Art?

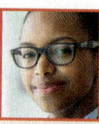

ACETAMINOPHEN, ASPIRIN, AND CAFFEINE

The combination of **acetaminophen**, **aspirin**, and **caffeine** may be effective for the treatment of headaches. In the United States, brand names include Anacin Advanced Headache Formula, Excedrin Extra Strength, Excedrin Migraine, and Goody's Extra Strength.

Pharmacokinetics

To understand the pharmacokinetics of acetaminophen, aspirin, and caffeine, it is important to review each medication individually. Acetaminophen reaches a peak of action in 0.5 to 2 hours and possesses a 1- to 3-hour half-life. It crosses the placental barrier and enters the breast milk. The drug is metabolized in the liver and excreted in the urine. Aspirin has an onset of action of 5 to 30 minutes, reaches a peak of action in 15 to 120 minutes, and has a duration of action of 3 to 6 hours. The half-life of aspirin is 15 minutes to 12 hours. The drug is absorbed in the stomach and metabolized in the liver. Caffeine has an onset of action of 15 minutes and reaches a peak of action in 15 to 45 minutes. It readily crosses the placental barrier and enters the breast milk. Like acetaminophen and aspirin, caffeine is metabolized in the liver. It is eliminated by the kidneys.

Action

Acetaminophen may act as an analgesic, and its mechanism of action is unknown. Aspirin has the ability to inhibit the synthesis of prostaglandins, which are a mediator of inflammation. Caffeine increases calcium permeability in the sarcoplasmic reticulum to promote the accumulation of cyclic adenosine monophosphate (cAMP) and block the adenosine receptors, stimulating the CNS, cardiac activity, gastric acid secretion, and diuresis. It causes a narrowing of the blood vessels, which is known as **vascular constriction**. Migraine headaches result from the vasodilation of blood vessels. In addition, caffeine increases the effectiveness of acetaminophen and aspirin by approximately 40%.

Use

Acetaminophen–aspirin–caffeine products are administered to reduce pain related to migraine or tension-type headache. Table 52.3 presents oral dosage of information for these combination products.

Patient-related variables specific to the use of acetaminophen–aspirin–caffeine include the following:

- Age:
  - Children younger than 18 years of age with suspicion of viral illness are identified on the Key Potentially Inappropriate Drugs in Pediatrics due to the risk of Reye syndrome.
  - Children older than 12 years of age may receive the adult dose of the combination agent.
  - The Beers Criteria identifies aspirin as an inappropriate medication and should be avoided in patients aged 65 years and older due to an increased risk of GI bleed.
- Reproduction, pregnancy, and lactation:
  - Fetal outcomes are influenced by the maternal dose of aspirin; low-dose aspirin is not associated with risks. High-dose aspirin may result in fetal mortality, intrauterine growth retardation, salicylate intoxication, bleeding abnormalities, and neonatal acidosis.

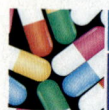

TABLE 52.3 DRUGS AT A GLANCE: Acetaminophen–Aspirin–Caffeine Combinations

Drug	Routes and Dosages	
	Adults	Children
Acetaminophen–aspirin–caffeine (Anacin Advanced Headache Formula, Excedrin Extra Strength, Excedrin Migraine, Vanquish Extra Strength Pain Reliever)	2 tablets PO once per 24 h (each tablet: aspirin 250 mg, acetaminophen 250 mg, caffeine 65 mg) (maximum of two tablets per 24 h)	>12 y: same as adults

- Use of aspirin close to delivery may cause premature closure of the ductus arteriosus.
- Do not use aspirin beginning at 20 weeks' gestation.
- Acetaminophen crosses the placenta, but an increased risk of congenital malformations has not been seen.
- Caffeine crosses the placenta, but usual dietary exposure does not pose a fetal risk.
- Salicylic acid is present in the breast milk.
- Breast-feeding is considered acceptable with acetaminophen and is the preferred initial treatment for acute migraine headaches in patients who are lactating.
- Caffeine is acceptable with breast-feeding.
- Abnormal kidney function and hepatic impairment:
  - People with hepatic impairment should not receive this combination agent on an ongoing basis. They may not metabolize acetaminophen in this combined medication effectively, leading to hepatotoxicity.

Adverse Effects

Each component of the combination medication has adverse effects, which will be addressed individually. Acetaminophen may result in headache, chest pain, dyspnea, myocardial damage with doses of 5 to 8 g/day, and hepatic impairment. Aspirin may lead to GI effects such as dyspepsia, heartburn, and epigastric discomfort as well as hematologic effects such as occult blood loss and hemostatic defects. Aspirin toxicity involves respiratory alkalosis, tachypnea, hemorrhage, excitement, confusion, seizures, tetany, cardiovascular collapse, and metabolic acidosis. Caffeine may result in excitement, insomnia, restlessness, tremors, headaches, and lightheadedness, as well as cardiovascular effects such as tachycardia, hypertension, extrasystole, and palpitations.

Contraindications

Contraindications to acetaminophen include a known allergy to the drug. Caution is necessary in impaired hepatic function, chronic alcoholism, pregnancy, and lactation. Contraindications to aspirin include a known hypersensitivity to the drug or other anti-inflammatory agents. Vigilance is warranted with abnormal kidney function. Contraindications to caffeine include duodenal ulcers, diabetes, and lactation. Caution is essential in pregnancy, abnormal kidney function and hepatic impairment, and cardiovascular disease.

Nursing Implications

People most commonly take the acetaminophen–aspirin–caffeine in the home setting. It is important to be familiar with all aspects of each medication to maintain medication safety.

Administering the Medication and Preventing Interactions

Administer the medication with food to avoid GI distress.

Several drug–drug interactions may occur with acetaminophen–aspirin–caffeine combinations. Alfalfa, anise, bilberry, and ginkgo biloba may enhance anticoagulant effects. Cannabinoid products increase the risk of tachycardia. The concomitant administration of caffeine and guarana, ma huang, and ephedra is not recommended.

Box 52.2 names the specific medications that increase or decrease the effects of each of the medications in the combined drug. Other drug–drug interactions include the following:

- Oral anticoagulants combined with acetaminophen increase hypothrombinemic effects.
- Aspirin combined with sulfonylureas and insulin results in greater glucose-lowering effects.
- Valproic acid combined with aspirin puts patients at risk for seizure activity secondary to protein receptor site displacement.
- Spironolactone or furosemide combined with aspirin leads to decreased diuretic effects.
- Theophylline or clozapine combined with caffeine increases the serum levels of theophylline or clozapine.

Assessing for Therapeutic Effects

Following the administration of the acetaminophen–aspirin–caffeine combination, the patient should exhibit diminished pain. The nurse assesses for pain using a pain scale.

Assessing for Adverse Effects

The nurse assesses for hepatotoxicity, allergic reaction, fluid and electrolyte imbalance, hypoglycemia, agitation, and cardiovascular effects.

Patient Teaching

Box 52.3 identifies patient teaching guidelines for acetaminophen–aspirin–caffeine combinations.

BOX 52.2 Drug Interactions: Acetaminophen, Aspirin, and Caffeine

Drugs That Increase the Effects of Acetaminophen
- Alcohol, barbiturates, carbamazepine, hydantoins, rifampin, sulfinpyrazone
  Increase the risk of hepatotoxicity

Drugs That Increase the Effects of Aspirin
- Alcohol, anticoagulants, NSAIDs
  Increase the bleeding risk
- Carbonic anhydrase inhibitors
  Increase the risk of salicylate toxicity

Drugs That Increase the Effects of Caffeine
- Cimetidine, hormonal contraceptive, disulfiram, ciprofloxacin, mexiletine
  Increase the central nervous system effects

Drugs That Decrease the Effects of Aspirin
- Acetazolamide, methazolamide, antacids, alkalinizers
  Decrease the salicylate levels

Drugs That Decrease the Effects of Caffeine
- Nicotine
  Produces vasoconstriction

BOX 52.3 Patient Teaching Guidelines for Acetaminophen–Aspirin–Caffeine Combinations

- Never exceed the recommended dosage of acetaminophen–aspirin–caffeine combinations.
- Avoid the use of over-the-counter and prescription forms of medications that contain acetaminophen.
- Take the drug with food or after meals if possible.
- Do not stop caffeine abruptly.
- Do not consume foods high in caffeine.
- Report the following conditions to your healthcare provider:
  - Any signs and symptoms of bleeding
  - Ringing in the ears, dizziness, confusion, abdominal pain, dyspnea, nausea, and vomiting
  - Abnormal heart rate and palpitations

NCLEX Success

1. An adolescent patient is suffering from migraine headaches and the healthcare provider orders a combination of acetaminophen, aspirin, and caffeine. Prior to the administration of the medication, it is necessary to assess for which of the following?
   A. anxiety and depression
   B. history of smoking
   C. family history of migraines
   D. antacid use

ERGOT ALKALOIDS

The ergotamine preparations are administered for abortive therapy for migraine headaches, although they have been largely replaced by the triptans (see later discussion). Clinical studies have shown that oral ergotamine plus caffeine is less effective than triptans for acute migraine. The prototype medication is ⓟ **ergotamine tartrate** (Ergomar), an alpha-adrenergic antagonist.

Pharmacokinetics

Ergotamine has a variable rate of absorption and onset of action. The peak of action is 0.5 to 3 hours. The half-life of ergotamine is 2 hours, but the effects of the medication can continue for 24 hours. The medication is metabolized by the cytochrome P450 enzyme CYP3A4 in the liver and excreted in the bile. Ergotamine is excreted in the breast milk and may cause vomiting, diarrhea, and changes in heart rate and blood pressure in the nursing infant. It has caused fetal growth retardation in animal studies.

Action

Ergotamine produces stimulation of the cranial and peripheral vascular smooth muscles while depressing the effects of the central vasomotor centers. It is a partial agonist and antagonist that act against tryptaminergic, dopaminergic, and alpha-adrenergic receptors to constrict the cranial and peripheral blood vessels.

Use

Prescribers order ergotamine individually or in combination with caffeine to prevent or stop migraine, cluster, or vascular headaches. Table 52.4 gives dosage information for the ergot alkaloids.

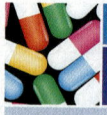

TABLE 52.4 DRUGS AT A GLANCE: Ergot Alkaloids

Drug	Routes and Dosages	
	Adults	**Children**
ⓟ **Ergotamine tartrate** (Ergomar)	1–2 mg sublingual followed by 1–2 mg every 30 min until headache abates or until maximum dosage of 6 mg/24 h or 10 mg/wk	2 mg sublingual at the first sign of a headache, then 2 mg every 30 min as tolerated; maximum dose 6 mg in 24 h
Dihydroergotamine mesylate (Trudhesa Migranal; 🍁 Migranal)	1 mg may be repeated at 1-h intervals to a total of 3 mg IM or 2 mg IV or SC (maximum dosage of 6 mg/wk) 1 spray (0.5 mg) in each nostril, may repeat with additional spray in 15 min if no relief (maximum of 4 sprays/attack); wait 6–8 h before treating another attack (maximum of sprays, 8 sprays/24 h, 24 sprays/wk)	Low-dose regimen: 6 to <10 y: 0.1 mg/dose IV every 6 h; 10–12 y: 0.15 mg/dose IV every 6 h; <16 y: 0.2 mg/dose every 6 h; maximum dose for all ages: 8 doses per episode High-dose regimen: 6–9 y: 0.5 mg/dose IV every 8 h; ≥10 y: 1 mg/dose every 8 h; maximum 15 doses per episode

Patient-related variables specific to the use of ergotamine include the following:

- Age:
  - Ergotamine is not routinely used in children but can be used in adolescents.
  - Ergotamine is not recommended for older adults due to vasoconstrictive properties.
- Reproduction, pregnancy, and lactation:
  - Ergotamine is contraindicated in pregnancy and lactation.
  - Ergotamine is excreted in the breast milk. It may cause vomiting, diarrhea, weak pulse, and unstable blood pressure in the nursing infant.
- Abnormal kidney function and hepatic impairment:
  - Ergotamine is contraindicated in patients with impaired kidney or hepatic function.

Adverse Effects

The cardiovascular adverse effects of ergotamine include absence of pulse, bradycardia, cardiac valvular fibrosis, cyanosis, edema, heart rhythm changes, gangrene, hypertension, ischemia, precordial distress, chest pain, tachycardia, and vasospasm. Musculoskeletal adverse effects include muscle pain, numbness, paresthesia, and weakness. Other side effects may include vertigo, nausea, vomiting, itching, pulmonary fibrosis, and genitourinary retroperitoneal fibrosis.

Contraindications

Contraindications of ergotamine include a known hypersensitivity reaction to the drug or its components. Additional contraindications are the existence of peripheral vascular disease, hepatic and kidney disease, coronary artery disease, hypertension, and sepsis. The FDA has issued a **BOXED WARNING** ◆ stating that ergotamine is contraindicated with potent inhibitors of CYP3A4 medications. These drugs include the protease inhibitors, azole antifungals, and some macrolide antibiotics. Concomitant use of these medications results in the risk of vasospasm, producing serious or life-threatening cerebral and limb ischemia. Pregnancy and lactation are also contraindications to the use of ergotamine.

Nursing Implications

Preventing Interactions

Ergot derivatives may increase the hypertensive effects of alpha 1 agonists. Ergotamine is metabolized by the cytochrome P450 enzyme CYP3A4 in the liver; therefore, it is important to avoid all CPY3A4 inhibitors. Cola, coffee, tea, and grapefruit juice increase the serum drug concentrations of ergotamine. In addition, many medications interact with ergotamine, increasing its effects (Box 52.4).

Administering the Medication

Administration of ergotamine is sublingual, and the tablet should be dissolved under the tongue. It is important that tablets not be crushed, chewed, or swallowed whole. Patients should not drink, eat, or smoke while the medication is being dissolved.

Assessing for Therapeutic Effects

The nurse assesses for a decrease in headache pain.

BOX 52.4 Drug Interactions: Ergotamine

Drugs That Increase the Effect of Ergotamine

- Alpha- and beta-adrenergic blockers, sympathomimetics
  Have additive vasoconstrictive effects
- Erythromycin, troleandomycin
  Increase the risk of peripheral vasospasm
- Rizatriptan, sumatriptan, zolmitriptan
  Increase the risk of coronary ischemia
- Azole antifungals, nefazodone, fluoxetine, fluvoxamine, amprenavir, delavirdine, efavirenz, indinavir, nelfinavir, ritonavir, saquinavir
  Inhibit ergotamine metabolism and increase toxicity
- Sibutramine, dexfenfluramine, nefazodone, fluvoxamine
  Increase the risk of muscle rigidity also known as serotonin rigidity
- Clarithromycin, boceprevir, cobicistat, crizotinib, posaconazole
  Increase the serum concentration of ergotamine

Assessing for Adverse Effects

Following administration of ergotamine, the nurse assesses for cardiovascular adverse effects. Measurement of pulse and blood pressure is essential. The nurse also assesses for vertigo, muscle pain, numbness, paresthesia, and weakness, as well as for signs and symptoms of a hypersensitivity reaction to ergotamine. It is important to assess the patient's fluid and electrolyte status if the patient is suffering from nausea and vomiting. In addition, the nurse assesses the patient's urinary elimination due to the adverse effect of retroperitoneal fibrosis in which the patient develops an obstruction of the ureters.

Patient Teaching

Box 52.5 identifies patient teaching guidelines for ergotamine.

Other Drugs in the Class

Dihydroergotamine mesylate reduces the rate of serotonin-induced platelet aggregation and has a weaker vasoconstrictive action than ergotamine. It has a greater adrenergic blocking activity to relieve migraine headaches.

NCLEX Success

2. For the patient with migraine headaches who receives a prescription for an ergot alkaloid as abortive therapy, which of the following is a priority nursing intervention for patient education?

   A. Notify the prescriber if an aura precedes the migraine headache.
   B. Administer the medication with food.
   C. Seek emergency help if cardiac changes occur.
   D. Administer the medication with caffeinated beverages.

BOX 52.5 — Patient Teaching Guidelines for Ergotamine

- Take ergotamine or ergot alkaloids at the onset of the migraine headache.
- Notify the prescriber if the migraine attacks occur more frequently or are not relieved.
- Rest in a dark room for 2 to 3 hours after taking the medication.
- Provide information on adverse effects and notify the prescriber if muscle pain, weakness of extremities, changes in heart rate, nausea, or vomiting develops.
- Never crush, swallow, or chew tablets.
- Do not increase dose unless indicated by the prescriber.

TRIPTANS

Triptans are serotonin 5-HT_{1B} and 5-HT_{1D} agonists that affect the pathophysiologic mechanism of migraine or cluster headaches, thus relieving the associated symptoms. The mechanism of action of the triptans, although similar to that of the ergot alkaloids, has a more selective serotonin agonist receptor profile, and it does not interact with adrenergic and dopaminergic receptors. In addition, the advantage of the administration of triptans over the ergot alkaloids is that these medications can be easily taken by patients during their daily lives. The prototype triptan is **sumatriptan** (Imitrex, Onzetra Xsail, others).

Pharmacokinetics

The oral preparation of sumatriptan has an onset of action of 60 to 90 minutes and a peak of action of 2 to 4 hours. The onset of action of intranasal sumatriptan is rapid, with a peak of action of 90 minutes. The onset of action of subcutaneous sumatriptan varies, with a peak of action of 5 to 20 minutes. Sumatriptan is widely distributed and is 10% to 20% protein bound. Its therapeutic half-life is 115 minutes. Metabolism occurs in the liver. Excretion is in the urine, with excretion of the oral preparation in the feces. Sumatriptan crosses the placenta and enters the breast milk.

Action

Sumatriptan binds to the serotonin receptors 5-HT_{1D}, producing vascular constriction of the cranial blood vessels and relieving the pain of a migraine headache. It also relieves the nausea, vomiting, photophobia, and phonophobia that accompany the migraine headache. Figure 52.1 shows the site of action of triptans, including sumatriptan, in the relief of a migraine.

Use

Healthcare providers use sumatriptan to treat acute migraine headache pain with or without an aura. They also use it to treat cluster headaches. Older adults should not take sumatriptan and other triptans. Table 52.5 gives dosage information for the triptans.

Patient-related variables specific to the use of sumatriptan include the following:

- Reproduction, pregnancy, and lactation:
  - An increased risk of congenital malformations was not seen with sumatriptan.
  - Breast-feeding is considered acceptable with sumatriptan.
- Abnormal kidney function and hepatic impairment:
  - There are no dosage adjustments according to the manufacturer's labeling of sumatriptan, but dosage adjustments are not expected due to the metabolism of the drug to inactive agents.

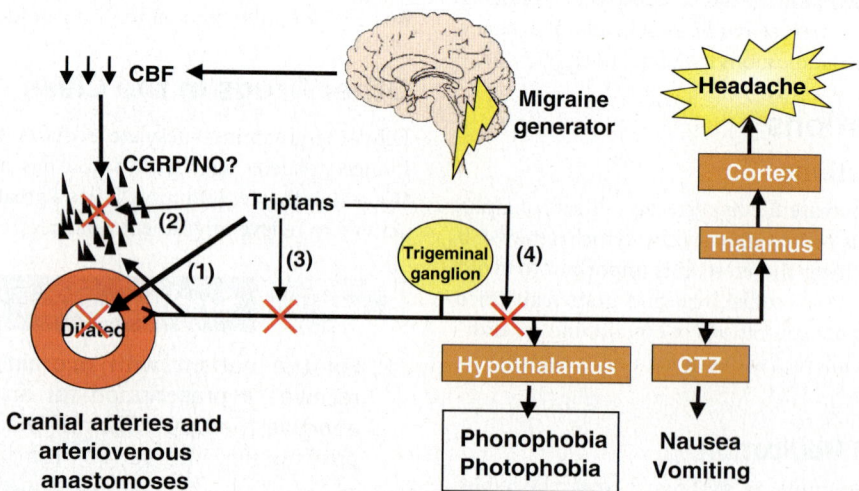

Figure 52.1. Site of action of migraine drugs. The site of action of triptans in aborting migraine attack include the following: (1) a direct contraction of dilated cranial extracerebral blood vessels; (2) suppression of neuropeptide (mainly calcitonin gene–related peptide or CGRP) release from peripheral nerve endings around blood vessels; (3) inhibition of impulse transmission centrally in the trigeminal nucleus caudalis; and (4) presynaptic blockade of synaptic transmission between axon terminals of the peripheral trigeminovascular neurons and cell bodies of their central counterparts. (Adapted with permission from Olesen, J., Tfelt-Hansen, P., Welch, K. M. A., Goadsby, P. J., & Ramadan, N. M. [2006]. *The headaches* [3rd ed., Fig. 51.4]. Wolters Kluwer.)

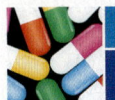

TABLE 52.5
DRUGS AT A GLANCE: Triptans

Drug	Routes and Dosages	
	Adults	**Children**
ⓟ Sumatriptan (Imitrex, Onzetra Xsail, others; ❋ Imitrex, Sumatriptan DF)	25, 50, or 100 mg PO; additional doses may be repeated in 2 h or more (maximum dosage 200 mg/d) 6 mg SC may be repeated in ≥1 h (maximum dosage 12 mg/24 h) 22 mg intranasally, half into each nostril or 10 mg divided doses of 5 mg, one in each nostril; may be repeated once after 2 h (maximum dosage 44 mg/24 h) 1 patch (6.5 mg/4 h) transdermal; may be repeated in ≥2 h (maximum 2 patches/24 h)	5–12 y: 5, 10, 20 mg intranasal in one nostril as a single dose as soon as possible with the onset of migraine; ≥12 y and adolescents: 10–20 mg intranasal in one nostril as a single dose as soon as possible with the onset of migraine
Almotriptan (❋ Axert, Mylan-Almotriptan, Sandoz Almotriptan)	612.5 mg PO repeat after 2 h if necessary (maximum 2 doses/24 h)	≥12 y: 6.25–12.5 mg PO repeat after 2 h if necessary (maximum 2 doses/24 h)
Eletriptan (Relpax; ❋ Relpax)	40 mg PO as a single dose, repeat after 2 h if necessary (maximum dose 80 mg/d)	Safety and efficacy have not been established
Frovatriptan (Frova; ❋ Frova)	2.5 mg PO; repeat after 2 h if necessary (maximum dose 7.5 mg)	Safety and efficacy have not been established
Naratriptan ❋ Amerge)	1–2.5 mg PO as a single dose; repeat in 4 h if necessary (maximum dose 5 mg/d)	Safety and efficacy have not been established
Rizatriptan (Maxalt, Maxalt-MLT; ❋ Maxalt, Maxalt RPD)	5–10 mg PO as a single dose; repeat after 2 h if necessary (maximum dose 30 mg/d)	≥6 y: <40 kg 5 mg PO as a single dose; ≥40 kg 10 mg as a single dose; safety and efficacy of multiple doses in a 24-h period have not been established
Zolmitriptan (Zomig; ❋ Zomig, Zomig Nasal Spray, Zomig Rapimelt)	1.25–2.5 mg PO as a single dose; may repeat after 2 h if necessary (maximum dose 10 mg/d) 2.5 mg intranasal by unit-dose spray device (maximum dose 5 mg/d) Orally disintegrating tablets (Zomig ZMT) 2.5–5 mg as a single dose; may repeat after 2 h if necessary (maximum dose 10 mg/d)	≥12 y: nasal inhalation, same as adult dosing
Sumatriptan and naproxen (Treximet; ❋Suvexx)	1 tablet (sumatriptan 85 mg and naproxen 500 mg) PO; if migraine is not relieved in 2 h, a second dose may be administered (maximum dose 2 tablets/24 h)	≥12 y: 1 tablet (sumatriptan 10 mg and naproxen 60 mg) PO (maximum dose 85 mg naproxen/naproxen 500 mg [single adult dose])

- In the oral form of sumatriptan, the bioavailability of the drug is increased with liver disease. If treatment is needed, do not exceed 50 mg.
- In the intranasal formulation of sumatriptan, no adjustment of dosage is required due to extensive nonhepatic metabolism to inactive agents.
- Oral, intranasal, and subcutaneous formulations are contraindicated in severe hepatic impairment.

Adverse Effects

CNS adverse effects of all sumatriptan preparations are dizziness, vertigo, headache, anxiety, malaise, myalgia, and fatigue. Cardiovascular adverse effects include alterations in blood pressure and chest pain as well as the most severe cardiovascular adverse effect, shock. The nasal administration of sumatriptan produces nausea, nasal and throat irritation, and a bad taste in the mouth. The injectable form of the drug may cause injection site discomfort.

Contraindications

Contraindications include a history of hypersensitivity reactions to the drug. Other contraindications are existing cerebrovascular or peripheral vascular syndromes. The oral, intranasal, and subcutaneous formulations of sumatriptan are contraindicated in sever hepatic impairment.

Nursing Implications

Preventing Interactions

Droxidopa, ergot derivatives, MAO inhibitors, and serotonergic agents enhance the effects of serotonin resulting in serotonin syndrome. Bromocriptine combined with triptans will place the patient at risk for triptan toxicity. St. John's wort combined with triptans will result in triptan toxicity.

> **Quality and Safety Alert: Safety**
>
> It is important to ask the patient about recent administration ergot alkaloids. The ergot alkaloids should not be given within 24 hours of the administration of triptans. The combination of ergot-containing drugs and the triptans results in cardiac ischemia.

Also, administration of monoamine oxidase (MAO) inhibitors leads to increased serum levels of sumatriptan and sumatriptan toxicity. Two weeks after an MAO inhibitor has been discontinued, it is permissible to give sumatriptan in combination with the MAO inhibitor.

Administering the Medication

It is important to administer sumatriptan at the onset of migraine symptoms. Although it is appropriate to administer a second dose of the oral preparation when symptoms return, this should not occur earlier than 2 hours after the first tablet is taken. Dosages should not exceed 100 mg in a single dose or 200 mg/day. It is necessary to administer the oral preparation with fluids and the intranasal preparation as a single dose of one spray in each nostril. With the subcutaneous preparation, administration just below the skin as soon as symptoms develop is best. If relief does not occur or if symptoms reappear, a second injection may follow 1 hour or longer after the first one. A person may have two injections in 24 hours. With the administration of all sumatriptan preparations, it is necessary to monitor the blood pressure for hypertension.

Assessing Therapeutic Effects

The nurse assesses for diminished pain and ultimate relief of migraine headaches.

Assessing for Adverse Effects

The nurse assesses for increased blood pressure, as well as chest pain, shock, dizziness, and vertigo. With subcutaneous administration, the nurse also assesses for irritation at the injection site.

Patient Teaching

Box 52.6 identifies patient teaching guidelines for sumatriptan.

Other Drugs in the Class

Almotriptan, eletriptan (Relpax), frovatriptan (Frova), naratriptan, rizatriptan (Maxalt, Maxalt-MLT), and zolmitriptan (Zomig) have similar action as sumatriptan. The triptans interact unfavorably with agents that produce increased serotonin effects, which can lead to serotonin syndrome.

BOX 52.6 Patient Teaching Guidelines for Sumatriptan

- Be sure that you understand how to administer subcutaneous sumatriptan or use the autoinjector.
- Do not administer more than two injections in 24 hours.
- Inject just below the skin as soon as symptoms are noted.
- Properly dispose of the autoinjector, syringes, and needles.
- Administer nasal spray as a single dose; repeat if necessary in 2 hours.
- Do not administer the medication if you are pregnant.
- Do not operate machinery after the administration of sumatriptan.
- Report symptoms of hypersensitivity such as heat, flushing, tiredness, and feeling sick to your healthcare provider.

Serotonin syndrome, and a potentially life-threatening reaction, may occur when two drugs that affect serotonin levels in the body are taken concurrently. Other symptoms of serotonin syndrome include restlessness, hallucinations, fever, loss of consciousness, tachycardia, and a rapid change in blood pressure. Naratriptan (Amerge) has a slow onset of action. Contraindications include a creatinine clearance (CrCl) less than 15 mL/min or severe hepatic impairment. Females of childbearing age should use barrier contraceptives due to the risk of serious congenital anomalies. Rizatriptan (Maxalt) is an oral preparation that can be swallowed or administered in a "melt-away" (orally disintegrating) formulation. It is effective in the treatment of acute migraine. The most common adverse effects are dizziness, fatigue, nausea, and somnolence. Patients with risk factors for coronary artery disease should receive the initial dose in a healthcare setting where their response can be evaluated. Zolmitriptan (Zomig) is a triptan that may be administered orally or intranasally. The onset of action of the oral drug is variable, whereas that of the intranasal preparation is 15 minutes. Zolmitriptan is effective for acute migraine therapy, with an optimal starting dose of 2.5 mg. The most commonly reported adverse effects were dizziness, nausea, somnolence, paresthesia, fatigue, and tightness of the throat or chest. With the administration of all triptans, do not administer them within 24 hours of receiving ergot alkaloids.

Sumatriptan–naproxen sodium (Treximet) is a combination drug that is administered orally. Patients should not divide, chew, or crush the tablets. This combination is effective in treating acute migraine and decreasing photophobia. The FDA has issued two **BOXED WARNING** ◆: (1) cardiovascular risk from sumatriptan, with an increased risk of adverse thrombotic events, including myocardial infarction and stroke, and (2) GI risk due to naproxen sodium, with an increased risk of GI irritation, inflammation, ulceration, bleeding, and perforation.

NCLEX Success

3. A patient has taken sumatriptan–naproxen sodium for an acute migraine. The patient has also taken over-the-counter ibuprofen for menstrual cramps. Which of the following adverse effects is the patient at risk for developing?
   A. bronchospasm
   B. urinary retention
   C. edema
   D. gastrointestinal bleeding

Clinical Application 52.3

Ms. Van Art is discharged from the ED following an acute migraine headache. Her prescriber orders sumatriptan (Imitrex) to be administered subcutaneously at the onset of an acute migraine headache.
- What education will Ms. Van Art receive prior to discharge?
- What information will Ms. Van Art need if subcutaneous medication administration is new to her?
- What medications are contraindicated with the administration of sumatriptan?

ESTROGEN

Estrogen in the form of **estradiol** is a treatment for menstrual migraines, which are most likely 2 days prior to menses through the 3rd day of bleeding. Perimenstrual estrogen supplementation is based on evidence that the natural decline in estrogen in the late luteal phase of the menstrual cycle, prior to menstruation, is associated with the increased risk of migraine.

Quality and Safety Alert: Patient-Centered Care

Patients who experience menstrual migraine without an aura can benefit from the use of estrogen–progestin containing contraceptives.

Pharmacokinetics

Metabolism of estradiol occurs in the liver. Excretion takes place in the urine. The drug crosses the placenta and enters the breast milk.

Action

Estradiol binds to intracellular receptors to form a complex that stimulates synthesis of proteins responsible for estrogenic effects. Prophylactic administration minimizes the premenstrual decline in estrogen that precipitates the development of the migraine headache.

Use

Transcutaneous administration of estradiol increases the estrogen levels in the late luteal phase of the menstrual cycle that contribute to the development of menstrual migraine headaches. Table 52.6 and Chapter 7 give dosage information for estradiol.

Patient-related variables specific to the use of estrogen include the following:

- Age
  - Safety and efficacy have not been established for treating migraines with estrogen in children.
- Reproduction, pregnancy, and lactation:
  - Treatment of migraine in pregnant patients is symptomatic rather than preventive so estrogen will not be prescribed.
  - Breast-feeding has a protective effect with more stable estrogen levels.
- Abnormal kidney function and hepatic impairment:
  - No dosage adjustments with abnormal kidney function.
  - Use is contraindicated with hepatic dysfunction.

Adverse Effects

The major adverse effect associated with the administration of estrogen preparations is thromboembolic disorders. Menstrual irregularity can occur because of the suppression of endogenous estrogen during treatment.

Contraindications

Contraindications include incomplete bone growth, which occurs in adolescents. Other contraindications are the presence of neoplasms, breast cancer, thromboembolic disorders, fibroids, endometriosis, thyroid disease, and pregnancy. The use of estrogen is contraindicated in hepatic dysfunction.

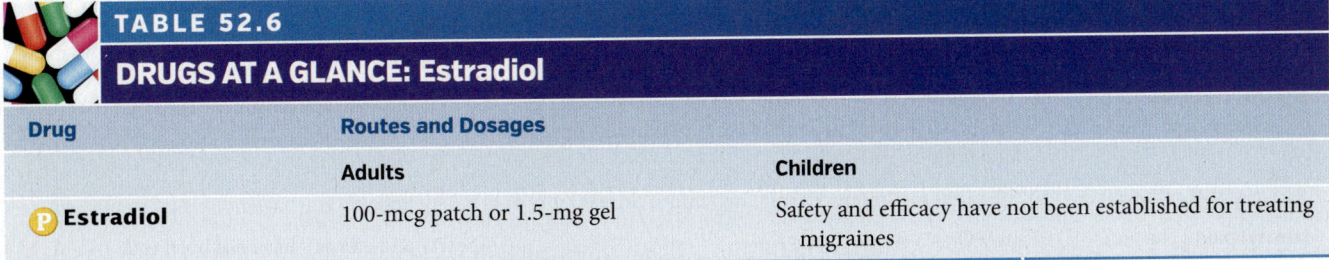

TABLE 52.6 DRUGS AT A GLANCE: Estradiol

Drug	Routes and Dosages	
	Adults	**Children**
Estradiol	100-mcg patch or 1.5-mg gel	Safety and efficacy have not been established for treating migraines

Nursing Implications

Preventing Interactions
Some drugs interact with estradiol, increasing or decreasing its effects (Box 52.7). In addition, the combination of estradiol and bromocriptine interferes with the effects of bromocriptine.

Administering the Medication
Prior to applying the transcutaneous preparation, it is necessary to clean and dry the skin area. It is important to apply the preparation to the trunk.

Assessing for Therapeutic Effects
The nurse assesses for the development of migraine headache in the later luteal phase of the menstrual cycle. If a headache does not develop, the dose is adequate.

Assessing for Adverse Effects
The nurse assesses for the development of leg pain or chest pain indicative of the development of thromboembolism. The patient is also assessed for breakthrough bleeding.

Patient Teaching
The patient should be instructed to notify the healthcare provider of intermittent breakthrough bleeding, spotting, or unexplained pain, especially calf or chest pain.

BOX 52.7 Drug Interactions: Estradiol

Drugs That Increase the Effects of Estradiol
- Cyclosporine, theophylline, tricyclic antidepressants
  Increase serum levels

Drugs That Decrease the Effects of Estradiol
- Phenytoin and rifampin
  Decrease serum levels
- Nicotine
  Reduces or cancels efficacy

CALCITONIN GENE–RELATED PEPTIDE RECEPTOR ANTAGONIST (GEPANTS)

The calcitonin gene–related peptide receptor antagonist agents are indicated for the treatment of episodic migraine headaches. **Ubrogepant** (Ubrelvy) was approved by the FDA in 2019, followed by rimegepant (Nurtec) in 2020 and atogepant (Qulipta) in 2021.

Pharmacokinetics
Ubrogepant has delayed absorption with a high-fat meal. The high-fat meal will delay absorption by 2 hours and reduces the concentration of the medication by 22%. The drug is 87% protein bound and metabolized primarily by CYP3A4. The half-life is approximately 5 to 7 hours with peak of action in 1.5 hours. It is excreted 42% unchanged in the feces and 6% unchanged in the urine.

Action and Use
Ubrogepant causes antagonism of the calcitonin gene–related peptide receptor and is used as a treatment of moderate to severe, episodic migraine headaches with or without an aura. Table 52.7 gives dosage information for the calcitonin gene–related peptide receptor antagonist medications.

Patient-related variables specific to the use of ubrogepant include the following:

- Age:
  - In older adults, the dosage of ubrogepant should be initiated at the lower end of the dosage range.
- Reproduction, pregnancy, and lactation:
  - Based on animal reproduction studies, ubrogepant may cause fetal harm. Based on available data, other agents for preventing migraine may be preferred for pregnant patients.
  - It is unknown if ubrogepant is present in the breast milk. The manufacturer does not recommend use with lactation.
- Abnormal kidney function and hepatic impairment:
  - Avoid use in patients with a CrCl less than 15 mL/min.
  - In patients with severe hepatic impairment, the maximum dose is 100 mg/24 hours.

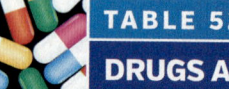

TABLE 52.7
DRUGS AT A GLANCE: Calcitonin Gene-Related Peptide Antagonist (Gepants)

Drug	Routes and Dosages	
	Adults	**Children**
Ubrogepant (Ubrelvy)	50–100 mg PO as a single dose; if symptoms persist or return, may repeat dose after >2 h; maximum dose 200 mg per 24 h	Safety and efficacy have not been established
Atogepant (Qulipta)	10, 30, or 60 mg PO once daily; maximum dose 60 mg/d	Safety and efficacy have not been established
Rimegepant (Nurtec)	75 mg PO as a single dose Preventive: 75 mg PO every other day	Safety and efficacy have not been established

Adverse Effects and Contraindications

The known adverse effects of ubrogepant are drowsiness, nausea, and xerostomia. The drug is contraindicated with concomitant use of strong CYP3A4 inhibitors, such as atazanavir, chloramphenicol, clofazimine, cobicistat, ketoconazole, itraconazole, clarithromycin, lopinavir, and nirmatrelvir/ritonavir.

Nursing Implications

Administering the Medication

Administer ubrogepant with or without food and avoid high-fat foods. Patients should not consume grapefruit juice with ubrogepant.

Assessing for Therapeutic Effects

Assess the patient to determine relief of migraine headache pain and related symptoms.

Assessing for Adverse Effects

Assess the patient regarding signs and symptoms of nausea, dizziness, and xerostomia.

Patient Teaching

Box 52.8 identifies patient teaching guidelines for ubrogepant.

Other Drugs in the Class

Rimegepant (Nurtec) and atogepant (Qulipta) are used for acute treatment of moderate to severe migraine and migraine prevention. The action of these medications is the same as ubrogepant. Rimegepant is packed in a foil individual dose pack. The patient should be instructed to use clean, dry hands and peel the foil covering blister to remove the tablet. The tablet should not be pushed through the foil. The tablet is placed under the tongue and disintegrates. Adverse effects of rimegepant are skin rash, hypersensitivity, and dyspnea. Atogepant is used for migraine prevention. It should be avoided in patients with recent cardiovascular or cardiovascular ischemic events. The use of atogepant should be limited to patients with less than 15 headaches per month and those with significant disability from frequent headaches who are unable to tolerate or do not respond to other preventive therapies. Adverse effects of atogepant include weight loss, decreased appetite, constipation, nausea, drowsiness, and increases serum hepatic enzymes.

BOX 52.8 *Patient Teaching Guidelines for Ubrogepant*

- Do not consume grapefruit or grapefruit juice.
- Do not take drugs used for human immunodeficiency virus (HIV), infections, or seizures with ubrogepant.
- Report signs and symptoms of a rash immediately to the prescriber.
- Take the medication with or without food.
- Administer the drug at the onset of the migraine.
- Store this medication at room temperature, not in the bathroom.

PREVENTIVE THERAPY FOR MIGRAINE HEADACHES

Preventive therapy is the administration of medications to prevent the onset of migraines. These medications are primarily administered for the treatment of other conditions and are thoroughly covered in other chapters. Their use in the prevention of migraines medications is discussed briefly. For complete information about these drugs, one may review the information in the chapters indicated.

Carboxylic Acid Derivative

Valproic acid (see Chapter 53) is a carboxylic acid derivative that is most commonly administered to control seizures. However, it has proved effective in the prevention of migraine headaches. Valproic acid is available in two forms. The dosage for valproic acid tablets is 250 mg orally two times per day, with a maximum dosage of 1,000 mg. The dosage of the extended-release preparation is 500 mg orally once per day. Limited data suggest that valproic acid is safe for children as young as 7 years of age, and extended-release valproic acid is well tolerated by adolescents with migraine headaches. The risk of hepatotoxicity with valproic acid in children younger than 2 years has been reported.

Gamma-Aminobutyric Acid

Gabapentin (Neurontin; see Chapter 53) is a gamma-aminobutyric acid medication commonly administered to control neuropathic pain and as an adjunctive agent for control of seizures. Studies have shown that gabapentin is effective in reducing the frequency of migraines. At the end of 12 weeks, 46% of patients who received 2,400 mg/day had a 50% reduction in the 4-week rate of migraine. The most commonly reported adverse effects were dizziness and somnolence.

Sulfamate-Substituted Monosaccharide

Topiramate (Topamax) is a sulfamate-substituted monosaccharide agent used most commonly as an antiepileptic agent (see Chapter 53). In clinical trials, the mean monthly migraine frequency decreased significantly with either 100 or 200 mg/day compared with placebo. However, with 50 mg/day, there was no statistically significant reduction in migraine frequency. The most commonly reported adverse effects include paresthesia, fatigue, anorexia, diarrhea, weight loss, altered memory, difficulty concentrating, and nausea. Limited data from comparative trials suggest that topiramate is as effective as the beta-adrenergic blocking agent propranolol; however, topiramate is much more expensive than propranolol.

Beta-Adrenergic Blocking Agents

The most common beta-adrenergic blocking agent administered prophylactically for migraine headaches is propranolol (Inderal) (see Chapter 27). The recommended dosage is two divided doses, starting at 40 mg daily. The maintenance dosage may be increased to 160 to 240 mg/day. Studies have shown that propranolol is effective in reducing migraine frequency.

In addition, two other beta-adrenergic blockers, metoprolol (50 mg daily in two divided doses, ranging to 200 mg daily) and timolol (5 mg once daily, ranging from 10 to 30 mg daily in two divided doses), are effective for migraine prophylaxis. It takes several weeks for these drugs to become effective, and it is necessary to titrate the dose for at least 3 months to ascertain effectiveness. A concern related to the use of beta-adrenergic blockers is the increased risk of stroke and other cardiovascular events, which limits their use in patients older than 60 years of age and in those who smoke.

Calcium Channel Blockers

Verapamil is the calcium channel blocker of choice for migraine prophylaxis. It takes several weeks for benefits of the medication to be noted. It seems to be the most effective calcium channel blocker for migraine prevention. It is necessary to take 120 mg in three divided doses.

Studies have also noted that tolerance may develop with calcium channel blockers. Tolerance to the medication can be overcome by increasing the dosage or switching to a different calcium channel blocker. Calcium channel blocking agents such as nifedipine (Procardia) (see Chapter 28) have been used for prevention of migraine headache. However, data supporting the efficacy of calcium channel blockers are weak and conflicting.

Angiotensin-Converting Enzyme Inhibitors

As Chapter 26 points out, enalapril maleate is the prototype angiotensin-converting enzyme (ACE) inhibitor, but clinical trials have shown that lisinopril seems to be more effective in the prevention of migraine headaches. A study has shown that a dose of 10 mg/day for 1 week and then 20 mg/day reduced the number of hours and days with headache and headache severity compared to a placebo. However, the small sample size and design of this clinical trial and another performed by the same investigators limits any definitive conclusions regarding the use of ACE inhibitors in migraine prevention. These drugs are not widely used in migraine management. An adverse effect with ACE inhibitors is the development of a cough, which is the result of an interference with bradykinin, substance P, or tachykinin metabolism.

Angiotensin II Receptor Blockers

Angiotensin II receptor blockers (see Chapter 26) can be effective in the prevention of migraine headache but are not commonly used. Studies on the effectiveness of candesartan have revealed that it produces favorable results in the prevention of migraine headaches. It is necessary to inform females of childbearing age that barrier contraceptives are required with this medication. The FDA has issued a **BOXED WARNING** stating that fetal injury and death have been reported with candesartan.

Olmesartan is effective and well tolerated as a migraine prophylactic agent for patients with comorbid hypertension and prehypertension. Researchers have studied patients with hypertension and prehypertension to determine the effectiveness of this medication.

Tricyclic Antidepressants

Imipramine (Tofranil) and other tricyclic antidepressants (see Chapter 54) are effective in the prevention of migraine and tension headaches. Amitriptyline 10 to 50 mg at bedtime is also effective for migraine prophylaxis. Tricyclic antidepressants have a sedative effect, and to minimize this, it helps to administer the drugs at bedtime. Other side effects of tricyclic antidepressants include dry mouth, constipation, tachycardia, palpitations, orthostatic hypotension, weight gain, and urinary retention.

Herbal and Vitamin Supplements

People with migraines may use herbal supplements to treat these headaches. Several herbs, including feverfew and butterbur, and vitamins, such as magnesium and riboflavin, have shown modest efficacy for migraine prevention. In general, it is necessary to encourage patients to try standard methods of preventing and treating migraine before taking products with uncertain benefits and risks.

Feverfew, an herbal medicine, is most widely studied for migraine prevention, but evidence of its benefit is conflicting. The main active ingredient of feverfew is thought to be parthenolide, which functions by inhibiting platelet aggregation, prostaglandin synthesis, and the release of inflammatory mediators such as histamine. Its exact mechanism in migraine prophylaxis is unknown. Study results have not established that feverfew is more effective than placebo for the prevention of migraine. Contraindications include pregnancy and lactation. The safety of the herb is unknown.

Butterbur is an extract of a perennial shrub. Two small clinical trials have shown limited efficacy in migraine prophylaxis. Concerns that the pyrrolizidine alkaloids in feverfew are hepatotoxic and potentially carcinogenic have raised concerns about their long-term safety. The most common adverse effect in the trials was burping.

Magnesium may be successful in treating and preventing migraine headaches in pregnant people. Adverse effects include diarrhea and GI discomfort.

Riboflavin, vitamin B_2, has demonstrated statistically significant benefit in the reduction in the frequency of headaches, the number of headache days per month, and mean headache severity. Its use is well tolerated. Riboflavin is inexpensive and produces minimal side effects. However, the benefits of the vitamin are not realized for up to 3 months of therapy. Without additional studies, it is uncertain who would most likely benefit from the administration of riboflavin and what dose produces optimal benefits.

NCLEX Success

4. Which of the following factors prevents the use of estradiol for the treatment of menstrual migraines for a 14-year-old patient?
    A. breakthrough bleeding
    B. leg pain
    C. incomplete long bone growth
    D. anxiety

5. A 16-year-old patient develops migraine headaches. Which of the following medications is safe and effective for the treatment of migraine headaches?

    A. sumatriptan
    B. ergotamine
    C. topiramate
    D. valproic acid
    E. gabapentin

ADJUVANT MEDICATIONS FOR MIGRAINE HEADACHES

Adjuvant medications administered for severe migraine headaches include antiemetics and opioids. Antiemetic agents are adjuvant medications administered to control the symptoms of nausea and vomiting related to migraine, tension, and cluster headaches. Table 52.8 gives dosage information for the antiemetics. Opioid use is controversial because these agents can contribute to the development of chronic daily headache and interference with preventive therapy. Opioids are not discussed in this section but are reviewed in Chapter 49.

Antiemetic agents may be useful for the treatment of symptoms related to migraine headache. **Chlorpromazine hydrochloride** (see Chapter 56) is a phenothiazine that has been shown to be effective in treating both the headache itself and the associated nausea and vomiting. Investigators have also shown that antiemetic drugs decrease the photophobia and phonophobia that may accompany the migraine headache. The mechanism of action involved in the decrease of nausea and vomiting is related to the suppression of the chemoreceptor zone. Besides chlorpromazine, related antiemetics include metoclopramide and prochlorperazine. Parenteral preparations of these drugs appear more effective than oral preparations. When administering the antiemetic agents, it is necessary to assess the patient for relief of headache, nausea, and vomiting. Chlorpromazine also depresses the CNS, so it is important to assess the patient's level of consciousness.

Metoclopramide is a GI stimulant that is effective in reducing headache, nausea, and vomiting. It is less effective than chlorpromazine in reducing symptoms. Metoclopramide is a potent central dopamine receptor antagonist that increases esophageal sphincter tone and elevates the chemoreceptor zone threshold. Although the drug can be administered by numerous routes, the American Headache Society guidelines prefer the intravenous route for migraine relief (see Table 52.8).

Prochlorperazine has the same antiemetic action as chlorpromazine and metoclopramide. When taking prochlorperazine orally, it is important to swallow it whole and not chew or crush the tablets. When administering the medication parenterally, it is necessary to give it intramuscularly (deep) and never subcutaneously. When administering metoclopramide and prochlorperazine, it is necessary to assess the patient for signs and symptoms of dystonia, which is indicative of a hypersensitivity reaction. If the patient develops dystonia, it is necessary to administer diphenhydramine to counteract this reaction. With all of these medications, the patient should be assessed for urinary retention due to the anticholinergic effects.

TABLE 52.8

DRUGS AT A GLANCE: Antiemetics Used for the Treatment of Headaches

Drug	Routes and Dosages	
	Adults	Children
Chlorpromazine hydrochloride (TEVA-Chlorpromazine)	10–25 mg PO every 4–6 h; 50–100-mg suppository rectally every 6–8 h; 25–50 mg IM/IV every 4–6 h	>6 mo: 0.55 mg/kg PO every 4–6 h PRN up to 500 mg/d >6 mo: 0.55 mg/kg IM/IV every 6–8 h
Metoclopramide (Reglan; Metoclopramide Hydrochloride Injection, Metoclopramide Omega, Metonia)	10–20 mg PO as a single dose; 10 mg IM/SC as a single dose; 10–20 mg IV as a single dose	2 mg/kg IM/IV
Prochlorperazine (Compro)	5–10 mg PO 3–4 2/d sustained release; 10–15 mg every 12 h; 5–10 mg IM every 3–4 h (maximum dose 40 mg); 2.5–10 mg IV every 3–4 h (maximum dose 40 mg); 25 mg per rectum two times per day	2.5 mg PO or per rectum 1–3 times per day or 5 mg two times per day (maximum dose 15 mg/d; 0.13 mg/kg IM every 3–4 h)

THE NURSING PROCESS

A concept map outlines the nursing process related to drug therapy considerations in this chapter. Additional nursing implications related to the disease process should also be considered in care decisions.

Assessment
- Assess the severity, patterns (including frequency), and occurrences of cluster, tension, or migraine headaches. Include any additional symptoms such as photophobia, aura, alterations in vision (e.g., flashing lights, unilateral vision loss), and nausea or vomiting.

Outcomes of Therapy
The patient will
- Take medications as prescribed to routinely prevent headache.
- Take medications to abort and/or treat acute migraine with the onset of symptoms or aura.
- Avoid trigger factors that contribute to headache symptoms.
- Experience fewer and less severe attacks of migraine, tension, or cluster headaches.

Nursing Interventions
- Implement measures to minimize and prevent the symptoms of headache.
- Instruct the patient on medications to treat acute migraine headache pain.
- Instruct the patient on the trigger points related to migraine and strategies to decrease trigger points.
- Instruct the patient on medications to prevent migraine headaches.
- Administer medications to treat acute migraine headaches.
- Administer medications to prevent migraine headaches.
- Administer antiemetic agents to reduce nausea and vomiting during acute episodes.

Evaluation
- Interview and observe patient for relief of symptoms.
- Interview and observe patient's ability to provide self-care.
- Interview and observe patient regarding safe, effective use of the medications for acute and preventive treatment.
- Interview and assess patient for medication adherence.

Visit thePoint* at http://thePoint.lww.com/Frandsen13e for answers to NCLEX Success questions (in Appendix A), answers to Clinical Application Case Studies (in Appendix B), additional information on the pathophysiology of headaches, and more!

REFERENCES AND RESOURCES

Cutrer, F. M. (2022). Pathophysiology, clinical manifestations, and diagnosis of migraine in adults. *UpToDate*. Lexi-Comp, Inc.

Hartford, E. A., Blume, H., Barry, D., Chatterjee, J. H., & Law, E. (2022). Disparities in the emergency department management of pediatric migraine by race, ethnicity, and language preference. *Academic Emergency Medicine A Global Journal of Emergency Care*, 29(9), 1057–1066. https://doi-org.proxy.library.maryville.edu/10.1111/acem.14550

Lippincott Advisor. (2022). *Drug information*. Wolters Kluwer.

Mack, K. J. (2022). Acute treatment of migraine in children. *UpToDate*. Lexi-Comp, Inc.

May, A. (2022). Cluster headache: Treatment and prognosis. *UpToDate*. Lexi-Comp, Inc.

O'Neal, M. A. (2022). Estrogen-associated migraine, including menstrual migraine. *UpToDate*. Lexi-Comp, Inc.

Schwedt, T. J., & Garza, I. (2022). Acute treatment of migraine in adults. *UpToDate*. Lexi-Comp, Inc.

UpToDate. (2022). *Drug information*. Lexi Comp, Inc.

CHAPTER 53

Drug Therapy for Seizure Disorders and Skeletal Muscle Disorders

LEARNING OBJECTIVES

After studying this chapter, you should be able to:

1. Identify types of seizures as well as the clinical considerations and manifestations of seizures.
2. Identify factors that influence the choice of antiepileptic medications in treating seizure disorders.
3. Identify the prototypes and describe the actions, uses, adverse effects, contraindications, and nursing implications for antiepileptic drugs in all classes.
4. Describe strategies for prevention and treatment of status epilepticus.
5. Implement the nursing process in the care of patients undergoing drug therapy for seizure disorders.
6. Discuss the common symptoms and disorders for which skeletal muscle relaxants are used.
7. Identify the prototypes and describe the actions, uses, adverse effects, contraindications, and nursing implications for the skeletal muscle relaxants.
8. Implement the nursing process in the care of patients undergoing drug therapy for muscle spasms and spasticity.

CLINICAL APPLICATION CASE STUDY

Two days ago, Andrew Cummings, a 7-year-old boy, was at home playing and experienced a tonic–clonic seizure, which was witnessed by his mother. On questioning the mother, a pediatric neurologist at the hospital where the boy was admitted determined that the seizure was unprovoked and had a generalized onset. The mother stated that it lasted approximately 3 minutes. The neurologist diagnoses a seizure disorder. Andrew is now taking carbamazepine (Tegretol) 50 mg orally four times per day and valproate (Depakene Syrup) 20 mg/kg/d.

KEY TERMS

Antiepileptic drugs: drugs used to control seizures or convulsions; also referred to as antiseizure medications or anticonvulsants

Clonic: spasms that alternate between contraction and relaxation

Clonic phase: rapid rhythmic and symmetric jerking movements of the body

Convulsion: tonic–clonic type of seizure characterized by spasmodic contractions of involuntary muscles

Epilepsy: a condition or disease where the patient has repetitive seizures

Gingival hyperplasia: overgrowth of the gums related to long-term administration of phenytoin

Malignant hyperthermia: rare but life-threatening complication of anesthesia characterized by hypercarbia, metabolic acidosis, skeletal muscle rigidity, fever, and cyanosis

Muscle spasm: sudden, involuntary, painful muscle contraction that occurs with musculoskeletal trauma or inflammation

Seizure: brief episode of abnormal electrical activity in nerve cells of the brain that may or may not be accompanied by visible changes in appearance or behavior

Spasticity: caused by nerve damage in the brain and spinal cord, it is a permanent condition that may be painful and disabling; involves increased muscle tone or contraction and stiff, awkward movements

Status epilepticus: repeated seizures or a seizure that lasts at least 30 minutes; may be convulsive, nonconvulsive, or partial

Tonic: muscle spasms with sustained contraction

Tonic–clonic: most common type of seizure; often referred to as a major motor seizure

Tonic phase: sustained contraction of skeletal muscles; abnormal postures, such as opisthotonos; and absence of respirations, during which the person becomes cyanotic

INTRODUCTION

The first part of this chapter introduces the condition or disease known as **epilepsy**, which is characterized by repetitive seizures, and discusses the pharmacologic care of the patient who is experiencing a **seizure**. Although the terms seizure and convulsion may be used interchangeably, they have different meanings. A seizure involves a brief episode of abnormal electrical activity in nerve cells of the brain that may or may not be accompanied by visible changes in appearance or behavior. It refers to all types of epileptic occurrences. A **convulsion** is a **tonic–clonic** type of seizure characterized by spasmodic contractions of involuntary muscles.

The second part of this chapter describes the role skeletal muscle relaxants play in decreasing seizures and reducing muscle spasms and spasticity associated with neurologic and musculoskeletal injuries. A **muscle spasm** is a sudden, involuntary, painful muscle contraction that occurs with musculoskeletal trauma (e.g., overuse or injury of skeletal muscle, twisting a joint, or tearing a ligament as with a sprain) or inflammation (e.g., bursitis, arthritis). Muscle spasm also occurs with acute and chronic low back pain. Spasms may be **clonic** (alternating contraction and relaxation) to **tonic** (sustained contraction). Muscle spasms commonly occur, sometimes causing significant disability with inflammation, edema, and poor coordination and mobility.

Spasticity involves increased muscle tone or contraction and stiff, awkward movements. It occurs in neurologic disorders such as multiple sclerosis, spinal cord injury, traumatic brain injury, cerebral palsy, and poststroke syndrome. Because spasticity is caused by nerve damage in the brain and spinal cord, it is a permanent condition that may be painful and disabling.

In patients with spinal cord injury, spasticity requires treatment when it impairs safety, mobility, and the ability to perform activities of daily living (e.g., self-care in hygiene, eating, dressing, and work or recreational activities). Stimuli that precipitate spasms vary from one individual to another and may include muscle stretching, bladder infections or stones, constipation and bowel distention, or infections. It is necessary to assess each person for personal precipitating factors, so that these factors can be avoided if possible. Treatment measures include passive range-of-motion and muscle-stretching exercises and antispasmodic medications (e.g., baclofen, dantrolene).

OVERVIEW OF EPILEPSY

Sudden, abnormal, hypersynchronous firing of neurons is characteristic of epilepsy. Signs and symptoms of seizure activity lead to the diagnosis. On the electroencephalogram (EEG), abnormal brain wave patterns are present.

Seizures may occur as single events in response to hypoglycemia, fever, electrolyte imbalances, overdoses of numerous medications (e.g., amphetamine, cocaine, isoniazid, lidocaine, lithium, methylphenidate, antispasmodics, theophylline), and withdrawal from alcohol or sedative–hypnotic drugs. Alternatively, seizures may be idiopathic (having no discernible cause) or attributable to a secondary cause. Authorities also classify seizures as unprovoked (idiopathic) or provoked (secondary). Secondary causes in infancy include developmental defects, metabolic disease, or birth injury. Fever is a common secondary cause in late infancy and early childhood. Inherited forms of epilepsy usually begin in childhood or adolescence. When epilepsy begins in adulthood, it is often caused by an acquired neurologic disorder (e.g., head injury, stroke, brain tumor) or alcohol and other drug effects. Toxemia is a secondary cause of seizures in pregnancy.

Some of the identified specific causes of seizures include alterations in cell membrane permeability or the distribution of ions across the neuronal cell membranes. Genetic mutations have also been linked to epilepsy. In addition, a decrease in the inhibition of thalamic or cortical neuronal activity is a cause. Finally, imbalances in the neurotransmitters gamma-aminobutyric acid (GABA) or acetylcholine excess result in seizure disorders.

Clinical Considerations and Manifestations

Experts broadly classify seizures as partial or generalized. Partial seizures begin in a specific area of the brain and often indicate a localized brain lesion such as birth injury, trauma, stroke, or tumor. They produce symptoms ranging from simple motor and sensory manifestations to more complex abnormal movements and bizarre behavior. Movements are usually automatic, repetitive, and inappropriate to the situation, such as chewing, swallowing, or aversive movements (automatisms). In simple partial seizures, consciousness is not impaired; in complex partial seizures, the level of consciousness is decreased.

Generalized seizures are bilateral and symmetric and have no discernible point of origin in the brain. The most common type is the tonic–clonic or major motor seizure. The **tonic phase** involves sustained contraction of skeletal muscles; abnormal postures, such as opisthotonos; and absence of respiration, during which the person becomes cyanotic. The **clonic phase** is characterized by rapid rhythmic and symmetric jerking movements of the body. Tonic–clonic seizures are sometimes preceded by an aura—a brief warning, such as a flash of light or a specific sound or smell. In children, febrile seizures (i.e., tonic–clonic seizures that occur with fever in the absence of other identifiable causes) are the most common form of epilepsy.

The absence seizure, which is characterized by abrupt alterations in consciousness that last only a few seconds, is a kind of generalized seizure. Other types of generalized seizures include the myoclonic type (contraction of a muscle or group of muscles) and the akinetic type (absence of movement). Some people are subject to mixed seizures.

Status epilepticus is repeated seizures or a seizure that lasts at least 30 minutes. It may be convulsive, nonconvulsive, or partial. It is a life-threatening emergency. The generalized tonic–clonic convulsion lasts several minutes or occurs in close intervals. During this time, the patient does not regain consciousness. Hypotension, hypoxia, and cardiac dysrhythmias may also occur. There is a high risk of permanent brain damage and death unless prompt, appropriate treatment is instituted. In a person taking medications for a diagnosed seizure disorder, the most common cause of status epilepticus is abruptly stopping **antiepileptic drugs** (AEDs). Antiepileptic drugs are used to control seizures or convulsions. AEDs are also referred to as antiseizure medications or anticonvulsants. In other patients, regardless of whether they have a diagnosed seizure disorder, causes of status epilepticus include brain trauma or tumors, systemic or central nervous system (CNS) infections, alcohol withdrawal, and overdoses of drugs (e.g., cocaine, theophylline).

Drug Therapy

Treatment of the underlying cause or use of an AED may relieve seizures. AEDs can usually control seizure activity but do not cure the underlying disorder. Numerous difficulties, for both clinicians and patients, have been associated with AED therapy, including trials of different drugs; consideration of monotherapy (using a single drug) versus combination therapy (using two or more drugs); the need to titrate dosage over time; lack of seizure control while drugs are being selected and dosages adjusted; social stigma and adverse drug effects, often leading to poor patient adherence; and undesirable drug interactions among AEDs and between AEDs and other medications.

The AEDs used in the prevention and treatment of seizures have evolved over the years. In recent years, the U.S. Food and Drug Administration (FDA) has approved newer medications in the treatment of seizure disorders. The FDA most often classifies these medications as newer or miscellaneous drugs. The medication tables identify the newer drugs primarily as derivatives. Table 53.1 summarizes the drug classes. For specific drugs, other tables identify the AEDs administered, the dosage, the type of seizure they are used to treat, and the therapeutic serum drug levels. The therapeutic serum drug level is very important because of the risk of drug toxicity.

> **Quality and Safety Alert: Safety**
>
> When administering AEDs requiring dosage calculation, two nurses should calculate the dosage, checking for accuracy.

Clinical Application 53.1

- According to Andrew's medical record, he should receive carbamazepine (Tegretol) 50 mg four times per day. The elixir is 100 mg/5 mL. The boy weighs 56 lb. How much carbamazepine does the nurse administer?
- The physician has ordered valproate (Depakene) 20 mg/kg/d for Andrew. The elixir is 250 mg/5 mL. How much valproate does the nurse administer?

NCLEX Success

1. A patient is admitted to the emergency department with repeated tonic-clonic seizures. Tonic-clonic seizures may be attributed to which of following drugs?
   A. ciprofloxacin hydrochloride
   B. cimetidine
   C. cocaine
   D. morphine sulfate

DRUGS USED TO TREAT SEIZURE DISORDERS

BARBITURATES

Phenobarbital is the prototype AED of the barbiturate class. Since its development in 1912, it has been used as an antiepileptic or sedative.

Pharmacokinetics

Phenobarbital, like all barbiturates, is absorbed rapidly through the gastrointestinal (GI) tract, usually within 1 hour. The oral drug has an onset of action of greater than 60 minutes and a duration of 10 to 12 hours. The intravenous (IV) form begins to act in 5 minutes and lasts approximately 6 hours. Phenobarbital has a half-life of 53 to 118 hours. In children, the half-life is 60 to 180 hours. The drug takes approximately 2 to 3 weeks to reach therapeutic serum levels and 3 weeks to reach a steady-state concentration. It is also lipid bound, which means that it crosses the placenta and is present in breast milk. Phenobarbital is metabolized in the liver and excreted by the kidney system.

TABLE 53.1

Drugs Administered for Seizures (Antiepileptic Drugs)

Drug Class	Prototype	Other Drugs in the Class
Drugs Used to Treat Seizure Disorders		
Barbiturates	Phenobarbital	Pentobarbital (Nembutal) Primidone (Mysoline)
Benzodiazepines	Diazepam (Valium, Diastat, Acudial, Pediatric Diazepam Intensol)	Clobazam (Onfi, Sympazan) Clonazepam (Klonopin) Clorazepate (Tranxene) Lorazepam (Ativan, LORazepam Intensol)
GABA structural analogs	Gabapentin (Neurontin)	Pregabalin (Lyrica, Lyrica CR) Tiagabine hydrochloride (Gabitril) Vigabatrin (Sabril)
Hydantoins	Phenytoin (Dilantin)	Fosphenytoin (Cerebyx)
Iminostilbenes	Carbamazepine (Tegretol, TEGretol-SR)	Eslicarbazepine (Aptiom) Oxcarbazepine (Oxtellar XR, Trileptal)
Other Antiepileptic Drugs (AEDs)		
Carbonic anhydrase inhibitor	Acetazolamide	
Succinimide	Ethosuximide (Zarontin)	
Sulfonamide	Zonisamide (Zonegran)	
Histone deacetylase inhibitor	Valproate (Depakote, Depakote ER, Depakote Sprinkles)	
Functionalized amino acids	Lacosamide (Vimpat)	
Mineral electrolytes	Magnesium sulfate	
Phenyltriazine derivatives	Lamotrigine (LaMICtal)	
	Levetiracetam (Keppra)	
Pyrrolidine derivatives	Brivaracetam (Brivlera)	
AMPA glutamate receptor antagonist	Perampanel (Fycompa)	
Sulfamate-substituted monosaccharides	Topiramate (Topamax)	
Tetrazole alkyl carbamate derivative	Cenobamate (Xcopri)	
Triazole derivatives	Rufinamide (Banzel)	
	Felbamate (Felbatol)	
Other Miscellaneous Antiepileptic Agents	Stiripentol (Diacomit)	

Action

Phenobarbital depresses the CNS by inhibiting the conduction of impulses in the ascending reticular activating system, thus depressing the cerebral cortex and cerebellar function. Figure 53.1 indicates the site of action of barbiturates, along with other AEDs.

Use

Prescribers order oral phenobarbital as a sedative and antiepileptic agent in the treatment of generalized tonic–clonic and partial seizures. Clinicians use the parenteral form to control acute seizures. Table 53.2 gives route and dosage information for phenobarbital and other barbiturates.

Patient-related variables specific to the use of phenobarbital include the following:

- Age:
  - Pediatric patients may be at increased risk of vitamin D deficiency with chronic therapy.
  - In pediatric patients, rapid IV administration may cause respiratory depression, apnea, laryngospasm, or hypotension.
  - Pediatric patients being treated for status epilepticus may experience CNS depression; respiratory support should be available.
  - In older adults, decreased absorption and altered metabolism and kidney excretion will result in greater sedation and increased risk of adverse drug reactions.

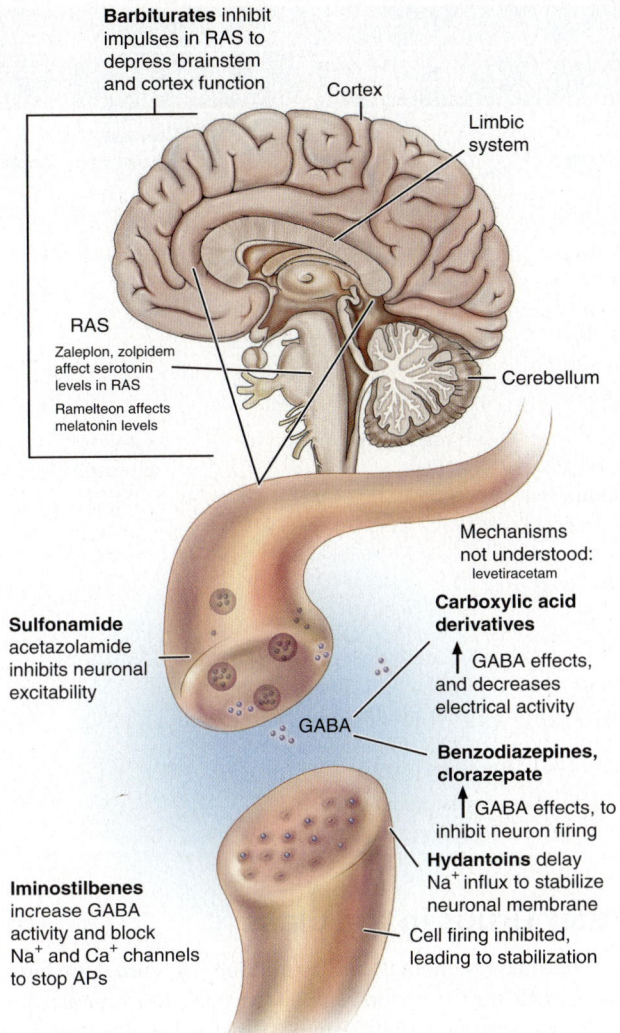

Figure 53.1. Sites of action of antiepileptic drugs. AP, action potential; GABA, gamma-aminobutyric acid; RAS, reticular activating system [Adapted with permission from Karch, A. M. (2020). *Focus on nursing pharmacology* (8th ed., Fig. 23.2). Wolters Kluwer.]

- Reproduction, pregnancy, and lactation:
  - Phenobarbital crosses the placenta. It can be detected in the placenta, fetal liver, and fetal brain.
  - Phenobarbital administered in the third trimester of pregnancy may result in neonatal abstinence syndrome (NAS) (Chapter 49). The symptoms of NAS include seizures and hyperirritability in the neonate.
  - Use of phenobarbital should be avoided in pregnancy.
  - Pregnant patients should be enrolled in North American Antiepileptic Drug Pregnancy Registry.
  - Phenobarbital is excreted in breast milk.
- Abnormal kidney function and hepatic impairment:
  - Patients who have decreased creatinine clearance (CrCl) may not be able to excrete phenobarbital adequately.
  - Patients with hepatic impairment require a lower dose to prevent adverse effects associated with the drug.
- Specific healthcare environments
  - Administration of parenteral phenobarbital should be done in a critical care unit to monitor for drug effects and provide early resuscitation in the event of a respiratory arrest.

Adverse Effects

As with all AEDs, CNS depression, possibly cognitive impairment with sedation, is the most common adverse effect. Other reported conditions include somnolence, agitation, confusion, vertigo, and nightmares. The most severe adverse effect is Stevens–Johnson syndrome, a hypersensitivity reaction. Respiratory problems may occur, particularly with parenteral phenobarbital. Sudden withdrawal of the medication places the patient at risk of status epilepticus. The FDA has issued a **BOXED WARNING** ◆ for phenobarbital. Patients who take phenobarbital are at risk of suicidal ideation. It is important to monitor the patient for statements that indicate depression and suicide.

Contraindications

Contraindications to phenobarbital include a known hypersensitivity to barbiturates. Other contraindications include liver failure, nephritis, porphyria, respiratory depression, or addiction to barbiturates. The administration of phenobarbital should be avoided during pregnancy. Caution is necessary in acute or chronic pain, lactation, fever, hyperthyroidism, diabetes, decreased liver kidney function, and pulmonary and cardiac disease.

Nursing Implications

Preventing Interactions

Several drugs interact with phenobarbital, increasing its effects (Box 53.1). Opioid analgesics combined with phenobarbital result in enhanced CNS depression. When administered with phenobarbital, corticosteroids, doxycycline, estrogens, hormonal contraceptives, oral anticoagulants, and tricyclic antidepressants have an increased metabolism and a decreased effect. Oil of primrose increases the effects of phenobarbital. Combined with vitamin D, phenobarbital increases the hepatic metabolism of the vitamin. In addition, it reduces calcium absorption. Because of this, it may be necessary to take supplemental vitamin D and calcium.

Administering the Medication

Oral administration of phenobarbital may occur without regard to food. Parenteral administration may involve combining the medication with dextrose, lactated Ringer's, or normal saline. However, if a precipitate forms, administration should not take place. Also, the drug is incompatible with acidic solutions, amphotericin B, chlorpromazine, diphenhydramine, insulin, and vancomycin. The nurse always injects IV phenobarbital into large veins at an infusion rate no faster than 60 mg per minute. Inadvertent intra-arterial injection can cause spasm of the artery and gangrene. When administering the intramuscular (IM) drug, the nurse uses a large needle and injects into deep muscle.

Assessing for Therapeutic Effects

The ultimate goal of therapy with phenobarbital is to decrease seizure effects. The patient's EEG reveals decreased brain waves consistent with seizure activity.

Assessing for Adverse Effects

The nurse assesses for increases in CNS activity consistent with paradoxical excitation, as noted most often in older adults. It is essential to assess respiratory problems such as

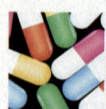

TABLE 53.2 DRUGS AT A GLANCE: Barbiturates

Drug	Type of Seizure Treated	Routes and Dosage Ranges		Therapeutic Serum Drug Level
		Adults	Children	
Phenobarbital	Generalized tonic–clonic and partial seizures	Status epilepticus: IV 20 mg/kg infused 50–100 mg/min; may repeat once after 10 min with an additional 5–10 mg/kg 60–200 mg or 50–100 mg PO daily in 2–3 divided doses	Status epilepticus: IV 20 mg/kg infused 50–100 mg/min; may repeat once after 10 min with an additional 5–10 mg/kg 3–6 mg/kg PO per day	10–40 mcg/mL
Pentobarbital (Nembutal)	Acute seizure episodes associated with anesthesia, eclampsia, meningitis, tetanus, and status epilepticus	Initial dose, 5–15 mg/kg administered at a rate of ≤50 mg/kg; may give an additional 5–10 mg/kg; follow with a continuous infusion Continuous infusion: 0.5–5 mg/kg	2–6 mg/kg; maximum 100 mg	Has not been determined
Primidone (Mysoline)	Tonic–clonic, psychomotor, and focal seizures	100–125 mg PO at bedtime; gradually increase dosage until satisfactory dosage is attained	>8 y, adult dosage <8 y, day 1–3, 50 mg PO at bedtime; day 4–6, 50 mg PO 2 times/d; day 7–9, 100–125 mg PO 2 times/d; maintenance dose, 125–250 mg PO 3 times/d	5–12 mcg/mL

hypoventilation, apnea, respiratory depression, laryngospasm, bronchospasm, and circulatory collapse, particularly in patients receiving parenteral phenobarbital. In addition, it is necessary to:

- Assess for bradycardia, hypotension, and syncope
- Assess the serum drug level for signs of toxicity or inadequate seizure treatment
- Assess for changes in the integumentary system indicative of the onset of Stevens–Johnson syndrome
- Assess complete blood count (CBC) and differential
- Assess blood urea nitrogen (BUN) and creatinine

Patient Teaching

Box 53.2 identifies patient teaching guidelines for phenobarbital.

BOX 53.1 Drug Interactions: Phenobarbital

Drugs That Increase the Effects of Phenobarbital
- Alcohol, chloramphenicol, diazepam, and monoamine oxidase inhibitors
  May increase central nervous system and respiratory depression
- Gabapentin and valproate
  Increase serum level
- Mephobarbital and primidone
  May increase serum level

Other Drugs in the Class

Pentobarbital (Nembutal) and primidone (Mysoline) are barbiturates with similar action as phenobarbital. Both medications exhibit antiseizure activity. Pentobarbital is listed in the Beers Criteria as a drug to be avoided in patients aged 65 years and over because of the risk of dependence and increased risk of overdosage in low doses. Primidone has significant hematologic

BOX 53.2 Patient Teaching Guidelines for Phenobarbital

- Understand that this drug is administered long term for the treatment of seizure activity.
- Do not stop the medication abruptly.
- Have regular tests to determine serum levels of the drug.
- Change positions slowly. This drug may cause drowsiness or syncope.
- Do not drive or operate machinery with central nervous system depression.
- If you are sexually active and able to become pregnant, use two forms of contraception.
- Notify your prescriber about the development of rashes or skin eruptions.
- Wear a medical alert bracelet or necklace stating that you have a seizure disorder and naming the medications you take.

adverse effects, including agranulocytosis, granulocytopenia, and megaloblastic anemia. It is important to obtain a baseline CBC before initiating therapy and at 6-month intervals. The drug is also associated with delayed hypersensitivity reactions ranging from maculopapular rash to Stevens–Johnson syndrome with toxic epidermal necrosis.

BENZODIAZEPINES

Drugs belonging to this class have a broad range of uses; they may act as antidepressants, antiepileptics, or skeletal muscle relaxants. The benzodiazepines potentiate the effects of GABA by increasing the attraction to the receptor sites. The prototype of this class is ⓟ **diazepam** (Valium, Diastat). See Figure 53.1 for the increased effects of GABA by benzodiazepines.

Pharmacokinetics

This varies with the preparation of diazepam. For the IV drug, the onset of action is 1 to 5 minutes, with a peak of 30 minutes and a duration of 15 to 60 minutes. For the oral drug, the onset of action is 30 to 60 minutes, with a peak of 1 to 2 hours and a duration of 3 hours. For the IM drug, the onset of action is generally within 15 to 30 minutes, with a peak of 30 to 45 minutes and a duration of 3 hours. For the rectal drug, the onset is rapid, with a peak of 1.5 hours and a duration of 3 hours. Its half-life, which is longer in newborns and older adults, is 20 to 80 hours. It is metabolized in the liver and excreted by the kidneys. In patients with a BMI > 30 there may be a prolonged action when discontinued.

Action

The exact mechanism of action of diazepam is unknown. However, authorities believe that the drug acts primarily on the limbic system and reticular formation to produce skeletal muscle relaxation. It potentiates the effect of GABA by increasing the attraction of the medication to the receptor sites.

Use

IV diazepam is an adjunctive skeletal muscle relaxant administered for the treatment of severe recurrent convulsive seizures and status epilepticus. Oral diazepam is an adjunctive agent used for seizure disorders. Clinicians also order benzodiazepines such as diazepam for treatment of Lennox–Gastaut syndrome, a mixed seizure disorder that presents at approximately 2 years of age. Table 53.3 gives route and dosage information for diazepam and other benzodiazepines.

Patient-related variables specific to the use of diazepam include the following:

- Age:
  - IV diazepam is recommended for use in children aged 1 month or older. Newborns require a lower dose.
  - Oral diazepam is recommended for children older than 6 months of age.
  - Rectal administration is not recommended in children younger than 2 years of age.
- In older adults, it is necessary to reduce the dosage of diazepam because the drug has an extended half-life in this population.
- Reproduction, pregnancy, and lactation:
  - Diazepam crosses the placenta, and teratogenic effects have been observed.
  - Increased risk of premature birth and low birth weight has been noted following the use of diazepam and other benzodiazepines.
  - Diazepam and its metabolites are present in breast milk.
- Abnormal kidney function and hepatic impairment:
  - Diazepam is excreted by the kidneys after being metabolized in the liver. Thus, patients with abnormal kidney function or hepatic impairment should take reduced dosages of diazepam.
- Specific healthcare environments:
  - Patients with critical illness or those in debilitated states should take reduced dosages of diazepam. During IV administration, patients should receive oxygen.

Adverse Effects

CNS adverse effects of diazepam include depression, disorientation, restlessness, and confusion. In the first 2 weeks of treatment, paradoxical excitatory reactions may occur. The most serious cardiovascular adverse effect is cardiovascular collapse with bradycardia and hypotension. Also, potentially life-threatening tachycardia may occur. In addition, the FDA issued a **BOXED WARNING** . The combination of a benzodiazepine such as diazepam and an opioid medication depresses the CNS, resulting in serious adverse effects, including respiratory depression or death. Other reported problems include constipation, diarrhea, incontinence, urinary retention, and changes in libido.

Contraindications

Patients with known hypersensitivity to benzodiazepines should not receive diazepam. Contraindications also include acute narrow-angle glaucoma, shock, coma, acute alcohol intoxication, and pregnancy.

Nursing Implications

Preventing Interactions

Many medications interact with diazepam, decreasing or increasing its effects (Box 53.3). The herbal supplements kava and valerian increase the effects of diazepam, as does grapefruit juice.

> **❗ Quality and Safety Alert: Safety**
>
> A review by the FDA has shown that the combination of (1) an opioid medication and (2) a benzodiazepine or any drug that suppresses the CNS results in serious adverse effects.

Administering the Medication

When preparing diazepam, the nurse does not mix the drug in plastic bags or tubing or combine it with other solutions. During administration, it is important to monitor pulse, blood pressure, and respiration. During parenteral administration, it is

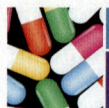

TABLE 53.3
DRUGS AT A GLANCE: Benzodiazepines

Drug	Type of Seizure Treated	Routes and Dosage Ranges		Therapeutic Serum Drug Level
		Adults	**Children**	
Diazepam (Valium, Diastat Acudial, Diazepam, Diastat Pediatric, Diazepam Intensol; ✹ BIO-Diazepam, Diastat Pediatric, Valium)	Status epilepticus	Seizure control: 2–10 mg PO 3–4 times/d Status epilepticus: 5–10 mg IV slowly administered; may repeat every 5–10 min; maximum dose of 30 mg	Status epilepticus: older than 1 mo and younger than 5 y, 0.2–0.5 mg slowly IV every 2–5 min up to a maximum dose of 5 mg 5 y and older, 1 mg IV every 2–5 min up to a maximum dose of 10 mg	Has not been determined
Clobazam (Onfi, Sympazan; ✹ Apo-Clobazam, Clobazam-10, TEVA-Clobazam)	Lennox–Gastaut, epilepsy (adjunctive)	Lennox–Gastaut: PO ≤30 kg; initial 5 mg once daily; then increase to 5 mg twice daily for ≥1 wk; then increase to 10 mg twice daily thereafter >30 kg: initial 5 mg twice daily for ≥1 wk, then increase to 5 mg twice daily for ≥1 wk, and then increase to 10 mg twice daily; after ≥1 wk, may increase to 20 mg twice daily Epilepsy: PO; initial 5–15 mg/d; dosage may be gradually adjusted based on tolerance and seizure control to a maximum dose of 80 mg/d	Lennox–Gastaut: ≥2 y through adolescence: refer to adult dosing Epilepsy: <2 y; initial 0.5–1 mg/kg/d 2–16 y: initial 5 mg daily; may be increased (no more frequently than every 5 d) to a maximum of 40 mg daily; daily doses of up to 30 mg may be taken as a single dose at bedtime; higher doses should be divided	30–300 ng/mL
Clonazepam (Klonopin; ✹ Apo-Clonazepam, Clonapen)	Myoclonic or akinetic seizures, alone or with other antiepileptic drugs (AEDs); possibly effective in generalized tonic, clonic, and psychomotor seizures	1.5 mg PO daily increased by 0.5 mg/d every 3–7 d if necessary; maximum dose, 20 mg/d	0.01–0.03 mg/kg/d PO, increased by 0.25–0.5 mg/d every 3–7 d if necessary; maximum dose, 0.2 mg/kg/d	20–80 ng/mL
Clorazepate (Tranxene-T)	Partial seizures, with other AEDs	7.5 mg PO three times daily maximum initial dose; increased by 7.5 mg every wk, if necessary; maximum dose 90 mg/d	>12 y, same as adults 9–12 y, 7.5 mg PO two times daily maximum initial dose; increased by 7.5 mg every wk, if necessary; maximum dose 60 mg/d	Has not been determined
Lorazepam (Ativan, LORazepam, Intensol, Loreev XR; ✹ APO-LORazepam, Ativan, TEVA-LORazepam)	Status epilepticus	18 y and older, 4 mg IV slowly at 2 mg/min; may give another 4 mg after 10–15 min if needed	Not recommended in children younger than 12 y	Has not been determined

AED, antiepileptic drug.

> **BOX 53.3 Drug Interactions: Diazepam**
>
> **Drugs That Increase the Effect of Diazepam**
> - Alcohol and omeprazole
>   *Increase central nervous system depression*
> - Cimetidine, disulfiram, and hormonal contraceptives
>   *Increase pharmacologic effects*
>
> **Drugs That Decrease the Effects of Diazepam**
> - Theophylline and ranitidine
>   *Decrease pharmacologic effects*

necessary to administer oxygen as well as to put the patient on bed rest for 3 hours. The nurse injects the IV form of the drug slowly into a large vein at 1 mL/minute—over at least 3 minutes in children—never intra-arterially or into small veins. Intra-arterial administration results in arterial spasm.

Assessing for Therapeutic Effects

When administering diazepam for a seizure disorder, the goal of therapy is to control seizure activity. When administering drug for status epilepticus, the goal is to eliminate the seizure activity.

Assessing for Adverse Effects

The nurse assesses for changes in cardiovascular status that could indicate hypotension, bradycardia, or tachycardia. The patient's CNS response is closely monitored. In addition, the nurse assesses for alterations in elimination patterns.

Patient Teaching

Box 53.4 identifies patient teaching guidelines for diazepam.

> **Clinical Application 53.2**
> - During a hospitalization, Andrew has an episode of status epilepticus. His neurologist orders diazepam (Valium) 1 mg IV every 2 to 5 minutes, with a maximum dosage of 10 mg. How does the nurse administer the medication?
> - What assessments and interventions are necessary to implement before, during, and after the administration of diazepam?

Other Drugs in the Class

Clobazam (Onfi, Sympazan), clonazepam (Klonopin), clorazepate (Tranxene-T), and lorazepam (Ativan) are all benzodiazepines. Clobazam, clorazepate, and lorazepam potentiate the action of GABA. The neuronal permeability is enhanced, allowing greater permeability to the chloride ions. This action results in decreased excitability in the brain. The action of clonazepam is unknown. Clobazam can be administered with or without food. The tablets can be crushed and placed in applesauce. The suspension should be shaken well and administered with an oral dosing syringe. Clonazepam is supplied in an orally disintegrating tablet. The patient should be instructed to open the pouch and peel back the foil. The patient's hands should be

> **BOX 53.4 Patient Teaching Guidelines for Diazepam**
>
> - Do not skip doses or stop therapy.
> - Do not use alcohol or smoke. Alcohol is more potent when combined with diazepam. Smoking may constrict blood vessels, resulting in reduced elimination of the drug.
> - Obtain instructions about the administration of rectal diazepam.
> - Use two types of contraceptives if you are sexually active and able to become pregnant.
> - Ask your prescriber about safety and central nervous system (CNS) depression. Protect yourself from falls. Do not drive or operate machinery if you have CNS depression.
> - Wear a medical alert bracelet or necklace stating that you have a seizure disorder and naming the medications you take.

very dry when removing the tablet. Somnolence is an adverse effect of this medication, which can be reduced by administering the medication at bedtime. Patients routinely receiving benzodiazepines should have routine monitoring of the CBC, liver enzymes, creatinine, BUN, and lactate.

> **NCLEX Success**
>
> 2. A patient is taking phenobarbital for a seizure disorder. Which of the following statements indicates that the patient should be seen by a healthcare provider immediately?
>   A. "I have a rash that started on my trunk, and now it is on my arms and legs."
>   B. "I will rest if I feel tired."
>   C. "I take my medication routinely and do not skip doses."
>   D. "I have my blood levels checked if my breathing decreases."

GAMMA-AMINOBUTYRIC ACID STRUCTURAL ANALOGS

In 1993, the FDA approved **gabapentin** (Neurontin) for treatment of partial seizures. In May of 2002, the FDA approved it for treatment of postherpetic neuralgia pain.

Pharmacokinetics and Action

Gabapentin reaches its peak in 1 hour. It binds to sites in the brain that have a high affinity for gabapentin. The drug crosses the placenta and may enter the breast milk. Metabolism occurs in the liver and elimination takes place in the urine. Structurally, gabapentin is related to GABA. Its antiepileptic action is related to its ability to inhibit postsynaptic responses and block postte-tanic potentiation.

Use

Prescribers order gabapentin as an adjunctive treatment for partial seizures and postherpetic neuralgia. There are many off-label uses, some of which include alcohol withdrawal, chronic refractory cough, generalized anxiety disorder, fibromyalgia, hiccups, neuropathic pain, and restless leg syndrome. Table 53.4 gives route and dosage information for gabapentin and other GABA structural analogs.

Patient-related variables specific to the use of gabapentin include the following:

- Age:
  - In infants, abrupt discontinuation of gabapentin will result in tachycardia, emesis, and irritability.
- Reproduction, pregnancy, and lactation:
  - Patients taking gabapentin should be prescribed folic acid supplementation prior to pregnancy.
  - Gabapentin crosses the placenta.
  - Patients exposed to gabapentin during pregnancy are encouraged to enroll in the North American Antiepileptic Drug Pregnancy Registry.
- Abnormal kidney function and hepatic impairment:
  - Use caution in patients with abnormal kidney function. See Table 53.4 for the gabapentin dosages based on the creatinine clearance.
  - Patients with impaired liver function require monitoring for elevated liver enzymes but do not require a dosage adjustment.

TABLE 53.4

DRUGS AT A GLANCE: Gamma-Aminobutyric Acid Structural Analogs

Drug	Type of Seizure Treated	Routes and Dosage Ranges		Therapeutic Serum Drug Level
		Adults	**Children**	
Gabapentin (Neurontin, Gralise; AG-Gabapentin, Auro-Gabapentin, Apo-Gabapentin, TARO-Gabapentin, Teva-Gabapentin)	Partial seizures	Epilepsy: 300 mg PO 3 times/d initially Maintenance: 900–1,800 mg/d PO in divided doses 3 times/d; maximum interval between doses should not exceed 12 h; up to 2,400–3,600 mg/d has been used Postherpetic neuralgia: 300 mg/d PO initially; 300 mg PO 2 times/d on day 2, 300 mg PO 3 times/d on day 3 Abnormal kidney function: creatinine clearance (CrCl) > 60 mL/min, 400 mg three times daily (1,200 mg/d); CrCl 30–60 mL/min, 300 mg two times daily (600 mg/d); CrCl 15–30 mL/min, 300 mg once daily; CrCl < 15 mL/min, 300 mg every other day. Patients on hemodialysis: 200–300 mg after each 4 h of hemodialysis	3–12 y, initially 10–15 mg/kg/d PO in three divided doses; 3–4 y, 40 mg/kg/d in three divided doses; doses up to 50 mg/kg/d were well tolerated; 5 y and older, adjust upward over about 3 d to 25–35 mg/kg daily in three divided doses Maximum dose: Children > 12 y, 300 mg three times per day; usual maintenance dose 900–1,900 mg/d	Clinical trial data indicate that monitoring serum levels is not necessary for safe use
Pregabalin (Lyrica, Lyrica CR; AG-Pregabalin, APO-Pregabalin, Auro-Pregabalin, Dom-Pregabalin, JAMP Pregabalin, SANDOZ-Pregabalin)	Partial-onset seizures with other AEDs	Epilepsy: 150–600 mg/d PO 2–3 times/d Fibromyalgia: 75–150 mg PO 2 times/d; maximum dose, 450 mg/d Postherpetic pain: 75–150 mg PO 2 times/d; maximum dose, 600 mg/d	Safety and efficacy not established	Has not been determined
Tiagabine (Gabitril)	Partial seizures, with other AEDs	4 mg PO daily for 1 wk; increased by 4–8 mg/wk until desired effect; maximum dose 56 mg/d in 2–4 divided doses	<12 y, not recommended 12–18 y, 4 mg PO daily for 1 wk; increased to 8 mg/d in 2 divided doses for 1 wk; then increased by 4–8 mg/wk up to a maximum of 32 mg/d in 2–4 divided doses	Has not been determined

TABLE 53.4

DRUGS AT A GLANCE: Gamma-Aminobutyric Acid Structural Analogs (Continued)

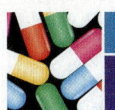

Drug	Type of Seizure Treated	Routes and Dosage Ranges		Therapeutic Serum Drug Level
		Adults	Children	
Vigabatrin (Sabril, Vigadrone; ✦ Sabril)	Infantile spasms Refractory complex partial seizures	500 mg PO twice daily; increase daily dose by 500 mg increments at weekly intervals based on response and tolerability Recommended dose: 1.5 g/d	Infantile spasms: 1 mo–2 y; PO 50 mg/kg divided twice daily; may titrate up to 25–50 mg/kg/d increments every 3 d to a maximum of 150 mg/kg/d divided twice daily Refractory complex partial seizures: children 10–<17 y and to 25–60 kg; PO 250 mg twice daily; increase dose by 500 mg increments at weekly intervals based on response. Recommended dose: 1000 mg twice daily	Has not been determined

AED, antiepileptic drug.

Adverse Effects

The most common adverse effects of gabapentin are associated with CNS depression and include dizziness, somnolence, insomnia, and ataxia. Other reported adverse effects are pruritus, dry mouth, dyspepsia, nausea, vomiting, and suicidal ideation.

Contraindications

Contraindications to gabapentin include a known hypersensitivity to the medication.

Nursing Implications

Preventing Interactions

Antacids do not affect the serum level, but they decrease absorption of gabapentin when administered at the same time. The herb *Ginkgo biloba* decreases the effect of the drug.

Administering the Medication

The nurse ensures that gabapentin is taken orally. People may take the drug with food to prevent GI upset. Extended-release tablets should be swallowed whole and not crushed or chewed. Do not administer within two hours of magnesium or aluminum containing antacids. For pediatric patients, the capsule can be opened and mixed with juice or applesauce.

Assessing for Therapeutic and Adverse Effects

The nurse assesses for the absence of partial seizures, the most important therapeutic effect.

It is also necessary to assess changes in mood and personality in patients receiving gabapentin, as with all antiepileptic medications, because suicidal ideation is the result of CNS depression. The nurse assesses for CNS depression that could affect patient safety.

Patient Teaching

Box 53.5 identifies patient teaching guidelines for gabapentin.

Other Drugs in the Class

Pregabalin (Lyrica) is administered for partial-onset seizures, postherpetic neuralgia, neuropathic pain, and neuropathic pain associated with diabetes. The drug increases the neuronal GABA and decreases calcium currents in the neuronal calcium channels to stabilize and decrease excitability. This action exerts anticonvulsant activity. It is necessary to instruct the patient to monitor his or her weight because of the increased risk of peripheral edema.

Tiagabine (Gabitril) is an adjunctive therapy for partial seizures. It is an inhibitor of GABA uptake in the presynaptic neurons. This action allows for an increase of GABA in the postsynaptic neurons. Patients should understand that the

> **BOX 53.5 Patient Teaching Guidelines for Gabapentin**
>
> - Do not stop taking the medication abruptly.
> - Take the medication with food to decrease gastrointestinal discomfort.
> - Do not cut, crush, or chew extended-release capsules. If swallowing is difficult, sprinkle the contents of the capsule over soft food.
> - Notify your prescriber if seizure activity occurs.
> - Be aware that you may experience nausea, vomiting, insomnia, fatigue, and confusion.
> - Do not drive or operate machinery with central nervous system depression.
> - Report severe nausea and vomiting, changes in stool or urine color, diarrhea, or changes in neurologic function to the prescriber.

herb *G. biloba* will decrease tiagabine effectiveness, placing the patient at risk of seizures.

Vigabatrin (Sabril) received FDA approval for treatment of infantile spasms and as adjunctive therapy in adults who experience refractory focal seizures. The FDA issued a **BOXED WARNING** ◆ for vigabatrin because it can cause permanent bilateral concentric visual field constriction. This damage can include tunnel vision, damage to the central retina, and decrease visual acuity. The loss of vision can occur within weeks of beginning therapy. This adverse effect has limited the availability of the drug in the United States. The drug is part of the Share (Support, Help, and Resources for Epilepsy) Program. Participating physicians and pharmacies can provide vigabatrin to patients who are deemed to need this medication. Visual field testing should be completed before beginning the medication and every 6 months.

HYDANTOINS

The prototype antiepileptic of the hydantoin class is **phenytoin** (Dilantin). The oldest and most widely used AED, it is often the initial drug of choice, especially in adults. In addition to its use in the treatment of seizures, phenytoin has off label uses in the prevention of posttrauma, trigeminal neuralgia, and rescue treatment. Rescue treatment is also known as salvage therapy and is treatment administered after patients with cancer do not respond to other treatments.

Pharmacokinetics

Phenytoin is highly bound (90%) to plasma proteins, and only the free drug (the fraction not bound to plasma albumin) is therapeutically active. The oral preparation, absorbed by the GI tract, has a slow onset of action, with a peak of 2 to 12 hours and a duration of 6 to 12 hours. The IV preparation has an onset of action of 1 to 2 hours with a rapid peak and a duration of 12 to 24 hours. The drug is metabolized by the liver and excreted in the urine.

Action

Phenytoin stabilizes the neuronal membrane by delaying the influx of sodium ions into the neurons and preventing the excitability caused by excessive stimulation. See Figure 53.1 for the site of action of hydantoins.

Use

Clinicians use phenytoin to control tonic–clonic seizures, psychomotor seizures, and nonepileptic seizures. They also use it to prevent seizure activity in patients during and following neurosurgery and brain injury. Table 53.5 gives route and dosage information for phenytoin and the other hydantoins.

Patient-related variables specific to the use of phenytoin include the following:

- Age:
  - When used for status epilepticus in pediatric patients, the IV phenytoin dose is determined according to the weight of the child. The recommended dosage is 15 to 20 mg/kg.
  - Chronic use of phenytoin has been associated with decreased bone mineral density in children.
  - In older adults, phenytoin must be administered cautiously. Older patients may have altered albumin levels, decreasing the affinity of phenytoin for albumin and causing displacement of the drug.
- Reproduction, pregnancy, and lactation:
  - Effective contraception is recommended for patients of reproductive potential.
  - Phenytoin may decrease the effectiveness of contraceptive agents.
  - Phenytoin crosses the placenta, and an increased risk of congenital malformations and adverse fetal outcomes may occur following utero phenytoin exposure.
  - Phenytoin is excreted in breast milk.
- Abnormal kidney function and hepatic impairment:
  - Abnormal kidney function or failure also causes displacement of the drug, placing the patient at risk of toxicity.
  - Hepatic impairment results in altered albumin levels, decreasing the affinity of phenytoin for albumin and causing displacement of the drug.
- Specific healthcare environments:
  - In critically ill patients, the IV administration of phenytoin can result in cardiovascular collapse. It is important to assess blood pressure, pulse, and respirations. Monitoring the patient's cardiovascular status is necessary with the use of telemetry.

Adverse Effects

The most common adverse effects of phenytoin affect the CNS (e.g., ataxia, drowsiness, lethargy) and GI tract (e.g., nausea, vomiting). **Gingival hyperplasia**, an overgrowth of gum tissue, is also common, especially in children. It is related to long-term administration of phenytoin. Long-term use may lead to an increased risk of osteoporosis because of its effect on vitamin D metabolism. Serious reactions are uncommon but may include allergic reactions, hepatitis, nephritis, bone marrow depression, and mental confusion.

Contraindications

Contraindications to phenytoin include a known hypersensitivity to the hydantoins. Other conditions that require caution are seizures related to hypoglycemia, sinus bradycardia, heart

TABLE 53.5
DRUGS AT A GLANCE: Hydantoins

Drug	Type of Seizure Treated	Routes and Dosage Ranges		Therapeutic Serum Drug Level
		Adults	**Children**	
Phenytoin (Dilantin, Dilantin Infatabs, Phenytek, Phenytoin Infatabs; ✹, Dilantin, Dilantin Infatabs, Tremytoine TARO-Phenytoin)	Generalized tonic–clonic and some partial seizures Prevention and treatment of seizures occurring during or after neurosurgery	Status epilepticus: loading dose IV 20 mg/kg at a maximum rate of 50 mg/min 100 mg PO three times daily initially; 300 mg (long acting) once daily as maintenance	Status epilepticus: loading dose IV 20 mg/kg at a maximum rate of 1 mg/kg/min 5–10 mg/kg 10 min after the loading dose Children and adolescents Immediate release: PO 5 mg/kg/d in 2–3 divided doses, individualize dose with dosage adjustments at no <7–10 d intervals; maintenance dose, 4–8 mg/kg/d Extended release: 5 mg/kg/d in 2–3 equally divided doses	5–20 mcg/mL (40–80 µmol/L)
Fosphenytoin (Cerebyx; ✹ Cerebyx)	Status epilepticus	Status epilepticus: IV loading dose 20 mg PE/kg administered at 100–150 PE/min	Not recommended	

PE, phenytoin equivalent.

block, and Stokes–Adams syndrome. In patients exhibiting seizures related to hypoglycemia, the primary treatment involves interventions to increase blood glucose (not the use of AEDs). Given the sedative effects associated with phenytoin, the patient is at risk of decreased heart rate; thus, frequent assessment of cardiac output is required if phenytoin is administered to these patients. Caution is also required when administering phenytoin during pregnancy. The risk of birth defects is a significant adverse effect.

Nursing Implications

Preventing Interactions
Several medications interact with phenytoin, increasing or decreasing its effects (Box 53.6). The effectiveness of corticosteroids, oral contraceptives, and nisoldipine is reduced when combined with phenytoin. Absorption of folic acid, calcium, and vitamin D is decreased with the administration of phenytoin. The herb *G. biloba* decreases the effect of the drug.

Administering the Medication
Phenytoin is available in several forms: a capsule (Dilantin), chewable tablet, oral suspension, and injectable solution. Patients should not switch between generic and trade name formulations because of differences in absorption and bioavailability. If a patient becomes stable on a generic drug and then switches to Dilantin, there is a risk of higher serum phenytoin levels and toxicity. If a patient becomes stable on Dilantin and then switches to a generic drug, there is a risk of lower serum phenytoin levels, loss of therapeutic effectiveness, and seizures. (There may also be differences in bioavailability among generic formulations manufactured by different companies.) The injectable solution is highly irritating to tissues. Therefore, when giving the drug intravenously, it is necessary to use special techniques.

Assessing for Therapeutic and Adverse Effects
The nurse assesses for the absence of tonic–clonic and psychomotor seizures.

The nurse assesses for the presence of a rash or skin eruption indicative of a hypersensitivity reaction; the presence of a

---

BOX 53.6 *Drug Interactions: Phenytoin**

Drugs That Increase the Effects of Phenytoin
- Alcohol, amiodarone, chloramphenicol, omeprazole, and ticlopidine
  Increase phenytoin levels

Drugs That Decrease the Effects of Phenytoin
- Enteral feedings
  Decrease phenytoin absorption

*Complex interactions and effects may occur when phenytoin and valproate are taken together. Phenytoin toxicity may result with apparently normal serum phenytoin levels.

BOX 53.7 Patient Teaching Guidelines for Phenytoin

- Do not stop taking the drug abruptly.
- Take the medication with food to prevent gastric upset.
- Have serum drug levels checked as ordered by your prescriber.
- Maintain good oral hygiene (regular brushing and flossing) to prevent gum disease.
- Have regular dental checkups.
- Use contraception if you are sexually active and able to become pregnant.
- Wear a medical alert bracelet or necklace stating that you have a seizure disorder and naming the medications you take.

NCLEX Success

3. Which of the following places the patient at risk of toxicity following the administration of phenytoin?
   A. The patient skips a dose of phenytoin.
   B. The patient takes a different brand of phenytoin.
   C. The patient switches to a different antiepileptic agent.
   D. The patient receives phenytoin in an enteral feeding.

skin eruption could be indicative of Stevens–Johnson syndrome. In addition, the nurse assesses for cardiovascular collapse with IV administration.

Patient Teaching

Box 53.7 identifies patient teaching guidelines for phenytoin.

Other Drugs in the Class

Fosphenytoin (Cerebyx) is administered intravenously, and the rate should not exceed 150 mg because of the risk of severe hypotension and cardiac dysrhythmias. During administration, the patient's cardiac function should be monitored. The patient's CBC, aspartate aminotransferase, alanine aminotransferase, and serum phenytoin level should be measured.

IMINOSTILBENES

The AEDs classified as the iminostilbenes include the prototype **P carbamazepine** (Tegretol).

Pharmacokinetics

Carbamazepine is administered orally and absorbed by the GI tract. The onset of action is slow in both the oral and oral extended-release preparations. The regular oral preparation peaks in 4 to 5 hours, whereas the oral suspension peaks in 1.5 hours. The extended-release preparation peaks in 3 to 12 hours. The half-life of the drug is 12 to 17 hours. Carbamazepine induces the liver enzymes to increase metabolism and shorten the half-life over time. The variability of the half-life is related to autoinduction, which is usually complete in 3 to 5 weeks. The drug is metabolized by the liver and excreted in the feces and urine. It crosses the placenta and enters breast milk.

Action

The mechanism of action of carbamazepine is not understood, but its antiepileptic activity may be related to inhibition of polysynaptic responses that block posttetanic potentiation. Like the tricyclic antidepressants, the drug affects sodium channels within the cortical neurons. It has the ability to decrease action potential of the cell by inhibiting the influx of sodium into the cell. See Figure 53.1 for the site of action of the iminostilbenes.

Use

Clinicians use carbamazepine to prevent partial seizures with complex symptoms, as in patients with psychomotor and temporal lobe epilepsy. Prescribers order the drug for generalized tonic–clonic and mixed seizures, either partial or generalized. Patients who have uncontrolled seizures or CNS depression on other AEDs use it commonly. Table 53.6 presents route and dosage information for carbamazepine and other iminostilbenes.

Patient-related variables specific to the use of carbamazepine include the following:

- Age:
  - In pediatric patients with HLA-B* allele, there is an increased risk of Stevens–Johnson syndrome and/or toxic epidermal necrolysis.
  - In older adults, it is necessary to assess patient safety when using carbamazepine as this medication may result in increased sedation and confusion.
- Reproduction, pregnancy, and lactation:
  - Carbamazepine may decrease serum plasma concentrations of contraceptive agents.
  - Carbamazepine may interfere with pregnancy tests.
  - Carbamazepine may be associated with teratogenic effects, such as spina bifida, craniofacial defects, and cardiovascular malformations.
  - Carbamazepine is detected in serum of breastfed infants, which may result in respiratory depression, seizures, nausea, vomiting, diarrhea, and/or decreased feeding in some neonates.
- Abnormal kidney function and hepatic impairment:
  - Caution is necessary with carbamazepine in patients with abnormal kidney function or hepatic impairment. The drug may cause hepatic cellular necrosis.

Adverse Effects

Carbamazepine may have serious adverse effects. The FDA has issued a **BOXED WARNING** for carbamazepine concerning aplastic anemia and agranulocytosis. An additional FDA **BOXED WARNING** has been issued due to the serious and sometimes fatal dermatologic reaction, including toxic epidermal necrolysis and Stevens–Johnson syndrome. Patients of Asian ancestry should be screened for the variant HLA-B*1502 allele prior to initiating therapy. The genetic variant has been associated with a significantly increased risk of developing Stevens–Johnson syndrome and/or toxic epidermal necrolysis. Other adverse effects include heart block, cardiac

TABLE 53.6
DRUGS AT A GLANCE: Iminostilbenes

Drug	Type of Seizure Treated	Routes and Dosage Ranges		Therapeutic Serum Drug Level
		Adults	Children	
ⓟ Carbamazepine (Carbatrol, Epitol, Equetro, TEGretol, TEGretol-SR; 🍁 APO-CarBAMazepine, DOM-CarBAMazepine, DOM-CarBAMazepine CR)	Partial, generalized tonic–clonic, and mixed seizures	Epilepsy: 200 mg PO twice daily, increased gradually to 600–1,200 mg daily if needed, in 3 or 4 divided doses Trigeminal neuralgia: 200 mg PO daily, increased gradually Bipolar disorder: 400 mg PO in divided doses, increased gradually to 1,600 mg if necessary	Epilepsy: 6–12 y, 100 mg PO twice daily (tablet) or 50 mg four times daily (suspension), increase to 1,000 mg daily if necessary in 3–4 divided doses; >12 y, 200 mg PO twice daily, increase to 1,000 mg daily for children 12–15 y and 1,200 mg for children older than 15 y	4–12 mcg/mL
Eslicarbazepine (Aptiom; 🍁 Aptiom)	Partial-onset seizures	Monotherapy: PO Initial: 400 mg once daily; may initiate treatment at 800 mg once daily; if seizure reduction outweighs risk, dosage can be increased in increments of 400–600 mg Maintenance dose: 800–1,600 mg daily	Dosage not established	No established range
Oxcarbazepine (Oxtellar XR, Trileptal; 🍁 APO-OXcarbazepine, Trileptal)	Partial seizures, as monotherapy or with other AEDs in adults, with other AEDs in children 4–16 y old	600 mg PO twice daily (1,200 mg/d); maximum dose, 2,400 mg/d Severe abnormal kidney function creatinine clearance (CrCl < 30 mL/min): 300 mg PO twice daily (600 mg/d) and increased slowly until response achieved	With other AEDs, 8–10 mg/kg/d PO, not to exceed 600 mg twice daily; titrate to reach target dose over 2 wk	Monitor serum sodium levels prior to beginning therapy and periodically during drug therapy

AED, antiepileptic drug.

failure, sinus tachycardia, respiratory depression, hepatitis, massive hepatic cellular necrosis with total loss of intact liver tissue, and suicidal ideation. Carbamazepine may cause syndrome of inappropriate antidiuretic hormone secretion (SIADH) secretion and hyponatremia.

Contraindications

Contraindications include a hypersensitivity reaction to carbamazepine or tricyclic antidepressants as well as administration of monoamine oxidase inhibitors. Caution is warranted in patients with a history of increased intraocular pressure; adverse hematologic reaction to other medications; cardiac, hepatic, or kidney damage; and latent psychosis.

Nursing Implications
Preventing Interactions

Some medications interact with carbamazepine, increasing or decreasing its effects (Box 53.8). Warfarin combined with

BOX 53.8 Drug Interactions: Carbamazepine

Drugs That Increase the Effects of Carbamazepine
- Erythromycin, troleandomycin, cimetidine, danazol, isoniazid, propoxyphene, and verapamil
  Increase serum levels and manifestations of toxicity
- Lithium
  Increases central nervous system (CNS) toxicity
- Isoniazid
  Increases the risk of hepatotoxicity

Drugs That Decrease the Effects of Carbamazepine
- Barbiturates
  Decrease serum levels
- Phenytoin and primidone
  Increase drug metabolism without changing seizure control

carbamazepine produces greater anticoagulant effects. The herb *G. biloba* decreases the effect of the drug.

Administering the Medication

It is essential that carbamazepine not be administered within 14 days of use of a monoamine oxidase inhibitor. The nurse should tell patients never to crush or chew extended-release tablets. When administering carbamazepine suspension, the nurse never mixes the preparation with other liquid medications because a precipitate may develop. The nurse ensures that the medication is taken with food to prevent GI upset.

Assessing for Therapeutic Effects

The nurse assesses the patient for absence of partial, tonic–clonic, and mixed seizures.

Assessing for Adverse Effects

There is a risk of aplastic anemia with the administration of carbamazepine, and hematologic assessments are most important. The nurse also assesses the integumentary system for Stevens–Johnson syndrome. Hepatic function must be assessed to check for hepatic adverse effects, including hepatic failure. The nurse also monitors serum sodium levels due to SIADH.

In addition, to prevent toxicity, the nurse assesses serum levels as ordered.

Patient Teaching

Box 53.9 identifies patient teaching guidelines for carbamazepine.

Other Drugs in the Class

Eslicarbazepine (Aptiom) is administered as monotherapy with partial-onset seizures and as an adjunctive therapy. The action is not precisely known, but it is thought to inhibit voltage-gated sodium channels. Oxcarbazepine (Trileptal) has two mechanisms of action that block the voltage-sensitive sodium channels to stabilize the excitability in the brain and control the seizure spread. It is important to monitor the serum sodium and chloride levels. The symptoms of hyponatremia can result. Patients with hyponatremia have an increased risk of seizure activity and seizure frequency. Also, the patient and family should monitor for suicidal ideations.

> **Clinical Application 53.3**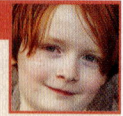
> - If Andrew receives a carbamazepine suspension at 9:00 a.m., when will the peak serum level be reached?
> - At 10 years of age, Andrew develops petechiae on his face and bruising on his arms and legs. His mother calls the pediatric nurse practitioner. What does this nurse suspect is the cause of the bruising?

OTHER ANTIEPILEPTIC DRUGS

CARBONIC ANHYDRASE INHIBITOR

The carbonic anhydrase inhibitor **acetazolamide** controls fluid secretion in the CNS. A diuretic, it is useful in the treatment of seizures as an adjuvant medication.

Pharmacokinetics and Action

Acetazolamide is absorbed by the GI tract. For regular tablets, the onset of action is 1 hour, the peak is 2 to 4 hours, and the duration of action is 6 to 12 hours. For sustained-release tablets, the onset of action is 2 hours, the peak is 3 to 6 hours, and the duration of action is 6 to 12 hours. The half-life of the drug is 5 to 6 hours. Acetazolamide is concentrated in the red blood cells, plasma, and kidneys. The drug is excreted by the kidneys and eliminated in the urine. It crosses the placenta.

The antiepileptic action of acetazolamide is unclear, but it is thought to inhibit CNS carbonic anhydrase to decrease neuronal excitability.

Use

Clinicians use acetazolamide for short-term control of absence and tonic–clonic seizures. Table 53.7 presents route and dosage information for acetazolamide.

Patient-related variables specific to the use of acetazolamide include the following:

- Age:
  - In older adults, acetazolamide must be used cautiously because of an increased risk of diuresis.
- Reproduction, pregnancy, and lactation:
  - Limited data are available on the use of acetazolamide during pregnancy. Pregnant patients administered acetazolamide for seizure treatment should be enrolled in the AED Pregnancy Registry.
- Abnormal kidney function and hepatic impairment:
  - In patients with a glomerular filtration rate greater than 50 mL/minute, administration of acetazolamide should occur every 6 hours. If the glomerular filtration rate is 10 to 50 mL/

BOX 53.9 Patient Teaching Guidelines for Carbamazepine

- Take the medication with food.
- Do not chew or crush extended-release tablets.
- Do not stop taking the medication abruptly.
- Avoid alcohol, sleep agents, or over-the-counter medications.
- Have hematologic testing as ordered by your prescriber.
- Use contraceptives if you are sexually active and able to become pregnant. Carbamazepine may decrease plasma concentrations of hormonal contraceptives (estrogen derivatives) so alternative or back-up methods of contraception should be considered.
- Wear medical alert bracelet or necklace stating that you have a seizure disorder and naming the medications you take.
- Report symptoms of bruising or bleeding immediately to your prescriber.

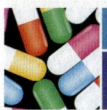

TABLE 53.7
DRUGS AT A GLANCE: Other Antiepileptic Drugs

Drug	Type of Seizure Treated	Routes and Dosage Ranges		Therapeutic Serum Drug Level
		Adults	**Children**	
Acetazolamide	Absence and tonic–clonic seizures	8–30 mg/kg/d PO in divided doses given in combination with other antiepileptics; starting dose 250 mg	8–30 mg/kg/d PO in divided doses given in combination with other AEDs; starting dose 250 mg	Has not been determined
Ethosuximide (Zarontin; 🍁 Zarontin)	Absence seizures, myoclonic, and akinetic epilepsy	500 mg/d PO initially, increased by 250 mg weekly until seizures are controlled or toxicity occurs; maximum dose, 1,500 mg/d	250 mg/d PO initially, increased at weekly intervals until seizures are controlled or toxicity occurs; maximum dose, ≈750–1,000 mg/d	40–100 mcg/mL
Zonisamide (Zonegran, Zonisade)	Partial seizures, with other AEDs	100–200 mg PO daily as a single dose or as 2–3 divided doses; increase by 100 mg/d every 1–2 wk if necessary; maximum dose, 600 mg daily	<16 y, 1–2 mg/kg PO given once daily or in divided doses twice daily; increase by 0.5–1 mg/kg/d only every 1–2 wk; target range is 4–8 mg/kg/d	10–20 mcg/mL
Valproate (Depakote, Depakote ER, Depakote Sprinkles; 🍁 APO-Divalproex, APO-Valproic, Depakene, DOM-Divalproex, DOM-Valproic acid)	Absence, mixed, and complex partial seizures	PO: 10–15 mg/kg/d, increase weekly by 5–10 mg/kg/d, until seizures controlled, adverse effects occur, or maximum dose (60 mg/kg/d) is reached; give amounts >250 mg/d in divided doses; usual daily dose, 1,000–1,600 mg, in divided doses IV: usual dose, diluted in 5% dextrose or 0.9% sodium chloride injection	>5 y: 10–15 mg/kg in two divided doses PO; maximum dose 1,000 mg/d ≥17 y: Depakote: 250 mg PO twice daily Depakote ER: ≥ 12 y 500 mg once daily for 15 d, may increase to 1,000 mg once daily	50–100 mcg/mL (350–700 µmol/L)
Lacosamide (Vimpat; 🍁 APO-Lacosamide, Auro-Lacosamide, MINT-Lacosamide, Pharma-Lacosamide, SANDOZ Lacosamide)	Adjunctive therapy for partial seizures and generalized tonic–clonic seizures	17 y and older, initially 50 mg PO twice daily; increase at weekly intervals to a maximum daily dosage of 100–200 mg twice daily; IV administration when PO route is not feasible Hepatic impairment: 300 mg maximum dosage	1–2 mg/kg/d PO in divided doses (maximum initial dose 50 mg/dose)	Not available
Magnesium sulfate	Preeclampsia and eclampsia paroxysms	Eclampsia, severe preeclampsia: total initial 10–14 g; may infuse 4–5 g in 250 mL of 5% dextrose while giving IM doses up to 10 g or may give initial dose of 4 g IV over 3–4 min; then inject 405 g IM into alternate buttocks every 4 h as needed depending on patellar reflex and respiratory function OR, after initial IV dose, 1–2 g/h by constant IV infusion; continue until paroxysms stop; do not exceed 30–40 g in 24 h		6 mg/100 mL

(Continued on page 970)

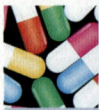

TABLE 53.7
DRUGS AT A GLANCE: Other Antiepileptic Drugs (Continued)

Drug	Type of Seizure Treated	Routes and Dosage Ranges		Therapeutic Serum Drug Level
		Adults	**Children**	
Lamotrigine (LaMICtal, LaMICtal ODT, LaMICtal XR, Subvenite; APO-LamoTRIgine, Auro-LamoTRIgine, LaMICtal, Mylan-Lamotrigine, PMS-LamoTRIgine, RATIO-Lamotrigine, Teva-Lamotrigine)	Partial seizures, with other AEDs Lennox–Gastaut syndrome, with other AEDs	With AEDs, other than valproic acid: 50 mg PO once daily for 2 wk, then 50 mg twice daily (100 mg/d) for 2 wk, then increase by 100 mg/d at weekly intervals to a maintenance dose; usual maintenance dose, 300–500 mg/d in 2 divided doses. With AEDs, including valproic acid: 25 mg PO every other day for 2 wk, then 25 mg once daily for 2 wk, then increase by 25–50 mg/d every 1–2 wk to a maintenance dose; usual maintenance dose, 100–150 mg/d in 2 divided doses	2–12 y, with enzyme-inducing AEDs, initially, PO 0.15 mg/kg/d in 1 or 2 doses for 2 wk; if calculated dose is 2.5–5 mg, give 5 mg on alternate days for 2 wk, and then 0.3 mg/kg/d in 1 or 2 doses, rounded to nearest 5 mg, for 2 wk; maintenance dose, PO 5–15 mg/kg/d in 2 divided doses >12 y, with enzyme-inducing AEDs, initially, PO 25 mg every other day for 2 wk, then 25 mg daily for 2 wk; maintenance dose, PO 100–400 mg daily in 1 or 2 divided doses; with valproic acid, PO 50 mg daily for 2 wk, then 100 mg daily in 2 divided doses for 2 wk; maintenance dose, PO 300–500 mg daily in 1 or 2 doses	Has not been determined
Levetiracetam (Elepsia XR, Keppra, Keppra XR, Roweepra, Roweepra XR, Spritam; Apo-Levetiracetam, Auro-Levetiracetam, Dom-Levetiracetam, JAMP-Levetiracetam, Keppra, PMS-Levetiracetam, PRO-Levetiracetam) Brivaracetam (Briviact; Briviact)	Myoclonic, tonic–clonic, partial seizures Partial-onset seizures	Partial-onset and tonic–clonic seizures: 500 mg PO twice daily initially, increased by 500 mg/d every 2 wk, if necessary; maximum dose, 1,500 mg twice daily Extended release: 1,000 mg once daily; increase every 2 wk by 1,000 mg/d to a maximum dose of 3,000 mg once daily IV 500 mg twice daily; increase every 2 wk by 500 mg/dose to a maximum of 1,500 mg twice daily Abnormal kidney function: creatinine clearance (CrCl > 80 mL/min), 500–1,500 mg; CrCl 50–80 mL/min, 500–1000 mg; CrCl 30–50 mL/min, 250–750 mg; CrCl < 30 mL/min, 250–500 mg Kidney failure with replacement therapy, on hemodialysis: 500–1,000 mg, with a supplemental dose of half the total daily dose (250–500 mg) PO or IV: 50 mg twice daily; may decrease to 25 mg twice daily or increase to 100 mg twice daily based on patient response	Myoclonic: PO immediate-release tablet or oral solution; ≥12 y, refer to adult dosing Partial seizures or refractory seizures (adjunctive treatment); 1 mo–<6 mo, 7 mg/kg/dose twice daily; increase every 2 wk to a recommended dose of 21 mg/kg/dose twice daily 6 mo–<4 y: initial 10 mg/kg/dose twice daily; increase every 2 wk by 10 mg/kg/dose to a recommended dose of 25 mg/kg/dose twice daily 4–5 y, 10 mg/kg PO twice daily; can increase the daily dose every 2 wk by increments of 10 mg/kg to recommended dose of 30 mg/kg twice daily (60 mg/kg/d) <11 kg: initial: 0.75 mg/kg/dose twice daily; maximum: 4.5 mg/kg/d in 2 divided doses 11–<20 kg: initial: 0.5 mg/kg/dose twice daily; maximum: 4 mg/kg/d in 2 divided doses 20–<50 kg: initial 0.5 mg/kg/dose twice daily; maximum: 3 mg/kg/d in 2 divided doses ≥50 kg: initial: 25 mg twice daily; maximum dose: 150 mg/kg/d in 2 divided doses Adolescents ≥16 y: Oral, IV: initial 25 mg twice daily; maximum 150 mg/d in 2 divided doses	Has not been determined

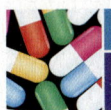

TABLE 53.7
DRUGS AT A GLANCE: Other Antiepileptic Drugs (Continued)

Drug	Type of Seizure Treated	Routes and Dosage Ranges		Therapeutic Serum Drug Level
		Adults	Children	
Perampanel (Fycompa; ✽ Fycompa)	Partial seizures	Patients not taking enzyme-inducing AED regimens: 2 mg PO once daily at bedtime; may increase dose by 2 mg at weekly intervals based on response and tolerability Recommended dose: 8–12 mg once daily Patients taking enzyme-inducing AED regimens: 4 mg PO once daily at bedtime; may increase dose by 2 mg at weekly intervals based on response and tolerability Recommended dose: 8–12 mg once daily at bedtime	Partial-onset seizures: adjunct ≥12 y 2 mg PO at bedtime; may increase daily dose by 2 mg increments at no more frequent than weekly intervals; recommended dose, 8–12 mg once daily at bedtime; 12 mg has shown greater efficacy for reduction of seizure rate than 8 mg; 12 mg is associated with higher adverse effects	
Topiramate (Eprontia, Topamax, Qudexy XR, Topamax Sprinkles, Trokendi XR; ✽ AG Topiramate, Apo-Topiramate, Auro-Topiramate, Dom-Topiramate)	Initial monotherapy for partial seizures or generalized tonic–clonic seizures; partial seizures, generalized tonic–clonic, and Lennox–Gastaut syndrome with other AEDs	25–50 mg PO daily, increased by 25–50 mg/wk until response; usual dose, 400 mg daily in 2 divided doses	2–16 y, week 1, 25 mg PO every PM, increase by 1–3 mg/kg/d at 1- or 2-wk intervals until response; usual dose 5–9 mg/kg/d, in 2 divided doses Monotherapy: 10 y and older, 25 mg PO twice daily, titrating to maintenance dose of 200 mg PO twice daily over 6 wk Week 1: 25 mg twice daily Week 2: 50 mg twice daily Week 3: 75 mg twice daily Week 4: 100 mg twice daily Week 5: 150 mg twice daily Week 6: 200 mg twice daily Check package insert for dosages of extended-release brands	Has not been determined
Cenobamate (Xcopri)		PO: initial weeks 1 and 2; 12.5 mg once daily; increase based on response and tolerance; weeks 3–4: 25 mg once daily; weeks 5–6: 50 mg once daily; weeks 7–8: 2 mg once daily; weeks 9–10: 150 mg once daily; weeks 11–12 and thereafter: 200 mg once daily; maximum dose 400 mg daily		Has not been determined

(Continued on page 972)

TABLE 53.7

DRUGS AT A GLANCE: Other Antiepileptic Drugs (Continued)

Drug	Type of Seizure Treated	Routes and Dosage Ranges		Therapeutic Serum Drug Level
		Adults	**Children**	
Ⓟ Rufinamide (Banzel; 🍁 Banzel)	Adjunctive treatment of seizures caused by Lennox–Gastaut syndrome	400–800 mg PO in 2 divided doses; maximum dosage 3,200 mg/d	<17 y: initial 10 mg/kg/d in 2 equally divided doses; increase dose by 10 mg/kg every other day to a maximum dose of 45 mg/kg/d, not to exceed 3,200 mg daily in 2 equally divided doses	Not available
Felbamate (Felbatol)	Focal seizures (partial onset) Lennox–Gastaut syndrome Partial seizures	1.2 g/d PO in 3 or 4 divided doses; may increase in increments of 1.2 g/d at weekly intervals based on response; maximum dosage 3.6 g/d in divided doses	Lennox–Gastaut: 2–14 y: PO 15 mg/kg/d in 3 or 4 divided doses; increase dose by 15 mg/kg/d increments at weekly intervals; maximum daily dose: 45 mg/kg/d or 3,600 mg/d whichever is less Partial seizures: Adolescents ≥14 y: PO 1,200 mg/d in 3 or 4 divided doses; increase dose in 1,200 mg/d increments at weekly intervals; maximum daily dose: 3,600 mg/d.	Not available
Stiripentol (Diacomit; 🍁 Diacomit)	Dravet syndrome associated seizures	PO: 50 mg/kg/d given in 2 or 3 divided doses; target dose of 50 mg/kg/d over 2–4 wk	Infants ≥ 6 mo weighing ≥7 kg: PO 50 mg/kg/d in 2 divided doses; ≥10 kg PO 50 mg/kg/d in 2–3 divided doses	Not available

minute, administration should occur every 12 hours. With a glomerular filtration rate of less than 10 mL/minute, the drug is not effective, and the patient should not receive it.
- Patients with hepatic impairment should not take acetazolamide.

Adverse Effects

The adverse effects of acetazolamide include excessive diuresis, Stevens–Johnson syndrome, CNS depression, aplastic anemia, leukopenia, thrombocytopenia, hypokalemia, asymptomatic hyperuricemia, and hyperchloremic acidosis.

Contraindications

Contraindications to acetazolamide include hypersensitivity to the drug, hyponatremia, hypokalemia, abnormal kidney function or hepatic insufficiency, and chronic noncongestive angle-closure glaucoma. Administration with thiazide diuretics or antibacterial sulfonamides should not occur.

Nursing Implications

Preventing Interactions

Several medications interact with acetazolamide. There is decreased kidney excretion of quinidine, amphetamine, procainamide, and tricyclic antidepressants with acetazolamide. Salicylates and lithium administered with acetazolamide result in diminished kidney excretion of these drugs. There is also a risk of salicylate toxicity related to metabolic acidosis with acetazolamide.

Administering the Medication

To prevent GI upset, the nurse ensures that the drug is taken with food. When administering to children, the drug can be crushed and mixed in cherry or chocolate syrup to mask the bitter taste. Crushing or chewing of regular tablets is permissible, but patients must swallow sustained-release tablets whole. It is necessary to store the oral preparation in a container with a tight-fitting lid at 59 to 86°F. Parenteral IV push is administered at a rate of 500 mg over 3 minutes.

Assessing for Therapeutic and Adverse Effects

The patient should be without symptoms of absence or tonic–clonic seizures.

The nurse assesses the integumentary system for any sign of skin rash or eruption and fluid and electrolyte levels for metabolic acidosis. The patient should have annual eye examinations to determine if there has been an increase in intraocular pressure.

Patient Teaching

Box 53.10 identifies patient teaching guidelines for acetazolamide.

BOX 53.10	**Patient Teaching Guidelines for Acetazolamide**

- Take the medication with food to prevent gastric upset.
- Have annual eye examinations to assess intraocular pressure.
- Report any changes in weight, unusual bruising or bleeding, pain, or rash to your prescriber.

SUCCINIMIDES

Ethosuximide (Zarontin) is a succinimide antiepileptic agent. The frequency of absence seizures is reduced through the depression of the motor cortex.

Pharmacokinetics and Action

Ethosuximide is rapidly and completely absorbed orally. The drug increases the seizure threshold to suppress the paroxysmal spike and wave pattern noted in absence seizures. The half-life for children is 30 hours and 50 to 60 hours for adults. The medication reaches a peak level in 1 to 7 hours. It is metabolized by the liver into three active metabolites and excreted slowly in the urine. Ethosuximide increases the seizure threshold to suppress the paroxysmal spike and wave pattern noted in absence seizures.

Use

Ethosuximide is used for absence seizures or in combination with other antiepileptic agents in patients with mixed type seizures. No dosage adjustments are required in patients with diminished kidney or hepatic function. Table 53.7 gives route and dosage information for ethosuximide.

Patient-related variables specific to the use of ethosuximide include the following:

- Reproduction, pregnancy, and lactation:
  - Patients with epilepsy who are planning to become pregnant should have baseline serum concentrations once or twice prior to pregnancy when seizure control is optimum.
  - Ethosuximide crosses the placenta. Congenital malformations have been reported in infants.
  - Ethosuximide is present in breast milk. The Canadian label recommends against breast-feeding while taking ethosuximide.

Adverse Effects and Contraindications

The most serious adverse effects of ethosuximide are its hematologic effects. Eosinophilia, leukopenia, thrombocytopenia, agranulocytosis, pancytopenia, and aplastic anemia have been reported. In the event of eosinophilia, multiorgan hypersensitivity, a potentially serious and often fatal drug reaction, can occur. Other adverse effects include anorexia, epigastric distress, abdominal pain, weight loss, diarrhea, constipation, and gingival hyperplasia. CNS effects are impaired physical and mental abilities, CNS depression, anxiety, and hyperactivity. Stevens–Johnson syndrome can result within 28 days of the onset of therapy. At the first sign of rash, the prescriber should be notified, and the medication discontinued.

Ethosuximide is contraindicated in patients who experience a hypersensitivity reaction.

Nursing Implications

Preventing Interactions

Carbamazepine and isoniazid will decrease the serum levels of ethosuximide, placing the patient at risk of seizures. *G. biloba* will decrease the seizure threshold. Cannabis will increase CNS depression.

Administering the Medication

Administer ethosuximide with food to decrease GI distress. The medication should be stored at 15°C to 30°C or 59°F to 86°F.

Assessing for Therapeutic and Adverse Effects

Good control with ethosuximide is indicated by the lack of seizure activity. Assess the patient's weight on a weekly basis because of anorexia and normal weight loss. Check the drug level, which should be in the therapeutic range. Assess the patient for changes in sensorium or increased seizure activity with dosage changes. Assess CBC monthly to determine signs and symptoms of eosinophilia.

Patient Teaching

Box 53.11 identifies patient teaching guidelines for ethosuximide.

SULFONAMIDE

 Zonisamide (Zonegran) is a sulfonamide antiepileptic medication. Prescribers administer it as adjunctive therapy for partial seizures.

> **! Quality and Safety Alert: Evidence-Based Practice**
>
> There are very few studies on the major congenital malformation rate of patients exposed to zonisamide during pregnancy. McCluskey et al. (2021) published a study on the safety of zonisamide in pregnancy. The data were collected from the United Kingdom and Ireland epilepsy and pregnancy registry. The background animal data of the study indicate that teratogenic effects with zonisamide exist and there is a risk of pregnancy loss. The human data suggest a low risk of malformation with an elevated risk of low birth weight. From December 1996 through July 2020, there were 112 cases of first trimester exposure to zonisamide, including 26 monotherapy cases. The median birth weight was on the 71st percentile for monotherapy and 44th percentile for polytherapy; there was a high rate of infants born small for the gestational age.

BOX 53.11	**Patient Teaching Guidelines for Ethosuximide**

- Report a skin rash or any hypersensitivity to the prescriber.
- Have monthly complete blood count or as ordered.
- Do not drive or operate machinery with central nervous system depression.
- Report any changes in behavior.

Pharmacokinetics and Action

Zonisamide is rapidly and completely absorbed. It is highly concentrated in erythrocytes and 40% protein bound. The hepatic cytochrome P450 isoenzyme CYP3A4 is responsible for the metabolism of zonisamide. Zonisamide does not affect GABA. Its action stabilizes the neuronal membranes. It accelerates the dopamine and serotonin neurotransmitters.

Use

Zonisamide is used for a variety of seizures but primarily adjunctive therapy for absence seizures or partial seizures. Infantile spasms are treated with zonisamide. The titration of the medication is faster with infantile spasms. Table 53.7 gives route and dosage information for zonisamide.

Patient-related variables specific to the use of zonisamide include the following:

- Age:
  - Oligohydrosis is an adverse effect commonly seen in children. It will often result in heat stroke and hyperthermia. The child should maintain hydration and protection from increased temperatures.
- Reproduction, pregnancy, and lactation:
  - Patients of childbearing potential should use effective contraception during therapy and for 1 month after discontinuation.
  - Zonisamide crosses the placenta and can be detected in the newborn after birth. Breast-feeding during zonisamide therapy is not recommended.
- Abnormal kidney function and hepatic impairment:
  - Patients with a GFR <50 mL/minute should not be administered zonisamide.

> **Quality and Safety Alert: Safety**
>
> When administering zonisamide, instruct the patient and family on the signs of heat stroke and to maintain adequate hydration. In addition, patients living in warm climates should pay particular attention to increases in body temperature.

Adverse Effects and Contraindications

CNS depression with dizziness and drowsiness has been reported. The most severe adverse effect is the development of toxic epidermal necrolysis and Stevens–Johnson syndrome. Oligohydrosis and heat stroke have been reported in adolescents receiving zonisamide therapy. Metabolic acidosis, abdominal pain, weight loss, constipation, agranulocytosis, and aplastic anemia have also been reported. The FDA has established a warning that zonisamide is contraindicated with all other sulfonamide drug classes. Zonisamide is contraindicated with a known hypersensitivity to sulfonamides.

Nursing Implications

Preventing Interactions

The half-life of zonisamide is decreased when combined with carbamazepine, phenobarbital, phenytoin, and valproate. Administration with kava kava may increase CNS depression.

Administering the Medication

The medication should be stored at room temperature and protected from light and moisture. The capsules should be swallowed whole with a full glass of water or other fluid. Administer without regard to food; however, the presence of food will delay maximum concentration. Patients receiving chronic therapy who are being withdrawn from zonisamide should have the drug withdrawn gradually to minimize seizure frequency. Zonisamide is a hazardous agent. The nurse should use appropriate precautions for handling the medication and should adhere to the health center guidelines for handling hazardous medications. The dosage information is in Table 53.7.

Assessing for Therapeutic and Adverse Effects

Assess the patient's response to the medication and decrease in seizure activity. Assess for metabolic acidosis with the onset of lethargy, confusion, headache, and weakness. If acidosis is suspected, assess arterial blood gases. Assess the patient's intake and output.

Patient Teaching

The patient should be instructed to maintain adequate hydration and protection in warm climates. The patient should avoid the consumption of alcoholic beverages. The medication should be tapered when discontinuing and not abruptly stopped.

HISTONE DEACETYLASE INHIBITOR

Valproate (Depakote, Depakote ER), a histone deacetylase inhibitor, has been in use for approximately 40 years. A researcher identified its antiseizure ability while studying laboratory rats. The drug is synthesized from valeric acid, which is found in the herb valerian.

Pharmacokinetics

The onset of action for oral and parenteral valproate varies, and it reaches its peak in serum in 15 minutes to 4 hours. Parenteral valproate reaches a peak of action in 1 hour. The drug is metabolized by the liver and excreted by the kidneys. It crosses the placenta and enters breast milk. See Figure 53.1 for the site of action of the carboxylic acid derivatives.

Action

The action of valproate is not understood, but it is thought to produce antiepileptic activity by increasing GABA effects, thus decreasing electrical activity.

Use

Clinicians use valproate alone or in combination with other AEDs for the treatment of simple and complex absence seizures, and prescribers also order the drug for the treatment of seizures related to Lennox–Gastaut syndrome. Table 53.7 presents route and dosage information for valproate.

Patient-related variables specific to the use of valproate include the following:

- Age:
  - Use in children younger than 12 years of age requires extreme caution. Fatal hepatotoxicity has occurred, and children

younger than 2 years of age are at greatest risk of hepatic failure within the first 6 months of drug administration.
- Pediatric patients require close monitoring of liver function. In addition, caution is warranted in children younger than 18 months of age and those younger than 2 years of age with congenital abnormalities and severe mental disability.
- When administering valproate to older adults, it is necessary to adjust the dosage slowly.
- Reproduction, pregnancy, and lactation:
  - Valproate should not be administered to patients of childbearing potential.
  - Valproate crosses the placenta and causes major congenital malformations.
  - Valproate is present in breast milk.
- Abnormal kidney function and hepatic impairment:
  - Valproate should be administered cautiously in abnormal kidney function or hepatic impairment.

> **BOX 53.12** **Drug Interactions: Valproate**
>
> **Drugs That Increase the Effects of Valproate**
> - Alcohol and central nervous system depressants
>   *Increase sedation*
> - Chlorpromazine, cimetidine, erythromycin, felbamate, and salicylates
>   *Increase serum levels and toxicity*
>
> **Drugs That Decrease the Effects of Valproate**
> - Carbamazepine, charcoal, and rifampin
>   *Decrease drug levels*
> - Fosphenytoin, phenytoin
>   *Valproate will decrease the protein binding of fosphenytoin and phenytoin. This leads to increase in fosphenytoin and phenytoin concentrations.*

Adverse Effects

The most life-threatening adverse effects associated with valproate are pancreatitis and hepatic failure. Other significant adverse effects include altered bleeding time, thrombocytopenia, bruising, and hemorrhage. The most common GI adverse effects are nausea, vomiting, indigestion, diarrhea, and abdominal cramps. CNS adverse effects include sedation, tremor, emotional upset, weakness, and suicidal ideation, as well as brain atrophy.

The FDA has issued several **BOXED WARNING** ◆ for valproate. The first instructs patients to discontinue valproate at any sign of pancreatitis. The development of this condition is life threatening. The second points out that valproate is a teratogenic medication. Patients of childbearing age should not take the drug without using two forms of birth control. Valproate can cause major congenital malformations, particularly neural tube defects. The third instructs the patient to check for signs of bleeding or bruising. Altered bleeding times may occur. The nurse should tell the patient to have platelet counts, bleeding time determination, and clotting times according to the prescriber's orders. Hepatic failure results in death with valproate. Patients with mitochondrial disease are at increased risk of acute liver failure and death.

Contraindications

Contraindications to valproate include significant hepatic impairment as well as a hypersensitivity reaction to the drug.

Nursing Implications

Preventing Interactions

Certain medications interact with valproate, decreasing or increasing its effects (Box 53.12). Serum levels of phenobarbital, primidone, ethosuximide, diazepam, lamotrigine, and zidovudine may increase when these drugs are combined with valproate. The herb *G. biloba* decreases the effect of the drug. Kava kava and valerian may enhance CNS depression.

Administering the Medication

The nurse dilutes the vial in 5% dextrose, 0.9% sodium chloride, or lactated Ringer solution for IV administration. The reconstituted medication is stable for 24 hours and does not need to be refrigerated. Infusion should occur over 1 hour, no faster than 20 mg per minute. IV administration is permissible only for 14 days, and a switch to an oral preparation is necessary. When administering Depakote to children, the nurse may open the tablets and sprinkle the contents on applesauce or pudding. It is important to note that Depakote ER should be swallowed whole and never crushed or chewed.

Assessing for Therapeutic Effects

The absence of simple and complex absent seizures is indicative that the therapeutic effects of the valproate have been attained.

Assessing for Adverse Effects

The nurse assesses the patient for signs and symptoms of pancreatitis, which include severe abdominal pain and back pain (Hinkle et al., 2021). The patient is also assessed for bleeding and bruising. In addition, the nurse needs to assess the patient's liver function tests routinely. Finally, it is necessary to assess the patient's motor and cognitive function because of brain atrophy.

Patient Teaching

Box 53.13 identifies patient teaching guidelines for valproate.

FUNCTIONALIZED AMINO ACIDS

Ⓟ Lacosamide (Vimpat) is an AED that is available in oral and IV preparations.

Pharmacokinetics

Lacosamide is rapidly absorbed. The oral preparation reaches its peak in 1 to 4 hours, and the IV preparation reaches its peak at the end of the infusion. The half-life of the medication is 13 hours. The drug is metabolized by the CYP3A4, CYP2C9, and CYP2C19 enzymes in the liver and excreted in the urine. It crosses the placenta and may enter the breast milk.

Action

The drug inhibits the voltage-sensitive sodium channels, producing stabilization of the neuronal membrane and inhibition of the repetitive firing of the neuron.

| BOX 53.13 | **Patient Teaching Guidelines for Valproate** |

- Take medication at regular intervals, do not skip a dose, and do not stop abruptly.
- Do not chew or crush extended-release tablets.
- Avoid alcohol and over-the-counter sleep aids.
- Keep follow-up appointments with your prescriber.
- Keep follow-up appointments for serum blood levels, platelet counts, bleeding and clotting times, liver function, and kidney function.
- Use two types of birth control if you are sexually active and able to become pregnant. Notify your prescriber if you become pregnant.
- Do not operate machinery with central nervous system (CNS) depression. You may have sedation, tremors, emotional upset, weakness, or suicidal ideation.
- Know the signs and symptoms of pancreatitis, such as upper abdominal pain and nausea and vomiting, which often begins or worsens after eating.
- If you have diabetes, be aware that this medication interferes with ketones.
- Report any unusual bleeding or bruising.
- Wear a medical alert bracelet or necklace stating that you have a seizure disorder and naming the medications you take.

Use

Indications for oral lacosamide include mono and adjunctive therapy for partial-onset seizures and adjunctive therapy for primary generalized tonic–clonic seizures. Clinicians use the IV drug on a short-term basis when oral administration is prohibited. Table 53.7 gives route and dosage information for lacosamide.

Patient-related variables specific to the use of lacosamide include the following:

- Age:
  - Pediatric patients who are on a single AED and converting to lacosamide monotherapy should be maintained on the maintenance dose for 3 days before withdrawing the concomitant AED.
  - In older adults, dosage reduction is not necessary unless abnormal kidney function is apparent. It is important to determine the dosage based on the patient's hepatic and kidney function.
- Reproduction, pregnancy, and lactation:
  - Lacosamide crosses the placenta.
  - Lacosamide is present in breast milk, and causes drowsiness and poor feeding in breastfed infants.
- Abnormal kidney function and hepatic impairment:
  - Kidney function regulates dosage, because the drug is eliminated in the urine. Patients with a CrCl of 30 mL/minute or less should receive 300 mg/day as the maximum dosage. In those with kidney failure with replacement therapy, the maximum dosage should be 300 mg daily or less.
  - In patients with mild to moderate hepatic impairment, it is necessary to titrate the dosage. The maximum dosage is 300 mg/day. Experts do not recommend use of the drug in patients with severe hepatic impairment, because the drug possesses hepatotoxic adverse effects.
- Specific healthcare environments:
  - Critically ill patients should receive lacosamide intravenously when oral preparation is prohibited. Caution is necessary in the presence of cardiac conduction abnormalities, myocardial ischemia, and heart failure.

Adverse Effects and Contraindications

The adverse effects of lacosamide include a prolonged PR interval, dizziness, ataxia, diplopia, somnolence, suicidal ideation, headache, nausea, and vomiting.

Contraindications include a known hypersensitivity to the drug.

Nursing Implications

Preventing Interactions

It is important that lacosamide not be combined with any medication that prolongs the PR interval. Patients should not take this drug in combination with alcohol.

Administering the Medication

The nurse may give IV lacosamide in 0.9% sodium chloride, 5% dextrose, or lactated Ringer solution. The period of infusion is 30 to 60 minutes. Administration of lacosamide should not occur in the same IV line with other medications. The Neurocritical Care Society recommends the IV administration rate at 200 mg over 15 minutes. The preparation is stable at room temperature for 24 hours.

Assessing for Therapeutic and Adverse Effects

The nurse assesses the patient for CNS depression and diminished partial-onset seizure activity.

The greatest risks associated with lacosamide are suicidal ideation and cardiac conduction abnormalities. The nurse assesses the patient for sudden personality changes, signs of aggression, and severe nausea and vomiting. During parenteral administration, the nurse assesses for signs of a prolonged PR interval.

Patient Teaching

Box 53.14 identifies patient teaching guidelines for lacosamide.

| BOX 53.14 | **Patient Teaching Guidelines for Lacosamide** |

- Do not discontinue the drug abruptly. If you need to stop taking it, taper the dosage.
- Report any mood changes to the prescriber.
- Keep follow-up appointments to monitor drug response and assessment of adverse effects.
- Do not drink alcohol because of the increased risk of central nervous system depression.
- If you are sexually active and able to become pregnant, use of a contraceptive is recommended.

MINERAL ELECTROLYTES: MAGNESIUM SULFATE

It is important to understand the use and administration of the mineral electrolyte ⓟ **magnesium sulfate** because of the fetal neuroprotection it can give to pregnant patients. This medication provides the opportunity to improve neurodevelopmental outcomes in infants by delaying preterm birth and decreasing maternal seizure risk. Table 53.7 contains some dosage information about this agent. Chapter 6 discusses the use of magnesium sulfate more fully.

PHENYLTRIAZINE DERIVATIVES

ⓟ **Lamotrigine** (LaMICtal) is used for adjunctive therapy in the treatment of partial seizures.

Pharmacokinetics

Lamotrigine is administered orally. It is absorbed by the GI tract with a rapid onset of action. Lamotrigine is metabolized by the liver and excreted in the urine. It crosses the placenta and enters the breast milk. The medication is 55% protein bound and has a 25- to 30-hour half-life.

Action

Lamotrigine inhibits the release of glutamate, an excitatory neurotransmitter, in the brain. The neurotransmitter is sensitive to sodium channels, thus decreasing seizure activity.

Use

Clinicians use lamotrigine for focal partial seizures as well as for generalized tonic–clonic, absence, or myoclonic seizures. Other uses include bipolar disorder. Table 53.7 gives route and dosage information for lamotrigine.

Patient-related variables specific to the use of lamotrigine include the following:

- Age:
  - Children should receive lamotrigine in combination with valproate and other AEDs.
  - Tablets administered to children should not be split; whole tablets should be used for dosing; round calculated dose down to the nearest whole tablet.
- Reproduction, pregnancy, and lactation:
  - Patients of childbearing age who plan to become pregnant and are being treated for epilepsy with lamotrigine should have baseline serum concentrations before pregnancy and during pregnancy when seizure control is adequate.
  - Lamotrigine crosses the placenta.
  - Patients should enroll in the North American Antiepileptic Drug Pregnancy Registry.
  - Lamotrigine is present in breast milk.
  - Breastfed infants of patients treated with lamotrigine may present with apnea, poor sucking, thrombocytosis, drowsiness, and rash.
- Abnormal kidney function and hepatic impairment:
  - Patients with CrCl <30 mL/minute may require dosage adjustment.
  - Moderate to severe hepatic impairment decreases the initial dose and adjusts based on clinical response and patient tolerance.

Adverse Effects

Adverse effects of lamotrigine include dizziness, drowsiness, headache, ataxia, blurred or double vision, nausea and vomiting, and weakness. The FDA has issued a **BOXED WARNING** ◆ related to the potential development of serious dermatologic reactions. Because a serious skin rash may occur, especially in children, lamotrigine should be administered cautiously to children younger than 16 years of age and should be discontinued at the first sign of skin rash in an adult. Skin rash is more likely to occur with concomitant valproate therapy, high lamotrigine starting dose, and rapid titration rate. It may resolve if lamotrigine is discontinued, but it progresses in some patients to more severe forms, such as Stevens–Johnson syndrome or toxic epidermal necrosis.

Contraindications

Contraindications to lamotrigine include any hypersensitivity to the drug. Patients who have signs and symptoms of suicide, as well as those who are pregnant or lactating, should not take it.

Nursing Implications

Preventing Interactions

Several medications interact with lamotrigine, increasing or decreasing its effects (Box 53.15). *G. biloba* and oil of primrose decrease the effects of lamotrigine.

Administering the Medication

The nurse should ensure that chewable tablets are chewed or crushed, not swallowed. If the drug is discontinued, it is essential to taper the medication over a 2-week period.

Assessing for Therapeutic and Adverse Effects

The nurse should assess for the lack of generalized focal, myoclonic, and absence seizures.

The nurse assesses the integumentary system daily for the onset of skin eruptions. The patient is also questioned about ophthalmologic changes.

BOX 53.15   *Drug Interactions: Lamotrigine*

Drugs That Increase the Effects of Lamotrigine

- Valproate
  Significantly increases plasma concentration

Drugs That Decrease the Effects of Lamotrigine

- Carbamazepine, fosphenytoin, oral contraceptives, phenobarbital, primidone, and phenytoin
  Decrease serum concentration

BOX 53.16	Patient Teaching Guidelines for Lamotrigine

- Call your prescriber if a skin rash develops.
- Use protection from sunlight.
- Do not operate machinery if you have central nervous system depression.
- Use a contraceptive if you are sexually active and able to become pregnant.
- Schedule eye examinations annually.
- Do not stop the medication abruptly.

Patient Teaching

Box 53.16 identifies patient teaching guidelines for lamotrigine.

PYRROLIDINE DERIVATIVES

Ⓟ Levetiracetam (Keppra) is an AED that is effective in the treatment of a wide variety of seizure disorders. The use of levetiracetam has increased in treating seizure disorders in adults and children. It is approved for use in patients with myoclonic, tonic–clonic, and partial seizures. In the United States, an unlabeled use of levetiracetam is status epilepticus.

Pharmacokinetics

Levetiracetam is administered orally or intravenously and is rapidly absorbed, reaching its peak in 1 hour. It is 10% protein bound with minimal hepatic metabolism. It is excreted in the urine and has a 7.1-hour half-life. The half-life in older adults is 9.6 hours.

Action

Levetiracetam is chemically unrelated to other AEDs, and its mechanism of action is unknown. It inhibits abnormal neuronal firing but does not affect normal neuronal excitability or function.

Use

Clinicians use levetiracetam as adjunctive therapy for partial-onset and generalized tonic–clonic seizures. Table 53.7 presents route and dosage information for levetiracetam.

Patient-related variables specific to the use of levetiracetam include the following:

- Age:
  - In infants and children ≤ 20 kg, use the oral solution of levetiracetam.
  - In older adults, the dose should be lowered by 30% to 50% and increased gradually.
- Abnormal kidney function and hepatic impairment:
  - It is essential to reduce the dose in patients with impaired kidney function, because the kidneys eliminate the majority of a dose (66%).
- Reproduction, pregnancy, and lactation:
  - Levetiracetam crosses the placenta and can be detected in the newborn.
  - Levetiracetam is present in breast milk.

Adverse Effects and Contraindications

Common adverse effects of levetiracetam include drowsiness, dizziness, and fatigue. Others include decreases in red and white blood cell counts, double vision, amnesia, anxiety, ataxia, emotional lability, hostility, nervousness, paresthesia, pharyngitis, and rhinitis. Postmarketing research noted that there is a risk of hepatic failure, acute kidney failure, and multiorgan failure. There is also a risk of development of Stevens–Johnson syndrome.

Contraindications include a known hypersensitivity to the medication, pregnancy, lactation, and suicidal ideation.

Nursing Implications

Preventing Interactions

CNS depressants combined with levetiracetam may increase symptoms of sedation.

Administering the Medication

It is essential that the IV preparation of levetiracetam be administered only on a short-term basis. The nurse tells patients not to crush extended-release forms of the drug. To prevent GI upset, the nurse administers the oral preparation with food. Although food may delay absorption, it does not affect the degree of absorption. The nurse monitors patients for psychosis and depression.

Assessing for Therapeutic and Adverse Effects

The nurse assesses the patient for symptoms of partial-onset and generalized tonic–clonic seizures, which should be absent.

The nurse assesses the patient for ocular changes, CNS depression, and hematologic changes.

Patient Teaching

Box 53.17 identifies patient teaching guidelines for levetiracetam.

Other Drugs in the Class

Brivaracetam (Briviact) is used to treat partial-onset seizures in monotherapy or adjunctive therapy. The mechanism of action is unknown. It is rapidly absorbed and should not be administered with a high fat meal. The patient's CBC, differential, AST, ALT, BUN, and creatinine should be monitored. Also, the patient should be assessed for suicidal ideations.

AMPA GLUTAMATE RECEPTOR ANTAGONIST

Ⓟ Perampanel (Fycompa) is an α-amino-3-hydroxy-5-methyl-4-isoxazolepropionic acid (AMPA) glutamate receptor antagonist, which is considered a miscellaneous antiepileptic agent.

> **BOX 53.17** **Patient Teaching Guidelines for Levetiracetam**
>
> - Do not crush or chew extended-release tablets.
> - Do not stop taking the medication abruptly.
> - Use a contraceptive if you are sexually active and able to become pregnant.
> - Schedule eye examinations annually.
> - Do not operate machinery if you have central nervous system depression.

Pharmacokinetics and Action

Perampanel is rapidly absorbed, but the presence of food will slow the absorption. It is 95% to 96% protein bound by albumin and alpha$_1$ acid glycoprotein. Metabolism occurs in the liver by primary oxidation with the isoenzymes CYP3A4, CYP3A5, CYP1A2, and CYP2B6 and subsequent glucuronidation.

This medication exerts an unknown antiseizure activity.

Use

Prescribers use perampanel for adjuvant treatment of partial-onset seizures with or without generalized seizures in individuals 12 years and older. Table 53.7 gives route and dosage information for perampanel.

Patient-related variables specific to the use of perampanel include the following:

- Age:
  - In pediatric patients, the oral dose is administered at bedtime.
  - Perampanel is administered cautiously in older adult patients due to the risk of dizziness, altered coordination, somnolence, and fatigue. Older adults are at risk of falls.
- Reproduction, pregnancy, and lactation:
  - Pregnant patients treated with perampanel should be enrolled in the North American Pregnancy Registry.
  - It is unknown if perampanel is present in breast milk.
- Abnormal kidney function and hepatic impairment:
  - Perampanel is not recommended in patients with severe abnormal kidney function.
  - Perampanel is not recommended in patients with severe hepatic impairment.

Adverse Effects and Contraindications

The most serious adverse effect of perampanel is hostile behavior. The FDA issued a **BOXED WARNING** ◆ that serious or life-threatening psychiatric and behavioral adverse reactions such as aggression, hostility, anger, and homicidal ideations can occur.

Other adverse effects in multiorgan hypersensitivity referred to as DRESS syndrome. DRESS is a drug reaction with eosinophilia and systemic symptoms that is life threatening. The reaction includes atypical lymphocytosis, lymphadenopathy, a skin eruption, and multiorgan failure. The metabolic adverse effect is hyponatremia and weight gain. Other less severe adverse effects are as follows: skin rash, abdominal pain, constipation, nausea, vomiting, urinary tract infection, bruising, blurred vision, diplopia, upper respiratory infection, lacerations, head trauma, and limb injury. According to the manufacturer's labeling, there are no contraindications to perampanel.

Nursing Implications

Preventing Interactions and Administering the Medication

According to the manufacturer, potential interactions may exist requiring a dosage or frequency adjustment. It is important to monitor the outcomes of therapy. Medications that alter CNS effects have a potential to cause enhanced adverse effects, particularly CNS depression. St. John's wort or kava kava combined with perampanel also produces and increases CNS depression.

The oral formulation should be administered at bedtime.

Assessing for Therapeutic and Adverse Effects

The nurse assesses the patient's response to the medication, including seizure activity, duration, and frequency. Also, the nurse assesses for aggressive, hostile, and homicidal behavior. In addition, it is necessary to assess serum sodium level and for changes in weight.

Patient Teaching

Box 53.18 identifies patient teaching guidelines for perampanel.

SULFAMATE-SUBSTITUTED MONOSACCHARIDES

P Topiramate (Topamax) is a sulfamate-substituted monosaccharide that was identified during a research project to develop a new antidiabetic agent. The drug has many unlabeled uses, including cluster headache prophylaxis, alcohol dependence, and weight loss.

Pharmacokinetics

Topiramate is absorbed in the GI tract and produces peak plasma levels about 2 hours after oral administration. The average

> **BOX 53.18** **Patient Teaching Guidelines for Perampanel**
>
> - Observe for hostile, aggressive, and homicidal behavior.
> - Report serious psychiatric and behavioral reactions.
> - Administer the medication at bedtime.
> - Monitor changes in weight.
> - Have serum sodium levels drawn as ordered.

half-life is about 21 hours, and steady-state concentrations are reached in about 4 days with normal kidney function. The drug is 20% bound to plasma proteins. Topiramate is not extensively metabolized and is primarily eliminated via the kidneys.

Action

The mechanism of action of topiramate is not understood, but the antiepileptic action may be related to the blockage of sodium channels in neurons with sustained depolarization. This action increases GABA activity at the receptors, potentiating the inhibition of the neurotransmitters blocking excitatory neurotransmitters at the neuron receptor sites.

Use

Clinicians use topiramate as monotherapy in partial-onset or primary generalized tonic–clonic seizures as well as in adjunctive therapy for partial-onset or primary generalized seizures. Lennox–Gastaut syndrome is also an indication. In addition, prescribers order the medication as a preventive for migraine headaches. Table 53.7 gives route and dosage information for topiramate.

Patient-related variables specific to the use of topiramate include the following:

- Age:
  - Necrotizing enterocolitis has been reported in neonates.
  - Pediatric patients <24 months may be at increased risk of topiramate-associated hyperammonemia, especially when administered with valproate. Monitor the patient for lethargy, vomiting, and mental status changes.
- Reproduction, pregnancy, and lactation:
  - Effective forms of contraception should be used with patients treated with topiramate.
  - Topiramate crosses the placenta and places the fetus at risk of cleft lip/palate and small for gestational age.
- Abnormal kidney function and hepatic impairment:
  - Patients with a CrCl less than 70 mL/minute should receive one-half of the usual dose.
  - Patients with elevated liver enzymes should receive reduced doses of topiramate, with the dosage increased slowly over time. It is necessary to monitor patients closely for increased hepatic effects.

Adverse Effects and Contraindications

Adverse effects of topiramate include CNS effects such as ataxia, somnolence, dizziness, and nystagmus as well as GI adverse effects such as nausea and dyspepsia. The metabolic adverse effects of topiramate are a decreased serum bicarbonate and weight loss. Kidney stones may develop. Other adverse effects are increased intraocular pressure and fatigue. A rare adverse effect is oligohydrosis, which is decreased sweating and hyperthermia. These adverse effects are more common in children and exposure to high environmental temperatures.

Contraindications include hypersensitivity to the drug and metabolic acidosis. Anticholinergic medications will increase the patient's risk of developing oligohydrosis and hyperthermia.

> **BOX 53.19** *Drug Interactions: Topiramate*
>
> **Drugs That Increase the Effects of Topiramate**
> - Alcohol
>   *Increases central nervous system (CNS) depression*
> - Carbonic anhydrase inhibitors
>   *Increase the risk of kidney stone development*
>
> **Drugs that Decrease the Effects of Topiramate**
> - Carbamazepine, phenytoin, and valproate
>   *Decrease serum levels*

Nursing Implications

Preventing Interactions

Several medications interact with topiramate, increasing or decreasing its effects (Box 53.19). The drug decreases the effectiveness of oral contraceptives. The herb *G. biloba* decreases the effect of topiramate. The ketogenic diet may increase the risk of acidosis and kidney stone development.

Administering the Medication

Topiramate has a very bitter taste. To prevent patients from tasting the bitterness, the nurse instructs them never to chew the medication. In addition, the nurse notes that it is necessary to store topiramate in a tightly closed container at 59°F to 86°F.

Assessing for Therapeutic and Adverse Effects

Patients are without symptoms of partial or generalized seizures. Those with Lennox–Gastaut syndrome have no seizure activity.

The nurse assesses the patient for pain or discomfort related to kidney stones. The patient should have an annual eye examination to determine the onset of increased intraocular pressure. Monitor the patient's temperature and diminished sweating when exposed to high environmental temperatures.

Patient Teaching

Box 53.20 identifies patient teaching guidelines for topiramate.

> **BOX 53.20** *Patient Teaching Guidelines for Topiramate*
>
> - Do not stop taking the medication abruptly.
> - Use two types of contraceptives if you are sexually active and able to become pregnant.
> - Do not operate machinery with central nervous system (CNS) depression.
> - Drink six to eight 8-oz glasses of water per day to decrease risk of kidney stone development.

TETRAZOLE ALKYL CARBAMATE DERIVATIVE

P Cenobamate (Xcopri) was approved by the FDA in 2019 for the treatment of partial-onset seizures in adults.

Pharmacokinetics and Action

Cenobamate is ≥88% absorbed and 60% protein bound primarily to albumin. It is metabolized hepatically by the CYP2A6, CYP2B6, CYP2E1, and UGT2B7 isoenzymes. The half-life is 50 to 60 hours and peak of action at 1 to 4 hours. It is excreted primarily in the urine and minimally in the feces. Cenobamate inhibits sodium channels to reduce the repetitive neuronal firing.

Use

As stated previously, cenobamate is used only in the adult population for focal onset seizures.

Patient-related variables specific to the use of cenobamate include the following:

- Reproduction, pregnancy, and lactation:
  - Cenobamate decreases the efficacy of oral contraceptives.
  - Adverse fetal effects have been noted in animal reproduction studies.
  - It is unknown whether cenobamate is present in breast milk.
- Abnormal kidney function and hepatic impairment:
  - Cenobamate is not recommended with severe abnormal kidney function or severe hepatic impairment.

Adverse Effects and Contraindications

CNS effects include cognitive dysfunction, fatigue, dizziness, vertigo, ataxia, aggressive behavior, hostility, and psychosis. Suicidal ideations and suicidal tendencies have been reported with cenobamate. Dermatologic adverse effects include maculopapular rash. The ECG changes include QT shortening related to the dosage administration. Higher doses increase the incidence of QT interval shortening.

Cenobamate is contraindicated in patients who experience hypersensitivity and familial QT syndrome.

Nursing Implications

Preventing Interactions

Cenobamate interacts with medications that are CYP3A4 inducers. The medications that are CYP3A4 inducers will have increased serum concentrations when combined with cenobamate. Some medications that are CYP3A4 inducers include atorvastatin, atazanavir, clarithromycin, clindamycin, corticosteroids, and immune modulators. Cannabis and cannabinoid products will result in increased CNS depression.

Administering the Medication

Cenobamate should be administered without regard to food. Tablets should not be crushed; they should be swallowed whole with liquid.

Assessing for Therapeutic and Adverse Effects

The nurse should assess for decreased seizure activity. It is important to assess for suicidal ideations and CNS depressant effects. The nurse should assess for skin rash indicating a hypersensitivity reaction.

Patient Teaching

Box 53.21 identifies patient teaching guidelines for cenobamate.

BOX 53.21 Patient Teaching Guidelines for Cenobamate

- Report skin eruptions to the primary care provider.
- Do not stop taking the medication abruptly.
- Use two types of contraceptives if you are sexually active and able to become pregnant.
- Do not operate machinery with CNS depression.
- Report familial QT interval shortening to the prescriber.

TRIAZOLE DERIVATIVES

Rufinamide (Banzel) is structurally unrelated to other AEDs. Rufinamide is effective in reducing the generalized tonic–clonic seizures related to Lennox–Gastaut syndrome.

Pharmacokinetics and Action

Rufinamide is absorbed slowly by the GI tract. Peak plasma concentrations occur between 4 and 6 hours. The drug is metabolized extensively without active metabolites. It is excreted by the kidneys.

Rufinamide decreases seizure activity by prolonging the inactive sodium channels in the cortical neurons.

Use

Clinicians use rufinamide in the treatment of seizures in patients with Lennox–Gastaut syndrome. Table 53.7 gives route and dosage information for rufinamide.

Patient-related variables specific to the use of rufinamide include the following:

- Age
  - Pediatric patients should be monitored closely for drug interactions, and may require dosage and frequency adjustments.
  - Administer to older adults cautiously. The initial doses should be reduced.
- Reproduction, pregnancy, and lactation:
  - Some hormonal contraceptives are not effective with rufinamide.
  - Adverse fetal changes have been observed in animal reproduction studies.
  - Patients exposed to rufinamide during pregnancy are encouraged to register with the North American Pregnancy Registry.
  - It is not known if rufinamide enters the breast milk.
- Abnormal kidney function and hepatic impairment:
  - It is necessary to administer rufinamide cautiously to patients with moderate hepatic impairment. Patients with severe hepatic impairment should not take the drug.

Adverse Effects and Contraindications

The most common adverse effects of rufinamide include fatigue, headache, somnolence, vomiting, and flulike symptoms. Dermatologic effects, including Stevens–Johnson syndrome, require immediate discontinuation of rufinamide. Decreased white blood cell counts may occur.

> **BOX 53.22 Drug Interactions: Rufinamide**
>
> **Drugs That Increase the Effect of Rufinamide**
> - Valproate
>   *Increases plasma concentration*
>
> **Drugs That Decrease the Effect of Rufinamide**
> - Primidone
>   *Decreases the serum concentration of rufinamide*
> - Carbamazepine, ethinyl estradiol, and norethindrone
>   *Decrease the effect of both drugs*
> - Phenobarbital and phenytoin
>   *May increase levels of these drugs as well as decrease rufinamide level*

> **BOX 53.23 Patient Teaching Guidelines for Rufinamide**
>
> - Take the medication with food.
> - Do not stop taking the medication abruptly.
> - Use two types of contraceptives if you are sexually active and able to become pregnant.

Contraindications include short QT syndrome, severe hepatic impairment, pregnancy, and lactation.

Nursing Implications

Preventing Interactions

Several drugs interact with rufinamide, increasing or decreasing its effects (Box 53.22).

Administering the Medication

To increase drug absorption, the nurse ensures that rufinamide is taken with food. It is acceptable to crush or split the medication for ease of administration.

Assessing for Therapeutic and Adverse Effects

The patient is without seizure activity related to Lennox–Gastaut syndrome.

It is important to assess the patient's CNS response to the medication. The nurse also assesses the patient for GI upset and flulike symptoms, as well as for hypersensitivity reactions such as Stevens–Johnson syndrome.

Patient Teaching

Box 53.23 identifies patient teaching guidelines for rufinamide.

MISCELLANEOUS ANTIEPILEPTIC DRUGS

Felbamate (Felbatol) is a miscellaneous antiseizure medication that is not first-line treatment of focal partial-onset seizures as monotherapy or adjunctive therapy.

Pharmacokinetics and Action

Felbamate is rapidly absorbed and is 22% to 48% protein bound. The half-life is 20 to 23 hours. It has a peak of action in 2 to 6 hours and excreted primarily in the urine. The action is unknown, but it affects the N-methyl-D-aspartate receptor antagonism, inhibition of sodium and calcium channels and potentiation of GABA.

Use

As previously stated, felbamate is administered to adults with focal partial-onset seizures. In pediatric patients, it is used as adjunctive therapy for Lennox–Gastaut syndrome and partial-onset seizures. It is also used as monotherapy for partial-onset seizures.

Patient-related variables specific to the use of felbamate include the following:

- Age:
  - For children ≥ 2 years and adolescents: The initial and maintenance dose should be reduced by 50%. A reduced dose may be required when used as adjunctive therapy with other antiseizure medications.
- Reproduction, pregnancy, and lactation:
  - Postmarketing reports in humans indicate fetal demise, genital malformations, anencephaly, and placental disorder
  - Felbamate is excreted in breast milk; thus, breast-feeding is not recommended.
- Abnormal kidney function and hepatic impairment:
  - In patients with CrCL 10 to 50 mL/minute, administer doses by 50% to 75%; for CrCL <10 mL/minute, administer doses by 50%.
  - Felbamate is contraindicated in hepatic impairment.

Adverse Effects and Contraindications

The FDA has placed three **BOXED WARNING** ◆ on felbamate. There is an increased risk of aplastic anemia, hepatic failure, and suicidal ideations. Other adverse effects include CNS depression, anorexia, upper respiratory infection, chest pain, electrolyte changes, leukopenia, increase liver enzymes, and serum alkaline phosphatase. Felbamate is contraindicated in patients with hypersensitivity reactions to the medication, history of blood dyscrasias, and hepatic dysfunction.

Nursing Implications

Preventing Interactions

All CNS depressant medication combined with felbamate will increase CNS depression. The herbal supplements cannabis, St. John's wort, and kava kava will increase CNS depression. Alcohol combined with felbamate will increase CNS depression.

Administering the Medication

Felbamate can be administered with or without food. The oral suspension should be well shaken before administration.

Assessing for Therapeutic and Adverse Effects

The nurse assesses the patient for diminished seizure activity. The AST, ALT, creatinine, BUN, and alkaline phosphatase are also monitored. The nurse assesses for suicidal ideations or changes in the patient's mood. In addition, the nurse should check for purpura, which indicates blood dyscrasias. The patient's skin integrity is assessed for rash.

BOX 53.24	**Patient Teaching Guidelines for Felbamate**

- Report increased bleeding or bruising to the primary care provider.
- Report rash or changes in mood to the primary care provider.
- Do not operate machinery with CNS depression.
- Do not consume alcohol or combine with cannabis.
- If you are sexually active and able to become pregnant, use two forms of birth control due to diminished oral contraceptive effects.

Other Drugs in the Class

Stiripentol (Diacomit) is used for Dravet syndrome seizures. Dravet syndrome is a rare pediatric genetic epilepsy with alterations in neurologic development. Clobazam, fenfluramine, and stiripentol are second-line therapy for treating Dravet syndrome. The action of stiripentol is not known, but it enhances $GABA_A$ receptor and indirect effect on P450 activity to increase blood levels of clobazam. Use cautiously with CNS depressants due to enhanced somnolence, agitation, fatigue, or fever. Do not administer with St. John's wort. The neutrophil and platelet count may decrease with the medication and should be monitored.

Patient Teaching

Box 53.24 identifies patient teaching guidelines for felbamate.

OVERVIEW OF SPINAL CORD INJURY

Spinal cord injuries are classified by the spinal level at which the injury occurs. Tetraplegia, or quadriplegia, is the impairment of motor and sensory function in the arms, trunk, legs, and pelvic organs. Paraplegia is the impairment of motor and sensory function in the thoracic, lumbar, and sacral segments of the spinal cord. Upper motor neuron injuries result in spastic paralysis with hyperreflexia, preventing purposeful movement. Lower motor neuron injuries result in the flaccidity of muscles and muscle atrophy. Following a spinal cord injury, the muscles below the injury become spastic due to a miscommunication between the muscle and the brain.

Spinal cord injury is a result of damage to the cord by trauma. The damage to the cord is related to indirect injury from vertebral fractures or contusions. The direct cause of spinal cord injury is from a penetrating wound. The indirect cause of spinal cord injury is the result of a vertebral fracture, fracture dislocations, or spinal subluxation.

Clinical Manifestations

The clinical manifestations of a spinal cord injury are the result of the type and level of the injury. The level of the spinal cord injury produces greater loss of function and sensation. Clinical manifestations of complete spinal cord injury are irreversible with loss of autonomic, neural, and motor function. Incomplete spinal cord injuries vary in the severity of neurologic loss according to the severity of the damage. Changes in the autonomic nervous system affect temperature regulation, bowel and bladder function, and hypotension.

Drug Therapy

All skeletal muscle relaxants except dantrolene are centrally acting drugs. Pharmacologic action is usually attributed to general depression of the CNS but may involve blockage of nerve impulses that cause increased muscle tone and contraction. It is unclear whether relief of pain results from muscle relaxation or sedative effects. In addition, although parenteral administration of some drugs (e.g., diazepam, methocarbamol) relieves pain associated with acute musculoskeletal trauma or inflammation, it is uncertain whether oral administration of usual doses exerts a beneficial effect in acute or chronic disorders.

Baclofen and diazepam increase the effects of GABA, an inhibitory neurotransmitter. Tizanidine inhibits motor neurons in the brain. Dantrolene is the only skeletal muscle relaxant that acts peripherally on the muscle itself; it inhibits the release of calcium in skeletal muscle cells, thereby decreasing the strength of muscle contraction.

Table 53.8 summarizes the drug classes of skeletal muscle reactants, naming the prototype drug.

Clinical Application 53.4

- Andrew is now a 20-year-old college student. While living in the dorm, he has not been consistently taking his antiepileptic medications. On his trip home for the holidays, he suffers a seizure and has an automobile accident that leaves him paralyzed. The site of the spinal cord injury is T12. This injury results in muscle spasticity. Why is muscle spasticity so severe with spinal cord injuries?

TABLE 53.8

Drugs Administered for the Treatment of Spasticity and to Relax Skeletal Muscles

Drug Class	Prototype	Other Drugs in the Class
Carbamate derivatives	Carisoprodol (Soma)	
Centrally acting skeletal muscle relaxants	Methocarbamol	
GABA derivatives	Baclofen (Gablofen, Lioresal)	
Direct-acting skeletal muscle relaxant	Dantrolene sodium (Dantrium, Revonto, Ryanodex)	
Tricyclic antidepressant derivatives	Cyclobenzaprine hydrochloride (Amrix, Fexmid)	Chlorzoxazone (Lorzone) Orphenadrine Citrate
Imidazole derivatives	Tizanidine hydrochloride (Zanaflex)	

DRUGS USED TO TREAT MUSCLE SPASMS AND SPASTICITY

CARBAMATE DERIVATIVES

Carisoprodol (Soma) is a centrally acting skeletal muscle relaxant. It is chemically related to meprobamate, which inhibits multineuronal spinal reflexes.

Pharmacokinetics

The onset of action of carisoprodol is 30 minutes, with a peak in 1 to 2 hours and a duration of 4 to 6 hours. The half-life is 8 hours. The drug is metabolized in the liver by the enzyme CYP2C19 and excreted in the urine. It crosses the placenta and is present in breast milk.

Action

The action of carisoprodol is not known, but animal studies have shown that the drug inhibits interneuronal activity in the descending reticular formation and spinal cord. It does not act directly to relax the skeletal muscles.

Use

Clinicians use carisoprodol in the relief of discomfort associated with acute painful musculoskeletal conditions in which relief was not attained by rest, physical therapy, or alternative measures. Table 53.9 gives route and dosage information for carisoprodol.

Patient-related variables specific to the use of carisoprodol include the following:

- Age:
  - Carisoprodol is identified in the Beers Criteria as a potentially inappropriate medication and should be avoided in patients age 65 years and older.
- Reproduction, pregnancy, and lactation:
  - Postmarketing data have not shown a risk of major congenital malformations.
  - Carisoprodol is present in breast milk. The effects of long-term development in the infant is not known.

Adverse Effects

CNS adverse effects of carisoprodol include dizziness, drowsiness, vertigo, ataxia, tremor, agitation, and irritability. Initially, after the first, second, third, or fourth dose, patients may exhibit an allergic or idiosyncratic reaction with rash, erythema multiforme, pruritus, eosinophilia, hypotension, bronchospasm, vision and speech alterations, and the most severe adverse effect, anaphylactoid shock.

Contraindications

Contraindications to carisoprodol include an allergic response to the drug or acute intermittent porphyria. Other contraindications are pregnancy and lactation.

Nursing Implications

Preventing Interactions

CNS system depressants and alcohol combined with carisoprodol increase CNS depression.

Administering the Medication

The nurse administers carisoprodol with food to prevent GI upset, giving the last dose of medication at bedtime. It is necessary to store the mediation in a container with a tight-fitting lid.

Assessing for Therapeutic Effects

The nurse assesses the musculoskeletal area for relief of pain and spasms associated with the musculoskeletal injury.

Assessing for Adverse Effects

The nurse assesses the integumentary system for signs and symptoms of an idiosyncratic reaction after the fourth to fifth doses of carisoprodol. It is also important to observe for visual changes, speech difficulties, bronchospasm, hypotension, and anaphylaxis. Carisoprodol is habit forming and should not be stopped abruptly. Abrupt withdrawal results in headache, nausea, insomnia, and abdominal cramping.

Patient Teaching

Box 53.25 identifies patient teaching guidelines for carisoprodol.

GAMMA-AMINOBUTYRIC ACID DERIVATIVES

The GABA derivative **baclofen** (Gablofen, Lioresal) is an agonist-specific inhibitor to $GABA_B$ receptors located in the spinal cord. It restricts the influx of calcium to reduce the presynaptic neurotransmitter release in the excitatory spinal pathways.

Pharmacokinetics

Oral baclofen begins to act in 1 hour, peaks in 2 hours, and lasts 4 to 8 hours. It is metabolized in the liver and excreted in urine; its half-life is 3 to 4 hours. Intrathecal baclofen has an onset of action of 30 to 60 minutes, peaks in 4 hours, and, like oral baclofen, has a duration of action of 4 to 8 hours. The drug crosses the placenta and enters the breast milk.

BOX 53.25 Patient Teaching Guidelines for Carisoprodol

- Do not operate machinery with central nervous system (CNS) depression.
- Do not combine with other CNS depressants or alcohol.
- Take the medication with food.
- Do not combine with over-the-counter cold remedies without approval from the prescriber.
- Do not stop taking the medication abruptly.
- Know the idiosyncratic effects of the drug and how to maintain safety when CNS effects are evident.
- Report signs and symptoms of idiosyncratic adverse effects.

Action

The exact mechanism of action of baclofen is unknown. It appears to reduce impulse transmissions from the spinal cord to the skeletal muscle, thus decreasing muscle spasms.

Use

Clinicians use baclofen to alleviate signs and symptoms of spasticity in patients with multiple sclerosis. It is particularly effective against flexor spasms, concomitant pain, and muscular rigidity. Other indications include the treatment of spinal cord injuries and other diseases of the spinal cord. Table 53.9 gives route and dosage information for baclofen.

Patient-related variables specific to the use of baclofen include the following:

- Age:
  - In pediatric patients, dosage reduction should be gradual due to significant adverse effects or overdose-related emergencies. Abrupt discontinuation can result in severe adverse effects, including multiple organ failure.
  - Older adults who take baclofen require close monitoring. Dosage reduction to prevent excessive CNS depression may be necessary.
- Reproduction, pregnancy, and lactation:
  - Infants exposed to baclofen in utero may present with feeding difficulties, high-pitched cry, hyperthermia, hypertonicity, muscle rigidity, seizure activity, and loose stools.
- Abnormal kidney function and hepatic impairment:
  - Dosage reduction is necessary in patients with abnormal kidney function.

Adverse Effects and Contraindications

The most common adverse effects of baclofen are transient drowsiness, dizziness, weakness, fatigue, confusion, headache, insomnia, hypotension, and urinary frequency. Elevated blood sugar may occur, requiring the administration of an oral hypoglycemic agent.

Contraindications include known hypersensitivity to the drug and skeletal muscle spasms resulting from rheumatic disorders.

Nursing Implications

Preventing Interactions

When baclofen is combined with alcohol or other CNS depressants, patients experience increased CNS depression.

Administering the Medication

Administration of baclofen is oral or intrathecal. The nurse starts with a low dose that is increased slowly, using the smallest dose possible to achieve muscle tone without adverse effects. If the benefits of the medication are not evident during a trial period, then the medication is withdrawn gradually.

Intrathecal administration involves an implantable pump. It is best to consult the manufacturer's literature concerning the pump instructions and initiation of long-term infusions. Resuscitation equipment should be readily available.

Assessing for Therapeutic Effects

The nurse assesses the affected musculoskeletal region for decrease in symptoms of spasticity.

TABLE 53.9
DRUGS AT A GLANCE: Drugs Used to Relax Skeletal Muscles

Drug	Routes and Dosage Ranges	
	Adults	**Children**
ⓟ Carisoprodol (Soma)	12 y and older, 250–350 mg PO three times daily for maximum of 2–3 wk, with last dose at bedtime Geriatric patients and patients with abnormal kidney function or hepatic impairment: reduce dose and monitor closely	Not recommended for children younger than 12 y
ⓟ Baclofen (Gablofen, Lioresal, Ozobax; 🍁 AP-Baclofen, Dom-Baclofen, Lioresal, Lioresal Intrathecal, Mylan-Baclofen, Baclofen 10 or 20)	Start at a low dosage and increase gradually until optimum effect is achieved (40–80 mg/d); 5 mg PO for 3 d; 10 mg three times daily for 3 d; 15 mg three times daily for 3 d; 20 mg three times daily for 3 d; may increase to a maximum of 80 mg/d (20 mg four times daily) Intrathecal, refer to manufacturer's instructions; testing is usually done with 50 mcg/mL injected into intrathecal space over 1 min; patient is observed for 4–8 h, and then a dose of 75 mcg/1.5 mL is given and patient is observed for another 4–8 h; a final screening bolus of 100 mcg/2 mL is given 24 h later if response is still not adequate. Patients who do not respond to this dose are not candidates for the implant. Maintenance dose: 22–1,400 mcg/d (smallest dose to achieve muscle tone without adverse effects)	Safety in children younger than 12 y of age has not been established; orphan drug use to decrease spasticity in children with cerebral palsy is being studied

(Continued on page 986)

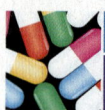

TABLE 53.9

DRUGS AT A GLANCE: Drugs Used to Relax Skeletal Muscles (Continued)

Drug	Routes and Dosage Ranges	
	Adults	**Children**
Dantrolene sodium (Dantrium, Revonto, Ryanodex; ❋ Dantrium)	Chronic spasticity: establish therapeutic goal before initiating therapy; titrate and individualize dosage, increasing until maximum performance is compatible to relieve dysfunction; initially 25 mg daily; increase to 25 mg three times daily for 7 d; then to 50 mg three times daily, and, if necessary, to 100 mg three times daily; most patients respond to 400 mg/d or less; maintain each dosage level for 4–7 d to evaluate response; discontinue after 45 d if benefits are not evident Preoperative prophylaxis of malignant hyperthermia: 4–8 mg/kg/d PO in 3–4 divided doses for 1–2 d prior to surgery; give the last dose 3–4 h before scheduled surgery with minimum amount of water; adjust dose to prevent incapacitation due to drowsiness and excessive GI irritation Postcrisis follow-up: 4–8 mg/kg/d PO in 4 divided doses for 1–3 d to prevent recurrence Parenteral administration for malignant hyperthermia: discontinue all anesthetics as soon as problem is recognized; give dantrolene by continuous rapid IV push beginning at minimum dose of 1 mg/kg and continuing until symptoms subside or maximum cumulative dose of 10 mg/kg has been given; if physiologic and metabolic abnormalities reappear, repeat regimen; give continuously until symptoms subside Preoperative prophylaxis of malignant hyperthermia: 2.5 mg/kg IV 1 h before surgery infused over 1 h	Safety for children <5 y has not been established Chronic spasticity: initially 0.5 mg/kg once daily for 7 d, followed by 0.5 mg/kg three times daily for 7 d; then 1 mg/kg three times daily for 7 d; then 2 mg/kg three times daily if necessary; do not exceed 100 mg four times daily
Cyclobenzaprine hydrochloride (Amrix, Fexmid; ❋ Apo-Cyclobenzaprine, Auro-Cyclobenzaprine, Dom-Cyclobenzaprine, JAMP-Cyclobenzaprine, Mylan-Cyclobenzaprine)	5 mg PO three times daily up to 10 mg PO three times daily, not to exceed 60 mg/d; do not use longer than 2–3 wk; extended-release capsules: 15 mg daily; some patients may require 30 mg/d	Safety and efficacy not established in children younger than 15 y
Chlorzoxazone (Lorzone)	250–500 mg PO three times per day	20 mg/kg/d PO in 3–4 divided doses
Methocarbamol (Robaxin)	PO 1.5 g 3–4 times per day IM/IV: 1 g may repeat every 2–3 d (up to 8 g/d in severe conditions)	≥16 y: PO 1,500 mg for 2–3 d; maximum dose 8 g/d Tetanus: 15 mg/kg/dose every 6 h
Orphenadrine citrate	100 mg PO two times per day 60 mg IV or IM every 12 h	Safety and efficacy not established in children
Tizanidine hydrochloride (Zanaflex; ❋ Gen-Tizanidine, Pal-Tizanidine)	4 mg PO daily, increased in 2–4 mg increments as needed over 2–4 wk; usual maintenance dose, 8 mg PO every 6–8 h; maximum dose, 36 mg/d in divided doses; reduce dose in patients with abnormal kidney function	Safety and efficacy not established

Assessing for Adverse Effects

It is important to assess the degree of CNS depression. The nurse assesses the patient's blood pressure for hypotension, particularly with position changes. Genitourinary assessments include the patient's level of urinary frequency and dysuria. Other adverse effects noted are weight gain, increased aspartate aminotransferase, blood sugar, and alkaline phosphatase.

Patient Teaching

Box 53.26 identifies patient teaching guidelines for baclofen.

BOX 53.26 Patient Teaching Guidelines for Baclofen

- Do not stop taking the drug abruptly; abrupt discontinuation may cause hallucinations or other serious side effects.
- Avoid alcohol and other central nervous system depressants.
- Do not take if you are pregnant or breast-feeding.
- Do not operate machinery.
- Report painful or frequent urination, constipation, headache, insomnia, or confusion.

Clinical Application 53.5

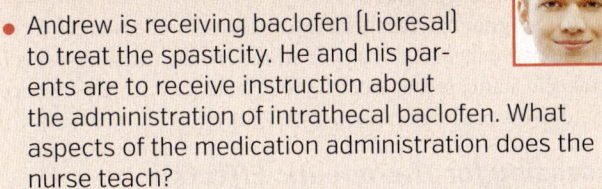

- Andrew is receiving baclofen (Lioresal) to treat the spasticity. He and his parents are to receive instruction about the administration of intrathecal baclofen. What aspects of the medication administration does the nurse teach?
- His parents ask the nurse why he is taking baclofen (Lioresal) and not diazepam (Valium), which he has taken in the past. What is the best response to this question?

NCLEX Success

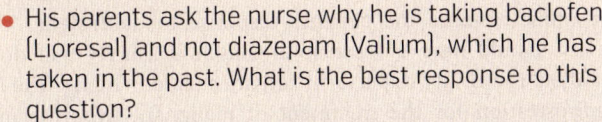

4. A patient is taking carisoprodol for back spasms related to an occupational injury. Which of the following is most important to teach the patient?
    A. to take the medication at 8:00 a.m., 2:00 p.m., and 8:00 p.m.
    B. to know the signs and symptoms of an idiosyncratic reaction
    C. to take the medication between meals
    D. to stop the medication with the first sign of abdominal cramping

5. A nurse administers baclofen to a young patient for a back injury. Which of the following interventions is most important related to the administration of baclofen?
    A. Assess heart rate.
    B. Assess for edema.
    C. Assess blood sugar.
    D. Assess for increased spasticity.

CENTRALLY ACTING SKELETAL MUSCLE RELAXANTS

Methocarbamol (Robaxin) is a centrally acting muscle relaxant often administered in conjunction with muscle rest, physical therapy, and other nonpharmacologic interventions for the relief of pain due to muscular spasticity.

Pharmacokinetics and Action

The onset of action of methocarbamol is approximately 30 minutes. It is 46% to 50% protein bound and metabolized in the liver. The half-life is 1 to 2 hours and excreted primarily in the urine. It invokes skeletal muscle relaxation by way of CNS depression.

Use

Methocarbamol is used in the treatment of muscle spasms and tetanus.

Patient-related variables specific to the use of methocarbamol include the following:

- Age:
  - Methocarbamol is identified in the Beers Criteria as a potentially inappropriate medication and should be avoided in patients age 65 years and older.
- Reproduction, pregnancy, and lactation:
  - The manufacturer notes that fetal and congenital abnormalities have been noted.
  - It is unknown if methocarbamol is present in breast milk.

Adverse Effects and Contraindications

The most common adverse effects of methocarbamol include CNS depression leading to an increased risk of falls or other accidental injuries.

Methocarbamol is contraindicated in patients with hypersensitivity to the drug. The IV formulation should not be administered in patients with abnormal kidney function.

Nursing Implications

Preventing Interactions

Medications that produce CNS depression combined with methocarbamol will enhance the depressant effect. Botulinum toxin will increase muscle weakness. Cannabis, alcohol, and kava kava will increase CNS depression

Administering the Medication

Oral tablets may be crushed or chewed. A maximum of 5 mL is administered IM, and 3 mL IV. When administering IV, monitor for extravasation.

Assessing for Therapeutic and Adverse Effects

Assess the patient for decrease in pain and muscle spasticity. Assess for signs and symptoms of rash.

Patient Teaching

Methocarbamol patient teaching should include the CNS depressive effects of the medication and to protect from accidental injury. Advise the patient to refrain from alcohol or the use of cannabinoid products.

DIRECT-ACTING SKELETAL MUSCLE RELAXANTS

Dantrolene sodium (Dantrium, Revonto, Ryanodex) is a drug administered for spasticity related to multiple sclerosis, cerebral palsy, spinal cord injury, and stroke.

Pharmacokinetics

Oral dantrolene is absorbed by the GI tract, reaching a peak in 4 to 6 hours. The duration of action is 8 to 10 hours, and the half-life is 9 hours. IV dantrolene has a rapid onset of action with a peak in 5 hours, a duration of action of 6 to 8 hours, and a half-life of 4 to 8 hours. The drug is metabolized by the liver and excreted in the urine. Dantrolene crosses the placenta and enters the breast milk.

Action

Dantrolene interferes with the release of calcium from the sarcoplasmic reticulum to relax skeletal muscle. It does not interfere with neuromuscular transmission or affect the surface membrane of the skeletal muscle.

Use

Dantrolene controls spasticity caused by upper motor neuron disorders, such as spinal cord injury, cerebrovascular accident, cerebral palsy, and multiple sclerosis. Clinicians may use it to prevent and manage **malignant hyperthermia**, a rare but life-threatening complication of anesthesia characterized by hypercarbia, metabolic acidosis, skeletal muscle rigidity, fever, and cyanosis. Table 53.9 gives route and dosage information for dantrolene.

Patient-related variables specific to the use of dantrolene include the following:

- Age:
  - Older adults have an increased risk of liver damage with the administration of dantrolene; this requires close monitoring of liver enzymes.
- Reproduction, pregnancy, and lactation:
  - Dantrolene crosses the placenta.
  - Breast-feeding is not recommended with the administration of dantrolene.
- Abnormal kidney function and hepatic impairment:
  - Patients with active liver disease should not receive dantrolene, as potentially fatal hepatocellular damage may occur.

Adverse Effects

Common adverse effects of dantrolene include drowsiness, dizziness, diarrhea, and fatigue. The most serious adverse effect is potentially fatal hepatitis, with jaundice and other symptoms that usually occur within 1 month of starting drug therapy. Liver function tests should be monitored periodically in all patients receiving dantrolene. These adverse effects do not occur with short-term use of IV drug for malignant hyperthermia. The FDA has issued a **BOXED WARNING** ♦ stating that the patient should have liver function tests and that dantrolene be discontinued at the first indication of hepatic impairment.

Contraindications

Contraindications to dantrolene include active liver disease. Other contraindications include spasticity used to maintain an upright position and balance with locomotion as well as spasticity from rheumatic conditions.

Nursing Implications

Preventing Interactions

The patient is at risk of hyperkalemia and myocardial depression if dantrolene is combined with verapamil. Alcohol, cannabis, and kava kava will increase CNS depression.

Administering the Medication

When administering dantrolene intravenously, the nurse monitors the injection sites and ensures that extravasation does not occur. Dantrolene is an alkaline agent that is irritating to the tissues.

When administering dantrolene orally, the nurse consults with other healthcare professionals to determine interventions that enhance mobility. Withdrawal of the oral medication should occur over 2 to 4 days. If diarrhea occurs, discontinuance of dantrolene is necessary.

If malignant hyperthermia develops, it is essential to discontinue all triggering drugs. In addition, the nurse assesses for metabolic acidosis and electrolyte imbalances. It may be necessary to use a cooling blanket.

Assessing for Therapeutic Effects

The nurse assesses the patient's response to dantrolene. The patient should have a decrease in muscle spasticity that does not affect the ability to perform activities of daily living. The IV administration for the treatment of malignant hyperthermia results in a reverse of symptoms, including decreased temperature and fluid and electrolyte balance without signs and symptoms of metabolic acidosis.

Assessing for Adverse Effects

It is necessary to check the patient's liver enzymes with the administration of oral dantrolene. The nurse assesses the patient for diarrhea, dizziness, and fatigue. Headache, anorexia, and nervousness are potentially serious adverse effects in people older than 35 years of age who have taken the drug for 60 days or longer. Females in this age group who take estrogens have the highest risk of developing these adverse effects. Hepatotoxicity can be prevented or minimized by administering the lowest effective dose, monitoring liver enzymes during therapy, and discontinuing the drug if no beneficial effects occur in 45 days.

Patient Teaching

Box 53.27 identifies the patient teaching guidelines for dantrolene.

BOX 53.27 Patient Teaching Guidelines for Dantrolene

- Do not alter positions when experiencing dizziness.
- Report gastrointestinal upset and eat small frequent meals.
- Avoid alcohol and other central nervous system depressants.
- Report severe diarrhea, headache, and anorexia.

TRICYCLIC ANTIDEPRESSANT DERIVATIVES

Cyclobenzaprine hydrochloride (Amrix, Fexmid) is a centrally acting skeletal muscle relaxant administered on a short-term basis for the relief of muscle spasm.

Pharmacokinetics

Cyclobenzaprine is administered orally and is well absorbed by the GI tract. The onset of action is 1 hour, with a peak in 3 to 8 hours, and the duration of action is 12 to 24 hours. The half-life is 1 to 3 days. The drug is highly protein bound. It is metabolized in the liver to inactive metabolites and is excreted in the urine, with some eliminated in the feces. Cyclobenzaprine crosses the placenta and is excreted in the breast milk.

Action

The mechanism of action of cyclobenzaprine is not known, but it appears to produce relaxation by acting at the brainstem and spinal cord to depress motor activity.

Use

Clinicians use cyclobenzaprine as an adjunctive to other measures such as physical therapy to relieve muscle spasm. Table 53.9 gives route and dosage information for cyclobenzaprine.

Patient-related variables specific to the use of cyclobenzaprine include the following:

- Age:
  - Cyclobenzaprine should not be administered to older adults. It is listed as an inappropriate medication on the Beers Criteria and should be avoided in patients age 65 years and older.
- Reproduction, pregnancy, and lactation:
  - There is limited information regarding cyclobenzaprine's effects on the fetus in utero.
  - Cyclobenzaprine is present in breast milk.
- Abnormal kidney function and hepatic impairment:
  - In moderate to severe hepatic impairment, cyclobenzaprine is not recommended.

Adverse Effects and Contraindications

Common adverse effects of cyclobenzaprine are drowsiness, dizziness, and anticholinergic effects (e.g., dry mouth, constipation, urinary retention, tachycardia).

Contraindications include known hypersensitivity to the drug. Other contraindications include acute myocardial infarction, dysrhythmia, heart block, conduction disturbances, heart failure, and hyperthyroidism. Caution is necessary with urinary retention, increased intraocular pressure, and mild hepatic impairment.

Nursing Implications

Preventing Interactions

Increased CNS depression occurs when cyclobenzaprine is combined with alcohol or other CNS depressants. When cyclobenzaprine is administered with one or more serotonergic agents, there is an increased risk of development of serotonin syndrome.

> **BOX 53.28** *Patient Teaching Guidelines for Cyclobenzaprine*
>
> - Avoid alcohol and other central nervous system (CNS) depressants.
> - Do not operate machinery with CNS depression.
> - Report effectiveness of therapy to prescriber.

Administering the Medication

Because of the risk of inconsistent doses, the nurse does not split the generic 10-mg tablets when administering cyclobenzaprine. Extended-release capsules are administered whole.

Assessing for Therapeutic and Adverse Effects

The nurse assesses the patient's response to the medication, which should indicate relief of the skeletal muscle spasm, decreased pain, and increased activity.

The nurse assesses for increased CNS depression, which will place the patient at risk of falls and injury. It is necessary to assess the patient's cardiovascular status, including pulse and blood pressure. The medication places the patient at risk of hypotension. Anticholinergic effects occur. The nurse assesses the patient for urinary retention.

Patient Teaching

Box 53.28 identifies patient teaching guidelines for cyclobenzaprine.

Other Drugs in the Class

Chlorzoxazone is a centrally acting skeletal muscle relaxant used to treat muscle spasms and pain associated with musculoskeletal conditions. It should be administered cautiously in patients with drug allergies, CNS depression, and altered liver and kidney function. Chlorzoxazone should be administered with food to prevent gastric upset. Do not combine with alcohol or CNS depressants. Assess the patient for injury due to CNS depression. Monitor the patient's liver function tests. Instruct the patient the medication may discolor urine orange or purple/red.

Orphenadrine citrate is also a centrally acting skeletal muscle relaxant that has tertiary amine anticholinergic effects. It is contraindicated in narrow angle glaucoma, duodenal obstruction, prostatic hypertrophy, and bladder neck obstruction. Use cautiously in older adults due to urinary hesitancy or retention.

IMIDAZOLINE DERIVATIVES

Tizanidine hydrochloride (Zanaflex) is a centrally acting $alpha_2$-adrenergic agonist administered for acute and intermittent management of increased muscle tone with spasticity.

Pharmacokinetics

Tizanidine is absorbed rapidly in the GI tract. The medication has an onset of action in 30 to 60 minutes, peak in 1 to 2 hours, and duration of action in 3 to 6 hours. It is metabolized by the liver with a 2.7- to 4.2-hour half-life, and the drug is excreted in the urine. Tizanidine crosses the placenta and enters the breast milk.

Action

Tizanidine is a centrally acting alpha$_2$-adrenergic agonist that produces antispasmodic effect as a result of indirect depression of postsynaptic reflexes by blocking the excitatory actions of spinal interneurons.

Use

Clinicians use tizanidine as indicated for use in patients who have acute and intermittent management of increased muscle tone associated with spasticity. Table 53.9 gives route and dosage information for tizanidine.

Patient-related variables specific to the use of tizanidine include the following:

- Age:
  - Older adults with potential organ impairment should be administered a reduced dose and less frequent administration.
- Reproduction, pregnancy, and lactation:
  - Oral contraceptive agents may decrease the clearance of tizanidine. Do not administer these medications together.
  - There is limited information on the effects of tizanidine in pregnancy.
  - It is not known if tizanidine is present in breast milk.

Adverse Effects and Contraindications

Common adverse effects of tizanidine include drowsiness, dizziness, constipation, dry mouth, and hypotension. Hypotension may be significant and occur at usual doses. The drug may also cause psychotic symptoms, including hallucinations.

Contraindications include hypersensitivity to the medication. Other contraindications include use of fluvoxamine and ciprofloxacin.

Nursing Implications

Preventing Interactions

The administration of alcohol, baclofen, or CNS depressants with tizanidine can increase the patient's susceptibility to symptoms of depression. Hormonal contraceptives may increase the plasma concentration of tizanidine. Administration with other alpha$_2$ agonists may have hypotensive effects. Kava and valerian may decrease the effect of the drug.

Administering the Medication

Patients may take tizanidine with or without food. However, consistent administration of the drug assists in absorption of the drug and its effect.

Assessing for Therapeutic and Adverse Effects

The nurse assesses the patient for a reduction of skeletal muscle spasms and decreased muscle tone.

The nurse assesses patients for somnolence, sedation, dizziness, and hallucinations. The cardiovascular patient's status is assessed for bradycardia and hypotension. In addition, it is necessary to assess the patient's liver and kidney function.

Patient Teaching

Box 53.29 identifies patient teaching guidelines for tizanidine.

BOX 53.29 **Patient Teaching Guidelines for Tizanidine**

- Do not alter positions when experiencing dizziness.
- Do not operate machinery.
- Report unusual sensory effects such as hallucinations or delusions.

THE NURSING PROCESS

A concept map outlines the nursing process related to drug therapy considerations in this chapter. Additional nursing implications related to the disease process should also be considered in care decisions.

Assessment

- Assess the patient status in relation to seizure activity and other factors.
  - Interview the patient about the seizure disorder and AEDs.
    - How long has the patient had the seizure disorder, and when was the last seizure?
    - What is the frequency of the seizures, and will something precipitate its development?
    - How does the seizure affect the patient (loss of consciousness, body part or parts affected, drowsiness after the seizure)?
    - What AEDs are prescribed, and what effect do they produce?
    - Does the patient take the AEDs as prescribed? What other medications have been prescribed?
    - What is the patient's attitude toward the seizure disorder?
  - Assess serum levels of AEDs.
  - Identify risk factors for seizure disorders (previous seizure activity, brain surgery, head injury, hypoxia, hypoglycemia, drug overdosage, withdrawal of AEDs or CNS depressants).
  - Observe and document seizure activity accurately; location (localized or general); and specific characteristics of abnormal movements or behavior, duration, and concomitant events (loss of consciousness, incontinence, and postseizure behavior).
  - Assess for risk of status epilepticus (recent changes in AED therapy, chronic alcohol ingestion, use of drugs known to cause seizures, and infection).

THE NURSING PROCESS (Continued)

Outcomes of Therapy

The patient will
- Take the medication as prescribed, and do not discontinue abruptly.
- Experience control of seizures, and avoid serious adverse effects.
- Verbalize knowledge of the disease process and treatment regimen.
- Keep follow-up appointments with the primary care provider.

Nursing Interventions

- Assist the patient in identifying the conditions under which seizures are likely to occur. Precipitating factors may include ingestion of alcoholic beverages or stimulant drugs; fever; severe physical or emotional stress; and sensory stimuli, such as flashing lights and loud noises. Identifying lifestyle changes (e.g., reducing stress, reducing alcohol and caffeine intake, increasing exercise, improving sleep, and diet) and treating existing disorders can reduce the frequency of seizures.
- Discuss the seizure disorder, the plan of treatment, and the importance of adhering to prescribed drug therapy with the patient and family members.
- Involve the patient in decision making when possible.
- Inform the patient and family that seizure control is not gained immediately when drug therapy is started.
- Protect the patient experiencing a generalized tonic–clonic seizure by
  - Placing a small pillow or piece of clothing under the head to prevent injury from the ground or floor. Never restrain the patient's movements; fractures may result.
  - Loosening tight clothing, especially around the neck and chest, to promote respirations.
  - Turning the patient to one side so that accumulating secretions can drain from the mouth and throat when paroxysms stop. Most of these seizures subside within 3 to 4 minutes, and the patient starts responding and regaining normal skin color. If the patient has one seizure after another (status epilepticus), has trouble breathing or continued cyanosis, or has sustained an injury, further care is needed, and a physician should be notified immediately.
- If an aura or smell is noted prior to the onset of seizure, be sure the patient notifies a nurse.

Evaluation

- Interview and observe for decrease in or absence of seizure activity.
- Interview and observe for avoidance of adverse drug effects, especially those that impair safety.
- When available, check laboratory reports of serum drug levels for the therapeutic ranges or evidence of underdosing or overdosing.

Visit thePoint at **http://thePoint.lww.com/Frandsen13e** for answers to NCLEX Success questions (in Appendix A), answers to Clinical Application Case Studies (in Appendix B), and more!

REFERENCES AND RESOURCES

Abrams, G. M., & Wakasa, M. (2022). Chronic complications of spinal cord injury and disease. In *UpToDate*. Lexi-Comp, Inc.

Hinkle, J. H., Cheever, K. H., & Overbaugh, K. J. (2021). *Brunner & Suddarth's textbook of medical-surgical nursing* (15th ed.). Wolters Kluwer.

Lippincott Advisor. (2022a). *Drug information*. Wolters Kluwer.

Lippincott Advisor. (2022b). *Drug information*. Wolters Kluwer.

McCluskey, G., Kinney, M. O., Russell, A., Smithson, W. H., Parsons, L., Morrison, P. J., Bromley, R., MacKillop, L., Heath, C., Liggan, B., Murphy, S., Delanty, N., Irwin, B., Campbell, E., Morrow, J., Hunt, S. J., Craig, J. J. (2021). Zonisamide safety in pregnancy: Data from the UK and Ireland epilepsy and pregnancy register. *Seizure: European Journal of Epilepsy*, 91, 311–315. www.elsivier.com/locate/seizure 10.1016/j.seizure.2021.07.002

Norris, T. L. (2019). *Porth's pathophysiology concepts of altered health states* (10th ed.). Wolters Kluwer.

Schachter, S. (2022). Antiseizure drugs: Mechanism of action, pharmacology, and adverse effects. In *UpToDate*. Lexi-Comp, Inc.

UpToDate. (2022). *Drug information*. Lexi-Comp, Inc.

CHAPTER 54

Drug Therapy for Anxiety and Insomnia

LEARNING OBJECTIVES

After studying this chapter, you should be able to:

1. Understand anxiety and its clinical manifestations.
2. Understand insomnia and its clinical manifestations.
3. Identify the prototype and describe the action, use, adverse effects, contraindications, and nursing implications for the benzodiazepines.
4. Discuss the various nonbenzodiazepines used to reduce anxiety and produce hypnosis in terms of their action, use, contraindications, adverse effects, and nursing implications.
5. Identify the prototype and describe the action, use, adverse effects, contraindications, and nursing implications for the dual orexin receptor antagonists.
6. Implement the nursing process in the care of the patient being treated for anxiety and insomnia.

CLINICAL APPLICATION CASE STUDY

Lorraine Terrence, an 83-year-old widow who has lived alone since her husband died 6 months ago, is in the early stages of Alzheimer disease. She has a history of cardiovascular disease and hypertension and has been admitted to the local hospital for observation after complaints of chest pain. At present, she is very anxious and agitated. The admitting nurse received a telephone call from Mrs. Terrence's daughter, who lives out of town. The daughter states that her mother has experienced anxiety and depression for many years and her symptoms have worsened since her father died. The daughter does not know what medications her mother currently takes, and she is concerned that her mother lives alone and wants her to move to a nursing home. The provider orders the following medications: alprazolam for anxiety, citalopram for depression, and zolpidem for sleep.

KEY TERMS

Anterograde amnesia: short-term memory loss

Anxiety: common disorder that may be referred to as nervousness, tension, worry, or other terms that denote an unpleasant feeling

Anxiety disorder: severe anxiety that is prolonged and impairs the ability to function in usual activities of daily living

Anxiolytics: antianxiety drugs

Hypnotics: drugs that produce sleep

Insomnia: prolonged difficulty in going to sleep or staying asleep long enough to feel rested

Sedatives: drugs that promote relaxation and ease agitation

INTRODUCTION

This chapter introduces the pharmacologic care of the patient who is experiencing **anxiety** and/or **insomnia**. Antianxiety and sedative–hypnotic drugs are central nervous system (CNS) depressants that have similar effects. **Anxiolytics** are antianxiety drugs, **sedatives** promote relaxation and ease agitation, and **hypnotics** produce sleep. The difference between the effects depends largely on dosage. Large doses of antianxiety and sedative drugs produce sleep, and small doses of hypnotics have anxiolytic or sedative effects. Also, therapeutic doses of hypnotics taken at bedtime may have residual sedative effects ("morning hangover") the following day. Because these drugs produce varying degrees of CNS depression, some are also used as anticonvulsants and anesthetics.

OVERVIEW OF ANXIETY

To promote understanding of the uses and effects of both benzodiazepines and nonbenzodiazepines, anxiety and insomnia are described in the following sections. The clinical manifestations of these disorders are similar and overlapping; that is, daytime anxiety may be manifested as nighttime difficulty in sleeping because the person cannot "turn off" worries, and difficulty in sleeping may be manifested as anxiety, fatigue, and decreased ability to function during usual waking hours. Many individuals with an anxiety disorder often go unidentified and untreated. Anxiety is a common disorder that may be referred to as nervousness, tension, worry, or other terms that denote an unpleasant feeling. An **anxiety disorder** is severe anxiety that is prolonged and impairs the ability to function in usual activities of daily living. Posttraumatic stress disorder (PTSD) is a condition that is a stress-related disorder that has mutual clinical manifestations, drug therapy, and nursing conditions with anxiety disorders. Thus, PTSD has been included in this chapter, along with generalized anxiety disorder (GAD). For further details on the etiology and pathophysiology of anxiety, visit thePoint® http://thePoint.lww.com/Frandsen13e.

Concept Mastery Alert

Anxiety disorders have distinctive characteristics, but all involve an excessive and irrational fear and dread. Some patients, but not all, experience physiologic symptoms, lack insight into their worrying, or have difficulty identifying the source and trigger for their anxiety.

Clinical Manifestations

The clinical manifestations of anxiety include motor tension, such as muscle tension, restlessness, trembling, and fatigue; they also include overactivity of the autonomic nervous system, such as dyspnea, palpitations, tachycardia, sweating, dry mouth, dizziness, nausea, and diarrhea. Other clinical manifestations include increased vigilance, such as feeling fearful, nervous, or keyed up; difficulty concentrating; irritability; and insomnia. Box 54.1 summarizes the clinical manifestations of specific anxiety disorders.

Drug Therapy

Benzodiazepines are widely used to treat anxiety disorders (Table 54.1). These drugs are useful in the short-term treatment of symptoms of acute anxiety in response to stressful situations. However, they may not be appropriate in all cases (see the discussion of benzodiazepines for more details). Antidepressants (i.e., selective serotonin reuptake inhibitors, tricyclic antidepressants, and newer miscellaneous drugs) are preferred as first-line drugs for long-term treatment of most chronic anxiety disorders, with benzodiazepines considered second-line drugs. Chapter 55 discusses antidepressant medications in more detail.

The barbiturates, a historically important group of CNS depressants, are obsolete for most uses, including treatment of anxiety and insomnia. A few may find use as intravenous (IV) general anesthetics (see Chapter 51), as treatment for seizure disorders (phenobarbital; see Chapter 53), and as drugs of abuse (see Chapter 58).

OVERVIEW OF SLEEP AND INSOMNIA

Sleep is a recurrent period of decreased mental and physical activity during which a person is relatively unresponsive to sensory and environmental stimuli. Normal sleep allows rest, renewal of energy for performing activities of daily living, and alertness on awakening. **Insomnia**, prolonged difficulty in going to sleep or staying asleep long enough to feel rested, is the most common sleep disorder. Occasional sleeplessness is a normal response to many stimuli and is not usually harmful. Insomnia is said to be chronic when it lasts longer than 1 month. As in anxiety, several neurotransmission systems are apparently involved in regulating sleep–wake cycles and producing insomnia. Chronic insomnia affects 57% of older adults in the United States and impairs quality of life and health. Older adults with poor sleep quality have almost twice the mortality rate from stroke, cancer, and heart disease than those who sleep well. For further details on the etiology and pathophysiology of insomnia, visit thePoint® http://thePoint.lww.com/Frandsen13e.

Clinical Manifestations

The clinical manifestations of insomnia include fatigue, lack of energy, and irritability. Patients with insomnia report diminished work performance and decreased concentration. Generally, patients with insomnia do not complain of daytime sleepiness. They tend to be overconcerned about their inability to fall asleep; the more they try to sleep, the more agitated they become, and the less they are able to fall asleep.

Drug Therapy

The main drugs used to treat insomnia are the benzodiazepines, nonbenzodiazepine hypnotics, and the dual orexin receptor antagonists (see Table 54.1). However, it is important to note that drug companies market only a few benzodiazepines for the

BOX 54.1 Types of Anxiety Disorders

Generalized Anxiety Disorder

Major diagnostic criteria for generalized anxiety disorder (GAD) include excessive and exaggerated anxiety and worry about everyday life circumstances and multiple symptoms for 6 months or more after elimination of disease processes or drugs as possible causes. The frequency, duration, or intensity of the worry is unrealistic or out of proportion to the actual situation. Symptoms are related to motor tension (e.g., muscle tension, restlessness, trembling, fatigue), overactivity of the autonomic nervous system (e.g., dyspnea, palpitations, tachycardia, sweating, dry mouth, dizziness, nausea, diarrhea), and increased vigilance (feeling fearful, nervous, or keyed up, difficulty concentrating, irritability, insomnia, being easily startled).

Symptoms of anxiety occur with many disease processes, including medical disorders (e.g., hyperthyroidism, cardiovascular disease, cancer) and psychiatric disorders (e.g., mood disorders, schizophrenia, substance use disorders). They also frequently occur with drugs that affect the CNS. With CNS stimulants (e.g., nasal decongestants, antiasthma drugs, nicotine, caffeine), symptoms occur with drug administration; with CNS depressants (e.g., alcohol, benzodiazepines), symptoms are more likely to occur when the drug is stopped, especially if stopped abruptly.

When the symptoms are secondary to medical illness, they may decrease as the illness improves. However, most people with GAD experience little relief when one stressful situation or problem is resolved. Instead, they quickly move on to another worry. Additional characteristics of GAD include its chronicity, although the severity of symptoms fluctuates over time; its frequent association with somatic symptoms (e.g., headache, gastrointestinal complaints, including irritable bowel syndrome); and its frequent coexistence with depression, other anxiety disorders, and substance use disorder or dependence.

Obsessive–Compulsive Disorders and Related Conditions

An obsession involves an uncontrollable desire to dwell on recurring, unwanted thoughts, ideas, or sensations; a compulsion involves repeated performance of some act to relieve the fear and anxiety associated with an obsession. Obsessive–compulsive disorder is characterized by obsessions or compulsions that are severe enough to be time consuming (e.g., take more than an hour per day), cause major distress, or impair the person's ability to function in usual activities or relationships. The compulsive behavior provides some relief from anxiety but is not pleasurable. Many people recognize that the obsessions or compulsions are not true; others may think that their obsessions could be true (known as poor insight). Even if people know their obsessions are not true, people have a hard time keeping their focus off the obsessions or stopping the compulsive actions. When patients resist or are prevented from performing the compulsive behavior, they experience increasing anxiety and often abuse alcohol or antianxiety, sedative-type drugs in the attempt to relieve anxiety.

Panic Disorder

Panic disorder involves acute, sudden, and recurrent attacks of anxiety, with feelings of intense fear, terror, or impending doom. It may be accompanied by such symptoms as palpitations, sweating, trembling, shortness of breath or a feeling of smothering, chest pain, nausea, or dizziness. Symptoms usually build to a peak over about 10 minutes and may require medication to be relieved. Afterward, the person usually lives in fear of another attack and may avoid places where an attack has occurred. For some people, the fear takes over their lives, and they cannot leave their homes.

A significant number (50% to 65%) of patients with panic disorder are thought to also have major depression. In addition, some patients with panic disorder also develop agoraphobia, a fear of having a panic attack in a place or situation where one cannot escape or get help. Combined panic disorder and agoraphobia often involves a chronic, relapsing pattern of significant functional impairment and may require lifetime treatment.

Posttraumatic Stress Disorder

Posttraumatic stress disorder (PTSD) is a trauma- and stress-related disorder that associates the condition with highly stressful events that may involve actual or threatened death or serious injury (e.g., natural disasters, military combat, violent acts such as rape or murder, explosions or bombings, serious automobile accidents). The person responds to such an event with thoughts and feelings of intense fear, helplessness, or horror and develops symptoms such as hyperarousal, irritability, outbursts of anger, difficulty sleeping, difficulty concentrating, and an exaggerated startle response. These thoughts, feelings, and symptoms persist as the traumatic event is relived through recurring thoughts, images, nightmares, or flashbacks in which the actual event seems to be occurring. The intense psychic discomfort leads people to avoid situations that remind them of the event, become detached from other people, have less interest in activities they formerly enjoyed, and develop other disorders (e.g., anxiety disorders, major depression, alcohol, or substance abuse disorders).

The response to stress is highly individualized and the same event or type of event might precipitate PTSD in one person and have little effect in another. Thus, most people experience major stresses and traumatic events during their lifetimes, but many do not develop PTSD. This point needs emphasis because many people seem to assume that PTSD is the normal response to a tragic event and that intensive counseling is needed. For example, counselors converge on schools in response to events that are perceived to be tragic or stressful. Some authorities take the opposing view, however, that talking about and reliving a traumatic event may increase anxiety in some people and thereby increase the likelihood that PTSD will occur. It is also important to note that many PTSD sufferers who need medical attention do not seek treatment.

Social Anxiety Disorder

Social anxiety disorder (SAD) involves excessive concern about scrutiny by others, which may start in childhood and be lifelong. Affected people are afraid that they will say or do something that will embarrass or humiliate them or that will cause them to be judged, negatively evaluated, or rejected. As a result, they try to avoid certain situations (e.g., public speaking) or experience considerable distress if they cannot avoid them. Many with SAD experience physical symptoms including tachycardia, nausea, and sweating. They are often uncomfortable around other people or experience anxiety in many social situations. SAD may be inherited; there is a threefold increase in the occurrence of SAD in related family members.

TABLE 54.1

Drugs Administered to Reduce Anxiety and Produce Hypnosis

Drug Class	Prototype	Other Drugs in the Class
Benzodiazepines	Diazepam (Diastat Acudial, Diazepam Intensol, Valium, Valtoco)	Alprazolam (Alprazolam Intensol, Xanax, Xanax XR) Clonazepam (Klonopin) Chlordiazepoxide Clorazepate Estazolam Flurazepam Lorazepam (Ativan, Lorazepam Intensol, Loreev XR) Midazolam (Nayzilam) Oxazepam Quazepam (Doral) Temazepam (Restoril) Triazolam (Halcion)
Sedative–hypnotics		Eszopiclone (Lunesta) Ramelteon (Rozerem) Suvorexant (Belsomra) Tasimelteon (Hetlioz, Hetlioz LQ) Zaleplon Zolpidem (Ambien, Ambien CR, Edluar, Zolpimist)
Dual Orexin Receptor Antagonists	Suvorexant (Belsomra)	Daridorexant (Quviviq) Lemborexant (DayVigo)

treatment of insomnia, although all are effective sedative–hypnotics. People also use over-the-counter (OTC) medications as sleep aids; these medications include antihistamines alone or in combination with pain relievers. Suvorexant (Belsomra) and other dual orexin receptor antagonist are approved to treat sleep onset and sleep maintenance insomnia. Along with OTC medications, many herbal supplements are consumed to decrease stress and anxiety and induce sleep. Box 54.2 summarizes herbal supplements that are commonly taken and may interact with other prescription medications administered for anxiety and sleep induction. In addition, contamination with undesirable substances may make such herbal remedies less trustworthy.

> **! Quality and Safety Alert: Evidence-Based Practice**
>
> Tachibana et al. [2021] conducted a study of the use of suvorexant as the first-line hypnotic agent used in older adult patients. The administration of suvorexant replaced the use of benzodiazepines to aid in sleep. The aim of the study was to determine whether suvorexant decreased the referrals for delirium in older patients. The study results showed that the number of delirium referral cases decreased significantly every year since 2016 in patients changed from benzodiazepines to suvorexant.

Clinical Application 54.1

- Mrs. Terrence's two sons come to visit her in the hospital. They complain to the nurse that their mother seems oversedated. In denial about her mental status, the sons request that their mother's medication be discontinued, but the nurses are concerned that if she is agitated, she may pull out her IV lines and Foley catheter as well as possibly strike out at staff. How does the nurse handle this situation while respecting the family's concerns?

BENZODIAZEPINES

Benzodiazepines are widely used for anxiety and insomnia and are also used for several other indications. These drugs have a wide margin of safety between therapeutic and toxic doses, and they are rarely fatal, even in overdose, unless combined with other CNS depressant drugs, such as alcohol. Practitioners have used benzodiazepines to manage the anxiety and hyperarousal caused by PTSD, but research does not support their efficacy. With the high prevalence of substance use disorder in patients with PTSD, judicious monitoring and consideration of alternate drug therapy would enhance safety in patients with a history of substance use. In addition, limited data suggest that benzodiazepines may impair the therapeutic effects of certain behavioral therapies, such as exposure therapy.

Benzodiazepines are Schedule IV drugs under the Controlled Substances Act. Drugs of abuse, they may cause physiologic dependence; therefore, withdrawal symptoms occur if these drugs are stopped abruptly. To avoid withdrawal symptoms, it is necessary to taper benzodiazepines gradually before discontinuing them completely. The Food and Drug Administration (FDA) has issued a **BOXED WARNING** ◆ for the combined use of benzodiazepines and opioid analgesics. The risk of serious adverse reactions, including slowed or difficult breathing and deaths, has been reported.

Although benzodiazepines are effective anxiolytics, long-term use is associated with concerns over tolerance, dependency, withdrawal, lack of efficacy for treating the depression that often accompanies anxiety disorders, and the need for multiple daily dosing with some agents. These drugs differ mainly in their plasma half-lives, production of active metabolites, and clinical uses. **Diazepam** (Diastat Acudial, Diazepam Intensol, Valium, Valtoco) is the prototype benzodiazepine.

Pharmacokinetics

Diazepam has a long half-life (20 to 100 hours) if the contribution from metabolites is included. The drug requires 5 to 7 days to reach steady-state serum levels. It is well absorbed, highly lipid soluble, widely distributed in body tissues, and highly bound to plasma proteins (85% to 98%). The high lipid solubility allows the drug to easily enter the CNS and perform its actions. After IV injection, diazepam may act within 1 to 5 minutes. However, the duration of action of a single IV dose is short (30 to 100 minutes). Thus, the pharmacodynamic effects (e.g., sedation) do not correlate with plasma drug levels because the

BOX 54.2 Herbal Supplements Commonly Used to Reduce Anxiety and Insomnia

Kava

This supplement is derived from the root of a shrub found in many South Pacific islands. The major active ingredients of kava extract are kavalactones, which have psychoactive properties. The extract is claimed to be useful in numerous disorders and has been used or studied most often for treatment of anxiety, stress, and restlessness. Although the mechanism of action is not known, it is believed that the herb modulates gamma-aminobutyric acid (GABA) activity and inhibits noradrenaline and dopamine reuptake. Effects include analgesia, sedation, diminished reflexes, impaired gait, and pupil dilation. Multiple research studies have demonstrated that the herb has reduced anxiety in patients with increased symptom levels. However, additional high-quality studies are needed because most of the clinical trials had methodologic flaws, with small sample sizes, and there were conflicts of interest. Limited clinical trials have shown that kava is not effective in the treatment of insomnia.

Adverse effects of kava include impaired thinking, judgment, motor reflexes, and vision. Serious adverse effects may occur with long-term, heavy use, including decreased plasma proteins, decreased platelet and lymphocyte counts, dyspnea, and pulmonary hypertension. The extract should not be taken concurrently with other CNS depressant drugs (e.g., benzodiazepines, ethanol), antiplatelet drugs, or levodopa (increases Parkinson symptoms). Kava may increase the sedative effects of anesthetics and should be discontinued at least 24 hours prior to surgery. In addition, it should not be taken during pregnancy or lactation or by children under 12 years of age. Finally, it should be used cautiously by patients with kidney disease, thrombocytopenia, or neutropenia. The U.S. Food and Drug Administration issued a warning that products containing kava have been implicated in many cases of severe liver toxicity (e.g., hepatitis, cirrhosis, liver failure).

Melatonin

This hormone is produced by the pineal gland, an endocrine gland in the brain. Endogenous melatonin is derived from the amino acid tryptophan, which is converted to serotonin, which is then enzymatically converted to melatonin in the pineal gland. Exogenous preparations are produced synthetically and may contain other ingredients. Melatonin products are widely available. Recommended doses on product labels usually range from 0.3 to 5 mg.

Melatonin influences sleep–wake cycles; it is released during sleep, and serum levels are very low during waking hours. Prolonged intake of exogenous melatonin can reset the sleep–wake cycle. As a result, it is widely promoted for prevention and treatment of jet lag (considered a circadian rhythm disorder) and treatment of insomnia. It is thought to act similarly to the benzodiazepines in inducing sleep. In several studies of patients with sleep disturbances, those taking melatonin experienced modest improvement compared with those taking a placebo. Other studies suggest that melatonin supplements improve sleep in older adults with melatonin deficiency and decrease weight loss in people with cancer. Large, controlled studies are needed to determine the effects of long-term use and the most effective regimen when used for jet lag.

Melatonin supplements are contraindicated in patients with hepatic insufficiency because of reduced clearance. They are also contraindicated in people with a history of cerebrovascular disease, depression, or neurologic disorders. They should be used cautiously by people with abnormal kidney function and those taking benzodiazepines or other CNS depressant drugs. Adverse effects include altered sleep patterns, confusion, headache, hypothermia, pruritus, sedation, and tachycardia.

Valerian

This herb is a perennial flowering plant, and the root has been used for centuries as a treatment for anxiety and insomnia. It is believed that valerian increases the amount of GABA in the brain, probably by inhibiting the transaminase enzyme that normally metabolizes GABA. Increasing GABA, an inhibitory neurotransmitter, results in calming, sedative effects. Shinjyo et al. (2020) reviewed 60 studies that examined the effectiveness of valerian for sleep problems. The results of these studies indicated that the inconsistency in the quality and production of valerian extracts contributed to ineffective improvement in sleep quality. Bystritsky (2022) reviewed other studies conducted on valerian and found that it did not reduce anxiety compared with placebo.

Adverse effects with acute overdose or chronic use of valerian include blurred vision, cardiac disturbance, excitability, headache, hypersensitivity reactions, insomnia, and nausea. There is a risk of hepatotoxicity from overdosage and from using combination herbal products containing valerian. Valerian should not be taken by people with hepatic impairment (risk of increased liver damage) or during pregnancy or lactation (effects are unknown). The herb should not be taken concurrently with any other sedatives, hypnotics, alcohol, or CNS depressants because of the potential for additive CNS depression.

---

drugs move in and out of the CNS rapidly. This redistribution allows a patient to awaken even though the drug may remain in the blood and other peripheral tissues for days or weeks before it is completely eliminated.

Diazepam is mainly metabolized in the liver by the cytochrome P450 enzymes (CYP3A4 subgroup) and glucuronide conjugation. Metabolites are excreted through the kidneys.

Action

Diazepam enhances the inhibitory effect of gamma-aminobutyric acid (GABA) to relieve anxiety, tension, and nervousness and to produce sleep. The decreased neuronal excitability also accounts for its usefulness as a muscle relaxant, hypnotic, and anticonvulsant.

Use

Healthcare providers mainly use diazepam for antianxiety, hypnotic, and anticonvulsant purposes. They also give the drug for preoperative sedation, prevention of agitation and delirium tremens in acute alcohol withdrawal, and treatment of anxiety symptoms associated with depression, acute psychosis, or mania. Thus, patients often take it concurrently with antidepressants,

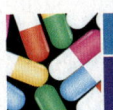

TABLE 54.2
DRUGS AT A GLANCE: Benzodiazepines

Drug	Routes and Dosage Ranges — Adults	Children
ⓟ **Diazepam** (Diastat AcuDial, Diazepam Intensol, Valium, Valtoco; 🍁 Diastat, Valium)	2–10 mg PO 2–4 times daily; 5–10 mg IM or IV. Give IV slowly, no faster than 5 mg (1 mL)/min repeated in 3–4 h if necessary Older or debilitated adults: 2–5 mg PO once or twice daily. Increased gradually if needed and tolerated	0.12–0.8 mg/kg/d in divided doses every 6–8 h
Alprazolam (Xanax, Xanax XR; 🍁 Jamp-Alprazolam, Xanax)	Anxiety: 0.25–0.5 mg PO three times daily; maximum 4 mg daily in divided doses. Older or debilitated adults: 0.25 mg PO 2–3 times daily. Increased gradually if necessary Panic disorder: 0.5 mg PO three times daily initially. Gradually increase to 4–10 mg daily Xanax XR, 0.5–1 mg PO daily; gradually increase PRN to a maximum dose of 3–6 mg daily	<18 y: dosage not established ≥18 y: same as adult dosage
Chlordiazepoxide	Anxiety: 5–10 mg PO daily in 3–4 divided doses Older or debilitated adults: 5 mg PO 2–4 times daily	<6 y: not recommended ≥6 y: 5 mg PO 2–4 times daily. Dose may be increased to 10 mg 2–3 times daily
Clonazepam (Klonopin; 🍁 APO-Clonazepam, Teva-Clonazepam)	Panic disorder: 0.25 mg PO two times daily, increasing to 1 mg daily after 3 d; max 4 mg/d	>10 y: same as adult dosage
Clorazepate	30 mg PO in divided doses or 15 mg PO at bedtime; dose adjusted based on response; range 15–60 mg daily; max 90 mg/d	9–12 y: 7.5 mg PO two times daily, increased by no more than 7.5 mg/wk; maximum 60 mg daily <9 y: not recommended
Estazolam	1 mg PO at bedtime; as needed; may increase to 2 mg	Not recommended for children
Flurazepam	15–30 mg PO at bedtime	Not for use in children <15 y of age
Lorazepam (Ativan, Lorazepam Intensol, Loreev XR; 🍁 Apo-Lorazepam, Ativan)	0.5–1 mg 2–3 times/d may increase in increments of 1 mg every 2–3 d up to 6 mg/d PO; 0.05 mg/kg IM to a maximum of 4 mg; 2 mg IV, diluted with 2 mL of sterile water, sodium chloride, or 5% dextrose injection. Do not exceed 2 mg/min; older or debilitated adults, 1–2 mg/d PO in divided doses	<12 y: PO, IV 0.05 mg/kg/dose, maximum 2 mg dose every 4–6 h ≥12 y: PO 0.25–2 mg/dose 2–3 times daily, maximum 2 mg/dose
Midazolam (Nayzilam)	Preoperative sedation: 0.05–0.08 mg/kg IM ~1 h before surgery Prediagnostic test sedation: 0.1–0.15 mg/kg IV or up to 0.2 mg/kg IV initially; maintenance dose, ~25% of initial dose; reduce dose by 25–30% if an opioid analgesic is also given Induction of anesthesia: 0.3–0.35 mg/kg IV initially, then reduce dose as above for maintenance; reduce initial dose to 0.15–0.3 mg/kg if a narcotic is also given	Preoperative or preprocedure sedation and induction of anesthesia: syrup 0.25–1 mg/kg PO; maximum of 20 mg as a single dose
Oxazepam (🍁 APO-Oxazepam, DOM-Oxazepam)	10–15 mg PO 3 times/d may increase in increments of 15–30 mg to a daily dose of 30–120 mg/d in 3–4 divided doses	Not for use in children <12 y of age
Quazepam (Doral)	7.5 mg at bedtime as needed	Not for use in children
Temazepam (Restoril)	7.5–15 mg PO at bedtime; may increase to 30 mg	Not for use in children <18 y of age
Triazolam (Halcion)	0.125–0.25 mg PO at bedtime	Not for use in children <18 y of age

antipsychotics, and mood stabilizers. However, use of diazepam contraindicates the use of some antidepressants. Experts do not advise using the drug for long periods, because it may cause excessive sedation and respiratory depression.

Investigators have extensively studied diazepam, and it has more approved uses than other drugs in its class. Table 54.2 gives route and dosage information for diazepam and the other benzodiazepines. Larger-than-usual doses may be necessary for patients who are severely anxious or agitated. Also, large doses are usually required to relax skeletal muscle, control muscle spasm, control seizures, and provide sedation before surgery, cardioversion, endoscopy, and angiography. When using benzodiazepines with opioid analgesics, it is important to reduce the analgesic dose initially and increase it gradually to avoid excessive CNS depression.

Patient-related variables specific to the use of diazepam include the following:

- Age:
  - Diazepam or low-dose clonazepam may be used in children who suffer from parasomnias, including sleepwalking. Use cautiously in children due to the increased risk of mental status changes.
  - Children may have unanticipated or variable responses, including paradoxical CNS stimulation and excitement rather than CNS depression and calming.
  - Children should take diazepam and other benzodiazepines only when clearly indicated, in the lowest effective dose, and for the shortest effective time.
  - Diazepam should not be used in children younger than 1 month of age.
  - In older adults, most benzodiazepines are metabolized more slowly, and half-lives are longer than in younger adults. Caution is necessary. Older adults may be sensitive to the drug's effects, especially drowsiness, poor coordination, and mental and/or mood changes.
  - Adverse effects in older adults may contribute to falls and other injuries unless patients are carefully monitored and safeguarded. It is important to make the initial dose of any antianxiety or sedative–hypnotic drug small and to increase doses gradually.
  - Diazepam and other benzodiazepines may produce paradoxical excitement and aggression in adults older than 50 years of age who have a history of psychosis.
  - Research studies suggest a relationship between benzodiazepine use and cognitive declines.
- Reproduction, pregnancy, and lactation:
  - Diazepam passes easily through the placenta with the greatest transfer amounts occurring in the third trimester. A wide range of congenital abnormalities have been reported.
  - Use during late pregnancy is associated with hypothermia and respiratory problems in the infant. Some studies suggest benzodiazepine use may be related to the occurrence of ectopic pregnancy.
  - Although benzodiazepines have been shown to be transferred into breast milk, the amount is small.
- Abnormal kidney function and hepatic impairment:
  - In impaired kidney excretion, active metabolites may accumulate, causing excessive sedation and respiratory depression.
  - Hepatic impairment also rules out use of diazepam.
- Specific healthcare environments
  - In critically ill patients, antianxiety and sedative–hypnotic drugs are often useful to relieve stress, anxiety, and agitation. Their calming effects decrease cardiac workload (e.g., heart rate, blood pressure, force of myocardial contraction, myocardial oxygen consumption) and respiratory effort.
  - Additional benefits include improving tolerance of treatment measures (e.g., mechanical ventilation); keeping patients who are confused from harming themselves by pulling out IV catheters, feeding or drainage tubes, wound drains, and other treatment devices; and allowing more rest or sleep. In addition to sedation, the drugs often induce amnesia, which may be a desirable effect in patients who are critically ill.
  - Caution is necessary with the use of diazepam in patients with critical illness.
  - Most patients take diazepam at home, and the home care nurse shares the responsibility for teaching patients how to use the drug effectively and how to recognize medication responses that should be reported to the healthcare provider.

Adverse Effects

Both therapeutic effects and adverse effects of diazepam are more likely to occur after 2 or 3 days of therapy than initially. Such effects accumulate with chronic usage and persist for several days after the drug is discontinued. Many of the adverse effects associated with diazepam are related to its CNS depressant effects. They include drowsiness, problems with memory, confusion, disinhibition, depressed mood with or without suicidal ideation, slurred speech, dizziness, shallow breathing, restlessness, irritability, loss of bladder control, and diminished sexual interest. Other effects may include new or worsening seizures, nausea, constipation, drooling or dry mouth, mild skin rash, and itching. Diazepam and other benzodiazepines exert effects on the GABA receptors and can lead to overdose. Signs of overdose include blurred or double vision, labored breathing, weakness, stupor, and coma. Flumazenil is a benzodiazepine antagonist that interacts with the GABA receptors to reverse overdose (see Chapter 58).

Contraindications

Contraindications to diazepam include severe respiratory disorders, such as chronic obstructive pulmonary disease or sleep apnea, severe liver or kidney disease, hypersensitivity reactions, and a history of alcohol or other drug abuse. People with narrow-angle glaucoma or who are pregnant or breast-feeding should not take diazepam. The concurrent use of diazepam and any other CNS depressants warrants caution.

NCLEX Success

1. Which baseline laboratory tests should a patient receive prior to starting a benzodiazepine?

    A. blood glucose level
    B. liver enzymes
    C. lipid profile
    D. thyroid panel

Nursing Implications

Preventing Interactions

Smaller-than-usual doses of diazepam and other benzodiazepines may be necessary in patients receiving cimetidine or other drugs that decrease the hepatic metabolism of benzodiazepines. Rhodiola rosea, Bacopa monnieri, 5-hydrocytriptophan, and St. John's wort are supplements that when combined with benzodiazepines increase the risk of serotonin syndrome.

Administering the Medication

There are various preparations of diazepam, for both oral and parenteral use. The nurse adheres to the following guidelines:

- Ensure that the patient has swallowed sustained-release tablets whole. It is important not to chew these tablets.
- Ensure that the patient consumes the entire dose of medication.
- Do not abruptly withdraw the medication. This places the patient at risk of alterations in mood.
- Administer the intramuscular preparation in a large muscle. Inject it slowly and rotate injection sites.
- Administer the IV form undiluted IV push at a rate of 5 mg/min. In children, inject it at a rate of 0.25 mg/kg over 3 minutes.

Assessing for Therapeutic Effects

The nurse observes for a relaxed, but easily aroused, appearance. The nurse interviews the patient to assess response to the medication. For example, the patient should verbalize that they feel less worried and more relaxed. Nonverbal behavior is important; response to the medication includes decreased heart rate and blood pressure and a relaxed posture. It is necessary to assess the level of drowsiness and sleep pattern.

Assessing for Adverse Effects

The nurse monitors the patient's blood pressure. It is necessary to make sure that the patient does not experience paradoxical responses, which include anger, aggression, and hallucinations, to the diazepam.

The nurse assesses for symptoms of diazepam dependence, overdose, and withdrawal. The presence of withdrawal symptoms when the drug is stopped indicates physical dependence, which is associated with longer use and higher doses. Common signs and symptoms of withdrawal include increased anxiety, psychomotor agitation, insomnia, irritability, headache, tremor, and palpitations. Less common but more serious signs include confusion, abnormal perception of movement, depersonalization, psychosis, and seizures. Symptoms usually occur 4 to 5 days after stopping a long-acting drug such as diazepam. Relief requires administration of a benzodiazepine.

Patient Teaching

Box 54.3 identifies guidelines for teaching patients who are taking diazepam and other benzodiazepines for anxiety and insomnia.

Other Drugs in the Class

Alprazolam (Alprazolam Intensol, Xanax, Xanax XR) is administered orally to reduce anxiety and panic disorders. Older adult patients are more sensitive to the effects of the drug and may experience ataxia and oversedation. Lorazepam (Ativan) is the benzodiazepine drug of choice to combat anxiety and depression as well as stress-related insomnia. Oxazepam is administered for anxiety and depression and alcohol withdrawal. Respiratory depression may occur with oxazepam, so respiratory and cardiovascular status should be assessed.

Chlordiazepoxide is most commonly administered for the control of withdrawal symptoms related to acute alcoholism. Clorazepate has a longer onset of action than diazepam. This drug is commonly administered for anxiety, alcohol withdrawal, and epilepsy.

> **Quality and Safety Alert: Safety**
>
> It is important not to confuse clorazepate with clonazepam; both drugs are used to control seizure activity, but dosages differ significantly. For instance, in adults the maximum daily dosage of clorazepate is 90 mg; with clonazepam, the maximum daily dosage is 4 mg.

Lorazepam (Ativan, Lorazepam Intensol, Loreev XR) is probably the benzodiazepine of first choice. The drug provides rapid tranquilization of patients experiencing agitation. Administered intravenously, it reduces nausea and vomiting as well as anxiety and induces procedural amnesia. Administered orally, it helps combat anxiety disorders and the anxiety associated with depressive symptoms or anxiety- or stress-associated insomnia. Flurazepam is administered on a short-term basis for the treatment of insomnia. Quazepam (Doral) is used for insomnia. Due to the risk of next day impairment and drug dependence it should only be administered when safer therapies have failed. Temazepam (Restoril) appears to act at the subcortical levels of the CNS. The drug's main site of action is the limbic system and mesencephalic reticular formation. It potentiates the effects of GABA. Temazepam is eliminated by conjugation and excreted through the kidneys. Thus, it is the drug of choice for older adult patients, those patients who have liver disease, or those who take medications that interfere with hepatic drug–metabolizing enzymes. The most severe adverse effect of temazepam is cardiovascular collapse. Triazolam (Halcion) has a very rapid onset of action, and it is necessary to administer the drug while patients are in bed. Cirrhosis of the liver or hepatic insufficiency is a contraindication. In addition, the hematocrit levels should be monitored due to the adverse effect of blood dyscrasias. Patients should not combine triazolam with ketoconazole or itraconazole.

Midazolam is discussed in detail in Chapter 51. The FDA has issued a for midazolam because of profound respiratory depression that may result in hypoxia, brain damage, or death. Rapid IV administration to neonates has resulted in hypotension and seizures. It is essential to titrate midazolam carefully according to age and medical conditions. Following administration of midazolam, continuous monitoring of respiratory depression is required; and if necessary, age-specific resuscitative measures should be implemented. The benzodiazepine antagonist flumazenil reverses the effects of midazolam.

> **Quality and Safety Alert: Safety**
>
> All benzodiazepines produce central nervous system depression and decreased blood pressure. Safety in ambulation is necessary with the administration of benzodiazepines.

BOX 54.3 Patient Teaching Guidelines for Benzodiazepines

- Medications to relieve anxiety or promote sleep can relieve symptoms temporarily, but they do not cure or solve the underlying problems. With rare exceptions, these drugs are recommended only for short-term use. For long-term relief, counseling or psychotherapy may be more beneficial because it can help you learn other ways to decrease your anxiety.
- Try to identify and avoid factors that cause anxiety, such as caffeine-containing beverages and stimulant drugs. This may prevent or decrease the severity of nervousness. If the drugs are used, these factors can cancel or decrease the drugs' effects. Stimulant drugs include asthma and cold remedies and appetite suppressants.
- Most pills to control anxiety belong to the same chemical group and have similar effects, including the ability to decrease nervousness, cause drowsiness, and cause dependence. Thus, there is no logical reason to take a combination of the drugs for anxiety or to take one drug for daytime sedation and another for sleep. Xanax, Ativan, and Restoril are commonly used examples of this group, but there are several others as well.
- Inform all healthcare providers when taking a sedative-type medication, preferably by the generic and trade names. This helps avoid multiple prescriptions of drugs with similar effects and reduces the risk of serious adverse effects from overdose.
- Do not perform tasks that require alertness if drowsy from medication. The drugs often impair mental and physical functioning, especially during the first several days of use, and thereby make routine activities potentially hazardous. Avoid smoking, ambulating without help, driving a car, operating machinery, bathing, and other potentially hazardous tasks. These activities may lead to falls or other injuries if undertaken while alertness is impaired.
- Avoid alcohol and other depressant drugs (e.g., over-the-counter [OTC] antihistamines and sleeping pills, narcotic analgesics, sedating herbs such as kava and valerian, and the dietary supplement melatonin) while taking any antianxiety or sedative–hypnotic drugs (except buspirone). An antihistamine that causes drowsiness is the active ingredient in OTC sleep aids (e.g., Compoz, Nytol, Sominex, Unisom) and in many pain reliever products with "PM" as part of their names (e.g., Tylenol PM). Because these drugs depress brain functioning when taken alone, combining them produces additive depression and may lead to excessive drowsiness, difficulty breathing, traumatic injuries, and other potentially serious adverse drug effects.
- Store drugs safely, out of reach of children and adults who are confused or less than alert. Accidental or intentional ingestion may lead to serious adverse effects. Also, do not keep the drug container at the bedside, because a person sedated by a previous dose may take additional doses.
- Do not share these drugs with anyone else. These mind-altering, brain-depressant drugs should be taken only by those people for whom they are prescribed.
- Do not stop taking a diazepam-related drug abruptly. Withdrawal symptoms can occur. When being discontinued, dosage should be gradually reduced, as directed by and with the supervision of a healthcare provider.
- Follow instructions carefully about how much, how often, and how long to take the drugs. These drugs produce more beneficial effects and fewer adverse reactions when used in the smallest effective doses and for the shortest duration feasible in particular circumstances. Omit one or more doses if excessive drowsiness occurs to avoid difficulty breathing, falls, and other adverse drug effects.
- Take oral benzodiazepines with a glass of water. Take them with food if stomach upset occurs.
- Take Xanax XR once daily, preferably in the morning. Take the tablet intact; do not crush, chew, or break it.

Clinical Application 54.2

Mrs. Terrence receives alprazolam 0.25 mg PO at 2:00 p.m. Later, when the nurse brings in her supper tray, the patient seems relaxed. The supper tray contains roast beef, salad, chocolate pie, and hot tea. Visitors arrive at 5:00 p.m. and remark to the nurse that Mrs. Terrence is agitated and wringing her hands. She says that she is afraid to verbalize her anxiety to the nursing staff. The nurse prepares to give Mrs. Terrence another dose of medication.
- What does the nurse prepare and why?
- What foods on the supper tray contribute to the patient's anxiety?
- What patient teaching is necessary?

NCLEX Success

2. Oxazepam can be used in the treatment of patients who have which conditions? (Select all that apply.)
   A. severe agitation
   B. schizophrenia with hallucinations
   C. anxiety with depression
   D. opioid dependence
   E. alcoholism

3. Benzodiazepines are thought to work through which action?
   A. exciting the central nervous system
   B. stimulating the reticular activating system
   C. increasing inhibitory feelings
   D. enhancing the effects of gamma-aminobutyric acid

NONBENZODIAZEPINE SEDATIVE–HYPNOTIC AGENTS

The nonbenzodiazepine sedative–hypnotics produce sleep. People may receive them prior to diagnostic or surgical procedures or take them nightly. Table 54.1 lists the most commonly administered nonbenzodiazepines that produce sleep. This classification lacks a specific prototype, so each drug in the class will be discussed individually.

In general, people should use sedative–hypnotics only when insomnia causes significant distress and resists management by nonpharmacologic means. The drugs are not indicated for occasional sleeplessness. The goal of treatment is to relieve anxiety or sleeplessness without permitting sensory perception, responsiveness to the environment, or alertness to drop below safe levels. The drugs of choice for most patients are the benzodiazepines and the nonbenzodiazepine hypnotics, eszopiclone, ramelteon, zaleplon, and zolpidem. However, for patients with insomnia associated with major depression, antidepressants are preferred (see Chapter 55).

The use of sedative–hypnotics every night should not occur unless absolutely necessary. Intermittent administration helps maintain drug effectiveness and decreases the risks of drug abuse and dependence. It also decreases disturbances of normal sleep patterns. For chronic insomnia, only eszopiclone is recommended for long-term treatment (≤12 months). To restore the sleep-producing effect, administration of the hypnotic drug must be interrupted for 1 to 2 weeks. Table 54.3 gives route and dosage information for the sedative–hypnotics. Box 54.4 identifies guidelines for teaching patients who are taking sedative–hypnotics for anxiety and insomnia.

Eszopiclone

Eszopiclone (Lunesta) is the first oral nonbenzodiazepine hypnotic to receive FDA approval for long-term use (≤12 months). During testing, researchers did not observe tolerance to the hypnotic benefits of the drug over a 6-month period. It increases total sleep time and reduces the amount of time needed to fall asleep. Studies show that eszopiclone does not reduce nighttime awakenings. The drug is a Schedule IV controlled substance.

Supposedly, the hypnotic effect of eszopiclone is due to interaction with the $GABA_A$ receptor at a location close to or coupled with the benzodiazepine receptors. The drug is rapidly absorbed after oral administration, reaching peak plasma levels 1 hour after administration. It has a half-life of 6 hours. It is metabolized in the liver and eliminated primarily by the kidney system.

People should take eszopiclone immediately prior to going to bed due to its rapid onset of action.

> **! Quality and Safety Alert: Safety**
>
> It is important to instruct patients not to engage in any activities following the administration of the medication.

Also, people should not take the medication following a high-fat meal, because the onset of action may be delayed by approximately 1 hour, or prior to bathing. In addition, geriatric people should not use the drug, according to the Beers Criteria.

Adverse reactions to eszopiclone include behavioral changes such as reduced inhibition, aggression or bizarre behavior, worsening depression and suicidal ideation, hallucinations, and **anterograde amnesia** (short-term memory loss). A commonly reported reaction to the drug is an unpleasant taste. Contraindications include hypersensitivity reaction. Caution is necessary during pregnancy and lactation, in depression, and with impaired hepatic or respiratory function. Older adult patients, those with hepatic impairment or debilitating conditions, and those taking drugs that inhibit CYP3A4 enzymes (e.g., antidepressants, antifungals, erythromycin, grapefruit, protease inhibitors, others) require lower dosages

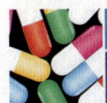

TABLE 54.3
DRUGS AT A GLANCE: Sedative–Hypnotics

Drug	Routes and Dosage Ranges	
	Adults	**Children**
Eszopiclone (Lunesta; 🍁 Lunesta)	1–2 mg PO at bedtime; may be increased to 3 mg if needed; for initial dose, debilitated patients, and those with hepatic impairment, 1 mg PO at bedtime; may be increased to 2 mg if needed	Not recommended
Ramelteon (Rozerem)	8 mg PO at bedtime	Not recommended
Tasimelteon (Hetlioz, Hetlioz LQ)	20 mg PO before bedtime at the same time each night	Dosage not established
Zaleplon	5–10 mg PO at bedtime; 5 mg for adults who are older and of low weight or have mild to moderate hepatic impairment	Dosage not established
Zolpidem (Ambien, Ambien CR, Edluar, Zolpimist; 🍁 APO-Zolpidem, Sublinox)	Immediate-release tablet, spray 5 mg (females) or 5–10 mg (males) PO at bedtime Extended-release tablet, 6.25 mg (females) or 6.25–12.5 mg (males) PO at bedtime	≥18 y, same as adult dosage

to reduce adverse effects. People who take eszopiclone should not take alcohol or other CNS depressants to avoid additive effects.

Ramelteon

Ramelteon (Rozerem), a melatonin agonist, is used for the long-term treatment of insomnia characterized by difficulty with sleep onset. Unlike other nonbenzodiazepine hypnotics, which bind to $GABA_A$ receptors, ramelteon binds to melatonin receptors in the CNS. Stimulation of melatonin receptors by ramelteon, like endogenous melatonin, is thought to play a role in the maintenance of the circadian rhythm, which helps regulate the normal sleep–wake cycle. Ramelteon does not appear to cause rebound insomnia posttreatment. Because it does not produce physical dependence, ramelteon is not classified as a controlled substance.

Ramelteon is rapidly absorbed orally, reaching peak plasma levels in about 45 minutes. Ramelteon is moderately protein bound (82%) and undergoes rapid hepatic first-pass metabolism by cytochrome P450 enzyme systems, including CYP3A4. Ramelteon is excreted primarily in the urine and does not accumulate in the body due to the short half-life of the drug (1 to 2.6 hours). Patients should avoid taking ramelteon with a high-fat meal because food may delay the onset of action.

Common adverse effects of ramelteon include headache, fatigue, dizziness, nausea, diarrhea, arthralgia/myalgia, and taste changes. The drug may affect endocrine hormones, resulting in decreased testosterone levels, increased prolactin levels, and decreased cortisol levels. Contraindications include severe hepatic impairment if combined with fluvoxamine. Caution is warranted in depression or impaired respiratory function. People should not take ramelteon with alcohol because of resulting excessive sedation and respiratory depression.

Tasimelteon

Tasimelteon (Hetlioz, Hetlioz LQ), a drug in the same class as ramelteon, has been approved for the treatment of non–24-hour sleep–wake disorder in adults, a circadian sleep–wake rhythm disorder that occurs primarily affecting blind individuals.

Zaleplon

Zaleplon is an oral, nonbenzodiazepine hypnotic approved for the short-term treatment (7 to 10 days) of insomnia. Overall, this drug is effective in helping people get to sleep and has several advantages as a hypnotic, including the rapid onset, absence of active metabolites, absence of clinically significant CYP450 drug interactions, rapid clearance from the body, and absence of major memory impairments. However, it may not increase total sleep time or decrease the number of awakenings during sleeping hours.

Zaleplon is well absorbed, but bioavailability is only about 30% because of extensive presystemic or first-pass hepatic metabolism. Onset of action is rapid, with a peak in 1 hour. A high-fat, heavy meal slows absorption and may reduce the drug's effectiveness in inducing sleep. It is 60% bound to plasma proteins, and its half-life is 1 hour. The drug is metabolized mainly in the liver to inactive metabolites. The metabolites and a small amount of unchanged drug are excreted in the urine.

Zaleplon apparently enhances the inhibitory effects of GABA, as do the benzodiazepines. A few studies indicate that it has abuse potential similar to that of the benzodiazepines; zaleplon is a Schedule IV controlled substance.

No dosage adjustment with zaleplon is necessary in mild to moderate abnormal kidney function. However, to reduce the risk of adverse effects, it is necessary to decrease the dosage in mild to moderate hepatic impairment and avoid using the drug in severe hepatic impairment. It is also important to decrease the dosage in older adults.

Adverse effects associated with zaleplon include depression, drowsiness, nausea, dizziness, headache, hypersensitivity, impaired coordination, and short-term memory impairment. Contraindications include hypersensitivity reactions and lactation. Caution is warranted during pregnancy and in impaired hepatic or respiratory function.

Use of zaleplon with alcohol or other CNS depressant drugs should not occur because of the increased risk of excessive sedation and respiratory depression. There is also a risk of increased serum zaleplon levels if people take the hypnotic concurrently with cimetidine. It is very important that patients taking zaleplon be taught about this interaction because cimetidine is available without prescription, and the patient may not inform the healthcare provider who prescribes zaleplon about taking cimetidine.

Zolpidem

Zolpidem (Ambien, Ambien CR, Edluar, Zolpimist) is a nonbenzodiazepine hypnotic that differs structurally from the benzodiazepines but produces similar effects. This drug is a Schedule IV drug approved for short-term treatment (7 to 10 days) of insomnia. It is well absorbed with oral administration and has a rapid onset of action, usually within 20 to 30 minutes. The half-life of zolpidem is 2.5 hours, and its hypnotic effects last 6 to 8 hours. A newer controlled-release form (Ambien CR) contains a rapid-releasing layer, which promotes falling asleep, and a slow-releasing layer, which promotes sleep all night. The drug is metabolized to inactive metabolites in the liver; these are then eliminated by kidney excretion.

Dosage reductions with zolpidem are not necessary in abnormal kidney function, but this condition requires close monitoring. Increased bioavailability, peak plasma concentration, and half-life occur in older adults and in patients with impaired hepatic function. Thus, dosage reduction is essential for these groups. People should not take zolpidem concurrently with alcohol or other CNS depressant drugs because of the increased risk of excessive sedation and respiratory depression.

Adverse effects of zolpidem include daytime drowsiness, dizziness, nausea, diarrhea, and anterograde amnesia. Hallucinations have been reported in some patients. Older adults may experience headache, somnolence, and dizziness. Caution is necessary with signs and symptoms of major depression because of increased risk of intentional overdose. Rebound insomnia may occur for a night or two after stopping the drug, and withdrawal symptoms may occur if it is stopped abruptly after approximately a week of regular use.

NCLEX Success

4. Zolpidem is the most appropriate choice for patients with which condition?
   A. difficulty in initiating and maintaining sleep
   B. morning awakening
   C. agitation and violent outbursts
   D. obstructive sleep apnea and respiratory problems

5. When a patient receives a prescription for zolpidem, which teaching point is most important?
   A. Take the medication with a high-fat meal.
   B. Only take the medication if acetaminophen PM does not produce sleep.
   C. Go to bed immediately after taking the medication.
   D. Take the medication if nondrug relaxation has not produced sleep.

DUAL RECEPTOR ANTAGONISTS

Suvorexant (Belsomra) is the prototype in the dual orexin receptor antagonist class. It was approved by the FDA in 2014. Daridorexant (Quviviq) was approved in January of 2022, and lemborexant (DayVigo) was approved in December 2019. Table 54.4 identifies the Dual Orexin Receptor Antagonists.

Pharmacokinetics

The onset of action of suvorexant is approximately 30 minutes. The drug reaches its peak in 2 hours, and the half-life is approximately 12 hours. It has decreased absorption in higher doses. The drug is greater than 99% protein bound. Suvorexant is primarily metabolized by the hepatic enzyme CYP3A4. Less metabolism takes place with the hepatic enzyme CYP2C9. The excretion of the drug takes place in the feces (66%) and urine (23%).

Action

Suvorexant blocks the binding of the wake-promoting peptides orexin A and orexin B to receptors OX1R and OX2R. It is thought that this action suppresses the wake drive. The antagonism of orexin receptors may also be the basis for potential adverse effects such as signs of narcolepsy or cataplexy.

Use

Suvorexant is used to treat insomnia and maintain sleep.

Patient-related variables specific to the use of suvorexant include the following:

- Age:
  - In children use the lowest recommended dosage.
  - In older adults no dosage adjustments are needed.
- Reproduction, pregnancy, and lactation:
  - Adverse fetal effects have been observed in animal studies.
  - It is unknown if suvorexant is present in breast milk.
- Abnormal kidney function and hepatic impairment:
  - There are no specific changes to dosage or administration in the presence of abnormal kidney function or hepatic impairment.

Adverse Effects and Contraindications

Suvorexant can produce abnormal dreams, dizziness, drowsiness, and headaches. These adverse effects are more common in females. Hypnogenic hallucinations, sleep paralysis, depression, sleep paralysis and suicidal ideations have been reported. Some patients have been diagnosed with hypercholesterolemia with suvorexant. In postmarketing studies, palpitations, tachycardia, pruritus, nausea, vomiting, and complex sleep-related disorders have been documented.

Suvorexant is contraindicated in patients diagnosed with narcolepsy.

Nursing Implications

Preventing Interactions

Alizapride, Azelastine nasal spray, Blonanserin, Bromopride, chlormethiazole, clofazimine, droperidol, magnesium sulfate, minocycline, olopatadine nasal spray, rufinamide, and all CNS depressants enhance the depressant effects of suvorexant. Drugs that induce CYP3A4 will increase the concentration of suvorexant. Grapefruit juice will increase the serum concentration of suvorexant. The suvorexant dosage should be reduced with the initial dose when combined with grapefruit juice. Kava kava, cannabinoid products, and valerian combined with suvorexant will increase CNS depression.

TABLE 54.4 DRUGS AT A GLANCE: Dual Orexin Receptor Antagonists

Drug	Routes and Dosage Ranges	
	Adults	Children
Suvorexant (Belsomra)	25–50 mg PO within 30 min of bedtime	Children ≥10 y and adolescents: 10–20 mg PO at bedtime
Daridorexant (Quviviq)	25–50 mg PO once daily within 30 min of bedtime	Not approved for use in children
Lemborexant (DayVigo; Frandsen13e-DayVigo)	5 mg PO immediately before bedtime	Not approved for use in children

Administering the Medication

Suvorexant should not be administered with a meal, as a full stomach will decrease absorption. Female patients with a body mass index (BMI) greater than 30 are at increased risk of adverse effects; increasing the drug's dosage should be done with caution in these patients. Suvorexant should be administered with 30 minutes of bedtime. Adults should have ≥7 hours of sleep before planned awakening. Pediatric patients should have at least 7 hours of sleep before planned awakening.

Assessing for Therapeutic Effects

The nurse interviews the patient to determine the effectiveness of the medication. The nurse observes the patient for a relaxed, easily arousable appearance following at least 7 hours of sleep.

Assessing for Adverse Effects

The nurse interviews the patient about abnormal dreaming, dizziness, drowsiness, and headaches. The patient is assessed for hallucinations, depression, depressive thoughts, and suicidal ideations.

Patient Teaching

Box 54.4 identifies guidelines for teaching patients who are taking nonbenzodiazepine and dual orexin receptor antagonists sedative hypnotics.

Other Drugs in the Class

Daridorexant (Quviviq) and Lemborexant (DayVigo) have the same mechanism of action as suvorexant. Daridorexant's pharmacokinetic properties are similar to suvorexant. Daridorexant has a slightly shorter half-life at 8 hours, but the onset of action is similar at 35 to 40 minutes. It should be used cautiously in patients experiencing depression, as the CNS depressant effects can worsen the patient's depression and increase the risk of suicidal ideations. It also should be used cautiously in older adults. There are no recommendations for patients with a BMI greater than 30. Lemborexant (DayVigo) has a more rapid onset of action at 15 to 20 minutes. The half-life of lemborexant is 17 to 19 hours. Next day drowsiness can impair the patient's physical and mental abilities.

BOX 54.4 Patient Teaching Guidelines for Nonbenzodiazepine Sedative–Hypnotics and Dual Orexin Receptor Antagonists

- Sleeping pills, like antianxiety drugs, can relieve symptoms temporarily, but they do not cure or solve the underlying problems. With rare exceptions, these drugs are recommended only for short-term use. For long-term relief, counseling or psychotherapy may be more beneficial because it can help you learn other ways to decrease your difficulty in sleeping.
- Avoid alcohol and other depressant drugs (e.g., OTC antihistamines and sleeping pills, narcotic analgesics, sedating herbs such as kava and valerian, and the dietary supplement melatonin) while taking sedative–hypnotic drugs and dual orexin receptor antagonists. An antihistamine that causes drowsiness is the active ingredient in OTC sleep aids (e.g., Compoz, Nytol, Sominex, Unisom) and in many pain reliever products with "PM" as part of their names (e.g., Tylenol PM). Because these drugs depress brain functioning when taken alone, combining them produces additive depression and may lead to excessive drowsiness, difficulty breathing, traumatic injuries, and other potentially serious adverse drug effects.
- Do not perform tasks that require alertness if drowsy from medication. The drugs often impair mental and physical functioning, especially during the first several days of use, and thereby make routine activities potentially hazardous. Avoid smoking, ambulating without help, driving a car, operating machinery, bathing, and other potentially hazardous tasks. These activities may lead to falls or other injuries if undertaken while alertness is impaired.
- Store drugs safely, out of reach of children and adults who are confused or less than alert. Accidental or intentional ingestion may lead to serious adverse effects. Also, do not keep the drug container at the bedside, because a person sedated by a previous dose may take additional doses.
- Take nonbenzodiazepine hypnotics on an empty stomach, at bedtime, because fatty heavy meals delay onset of action.
- Do not take herbal supplements with nonbenzodiazepine sedative–hypnotics.
- Do not take most "sleeping pills" every night. Many sleeping pills lose their effectiveness in 2 to 4 weeks if taken nightly and cause sleep disturbances when stopped. If longer drug therapy for insomnia is needed, eszopiclone and ramelteon are approved for long-term use.
- If you are taking either suvorexant (Belsomra) or lemborexant (DayVigo), which are dual orexin receptor antagonists, do not increase the dosage. Ensure protection from falls related to increased drowsiness and report suicidal ideations to the prescriber. Administer the drug 30 minutes prior to bedtime and ensure at least 7 hours of sleep. Take the medication with or without food.
- Use nondrug measures to promote relaxation, rest, and sleep when possible. Physical exercise, reading, craft work, stress management, and relaxation techniques are safer than any drug.
- Take sleeping pills just before going to bed so that you are lying down when the expected drowsiness occurs.
- Do not take zolpidem concurrently with alcohol or other CNS depressant drugs because of increased risk of excessive sedation and respiratory depression.
- Prime zolpidem oral spray prior to initial use. Compress the container five times, hold the container upright, and aim it directly into the mouth.
- Report adverse effects such as hypersensitivity reactions, complex sleep-related behaviors, or thoughts of suicide to the prescriber.

THE NURSING PROCESS

A concept map outlines the nursing process related to drug therapy considerations in this chapter. Additional nursing implications related to the disease process should also be considered in care decisions.

Assessment
- Assess the patient's subjective and objective data regarding anxiety and insomnia.
- Assess the patient's sleep patterns.
- Assess physiological aspects of anxiety (e.g., increased heart rate and respiratory rate).
- Obtain a careful drug history, including the use of alcohol and sedative–hypnotic drugs, and assess the likelihood of drug abuse and dependence.
- Assess for use of CNS stimulants (e.g., appetite suppressants, bronchodilators, nasal decongestants, caffeine, cocaine) and herbs (e.g., St John's wort, ephedra).
- Identify coping mechanisms used in managing previous situations of stress, anxiety, and insomnia.

Outcomes of Therapy

The patient will
- Feel more calm, relaxed, and comfortable with anxiety; experience improved quantity and quality of sleep with insomnia.
- Be monitored for excessive sedation and impaired mobility to prevent falls or other injuries (in health care settings).
- Verbalize and demonstrate nondrug activities to reduce or manage anxiety or insomnia.
- Demonstrate safe, accurate drug usage.
- Notify a health care provider if he or she wants to stop taking a benzodiazepine; agree to not stop taking a benzodiazepine abruptly.
- Avoid preventable adverse effects, including abuse and dependence.

Nursing Interventions
- Use nondrug measures to relieve anxiety or to enhance the effectiveness of antianxiety drugs.
  - Assist patients to identify and avoid or decrease situations that cause anxiety and insomnia, when possible. In addition, help them to understand that medications do not solve underlying problems.
  - Implement therapeutic communication skills.
  - Instruct on the overall treatment plan, including medical treatments, diagnostic tests, medication and treatment measures, and any aspects of care.
  - When a benzodiazepine is used with diagnostic tests or minor surgery, provide instructions for postprocedure care to the patient or to family members, preferably in written form.
- Implement measures to decrease the need for or increase the effectiveness of sedative-hypnotic drugs, such as the following:
  - Modify the environment to promote rest and sleep (e.g., reduce noise and light).
  - Plan care to allow uninterrupted periods of rest and sleep, when possible.
  - Relieve symptoms that interfere with rest and sleep. Drugs such as analgesics for pain or antitussives for cough are usually safer and more effective than sedative–hypnotic drugs. Nondrug measures, such as positioning, exercise, and back rubs, may be helpful in relieving muscle tension and other discomforts. Allowing the patient to verbalize concerns, providing information so that he or she knows what to expect, or consulting other personnel (e.g., social worker, chaplain) may be useful in decreasing anxiety.
  - Help the patient modify lifestyle habits to promote rest and sleep (e.g., limiting intake of caffeine-containing beverages, limiting intake of fluids during evening hours if nocturia interferes with sleep, avoiding daytime naps, having a regular schedule of rest and sleep periods, increasing physical activity, not trying to sleep unless tired or drowsy).
- Boxes 54.3 and 54.4 present patient teaching guidelines for antianxiety medications and sedative-hypnotics.

Evaluation
- Decreased symptoms of anxiety or insomnia and increased rest and sleep are reported or observed.
- Excessive sedation and motor impairment are not observed.
- The patient reports no serious adverse effects.
- Monitoring of prescriptions (e.g., "pill counts") does not indicate excessive use.

Visit thePoint® *at* **http://thePoint.lww.com/ Frandsen13e** *for answers to NCLEX Success questions (in Appendix A), answers to Clinical Application Case Studies (in Appendix B), additional information on the etiology and pathophysiology of anxiety and insomnia, and more!*

REFERENCES AND RESOURCES

Bystritsky, A. (2022). Complementary and alternative treatments for anxiety symptoms and disorders: Herbs and medications. *UpToDate*. Lexi Comp, Inc.

Neubauer, D. N. (2022). Pharmacotherapy for insomnia in adults. *UpToDate*. Lexi Comp, Inc.

Shinjyo, N., Waddel, G., & Green, J. (2020). Valerian root treating sleep problems and associated disorders—A systematic review. *Journal of Evidence-Based Integrative Medicine*. 2020;1–31. https://doi.org/10.1177/2515690X20967323

Tachibana, M., Inada, T., Ichida, M., Lojima, S., Arai, T., Naito, K., & Ozaki, N. (2021). Significant decrease in delirium referrals after changing hypnotic from benzodiazepine to suvorexant. *Japanese Psychogeriatric Society.*, 21, 324–332. https://doi.org/10.1111/psyg.12672

UpToDate (2022). *Drug information*. Lexi-Comp, Inc.

Varanasi, S. (2021). Anxiety medication interactions: Which herbal supplements should I avoid? *GoodRX Health*. https://www.goodrx.com/conditions/generalized-anxiety-disorder/interactions-with-anxiety-medications

Winkelman, J. W. (2022). Overview of the treatment of insomnia in adults. *UpToDate*. Lexi-Comp, Inc.

Wyatt, S. A. Understanding benzodiazepines commonly prescribed but caution advised. *Psychiatric Times*, 4, 32–35. NLM UID: 9014543.

CHAPTER 55

Drug Therapy for Depression and Mood Disorders

LEARNING OBJECTIVES

After studying this chapter, you should be able to:

1. Describe the major features of various mood disorders.
2. Compare and contrast the different categories of antidepressants: tricyclic antidepressants, selective serotonin reuptake inhibitors, mixed serotonin–norepinephrine reuptake inhibitors, monoamine oxidase inhibitors, and other atypical antidepressants.
3. Discuss the drugs used to treat depression in terms of prototype, action, indications for use, adverse effects, and nursing implications.
4. Discuss the drugs used to treat bipolar disorder in terms of prototype, action, indications for use, adverse effects, and nursing implications.
5. Discuss the use of ketamine in the treatment of depression.
6. Implement the nursing process in the care of patients undergoing drug therapy for mood disorders.

CLINICAL APPLICATION CASE STUDY

While in the hospital, Carl Mehring, a 70-year-old man, receives a diagnosis of chronic depression secondary to chronic heart failure, hypertension, diabetes mellitus, and abnormal kidney function. As his health has declined, so has his interest in his family, friends, and hobbies. His physician prescribes sertraline 50 mg orally at bedtime.

KEY TERMS

Antidepressant discontinuation syndrome: condition that occurs with sudden termination of most antidepressant drugs. Typical symptoms may occur more rapidly and may be more intense with drugs that have a short half-life and/or are used for long periods

Bipolar disorder: mood disorder in which people alternate between periods of depression and overexcitement or mania

Cyclothymia: mild type of bipolar disorder involving periods of hypomania and depression that do not meet the criteria for mania and major depression

Depression: most common mental illness, which is characterized by depressed mood, feelings of sadness, or emotional upset; occurs in people of all ages

Dysthymia: chronically depressed mood and at least two other symptoms of depression for 2 years

Enuresis: bed wetting or involuntary urination resulting from a physical or psychological disorder

Hypomania: persistent irritable mood but absence of psychotic symptoms characteristic of true mania

Mania: emotional disorder characterized by euphoria or irritability

Postpartum depression: major depressive episode occurring after the birth of a child

Seasonal affective disorder: episodes of major depression, mania, or hypomania that occur during a particular season

Serotonin syndrome: a serious and sometimes fatal reaction characterized by hypertensive crisis, hyperpyrexia, extreme agitation progressing to delirium and coma, muscle rigidity, and seizures, may occur due to combined therapy with a selective serotonin reuptake inhibitor (SSRI) and a monoamine oxidase (MAO) inhibitor or another drug that potentiates serotonin neurotransmission

INTRODUCTION

Mood disorders include depression (Box 55.1), dysthymia, bipolar disorder, and cyclothymia. Major depressive disorder is relatively common in adults, and it also occurs in children and adolescents. This chapter focuses on depression and antidepressant drugs as well as bipolar disorder and mood-stabilizing drugs.

OVERVIEW OF DEPRESSION

Depression, the most common mental illness, is characterized by depressed mood, feeling of sadness, or emotional upset. It occurs in people of all ages. The symptoms of depression interfere with everyday life for several weeks or longer. In 2020, the prevalence rate of a major depressive episode among U.S. adults age 18 years or older was 21 million individuals, which represented 8.4% of all U.S. adults (National Institutes of Health, 2020). The prevalence of depression among females is 10.5% compared to males at 6.2%. The most common age range of individuals with a major depressive episode is 18 to 25 years with a 17% prevalence. It is difficult to determine the overall incidence of depression in the United States, because only 50% of the people who meet the criteria for depression (see Box 55.1) seek help. Depression is not a normal part of aging, and it is a common problem among older adults. Life changes are great contributors to depression in the older adult—for example, acute and chronic health problems, or the death of a spouse, significant others, relatives, or close friends. Depression has no particular racial affinity. For further details on the etiology and pathophysiology of depression, visit thePoint® http://thePoint.lww.com/Frandsen13e.

Clinical Manifestations

Box 55.1 outlines the clinical manifestations of depression. Behavioral changes, especially anxiety, agitation, panic attacks, insomnia, irritability, hostility, impulsivity, akathisia, hypomania, and mania, may indicate worsening depression or suicidality.

BOX 55.1 *Types and Symptoms of Mood Disorders*

Depression

Mild depression occurs in everyone as a normal response to life stresses and losses and usually does not require treatment; severe or major depression is a psychiatric illness and requires treatment. Major depression also is categorized as unipolar, in which people of usually normal moods experience recurrent episodes of depression.

Major Depression, Seasonal Affective Disorder, and Postpartum Depression

Major depression is noted to be present for 2 weeks with the patient having a distinct change in the previous level of functioning. The symptoms of depression include

- Feelings of hopelessness or sadness
- Lack of interest in daily activities
- Loss of sleep or excessive sleep
- Weight loss or weight gain
- Fear and anxiousness
- Lack of self-worth
- Agitation
- Unexplained physiologic symptoms
- Suicidal ideations

Seasonal affective disorder is episodes of major depression, mania, or hypomania that occurs during a particular season. Most commonly, this occurs in winter and resolves in spring and summer. However, it can also occur in spring and summer. Treatment generally involves the use of psychotherapy and/or antidepressants.

- Fall and winter onset: The patient experiences increased sleep and appetite with carbohydrate craving and increase weight.
- Spring and summer onset: The patient experiences insomnia, decreased sleep, decreased appetite, and weight loss.

Postpartum depression is a major depressive episode occurring after the birth of a child. This is a condition in which a postpartum parent develops depressive symptoms. These symptoms can be mild and termed the baby blues or present as major depression. Risk factors for postpartum depression include previous depression, antenatal depression, and high levels of postnatal stress. Additional factors that can contribute to postpartum depression are stressful life events, such as marital conflict, single parenting, multiparity, intimate partner violence, lack of financial and social support, or unwanted pregnancy. Treatment for postpartum depression is psychotherapy and antidepressants.

Bipolar Disorder

Bipolar disorder involves episodes of depression alternating with episodes of mania. The chapter section *Overview of Bipolar Disorder* provides greater detail about the symptoms and subtypes of this disorder.

Drug Therapy

Antidepressant therapy may be indicated if depressive symptoms persist at least 2 weeks, impair social relationships or work performance, and occur independently of life events. Antidepressants are used to regulate mood specifically affecting serotonin, norepinephrine, and dopamine. Antidepressant effects are attributed to changes in receptors rather than changes in neurotransmitters. Although some of the drugs act more selectively on one neurotransmission system than another initially, this selectivity seems to be lost with chronic administration. Drugs used in the pharmacologic management of depressive disorders are derived from several chemical groups. Older antidepressants include the tricyclic antidepressants (TCAs) and the monoamine oxidase (MAO) inhibitors. The selective serotonin reuptake inhibitors (SSRIs), the serotonin–norepinephrine reuptake inhibitors (SNRIs), and several adjuvant atypical antidepressant drugs that differ from TCAs and MAO inhibitors are more commonly prescribed. As the name implies, reuptake inhibitors block the reuptake of certain neurotransmitters (serotonin with the SSRIs and serotonin and norepinephrine with the SNRIs). Table 55.1 lists the drugs used to treat depression. The mood-stabilizing section lists some atypical antipsychotics.

General characteristics of antidepressants include the following:

- All are effective in relieving depression, but they differ in their adverse effects.
- People must take them for 2 to 4 weeks before depressive symptoms improve.
- Administration is oral. Absorbed from the small bowel, they enter the portal circulation and circulate through the liver, where they undergo extensive first-pass metabolism before reaching the systemic circulation.
- Metabolism is by the cytochrome P450 (CYP) enzymes in the liver. Thus, antidepressants may interact with each other and with a wide variety of drugs that are normally metabolized by the same subgroups of enzymes. Additionally, there is a documented ethnic variation (pharmacogenomics or pharmacoethnicity) in response to antidepressants (Box 55.2).

TABLE 55.1 Drugs Administered for the Treatment of Depression

Drug Class	Prototype	Other Drugs in the Class
Antidepressants		
Tricyclic antidepressants	Imipramine	Amitriptyline Amoxapine Clomipramine (Anafranil) Desipramine (Norpramin) Doxepin (Silenor) Nortriptyline (Pamelor) Protriptyline hydrochloride Trimipramine
Selective serotonin reuptake inhibitors (SSRIs)	Fluoxetine (PROzac)	Citalopram (Celexa) Escitalopram (Lexapro) Fluvoxamine (Luvox) Paroxetine (Paxil, Paxil CR, Brisdelle, Pexeva) Sertraline (Zoloft) Vilazodone (Viibryd, Viibryd Starter Pack)
Serotonin–norepinephrine reuptake inhibitors (SNRIs)	Venlafaxine (Effexor XR)	Desvenlafaxine (Pristiq) Duloxetine (Cymbalta, Drizalma Sprinkle) Levomilnacipran (Fetzima, Fetzima Titration) Milnacipran (Savella, Savella Titration Pack) Nefazodone
Monoamine oxidase (MAO) inhibitors	Phenelzine (Nardil)	Isocarboxazid (Marplan) Selegiline hydrochloride (Emsam, Zelapar) Tranylcypromine (Parnate)
Atypical antidepressants		Bupropion (Aplenzin, Wellbutrin SR, Wellbutrin XL) Mirtazapine (Remeron) Trazodone
Mood-stabilizing agents	Lithium carbonate (Lithobid)	Aripiprazole (Abilify, Abilify Maintena, Abilify MyCite) Ketamine (Ketalar) Olanzapine (ZyPREXA, ZyPREXA Relprevv, ZyPREXA Zydis) Quetiapine (Seroquel) Olanzapine–fluoxetine (Symbyax) Risperidone (Perseris, RisperDAL, RisperDAL Consta) Ziprasidone (Geodon)

BOX 55.2 — Genetic and Ethnic Differences in Response to Antidepressant Drug Therapy

Genetic factors are known to influence metabolism of antidepressant agents. This pharmacokinetics can affect the dose required to achieve a therapeutic antidepressant serum concentration. Genetic or ethnic variations in the cytochrome P450 2D6 (CYP2D6) may be attributed to greater rates of metabolism of antidepressants. Rush (2023) reported the following pharmacogenomic information of patients who may metabolize rapidly due to the genetic polymorphisms of hepatic enzymes and who thus require larger doses of antidepressants:

- African Americans: 5%
- Asian Americans: rarely seen
- Ethiopians (Black population): 16% to 29%
- Saudi Arabians: 20%
- White population:
  - Spain: 7% to 10%
  - Sweden: 1% to 2%
  - United States: 4%

Because the available drugs have similar efficacy in treating depression, the choice of an antidepressant depends on the patient's age; medical condition; previous history of drug response, if any; and the specific drug's adverse effects. Also, prescribers often use the side effect profile to help determine the best choice for a specific patient. In addition, cost is a factor to consider. Although the newer drugs are much more expensive than the TCAs, they may be more cost-effective overall because TCAs are more likely to cause serious adverse effects, they require monitoring of plasma drug levels and electrocardiograms (ECGs), and patients are more likely to stop taking them.

It is important to note that sudden termination of most antidepressants results in **antidepressant discontinuation syndrome**. The typical symptoms may occur more rapidly and may be more intense with drugs that have a short half-life and/or used for long periods of time. In general, symptoms include flulike symptoms, insomnia, nausea, imbalance, sensory disturbances, and hyperarousal. To avoid this syndrome, it is essential to taper the dosage of the antidepressant and discontinue it gradually, over 6 to 8 weeks, unless severe drug toxicity, anaphylactic reaction, or another life-threatening condition is present. The occurrence of withdrawal symptoms may indicate skipped doses or abrupt discontinuation of the drug.

Quality and Safety Alert: Evidence-Based Practice

Marasine et al. (2021) examined the use of antidepressants for the treatment of depression. Depression is a major global problem that can result in a lifetime of symptoms and resulting disability. The researchers examined and summarized studies on antidepressant use among patients diagnosed with depression from the following journals: *Method, PubMed, Embase, Web of Science, Scopus,* and *Google Literature* (2000 to 2019). The researchers found that females were the primary users of antidepressants. Since females were more likely to use antidepressants, the examined studies ascertain that alterations in hormone regulation cause a dysregulation of response to stress. In addition, females play multiple roles in both the family and society, thus increasing stress. The selective serotonin reuptake inhibitors (SSRIs) were the antidepressant agents primarily used. The SSRIs are preferred over other drug classes because of fewer side effects and greater tolerability.

OVERVIEW OF BIPOLAR DISORDER

Bipolar disorder is a mood disorder in which people alternate between periods of depression and overexcitement or mania. There are two subtypes of this disorder, which are defined by the presentation of the mood disorder. Bipolar disorder type I is characterized by episodes of major depression plus mania. **Mania** is an emotional disorder characterized by euphoria or irritability. Bipolar disorder type I with mania occurs equally in males and females. Bipolar disorder type II is characterized by episodes of major depression plus episodes of hypomania. **Hypomania** is a persistent irritable mood with the absence of psychotic symptoms characteristic of true mania. Hypomania occurs more frequently in females. Bipolar spectrum disorder broadens the definition of bipolar disorder to include conditions such as cyclothymia. **Cyclothymia** is a mild type of bipolar disorder involving periods of hypomania and depression that do not meet the criteria for mania and major depression. **Dysthymia** is a chronically depressed mood and at least two other symptoms of depression (e.g., depressed mood, feelings of sadness, or emotional upset) for 2 years. Dysthymia occurs in people of all ages. The prevalence of bipolar disorder in adults is dependent on the population and area in which it is studied. Stovall (2022) reported that, on a nationally representative sample of adults, the estimated lifetime prevalence of bipolar I was 1% and bipolar II was 1.1%. The mean age of onset for bipolar I and II is 18 to 20 years of age.

Clinical Manifestations

Bipolar disorder manifests with unpredictable mood swings. In the manic phase, clinical manifestations include excessive happiness and energy, excitement, racing thoughts, restlessness, decreased need for sleep, high sex drive, and a tendency to make grandiose statements and unattainable plans. During a depressive episode, manifestations include sadness, lack of energy, increased need for sleep, uncontrollable crying, changes in appetite, and thoughts of suicide.

Drug Therapy

Research has shown that mood-stabilizing drugs such as lithium stimulate neuronal growth and reduce brain atrophy in people with long-standing mood disorders. Table 55.1 lists some mood-stabilizing drugs.

TRICYCLIC ANTIDEPRESSANTS

TCAs are the oldest antidepressants, although they are now second-line drugs for the treatment of depression. **Imipramine** is the prototype. A patient's previous response or susceptibility to adverse effects may be the basis for initial selection of TCAs. For example, if a patient (or a close family member) once responded well to a particular drug, that drug is probably the drug of choice for repeated episodes of depression. The response of family members to individual drugs may be significant because there is a strong genetic component to depression and drug response. If therapeutic effects do not occur within 4 weeks, it is probably necessary to discontinue or change the TCA, because some patients tolerate or respond better to one TCA than to another. For patients with suicidal tendencies, beginning an SSRI or another newer drug is preferred over a TCA due to the safety profile.

Pharmacokinetics

Imipramine is well absorbed after oral administration, and the drug is widely distributed in body tissues. Peak levels occur in 2 to 6 hours, and the duration of action is unknown. Its half-life is 8 to 21 hours. Imipramine is metabolized in the liver by CYP2D6 enzymes to the active metabolite, desipramine, and inactive metabolites. It goes through significant first-pass metabolism. Imipramine is excreted primarily in the urine as metabolites.

Action

Imipramine blocks the reuptake of norepinephrine and serotonin at the presynaptic nerve endings, increasing the action of both neurotransmitters. The drug's use in enuresis may be due to the fact that imipramine also blocks acetylcholine receptors.

Use

Imipramine may be useful in the treatment of depression. Prescribers may order it for children and adolescents in the management of **enuresis** (bed wetting or involuntary urination resulting from a physical or psychological disorder) after physical causes (e.g., urethral irritation, excessive intake of fluids) have been ruled out. Table 55.2 contains route and dosage information for imipramine and the other TCAs.

Patient-related variables specific to the use of imipramine include the following:

- Age:
  - TCAs are more toxic in overdose than other antidepressants, and suicide is a leading cause of death in adolescents. The U.S. Food and Drug Administration (FDA) has issued a **BOXED WARNING** ◆ alerting healthcare providers to the increased risk of suicidal ideation in children, adolescents, and young adults 18 to 24 years of age who are taking antidepressants, including imipramine.
  - Clinical trials have shown imipramine and other TCAs have not been superior to placebo for the treatment of depression in children and adolescents. TCAs are not recommended as first-line agents, although they may be beneficial in patients with attention deficit hyperactivity disorder or enuresis.
  - Imipramine is identified on the Key Potentially Inappropriate Drugs in Pediatrics and should be used with caution due to the risk of sudden cardiac arrest.
  - In older adults, the dosage of imipramine should be reduced to 10 to 25 mg/day.
  - Imipramine may cause or aggravate conditions common in older adults (e.g., cardiac conduction abnormalities, urinary retention, narrow-angle glaucoma). In addition, impaired compensatory mechanisms make older adults more likely to experience anticholinergic effects, confusion, orthostatic hypotension, and sedation. It is important to monitor vital signs, serum drug levels, and ECGs regularly.
- Reproduction, pregnancy, and lactation:
  - Congenital abnormalities have been reported in humans.
  - TCAs may be associated with irritability, jitteriness, and convulsions in the neonate.
  - Pregnant patients exposed to TCAs should be enrolled in the National Pregnancy Registry for Antidepressants.
  - Imipramine use during breast-feeding would usually not be expected to cause adverse effects in breastfed infants, especially if the infant is older than 2 months (2022a).
- Abnormal kidney function and hepatic impairment:
  - Use with caution in patients with abnormal kidney function or hepatic impairment. No dosage adjustments are recommended by the manufacturer.
- Specific healthcare environments:
  - Surgery: Antidepressants, including imipramine, warrant very cautious use perioperatively because of the risk of serious adverse effects and interactions with anesthetics and other commonly used drugs. It is necessary to discontinue imipramine several days before elective surgery and resume it several days after surgery.
  - Critical Care: Adverse effects common with imipramine use (e.g., confusion, dysrhythmias, tachycardia, orthostatic hypotension, urinary retention) are a concern and may further compromise patients who are critically ill.
  - Home Care: The nurse who sees a patient taking imipramine in the home setting should assess the patient for improvement of symptoms, appropriate administration of the drug, and management of adverse effects, particularly safety factors. A nurse visiting the home for other reasons should observe for signs of depression; health concerns may precipitate symptoms.

Adverse Effects

Adverse effects of imipramine include sedation, orthostatic hypotension, cardiac dysrhythmias, anticholinergic symptoms (e.g., blurred vision, dry mouth, constipation, urinary retention), and weight gain. Symptoms of TCA overdose occur 1 to 4 hours after drug ingestion. They consist primarily of CNS depression and cardiovascular effects (e.g., nystagmus, tremor, restlessness, seizures, hypotension, dysrhythmias, myocardial depression). Death usually results from cardiac, respiratory, and circulatory failure.

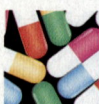

TABLE 55.2
DRUGS AT A GLANCE: Tricyclic Antidepressants

Drug	Routes and Dosage Ranges	
	Adults	**Children**
ⓟ Imipramine	75 mg PO daily initially in divided doses or a single bedtime dose, gradually increased to 150 mg daily if necessary; maintenance dose, 5–150 mg PO daily; max dosage of 200 mg daily Older adults: PO 10–25 mg daily at bedtime	≥8 y: 1.5 mg/kg/d in 2–3 divided doses; max daily dosage 5 mg/kg/d Adolescents: 25–50 mg PO daily in divided doses, increased to max dosage of 100 mg daily if necessary Children >6 y (enuresis): 25–50 mg PO 1 h before bedtime
Amitriptyline (✦ AG-Amitriptyline, Amitriptyline-10, Amitriptyline-25, APO-Amitriptyline, JAMP-Amitriptyline)	25–50 mg PO initially once daily at bedtime or in divided doses, gradually increased to 100–300 mg daily if necessary Older adults: 10–25 mg PO at bedtime; increase dose gradually based on response and tolerability to 25–50 mg increments at intervals of ≥1 week up to usual dose of 100–300 mg/d	Children: 9 to <12 y: 1 mg/kg/d in three divided doses after 3 days, dose may be increased to 1.5 mg/kg/d in three divided doses Adolescents: 10 mg PO three times daily and 20 mg at bedtime
Amoxapine	25–50 mg PO three times daily; may be increased to 100 mg 2–3 times daily by the end of the first week based on response and tolerability; may be titrated to 600 mg daily in divided doses	Not approved for use in children
Clomipramine (Anafranil; ✦ Anafranil)	Obsessive–compulsive disorder: 25 mg PO daily, increased to 100 mg daily by end of 2 wk, in divided doses, with meals; give maintenance dose in a single dose at bedtime; max dose 250 mg daily	≥10 y: 25 mg PO initially daily, increased to 3 mg/kg/d or 200 mg/d, whichever is less, over 2 wk. Give maintenance dose in a single dose at bedtime. Max dose 3 mg/kg or 200 mg, whichever is less
Desipramine (Norpramin; ✦ Dom-Desipramine, Nu-Desipramine)	25–50 mg PO daily in divided doses or as a single daily dose; usual maintenance dose 100–200 once daily or in divided doses; max dose 300 mg/d Older adults: 25–100 mg PO daily in divided doses or as a single daily dose; max dose 150 mg/d	6–12 y: 1–3 mg/kg/d PO in divided doses; monitor carefully with doses >3 mg/kg/d; maximum daily dose: 5 mg/kg/d Adolescents: 25–100 mg PO daily in divided doses or as a single daily dose; max dose 150 mg/d
Doxepin (Silenor; ✦ NOVO-Doxepin, Silenor, SINEquan)	Depression: 25–50 mg PO initially daily in divided doses or a single dose at bedtime; max dose 300 mg/d Insomnia: 3–6 mg PO once daily 30 min before bedtime	7–11 y: 1–3 mg/kg/d in single or divided doses ≥12 y: 25–75 mg/d PO initially at bedtime or in 2–3 divided doses; max single dose 150 mg or 300 mg daily
Nortriptyline (Pamelor; ✦ APO-Nortriptyline, Aventyl)	25 mg PO three or four times daily or in a single dose (75–100 mg) at bedtime; max dose 150 mg/d Older adults: 30–50 mg/d PO in divided doses or a single dose once daily	Depression: 6–12 y: 1–3 mg/kg/d in 4 divided doses; max dose 150 mg/d Depression: Adolescents: 30–50 mg/d PO in 3–4 divided doses or a single dose once daily; max dose 150 mg/d Enuresis: ≥6–12 y: 10–20 mg PO per day; maximum dose: 40 mg/d
Protriptyline hydrochloride	10–20 mg PO divided in 3–4 doses; gradually increase based on response	Adolescents: 5 mg PO three times per day; gradually titrate based on response; maximum dose 60 mg/d
Trimipramine (✦ APO-Trimipramine)	25–50 mg PO daily at bedtime or in divided doses; initial doses 100 mg PO daily for hospitalized patients	Adolescents: ≤50 mg daily at bedtime or in divided doses; gradually increase based on tolerability; maximum dose: 100 mg/d

TCAs are associated with clearly defined withdrawal syndromes, and these drugs also have strong anticholinergic effects. When they are abruptly discontinued, cholinergic rebound may occur. Symptoms include hypersalivation, diarrhea, urinary urgency, abdominal cramping, and sweating.

Contraindications

Contraindications to imipramine include known sensitivity to the drug and immediately postacute myocardial infarction.

Nursing Implications

Preventing Interactions

Several drugs interact with imipramine. The drug may inhibit the metabolism of other drugs, including antidepressants, phenothiazines, carbamazepine, flecainide, and propafenone. The use of imipramine and MAO inhibitors concurrently may have serious effects, including severe seizures and death. Alcohol may increase the sedative effects of imipramine. The herb St. John's wort may reduce the blood levels of imipramine and other TCAs. St. John's wort and yohimbe increase the patient's risk of developing serotonin syndrome. Grapefruit juice can inhibit the metabolism of imipramine and other TCAs.

Administering the Medication

People should take imipramine at bedtime to aid sleep and decrease daytime sedation. Overall, with TCAs, it is best to begin with small doses, which are increased to the desired dose over 1 to 2 weeks. Administration once or twice daily is possible because the drug has a long elimination half-life. Measurement of plasma levels is helpful in adjusting drug dosages.

Assessing for Therapeutic Effects

The nurse is aware of patient statements about feeling better or less depressed. The nurse observes for increased appetite, physical activity, and interest in surroundings; improved sleep patterns; improved appearance; decreased anxiety; and decreased somatic complaints. Mood elevation may take 2 to 3 weeks or longer. Note that it may even take 4 to 8 weeks of treatment before a patient may experience a response, partial response, or no response to imipramine.

Assessing for Adverse Effects

The nurse observes for CNS effects, gastrointestinal (GI) effects, cardiovascular effects, and other effects. Because imipramine may have adverse effects on the heart, especially in overdose, experts recommend baseline and follow-up ECGs for all patients. In addition, it is important to assess for suicidal thoughts or plans, especially at the beginning of therapy or when dosages are increased or decreased.

Patient Teaching

Box 55.3 presents patient teaching guidelines for the antidepressants, including the TCAs.

Other Drugs in the Class

Commonly used TCAs include amitriptyline, clomipramine (Anafranil), desipramine (Norpramin), doxepin (Silenor), and nortriptyline (Pamelor). Amitriptyline, desipramine, and nortriptyline are the TCAs most commonly prescribed to treat depression in children older than 12 years of age although they are not first-line agents. The FDA has approved clomipramine for treatment of obsessive–compulsive disorder in children. In general, amitriptyline, clomipramine, desipramine, doxepin, and nortriptyline are similar to imipramine in terms of adverse effects. Amitriptyline and doxepin are more likely to cause weight gain. Desipramine is more likely to cause drowsiness. These TCAs are effective; however, antidepressants that produce fewer adverse effects are increasingly replacing them.

Amoxapine is used to relieve symptoms of depression in patients with reactive or neurotic disorders. It is also effective in treating endogenous and psychotic disorders. According to the Beers Criteria, amoxapine should be avoided in patients older than 65 years because this drug has strong anticholinergic properties that produce sedation and orthostatic hypotension.

Trimipramine is used for depression in adults. This drug also has strong anticholinergic properties. It can be used in the geriatric population; the dose is 50 mg daily, which can be increased to 100 mg daily. The lowest effective dose should be administered at bedtime. It is necessary to monitor blood pressure and pulse rate with initial therapy.

NCLEX Success

1. Which of the following adverse effects of imipramine is considered the most serious?
   A. dry mouth
   B. constipation
   C. urinary retention
   D. orthostatic hypotension

SELECTIVE SEROTONIN REUPTAKE INHIBITORS

SSRIs, of which **fluoxetine** (PROzac, Sarafem) is the prototype, produce fewer serious adverse effects than the TCAs. (SSRIs are called "selective" because they seem to primarily affect serotonin and not other neurotransmitters.) The drugs of first choice in the treatment of depression, SSRIs are effective and usually produce fewer and milder adverse effects than other antidepressants. There are no guidelines for choosing one SSRI over another.

Pharmacokinetics

Fluoxetine is well absorbed with oral administration, with a peak of action of 6 to 8 hours. The half-life of elimination for the parent drug is 2 to 3 days; this may lead to accumulation with chronic administration. (An active metabolite has a half-life of 7 to 9 days.) Thus, steady-state blood levels are achieved slowly,

BOX 55.3 Patient Teaching Guidelines for Antidepressants

General Considerations

- Do not alter doses of antidepressants when symptoms subside; these drugs are usually given for several months, perhaps years.
- Be aware that therapeutic effects (relief of symptoms) may not occur for 2 to 4 weeks after drug therapy is started. As a result, it is very important not to think the drug is ineffective and stop taking it prematurely. Continue to take the drug even if you feel better to prevent the return of depression.
- Do not take other prescription or over-the-counter drugs, including cold remedies, without consulting a healthcare provider. Potentially serious drug interactions may occur.
- Do not take the herbal supplement St. John's wort while taking a prescription antidepressant. Serious interactions may occur.
- Inform any physician, surgeon, dentist, or nurse practitioner about the antidepressants being taken. Potentially serious adverse effects or drug interactions may occur if certain other drugs are prescribed.
- Avoid activities that require alertness and physical coordination (e.g., driving a car, operating other machinery) until reasonably sure the medication does not make you drowsy or impair your ability to perform the activities safely.
- Avoid alcohol and other CNS depressants (e.g., any drugs that cause drowsiness). Excessive drowsiness, dizziness, difficulty breathing, and low blood pressure may occur, with potentially serious consequences.
- Learn the name and type of the prescribed antidepressant to help avoid undesirable interactions with other drugs or a physician prescribing other drugs with similar effects. There are several different types of antidepressants, with different characteristics and precautions for safe and effective usage.
- Do not stop taking any antidepressant without discussing it with a healthcare provider. If a problem occurs, the type of drug, the dose, or other aspects may be changed to solve the problem and allow continued use of the medication.
- Understand that counseling, support groups, relaxation techniques, and other nonpharmacologic treatments are recommended along with drug therapy.
- Notify your physician if you become pregnant or intend to become pregnant during therapy with antidepressants.

Self- or Caregiver Administration

- With a tricyclic antidepressant (e.g., amitriptyline), take at bedtime to aid sleep and decrease adverse effects. Also, report urinary retention, fainting, irregular heartbeat, seizures, restlessness, and mental confusion. These are potentially serious adverse drug effects.
- With a selective serotonin reuptake inhibitor, take the drug in the morning because it may interfere with sleep if taken at bedtime.
  - In addition, notify a healthcare provider if a skin rash or other allergic reaction occurs. Allergic reactions are uncommon but may require that the drug be discontinued.
  - Recognize the importance of follow-up and seeking professional help for the signs of dizziness or insomnia or other symptoms that negatively affect your life.
  - Do not combine fluoxetine with dextromethorphan cough suppressant due to the risk of visual hallucinations.
- Realize that escitalopram (Lexapro) is a derivative of citalopram (Celexa). The two medications should not be taken concomitantly.
- With venlafaxine (Effexor), take as directed or ask for instructions. This drug is often taken twice daily. Notify a healthcare provider if a skin rash or other allergic reaction occurs. An allergic reaction may require that the drug be discontinued.
- With venlafaxine, use effective birth control methods while taking this drug. Pregnancy is a contraindication.
- With duloxetine and desvenlafaxine, swallow the medication whole; do not crush, chew, or sprinkle capsule contents on food.
- With phenelzine and other monoamine oxidase inhibitors, avoid foods that contain tyramine or tyrosine to prevent the risk of hypertensive crisis. This includes aged cheeses, coffee, chocolate, wine, bananas, avocados, fava beans, and most fermented and pickled foods.
- Bupropion is a unique drug prescribed for depression (brand name, Wellbutrin) and for smoking cessation (brand name, Zyban). It is extremely important not to increase the dose or take the two brand names at the same time (as might happen with different physicians or filling prescriptions at different pharmacies). Overdoses may cause seizures as well as other adverse effects. When used for smoking cessation, Zyban is recommended for up to 12 weeks if progress is being made. If significant progress is not made by approximately 7 weeks, it is considered unlikely that longer drug use will be helpful.
- Know that there are short-, intermediate-, and long-acting forms of bupropion that are taken three times, two times, or one time per day, respectively. Be sure to take your medication as prescribed.
- Make sure that you and the people you live with are familiar with the signs and symptoms of worsening depression and know how to seek help for signs of overdose.

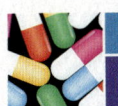

TABLE 55.3
DRUGS AT A GLANCE: Selective Serotonin Reuptake Inhibitors (SSRIs)

Drug	Routes and Dosage Ranges	
	Adults	**Children**
Fluoxetine (PROzac, AG-Fluoxetine, APO-Fluoxetine)	20 mg PO once daily in the morning, increased after several weeks if necessary. Give doses larger than 20 mg once in the morning or in two divided doses, morning and noon. Max daily dose 60 mg Prozac weekly (delayed-release capsules) 90 mg PO once each week, starting 7 d after the last 20-mg dose	8 to <12 y for depression: 5–10 mg/d PO; may increase to 20 mg/d after 1 wk if necessary >12 y and adolescents 10–20 mg PO may increase in 10–20 mg increments every 1–2 weeks; usual effective dose: 20–40 mg; maximum dose: 60 mg
Citalopram (Celexa; ACCEL-Citalopram, ACT-Citalopram, AG-Citalopram, AURO-Citalopram)	20 mg PO initially once daily, morning or evening, increased to max dose of 40 mg daily in 1 wk, if necessary Older adults/hepatic impairment: 20 mg PO daily	≥7 y: 10 mg PO once daily; increase dose slowly by 10 mg/d every 1–2 weeks as clinically needed; maximum dose 40 mg
Escitalopram (Lexapro; ACH-Escitalopram, Cipralex)	10 mg PO once daily; may increase to max dose of 20 mg after minimum of 1 wk of therapy	≥12 y: 10 mg PO once daily; may increase to max dose of 20 mg if symptoms do not lessen within 3 wk of therapy
Paroxetine (Paxil, Paxil CR, Pexeva; ACT-PARoxetine, AG-Paroxetine, APO-PARoxetine, Auro-PARoxetine, DOM-PARoxetine, Paxil, Paxil CR, Sandoz PARoxetine)	20 mg PO once daily in the morning, increased at 1 wk or longer intervals, if necessary; usual range 20–50 mg/d; max dose 50 mg/d Controlled-release (CR) tablets: 25 mg PO once daily in the morning, increase up to 62.5 mg/d max if necessary Older or debilitated adults: 10 mg PO once daily, increase if necessary; maximum dose 40 mg Severe abnormal kidney function or hepatic impairment: same as for older adults	OCD: 7–17 y: immediate release: 10 mg PO once daily; titrate every 7–14 days in 10 mg/d increments; maximum dose: 60 mg/d
Sertraline (Zoloft; AG-Sertraline, APO-Sertraline, Auro-Sertraline MINT-Sertraline, Mylan-Sertraline, Zoloft)	Depression, OCD: 50 mg PO once daily morning or evening, increase at 1-wk or longer intervals to a max daily dose of 200 mg Panic disorder, PTSD: 25 mg PO once daily, increase after 1 wk to 50 mg once daily; max dosage 200 mg daily	OCD: ≥6 y, 25 mg PO once daily, increase dose in increments of 25–50 mg to a max daily dose of 200 mg Adolescents: 50 mg PO once daily, increase dose in increments of 25–50 mg to a max daily dose of 200 mg
Vilazodone (Viibryd, Viibryd Starter Pack; Viibryd, Viibryd Starter Pack)	Major depressive disorder: 10 mg PO once daily for 7 days, then increase to 20 mg once daily, maximum dose: 40 mg once daily	Not approved in children

OCD, obsessive–compulsive disorder; PTSD, posttraumatic stress disorder.

over several weeks, and drug effects decrease slowly (over 2 to 3 months) when fluoxetine is discontinued. The drug is present in breast milk. Metabolism takes place in the liver, and excretion predominately occurs in the kidneys.

Action

Fluoxetine blocks the reabsorption of the neurotransmitter serotonin in the brain. This helps elevate the patient's mood. Fluoxetine has no effect on the norepinephrine or dopamine.

Use

Uses for fluoxetine include the treatment of depression and its associated anxiety, obsessive–compulsive disorder, bulimia nervosa, and premenstrual dysphoric disorder. Table 55.3 gives the route and dosage information for fluoxetine and other SSRIs.

Patient-related variables specific to the use of fluoxetine include the following:

- Age:
  - The FDA has issued a **BOXED WARNING** alerting healthcare providers to the increased risk of suicidal ideation in children, adolescents, and young adults 18 to 24 years of age when taking antidepressant medications, including fluoxetine.
  - Children with abnormal kidney function or hepatic impairment have an increased risk of adverse drug effects.
  - In older adults, fluoxetine and other SSRIs are the drugs of choice because they produce fewer sedative,

- anticholinergic, cardiotoxic, and psychomotor adverse effects than the TCAs and related antidepressants.
  - Elimination may be slower, and smaller or less frequent doses may be prudent in older adults.
  - Weight loss is often associated with SSRIs and may be undesirable in older adults.
  - Use of maintenance antidepressant therapy is beneficial to prevent recurrence of depression in older adults.
- Reproduction, pregnancy, and lactation:
  - Use cautiously during pregnancy and only if the benefit outweighs the risk to the fetus.
  - Fluoxetine is present in breast milk. Breast-feeding is not recommended.
- Abnormal kidney function and hepatic impairment:
  - No dosage adjustments with abnormal kidney function.
  - Hepatic impairment leads to reduced first-pass metabolism of fluoxetine and most antidepressant drugs, resulting in higher plasma levels. Thus, caution is warranted in severe liver impairment.
- Specific healthcare environments:
  - Patients who are critically ill may need a drug to combat the depression that often develops with major illness. The decision to start fluoxetine should involve a thorough assessment of the patient's condition, other drugs being given, and potential adverse drug effects.
  - Antidepressants, including fluoxetine, warrant caution perioperatively because of the risk of serious adverse effects and adverse interactions with anesthetics and other commonly used drugs.

Adverse effects of fluoxetine include a high incidence of GI symptoms (e.g., nausea, diarrhea, and weight loss) and sexual dysfunction (e.g., delayed ejaculation in males, impaired orgasmic ability in females). Most SSRIs also cause some degree of CNS stimulation (e.g., anxiety, nervousness, insomnia), which is most prominent with fluoxetine. These drugs are also associated with increased risk of GI bleeding. For patients with diabetes mellitus, SSRIs may have a hypoglycemic effect.

Serotonin syndrome, a serious and sometimes fatal reaction characterized by hypertensive crisis, hyperpyrexia, extreme agitation progressing to delirium and coma, muscle rigidity, and seizures, may occur due to combined therapy with an SSRI and an MAO inhibitor or another drug that potentiates serotonin neurotransmission. It is important not to take an SSRI or SNRI and an MAO inhibitor concurrently or within 2 weeks of each other. In most cases, if a patient taking an SSRI is transferred to an MAO inhibitor, it is necessary to discontinue the SSRI at least 14 days before starting the MAO inhibitor. However, the patient should discontinue fluoxetine at least 5 weeks before starting an MAO inhibitor due to the prolonged half-life.

As previously discussed, antidepressant discontinuation syndrome can occur with sudden termination of the SSRIs. Withdrawal symptoms include dizziness, GI upset, lethargy or anxiety/hyperarousal, dysphoria, sleep problems, and headache, which can last from several days to several weeks. More serious symptoms may include aggression, hypomania, mood disturbances, and suicidal tendencies. Fluoxetine, with its long half-life, has not been associated with withdrawal symptoms.

Contraindications

Contraindications to fluoxetine include known sensitivity to the drug as well as the use of MAO inhibitors or thioridazine.

Quality and Safety Alert: Safety

People of any age who have attempted suicide should not receive fluoxetine.

Nursing Implications

Preventing Interactions

Because fluoxetine and other SSRIs are highly bound to plasma proteins, they compete with endogenous compounds and other medications for binding sites, resulting in drug interactions. Several drugs increase the effects of fluoxetine (Box 55.4). Also, CYP2D6 enzymes metabolize fluoxetine; therefore, the drug may cause accumulation of other drugs using this enzyme system (e.g., amitriptyline, imipramine, desipramine, thioridazine). Kava kava, St. John's wort, tryptophan, and valerian may increase sedative and hypnotic effects. They also increase the risk of serotonin syndrome.

Quality and Safety Alert: Safety

Fluoxetine can prevent the conversion of codeine to its active form, resulting in lack of pain relief when the drugs are used concurrently.

Administering the Medication

People typically take SSRIs, including fluoxetine, once daily in the morning to prevent interference with sleep. They may take the drug with food to avoid GI upset. The nurse advises the patient to use sugar-free gum or hard candies to counteract dry mouth.

BOX 55.4 Drug Interactions: Fluoxetine

Drugs That Increase the Effects of Fluoxetine

- Alcohol
  Increases the sedative effect
- Amiodarone, cimetidine, ciprofloxacin, cytochrome P450 2D6 inhibitors (e.g., opioid analgesics, beta-adrenergic blockers, promethazine), and macrolide antibiotics
  Increase the risk of toxicity
- Anticoagulants
  Increase risk of bleeding
- Blood glucose lowering agents
  Increase risk of lowered blood glucose
- Antipsychotics
  Increase risk of serotonin syndrome
- Haloperidol
  Increases the risk of neurologic toxicity
- 5-Hydroxytryptophan
  Increases the risk of serotonin syndrome

Assessing for Therapeutic Effects

The nurse assesses for statements of improved depression. The patient is assessed for improvement in appetite, physical activity, and interest in surroundings; improved sleep patterns; improved appearance; decreased anxiety; and reduced somatic complaints. The patient response to fluoxetine can significantly vary from patient to patient. The full response of the medication may not be seen for 8 to 12 weeks. Therapeutic serum levels of fluoxetine range from 100 to 800 ng/mL.

Assessing for Adverse Effects

The nurse assesses for dizziness, headache, nervousness, insomnia, nausea, diarrhea, dry mouth, sedation, skin rash, and sexual dysfunction.

> **! Quality and Safety Alert: Safety**
>
> It is essential to assess for suicidal thoughts or plans, especially at the beginning of therapy or when dosages are increased or decreased.

Patient Teaching

Box 55.3 contains patient teaching guidelines for the antidepressants, including the SSRIs.

Other Drugs in the Class

Other SSRIs include citalopram (Celexa), escitalopram (Lexapro), paroxetine (Paxil), sertraline (Zoloft), and vilazodone (Viibryd, Viibryd Starter Pack).

Sertraline and citalopram also have active metabolites, but paroxetine, like fluoxetine, is more likely to accumulate. Escitalopram, paroxetine, and sertraline reach steady-state concentrations in 1 to 2 weeks. People may take the drugs in the morning or evening (but at the same time each day). An evening dose may interfere with sleep. The SSRIs are strong inhibitors of the CYP enzyme system, which metabolizes many drugs. As a result, serum drug levels and risks of adverse effects are greatly increased. Most significantly, fluoxetine, paroxetine, and sertraline slow metabolism of bupropion, codeine, desipramine, dextromethorphan, flecainide, metoprolol, nortriptyline, phenothiazines, propranolol, risperidone, and timolol. Vilazodone can produce discontinuation syndrome; its abrupt discontinuation or interruption will produce symptoms including nausea, vomiting, diarrhea, headache, lightheadedness, sweating, chills, tremors, paresthesias, somnolence, and sleep disturbances. Discontinuation of antidepressant treatment should last for greater than 3 weeks.

> **! Quality and Safety Alert: Safety**
>
> With citalopram and escitalopram, poor metabolizers of CYP2C19 or concurrent use of moderate-to-strong CYP2C19 inhibitors (e.g., cimetidine, chloramphenicol, omeprazole) should receive half the maximum dose (20 mg) daily.

Paroxetine, which has a half-life of approximately 24 hours and does not produce active metabolites, may be associated with antidepressant discontinuation syndrome even when discontinued gradually, over 7 to 10 days. Symptoms may include a flulike syndrome with nausea, vomiting, fatigue, muscle aches, dizziness, headache, and insomnia.

> **Clinical Application 55.1**
>
> - Mr. Mehring visits the physician again 2 weeks later. His wife complains that she sees no improvement in her husband's mood and that he is taking too many drugs. How should the nurse respond?

SEROTONIN–NOREPINEPHRINE REUPTAKE INHIBITORS

Like the SSRIs, the SNRIs, of which **venlafaxine** (Effexor XR) is the prototype, inhibit the neuronal uptake of serotonin. In addition, they inhibit the uptake of norepinephrine, increasing the activity of these neurotransmitters in the brain. The SNRIs are similar to SSRIs in terms of therapeutic effects.

Pharmacokinetics and Action

Venlafaxine is well absorbed, extensively metabolized in the liver, and excreted in urine. It crosses the placenta and may enter breast milk.

The drug increases the levels of serotonin and norepinephrine in the brain by preventing the reuptake of these neurotransmitters known to play an important part in mood. The drug also weakly inhibits dopamine reuptake.

Use

SNRIs are a standard first-line treatment for depression and anxiety disorders. Uses for venlafaxine include the treatment of depression, as well as generalized anxiety disorder, social anxiety disorder, and panic disorder. Table 55.4 gives route and dosage information of venlafaxine and the other SNRIs.

Patient-related variables specific to the use of venlafaxine include the following:

- Age:
  - The FDA has issued a **BOXED WARNING** alerting healthcare providers to the increased risk of suicidal ideation in children, adolescents, and young adults 18 to 24 years of age when taking antidepressant medications, including venlafaxine. Children who take the drug are quite likely to experience weight loss.
  - Venlafaxine and other SNRIs are suitable for use in older people, although the weight loss often associated with these drugs may be undesirable. Authorities recommend using smaller initial doses and dosing increments. In addition, there is an increased risk of the syndrome of inappropriate antidiuretic hormone or hyponatremia in older adults; thus, it is necessary to monitor sodium levels frequently.
- Reproduction, pregnancy, and lactation:
  - For patients planning to become pregnant, other antidepressant agents should be considered and venlafaxine should not be administered.

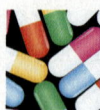

TABLE 55.4
DRUGS AT A GLANCE: Serotonin–Norepinephrine Reuptake Inhibitors

Drug	Routes and Dosage Ranges	
	Adults	**Children**
ⓟ **Venlafaxine** (Effexor XR; 🍁 ACT-Venlafaxine, APO-Venlafaxine XR, Auro-Venlafaxine, DOM-Venlafaxine XR, MYLAN-Venlafaxine XR)	Immediate-release tablets: 37.5–75 mg/d PO initially in 2–3 divided doses with food; increase by ≤75 mg/d (4 d or longer between increments); usual dosage 75–225 mg/d; max dose 375 mg/d Extended-release (XR) capsules: initially, 37.5 or 75 mg/d PO in a single dose, morning or evening; increase by ≤75 mg/d (4 d or longer between increments) usual dosage 75–225 mg/d; max dose 225 mg/d Hepatic or abnormal kidney function: reduce dose by 50% and increase very slowly	≥12 y and Adolescents: 37.5 mg once daily for week 1 then titrate with once daily dosing by the following: increase to 75 mg/d for week 2; increase to 112.5 mg/d for week 3; increase to 150 mg/d for weeks 4–6; if no response after week 6 increase to 225 mg/d.
Desvenlafaxine (Pristiq; 🍁 APO-Desvenlafaxine, Pristiq)	50 mg PO once daily; increases >100 mg daily not recommended	Not approved for use in children and adolescents
Duloxetine (Cymbalta, Drizalma Sprinkle; 🍁 AG-Duloxetine, APO-Duloxetine, Auro-Duloxetine, Cymbalta, JAMP-Duloxetine)	40–60 mg PO daily. Dose may be divided. Increase to 60 mg once daily; max daily dose 120 mg daily Abnormal kidney function: decrease doses	7–17 y: 30 mg once daily; increase to 60 mg once daily; max daily dose 120 mg daily
Levomilnacipran (Fetzima Titration; 🍁 Fetzima)	20 mg PO once daily for 2 days; increase to 40 mg once daily; may then be increased in increments of 40 mg at intervals of 2 or more days Maintenance: 40–120 mg once daily Maximum dose: 120 mg daily	Not approved for use in children and adolescents
Milnacipran (Savella, Savella Titration Pack)	50 mg PO twice daily Titration schedule: 12.5 mg once on day 1; 12.5 mg twice daily on days 2–3; 25 mg twice daily on days 4–7; then, 50 mg twice daily thereafter. Dose may be increased to 100 mg twice daily, based on individual response	Not approved for use in children and adolescents
Nefazodone	Depression: 100 mg PO twice daily, alternatively, depression treatment guidelines suggest starting doses of 50–100 mg/d; gradually increase dose in increments of 100–200 mg/d (in two divided doses) and intervals ≥1 week to a usual dose of 150–600 mg in two divided doses	Not approved for use in children

- Nonteratogenic adverse effects have been observed with venlafaxine or other SSRIs/SNRIs when used in pregnancy.
- Cyanosis, apnea, respiratory distress, seizures, temperature instability, feeding difficulty, vomiting, hypoglycemia, hyper-reflexia, jitteriness, irritability, and constant crying have been reported in the neonate after delivery when exposed in utero in the third trimester of pregnancy.
- Cases of galactorrhea and elevated serum prolactin have been reported. The prolactin level in a patient with established lactation may not affect breast-feeding ability.
- Abnormal kidney function and hepatic impairment:
  - Venlafaxine is excreted by the kidneys; thus, dosage adjustment is necessary in patients with abnormal kidney function.
  - Caution is warranted in patients with hepatic impairment. Prescribers should consider lower doses, longer intervals between doses, and slower dose increases than usual.
- Specific healthcare environments:
  - Patients who are critically ill may need a drug such as venlafaxine to combat the depression that often develops with major illness. It is necessary to make a thorough assessment of the patient's condition, other drugs being given, potential adverse drug effects, and other factors before starting the drug.

Adverse Effects

Adverse effects of venlafaxine, which may be greater than with the SSRIs, include the following:

- CNS effects: anxiety, dizziness, dreams, insomnia, nervousness, somnolence, and tremors
- GI effects: anorexia, weight loss, nausea, vomiting, constipation, and diarrhea

- Cardiovascular effects: hypertension, tachycardia, and vasodilation
- Genitourinary effects: abnormal ejaculation, impotence, and urinary frequency. (The negative effect of venlafaxine on sexual function is less than that reported with the SSRIs.)
- Dermatologic effects: sweating, rash, and pruritus

Contraindications

Contraindications to venlafaxine include known sensitivity to the drug, use of an MAO inhibitor, and pregnancy.

Nursing Implications

Preventing Interactions

Venlafaxine and other SNRIs interact with MAO inhibitors, leading to increased serum levels and the risk of serotonin syndrome. It is necessary to discontinue the MAO inhibitor at least 14 days before starting venlafaxine. St. John's wort combined with venlafaxine will increase the development of serotonin syndrome.

Administering the Medication

People should take venlafaxine with food to decrease its GI effects (e.g., nausea and vomiting). They should take the extended-release formulation in the morning and evening, at approximately the same time. For patients who have difficulty swallowing extended-release capsules, they can be opened and sprinkled on applesauce. The nurse instructs patients to swallow the applesauce and medication without chewing and to follow this by drinking a glass of water. This will ensure all pellets are swallowed.

Assessing for Therapeutic Effects

The nurse assesses for improvement in mood, including improvement in anxiety level, reduced agitation or irritability episodes, decreased number of panic attacks, and ability to sleep through the night.

Assessing for Adverse Effects

The nurse observes for dizziness, headache, nervousness, insomnia, nausea, diarrhea, dizziness, dry mouth, sedation, and skin rash. Also, it is necessary to assess for altered sexual function and provide options and resources for the patient and the significant other. In addition, the nurse evaluates for the occurrence of weight loss. Finally, it is important to monitor for signs of suicidal ideation and hostility.

Patient Teaching

Box 55.3 presents patient teaching guidelines for the antidepressants, including the SNRIs.

Other Drugs in the Class

Desvenlafaxine (Pristiq) and duloxetine (Cymbalta, Drizalma Sprinkle) inhibit the neuronal uptake of serotonin. Desvenlafaxine, a synthetic form of the major active metabolite of venlafaxine, is used to treat major depressive disorder in adults. Duloxetine is commonly used in the treatment of neuropathic pain and relieves painful physical symptoms (e.g., overall pain, backache, shoulder pain) associated with depression, thereby reducing remission rates, and reducing depression-associated anxiety. Levomilnacipran (Fetzima, Fetzima Titration) is administered with or without food at the same time every day. Its primary use is the treatment of major depressive disorder. If a patient is taking nonsteroidal anti-inflammatory drugs or any anticoagulants with levomilnacipran, the nurse instructs the patient that the risk of bleeding is increased. Also, because levomilnacipran has the potential to increase blood pressure and pulse rate, pulse and blood pressure must be monitored closely. If hypertension and tachycardia occur, a dosage reduced is warranted. Milnacipran (Savella, Savella Titration Pack) is a potent inhibitor of norepinephrine and serotonin reuptake. As with other drugs in this class, it is important to monitor blood pressure and pulse rate. In addition, it is necessary to check periodically for increases in intraocular pressure in any patient who has a history of intraocular pressure elevation or glaucoma.

Nefazodone is administered for depression. It can cause life-threatening hepatic failure, resulting in death or transplant, in 1 out of 250,000 to 300,000 patients treated with nefazodone. The patient must be instructed on the risk of liver dysfunction. Nefazodone may be administered with or without food. However, administration with food may decrease absorption and the effectiveness of the medication. In patients who have a history of orthostatic hypotension, the administration of nefazodone may result in transient hypotensive episodes. Instruct patients to use caution when changing positions.

MONOAMINE OXIDASE INHIBITORS

MAO inhibitors are third-line agents for the treatment of depression and are rarely used in clinical practice today, mainly because they may interact with some foods and drugs to produce severe hypertension and possible heart attack or stroke. Prescribers are most likely to order MAO inhibitors when a patient does not respond to other antidepressant drugs or when electroconvulsive therapy is refused or contraindicated. The prototype MAO inhibitor is **P phenelzine** (Nardil).

Pharmacokinetics and Action

Phenelzine is well absorbed and widely distributed. The drug reaches peak levels in 2 to 4 hours, but mood elevation may take 2 to 8 weeks. It is metabolized in the liver and excreted by the kidneys. The drug improves mood by binding irreversibly to MAO, increasing the concentrations of epinephrine, norepinephrine, serotonin, and dopamine in the CNS.

Use

Phenelzine is used to treat depression when other antidepressants have been unsuccessful in symptom management. Table 55.5 gives route and dosage information for this drug and other MAO inhibitors.

Patient-related variables specific to the use of phenelzine include the following:

- Age:
  - Phenelzine and other MAO inhibitors may be more likely to cause hypertensive crises in older adults because their cardiovascular, kidney, and hepatic functions are often diminished.

TABLE 55.5
DRUGS AT A GLANCE: Monoamine Oxidase Inhibitors

Drug	Routes and Dosage Ranges	
	Adults	**Children**
Phenelzine (Nardil; ❋ Nardil)	15 mg PO three times daily; not to exceed 90 mg/d	Not approved for use in children and adolescents
Selegiline (Emsam, Zelapar; ❋ APO-Selegiline, TEVA-Selegiline)	Depression: 6 mg/24 h transdermal, target dose 6 mg/24 h once daily; may titrate based on clinical response in increments of 3 mg/d every 2 weeks up to a maximum of 12 mg/24 h Parkinson disease: 5 mg PO twice daily at breakfast and lunch with concomitant carbidopa/levodopa therapy; maximum 10 mg/d	Depression: Adolescents >17 y: Same as adult dosing
Isocarboxazid (Marplan)	10 mg PO 2–4 times daily; increase to 40 mg by the end of the first week to a max daily dose of 60 mg/d	Not approved for use in children and adolescents
Tranylcypromine (Parnate; ❋ Parnate)	10 mg PO initially; increase in 10-mg intervals every 1–3 wk; usual dosage range 30–60 mg PO daily in divided doses, not to exceed 60 mg/d	Younger than 16 y: not recommended 16 y of age or older: same as adults

- Reproduction, pregnancy, and lactation:
  - Adverse fetal effects have been noted in animal reproduction studies.
  - It is not known if phenelzine is excreted in breast milk.
- Abnormal kidney function and hepatic impairment:
  - The use of phenelzine is contraindicated in patients with abnormal kidney function or hepatic impairment
- Specific healthcare environments:
  - Critical Care: Phenelzine interacts with numerous drugs and could potentially complicate the condition of patients with critical illness. If it is necessary to continue phenelzine, its use must be cautious and slow and careful monitoring of patients' responses is warranted; patients with critical illness are often frail and unstable, with multiple organ dysfunctions.
  - Surgery: Phenelzine use within 10 days prior to elective surgery is contraindicated.

Adverse Effects

The most serious adverse effect associated with phenelzine is hypertensive crisis, which can be precipitated by intake of foods containing tyramine. Other reported effects include dysrhythmias, drowsiness, dizziness, sexual dysfunction, and orthostatic hypotension.

Contraindications

Contraindications to phenelzine include known sensitivity to the drug. Patients should not have elective surgery requiring general anesthesia or spinal anesthesia or use local anesthesia containing sympathomimetic vasoconstrictors. Patients diagnosed with abnormal kidney function or hepatic impairment should not be prescribed phenelzine. Patients who take other MAO inhibitors or weight-reduction and over-the-counter cold or hay fever preparations containing vasoconstrictors should not take phenelzine.

Nursing Implications

Preventing Interactions

Phenelzine interacts with many drugs (Box 55.5) and some herbs and foods, increasing its effects. It is important that SSRIs and phenelzine are not taken concurrently or close together because serious and fatal reactions may occur. Other critical interactions occur with foods that contain tyramine, a monoamine precursor of norepinephrine. Normally, tyramine is deactivated in the GI tract and liver, so that large amounts do not reach the systemic circulation. When deactivation is blocked by MAO inhibitors,

BOX 55.5 Drug Interactions: Phenelzine

Drugs That Increase the Effects of Phenelzine

- Alcohol (red wine, beer)
  Increases central nervous system depression
- Altretamine
  Increases the risk of orthostatic hypotension
- Antidepressants (tricyclic antidepressants, selective serotonin reuptake inhibitors, serotonin–norepinephrine reuptake inhibitors), buspirone, carbamazepine, dextromethorphan, 5-hydroxytryptophan
  Increase the risk of serotonin syndrome
- Levodopa
  Increases the risk of hypertensive reactions
- Monoamine oxidase inhibitors
  Increase the risk of serotonin syndrome and hypertensive crisis
- Narcotic analgesics
  Increase the risk of hypotension, respiratory depression, or coma
- Selegiline, sibutramine, tramadol
  Increase the risk of hypertensive crisis

tyramine is absorbed systemically and transported to adrenergic nerve terminals, where it causes a sudden release of large amounts of norepinephrine. Caffeine, kava kava, phenylalanine, St. John's wort, and valerian increase the effects of phenelzine. Patients should not consume game meats, soy products, seaweed, sesame seeds, aged cheeses and meats, brewer's yeast, sauerkraut, and fava beans as these foods contain tryptophan which will lead to hypertensive crisis. In addition, tyrosine containing foods (e.g., meats, seafood, wheat products, and oatmeal) will also contribute to the development of hypertensive crisis. High protein foods and those that have undergone aging, fermentation, pickling, smoking, and bacterial contamination should be avoided.

Administering the Medication

Phenelzine is taken orally three times a day, which may require a reminder system for accurate administration. The drug may be crushed and mixed with fluids or food for patients with difficulty swallowing.

Assessing for Therapeutic and Adverse Effects

The nurse assesses for improvement in symptoms of depression, including improvement in anxiety level, reduced agitation or irritability episodes, decreased number of panic attacks, and ability to sleep through the night. It is important to monitor the patient for severe headache, nausea, vomiting, neck stiffness, photophobia, and sweating.

In addition, it is necessary to observe for blurred vision, constipation, dizziness, dry mouth, hypotension, urinary retention, and hypoglycemia. If the patient eats any foods containing tyramine, hypertensive crisis may occur. The treatment for hypertensive crisis is phentolamine.

Patient Teaching

Box 55.3 contains patient teaching guidelines for the antidepressants, including the MAO inhibitors.

Other Drugs in the Class

Isocarboxazid, selegiline, and tranylcypromine have the same adverse effects as phenelzine, and they interact with drugs and foods in the same way.

Selegiline, an MAO inhibitor, is an antiparkinsonian drug (Chapter 48). For depression, the transdermal preparation can be prescribed. The initial dose is 6 mg/24 hours once daily, with a maximum dose of 2.5 mg/day. It is a potent, irreversible monoamine oxidase inhibitor with a great affinity for MAO-B in the brain. Selegiline increases dopaminergic activity by interfering with dopamine reuptake at the synapse. The metabolites of amphetamine and methamphetamine are also affected and interfere with neuronal uptake and enhance the release of the neurotransmitters, norepinephrine, dopamine, and serotonin.

NCLEX Success

2. Fluoxetine achieves its effects by
   A. blocking the uptake of monoamines
   B. inhibiting monoamine oxidase A (MAO-A) enzyme in nerve terminals
   C. selectively inhibiting serotonin reuptake
   D. directly stimulating serotonin receptors

ATYPICAL ANTIDEPRESSANTS

Other drugs used to treat depression include bupropion, mirtazapine, and trazodone. Table 55.6 gives route and dosage information for these drugs. People also use the herbal preparation St. John's wort as an antidepressant (Box 55.6).

Bupropion

Bupropion (Aplenzin, Wellbutrin SR, Wellbutrin XL, Zyban) inhibits the reuptake of dopamine, norepinephrine, and serotonin. After an oral dose, peak plasma levels are reached in about 2 hours. The drug is metabolized in the liver and excreted primarily in the urine. Several metabolites are pharmacologically active. Bupropion is useful in the treatment of depression, seasonal affective disorder (SAD) (see Box 55.1), and smoking cessation. Prescribers often add it to a drug regimen when an SSRI does not provide a complete response. Acute episodes of depression usually require several months of drug therapy. It is necessary to reduce the dosage in patients with impaired hepatic or kidney function. Bupropion and its metabolites cross the placenta and are present in breast milk. There is an increased risk of overall congenital malformations following maternal use of bupropion during pregnancy.

Bupropion may have significant adverse effects. Seizures are likely to occur with doses above 450 mg/day and in patients known to have a seizure disorder. The drug has few adverse effects on cardiac function and does not cause orthostatic hypotension or sexual dysfunction. However, in addition to seizures, the drug has CNS stimulant effects (agitation, anxiety, excitement, increased motor activity, insomnia, restlessness) that may require a sedative during the first few days of administration. These effects may increase the risk of abuse. Other common adverse effects include dry mouth, headache, nausea and vomiting, and constipation. The FDA has issued a **BOXED WARNING** ◆ for bupropion, because serious neuropsychiatric reactions have been reported with the administration of the drug for smoking cessation. These reactions are more common with the discontinuation of the medication.

Mirtazapine

Mirtazapine (Remeron), another atypical antidepressant and alpha-2 antagonist, blocks presynaptic $alpha_2$-adrenergic receptors (which increase the release of norepinephrine), serotonin receptors, and histamine H_1 receptors. Consequently, the drug decreases anxiety, agitation, insomnia, and migraine headaches as well as depression.

Mirtazapine is well absorbed after oral administration, and it is metabolized in the liver, mainly to inactive metabolites. Common adverse effects include drowsiness (with accompanying cognitive and motor impairment), increased appetite, weight gain, dizziness, dry mouth, and constipation. The drug does not cause sexual dysfunction. Mirtazapine should not be taken concurrently with other CNS depressants (e.g., alcohol, benzodiazepine, antianxiety, or hypnotic agents) because of additive sedation. In addition, it should not be taken concurrently with an MAO inhibitor.

It is necessary to monitor patients for agranulocytosis or severe neutropenia. Patients should report sore throat, stomatitis, or any signs of an infection to the prescriber. Mirtazapine

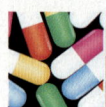

TABLE 55.6
DRUGS AT A GLANCE: Atypical Antidepressants

Drug	Routes and Dosage Ranges	
	Adults	Children
Bupropion (Aplenzin, Wellbutrin SR, Wellbutrin XL; ✽ ACT-BuPROPion XL MYLAN-BuPROPion XL, PMS-BuPROPion SR, SANDOZ-BuPROPion, Wellbutrin SR, Wellbutrin XL, Zyban)	Immediate-release tablets: 100 mg PO twice daily; increase to 100 mg three times daily (at least 6 h apart) if necessary; max single dose 450 mg daily Sustained-release (SR) tablets: 150 mg PO once daily in the morning; increase to 150 mg twice daily (at least 8 h apart); max daily dose 200 mg twice daily Wellbutrin XL: 150 mg PO once daily in the morning; may increase to target dose of 300 mg on or after 4th day of therapy; max single dose 450 mg	≥8 y and adolescents: 37.5 mg PO twice daily; titrate intervals of every 1–2 weeks to 100–300 mg/d in divided doses; maximum dose: 400 mg/d ≥11 y and adolescents: 12-h sustained release: 2 mg/kg PO once daily up to 100 mg administered as a morning dose; may titrate as needed every 2–3 weeks using the following titration schedule: Step 2: increase up to 3 mg/kg every morning Step 3: Increase to 3 mg/kg every morning and 2 mg/kg at 5 pm Step 4: Increase up to 3 mg/kg/dose twice daily; maximum dose: 150 mg (2.2 mg/kg in the morning and 1.7 mg/kg in the afternoon) 24-h extended release: ≥12 y–adolescents: 150 mg PO once daily; titrate up every two weeks to 300 mg once daily; maximum dose: 400 mg/d
Mirtazapine (Remeron, Remeron Sol, Tab; ✽ Remeron, Teva-Mirtazapine, ZYM-Mirtazapine)	15 mg/d PO initially, not to exceed 45 mg/d; usual dosage range 15–45 mg daily	Not recommended for use in children
Trazodone (✽ APO-TraZODone, APO-TraZODone D, DOM-TraZODone, TraZODone-50, TraZODone-100, TraZODone-150)	150 mg PO initially daily in divided doses; increase to a max dose of 600 mg daily if necessary	Insomnia: 18 mo to <3 y: 1–2 mg/kg/dose PO at bedtime: maximum dose: 25 mg/dose 3–5 y: 1–2 mg/kg PO at bedtime: maximum dose: 50 mg/dose >5 y: 0.75–1 mg/kg/dose PO at bedtime; maximum dose: 200 mg/dose

crosses the placenta. There has not been a significant increase in major teratogenic effects during pregnancy, but the information related to this is limited. Mirtazapine is present in breast milk.

Trazodone

Trazodone is used more often for sedation and sleep than for depression because high doses (greater than 300 mg/day) are required for antidepressant effects, and these amounts cause excessive sedation in many patients. The drug is often given concurrently with a stimulating antidepressant, such as bupropion, fluoxetine, sertraline, or venlafaxine.

Trazodone should be administered with food for maximum absorption. The drug is metabolized in the liver and excreted primarily by the kidneys. Adverse effects include sedation, dizziness, edema, cardiac dysrhythmias, and priapism (prolonged and painful penile erection). Trazodone crosses the placenta and can be detected in cord blood. Based on the data, an increased risk of adverse pregnancy outcomes has not been observed following the use of trazodone during pregnancy. Trazadone is present in breast milk,

BOX 55.6 Use of St. John's Wort as an Antidepressant

St. John's wort (*Hypericum perforatum*) is an herb that is widely used for depression. However, evidence for the efficacy of St. John's wort is modest at best. Most authorities agree that there is insufficient evidence to support the use of St. John's wort for mild to moderate depression and that more studies are needed to confirm the safety and effectiveness of this herb.

Drug interactions may be extensive. People should not combine St. John's wort with alcohol, antidepressants, nasal decongestants, or other over-the-counter cold and flu medications, bronchodilators, opioid analgesics, or amino acid supplements containing phenylalanine and tyrosine. All of these interactions may result in hypertension, possibly severe.

For patients who report use of St. John's wort, it is necessary to teach them to purchase products from reputable sources; to avoid taking antidepressant drugs, alcohol, and cold and flu medications while taking the herb; to avoid using the herb during pregnancy because effects are unknown; and to use sunscreen lotions and clothing to protect themselves from sun exposure.

MOOD-STABILIZING AGENTS: DRUGS USED TO TREAT BIPOLAR DISORDER

Lithium carbonate (Lithobid), the prototype, is a naturally occurring metallic salt that is used in patients with bipolar disorder, mainly to treat and prevent manic episodes. When used therapeutically, lithium is effective in controlling mania in 65% to 80% of patients. When used prophylactically, the drug decreases the frequency and intensity of manic cycles.

Pharmacokinetics

Lithium is well absorbed after oral administration, with peak serum levels in 1 to 3 hours after a dose and steady-state concentrations in 5 to 7 days. The drug is not metabolized; it is entirely excreted by the kidneys.

Action

The exact mechanism of action of lithium is unknown. However, the drug is known to affect the synthesis, release, and reuptake of several neurotransmitters in the brain, including acetylcholine, dopamine, GABA, and norepinephrine. It also stabilizes postsynaptic receptor sensitivity to neurotransmitters, probably by competing with calcium, magnesium, potassium, and sodium ions for binding sites. Lithium may also stimulate neuronal growth, exerting a neuroprotective effect on areas of the brain involved with mood.

Use

Lithium is the drug of choice for use in the treatment of manic episodes of bipolar disorder and as a maintenance treatment to decrease the number and intensity of manic episodes. Long-term therapy is the usual practice because of the high recurrence rate of bipolar disorder if the drug is discontinued. The prescriber may add an antiepileptic agent to the regimen.

Patient-related variables specific to the use of lithium include the following:

- Age:
  - Older adult patients should be administered the lowest doses. The guidelines for administration recommend target serum concentrations at 0.4 to 0.8 mEq/L.
- Reproduction, pregnancy, and lactation:
  - Lithium crosses the placenta.
  - For planned pregnancies, use of lithium should be avoided in the first trimester of pregnancy. If lithium is needed during pregnancy, the minimum effective dosage should be prescribed. The maternal lithium concentrations should be monitored at the start of therapy and after the period of fetal production and the development of organs (organogenesis).
  - Lithium should be suspended 24 to 48 hours prior to delivery or at the onset of labor when delivery is spontaneous.
  - Cardiac malformations in the infant have been noted when lithium is administered in the first trimester of pregnancy.
  - Lithium is present in breast milk.
- Abnormal kidney function and hepatic impairment:
  - Adequate kidney function is a prerequisite for lithium therapy. The proximal kidney tubules reabsorb approximately 80% of a lithium dose, and the amount of reabsorption depends on the concentration of sodium in the tubules. A sodium deficit causes more lithium to be reabsorbed and increases the risk of lithium toxicity. A sodium excess causes more lithium to be excreted (i.e., lithium diuresis) and may lower serum lithium levels to nontherapeutic ranges.
  - Caution is necessary when lithium is used in patients with hepatic impairment.
- Specific healthcare environments:
  - Critical Care: Lithium warrants caution in patients with critical illness. Lower doses are necessary in patients with conditions that impair lithium excretion (e.g., diuretic drug therapy, dehydration, low-salt diet, abnormal kidney function, decreased cardiac output).
  - Surgery: It is necessary to discontinue lithium 1 to 2 days before surgery and resume it when full oral intake of food and fluids is allowed.

Quality and Safety Alert: Safety

Gradually tapering the lithium dose over 2 to 4 weeks delays the recurrence of symptoms.

It is important to note that doses should be relatively low initially and may increase gradually according to regular measurements of serum drug levels. Dosage is based on serum drug levels, control of symptoms, and occurrence of adverse effects. Measurements of serum levels are required for two reasons: (1) therapeutic doses are only slightly lower than toxic doses and (2) patients vary widely in rates of lithium absorption and excretion. Thus, a dose that is therapeutic in one patient may be toxic in another.

Table 55.7 gives route and dosage information for lithium and other mood-stabilizing drugs.

Quality and Safety Alert: Safety

If a patient with abnormal kidney function or unstable kidney function receives lithium, it is essential that the dose be markedly reduced and that plasma serum levels be closely monitored.

Quality and Safety Alert: Safety

Lithium may prolong the effects of anesthetics and neuromuscular blocking drugs.

Adverse Effects and Contraindications

Common adverse effects of lithium include metallic taste, hand tremors, nausea, polyuria, polydipsia, diarrhea, muscular weakness, fatigue, edema, and weight gain.

Cardiac malformations are a common anomaly when lithium is administered in the first trimester.

Nursing Implications

Preventing Interactions

Several drugs interact with lithium, increasing or decreasing its effects (Box 55.7). No herbal interactions exist.

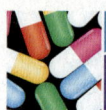

TABLE 55.7 DRUGS AT A GLANCE: Mood-Stabilizing Agents

Drug	Routes and Dosage Ranges	
	Adults	**Children**
ⓟ **Lithium carbonate** (Lithobid; 🍁 APO-Lithium Carbonate, DOM-Lithium Carbonate Carbolith, Lithane, PMS-Lithium Carbonate)	Immediate-release: 300 mg PO three times daily or less; usual dosage 900–1,800 mg PO daily in 3–4 divided doses Extended-release: 450 mg two times daily or less; usual dosage 900–1800 mg PO daily in 2 divided doses. Maintain a serum lithium level of 0.6–1.2 mEq/L	≥6 y: <30 kg initially 300 mg PO twice daily; ≥30 kg 300 mg PO three or four times daily >12 y: same as adults Maintenance dose: 15–60 mg/kg/d PO three times daily Maximum daily dose 40 mg/kg/d Maintain a serum lithium level <1.4 mEq/L
Aripiprazole (Abilify, Abilify Maintena, Abilify MyCite; 🍁 Abilify, APO-ARIPiprazole, Abilify Maintena, AURO-ARIPiprazole)	30 mg PO daily	Mania: ≥10–17 y, 2 mg PO daily for 7 days and then 5 mg daily for 2 days to 10 mg daily, not to exceed 30 mg daily; close monitoring in children with depression
Olanzapine (ZyPREXA, ZyPREXA Relprevv, ZyPREXA Zydis; 🍁 ACT-OLANZapine, JAMP-OLANZapine ODT, Teva-OLANZapine, Zyprexa, XyPEXA Zyds)	10–15 mg/d PO initially; may increase by 5 mg daily at no <24 intervals to max dose of 20 mg/d Older or debilitated adults: 5 mg/d PO	13–17 y: 2.5–5 mg/d PO initially; may increase by 2.5–5 mg daily to max dose of 20 mg/d
Quetiapine (Seroquel, SEROquel XR; 🍁 Dom-Quetiapine, Seroquel, Seroquel QR, ZyPREXA Zyds)	Acute mania: 50 mg PO twice daily on day 1; 100 mg PO twice daily on day 2; 150 mg PO twice daily on day 3; 200 mg PO twice daily on day 4. If needed, may continue to increase max dose 800 mg/d. Depressive episodes: 50 mg PO at bedtime; may increase by 50 mg/d to max dose 600 mg at bedtime	13–17 y: 25 mg PO twice daily on day 1; 50 mg PO twice daily on day 2; 100 mg PO twice daily on day 3; 150 mg PO twice daily on day 4; 200 mg PO twice daily on day 5. If needed, may continue to increase in increments of no >100 mg/d to max dose 400–600 mg/d
Olanzapine–fluoxetine (Symbyax)	Depressive episodes: 6 mg/25 mg PO in evening; usual dose 6–12 mg/25–50 mg; may increase to max 18 mg/75 mg daily	10–17 y: 3 mg/25 mg PO in evening; usual dose 6–12 mg/25–50 mg daily
Risperidone (Perseris, RisperDAL, RisperDAL Consta; 🍁 AG-Risperidone, RAN-Risperidone, RisperDAL, RisperDAL Consta)	Acute mania: 2–3 mg/d PO initially; may increase 1 mg/d to max dose of 6 mg/d Older or debilitated adults: 0.5 mg/d PO initially, may increase by 0.5–3 mg/d, and then may increase by 1 mg/wk to max dose of 6 mg/d Maintenance (RisperDAL Consta): 25 mg IM every 2 wk; max dose 50 mg every 2 wk	10–17 y: 0.5 mg/d PO initially; titrate 0.5–1 daily to a target dose of 2.5 mg/d; dosage range 0.5–6 mg/d
Ziprasidone (Geodon; 🍁 AURO-Ziprasidone, Zeldox)	Acute mania: 40 mg PO initially twice daily; usual dose 40–80 mg twice daily; max dose 80 mg twice daily	Not recommended for use in children with bipolar disorder

Administering the Medication

Before beginning lithium therapy, it is important to obtain baseline studies of kidney, cardiac, and thyroid status because adverse drug effects involve these organ systems. Baseline electrolyte studies are also necessary.

When lithium therapy begins, it is necessary to measure the serum drug concentration two or three times weekly in the morning, 12 hours (trough) after the last dose of the drug. For most patients, the therapeutic range of serum drug levels is 0.5 to 1.2 mEq/L (SI units, 0.5 to 1.2 mmol/L). Serum lithium levels should not exceed 1.5 mEq/L because of the risk of serious drug toxicity. Doses of lithium should decrease after mania is controlled. During long-term maintenance therapy, it is necessary to measure serum lithium levels at least every 3 months.

People should take lithium with food to decrease the risk of nausea and vomiting.

Assessing for Therapeutic and Adverse Effects

The nurse observes for decreases in manic behavior and stability in mood swings. Therapeutic effects do not occur until approximately 7 to 10 days after therapeutic serum drug levels are attained (1 to 1.5 mEq/L with acute mania; 0.6 to 1.2 mEq/L for maintenance therapy). In mania, a person usually takes a benzodiazepine or an antipsychotic drug to reduce agitation and control behavior until the lithium takes effect.

Chapter 55 • Drug Therapy for Depression and Mood Disorders 1027

THE NURSING PROCESS

A concept map outlines the nursing process related to drug therapy considerations in this chapter. Additional nursing implications related to the disease process should also be considered in care decisions.

Assessment
- Identify patients at risk for current or potential depression. Areas to assess include health status, family and social relationship, and work status. Severe or prolonged illness, impaired interpersonal relationships, inability to work, and job dissatisfaction may precipitate depression. Depression also occurs without an identifiable cause.
- Observe for signs and symptoms of depression. Clinical manifestations are nonspecific and vary in severity. For example, fatigue and insomnia may be caused by a variety of disorders and range from mild to severe. When symptoms are present, try to determine their frequency, duration, and severity.
- When a patient appears depressed or has a history of depression, assess for suicidal thoughts and behaviors. Statements indicating a detailed plan, accompanied by the intent, ability, and method for carrying out the plan, place the patient at high risk for suicide.
- Identify the patient's usual coping mechanisms for stressful situations. Coping mechanisms vary widely, and behavior that may be helpful to one patient may not be helpful to another. For example, one person may prefer being alone or having decreased contact with family and friends, whereas another may find increased contact desirable.

Outcomes of Therapy
The patient will
- Experience improvement of mood and depressive state.
- Receive or self-administer the drugs correctly.
- Identify signs and symptoms of suicidal ideation (or caretakers will). If present, caretakers will implement safety measures.
- Show improvement in activities of daily living, nutrition, exercise habits, and social interaction by the end of the hospital stay.
- Maintain self-care activities after discharge.
- Identify preventable adverse drug effects. If present, patients and/or caregivers can take action.

Nursing Interventions
The nurse will use general measures to prevent or decrease the severity of depression such as supportive psychotherapy and reduction of environmental stress. Specific measures include the following:
- Support the patient's usual mechanisms for handling stressful situations, when feasible. Helpful actions may involve relieving pain or insomnia, scheduling rest periods, and increasing or decreasing socialization.
- Call the patient by name, encourage self-care activities, allow him or her to participate in setting goals and making decisions, and praise efforts to accomplish tasks. These actions promote a positive self-image.
- When signs and symptoms of depression are observed, initiate treatment before depression becomes severe.
- Provide patient teaching regarding drug therapy (see Boxes 55.3 and 55.8).

Evaluation
- Observe for behaviors indicating lessened depression.
- Interview regarding feelings and mood.
- Observe and interview regarding adverse drug effects.
- Observe and interview regarding suicidal thoughts and behaviors.

Unfolding Patient Stories: Jermaine Jones • Part 2

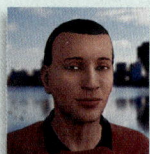

Remember from Chapter 35 Jermaine Jones, a 34-year-old male diagnosed with depression. He is prescribed sertraline 50 mg PO daily and states that he drinks a beer occasionally and will take one of his wife's prescription alprazolam for sleep. What patient education would the nurse provide on the adverse effects of these medications when taken with alcohol? When comparing sertraline with other antidepressant drugs, how would the nurse differentiate drug classifications, actions, and adverse effects? What patient education would the nurse provide regarding sharing prescription medication?

Care for Jermaine and other patients in a realistic virtual environment: vSim for Nursing (thepoint.lww.com/vSimPharm). Practice documenting these patients' care in DocuCare (thepoint.lww.com/DocuCareEHR).

Visit thePoint at http://thePoint.lww.com/Frandsen13e for answers to NCLEX Success questions (in Appendix A), answers to Clinical Application Case Studies (in Appendix B), additional information on the etiology and pathophysiology of depression and bipolar disorder, and more!

REFERENCES AND RESOURCES

Avery, D. (2022). Seasonal affective disorder: Treatment. *UpToDate*. Lexi-Comp, Inc.

Boyd, M. A. (2018). *Psychiatric nursing: Contemporary practice* (6th ed.). Wolters Kluwer.

Hirsch, M., & Birnbaum, R. J. (2022a). Selective serotonin reuptake inhibitors: Pharmacology, administration, and side effects. *UpToDate*. Lexi-Comp, Inc.

Hirsch, M., & Birnbaum, R. J. (2022b). Tricyclic and tetracyclic drugs: Pharmacology, administration, and side effects. *UpToDate*. Lexi-Comp, Inc.

Holtzheimer, P. E. (2022). Bipolar disorder in adults: Overview of neuromodulation procedures. *UpToDate*. Lexi-Comp, Inc.

Marasine, N. R., Sankhi, S., Lamichhane, R., Marasini, N. R., & Dangi, N. B. (2021). Use of antidepressants among patients diagnosed with depression: A scoping review. *BioMed Research International*, 2021, 1–8. 10.1155/2021/6999028

National Institutes of Health. (2020). Major depression. *Transforming the Understanding and Treatment of Mental Illness* Retrieved from: https://www.nimh.nih.gov/health/statistics/major-depression

National Institutes of Health. (2022a). *Drugs and lactation database*. National Library of Medicine. Retrieved from: https://www.ncbi.nlm.nih.gov/books/NBK501180/#:~:text=Summary%20of%20Use%20during%20Lactation&text=Imipramine%20use%20during%20breastfeeding%20would,to%20be%20possible%20during%20breastfeeding

National Institutes of Health. (2022b). Depression and older adults. National Institute on Aging. Retrieved from: https://www.nia.nih.gov/health/depression-and-older-adults

Nelson, C. (2020). *Serotonin-norepinephrine reuptake inhibitors (SNRIs): Pharmacology, administration, and side effects. UpToDate*. Lexi-Comp, Inc.

Rush, A. J. (2023). Unipolar major depression in adults: Choosing initial treatment. *UpToDate*. Lexi-Comp, Inc.

Stovall, J. (2022). Bipolar disorder in adults: Epidemiology and pathogenesis. *UpToDate*. Lexi-Comp, Inc.

UpToDate. (2022). *Drug information*. Lexi-Comp, Inc.

Viguera, A. (2022). Postpartum unipolar major depression: Epidemiology, clinical features, assessment, and diagnosis. *UpToDate*. Lexi-Comp, Inc.

CHAPTER 56

Drug Therapy for Psychotic Disorders

LEARNING OBJECTIVES

After studying this chapter, you should be able to:

1. Discuss clinical considerations and common manifestations of psychotic disorders, including schizophrenia.
2. Identify the prototype and describe the action, use, adverse effects, contraindications, and nursing implications for the first-generation antipsychotics.
3. Recognize the significance of the level of potency of first-generation antipsychotics.
4. Identify the prototype and describe the action, use, adverse effects, contraindications, and nursing implications for the second-generation antipsychotics.
5. Implement the nursing process in the care of the patient being treated with antipsychotics.

CLINICAL APPLICATION CASE STUDY

Caroline Jones, a 20-year-old college student, is brought to the university's mental health clinic by a friend. The friend says that Caroline has been talking to the television set and has complained that the voices from the television are telling her that she is ugly. In addition, she has become more withdrawn and reclusive. Caroline has not taken care of her personal hygiene for some time, and she looks disheveled. She receives a diagnosis of psychosis. The treatment plan involves supportive psychotherapy and haloperidol 10 mg twice daily.

KEY TERMS

Akathisia: motor restlessness and inability to be still, usually occurs in the first few months of treatment with antipsychotic agents

Alogia: poverty or lack of speech

Anhedonia: inability to experience pleasure

Asociality: social withdrawal

Avolition: lack of motivation

Catatonia: grossly disorganized or abnormal motor behavior

Delusions: false beliefs that persist in the absence of reason or evidence

Disorganized thinking: speech so disorganized that it substantially impairs communication

Drug-induced parkinsonism: loss of muscle movement, muscular rigidity and tremors, shuffling gait, masked facies, and drooling

Dystonias: uncoordinated, twisting, and repetitive movements

Extrapyramidal effects: movement disorders such as tardive dyskinesia, akathisia, dystonia, and drug-induced parkinsonism that may occur with usage of antipsychotic drugs

Hallucinations: sensory perceptions of people or objects that are not present in the external environment

Neuroleptic malignant syndrome: a rare but potentially fatal adverse effect; characterized by rigidity, severe hyperthermia, respiratory failure, and acute kidney failure

Paranoia: belief that other people control their thoughts, feelings, and behaviors or seek to harm them

Psychosis: severe mental disorder characterized by disorganized thought processes, hallucinations, and delusions

Tardive dyskinesia: irreversible late extrapyramidal effects of some antipsychotic drugs that include lip smacking, tongue protrusion, facial grimaces, and choreic movements of trunk and limbs

INTRODUCTION

This chapter introduces the pharmacologic care of the patient who is experiencing **psychosis**. Psychosis is a severe mental disorder characterized by disorganized thought processes, hallucinations, and delusions. Emotional responses may be blunted or inappropriate. Behavior may be bizarre and range from hypoactivity to hyperactivity with agitation, aggressiveness, hostility, and combativeness; it also may involve social withdrawal in which a person pays less than normal attention to the environment and other people, deterioration from previous levels of occupational and social functioning (poor self-care and interpersonal skills), hallucinations, and paranoid delusions. This chapter focuses primarily on schizophrenia as a chronic psychosis.

Several features are characteristic of psychosis. **Hallucinations** are sensory perceptions of people or objects that are not present in the external environment. More specifically, people see, hear, or feel stimuli that are not visible to external observers, and they cannot distinguish between these false perceptions and reality. Hallucinations occur in delirium, dementias, schizophrenia, and other psychotic states. In schizophrenia or bipolar affective disorder, they are usually auditory; in delirium, they are usually visual or tactile; and in dementia, they are usually visual. **Delusions** are false beliefs that persist in the absence of reason or evidence. Deluded people are often fearful and exhibit **paranoia**, the belief that other people control their thoughts, feelings, and behaviors or seek to harm them. Delusions indicate severe mental illness. Although they are commonly associated with schizophrenia, delusions also occur with delirium, dementias, and other psychotic disorders.

OVERVIEW OF PSYCHOSIS

Psychosis may be acute or chronic. Acute episodes, also called confusion or delirium, have a sudden onset over hours to days and may be precipitated by physical disorders (e.g., brain damage related to cerebrovascular disease or head injury, metabolic disorders, infections); drug intoxication with adrenergics, antidepressants, some anticonvulsants, amphetamines, cocaine, and others; and drug withdrawal after chronic use (e.g., alcohol, benzodiazepine antianxiety, or sedative–hypnotic agents). In addition, acute psychotic episodes may be superimposed on chronic dementias and psychoses, such as schizophrenia.

Clinical Considerations

There is evidence of abnormal neurotransmission systems in the brains of people with schizophrenia, especially in the dopaminergic, serotonergic, and glutamatergic systems. There is also evidence of extensive interactions among neurotransmission systems. In addition, illnesses or drugs that alter neurotransmission in one system are likely to alter neurotransmission in other systems. The dopaminergic, serotonergic, and glutamatergic systems have been the focus of the most studies.

Stimulation of dopamine can initiate psychotic symptoms or exacerbate an existing psychotic disorder. Two findings further support the importance of dopamine: (1) antipsychotic drugs exert their therapeutic effects by decreasing dopamine activity (i.e., blocking dopamine receptors) and (2) drugs that increase dopamine levels in the brain (e.g., bromocriptine, cocaine, levodopa) can cause signs and symptoms of psychosis.

Experts also believe that underactivity of dopamine$_1$ (D_1) receptors in the prefrontal cortex accounts for associated negative symptoms including inability to experience pleasure (**anhedonia**), lack of motivation (**avolition**), diminished emotional expression, poor grooming and hygiene, poor social skills, poverty or lack of speech (**alogia**), and social withdrawal (**asociality**).

The serotonergic system, which is widespread in the brain, is mainly inhibitory in nature. In schizophrenia, serotonin apparently decreases dopamine activity in the part of the brain associated with negative symptoms, causing, or aggravating these symptoms.

Clinical Manifestations

Symptoms of psychosis may begin gradually or suddenly, usually during adolescence or early adulthood. The American Psychiatric Association's (2022) *Diagnostic and Statistical Manual of Mental Disorders, 5th Edition, Text Revision*: *DSM-5-TR* stipulates that characteristic psychotic symptoms must have been present during a 1-month period, with presence of some overt psychotic symptoms for at least 6 months, before schizophrenia can be diagnosed. There are five domains that comprise the clinical features of psychotic disorders: delusions, hallucinations, disorganized speech that impairs communication (**disorganized thinking**), grossly disorganized or abnormal motor behavior (**catatonia**), and negative symptoms. Two negative symptoms most often seen with schizophrenia include diminished emotional expression and avolition. Criteria changes for substance use disorders in the *DSM-5-TR* provide for the ability to assign a diagnosis (unspecified schizophrenia spectrum and other psychotic disorder) to individuals who are experiencing symptoms of schizophrenia or other psychotic symptoms but do not meet the full diagnostic criteria for schizophrenia or another more specific psychotic disorder. Antipsychotic drugs are generally more effective in treating positive symptoms than negative symptoms, although the newer, atypical medications have been effective at treating the negative symptoms.

Drug Therapy

Overall, the goal of drug treatment is to relieve symptoms with minimal or tolerable adverse effects. In patients with acute psychosis, the goal during the first week of treatment is to decrease symptoms (e.g., aggression, agitation, combativeness, hostility) and normalize patterns of sleeping and eating. The next goals may be increased ability for self-care and increased socialization. Therapeutic effects usually occur gradually, over 1 to 2 months. Long-term goals include increasing the patient's ability to cope with the environment, promoting optimal functioning in self-care and activities of daily living, and preventing acute episodes and hospitalizations. With drug therapy, patients often can participate in psychotherapy, group therapy, or other treatment modalities; return to community settings; and return to their preillness level of functioning.

Schizophrenia in children and adolescents is often characterized by more severe symptoms and a more chronic course than in adults. Drug therapy for psychosis in children has been often prescribed off-label to manage other problems (aggression, hyperactivity, anxiety, irritability, sleep) and given longer than recommended. However, research establishing an evidence base for treatment decisions in children and adolescents is growing. Dosage regulation is difficult because children may require lower plasma levels for therapeutic effects, but they also metabolize antipsychotic drugs more rapidly than do adults. Much is still not known about the efficacy, tolerability, and long-term safety of these drugs in young people.

BOX 56.1 Recommendations for the Use of Antipsychotic Medications in Children and Adolescents

Before starting therapy:
- Assess the general mental health of the family.
- Conduct a thorough psychiatric and physical examination.
- Confirm that other recommended psychosocial or psychopharmacological treatment options are attempted and found insufficient.
- Explore strategies for pharmacologic and psychosocial treatment based on the best evidence.
- Choose a drug based on potency, adverse effect profile, and the patient's response.
- Avoid the use of prescribing multiple antipsychotic drugs simultaneously.
- Educate the child and family about the treatment and monitoring plan, including the importance of lifestyle modifications, and the need to regularly attempt discontinuation.
- Explain all risks and benefits of the treatment plan to the parents.
- Clarify any questions or concerns the parents or patient may have.
- Document the consent of the parents to the treatment plan.
- Assess the response to treatment and discuss with the patient and family the ongoing treatment plan.

Multiple national and international organizations advocate the appropriate use of antipsychotic medications and high quality assessment of the pediatric population to enhance safety. Box 56.1 lists major national and international recommendations.

Drugs used in the treatment of psychosis, also known as neuroleptics because of the increased risk of extrapyramidal neurologic effects with their use, are summarized in Table 56.1. As a class, antipsychotics are also effective in the treatment of

TABLE 56.1 Drugs Administered for the Treatment of Psychosis

Drug Class	Prototype	Other Drugs in the Class
First-generation (typical) antipsychotics	Chlorpromazine Haloperidol (Haldol)	Fluphenazine Loxapine Perphenazine Pimozide Thioridazine Trifluoperazine Thiothixene
Second-generation (atypical) antipsychotics	Clozapine (Clozaril, Versacloz)	Aripiprazole (Abilify, Abilify Maintena) Asenapine (Saphris, Secuado) Iloperidone (Fanapt) Lurasidone (Latuda) Olanzapine (Zyprexa, Zyprexa Relprevv) Paliperidone (Invega, Invega Sustenna, Invega Trinza) Quetiapine (Seroquel, Seroquel XR) Risperidone (Risperdal, Perseris, Risperdal Consta) Ziprasidone (Geodon)

acute agitation, bipolar mania, and other psychiatric conditions. These drugs may be broadly categorized as (1) "typical," "conventional," or first-generation agents and (2) "atypical" or second-generation agents. Typical antipsychotic drugs fall into five different major chemical categories, including two that are discussed in this chapter—the phenothiazines, such as chlorpromazine, and older nonphenothiazines, such as haloperidol. In addition, the typical, first-generation drugs can be classified by potency. The level of potency refers to the size of the dose needed to produce a given response; all first-generation antipsychotics have the same ability to relieve symptoms of psychosis.

- Low potency: chlorpromazine, thioridazine
- Medium potency: loxapine, perphenazine
- High potency: fluphenazine, haloperidol, pimozide, thiothixene, trifluoperazine

> **Quality and Safety Alert: Safety**
>
> Although the atypical antipsychotic agents have replaced the typical agents in the treatment of psychiatric disorders, they remain widely used in the treatment of nausea. See Chapter 38 for additional information.

Second-generation drugs, including clozapine and other related drugs, generally have lower risk of extrapyramidal adverse effects and tardive dyskinesia compared with the typical first-generation antipsychotics. Antipsychotic effects may not occur until the drugs have been given for a few weeks.

Prescribers caring for patients with psychosis have a greater choice of drugs than ever before. Some general factors to consider include the patient's age and physical condition, the severity and duration of illness, the frequency and severity of adverse effects produced by each drug, the patient's use of and response to antipsychotic drugs in the past, the supervision available, and the prescriber's experience with a particular drug.

> **Quality and Safety Alert: Safety**
>
> All antipsychotics are identified in the Beers Criteria as potentially inappropriate medications in patients 65 years and older with dementia. Antipsychotics should be avoided because they increase the risk of mortality and cerebrovascular accidents as well as lead to a greater rate of cognitive decline.

People with schizophrenia usually need to take antipsychotics for years because there is a high rate of relapse (acute psychotic episodes) when drug therapy is discontinued, most often by patients who become unwilling or unable to continue taking their medication. With wider use of maintenance therapy and the newer, better-tolerated antipsychotic drugs, patients may experience fewer psychotic episodes and hospitalizations.

Most antipsychotics are available in oral formulations. Patients who are unable or unwilling to take daily doses of an antipsychotic may receive periodic injections of long-acting forms of aripiprazole, fluphenazine, haloperidol, olanzapine, risperidone, or paliperidone. These long-acting injectable (LAI) antipsychotics may be an important therapeutic option for patients with schizophrenia; it allows a prescriber to tailor pharmacotherapy to each patient's needs. The LAI form may serve to replace oral medications for patients who may have difficulty with medication adherence. These first- and second-generation antipsychotic LAIs are administered via "depot" injections. Depot refers to the way the drug is deposited and stored in the muscle before being absorbed. The injected drug takes time to move out of the muscle into the bloodstream, extending its action. However, extrapyramidal effects may be more problematic with depot injections of antipsychotics. Although some LAIs are expensive because they have been recently approved for use, they potentially reduce the financial burden of schizophrenia and improve quality of life.

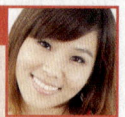

> **Clinical Application 56.1**
>
> - Describe the positive and negative symptoms that Caroline is experiencing.
> - What neurotransmitter system is involved in Caroline's psychosis?
> - How do antipsychotic drugs decrease Caroline's psychotic symptoms?

FIRST-GENERATION ANTIPSYCHOTICS

Healthcare providers have used the first-generation antipsychotics, including phenothiazines and nonphenothiazines, to treat psychosis since the 1950s. Although these drugs are historically significant, their usage and clinical importance have waned in recent years. Two drugs are identified as prototypes in this chapter. **Chlorpromazine hydrochloride** is the prototype drug of the phenothiazine groups, and **haloperidol** (Haldol) is the prototype nonphenothiazine first-generation antipsychotic. Table 56.2 gives route and dosage information for the first-generation typical antipsychotics.

Pharmacokinetics

Chlorpromazine is well absorbed and distributed to most body tissues, and it reaches high concentrations in the brain. After oral administration, the onset of action is 30 to 60 minutes, with a peak of 2 to 4 hours and a duration of 4 to 6 hours. After intramuscular (IM) administration, the onset of action is 10 to 15 minutes, with a peak at 15 to 20 minutes and a duration of 4 to 6 hours. The half-life is 2 to 30 hours. The drug is metabolized in the liver and excreted in urine.

Action

The mechanism of action of chlorpromazine is not fully understood. When the drug produces antipsychotic effects, it blocks the postsynaptic dopamine receptors in the brain.

Use

The major clinical indication for chlorpromazine and other phenothiazine antipsychotics is schizophrenia. Chlorpromazine is not approved for the treatment of patients with dementia-related psychosis.

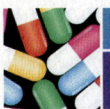

TABLE 56.2
DRUGS AT A GLANCE: First-Generation Typical Antipsychotics

Drug	Routes and Dosage Ranges	
	Adults	**Children**
ⓟ Chlorpromazine (✦ Teva-Chlorpromazine)	Excessive anxiety, agitation in psychiatric patients: 25 mg IM; may repeat in 1 h; increase dosage gradually in inpatients up to 400 mg every 4–6 h; max daily dosage 2000 mg/d; as soon as possible, switch to an oral dosage of 25–50 mg PO 3 times/d Initial oral dosage: 10 mg PO 3–4 times/d or 25 mg PO 2–3 times/d; increase daily dose by 20–50 mg semiweekly until optimum dosage is reached; dosages of 200–800 mg can be administered in discharged mental patients	Generally not used in children younger than 6 mo Psychiatric outpatients: 0.55 mg/kg PO every 4–6 h, 1 mg/kg rectally every 6–8 h not to exceed 40 mg/d (up to 5 y), or 75 mg/d (5–12 y) Psychiatric inpatients: 50–100 mg PO per day; max dosage 40 mg IM per day for children up to 5 y; 75 mg/d IM for children 5–12 y
ⓟ Haloperidol (Haldol, Haldol decanoate; ✦ Novo-Peridol, PMS-Haloperidol, PMS-Haloperidol LA)	Acute psychosis: 1–15 mg PO daily initially in divided doses; gradually increase to 100 mg daily, if necessary; usual maintenance dose, 5–20 mg daily Chronic schizophrenia: 6–15 mg PO daily; max 100 mg daily; dosage is reduced for maintenance, usually 15–20 mg daily. Haloperidol decanoate IM, initial dose up to 100 mg, depending on previous dose of oral drug, then titrated according to response; usually given every 4 wk	Acute psychosis: 3–12 y, 0.05–0.15 mg/kg/d PO in 2–3 divided doses Acute psychosis, chronic refractory schizophrenia, Tourette syndrome, mental retardation with hyperkinesia: 13 y and older, same as adults Chronic refractory schizophrenia: dosage not established Tourette syndrome: 1.5–6 mg PO daily initially in divided doses; usual maintenance dose, 1.5 mg daily Mental retardation with hyperkinesia: 1.5 mg PO initially, in divided doses, gradually increase to a max of 15 mg daily, if necessary; when symptoms are controlled, dosage is gradually reduced to the minimum effective level; IM dosage not established
Fluphenazine (✦ Apo-Fluphenazine, Fluphenazine Omega)	2.5–10 mg PO initially, gradually reduced to a maintenance dose of 1–5 mg (doses above 3 mg are rarely necessary) Acute psychosis: 1.25 mg initially, increased gradually to 2.5–10 mg daily in 3–4 divided doses	5–12 y, 0.75–10 mg PO daily; no IM dosage established
Loxapine (✦ Loxapac, PHL-Loxapine, Xylac)	Schizophrenia, 10 mg PO twice daily; usual dosage 60–100 mg daily in divided doses 2–4 times daily; max dosage not to exceed 250 mg daily Acute agitation with schizophrenia or bipolar disorder, 10 mg once daily; max dosage 10 mg in 24-h period	Safety and efficacy not established
Perphenazine (✦ Apo-Perphenazine)	Outpatients: 4–8 mg PO 3 times/d; reduce dose as soon as possible to minimum effective dosage; max dosage 64 mg/d Inpatients: 8–16 mg PO 2–4 times/d; max dosage 64 mg/d	4 mg PO 2–4 times/d; max dosage 16 mg/d
Pimozide (✦ Apo-Pimozide, Orap)	1–2 mg PO daily initially; max dosage 10 mg daily or 0.2 mg/kg/d (whichever is less)	2–12 y, 0.05 mg/kg PO initially at bedtime; usual dosage 2–4 mg daily; max dosage 0.2 mg/kg/d not to exceed 10 mg daily
Thioridazine	50–100 mg PO initially three times daily; usual dosage 300–5,800 mg in 2–4 divided doses; max dosage 800 mg daily	≥6 y: 0.5 mg/kg/d PO; max daily dose 3 mg/kg/d
Thiothixene (✦ Navane)	6–10 mg PO daily in divided doses; usual dosage 20–30 mg daily; max 60 mg daily Older or debilitated adults, PO one third to one half the usual adult dosage	<12 y, dosage not established ≥12 y, same as adults
Trifluoperazine	2–5 mg PO initially daily in divided doses; usual dosage 15–20 mg daily; max dosage 50 mg daily	6–12 y: 1 mg initially 1–2 times daily; max dosage 15 mg daily Adolescents: same as adults

It is necessary to individualize the dosage and route of administration of chlorpromazine according to the patient's condition and response; as mentioned, prescribers may exceed the recommended maximum dosage approved by the U.S. Food and Drug Administration (FDA).

Patient-related variables specific to the use of chlorpromazine include the following:

- Age:
  - In children, first-generation antipsychotics have generally been replaced by second-generation agents.
  - In older adults, the dosage of chlorpromazine should be started at one fourth to one third of the level for younger adults.
  - The FDA has issued a **BOXED WARNING** ◆ related to the increased risk of death in older adult patients with dementia-related psychosis treated with antipsychotic drugs.
- Reproduction, pregnancy, and lactation:
  - Jaundice and hyper- or hyporeflexia have been reported in newborn infants following maternal use of phenothiazines.
  - If used during the third trimester of pregnancy, there is a risk of abnormal muscle movements (extrapyramidal effects [EPS]) and withdrawal symptoms in newborns following delivery.
  - Following maternal use, newborns may manifest symptoms that include agitation, hypertonia or hypotonia, respiratory distress, somnolence, tremor, and feeding disorders.
  - Drowsiness and lethargy were observed in breastfed infants with use of chlorpromazine.
- Abnormal kidney function and hepatic impairment:
  - Since chlorpromazine is excreted in the kidneys, monitor kidney function periodically in patients with abnormal kidney function during long-term therapy and lower the dosage or discontinue the drug altogether if test results (e.g., blood urea nitrogen) become abnormal.
  - With hepatic impairment, metabolism may be slowed and drug elimination half-lives prolonged, with resultant accumulation and increased risk of adverse effects.
- Specific healthcare environments:
  - In critically ill patients, the undesirable adverse effects (anticholinergic symptoms, hypotension, tachycardia, cardiac dysrhythmias, extrapyramidal effects) and the drug's ability to lower the seizure threshold limit its use.

Adverse Effects

Chlorpromazine has several adverse effects, including

- Central nervous system (CNS) effects: excessive sedation, drowsiness, lethargy, fatigue, slurred speech, impaired mobility, and impaired mental processes. **Extrapyramidal effects** may also occur. Symptoms include movement disorders such as tardive dyskinesia, akathisia, dystonia, and drug-induced parkinsonism.
  - **Tardive dyskinesia** occurs as the result of long-term chlorpromazine use. Patients may experience lip smacking, tongue protrusion, and facial grimaces and may have choreic movements of trunk and limbs. This condition is usually irreversible, and there is no effective treatment.
  - **Akathisia** (motor restlessness and inability to be still), the most common extrapyramidal reaction, may occur about 5 to 60 days from the start of drug therapy.
  - **Dystonias** are uncoordinated, twisting, and repetitive movements of the neck, face, eyes, tongue, trunk, or extremities. These adverse effects may occur suddenly 1 to 5 days after drug therapy is started and may be misinterpreted as seizures or other disorders.
  - **Drug-induced parkinsonism** is loss of muscle movement (akinesia), muscular rigidity and tremors, shuffling gait, masked facies, and drooling.
  - **Neuroleptic malignant syndrome** is a rare but potentially fatal reaction, which may occur hours to months after initial drug use. Symptoms of fever, muscle rigidity, respiratory failure, acute kidney failure, and confusion develop rapidly.
- Cardiovascular effects: prolonged QT and PR interval, T-wave blunting, and depression of the ST interval.
- Hematologic effects: agranulocytosis and pancytopenia.
- Other effects: antiadrenergic effects, such as hypotension, dizziness, fatigue, and faintness, as well as respiratory depression, endocrine effects, photosensitivity, and difficulty with temperature regulation.

In addition, children may demonstrate weight gain, extrapyramidal effects, development of diabetes, and increased prolactin levels.

Contraindications

Contraindications to phenothiazines include hypersensitivity to the drug, concomitant use with large amounts of CNS depressants (e.g., alcohol, barbiturates, opioids); and comatose states. Because of wide-ranging adverse effects, chlorpromazine may cause or aggravate several conditions so it must be used with precaution in liver damage, coronary artery disease, cerebrovascular disease, parkinsonism, bone marrow depression, severe hypotension or hypertension, coma, and severely depressed states. Caution also is warranted in seizure disorders, diabetes mellitus, glaucoma, prostatic hypertrophy, peptic ulcer disease, and chronic respiratory disorders, as well as in pregnancy, especially during the first trimester.

Nursing Implications

Preventing Interactions

Many medications interact with chlorpromazine, increasing or decreasing its effects (Box 56.2). The combination of the herbal supplement with kava results in increased dystonia.

Administering the Medication

For acute psychotic episodes, therapy with chlorpromazine may require IM administration and hospitalization. Control of symptoms usually occurs within 48 to 72 hours, after which the person takes the oral drug. It is necessary to obtain a baseline electrocardiogram (ECG) prior to administering the drug, because of associated risk of alterations in the cardiac rhythm. The nurse needs to check doses carefully, especially when starting or stopping an antipsychotic drug or substituting one for another. The dosages are often changed during the course of treatment. When the drug

> **BOX 56.2 Drug Interactions: Chlorpromazine**
>
> **Drugs That Increase the Effects of Chlorpromazine**
> - Barbiturates, lithium
>   *May decrease phenothiazine effect*
> - Central nervous system (CNS) depressants, narcotics
>   *produce additive CNS depression and hypotension*
> - Anticholinergic drugs
>   *Increase anticholinergic effects such as decreased secretions and urinary retention*
> - Beta-adrenergic blockers, centrally acting hypertensives
>   *Produce tachycardia, may decrease antihypertensive effect*
> - Epinephrine, norepinephrine
>   *Produce hypotension*
>
> **Drugs That Decrease the Effects of Chlorpromazine**
> - Antacids
>   *Decrease absorption*
> - Anticholinergic drugs
>   *Decrease antipsychotic effects*

is started, it is usually necessary to titrate initial doses upward over days or weeks and then reduce them for maintenance. Discontinuation of the drug requires a gradual reduction in dosage.

For IM administration, the nurse adheres to the following guidelines:

- Determine the dose, which is approximately half of an oral dose. IM doses avoid first-pass metabolism and produce serum drug levels approximately double those of oral doses.
- Change the needle after filling the syringe with the injectable medication.
- Give the injection in the ventrogluteal muscle with a 1½-in needle.
- Have the patient lie down for 30 to 60 minutes after the injection to prevent orthostatic hypotension.
- Watch for idiopathic edema and muscle necrosis, which may occur with IM administration.

For oral administration, the nurse adheres to the following guidelines:

- Give doses 1 to 2 hours before bedtime; peak sedation occurs in about 2 hours.
- Mix liquid concentrations with at least 60 mL of fruit juice. Avoid contact with skin because the liquid forms can cause contact dermatitis.
- Administer the oral preparation with food to reduce gastric upset.
- Use divided doses.

Assessing for Therapeutic Effects

With acute psychotic episodes, the nurse observes for decreased agitation, combativeness, and psychomotor activity. The sedative effects of chlorpromazine, considered to be therapeutic, occur within 48 to 72 hours. With acute or chronic psychosis, the nurse observes for decreased psychotic behaviors, such as decreased hallucinations and delusions.

Assessing for Adverse Effects

The nurse assesses the fluid and electrolyte status for a possible fluid volume deficit. It is also necessary to measure the patient's weight daily and assess for signs of dehydration. In addition, the nurse assesses for increased anticholinergic effects, such as diminished fluid status and urinary retention.

The nurse assesses for aspiration related to depressed cough reflex. It is important to monitor kidney and hepatic function along with the complete blood count. A depression in white blood cell count requires discontinuation of the medication.

The nurse monitors for increased CNS depression that could result in falls or altered safety. The nurse also assesses for extrapyramidal effects such as dystonia, tardive dyskinesia, and akathisia.

Patient Teaching

Box 56.3 identifies patient teaching guidelines for chlorpromazine.

Other Drugs in the Class

Although other first-generation antipsychotics have similar indications, their safety profiles and their degree of efficacy and tolerability differ.

Fluphenazine is a high-potency antipsychotic used in the management of schizophrenia. The most common adverse effect seen is extrapyramidal effects. Other effects include menstrual irregularities, gynecomastia, and galactorrhea. Relative to other antipsychotics, fluphenazine has a low potential of anticholinergic effects (constipation, xerostomia, blurred vision, urinary retention). The drug can be administered orally or intramuscularly. Two injectable preparations are available; the decanoate injection is a depot preparation and intended for use in the management of patients who require prolonged therapy.

> **BOX 56.3 Patient Teaching Guidelines for Chlorpromazine**
>
> - Do not combine the medication with over-the-counter medications or alcohol.
> - Be sure to drink enough fluids, especially during hot weather.
> - If you go outdoors, wear protective clothing, and use sunscreen.
> - Use caution when changing positions. It may be necessary to lie down for approximately an hour after taking your medication, because faintness and dizziness may occur.
> - Do not overexercise and reduce body fluids.
> - Do not drive a car or operate dangerous machinery. Dizziness or decreased mental alertness may occur.
> - Report dark urine, pale stools, and yellowing of the eyes or skin to a healthcare provider.
> - Discuss chlorpromazine use with a healthcare provider if you intend to become pregnant.

Pimozide is a high-potency agent approved only for the treatment of Tourette syndrome. The drug suppresses severe motor and phonic tics that have not responded to standard treatment. Adverse effects include sedation, akathisia, drowsiness, akinesia, and visual disturbances. More rarely, neuroleptic malignant syndrome and prolongation of the QT interval can occur. Pimozide can also prolong the QT interval on the ECG, which increases the risk of fatal dysrhythmias. Concurrent administration with citalopram (Celexa), escitalopram (Lexapro), or sertraline (Zoloft) should be avoided because the combination can increase the risk of dysrhythmias. An ECG should be performed baseline and periodically thereafter, especially during dosage adjustment to observe for prolongation of the QT interval.

Because the drug is highly metabolized by CYP1A2, CYP2D6, and CYP3A4 of the cytochrome P450 system, major drug interactions are possible.

> **Quality and Safety Alert: Safety**
>
> In adults and children, if drug therapy with pimozide exceeds a dose of 4 mg/day, CYP2D6 genomic testing is recommended. Patients who are poor metabolizers of CYP2D6 should receive incremental dose changes over greater time (14 days) and should not receive doses in excess of 4 mg/day.

Trifluoperazine is a high-potency antipsychotic that is used to treat schizophrenia and other psychotic disorders. The drug leads to early extrapyramidal effects most commonly, and it has a moderate potential for anticholinergic effects.

Perphenazine and loxapine are medium-potency agents used to treat schizophrenia. Perphenazine is also used to manage other psychotic disorders. The adverse effect profile of both drugs is similar to fluphenazine.

Thioridazine is a low-potency antipsychotic that is now reserved for use in patients with schizophrenia who have not responded to an adequate course of treatment with safer agents. The FDA has issued a **BOXED WARNING** regarding concerns with prolonged QT interval, which increases the risk of fatal dysrhythmias in using thioridazine. Common adverse effects relate to its anticholinergic effects. Weight gain and inhibition of ejaculation may also occur.

NCLEX Success

1. A patient who is hospitalized because of a relapse of their psychotic disorder states, "I quit taking my medicines because I always forget to take them at least one time a day." Which of the following regimens for the patient's antipsychotic medications will increase medication adherence?
    A. monthly injection by a home care nurse
    B. low-dose daily therapy
    C. daily visits to the clinic to receive the medications
    D. once-a-week drug therapy

2. A patient taking chlorpromazine develops a high fever, respiratory depression, and diminished level of consciousness. Given what the nurse recognizes as adverse effects of chlorpromazine, what condition do the symptoms suggest that the patient has developed?
    A. neuroleptic malignant syndrome
    B. dystonia
    C. anhedonia
    D. akathisia

3. A 68-year-old patient is seen by a home care nurse. The patient has been taking chlorpromazine for 40 years for schizophrenia. Which of the following adverse effects are most seen after use of chlorpromazine for a long period?
    A. lethargy
    B. amnesia
    C. tardive dyskinesia
    D. dystonia

FIRST-GENERATION NONPHENOTHIAZINES

Nonphenothiazines include the first-generation antipsychotics, which are similar to phenothiazines in many ways. They were introduced approximately 50 years ago and are effective in treating acute psychosis, chronic psychotic disorders, and other psychiatric conditions. They are effective in treating both psychotic disorders and nonpsychotic depression.

The first-generation antipsychotic medication **haloperidol** (Haldol) is the prototype "typical" nonphenothiazine. This butyrophenone is a frequently used, long-acting antipsychotic.

Pharmacokinetics

Haloperidol is well absorbed after oral or IM administration. For the oral drug, the onset of action is 2 hours, with a peak of 2 to 6 hours and a duration of 8 to 12 hours. For the IM drug, the onset of action is 20 to 30 minutes, with a peak of 30 to 45 minutes and a duration of 4 to 8 hours. The half-life of the drug is 21 to 24 hours. It is metabolized in the liver and is excreted in urine and bile.

Action

The mechanism of action of haloperidol is not fully understood, but experts believe that the drug produces antipsychotic effects by blocking the postsynaptic dopamine receptors in the brain.

Use

Prescribers order haloperidol to control the symptoms of schizophrenia and psychotic disorders.

Patient-related variables specific to the use of haloperidol and other second-generation antipsychotic drugs include the following:

- Age:
  - The FDA has issued a **BOXED WARNING** ♦ regarding extrapyramidal and withdrawal symptoms in newborns who have been exposed to haloperidol. Withdrawal symptoms occur in newborns when haloperidol is taken during the third trimester of pregnancy.
  - The FDA has not approved haloperidol for treatment of dementia-related psychosis. A **BOXED WARNING** ♦ alerts healthcare practitioners that older patients who suffer from dementia and dementia-related psychosis and receive haloperidol have an increased risk of death compared with those patients who receive a placebo. (The deaths were related to cardiovascular or infectious diseases.)
- Reproduction, pregnancy, and lactation:
  - Haloperidol is preferred over first-generation antipsychotics during pregnancy.
  - Taking haloperidol during the third trimester of pregnancy has a risk following delivery for abnormal muscle movements (extrapyramidal effects) and withdrawal symptoms in newborns.
  - Breast-feeding is not recommended as adverse effects have been reported.
  - Galactorrhea and gynecomastia are adverse effects.
- Abnormal kidney function and hepatic impairment:
  - It is necessary to monitor kidney function periodically during long-term therapy and lower the dosage or discontinue the drug altogether if test results (e.g., blood urea nitrogen) become abnormal.
  - Since haloperidol undergoes extensive hepatic metabolism, hepatic impairment may case resultant accumulation of the drug and increased risk of adverse effects.

Adverse Effects

Haloperidol has several adverse effects, including

- Cardiovascular effects: abnormal T waves, prolonged ventricular depolarization, QT prolongation, torsade de pointes, tachycardia, and sudden death
- CNS effects: akathisia, hyperthermia, dystonia, extrapyramidal effects, neuroleptic malignant syndrome, parkinsonism, seizures, and vertigo
- Dermatologic effects: photosensitivity, hyperpigmentation, contact dermatitis, and alopecia
- Genitourinary effects: anticholinergic adverse effects such as urinary retention, sexual dysfunction, amenorrhea, breast engorgement and galactorrhea (women), and priapism and gynecomastia (men)
- Metabolic effects: hyperglycemia, hypoglycemia, and hyponatremia
- Respiratory effects: bronchospasm or laryngospasm

Contraindications

Contraindications to haloperidol include Parkinson disease, seizure disorders, and severe mental depression.

Nursing Implications

Preventing Interactions

Many medications interact with haloperidol (Box 56.4), increasing or decreasing its effects. In addition, several herbs increase the effects of haloperidol, including American and Asian ginseng, kava, gotu kola, Scotch broom, St. John's wort, valerian, and yohimbine.

Administering the Medication

Oral administration of haloperidol tablets requires taking the tablets with a full glass of water or milk. People should take them with food to decrease gastric upset. IM administration of haloperidol decanoate requires that the nurse gives the drug intramuscularly deep in the ventrogluteal muscle. (The amount injected should not exceed 3 mL.) During administration of the IM preparation, the patient should be in the recumbent position and remain recumbent for 1 hour following the administration. It is necessary to keep the preparation in a light-protected container.

When discontinuing haloperidol, it is essential to taper the dosage to prevent extrapyramidal effects. If the medication is abruptly discontinued, the patient is at risk of this condition.

Assessing for Therapeutic Effects

When haloperidol is given for acute psychotic episodes, the nurse observes for sedation, decreased agitation, combativeness, and psychomotor activity. When the drug is given for acute or chronic psychosis, the nurse observes for decreased psychotic behaviors, such as decreased hallucinations and delusions.

BOX 56.4 *Drug Interactions: Haloperidol*

Drugs That Increase the Effects of Haloperidol

- Alcohol, central nervous system depressants, anticholinergic drugs, antidepressants, antihistamines
  Increase sedation and anticholinergic effects
- Nonsteroidal anti-inflammatory drugs
  Increase drowsiness and confusion
- Propranolol and angiotensin-converting enzyme inhibitors, lithium
  Enhance neurotoxic effect of antipsychotics and increase extrapyramidal effects
- Antifungals, buspirone, macrolides
  May increase haloperidol level

Drugs That Decrease the Effects of Haloperidol

- Antacids
  Inhibit absorption
- Carbamazepine, rifampin
  May decrease haloperidol level

BOX 56.5 Patient Teaching Guidelines for Haloperidol

- Report sore throat or fever to the prescriber.
- Notify the prescriber of any adverse effects such as tardive dyskinesia, dystonia, or akathisia.
- Do not drive a car or operate dangerous machinery. Dizziness or decreased mental alertness may occur.
- If you go outdoors, wear protective clothing and use sunscreen.
- Maintain adequate hydration.
- Use lozenges to counteract anticholinergic effects.
- Realize that dark-colored urine (pink or red-brown) is normal.
- Discuss haloperidol use with a healthcare provider if you intend to become pregnant.

Assessing for Adverse Effects

The nurse assesses the ECG for tachycardia and other abnormalities. The patient's temperature is assessed for the onset of neuroleptic malignant syndrome. In addition, the nurse assesses for laryngospasm. Finally, it is necessary to monitor for the development of parkinsonism and extrapyramidal signs and symptoms, most notably tardive dyskinesia.

Patient Teaching

Box 56.5 identifies patient teaching guidelines for haloperidol.

Other Drugs in the Class

Thiothixene is a high-potency antipsychotic used in the management of schizophrenia. The most common adverse effect seen is extrapyramidal effects. Other effects include menstrual irregularities, gynecomastia, and galactorrhea. Use with other anticholinergic agents or drugs that are CNS depressants can enhance adverse effects.

Clinical Application 56.2

- After 6 weeks of therapy, Caroline has far fewer symptoms. She has withdrawn from her university classes to focus on her treatment and recovery. However, her friends observe that she has a gradual loss of muscle movement and a shuffling gait. What adverse reaction is likely to be occurring?
- Caroline has decided that she no longer wants to take the medication because of the adverse effects, despite experiencing a decrease in psychotic thinking. How would the nurse handle this situation?

SECOND-GENERATION "ATYPICAL" ANTIPSYCHOTICS

The "atypical" antipsychotics are the drugs of choice, especially for patients who are newly diagnosed with schizophrenia. These second-generation antipsychotics differ from first-generation agents in that they have a broader range of action due to their effects on the serotonergic, noradrenergic, and dopaminergic systems. They may be more effective in relieving some symptoms, they usually produce milder adverse effects, and patients seem to take them more consistently. Better adherence to the drug regimen helps prevent acute episodes of psychosis and repeated hospitalizations, thereby reducing the overall cost of healthcare, according to studies. A major drawback is the high cost of these drugs, which may preclude their use in some patients. **Ⓟ Clozapine** (Clozaril, Versacloz) is the prototype "atypical" antipsychotic.

Pharmacokinetics

Clozapine is an oral drug. Its onset of action is unknown, with a peak of 1 to 6 hours and a duration of weeks. The half-life is 12 hours. Clozapine crosses the placenta and enters the breast milk. The drug is metabolized in the liver, and it is excreted in the urine and in the feces.

Action

The mechanism of action of clozapine is not clearly understood. Apparently, the drug blocks the dopamine receptors in the brain, depressing the reticular activating system. It also blocks the serotonin and glutamate receptors. In addition, clozapine has anticholinergic, antihistamine, and alpha-adrenergic blocking activity.

Use

Clinicians consider clozapine and other "atypical" antipsychotics to be first-line therapy for schizophrenia. Prescribers use the drug to manage patients with severe schizophrenia who have not responded to standard antipsychotic medications. Other uses in psychosis include reducing the risk of recurrent suicidal behavior in patients with schizophrenia or with schizoaffective disorder. Clozapine is available only through a distribution system that ensures monitoring of white blood cell count and absolute neutrophil count. Table 56.3 presents route and dosage information for atypical antipsychotics, including clozapine.

Patient-related variables specific to the use of clozapine and other second-generation antipsychotics include the following:

- Age:
  - The use of clozapine has been reserved for treatment-resistant children and adolescents because of its greater propensity to cause serious hematologic adverse events (agranulocytosis) compared with other first- and second-generation antipsychotic medications.
  - The safety and effectiveness of clozapine in children have not been established.
  - The FDA has issued a **BOXED WARNING** ◆ related to the administration of clozapine and other second-generation antipsychotics to older adult patients with dementia. The risk of death is increased in these patients.
  - The FDA has not approved the drug for use in dementia-related psychosis.

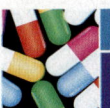

TABLE 56.3
DRUGS AT A GLANCE: Atypical Antipsychotics

Drug	Routes and Dosage Ranges	
	Adults	**Children**
Ⓟ Clozapine (Clozaril, Versacloz; ✚ Clozaril, AA-Clozapine, GEN-Clozapine)	12.5 mg PO once or twice daily; increase by 25–50 mg daily every 3–7 d up to a max dose of 900 mg daily.	≥6 y, 6.25–12.5 mg once daily Adolescents, 12.5 mg PO initially once or twice daily; increase to a target dose of 125–475 mg/d in divided doses
Aripiprazole (Abilify, Abilify Maintena; ✚ Abilify, Abilify Maintena, TEVA-ARIPiprazole)	Acute agitation: 9.75 mg PO initially as a single dose; range 5.25–15 mg PO daily initially; repeat doses may be given at ≥2-h intervals to a maximum of 30 mg daily Schizophrenia: 10–15 mg once daily; may be increased to a max dosage of 30 mg once daily; extended release 400 mg IM once monthly Older adults: 12.5–25 mg PO daily, increase in 2.5-mg increments to desired response	≥8 y, 10–15 mg PO once daily initially; efficacy has not been established above 10–15 mg daily
Asenapine (Saphris, Secuado; ✚ Saphris)	Schizophrenia: 5 mg SL 2 times/d Secuado (patch): 3.8 mg/24 h once daily; may increase to 5.7 mg/24 h or 7.6 mg/24 h after 1 wk Bipolar disorder: 10 mg SL 2 times/d; may be decreased to 5 mg/d as needed	≥10 y, 2.5 mg SL 2 time/daily, maximum 20 mg/d
Iloperidone (Fanapt)	12–24 mg PO daily; titrate based on orthostatic hypotension tolerance; initially 1 mg PO 2 times/d then 2, 4, 6, 8, 10, and 12 mg PO 2 times/d on days 2, 3, 4, 5, 6, and 7, respectively	Safety and efficacy not established
Lurasidone (Latuda; ✚ Latuda)	40 mg PO initially once daily; max recommended dose is 160 mg/d; take with food (≥350 calories) Older adults: do not give to older patients with dementia-related psychosis	13–17 y, 40 mg PO initially once daily; max recommended dose is 80 mg/d >17 y, same as adult
Olanzapine (Zyprexa; ✚ Teva-Olanzapine ODT, APO-Olanzapine, Zyprexa)	5–10 mg PO initially once daily at bedtime; increase over several weeks to 20 mg daily, if necessary	4 to <6 y, 1.25 mg PO once daily titrated to target of 10 mg/d 6–12 y, 2.5 mg PO once daily titrated to target of 10 mg/d Adolescents, initial: 2.5–5 mg PO once daily titrated to a target of 10 mg/d once daily
Paliperidone (Invega, Invega Sustenna, Invega Trinza; ✚ Invega, Invega Sustenna, Invega Trinza)	6 mg PO daily in the morning; may be increased over several weeks to a max of 12 mg daily Maintenance dose of 39–234 mg (as palmitate) or 25–150 mg (as base) every month IM monthly (Invega Sustenna) or every 3 mo (Invega Trinza)	≤18 y, 6 mg PO once daily or 78–234 mg IM monthly
Quetiapine (Seroquel, Seroquel XR; ✚ Dom-Quetiapine, Seroquel, Seroquel XR, BIO-Quetiapine)	25 mg PO 2 times/d initially; increase by 25–50 mg two or three times daily on 2nd and 3rd days, as tolerated, to 300–400 mg, in two or three divided doses on the 4th day; additional increments or decrements can be made at 2-d intervals; max dose 800 mg/d Older or debilitated adults: use lower initial doses and increase more gradually, to a lower target dose than for other adults Hepatic impairment: same as for older or debilitated adults	≥10 y, titrate 25 mg PO 2 times/d until clinical response 25 mg PO 2 times/d initially; increase by 25–50 mg two or three times daily on 2nd and 3rd days, as tolerated, to usual dose range 200–300 mg, in two or three divided doses on the 4th day; additional increments or decrements can be made at 2-d intervals; max dose 600 mg/d

(Continued on page 1040)

TABLE 56.3

DRUGS AT A GLANCE: Atypical Antipsychotics (Continued)

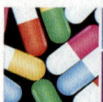

Drug	Routes and Dosage Ranges	
	Adults	**Children**
Risperidone (Risperdal, Perseris; ✚ APO-Risperidone, DOMRisperidone, MINT-Risperidone)	1 mg twice daily PO, initially; increase to 2 mg/d twice daily on the 2nd day; increase to 3 mg twice daily on the 3rd day, if necessary; usual maintenance dose, 4–8 mg/d; after initial titration, dosage increases or decreases should be made at a rate of 1 mg/wk Older or debilitated adults: initially 0.5 mg twice daily; increase in 0.5-mg increments to 1.5 mg twice daily Abnormal kidney function or hepatic impairment: same as for older or debilitated adults	Schizophrenia 13–17 y, initially 0.5 mg/d PO; increase 0.5–1 mg/d for a target dose of 3 mg/d; dose range is 0.5–3 mg daily Bipolar mania: 10–17 y, initially 0.5 mg/d PO; increase 0.5–1 mg/d for a target dose of 1–2.5 mg/d; dosage range is 1–6 mg/d Autism spectrum disorder, <20 kg, 0.25 mg PO initially, and increased to a maintenance dose of 0.5 mg daily ≥20 kg, 0.5 mg PO initially, and increased to a maintenance dose of 1.0 mg daily
Risperidone (Risperdal Consta; ✚ Risperdal Consta)	25 mg IM every 2 wk; max dose not to exceed 50 mg/2 wk; oral risperidone should be continued for first 3 wk of therapy to ensure adequate blood levels are maintained	<18 y, dosage not established
Ziprasidone (Geodon; ✚ Zeldox, Auro-Ziprasidone)	20 mg PO twice daily with food, initially; gradually increased up to 80 mg twice daily, if necessary Acute agitation in schizophrenia: 10–20 mg IM every 4 h up to a max of 40 mg/d, not to exceed 3 d	Schizophrenia (acute agitation): 5–11 y, 10 mg IM 12 y 10–20 mg Autism: ≥8 y, 20–160 mg/d divided twice daily

- Reproduction, pregnancy, and lactation:
  - Routine use of atypical antipsychotics during pregnancy is not recommended as safety data are limited so treatment is guided by considering the risk versus benefits.
  - Although other antipsychotics are preferred for use during pregnancy, clozapine may be considered in those who cannot be changed to recommended antipsychotics.
  - Clozapine is not recommended in breast-feeding due to the potential for adverse effects to an infant.
- Abnormal kidney function and hepatic impairment:
  - In patients with impaired kidney functioning, dose reduction may be necessary; the drug should not be used in patients with severe kidney disorders.
  - For patients with significant hepatic impairment, dose reduction may be warranted because clozapine is extensively metabolized by the liver, partially via the cytochrome P450 system.
  - Clozapine should not be given to patients with active liver disease associated with nausea, loss of appetite or jaundice, or worsening liver disease or liver failure.
- Gastrointestinal effects: The patient is at risk of severe constipation.
- CNS effects: increased risk of seizures in patients with a known seizure disorder. An FDA-issued **BOXED WARNING** ◆ alerts users of clozapine that the drug increases the risk of seizure activity as the dose increases.
- Hematologic effects: agranulocytosis. Clozapine can decrease the number of neutrophils, a type of white blood cell, that function in the body to fight off infections. When neutrophils are significantly decreased, severe neutropenia may result and the body may become prone to infections. Also, the FDA has issued a **BOXED WARNING** ◆ regarding the potential risk of fatal agranulocytosis in patients who take clozapine.
- Metabolic effects: hyperglycemia and weight gain. The FDA has issued a **BOXED WARNING** ◆ regarding the risk of hyperglycemia in patients who take clozapine. (In some extreme cases, there have been reports of ketoacidosis, hyperosmolar coma, and death.)

Adverse Effects

Clozapine has several adverse effects, including

- Cardiovascular effects: orthostatic hypotension, tachycardia, ECG changes, and increased risk of myocarditis (greatest during the 1st month of treatment). The patient is also at risk of myocardial infarction, pericarditis, cardiomyopathy, mitral insufficiency, heart failure, and pericardial effusion.

Contraindications

Contraindications to clozapine include a known hypersensitivity to the drug (e.g., photosensitivity, vasculitis, erythema multiforme, or Stevens–Johnson syndrome). Caution is warranted in cardiovascular disease, narrow-angle glaucoma, diabetes mellitus, CNS depression, and a history of seizure disorders, and/or pulmonary disease.

Clinical Application 56.3

- Caroline's family has read some literature about the newer atypical antipsychotic medications and the success they have had in treating patients with positive and negative symptoms of schizophrenia. Consequently, her physician has prescribed clozapine 12.5 mg twice daily. What safety patient teaching should the nurse conduct?

Nursing Implications

Preventing Interactions

Many medications interact with clozapine, increasing or decreasing its effects (Box 56.6). In addition, several herbs increase the effects of clozapine, including American and Asian ginseng, guarana, gotu kola, kava, St. John's wort, valerian, yerba mate, and yohimbine.

Administering the Medication

Prior to beginning the administration of clozapine, it is necessary to obtain a baseline white blood cell count and neutrophil count. Also, it is important to monitor the blood glucose level regularly for hyperglycemia, especially if signs and symptoms of diabetes mellitus or risk factors are present.

If clozapine is to be discontinued, gradual tapering over a 2-week period is essential. If the drug is discontinued abruptly, the nurse monitors for symptoms of acute psychosis.

Assessing for Therapeutic Effects

When clozapine is given for acute psychotic episodes, the nurse observes for sedation, decreased agitation, combativeness, and psychomotor activity. When the drug is given for acute or chronic psychosis, the nurse observes for decreased psychotic behaviors, such as decreased hallucinations and delusions.

Assessing for Adverse Effects

The nurse implements a thorough assessment of the cardiovascular and cardiopulmonary status to check for orthostatic hypotension, heart failure, and cardiovascular adverse events. It is essential to monitor the complete blood count due to the risk of fatal agranulocytosis. Also, it is necessary to monitor the intraocular pressure for increased pressure and potential development of glaucoma. In January 2020, the FDA strengthened an existing safety warning that constipation caused by clozapine can progress to serious bowel complications, such as intestinal ischemia and necrotizing colitis, which could require hospitalization or lead to death.

Patient Teaching

Box 56.7 identifies patient teaching guidelines for clozapine.

Other Drugs in the Class

Aripiprazole (Abilify, Abilify Maintena) is the first of a new class of drugs called the dopamine system stabilizers. In its oral form, the drug is used to treat schizophrenia, bipolar disorder, major depressive disorder, irritability associated with autistic disorder, and Tourette syndrome; the injectable immediate-release formulation is used to treat agitation associated with schizophrenia or bipolar mania, and the extended-release injection (Abilify Maintena) is used to treat schizophrenia. The injectable products are not interchangeable. Aripiprazole may not be as effective as other agents. Adverse effects include headache, extrapyramidal reaction, drowsiness, akathisia, sedation, agitation, weight gain, nausea, vomiting, constipations, and tremors. The drug does not prolong the QT interval. The FDA has announced a safety alert, confirming that compulsive or uncontrollable urges to gamble, binge eat, shop, and have sex have been reported with the use of aripiprazole.

BOX 56.6 Drug Interactions: Clozapine

Drugs That Increase the Effects of Clozapine

- Alcohol
  Increases central nervous system depression
- Cimetidine, caffeine, other cytochrome P450 inhibitors (SSRIs), ritonavir
  Increase the risk of toxicity
- Anticholinergics
  May potentiate the anticholinergic effects of clozapine

Drugs That Decrease the Effects of Clozapine

- Phenytoin, ethotoin, other cytochrome P450 inducers
  Decrease the serum concentration

BOX 56.7 Patient Teaching Guidelines for Clozapine

- Obtain weekly blood tests to determine the safe and effective dosage.
- Keep appointments for white blood cell count monitoring.
- Keep counseling appointments.
- Be aware that only 1 week of medication will be dispensed at a time.
- Do not drive a car or operate dangerous machinery. Dizziness or decreased mental alertness may occur.
- Do not stop the medication abruptly.
- You may experience drowsiness, dizziness, and decreased alertness.
- You may experience constipation and a stool softener may need to routinely be administered if constipation occurs.
- Discuss clozapine use with a healthcare provider if you intend to become pregnant.
- Notify the prescriber of increased heart rate.
- Report lethargy, weakness, or flulike symptoms to the prescriber.

Quality and Safety Alert: Safety

Numerous drug interactions are possible with aripiprazole because the drug and its metabolite are metabolized hepatically by CYP2D6 and CYP3A4 enzymes of the cytochrome P450 system, respectively. Drugs that inhibit CYP2D6 (e.g., quinidine, paroxetine, fluoxetine) and CYP3A4 (e.g., erythromycin, fluconazole, ketoconazole, itraconazole) can raise the drug's serum level, increasing the risk of adverse effects. Drugs that induce CPY3A4 (e.g., barbiturates, carbamazepine, phenytoin, rifampin) can speed up the metabolism of aripiprazole and can lower the serum level, reducing the efficacy of the drug at that dosage.

Asenapine (Saphris) is used to manage acute and chronic schizophrenia and manic or mixed episodes of bipolar disorder. The risk of dyslipidemia, diabetes, or weight gain is low. Adverse effects include drowsiness, insomnia, and increased creatine phosphokinase. Few drug interactions are noted. Sublingual tablets should be allowed to completely dissolve and should not be split, crushed, chewed, or swallowed. Patients should not eat or drink for at least 10 minutes after taking asenapine; this decreases the bioavailability of the drug.

Iloperidone (Fanapt) is used to treat schizophrenia in adults. The drug is better tolerated than some, but common adverse effects include prolonged QT interval, hypotension, and weight gain. Other dose-related adverse effects include tachycardia, dry mouth, fatigue, drowsiness, and increased serum prolactin level. The drug is metabolized by the liver by the CYP2D6 and CYP3A4 enzymes, so numerous drug interactions are possible.

Quality and Safety Alert: Safety

The dose of iloperidone should by decreased by 50% in patients while concurrently taking strong CYP2D6 inhibitors (e.g., paroxetine, fluoxetine, quinidine) or strong CYP3A4 inhibitors (e.g., ketoconazole, clarithromycin) because the drugs can increase levels of iloperidone and increase adverse effects, including prolongation of the QT interval. In addition, a decrease in iloperidone dose by 50% is necessary in patients who are poor metabolizers of CYP2D6.

Olanzapine (Zyprexa) is also used to manage schizophrenia and manic or mixed episodes of bipolar disorder. The drug can cause leukopenia and neutropenia, which increases the risk of infection. Other adverse effects include drowsiness, extrapyramidal effects, akathisia, Parkinson-like syndrome, dizziness, headache, increased serum prolactin, increased appetite, xerostomia, increased serum aspartate aminotransferase (AST), decreased serum bilirubin, and increased serum alanine aminotransferase (ALT). The drug is highly metabolized by CYP1A2 and CYP2D6 of the cytochrome P450 system. About 40% of the drug is removed via first-pass metabolism. Drug interactions are likely with drugs that induce CYP1A2 (e.g., nafcillin, omeprazole, modafinil) or inhibit this enzyme (e.g., ciprofloxacin, verapamil, cimetidine). In addition, vegetables such as char-grilled meat, cabbages, broccoli, and cauliflower are known to increase levels of CYP1A2. Conversely, St. John's wort, echinacea, peppermint, German chamomile, and dandelion teas, as well as tobacco, are inhibitors of CPY1A2. Drugs that induce (e.g., haloperidol, dexamethasone, glutethimide) or inhibit (e.g., quinidine, paroxetine, fluoxetine) CYP2D6 are known to interact with olanzapine.

Lurasidone (Latuda) is used to treat schizophrenia and bipolar depression. The FDA has issued a **BOXED WARNING** ◆ stating that older patients who suffer from dementia and dementia-related psychosis treated with lurasidone have an increased risk of death. The drug is not approved for the treatment of dementia-related psychosis. Administering the drug with food greatly increases absorption. Reported adverse effects include somnolence, Parkinson syndrome, and akathisia. The drug does not cause prolonged QT interval, orthostatic hypotension, or cholinergic effects. Because lurasidone is metabolized by CYP3A4, drug interactions will occur with concurrent use of drugs that are strong inhibitors of CYP3A4 (ketoconazole), and strong inducers (rifampin) are contraindicated.

Risperidone (Risperdal, Perseris) is prescribed for the treatment of schizophrenia and acute bipolar mania. The drug is also used to manage children with autism spectrum disorders to reduce irritability-associated symptoms, including self-injury, aggression, tantrums, and mood swings. In schizophrenia, relief of positive and negative symptoms and improved cognitive function may occur in as little as 1 week. Generally, adverse effects are mild and include weight gain, diabetes, and dyslipidemia. A dose-related increase in extrapyramidal effects may occur with increased oral doses and the long-term formulation (Risperdal Consta), a depot preparation.

Paliperidone (Invega) is used in the treatment of schizophrenia and other psychoses. As major active metabolite of risperidone, it has the same therapeutic and adverse effects. The drug is available in three forms, a short-acting oral form (Invega), a LAI form (Invega Sustenna; to be taken monthly), and a LAI form (Invega Trinza; to be taken every 3 months). Common adverse effects include akathisia, headache, Parkinson-like syndrome, dystonia, and tremor.

Quetiapine (Seroquel, Seroquel XR) is prescribed to treat schizophrenia, depressive disorder, and manic episodes with bipolar disorder. Extended-release Seroquel XR is for use only in adults and should not be given to patients younger than 18 years old. Adverse effects include tachycardia, increased systolic and/or increased systolic and diastolic blood pressure, drowsiness, headache, agitation, dizziness, weight gain, increased serum total cholesterol, low-density cholesterol, triglycerides, and decreased high-density cholesterol, as well as xerostomia, constipation, and increased appetite. As with many atypical antipsychotic agents, the potential for clinically relevant drug interactions exists because the drug is metabolized by CYP2D6 and CYP3A4.

Quality and Safety Alert: Evidence-Based Practice

Kishimoto et al. (2019) completed a systematic review and meta-analysis of 59 randomized trials and 45,787 participants comparing drug effectiveness and safety in two or more second-generation antipsychotics (SGAs) in the long-term treatment of schizophrenia. No one SGA proved superior over another in terms of overall effectiveness and tolerability. However, clozapine, olanzapine, and risperidone demonstrated less all-cause discontinuation while quetiapine more frequently required termination as compared to other SGAs. Since there were limited trials that directly compared an SGA to an existing standard of care, the results must be interpreted cautiously. The use of a specific SGA needs to be tailored to optimize the individual patient's treatment outcomes.

Ziprasidone (Geodon) is indicated for schizophrenia, bipolar mania, and autism spectrum disorder in children. The drug produces fewer extrapyramidal effects than other second-generation agents and reportedly leads to improvement in positive and negative symptoms and cognitive function. Because ziprasidone prolongs the QT interval, the drug should not be administered with other drugs (e.g., tricyclic antidepressants that have the potential to prolong QT interval). Like olanzapine, ziprasidone can cause leukopenia and neutropenia that increases the risk of infection. Numerous drug interactions are possible with ziprasidone as the drug and its metabolite are metabolized hepatically by CYP2D6 and CYP3A4, respectively. Drugs that inhibit CYP2D6 (e.g., quinidine, paroxetine, fluoxetine) and CYP3A4 (e.g., erythromycin, fluconazole, ketoconazole, itraconazole) can raise the drug's serum level, increasing the risk of adverse effects. Drugs that induce CPY3A4 (e.g., barbiturates, carbamazepine, phenytoin, rifampin) can speed up the metabolism of aripiprazole and can lower the serum level, reducing the efficacy of the drug at that dosage.

Clinical Application 56.4

Caroline has not adhered to her daily antipsychotic regimen. She states that she feels her symptoms are under control, and because she feels "normal" again, she no longer needs to take the medication. She has dropped out of the university and has moved home with her parents. She spends her free time in her room and she is isolating herself again.

- What does the nurse discuss with the patient and her family?
- What medication alternatives does the nurse suggest at this point, considering Caroline's history of nonadherence?

NCLEX Success

4. A patient reports to the prescriber that fever, sore throat, and malaise have developed after starting clozapine therapy. Which of the following interventions is most important?

   A. Treat the patient with a broad-spectrum antibiotic.
   B. Discontinue the clozapine and obtain a complete blood count with differential.
   C. Inform the patient that this is normal when taking clozapine.
   D. Assess the patient for diminished mental alertness.

5. Which statement made by a patient indicates that further patient teaching regarding adherence to the medication regimen is required?

   A. "If I experience muscle spasms in my neck, I must report that to the health care provider."
   B. "If I experience sudden fever and difficulty breathing, I must report that to the health care provider."
   C. "If I experience sedation, I must cut down on my medication."
   D. "If I experience dizziness, I must report that to the healthcare provider."

Clinical Application 56.5

- Caroline has been taking clozapine for 6 months, and she has all the necessary blood tests for white blood cell count monitoring. Her psychotic symptoms have decreased. Adverse effects have been minimal. Caroline is eager to return to the university next semester and asks how long she needs to take this medication. What response is appropriate?

THE NURSING PROCESS

A concept map outlines the nursing process related to drug therapy considerations in this chapter. Additional nursing implications related to the disease process should also be considered in care decisions.

Assessment
- Assess the patient's mental health status, history of psychotic behavior, need for antipsychotic drugs, and response and compliance to drug therapy. Some assessment directives include the following:
  - Interview the patient and family members. Attempts to interview an acutely psychotic person will yield little useful information.
  - Assess the patient's level of orientation and presence of positive and negative symptoms and cognitive status, if possible.
  - Determine from family members what predisposing factors precipitated the event (e.g., increased environmental stress, ingestion of alcohol or drugs).
  - Ask the family if the patient seems to be a hazard to self or others.
  - Have the family provide some description of preillness personality traits, level of social interaction, and ability to function in usual activities of daily living.

Outcomes of Therapy

The patient will
- Become less agitated within a few hours of the start of drug therapy, and less psychotic within 1 to 3 weeks.
- Be kept safe while sedated from drug therapy.
- Be cared for by staff in areas of nutrition, hygiene, exercise, and social interactions when unable to provide self-care.
- Improve in ability to participate in self-care activities.
- Avoid preventable adverse drug effects, especially those that impair safety.
- Be helped to take medications as prescribed and return for follow-up appointments with health care providers.

Nursing Interventions
- Use nondrug measures when appropriate to increase the effectiveness of drug therapy and to decrease adverse reactions.
- Answer questions or provide information about drug therapy and other aspects of the treatment plan.
- Devise a schedule of administration times that is as convenient as possible for the patient.
- Assist the patient or caregiver in preventing or managing adverse drug effects through patient education (see Boxes 56.3, 56.5, and 56.7).
- Supervise ambulation to prevent falls or other injuries if the patient is drowsy or elderly or has postural hypotension.
- Instruct the patient to lie down for approximately 1 hour after a large oral dose or an injection of antipsychotic medication.
- Apply elastic stockings, and instruct the patient to change positions gradually, elevate legs when sitting, avoid standing for prolonged periods, and avoid hot baths (hot baths cause vasodilation and increase the incidence of hypotension).
- Instruct the patient on oral hygiene. The effects of the medications can lead to dry mouth and oral infections.
- Instruct the patient about strategies to decrease dry mouth such as chewing sugarless gum, frequently brushing teeth, and rinsing the mouth with water.
- Instruct the patient about measures to increase fluid intake, dietary fiber, and exercise, which can help prevent constipation.
- Instruct the patient regarding the importance of keeping medical appointments and taking medications as prescribed.

Evaluation
- Interview the patient to determine the presence and extent of hallucinations and delusions.
- Observe the patient for decreased signs and symptoms.
- Document abilities and limitations in self-care.
- Note whether any injuries have occurred during drug therapy.
- Interview the caregiver about the patient's behavior, medication response, and compliance with drug therapy and follow-up care.

Visit thePoint® at http://thePoint.lww.com/Frandsen13e for answers to NCLEX Success questions (in Appendix A), answers to Clinical Application Case Studies (in Appendix B), additional information on the etiology and pathophysiology of schizophrenia, and more!

REFERENCES AND RESOURCES

American Psychiatric Association. (2022). *Diagnostic and statistical manual of mental disorders* (5th ed., Text Revision ed.).

Arango, C., Ng-Mak, D., Finn, E., Byrne, A., & Loebel, A. (2019). Lurasidone compared to other atypical antipsychotic monotherapies for adolescent schizophrenia: A systematic literature review and network meta-analysis. *European Child & Adolescent Psychiatry*. https://doi.org/10.1007/s00787-019-01425-2

Dinnissen, M., Dietrich, A., van der Molen, J. H., Verhallen, A. M., Buiteveld, Y., Jongejan, S., Troost, P. W., Buitelaar, J. K., Hoekstra, P. J., & van den Hoofdakker, B. J. (2020). Prescribing antipsychotics in child and adolescent psychiatry: Guideline adherence. *European Child & Adolescent Psychiatry*, 29(12), 1717–1727. https://doi.org/10.1007/s00787-020-01488-6

Fischer, B. A., & Buchanan, R. W. (2020). Schizophrenia in adults: Clinical manifestations, course, assessment, and diagnosis. *UpToDate*. Lexi-Comp, Inc.

Jibson, M. (2020). First generation antipsychotic medications: Pharmacology, administration, and comparative side effects. *UpToDate*. Lexi-Comp, Inc.

Kealey, E., Scholle, S. H., Byron, S. C., Hoagwood, K., Leckman-Westin, E., Kelleher, K., & Finnerty, M. (2014). Quality concerns in antipsychotic prescribing for youth: A review of treatment guidelines. *Academic Pediatrics*, 14(Suppl. 5), S68–S75. https://doi.org/10.1016/j.acap.2014.05.009

Kishimoto, T., Hagi, K., Nitta, M., Kane, J. M., & Currell, C. U. (2019). Long-term effectiveness of oral second-generation antipsychotics in patients with schizophrenia and related disorders: A systematic review and meta-analysis of direct head-to-head comparisons. *World Psychiatry*, 18(2), 208–224. https://doi.org/10.1002/wps.20632

Lippincott Advisor. (2022). Retrieved from http://advisor.lww.com

Lippincott Williams & Wilkins. (2022). *Nursing 2023 drug handbook* (43rd ed.). Wolters Kluwer.

Lorberg, B., Davico, C., Martsenkovskyi, D., & Vitiello, B. (2019). Principles in using psychotropic medication in children and adolescents. In J. M. Rey & A. Martin (Eds.), *IACAPAP e-textbook of child and adolescent mental health*. International Association for Child and Adolescent Psychiatry and Allied Professions.

Rikinkumar, P., Velunm, N., Patel, J., Manchado, T., & Diler, R. (2021). Second-generation antipsychotics (SGA) in the management of acute pediatric bipolar depression: A systematic review and meta-analysis. *Psychopharmacology*, 60(10) supplement, 214.

Stone, J. M., Roux, S., Taylor, D., & Morrison, P. D. (2018). First-generation *versus* second-generation long-acting injectable antipsychotic drugs and time to relapse. *Therapeutic Advances in Psychopharmacology*, 8(12), 333–336. https://doi.org/10.1177/2045125318795130

Zaim, N., Findling, R. L., & Sun, A. (2020). Antipsychotics for treatment of adolescent onset schizophrenia: A review. *Current Treatment Options in Psychiatry*, 7, 23–38. https://doi.org/10.1007/s40501-020-00198-9

CHAPTER 57

Drug Therapy for Attention Deficit Hyperactivity Disorder and Narcolepsy

LEARNING OBJECTIVES

After studying this chapter, you should be able to:

1. Recognize the clinical manifestations of attention deficit hyperactivity disorder.
2. Recognize the clinical manifestations of narcolepsy.
3. Identify the prototypes and discuss the action, use, adverse effects, contraindications, and nursing implications for the stimulants used in the treatment of attention deficit hyperactivity disorder and narcolepsy.
4. Implement the nursing process in the care of patients who take central nervous system stimulants for attention deficit hyperactivity disorder and narcolepsy.

CLINICAL APPLICATION CASE STUDY

Brian Connor received a diagnosis of attention deficit hyperactivity disorder at 7 years of age. He is now 9 years old and is taking methylphenidate (Ritalin) 15 mg daily, which he takes each morning before school. With drug therapy and individual counseling, his attention span and school performance have improved. However, Brian's most recent physical examination shows that his height and weight are less than normal for his age and that he has lost weight since his examination last year. The school nurse talks with Brian's teachers, who report that he seems more restless in class after lunch. He has had more difficulty getting along with his classmates due to his impulsive behaviors.

KEY TERMS

Attention deficit hyperactivity disorder: relatively common disorder of childhood onset characterized by inattention, impulsiveness, and overactivity

Cataplexy: episodic, sudden loss of muscle tone ranging from slight weakness to complete body collapse in response to strong emotion

Drug holiday: temporary drug-free period to allow some return of normal functions, to maintain sensitivity to a drug, and to reduce the likelihood of adverse effects

Hypnagogic hallucinations: vivid, often frightening, dreamlike experiences that occur while dozing, falling asleep, or awakening

Narcolepsy: a clinical condition of daytime sleepiness with cataplexy, hypnagogic hallucinations, and sleep paralysis

INTRODUCTION

This chapter introduces the pharmacologic care of attention deficit hyperactivity disorder (ADHD) and narcolepsy. Clinicians use drugs that stimulate the central nervous system (CNS) to treat these disorders.

OVERVIEW OF ATTENTION DEFICIT HYPERACTIVITY DISORDER

To adequately understand the pharmacologic treatment of **attention deficit hyperactivity disorder**, or ADHD, it is important to understand the clinical manifestations of ADHD. For further details on the etiology and pathophysiology of ADHD, visit thePoint http://thePoint.lww.com/Frandsen13e. ADHD is a relatively common disorder of childhood characterized by inattention, impulsiveness, and overactivity.

Clinical Manifestations

Clinical manifestations of ADHD usually occur in various or multiple environments in a child's life, including school, home, place of worship, or recreational activities. The level of problems typically varies, but symptoms generally worsen in situations that require sustained attention, such as listening to a teacher, performing repetitive tasks, or reading lengthy materials.

Hyperactivity in children presents as fidgeting or squirming in their seats, excessive running or climbing when it is dangerous or inappropriate, disruptive playing during quiet activities, and demonstrating a driven verbal or motor quality. Impulsivity manifests as impatience, blurting out answers, and frequently interrupting others. Inattention manifests as messy work, careless mistakes, and appearance of daydreaming. Based on the behaviors associated with ADHD, people with the disorder also may have low self-esteem and strained peer relations. Early diagnosis and treatment are essential. Evidence suggests that behavior management combined with pharmacotherapy yields the best outcomes.

Drug Therapy

Drug therapy is indicated when symptoms are moderate to severe; are present for several months; and interfere in social, academic, or behavioral functioning. Counseling and psychotherapy (e.g., parental counseling, family therapy) are recommended along with drug therapy for effective treatment and realistic expectations of outcomes. Young children may not require treatment until starting school. Then, the goal of drug therapy is to control symptoms, facilitate learning, and promote social development. Table 57.1 summarizes the drugs used in the treatment of ADHD, and Figure 57.1 identifies the mechanisms of action of these drugs. Treatment is based on individual signs and symptoms.

OVERVIEW OF NARCOLEPSY

To adequately understand the pharmacologic treatment of narcolepsy, it is important to understand the clinical manifestations of the disorder. For further details on the etiology and pathophysiology of narcolepsy, visit thePoint http://thePoint.lww.com/Frandsen13e. **Narcolepsy** is a clinical condition of daytime sleepiness with cataplexy, hypnagogic hallucinations, and sleep paralysis. This condition is characterized by excessive sleepiness and sleep attacks at inappropriate times, such as at work. Narcolepsy affects males and females equally and usually begins during the teenage or young adult years. Nearly half of patients with narcolepsy report that the sleepiness substantially interferes with their daily lives, including school, work, marriage, and social life.

TABLE 57.1

Drugs Administered for the Treatment of Attention Deficit Hyperactivity Disorder and Narcolepsy

Drug Class	Prototype	Other Drugs in the Class
Amphetamines	Dextroamphetamine (Dexedrine, ProCentra, Zenzedi)	Dextroamphetamine and amphetamine (Adderall XR, Adderall, Mydayis) Lisdexamfetamine (Vyvanse) Methamphetamine (Desoxyn)
Amphetamine-related CNS stimulants	Methylphenidate (Adhansia XR, Aptensio, Concerta, Cotempla XR-ODT, Daytrana, Jornay PM, Concerta, Daytrana, Methylin, QuilliChew ER, Quillivant XR, Relexxiii, Ritalin, Ritalin LA)	Dexmethylphenidate (Focalin, Focalin XR) Armodafinil (Nuvigil) Modafinil (Provigil) Serdexmethylphenidate-dexmethylphenidate (Azstarys)
Selective norepinephrine reuptake inhibitors	Atomoxetine (Strattera)	
Sympatholytics	Guanfacine (Intuniv)	
CNS depressant	Sodium oxybate (Xyrem)	

CNS, central nervous system.

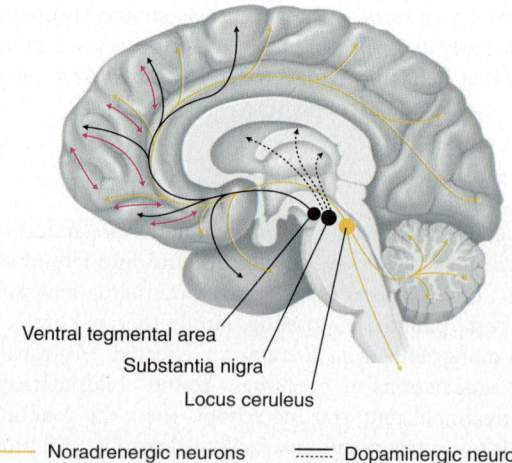

- Ventral tegmental area
- Substantia nigra
- Locus ceruleus

— Noradrenergic neurons   ---- Dopaminergic neurons
— Postsynaptic neuron receptors that receive noradrenergic innervation

Figure 57.1. Mechanisms of action for commonly used drugs to treat ADHD. Amphetamine, amphetamine-related CNS stimulants, and selective norepinephrine reuptake inhibitors act on noradrenergic neurons originating in the locus ceruleus and projecting throughout the cerebral cortex, hypothalamus, cerebellum, and spinal cord (*yellow*). Amphetamine also acts on dopaminergic neurons originating in the ventral tegmental area and projecting to the cerebral cortex, hypothalamus, and nucleus accumbens (*black solid lines*). Other dopaminergic neurons originating in the substantia nigra and projecting to the striatum (*black dashed lines*) help initiate intended movement. Sympatholytics, such as guanfacine, preferentially bind postsynaptic alpha$_{2A}$-adrenoreceptors in the prefrontal cortex (*pink solid lines*), which is theorized to improve delay-related firing of prefrontal cortex neurons, improving symptoms associated with ADHD. (Adapted with permission from Golan, D. E., Tashjian, A. H., & Armstrong, E. J. (2008). *Principles of pharmacology: The pathophysiologic basis of drug therapy* (2nd ed., Fig. 17.9). Wolters Kluwer Health.)

Clinical Manifestations

People with narcolepsy often experience disturbed nocturnal sleep and an abnormal daytime sleep pattern; it is important not to confuse this pattern with insomnia. Excessive daytime drowsiness (even after an adequate night's sleep) and fatigue are characteristic. People are likely to become drowsy or fall asleep or just be very tired. The hazards of drowsiness during normal waking hours and suddenly going to sleep in unsafe environments restrict activities of daily living.

Cataplexy is an episodic, sudden loss of muscle tone ranging from slight weakness to complete body collapse in response to strong emotion. These episodes may be triggered by emotional reactions such as laughter, anger, or fear, lasting from a few seconds to minutes. Cataplexy can cause an affected person to fall, which may lead to injury. Episodes of cataplexy vary in frequency from several times a day to a few times a year. Other signs and symptoms of narcolepsy include hypnagogic hallucinations and sleep paralysis. **Hypnagogic hallucinations** are vivid, often frightening, dreamlike experiences that occur while dozing, falling asleep, or awakening. Sleep paralysis is the temporary inability to move or talk on waking.

Drug Therapy

Treatment of narcolepsy is based on individual symptoms and therapeutic response. In addition to drug therapy, prevention of sleep deprivation, regular sleeping and waking times, avoiding shift work, and short naps may be helpful in reducing daytime sleepiness. Also, avoiding large meals, alcohol, and caffeine-containing beverages before bedtime may enhance sleep quality. However, even adequate amounts of nighttime sleep do not produce full alertness. Table 57.1 summarizes the medications used in the treatment of narcolepsy.

Clinical Application 57.1

Brian has been disrupting class, most notably after lunch. The teachers have contacted his parents regarding this situation. His parents have made an appointment with his healthcare provider, who changed his medication to methylphenidate XR (Ritalin LA). This new medication comes in capsule form, and Brian and his parents are afraid that he cannot swallow the large capsule.
- Is this an appropriate medication change?
- Brian's mother asks if she can empty the contents of the capsule in applesauce. What patient teaching should the nurse implement?
- What strategies might the nurse suggest to Brian and his parents to help him with taking this new medication?

NCLEX Success

1. For a patient taking methylphenidate every morning which of the following behaviors is most important for a child to demonstrate?
   A. sitting and playing with toys for 90 minutes
   B. getting along well with peers
   C. expressing anger in an appropriate manner
   D. not throwing toys across the room

STIMULANTS

CNS stimulants act by facilitating initiation and transmission of nerve impulses that excite other cells. The drugs are somewhat selective in their actions at lower doses but tend to involve the entire CNS at higher doses. Stimulant drugs and stimulant-like drugs (e.g., methylphenidate) are generally the first-line treatment for ADHD in school-aged children and adolescents. These drugs are generally available in short-, intermediate-, and long-acting formulations. In addition to the aforementioned formulations, transdermal medications for ADHD have become popular. This formulation improves adherence to the treatment. In ADHD, the drugs improve academic performance, behavior, and interpersonal relationships. In narcolepsy, stimulants significantly improve the performance of daily activities. The major groups of stimulants are amphetamines, amphetamine-related drugs, and xanthines.

The main goal of therapy with CNS stimulants is to relieve symptoms of the disorders for which they are given. A secondary goal is to have patients use the drugs appropriately. Misuse of stimulants often occurs when people who want to combat fatigue and delay sleep, such as long-distance drivers, students, and athletes, take the drugs. College students reportedly use stimulants as study aids; this is not justified. These drugs are dangerous for drivers and those involved in similar activities, and they have no legitimate use in athletics.

When a prescriber orders a CNS stimulant, the dose starts low and then increases as necessary, usually at weekly intervals, until the drug becomes effective or the dose reaches a maximum. It is also necessary to limit the number of doses that can be obtained with one prescription. This action reduces the likelihood of drug dependence or misuse of prescription drugs for purposes not intended as prescribed. For additional information on substance abuse and diversion, see Chapter 49.

Overdoses may occur with acute or chronic ingestion of large amounts of a single stimulant, combinations of stimulants, or concurrent ingestion of a stimulant and another drug that slows the metabolism of the stimulant. Signs of toxicity may include severe agitation, cardiac dysrhythmias, combativeness, confusion, delirium, hallucinations, high body temperature, hyperactivity, hypertension, insomnia, irritability, nervousness, panic states, restlessness, tremors, seizures, coma, circulatory collapse, and death.

AMPHETAMINES

Amphetamines produce mood elevation or euphoria, increasing mental alertness and capacity for work, decreasing fatigue and drowsiness, and prolonging wakefulness. They are prescribed as single salts (dextroamphetamine) or mixed dextroamphetamine–amphetamine salts. Large doses can lead to signs of excessive CNS stimulation (e.g., agitation, confusion, hyperactivity, difficulty concentrating on tasks, hyperactivity, nervousness, restlessness) and sympathetic nervous system stimulation (e.g., increased heart rate and blood pressure, pupil dilation, slowed gastrointestinal [GI] motility, and other symptoms). Overdoses can result in psychosis, convulsions, stroke, cardiac arrest, and death. Amphetamines are schedule II drugs under the Controlled Substances Act; they have a high potential for drug abuse and dependence. Widely sold on the street, they are commonly misused. ⓟ **Dextroamphetamine** (Dexedrine, ProCentra, Zenzedi) is the prototype amphetamine.

Pharmacokinetics

Dextroamphetamine has a rapid absorption and onset of action. The drug reaches its peak in 1 to 5 hours, and the duration is between 8 and 10 hours. It is metabolized by the liver and excreted in the urine. Dextroamphetamine may cross the placenta and has been found in breast milk.

Action

Dextroamphetamine acts in the CNS to release norepinephrine from nerve terminals and increases the amounts of norepinephrine, dopamine, and possibly serotonin in the brain. Dopamine is released in higher doses. Dextroamphetamine suppresses appetite, increases alertness, elevates mood, and improves physical performance. The drug's effectiveness and efficacy in ADHD are paradoxical, and its action is not well understood.

Use

The clinical indications for use of dextroamphetamine include the management of ADHD and narcolepsy. Amphetamines are useful in both acute and chronic conditions. Table 57.2 summarizes the route and dosage information for dextroamphetamine and other amphetamines.

Patient-related variables specific to the use of dextroamphetamine include the following:

- Age:
  - In children, the administration of dextroamphetamine results in suppression of weight and height (e.g., less than the estimated average of 2 inches per year), so regular monitoring is required.
  - In children with psychosis or Tourette syndrome, CNS stimulants may exacerbate symptoms.
  - In children and adolescents with preexisting heart disease, usual doses of dextroamphetamine may cause sudden death.
  - In ADHD, careful documentation of baseline symptoms over approximately 1 month is necessary to establish the diagnosis and evaluate outcomes of treatment. This may involve videotapes of behavior, observations and ratings by clinicians familiar with the condition, and interviewing the child, parents, or caretakers. Some authorities believe that ADHD is overdiagnosed and that stimulant drugs are prescribed unnecessarily. Kazda, Bell, and Thomas (2021) conducted a systematic scoping review of 334 published studies in children and adolescents with ADHD. The researchers found convincing evidence of the overdiagnosis of ADHD in children and adolescents.
  - In older adults, the use of dextroamphetamine warrants caution. As with most other drugs, slowed metabolism and excretion increase the risks of accumulation and toxicity. Older adults are likely to experience anxiety, confusion, insomnia, and nervousness from excessive CNS stimulation. Older adults often have cardiovascular disorders (e.g., angina, dysrhythmias, hypertension) that may be aggravated by the cardiac-stimulating effects of the drug.
- Reproduction, pregnancy, and lactation:
  - The use of amphetamine/methamphetamine during pregnancy may lead to an increased risk of premature birth and low birth weight.
  - Breast-feeding is not recommended according to the American Academy of Pediatrics.
- Abnormal kidney function and hepatic impairment:
  - Dextroamphetamine is excreted by the kidneys after being metabolized in the liver. Thus, caution is necessary in patients with Abnormal kidney function and/or hepatic impairment. The nurse monitors such patients for adverse effects and helps ensure that lower doses are used.

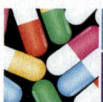

TABLE 57.2
DRUGS AT A GLANCE: Amphetamines

Drug	Routes and Dosage Ranges	
	Adults	**Children**
Dextroamphetamine (Dexedrine, ProCentra, Zenzedi, Xelstrym transdermal ❋ ACT Dextroamphetamine SR, Dexedrine)	Narcolepsy: start with 10 mg/d PO in divided doses; increase in increments of 10 mg/d at weekly intervals. Reduce dose if adverse effects occur. Usual dose is 5–60 mg/d PO in divided doses. Long-acting forms can be given once daily	ADHD, 3–5 y, start with 2.5 mg/d PO; increase in increments of 2.5 mg/d at weekly intervals until optimal response is obtained ≥6 y, start with 5 mg PO twice daily; increase in increments of 5 mg/d until optimal response is obtained; dosage will rarely exceed 40 mg/d; long-acting forms may be used once a day Extended Release: >6 y: 5 mg PO once or twice per day with first dose in the morning; increase in increments of 5 mg/d until optimal dose is obtained: usual range 5–20 mg/d; maximum dose 40 mg/d in 1–2 divided doses Xelstrym transdermal: >6 y and <18 y: 4.5 mg/9 h topical applied 2 h before effect is desired and remove within 9 h after application; may titrate in 4.5 mg increments at weekly intervals based on clinical response; maximum dose 18 mg/9 h Narcolepsy, 6–12 y, start with 5 mg/d PO; increase in increments of 5 mg at weekly intervals until optimal response is obtained; max dose 60 mg daily ≥12 y: same as adults
Dextroamphetamine and amphetamine (Adderall XR, Adderall, Mydayis; ❋ Adderall, Adderall XR, APO Amphetamine XR, SANDOZ Amphetamine XR)	Narcolepsy, 10 mg/d PO initially, increased if necessary ADHD, extended-release 20 mg/d	ADHD, 3–5 y, 2.5 mg/d PO; increased if necessary 6–12 y, 5 mg PO 1–2 times daily; increased if necessary; max dose 40 mg/d in 1–3 divided doses; extended-release 5–10 mg/d PO, increase at weekly intervals if necessary; max dose 30 mg/d 13–17 y, 10 mg PO once daily; increase to 20 mg if necessary
Lisdexamfetamine (Vyvanse; ❋ Vyvanse)	ADHD, 30 mg PO once daily in morning; increased if necessary; max dose 70 mg daily	ADHD, ≥6 y, 30 mg PO once daily; increased if necessary; max dose 70 mg/d
Methamphetamine (Desoxyn)	Narcolepsy, 20–60 mg PO administered within 1 h of awakening	≥6 y, 5 mg PO 1–2 times daily initially, increased if necessary; usual dose 20–25 mg/d, in 2 divided doses

Adverse Effects

Dextroamphetamine has several adverse effects.

- Cardiovascular effects: tachycardia, other dysrhythmias, and hypertension. A **BOXED WARNING** ◆ issued by the U.S. Food and Drug Administration (FDA) makes users aware of the drug's high potential for misuse; misuse may cause sudden death or serious cardiovascular events. It is essential to obtain a baseline electrocardiogram (ECG) and blood pressure reading.
- CNS effects: excessive CNS stimulation. Possible anxiety, hyperactivity, nervousness, insomnia, tremors, convulsion, and psychotic behavior may occur. These reactions are more likely with larger doses.
- GI effects: gastritis, nausea, diarrhea, and constipation
- Other effects: anorexia and weight loss

Contraindications

Contraindications to dextroamphetamine include cardiovascular disorders (e.g., angina, dysrhythmias, hypertension), which are likely to be aggravated by the drug. Other contraindications include anxiety or agitation, glaucoma, and hyperthyroidism, as well as a history of drug misuse, pregnancy, or lactation. The Canadian labeling of dextroamphetamine indicates that people with Tourette syndrome and children with motor tics should not take the drug. This labeling does not exist in the United States.

Nursing Implications

Preventing Interactions

Many medications interact with dextroamphetamine, increasing or decreasing its effects (Box 57.1). In addition, the use of the herb ephedra increases the effect of dextroamphetamine, while caffeine and acidic foods and juices decrease the drug's effect.

Administering the Medication

Dextroamphetamine dosage should be titrated carefully to avoid excessive CNS stimulation, anorexia, and insomnia. The first dose of dextroamphetamine should be administered on awakening or early in the day and the last dose at least 6 hours before bedtime. Children with ADHD should take the drug 30 to 45 minutes before meals to minimize the appetite-suppressing effects. It is important not to crush, chew, or bite the long-acting form; this destroys the extended-release feature and may result in an overdose. For young children who have difficulty swallowing pills, the capsules may be opened and taken with pudding or ice cream. The drug beads should not be chewed.

With the transdermal system, the protective pouch is removed and the medication applied to the hip, upper arm, chest, flank, or hip. Tight clothing should be avoided. Each application requires a different site, and heat should not be applied to the site. The site should be checked often to make sure it remains intact and attached to the skin. If the patch is not attached, firm pressure should be applied. If the patch comes off, a new patch can be applied, but total wear time of the patch should not exceed 9 hours. Thorough hand washing is required after applying the patch. Do not use oil-based products or hand sanitizer under the site of application.

Dextroamphetamine often causes loss of appetite, and the healthcare provider may stop the medication during the months when the child is not in school. This temporary drug-free period, called a **drug holiday,** allows some return of normal functions, to maintain sensitivity to a drug, and to reduce the likelihood of adverse effects. A drug holiday from dextroamphetamine helps decrease weight loss and growth suppression in children. It may not be appropriate for every child.

Assessing for Therapeutic Effects

For patients with ADHD, the nurse assesses for improved behavior and performance of cognitive and psychomotor tasks. For patients with narcolepsy, the nurse assesses for fewer sleep attacks, increased mental alertness, and decreased mental fatigue.

Assessing for Adverse Effects

The nurse assesses for signs and symptoms of excessive CNS stimulation as evidenced by an inability to complete tasks due to nervousness and hyperactivity. It is necessary to check the patient's cardiovascular status for tachycardia and elevation in blood pressure. The nurse assesses the patient's diet for inability to eat and the patient for loss of weight. The patient's growth should be monitored regularly. It is also important to assess the GI system for constipation or diarrhea.

Patient Teaching

Box 57.2 identifies patient teaching guidelines for drugs used in ADHD or narcolepsy.

Other Drugs in the Class

Dextroamphetamine–amphetamine (Adderall, Adderall XR, Mydayis) is a mixed salt drug that is available in immediate- and sustained-release preparations. The immediate-release form has an onset of action of 20 to 60 minutes and a duration of up to 6 hours. The extended-release form extends the duration to at least 10 hours. Lisdexamfetamine (Vyvanse) is a prodrug of dextroamphetamine that is pharmacologically activated after oral ingestion and was designed to discourage drug misuse. Lisdexamfetamine has an onset of action within 60 minutes and lasts up to 10 hours. The adverse effects of both medications are the same as the prototype drug, dextroamphetamine.

BOX 57.1 Drug Interactions: Dextroamphetamine

Drugs That Increase the Effects of Dextroamphetamine
- Albuterol, pseudoephedrine, tricyclic antidepressants
  Increase stimulant effects of dextroamphetamine
- Antacids
  Decrease the excretion of amphetamines
- Monoamine oxidase inhibitors
  Enhance the hypertensive effects of amphetamines

Drugs That Decrease the Effects of Dextroamphetamine
- Ammonium chloride
  Decreases the serum concentration of dextroamphetamine
- Antipsychotics, lithium, alcohol
  Diminish the stimulant effect of dextroamphetamine
- Gastrointestinal acidifying agents
  Decrease the serum concentration of dextroamphetamine

NCLEX Success

2. Which finding is indicative of an adverse effect of dextroamphetamine?
   A. increased appetite
   B. respiratory depression
   C. sedation
   D. cardiac dysrhythmias

BOX 57.2 Patient Teaching Guidelines for Drugs Used in Attention Deficit Hyperactivity Disorder and Narcolepsy

General Considerations

- When diagnosed with ADHD and before taking any medication for it, adult patients and parents of children with ADHD should inform the healthcare provider about any other stimulant drugs being taken, involvement in strenuous activities of any kind, any heart disease, or any family history of sudden cardiac death. All drugs for ADHD stimulate the heart and blood vessels. The effects are usually a faster heartbeat and increased blood pressure, but cardiac arrest, stroke, or sudden death may occur.
- Use caution while driving or performing other tasks requiring alertness. These drugs may mask symptoms of fatigue, impair physical coordination, and cause dizziness or drowsiness.
- Notify a healthcare provider of nervousness, insomnia, heart palpitations, vomiting, fever, or skin rash. These are adverse drug effects and dosage may need to be reduced.
- Avoid other stimulants, including caffeine.
- Record weight at least weekly; report excessive losses.
- The drugs may cause weight loss; caloric intake (of nutritional foods) may need to be increased, especially in children.
- Insufficient intake of long-chain polyunsaturated fatty acids plays a role in the development of ADHD. Zinc, iron, and magnesium supplementation may reduce symptoms of ADHD in children.
- Take stimulant drugs only as prescribed:
  - Accurate dosing is important because underuse may cause the recurrence of symptoms and overuse may cause toxicity.
- Do not increase the dosage without consulting with your healthcare provider. These drugs have a high potential for misuse. The risks of serious health problems and drug dependence are lessened if they are taken correctly. The likelihood of medical problems is greatly increased when ADHD medication is used improperly or in combination with other drugs.
- Get adequate rest and sleep. Do not take stimulant drugs to delay fatigue and sleep; these are normal, necessary resting mechanisms for the body.
- Keep these medications away from children, preferably in a locked cabinet. Parents (or a school nurse) need to dispense each dose and to be sure the drug is taken only by the child for whom it was prescribed.

Self- or Parental Administration

- Take (or give) regular tablets approximately 30 to 45 minutes before meals.
- Take (or give) the last dose of the day in the afternoon, before 6:00 PM, to avoid interference with sleep.
- Ensure that long-acting/extended-release CNS stimulants are swallowed whole, without crushing or chewing.
- Apply the Daytrana skin patch to the hip area as prescribed. Patch should be removed after 9 hours; alternate hips. See the manufacturer's instructions for opening, applying, removing, and disposing of the skin patch.
- If excessive weight loss, nervousness, or insomnia develops, ask the prescriber if the dose can be reduced or taken on a different schedule to relieve these adverse effects.

AMPHETAMINE-RELATED DRUGS

Amphetamine-related drugs, which resemble amphetamines, have essentially the same stimulant effects as the amphetamines and are also schedule II drugs. **Methylphenidate** (Ritalin, others) is the prototype. This drug, marketed under generic and trade names, is available in several dosage forms, including immediate-release and chewable tablets, extended-release capsules, and a transdermal patch. These dosage forms are not interchangeable.

The U.S. FDA has issued a **BOXED WARNING** regarding the risk of drug dependence with amphetamine-related drugs. Methylphenidate has become a drug of misuse, and its nonmedical use, alone or with other drugs, has been associated with increased visits for emergency departments by adolescents and young adults.

Pharmacokinetics

Methylphenidate is well absorbed after oral administration. Depending on the formulation, the onset of action varies, with a peak in 1 to 8 hours and a duration of action of 3 to 12 hours (longer for transdermal and long-acting preparations). The drug is mostly metabolized in the liver and excreted in the urine.

Action

Methylphenidate is a mild cortical stimulant. It blocks the reuptake of norepinephrine and dopamine into the presynaptic neurons resulting in the stimulation of the cerebral cortex. The drug suppresses appetite, increases alertness, elevates mood, and improves physical performance. The efficacy in ADHD is paradoxical and not well understood.

Use

The clinical indications for use of methylphenidate include the management of ADHD and narcolepsy. The drug may be useful for the treatment of both acute and chronic conditions. Table 57.3 gives route and dosage information for methylphenidate and other amphetamine-related drugs.

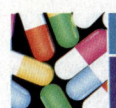

TABLE 57.3
DRUGS AT A GLANCE: Amphetamine-Related Central Nervous System Stimulants

Drug	Routes and Dosage Ranges	
	Adults	**Children**
Methylphenidate (Adhansia XR, Aptensio, Concerta, Cotempla XR-ODT, Daytrana, Jornay PM, Concerta, Daytrana, Methylin, QuilliChew ER, Quillivant XR, Relexxii, Ritalin, Ritalin LA, Biphentin, ACT Methylphenidate ER, APO-Methylphenidate, APO-Methylphenidate SR, Concerta, Foquest)	ADHD, 10–60 mg/d PO two or three times daily, preferably 30–45 min before meals. If insomnia is a problem, drug should be taken before 6:00 p.m. Timed-release tablets (duration of 8 h) may be used. ER forms (Concerta), 18 mg PO daily in the morning; may be increased by 18 mg/d at 1-wk intervals to a max of 54 mg/d (Aptensio XR); increments of 10 mg/d to a max of 60 mg/d (Ritalin LA) Narcolepsy: immediate release 5 mg twice daily; increase in increments of 5–10 mg/d to a max of 60 mg/d Extended and sustained release may be given in place of immediate release tab when dosage amount corresponds to max of 60 mg/d	ADHD, 6–12 y, start with 5 mg PO before breakfast and lunch with gradual increase 13–17 y, start in the morning without regard to food. Titrate to a max of 72 mg/d. Do not exceed 2 mg/kg/d Transdermal patch (Daytrana) 10–30 mg/d. Apply patch 2 h before effect needed and remove after 9 h in increments of 5–10 mg/wk. Daily dosage exceeding 60 mg/d is not recommended. Discontinue use after 1 mo if no improvement Extended release forms consult manufacturer's dosing guidelines
Dexmethylphenidate (Focalin, Focalin XR)	5–10 mg/d PO, increased if necessary, max dose 20 mg/d	6 y and older, 2.5–5 mg/d PO, increased if necessary, max dose 20 mg/d
Serdexmethylphenidate-dexmethylphenidate (Azstarys)	ADHD, Serdexmethylphenidate 39.2 mg/dexmethylphenidate 7.8 mg once daily in the morning; after 1 week, may increase dose to serdexmethylphenidate 52.3 mg/dexmethylphenidate 10.4 mg once daily; maximum dose: serdexmethylphenidate 52.3 mg/serdexmethylphenidate 10.4 mg once daily. Reduce dose if paradoxical aggravation of symptoms is noted	Children >6 y: Serdexmethylphenidate 39.2 mg/dexmethylphenidate 7.8 mg once daily in the morning; after 1 week, may increase dose to serdexmethylphenidate 52.3 mg/dexmethylphenidate 10.4 mg once daily; maximum dose: serdexmethylphenidate 52.3 mg/serdexmethylphenidate 10.4 mg once daily. Reduce dose if paradoxical aggravation of symptoms is noted
Armodafinil (Nuvigil)	Narcolepsy, 150–250 mg once daily in the morning	Safety and effectiveness not established in children
Modafinil (Provigil, Alertec, Auro-Modafinil)	Narcolepsy, 200 mg once daily in the morning ADHD, 100–400 mg once daily	Safety concerns in children reported

Patient-related variables specific to the use of methylphenidate include the following:

- Age:
  - Use cautiously in preschool-age children due to higher rates of adverse effects in this age group.
- Reproduction, pregnancy, and lactation:
  - There is limited information on the use of methylphenidate during pregnancy. UpToDate (2022) reports a study conducted in 2015 stated that methylphenidate used during pregnancy to treat ADHD or narcolepsy can be considered, but pregnancy and fetal outcomes must be assessed.
  - Breast-feeding is acceptable if relevant infant dose (RID) of a medication is less than 10%.
- Abnormal kidney function and hepatic impairment:
  - No dosage reductions are needed in abnormal kidney function or hepatic impairment.

> **Quality and Safety Alert: Evidence-Based Practice**
>
> Roche et al. (2021) conducted a study on the use of methylphenidate to treat ADHD in children with Down syndrome. This retrospective study of 21 children examined the efficacy and safety of methylphenidate. The observation of the children involved study of the two main symptoms of ADHD, attention and concentration, along with hyperactivity and impulsivity. Twelve of the 21 children experienced adverse effects of methylphenidate, but only three participants of the study required the drug to be discontinued. Sixteen of the 21 students showed improvement of attention and reduction in hyperactivity while taking methylphenidate. The most common adverse effects noted in the study were loss of appetite and insomnia. In conclusion, methylphenidate was safe and effective in 76% of the cases studied.

Adverse Effects

The adverse effects of methylphenidate include tachycardia, dysrhythmias, hypertension, anxiety, hyperactivity, nervousness, insomnia, tremors, convulsion, psychosis, gastritis, nausea, diarrhea, constipation, rash, alopecia, exfoliative dermatitis, leukopenia, anemia, anorexia, and weight loss. Priapism is associated with methylphenidate and other neurostimulants. It can range from severe with dosage changes, medication withdrawal, or changes in medication brands.

Contraindications

Contraindications to methylphenidate include cardiovascular conditions (e.g., angina, dysrhythmias, hypertension) that are likely to be aggravated by the drug. Other contraindications are anxiety or agitation, glaucoma, or hyperthyroidism. Conditions such as a history of drug abuse or pregnancy or lactation usually preclude use of the drug. However, if it is administered during pregnancy or lactation, fetal and infant outcomes must be assessed. Caution is necessary with seizure disorders.

Nursing Implications

Preventing Interactions

Methylphenidate may increase effects of phenytoin, tricyclic antidepressants, selective serotonin reuptake inhibitors, and oral anticoagulants. Also, methylphenidate may decrease effects of antihypertensive drugs. In patients with chronic alcohol use disorder, administration of methylphenidate has an increased risk of medication tolerance and psychological dependence. The combination of methylphenidate with cannabis will increase dizziness.

Administering the Medication

People should take the first dose of methylphenidate on awakening or early in the day, and they should take the last dose at least 6 hours before bedtime. Children with ADHD should take the drug 30 to 45 minutes before meals to minimize the appetite-suppressive effects. It is important not to crush, chew, or bite the long-acting form of methylphenidate; this destroys the extended-release feature and may result in an overdose. Extended-release tablets (Concerta) are coated with immediate-release methylphenidate (for initial dosing) and use an osmotic pump to gradually release methylphenidate to approximate a three-times-a-day dosing schedule. They, too, should be taken whole. Like dextroamphetamine, methylphenidate often causes loss of appetite. Thus, the healthcare provider may stop the medication during the months when the child is not in school. A drug holiday helps decrease weight loss and growth suppression. It may not be appropriate for every child.

Assessing for Therapeutic Effects

For patients with ADHD, the nurse assesses for improved behavior and performance of cognitive and psychomotor tasks. For patients with narcolepsy, the nurse assesses for fewer sleep attacks, as well as for increased mental alertness and decreased mental fatigue.

Assessing for Adverse Effects

The nurse assesses the blood pressure and pulse for hypertension and tachycardia related to the stimulant effects. It is necessary to assess the patient's CNS response for increased anxiety and hyperactivity that impairs the ability to perform activities of daily living. The nurse checks the patient's sleep patterns and inability to sleep restfully. It is also important to assess the patient's GI status for reflux and pain leading to gastritis. In addition, the nurse checks the complete blood count and platelet count for the onset of anemia.

Patient Teaching

Box 57.2 identifies patient teaching guidelines for medications administered for the treatment of ADHD or narcolepsy.

Clinical Application 57.2

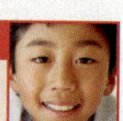

Brian has been taking methylphenidate XR (Ritalin LA) every morning for 2 months, and the teachers have noticed that his concentration and his behavior have improved after lunch. However, his appetite has decreased dramatically, and he has lost 4 lbs. The teachers have noticed that he does not eat his lunch and skips his afternoon snack. His parents are concerned and schedule a visit to the healthcare provider. The healthcare provider is hesitant to change Brian's medication regimen because his behavior at school has improved.

- What patient teaching can the school nurse provide to Brian and his parents to increase his weight?

Clinical Application 57.3

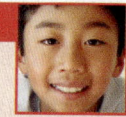

Brian has been maintaining his weight with his current dosage of methylphenidate and continues to drink two nutritional supplement drinks per day. It is now late spring, and his healthcare provider wants to try a drug holiday in the summer. Brian's parents are concerned about their son's being able to function at summer camp without any pharmacologic intervention. They voice their worries to the school nurse.

- What information should the school nurse provide to Brian's parents? What are the advantages and disadvantages of their decision to support a drug holiday?

Other Drugs in the Class

Dexmethylphenidate (Focalin, Focalin XR) is a CNS stimulant that blocks the reuptake of norepinephrine and dopamine to increase their release in extraneuronal space. The drug has a high abuse potential. The FDA has issued a **BOXED WARNING** regarding caution with the use of dexmethylphenidate in patients with a history of drug dependence or alcoholism. Chronic, abusive use can lead to marked tolerance and psychological dependence with varying degrees of abnormal behavior. Serdexmethylphenidate and dexmethylphenidate (Azstarys) also blocks the reuptake of norepinephrine and dopamine to increase their release in the extraneuronal space. The action of serdexmethylphenidate is unknown. Serdexmethylphenidate and dexmethylphenidate possesses a similar drug profile to dexmethylphenidate and high misuse potential. Modafinil (Provigil) and armodafinil (Nuvigil) are used to treat narcolepsy and to improve wakefulness in other sleep disorders (e.g., obstructive sleep apnea/hypopnea syndrome, shift work sleep disorder). Modafinil is also used to treat ADHD and to decrease the fatigue associated with multiple sclerosis and other disorders. Armodafinil is the R-enantiomer of modafinil, which means that both drugs have identical chemical and physical properties but may interact differently in the body. The FDA requires that a specific warning against the use of modafinil in children be included on the label as serious dermatologic adverse effects and psychiatric events have been reported.

> ### NCLEX Success
>
> 3. Which of the following are expected adverse effects of amphetamine sulfate? (Select all that apply.)
>   A. weight loss
>   B. anorexia
>   C. dry mouth
>   D. bradycardia
>   E. constipation
>
> 4. A child comes to the school nurse's office and states, "I did not take my Ritalin today." Which of the following is the most appropriate nursing intervention?
>   A. Call the child's parent or guardian to try to find out if the child has taken the medicine.
>   B. Give the child the morning dose of medication because it is in the office.
>   C. Send the child back to class and say that it is not necessary to take the medication.
>   D. Call the child's physician to obtain a one-time dose of methylphenidate.

OTHER MEDICATIONS USED TO TREAT ATTENTION DEFICIT HYPERACTIVITY DISORDER AND NARCOLEPSY

Three other drugs are commonly administered for the treatment of ADHD or narcolepsy. These drugs include the selective norepinephrine reuptake inhibitor atomoxetine and the antihypertensive drug guanfacine. Table 57.4 gives route and dosage information for these medications.

Atomoxetine (Strattera), a second-line drug for the treatment of ADHD in children and adults, acts to inhibit reuptake of norepinephrine in nerve synapses. It has a low risk of misuse and dependence compared with the other drugs used for ADHD and is not a controlled substance. The drug is rapidly absorbed with oral administration, with peak plasma levels in 1 to 2 hours. Atomoxetine is metabolized in the liver and is excreted mainly in urine. People may take the drug with or without food. Dosage adjustment is necessary in patients receiving strong CYP2D6 inhibitors (e.g., paroxetine, fluoxetine, quinidine) or patients known to be CYP2D6 poor metabolizers. Common adverse effects include weight loss, abdominal pain, anorexia, cough, dry mouth, headache, insomnia, irritability, nausea, and vomiting. A **BOXED WARNING** ◆ advises that suicidal ideation may occur in children and adolescents with ADHD who take atomoxetine; it is necessary to balance risk with clinical need.

Guanfacine (Intuniv), a selective alpha$_{2A}$-adrenoreceptor agonist used in ADHD, preferentially binds postsynaptic alpha$_{2A}$-adrenoreceptors in the prefrontal cortex. The drug is thought to improve delay-related firing of prefrontal cortex neurons affecting underlying working memory and behavioral inhibition. In addition, guanfacine reduces sympathetic nerve impulses resulting in reduced sympathetic outflow and a subsequent decrease in vasomotor tone and heart rate, making it useful in the treatment of hypertension. It is available in an extended-release form that is usually reserved for children and adolescents in whom atomoxetine has not been effective or produces unacceptable adverse effects. No response may occur for up to 2 weeks. Guanfacine is metabolized by the liver and excreted in the urine. It crosses the placenta and enters the breast milk. Adverse effects include sedation, weakness, dizziness, vision disturbance, and headache, as well as cardiovascular conditions (bradycardia and hypotension) and GI problems (dry mouth, constipation, and abdominal pain). Caution is necessary in cardiovascular disease, in hepatic and abnormal kidney function, and in pregnancy or during lactation. The extended-release and immediate-release forms are not interchangeable on a milligram-per-milligram basis because of differences in bioavailability.

Sodium oxybate (Xyrem), the sodium salt of gamma hydroxybutyrate (GABA), is prescribed to treat cataplexy and excessive daytime sleepiness in individuals with narcolepsy. The drug is a CNS depressant that can cause significant respiratory depression and decreased level of consciousness. The FDA has issued a **BOXED WARNING** ◆ regarding the risk of CNS depression and possible abuse and misuse. Because of the risks, the drug is available only through a restricted Risk Evaluation and Mitigation Strategy program.

> ### NCLEX Success
>
> 5. An 8-year-old child has been taking dexmethylphenidate 5 mg daily for 3 months. The child's mother is concerned that this dosage is not adequately treating the symptoms of attention deficit hyperactivity disorder. Which of the following behaviors would support the mother's concerns?
>   A. increased concentration during school
>   B. weight gain of 8 lbs over the past 3 months
>   C. increased activity
>   D. bradycardia

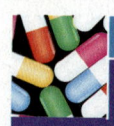

TABLE 57.4
DRUGS AT A GLANCE: Other Drugs Administered for Attention Deficit Hyperactivity Disorder

Drug	Routes and dosage ranges	
	Adults	**Children**
Selective norepinephrine reuptake inhibitors		
Atomoxetine (Strattera; ❋ Teva-Atomoxetine, Strattera)	Adults and children more than 70 kg: start with 40 mg/d PO; increase after a minimum of 3 d to a target daily dose of 80 mg PO daily given as a single dose in the morning or 2 evenly divided doses during the day. Dosage may be increased to 100 mg/d after 2–4 wk if needed	32 kg or less, start with 0.5 mg/kg/d PO and increase after a minimum of 3 d to a target daily dose of 1.2 mg/kg/d as a single daily dose in the morning; may be given in 2 evenly divided doses throughout the day. Do not exceed 1.4 mg/kg/d or 100 mg/d, whichever is less ≥6 y and ≤70 kg: start with 0.5 mg/kg/d increase after a minimum of 3 d to 1.2 mg/kg/d
Sympatholytics		
Guanfacine (Intuniv; ❋ APO Guanfacine XR, Intuniv XR)		ADHD, 6–12 4 mg/d 13–17 y, 7 mg/d >17 y, 1 mg/kg/d PO in ER tablet; increase by 1 mg/d/wk to a max of 4 mg/d
Central nervous system depressant		
Sodium oxybate (Xyrem; ❋ Xyrem)	Narcolepsy, PO 2.25 g at bedtime initially after the patient is in bed, and 2.25 g 2.5–4 h later (4.5 g per night). Titrate dose by 1.5 g per night (0.75 g at bedtime and 0.75 g 2.5–4 h later) in weekly intervals (max dose: 9 g per night)	Narcolepsy, ≥7 y 20 to <30 kg: PO, up to 1 g at bedtime initially after the patient is in bed, and up to 1 g 2.5–4 h later (up to 2 g per night). Titrate dose by 1 g per night (0.5 g at bedtime and 0.5 g 2.5–4 h later) in weekly intervals; max dose, 3 g/dose; 6 g per night 30 to <45 kg, PO, up to 1.5 g at bedtime initially after the patient is in bed, and up to 1.5 g 2.5–4 h later (up to 3 g per night). Titrate dose by 1 g per night (0.5 g at bedtime and 0.5 g 2.5–4 h later) in weekly intervals; maximum dose; 3.75 g/dose; 7.5 g per night ≥45 kg, PO up to 2.25 g at bedtime initially after the patient is in bed, and up to 2.25 g 2.5–4 h later (up to 4.5 g per night). Titrate dose by 1.5 g per night (0.75 g at bedtime and 0.75 g 2.5–4 h later) in weekly intervals; max dose, 4.5 g/dose; 9 g per night

THE NURSING PROCESS

A concept map outlines the nursing process related to drug therapy considerations in this chapter. Additional nursing implications related to the disease process should also be considered in care decisions.

Assessment
- Assess use of stimulant and depressant drugs (prescribed, over-the-counter, or street drugs).
- Assess caffeine intake as a possible cause of anxiety, nervousness, insomnia, or tachycardia, alone or in combination with other CNS stimulants. Heavy users of caffeine may also be taking other psychoactive medications, especially CNS depressants such as antianxiety and sedative-hypnotic drugs.
- Try to identify potentially significant sources of caffeine intake.
- Assess for conditions that are aggravated by CNS stimulants.
- For a child with possible ADHD, assess behavior as specifically and thoroughly as possible.
- For any patient receiving amphetamines or methylphenidate, assess behavior for signs of tolerance and abuse.

Outcomes of Therapy

The patient will
- Take CNS stimulants safely and accurately.
- Improve attention span and task performance (children and adults with ADHD) and decrease hyperactivity (children with ADHD).
- Function appropriately in social interactions with other children.
- Maintain appropriate height and weight for age.
- Have fewer sleep episodes during normal waking hours (for patients with narcolepsy).

Nursing Interventions
- For a child receiving a CNS stimulant, assist parents in scheduling drug administration to increase beneficial effects and help prevent drug dependence and stunted growth. In addition, ask parents to control drug distribution and monitor the number of pills or capsules available and the number prescribed. The goals are to prevent overuse by the child for whom the drug is prescribed and to prevent the child from sharing his medication with other children who wish to take the drug for nonmedical purposes.
- Record weight at least weekly.
- Promote nutrition to avoid excessive weight loss.
- Provide information about the condition for which a stimulant drug is being given and the potential consequences of overusing the drug.

Evaluation
- Ask parents and teachers of children with ADHD to report on behavior and academic performance.
- For adolescents and adults with ADHD, ask the patient or family about the patient's ability to function in work, school, or social environments.
- Ask parents and older children about weight loss and decreased nutritional status.
- Assess for decreased inappropriate sleep episodes in patients with narcolepsy.

Visit thePoint at http://thePoint.lww.com/Frandsen13e for answers to NCLEX Success questions (in Appendix A), answers to Clinical Application Case Studies (in Appendix B), additional information on the etiology and pathophysiology of attention deficit hyperactivity disorder (ADHD) and narcolepsy, and more!

REFERENCES AND RESOURCES

Boyd, M. A., & Luebbert, R. (2022). *Psychiatric nursing* (7th ed.). Wolters Kluwer Health/Lippincott, Williams, & Wilkins.

Centers for Disease Control and Prevention. (2022). *Attention-deficit/Hyperactivity disorder. What is ADHD*. December 2, 2022. https://www.cdc.gov/ncbdd/adhad/facts.html

Kazda, L., Bell, K, Thomas, R., McGeechan, K., Sims, R., & Barratt, A. (2021). Overdiagnosis of attention-deficit/hyperactivity disorder in children and adolescents a systematic scoping review. *Journal of the American Medication Association Network Open*, 4(4), e215335. https://doi.org/10.1001/jamanetworkopen.2021.5335

Krull, K. R. (2022a). Attention deficit hyperactivity disorder in children and adolescents: Epidemiology and pathogenesis. *UpToDate*. Lexi Comp, Inc.

Krull, K. R. (2022b). Attention deficit hyperactivity disorder in children and adolescents: Overview of treatment and prognosis. *UpToDate*. Lexi Comp, Inc.

Roche, M., Mircher, C., Toulas, J., Prioux, E., Conte, M., Ravel, A., Falquero, S., Labidi, A., Stora, S., Durand, S., Megarbane, A., & Cieuta-Walti, C. (2021). Efficacy and safety of methylphenidate on attention deficit hyperactivity disorder in children with Down syndrome. *Journal of Intellectual Disability*, 65(8), 795–800. https://doi.org/10.1111/jir.12832

Scammell, T. E. (2022). Treatment of narcolepsy in adults. *UpToDate*. Lexi Comp, Inc.

UpToDate. (2022). *Drug information*. Lexi Comp, Inc.

CHAPTER 58

Drug Therapy for Substance Use Disorders

LEARNING OBJECTIVES

After studying this chapter, you should be able to:

1. Describe the clinical considerations and manifestations of substance use disorders.
2. Identify the central nervous system (CNS) depressants of abuse.
3. Categorize the prototypes and describe the action, use, adverse effects, contraindications, and nursing implications for the treatment of alcohol withdrawal and for the maintenance of sobriety.
4. Identify commonly misused CNS stimulants.
5. Identify commonly misused psychoactive medications.
6. Implement the nursing process for patients who may be misusing CNS depressants, CNS stimulants, or other psychoactive substances.

CLINICAL APPLICATION CASE STUDY

Bryan Wilson is a 24-year-old man who regularly uses marijuana, alcohol, and tobacco. He was involved in a physical altercation at a local nightclub, and the owner called the police. The police brought Mr. Wilson to the emergency department, where he received a diagnosis of acute alcohol intoxication. He is admitted for treatment of alcohol withdrawal.

KEY TERMS

Intoxication: development of a reversible substance-specific syndrome caused by the recent ingestion of or exposure to a substance

Physical dependence: physiologic adaptation to chronic use of a drug so that withdrawal occurs when the drug is stopped, when its action is antagonized by another drug, or when its dosage is decreased

Psychological dependence: a mental cycle of reliance on taking a particular drug for the reinforcement of feelings of satisfaction it provides

Substance dependence: overwhelming desire to repeat the use of drugs to produce pleasure or avoid discomfort even when significant problems related to use have developed

Substance use disorder: maladaptive pattern of substance use manifested by recurrent and significant adverse consequences related to repeated use of the substance

Tolerance: decreased effect from original response to a drug that requires a higher dose of the drug to achieve the same level of response reached initially

Withdrawal: development of a substance-specific maladaptive behavioral change, with physiologic and cognitive concomitants due to the cessation of or reduction in heavy and prolonged substance use

INTRODUCTION

This chapter introduces the pharmacologic management of patients who are experiencing substance use disorders, which include the conditions of substance abuse and substance dependence in the *Diagnostic and Statistical Manual of Mental Disorders, 5th Edition, Text Revision*: DSM-5-TR (2022). It describes commonly misused substances, characteristics of substance-related disorders, and drugs used to treat substance-related disorders. A **substance use disorder** is a maladaptive pattern of substance use, leading to clinically significant impairment or distress. This misuse involves self-administration of a drug for prolonged periods or in excessive amounts. It produces physical or psychological dependence, impairs functions of body organs, reduces the ability to function in usual activities of daily living, and decreases the ability and motivation to function as a productive member of society.

Substance use disorder is a significant health, social, economic, and legal problem. It is often associated with substantial damage to the user and society (e.g., crime, child and spouse abuse, traumatic injury, chronic health problems, death).

OVERVIEW OF SUBSTANCE USE

Most drugs associated with substance use disorder are those that affect the central nervous system (CNS) and alter the state of consciousness. Commonly used drugs include CNS depressants (e.g., alcohol, antianxiety and sedative–hypnotic agents, opioid analgesics), CNS stimulants (e.g., cocaine, methamphetamine, methylphenidate, nicotine), and other mind-altering drugs (e.g., marijuana, "ecstasy"). The overwhelming desire to repeat the use of drugs to produce pleasure or avoid discomfort even when significant problems related to its use have developed is known as **substance dependence**. Many of these commonly misused drugs have clinical usefulness and are discussed elsewhere: anxiolytics and sedative–hypnotics (see Chapter 54), opioids (see Chapter 49), and CNS stimulants (see Chapter 57). Although they produce different effects, they are associated with feelings of pleasure, positive reinforcement, and compulsive self-administration.

Psychological dependence involves feelings of satisfaction and pleasure from taking a drug. These feelings, perceived as extremely desirable by the person misusing the drug, contribute to acute **intoxication** (symptoms caused by recent ingestion of or exposure to a substance), development and maintenance of patterns of substance use disorder, and return to such behavior after periods of abstinence.

Physical dependence involves physiologic adaptation to chronic use of a drug so that **withdrawal** or unpleasant symptoms occur when the drug is stopped, when its action is antagonized by another drug, or when its dosage is decreased. Withdrawal or abstinence produces specific manifestations according to the type of drug and does not occur as long as adequate dosage is maintained. Attempts to avoid withdrawal symptoms reinforce psychological dependence and promote continuing drug use.

Characteristics of drug dependence include craving a drug, often with unsuccessful attempts to decrease its use; compulsive drug-seeking behavior; physical dependence; and continuing to take a drug despite adverse consequences (e.g., drug-related illnesses, mental or legal problems, job loss or decreased ability to function in an occupation, impaired family relationships). Box 58.1 describes other characteristics of substance use disorders.

Tolerance, which may be associated with many drugs if used repeatedly, is often an element of drug dependence. Increasing doses are required to obtain psychological effects or avoid physical withdrawal symptoms than were originally required. The body "adjusts" to the drugs, and higher doses are

---

> **BOX 58.1** *Characteristics of Substance Use Disorders*
>
> - Substance use disorders involve all socioeconomic levels and affect all age groups. Substance use disorders are especially prevalent among adolescents and young adults. Patterns of use may vary by age group. For example, adolescents and young adults are more likely to use illicit drugs, and older adults are more likely to abuse alcohol and prescription drugs. Healthcare professionals (e.g., physicians, pharmacists, nurses) are also considered at high risk of development of substance use disorders, at least partly because of easy access.
> - A person who misuses one drug is likely to misuse others.
> - Multiple drugs are often used concurrently. Alcohol, for example, is often used with other drugs, probably because it is legal and readily available. In addition, alcohol, marijuana, opioids, and sedatives are often used to combat the anxiety and nervousness induced by cocaine, methamphetamine, and other CNS stimulants.
> - Individuals who use alcohol and other drugs are not reliable sources of information about the types or amounts of drugs used. Most people with substance use disorders understate the amount and frequency of substance use; people who use heroin may overstate the amount used in attempts to obtain higher doses of methadone. In addition, those who use illegal street drugs may not know what they have taken because of varying purity, potency, additives, contaminants, names, and substitutions of one drug for another.
> - People with substance use disorders rarely seek healthcare unless circumstances force the issue. Thus, most substance use comes to the attention of healthcare professionals when the individual experiences a complication such as acute intoxication, withdrawal, or serious medical problems resulting from chronic drug misuse.
> - Smoking or inhaling drug vapors is a preferred route of administration for cocaine, marijuana, and nicotine because the drugs are rapidly absorbed from the large surface area of the lungs. Then, they rapidly circulate to the heart and brain without dilution by the systemic circulation or metabolism by enzymes.
> - People with substance use disorders who inject drugs intravenously may experience serious problems because they use impure drugs of unknown potency, contaminated needles, poor hygiene, and other dangerous practices. Specific problems include overdoses, death, and numerous infections (e.g., hepatitis, human immunodeficiency virus infection, endocarditis, phlebitis, cellulitis at injection sites).

needed to achieve feelings of pleasure ("reward") or to stave off withdrawal symptoms ("punishment"). Both reward and punishment serve to reinforce continued substance use.

Clinical Considerations

Drug dependence is a complex phenomenon. Although the cause is unknown, one theory is that drugs stimulate or inhibit neurotransmitters in the brain to produce pleasure or reward system or to decrease unpleasant feelings such as anxiety. For example, dopaminergic neurons in the limbic system are associated with the brain's reward system and are thought to be sites of action of alcohol, amphetamines, cocaine, nicotine, and opiates. These major drugs of intentional misuse increase dopaminergic transmission and the availability of dopamine. These actions are believed to stimulate the brain's reward system and lead to compulsive drug administration and substance misuse.

The noradrenergic neurotransmission system, which uses norepinephrine as its neurotransmitter, is often involved as well as the dopaminergic system. Noradrenergic neurons innervate the limbic system and cerebral cortex and are important in setting mood and affect. Drugs that alter noradrenergic transmission have profound effects on mood and affect. Amphetamines and cocaine increase noradrenergic transmission, as with dopaminergic transmission, by promoting the release of norepinephrine and/or inhibiting its reuptake. Increased norepinephrine leads to mood elevation and euphoria, which promotes continued drug abuse. Increased norepinephrine also leads to major adverse effects of amphetamines and cocaine, including myocardial infarction, severe hypertension, and stroke, as well as profound mood swings from euphoria to depression. Prolonged substance use damages nerve cells in the brain and alters brain functions. The damage is long lasting.

Clinical Manifestations

Drug effects vary according to the type of substance intentionally being misused, the amount, route of administration, duration of use, and phase of substance use (e.g., acute intoxication, withdrawal syndromes, organ damage, medical illness). Thus, acute intoxication often produces profound behavioral changes, and chronic misuse often leads to serious organ damage and impaired ability to function in work, family, or social settings. Withdrawal symptoms are characteristic of certain types of drugs and are usually opposite to the effects originally produced. For example, withdrawal symptoms of alcohol and sedative-type drugs are mainly agitation, nervousness, and hyperactivity.

Therapy

General Approach

The major goals of treatment for substance use disorder are detoxification, initiation of abstinence, and prevention of relapse. Patients who are likely to benefit from treatment are those who recognize that substance use is negatively influencing their problems and causing significant problems in their ability to function. Despite advances in treatment and the many adverse consequences of substance use, relapses to drug-taking behavior are common among people who have been detoxified or even abstinent for varying periods of time.

Treatments for substance use are limited but increasing, and more treatment facilities are needed. For most health professionals, contact with patients with substance use disorder is more likely to occur in acute situations, such as with intoxication or overdose, withdrawal syndromes, or various medical–surgical illnesses associated with the substance use. In general, treatment depends on the type, extent, and duration of drug-taking behavior and the situation for which treatment is needed.

Psychological rehabilitation efforts should be part of any treatment program for a person with substance use disorder. Several approaches may be useful, including inpatient and outpatient psychotherapy, voluntary self-help groups (e.g., Alcoholics Anonymous, Narcotics Anonymous), and other types of emotional support and counseling.

Quality and Safety Alert: Evidence-Based Practice

Stellern et al. (2023) conducted a systematic review and meta-analysis of existing findings that compared a substance use disorders group (total N = 1936) with a control group (total N = 1567) from 22 cross-sectional studies using the Difficulties in Emotion Regulation Scale (DERS), an instrument that measures problems with emotion regulation. The 36-items self-report scale, the predominant instrument in the literature, asks individuals how they relate to their emotions to produce scores on six subscales (nonacceptance of emotional responses, difficulty engaging in goal-directed behavior, impulse control difficulties, lack of emotional awareness, limited access to emotion regulation strategies, and lack of emotional clarity). Compared to the control group, individuals with substance use disorders had significantly greater DERS that remained significant even after removing outliers and studies with high risk of bias. Individuals with substance use disorders demonstrated poorer emotion regulation on each subscale of the DERS, with the largest deficits in the Strategies and Impulse subscales. In these studies, individuals with substance use disorders appeared to have greater difficulties in emotion regulation than people without substance use disorders.

Since the ability to regulate emotions effectively has been associated with resilience to psychopathology and emotional regulation is a skill that can be developed, this study suggests that individuals with substance use disorders may benefit from therapy that strengthens skill mastery of emotional regulation as an important mechanism for symptom reduction in successful treatment outcomes.

Use of Drugs

Drug therapy for treatment of drug dependence is limited for several reasons. First, specific antidotes are available only for benzodiazepines (flumazenil) and opioid narcotics (naltrexone). Second, there is a high risk of substituting one abused drug for another. Third, there are significant drawbacks to giving CNS stimulants to reverse effects of CNS depressants and vice versa. Fourth, there is often inadequate information about the types and amounts of drug taken. Two of the more successful drug therapy regimens are methadone administration for heroin dependence and nicotine replacement (or other drugs [e.g., bupropion or varenicline]) for nicotine dependence. With both treatments, however, a combination of drug therapy and counseling is more effective than either method alone. Treatment

TABLE 58.1 Drugs Administered for the Treatment of Substance Use Disorders

Drug Class	Representative Drugs
Antialcoholic drug; enzyme inhibitor	Disulfiram
Benzodiazepine	Chlordiazepoxide (Librium) Lorazepam (Ativan)
GABA agonist/glutamate antagonist	Acamprosate
Centrally acting alpha-agonist antihypertensive	Clonidine (Catapres)
Benzodiazepine receptor antagonist	Flumazenil
Opioid antagonist	Naloxone (Narcan)
Opioid antagonist	Naltrexone (Vivitrol)
Opioid agonist–antagonist analgesic	Buprenorphine (Buprenex, Belbuca, Butrans, Sublocade) Naltrexone–buprenorphine (Suboxone)
Opioid agonist analgesic	Methadone (Methadose)
Antipsychotic; dopamine blocker	Haloperidol (Haldol)
Nicotine receptor agonist	Varenicline (Chantix)
Atypical antidepressant; smoking deterrent	Bupropion (Zyban, Wellbutrin SR, Contrave)
Smoking deterrent	Nicotine (Nicoderm CQ, Nicorette mini, Nicotrol NS)

programs for substance use emphasize sobriety, which is complete abstinence from substance use. Combined with psychotherapy, there are pharmacologic interventions that can assist the patient with sobriety. Table 58.1 lists the specific drugs that may be used to treat substance-related disorders.

CENTRAL NERVOUS SYSTEM DEPRESSANT USE: DRUG THERAPY

CNS depressants are drugs that slow down or "depress" brain activity. These drugs can induce varying degrees of CNS depression ranging from tranquilizing relief of anxiety to anesthesia, coma, and even death. Effects produced by these substances depend on the size of the dose and potency of the drug administered. These drugs include alcohol, benzodiazepines (antianxiety drugs), and opioids. For further details on these substances, visit thePoint® http://thePoint.lww.com/Frandsen13e.

BENZODIAZEPINES FOR TREATMENT OF ALCOHOL WITHDRAWAL

Benzodiazepines are the drugs of choice for treating withdrawal from alcohol and other CNS depressants. **Ⓟ Chlordiazepoxide** (Librium), the prototype benzodiazepine for treatment of such substance use, provides adequate sedation and has a significant anticonvulsant effect. The drug may also make it easier for the patient to participate in rehabilitation programs and allow for the gradual reduction and discontinuation of the misused substance.

Pharmacokinetics

The oral form of chlordiazepoxide has a rapid onset of action, with a peak of 1 hour. The intramuscular (IM) form has an onset of action within 10 to 15 minutes and peaks within 15 to 30 minutes. The IV form has an immediate onset of action and peaks within 30 minutes. For all forms, the duration is 48 to 72 hours. Metabolism occurs in the liver, and excretion is in the urine.

Action

The exact mechanism of action of chlordiazepoxide is not understood; however, the drug acts mainly at the subcortical levels of the CNS. The main sites of action may be the limbic system and reticular formation.

Use

Prescribers may order chlordiazepoxide for acute alcohol withdrawal as well as for the management of anxiety disorders. The drug is useful in symptomatic relief of acute agitation, tremors, and delirium tremens. Treatment with chlordiazepoxide for alcohol withdrawal should begin as soon as the clinician identifies that the patient needs it. Table 58.2 gives route and dosage information for chlordiazepoxide and other drugs used to treat substance use.

Patient-related variables specific to the use of chlordiazepoxide include the following:

- Reproduction, pregnancy, and lactation:
  - Chlordiazepoxide crosses the placenta and fetal serum concentrations are comparable to those in the mother.
  - Pregnancy should be avoided during therapy with chlordiazepoxide.
  - Pregnancy testing is recommended before treating acute alcohol withdrawal symptoms with chlordiazepoxide in females of child-bearing age.
  - Data related to long-term maternal use on neurodevelopment of a developing fetus are inconclusive and newborns exposed to chlordiazepoxide in utero should be monitored for feeding problems, respiratory depression, sedation, and withdrawal.
- Abnormal kidney function and hepatic impairment:
  - Since chlordiazepoxide is excreted in the urine after being metabolized in the liver, caution is warranted in patients with abnormal kidney function or hepatic impairment.
- Specific healthcare environments:
  - Alcohol detoxification through pharmacologic means may occur in the home.
  - The home care nurse should teach patients and caregivers to recognize signs and symptoms of alcohol withdrawal and assist them to understand the pharmacologic treatment regimen.

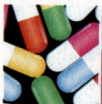

TABLE 58.2

DRUGS AT A GLANCE: Drugs Used to Treat Substance Use Disorders

Drug	Routes and Dosage Ranges	
	Adults	**Children**
Ⓟ Chlordiazepoxide (Librium)	50–100 mg PO followed by repeated doses up to 300 mg/d; subsequent doses reduced to lowest effective dose	Not recommended in children younger than 6 y ≥6 y, 5 mg PO two to four times daily; may be increased to 10 mg PO two to three times daily
Ⓟ Disulfiram	Initially, 500 mg/d PO once daily for 1–2 wk (maximum 500 mg daily) Maintenance: 125–500 mg PO daily (maximum 500 mg daily)	Safety and efficacy in patients younger than 18 y not established
Acamprosate (🍁 Campral)	666 mg PO 3 times daily	Safety and efficacy not established in children
Buprenorphine (Buprenex, Belbuca, Butrans, Sublocade; 🍁 Butrans)	12–16 mg/d SL; use as induction with switch to Suboxone for maintenance (same dosage)	Neonatal abstinence syndrome: Full-term infant, sublingual solution (0.075 mg/mL); Initial: 5.3 mcg/kg/dose every 8 h Ages 2–12 y, 2–6 mcg/kg IM or slow IV injection every 4–6 h ≥13 y, same as adult dosage
Buprenorphine–naloxone (Suboxone, Bunavail, Zubsolv; 🍁 Mylan-Buprenorphine/ Naloxone, Suboxone)	Short-acting opioid dependency: Suboxone film, day 1, initial buprenorphine 2–4 mg/naloxone 0.5–1.0 mg film sublingually approximately every 2 h to control acute withdrawal symptoms up to total dose of buprenorphine 8 mg/naloxone 2 mg; day 2 up to buprenorphine 16 mg/naloxone 4 mg Zubsolv, day 1, initial sublingual tablet, buprenorphine 1.4 mg/naloxone 0.36 mg and to control withdrawal symptoms increase in those increments every 1.5–2 h to a total day 1 dose up to buprenorphine 5.7 mg/naloxone 1.4 mg; day 2, up to buprenorphine 4.2 mg/naloxone 2.9 mg once daily Maintenance: Bunavail, buccal film, buprenorphine 8.4 mg/naloxone 1.4 mg	≥16 y, same as adult dosage
Bupropion (Zyban, Wellbutrin SR, Contrave; 🍁 Bupropion SR, Zyban)	Smoking cessation: 150 mg PO once daily for 3 d, then increase to 150 mg twice daily, at least 8 h apart; maximum dose, 300 mg/d; treat for 7–12 wk	Safety and efficacy in patients younger than 18 y not established
Clonidine (Catapres; 🍁 Catapres, Novo-Clonidine)	Methadone withdrawal: 0.1 mg PO three times daily up to a maximum of 1 mg daily Nicotine withdrawal: 0.1 mg PO twice daily, increased by 0.1 mg daily every 7 d 0.1 mg/24 patch transdermal applied once every 7 d, increased by 0.1 mg daily at 1-wk intervals	Neonatal abstinence syndrome (opioid withdrawal; limited data available): GA < 35 wk, 0.5–1.0 mcg/kg/dose PO every 6 h until stable and tapered as tolerated GA ≥ 35 wk, 0.5–1.0 mcg/kg/dose PO every 4–6 h until stable and tapered as tolerated
Flumazenil	Suspected benzodiazepine overdose: 0.2 mg IV over 30 s; repeat with 0.3 mg IV every 30 s to maximum dose of 3 mg	Reversal of benzodiazepine when used in conscious sedation: ≥1 y, 0.01 mg/kg IV over 15 s to maximum 0.2 mg; repeated as needed at 1-min intervals to maximum 4 doses or 1 mg or 0.05 mg/kg, whichever lower

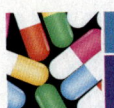

TABLE 58.2
DRUGS AT A GLANCE: Drugs Used to Treat Substance Use Disorders (Continued)

Drug	Routes and Dosage Ranges	
	Adults	**Children**
Haloperidol (Haldol; ❋ PMS-Haloperidol, Novo-Peridol)	0.5–2 PO mg two to three times daily with moderate symptoms, 3–5 mg PO two to three times daily for more resistant patients, 2–5 mg IM daily every 60 min or 4–8 h as needed	3–12 y or 15–40 kg, 0.5 mg/d (25–50 mcg/kg/d) as initial dose; may increase in 0.5-mg increments
Lorazepam (Ativan; ❋ Apo-Lorazepam)	Alcohol withdrawal hallucinations or seizures: 1–4 mg IV, every 5–15 min until calm, repeat as necessary 1–4 mg IM, every 30–50 min until calm, repeat as necessary Benzodiazepine withdrawal: 2 mg PO every 6–8 h initially, then tapered over 1–2 wk	No recommendations for treatment of withdrawal in children
Methadone (Methadose; ❋ Metadol, Methadose)	Withdrawal: 20–30 mg daily initially PO or parenteral; increase dose to suppress withdrawal signs; 40 mg/d in single or divided doses is an adequate stabilizing dose; gradually reduce dosage every day after 2–3 d of stabilization dose Maintenance: 20–120 mg PO daily	Neonatal abstinence syndrome: Initial: 0.05–0.1 mg/kg/dose PO, IV every 6 h or 0.05–0.1 mg/kg/dose PO, IV every 4 h
Naloxone (NarcanZimhi; ❋ Naloxone hydrochloride injection)	Overdose: 0.4–2 mg IV; additional doses may be repeated at 2–3-min intervals; if no response after 10 mg, question the diagnosis; IM, subcutaneous, endotracheal routes may be used if IV route is unavailable Narcan nasal spray: 4 or 8 mg (contents of 1 nasal spray) as single dose; may repeat every 2–3 min in alternating nostrils until medical assistance available (4 mg nasal spray available without prescription)	Birth to 5 y or ≤20 kg, 0.1 mg/kg/dose IV; additional 0.1 mg/kg every 2–3 min as needed; may be given intraosseous or endotracheally ≥5 y or >20 kg, 2 mg IV, may repeat every 2–3 min; IM, subcutaneous, endotracheal routes may be used if IV route is unavailable
Naltrexone (Vivitrol; ❋ APO-Naltrexone, ReVia)	Alcohol dependence: 50 mg PO daily or 380 mg IM every 4 wk Opioid dependence: initial dose, 25 mg PO; observe for 1 h; if no signs or symptoms are seen, complete dose with 25 mg PO; usual maintenance dose is 50 mg/24 h; flexible dosing can include 100 mg PO every other day or 150 mg PO every 3 d or 380 mg IM every 4 wk	Not approved for use in children <18 y. Safety and efficacy not established
Nicotine (Nicoderm CQ, Nicorette mini, Nicotrol NS; ❋ Habitrol, Nicoderm, Nicorette, Nicotrol)	Transdermal, apply system (5–21) mg once every 24 h; dosage based on response and stage of withdrawal Nicotine chewing gum, 1 piece (2 or 4 mg) every 1–2 h for wk 1–6 with an urge to smoke; gradual reduction over next 6 wk Nasal lozenge, 2 mg or 4 mg dose within 30 min of awakening, then every 1–2 h for wk 1–6; gradual reduction over next 6 wk (max 5 lozenges every 6 h or 20 lozenges daily) Nasal spray, 1–2 sprays each hour, up to 10 sprays/h or 80 total sprays per day Nasal inhaler, 6–16 cartridges daily for first 6–12 wk, then gradual reduction over next 6–12 wk	Safety and efficacy in patients younger than 18 y who smoke not established
Varenicline (Chantix; ❋ Champix)	Patient should pick a date to stop smoking and begin drug therapy 1 wk before that date; d 1–3, 0.5 mg/d PO; d 4–7, 0.5 mg PO twice daily; d 8 until the end of treatment, 1 mg PO twice daily; treatment should last 12 wk	Not recommended for children younger than 18 y

GA, gestational age.

Adverse Effects

CNS adverse effects of chlordiazepoxide include sedation, depression, lethargy, disorientation, and delirium. Patients taking high dosages may experience paradoxical excitatory reactions during the first few weeks of treatment. Other adverse effects include alterations in pulse and blood pressure, urticaria, constipation, diarrhea, dry mouth, jaundice, changes in libido, and blood dyscrasias.

The U.S. Food and Drug Administration (FDA) has issued a BOXED WARNING ◆ for the combined use of benzodiazepines and opioid analgesics. Serious adverse reactions, including slowed or difficult breathing and death, have been reported.

Contraindications

Contraindications to chlordiazepoxide include hypersensitivity to benzodiazepines, psychosis, acute narrow-angle glaucoma, shock, coma, and acute alcoholic intoxication with depression of vital signs.

Nursing Implications

Preventing Interactions

Some medications interact with chlordiazepoxide, increasing its effects (Box 58.2). In addition, kava and valerian are herbs known to increase the effects of chlordiazepoxide.

Administering the Medication

Chlordiazepoxide is available in capsule form for oral use and powder form for parenteral use. For adults, the dosage is individualized and is often based on an institution-specific protocol. It is necessary to increase the dosage carefully to avoid adverse effects. The nurse gives IM injections slowly in the upper outer quadrant of the gluteus muscle. The nurse should take the patient's vital signs regularly during this period, especially when giving the IV form of the drug, as well as observe and document subjective and objective reports by the patient. It is important to taper the drug gradually based on the patient's response to treatment.

Assessing for Therapeutic Effects

The nurse assesses the patient's vital signs; they should stabilize to within normal parameters. In addition, the nurse observes for the presence of cognitive impairment and/or thought disturbances and assesses for signs and symptoms of agitation and/or restlessness. The patient should not appear restless or confused and should not complain of thought disturbances.

BOX 58.2 Drug Interactions: Chlordiazepoxide

Drugs That Increase the Effect of Chlordiazepoxide
- Antiepileptic drugs, central nervous system depressants, cimetidine, phenytoin
  Increase central nervous system depression
- Levodopa
  Increases parkinsonian symptoms

Assessing for Adverse Effects

The nurse assesses the patient for signs and symptoms of CNS depression. It is necessary to check the blood pressure for fluctuations from hypertension to hypotension. The nurse assesses the skin for redness, itching, and signs of bruising as well as the skin and sclera for jaundice. It is also necessary to interview the patient regarding the following:

- Frequency and amount of bowel movements
- Desire for sexual intercourse

Clinical Application 58.1

Mr. Wilson admits to the nurse in the emergency department that he consumes alcohol daily. He admits to smoking tobacco in the form of cigarettes (one pack per day) and to smoking marijuana (average, two times per week). The healthcare providers in the emergency department are concerned that he may experience alcohol withdrawal, and a physician subsequently prescribes a short-acting benzodiazepine.
- Is a benzodiazepine the pharmacologic treatment of choice for this condition?
- What are some symptoms for which the nurse should monitor?

Patient Teaching

With chlordiazepoxide, it is necessary to instruct the patient and/or caregiver to take the drug as prescribed and not to stop taking it without consulting the healthcare provider.

ENZYME INHIBITORS FOR MAINTENANCE OF ALCOHOL SOBRIETY

Drug therapy for maintenance of sobriety is limited, mainly because of poor adherence. One of the drugs approved for this purpose is **P disulfiram**.

Pharmacokinetics and Action

Disulfiram is quickly absorbed in the gastrointestinal tract. It has a slow onset of action, with a peak of up to 12 hours and a duration of 1 to 2 weeks. The medication is deposited in fat. It is metabolized slowly by the liver and excreted by the lungs and in the feces.

Disulfiram inhibits the enzyme aldehyde dehydrogenase to block the oxidation of alcohol. This allows acetaldehyde to accumulate in the blood to concentrations that are 5 to 10 times higher than normally achieved during alcohol metabolism. This accumulation of acetaldehyde produces an unpleasant reaction when disulfiram is consumed with alcohol.

Use

Prescribers order disulfiram for people with alcohol use disorder to maintain a state of sobriety. Table 58.2 gives route and dosage information for disulfiram and other drugs used to treat substance use disorders.

Patient-related variables specific to the use of disulfiram include the following:

- Age:
  - Disulfiram is not approved for use in children.
- Reproduction, pregnancy, and lactation:
  - Safe use during pregnancy has not been established.
  - It is uncertain if disulfiram enters breast milk; however, its use during breast-feeding is not recommended.
- Abnormal kidney function and hepatic impairment:
  - Hepatitis and hepatic failure may occur with disulfiram. This reaction may be severe, resulting in death in patients with hepatic impairment.

Adverse Effects

The combination of disulfiram with alcohol may result in headaches, confusion, seizures, chest pain, flushing, palpitations, hypotension, sweating, blurred vision, nausea, vomiting, and a garliclike aftertaste. More severe effects (with alcohol) include dysrhythmias, cardiovascular collapse, heart failure, myocardial infarction, and death.

Contraindications

Contraindications to disulfiram include use with alcohol, metronidazole, or paraldehyde, as well as multiple drug dependence. A **BOXED WARNING** states that the drug should not be given to a patient who has consumed alcohol in the past 12 hours or without their full knowledge. It is important that disulfiram never be administered to patients with myocardial disease, coronary occlusion, or psychosis. Patients who are known to be allergic to the drug should not take it.

Nursing Implications

Preventing Interactions

Nitroglycerin, paraldehyde, metronidazole, and cotrimoxazole produce a reaction similar to that of alcohol; the accumulation of acetaldehyde produces an unpleasant reaction accompanied by nausea and vomiting. Isoniazid and disulfiram produce neurologic effects such as changes in behavior and coordination. Warfarin, paraldehyde, and phenytoin combined with disulfiram result in increased serum blood levels of the drugs.

Administering the Medication

Administration of disulfiram at bedtime allows the patient to sleep, because the drug has a sedative effect.

Assessing Therapeutic and Adverse Effects

The nurse determines whether the patient has remained sober. In the event disulfiram is consumed with alcohol, the nurse assesses for cardiovascular effects. In a patient who presents with a severe reaction, it is essential to monitor for shock and hypokalemia.

Patient Teaching

With disulfiram, it is necessary to instruct the patient to

- Take the medication daily—at bedtime if dizziness and drowsiness occur.
- Never consume alcohol in any form, including liniments, mouthwash, over-the-counter cough and cold aids, vinegars, sauces, and colognes.
- Not take the medication if alcohol has been consumed.
- Have periodic liver function tests.
- Wear a medical alert bracelet.

DRUGS USED TO REDUCE CRAVINGS IN ALCOHOL USE

Acamprosate and oral naltrexone (Vivitrol) are used for relapse prevention and are considered anticraving agents. These drugs have different mechanisms of action and target different neurotransmitter systems that may provide effectiveness for different aspects of alcohol use behavior. In treatment for alcohol use disorders, acamprosate has been found to be slightly more effective in promoting abstinence and naltrexone slightly more effective in reducing heavy drinking and craving.

Alcohol use stimulates opioid receptors and releases endorphins in the brain, and naltrexone, an opioid antagonist, is thought to reduce the incentive to drink and decrease craving by blocking the rewarding effect of alcohol. Acamprosate is a GABA agonist/glutamate antagonist used in the treatment of alcohol abuse. Although the exact mechanism is unclear, the drug is thought to normalize the dysregulation of N-methyl-D-aspartate (NMDA)-mediated glutamatergic excitation that occurs in alcohol withdrawal and early abstinence, restoring balance to GABA and glutamate. Unlike naltrexone, acamprosate does not appear to affect alcohol consumption after the first drink and does not cause a disulfiram-like reaction following alcohol ingestion. Among the two, acamprosate has low abuse potential, is better tolerated, and is safer in overdose.

NCLEX Success

1. The nurse caring for a patient with alcohol use disorder may expect to see what symptom as the patient enters withdrawal?
   A. sleep
   B. muscle relaxation
   C. euphoria
   D. agitation

2. A patient is admitted to the chemical dependence unit with alcohol use disorder. For which of the following symptoms does the nurse assess during alcohol withdrawal?
   A. euphoria, hyperactivity, and insomnia
   B. depression, suicidal ideation, and hypersomnia
   C. diaphoresis, nausea, vomiting, and tremors
   D. unsteady gait, nystagmus, and profound disorientation

3. Which of the following medications is the healthcare provider most likely to prescribe for a patient who is experiencing alcohol withdrawal?
   A. haloperidol
   B. chlordiazepoxide
   C. propoxyphene
   D. phenytoin

Clinical Application 58.2

Mr. Wilson is scheduled to be discharged after completing an alcohol withdrawal protocol for several days. After discharge, he is scheduled to attend outpatient chemical dependency treatment. His healthcare provider has prescribed disulfiram for the patient to take on an outpatient basis.

- Is this an appropriate treatment choice for the patient?
- What symptoms will Mr. Wilson have if he drinks alcohol and takes disulfiram?
- What patient teaching should the nurse provide to Mr. Wilson regarding his treatment plan with disulfiram?

OPIOID AGONISTS AND ANTAGONISTS FOR TREATMENT OF OPIOID USE DISORDER

Ideally, the goal of treatment for opioid use disorder is abstinence from further opioid use. However, because patients who use opioids rarely meet this goal, long-term drug therapy may be used to treat heroin dependence.

The first option uses opioid substitutes to prevent withdrawal symptoms and improve a lifestyle that revolves around obtaining, using, and recovering from a drug. The substitute is methadone, an agonist at specific opioid receptors in the CNS. This drug has long been used as a detoxification and/or as maintenance therapy for opioid addiction. It is usually given in a single, daily oral dose at an outpatient methadone clinic. The FDA has issued a **BOXED WARNING** concerning methadone, stating that it should be part of an approved program for opioid use disorder. Deaths have been reported during the initiation of treatment. It is essential that emergency services be on standby. Another **BOXED WARNING** for methadone stipulates that monitoring for QT interval prolongation on an electrocardiogram is necessary. Methadone is also used in the treatment of neonatal abstinence syndrome. However, the long elimination half-life makes tapering difficult, and an alternate drug should be considered.

Proponents say that methadone blocks the euphoria produced by heroin, acts longer, and reduces preoccupation with drug use. This effect allows a more normal lifestyle for the patient and reduces morbidity and mortality associated with the use of illegal and injected drugs. Opponents say that methadone maintenance only substitutes one type of drug dependence for another. In addition, a substantial percentage of those people receiving methadone maintenance therapy misuse other drugs, including cocaine.

A second option uses naltrexone, a pure opioid antagonist that blocks opioids from occupying receptor sites, thereby preventing their physiologic effects. (As discussed previously, this drug is also used to combat alcohol use disorder.) Used to maintain opioid-free states in the person dependent on opioids, it is recommended for use in conjunction with psychological counseling to promote patient motivation and adherence.

If the patient taking naltrexone has mild or moderate pain, they should receive a nonopioid analgesic (e.g., acetaminophen or a nonsteroidal anti-inflammatory drug). If the patient has severe pain and requires an opioid, administration of the naltrexone should occur in a setting staffed and equipped for cardiopulmonary resuscitation because respiratory depression may be deeper and more prolonged than usual. The FDA has issued a **BOXED WARNING** about naltrexone and the risk of hepatocellular injury. It is necessary to obtain periodic liver function tests during therapy and discontinue the drug at signs of increasing hepatic impairment.

A third option is buprenorphine (Buprenex, Belbuca, Butrans, Sublocade), an opioid agonist–antagonist analgesic that is occasionally injected therapeutically to relieve moderate to severe pain. The drug is given sublingually to treat opioid dependence. It is essential that the pill or film be dissolved under the tongue and not swallowed. Serious and potentially deadly adverse effects may occur if a patient combines this drug with other CNS depressant medications. Suboxone, a buprenorphine–naloxone combination, is preferred therapy over buprenorphine alone for induction treatment and for maintenance therapy for short-acting opioid dependence. Naloxone has poor transmucosal bioavailability, but if the combination product is injected, naloxone will compete with buprenorphine at the receptor and reduce any euphoric effects of the injection. However, naloxone's action of shutting off opioid receptors and signals in the body can trigger withdrawal symptoms in people who are currently taking an opioid. Naloxone administration places individuals with chronic misuse of an opioid agonist (such as heroin) at risk of developing seizures and respiratory failure, which can be fatal.

> **! Quality and Safety Alert: Safety**
>
> The FDA has issued a safety warning about the risks of dental problems associated with transmucosal (buccal, sublingual) buprenorphine-containing medicines, including decay, abscess, and tooth loss.

Physicians who prescribe buprenorphine for outpatient use must meet several restrictions and are required to have special training. The FDA has issued a **BOXED WARNING** for buprenorphine because use of buccal and transdermal routes increases the risk of substance use disorder and the risk of life-threatening respiratory depression. In addition, there is a risk of fatal overdose with accidental exposure by children of buprenorphine administered by buccal film or a transdermal patch. Also, prolonged use of the buccal or transdermal routes of buprenorphine during pregnancy has been known to cause neonatal abstinence syndrome.

> **! Quality and Safety Alert: Safety**
>
> Opioids should not be abruptly discontinued in a patient who is physically dependent. Patients taking opioid pain medications long term should be instructed not to stop taking their medicine suddenly; they should first develop a plan with their healthcare prescriber for how to slowly decrease the dose of the opioid while continuing to manage their pain.

CENTRAL NERVOUS SYSTEM STIMULANT ABUSE: DRUG THERAPY

CNS stimulants are identified by the behavioral stimulation and psychomotor agitation that they produce. The amount of CNS stimulation caused by a certain drug depends on both the area in the brain or spinal cord that is affected by the drug and the cellular mechanism fundamental to the increased excitability. CNS stimulants include amphetamines and related drugs, caffeine (discussed in Chapter 57), cocaine, and nicotine. A detailed description of these substances is found on thePoint http://thePoint.lww.com/Frandsen13e. For the most part, few proven pharmacologic treatments are effective in the treatment of CNS stimulant use, because most of the cravings patients experience are psychological in nature.

NCLEX Success

4. What is the most common cause of death from opioids?
   A. hypertension
   B. central nervous system stimulation
   C. respiratory depression
   D. myocardial infarction

5. A nurse working in the emergency department is caring for a patient who has been brought in with suspected opioid overdose. What is the appropriate treatment to administer?
   A. disulfiram
   B. naloxone
   C. amitriptyline
   D. chlordiazepoxide

PSYCHOACTIVE SUBSTANCE USE: DRUG THERAPY

Other psychoactive substances include marijuana, hallucinogens, "club" and "date-rape" drugs, and inhalants. Few proven pharmacologic treatments are effective in the treatment of psychoactive substance misuse and dependence. For further details on other psychoactive medications of abuse, visit thePoint http://thePoint.lww.com/Frandsen13e.

THE NURSING PROCESS

A concept map outlines the nursing process related to drug therapy considerations in this chapter. Additional nursing implications related to the disease process should also be considered in care decisions.

Assessment
- Interview the patient regarding alcohol and other drug use to help determine immediate and long-term nursing care needs.
- Assess behavior that may indicate drug misuse, such as alcohol on the breath, altered speech patterns, staggering gait, and other signs of excessive CNS depression or stimulation.
- Assess for disorders that may be caused by substance misuse. These disorders may include infections, liver disease, accidental injuries, and psychiatric problems of anxiety or depression.
- Assess liver function, complete blood count (hypocalcemia, hypomagnesemia, and acidosis are common in people who misuse alcohol), and alcohol and drug levels in the blood.

Outcomes of Therapy

The patient will
- Maintain safety if impaired by alcohol and drug misuse.
- Remain current on information regarding drug effects and treatment resources.
- Maintain efforts toward stopping drug usage be recognized and reinforced.

Nursing Interventions
- Decrease environmental stimuli for the person undergoing drug withdrawal.
- Record vital signs; cardiovascular, respiratory, and neurologic functions; mental status; and behavior at regular intervals.
- Support use of resources for stopping drug misuse (psychotherapy, treatment programs).
- Request patient referrals to psychiatric/mental health physicians, nurse clinical specialists, or self-help programs when indicated.
- Use therapeutic communication skills to discuss alcohol or other drug-related health problems, health-related benefits of stopping substance use, and available services or treatment options.
- Teach nondrug techniques for coping with stress and anxiety.
- Provide positive reinforcement for efforts toward quitting substance misuse.
- Inform smokers with young children in the home that cigarette smoke can precipitate or aggravate asthma and upper respiratory disorders in children.
- Inform smokers with nonsmoking spouses or other members of the household that secondhand smoke can increase the risks of cancer and lung disease in the nonsmokers as well as in the person who smokes.
- For those who smoke and are concerned about weight gain if they quit smoking, emphasize that the health benefits of quitting far outweigh the disadvantages of gaining a few pounds and discuss ways to control weight without smoking.

Evaluation
- Observe for improved behavior (e.g., less impulsiveness, improved judgment and thought processes, commits no injury to self or others).
- Observe for use or avoidance of nonprescribed drugs while hospitalized.
- Interview to determine the patient's insight into personal problems stemming from drug misuse.
- Verify enrollment in a treatment program.
- Observe for appropriate use of drugs to decrease misuse of other drugs.

Visit **thePoint** at **http://thePoint.lww.com/Frandsen13e** for answers to NCLEX Success questions (in Appendix A), answers to Clinical Application Case Studies (in Appendix B), additional information on the etiology of substance use disorder, CNS system depressants and stimulants that are commonly misused, other psychoactive medications that are misused, and more!

REFERENCES AND RESOURCES

American Psychiatric Association. (2022). *Diagnostic and statistical manual of mental disorders—Text revision* (5th ed.).

Boson, K., Anderberg, M., Melander Hagborg, J., Wennberg, P., & Dahlberg, M. (2022). Adolescents with substance use problems in outpatient treatment: A one-year prospective follow-up study focusing on mental health and gender differences. *Substance Abuse Treatment, Prevention, and Policy, 17*(1), 1–10. https://doi.org/10.1186/s13011-022-00482-2

Bukstein, O. (2023). Approach to treating substance use disorder in adolescents. *UpToDate*. Lexi-Comp, Inc.

Castells, X., Cunill, R., Perez-Mana, C., & Capella, D. (2016). Psychostimulants drugs for cocaine dependence. *Cochrane Database of Systematic Reviews, 9*, CD007380. https://doi.org/10.1002/14651858.CD007380.pub4

Cullen, K. A., Liu, S. T., Bernat, J. K., Slavit, W. I., Tynan, M. A., King, B. A., & Neff, L. J. (2019). Flavored tobacco product use among middle and high school students—United States, 2014-2018. *MMWR Morbidity and Mortality Weekly Report, 68*(39), 839.

Dogosh, K. L., Cacciola, J. S., & Jarvis, M. E. (2019). Clinical assessment of substance use disorders. *UpToDate*. Lexi-Comp, Inc.

Lippincott Advisor. (2023). http://advisor.lww.com

Lippincott Williams & Wilkins. (2022). *Nursing 2023 drug handbook* (43th ed.). Wolters Kluwer.

McCarty, D. A. (2019). Changing landscape for treatment of alcohol and drug use disorders. *American Journal of Public Health, 109*(6), 838–839. https://doi.org/10.2105/AJPH.2019.305080

Stellern, L., Xiao, K. B., Sanches, M., Gowin, J. L., & Sloan, M. E. (2023). Emotional regulation in substance use disorders: A systematic review and meta-analysis. *Addiction, 118*(1), 30–47.

Clinical Judgment in Practice: Section 9: Drugs Affecting the Autonomic and Central Nervous System

The family of a 68-year-old patient has noted that the patient has decreasing memory. Their symptoms include losing keys, having difficulty with directions, and most recently being unable to recognize street signs. Last week at the department of motor vehicles, the patient could not identify the street signs while being examined for their motor vehicle license. The patient's spouse then tried to teach the patient the signs without success.

The patient's family made an appointment with the primary care provider. During the visit, memory tests were conducted in which the patient could not identify the current President of the United States or successfully complete other significant memory-related exercises. The primary care provider diagnosed the patient with early-onset Alzheimer disease. The patient was prescribed donepezil 5 mg PO at bedtime.

For the past 6 months, the patient's memory has begun to decline with periods of agitation. According to the patient's family, the patient's mood changes from manic to periods of quietness and depression. You are the patient's home care nurse. After you consult with the patient's primary care provider, an additional medication is recommended to slow the progression of the patient's Alzheimer disease. The patient is prescribed donepezil–memantine 7 mg/10 mg, to be taken orally every evening.

Step 1: Recognize Cues
Identify the relevant and important information from different sources, such as the medical history or subjective and objective data.

Answer: *The patient's family has noted a decrease in the patient's memory. The patient was unable to identify the street signs at the department of motor vehicles. The patient could not identify the President of the United States or accurately answer the memory tests administered by the primary care provider.*

After 6 months of treatment with donepezil, the patient's memory declines and the family describes mood changes. The patient has periods of mania and depression. As the disease process progresses, the patient will become more confused, depressed, fearful, and anxious.

Step 2: Analyze Cues
Organize and link the recognized cues to the patient's clinical presentation.

Answer: *You link the clustered symptoms of the patient's decreasing memory to the need for a change in the medication regime. Donepezil routinely delays the progression of Alzheimer disease symptoms for up to 55 weeks. The patient's memory began to decline after 6 months. In addition, agitation and depressive mood resulted.*

Step 3: Prioritize Hypotheses
Evaluate hypotheses and rank them according to priority, such as urgency, likelihood, risk, difficulty, and/or time. Cluster your findings to generate a list of problems (actual or potential) you believe the patient is experiencing or may experience and determine the level of urgency. Which problem is of the greatest concern?

Answer: *You prioritize the needs of the patient. The increasing signs of dementia, loss of memory, and mood changes place the patient at risk for injury. The family must be instructed on strategies to protect the patient from injury. Due to the changes in the patient's behavior and memory, it becomes more difficult to assess the patient for adverse effects of the medication.*

Step 4: Generate Solutions
Identify expected outcomes and use hypotheses to define a set of interventions for the expected outcomes.

Answer: *The patient will remain safe in the home environment. As the home care nurse, you consult with the family to identify potential hazards to the patient's safety. The patient is able to open the doors of the home and has been found wandering the neighborhood. The family must work outside of the home and the patient must not be left alone.*

Step 5: Take Actions
Implement the solutions that address the highest priorities.

Answer: *The family installs door alarms to protect the patient from leaving the home unattended. The family removes obstructed areas in the home to prevent falls. You assist the family in developing a consistent daily plan of care. The family will utilize adult day care when at work. The patient will not be left alone. The patient will not use major appliances, particularly the stove and oven. You instruct the family on safety in the bathroom. An elevated toilet seat will be installed. A shower chair and any ambulation devices will be utilized. You will assess for adverse effects of donepezil–memantine. You and family will report changes in memory and mood to the primary care provider.*

Step 6: Evaluate Outcomes
Compare observed outcomes against expected outcomes.

Answer: The patient has been taking donepezil–memantine for 2 weeks. The primary care provider has determined the dosage should be increased to aid in decreasing memory loss. The dosage was increased to 28 mg/10 mg to be administered with the evening meal. Prior to the increased dosage, the patient's blood pressure was 128/86, pulse 72, respiration 22, and temperature 98.4°F. The patient's mood has been less combative with increasing interest in word search puzzles and increased socialization with family. The family understands all safety devices to be used.

SECTION 10

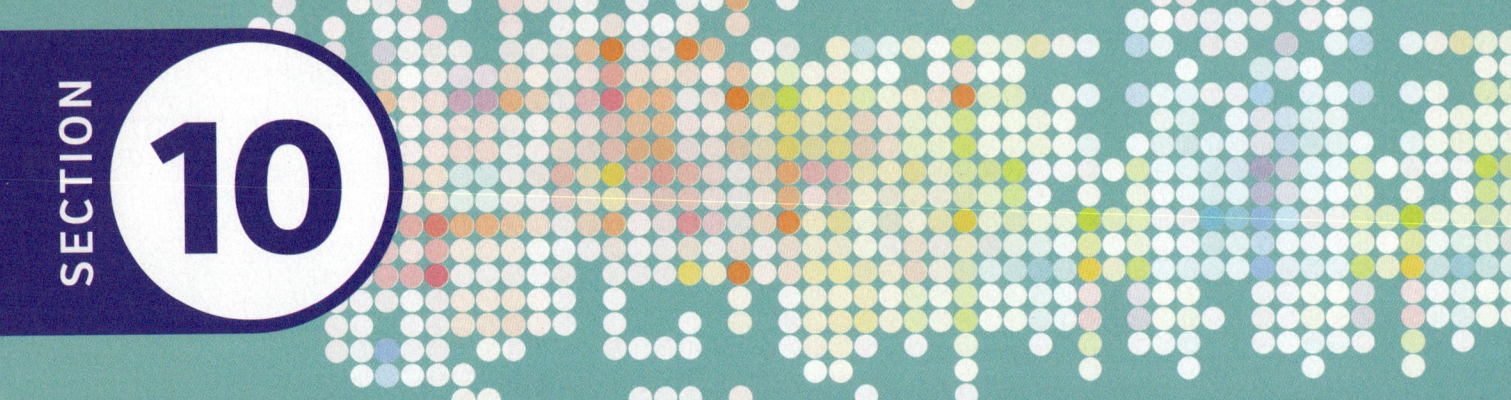

Drugs Affecting the Eye, Ear, and Skin

Chapter 59 Drug Therapy for Disorders of the Eye
Chapter 60 Drug Therapy for Disorders of the Ear
Chapter 61 Drug Therapy for Disorders of the Skin

CHAPTER 59

Drug Therapy for Disorders of the Eye

LEARNING OBJECTIVES

After studying this chapter, you should be able to:

1. Describe the basic structures and functions of the eye.
2. Describe the specific disorders of the eye and the clinical manifestations of the disorders.
3. Identify the prototypes and describe the action, use, adverse effects, contraindications, and nursing implications for medications administered for diagnosis and treatment of ocular disorders.
4. Identify the prototypes and describe the action, use, adverse effects, contraindications, and nursing implications for medications administered for glaucoma.
5. Identify the prototypes and describe the action, use, adverse effects, contraindications, and nursing implications for medications administered for ocular infections and inflammation.
6. Implement the nursing process in the care of the patient with an ocular disorder.

CLINICAL APPLICATION CASE STUDY

Irene Molnar is a 75-year-old woman who has open-angle glaucoma. Her physician has prescribed the following: acetazolamide (Diamox), 250 mg orally, every 6 hours; timolol (Timoptic), one drop in each eye, twice daily; and pilocarpine (Isopto Carpine), one drop of 2% solution in each eye, three times daily. You are a home care nurse visiting Mrs. Molnar.

KEY TERMS

Blepharitis: chronic infection of glands and lash follicles on the margins of the eyelids

Conjunctiva: mucous membrane lining the eyelids

Conjunctivitis: inflammation of the conjunctiva

Glaucoma: group of diseases characterized by optic nerve damage and changes in visual fields, which is characterized by increased intraocular pressure (IOP) (greater than 22 mm Hg), although it may also occur with normal IOP (less than 21 mm Hg); one of the leading causes of blindness in the United States

Intraocular pressure (IOP): pressure inside the eye; normally less than 21 mm Hg (average 15 to 16 mm Hg)

Keratitis: inflammation of the cornea

Lacrimation: production of tears

Miosis: pupil constriction

Mydriasis: pupil dilation

Nasolacrimal occlusion: application of pressure to the tear duct

Refraction: deflection of light rays in various directions according to the density of the ocular structures through which they pass

Tonometry: diagnostic test to measure the pressure inside the eye to determine the diagnosis of glaucoma

INTRODUCTION

This chapter introduces the eye and its disorders. It addresses the drug therapy implemented to enhance visualization of the eye for eye examination and the drug therapy for ocular disorders, including glaucoma, ocular infection, and ocular inflammation.

BASIC STRUCTURE AND FUNCTION OF THE EYE

The eye is the major sensory organ through which a person receives information about the external environment. Extensive discussion of vision and ocular anatomy is beyond the scope of this chapter, but some characteristics and functions are described to facilitate understanding of ocular drug therapy.

The eyelids and lacrimal system function to protect the eye. The eyelid is a barrier to the entry of foreign bodies, strong light, dust, and other potential irritants. The **conjunctiva** is the mucous membrane lining the eyelids. The canthi (singular, canthus) are the angles where the upper and lower eyelids meet. The lacrimal system produces a fluid that constantly moistens and cleanses the anterior surface of the eyeball. The fluid drains through two small openings in the inner canthus and flows through the nasolacrimal duct into the nasal cavity. When the conjunctiva is irritated or certain emotions are experienced (e.g., sadness), the lacrimal gland produces more fluid than the drainage system can accommodate. The excess fluid overflows the eyelids and becomes tears. Production of tears is known as **lacrimation**.

The eyeball is a spherical structure composed of the sclera, cornea, choroid, and retina, plus special refractive tissues. The sclera is a white, opaque, fibrous tissue that covers the posterior five sixths of the eyeball. The cornea is a transparent, special connective tissue that covers the anterior sixth of the eyeball. It contains no blood vessels. The choroid, composed of blood vessels and connective tissue, continues forward to form the iris. The iris is composed of pigmented cells, the opening called the pupil, and muscles that control the size of the pupil by contracting or dilating in response to stimuli. Pupil constriction is called **miosis**, and pupil dilation is called **mydriasis**. The retina is the innermost layer of the eyeball.

For vision to occur, light rays must enter the eye through the cornea; travel through the pupil, lens, and vitreous body (discussed below); and be focused on the retina. Light rays do not travel directly to the retina. Instead, they are deflected in various directions according to the density of the ocular structures through which they pass. This process, called **refraction**, is controlled by the aqueous humor, lens, and vitreous body. The optic disk is the area of the retina where ophthalmic blood vessels and the optic nerve enter the eyeball.

The structure and function of the eyeball are further influenced by the lens, aqueous humor, and vitreous body. The lens is an elastic, transparent structure; its function is to focus light rays to form images on the retina. It is located behind the iris and is held in place by ligaments attached to the ciliary body. The aqueous humor is a clear fluid produced by capillaries in the ciliary body. Most of the fluid flows through the pupil into the anterior chamber (between the cornea and the lens and anterior to the iris). A small amount flows into a passage called Schlemm canal, from which it enters the venous circulation.

Nearly 60% to 80% of the aqueous humor is drained through the trabecular meshwork outflow pathways, as seen in Figure 59.1. In the healthy eye, the pressure inside the eye, **intraocular pressure (IOP)**, is maintained through a balance between the amount of aqueous humor produced in the ciliary body epithelium and the amount drained from the anterior chamber. Impaired drainage of aqueous humor causes increased IOP. IOP is normally less than 21 mm Hg, with an average of 15 to 16 mm Hg. The vitreous body is a transparent, jellylike mass located in the posterior portion of the eyeball. It functions to refract light rays and maintain the normal shape of the eyeball.

OVERVIEW OF DISORDERS OF THE EYE

The eye is subject to many disorders that threaten its structure, function, or both. Some disorders in which ophthalmic drugs play a prominent role are discussed in this section. For in-depth information on the etiology and pathophysiology of disorders of the eye, visit thePoint http://thePoint.lww.com/Frandsen13e.

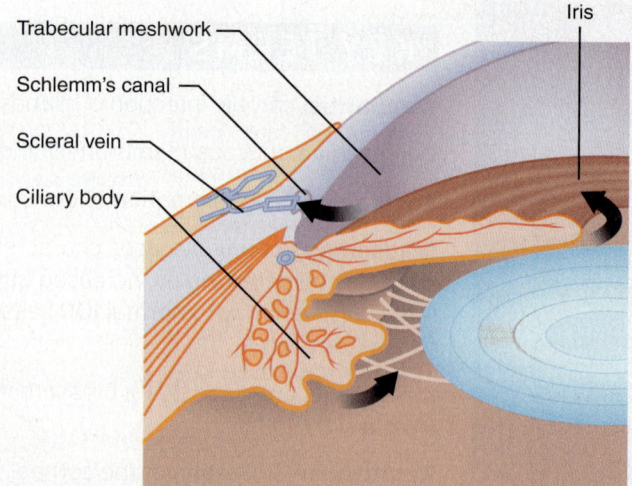

Figure 59.1. Ocular anatomy concerned with control of intraocular pressure. [Reprinted with permission from Barash, P. G., Cullen, B. F., Stoelting, R. K., et al. (2017). *Clinical anesthesia* (8th ed.). Wolters Kluwer.]

Specific Disorders of the Eye

Refractive Errors

Refractive errors include myopia (nearsightedness), hyperopia (farsightedness), presbyopia, and astigmatism. These conditions impair vision by interfering with the eye's ability to focus light rays on the retina. Ophthalmic drugs are used only in the diagnosis of the conditions; treatment involves prescription of eyeglasses or contact lenses.

Glaucoma

Glaucoma is one of the leading causes of blindness in the United States and the most common cause of blindness in African Americans. It is a group of diseases characterized by optic nerve damage and changes in visual fields. It is often characterized by increased IOP (above 22 mm Hg) but may also occur with normal IOP (below 21 mm Hg; average 15 to 16 mm Hg). Diagnostic tests for glaucoma include ophthalmoscopic examination of the optic disk; measurement of IOP, or **tonometry** (the diagnostic test to measure the pressure inside the eye); and testing of visual fields.

Ocular Infections and Inflammation

Ocular infections may result from foreign bodies, contaminated hands, contaminated eye medications, or infections in contiguous structures (e.g., nose, face, sinuses). Causes of ocular inflammation include bacteria, viruses, allergic reactions, and irritating chemicals. These conditions include the following:

- **Conjunctivitis**, which is inflammation of the conjunctiva
- **Blepharitis**, which is a chronic infection of glands and lash follicles on the margins of the eyelids
- **Keratitis**, which is inflammation of the cornea
- Corneal ulcers
- Fungal infections

Clinical Manifestations

Refractive errors are manifested by loss of near or far vision. Glaucoma is characterized by blurred vision, halos around lights, difficulty focusing, difficulty adjusting to low lighting, loss of peripheral vision, headache, and aching around the eye. Conjunctivitis involves redness, tearing, itching, edema, and burning or gritty sensations. Blepharitis is an inflammation of the anterior or posterior structures of the eyelids. Anterior blepharitis presents with burning, redness, and itching of the anterior eyelids. Posterior blepharitis is eyelid inflammation with inflammation of the meibomian glands. An infected sebaceous gland is noted as a hordeolum or stye-producing pain, redness, and swelling of the site. Keratitis is characterized by irritation, increased tear production, and photophobia. Corneal ulcers and fungal infections also produce eye pain, discharge, changes in vision, swelling, and redness.

> **Clinical Application 59.1**
> - Mrs. Molnar has been diagnosed with open-angle glaucoma. What is the normal intraocular pressure?
> - What is the intraocular pressure that is diagnostic of open-angle glaucoma?
> - If untreated, what is the outcome of this disease?

> **NCLEX Success**
> 1. When applying mascara, a patient may have scratched the cornea. The patient states they do not have time to go to the ophthalmologist. What ocular disorder could this result in?
>   A. corneal redness
>   B. corneal ulceration
>   C. blepharitis
>   D. conjunctivitis

Drug Therapy

Drug therapy of ophthalmic conditions is unique because of the location, structure, and function of the eye. Many systemic drugs are unable to cross the blood–eye barrier and achieve therapeutic concentrations in ocular structures. In general, penetration is greater if the drug achieves a high concentration in the blood, is fat soluble, and is poorly bound to serum proteins and if inflammation is present.

Because of the difficulties associated with systemic therapy, various methods of administering drugs locally have been developed. The most common and preferred method is topical application of ophthalmic solutions or suspensions (eyedrops) to the conjunctiva. Drugs are distributed through the tear film covering the eye and may be used for superficial disorders (e.g., conjunctivitis) or for relatively deep ocular disorders (e.g., glaucoma). Topical ophthalmic ointments may also be used. In addition, ophthalmologists may inject medications (e.g., antibiotics, corticosteroids, local anesthetics) into or around various eye structures. A major use of topical ophthalmic drugs in children is to dilate the pupil and paralyze accommodation for ophthalmoscopic examination. As a general rule, practitioners prefer the short-acting mydriatics and cycloplegics (e.g., cyclopentolate, tropicamide) because they cause fewer systemic adverse effects than atropine. In addition, children usually receive lower drug concentrations (given empirically) because of their smaller size and the potential risk of systemic adverse effects.

DRUG THERAPY FOR THE DIAGNOSIS AND TREATMENT OF OCULAR DISORDERS

Drugs used to diagnose or treat ophthalmic disorders represent numerous therapeutic classifications, most of which are discussed in other chapters. This chapter describes the major classes of drugs used in ophthalmology. Later, the chapter discusses drugs used in the treatment of glaucoma. Table 59.1 summarizes the medications used to diagnose and treat some ocular disorders. Ocular medications are administered topically with limited systemic effects.

ANTICHOLINERGIC DRUGS

Anticholinergic drugs dilate the pupil to provide greater observation of the inner aspect of the eye. The prototype of this class is **atropine sulfate** (Isopto Atropine: ophthalmic).

TABLE 59.1
Drugs Administered for Diagnosis and Treatment of Ocular Disorders

Drug Class	Prototype	Other Drugs in the Class
Anticholinergic drugs	Atropine sulfate (Isopto Atropine)	Cyclopentolate (Cyclogyl) Homatropine (Homatropaire) Tropicamide (Mydriacyl)
Adrenergic agonists	Phenylephrine hydrochloride (Altafrin)	
Local anesthetic drugs	Lidocaine (Akten)	Proparacaine (Alcaine) Tetracaine (Altacaine, Tetcaine, TetraVisc)

Pharmacokinetics and Action

The onset of action of atropine (ophthalmic) is 5 to 10 minutes, with a peak of action in 30 to 40 minutes and a duration of action of 7 to 14 days. Metabolism occurs in the liver, and excretion takes place in the urine.

Atropine (ophthalmic) blocks the effects of acetylcholine in the central nervous system (CNS). It produces mydriatic effects by relaxing the pupil of the eye and prevents accommodation of near vision.

Use

Diagnostic use of atropine (ophthalmic) involves production of mydriasis and cycloplegia–pupillary dilation in acute and inflammatory conditions of the iris and uveal tract. Other uses include measurement of refractive errors and treatment of uveitis. Table 59.2 presents route and dosage information for atropine and related drugs in adults and children.

Patient-related variables specific to the use of atropine ophthalmic include the following:

- Reproduction, pregnancy, and lactation:
  - If administered in pregnancy the lowest effective dosage should be administered.
  - It is unknown if atropine is excreted in breast milk.
- Abnormal kidney function and hepatic impairment:
  - Use cautiously with abnormal kidney function. The dosage may need to be lowered with impaired kidney function.

Adverse Effects and Contraindications

Atropine (ophthalmic) may cause local transient stinging. The systemic effects of this medication depend on the amount of medication absorbed and rarely lead to an inhibition of vagal stimulation affecting the heart or diminished bronchial or gastric secretions.

Contraindications to atropine (ophthalmic) include the presence of glaucoma or the tendency to this condition.

Nursing Implications
Administering the Medication

For uveitis, it is necessary to instill one to two drops of atropine (ophthalmic) in the eye 1 hour prior to examination or three times per day to decrease inflammation of the iris and uveal tract. The nurse uses **nasolacrimal occlusion** to prevent the systemic absorption of the ophthalmic medication. In this process, the nurse applies finger pressure over the lacrimal sac for 1 to 2 minutes after instillation to decrease the risk of absorption and systemic effects. Box 59.1 presents general nursing guidelines for the topical administration of eye medications.

Assessing for Therapeutic and Adverse Effects

One hour following administration, the ophthalmologist uses an ophthalmic scope to assess the ability to visualize the inner aspect of the eye. In the treatment of uveitis, the nurse assesses for diminished blurred vision and diminished photophobia.

It is necessary to assess for pain and stinging. In addition, the nurse assesses for blurred vision and sensitivity to light. These effects should diminish and are reversible over time.

Patient Teaching

The nurse instructs patients about the effects of the medication such as photophobia and stinging on administration. It is essential to tell patients not to drive if their vision is impaired. The nurse should tell them to wear sunglasses. Box 59.2 presents additional patient teaching guidelines for ophthalmic medications, including atropine.

Other Drugs in the Class

Cyclopentolate (Cyclogyl) is useful when given prior to ophthalmic examinations that involve diagnostic testing. It increases the papillary size so the fundus of the eye can be thoroughly examined. Five minutes before the examination, the ophthalmologist or nurse administers the drug (2% solution) to patients who have a heavily pigmented iris. To avoid excessive systemic absorption, it is necessary to use nasolacrimal occlusion during and for 1 to 2 minutes following administration. Patients who have uveitis should receive cyclopentolate in combination with atropine (ophthalmic). Caution is important in the older adults due to increased IOP. Psychotic reactions and behavioral disturbances have occurred in children. It is important to withhold infant feeding for 4 hours after ophthalmic examination due to feeding intolerance.

NCLEX Success

2. An older adult patient is receiving cyclopentolate for visualization of the eye. What is the patient at risk of developing?
   A. cataracts
   B. retinal detachment
   C. increased intraocular pressure
   D. cerebral edema

ADRENERGIC AGONIST

Phenylephrine (Altafrin), the prototype ophthalmic adrenergic agonist, is used for its mydriatic effects. Unlike anticholinergic drugs, it does not produce cycloplegic effects.

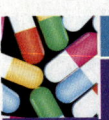

TABLE 59.2

DRUGS AT A GLANCE: Drugs for the Diagnosis and Treatment of Ocular Disorders

Drug	Routes and Dosage Ranges	
	Adults	**Children**
Anticholinergic Drugs		
ⓟ Atropine sulfate (ophthalmic) (Isopto Atropine; 🍁 Isopto Atropine, Minims Atropine Sulfate, Odan-Atropine)	Prior to evaluation: 1–2 drops of 1.0% solution 1 h before procedure	≥3 mo: 1 drop of 1.0% solution 40 min before procedure ≥3 y: 1–2 drops of 1.0% solution 40 min before procedure
Cyclopentolate (Cyclogyl; 🍁 Cyclogyl, Minims Cyclopentolate HC, Odan-Cyclopentolate)	1–2 drops of 0.5%, 1%, or 2% solution; may repeat in 5–10 min; instill 2% in heavily pigmented iris	Infants: 1 drop of 0.5% solution as a single-dose cyclopentolate and phenylephrine combination formulation is the preferred agent for use in infants Children and adolescents: 1–2 drops of 0.5%, 1%, or 2% solution; may repeat with 0.5% or 1% solution in 5–10 min
Homatropine	1–2 drops of 2% or 5% solution; may repeat in 5–10 min if necessary before refraction Uveitis: 1–2 drops of 2% or 5% solution every 3–4 h	≥3 mo: same as for adults
Tropicamide (Mydriacyl; 🍁 Mydriacyl, Odan-Tropicamide)	Cycloplegia: 1–2 drops of 1% solution 20–30 min before refraction Mydriasis: 1–2 drops of 0.5% solution 15–20 min before	Cycloplegia, mydriasis, same as adult dosage
Adrenergic Agonists		
ⓟ Phenylephrine (Altafrin; 🍁 Minims Phenylephrine HCl)	Mydriasis, 1 drop of 2.5% or 10% solution every 3–5 min as needed (max 3 drops per eye)	Mydriasis: Infants 1 drop of 2.5% solution every 3–5 min as needed (max 3 drops per eye) Children and adolescents: same as adult dosage
Local Anesthetic Drugs		
ⓟ Lidocaine (Akten)	Anesthesia, 2 drops to ocular surface in the area of procedure; may repeat to maintain effect	Refer to adult dosage
Proparacaine (Alcaine)	Ophthalmic surgery: 1 drop of 0.5% solution in the eye every 5–10 min for 5–7 doses Tonometry, gonioscopy, suture removal: 1 drop of 0.5% solution in the eye prior to the procedure	Same as adult dosage
Tetracaine (Altacaine, Tetcaine, TetraVisc)	Short-term anesthesia: 1–2 drops in the affected eye before examination Minor surgical procedure: 1–2 drops every 5–10 min for up to 3 doses Prolonged surgical procedure: 1–2 drops every 5–10 min for up to 5 doses	Safety and efficacy not established

BOX 59.1 General Nursing Guidelines for the Administration of Topical Ophthalmic Medications

- Topical application is the most common route of administration for ophthalmic drugs, and correct administration is essential for optimal therapeutic effects.
- Systemic absorption of eyedrops can be decreased by closing the eye and applying pressure over the tear duct (nasolacrimal occlusion) for 3 to 5 minutes after instillation.
- When multiple eyedrops are required, there should be an interval of 5 to 10 minutes between drops because of limited eye capacity and rapid drainage into tear ducts.
- Absorption of eye medications is increased in eye disorders associated with hyperemia and inflammation.
- Many ophthalmic drugs are available as eyedrops (solutions or suspensions) and ointments. Ointments are administered less frequently than drops and often produce higher concentrations of drug in target tissues. However, they also cause blurred vision, which limits their daytime use, at least for ambulatory patients. For some patients, drops may be used during waking hours and ointments at bedtime.
- Topical ophthalmic medications should not be used after the expiration date; cloudy, discolored solutions should be discarded.
- Topical eye medications contain a number of inactive ingredients, such as preservatives, buffers, tonicity drugs, and antioxidants. Some contain sulfites, to which some people may have an allergic reaction.
- Some eyedrops contain benzalkonium hydrochloride, a preservative, which is absorbed by soft contact lenses. The medications should not be applied while wearing soft contacts and should be instilled 15 minutes or longer before inserting soft contacts.
- To increase safety and accuracy of ophthalmic drug therapy, the labels and caps of eye medications are color coded.

BOX 59.2 Patient Teaching Guidelines for Topical Eye Medications

General Considerations

- Prevent eye disorders, when possible. For example, try to avoid long periods of reading and computer work; minimize exposure to dust, smog, cigarette smoke, and other eye irritants; and wash hands often and avoid touching the eyes to decrease risk of infection. Use protective eyewear when indicated.
- Do not use nonprescription eyedrops (e.g., Murine, Visine) on a regular basis for longer than 48 to 72 hours. Report persistent eye irritation and redness to a healthcare provider.
- Have regular eye examinations and testing for glaucoma after 40 years of age.
- Be aware that eyedrop preparations often contain sulfites, which can cause allergic reactions in some people.
- If you have glaucoma, do not take any drugs without your ophthalmologist's knowledge and consent. Many drugs given for purposes other than eye disorders may cause or aggravate glaucoma. Also, wear a medical alert bracelet or carry identification that states you have glaucoma. This helps avoid administration of drugs that aggravate glaucoma or to maintain treatment of glaucoma, in emergencies.
- If you have an eye infection, wash your hands before and after contact with the infected eye to avoid spreading the infection to the unaffected eye or to other people. Also, avoid touching the unaffected eye.
- If you wear contact lenses, wash your hands before inserting them and follow instructions for care (e.g., cleaning, inserting, or removing, and duration of wear). Improper or infrequent cleaning may lead to infection. Overwearing is a common cause of corneal abrasions and should be avoided to prevent the development of ulcers.
- If you wear soft contact lenses, do not use any eye medication without consulting a specialist in eye care. Some eyedrops contain benzalkonium hydrochloride, a preservative, which is absorbed by soft contacts. The medication should not be applied while wearing soft contacts and should be instilled 15 minutes or longer before inserting soft contacts.
- Never use eye medications used by someone else and never allow your eye medications to be used by anyone else. These preparations should be used by one person only, and they are dispensed in small amounts for this purpose. Single-person use minimizes cross-contamination and risks of infection.
- Know that many eyedrops and ointments cause temporary blurring of vision. Do not use such medications just before driving or operating potentially hazardous machinery.
- Avoid straining at stool (use laxatives or stool softeners if necessary), heavy lifting, bending over, coughing, and vomiting when possible. These activities increase IOP, which may cause eye damage in glaucoma and after eye surgery.

Self-Administration

- If using more than one eye medication, be sure to administer the correct one at the correct time. Benefits depend on accurate administration.
- Check expiration dates; do not use any eye medication after the expiration date and do not use any liquid medication that has changed colors or contains particles.
- Shake the container if instructed on the label to do so. Suspensions should be shaken well to ensure the drug is evenly dispersed in the liquid and not settled in the bottom of the container.
- Wash hands thoroughly.
- Tilt the head back or lie down and look up.
- Pull the lower lid down to expose the conjunctiva (mucous membrane).
- Place the dropper directly over the eye. Avoid contact of the dropper with the eye, finger, or any other surface. Such contact contaminates the solution and may cause eye infections and serious damage to the eye, with possible loss of vision.
- Look up just before applying a drop; look down for several seconds after applying the drop.
- Release the eyelid, close the eyes, and press the inside corner of the eye with a finger for 3 to 5 minutes. Closing the eyes and blocking the tear duct helps the medication be more effective by slowing its drainage out of the eye.
- Do not blink for 30 seconds after the administration of eye medications and during the eye examination.
- Do not rub the eye; do not rinse the dropper.
- If more than one eyedrop is ordered, wait 10 minutes before instilling the second medication.
- Use the same basic procedure to insert eye ointments.

Pharmacokinetics and Action

The mydriatic effects of phenylephrine (ophthalmic) occur 15 to 30 minutes after administration. Peak plasma effects occur in less than 20 minutes, and the duration of action is 1 to 3 hours. Systemic absorption is minimal.

Phenylephrine (ophthalmic) causes contraction of the dilator muscles of the pupil. It produces mydriasis, vasoconstriction, and increased outflow of aqueous humor.

Use

Uses of phenylephrine (ophthalmic) include mydriasis prior to ophthalmic procedures and therapy of wide-angle glaucoma. It can also provide relief of redness with eye irritation. Table 59.2 presents route and dosage information for phenylephrine.

Patient-related variables specific to the use of phenylephrine include the following:

- Age:
  - The 10% solution should not be used in infants <1 year.
  - Neonates and young infants are susceptible to systemic blood pressure effects with ophthalmic products.
- Reproduction, pregnancy, and lactation:
  - Animal reproduction studies have not been conducted on phenylephrine ophthalmic.
  - It is unknown if phenylephrine ophthalmic enters breast milk.

Adverse Effects and Contraindications

With phenylephrine (ophthalmic), systemic adverse effects are rare, but dysrhythmia, hypertension, myocardial infarction, syncope, and subarachnoid bleeding may occur. Ocular effects are reversible and include burning, irritation, visual changes, floaters, and rebound miosis.

Contraindications include hypersensitivity reactions, hypertension, ventricular tachycardia, and narrow-angle glaucoma.

Nursing Implications

Preventing Interactions

Phenylephrine combined with atomoxetine enhances the effects of hypertension and tachycardia. Taking phenylephrine with monoamine oxidase (MAO) inhibitors and sympathomimetic drugs also contributes to the effects of hypertension.

Administering the Medication

Box 59.1 lists general nursing guidelines for the administration of ophthalmic medications. Patients should take phenylephrine for no longer than 72 hours. To administer the ophthalmic solution, the nurse has the patient lie down with the head tilted back. Then the nurse takes the following steps:

- Hold the dropper above the eye and drop the medication inside the lower lid, without touching the dropper to the eye
- Has the patient keep the eye open and avoid blinking for 30 seconds
- Applies pressure to the inside corner of the eye for 1 minute

Assessing for Therapeutic and Adverse Effects

The nurse assesses whether the inner aspect of the eye can be visualized 15 minutes after administration.

The nurse measures the blood pressure and the heart rate and checks for hypertension and dysrhythmia. The nurse also asks the patient about visual floaters. In addition, it is necessary to assess for burning and irritation of the eye.

Patient Teaching

Box 59.2 presents patient teaching guidelines for topical ophthalmics, including phenylephrine.

NCLEX Success

3. The nurse instructs a patient on the procedure to occlude the tear ducts for 5 minutes after administering eyedrops. What is the purpose of this patient teaching?
   A. It prevents eye infections.
   B. It prevents systemic absorption of the medication.
   C. It makes self-administration easier.
   D. It allows for the administration of a smaller dose.

LOCAL ANESTHETIC DRUGS

P **Lidocaine** (Akten) is the prototype local anesthetic drug for ophthalmic use.

Pharmacokinetics and Action

The onset of action of lidocaine is 20 seconds to 5 minutes, with a median onset of 40 seconds. The duration of action is 5 to 30 minutes, with a median of 15 minutes.

Lidocaine blocks the initiation and conduction of nerve impulses. It decreases the neuronal membrane's permeability to sodium ions, resulting in an inhibition of depolarization and blocking of conduction.

Use

Lidocaine produces local anesthesia of the ocular surface during ophthalmic procedures such as surgery, tonometry, and gonioscopy. Table 59.2 presents route and dosage information for lidocaine and other ophthalmic local anesthetics.

Patient-related variables specific to the use of lidocaine include reproduction, pregnancy, and lactation. No adverse effects have been observed in animal reproduction studies. In patients who are breast-feeding, no systemic exposure has been shown with ophthalmic lidocaine.

Adverse Effects

Local adverse effects of lidocaine include burning. Specific ocular effects include conjunctival hyperemia, corneal epithelial changes, diplopia, and changes in vision.

Nursing Implications

Administering the Medication

It is important not to administer solution if it is crystallized. The nurse is certain not to touch the eye with the tip of the applicator.

Assessing for Therapeutic and Adverse Effects

The physician performing the procedure assesses for adequate anesthesia. The nurse may assess for opacity of the lens and loss of vision with prolonged use.

DRUG THERAPY FOR THE TREATMENT OF GLAUCOMA

At present, the goal of drug therapy for chronic open-angle glaucoma is to slow disease progression by reducing IOP. For monotherapy, the prostaglandin analogs and beta-adrenergic blockers are first-line drugs. The prostaglandin analogs may be preferred because they are generally more effective at lowering IOP, show a better tolerated adverse effect profile than nonselective drugs, and offer a once-daily dosing regimen. Older drug classes, including the beta-adrenergic blockers, alpha agonists, and carbonic anhydrase inhibitors, lower IOP by decreasing the production of aqueous humor. These drugs are commonly used either alone or in combination for the treatment of chronic open-angle glaucoma and are outlined in Table 59.3.

PROSTAGLANDIN ANALOGS

The prostaglandin analogs are the most widely prescribed glaucoma drugs, and lower IOP by increasing the aqueous drainage by a mechanism of action different from other drugs, namely, by increasing the uveoscleral outflow; aqueous inflow is not affected. Of the prostaglandin analogs, **bimatoprost** (Durysta, Latisse, Lumigan) is the prototype. Bimatoprost is classified as a prostamide, whereas latanoprost, travoprost, and tafluprost are prostanoids.

Pharmacokinetics

The onset of action of bimatoprost is approximately 4 hours, with maximum reduction of IOP in 8 to 12 hours. It is 88% protein bound and undergoes oxidation, *N*-deethylation, and glucuronidation after reaching systemic circulation to form metabolites. Excretion is primarily in the urine, with 25% excreted in the feces.

Action

Bimatoprost produces ocular hypotensive effects to decrease IOP and to increase outflow of aqueous humor. (Latisse formulation can also increase the percent and duration of hairs in the growth phase to increase eyelash growth.)

Use

In patients with open-angle glaucoma and ocular hypertension, healthcare providers use bimatoprost to reduce IOP. Treatment of hypotrichosis of the eyelashes is another use. Table 59.4 contains route and dosage information for bimatoprost and other prostaglandin analogs.

Patient-related variables specific to the use of bimatoprost include reproduction, pregnancy, and lactation. Ophthalmic prostaglandins such as bimatoprost have an increased risk of miscarriage and major congenital anomalies.

Adverse Effects and Contraindications

Ocular adverse effects of bimatoprost include iris and eyelid hyperpigmentation and eyelash changes. Use of the Latisse formulation may result in erythema of the eyelid, allergic conjunctivitis, blepharitis, burning, cataract formation, conjunctival edema, pain, photophobia, tearing, and visual disturbances.

Contraindications include hypersensitivity.

TABLE 59.3

Drugs Administered for the Treatment of Open-Angle Glaucoma

Drug Class	Prototype	Other Drugs in the Class
Prostaglandin analogs	Bimatoprost (Durysta, Latisse, Lumigan)	Latanoprost (Xelpros, Xalatan) Tafluprost (Zioptan) Travoprost (Travatan Z) Latanaprostene bunod
Beta-adrenergic blocking drugs	Timolol maleate (Betamol, Istalol, Timoptic, Timoptic Ocudose, Timoptic-XE)	Betaxolol (Betoptic S) Carteolol Levobunolol Metipranolol
Alpha$_2$-adrenergic agonists	Brimonidine (Alphagan P, Lumify)	Apraclonidine hydrochloride (Iopidine)
Cholinergic drugs	Pilocarpine (Isopto Carpine) Pilocarpine Ocular System (Ocusert Pilo-20 or Pilo-40)	
Carbonic anhydrase inhibitors	Acetazolamide	Brinzolamide (Azopt) Dorzolamide (Trusopt)
Combination Medications for the Treatment of Open-Angle Glaucoma		Brimonidine and timolol (Combigan) Brinzolamide and Brimonidine (Simbrinza) Dorzolamide and timolol (Cosopt, Cosopt PF) Netarsudil and latanoprost (Rocklatan)
Osmotic drugs	Mannitol (Osmitrol)	

TABLE 59.4

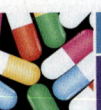

DRUGS AT A GLANCE: Antiglaucoma Drugs

Drug	Routes and Dosage Ranges	
	Adults	**Children**
Prostaglandin Analogs		
ⓟ **Bimatoprost** (Durysta, Latisse, Lumigan; 🍁 Latisse, Lumigan RC, Vistitan)	Glaucoma: 1 drop at bedtime Hypotrichosis of eyelashes: 1 drop on applicator applied evenly along the skin of the upper eyelid at the base of the eyelashes at bedtime	≥16 y: IOP reduction (Lumigan), refer to adult dosage. Not recommended under age of 16 due to hyperpigmentation ≥5 y, hypotrichosis of eyelashes (Latisse). Same as adult dosage
Latanoprost (Xalatan, Xelpros; 🍁 APO Latanoprost, GD Latanoprost, JAMP Latanoprost, MED-Latanoprost, Xalatan)	Elevated IOP: 1 drop at bedtime Elevated IOP: 1 drop into affected eye in the evening	1 drop in the affected eye every evening >16 years refer to adult dosage
Latanoprostene bunod (Vyzulta)		
Tafluprost (Zioptan)	Elevated IOP: 1 drop at bedtime	Safety and efficacy not established
Travoprost (Travatan Z; 🍁 APO-Travoprost, Sandoz-Travoprost, Travatan Z)	Elevated IOP: 1 drop at bedtime	Children ≥2 months limited data; 1 drop into the affected eye in the evening ≥16 y: elevated IOP: refer to adult dosage.
Beta-Adrenergic Blocking Drugs		
ⓟ **Timolol maleate** (Betamol, Istalol, Timolol Maleate Ocudose, Timoptic, Timoptic Ocudose, Timoptic-XE; 🍁 APO-Timop, SANDOZ-Timolol, Timoptic, Timoptic-XE)	Solution, 1 drop of 0.25% solution twice daily; mat increase to 1 drop of 0.5% solution twice daily if response inadequate Gel, 1 drop of 0.25% or 0.5% solution once daily	Same as for adults
Betaxolol (Betoptic S; 🍁 Betoptic S)	Solution and suspension, 1 or 2 drops twice daily	Suspension, 1 drop twice daily
Carteolol	1 drop twice daily	Safety and efficacy not established
Levobunolol (🍁 APO-Levobunolol, Betagen)	1 or 2 drops of 0.25% solution twice daily; 1 or 2 drops of 0.5% solution once daily (doses >1 drop of 0.5% solution twice daily are generally not more effective)	Safety and efficacy not established
Metipranolol	Glaucoma, 1 drop twice daily	Safety and efficacy not established
Alpha₂-Adrenergic Agonists		
ⓟ **Brimonidine** (Alphagan P, Lumify; 🍁 Alphagan P, Brimonidine P)	1 drop 3 times daily, every 8 h	≥2 y: same as for adults
Apraclonidine hydrochloride (Iopidine; 🍁 Iopidine)	Open-angle glaucoma: 1 drop 0.5% solution every 12 h Intraoperative and postoperative increased IOP: 1–2 drops of 1% solution 1 h before surgery and immediately after surgery	Safety and efficacy not established
Cholinergic Drugs		
ⓟ **Pilocarpine** (🍁 Isopto Carpine, Odan-Pilocarpine)	Elevated IOP: 1 drop of 1% or 2% solution up to 4 times daily Glaucoma: 1 drop of 1% or 2% solution up to 3 times over a 30-min period Miosis: 1 drop (or 2 drops 5 min apart)	<2 y: 1 drop of 1% solution up to 3 times daily ≥2 y: same as for adults
Pilocarpine Ocular System (Ocusert Pilo-20 or Pilo-40)	Miosis: one system in conjunctival sac per week	Same as for adults
Rho Kinase Inhibitor		
Netarsudil (Rhopressa)	Increased IOP; Instill 1 drop into affected eye(s) each pm	

TABLE 59.4

DRUGS AT A GLANCE: Antiglaucoma Drugs (Continued)

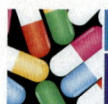

Drug	Routes and Dosage Ranges	
	Adults	**Children**
Carbonic Anhydrase Inhibitors		
Ⓟ Acetazolamide	Glaucoma: 250 mg PO 1–4 times daily; preoperatively: 5–10 mg/kg/d IV, IM in divided doses, every 6 h	<12 y, glaucoma: 10–30 mg/kg/d PO divided every 6–8 h (max 1,000 mg/d); preoperatively: 5–10 mg/kg IV every 6 h
Brinzolamide (Azopt; 🍁 Azopt)	IOP reduction: 1 drop 3 times daily	Safety and efficacy not established
Dorzolamide (Trusopt; 🍁 APO-Dorzolamide, JAMP-Dorzolamide, RIVA-Dorzolamide, Trusopt, SANDOZ-Dorzolamide)	IOP reduction: 1 drop 3 times daily	Same as adults
Combination Medications for the Treatment of Open-Angle Glaucoma		
Brimonidine and timolol (Combigan; Combigan)	IOP: 1 drop in each eye(s) every 12 h	
Brinzolamide and brimonidine (Simbrinza; 🍁 Simbrinza)	IOP: 1 drop in each eye(s) 2–3 times per day	
Dorzolamide and timolol (Cosopt, Cosopt PF; 🍁 ACT Dorzotimolol, APO-Dorzo-Timop)	IOP: 1 drop in each eye(s) twice daily	
Netarsudil and latanoprost (Rocklatan)	IOP: 1 drop in each eye(s) every evening	
Osmotic Drugs		
Ⓟ Mannitol (Osmitrol; 🍁 Osmitrol, Resectisol)	IOP reduction: 1.5–2 g/kg as a 20% solution over 45 min twice daily for IOP > 35 mm Hg	Infants, children, adolescents: 1–2 mg IV over 20–30 min

IOP, intraocular pressure.

Nursing Implications

Preventing Interactions

Latanoprost combined with nonsteroidal anti-inflammatory drugs (NSAIDs) may increase intraocular pressure.

Administering the Medication

When applying Latisse to the eyelid, patients who are wearing contacts should remove them; in addition, it is necessary to remove makeup and wash the face thoroughly with soap and water. Patients should apply the medication with a sterile applicator and use a new applicator for each eye. It is important that contacts not be reinserted for 15 minutes.

Assessing for Therapeutic and Adverse Effects

It is important to assess IOP. In patients taking the medication for hypertrichosis of the eyelashes, the nurse assesses for increased growth of eyelashes.

The nurse assesses for ocular changes, including pruritus, blepharitis, and visual disturbances.

Patient Teaching

The nurse instructs the patient about the importance of keeping regularly scheduled medical appointments to check IOP. Box 59.2 contains additional patient teaching information.

Other Drugs in the Class

Other prostaglandin analogs include latanoprost (Xalatan), latanoprostene bunod (Vyzulta), travoprost (Travatan Z), and tafluprost (Zioptan). Like bimatoprost, they act to lower IOP. Tafluprost is the only topical prostaglandin analog that does not contain the widely used preservative, benzalkonium chloride.

> **❗ Quality and Safety Alert: Evidence-Based Practice**
>
> Medications for the treatment of open-angle glaucoma are often very expensive. Delavar et al. (2022) conducted a research study of patients enrolled in the National Institutes of Health All of Us Research Program. The research study was conducted to determine how race and ethnicity affect the ability to pay for glaucoma medications among patients with glaucoma. Participants included 3,826 patients with glaucoma, of whom 481 were African American, 119 were non-Hispanic Asian, 351 were Hispanic, and 2,875 were non-Hispanic White. Non-Hispanic African American and Hispanic individuals were more likely than non-Hispanic White individuals to report an inability to afford glaucoma medications. In addition, non-Hispanic White individuals were equally as likely to ask for low-cost medication from their prescribers as were those of racial and ethnic minority groups. In conclusion, clinicians should be proactive and discuss the cost of medications to promote better medication adherence and health equity among patients diagnosed with glaucoma.

BETA-ADRENERGIC BLOCKING DRUGS

The purpose of the administration of beta-adrenergic blocking drugs is to decrease the IOP. Although the prototype medication in this class is propranolol (see Chapter 26), it is not formulated in an ophthalmic preparation. The drug **timolol maleate** (Betamol, Istalol, Timolol Maleate Ocudose, Timoptic, Timoptic Maleate-EX, Timoptic-XE) was the first drug developed in this class for the treatment of open-angle glaucoma.

Pharmacokinetics and Action

The onset of action of timolol is 30 minutes, with a peak action in 1 to 2 hours. The duration of action for intraocular effects is 24 hours.

Timolol blocks the $beta_1$- and $beta_2$-adrenergic receptors to reduce the IOP by reducing aqueous humor production and increasing outflow.

Use

Uses for timolol include chronic open-angle glaucoma, aphakic glaucoma, secondary glaucoma, and ocular hypertension. Table 59.4 presents route and dosage information for timolol and other beta-adrenergic blocking drugs.

Patient-related variables specific to the use of timolol include reproduction, pregnancy, and lactation. Decreased fetal heart rate has been noted with maternal use of timolol during pregnancy. If timolol is needed to treat glaucoma during pregnancy, the minimum effective dose should be used in combination with punctal occlusion to decrease fetal exposure. Punctal occlusion is accomplished by closing off the small funnel-like drain hole at the inner canthus of the eye. The minimum effective doses should be administered with breast-feeding. Due to the cardiorespiratory problems that can result in breast-fed infants, they should be monitored for the adverse effects of timolol. It is important to apply punctal occlusion with the instillation of timolol eyedrops. The manufacturer recommends breast-feeding be discontinued with the use of timolol; the prescriber must take into account the importance of treatment to the mother.

Adverse Effects and Contraindications

The most common adverse effects associated with timolol are burning and stinging. Most adverse effects of systemic beta-adrenergic blockers may also occur with ophthalmic preparations, and patients with respiratory or cardiac disease may not be able to take them.

Contraindications include asthma and chronic obstructive pulmonary disease, as well as heart failure, bradycardia, atrioventricular block, left ventricular dysfunction, and cardiogenic shock. Known hypersensitivity to timolol is also a contraindication.

Nursing Implications

Preventing Interactions

Box 59.3 lists the drug interactions with timolol. Garlic, ginger, ginseng, goldenseal, and nettle will increase the effects of timolol.

BOX 59.3 Drug Interactions: Timolol

Drugs That Increase the Effect of Timolol
- Amifostine, amiodarone, antihypertensives, beta-adrenergic blockers, calcium channel blockers, cardiac glycosides, monoamine oxidase inhibitors, reserpine
  Increase hypotensive and bradycardic effects

Administering the Medication

Administration of the ophthalmic form of timolol necessitates the following:

- Have patients who wear contact lenses remove the lenses prior to administration.
- When administering more than one ophthalmic medication, wait 10 minutes between each medication.
- Use good hand hygiene before administering ophthalmic drugs.
- Always invert the bottle of timolol and shake it before use.
- Have the patient tilt the head back. Use the index finger of one hand to pull the lower lid down to form a pocket for the eyedrop. Place the dispenser tip close to the eye and gently squeeze the bottle to administer one drop.
- Have patients who wear contact lenses wait 15 minutes before inserting them. The product can contain benzalkonium chloride, which can be absorbed into the soft contact lens.

Assessing for Therapeutic and Adverse Effects

The nurse helps ensure that the patient keeps regularly scheduled appointments with the ophthalmologist to assess the IOP. In addition, the nurse asks the patient about stinging and burning of the eyes.

Patient Teaching

Box 59.2 contains additional patient teaching information for topical ophthalmic medications, including timolol.

Clinical Application 59.2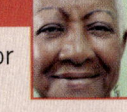

- Mrs. Molnar has received prescriptions for timolol and pilocarpine eyedrops. What patient teaching regarding these medications should the nurse provide?
- What is the action of timolol?

ALPHA$_2$-ADRENERGIC AGONISTS

Alpha$_2$-adrenergic agonists are administered when a patient's IOP is not lowered adequately with a beta-adrenergic blocker or when a beta-adrenergic blocker is contraindicated. **Brimonidine** (Alphagan P, Lumify) is the prototype. Practitioners, who consider this group of medications to be as effective as timolol, use it in conjunction with other antiglaucoma drugs such as beta-adrenergic blockers or carbonic anhydrase inhibitors when multiple drugs are required.

Pharmacokinetics and Action

Brimonidine has a rapid onset of action, with a half-life of 2 hours. Extensive metabolism occurs in the liver. The drug reduces aqueous humor production and increases uveoscleral outflow.

Use

Brimonidine is used to lower IOP in patients with open-angle glaucoma or ocular hypertension. It has also been approved for the relief of ocular redness. Table 59.4 presents route and dosage information for brimonidine and the other alpha$_2$-adrenergic agonists.

Patient-related variables specific to the use of brimonidine include the following:

- Age
  - Administration to children can result in a higher risk of adverse effects. Children are at greatest risk of CNS depression from brimonidine, with somnolence and diminished alertness.
- Reproduction, pregnancy, and lactation:
  - Teratogenic effects have not been observed in animal reproduction studies.
  - It is unknown if brimonidine is present in breast milk.

Adverse Effects

Several adverse effects may occur with brimonidine use. Cardiovascular effects include hypertension, bradycardia, hypotension, and tachycardia. CNS effects include headache, dizziness, somnolence, diminished attention and alertness, and insomnia. Respiratory effects are bronchitis, cough, dyspnea, sinusitis, nasal dryness, and apnea. Local reactions such as stinging and burning of the eye may occur. Other ocular effects are blepharitis, conjunctival edema, conjunctival hemorrhage, dryness, irritation, and eye pain. In addition, allergic conjunctivitis, hyperemia, and pruritus affect approximately 10% to 20% of patients.

Contraindications

Contraindications to brimonidine include known hypersensitivity to the drug or use within 14 days of an MAO inhibitor. Caution is warranted in patients with advanced cardiovascular disease.

Nursing Implications

Preventing Interactions

Box 59.4 lists the medications that interact with brimonidine. Bayberry, blue cohosh, cayenne, ephedra, ginger, ginseng, and licorice will increase the effects of brimonidine. Black cohosh, California poppy, coleus, goldenseal, hawthorne, and mistletoe will decrease the effects of brimonidine.

Administering the Medication

Box 59.1 lists general guidelines for the administration of topical ophthalmic medications.

BOX 59.4 *Drug Interactions: Brimonidine*

Drugs That Increase the Effects of Brimonidine
- Hypotensive drugs, monoamine oxidase inhibitors
  Increase hypotensive effects
- Hydroxyzine, selective serotonin reuptake inhibitors, central nervous system (CNS) depressants
  Increase CNS depression

Assessing for Therapeutic and Adverse Effects

It is necessary to assess the IOP.

The nurse monitors the blood pressure and assesses for hypertension and hypotension; the nurse also checks the heart rate and monitors for bradycardia or tachycardia. The nurse assesses the CNS for depressive effects such as dizziness, somnolence, and diminished alertness. In addition, the nurse assesses the respiratory status for cough and dyspnea and checks for nasal dryness, sinus infection, and sinusitis. It is necessary to assess for hypersensitivity reactions as well.

Patient Teaching

The nurse ensures that the patient keeps regularly scheduled appointments with the ophthalmologist to assess the IOP. Box 59.2 contains additional patient teaching information for the topical ophthalmic medications, including brimonidine.

CHOLINERGIC DRUGS

Ophthalmic cholinergic drugs increase the outflow of aqueous humor to reduce IOP. The prototype of this class is **P** **pilocarpine** (Vuity), which is administered for glaucoma and as a miotic drug.

Pharmacokinetics and Action

Following administration of pilocarpine, miosis begins in 10 to 30 minutes, with reduction in IOP in 1 hour. The miotic duration of action is 4 to 8 hours. Metabolism occurs in the liver.

Pilocarpine stimulates the cholinergic receptors in the eye, causing miosis, loss of accommodation, and lowering of the IOP.

Use

Pilocarpine is used for chronic simple glaucoma as well as for chronic and acute angle-closure glaucoma. Table 59.4 gives route and dosage information for pilocarpine.

Patient-related variables specific to the use of pilocarpine include reproduction, pregnancy, and lactation. Animal reproduction studies have not been conducted. It is unknown if pilocarpine is excreted in breast milk.

Adverse Effects

Several adverse effects may occur with pilocarpine. Ocular conditions include burning, ciliary spasm, conjunctival vascular congestion, lacrimation, lens opacity, retinal detachment, myopia, and diminished visual acuity. CNS problems may include headache. Cardiopulmonary manifestations are hypertension, tachycardia, bronchial spasm, and pulmonary edema. Gastrointestinal (GI) effects include nausea, vomiting, diarrhea, and increased salivation.

Contraindications

Contraindications include known hypersensitivity to the drug or acute inflammation of the anterior chamber of the eye.

Nursing Implications

Preventing Interactions

Acetylcholinesterase inhibitors may enhance the adverse effects of pilocarpine.

Administering the Medication

If the solution and gel have been prescribed together, it is necessary to administer the solution first and then give the gel 5 minutes later. Following the administration of the solution, the nurse or patient should provide pressure on the lacrimal sac for 1 to 2 minutes. Box 59.1 lists general guidelines for the administration of topical ophthalmic medications.

Assessing for Therapeutic and Adverse Effects

It is necessary to check the IOP.

The nurse assesses for ocular burning, lens opacity, diminished visual acuity, and headache over the affected eye. The nurse monitors the patient's blood pressure and heart rate and assesses for signs of hypertension and tachycardia. The nurse also assesses for bronchial spasm and pulmonary edema as well as for nausea, vomiting, diarrhea, and increased salivation.

Patient Teaching

The nurse helps ensure that the patient keeps regularly scheduled appointments with the ophthalmologist to assess the IOP. Box 59.2 provides patient teaching information for pilocarpine.

RHO KINASE INHIBITOR

Netarsudil (Rhopressa) was approved by the FDA in 2017.

Action and Use

Netarsudil (Rhopressa) is a rho kinase inhibitor. The exact action is unknown, but it may reduce IOP by increasing the outflow of aqueous humor through the trabecular meshwork. It is used to lower IOP in patients with open angle or ocular hypertension.

Patient-related variables specific to the use of netarsudil include reproduction, pregnancy, and lactation. Adverse effects have not been observed in animal reproduction studies. It is unknown whether netarsudil enters the breast milk.

Adverse Effects and Contraindications

The adverse effects of netarsudil include conjunctival hyperemia, conjunctival hemorrhage, and corneal deposits. The patient may experience erythema of the eye, blurred vision, decreased visual acuity, increased lacrimation, and corneal staining. There are no contraindications noted with netarsudil.

Nursing Implications

Preventing Interactions

There are no reported drug or herbal interactions with netarsudil.

Administering the Medication

If administering netarsudil with additional eye medications, wait at least 5 minutes between medication applications. Remove contact lenses prior to administration and wait at least 15 minutes after administration to reinsert contact lenses. Avoid touching the eye dropper tip with the fingers, eyelid, or surrounding eye areas.

Assessing for Therapeutic and Adverse Effects

The nurse helps to ensure that the patient keeps regularly scheduled appointments with the ophthalmologist to assess IOP. The nurse should assess the eye for redness or erythema. Any changes in vision should be reported to the prescriber.

Patient Teaching

Box 59.2 contains patient teaching information for topical ophthalmic medications, including netarsudil.

NCLEX Success

4. A patient with Parkinson disease is taking selegiline hydrochloride. The patient receives a diagnosis of increased IOP and the ophthalmologist prescribes brimonidine drops. What recommendation does the nurse make to the prescriber?
   A. Stop the selegiline hydrochloride for 2 weeks before starting the brimonidine.
   B. Suggest that because administration of brimonidine increases blood pressure, another alpha$_2$-adrenergic agonist should be prescribed.
   C. Ask the prescriber whether levobunolol would be more stable and cause fewer adverse effects.
   D. Increase the selegiline hydrochloride to prevent the increase in Parkinson-related symptoms.

CARBONIC ANHYDRASE INHIBITORS

P **Acetazolamide**, the prototype ocular carbonic anhydrase inhibitor, is an oral drug. Prescribers use it for the management of glaucoma.

Pharmacokinetics and Action

Oral acetazolamide has an onset of action in 1 hour. Absorption occurs in the GI tract. Intravenous (IV) administration has an onset of action of 15 minutes. Distribution takes place throughout the body, concentrating in the red blood cells, plasma, and kidneys. Elimination is in the urine.

Acetazolamide inhibits carbonic anhydrase in the eye to reduce the rate of aqueous humor formation and lower the IOP.

Use

Uses for acetazolamide include open-angle glaucoma and secondary glaucoma. Practitioners also use it preoperatively for the treatment of acute closed-angle glaucoma. Table 59.4 presents route and dosage information for acetazolamide and other carbonic anhydrase inhibitors.

Patient-related variables specific to the use of acetazolamide include the following:

- Age:
  - Growth retardation has been reported in children receiving acetazolamide and antiseizure medications (Chapter 53).
  - In older adults, it is important to start acetazolamide at the low end of the dosing range because of age-related decreases in hepatic, kidney, and cardiac function and concomitant disease and polypharmacy.
  - Older adults with diabetes or kidney impairment have an increased risk of metabolic acidosis when prescribed acetazolamide.
- Reproduction, pregnancy, and lactation:
  - There are limited data on the effects of acetazolamide during pregnancy.
  - Acetazolamide is present in breast milk.
- Abnormal kidney function and hepatic impairment:
  - Acetazolamide should not be administered to patients with severe abnormal kidney function.

Adverse Effects

The major adverse effects associated with acetazolamide are Stevens–Johnson syndrome, flaccid paralysis, agranulocytosis, hemolytic anemia, aplastic anemia, leukopenia, pancytopenia, and metabolic acidosis.

Contraindications

Contraindications to acetazolamide include known hypersensitivity to carbonic anhydrase inhibitors, kidney and hepatic disease, and Addison disease, as well as electrolyte imbalance. Caution is necessary in older adults. Specialists do not recommend the drug for the treatment of chronic noncongestive angle-closure glaucoma.

Nursing Implications

Preventing Interactions

The medications that interact with acetazolamide are listed in Box 59.5. The use of garlic, ginger, ginseng, goldenseal, or nettle will increase the effects of acetazolamide.

Administering the Medication

To reduce GI upset, it is necessary to administer acetazolamide with food or meals. Patients should not crush or chew sustained-release preparations.

> **BOX 59.5 Drug Interactions: Acetazolamide**
>
> **Drugs That Increase the Effect of Acetazolamide**
> - Alcohol, central nervous system (CNS) depressants, droperidol, hydroxyzine, selective serotonin reuptake inhibitors
>   *Enhance CNS depression*
> - Alfuzosin, amifostine, antihypertensives, diazoxide, pentoxifylline, phosphodiesterase five inhibitors (sildenafil), prostacyclin analogs (treprostinil)
>   *Enhance antihypertensive effects*
> - Salicylates
>   *Act by unknown mechanism*

Assessing Therapeutic and Adverse Effects

It is necessary to assess the IOP.

The nurse assesses the patient's skin for signs of redness, blisters, or swelling that may indicate Stevens–Johnson syndrome. In addition, the nurse checks the complete blood count for signs of anemia and the electrolytes for signs of acidosis.

Patient Teaching

The nurse helps ensure that the patient keeps regularly scheduled appointments with the ophthalmologist to assess the IOP. Box 59.6 presents patient teaching guidelines for acetazolamide.

Other Drugs in the Class

Brinzolamide (Azopt) reduces IOP in patients with ocular hypertension or open-angle glaucoma. The drug is contraindicated in patients with a known hypersensitivity to brinzolamide, sulfonamides, or any component of the formulation. It reaches peak effect in 2 hours and has an 8- to 12-hour duration of action. It can be absorbed in the systemic circulation and accumulates in the red blood cells. It is excreted unchanged in the urine.

Dorzolamide hydrochloride (Trusopt) is a carbonic anhydrase inhibitor administered for increased IOP or open-angle glaucoma. One drop is inserted into each eye three times per day. It decreases the aqueous humor secretion by slowing bicarbonate ions to reduce sodium and fluid transport, thus reducing IOP. Adverse reactions are bitter taste, ocular burning and stinging, photophobia, and superficial punctuate keratitis.

> **BOX 59.6 Patient Teaching Guidelines for Acetazolamide**
>
> - Maintain regularly scheduled medical appointments to monitor laboratory values and IOP.
> - Maintain a fluid intake of 1.5 to 2.5 L per 24 hours as well as a diet high in potassium. Good sources of potassium are milk and other dairy products, meat, poultry, fish, eggs, and nuts.
> - Report numbness, tingling, burning, drowsiness, and visual disturbances to the prescriber.

COMBINATION MEDICATIONS FOR OPEN-ANGLE GLAUCOMA

Currently, several combination drug products have been developed for the treatment of open-angle glaucoma. It is important to understand the action, adverse effects, contraindications, and nursing implications for each drug combination. Several combination products are briefly introduced below; however, it is important to review the in-depth information on each drug presented previously in the chapter.

Brimonidine and timolol (Combigan) is an alpha$_2$ agonist and beta blocker. It is administered every 12 hours. Brimonidine reduces the aqueous humor and increases uveoscleral outflow. Timolol blocks beta$_1$- and beta$_2$-adrenergic receptors to reduce intraocular pressure and aqueous humor production. The adverse ocular effects of this combination medication are allergic conjunctivitis, conjunctival hyperemia, and eye pruritus.

Brinzolamide and brimonidine (Simbrinza) is an anti-glaucoma medication that combines an alpha$_2$ agonist and carbonic anhydrase inhibitor ophthalmic agent. The action of brinzolamide inhibits carbonic anhydrase, leading to a decrease in aqueous humor secretion. Brimonidine is the alpha$_2$-adrenergic receptor agonist that reduces aqueous humor formation and increases uveoscleral outflow. The combination of two agents enhances the ability to reduce IOP better than with one agent alone. Hypersensitivity reactions of the eye have been noted, along with blurred vision and eye irritation.

Dorzolamide and timolol (Cosopt, Cosopt PF) is a beta blocker and non-selective carbonic anhydrase inhibitor. The inhibition of carbonic anhydrase in the ciliary process of the eye decreases the bicarbonate ion formation to decrease sodium and fluid and decrease aqueous humor. Timolol is a beta blocker that reduces aqueous humor promoting the outflow of fluid.

Netarsudil and latanoprost (Rocklatan) combine a prostaglandin and rho kinase inhibitor. The exact action of these medications is not specifically known, but it is suspected that they increase the outflow of aqueous humor. This formulation is known to cause ocular inflammation. It should be used with caution in patients with a history of iritis or uveitis.

OSMOTIC DRUGS

Osmotic diuretics are used to reduce IOP when the pressure cannot be lowered by other means. The drugs in this class are especially useful for treating acute episodes of angle-closure, absolute, or secondary glaucoma and for lowering IOP prior to intraocular surgery. Chapter 34 provides additional information on the prototype osmotic diuretic **mannitol** (Osmitrol), which is discussed in this section as it relates to reducing IOP.

Pharmacokinetics and Action

After IV administration of mannitol, absorption is immediate, and the drug begins to work in 15 to 30 minutes. When used preoperatively to reduce IOP, administration 60 to 90 minutes prior to surgery allows the drug to reach its peak of action to achieve maximum IOP reduction. The drug's half-life is approximately 1 to 1.6 hours. Excretion is primarily as unchanged drug in the urine. Mannitol reduces the IOP by creating an osmotic gradient in between the plasma and ocular fields.

Use

Mannitol temporarily reduces IOP in acute attacks of glaucoma. Prescribers also order it for reduction of IOP prior to surgery. Table 59.4 contains route and dosage information for mannitol.

Patient-related variables specific to the use of mannitol include the following:

- Age:
  - In pediatric patients, mannitol may increase cerebral blood flow, increasing the risk of postoperative bleeding in neurosurgical patients and thus worsening intracranial hypertension.
  - In older adults, it is important to start mannitol at the low end of the dosing range because of age-related decreases in hepatic, kidney, and cardiac function and concomitant disease and polypharmacy.
- Reproduction, pregnancy, and lactation:
  - Mannitol crosses the placenta.
  - It is not known if mannitol is present in breast milk.
- Abnormal kidney function and hepatic impairment:
  - Mannitol is contraindicated in severe abnormal kidney function.

Adverse Effects and Contraindications

Adverse effects of mannitol relate to decreased fluid volume. The most serious of these conditions is hyperosmolar nonketotic coma. Other adverse effects include confusion, headache, syncope, cardiac dysrhythmias, nausea, vomiting, and severe dehydration.

Contraindications include severe dehydration, abdominal pain, appendicitis, pulmonary edema, and severe cardiac decompensation.

Nursing Implications

Assessing for Therapeutic and Adverse Effects

It is important to check for therapeutic effects, indicated by a reduction in IOP. In addition, the nurse checks fluid and electrolytes and assesses for signs and symptoms of dehydration. Blood pressure, pulse, and respirations are monitored. The nurse assesses for hyperglycemia, adventitious breath sounds, and pupillary reflexes. It is also necessary to assess for hypersensitivity to mannitol.

> **Quality and Safety Alert: Safety**
>
> If extravasation occurs at the injection site, stop the infusion of mannitol and leave the IV cannula in place. Aspirate the IV line gently, and initiate the antidote, hyaluronidase, as per the institutional protocol.

Patient Teaching

The nurse instructs the patient about the importance of keeping regularly scheduled medical appointments to check IOP. In addition, the nurse reminds the patient to report severe headache, chest pain, confusion, rapid respirations, and violent diarrhea to his or her prescriber. Box 59.2 contains additional patient teaching information for the ophthalmologic medications.

NCLEX Success

5. A 14-year-old student visits the school nurse's office. The student wants longer eyelashes after watching a commercial for Latisse. What information should the school nurse provide the student regarding this form of bimatoprost?
   A. "This medication is only given to patients with glaucoma."
   B. "This medication is not recommended for anyone under the age of 16."
   C. "You do not need this medication—your eyelashes are long enough."
   D. "You should talk to your guidance counselor about ways to build your self-esteem."

DRUG THERAPY FOR OCULAR INFECTIONS AND INFLAMMATION

Previous chapters have presented information about the medications administered to treat viral, fungal, and bacterial infections and the inflammation that often accompanies an infection. This section of the chapter addresses the anti-infective medications administered for the treatment of ocular infections and the anti-inflammatory drugs used to decrease inflammation.

The nonsteroidal anti-inflammatory drugs (NSAIDs) and corticosteroids are administered to decrease the inflammatory response. Table 59.5 lists the drugs administered to treat ocular infections and to reduce ocular inflammation.

ANTIBACTERIAL DRUGS

Various antibacterial drugs have ophthalmic uses. The most common prescribed drug is the prototype fluoroquinolone **ⓟ ciprofloxacin** (Ciloxan).

Pharmacokinetics and Action

The amount of ciprofloxacin absorbed by the body is so small that its pharmacokinetic properties are inconsequential. Ciprofloxacin ophthalmic inhibits DNA gyrase and the relaxation of supercoiled DNA, which promotes breakage of double-stranded DNA in the target bacteria.

Use

Uses of ciprofloxacin include the treatment of corneal ulcer and bacterial conjunctivitis. It is essential that contact lenses not be worn during drug therapy. Table 59.6 presents route and dosage information about ciprofloxacin and other antibacterial ophthalmic drugs.

Patient-related variables specific to the use of ciprofloxacin include reproduction, pregnancy, and lactation. The amount

TABLE 59.5

Drugs Administered for the Treatment of Ocular Infections and Inflammation

Drug Class	Prototype	Other Drugs in the Class
Antibacterial drugs	Ciprofloxacin ophthalmic (Ciloxan)	Erythromycin 5% ointment Gatifloxacin (Zymaxid) Gentamicin 3 mg/mL solution or 3 mg/g ointment (Gentak) Levofloxacin 5 mg/mL solution Moxifloxacin (Vigamox) Ofloxacin (Ocuflox) Sulfacetam Tobramycin (0.3% solution and 3 mg/g ointment) (Tobrex)
Antiviral drugs	Trifluridine 1% solution	Ganciclovir (Zirgan)
Antifungal drugs	Natamycin 5% suspension (Natacyn)	
Antiallergic drugs	Cromolyn	Lodoxamide (Alomide)
H_1-receptor antagonists: second generation	Emedastine difumarate	Azelastine Epinastine (Elestat) Ketotifen (Alaway Children's Allergy, Claritin Eye, Zaditor) Olopatadine (Pataday, Pazeo)
Corticosteroids	Dexamethasone (Dextenza, Dexycu, Maxidex, Ozurdex)	Fluorometholone (Flarex, FML, Liquifilm) Loteprednol (Alrex) Prednisolone (Pred Forte) Rimexolone
Anti-inflammatory drugs	Diclofenac	Flurbiprofen (Ocufen) Ketorolac (Acular, Acuvail)
Immunosuppressants	Cyclosporine emulsion (Cequa, Restasis, Restasis MultiDose, Verkazia)	

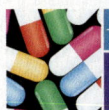

TABLE 59.6

DRUGS AT A GLANCE: Antimicrobial Drugs

Drug	Routes and Dosage Ranges	
	Adults	**Children**
Antibacterial Drugs		
Ⓟ **Ciprofloxacin** Ophthalmic (Ciloxan; 🍁 Ciloxan)	Corneal ulcer: day 1, 2 drops every 15 min for 6 h, then every 30 min for rest of day; day 2, 2 drops every hour; day 3–14, 2 drops every 4 h Conjunctivitis: 1 or 2 drops every 2 h while awake for 2 d, then 1 or 2 drops every 4 h while awake for 5 d	Safety and efficacy not established in infants <1 y ≥1 y: same as for adults
Erythromycin 5% ointment (🍁 EURO-Erythromycin, PDP-Erythromycin)	Ocular infection: instill 1 cm ribbon up to 6 times daily	Ocular infection: same as adult dosage Prevention of neonatal gonococcal or chlamydial conjunctivitis: 1 cm in each lower conjunctival sac
Gatifloxacin (Zymaxid; 🍁 Zymar)	Conjunctivitis: 1 drop every 2 h while awake, up to 8 times daily for 2 d, then 1 drop up to 4 times daily while awake for 5 d	≥1 y: same as for adults
Gentamicin 3 mg/mL solution or 3 mg/g ointment (Gentak; 🍁 Odan-Gentamicin)	Infection: Solution, 1–2 drops every 4 h up to 2 drops every hour for severe infections Ointment, apply 0.5 in, 2 or 3 times daily to every 3–4 h	Same as for adults
Levofloxacin 5 mg/mL solution	Conjunctivitis: 1 or 2 drops every 2 h up to 8 doses/d for 1 or 2 d, then every 4 h up to 4 doses/d for 5 d	Conjunctivitis: ≥1 y, same as adult dosage Corneal ulcer: ≥6 y, 1.5% solution, 1 or 2 drops every 30 min to 2 h while awake and 4 and 6 h after retiring, then on day 4 through completion 1 or 2 drops every 4 h while awake
Moxifloxacin (Vigamox; 🍁 PMS-Moxifloxacin, Vigamox)	Conjunctivitis: Vigamox, 1 drop 3 times daily for 7 d Moxeza, 1 drop 2 times daily for 7 d	Conjunctivitis: ≥1 y: Vigamox, same as for adults ≥4 mo: Moxeza, same as for adults
Ofloxacin (Ocuflox; 🍁 APO-Ofloxacin, Ocuflox)	Conjunctivitis: 1 or 2 drops every 2–4 h while awake for 2 d and then 4 times daily for 3–5 d Corneal ulcer: 1 or 2 drops every 30 min while awake, every 4–6 h during sleep for 1–2 d, then every hour while awake for 4–6 d, and then every 4 h while awake until healed	Conjunctivitis, corneal ulcer: ≥1 y, same as for adults
Sulfacetamide (🍁 Odan-Sulfacetamide)	Conjunctivitis, corneal ulcers, or other superficial infections caused by susceptible organisms: 1 or 2 drops every 2–3 h or 0.5-in ointment 3 or 4 times daily and at bedtime for 7–10 d	≥2 mo: same as for adults
Tobramycin (0.3% solution and 3 mg/g ointment) (Tobrex; 🍁 Tobrex, SANDOZ-Tobramycin)	Infection: Solution, 1 or 2 drops every 4 h, up to 2 drops every hour Ointment, 0.5-in ribbon 2–3 times daily, up to every 3–4 h until improvement	Infection: ≥2 mo, same as for adults
Antiviral Drugs		
Ⓟ **Trifluridine** (🍁 APO-Trifluridine, Viroptic)	Keratoconjunctivitis or corneal ulcers caused by herpes simplex virus: 1 drop every 2 h while awake (maximum, 9 drops/d) until corneal ulcer heals and then 1 drop every 4 h (minimum, 5 drops/d), for 7 d	≥6 y: same as for adults
Ganciclovir (Zirgan)	Herpetic keratitis: 1 drop every 3 h while awake (maximum, 5 drops/d) until corneal ulcer heals and then 1 drop 3 times daily for 7 d	≥2 y: same as adults
Antifungal Drugs		
Natamycin 5% suspension (Natacyn)	1 drop every 1–2 h for 3–4 d and then every 3–4 h for 14–21 d	Safety and efficacy not established

of ciprofloxacin absorbed topically with ophthalmic solution is minimal. The manufacturer recommends the lowest possible dose. It is unknown if ciprofloxacin is detected in breast milk.

Adverse Effects

Ciprofloxacin ophthalmic has adverse effects that include hypersensitivity reactions and superinfection. When ciprofloxacin ophthalmic is administered concurrently with any of the quinolones, hypersensitivity reactions, tendon inflammation, and tendon rupture may occur. There have been reports of superinfections with prolonged use, with possible fungal or bacterial infections.

Contraindications

Patients with a known hypersensitivity to ciprofloxacin or any quinolone should not receive the drug.

Nursing Implications

Preventing Interactions

The only interaction identified with ciprofloxacin ophthalmic is anaphylaxis when administered with quinolones.

Administering the Medication

Ciprofloxacin ophthalmic is for topical use only. It is important not to contaminate the tip of the applicator.

Assessing for Therapeutic Effects

The nurse assesses for decreased conjunctival redness and eye drainage.

Patient Teaching

Box 59.2 contains patient teaching information for topical ophthalmic medications.

Other Drugs in the Class

An ophthalmic form of erythromycin can produce edema, urticaria, dermatitis, and angioneurotic edema. Most ophthalmic agents in this class produce a burning sensation and eye irritation. Long-term topical use of antibacterial agents may lead to superinfection, and patients with viral, fungal, or mycobacterial infections of the eye should not use this drug.

ANTIVIRAL DRUGS

The prototype **P trifluridine** is the most commonly administered antiviral ophthalmic drug. A locally active drug, it is available as an ophthalmic ointment.

Pharmacokinetics and Action

Systemic absorption of trifluridine is negligible. The drug does not affect liver or kidney function.

Trifluridine interferes with viral replication. It incorporates viral DNA in place of thymidine to inhibit thymidylate synthetase, causing formation of defective viral proteins.

Use

Uses of trifluridine include treatment of primary keratoconjunctivitis and recurrent epithelial keratitis caused by herpes simplex virus types 1 and 2. Table 59.6 presents route and dosage information for trifluridine.

Patient-related variables specific to the use of trifluridine include reproduction, pregnancy, and lactation. No adverse fetal effects have been noted in animal studies. The amount of trifluridine in breast milk is negligible.

Adverse Effects and Contraindications

The most common adverse effects associated with trifluridine are burning and stinging. Rare adverse effects include epithelial keratopathy, increased IOP, palpebral edema, and stromal edema.

Contraindications include known hypersensitivity to trifluridine or its components.

Nursing Implications

Administering the Medication

Trifluridine is a hazardous drug, and it is important to wear gloves when administering the medication. If trifluridine is being used with other ophthalmic medications, it is necessary to wait several minutes between applications. Storage of the medication in the refrigerator at 2°C to 8°C or 36°F to 48°F is required. Disposal in accordance with biohazard procedures should occur.

Assessing for Therapeutic and Adverse Effects

It is necessary to assess for decreased erythema of the conjunctiva. Complete healing of the corneal ulcer should occur in 1 to 2 weeks.

The nurse assesses for transient burning, stinging, and irritation of the eye. The nurse also assesses for photophobia, increased IOP, epithelial keratopathy, keratitis, palpebral edema, and stromal edema.

Patient Teaching

The nurse provides instruction to the patient on medication administration, including safe handling of the drug. The patient is also taught about the importance of keeping regularly scheduled medical appointments for eye examinations. In addition, the nurse tells the patient that herpetic eye infections often recur and, if not treated, lead to damage of the cornea. Box 59.2 contains additional patient teaching information.

Other Drugs in the Class

Ganciclovir (Zirgan) is an antiviral ophthalmic agent used to treat herpetic keratitis. Gloves and a protective gown should be worn for administering the drug topically. Current guidelines for the use of antiretroviral agents in HIV-1–infected adults and adolescents (Department of Health and Human Services, 2021) include recommendations on the HIV-related uses of ganciclovir for progressive outer retinal necrosis and acute retinal necrosis both of which are infections and necrotizing inflammation associated with a high rate of blindness.

ANTIFUNGAL DRUGS

Natamycin (Natacyn) is the prototype ophthalmic antifungal drug.

Pharmacokinetics and Action

Approximately 2% of natamycin administered topically is absorbed systemically. It is distributed by adhering to the cornea and is retained in the conjunctival fornices. It does not affect intraocular fluid concentrations.

Natamycin increases cellular permeability to susceptible fungi.

Use

Uses of natamycin include the treatment of blepharitis, conjunctivitis, and keratitis. It is effective against common fungi such as *Aspergillus, Candida, Cephalosporium, Fusarium,* and *Penicillium.* Table 59.6 presents route and dosage information for natamycin.

Patient-related variables specific to the use of natamycin include reproduction, pregnancy, and lactation. No animal reproduction studies have been conducted on natamycin. It is unknown if natamycin is excreted in breast milk.

Adverse Effects

Reported adverse effects of natamycin may be numerous. These conditions may include hypersensitivity and allergic reactions, chest pain, opacity of the cornea, eye pain, edema, dyspnea, hyperemia, irritation, foreign body sensation of the eye, paresthesia, tearing, and alteration in visual acuity.

Contraindications

Patients who have exhibited a hypersensitivity reaction to natamycin should not take the drug.

Nursing Implications

Administering the Medication

It is important that contact lenses are not worn when signs and symptoms of the fungal infection are visible. In any case, the natamycin solution contains benzalkonium chloride, which can be absorbed by the lens; thus, it is necessary to remove the lenses prior to administration of the medication. Reinsertion of the lenses should not occur for 15 minutes. The nurse shakes the medication well and then administers it without touching the applicator tip to the eye.

Assessing for Therapeutic and Adverse Effects

The nurse assesses for decreased eye pain, redness, and tearing. Also, the patient should also have increased visual acuity with a decrease in blurring and cloudiness.

It is also necessary to assess for signs and symptoms of a hypersensitivity reaction such as hyperemia, dyspnea, edema, or chest pain. The nurse also assesses for paresthesia and visual changes.

Patient Teaching

The nurse tells the patient to discontinue wearing contacts during the acute phase of the fungal infection. Also, the nurse emphasizes that even when the patient is wearing contacts, they should not reinsert them for 15 minutes after instillation of the medication. In addition, it is important to maintain good hand hygiene and prevent contamination of the applicator tip. Box 59.2 contains additional patient teaching information.

ANTIALLERGIC DRUGS

Cromolyn sodium is the prototype antiallergic ophthalmic drug.

Pharmacokinetics and Action

The onset of action varies. The half-life of the drug is 80 to 90 minutes. Cromolyn is excreted unchanged in the urine and feces with small amounts in exhaled gases.

Cromolyn reduces the release of leukotrienes, thus decreasing or stopping the body's reaction to an allergen.

Use

Uses of cromolyn include the treatment of vernal keratitis, vernal conjunctivitis, and vernal keratoconjunctivitis. Table 59.7 presents route and dosage information for cromolyn and other ophthalmic antiallergy medications.

Patient-related variables specific to the use of cromolyn include reproduction, pregnancy, and lactation. Adverse fetal effects have not been observed with cromolyn ophthalmic. It is not known if cromolyn is excreted in breast milk.

Adverse Effects and Contraindications

Cromolyn is associated with several adverse effects, including hypersensitivity reactions. Eye effects include edema, dryness, irritation, itching, puffiness, rash, and tearing. Styes may also develop.

Contraindications include a known hypersensitivity to the drug or its formulations.

Nursing Implications

Assessing for Therapeutic Effects

The nurse assesses for a reduction in allergic conjunctivitis, keratitis, or keratoconjunctivitis. Response to treatment with cromolyn may occur in a few days. However, treatment for up to 6 weeks is routinely necessary.

Assessing for Adverse Effects

The nurse assesses for hypersensitivity response to the medication as well as ocular effects that include edema, dryness, irritation, itching, swelling, rash, or tearing. It is necessary to ask the patient about feelings of a foreign body, which could indicate a stye. Withdrawal may result in the exacerbation of symptoms.

Patient Teaching

Box 59.2 contains additional patient teaching information.

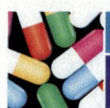

TABLE 59.7
DRUGS AT A GLANCE: Anti-inflammatory Drugs

Drug	Routes and Dosage Ranges	
	Adults	**Children**
Antiallergic Drugs		
Ⓟ **Cromolyn sodium**	1–2 drops in each eye 4–6 times per day	≥4 y, same as for adults
Lodoxamide (Alomide; 🍁 Alomide)	1–2 drops 4 times a day for up to 3 mo	≥2 y, same as for adults
H₁-Receptor Antagonists: Second Generation		
Azelastine	1 drop twice daily	≥3 y, same as for adults
Epinastine	1 drop 2 times per day even when symptoms subside	≥3 y, same as for adults
Ketotifen (Alaway, Claritin Eye, Zaditor; Zaditor)	1 drop 2 times a day at least 8 h apart	≥3 y, same as for adults
Olopatadine (Pataday, Patanol, Pazeo; ACT-Olopatadine, Pataday, Patanol)	Patanol, 1 drop 2 times per day at least 6 h between doses Pataday and Pazeo, 1 drop once daily	Patanol, ≥3 y, same as adult dosage Pataday, ≥2 y, same as adult dosage
Corticosteroids		
Ⓟ **Dexamethasone** (Dextenza, Dexycu, Maxidex, Ozurdex; 🍁 Maxidex, Ozurdex)	Ophthalmic solution, 1–2 drops into conjunctival sac every hour during the day and every other hour during the night; gradually reduce dose to 1 drop every 3–4 times per day Ophthalmic suspension, 1–2 drops into conjunctival sac 4–6 times per day; may use hourly in severe disease; taper dose during discontinuation Macular edema or noninfective uveitis: Ophthalmic injection, ocular implant with Ozurdex, intravitreal 0.7-mg implant injected in the affected eye	Ophthalmic solution, 1–2 drops into conjunctival sac every hour during the day and every other hour during the night; gradually reduce dose to every 3–4 h, then 3–4 times per day Ophthalmic suspension, 1–2 drops into conjunctival sac up to 4–6 times per day; may use hourly in severe disease in older children; taper dose during discontinuation; following strabismus surgery: 2–4 times per day
Fluorometholone (Flarex, FML ForteFMLLiquifilm; 🍁 Flarex, SANDOZ-Fluorometholone)	Ointment, 1/2-in ribbon to conjunctival sac 1–3 times daily; may increase to every 4 h during the initial 24–48 h Suspension, 1 drop into the conjunctival sac 2–4 times per day	≥2 y of age, same as for adults
Loteprednol (Lotemax, Alrex; 🍁 Alrex Lotemax)	Seasonal allergic conjunctivitis: 0.2% suspension 1 drop 4 times per day Inflammatory conditions: 0.5% suspension 1–2 drops into the conjunctival sac 4 times per day; during the first week the dose may be increased by 1 drop every hour; do not discontinue therapy prematurely; if signs and symptoms do not improve in 2 d, the patient should be reevaluated Postoperative inflammation: 0.5% suspension 1–2 drops into the conjunctival sac 4 times per day beginning 24 h after surgery and continue for 2 wk	Safety and efficacy not established
Prednisolone (Pred Forte, Pred Mild; 🍁 PMS-Prednisolone, Pred Forte, Sandoz Prednisolone)	1–2 drops into conjunctival sac 2–4 times daily; dosing frequency first 48 h may be increased if necessary	1–2 drops into conjunctival sac 3–6 times daily

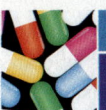

TABLE 59.7
DRUGS AT A GLANCE: Anti-inflammatory Drugs (Continued)

Drug	Routes and Dosage Ranges	
	Adults	**Children**
Anti-inflammatory Drugs		
ⓟ Diclofenac (✳APO-Diclofenac, MINT-Diclofenac)	Cataract surgery: 1 drop 4 times per day beginning 24 h after surgery and continuing for 2 wk Corneal refractive surgery: 1–2 drops within the hour prior to surgery and continuing 4 times daily for up to 3 d	Safety and efficacy of ophthalmic preparation not established
Flurbiprofen	1 drop every 30 min starting 2 h prior to surgery (total of 4 drops to each affected eye)	Same as for adults
Ketorolac (Acular, Acuvail, Acular LS; ✳ Acular, Acuvail, Acular LS)	Seasonal allergic conjunctivitis: 1 drop 4 times per day Postoperative inflammation: 1 drop 4 times per day starting 24 h after cataract surgery and through 14 d after surgery Postoperative pain: 1 drop times per day as needed up to 4 d after corneal refractive surgery Postoperative pain and photophobia: 1 drop 2 times per day as needed beginning 24 h before and for up to 2 wk after incisional refractive surgery	Seasonal allergic conjunctivitis: ≥2 y, same as adult dosage Postoperative ocular pain: ≥3 y, same as for adults Postoperative pain: ≥3 y, same as for adults
Immunosuppressants		
ⓟ Cyclosporine emulsion (Cequa, Restasis, Verkazia; Restasis MultiDose; ✳ Restasis, Restasis MultiDose, TEVA-CycloSPORINE, Verkazia)	1 drop every 12 h	≥16 y, same as for adults

H_1-RECEPTOR ANTAGONISTS: SECOND GENERATION

Azelastine ophthalmic will be discussed in place of the prototype of this class emedastine difumarate, which has been discontinued. Allergic rhinitis produces ocular pruritus. The second-generation antihistamines block the H_1 receptors to relieve ocular pruritus or allergic conjunctivitis.

Pharmacokinetics, Action, and Use

Azelastine is a selective histamine H_1-receptor antagonist for topical ophthalmic use. It competes with histamine for the H_1 receptor sites on the effector cells and inhibits the release of histamine and other mediators that are producing the allergic response. It is used for adult and pediatric patients to relieve seasonal allergic conjunctivitis.

Adverse Effects and Contraindications

Azelastine produces a headache in 15% of the patients Thirty percent of patients have reported ocular burning and stinging. Other adverse effects are fatigue, pruritus, temporary blurring of vision, asthma, and shortness of breath. Azelastine is contraindicated in patients who exhibit signs and symptoms of hypersensitivity.

Nursing Implications
Administering the Medication

Check the solution for clarity before administering it. Prior to and following the administration of the medication, wash hands for a minimum of 20 seconds. Instill one drop in the conjunctival sac. Never touch the eye with the eye dropper tip. The patient should close the eye for 1 to 2 minutes after instillation. Wait 10 minutes to insert contact lenses.

Assessing for Therapeutic and Adverse Effects

Assess the patient for decreased ocular redness, watering, and inflammation. Adverse effects of azelastine include a hypersensitivity reaction with increased redness, edema, and pruritus.

Patient Teaching

The patient should be taught to wash hands for 20 seconds prior to and following the administration of azelastine. Instill the medication in the conjunctival sac without touching the medication tip to the eye. The patient should close the eye for 1 to 2 minutes after the medication administration. Contact lenses should not be inserted for a minimum of 10 minutes after instillation. Instruct the patient on the signs and symptoms of hypersensitivity.

Other Drugs in the Class

Other drugs in the class including epinastine, ketotifen (Alaway Children's Allergy, Claritin Eye, Zaditor), and olopatadine (Pataday, Pazeo) treat allergic conjunctivitis. Each medication has a similar action and adverse effects.

CORTICOSTEROIDS

The prototype corticosteroid ophthalmic drug is **dexamethasone** (Dextenza, Dexycu, Maxidex, Ozurdex).

Pharmacokinetics

The onset of action of dexamethasone ophthalmic drops is unknown. The half-life and duration of action are unknown. The onset of action of the implant is 20% to 30% within the first 2 months following intravitreal injection. The duration of action is 1 to 3 months.

Action

Dexamethasone decreases inflammation by suppressing the migration of neutrophils and decreasing the production of the mediators of inflammation. It reverses the increase in capillary permeability and suppresses the normal immune response.

Use

Uses of dexamethasone include a decrease of symptoms of allergic conjunctivitis, iritis, and cyclitis. It is a treatment of corneal injury from chemical, radiation, and thermal burns or penetrating foreign bodies. Dexamethasone in the form of an intravitreal implant (Ozurdex) is used for the treatment of macular edema following retinal vein occlusion or central retinal vein occlusion, as well as for noninfective uveitis. Table 59.7 presents dosage information for the corticosteroid ophthalmic drugs.

Patient-related variables specific to the use of dexamethasone include reproduction, pregnancy, and lactation. Systemic exposure in pregnancy is negligible. It is unknown if there are detectable concentrations of dexamethasone in breast milk.

Adverse Effects

Ocular adverse effects associated with dexamethasone include blurred vision, increased IOP, photophobia, vitreous detachment, conjunctival edema, corneal edema, eye pain, dryness, irritation, and eye discharge.

Contraindications

Contraindications to dexamethasone include corneal or conjunctival viral disease caused by herpes simplex, vaccinia, or varicella. Also, other contraindications are mycobacterial and fungal infection of the eye as well as advanced glaucoma and hypersensitivity to corticosteroids. In addition, patients who are taking corticorelin, a synthetic hormone that is administered to diagnose Cushing disease, should not receive ophthalmic forms of dexamethasone.

Nursing Implications

Preventing Interactions

The dexamethasone decreases the therapeutic effects of corticorelin. If patients who are taking the chelating drug deferasirox combine it with corticosteroids, there is an increased risk of GI ulceration, irritation, and bleeding.

Administering the Medication

> **! Quality and Safety Alert: Safety**
> It is important to double check medications before administration. The nurse should not confuse medications with similar names. For example, it is easy to confuse dexamethasone (Maxidex) with triamterene/hydrochlorothiazide (Maxzide).

The solution and suspension contain benzalkonium chloride. Thus, a nurse may administer dexamethasone solutions and suspensions, but an ophthalmologist gives the implant (Ozurdex) under aseptic conditions. Prior to injection of Ozurdex, a broad-spectrum bactericidal drug is administered. If administered to both eyes, a different applicator is used for each application. Box 59.1 lists general guidelines for the administration of topical ophthalmic medications.

Assessing for Therapeutic Effects

The nurse assesses for decreased pain, irritation, redness, and eye drainage. An ophthalmologist evaluates patients who have received Ozurdex for decreased macular edema and inflammation of the uveal tract.

Assessing for Adverse Effects

The nurse assesses for eye pain, blurred vision, photophobia, increased IOP, photophobia, vitreous detachment, conjunctival edema, eye dryness, or eye discharge.

Patient Teaching

For patients who use the ophthalmic implant (Ozurdex), it is important to instruct them about the sterile procedure for administration and the rationale for the implant. Box 59.2 contains additional patient teaching information.

ANTI-INFLAMMATORY DRUGS

The prototype ophthalmic NSAID is **diclofenac**, an analgesic, non-narcotic drug.

Pharmacokinetics and Action

Very little systemic absorption of diclofenac occurs. Mainly, it has local effects.

This cyclooxygenase 1 and 2 inhibitor decreases the formation of prostaglandin, thus resulting in an anti-inflammatory action.

Use

Diclofenac reduces inflammation following cataract extraction. It is administered to relieve pain and photophobia associated with corneal refractive surgery. Table 59.7 provides route and dosage information about diclofenac and other NSAIDs.

Patient-related variables specific to the use of diclofenac include reproduction, pregnancy, and lactation. Systemic exposure in pregnancy is negligible. It is unknown if there are detectable concentrations of diclofenac in breast milk.

Adverse Effects

Diclofenac may produce facial edema, dizziness, fever, headache, pain, and insomnia. Associated ocular adverse effects are burning, stinging, increased IOP, keratitis, and lacrimation. Less frequently occurring ocular conditions include disturbances in vision, inflammation, corneal deposits and edema, corneal lesions or opacity, discharge, swelling, iritis, itching, and allergy. In addition, rhinitis, muscle pain and weakness, abdominal pain, nausea, vomiting, and viral infection may follow use.

Contraindications

Contraindications to diclofenac include hypersensitivity to any NSAID.

Nursing Implications

Preventing Interactions

Any ophthalmic NSAID combined with latanoprost diminishes the therapeutic effect of latanoprost.

Administering the Medication

As with other ophthalmic medications, it is necessary to prevent contamination of the applicator tip. In addition, it is important to wait at least 5 minutes before administering any other eyedrops. In the postoperative phase of drug administration, 2 bottles of diclofenac should be used and labeled appropriately left and right to prevent the risk of cross-contamination.

Assessing for Therapeutic and Adverse Effects

The nurse assesses for decreased inflammation and pain related to surgery.

In addition, the nurse assesses for tearing, inflammation, and pain or discomfort of the eye, as well as for facial edema and rhinitis. It is necessary to assess for increased IOP. Also, the nurse assesses for GI conditions and viral infections.

Patient Teaching

Box 59.2 contains patient teaching information.

IMMUNOSUPPRESSANTS

The prototype ophthalmic immunosuppressant drug is **cyclosporine emulsion** (Cequa, Restasis, Restasis MultiDose, Verkazia).

Pharmacokinetics and Action

No systemic concentrations of cyclosporine are detected in blood samples.

The drug increases tear production.

Use

Cyclosporine emulsion increases tear production in keratoconjunctivitis sicca, which is an ocular inflammation. Table 59.7 presents route and dosage information for the cyclosporine emulsion.

Patient-related variables specific to the use of cyclosporine include reproduction, pregnancy, and lactation. Systemic exposure in pregnancy is negligible. Cyclosporine is present in breast milk. The decision to continue breast-feeding should be made by the prescriber.

Adverse Effects and Contraindications

The adverse effects of cyclosporine emulsion are burning, hyperemia, ocular pain, and pruritus.

Contraindications include active eye infections or hypersensitivity to the medication.

Nursing Implications

Administering the Medication

It is important to invert the medication bottle to mix the emulsion adequately prior to administration. In addition, patients should remove contact lenses before administration and not reinsert them for 15 minutes. The instillation of other ocular medications should occur at 15-minute intervals.

Assessing for Therapeutic and Adverse Effects

The nurse interviews the patient to determine if the dryness of the eye has resolved.

In addition, the nurse assesses for discomfort of the eye, pruritus, and hyperemia.

Patient Teaching

It is important to instruct the patient about medication administration, including inversion of the bottle to mix the medication, removal of contacts, and waiting 15 minutes between the administration of other ocular medications. Box 59.2 contains additional patient teaching information.

THE NURSING PROCESS

A concept map outlines the nursing process related to drug therapy considerations in this chapter. Additional nursing implications related to the disease process should also be considered in care decisions.

Assessment
- Assess visual acuity and the ability to complete activities of daily living and work-related activities.
- Identify risk factors for eye disorders. These include trauma, allergies, infection in one eye (a risk factor for infection in the other eye), use of contact lenses, infections of facial structures or skin, and occupational exposure to chemical irritants or foreign bodies.
- Assess subjective and objective data related to eye pain, inflammation of the eye, purulent or mucous discharge from the eye, pruritus, or photosensitivity.

Outcomes of Therapy

The patient will
- Administer ophthalmic medications as prescribed.
- Follow safety precautions to protect eyes from trauma and disease.
- Experience improvement in signs and symptoms (e.g., decreased drainage with infections, decreased intraocular pressure with glaucoma).
- Avoid injury from impaired vision (e.g., falls).
- Avoid systemic effects of ophthalmic drugs.
- Have regular eye examinations.

Nursing Interventions
- Instruct the patient to have regular eye examinations; including annual monitoring of intraocular pressure at the age of 40 years.
- Instruct patients who have glaucoma not to take any medications without a prescriber's knowledge. Many drugs given for purposes other than eye disorders may cause or aggravate glaucoma. Also, suggest that patients wear a medical alert bracelet stating that they have glaucoma.
- Assist patients at risk of eye damage from IOP (e.g., those with glaucoma; those who have had intraocular surgery, such as cataract removal) to avoid straining at stool (use laxatives or stool softeners if needed), heavy lifting, bending over, coughing, and vomiting when possible.
- Promote handwashing and keeping hands away from eyes to prevent eye infections.
- Cleanse contact lenses or assist patients in lens care, when needed.
- Apply warm, wet compresses; they are often useful in ophthalmic inflammation or infections.

Evaluation
- Observe and interview for compliance with instructions regarding drug therapy and follow-up care.
- Observe and interview for relief of symptoms.
- Observe for systemic adverse effects of ophthalmic drugs (e.g., tachycardia and dysrhythmias with adrenergic drugs; bradycardia or bronchoconstriction with beta-adrenergic blockers).

Visit **thePoint** *at* **http://thePoint.lww.com/Frandsen13e** *for answers to NCLEX Success questions (in Appendix A), answers to Clinical Application Case Studies (in Appendix B), additional information on etiology and pathophysiology of eye disorders, and more!*

REFERENCES AND RESOURCES

Delavar, A., Saseendrakumar, B., Weinreb, R. N., & Baxter, S. L. (2022). Racial and ethnic disparities in cost-related barriers to medication adherence among patients with glaucoma enrolled in the National Institutes of Health *All of Us* research program. *Journal of American Medical Association Ophthalmology, 140*(4), 354–361. https://doi.org/10.100/jamaophthalmol.2022.0055

DHHS Panel on antiretroviral guidelines for adults and adolescents. (2021). *Guidelines for the use of antiretroviral agents in HIV-1-infected adults and adolescents.* Department of Health and Human Services. Retrieved from https://clinicalinfo.hiv.gov/sites/default/files/guidelines/archive/AdultandAdolescentGL_2021_08_16.pdf

Hinkle, J. H., Cheever, K. H., & Overbaugh, K. J. (2021). *Brunner & Suddarth's textbook of medical-surgical nursing* (15th ed.). Wolters Kluwer.

Jacobs, D. S. (2022). Open-angle glaucoma: Treatment. *UpToDate*. Lexi-Comp, Inc.

Norris, T. L. (2019). *Porth's pathophysiology concepts of altered health states* (10th ed.). Wolters Kluwer.

Reynolds, J. D., & Reynolds, A. L. (2022). Overview of glaucoma in infants and children. *UpToDate*. Lexi-Comp, Inc.

UpToDate. (2020). *Drug information.* Lexi-Comp, Inc.

CHAPTER 60

Drug Therapy for Disorders of the Ear

LEARNING OBJECTIVES

After studying this chapter, you should be able to:

1. Describe the characteristics of acute otitis externa, necrotizing otitis externa, and otitis media.
2. Identify the prototype and describe the action, use, adverse effects, contraindications, and nursing implications for topical medications used to treat otitis externa.
3. Identify the prototype and describe the action, use, adverse effects, contraindications, and nursing implications for systemic medications used to treat necrotizing otitis externa.
4. Identify the prototype and describe the action, use, adverse effects, contraindications, and nursing implications for systemic medications used to treat otitis media.
5. Identify the adjuvant drugs used to treat otitis externa and otitis media.
6. Implement the nursing process in the care of the patient with otitis externa or otitis media.

CLINICAL APPLICATION CASE STUDY

Derrick Washington is a member of the high school swim team. He has been swimming two times per day for the past 3 months. The swim team has been very successful this season; it has qualified for the state finals. One morning well before the state meet, Derrick awakens with a severe earache. His mother makes an appointment with a pediatric nurse practitioner, who diagnoses acute otitis externa (swimmer's ear). The nurse prescribes neomycin–polymyxin B–hydrocortisone suspension.

KEY TERMS

Necrotizing otitis externa: invasive soft tissue infection of the external auditory canal and skull; also called malignant external otitis

Otalgia: ear pain

Otic: relating to the ear

Otitis externa: inflammation of the external ear that occurs as a mild allergic dermatitis or as a severe cellulitis

Otitis media: inflammation of the middle ear

Otorrhea: any discharge from the ear (clear to purulent) following perforation of the tympanic membrane

INTRODUCTION

This chapter discusses selected ear-related disorders and their pharmacologic treatment. Infections, whether bacterial or fungal, or allergic reactions result in ear pain–related inflammation.

OVERVIEW OF DISORDERS OF THE EAR

Otitis externa is a disorder of the external ear that produces inflammation. This condition, most commonly known as swimmer's ear, is more likely to occur in the summer months. People whose ears are frequently exposed to moisture are more prone to the development of this disorder. **Necrotizing otitis externa** is an invasive soft tissue infection of the external auditory canal and skull. Malignant necrotizing otitis externa (also called malignant otitis externa) most commonly affects older adult patients with diabetes mellitus and patients with the human immunodeficiency virus. The disease is rare in children. **Otitis media** is an acute infection or inflammation of the middle ear. Acute otitis media is the most common ailment for which anti-infective agents are prescribed in children.

The pharmacologic therapy of choice for disorders of the ear is **otic** preparations. These medications, which are discussed elsewhere in this book, have special uses in the treatment of ear conditions.

Clinical Manifestations

Otitis Externa

In acute otitis externa, the patient complains of **otalgia** (ear pain) and **otorrhea** (drainage from the external auditory canal). The discharge may be yellow or green, with a foul odor most likely due to *Pseudomonas aeruginosa*. The patient may also report a feeling of "fullness" in the ear, decreased hearing, and pruritus.

In necrotizing otitis externa, the presenting symptoms are otalgia and otorrhea with purulent drainage. The pain is primarily experienced at night and may extend to the temporomandibular joint when chewing. The advancement of the infection results in osteomyelitis of the skull and temporomandibular joint that can be associated with cranial nerve palsies.

Otitis Media

In acute otitis media, marked fluid and inflammation in the mucosa lining the middle ear space are present (Fig. 60.1). These cause pain and general symptoms of illness such as fever, irritability, and problems feeding and sleeping. Otalgia and diminished hearing occur. An upper respiratory tract infection or seasonal allergic rhinitis commonly precedes acute otitis media. Changes in equilibrium may occur. If the tympanic membrane ruptures, patients report a reduction or relief of ear pain.

Drug Therapy

Table 60.1 lists the various drugs used to treat ear disorders.

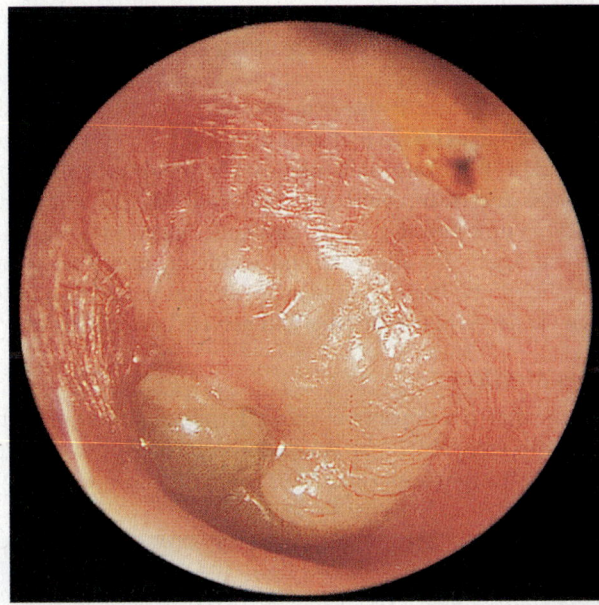

Figure 60.1. Acute otitis media. (Reprinted with permission from Weber, J., & Kelly, J. H. (2014). *Health assessment in nursing* (6th ed., Image in Abnormal Findings 17-2 table). Wolters Kluwer Health | Lippincott Williams & Wilkins.)

Otitis Externa

For acute otitis externa, use of topical agents, as opposed to systemic agents, is more common. Systemic medications are indicated only if a deep tissue infection develops outside the external canal or if immunocompromised status is an issue. Topical drugs are more effective because they deliver higher concentrations of medication to the infected, inflamed tissue. The use of these agents also reduces adverse effects. Acute otitis externa caused by *P. aeruginosa* or *Staphylococcus aureus* is treated with ciprofloxacin hydrochloride otic solution. The otic solution is instilled in the affected ear (Table 60.3).

TABLE 60.1

Drugs Administered for the Treatment of Disorders of the Ear

Drug Class	Prototype	Other Drugs in the Class
Acute otitis externa		
Anti-infective, antiseptic, glucocorticoid, and acidifying agents	Neomycin–polymyxin B–hydrocortisone	Coly-Mycin S Otic Cipro HC Otic Ofloxacin
Necrotizing otitis externa		
Fluoroquinolones	Ciprofloxacin (Cipro)	
Acute otitis media		
Penicillin	Amoxicillin	

When the infection extends to the pinna, prescribers order oral anti-infective agents. For necrotizing otitis externa, the primary treatment is systemic antipseudomonal antimicrobial agents. Ciprofloxacin is the drug of choice for adults, whereas cephalexin (Keflex) is the preferred drug for children (see Chapters 18 and 19). The otic solutions most commonly prescribed for acute otitis externa are combination solutions. These medications contain an anti-infective agent, antiseptic, glucocorticoid, and acidifying agent. The antiseptic and acidifying agents have bacteriostatic effects. These agents contain alcohol and acetic acid to loosen the debris in the ear canal and prevent bacterial growth.

Otitis Media

Oral amoxicillin is the drug of choice for the treatment of acute otitis media (see Table 60.3). Patients who are allergic to penicillins may take cephalosporins.

> **! Quality and Safety Alert: Evidence-Based Practice**
>
> A Cochrane Review (2020) explored whether topical antibiotics are effective in treating chronic necrotizing otitis externa and whether one type of topical antibiotic treatment is more effective than any other. It is unclear whether topical antibiotics contribute to the resolution of ear discharge in patients with chronic otitis media. Some evidence indicates that using topical antibiotics may be effective when compared to a placebo or when added to treatment with a systemic antibiotic, but certainty of evidence is very low. In addition, the type of topical antibiotic that would be the most effective is unclear.

ANTI-INFECTIVE, ANTISEPTIC, GLUCOCORTICOID, AND ACIDIFYING AGENTS

Healthcare providers use the combination drug **neomycin–polymyxin B–hydrocortisone** for the treatment of acute external otitis media. Neomycin and polymyxin B are antibiotics, which combat bacterial infections. Hydrocortisone is a steroid, which reduces the actions of chemicals in the body that cause inflammation, redness, and swelling.

Pharmacokinetics

The metabolism and transport effects of polymyxin and neomycin are unknown. Hydrocortisone is metabolized in the liver, and excretion occurs in the urine.

Action

Each component of neomycin–polymyxin B–hydrocortisone suspension has its own mechanism of action. Neomycin, an aminoglycoside, inhibits bacterial protein synthesis by irreversibly binding to the 30S ribosome of the susceptible bacteria. Polymyxin B, a miscellaneous anti-infective agent, binds to the lipid phosphates in the bacterial cell membrane, which changes the membrane permeability to prevent leakage of cytoplasm from the bacterial cell wall, contributing to cell death. Hydrocortisone, a steroid, decreases inflammation by stabilizing the leukocyte lysosome membrane, inhibiting phagocytosis and release of allergic substances.

Use

Healthcare providers use neomycin–polymyxin B–hydrocortisone suspension for the treatment of acute otitis externa caused by *P. aeruginosa*, *Proteus*, and *S. aureus*. Table 60.2 presents route and dosage information for neomycin–polymyxin B–hydrocortisone suspension.

Patient-related variables specific to the use of neomycin–polymyxin B–hydrocortisone suspension include the following:

- Age:
  - In children, neomycin–polymyxin B–hydrocortisone suspension is recommended only for bacterial infections of the external auditory canal due to the adverse

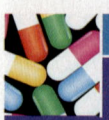

TABLE 60.2

DRUGS AT A GLANCE: Anti-Infective, Antiseptic, Glucocorticoid, and Acidifying Drugs

Drug	Routes and Dosage Ranges	
	Adults	**Children**
Neomycin–polymyxin B–hydrocortisone (✱ Odan-Spor-HC)	Instill 4 drops three to four times daily for no more than 10 d	6 mo and older, 3 drops into affected ear three to four times daily for no more than 10 d
Neomycin–colistin–hydrocortisone–thonzonium (Coly-Mycin S Otic)	5 drops in affected ear three to four times daily for no more than 10 d	4 drops in affected ear three to four times daily for no more than 10 d
Ciprofloxacin–hydrocortisone (Cipro HC Otic; ✱ Cipro HC)	3 drops in affected ear twice daily for 7 d	≥1 y, 3 drops in affected ear twice daily for 7 d
Ofloxacin	Otitis media, chronic suppurative: 10 drops into affected ear twice daily for 14 d	1–12 y, 5 drops into affected ear twice daily for 10 d
	Otitis externa: 10 drops into affected ear twice daily for 7 d	≥13 y, same as adult

effect of ototoxicity. The hydrocortisone may cause suppression of the hypothalamic–pituitary–adrenal axis in younger children.
- Reproduction, pregnancy, and lactation:
  - No animal reproduction studies have been conducted.
  - It is unknown if systemic absorption following topical administration is detectable in breast milk.

Adverse Effects and Contraindications

Adverse effects of neomycin–polymyxin B–hydrocortisone suspension include burning, stinging, and ototoxicity.

Contraindications include a known hypersensitivity to the drug's components. Prescribers should not order it for viral, fungal, or mycobacterial infections.

Nursing Implications

Preventing Interactions

Neomycin–polymyxin B–hydrocortisone suspension is associated with no significant drug or herbal interactions.

Administering the Medication

Administration of neomycin–polymyxin B–hydrocortisone suspension is directly in the external ear canal. Prior to administering the otic suspension, it is necessary to shake the medication well. In addition, if cerumen is present, cleaning of the ear canal with a cotton swab is important.

> **Quality and Safety Alert: Safety**
>
> It is necessary to assess the tympanic membrane with an otoscope before inserting neomycin–polymyxin B–hydrocortisone suspension. If the tympanic membrane is torn, then this medication should not be inserted because it will be absorbed directly by the inner ear, leading to hearing loss.

The proper administration of eardrops requires tilting the head toward the opposite shoulder, pulling the superior aspect of the auricle upward, and instilling the eardrops into the ear canal. The patient should then lie on the side opposite the side of administration for 20 minutes. To maximize medication absorption, the patient should have a cotton ball placed in the ear canal.

Assessing for Therapeutic and Adverse Effects

The nurse assesses for decreased ear pain and itching as well as for decreased drainage from the ear canal.

It is also necessary to assess for signs of hearing loss due to ototoxicity. The nurse also assesses for burning and stinging.

Patient Teaching

Box 60.1 lists patient teaching guidelines for Cortisporin.

Other Drugs in the Class

The otic drug Coly-Mycin, a combination of neomycin, colistin, hydrocortisone, and thonzonium, is an antibiotic and corticosteroid administered for ear inflammation and infection. Contraindications include a known hypersensitivity to aminoglycosides as well as the presence of herpes simplex,

---

BOX 60.1 *Patient Teaching Guidelines for Neomycin–Polymyxin B–Hydrocortisone Suspension*

- Prior to administering the otic suspension, shake the medication well. If any earwax is present, use a cotton swab to remove it.
  - Tilt your head toward the opposite shoulder, pull the top of your outer ear upward, and put the eardrops into the ear canal.
  - Then lie on the side opposite the side of administration for 20 minutes. To maximize medication absorption, place a cotton ball in your ear for that time.
- Refrain from inserting anything in the ear canal.
- Do not let water enter the ear canal during the treatment period. If you swim, use ear plugs, shake the ear dry after swimming, and use a blow dryer on the low setting 12 inches away to dry the ear canal.
- Stop using the medication after 10 days.
- Have a follow-up assessment in 1 to 2 weeks.

---

vaccinia, or varicella. The neomycin may cause cutaneous sensitization, with itching, redness, edema, and diminished healing.

The combination drug Cipro HC contains ciprofloxacin and hydrocortisone. Its twice-daily administration makes it more convenient for parents with young children.

Ofloxacin (otic form), used for treatment of otitis externa and otitis media, is suitable for administration to a patient with a perforated tympanic membrane. This medication does not contain neomycin; therefore, there is no risk of ototoxicity.

Clinical Application 60.1

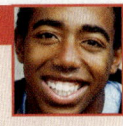

- What does the nurse tell Derrick and his mother about the pathophysiology of otitis externa?
- What is the reason for the development of otitis externa in this case?
- What signs and symptoms of otitis externa does the nurse expect Derrick to present?

NCLEX Success

1. Which of the following patients are at risk for the development of otitis externa?
   - A. a patient who wears ear plugs while swimming
   - B. a patient who has hearing loss
   - C. a patient who wears a hearing aid
   - D. a patient with labyrinthitis

2. What is the duration of therapy for neomycin–polymyxin B–hydrocortisone?
   - A. 5 days
   - B. 8 days
   - C. 10 days
   - D. 14 days

> **Clinical Application 60.2**
> - What patient teaching does the nurse need to provide to Derrick and his mother?
> - The state swim meet is in 2 weeks. Will Derrick be able to participate?
> - What does the school nurse need to teach the swim coach to prevent further outbreaks of otitis externa?

FLUOROQUINOLONE: CIPROFLOXACIN

The fluoroquinolone **ciprofloxacin** (Cipro) is the drug of choice for necrotizing otitis externa. Initially, administration is intravenous, until symptoms decrease; then it is oral. A suspension is available, as indicated.

Pharmacokinetics

The intravenous preparation has an onset of action in 10 minutes, with a peak of action in 30 minutes and duration of 4 to 5 hours. Onset of action for the oral preparation varies, with a peak of action in 60 to 90 minutes, and the same duration of action. The intravenous and oral preparations are absorbed rapidly and distributed to the kidneys, gallbladder, liver, lungs, gynecologic or prostate tissue, and cerebrospinal fluid. It is 20% to 40% protein bound, and partial metabolism takes place in the liver. The serum half-life is 3 to 5 hours with normal kidney function. The excretion of the drug occurs in the urine and feces.

Action

Ciprofloxacin inhibits DNA gyrase in susceptible organisms and inhibits the supercoiled DNA, promoting breakage of the double-stranded DNA.

Use

Healthcare providers use ciprofloxacin for the treatment of *P. aeruginosa* in patients with necrotizing otitis externa. The cure rate with fluoroquinolones is approximately 90%. (If the causative agent is *Aspergillus*, amphotericin B is the drug of choice [see Chapter 24].) Table 60.3 gives route and dosage information for ciprofloxacin and other oral anti-infective drugs.

Patient-related variables specific to the use of ciprofloxacin include reproduction, pregnancy, and lactation. No animal reproduction studies have been conducted with ciprofloxacin otic solution. When administered systemically, ciprofloxacin enters the breast milk. When administered topically, ciprofloxacin is found in significantly lower levels in breast milk than when administered systemically.

Adverse Effects

Patients generally tolerate ciprofloxacin well. The most frequent adverse effects are gastrointestinal (GI) and include nausea, vomiting, and abdominal discomfort. Dizziness and mild headache may occur. Allergic and skin reactions have also been reported. Photosensitivity can occur while taking ciprofloxacin with exposure to direct or indirect sunlight. Artificial light or sun lamps may also precipitate photosensitivity reactions. The U.S. Food and Drug Administration (FDA) has expanded the current **BOXED WARNING** ◆ for fluoroquinolones, including ciprofloxacin, not only alerting health professionals to the increased disabling risk of tendinitis and tendon rupture but also the significant risk of peripheral neuropathy, central nervous system and cardiac effects, and dermatologic and hypersensitivity reactions. The risk is greater for people older than 60 years of age; those with heart, kidney, and lung transplants; and those taking corticosteroid medications. Adverse effects can occur up to weeks after beginning fluoroquinolones and may potentially be permanent. Discontinuation of the drug is necessary with the development of adverse effects. Another **BOXED WARNING** ◆ exists for fluoroquinolones, including ciprofloxacin, because the drugs in this class may exacerbate muscle weakness in persons with myasthenia gravis; their use should be avoided in these patients. QT interval prolongation may occur, and the degree of severity varies by agent.

TABLE 60.3

DRUGS AT A GLANCE: Oral Anti-Infective Drugs

Drug	Routes and Dosage Ranges	
	Adults	**Children**
Amoxicillin (✦ Apo-Amoxi, JAMP-Amoxicillin, Pro-Amox-500)	250–500 mg PO every 8 h or 500–875 mg every 12 h	≥3 mo weighing <40 kg, 20–30 mg/kg/d PO in divided doses every 12 h Older than 3 mo, 20–45 mg/kg/d PO in divided doses every 8–12 h In severe case of acute otitis media, the dosage can be 80–100 mg/kg/d (immediate release) PO in divided doses every 8 h ≥12 y PO (extended release) same as adult dose
Ciprofloxacin (Cetraxal, Otiprio, Cipro; ✦ Cipro, Apo-Ciproflox, Priva-Ciprofloxacin)	200–400 mg IV every 12 h; then 250–750 mg PO every 12 h as symptoms decrease 0.5 mg of 0.2% otic solution into affected ear twice daily for 7 d 12 mg 6% otic suspension as a single dose	Not typically used in children as a first-line drug 15–20 mg/kg/dose PO twice daily; max dose 750 mg

Contraindications

Patients with a known sensitivity to ciprofloxacin should not receive the drug or any other fluoroquinolone. Administration of ciprofloxacin with tizanidine is contraindicated.

Nursing Implications

Preventing Interactions

Many medications, herbs, and foods interact with ciprofloxacin, increasing or decreasing its effects (see Box 19.3).

Administering the Medication

Parenteral administration of ciprofloxacin should occur over 60 minutes through a verified patent intravenous line. If signs and symptoms of hypersensitivity develop, it is important to discontinue the medication. Patients may take the oral preparation with food to reduce GI upset. However, they should not take it within 2 hours of eating dairy products, calcium-fortified juices, antacids, zinc, or iron. Enteral feedings should be discontinued for 1 to 2 hours prior to and after ciprofloxacin administration because drug absorption is decreased by more than 30% with enteral feedings.

Assessing for Therapeutic and Adverse Effects

The nurse assesses for diminished pain with chewing, otalgia, and otorrhea. The nurse also assesses the patient's kidney function during the course of treatment. It is also important to observe for any signs or symptoms of hypersensitivity to the medication.

Patient Teaching

Patient teaching guidelines for ciprofloxacin are listed in the Box 60.2.

> **BOX 60.2 Patient Teaching Guidelines for Ciprofloxacin**
>
> - Avoid exposure to sunlight and apply sunscreen during the course of drug treatment.
> - Do not operate machinery or drive if experiencing dizziness or light-headedness occurs.
> - Stay well hydrated during the course of treatment.
> - Do not drink calcium-fortified juices or dairy products while taking the drug.
> - Do not take antacids, zinc, or iron supplements during the course of drug treatment.
> - Report tendon pain to the primary care provider.
> - Report nausea, vomiting, or diarrhea.

> **NCLEX Success**
>
> 3. A 70-year-old patient has been diagnosed with necrotizing otitis media. What is the patient at risk for developing while being treated with ciprofloxacin?
>   A. edema
>   B. tendon rupture
>   C. decreased QT interval
>   D. chest pain

PENICILLIN: AMOXICILLIN

Amoxicillin, a penicillin, is the preferred antibacterial agent for the treatment of acute otitis media unless a child has received the drug within 30 days, also has purulent conjunctivitis, or is allergic to the drug. A consensus group convened by the Centers for Disease Control and Prevention recommended increasing the dose used for empiric treatment because of concerns about increasingly resistant strains of *Streptococcus pneumoniae*, which are theoretically susceptible to a higher dose. Combination of amoxicillin with clavulanic acid reestablishes amoxicillin's activity against beta-lactamase–producing bacteria, including *Haemophilus influenzae* and penicillinase-producing anaerobes.

Many people with acute otitis media do not benefit from antibiotics because the cause of their illness is not bacterial in origin, or their immune system clears the infection without the use of a drug. Unfortunately, no clinical criteria currently distinguish people with acute otitis media who require antibiotic therapy from those who do not.

Pharmacokinetics

Amoxicillin has a variable onset of action; it reaches a peak in 1 hour. The duration of action is 6 to 8 hours. The therapeutic half-life is 1 to 1.4 hours. Metabolism occurs in the liver, and excretion of unchanged drug is in the urine. Amoxicillin crosses the placenta and enters the breast milk, which is a consideration because penicillin agents are often given during pregnancy.

Action

Amoxicillin has bactericidal properties. It inhibits cell wall synthesis of sensitive organisms, resulting in cell death.

Use

Amoxicillin is administered for the treatment of acute otitis media. It is active against *S. pneumoniae*, *H. influenzae*, and *Streptococcus pyogenes*.

Patient-related variables specific to the use of amoxicillin include reproduction, pregnancy, and lactation. Penicillin antibiotics are considered compatible for use during pregnancy. Use these drugs cautiously when administered to patients who are breast-feeding.

Adverse Effects

The most common adverse effect is hypersensitivity to the medication, with the development of a rash or severe reactions with anaphylaxis. The most common GI adverse effects are glossitis, stomatitis, gastritis, sore throat, nausea, vomiting, abdominal pain, and diarrhea. Other adverse effects include the development of superinfections.

Contraindications

Contraindications to use of amoxicillin include a known hypersensitivity to penicillin, cephalosporin, or other allergens. In the event of a penicillin allergy without urticaria or anaphylaxis, prescribers order an antibiotic with additional beta-lactamase coverage (see Chapter 18).

Nursing Implications

Preventing Interactions

Potentially significant interactions with amoxicillin and other drugs may exist that may require dose or frequency modifications, additional monitoring, and/or alternate therapy. Amoxicillin may diminish or enhance the therapeutic effects of other drugs. Amoxicillin may diminish the therapeutic of several vaccines (i.e., cholera, bacillus Calmette-Guérin, and typhoid), mycophenolate, lactobacillus, and estriol. The drug may enhance the anticoagulant effects of vitamin K antagonists (e.g., warfarin) and methotrexate. Box 60.3 lists drugs that increase or decrease the effect of amoxicillin. No significant herbal interactions have been identified.

Administering the Medication

Amoxicillin is administered orally. It is necessary to take amoxicillin in divided doses around the clock within 1 hour of a meal. The patient should take the full course of antibiotics and not discontinue them, even if the otitis media seems to be improving.

Assessing for Therapeutic Effects

The nurse assesses for otalgia and otorrhea. Both pain and drainage may decrease with antibiotic therapy. It is also necessary to assess the patient's hearing. As the fullness of the tympanic membrane decreases, the patient reports improvement in hearing. The nurse inspects the tympanic membrane for bulging (see Fig. 60.1). As the infection resolves, the tympanic membrane becomes shiny gray with a visible cone of light from the otoscope (Fig. 60.2).

> **Quality and Safety Alert: Evidence-Based Practice**
>
> Van Uum et al. (2019) sought to clarify the reasons parents tend to be cautious about administering analgesics to their children suffering from acute otitis media. The qualitative study revealed that parents had difficulty recognizing earache and other symptoms related to ear infection. Parents stated that they consulted with the general practitioner and received insufficient information on the benefits of pain management. Parents who reported receiving an explanation about the use of antibiotics and specific information on pain management from the general practitioner were likely to use pain medication in the event of future episodes of acute otitis media. It is important that general practitioners and other members of the healthcare team assist caregivers in understanding the need for drug management of acute otitis media and pain management in children.

BOX 60.3 Drug Interactions: Amoxicillin

Drugs That Decreases the Effects of Amoxicillin
- Chloramphenicol and tetracycline
  Cause inhibition of the activity of amoxicillin

Drug That Increases the Effects of Amoxicillin
- Probenecid
  Prolongs the serum concentration and activity of amoxicillin

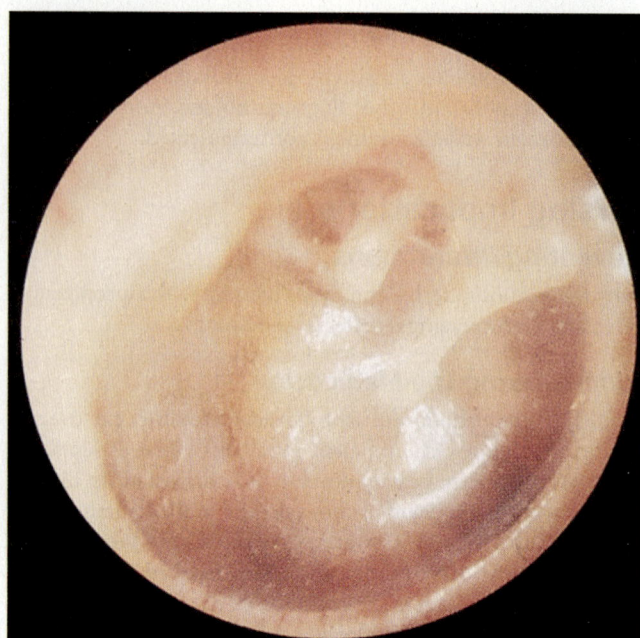

Figure 60.2. Normal tympanic membrane, after resolution of otitis media. (Adapted with permission from Moore, K. L., Dalley, A. F., & Agur, A. M. R. (2018). *Essential clinical anatomy* (8th ed., Fig. B8.42). Wolters Kluwer Health.)

Assessing for Adverse Effects

The nurse assesses the patient for signs and symptoms of hypersensitivity, with symptoms of wheezing, rash, or difficulty breathing. It is also important to assess for GI adverse effects such as nausea, vomiting, stomatitis, mouth irritation, sore throat, abdominal pain, and diarrhea. In addition, the nurse assesses for signs of superinfection.

Patient Teaching

Box 60.4 lists patient teaching guidelines for amoxicillin.

NCLEX Success

4. Which of the following assessment findings reveals that the amoxicillin is decreasing the symptoms of acute otitis media?
   A. retracted tympanic membrane
   B. otalgia
   C. otorrhea
   D. visible cone of light

5. A 76-year-old patient is receiving amoxicillin for acute otitis media. The patient also has gout. Which of the following antigout medications increases the effect of amoxicillin?
   A. allopurinol
   B. probenecid
   C. aspirin
   D. acetaminophen

| BOX 60.4 | **Patient Teaching Guidelines for Amoxicillin** |

Self- or Caregiver Administration
- Ensure that the child takes the entire course of the drug.
- Administer the drug around the clock.
- Take the medication within an hour of completing a meal.
- Report persistent ear pain or diminished hearing.

Unfolding Patient Stories: Toua Xiong • Part 2

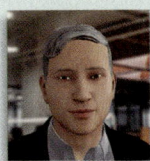

Think back to Toua Xiong, a 64-year-old male with emphysema from Chapter 33. He presents to the clinic with left ear pain and fever following an upper respiratory infection. The provider prescribes amoxicillin for acute otitis media. What patient education would the nurse provide on amoxicillin and the treatment options for fever and pain relief? How would the nurse differentiate a hypersensitivity reaction to amoxicillin from worsening respiratory symptoms associated with an acute exacerbation of emphysema?

Care for Toua and other patients in a realistic virtual environment: *vSim for Nursing* (thepoint.lww.com/vSimPharm). Practice documenting these patients' care in DocuCare (thepoint.lww.com/DocuCareEHR).

ADJUVANT MEDICATIONS TO TREAT PAIN AND FEVER RELATED TO INFECTIONS OF THE EAR

Infections of the ear produce pain and may result in fever. The adjuvant medications most commonly administered for relief of pain and fever include agents such as aspirin, acetaminophen (Tylenol), or ibuprofen (Motrin) (see Chapter 16).

Salicylates

Aspirin is the prototype of the salicylates. Children should not take this drug. Aspirin has the ability to inhibit prostaglandin synthesis (a cause of the inflammatory effect). Its role in fever reduction, or antipyretic action, is not understood. Experts believe that aspirin acts on the thermoregulatory center of the hypothalamus, blocking the effects of the endogenous pyrogens and inhibiting the synthesis of prostaglandins. Administration is oral or rectal. To prevent gastric irritation, it is necessary to take the oral preparation with food.

Nonnarcotic Analgesic Antipyretic

Acetaminophen is equivalent to aspirin in analgesic and antipyretic effects, and it possesses weak anti-inflammatory properties. This drug is safe for children. It acts directly on the hypothalamus to increase vasodilation and sweating. Although the primary mechanism of action of acetaminophen is not fully understood, it is believed to inhibit cyclooxygenase (COX), with a predominant effect on COX-2. Acetaminophen is oral or rectal. Alternating acetaminophen and ibuprofen every 4 hours over a 3-day period to control fever in young children (ages 6 to 36 months) has been shown to be more effective than monotherapy with either agent. A discussion of the prototype considerations is found in Chapter 16.

Propionic Acid Derivatives

Ibuprofen (Motrin, Advil) is a nonsteroidal anti-inflammatory agent that inhibits prostaglandin synthesis in both the central and peripheral nervous systems. There are two forms of cyclooxygenase, COX-1 and COX-2. Ibuprofen blocks prostaglandin synthesis and modulates T-cell production, inhibiting the chemotaxis of the inflammatory cells and increasing their destruction. The drug blocks COX-1 and COX-2 and is more selective with COX-1. It is administered to reduce pain, inflammation, and fever. Ibuprofen is administered orally or intravenously. For treatment of otalgia and fever, the drug is administered orally. Chapter 16 describes ibuprofen as a prototype.

THE NURSING PROCESS

A concept map outlines the nursing process related to drug therapy considerations in this chapter. Additional nursing implications related to the disease process should also be considered in care decisions.

Assessment
- Assess for diminished hearing and signs of ear infection.
- Inspect the external ear and palpate the auricle and surrounding tissue.
- Inspect for alterations in skin integrity of the outer ear.
- Inspect the tympanic membrane with an otoscope.
- Assess for fluid in the eardrum and absence of the cone of light.
- Interview the patient related to fullness of the ear, diminished hearing, or pain.
- Assess temperature.

Outcomes of Therapy
The patient will
- Take the entire course of anti-infective agents safely and accurately.
- Take anti-inflammatory/antipyretic agents as ordered to reduce pain and fever.
- Not insert any items in the ear.
- Use earplugs when swimming.
- Dry the ear carefully following bathing or swimming.

Nursing Interventions
- Instruct the patient on the administration of ear drops.
- Instruct on the medication regimen and about administration of anti-infective agents around the clock.
- Assess the tympanic membrane for signs of infection.
- Assess the lesion of the external ear for signs of healing.
- Instruct parents to never let a baby sleep drinking a bottle (this promotes the development of otitis media).
- Administer pain and fever reducers as needed.
- Assess for ear drainage.

Evaluation
- Interview the patient for relief of symptoms with the completion of the course of anti-infective agents.
- Interview the patient regarding compliance with the medication regimen.
- Assess the external and middle ear for signs of infection or inflammation.

Visit thePoint at http://thePoint.lww.com/Frandsen13e for answers to NCLEX Success questions (in Appendix A), answers to Clinical Application Case Studies (in Appendix B), additional information on etiology and pathophysiology, and more!

REFERENCES AND RESOURCES

Brennan-Jones, C. G., Head, K., Chong, L. Y., Burton, M. J., Schilder, A. G. M., & Bhutta, M. F. (2020). Topical antibiotics for chronic suppurative otitis media. *Cochrane Database of Systematic Reviews*, (1), CD013051. doi: 10.1002/14651858.CD013051.pub2

Gandis, J. R., & Yu, V. L. (2021). Malignant (necrotizing) external otitis. UpToDate. Lexi-comp, Inc.

Goguen, L. A. (2021). External otitis: Treatment. *UpToDate*. Lexi-comp, Inc.

Hinkle, J. H., Cheever, K. H., & Overbaugh, K. (2021). *Brunner & Suddarth's textbook of medical-surgical nursing* (15th ed.). Wolters Kluwer.

Limb, C. J., Lustig, L. R., & Durand, M. L. (2021). Acute otitis media in adults. *UpToDate*. Lexi-comp, Inc.

Lippincott Advisor for Education. (2021). *Drugs*. Lippincott Williams and Wilkins.

Norris, T. L. (2019). *Porth's pathophysiology: Concepts of altered health states* (10th ed.). Wolters Kluwer.

UpToDate. (2021). *Drug information*. Lexi-Comp, Inc.

Van Uum, R. T., Venekamp, R. P., Schilder, A. G. M., Damoiseaux, R. A. M. J., & Anthierens, S. (2019). Pain management in acute otitis media: A qualitative study of parents' view and expectations. *BMC Family Practice, 20*(18), 1–7. doi: 10.1186/s12875-019-0908-9

CHAPTER 61

Drug Therapy for Disorders of the Skin

LEARNING OBJECTIVES

After studying this chapter, you should be able to:

1. Understand the corticosteroid drug therapy used to treat pruritus, dermatoses, dermatitis, and plaque psoriasis.
2. Understand the antimicrobial drug therapy used to treat bacterial skin infections, rosacea, bacterial vaginosis, impetigo, and burn wounds.
3. Understand the antifungal drug therapy used to treat tinea pedis, cutaneous candidiasis, seborrheic dermatitis, and dandruff.
4. Understand the antiviral drug therapy used to treat herpes genitalis and herpes labialis.
5. Understand the drug therapy for miscellaneous skin disorders.
6. Understand the drug therapy for acne and acne vulgaris, including the prototype, action, use, adverse effects, contraindications, and nursing implications for the retinoids.
7. Implement the nursing process in the care of patients with disorders of the skin.

CLINICAL APPLICATION CASE STUDY

Gerard Aylward is a 16-year-old high school sophomore who has a history of asthma. As a child, he received allergy shots on a weekly basis. He now has a severe case of acne vulgaris. He has been taking tetracycline hydrochloride 500 mg orally every 12 hours. His acne remains severe, and his dermatologist has decided to discontinue the tetracycline and start isotretinoin 35 mg orally two times per day for 15 weeks.

KEY TERMS

Acne: a disorder of the hair follicles and sebaceous glands that become clogged. This leads to pimples and cysts. It is a common condition that usually develops during puberty due to hormonal changes. The condition is either superficial or deep

Acne vulgaris: a common chronic skin disease involving blockage and/or inflammation of hair follicles and sebaceous glands

Dermatitis: a general term denoting an inflammatory response of the skin to injuries, irritants, allergens, or trauma; also referred to as eczema

Erythema: redness of the skin

Pruritus: itching of the skin

Psoriasis: scaling, dry, erythematous skin eruptions on the elbows, knees, scalp, and trunk

Rosacea: chronic disease characterized by erythema, telangiectasis, and acnelike lesions of facial skin

Tinea pedis: common type of ringworm infection; also called athlete's foot

Toxic epidermal necrosis: widespread sloughing of the skin with severe mucositis

Urticaria: inflammatory response characterized by a skin lesion called a wheal, a raised edematous area with a pale center and red border, which itches intensely; also known as hives

INTRODUCTION

This chapter discusses the disorders of the skin and the treatment of these disorders with corticosteroids, antimicrobial, antifungal, antiviral, and miscellaneous drugs. In addition, it introduces acne and acne vulgaris and the drugs administered for their treatment.

OVERVIEW OF DRUG THERAPY FOR SKIN DISORDERS

Many different drugs are used to prevent or treat dermatologic disorders. **Dermatitis** is the inflammatory response of the skin to injuries, irritants, allergens, or trauma. It can also be referred to as eczema. The general treatment goals for many skin disorders are to relieve symptoms (e.g., dryness, pruritus, inflammation, infection), eradicate or improve lesions, promote healing and repair, restore skin integrity, and prevent recurrence. Specific goals often depend on the condition being treated. With acne, for example, treatment aims to minimize as many pathogenic factors as possible by reducing sebum production, preventing the formation of microcomedones, suppressing *Propionibacterium acnes*, and reducing inflammation that may lead to scarring.

Topical drugs are used primarily for local effects of skin and mucous membranes, and systemic absorption is undesirable. Major factors that increase systemic absorption of topical medications include damaged or inflamed skin, high concentrations of the drug, and application of the drug to the face or mucous membranes, to large areas of the body, or for prolonged periods. With topical medications, cautious use is recommended with infants and young children due to the fact they have more permeable skin and are more likely to absorb the topical drugs. Box 61.1 presents general patient teaching information for topical medications for skin disorders.

Corticosteroid Drug Therapy

Corticosteroids (see Chapter 17) are used to treat inflammation in many dermatologic conditions. They are most often applied topically but also may be given orally or parenterally. The choice of corticosteroid depends on the acuity, severity, location, and extent of the condition being treated. A general principle regarding the use of topical corticosteroids is to begin with the lowest potency and to apply the drug for the shortest duration of time.

The administration of corticosteroids can reduce **erythema** (redness of the skin). In addition, corticosteroids are administered to reduce psoriasis and seborrheic dermatitis. **Psoriasis** is a chronic skin condition with scaling, dry erythematous skin eruptions on the elbows, knees, scalp, and trunk. Seborrheic dermatitis is a chronic, relapsing disease involving the sebaceous glands. The simple form of seborrheic dermatitis is called dandruff.

The action of corticosteroids reduces itching of the skin known as **pruritus**. Table 61.1 identifies topical corticosteroids administered to relieve these symptoms. Topical corticosteroids have anti-inflammatory, antipruritic, and vasoconstrictive properties. They depress the inflammatory processes by suppressing the release of kinins, histamine, and prostaglandins. They are well absorbed through the skin to decrease the inflammatory process of dermatitis. The most common adverse effect of topical corticosteroids is hypersensitivity at the site of application. High potency corticosteroids, such as amcinonide, can produce Cushing syndrome with suppression of the hypothalamic–pituitary–adrenal (HPA) axis. This is a risk if an occlusive dressing is applied over the medication or with long-term use. The use of high potency topical corticosteroids should not exceed 4 weeks, but severe lesions can be treated for longer periods of time. Topical corticosteroids are not contraindicated in pregnancy. Topical corticosteroids should not be applied to the breast or areolar tissue until breast-feeding is stopped.

Concept Mastery Alert

Avoid applying a dressing over a topical corticosteroid. Covering the ointment, especially with an impervious dressing, increases the likelihood that localized adverse reactions will occur.

NCLEX Success

1. A patient has been prescribed amcinonide for pruritus. Which of the following interventions is contraindicated with this medication?
   A. Apply a thin layer to the pruritus 2–3 times per day.
   B. Cover the medication with a dressing.
   C. Clean the area with a mild soap prior to applying the cream.
   D. Report increased redness to the prescriber.

Antibacterial Drug Therapy

Bacterial skin infections are quite common and are most often caused by streptococci or staphylococci. Cellulitis is characterized by erythema, tenderness, and edema, which may spread to subcutaneous tissue, producing symptoms of generalized

BOX 61.1 Patient Teaching Guidelines for Topical Medications for Skin Disorders

General Considerations

- Promote healthy skin by consuming a balanced diet, taking personal hygiene measures, avoiding excessive exposure to sunlight, avoiding skin injuries, and lubricating dry skin. Healthy skin is less susceptible to inflammation, infections, and other disorders, and heals more rapidly.
- Prevent actinic keratosis and skin cancer beginning in childhood by minimizing sun exposure, wearing sun-protective clothing, and using sunscreen.
- Topical corticosteroids come in many vehicles (e.g., creams, lotions, ointments) that cannot be used interchangeably. In addition, they should not be covered with occlusive dressings unless instructed to do so.
- In the home care setting, when applying medication to wounds secondary to burns, the drugs are to be applied using sterile gloves or sterile applicators with cotton tips.
- Adverse effects of topical medications may involve the skin (e.g., irritation, infection) where the drug is applied or the entire body, when the drug is absorbed into the bloodstream. Systemic absorption is increased when the drug is highly potent; applied to inflamed skin, over a large surface area, or frequently; or covered with an occlusive dressing (e.g., plastic wrap). Systemic absorption is of most concern with corticosteroid preparations.
- Some ways to prevent or decrease skin disorders include the following:
  - Identifying and avoiding, when possible, substances that cause skin irritation and inflammation (e.g., harsh cleaning products, latex gloves, cosmetics, pet dander).
  - Bathing in warm water with a mild cleanser (e.g., Cetaphil), patting skin dry, and applying lotions or oils (e.g., Eucerin, mineral oil) to lubricate skin and decrease dryness.
  - Avoiding scratching, squeezing, or rubbing skin lesions. These behaviors cause additional skin damage and increase risks of infection. Fingernails should be cut short; cotton gloves can be worn at night.
  - Maintaining a cool environment; preventing sweating.
  - Applying cold compresses to inflamed, itchy skin.
  - Using baking soda or colloidal oatmeal (Aveeno) in bath water to relieve itching.
- If you are taking an oral antihistamine to relieve itching, take it on a regular schedule, around the clock, for greater effectiveness.
- Individuals can wear cosmetics over most topical medications. If unclear, ask a healthcare provider whether makeup is permissible. With acne, use noncomedogenic makeup, moisturizers, and sunscreens.

Self-Administration

- For topical application to skin lesions, cleanse the skin and remove previously applied medication to promote drug contact with the affected area of the skin.
- Wash the skin and pat it dry.
- Apply a small amount of the drug preparation and rub it in well. A thin layer of medication is effective and decreases the incidence and severity of adverse effects. With acne and rosacea, preventing skin lesions is easier than eliminating lesions that are already present. As a result, topical medications should be applied to the general area of involvement rather than individual lesions.
- Wash hands before and after application. Wash before to avoid infection; wash afterward to avoid transferring the drug to the face or eyes and causing adverse reactions.
- With azelaic acid (Azelex) for acne, use for the full prescribed period, do not use occlusive dressings or wrappings, and keep away from mouth, eyes, and other mucous membranes (if it gets into eyes, wash eyes with a large amount of water).
- With benzoyl peroxide for acne:
  - With cleansing solutions, wash affected areas once or twice daily. Wet skin areas to be treated before applying the cleanser. Rinse thoroughly and pat dry. Reduce use if excessive drying or peeling occurs.
  - With other dosage forms, apply once daily initially and gradually increase to two or three times daily if needed. Cleanse skin, let dry completely, and apply a small amount over the affected area. Reduce dosage if excessive drying, redness, or discomfort occurs. If excessive stinging or burning occurs after any single application, remove with mild soap and water and resume use the next day. Keep away from eyes, mouth, and inside of nose. Rinse with water if contact occurs with these areas. Avoid other sources of skin irritation (e.g., sunlight, sunlamps, other topical acne medications).

---

malaise, chills, and fever. Folliculitis is an infection of the hair follicles most often on the scalp or bearded areas of the face. Furuncles and carbuncles are infections usually caused by staphylococci. Impetigo is a superficial skin infection caused by streptococci or staphylococci. These infections are treated with antibacterial agents which are administered orally, parenterally, or topically to treat dermatologic infections. Topical antibacterials are used to treat superficial skin disorders such as acne and skin infections. Systemic antibacterials (e.g., cephalosporins; Chapter 18) are used for soft tissue infections such as cellulitis and postoperative wound infections. Tetracyclines (Chapter 20) are used for acne and rosacea. **Acne** is a disorder of the hair follicles and sebaceous glands that become clogged. This leads to pimples and cysts. It is a common condition that usually develops during puberty due to hormonal changes. The condition is either superficial or deep. **Rosacea** is a chronic disease characterized by erythema, telangiectasis, and acnelike lesions of facial skin. Fluoroquinolones (Chapter 19) (e.g., ciprofloxacin) may be used to treat soft tissue infections caused by gram-negative organisms. Table 61.2 identifies the antibacterial topical agents

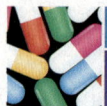

TABLE 61.1
DRUGS AT A GLANCE: Topical Corticosteroid Preparations

Drug	Indications	Route and Dosage Ranges
Amcinonide; TARO-Amcinonide	Inflammatory and pruritic manifestations of corticosteroid-responsive dermatoses	High potency corticosteroid cream, lotion, or ointment 0.1%: Apply thin film 2–3 times per day
Betamethasone, dipropionate (Luxiq, Sernivo); Betaderm, Beteflam, Celestoderm V, Diprolene, Rivasone Scalp, Rolene, Rosone, TARO-Sone, TEVA-Ectosone	Dermatoses; dermatoses of the scalp, and plaque psoriasis	Cream, gel, lotion, foam, or spray Cream, gel, or lotion: Apply sparingly to affected areas Foam: Invert the can and dispense a small amount on a saucer. Do not dispense directly into the hands. Massage small amounts until foam disappears. Plaque psoriasis (spray patch is approved in Canada for patients 18 y and older): Clean and dry area before applying the patch. Cut the patch to size. Peel off the adhesive and apply the medicated side to the affected area.
Clobetasol propionate (Clobetasol Propionate E, Clobetavix, Clobex, Clobex Spray, Clodan, Impeklo, Tovet; APO-Clobetasol, Clobex, Clobex Spray, Dermovate, TARO-Clobetasol, TARO-Clobetasol Topical)	Dermatoses, psoriasis	Foam, cream, spray, and shampoo Foam: Apply twice daily for 2 wk Cream: Apply twice daily for 2–4 wk Spray: Apply by spraying directly to affected area and gently rub daily for 2–4 wk Shampoo: Apply thin film to dry scalp once daily, leave in place 15 min, add water and lather, rinse thoroughly (limit treatment to 4 wk)
Desoximetasone (Topicort Spray; Desoxi, Topicort)	Dermatoses, plaque psoriasis	Cream, gel, ointment, spray Apply a thin layer to affected area twice daily
Diflorasone diacetate (ApexiCon E, Psorcon)	Dermatoses	Apply sparingly 1–3 times per day
Fluocinonide (Vanos; Lidex, Lyderm, Tiamol)	Acute dermatitis, Psoriasis	Cream, gel, ointment, solution Apply in a thin layer 2–4 times daily
Flurandrenolide (Cordran, Nolix)	Dermatoses	Cream, lotion, ointment: Apply a thin layer 2–3 times per day Tape: Apply 1–2 times per day
Halobetasol propionate (Halobetasol Propionate, Lexette, Ultravate; Bryhali, Ultravate)	Dermatoses, plaque psoriasis	Lotion, foam, cream, and ointment Lotion: Apply 0.01% in a thin layer to affected skin daily for up to 8 wk Foam: Apply 0.05% in a thin layer to affected skin twice daily for up to 2 wk Cream and Ointment: Apply sparingly 1–2 times daily, do not exceed 2 wk

commonly administered for the prevention and treatment of skin infections.

Trauma to the skin due to lacerations, abrasions, puncture wounds, surgical incisions, or burns can lead to the development of infection. Cutaneous ulcerations caused by trauma and impaired circulation may become inflamed or infected. The application of topical antibacterial agents such as neomycin, bacitracin, or polymyxin or a combination ointment has been shown to enhance healing particularly with sutured lacerations. For patients at greatest risk of the development of a postoperative infection, mupirocin can be prescribed to prevent a postoperative surgical infection.

> **Quality and Safety Alert: Safety**
>
> Mupirocin is administered for surgical prophylaxis in patients who are carriers of methicillin-resistant *Staphylococcus aureus* (MRSA). Intranasal mupirocin is administered twice daily for 5 days prior to surgery.

Burn injuries possess one of the greatest risks for the development of infection. Commonly, topical agents containing antimicrobial ointments, silver sulfadiazine, bismuth-impregnated petroleum gauze, mafenide, and chlorhexidine are applied to prevent infection. The silver containing agents release sliver into

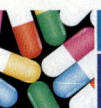

TABLE 61.2
DRUGS AT A GLANCE: Antimicrobial Drugs for Skin Disorders

Drug	Indications	Route and Dosage Ranges
Antibacterial Drugs		
Azelaic acid (Azelex, Finacea; ❋ Finacea)	Acne (20% cream) Rosacea (15% gel)	Children and Adults To lesions, twice daily
Bacitracin	Bacterial skin infections	Children and Adults To affected area, one to three times daily
Benzoyl peroxide (Acne-Clear, Benziq, others; ❋ Benzac W Wash 10 Nettoyant)	Acne	Children: ≥7 y and Adults To affected areas, once or twice daily
Clindamycin (Cleocin, Cleocin T, Clindamycin ETZ, Clindacin Pac, Clindacin-P, Clindagel, Clindesse, Evoclin; ❋, Dalacin Vaginal, TARO-Clindamycin)	Acne	Children: ≥7 y and Adults To affected areas, twice daily
Erythromycin (Ery, Erygel)	Acne	Children: ≥7 y and Adults To affected areas, twice daily
Gentamicin	Skin infections caused by susceptible organisms	Children and Adults To infected areas, three to four times daily
Metronidazole (MetroCream, MetroLotion, Noritate, Nuvessa Rosadan, Vandazole; ❋ Flagyl, Metrogel, Nidagel, Noritate)	Rosacea Bacterial Vaginosis	Children: ≥6 months and Adults To affected area, once or twice daily Children: >12 y and Adults One applicator full in the vaginal vault once daily at bedtime for 5 d
Mupirocin (Centany, Centany AT)	Impetigo caused by *Staphylococcus aureus*, beta-hemolytic streptococci, or *Streptococcus pyogenes* Eradication of nasal colonization with methicillin-resistant *S. aureus*	Children and Adults Impetigo: ointment, to affected areas, three times daily Other skin lesions: cream, three times daily for 10 d Eradication of nasal colonization: ointment from single-use tube, one half in each nostril, morning and evening for 5 d
Retapamulin (Altabax)	Impetigo	Children and Adults To affected area, twice daily for 5 d
Silver sulfadiazine (Silvadene; ❋ Flamazine)	Prevent or treat infection in burn wounds caused by *Pseudomonas* and many other organisms	Children and Adults To affected area, once or twice daily, using sterile technique
Bacitracin and polymyxin B (Polysporin)	Bacterial skin infections	Children and Adults To lesions, one to three times daily
Erythromycin/benzoyl peroxide (Benzamycin; ❋ Benzamycin)	Acne	Children: ≥7 y and Adults To affected areas, twice daily
Neomycin, polymyxin B, and bacitracin	Bacterial skin infections	Children and Adults To lesions, two or three times daily

the wound, providing broad-spectrum antimicrobial action and enhancing anti-inflammatory properties. In addition to burn injuries, it is important to understand **toxic epidermal necrolysis** and Stevens–Johnson syndrome. Toxic epidermal necrolysis is the widespread sloughing of skin and development of severe mucositis that is associated with a risk of sepsis. Stevens–Johnson syndrome is generalized blistering with skin sloughing very similar to that of burn injuries. The onset of toxic epidermal necrolysis is 4 days to 8 weeks after continuous use of a drug. Common drugs that result in Stevens–Johnson syndrome are allopurinol, lamotrigine, sulfasalazine, nevirapine, and oxicam. Amoxicillin and ampicillin have also been linked to Stevens–Johnson syndrome. The antibacterial treatment of the wounds is based on the culture results.

NCLEX Success

2. A patient is admitted to the emergency department with skin sloughing and pain. What is the priority question the nurse should ask the patient?
   A. Have you traveled out of the country?
   B. Have you been near someone with the same skin condition?
   C. Have you been taking any new medications in the last 4 days to 8 weeks?
   D. Have you been exposed to measles or Mpox?

Unfolding Patient Stories: Harry Hadley • Part 2

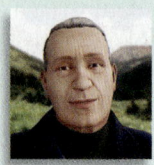

Recall Harry Hadley from Chapter 19, who is being treated for cellulitis of his right lower leg caused by a feral cat bite. Oral augmentin was changed to intravenous vancomycin when culture results identified MRSA. How would the nurse explain why the oral route was preferred over topical antibiotic application for the initial treatment of the feral cat bite and why the route of medication was subsequently changed from oral augmentin to intravenous vancomycin administration?

Care for Harry and other patients in a realistic virtual environment: *vSim for Nursing* (thepoint.lww.com/vSimPharm). Practice documenting these patients' care in DocuCare (thepoint.lww.com/DocuCareEHR).

Antifungal Drug Therapy

Fungal infections of the skin and mucus membranes are most often caused by *Candida albicans*. Oral candidiasis (thrush) involves mucus membranes of the mouth. It often occurs as a superinfection after the use of broad-spectrum antibiotics. Candidiasis of the vagina and vulva occurs with systemic antibiotic therapy and in females with diabetes mellitus. Intertrigo involves skin folds or areas where two skin surfaces are in contact. (e.g., groin, pendulous breasts). Tinea corporis infections are fungal infections of the skin, also known as body ringworm. These infections are found on the body or the face. **Tinea pedis**, commonly called athlete's foot, is a type of ringworm infection found on the foot and between the toes.

The treatment of antifungal infections, also referred to as dermatophyte infections, consists of topical or systemic antifungal agents. Table 61.3 identifies the most commonly prescribed antifungal agents. Nystatin (Chapter 24) is administered for candida albicans (thrush). It binds to the sterols in the fungal cell membrane, altering its cellular wall permeability to promote the leakage of the cellular contents. Dermatophyte infections are limited to the epidermis and are treated with butenafine, ciclopirox, clotrimazole, econazole, ketoconazole, miconazole, oxiconazole, terbinafine, or tolnaftate. Butenafine imparts a fungicidal activity on the dermatophytes, causing an inhibition of the ergosterol synthesis to weaken the fungal cell membrane. The azoles bind to the phospholipids in the fungal cell to alter the cell wall permeability and release intracellular elements.

Antiviral Drug Therapy

Viral infections of the skin include verrucae (warts) and herpes infections. There are two types of herpes infections: herpes simplex type 1 infections usually involve the face or neck (e.g., fever blisters or cold sores on the lips) and type 2 infections involve the genitalia. Other herpes infections include varicella (chickenpox) and herpes zoster (shingles). Acyclovir (Chapter 23) is administered topically. It is converted to acyclovir monophosphate and then to acyclovir triphosphate by other cellular enzymes. Acyclovir triphosphate inhibits DNA synthesis and viral replication to be incorporated in the viral DNA. Penciclovir is also a topical agent administered for the treatment of herpes simplex 1 or 2. Its action is similar to acyclovir by converting to penciclovir triphosphate to inhibit the herpes simplex virus polymerase to inhibit DNA synthesis and viral replication. Table 61.4 lists the topical antiviral agents.

Other Drugs Used for Skin Disorders

The other drugs used for skin disorders include enzymes, immunosuppressants, antihistamines, local anesthetic agents, emollients, and moisturizers. Table 61.5 lists these medications and preparations.

Enzymes

Enzymes such as trypsin, collagenase, papain, and bromelain are exogenous enzymatic agents used for wound debridement in patients who are not candidates for surgical debridement. The collagen in these products stimulates angiogenesis and increases epithelial tissue.

Immunosuppressant Drug Therapy

Immunosuppressants (see Chapter 13) may be used to treat inflammatory skin disorders. Two topical agents, tacrolimus (Protopic) ointment and pimecrolimus (Elidel) cream, are used for moderate to severe atopic dermatitis. However, the U.S. Food and Drug Administration (FDA) has issued **BOXED WARNING** ◆ for these drugs because both medications may cause a possible increased risk of skin cancer and lymphoma. Precautions include using them only when other drugs are ineffective and avoiding long-term use. Several systemic drugs, including alefacept (Amevive), etanercept (Enbrel), and infliximab (Remicade), are used for the treatment of severe psoriasis. The FDA has issued **BOXED WARNING** ◆ for these drugs concerning the increased risks of infection, and their long-term effects are unknown. In February 2022, tralokinumab was approved as an immunomodulator treatment for moderate to severe atopic dermatitis. In September

NCLEX Success

3. A patient diagnosed with atopic dermatitis receives a prescription for pimecrolimus cream. What is this patient at increased risk of developing?
   A. skin cancer
   B. infection
   C. papilledema
   D. joint pain

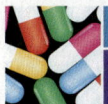

TABLE 61.3
DRUGS AT A GLANCE: Antifungal Drugs

Drug	Indications	Route and Dosage Ranges
Butenafine (Mentax)	Tinea pedis	Children and Adults To affected area, once daily for 2–4 wk
Ciclopirox (Ciclodan; ❋ APO-Ciclopirox, Penlac Nail Lacquer)	Tinea infections Cutaneous candidiasis	Children: ≥10 y and Adults To affected area, twice daily for 2–4 wk
Clotrimazole (Lotrimin AF, Shopko Athletes Foot; ❋ Canesten Topical, Clotrimaderm)	Tinea infections Cutaneous candidiasis	Children and Adults To affected areas, twice daily for 2–4 wk
Econazole (Ecoza, Zolpak)	Tinea infections Cutaneous candidiasis	Children and Adults To affected areas, once daily for tinea infections, twice daily for candidiasis
Ketoconazole (Extina, Xolegel; ❋ Ketoderm)	Tinea infections Cutaneous candidiasis Seborrheic dermatitis Dandruff	Adults Tinea infections and candidiasis: to affected areas, once daily for 2–4 wk Children: <2 y and Adults Seborrheic dermatitis: twice daily for 4 wk Shampoo: Apply to wet hair, lather, and rinse; Used every 3–4 d for 8 wk
Miconazole (Micatin, Podactin, others)	Tinea infections Cutaneous candidiasis	Children: >2 y and Adults To affected area, once daily for 2–4 wk
Naftifine (Naftin)	Tinea infections	Children: >12 y and Adults To affected areas, once daily with cream, twice daily with gel
Nystatin (Nyamyc, Nystop)	Candidiasis of skin and mucous membranes	Children and Adults To affected areas, two or three times daily until healed
Oxiconazole (Oxistat)	Tinea infections	Children: >12 y and Adults To affected areas, once or twice daily for 2–4 wk
Terbinafine (Lamisil; ❋ Lamisil)	Tinea infections	Children: >12 y and Adults To affected areas, twice daily for 1–4 wk
Tolnaftate (Dr. Gs Clear Gel, Podactin, Tinactin, and others)	Tinea infections	Children: >2 y and Adults To affected areas, twice daily for 2–4 wk

2022, dupilumab was approved as a treatment for atopic dermatitis and chronic rhinosinusitis. This medication is administered subcutaneously.

Antihistamines

Antihistamines (Chapter 32) are administered orally for the treatment of urticaria. **Urticaria** is an inflammatory response characterized by a skin lesion called a wheal, a raised edematous area with a pale center and red border, which itches intensely; also known as hives. The first-generation antihistamines include diphenhydramine, chlorpheniramine, and hydroxyzine. The second-generation antihistamines are less sedating. The drugs in this class include cetirizine, levocetirizine, loratadine, desloratadine, and fexofenadine.

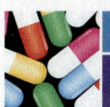

TABLE 61.4
DRUGS AT A GLANCE: Antiviral Drugs

Drug	Indications	Route and Dosage Ranges
Acyclovir (Sitavig, Zovirax; ❋ APO-Acyclovir, TEVA-Acyclovir, Zovirax)	Herpes genitalis Herpes labialis in patients who are immunosuppressed	Children: >12 y and Adults To lesions, every 3 h six times daily for 7 d
Penciclovir (Denavir)	Herpes labialis	Children: >12 y and Adults To lesions, every 2 h while awake for 4 d

TABLE 61.5

DRUGS AT A GLANCE: Other Drugs Used for Skin Disorders

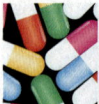

Drug	Indications	Route and Dosage Ranges
Enzymes		
Trypsin (TBC)	Debridement of infected wounds (e.g., decubitus and varicose ulcers)	Adults Topically by spray twice daily
Immunomodulators		
Dupilumab (Dupixent; 🍁 Dupixent)	Atopic dermatitis	Children: ≥6 months–<6 y: Atopic dermatitis (AD), moderate to severe: Note: May be used in combination with topical corticosteroids or topical calcineurin inhibitors. Infants ≥6 months and children <6 y: Note: Prefilled syringe may be used in ages ≥6 months; prefilled pen is only for use in ages ≥2 y. An initial loading dose is not necessary in pediatric patients <6 y 5 to <15 kg: Sub-Q: 200 mg every 4 weeks. 15 to <30 kg: Sub-Q: 300 mg every 4 weeks. Children ≥6 years and adolescents ≤17 years: Prefilled pen, prefilled syringe 15 to <30 kg: Sub-Q: Initial: 600 mg once (administered as two 300 mg injections), followed by a maintenance dose of 300 mg every 4 weeks 30 to <60 kg: Sub-Q: Initial: 400 mg once (administered as two 200 mg injections), followed by a maintenance dose of 200 mg every other week ≥60 kg: Sub-Q: Initial: 600 mg once (administered as two 300 mg injections), followed by a maintenance dose of 300 mg every other week Adolescents ≥18 y: Prefilled pen, prefilled syringe: Sub-Q: Initial: 600 mg once (administered as two 300 mg injections), followed by a maintenance dose of 300 mg every other week Adults: Sub-Q: 600 mg once (given as two 300 mg injections), followed by 300 mg once every other week
Pimecrolimus (Elidel; © C.A. Pilotti and P.D. Bridge 2023. Ganoderma Diseases of Tropical Crops (C.A. Pilotti and P.D. Bridge) Elidel)	Atopic dermatitis	Children >2 y and Adults Topically to affected skin, twice daily
Tacrolimus (Protopic; 🍁 Protopic)	Atopic dermatitis	Children ≥2–15 y: 0.03% ointment apply a thin layer topically twice daily Adults 0.03% or 0.1% Topically to affected skin, twice daily
Tralokinumab (Adbry)	Atopic dermatitis	Adults 600 mg subcutaneous (given as four 150 mg injections) once, followed by 300 mg (given as two 150 mg injections) once every other week. In patients with body weight <100 kg who achieve clear or almost clear skin after 16 wk of therapy, dosage should be reduced to 300 mg (given as two injections) every 4 wk.
Other Drugs		
Becaplermin (Regranex)	Diabetic skin ulcers	Children: ≥16 y and Adults Topically to ulcer; amount calculated according to size of the ulcer
Calcipotriene (Calcitrene, Dovonex, Sorilux; 🍁 Dovonex)	Psoriasis	Children: ≥2 y and Adults Topically to skin lesions twice daily
Capsaicin (Alivio, Allevess, Arthritis Pain Relief, Asperflex Hot Pain Reliever, Capsaicin HP, and others)	Relief of pain associated with rheumatoid arthritis, osteoarthritis, and neuralgias	Children: ≥12 y and Adults Topically to affected area, up to three or four times daily
Coal tar (Beta Care Betatar Gel, DSH Tar. Pentrax Gold, Psoriasin)	Psoriasis Dermatitis	Children and Adults Topically to skin, in various concentrations and preparations

TABLE 61.5

DRUGS AT A GLANCE: Other Drugs Used for Skin Disorders (Continued)

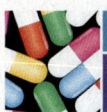

Drug	Indications	Route and Dosage Ranges
Colloidal oatmeal (Aveeno)	Pruritus	Children and Adults Topically as a bath solution (1 cup in bathtub of water)
Fluorouracil (Carac, Efudex, Fluoroplex, Tolak; 🍁 Efudex, Tolak)	Actinic keratoses Superficial basal cell carcinomas	Adults Topically to skin lesions twice daily for 2–6 wk
Salicylic acid (AcNesic, Bensal HP, Gordofilm, Clear Away One Step Wart Remover, Neutrogena Oil-Free Acne Wash, and others)	Removal of warts, corns, calluses Superficial fungal infections Seborrheic dermatitis Acne Psoriasis	Children and Adults Topically to skin lesions
Selenium sulfide (Anti-Dandruff)	Dandruff Tinea versicolor	Topically to scalp as shampoo once or twice weekly

Local Anesthetic Agents

Local anesthetic agents (benzocaine, dibucaine, pramoxine), astringents and protectants (witch hazel and zinc oxide), corticosteroids (hydrocortisone, Anusol-HC, Preparation H), and bulk forming laxatives to prevent constipation are used to treat symptomatic hemorrhoids in adults. For thrombosed external hemorrhoids, a pea-sized amount of nitroglycerin 0.2% to 0.5% can be prescribed. The patient should be instructed that the systemic adverse effect of headache can occur. Phenylephrine 0.25% (Preparation H, Rectacaine) ointment or suppository can be applied four times per day for the relief of acute symptoms of bleeding or pain on defecation.

Emollients and Moisturizers

Emollients and moisturizers (e.g., lanolin) are lubricants used to relieve dry skin and pruritus. Keratolytics are used to treat keratin-containing skin conditions. Alpha hydroxy acids (e.g., glycolic acid) are used to treat wrinkles and sun-changed skin. These acids are a component of many antiaging cosmetics and other products. Salicylic acid is used to remove warts, corns, and calluses. Sunscreens are used to protect the skin from the damaging effects of ultraviolet radiation, thereby decreasing skin cancer and signs of aging, including wrinkles. Dermatologists recommend sunscreen preparations that block both UVA and UVB and have a sun protection factor (SPF) of 30 or higher.

HERBAL PREPARATIONS FOR SKIN DISORDERS

Many supplements are promoted for use in skin conditions. Most of these formulations have not been tested adequately to ensure effectiveness. At the same time, however, topical use rarely causes adverse effects or drug interactions. Two topical agents for which there is some support of safety and effectiveness are aloe and oat preparations (Box 61.2).

ACNE VULGARIS

As stated earlier, acne is a disorder of the hair follicles and sebaceous glands that become clogged, leading to pimples and cysts; it usually develops during puberty. **Acne vulgaris** is a common chronic skin disease involving blockage and/or inflammation of hair follicles and sebaceous glands. Acne

BOX 61.2 Herbal Preparations Used in Skin Conditions

- Aloe is often used as a topical remedy for minor burns and wounds (e.g., sunburn, cuts, abrasions) to decrease pain, itching, and inflammation and to promote healing. Its active ingredients are unknown. Wound healing is attributed to moisturizing effects and increased blood flow to the area. Reduced inflammation and pain may result from inhibition of arachidonic acid metabolism and formation of inflammatory prostaglandins. Reduced itching may result from inhibition of histamine production.
- Commercial aloe products are available for topical use, but fresh gel from the plant may be preferred. When used for this purpose, a clear, thin, gel-like liquid can be squeezed directly from a plant leaf onto the burned or injured area several times daily if needed.
- Oats, a cereal, a good source of dietary fiber, and a well-documented cholesterol-lowering product, is also used topically to treat minor skin irritation and pruritus associated with common skin disorders. Oats contain gluten, which forms a sticky mass that has emollient effects and holds moisture in the skin when it is mixed with a liquid. Oats are contained in bath products, cleansing bars, and lotions (e.g., Aveeno products) that can be used topically once or twice daily. They should not be used near the eyes or on the inflamed skin. After use, it is important to wash bath products off with water.

lesions vary from small comedones to acne vulgaris, the most severe form, in which follicles become infected and irritating secretions leak into surrounding tissues to form inflammatory pustules, cysts, and abscesses. Most patients have a variety of lesion types at one time. At least four pathologic events take place within acne-infected hair follicles: (1) androgen-mediated stimulation of sebaceous gland activity; (2) abnormal keratinization leading to follicular plugging (comedone formation); (3) proliferation of the bacterium *P. acnes* within the follicle; and (4) inflammation.

Acne occurs most often on the face, upper back, and chest because there are large numbers of sebaceous glands in these areas. One etiologic factor is increased secretion of male hormones (androgens), which occurs at puberty in both sexes. This leads to increased production of sebum and proliferation of *P. acnes*, which depend on sebum for survival. *P. acnes* bacteria contain lipase enzymes that break down free fatty acids and produce inflammation in acne lesions. Other causative factors may include medications (e.g., phenytoin, corticosteroids) and stress (i.e., the stress mechanism may involve stimulation of androgen secretion).

> **Quality and Safety Alert: Safety**
>
> The development of acne is not related to a lack of facial hygiene. The use of harsh astringents, abrasives, or vigorous scrubbing can worsen acne and the likelihood of inflammation and scarring.

Scientists have explored the role of diet in acne development for decades. Several research trials have noted that a low dietary glycemic load provides superior reduction in the number of inflammatory acne lesions in teenagers. Previous studies found no evidence that the ingestion of certain foods or dietary constituents (e.g., chocolate, zinc, antioxidants) play a role in acne development. However, based on a variety of emerging data, there is renewed interest in reinvestigating the effects of diet on acne development and management (Graber, 2023).

Several prescription and nonprescription antiacne products are available for acne vulgaris.

Antimicrobial drugs include both topical and systemic agents. Topical drugs are indicated for mild to moderate acne, often in combination with a topical retinoid to maximize reduction in severity and number of lesions. The goal is to eliminate the *P. acnes* colonizing the skin, thus reducing the inflammatory response. The most commonly used topical antimicrobials include benzoyl peroxide, clindamycin, and erythromycin. Azelaic acid (Azelex) has antibacterial activity against *P. acnes* and is reportedly as effective as benzoyl peroxide, topical erythromycin, or tretinoin (a retinoid) in the treatment of acne vulgaris. Benzoyl peroxide is an effective topical agent that is available in numerous preparations (e.g., gel, lotion, cream, wash) and concentrations (e.g., 2.5% to 10%). Low-concentration forms and lotion and cream preparations are the least irritating. Clindamycin and erythromycin are also available in topical dosage forms. These drugs reduce *P. acnes* with comparable efficacy. Combination products of topical clindamycin or erythromycin and benzoyl peroxide are more effective than antibiotics alone, and the benzoyl peroxide also decreases the development of antibiotic resistance. Best results require 8 to 12 weeks of therapy, and maintenance therapy is usually required.

Adverse effects of topical antibiotics include erythema, peeling, dryness, and burning as well as development of resistant strains of *P. acnes*. Recommendations for reducing drug resistance include using topical retinoids or benzoyl peroxide or both when using topical antibiotics. It is important to avoid long-term use of topical or oral antibiotics when feasible. Benzoyl peroxide can also cause an irritant dermatitis and bleach hair, clothes, and bed linens.

Oral antibiotics are first-line treatment for patients with moderate to severe inflammatory acne because they produce more rapid clinical improvement than topical preparations. These drugs have both antimicrobial and anti-inflammatory effects. Tetracycline also has direct anti-inflammatory properties. It reduces *P. acnes* organisms and thereby inhibits production of *P. acnes*–induced inflammatory cytokines. Commonly used oral antibiotics include tetracycline, doxycycline, minocycline, trimethoprim–sulfamethoxazole, clindamycin, azithromycin, and erythromycin. Tetracycline, clindamycin, azithromycin, and erythromycin suppress leukocyte chemotaxis and bacterial lipase activity. Minocycline and doxycycline inhibit cytokines and proteinase enzymes that contribute to inflammation and tissue breakdown. Trimethoprim–sulfamethoxazole interferes with bacterial folic acid synthesis and inhibits dihydrofolic acid reduction to tetrahydrofolate, resulting in sequential inhibition of enzymes of the folic acid pathway. Resistance is commonly reported with erythromycin. Resistance to minocycline is rare but may be emerging in the United States. All oral antibiotics require at least 6 to 8 weeks of use. Although there are no established guidelines for duration of use, some clinicians encourage using the drugs for shorter periods and avoiding long-term use as maintenance therapy, to decrease the development of resistant *P. acnes* and the occurrence of adverse effects such as vaginal candidiasis and gastrointestinal (GI) distress.

Retinoids, in both systemic and topical forms, may be used for moderate to severe acne. All topical retinoids (isotretinoin, acitretin, adapalene, tazarotene) reduce acne lesions, usually within 12 weeks. Isotretinoin is often used with other products.

> **Quality and Safety Alert: Evidence-Based Practice**
>
> Acne is a dermatologic condition that affects a patient's psychosocial health and quality of life. Secrest et al. (2020) assessed quality of life using the Skindex-16 Scores among patients with acne who received isotretinoin treatment. The researchers conducted a longitudinal, retrospective case series study of Skindex-16 data collected at monthly visits from 57 patients receiving isotretinoin. Findings revealed that patients receiving isotretinoin treatment achieved a greater than 50% improvement in their quality of life by month two, and a 4- to 5-fold improvement with the full course of treatment.

Clinical Application 61.1

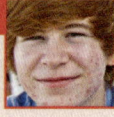

- Gerard first took tetracycline for his acne vulgaris. How does tetracycline work against this disorder?
- What are some topical applications that he could use to assist in clearing his acne vulgaris?

TABLE 61.6

DRUGS AT A GLANCE: Retinoids

Drug	Indications	Route and Dosage Ranges
Isotretinoin (Absorica, Accutane, Claravis, Amnesteem, Myorisan, Zenatane; ✦ Accutane, Clarus, Epuris)	Severe cystic acne Disorders characterized by excessive keratinization (e.g., pityriasis, ichthyosis) Mycosis fungoides	Children and Adults 1–2 mg/kg/d PO, in two divided doses, for 15–20 wk
Acitretin (✦ Soriatane, MINT-Acitretin, TARO-Acitretin)	Severe psoriasis	Adults 25–50 mg/d PO
Adapalene (Differin; ✦ Differin, Differin XP)	Acne vulgaris	Children: ≥7 y and Adults Topically to skin lesions once daily at bedtime
Tazarotene (Arazlo, Fabior, Tazorac; ✦ Arazlo, Tazorac)	Acne Psoriasis	Children: >9 y and Adults Topically to skin, after cleansing, once daily at bedtime

RETINOIDS

Retinoids are vitamin A derivatives that are active in proliferation and differentiation of skin cells. These drugs are commonly used to treat acne, psoriasis, aging and wrinkling of skin from sunlight exposure, and skin cancers. The prototype drug in this class is **isotretinoin** (Absorica, Accutane, Amnesteem, Claravis, Myorisan). The retinoids are listed in Table 61.6.

Pharmacokinetics

Isotretinoin dissolves slowly in the GI tract, and the drug is then absorbed rapidly. It crosses the placenta. Isotretinoin is metabolized in the liver and excreted in equal amounts in the feces and urine.

Action

The antiacne effects of isotretinoin include suppression of sebum production, inhibition of comedone formation, and inhibition of inflammation. The drug normalizes keratinization, reversibly decreases the size of sebaceous glands, and makes sebum less viscous and less likely to plug follicles. The decrease in sebum results in the inhibition of the sebum-dependent bacterium *P. acnes*, which is a key promoter of inflammation in acne vulgaris. Researchers have often found that isotretinoin also decreases cell proliferation and induces differentiation in neuroblastoma.

Use

Uses of isotretinoin include treatment of severe recalcitrant nodular acne that is unresponsive to other treatments in adolescents and adults.

Patient-related variables specific to the use of isotretinoin include the following:

- Reproduction, pregnancy, and lactation:
  - Isotretinoin may cause teratogenicity and has a structural or toxicity profile similar to hazardous medications.
  - Use of isotretinoin is contraindicated with pregnancy.
- Abnormal kidney function and hepatic impairment:
  - No dosage adjustments are required with kidney impairment.
  - No dosage adjustments are required with hepatic impairment; however, hepatotoxicity has been reported during treatment. Liver enzymes should be monitored during therapy.

Adverse Effects

Isotretinoin has severe adverse effects. Therefore, in the United States, the FDA has imposed restrictions on who may prescribe and distribute the drug. These adverse effects, which may limit its use, include:

- Reproductive effects: severe life-threatening congenital malformations and spontaneous abortions.
- Psychiatric effects (serious): depression, psychosis, aggressive or violent behavior, and changes in mood; rarely, suicidal thoughts and actions have been reported. It is important to observe closely all patients for symptoms of depression or suicidal thoughts; it may be necessary to discontinue therapy and make appropriate referrals to mental health professionals.
- Dermatologic effects (most common): dryness and swelling of the lips (cheilitis), dry skin and mucous membranes, nasal dryness, epistaxis, dry mouth, conjunctivitis, peeling skin, skin fragility, rash, and pruritus.
- GI effects (potential): nausea, vomiting, and, rarely, inflammatory bowel disease and pancreatitis.
- Musculoskeletal effects (common): arthralgia, myalgia (particularly with vigorous exercise), weakness, increased creatine phosphokinase (CPK), and back pain in some children as well as bone abnormalities, decreased bone mineral density, and premature epiphyseal closure.
- Metabolic effects: hyperlipidemia (elevated triglycerides in 45% of patients, elevated total cholesterol, and low-density lipoprotein in 30% of patients: usually transient elevations).
- Other effects: decreased night vision, corneal opacities, hepatotoxicity, and bone marrow suppression.

> **BOX 61.3** *iPLEDGE Program*
>
> - The iPLEDGE program is a risk management program designed to prevent fetal exposure to isotretinoin. Registration, activation, and additional information are provided at https://www.ipledgeprogram.com/iPledgeUI/home.u or by calling 866-495-0654. The program requires that
>   - All patients who are able to become pregnant or father a child must use two forms of birth control for at least 1 month prior to starting therapy, during therapy, and for 1 month after therapy. Patients are allowed to avoid the contraceptive requirements if they agree to abstain completely from sex; this commitment must be made in writing.
>   - All patients who are able to become pregnant must have two negative blood or urine pregnancy tests before receiving the initial prescription. It is essential that the second pregnancy test be conducted in a certified laboratory. During each month of therapy and 1 month after completing therapy, patients must see their healthcare provider for evaluation, counseling, and education. They must also have a negative pregnancy test in a certified laboratory monthly and 1 month after completing therapy.
>   - Every month, prescribers must document in the iPLEDGE system the results of the pregnancy test and the two forms of birth control in use. The prescriber must also document the counseling and education. All patients, even if not able to become pregnant, must be counseled about the iPLEDGE program and the risk of congenital anomalies.
>   - Healthcare providers can prescribe only a maximum 30-day supply at each monthly visit.
>   - Physicians must certify their expertise in the diagnosis and treatment of acne.

Contraindications

Contraindications to isotretinoin include hypersensitivity to the drug, parabens (used as a preservative), vitamin A, or other retinoids, as well as pregnancy. As reported earlier, the FDA has issued a **BOXED WARNING** ♦ stating that isotretinoin in pregnancy causes both spontaneous abortions and severe life-threatening congenital malformations. In addition, patients who can become pregnant should not take isotretinoin unless they have had two negative pregnancy test results before beginning therapy, will begin drug therapy on the 2nd or 3rd day of the next menstrual period, and will adhere to stringent contraceptive measures for 1 month before therapy, during therapy, and for 1 month after therapy. Box 61.3 describes the measures put in place by the iPLEDGE program developed by the FDA. The FDA has established a computer-based risk evaluation and mitigation strategy (REMS) to prevent fetal exposure to isotretinoin.

Cautious use is also advisable with a history of mental illness or a family history of psychiatric disorders. Other conditions that warrant caution are asthma, liver disease, diabetes, heart disease, osteoporosis, history of childhood osteoporosis, genetic predisposition for age-related osteoporosis, weak bones, anorexia nervosa, osteomalacia, and other disorders of bone metabolism.

Nursing Implications

Preventing Interactions

Many medications interact with isotretinoin, increasing its effects (Box 61.4). Isotretinoin may decrease the therapeutic effect of estrogen and progestin contraceptives. Microdosed progesterone-only preparations, in particular, may be ineffective.

Administering the Medication

Before starting isotretinoin, it is necessary to perform a complete blood cell count (CBC), a fasting lipid profile, and liver function tests to obtain a baseline. People should take the drug with or shortly after a meal to improve absorption. It is necessary to swallow capsules whole with a full glass of liquid. The contents of the capsule may irritate the esophagus if removed from the capsule. Patients who can become pregnant should have a pregnancy test and avoid coming in contact with the contents of the capsules because the drug is teratogenic.

Assessing for Therapeutic Effects

The nurse assesses for a decrease in total cyst count. The ideal value is a 70% decrease.

Assessing for Adverse Effects

With oral retinoids, the nurse observes for hypervitaminosis. Common signs include nausea and vomiting; headache; blurred vision, eye irritation, and conjunctivitis; skin disorders; musculoskeletal pain (any evidence of osteoporosis, osteopenia, or fractures); and depression and suicidal ideation. Although adverse effects commonly occur with usual doses, they are more severe with higher doses. Most adverse effects can be managed without stopping the drug.

Also, the nurse monitors laboratory tests. It is important to conduct repeat tests (CBC, lipid profile, liver function tests) at

> **BOX 61.4** *Drug Interactions: Isotretinoin*
>
> **Drugs That Increase the Effects of Isotretinoin**
> - Alcohol
>   *Increases triglycerides*
> - Corticosteroids
>   *Increases the risk of osteoporosis*
> - Phenytoin
>   *Increases the risk of osteomalacia*
> - Tetracycline
>   *Increases the risk of cerebri pseudotumor*
> - Vitamin A
>   *Produces toxic effects associated with isotretinoin*

BOX 61.5 Patient Teaching Guidelines for Isotretinoin

- Understand that acne is not caused by dirt, that washing does not improve acne, and that vigorous scrubbing may worsen acne lesions. There is also no evidence that acne is caused by eating chocolate or other foods.
- Know that all patients who are able to become pregnant or father a child must use two forms of birth control.
  - Adhere to mandatory pregnancy testing requirements.
- Take the drug with or shortly after meals.
- Report bone, muscle, or joint pain or visual disturbances immediately, as well as persistent headaches or GI pain.
- Report depression or suicidal thoughts immediately.
- Do not take oral vitamin A supplements.
- Avoid using abrasives, medicated soaps and cleansers, acne preparations containing peeling drugs, and topical products containing alcohol (e.g., cosmetics, aftershave). These products will exacerbate skin dryness and irritation.
- Avoid prolonged sun exposure. Use sun block.
- Do not donate blood during therapy and up to 1 month after therapy.

NCLEX Success

4. The mother of a child being treated for acne vulgaris asks a nurse why her child is being treated with doxycycline and a topical benzoyl peroxide agent. Which of the following is the best response the nurse can make to the patient's mother?
   A. "Benzoyl peroxide cannot be administered without doxycycline."
   B. "Doxycycline should be administered only until the acne vulgaris improves."
   C. "If your child's acne does not improve in 2 weeks, then one of the two agents will be stopped."
   D. "Doxycycline orally and benzoyl peroxide topically will provide better treatment of the acne vulgaris."

5. A patient with severe acne vulgaris is placed on isotretinoin. What are the adverse effects of isotretinoin? (Select all that apply.)
   A. Hyperlipidemia
   B. Pancreatitis
   C. Fragile skin
   D. Increased bone growth
   E. Cardiac dysrhythmia

4 and 8 weeks. If the repeat tests are normal and the dose is stable, monitoring is no longer necessary.

Patient Teaching

Box 61.5 identifies patient teaching guidelines for isotretinoin.

Clinical Application 61.2

- How does isotretinoin work to reduce acne vulgaris?
- Isotretinoin may cause severe psychiatric adverse effects, such as depression, psychosis, or violent behavior. What are some strategies the nurse can teach Gerard's parents about looking for psychosocial abnormalities?

Other Drugs in the Class

Adapalene and tazarotene are effective topical retinoids used to treat both noninflammatory and inflammatory acne. Adapalene is the only topical retinoid available without a prescription. A combination gel product (Epiduo, Epiduo Forte) containing adapalene and benzoyl peroxide is available by prescription. Traditionally, administration of most topical retinoids takes place at bedtime because of initial reports of drug instability in the presence of light; newer formulations are less affected by exposure to light.

THE NURSING PROCESS

A concept map outlines the nursing process related to drug therapy considerations in this chapter. Additional nursing implications related to the disease process should also be considered in care decisions.

Assessment

- When a skin rash is present, inspect the area and interview the patient to determine the following: location, appearance, distribution, accompanying symptoms, and history of development.
- Some etiologic factors include the following:
  - Drug therapy. Many commonly used drugs may cause skin lesions, including anti-infective agents, narcotic analgesics, and thiazide diuretics. Skin rashes due to drug therapy are usually generalized and appear abruptly.
  - Irritants or allergens that may cause contact dermatitis.
  - Communicable diseases (e.g., measles, chickenpox), which cause characteristic skin rashes and systemic signs and symptoms.
- When assessing the skin, consider the age of the patient. Infants are likely to have "diaper" dermatitis, miliaria (heat rash), and tinea capitis (ringworm infection of the scalp). School-aged children have a relatively high incidence of measles, chickenpox, and tinea infections. Adolescents often have acne. Older adults are more likely to have dry skin, actinic keratoses (lesions on sun-exposed skin formerly thought to be premalignant but now considered early-stage squamous cell cancer), and skin cancer.
- Assess for skin neoplasms. Basal cell carcinoma may initially appear as a pale nodule, most often on the head and neck. Squamous cell carcinomas may appear as actinic keratoses or ulcerated areas. Malignant melanoma is the most serious skin cancer. It involves melanocytes, the pigment-producing cells of the skin. Malignant melanoma may occur in pigmented nevi (moles) or previously normal skin. In nevi, malignant melanoma may be manifested by enlargement and ulceration. In previously normal skin, lesions appear as irregularly shaped.

Outcomes of Therapy

The patient will
- Apply topical drugs correctly.
- Experience relief of symptoms.
- Use techniques to prevent or minimize skin damage and disorders.
- Avoid scarring and disfigurement when possible.
- Be encouraged to express concerns about acute and chronic body-image changes.

Nursing Interventions

- Use measures to prevent or minimize skin disorders, including good personal hygiene.
- Maintain adequate nutrition, rest, and exercise.
- Practice safety measures to avoid injury to the skin. Injury with a disruption of skin integrity increases the likelihood of skin infections.
- Avoid known irritants or allergens such as:
  - Soaps and detergents
  - Toiletries or makeup containing preservatives
  - Antiseptic agents
  - Disinfectants
  - Acids and alkalis
  - Allergens: food, pollen, plants, latex
- Prevent pressure ulcers by avoiding trauma to the skin and prolonged pressure on any part of the body. Implement frequent position changes and correct lifting techniques. Daily inspection of the skin is needed for early detection and treatment of beginning pressure ulcers.
- Avoid excessive exposure to sunlight and other sources of UV light.
- Apply sunscreen daily.
- When skin rashes are present, cool, wet compresses or baths are often effective in relieving pruritus. A cool environment also tends to decrease pruritus. Keep the patient's fingernails cut short.
- For relief of severe itching, a systemic antihistamine may be needed.

Evaluation

- Observe and interview regarding use of dermatologic drugs.
- Observe for improvement in skin lesions and symptoms.
- Interview regarding use of measures to promote healthy skin and prevent skin disorders.

Visit thePoint® at **http://thePoint.lww.com/Frandsen13e** for answers to NCLEX Success questions (in Appendix A), answers to Clinical Application Case Studies (in Appendix B), additional information on etiology, pathophysiology, and more!

REFERENCES AND RESOURCES

Armstrong, D. G., & Meyr, A. J. (2022). Basic principles of wound management. *UpToDate*. Lexi-Comp, Inc.

Bleday, R., & Breen, E. (2022). Home and office treatment of symptomatic. *UpToDate*. Lexi-Comp, Inc.

Feldman, S. R. (2022). Treatment of psoriasis in adults. *UpToDate*. Lexi-Comp, Inc.

Fransway, A. F., & Reeder, M. (2022). Irritant contact dermatitis in adults. *UpToDate*. Lexi-Comp, Inc.

Graber, E. (2023). Acne vulgaris: Overview of management. *UpToDate*. Lexi-Comp, Inc.

Hinkle, J. H., Cheever, K. H., & Overbaugh, K. J. (2021). *Brunner & Suddarth's textbook of medical-surgical nursing* (15th ed.). Wolters Kluwer.

Howe, W. (2022). Treatment of atopic dermatitis (eczema). *UpToDate*. Lexi-Comp, Inc.

Hugh, W. A. (2022). Stevens-Johnson syndrome and toxic epidermal necrolysis: pathogenesis, clinical manifestations, and diagnosis. *UpToDate*.

Hull, C., & Zone, J. J. (2022). Approach to the patient with cutaneous blisters. In *UpToDate*.

iPLEDGE: Committed to Pregnancy Prevention. *U.S. Food and Drug Administration–approved program for use of isotretinoin*. Retrieved from http://www.ipledgeprogram.com.

Lippincott Advisor. (2022). *Drug information*. Wolters Kluwer.

Norris, T. L. (2019). *Porth's pathophysiology: Concepts of altered health states* (10th ed.). Wolters Kluwer.

Sasseville, D. (2022). Seborrheic dermatitis in adolescents and adults. *UpToDate*. Lexi-Comp, Inc.

Secrest, A., Hopkins, Z. H., Frost, Z. E., Taliercio, V. L., Edwards, L. D., Biber, J. E., Chen, S. C., Chren, M.-M., Ferris, L. K., Kean, J., Hess, R., & for the Dermatology PRO Consortium. (2020). Quality of life assessed using Skindex-16 Scores among patients with acne receiving isotretinoin treatment. *Journal of American Medicine Dermatology*, 156(10), 1098–1106. https://doi.org/10.1001/jamadermatol.2020.2330

UpToDate. (2022). *Drug information*. Lexi-Comp, Inc.

Weston, W. L., & Howe, W. (2022). Overview of dermatitis (eczematous dermatoses). *UpToDate*. Lexi-Comp, Inc.

Clinical Judgment in Practice: Section 10: Drugs Affecting the Eye, Ear, and Skin

A 16-year-old girl visiting the school guidance counselor states that she is having difficulty at home and in school. She feels depressed and unsure of herself. She also states that she may be pregnant. The guidance counselor sends her to see the school nurse practitioner (NP). The guidance counselor informs the NP about the statements the student has made regarding her difficulty at home and in school, that she feels depressed, and that she may be pregnant. The NP reviews the student's health record and notes that she is currently taking a birth control pill and isotretinoin for acne. When the student arrives for her appointment, the NP interviews her to acquire a more complete health history and to gather more subjective data related to her statement of depression and difficulties both at home and at school. The student states, "I cannot get along with my parents. They are very strict and will not let me go out with my friends. Recently, my parents were gone, and my boyfriend and I had sex. If they knew they would kill me!" Since she states she is depressed, the NP asks the student if she will hurt herself due to her depression. She states, "I just sleep a lot. I won't hurt myself, it is against my religion."

The NP asks the student what makes her think she is pregnant since she is taking the birth control pill. The NP also inquires if the student has done a pregnancy test. The student states, "I always forget to take the birth control pill. My period is ten days late. I have not had a pregnancy test."

Step 1: Recognize Cues
Identify the relevant and important information from different sources, such as the medical history or subjective and objective data.

Answer: *The student states she is depressed, denies being suicidal, and states that her difficulties in school and with her family have increased. She states she sleeps a lot. She states she may be pregnant but doesn't know since she has not had a pregnancy test. Her period is 10 days late. She is taking isotretinoin which is teratogenic, and she forgets to take the prescribed birth control pills.*

Step 2: Analyze Cues
Organize and link the recognized cues to the patient's clinical presentation.

Answer: *As the NP, you link the statements made by the student to develop the following plan of care:*

- *The student thinks she is pregnant but has not had a pregnancy test. Since you are the primary health provider for students of childbearing age, you have pregnancy tests in your office. You give the student a pregnancy test to use with her first void the next morning. The student will come to your office to report the results.*
- *You meet with the guidance counselor regarding the student's depression to plan care to support her mental health.*

Step 3: Prioritize Hypotheses
Evaluate hypotheses and rank them according to priority, such as urgency, likelihood, risk, difficulty, and/or time. Cluster your findings to generate a list of problems (actual or potential) you believe the patient is experiencing or may experience and determine the level of urgency. Which problem is of the greatest concern?

Answer: *The student has many priorities of actual and potential health problems. If it is confirmed she is pregnant, the fetus is at risk for congenital anomalies due to the teratogenic effects of her acne medication isotretinoin. Also, if pregnancy is confirmed, she will need to stop taking the acne medication and see both her dermatology and primary care provider. If she is not pregnant, she will need medication teaching on the risks of isotretinoin and the required administration of birth control to prevent pregnancy. In addition to the risk to the fetus, isotretinoin is also related to mental health issues that include depression and suicidal ideations. The student must be evaluated by you, the guidance counselor, and the primary care provider regarding her depressive symptoms. You should receive permission from the student to discuss the healthcare needs with her family.*

Step 4: Generate Solutions
Identify expected outcomes and use hypotheses to define a set of interventions for the expected outcomes.

Answer: *The student's pregnancy test is negative. Since her test is negative, you anticipate she will need increased patient teaching regarding the risk of teratogenic effects on the fetus if she becomes pregnant while taking isotretinoin.*

Regarding the student's statement of depression, her depression may be related to the adverse effects of isotretinoin. One adverse effect of isotretinoin is suicidal ideations. You suspect she will need to meet with the guidance counselor on a biweekly basis to discuss the difficulties she is having in school and with her family. In addition, the student will agree to discuss her mental health issues with her family and with you. The school's care team recognizes the need to intervene if her depressive symptoms increase. You also anticipate the need to increase healthcare teaching to the parents regarding the adverse effects of isotretinoin, particularly depression and suicidal ideations.

Step 5: Take Actions
Implement the solutions that address the highest priorities.

Answer: *You work with the student to develop a plan for her to remember to take her birth control pill; she agrees to use a calendar every morning to mark off the administration of the birth control pill. She will also check in with you every morning at school to report her medication adherence and will set her smartphone with a drug reminder alarm. In addition, you review the practice of safe sex with the student and the use of a condom to further protect from pregnancy and sexually transmitted diseases.*

The student meets with the guidance counselor two times per week. Together they are developing strategies to address mental health concerns. You meet with the student and family to discuss the student's mental health concerns and to educate them on the adverse effects of isotretinoin including depression and suicidal ideations.

Step 6: Evaluate Outcomes
Compare observed outcomes against expected outcomes.

Answer: *The student is adherent with her isotretinoin acne medication and her birth control pills. The student reports she is sleeping less and is less depressed. The student and family have begun seeing a family counselor. She denies suicidal ideations. The student's grades have improved.*

Index

Note: Page numbers followed by "*f*" indicate figures; "*t*", tables; "*b*", boxes.

A

abacavir, 432
abacavir sulfate (Ziagen), 432
abatacept (Orencia, Orencia ClickJect), 211*t*, 222*t*–224*t*, 227
abbreviations, 41, 41*t*
abciximab (ReoPro), 140*t*, 151*t*–152*t*, 154
Abelcet (amphotericin B lipid complex), 446–447, 448*t*, 449
Abenol (acetaminophen), 286, 288, 290, 290*t*, 294–297, 295*t*, 297*b*
Abilify (aripiprazole), 1009*t*, 1024*t*, 1025, 1031*t*, 1039*t*–1040*t*, 1041
Abilify Maintena (aripiprazole), 1009*t*, 1024*t*, 1025, 1031*t*, 1039*t*–1040*t*, 1041
Abilify MyCite (aripiprazole), 1009*t*, 1024*t*, 1025
abiraterone (Yonsa, Zytiga), 236*t*–238*t*, 260–263, 261*t*–263*t*
abnormal kidney function
    cyclosporine use in, 217
    mycophenolate mofetil uses in, 213
abortifacient, 93
abortive therapy, 937. *See also* migraine headaches
Abraxane (paclitaxel), 236*t*–245*t*
Abreva (docosanol), 416*t*, 417
Abrilada (adalimumab), 211*t*, 222*t*–224*t*, 227
abrocitinib (Cibinqo), 211*t*, 220*t*, 221
Absorica (isotretinoin), 1118–1119
absorption, 16–17
Abstral (fentanyl), 894*t*, 896*t*–897*t*, 902, 932*t*
abuse-deterrent formulations, 893–894
acamprosate (Vivitrol), 1061*t*–1063*t*, 1065
acarbose (Precose), 754*t*, 758, 763, 767–769, 768*t*, 769*b*, 777
ACCEL-Leflunomide (leflunomide), 211*t*, 216
Accolate (zafirlukast), 605*t*, 618*t*, 619
Accupril (quinapril), 482*t*, 485*t*, 488, 495*t*–496*t*
Accupril (quinapril hydrochloride), 754*t*
accuretic, 495*t*–496*t*
Accutane (isotretinoin), 1118–1119
ACE inhibitors. *See* angiotensin-converting enzyme (ACE) inhibitors
acebutolol (Sectral), 482*t*, 496*t*–498*t*, 511*t*, 512
Aceon (Perindopril erbumine), 754*t*
Acetadote (acetylcysteine), 574*t*, 581–582, 581*t*
acetaminophen (Tylenol, paracetamol, Abenol, Apo-Acetaminophen, Atasol, Novo-Gesic), 286, 288, 290, 290*t*, 294–297, 295*t*, 297*b*, 581–583, 583*t*, 1107
    abnormal kidney function and hepatic impairment, 296
    administration, 296
    adverse effects, 296–297
    contraindications, 296
    mechanism of action, 295
    metabolic pathway for, 295*f*
    nursing implications, 296–297
    patient teaching guidelines, 297, 297*b*
    pharmacokinetics, 295
    preventing interactions, 296, 296*b*
    reproduction, pregnancy, and lactation, 296
    therapeutic effects, 296
    toxicity, 297
    treatment of overdose, 297
acetaminophen–aspirin–caffeine (Excedrin), 940–941
    adverse effects, 941
    contraindications, 941
    dosage usage, 940–941
    in hepatic impairment, 941
    mechanism of action, 940
    nursing implications, 941
    patient teaching guidelines, 941, 942*b*
    pharmacokinetics, 940
    therapeutic effects, 941
acetazolamide, 956*t*, 968, 969*t*–972*t*, 1082*t*–1084*t*
acetic acid derivatives, 290*t*, 302–305, 302*t*–303*t*
    abnormal kidney function, 303
    administration of, 304
    adverse effects, 303
    contraindications, 303–304
    in hepatic impairment patients, 303
    indomethacin, 302, 302*t*–303*t*
    nursing implications, 304
    patient teaching guidelines, 304, 304*b*
    pharmacokinetics, 302
    preventing interactions, 304, 304*b*
    therapeutic effects, 304
acetylcholine, 845, 853
acetylcholinesterase drugs, 831, 853
acetylcholinesterase inhibitors (indirect-acting cholinergics), 855*t*
    abnormal kidney function and hepatic impairment, 854
    administration of, 856
    adverse effects, 855–856
    contraindications, 856
    drug interactions, 856*b*
    in lactation, 854
    mechanism of action, 854, 854*f*
    muscarine, 855
    neostigmine, 854
    nursing implications, 856
    patient teaching guidelines, 856, 856*b*
    pharmacokinetics, 854
    physostigmine, 855, 857
    in pregnancy, 854
    pyridostigmine, 854
    routes and dosage ranges, 854, 855*t*
    therapeutic effects, 856
    uses, 854–855
acetylcholinesterase–NMDA receptor antagonist, 859*t*
acetylcysteine (Acetadote), 574*t*, 581–582, 581*t*
acetylsalicylic acid (aspirin, Robaxisal), 754*t*, 778*t*
ACH-Alendronate (alendronate), 820*t*–821*t*
ACHBicalutamide (bicalutamide), 236*t*–238*t*, 261*t*–263*t*, 263
ACH-Letrozole (letrozole), 236*t*–238*t*, 260, 261*t*–263*t*
achlorhydria, 700
ACH-Mycophenolate (mycophenolate mofetil/ mycophenolate sodium), 213*t*
acid reflux, 602
acidifying agents, 1102–1104, 1102*t*
AcipHex (rabeprazole), 692*t*, 699*t*, 700
acitretin, 87*b*, 1119*t*
Aclasta (zoledronic acid), 820*t*–821*t*
acne, 1110–1112
acne vulgaris, 1117–1118
Acne-Clear (benzoyl peroxide), 1113*t*
AcNesic (salicylic acid), 1116*t*–1117*t*
acquired immunodeficiency syndrome, 324
acrivastine (Semprex-D), 590*t*, 595–596, 595*t*
acromegaly, 807
    abnormal kidney function and hepatic impairment, 808
    administration of, 808
    adverse effects, 808
    contraindications, 808
    lactation, 808
    lanreotide, 808
    mechanism of action, 807
    nursing implications, 808
    octreotide acetate, 807–808, 809*b*
    pasireotide, 808–809
    patient teaching guidelines, 808, 809*b*
    pharmacokinetics, 807
    in pregnancy patients, 808
    preventing interactions, 808
    therapeutic effects, 808
    uses, 808
ACT Alendronate (alendronate), 820*t*–821*t*
ACT Bortezomib (bortezomib), 236*t*–238*t*, 252*t*–257*t*, 259–260
ACT Celecoxib (celecoxib), 290*t*, 305–306, 305*t*, 306*b*
ACT Ciprofloxacin (ciprofloxacin), 358*t*
ACT Losartan/HCT (hyzaar), 495*t*–496*t*
ACT Olmesartan (benicar HCT), 495*t*–496*t*
ACT Raloxifene (raloxifene), 823*t*
ACT Ramipril (ramipril), 482*t*, 485*t*, 488
ACTAnastrozole (anastrozole), 236*t*–238*t*, 260, 261*t*–263*t*
ACTClarithromycin XL (clarithromycin), 378*t*
ACT-Dutasteride (dutasteride), 119*t*, 126, 126*t*
Actemra (tocilizumab), 222*t*–224*t*, 227
Actemra ACTPen (tocilizumab), 222*t*–224*t*, 227
ACT-Exemestane (exemestane), 236*t*–238*t*, 260, 261*t*–263*t*
ACTH (corticotropin), 802
Acthar (corticotropin), 800*t*–801*t*
ActHIB (haemophilus influenzae type b (Hib)), 194, 194*b*, 195*t*–199*t*
Acthrel (corticotropin), 799*t*
ACT-Imatinib (imatinib), 236*t*–238*t*, 252, 252*t*–257*t*, 258–259
Actimmune (interferon gamma-1b), 187*t*, 188
Actiq (fentanyl), 894*t*, 896*t*–897*t*, 902, 922*t*, 932
Activase (alteplase), 140*t*, 155–157, 155*t*
Activase rtPA (alteplase), 140*t*, 155–157, 155*t*
activated partial thromboplastin time (aPTT), 142–143
active antiretroviral therapy, 406*b*
active immunity, 193, 195*t*–199*t*
active tuberculosis, 389, 399*t*
Activella (estradiol/norethindrone), 112*t*
Actonel (risedronate), 820*t*–821*t*
Actonel DR (risedronate), 820*t*–821*t*
Actos (pioglitazone), 754*t*, 767*b*, 769, 769*t*, 777
ACT-Pramipexole (pramipexole dihydrochloride), 871*t*–872*t*
ACT-Ropinirole (ropinirole hydrochloride), 871*t*–872*t*
ACT-Solifenacin (solifenacin succinate), 887*t*
Acudial (diazepam), 956*t*
Acular (ketorolac), 1090*t*, 1094*t*–1095*t*
Acular LS (ketorolac), 1094*t*–1095*t*
acupressure, 719
acupuncture, 719
acute adrenal crisis, 828–829
acute adrenocortical insufficiency, 325–326
acute coronary syndromes, 522–523, 526
acute gouty arthritis, 288–290
acute GVHD, 210, 212, 220
acute hypotension, 540–541, 540*f*
acute inflammation, 272–273
    cellular stage, 272–273, 274*f*
    opsonization and phagocytosis, 273, 274*f*
    vascular stage, 272, 273*f*
acute lymphocytic leukemia, 239*t*–245*t*
acute myeloid leukemia, 239*t*–245*t*
acute pain, 901*b*
acute respiratory distress syndrome, 326
acute severe respiratory syndrome coronavirus 2 (SARS-CoV-2), 410–411, 411*b*
Acuvail (ketorolac), 1090*t*, 1094*t*–1095*t*

1127

acyclovir (Sitavig, Zovirax), 415–417, 416t, 1114, 1115t
Adacel (diphtheria, tetanus toxoids, and acellular pertussis (DTaP)), 195t–199t
Adalat (nifedipine), 524t, 531–533, 532t, 533b
Adalat CC (nifedipine), 482t, 492t
Adalat XL (nifedipine), 93, 93t
adalimumab (Humira, Humira Pediatric Crohn's Start, Humira Pen, Abrilada, Amgevita SureClick, Hadlima), 211t, 222t–224t, 227
adapalene, 1119t, 1121
Adbry (tralokinumab), 1116t–1117t
Adcirca (tadalafil), 124t
Adderall (dextroamphetamine and amphetamine), 1047t, 1050t, 1051
Adderall XR (dextroamphetamine and amphetamine), 1047t, 1050t, 1051
Addison disease
　adrenocorticoids/mineralocorticoids, 830
　　administration of, 831
　　adverse effects, 831
　　contraindications, 831
　　in lactation, 831
　　mechanism of action, 830
　　nursing implications, 831–832
　　patient teaching guidelines, 832, 832b
　　pharmacokinetics, 830
　　in pregnancy, 831
　　preventing interactions, 831, 831b
　　therapeutic effects, 831
　　uses, 830–831
　clinical considerations, 828–829
　clinical manifestations, 828–829
　diagnosis, 829
　drugs for, 830t
　mineralocorticoids, 832
　　abnormal kidney function, 832
　　administration of, 832
　　adverse effects, 832–833
　　contraindications, 832
　　in hepatic impairment patients, 832
　　in lactation, 832
　　mechanism of action, 832
　　nursing implications, 832–833
　　patient teaching guidelines, 833, 833b
　　pharmacokinetics, 832
　　in pregnancy, 832
　　preventing interactions, 832, 833b
　　therapeutic effects, 832–833
　　uses, 832
　overview of, 828–829
　treatment for, 830–833
addisonian crisis, 319, 828–829
Addison's disease, 315
additive effects, 22
adefovir dipivoxil (Hepsera), 408t–409t, 426, 426t
Adenocard (adenosine), 517–518
adenosine (Adenocard), 517–518
adenosine diphosphate (ADP) receptor antagonists, 150, 524t, 535
　abnormal kidney function, 151
　administration of, 152–153
　adverse effects, 152–153
　cangrelor, 150, 153
　contraindications, 152
　dosages and information, 150–151, 151t–152t
　drug interactions, 152b
　in hepatic impairment patients, 151
　mechanism of action, 150
　nursing implications, 152–153
　patient teaching guidelines, 153, 153b
　pharmacokinetics, 150
　prasugrel, 150, 152–153
　preventing interactions, 152
　therapeutic effects, 153
　ticagrelor, 150, 152–154

use, 150–151
adequate intake (AI), 646b
Adhansia XR (methylphenidate), 1047t, 1053t
Adipex-P (phentermine hydrochloride), 679t
adjuvant drugs, 922t
adjuvant medications, 211, 211t, 221–228
　in general anesthesia, 931–932, 932t
Adlarity (donepezil), 859t
Adlyxin (lixisenatide), 754t, 775t
administration of drugs
　clinical judgment in practice, 34b
　drug actions after, 19
　ear and eye solutions, 42t–43t
　ear medications, 57
　herbal and dietary supplements, 58–59, 59t–61t, 61b
　intramuscular injections
　　advantages and disadvantages of, 45t–46t
　　sites for, 56
　intravenous injections
　　administration technique, 45t–46t, 46b
　　advantages and disadvantages of, 45t–46t
　　continuous infusion, 46b
　　drug preparation for, 46b
　　equipment for, 46b
　　intermittent infusion, 46b
　　needleless systems, 46b
　　principles of, 46b
　　sites for, 48–50, 50f
　legal responsibilities, 34
　medication errors, 34–40
　medication systems, 39
　nasogastric tube, 55
　nursing actions for, 50–57
　oral, 45t–46t
　parenteral
　　ampules used in, 48
　　definition of, 42t–43t, 45
　　equipment for, 45, 47
　　injection sites, 48–50, 49f
　patient teaching guidelines, 52b, 53b
　pharmacokinetics affected by, 16–19
　principles of, 33–34
　psychological considerations, 24
　rectal suppositories, 42t–43t
　safety
　　administration of, 8–9
　　Beers criteria, 11
　　do not use list, 10
　　pregnancy categories, 11
　　QSEN, 10, 10b
　　targeted high-risk activities, 10–11
　subcutaneous injections
　　absorption after, 17
　　sites for, 48–50, 49f–50f
　　using IV line already established, 56–57
　　vaginal suppositories, 42t–43t
administration of record, 39
adolescents, 202. See also infants
ADP (adenosine diphosphate) receptor antagonists, 524t, 535
adrenal cortex disorders, 315–316
adrenal glands, 828, 828f
adrenal hyperplasia, 315
adrenal insufficiency, 319
Adrenalin (epinephrine), 541–542, 543t, 545–547, 605t, 607, 608t
adrenergic agonists, 1078t, 1078t–1079t
　adverse effects, 1081
　contraindications, 1081
　dose usage, 1081
　mechanisms of action, 1081
　nursing implications, 1081
　patient teaching guidelines, 1081
　pharmacokinetics, 1081
　preventing interactions, 1081

　therapeutic effects, 1081
adrenergic beta receptor
　signal transduction mechanism for, 846f
　structure and function of, 844–850
adrenergic drugs
　action, 541–542, 542t, 606–607
　administration of, 544, 607
　adverse effects, 543–544, 607
　albuterol, 606–610, 608t
　contraindications, 544, 607
　dobutamine, 543t, 547
　dopamine, 541–542, 543t, 546–547
　dosage ranges, 608t
　drug interactions, 544, 545b
　epinephrine, 541–542, 545–547, 605t, 607, 608t
　formoterol, 605t, 608t, 610, 621t
　isoproterenol, 542
　lactation, 543
　levalbuterol, 605t, 608t, 610
　metaproterenol, 605t, 608t, 610
　nursing implications, 544–545, 607
　patient teaching guidelines, 545, 546b, 607, 609b
　pharmacokinetics, 542, 606
　phenylephrine, 541–542, 547, 1078, 1079t
　pregnancy, 543
　preventing interactions, 544, 545b, 607
　pseudoephedrine, 542, 582
　reproduction, 543
　salmeterol, 605t, 608t, 610
　terbutaline, 605t, 608t, 610
　therapeutic effects, 544, 607
　use, 607
　uses, 542–543
adrenergics, 607
　fiber, 845
　receptors (beta1, beta2, and alpha), 541, 542t, 847–848
adrenocortical excess, 829
adrenocortical hyperfunction, 315–316
adrenocortical insufficiency, 319, 828–829
adrenocorticoids/mineralocorticoids, 830t
adrenocorticotropic hormone (ACTH), 802, 828–829
Adriamycin (doxorubicin), 235, 236t–245t, 239, 245–247, 248b, 251b, 264t
Aducanumab (Aduhelm), 855t, 859t, 861
Aduhelm (Aducanumab), 855t, 859t, 861
adult, 76
　development, testosterone, 119
Advagraf (tacrolimus), 211t, 212, 215b, 216, 218–219
Advair (fluticasone/salmeterol), 621, 621t
Advair Diskus (fluticasone/salmeterol), 621, 621t
Advair HFA (fluticasone/salmeterol), 621, 621t
adverse effects
　acetaminophen, 296–297
　acetaminophen–aspirin–caffeine, 941
　acetic acid derivatives, 303
　acetylcholinesterase inhibitors, 855–856
　acromegaly, 808
　adenosine diphosphate receptor antagonists, 152–153
　adrenergic agonist, 1081
　adrenergic drugs, 607
　adrenocorticoids/mineralocorticoids, 831
　5-alpha reductase inhibitors, 127
　alpha$_2$-adrenergic agonists, 1086
　alpha$_1$-adrenergic blockers, 128–129
　amebicides, 465
　amides, 914
　aminoglycosides, 354–357
　AMPA glutamate receptor antagonist, 979
　amphetamine-related drugs, 1054
　amphetamines, 1050
　angiotensin II receptor blockers, 489
　angiotensin-converting enzyme inhibitors, 486

anterior pituitary hormone drugs, 801
antiallergic drugs, 1093
antiamyloid monoclonal antibody, 861
antibacterial drugs, 1092
anticholinergic drugs, 611, 1078
antifungal drugs, 1093
antimalarials, 466, 468
antineoplastic drugs, 247–249
antineoplastics, 836–837
antitussives, 579
antiviral drugs, 1092
azoles, 452
barbiturates, 957
benzodiazepines, 959, 998, 1064
beta-adrenergic blocking drugs, 1085
bile acid sequestrants, 169
bisphosphonates, 821–822
calcitonin gene–related peptide receptor antagonist, 949
calcium channel blockers, 493
calcium preparations, 817
carbamate derivatives, 984
carbapenems, 348
carbonic anhydrase inhibitor, 972
carbonic anhydrase inhibitors, 1088
cathartics, 728
cephalosporins, 345
cholesterol absorption inhibitor, 172
cholinergic agonist, 862
cholinergic drugs, 1086–1087
cholinesterase inhibitor–N-methyl-D-aspartate receptor antagonist, 858–859
colchicine, 307
corticosteroids, 615, 1096
cyclosporine, 218
cytotoxic antineoplastic drugs, 247–249
11-deoxycortisol inhibitors, 834–835
direct factor Xa inhibitors, 149
direct thrombin inhibitors, 147
direct-acting skeletal muscle relaxants, 988
dual receptor antagonists, 1003
echinocandins, 455
enzyme inhibitors for maintenance, 1065
ergot alkaloids, 943
erythropoiesis-stimulating agents, 182
esters, 916
estradiol, 947
estrogen(s), 104–105
estrogen–progestin combinations, 104
exogenous corticosteroids, 327, 329
expectorants, 580
fibrates, 171
first-generation antipsychotics, 1034
first-generation nonphenothiazines, 1037
fluoroquinolone, 359–360, 1104
functionalized amino acids, 976
gamma-aminobutyric acid, 985
gamma-aminobutyric acid structural analogs, 963
granulocyte colony-stimulating factors, 184
heparin(s), 143
histone deacetylase inhibitor, 975
HMG-CoA reductase inhibitors, 166–167
hydantoins, 964
hypothalamic hormone drugs, 807
imidazoline, 990
iminostilbenes, 966–967
immunizations, 203
immunosuppressant drugs, 214
immunosuppressants, 1097
indirect-acting cholinergics, 855–856
inhalation anesthetics, 923–924
interferon(s), 186–187
intravenous general anesthetics, 927
isoniazid, 394
laxative(s), 725

leukotriene modifiers, 618
lipase inhibitors, 682
local anesthetic, 1081
loop diuretics, 633
macrolides, 377
mineralocorticoids, 832–833
miscellaneous antiepileptic drugs, 982
monoamine oxidase inhibitors, 1016
monobactams, 349–350
mood-stabilizing agents, 1023
mucolytics, 582
mycophenolate mofetil (CellCept, Myfortic), 214
nasal decongestants, 576
neuromuscular blocking agents, 929–930
N-methyl-D-aspartate receptor antagonist, 861
nonsteroidal anti-inflammatory drugs, 939
noradrenergic sympathomimetic anorexiants, 680
osmotic drugs, 1089
oxicam derivatives, 290t, 300–301, 301t
PCSK9 inhibitors, 174
penicillin, 1105
penicillin(s), 338–339
phenyltriazine derivatives, 977
phosphodiesterase type 5 inhibitors, 124
polyenes, 449
posterior pituitary hormone, 804
potassium-sparing diuretics, 639
progestin(s), 108
progestin–estrogen combinations, 104
propionic acid derivatives, 299–300
propylthiouracil, 788
prostaglandin analogs, 1082
proton pump inhibitors, 33
pyrimidine analog, 457
pyrrolidine derivatives, 978
retinoids, 1119
reversible indirect-acting cholinergics, 858–859
rho kinase inhibitor, 1087
rifamycins, 396
ruxolitinib (Jakafi), 221
salicylates, 293
second-generation "atypical" antipsychotics, 1040
selective COX-2 inhibitor, 290t, 305–306
selective serotonin reuptake inhibitors, 1016
serotonin-norepinephrine reuptake inhibitors, 1018–1019
sodium glucose cotransporter 2 inhibitors, 776
succinimides, 973
sulfamate-substituted monosaccharides, 980
sulfonamide, 974
sulphonamides, 370–371
testosterone, 121
tetracycline, 367–368
tetrazole alkyl carbamate derivative, 981
thiazide diuretics, 635
thrombolytic drugs, 156
thyroid drugs, 791
triazole derivatives, 981–982
tricyclic antidepressant(s), 989, 1011–1013
triptans, 945
uricosuric agents, 308
vitamin D, 819
warfarin, 145
xanthines, 613
Advil (ibuprofen), 290t, 293, 295–300, 298t–299t, 300b, 1107
Advil Allergy & Congestion Relief, 583t
Advil Cold and Sinus Tablets, 583t
afatinib (Gilotrif), 236t–238t, 252t–257t
Afeditab CR (nifedipine), 93, 93t
affinity, 845
Afinitor (everolimus), 211t, 219
Afinitor Disperz (everolimus), 211t, 219, 236t–238t, 252t–257t, 258

Afluria (influenza (IIV4)), 195t–199t
Afrezza, 753, 756t–757t
African Americans, antihypertensive drug actions in, 23–24
Afrin (oxymetazoline), 574t–575t, 576–578
afterload, 524–525, 534
AG-Celecoxib (celecoxib), 290t, 305–306, 305t, 306b
age-related changes, 76
Aggrastat (tirofiban), 151t–152t, 154, 156
Aggrenox (dipyridamole and aspirin), 151t–152t, 155
agonists, 845
alpha$_2$-adrenergic agonists (see alpha$_2$-adrenergic agonists)
opioid, 894–903, 896t–897t
partial, 942
Agriflu (influenza (IIV4)), 195t–199t
Agrylin (anagrelide), 151t–152t
AG-Sildenafil (sildenafil), 123, 124t
A-Hydrocort (hydrocortisone), 320t–323t
AirDuo RespiClick (fluticasone/salmeterol), 621t
Airomir (albuterol), 608t
airway hyper responsiveness, 602
AJ-PIP/TAZ (piperacillin/tazobactam), 335t–337t
akathisia, 1034
akinesia, 868–869
Akten (lidocaine), 1078t–1079t
Akynzeo (netupitant/palonosetron), 708t, 715t, 716
Ala Cort (hydrocortisone), 318t, 320t–323t
Ala Scalp (hydrocortisone), 318t, 320t–323t
alanine aminotransferase (ALT), 216, 383, 450
Alaway (ketotifen), 1094t–1095t
Alaway Children's Allergy (ketotifen), 1090t, 1096
albendazole, 464t
albiglutide (Tanzeum), 754t
albuterol, 606–610, 608t
Alcaine (proparacaine), 1078t–1079t
alcohol use, cravings in, 1065
alcohol withdrawal, benzodiazepines, 1061
aldactazide, 495t–496t, 631t, 641t
Aldactone (spironolactone), 482t, 495t–498t, 554t, 563, 631t, 637–640, 638t, 639b, 641t
aldesleukin (Proleukin), 188
aldosterone, 314–315
kidney functions of, 316b
aldosterone antagonists, 554t, 563
alemtuzumab (Campath, Lemtrada), 211t, 222t–224t, 225, 236t–238t, 252t–257t
alendronate (Fosamax), 815t, 820–822, 820t–821t
Aleve (naproxen sodium), 290t, 298t–299t, 938, 938t–939t
Alfenta (alfentanil), 932
alfentanil (Alfenta), 932
Alferon N (interferon alfa-3n), 187t, 188
alfuzosin (Uroxatral, Apo-Alfuzosin, Sandoz-Alfuzosin, Xatral), 128t, 129
alfuzosin (Uroxatral, Xatral), 119t
Alimta (pemetrexed), 236t–245t
Alinia (nitazoxanide), 464t, 738t, 741t, 742
alirocumab (Praluent), 164t, 173–174, 173t, 211t, 222t–224t, 225
aliskiren (Tekturna), 482t, 494, 496t–498t
Alivio (capsaicin), 1116t–1117t
Alkeran (melphalan), 236t–245t
Alkindi Sprinkle (hydrocortisone), 830–832, 830t, 832b
alkylating drugs, 236t–238t
Allegra Allergy (fexofenadine), 590t, 596–600, 596t, 597b
Aller-Chlor (chlorpheniramine), 590t–591t, 593
allergic asthma, 210, 226
allergic conjunctivitis, 1082
allergic contact dermatitis, 588, 588f
allergic disorders, 210
allergic drug reactions, 589

allergic rhinitis, 323, 588, 588f, 595–596
allergies, 589
Allergy-Time (chlorpheniramine), 590t–591t, 593
Allerject (epinephrine), 541–542, 543t, 545–547
Allevacaine (benzocaine), 912t, 916t
Allevess (capsaicin), 1116t–1117t
Alli (orlistat), 679t, 681–683, 682t
allopurinol (Zyloprim, Aloprim; Apo-Allopurinol, Apo-Allopurinol A), 292t, 308–310, 309t, 309b
Almotriptan, 946
almotriptan (Axert, Mylan-Almotriptan, Sandoz Almotriptan), 945t
alogliptin (Nesina), 754t, 772, 772t
Alomide (lodoxamide), 1090t, 1094t–1095t
alopecia, 239t–245t, 247, 248b, 252t–257t
Aloprim (allopurinol), 292t, 308–310, 309t, 309b
Alora (estradiol transdermal system), 103t
alosetron (Lotronex), 738t, 741t, 742–743
Aloxi (palonosetron), 708t, 714t
alpha and beta receptors, 847b
alpha$_2$-adrenergic agonists, 932, 1082t–1084t, 1085
　adverse effects, 1086
　contraindications, 1086
　dose usage, 1086
　drug interactions, 1086b
　mechanisms of action, 1086
　nursing implications, 1086
　patient teaching guidelines, 1086
　pharmacokinetics, 1086
　preventing interactions, 1086
　therapeutic effects, 1086
alpha$_1$-adrenergic blockers, 119t, 499
　administration, 129
　adverse effects, 128–129
　alfuzosin, 128t, 129
　contraindications, 128
　doxazosin, 128t, 129
　drug interactions, 129, 129b
　mechanism of action, 128
　patient education guidelines for, 127b, 129, 856b
　pharmacokinetics, 128
　routes and dosage ranges, 128t
　silodosin, 128t, 129
　terazosin, 128t, 129
　therapeutic effects, 129
alpha–beta-adrenergic blockers, 496t–498t
Alphagan P (brimonidine), 1082t–1084t, 1085
alpha-glucosidase inhibitors
　abnormal kidney function, 768
　administration, 768
　adverse effects, 768–769
　contraindications, 768
　drug interactions, 768, 769b
　in hepatic impairment patients, 768
　in lactation, 768
　mechanism of action, 768
　nursing implications, 768–769
　patient teaching guidelines, 769
　pharmacokinetics, 767–768
　in pregnancy patients, 768
　therapeutic effects, 769
　uses, 768
alprazolam (Alprazolam Intensol, Xanax, Xanax XR), 87b, 96b, 101, 995t, 999
Alprazolam Intensol (alprazolam), 995t, 999
alprostadil (Caverject aqueous, Caverject powder, Edex powder, Muse, Caverject), 119t, 125, 126b
Alrex (loteprednol), 1090t, 1094t–1095t
Altabax (retapamulin), 1113t
Altacaine (tetracaine), 912t, 1078t–1079t
Altace (ramipril), 482t, 485t, 488, 754t
Altafrin (phenylephrine hydrochloride), 1078, 1078t–1079t
Altavera, 110t–111t

alteplase (Activase, Cathflo Activase, Activase rtPA, Cathflo Activase), 140t, 155–157, 155t
altered immune function, 209–211
　clinical manifestations, 210
altered nutritional states
　abnormal kidney function, 654
　clinical considerations, 645–646
　clinical manifestations, 646
　drug therapy, 646–654
　electrolytes, 651t–653t
　in hepatic impairment patients, 654
　minerals, 651t–653t
　vitamins, 647t–650t, 654t–656t
alternate-day therapy, 328
Altoprev (lovastatin), 164t, 166t, 167, 754t
altretamine (Hexalen), 236t–238t
Alupent (metaproterenol), 605t, 608t, 610
Alvesco (ciclesonide), 605, 616t, 617
Alyacen, 110t–111t
Alymsys (bevacizumab), 236t–238t, 252t–257t, 257–258
Alzheimer disease
　drug therapy, 858
　nursing interventions, 865b
　nursing process, 865b
　overview of, 857–858
　symptoms, 857
Amabelz (estradiol/norethindrone), 112t
Amanita muscaria, 855, 881
amantadine hydrochloride, 422–423, 422t, 871t, 873
Amaryl (glimepiride), 754t, 763b, 765t, 767b, 777
Ambien (zolpidem), 995t, 1002
Ambien CR (zolpidem), 995t, 1002
AmBisome (liposomal amphotericin B), 446–447, 448t
amcinonide, 1112t
amebiasis, 463–464, 464t, 466
amebicides, 463–465, 464t
　action and use, 464–465, 464t
　adverse effects, 465
　contraindications, 465
　nursing implications, 465, 466b
　patient teaching guidelines, 465, 466b
　pharmacokinetics, 463–464
　therapeutic effects, 465
Amerge (naratriptan), 945t
American drug laws, 5–8, 6t–7t
American Geriatrics Society Beers Criteria, 11
Amethyst, 110t–111t
Ametop (tetracaine), 912t
Amgevita SureClick (adalimumab), 211t, 222t–224t, 227
Amicar (aminocaproic acid), 140t, 158, 158t
Amidate (etomidate), 835t, 836, 922t, 926t, 927
amides, 912t
　administration of, 914
　adverse effects, 914
　bupivacaine, 915
　contraindications, 914
　drugs, 913t
　in lactation, 913
　mechanism of action, 912–913
　mepivacaine, 915
　nursing implications, 914
　patient teaching guidelines, 914, 914b
　pharmacokinetics, 912–913
　in pregnancy, 913
　preventing interactions, 914, 914b
　route and dosage, 913t
　therapeutic effects, 914
　uses, 913
amifostine (Ethyol), 236t–238t, 264t
amikacin (Erfa-Amikacin, VPI-Amikacin), 353–354, 353t, 355t, 357
amiloride (Midamor), 96b, 482t, 496t–498t, 631t, 638t, 639–640
aminocaproic acid (Amicar), 140t, 158, 158t

aminoglycosides. See also specific drug
　abnormal kidney function, 354
　administration of, 356
　adverse effects, 354–357
　amikacin, 353–354, 353t, 355t, 357
　assessment, 362b
　contraindications, 356
　dosage information, 354, 355t
　drug interactions, 356, 356b
　evaluation, 362b
　in hepatic impairment patients, 354
　mechanism of action, 354
　neomycin, 353t, 355t, 357
　nursing implications, 356–357
　nursing interventions, 362b
　nursing process, 362b
　paromomycin, 353t, 355t, 357
　patient teaching guidelines, 357, 357b
　peak and trough level, 353–354
　pharmacokinetics, 354
　plazomicin, 353t, 355t, 357
　streptomycin, 353t, 355t, 357
　therapeutic effects, 356
　tobramycin, 353–354, 353t, 355t, 357
　uses, 354
aminopenicillins, 336t–337t, 339
amiodarone (Nexterone, Pacerone; Cordarone), 77, 513–515, 513t
Amitiza (lubiprostone), 724t, 732–733, 732t
amitriptyline, 1009t, 1012t
amitriptyline hydrochloride, 77
amlodipine (Norvasc; ACT AmLODIPine, DOMAmLODIPine), 482t, 491–494, 492t, 524t, 532t, 533
amnesia, 921
Amnesteem (isotretinoin), 1118–1119
amoxapine, 1009t, 1012t, 1013
amoxicillin (Amoxil, Larotid, Apo-Amoxi, Mylan-Amoxicillin, Novamoxin, NPR-Amoxicillin, Nu-Amoxi, PHL-Amoxicillin, Pro- Amox-250, Pro-Amox-500, Moxatag, Novamoxin), 4–5, 335t–337t, 339, 692t, 701t, 702, 1104t, 1105–1106
amoxicillin–clavulanate (Augmentin, Augmentin XR; Amoxi-Clav, Apo-Amoxi-Clav, Clavulin, Novo-Clavamoxin, ratio-Aclavulanate), 335t–337t, 338
Amoxi-Clav (amoxicillin-clavulanate), 335t–337t, 338
Amoxil (amoxicillin), 4–5, 335t
AMPA glutamate receptor antagonist, 956t, 978
　abnormal kidney function, 979
　adverse effects, 979
　contraindications, 979
　dose usage, 979
　hepatic impairment, 979
　mechanisms of action, 979
　nursing implications, 979
　patient teaching guidelines, 979b
　pharmacokinetics, 979
　preventing interactions, 979
　therapeutic effects, 979
amphetamine-related CNS stimulants, 1047t
amphetamine-related drugs, 1052–1055, 1053t
　abnormal kidney function, 1053
　adverse effects, 1054
　contraindications, 1054
　dose usage, 1052–1053
　hepatic impairment, 1053
　mechanisms of action, 1052
　nursing implications, 1054
　patient teaching guidelines, 1054
　pharmacokinetics, 1049
　preventing interactions, 1054
　therapeutic effects, 1054
amphetamines, 685, 1047t, 1049–1051, 1050t, 1060
　abnormal kidney function, 1049

adverse effects, 1050
contraindications, 1050
dose usage, 1049
drug interactions, 1051b
hepatic impairment, 1049
mechanisms of action, 1049
nursing implications, 1051
patient teaching guidelines, 1052b
pharmacokinetics, 1049
preventing interactions, 1051
therapeutic effects, 1051
amphojel, 692t
amphotericin B deoxycholate (Fungizone), 446–449, 447t–448t, 449b
ampicillin (Novo-Ampicillin), 335t–337t, 336–340, 338b
ampicillin–sulbactam (Unasyn), 335t–337t, 339
ampules, 48
Amrix (cyclobenzaprin), 77
Amrix (cyclobenzaprine hydrochloride), 983t, 985t–986t, 989
amylin analogs
 administration, 773
 adverse effects, 773
 contraindications, 773
 drug interactions, 773, 774b
 mechanism of action, 773
 nursing implications, 773
 patient teaching guidelines, 773
 pharmacokinetics, 773
 therapeutic effects, 773
 uses, 773
anabolic steroids, 119
 abuse of, 122–123
 administration, 121
 contraindications, 121
 fluoxymesterone, 120
 mechanism of action, 120
 methyltestosterone, 120t
 nursing implications, 121
 pharmacokinetics, 120
 route and dosage information, 120t
 therapeutic effects, 121
Anacaine (benzocaine), 912t, 916
Anafranil (clomipramine), 1009t, 1012t
anagrelide (Agrylin), 140t, 151t–152t
anakinra (Kineret), 211t, 222t–224t, 227
analgesia, 921
Anandron (nilutamide), 236t–238t, 261t–263t, 263
Anapen (epinephrine), 541–542, 543t, 545–547
anaphylactic shock, 541, 546, 546b
anaphylactoid reactions, 589
anaphylaxis, 587–589
Anaprox (naproxen sodium), 290t, 298t–299t
anasarca, 630
Anaspaz (hyoscyamine sulfate), 882t
anastrozole (Arimidex, ACTAnastrozole), 236t–238t, 260, 261t–263t
Anbesol (benzocaine), 916
Anbesol Cold Sore Therapy (benzocaine), 912t, 916t
Ancobon (flucytosine), 456–457, 456t, 457b
Andriol (testosterone cypionate, testosterone enanthate), 120t
Androderm (testosterone cypionate, testosterone enanthate), 120t
Androderm (testosterone transdermal systems), 120t
androgen deficiency, 118
 abuse of, 122–123
 assessment, 130b
 clinical considerations, 118
 clinical manifestations, 118
 evaluation, 130b
 nursing interventions, 130b
 nursing process, 130b
 outcomes of therapy, 130b
 testosterone (see testosterone)
androgen-producing tumor, 315
androgens, 119t
Android (methyltestosterone), 120t
androstenedione, 123
Anectine (succinylcholine), 922t, 929t, 931
anesthesia, general. See general anesthesia
Angeliq (estradiol/drospirenone), 112t
angina pectoris
 beta-adrenergic blockers (see beta-adrenergic blocker(s))
 calcium channel blockers (see calcium channel blockers)
 organic nitrates (see organic nitrates)
Angiomax (bivalirudin), 141t–142t, 147–148
angiotensin II receptor antagonists, 754t
angiotensin II receptor blockers, 488–489, 778, 950
 abnormal kidney function, 489
 action, 489
 administration of, 486
 adverse effects, 489
 azilsartan, 490
 candesartan, 482t, 490, 490t, 495t–496t
 contraindications, 489
 drug interactions, 491b
 in hepatic impairment patients, 489
 hydrocodone, 578–580
 irbesartan, 482t, 490–491, 490t, 495t–496t
 nursing implications, 489–490
 olmesartan, 482t, 490t, 491, 495t–496t
 patient teaching guidelines, 487b, 490
 pharmacokinetics, 489
 preventing interactions, 489
 telmisartan, 482t, 490t, 491, 495t–496t
 therapeutic effects, 489
 use, 489
 valsartan, 482t, 490t, 491, 494, 495t–496t
angiotensin receptor blockers (ARBs), 561, 562t
angiotensin receptor–neprilysin inhibitors (ARNI), 555–557, 556t, 556b
angiotensin-converting enzyme (ACE) inhibitors, 23–24, 484, 485t, 524t, 535, 560–561, 562t, 754t, 777–778, 950. See also specific drug
 abnormal kidney function, 486
 action, 484
 administration of, 486
 adverse effects, 486
 benazepril (Lotensin), 488
 contraindications, 486
 enalapril (Vasotec), 488
 fosinopril, 488
 in hepatic impairment patients, 486
 lisinopril (Zestril), 488
 moexipril, 488
 nursing implications, 486
 patient teaching guidelines, 486, 487b
 perindopril (Coversyl), 488
 pharmacokinetics, 484
 preventing interactions, 486
 quinapril (Accupril), 488
 ramipril (Altace), 488
 therapeutic effects, 486
 trandolapril, 488
 use, 484–486
anhedonia, 1030
anidulafungin (Eraxis), 447t, 455t, 456
Anjeso (meloxicam), 290t, 300–301, 301t, 301b, 302b
annual flu vaccination, 194b
anorexia, 248b
ANS. See autonomic nervous system (ANS)
antacids, 21
 abnormal kidney function, 692
 action, 691
 administration, 693
 adverse effects, 693
 calcium carbonate, 692
 contraindications, 693
 in hepatic impairment patients, 692
 lactation, 692
 nursing implications, 693
 patient teaching guidelines, 693, 694b
 pharmacokinetics, 691
 pregnancy, 692
 preventing interactions, 693
 products, 694t
 reproduction, 692
 therapeutic effects, 693
 use, 692–693
antagonists, 845, 1066
 adenosine diphosphate receptor (see adenosine diphosphate receptor)
Antara (fenofibrate), 164t, 170–171, 170t, 171b
anterior pituitary hormone drugs, 800t–801t
 abnormal kidney function and hepatic impairment, 801
 administration of, 802
 adverse effects, 801–802
 contraindications, 801–802
 corticotropin, 802
 follitropin alfa/beta, 803
 in lactation, 801
 mechanism of action, 799
 menotropins, 803
 nursing implications, 802
 patient teaching guidelines, 802, 802b
 pegvisomant, 803
 pharmacokinetics, 799
 in pregnancy, 801
 preventing interactions, 802
 recombinant hCG choriogonadotropin alpha, 803
 therapeutic effects, 802
 thyrotropin alfa, 803
 uses, 800–801
anterograde amnesia, 1001–1002
anthelmintics, 464t, 469–470, 470t, 470b
anthracycline agents, 236t–238t, 238–239, 245
antiadrenergic (sympatholytic) drugs, 499
antiallergic drugs, 1090t, 1093, 1094t–1095t
 adverse effects, 1093
 contraindications, 1093
 dose usage, 1093
 mechanisms of action, 1093
 nursing implications, 1093
 patient teaching guidelines, 1092
 pharmacokinetics, 1093
 therapeutic effects, 1093
antiamyloid monoclonal antibody, 855t, 859t, 861–862
 administration of, 861
 adverse effects, 861–862
 contraindications, 861
 mechanism of action, 861
 nursing implications, 861–862
 patient teaching guidelines, 862
 pharmacokinetics, 861
 in pregnancy, 861
 preventing interactions, 861
 therapeutic effects, 861–862
 use in, 861
antiandrogens, 236t–238t, 260–263, 261t–263t
antianxiety drugs. See benzodiazepines
antiasthmatic drugs
 adrenergics (see adrenergic drugs)
 anticholinergics (see anticholinergic drugs)
 corticosteroids (see corticosteroids)
 immunosuppressant monoclonal antibodies, 619–620
 leukotriene modifiers (see leukotriene modifiers)
 mast cell stabilizers, 620–621
 xanthines (see xanthines)

antibacterial drugs, 463, 464t, 1090, 1090t–1091t, 1110–1117
　adverse effects, 1092
　contraindications, 1092
　dose usage, 1090–1092
　mechanisms of action, 1090
　nursing implications, 1092
　patient teaching guidelines, 1092
　pharmacokinetics, 1090
　therapeutic effects, 1092
antibiotic resistance, 278–280, 278b
antibiotic-associated colitis, 739
antibiotics, 273, 278–282
antibodies, 193
antibody preparations, 211, 211t, 221–226, 222t–224t
anticholinergic drug scale (ADS), 78
anticholinergic drugs, 610, 1077, 1078t–1079t
　abnormal kidney function, 1078
　action, 610
　administration of, 611, 883
　adverse effects, 611, 883, 1078
　belladonna alkaloid and derivatives, 880–883, 882t
　benztropine mesylate, 883–885
　body system and indication, 879t
　body tissues and organs
　　antispasmodic effects, 880
　　bronchodilation and decreased respiratory tract secretions, 880
　　CNS stimulation, 880
　　cycloplegia, 880
　　mechanism of action, 880f
　　mydriasis, 880
　　parasympathetic (vagal) stimulation, 880
　clinical use, 879
　contraindications, 611, 883, 1078
　darifenacin (Enablex), 888
　dosage information, 611t
　dose usage, 1078
　drug interactions, 611b, 884
　drug therapy, 879–880
　flavoxate, 888
　gastrointestinal, 885–886
　hepatic impairment, 1078
　ipratropium, 610–612, 611t
　mechanism of action, 880f, 884
　mechanisms of action, 1078
　medications, 880, 881t
　nursing implications, 611, 883, 1078
　patient teaching guidelines, 609b, 611, 883, 883b, 1080b
　pharmacokinetics, 610, 884, 1078
　preventing interactions, 611
　solifenacin (Vesicare), 887t, 888
　therapeutic effects, 611, 883, 885, 1078
　tiotropium, 605t, 611–612, 611t
　tolterodine (Detrol and Detrol LA), 879t, 881t, 887t, 888
　trihexyphenidyl, 884–885, 884t
　trospium chloride, 879t, 881t, 887t, 888
　urinary antispasmodics, 886–888, 887t
　use, 610–611
anticholinergics, 692t, 693
anticipatory nausea and vomiting, 707
anticoagulant drugs
　direct factor Xa inhibitors, 148
　direct thrombin inhibitors, 141t–142t, 147
　　(see also direct thrombin inhibitors)
　heparin(s), 139
　　abnormal kidney function, 142
　　administration of, 143
　　adverse effects, 143
　　age, 140
　　contraindications, 143
　　drug interactions, 143b
　　endogenous and exogenous, 139
　　fondaparinux, 143–144

　　in hepatic impairment patients, 142
　　LMWHs, 142–143, 157
　　mechanism of action, 140
　　nursing implications, 143
　　patient teaching guidelines, 143, 144b
　　pharmacokinetics, 140
　　preventing interactions, 143
　　prototype, 140t
　　therapeutic effects, 143
　warfarin
　　administration, 145
　　adverse effects, 145
　　contraindications, 145
　　drug interactions, 145, 146b
　　mechanism of action, 144–145
　　nursing implications, 145–146
　　patient teaching guidelines, 144b, 146
　　patients with hepatic impairment, 145
　　pharmacokinetics, 144
　　preventing interactions, 146b
　　therapeutic effects, 145
anticoagulants, 831
Anti-Dandruff (selenium sulfide), 1116t–1117t
antidepressant discontinuation syndrome, 1010
antidepressant therapy, 1009
antidepressants, 96
　genetic and ethnic differences in, 1010b
　PMS and PMDD, 101
　St. John's Wort as an, 1022b
　weight gain caused by, 675b, 685
antidiabetic drugs, 760b
　actions of, 755f
　alpha-glucosidase inhibitors, 767–769, 768t, 769b
　amylin analogs, 773, 773t, 774b
　biguanides, 765–767, 766t, 767b
　dipeptidyl peptidase-4 inhibitors, 771–772, 772t, 772b
　glucagon-like peptide-1 receptor agonists (incretin mimetics), 774–776, 775t
　meglitinides, 769–770, 770t, 771b
　patient teaching guidelines for, 763b, 767b
　sodium glucose cotransporter 2 inhibitors, 776–777, 776t, 777b
　sulfonylureas, 764–765, 765t
　thiazolidinediones, 769, 769t
　weight gain secondary to, 675b
antidiarrheals
　antibacterial drugs, 741–743
　bile-binding drugs, 741–742
　bismuth salts, 741, 741t
　diphenoxylate with atropine for, 737–739, 738t, 740b
　enzymatic replacement therapy, 741, 741t
　octreotide acetate, 741–742, 741t
　patient teaching guidelines, 739, 740b
　polycarbophil, 741t, 742
　selective 5-HT$_3$ receptor antagonist, 738t, 741–743, 741t
antidote
　definition of, 22
　half-life of, 19
antidysrhythmic drugs, 507t–508t, 513, 515–516
　adenosine, 517–518
　assessment, 519b
　evaluation, 519b
　magnesium sulfate, 518
　nursing interventions, 519b
　patient teaching guidelines, 509b
　therapeutic serum drug level, 508t
　therapy, outcomes of, 519b
　unclassified, 507t, 517–518
antiepileptic drugs (AEDs), 955, 956t
　barbiturates, 955
　carbonic anhydrase inhibitor, 968
　functionalized amino acids, 975

　gamma-aminobutyric acid structural analogs, 961
　iminostilbenes, 966
　phenyltriazine derivatives, 977
　pyrrolidine derivatives, 978
　succinimides, 973
　sulfonamide, 973
　triazole derivatives, 981
　weight gain caused by, 675b
antiestrogens, 236t–238t, 252t–257t, 260, 261t–263t
antifolate, 236t–245t
antifungal drugs, 1090t–1091t, 1093, 1114
　adverse effects, 1093
　azoles, 450–454, 451t–452t
　caspofungin, 454–456, 455t, 455b
　contraindications, 1093
　dose usage, 1093
　mechanisms of action, 1093
　nursing implications, 1093
　patient teaching guidelines, 1093
　pharmacokinetics, 1093
　polyenes, 446–449, 447t–448t
　pyrimidine analog, 456–457, 456t, 457b
　supercial mycoses, 457–459, 458t, 458b, 459b
　therapeutic effects, 1093
antigout medication
　mechanism of action, 306
　mitotic agent, 292t, 306–307, 307t
　therapeutic effects, 307
　uricosuric agents, 290, 292t, 308–310, 309t
antihepaciviral nucleoside, 412b, 427–428
antihistamines, 582, 587, 1115. See also specific drug
　abnormal kidney function, 711
　action, 710
　adverse effects, 711
　as antiemetic agents, 710
　contraindications, 711
　dimenhydrinate, 711t, 712
　doxylamine and pyridoxine combination, 712
　in hepatic impairment patients, 711
　lactation, 710
　meclizine, 712
　multi-ingredient nonprescription, 583t
　nursing implications, 711–712
　oral administration, 711
　patient teaching guidelines, 710b, 712
　pharmacokinetics, 710
　pregnancy, 710
　preventing interactions, 711
　reproduction, 710
　therapeutic effects, 711
　uses, 710–711, 711t
　weight gain caused by, 675b
antihypertensive drugs, 524t, 534. See also specific drug
　in African Americans, 24
　sites of action of, 480, 481f
　weight gain caused by, 675b
anti-infective agents, 1102–1104, 1102t
anti-inflammatory drugs, 605, 1090t, 1094t–1095t, 1096
antimalarials, 465
　action and use, 466, 467t
　administration, 468
　adverse effects, 466, 468
　contraindications, 468
　drugs, 464t, 467t
　nursing implications, 468, 468b
　patient teaching guidelines, 466b
　pharmacokinetics, 465–466
　preventing interactions, 468, 468b
　therapeutic and adverse effects, 468
antimetabolites, 236t–238t
antimicrobial drugs, 1118. See also specific drug
　acute inflammation, 273
　antibiotic resistance pattern, 282

Index **1133**

antibiotic-resistant microorganisms, 278–280, 278b
   assessment, 284f
   bacterial resistance, 280
   chronic inflammation, 273
   clinical manifestations, 273, 280
   combination therapy, 283
   community-acquired vs. hospital-acquired infections, 278
   culture and sensitivity studies, 282
   description, 272
   drug therapy, 273
   empiric therapy, 282
   evaluation, 284f
   host defense mechanisms, 272, 277
   medication cost, 283
   microorganisms, 273–283
   normal flora, 277
   opportunistic pathogens, 277–278
   pathogen laboratory identification, 278
   pathophysiology, 273
   patient teaching guidelines, 281, 281b
   penetrate infected tissues, 283
   therapy outcomes, 284f
   toxicity and risk-to-benefit ratio, 283
antimicrotubules, 236t–238t
antineoplastic drugs. See specific drug
antineoplastic hormone inhibitors, 236t–238t, 260–264, 261t–263t, 261f
antineoplastics drugs, 835t
   abnormal kidney function and hepatic impairment, 246, 836
   administration of, 250–251
   adverse effects, 247–249, 836–837
   alkylating drugs, 235–238, 236t–238t
   antiandrogens, 236t–238t, 260–263, 261t–263t
   antiestrogens, 236t–238t, 252t–257t, 260, 261t–263t
   antimetabolites, 236t–238t, 238
   antitumor antibiotics, 236t–238t, 238–239
   aromatase inhibitors, 236t–238t, 260, 261t–263t
   biologic targeted, 252–260
   cell cycle, 232, 232f
   characteristics of, 235b
   classification of, 234
   contraindications, 249–250, 836
   cytoprotectant drugs, 236t–238t, 264, 264t
   description of, 232–233
   gonadotropin-releasing hormone agonists, 236t–238t, 261t–263t, 263–264
   growth factors, 258–259
   in hepatic-impaired patients, 246
   hormone inhibitor drugs, 236t–238t, 260–264, 261t–263t, 261f
   in lactation, 836
   mechanism of action, 836
   monoclonal antibodies, 257–258
   nitrosoureas, 235, 236t–245t, 238
   nursing implications, 250–251, 836–837
   nursing process for, 265
   patient teaching guidelines, 837, 837b
   pharmacokinetics, 836
   plant alkaloids, 236t–238t, 239
   platinum compounds, 235, 236t–245t, 238
   podophyllotoxins, 236t–245t
   in pregnancy, 836
   preventing interactions, 250, 836
   proteasome inhibitors, 236t–238t, 252t–257t, 259–260
   taxanes, 236t–238t, 239, 249–250
   therapeutic effects, 251, 836–837
   tyrosine kinase inhibitors, 236t–238t, 258–259
   uses, 836
   vinca alkaloids, 236t–245t, 239, 248b, 250
antiparasitic drugs, 466b
antiparkinson drugs, 871t–872t, 874, 877

anticholinergics (see anticholinergic drugs)
antiplatelet drugs, 779. See also adenosine diphosphate receptor antagonists
   adenosine diphosphate receptor antagonists, 150
   dipyridamole, 151t–152t, 155–156
   glycoprotein IIb/IIIa receptor antagonists, 154
   phosphodiesterase-3 enzyme inhibitor, 154
   thromboxane A_2 inhibitors, 154
antiprostaglandins, 286
antipsychotic drugs, 1061t. See also specific drug
   weight gain caused by, 675b
antipyretic agents, 291
antirejection agents, 216–219
antiseptic agents, 1102–1104, 1102t
antistaphylococcal penicillins, 336t–337t, 339
antithymocyte globulin (ATG) (Atgam, equine; Thymoglobulin, rabbit), 211t, 222t–224t, 224, 226
antithyroid drug, 786–789, 787t
antitumor antibiotics, 236t–238t
antitussives
   action, 578
   administration of, 579
   adverse effects, 579
   benzonatate, 574t, 579, 579t
   codeine, 579–580
   contraindications, 579
   dosage ranges, 578, 579t
   hydrocodone, 579–580
   lactation, 579
   multi-ingredient nonprescription, 583t
   nursing implications, 579
   patient teaching guidelines, 577b, 579
   pharmacokinetics, 578
   pregnancy, 579
   preventing interactions, 579
   reproduction, 579
   reproduction, pregnancy, and lactation, 579
   therapeutic effects, 579
   use, 578–579
Antivert, Dramamine Less Drowsy, Motion-Time (meclizine), 708t, 711t, 712
antiviral drugs, 1090t–1091t, 1092, 1114
   adverse effects, 1092
   contraindications, 1092
   dose usage, 1092
   mechanisms of action, 1092
   nursing implications, 1092
   patient teaching guidelines, 1092
   pharmacokinetics, 1092
   therapeutic effects, 1092
Anucort (hydrocortisone), 318t, 320t–323t
anuria, 633
Anusol (hydrocortisone), 318t, 320t–323t
anxiety
   clinical manifestations, 993
   drug therapy, 993
   and hypnosis
      benzodiazepines (see benzodiazepines)
      dual receptor antagonists, 1003–1004
      herbal supplements, 996b
      nursing process, 1005b
      sedative hypnotics (see nonbenzodiazepine sedative hypnotics)
   and insomnia, 993–995
      clinical manifestations, 993
      overview, 993–995
   overview of, 993
anxiety disorder, 993
anxiolytics, 993
Anzemet (dolasetron), 708t, 713, 714t
APAP (acetaminophen), 286, 288, 290, 290t, 294–297, 295t, 297b
ApexiCon E (diflorasone diacetate), 1112t
Apidra (insulin glulisine), 753, 754t, 756t–757t
apixaban (Eliquis), 140t–142t, 148–149

Aplenzin (bupropion), 1009t, 1021, 1022t
Apo- Napro-Na (naproxen sodium), 290t, 298t–299t
APO Selegiline (selegiline hydrochloride), 871t–872t
Apo-Acetaminophen (acetaminophen), 286, 288, 290, 290t, 294–297, 295t, 297b
Apo-Alfuzosin (alfuzosin), 128t, 129
Apo-Allopurinol, Apo-Allopurinol A (allopurinol), 292t, 308–310, 309t, 309b
Apo-Amoxi (amoxicillin), 336t–337t
Apo-Amoxi-Clav (amoxicillin-clavulanate), 335t–337t, 338
Apo-Azathioprine (azathioprine), 211t, 212, 216
Apo-Azithromycin Z (azithromycin), 378t
Apo-Beclomethasone (beclomethasone), 320t–323t, 605, 614–615, 616t
Apo-Cal (calcium carbonate precipitated), 816t
Apo-Candesartan HCTZ (atacand HCT), 495t–496t
Apo-Cefaclor (cefaclor), 336t–337t
Apo-Cefadroxil (cefadroxil), 342t–344t
Apo-Cefprozil (cefprozil), 336t–337t
Apo-Cefuroxime (cefuroxime), 342t–344t
Apo-Cephalex (cephalexin), 336t–337t
Apo-Clarithromycin (clarithromycin), 378t
Apo-Clarithromycin XL (clarithromycin), 378t
Apo-Clindamycin (clindamycin hydrochloride), 381t–382t
APO-Darifenacin (Darifenacin hydrobromide), 887t
Apo-Desmopressin (desmopressin), 804t
Apo-Dexamethasone (dexamethasone), 318t, 320t–323t, 324–325, 328–329
Apo-Diazepam (diazepam), 864t
Apo-Diclo (diclofenac potassium), 290t, 302t–303t
Apo-Diclo SR Voltaren (diclofenac potassium), 290t, 302t–303t
Apo-Diltiaz SR (diltiazem), 524t, 532t, 533–534
Apo-Doxazosin (Cardura), 128t, 129
Apo-Dutasteride (dutasteride), 119t, 126, 126t
APOExemestane (exemestane), 236t–238t, 260, 261t–263t
Apo-Fluconazole, 451t–452t
Apo-Fluticasone (fluticasone), 320t–323t
APOFluticasone HFa (fluticasone), 318t, 320t–323t
Apo-Hydroxyurea (hydroxyurea), 236t–245t, 238
Apo-Imatinib (imatinib), 236t–238t, 252, 252t–257t, 258–259
Apo-Indomethacin (indomethacin), 290t, 297, 302–305, 302t–303t, 304b
Apo-Ipravent Solution (ipratropium bromide), 611t, 882t
Apo-Ipravent Sterules (ipratropium bromide), 882t
Apo-Ketoconazole (ketoconazole), 451t–452t, 453, 835t
Apokyn (apomorphine hydrochloride), 871t–872t, 874
APOLeflunomide (leflunomide), 211t, 216
Apo-Letrozole (letrozole), 236t–238t, 260, 261t–263t
APO-Levocarb (Levodopa–carbidopa), 871t–872t
APO-Levocarb CR (Levodopa–carbidopa), 871t–872t
Apo-Linezolid (linezolid), 381t–382t
Apo-Meloxicam (meloxicam), 290t, 300–301, 301t, 301b, 302b
Apo-Methimazole (methimazole), 787t
Apo-MetroNIDAZOLE (metronidazole), 381t–382t
Apo-Mometasone (mometasone), 320t–323t, 605t, 616t, 617, 621t
APO-Mycophenolate (mycophenolate mofetil/mycophenolate sodium), 213t
Apo-Nabumetone (nabumetone), 290t, 298t–299t, 300, 302t–303t, 305
Apo-Oflox (ofloxacin), 353t, 358t, 360

APO-Oxybutynin (oxybutynin), 887t
Apo-Paclitaxel (paclitaxel (conventional)), 236t–245t
Apo-Pen VK (penicillin V), 336t–337t
Apo-Piroxicam (piroxicam), 290t, 301, 301t
APO-Pramipexole (pramipexole dihydrochloride), 871t–872t
Apo-Prednisone (prednisone), 317, 318t, 320t–323t, 324–326, 328–329, 815t
APO-Quinine, 464t, 467t, 468
Apo-Raloxifene (raloxifene), 823t
APO-Rasagiline (rasagiline), 871t–872t
Apo-Salvent-Ipravent Sterules (ipratropium/albuterol), 621t
Apo-Sulfatrim (trimethoprim-sulfamethoxazole), 370t
Apo-Sulin (sulindac), 290t, 302t–303t, 305
Apo-Tamox (tamoxifen), 236t–238t, 260, 261t–263t
APO-Tamsulosin CR (tamsulosin), 119t, 128, 128t
Apo-Terbinafine, 458t
Apo-theo LA (short-acting theophylline), 612t
APO-Tolterodine (Tolterodine tartrate), 887t
Apo-Triamcinolone AQ (triamcinolone acetonide), 320t–323t
Apo-Warfarin (warfarin), 141t–142t
Apprilon (doxycycline), 365t–366t, 367–368
apraclonidine hydrochloride (Iopidine), 1082t–1084t
aprepitant (Emend), 708t, 714t–715t, 715, 716b
Apri, 110t–111t
Aptensio (methylphenidate), 1047t, 1053t
Aptiom (eslicarbazepine), 956t, 967t, 968
AquaMEPHYTON (vitamin K), 158t
aqueous humor, 1076
arachidonic acid, 286
Aranelle, 110t–111t
Aranesp (darbepoetin alfa), 181t
Arava (leflunomide), 211t, 213t, 216, 222t–224t
Aredia (pamidronate), 820t–821t, 822
argatroban, 140t–142t, 142, 147–148
Aricept (donepezil), 855t, 858, 859t
Aricept RDT (donepezil), 859t
Arimidex (anastrozole), 236t–238t, 260, 261t–263t
aripiprazole (Abilify, Abilify Maintena, Abilify MyCite), 1009t, 1024t, 1025, 1031t, 1039t–1040t, 1041
Aristocort, Aristocort R (triamcinolone), 320t–323t
Arixtra (fondaparinux), 140, 141t–142t
armodafinil (Nuvigil), 1047t, 1053t, 1054–1055
Arnuity Ellipta (fluticasone), 318t, 320t–323t
Arnuity Ellipta (fluticasone aerosol), 616t
Aromasin (exemestane), 236t–238t, 260, 261t–263t
aromatase inhibitors, 236t–238t, 260, 261t–263t
Arranon (nelarabine), 236t–245t
artemether/lumefantrine (Coartem), 464t, 467t, 468
artemisinin-based combination therapies (ACTs), 468
arthritis, 323
    osteoarthritis, 676b
    psoriatic, 210, 216, 219, 220t
    rheumatoid, 210, 216–217, 219, 220t, 226–227
Arthritis Pain Relief (capsaicin), 1116t–1117t
Arzerra (ofatumumab), 236t–238t, 252t–257t, 257
Asaphen (aspirin), 151t–152t
ascariasis, 470, 470t
Asceniv (immune globulin (human) (IG; IGIM)), 200t–201t
ascites, 631, 638
ascorbic acid (vitamin C), 654t–656t
    administration, 661
    adverse effects, 661
    contraindications, 661
    nursing implications, 661
    patient teaching guidelines, 657b, 661
    pharmacokinetics, 660
    therapeutic effects, 661
    use, 660–661
Ascriptin (aspirin), 151t–152t
asenapine (Saphris, Secuado), 1031t, 1039t–1040t, 1042
Asmanex, Asmanex HFA (mometasone), 318t, 320t–323t
Asmanex HFA (mometasone), 605t, 616t, 617, 621t
Asmanex Twisthaler (mometasone), 605t, 616t, 617, 621t
asociality, 1030
asparaginase (Erwinaze), 236t–245t, 238, 246–247
aspartate aminotransferase (AST), 216, 383, 450
Asperflex Hot Pain Reliever (capsaicin), 1116t–1117t
aspirin, 272–273, 524t, 535, 1107
aspirin (acetylsalicylic acid), 286, 288, 290–295, 290t, 304–306, 308, 754t, 778t
aspirin (Aggrenox), 151t–152t, 155
aspirin (Ascriptin, Bayer, Ecotrin; Asaphen, Entrophen, Novasen, Praxis), 140t, 151t–152t
Astagraf XL (tacrolimus), 211t, 212, 215b, 216, 218–219
Astelin (azelastine), 590t, 595–596, 595t
Astepro Allergy (azelastine), 590t, 595–596, 595t
asthma, 323–324
    action, 606–607
    adjuvant medications, 605t, 620–621
    administration, 605, 605t
    adrenergics (see adrenergic drugs)
    anticholinergics (see anticholinergic drugs)
    assessment, 622b
    clinical judgment, 555b
    clinical manifestations, 602–603
    combination regimens, 621, 621t
    corticosteroids (see corticosteroids)
    drug therapy, 605–606
    evaluation, 622b
    immunosuppressant monoclonal antibody, 605
    leukotriene modifiers (see leukotriene modifiers)
    management, 603–606, 604b
    mast cell stabilizers, 620–621
    nonpharmacologic approaches, 603–605
    nursing interventions, 622b
    nursing process, 622b
    outcomes of therapy, 622b
    xanthines (see xanthines)
Asthmanefrin Refill (epinephrine), 608t
asystole, 505b
Atacand (Candesartan cilexetil), 754t
Atacand (candesartan, atacand HCT), 482t, 490, 490t, 495t–496t
atacand HCT (APO-Candesartan HCTZ, Atacand, DOMCandesartan), 495t–496t
Atarax (hydroxyzine pamoate), 589–590, 590t–591t, 593
Atasol (acetaminophen), 286, 288, 290, 290t, 294–297, 295t, 297b
atenolol (Tenormin), 96b, 482t, 496t–498t, 499, 524t, 529–531, 530t, 531b
Atgam (antithymocyte globulin (ATG)), 222t–224t, 224, 226
athlete's foot, 1114
Ativan (lorazepam), 717, 956t, 960t, 995t, 999, 1061t–1063t
atogepant (Qulipta), 948t, 949
atomoxetine (Strattera), 1047t, 1055, 1056t
atorvastatin (Lipitor), 87b, 96b, 164–167, 166t, 167b, 168b
Atorvastatin calcium (Lipitor), 754t
atovaquone/proguanil (Malarone), 464t, 467t, 468
Atracurium, 922t, 929t
atrial fibrillation, 505b
atrial flutter, 505b
Atriance (nelarabine), 236t–245t
AtroPen (atropine sulfate), 863, 864t, 880–883, 881t–882t, 883b

atropine, 518, 1078
atropine sulfate (AtroPen), 855, 864t, 880–883, 881t–882t, 883b
atropine sulfate (Isopto Atropine), 1077, 1078t–1079t
atropine sulfate (Sal-Tropine), 855, 864t
Atrovent (ipratropium), 605t, 610–612, 611t
Atrovent HFA (ipratropium bromide), 611t, 879t, 881t–882t, 883
attention deficit hyperactivity disorder (ADHD), 1047
    amphetamine-related drugs (see amphetamine-related drugs)
    amphetamines (see amphetamines)
    assessment, 1057b
    atomoxetine, 1055
    clinical manifestations, 1047
    drug therapy, 1047
    evaluation, 1057b
    guanfacine, 1055
    mechanisms of action, 1048f
    nursing interventions, 1057b
    nursing process, 1057b
    outcomes of therapy, 1057b
    overview of, 1047
    sodium oxybate, 1055
    stimulants, 1048–1049
    treatment of, 1047t
    xanthines (see xanthines)
atypical antidepressants, 1009t, 1021–1022, 1022t, 1061t
    bupropion, 1021
    mirtazapine, 1021–1022
    trazodone, 1022
Aubra EQ, 110t–111t
Augmentin (amoxicillin-clavulanate), 335t–337t, 338
Augmentin XR (amoxicillin-clavulanate), 335t–337t, 338
Aura, 936
Auri-Perindopril (perindopril), 482t, 485t, 488
AURO Tofacitinib (tofacitinib), 211t, 221
Auro-Cefixime (cefixime), 342t–344t
Auro-Cefprozil (cefprozil), 336t–337t
Auro-Cefuroxime (cefuroxime), 342t–344t
Auro-Galantamine ER (galantamine), 855t, 859, 859t
AURO-Indomethacin (indomethacin), 92–93, 93t
Auro-Meloxicam (meloxicam), 290t, 300–301, 301t, 301b, 302b
Auro-MetroNIDAZOLE (metronidazole), 381t–382t
Auro-Moxifloxacin (moxifloxacin), 358t
autoantigens, 209
autoimmune disorders, 784
    description of, 209
    immunosuppressants for, 210
automaticity (electrical impulse), dysrhythmias, 504
autonomic drugs, characteristics of, 850
autonomic nervous system (ANS)
    neurotransmitter, 844–845
    nursing process, 851b
    organization of, 845f
    structure and function, 844
autoregulation, 478
    of blood flow, 478
Ava-Clindamycin (clindamycin hydrochloride), 381t–382t
avalide (Irbesartan-HCT, Avalide), 495t–496t
Avamys (fluticasone), 616t
avanafil (Stendra), 119t, 124t, 125
Avandia (rosiglitazone), 754t, 767b, 769, 769t, 772t
Avapro (irbesartan), 482t, 490–491, 490t, 495t–496t, 754t
Avastin (bevacizumab), 211t, 225, 236t–238t, 252t–257t, 257–258

Avaxim (hepatitis A vaccine), 194–203, 195t–199t
Aveeno (colloidal oatmeal), 1116t–1117t
Avian influenza A (H5N1), 406b
Aviane-28, 110t–111t
Avodart (dutasteride), 119t, 126, 126t, 128
avolition, 1030
Avonex (interferon beta-1a), 187t, 188
Avsola (infliximab), 211t, 227
Avycaz (ceftazidime-avibactam), 335t, 342t–344t
Axert (almotriptan), 945t
Axid (nizatidine), 692t, 696t, 698
Axiron (testosterone enanthate, testosterone cypionate), 120t
axitinib (Inlyta), 236t–238t, 252t–257t
azacitidine (Vidaza), 236t–245t
Azactam (aztreonam), 335t, 349, 350b
Azasan (azathioprine), 211t, 212, 216
azathioprine (Azasan, Imuran; Apo-Azathioprine, Imuran, TEVA Azathioprine), 211t, 212, 213t, 216, 857
azelaic acid (Azelex, Finacea), 1113t, 1118
azelastine, 1090t, 1094t–1095t
azelastine (Astepro Allergy; Astelin), 590t, 595–596, 595t
Azelex (azelaic acid), 1113t, 1118
Azilect (rasagiline), 869t, 871t–872t, 874
azilsartan (Edarbi), 482t, 490, 490t
azilsartan medoxomil (Edarbi), 754t
azithromycin (Apo-Azithromycin Z, Azithromycin for Injection, Dom- Azithromycin, PRO-Azithromycin, Zithromax), 377, 378t, 379
 action of, 380
 adverse effects, 380
 warfarin, 380
Azmacort (triamcinolone), 605t
azoles
 abnormal kidney function, 450
 action, 450
 administration of, 452–453
 adverse effects, 452
 age, 450
 assessment, 453
 contraindications, 452
 drug administration, 450, 451t–452t, 453b
 fatal hepatic damage, 450
 in hepatic impairment, 450
 lactation, 450
 nursing implications, 452–453
 patient teaching guidelines, 453, 453b
 pharmacokinetics, 450
 pregnancy, 450
 preventing interactions, 452, 453b
 reproduction, 450
 therapeutic effects, 453
 use, 450–452
Azopt (brinzolamide), 1082t–1084t, 1088
azor, 491, 495t–496t
Azstarys (serdexmethylphenidate and dexmethylphenidate), 1047t, 1053t, 1054–1055
aztreonam (Azactam), 335t, 349, 350b
Azulfidine (sulfasalazine), 365t, 370t, 372
Azurette, 110t–111t

B
B cells, 216, 221, 225–226
Baby Anbesol (benzocaine), 912t, 916t
Bacillus anthracis, 358, 365
bacitracin (Polysporin), 1113t
baclofen (Gablofen, Lioresal, Ozobax), 983–984, 983t, 985t–986t
bacteria
 gram-negative (see gram-negative bacteria)
 gram-positive (see gram-positive bacteria)
bacteria, description of, 272–273
bacterial vaginosis, 464

bactericidal, 280–281
bacteriostatic, 280–281
Bacteroides, 275b, 277
Bacteroides fragilis, 275b
Bactrim (trimethoprim-sulfamethoxazole), 365t, 367, 369
bad cholesterol, 168
balanced anesthesia, 921
baloxavir marboxil (Xofluza), 412b, 422t, 424–425
Balziva-28, 110t–111t
Banzel (rufinamide), 956t, 969t–972t, 981
bar coding, 39
barbiturates, 955, 958t, 993
 abnormal kidney function, 957
 adverse effects, 957
 contraindications, 957
 dosage usage, 956–957
 hepatic impairment, 957
 mechanisms of action, 956, 957f
 nursing implications, 957–958
 patient teaching guidelines, 958, 958b
 pharmacokinetics, 955
 preventing interactions, 957
 therapeutic effects, 957
baricitinib (Olumiant), 211t, 220t, 221, 411t, 413–414
baroreceptors, 481f
Barriere-HC (hydrocortisone), 320t–323t
basal ganglia, 868
basiliximab (Simulect), 211t, 222t–224t, 224–225
Baxdela (delafloxacin), 353t, 358t
Bayer (aspirin), 151t–152t
BBW (black box warning), 25. *See also specific drug*
becaplermin (Regranex), 1116t–1117t
beclomethasone (Beconase AQ, QNASL, QNASL Children; Apo-Beclomethasone, Mylan-Beclo AQ, Rivanase AQ, QVAR RediHaler, QVAR), 320t–323t
beclomethasone (Qvar RediHaler Beconase AQ, QVAR), 605t, 614–615, 616t
Beconase AQ (beclomethasone), 318t, 320t–323t
Beers criteria, 76–77
 older adults medications, 11
belatacept (Nulojix), 211t, 222t–224t, 227–228
Belbuca (buprenorphine), 904t, 1061t–1063t, 1066
belladonna alkaloid and derivatives
 administration, 883
 adverse effects, 881–883
 contraindications, 883
 drug interactions, 883
 homatropine hydrobromide, 882t
 ipratropium (Atrovent HFA), 882t
 mechanism of action, 880
 nursing implications, 883
 patient teaching guidelines, 883, 883b
 pharmacokinetics, 880
 scopolamine, 882t, 883
 therapeutic effects, 883
 tiotropium bromide (Spiriva HandiHaler, Spiriva Respimat), 879t, 881t–882t, 883
 uses, 880–881
Belsomra (suvorexant), 995t, 1003t
benazepril (Lotensin), 482t, 485t, 488
benazepril hydrochloride (Lotensin), 754t
bendamustine (Bendeka, Treanda), 236t–245t
Bendeka (bendamustine), 236t–245t
Benicar (olmesartan), 482t, 490t, 491, 495t–496t
Benicar (olmesartan medoxomil), 754t
benicar HCT (Olmetec, ACT Olmesartan, RIVAOlmesartan), 491, 495t–496t
benign prostatic hypertrophy
 5-alpha reductase inhibitor (*see* 5-alpha reductase inhibitors)
 assessment, 130b
 clinical considerations, 118
 clinical manifestations, 118

 evaluation, 130b
 nursing interventions, 130b
 nursing process, 130b
 therapy, outcomes of, 130b
benralizumab (Fasenra), 605t, 619t, 620
Bensal HP (salicylic acid), 1116t–1117t
Bentyl (dicyclomine hydrochloride), 885–886, 886t
Benzamycin (erythromycin/benzoyl peroxide), 1113t
benzimidazole, 469
Benziq (benzoyl peroxide), 1113t
benzocaine (Allevacaine, Anacaine, Anbesol Cold Sore Therapy, Baby Anbesol, Benz-O-Sthetic, Blistex, Cepacol INSTAMAX, GoodSense Oral Pain Relief, HurriCaine One, Hurricaine, Hurricane Snap-n-Go, HurriPak Starter Kit, Instant Oral Pain Relief Max, Ivy-Rid, Dentapaine, LolliCaine, Ora-film, Zilactin Baby), 912t, 916, 916t, 1117
benzodiazepine antianxiety drugs, 717
benzodiazepine receptor antagonist, 1061t
benzodiazepines (flumazenil), 922, 931–932, 956t, 959, 960t, 993, 995–1000, 995t, 1060–1064, 1061t. *See also specific drug*
 abnormal kidney function, 959, 998, 1061
 adverse effects, 959, 998, 1064
 contraindications, 959, 998, 1064
 dose usage, 996–998, 1061
 drug interactions, 1064b
 hepatic impairment, 959, 998, 1061
 mechanisms of action, 959, 996, 1061
 nursing implications, 959–961, 999, 1064
 patient teaching, 1064
 patient teaching guidelines, 961b, 1000b
 pharmacokinetics, 959, 995–996, 1061
 preventing interactions, 959, 999, 1064
 therapeutic effects, 961, 999, 1064
benzonatate (Tessalon), 574t, 579, 579t
Benz-O-Sthetic (benzocaine), 912t, 916, 916t
benzoyl peroxide (Acne-Clear, Benziq), 1111b, 1113t
benzphetamine, 679t
benztropine mesylate (Benztropine Omega, PMS-Benztropine), 884t
benztropine mesylate (Cogentin), 883–885
Benztropine Omega (benztropine mesylate), 884t
benzylisoquinolinium nondepolarizing neuromuscular blocking agents, 931
Beriplex P/N (prothrombin complex concentrate, human), 158t
Beta Care Betatar Gel (coal tar), 1116t–1117t
beta-adrenergic blocker(s). *See also specific drug*
 abnormal kidney function, 529
 action, 529
 administration of, 524t, 530
 adverse effects, 530
 bisoprolol, 524t, 530t, 531
 cardioselectivity, 529
 contraindications, 530
 dosage ranges, 530t
 drug interactions, 530, 531b
 in hepatic impairment, 529
 lactation, 529
 metoprolol, 530t, 531
 nadolol, 529, 530t
 nursing implications, 530–531
 patient teaching guidelines, 528, 531
 pharmacokinetics, 529
 pregnancy, 529
 propranolol, 530t, 531
 reproduction, 529
 therapeutic effects, 530
 uses of, 529
beta-adrenergic blocking agents, 499, 562t, 563–564

beta-adrenergic blocking drugs, 949–950, 1082t–1084t, 1085
  adverse effects, 1085
  contraindications, 1085
  dose usage, 1085
  drug interactions, 1085b
  mechanisms of action, 1085
  nursing implications, 1085
  patient teaching guidelines, 1085
  pharmacokinetics, 1085
  preventing interactions, 1085
  therapeutic effects, 1085
beta-adrenergic–blocking agent, 787t, 789
Betaject (betamethasone acetate and sodium phosphate), 320t–323t
beta-lactam antibacterial agents
  assessment, 351b
  carbapenems (see carbapenems)
  cephalosporins (see cephalosporins)
  description of, 335
  evaluation, 351b
  monobactams, 335, 349
  nursing interventions, 351b
  nursing process, 351b
  outcomes of therapy, 351b
  penicillins (see penicillin)
beta-lactamases, 335
betamethasone (betamethasone acetate and sodium phosphate) (Celestone, Soluspan), 318t, 320t–323t
betamethasone acetate (betamethasone), 320t–323t
betamethasone, dipropionate (Luxiq, Sernivo), 1112t
Betamol (timolol maleate), 1082t–1084t, 1085
Betapace (sotalol), 511t, 513, 513t, 515
Betaseron (interferon beta-1b), 187t
betaxolol (Betoptic S), 1082t–1084t
bethanechol (Urecholine), 692t, 855t, 862–863
Betoptic S (betaxolol), 1082t–1084t
bevacizumab (Alymsys, Avastin, Mvasi, Zirabev), 236t–238t, 252t–257t, 257–258
bevacizumab (Avastin, Mvasi, Zirabev), 211t, 222t–224t, 225
Bexxar (tositumomab), 236t–238t, 252t–257t, 258
Beyaz, 110t–111t
bezlotoxumab (Zinplava), 211t, 222t–224t, 225
bicalutamide (Casodex, ACHBicalutamide, ACT Bicalutamide, Casodex, Com-Bicalutamide)), 236t–238t, 261t–263t, 263
Bicillin LA (penicillin G benzathine), 335t
BiCNU (carmustine), 235, 236t–238t, 238–239
BiDil (hydralazine), 482t, 499
bier block anesthesia, 911
biguanides
  abnormal kidney function, 766
  administration, 767
  adverse effects, 766
  contraindications, 766
  drug interactions, 766, 767b
  in hepatic impairment patients, 766
  in lactation, 766
  mechanism of action, 765
  nursing implications, 766–767
  patient teaching guidelines, 767
  pharmacokinetics, 765
  in pregnancy patients, 766
  therapeutic effects, 767
  uses, 765–766
Bijuva (estradiol/progesterone), 112t
bile acid sequestrants, 168–170
  abnormal kidney function, 169
  administration of, 169
  adverse effects, 169
  colesevelam, 169t, 170
  colestipol, 169t, 170
  contraindications, 169
  dosage information, 168, 169t

hepatic impairment patients, 169
  mechanism of action, 168
  nursing implications, 169–170
  patient teaching guidelines, 169–170
  pharmacokinetics, 168
  preventing interactions, 169
  therapeutic effects, 169
bilirubin, 383
bimatoprost (Durysta, Latisse, Lumigan), 1082t
Bio-Diazepam (diazepam), 864t
Bio-Letrozole (letrozole), 236t–238t, 260, 261t–263t
biologic antineoplastic drugs, 236t–238t
biologic response modifiers, 186, 211, 221
biologics license applications (BLAs), 76
biotin, 648t
biotransformation, 18
bipolar disorder, 1008b, 1010
  assessment, 1027b
  atypical antidepressants (see atypical antidepressants)
  clinical manifestations, 1008b, 1010
  drug therapy, 1010
  evaluation, 1027b
  ketamine, 1026
  medications, 1026
  monoamine oxidase inhibitors, 1019–1021 (see also atypical antidepressants)
  mood-stabilizing agents, 1023–1026 (see also atypical antidepressants)
  nursing interventions, 1027b
  nursing process, 1027b
  outcomes of therapy, 1027b
  overview of, 1010
  selective serotonin reuptake inhibitors, 1013–1017 (see also selective serotonin reuptake inhibitors)
  serotonin-norepinephrine reuptake inhibitors (see serotonin-norepinephrine reuptake inhibitors)
  serotonin–norepinephrine reuptake inhibitors, 1017–1019
birth control pills, 102
bisacodyl (Dulcolax), 724t, 728–730, 729t, 730b
bismuth subcitrate potassium, metronidazole, and tetracycline (Pylera), 692t
bismuth subsalicylate (Pepto-Bismol), 692t, 701t, 702–703, 738t, 741, 741t
bisoprolol, 482t, 524t, 529, 530t, 531
bisphosphonates
  abnormal kidney function, 820
  administration of, 822
  adverse effects, 821–822
  contraindications, 821
  in hepatic impairment patients, 820
  in lactation, 820
  mechanism of action, 820
  nursing implications, 822
  patient teaching guidelines, 822, 822b
  pharmacokinetics, 820
  in pregnancy, 820
  preventing interactions, 822
  therapeutic effects, 822
  uses, 820
bivalirudin, 140t
bivalirudin (Angiomax), 141t–142t, 147–148
Bivigam (immune globulin intravenous (IGIV), immune globulin (human (IG; IGIM)), 200t–201t, 203
black box warnings (BBW), 25. See also specific drug
black cohosh, 59t–61t
blastomycosis, 445
bleeding, 248b
  control, 157–158
Blenoxane (bleomycin), 236t–245t, 238–239, 246
bleomycin (Blenoxane), 236t–245t, 238–239, 246

blepharitis, 1077
blinatumomab (Blincyto), 236t–238t, 252t–257t
Blincyto (blinatumomab), 236t–238t, 252t–257t
Blistex (benzocaine), 912t, 916, 916t
Blocadren (timolol), 482t, 496t–498t, 499
blood glucose levels, 750, 829
blood glucose meters, 755–758
blood lipids, 162
blood pressure. See also hypotension
  classification of, 478b
  elevated (see hypertension)
  regulation of, 478
  vascular resistance, 478
blood test, for tuberculosis, 390, 390b
blood urea nitrogen (BUN), 360
blood-brain barrier, 70
body mass index (BMI), 674, 676b, 678b
body ringworm, 1114
body surface area (BSA), 68, 69t
body weight
  loss of (see weight loss)
  obesity (see obesity)
body weight, drug action affected by, 23
bone disorders
  bisphosphonates for, 820–822
  calcium and, 813b
  description of, 814
  osteoporosis, 814
bone marrow transplantation, 209–210, 216, 226
bone marrow/stem cell transplantation, 210
bone metabolism, 812
Boniva (ibandronate), 820t–821t
Bontril PDM (phendimetrazine), 679t
Boostrix (diphtheria, tetanus toxoids, and acellular pertussis (DTaP)), 195t–199t
bortezomib (Velcade, ACT Bortezomib, PMSBortezomib), 236t–238t, 252t–257t, 259–260
Bosulif (bosutinib), 236t–238t, 252t–257t, 258
bosutinib (Bosulif), 236t–238t, 252t–257t, 258
bradydysrhythmias, 504, 506
bradykinesia, 868–869
bradykinin, 288, 289b, 484
brain tumors, 235, 239t–245t
brand name, 4–5
breakthrough pain, 897
breast cancer, 239t–245t
Brenzys (etanercept), 211t, 215, 227
Brevibloc (esmolol), 524t
Brevicon, Brevicon 1/35, 110t–111t
Brevital (methohexital sodium), 928
Brevital sodium (methohexital), 922t, 926t
Brexafemme (ibrexafungerp), 458t, 459
brexanolone, 96b
Bricanyl Turbohaler (terbutaline), 608t
Bridion (sugammadex), 930
Brilinta (ticagrelor), 140t, 151t–152t, 152–153
brimonidine (Alphagan P, Lumify, Combigan), 1082t–1084t, 1085
brinzolamide (Simbrinza, Azopt), 1082t–1084t, 1088
Brisdelle (paroxetine), 1009t
brivaracetam (Briviact), 969t–972t, 978
brivaracetam (Brivlera), 956t
Briviact (brivaracetam), 969t–972t
Brivlera (brivaracetam), 956t
bromocriptine mesylate (Parlodel, Cycloset), 869t, 871t–872t, 874
bronchial secretions, 574
bronchoconstriction, 602, 621
bronchoconstrictive disorders, 603, 603b
bronchodilators, 605
bronchospasm, 605, 607, 610–613, 620
budesonide (Pulmicort Terbuhaler, Pulmicort Respules Rhinocort, Entocort EC), 605t, 606, 616t, 617

budesonide (Pulmicort, Pulmicort Flexhaler; Pulmicort Nebuamp, Pulmicort Turbuhaler, TEVABudesonide, Entocort EC; Cortiment, Entocort, Rhinocort Allergy; Mylan-Budesonide AQ, Rhinocort Aqua, Rhinocort Turbuhaler, Uceris), 318t, 320t–323t
budesonide/formoterol (Symbicort), 621t
bulk-forming laxative(s), 724, 724t, 726t
bumetanide (Bumex), 482t, 631t–632t, 635
bumetanide (Burinex), 632t
Bumex (bumetanide), 482t, 631t–632t, 635
Bunavail (buprenorphine/naloxone), 904t, 1062t–1063t
Bupivacaine (Bupivacaine Fisiopharma, Bupivacaine Spinal, Marcaine Preservative Free, Marcaine Spinal, Sensorcaine, Saracoll), 912t
Bupivacaine Fisiopharma (bupivacaine), 912t, 915
Bupivacaine Spinal (bupivacaine), 912t, 915
Buprenex (buprenorphine), 904t, 1061t–1063t, 1066
buprenorphine (Buprenex, Belbuca, Butrans, Sublocade), 904t, 1061t–1063t, 1066
buprenorphine (Subutex; BuTrans, Sublocade), 894t, 896t–897t
Buprenorphine/naloxone (Suboxone, Bunavail, Zubsolv; Mylan-Buprenorphine/Naloxone, Suboxone), 904t, 1062t–1063t
bupropion, 96b, 681, 685, 685t
bupropion (Aplenzin, Wellbutrin SR, Wellbutrin XL, Zyban, Contrave), 1009t, 1021, 1022t, 1061t–1063t
bupropion–naltrexone (Contrave), 679t, 685, 685t
Burinex (bumetanide), 631t–632t, 635
burns, 371–372, 1077
Buscopan (scopolamine), 882t
busulfan (Busulfex, Myleran), 236t–245t
Busulfex (busulfan), 236t–245t
butenafine (Mentax), 1114, 1115t
butoconazole (Gynazole-1), 447t
butorphanol, 903–905, 904t
Butrans (buprenorphine), 896t–897t, 904t, 1061t–1063t, 1066
butterbur, 950
Byetta (exenatide), 754t, 758b, 763b, 772b, 774–775, 775t, 777
Byfavo (remimazolam), 932

C

cabazitaxel (Jevtana), 236t–245t
cabergoline, 833–834, 835t
Cabometyx (cabozantinib), 236t–238t, 252t–257t, 258
cabozantinib (Cabometyx, Cometriq), 236t–238t, 252t–257t, 258
CAD. See coronary artery disease (CAD)
Caelyx (lipodox 50), 236t–238t
Calan (verapamil), 482t, 512b, 516–517, 516t
Calan SR (verapamil), 524t, 531–534, 532t
Calciferol (ergocalciferol), 814, 816t
Calciferol (vitamin D), 818–820
  abnormal kidney function, 819
  administration of, 819
  adverse effects, 819
  contraindications, 819
  in hepatic impairment patients, 819
  in lactation, 818
  mechanism of action, 818
  nursing implications, 819
  patient teaching guidelines, 819–820, 819b
  pharmacokinetics, 818
  in pregnancy, 818
  preventing interactions, 819, 819b
  therapeutic effects, 819–820
  uses, 818–819, 819t
Calcimar (calcitonin), 823, 823t
calcipotriene (Calcitrene, Dovonex, Sorilux), 1116t–1117t
calcitonin (Miacalcin), 813–814, 823, 823t
calcitonin gene–related peptide receptor antagonist, 948–949
  abnormal kidney function, 948
  adverse effects, 949
  contraindications, 949
  dosage usage, 948
  drugs, 949
  hepatic impairment, 948
  mechanism of action, 948
  nursing implications, 949
  patient teaching guidelines, 949, 949b
  pharmacokinetics, 948
  therapeutic effects, 949
Cal-Citrate (calcium citrate), 816t
Calcitrene (calcipotriene), 1116t–1117t
calcitriol (Rocaltrol), 814, 816t, 819
calcium acetate (PhosLo), 816t
calcium and bone disorders, 813b
calcium and bone metabolism
  assessment, 825b
  clinical manifestations, 814
  disorders of, 813b
  drug therapy, 814
  evaluation, 825b
  nursing interventions, 825b
  nursing process, 825b
  outcomes of therapy, 825b
  overview of, 813–814
  in serum, hormonal regulation of, 812, 812f
calcium carbonate, 815
calcium carbonate antacids, 692, 694t
calcium carbonate precipitated (Os-Cal, Tums, Apo-Cal), 816t
calcium channel blockers, 950. See also specific drug
  abnormal kidney function, 492, 532
  action, 491, 532
  administration of, 493, 524t, 533
  adverse effects, 493, 533
  for cardiovascular disorders treatment, 532–533
  contraindications, 493, 533
  dihydropyridines, 493, 531–534
  diltiazem, 482t, 491, 492t, 493
  drug interactions, 533, 533b
  isradipine, 482t, 492t, 494
  lactation, 532
  mechanism of action, 533
  nicardipine, 482t, 492t, 494, 531–533, 532t
  nifedipine, 482t, 492t, 493
  nisoldipine, 482t, 492t, 494
  nondihydropyridines, 531–534
  nursing implications, 493, 533
  patient teaching guidelines, 487b, 493, 527b, 533
  pharmacokinetics, 491, 532
  pregnancy, 532
  preventing interactions, 493
  reproduction, 532
  therapeutic effects, 493, 533
  use, 491–492
  uses, 532, 532t
  verapamil, 482t, 492t, 493–494
calcium chloride (Calciject), 518–519, 816t
calcium citrate (Cal-Citrate; Osteocit), 816t
calcium gluconate, 91, 668, 816t
calcium preparations
  abnormal kidney function, 817
  administration of, 817
  adverse effects, 817
  contraindications, 817
  drugs, 816t
  in hepatic impairment patients, 817
  in lactation, 817
  mechanism of action, 815
  nursing implications, 817–818
  oral calcium, 815
  patient teaching guidelines, 818, 818b
  pharmacokinetics, 815
  in pregnancy, 817
  preventing interactions, 817, 817b
  therapeutic effects, 817
  uses, 815–817
Calcium Sandoz (calcium gluconate), 816t
calories, 674, 683
Calphron (calcium acetate), 816t
Cambia (diclofenac potassium), 290t, 302t–303t
Camcevi (leuprolide acetate), 806t
Camila (norethindrone), 107t–108t
cAMP (cyclic adenosine monophosphate), 19–20
Campath (alemtuzumab), 211t, 225, 236t–238t, 252t–257t
Camptosar (irinotecan), 236t–245t, 246–247, 250
camptothecins, 236t–245t
Campylobacter jejuni, 385
canagliflozin (Invokana), 562t, 564, 776–777, 776t, 777b
cancer
  classification of, 234
  clinical considerations, 233–234
  clinical judgment in practice, 235b
  clinical manifestations, 234
  cytotoxic antineoplastic drugs (see Cytotoxic antineoplastic drugs)
  drug therapy, 234
  etiology, 232
  immunizations in patients with, 202
  immunosuppression-related, 216
  obesity, 676b
  pain, 898, 902
Cancidas (caspofungin), 454–456, 455t, 455b
candesartan (Atacand), 482t, 490, 490t, 495t–496t
candesartan cilexetil (Atacand), 754t
Candida albicans, 445, 1114
candidiasis, 445
cangrelor (Kengreal), 140t, 150, 151t–152t, 153
cannabinoids, 718
canthi, 1076
CAP (community-acquired pneumonia), 278
capecitabine (Xeloda), 236t–245t
Capoten (Captopril), 754t
capsaicin (Alivio, Allevess, Arthritis Pain Relief, Asperflex Hot Pain Reliever, Capsaicin HP), 1116t–1117t
capsaicin (Zostrix), 59t–61t
Capsaicin HP (capsaicin), 1116t–1117t
capsules, 41
captopril (Capoten), 482t, 484–488, 485t, 754t
Carac (fluorouracil), 1116t–1117t
Carafate (sucralfate), 692t, 701t, 702
carbamate derivatives, 984
  adverse effects, 984
  contraindications, 984
  dose usage, 984
  mechanisms of action, 984
  nursing implications, 984
  patient teaching guidelines, 984b
  pharmacokinetics, 984
  preventing interactions, 984
  therapeutic effects, 984
carbamazepine (Carbatrol, Epitol, Equetro, TEGretol, TEGretol-SR), 87b, 956t, 966, 967t
carbapenem–beta-lactamase inhibitor combinations, 347t
carbapenems
  abnormal kidney function and hepatic impairment, 348
  administration of, 348
  adverse effects, 348
  contraindications, 348
  mechanism of action, 347
  nursing implications, 348
  patient teaching guidelines, 348
  pharmacokinetics, 347
  preventing interactions, 348, 348b
  reproduction, pregnancy, and lactation, 347
  route and dosage information, 347, 347t
  therapeutic effects, 348

Carbatrol (carbamazepine), 967t
carbenicillin indanyl sodium, 335t
carbidopa (levodopa), 869–873, 869t
Carbocaine (mepivacaine), 912t, 915
Carbocaine Preservative Free (mepivacaine), 912t
carbohydrate metabolism, 316b, 751, 751b
carbonic anhydrase inhibitors, 956t, 968, 969t–972t, 1082t–1084t, 1087
  abnormal kidney function, 968
  adverse effects, 972, 1088
  contraindications, 972, 1088
  dose usage, 968–972, 1088
  drug interactions, 1088b
  hepatic impairment, 968
  mechanisms of action, 968, 1087–1088
  nursing implications, 972, 1088
  patient teaching guidelines, 973b, 1088b
  pharmacokinetics, 968, 1087–1088
  preventing interactions, 972, 1088
  therapeutic effects, 972, 1088
carboplatin (Paraplatin), 236t–245t, 238, 250, 258
carboprost tromethamine (Hemabate), 94t, 95
carboxylic acid derivative, 949
carcinomas, 234
Cardene (nicardipine), 524t, 532t, 533
cardiac dysrhythmias, 551
cardiac glycosides, 562t, 564–565
cardiac output, 494
cardiac transplantation, 213t
cardiogenic shock, 512, 514–515, 517, 540, 541t, 542, 546b
cardioselectivity, beta-adrenergic blocker(s), 529
cardiotonic-inotropic agents. See phosphodiesterase inhibitors
cardiovascular disorders, 24, 676b
cardiovascular effects, 785t–786t
cardiovascular system, 316b
  glucocorticoids' effect on, 316b
Cardizem (diltiazem), 516–517, 516t, 517b, 524t, 532t, 533–534
Cardizem CD (diltiazem), 482t
Cardura (doxazosin), 482t
Cardura (doxazosin, Apo-Doxazosin, Teva-Doxazosin) Doxazosin XL), 119t, 128t, 129
carfilzomib (Kyprolis), 236t–238t, 252t–257t, 260
Carimune NF (immune globulin (human) (IG; IGIM), immune globulin intravenous (IGIV)), 200t–201t, 203
carisoprodol (Soma), 983t, 984, 985t–986t
carmustine (BiCNU, Gliadel), 235, 236t–238t, 238–239
CaroSpir (spironolactone), 496t–498t, 637–640, 638t, 639b
carteolol, 1082t–1084t
Cartia XT (diltiazem), 482t, 524t, 532t, 533–534
carvedilol (Coreg), 482t, 524t
carvedilol (Coreg, Coreg CR), 496t–498t
Casodex (bicalutamide), 236t–238t, 261t–263t, 263
caspofungin (Cancidas), 454–456, 455t, 455b
castor oil, 724t, 729t, 730
cataplexy, 1048
Catapres (clonidine), 482t, 496t–498t, 1061t–1063t
catatonia, 1030–1031
catechol-O-methyltransferase (COMT) inhibitors
  abnormal kidney function, 876
  administration, 876
  adverse effects, 876
  contraindications, 876
  drug interactions, 876
  entacapone (Comtan), 876–877
  in hepatic impairment patient, 876
  in lactation, 876
  mechanism of action, 875
  nursing implications, 876
  patient teaching guidelines, 876, 877b
  pharmacokinetics, 875

in pregnancy, 876
therapeutic effects, 876
uses, 876
cathartics
  action, 728
  administration of, 728
  adverse effects, 728
  contraindications, 728
  definition of, 723, 728
  drug interactions, 724t, 728, 729t. 730b
  lactation, 728
  nursing implications, 728–730
  patient teaching guidelines, 727b, 729–730
  pharmacokinetics, 728
  pregnancy, 728
  reproduction, 728
  saline, 724t, 728, 729t, 730
  stimulant, 724t, 728, 729t, 730
  therapeutic effects, 728
  uses, 725t, 728
catheters
  description of, 46b
  peripherally inserted central, 46b
Cathflo Activase (alteplase), 140t, 155–157, 155t
Caverject (alprostadil), 125, 126b
Caverject aqueous (alprostadil), 119t
Caverject powder (alprostadil), 119t
Caziant, 110t–111t
CCR5 antagonists, 440–441, 440b
Ceclor (cefaclor), 336t–337t
cefaclor (Apo-Cefaclor, Ceclor, Novo-Cefaclor), 335t–337t
cefadroxil (Apo-Cefadroxil, PRO-Cefadroxil, Teva-Cefadroxil), 335t, 342t–344t
cefazolin, 335t, 340–341, 342t–344t, 345
cefdinir, 335t, 342t–344t, 346
cefditoren, 335t, 342t–344t
cefepime (Maxipime), 335t, 341, 342t–344t
cefiderocol (Fetroja), 335t, 341, 342t–344t
cefixime (Suprax; Auro-Cefixime, Suprax), 335t, 342t–344t
Cefotan (cefotetan), 340, 342t–344t
cefotaxime, 335t, 342t–344t
cefotetan (Cefotan), 335t, 340–341, 342t–344t, 346
cefoxitin (Mefoxin), 335t, 340–341, 342t–344t
cefpodoxime, 335t, 342t–344t, 346
cefprozil (Apo-Cefprozil, Auro-Cefprozil), 335t–337t
ceftaroline (Teflaro), 335t, 341, 342t–344t
ceftazidime (Fortaz, Tazicef), 335t, 340–341, 342t–344t
ceftazidime-avibactam (Avycaz), 335t, 342t–344t, 346
ceftibuten, 335t, 342t–344t
Ceftin (cefuroxime), 342t–344t
ceftolozane-tazobactam (Zerbaxa), 335t, 342t–344t, 346
ceftriaxone, 335t, 340–341, 342t–344t, 345
cefuroxime (Zinacef; Apo-Cefuroxime, Auro-Cefuroxime, Ceftin, cefuroxime for injection, PRO-Cefuroxime), 335t, 340, 342t–344t
ceiling threshold, 636
Celebrex (celecoxib), 290t, 305–306, 305t, 306b
celecoxib (Celebrex, ACT Celecoxib, AG-Celecoxib), 290t, 305–306, 305t, 306b
Celestone (betamethasone), 318t, 320t–323t
Celestone Soluspan (betamethasone acetate and sodium phosphate), 320t–323t
Celexa (citalopram), 1009t, 1017, 1036
CellCept (mycophenolate), 857
CellCept (mycophenolate mofetil/mycophenolate sodium), 213t
CellCept, CellCept Intravenous (mycophenolate mofetil IV), 212–216
cenobamate (Xcopri), 956t, 969t–972t
Centany (mupirocin), 1113t

Centany AT (mupirocin), 1113t
Centers for Disease Control and Prevention (CDC), 464
central nervous system (CNS), 377, 844, 844f
  depressant, 1061
  drug distribution into, 17
  effects, 785t–786t
  stimulant abuse, 1067
  stimulants (see specific drug)
  tumors, 324
central obesity, 676b
central precocious puberty
  abnormal kidney function and hepatic impairment, 807
  administration of, 807
  adverse effects, 807
  contraindications, 807
  drugs, 806t
  goserelin, 807
  histrelin, 807
  in lactation, 807
  leuprolide acetate, 805
  mechanism of action, 805
  nafarelin, 807
  nursing implications, 807
  patient teaching guidelines, 807, 807b
  pharmacokinetics, 805
  in pregnancy patients, 807
  preventing interactions, 807
  therapeutic effects, 807
  triptorelin, 807
  uses, 806–807
centrally acting alphaagonist antihypertensive, 1061t
centrally acting skeletal muscle relaxants, 987
Cepacol INSTAMAX (benzocaine), 912t, 916, 916t
cephalexin (Keflex; Apo-Cephalex, Dom-Cephalexin, PMS Cephalexin, Teva-Cephalexin), 335t–337t
cephalosporin–beta-lactamase inhibitor combinations, 342t–344t
cephalosporins
  abnormal kidney function and hepatic impairment, 345
  administration of, 345
  adverse effects, 345
  cefotetan, 335t, 340–341, 342t–344t, 346
  cephalosporin–beta-lactamase combinations, 342t–344t
  classification, 340–341
  contraindications, 348
  descriptions, 340
  fifth-generation, 341
  first-generation, 340
  fourth-generation, 341
  mechanism of action, 341
  nursing implications, 345
  oral, 345, 346b
  parenteral administration, 345
  patient teaching guidelines, 345, 346b
  pharmacokinetics, 341
  preventing interactions, 345, 345b
  second-generation, 340
  therapeutic effects, 345
  third-generation, 340–341
Cequa (cyclosporine emulsion), 1090t, 1094t–1095t, 1097
cerebrospinal fluid (CSF), 336
Cerebyx (fosphenytoin), 956t, 965t, 966
ceritinib (Zykadia), 236t–238t, 252t–257t, 258
certified medical assistants (CMAs), 34
certolizumab (Cimzia, Cimzia Prefilled, Cimzia Starter Kit; Cimzia), 211t, 222t–224t, 227
Cerubidine (daunorubicin), 236t–245t, 238–239, 247, 248b
Cervarix (human papillomavirus (HPV)), 194b, 195t–199t, 201

Cervidil (dinoprostone), 94, 94t
Cesamet (nabilone), 708t, 717t, 718
cetirizine (Zyrtec Allergy), 590t, 594–597, 595t
Cetraxal (ciprofloxacin), 1104t
cetuximab (Erbitux), 211t, 222t–224t, 225, 236t–238t, 252t–257t, 257, 259f
chamomile, 59t–61t
Chantix (varenicline), 1061t–1063t
Chateal, 110t–111t
chelating agents, 662t–664t, 667–668
chemoreceptor trigger zone (CTZ), 707
chemotaxis, 274f
chemotherapy
    adjuvant, 252–264
    complications, 248b
    definition, 232–233
    description, 232–233
    neoadjuvant, 232, 234
    palliative, 247
    patient teaching guidelines, 251, 251b
chemotherapy-induced emesis, 324
chickenpox vaccine, 194b
Chlamydia trachomatis, 368
chlorambucil (Leukeran), 236t–245t
chloramphenicol (Chloromycetin), 381–383
chloramphenicol (Chloromycetin Succinate), 381–383, 381t–382t
chlordiazepoxide (Librium), 995t, 999, 1061–1064, 1061t–1063t
Chloromycetin (chloramphenicol), 381–383
chloromycetin succinate, 381t–382t
Chloroprocaine (Clorotekal, Nesacaine, Nesacaine-MPF), 912t
Chloroprocaine hydrochloride (Clorotekal, Nesacaine, Nesacaine-MPF), 915–916, 916t, 916b
chloroquine phosphate, 464t, 465, 467t, 468, 468b
chloroquine with primaquine, 467t
chlorothiazide (Diuril), 482t, 631t, 635–637, 636t, 637b
chlorothiazide (Thalitone), 631t, 636t, 637
chlorpheniramine (Aller-Chlor, Allergy-Time), 582, 590t–591t, 593
chlorpromazine (Thorazine), 708t–709t, 710, 1031t, 1033t
chlorpromazine hydrochloride (TEVA-Chlorpromazine), 951, 951t, 1032
Chlorpropamide, 754t, 765t
chlorthalidone (APO-Chlorthalidone), 482t, 496t–498t
chlorthalidone (Thalitone), 631t, 636t, 637
chlorzoxazone (Lorzone), 985t–986t, 989
cholecalciferol (Delta-D, D-Vi-Sol; D-Tabs, EURO-D), 816t
cholestatic hepatitis, 123
cholesterol, 162
cholesterol absorption inhibitor
    abnormal kidney function and hepatic impairment, 172
    administration of, 172
    adverse effects, 172
    contraindications, 172
    dietary management, 172
    drug interactions, 172, 172b
    mechanism of action, 172
    niacin, 164t, 174–175, 174t
    nursing implications, 172–173
    patient teaching guidelines, 173
    pharmacokinetics, 172
    reproduction, pregnancy, and lactation, 172
    therapeutic effects, 172
cholesterol-lowering agents, 675b
cholestyramine (Prevalite; Olestyr, PMS-Cholestyramine, Questran, Novo-Cholamine), 164t, 168–170, 169t, 738t, 741t, 742
cholinergic agonist, 855t

    administration, 862
    adverse effects, 862
    contraindications, 862
    evaluation, 865b
    mechanism of action, 862
    nursing implications, 862–863
    nursing interventions, 865b
    patient teaching guidelines, 863, 863b
    pharmacokinetics, 862
    therapeutic effects, 862
    in use, 862
cholinergic drugs, 853, 1082t–1084t, 1086. *See also* specific drug
    adverse effects, 1086–1087
    contraindications, 1087
    dose usage, 1086
    mechanisms of action, 1086
    nursing implications, 1087
    patient teaching guidelines, 1087
    pharmacokinetics, 1086
    preventing interactions, 1087
    therapeutic effects, 1087
cholinergic fibers, 845
cholinergic receptors, 849, 853, 854f
cholinesterase inhibitor–*N*-methyl-D-aspartate receptor antagonist, 861
    abnormal kidney function, 858
    administration, 858–859
    adverse effects, 858–859
    contraindications, 858
    donepezil, 858
    drug interactions, 858, 859b
    galantamine hydrobromide, 859
    in hepatic impairment patients, 858
    mechanism of action, 858
    nursing implications, 858–859
    patient teaching guidelines for, 859, 860b
    pharmacokinetics, 858
    rivastigmine, 859, 859t
    routes and dosage ranges, 859t
    therapeutic effects, 859
    uses, 858
cholinesterase inhibitors, 855t, 858–860, 859t
cholinesterase–NMDA receptor antagonist, 855t
chondroitin, 59t–61t
choriogonadotropin alpha (Ovidrel), 803
chorionic gonadotropin (human chorionic gonadotropin), 803
choroid, 1076
chronic airflow limitation (CAL), 603b
chronic bronchitis, 603b
chronic GVHD, 210
chronic inflammation, 273
chronic myeloid leukemia, 252t–257t
chronic obstructive airway disease (COAD), 603b
chronic obstructive lung disease (COLD), 603b
chronic obstructive pulmonary disease (COPD), 325
chronic pain, 892, 894, 895, 898, 902–903
chronic renal rejection reactions, 210
chronic tophaceous gout, 288–290
chronotropic effect, 545–546
chronotropic medications, 506
Cialis (tadalafil), 119t, 124t, 125
Cibinqo (abrocitinib), 211t, 227
ciclesonide (Alvesco), 605, 616t, 617
Ciclodan (ciclopirox), 1115t
ciclopirox (Ciclodan), 1115t
ciclopirox (Loprox, Penlac), 447t
cilostazol, 140t, 151t–152t
Ciloxan (ciprofloxacin ophthalmic), 1090t
cimetidine (Tagamet), 692t, 693, 695–698, 696t
Cimzia (certolizumab), 211t, 227
Cimzia Prefilled (certolizumab), 211t, 227
Cimzia Starter Kit (certolizumab), 211t, 227
Cinqair (reslizumab), 605t, 619t, 620

Cipro (ciprofloxacin), 353t, 357–360, 358t, 359b, 1104t
Cipro HC Otic (ciprofloxacin-hydrocortisone), 1102
ciprofloxacin (Cetraxal, Otiprio, Cipro, ACT Ciprofloxacin, Ophthalmic), 353t, 357–360, 358t, 359b, 1104–1105, 1104t
ciprofloxacin ophthalmic (Ciloxan), 1090t
ciprofloxacin-hydrocortisone (Cipro HC Otic), 1102
Cisatracurium (Nimbex; Cisatracurium Omega), 922t, 929t, 931
Cisatracurium Omega (cisatracurium), 929t
cisplatin, 236t–245t, 238, 246, 248b, 250
citalopram, 1017
citalopram (Celexa), 1009t, 1017, 1036
Citrucel (methylcellulose), 724t, 726t
cladribine (Mavenclad), 236t–245t
Claforan (cefotaxime), 342t–344t
Claravis (isotretinoin), 1118–1119
Clarinex (desloratadine), 589–590, 590t, 596, 596t
clarithromycin (ACTClarithromycin XL, APOClarithromycin, APO-Clarithromycin XL, Biaxin, Biaxin BID, Dom-Clarithromycin, PMS Clarithromycin), 377, 378t, 380, 692t, 701t
    absorption of, 380
    administration, 380
    adverse effects, 380
Claritin (loratadine), 595t, 596
Claritin Eye (ketotifen), 1090t, 1094t–1095t, 1096
class IA sodium channel blockers, 506
    abnormal kidney function, 507
    action, 506
    administration of, 507t, 509
    adverse effects, 507
    contraindications, 507
    dosage of, 506–507, 507t
    drug interaction, 508t
    in hepatic impairment, 507
    mechanism of action, 506, 507t
    nursing implications, 508–509
    patient teaching guidelines, 509, 509b
    pharmacokinetics, 506
    preventing interactions, 509, 509b
    quinidine, 508t, 510
    therapeutic effects, 509
    use, 506–507
class IB sodium channel blockers, 507t–508t, 510
class IC sodium channel blockers, 507t–508t, 510
class II beta-adrenergic blockers
    action, 511
    administration of, 507t, 512
    adverse effects, 512
    contraindications, 512
    drug-drug interaction, 512, 512b
    effectiveness, 511
    lactation, 512
    nursing implications, 512
    patient teaching guidelines, 509b, 512
    pharmacokinetics, 511
    pregnancy, 512
    propranolol, 511–512, 511t, 512b
    reproduction, 512
    therapeutic effects, 512
    use, 511
class III potassium channel blockers
    abnormal kidney function, 514
    action, 513
    administration of, 507t, 514
    adverse effects, 514
    amiodarone, 513–515, 513t
    contraindications, 514
    dofetilide, 513t, 515
    electrophysiologic characteristics, 513
    in hepatic impairment, 514

class III potassium channel blockers (Continued)
  lactation, 514
  mechanism of action, 513
  nursing implications, 514–515
  patient teaching guidelines, 509b, 515
  pharmacokinetics, 513
  pregnancy, 514
  preventing interactions, 514
  reproduction, 514
  therapeutic effects, 514
  use of, 513–514
class IV calcium channel blockers
  action, 516
  administration of, 507t, 517
  adverse effects, 517
  contraindications, 517
  diltiazem, 516–517, 516t, 517b
  drugs, 516, 516t
  effectiveness, 516
  nursing implications, 517
  patient teaching guidelines, 509b, 517
  pharmacokinetics, 516
  pregnancy, 517
  preventing interaction, 517, 517b
  reproduction, 517
  therapeutic effects, 517
  use, 516–517
Clavulin (amoxicillin-clavulanate), 335t–337t, 338
Clear Away One Step Wart Remover (salicylic acid), 1116t–1117t
clemastine, 96b, 589–590, 590t–591t
Cleocin (clindamycin), 1113t
Cleocin (clindamycin hydrochloride), 381t–382t, 383
Cleocin T (clindamycin), 1113t
Climara (estradiol transdermal system), 103t
Climara Pro (estradiol/levonorgestrel), 112t
Clindacin Pac (clindamycin), 1113t
Clindacin-P (clindamycin), 1113t
Clindagel (clindamycin), 1113t
clindamycin (Cleocin, Cleocin T, Clindamycin ETZ, Clindacin Pac, Clindacin-P, Clindagel, Clindesse, Evoclin), 1113t
Clindamycin ETZ (clindamycin), 1113t
clindamycin hydrochloride (Cleocin; Apo-Clindamycin, Ava- Clindamycin, Clindamycin-150 or 300, Dalacin C, Dalacin C Palmitate, Riva Clindamycin,Teva-Clindamycin), 381t–382t, 383
Clindamycin-150 or 300 (clindamycin hydrochloride), 381t–382t
Clindesse (clindamycin), 1113t
"Clinical Guidelines on the Identification, Evaluation, and Treatment of Overweight and Obesity in Adults," 678b
clinical trials, 8
clobazam (Onfi, Sympazan), 956t, 960t
clobetasol propionate (Clobetasol Propionate E, Clobetavix, Clobex, Clobex Spray, Clodan, Impeklo, Tovet), 1112t
Clobetasol Propionate E (clobetasol propionate), 1112t
Clobetavix (clobetasol propionate), 1112t
Clobex (clobetasol propionate), 1112t
Clobex Spray (clobetasol propionate), 1112t
Clodan (clobetasol propionate), 1112t
clofarabine (Clolar), 236t–245t
Clolar (clofarabine), 236t–245t
Clomid (clomiphene citrate), 84, 85t
clomiphene citrate (Clomid, Serophene), 84, 85t
clomipramine (Anafranil), 1009t, 1012t
clonazepam (Klonopin), 956t, 960t, 995t
clonic, 954
clonic phase, 955

clonidine (Catapres), 482t, 496t–498t, 1061t–1063t
cloning, 4
clopidogrel (Plavix), 140t, 150, 151t–152t
clorazepate (Tranxene), 956t, 995t
clorazepate (Tranxene-T), 960t
Clorotekal (chloroprocaine hydrochloride), 912t, 915, 916t
clotrimazole (Lotrimin AF, Shopko Athletes Foot), 447t, 450, 451t–452t, 1115t
clozapine (Clozaril, Versacloz), 96b, 675b, 1031t, 1039t–1040t
Clozaril (clozapine), 1031t, 1039t–1040t
cluster headaches, 936
  clinical manifestations, 936
  drug therapy for
    ergot alkaloids, 938t, 942–943
    triptans, 944–947, 945t
  treatment of, 937
CMV immune globulin, intravenous, human (CMV-IGIV) (CytoGam; CytoGam), 200t–201t
CNS (central nervous system), 844, 844f
CNS depressant, 1047t
coagulation disorders
  assessment, 159b
  bleeding control, 157–158
  clinical manifestations, 138
  direct thrombin inhibitors (see direct thrombin inhibitors)
  drug therapy, 138–139, 139f, 140t
  evaluation, 159b
  nursing interventions, 159b
  nursing process, 159b
  outcomes of therapy, 159b
  thrombolytic drugs (see thrombolytic drugs)
  vitamin K antagonists (see vitamin K (Mephyton))
coal tar (Beta Care Betatar Gel, DSH Tar. Pentrax Gold, Psoriasin), 1116t–1117t
Coartem (artemether/lumefantrine), 464t, 467t, 468
cobicistat, 432–433
cocaine, 1060
coccidioidomycosis, 445
Cockroft-Gault method, 79
codeine (Codeine Contin, PMS-Codeine, Ratio-Codeine), 96b, 574t, 578–580, 579t, 894t, 896t–897t, 901–902, 902t
Codeine Contin (codeine, narcotic codeine), 574t, 578–580, 579t, 896t–897t, 901
Cogentin (benztropine mesylate), 883–885
Colace (docusate sodium), 724t, 726t
colchicine (Colcrys, Mitigare; JAMP-Colchicine, PMSColchicine, Sandoz Colchicine), 292t, 306–307, 307t, 308b
  abnormal kidney function and hepatic impairment, 307
  administration of, 307
  adverse effects, 307
  contraindications, 307
  nursing implications, 307
  patient teaching guidelines, 307, 308b
  pharmacokinetics, 306
  preventing interactions, 307
Colcrys (colchicine), 292t, 306–307, 307t, 308b
cold remedies, 582, 582b
colesevelam (WelChol, Lodalis), 164t, 169t, 170
Colestid (colestipol), 164t, 169t, 170, 738t, 741t, 742
Colestid Flavored (colestipol), 164t, 169t, 170
colestipol (Colestid, Colestid Flavored), 164t, 169t, 170, 738t, 741t, 742
colloidal oatmeal (Aveeno), 1116t–1117t
Colocort (hydrocortisone), 318t, 320t–323t
colon cancer, 233, 239t–245t
colonization, 274
colony-stimulating factors (CSF), 179

colorectal cancer, 252t–257t
Coly-Mycin S Otic (neomycin-colistin-hydrocortisone- thonzonium), 1102
CoLyte (polyethylene glycol-electrolyte solution), 724t, 729t
Combat Methamphetamine Epidemic Act of 2005, 582
Com-Bicalutamide (bicalutamide), 236t–238t, 261t–263t, 263
Combigan (brimonidine and timolol), 1082t–1084t
combination regimens, asthma, 621, 621t
CombiPatch (estradiol/norethindrone), 112t
Combivent Respimat (ipratropium/albuterol), 621t
Combivent UDV (ipratropium/albuterol), 621t
Cometriq (cabozantinib), 236t–238t, 252t–257t, 258
common cold, 574
  combination products, 582–585
  OTC formulations, 582–583
community-acquired infection, 278
community-acquired pneumonia (CAP), 278
compensated shock, 541
complement, 289b
compliance, 780b
Comprehensive Drug Abuse Prevention and Control Act, 7
Compro (prochlorperazine), 708–709, 708t–709t, 709b, 951t
computerized provider order entry (CPOE), 39
Comtan (entacapone), 869t, 876–877
Comtrex Severe Cold & Sinus Tablets, 583t
concentration-dependent bactericidal effects, 356
Concerta (methylphenidate), 1047t, 1053t
conductivity (electrical impulses), dysrhythmias, 504
confusion, 1030
congenital adrenogenital syndromes, 315
conjugated estrogen-medroxyprogesterone (Prempro), 109, 112t
conjugated estrogens (Premarin, synthetic conjugated), 101–105, 103t
conjugated estrogens/medroxyprogesterone acetate (Premphase, Premplus), 112t
conjunctivitis, 1077
constipation
  administration, 724t
  assessment, 734b
  clinical manifestations, 723
  defecation, 723
  definition, 723
  drug therapy for, 723–724
    cathartics (see cathartics; laxative(s))
  evaluation, 734b
  lactulose, 724t, 732, 732t
  lifestyle changes, 723
  linaclotide, 730–731, 731t
  lubiprostone, 724t, 732–733, 732t
  nursing interventions, 734b
  nursing process, 734b
  plecanatide, 724t, 731–732
  prucalopride, 724t, 732t, 733
  sorbitol, 723, 724t, 732t, 733
  tegaserod, 724t, 732t, 733
  therapy, outcomes of, 734b
Constulose (lactulose), 724t, 732, 732t
consumers, medication errors by, 35t–36t
Contac Day and Night Cold & Flu Caplets, 583t
continuous infusion, 46b
Contrave(bupropion–naltrexone), 679t, 685
Contrave (bupropion), 1061t–1063t
controlled substances, 7
Controlled Substances Act, 7, 7b
conventional antirejection agents, 211, 211t, 216–219
convoluted tubules, 630f, 635
convulsion, 954

ConZip (Oxymorphone Tramadol), 894t, 896t–897t, 902t, 903
Cordarone (amiodarone), 513–515, 513t
Cordran (flurandrenolide), 1112t
Coreg (carvedilol), 482t, 524t
Corgard (nadolol), 482t
Coricidin D Cold Flu & Sinus, 583t
Coricidin HBP Cold & Flu, 583t
Corlanor (ivabradine), 559–560, 560t, 560b
Corlopam (fenoldopam), 482t
cornea, 1076
corneal ulcers, 1077
coronary artery disease (CAD), 551
    assessment, 537b
    clinical considerations, 522
    clinical manifestations, 522–523
    drug therapy, 524, 524t
    etiology, 522
    evaluation, 537b
    nonpharmacologic management, 523–524
    nursing interventions, 537b
    outcomes of therapy, 537b
    risk factors for, 523
    stable angina, 522–523, 522f
coronary artery endothelial dysfunction, 551
coronary artery vasospasm, 522
coronary heart disease, 522
coronaviruses, 406b
Cortef (hydrocortisone), 320t–323t, 830–832, 830t, 832b
Cortenema (hydrocortisone), 318t, 320t–323t
corticosteroids, 221, 272–273, 314, 614–617, 715, 717, 829, 831–832, 1090t, 1094t–1095t, 1096
    abnormal kidney function, 615
    action, 614
    administration of, 615, 1110
    adrenal cortex disorders, 315–316
    adverse effects, 615, 1096
    assessment, 332b
    beclomethasone, 614–617, 616t
    budesonide, 605t, 616t, 617
    contraindications, 615, 1096
    dosage information, 616t
    dose usage, 1096
    drug therapy, 1110
    drugs, 616t
    endogenous, 314–315
    exogenous (see exogenous corticosteroids)
    fluticasone, 605t, 616t, 617
    in hepatic impairment patients, 615
    mechanisms of action, 1096
    methylprednisolone, 605t, 616t, 617
    mometasone, 605t, 616t, 617, 621t
    nursing implications, 615–617, 1096
    nursing process, 332b
    patient teaching guidelines, 617, 1096
    pharmacokinetics, 614, 1096
    prednisone, 605t, 616t, 617
    preventing interactions, 615
    therapeutic effects, 615–617, 1096
    triamcinolone acetonide, 605t, 617
    use, 614–615
    weight gain caused by, 675b
corticotropin, 829
corticotropin (Acthrel, HP Acthar Gel, ACTH), 799t–801t, 802
corticotropin-releasing hormone (CRH), 828
Cortifoam (hydrocortisone), 318t, 320t–323t
Cortifoam (hydrocortisone acetate), 320t–323t
Cortiment (budesonide), 320t–323t
cortisol, 314, 829–830
cortisone acetate, 318t, 320t–323t
Cortrosyn (cosyntropin), 799t–801t
Corvert (ibutilide), 513t, 515
corzide, 495t–496t

Cosmegen (dactinomycin), 236t–245t
Cosopt (dorzolamide and timolol), 1082t–1084t
Cosopt PF (dorzolamide and timolol), 1082t–1084t
cosyntropin (Cortrosyn), 799t–801t
Cotempla XR-ODT (methylphenidate), 1047t, 1053t
cough, 574
Coumadin (warfarin), 141t–142t, 144
Covera-HS (verapamil), 524t, 531–534, 532t
Coversyl (perindopril), 482t, 485t, 488
COVID-19 (Pfizer-BioNTech, Moderna, Johnson & Johnson), 79, 194, 194b, 195t–199t, 201–203, 202b, 892b
    drugs, 410–415
COX-1, 286
COX-2 inhibitors, 286
Cozaar (losartan), 482t, 490t, 561, 562t, 778, 778t
creatine, 59t–61t
Cresemba (isavuconazole), 447t, 451t–452t, 454
Crestor (rosuvastatin), 164t, 166t, 754t
Crinone (progesterone), 107t–108t
Crohn's disease, 209–210, 226–227
cromolyn (Nasalcrom), 605t, 620, 1090t
cromolyn sodium, 1093, 1094t–1095t
cross-allergenicity, 338
cross-tolerance, 25
crotamiton (Crotan), 464t, 471t
Crotan (crotamiton), 464t, 471t
cryptococcosis, 445, 447, 456
Cryptococcus neoformans, 445
Cryselle, 110t–111t
crystalluria, 371–372
Crystapen (penicillin G benzathine), 336t–337t
Cubicin (daptomycin), 381t–382t, 383–384
Cubicin RF (daptomycin), 381t–382t
culture, 282
Cushing's disease, 315–316
    antineoplastics (see anticholinergic drugs; antineoplastics)
    assessment of, 838b
    clinical considerations, 829
    clinical manifestations, 829
    11-deoxycortisol inhibitors (see 11-deoxycortisol inhibitors)
    diagnosis, 829–830
    drug therapy for, 833
    evaluation of, 838b
    nursing interventions, 838b
    nursing process, 838b
    outcomes of therapy, 838b
    overview of, 829–830
Cutaquig (immune globulin (human) (IG; IGIM)), 200t–201t
Cutivate (fluticasone topical), 318t, 320t–323t
Cuvitru (immune globulin (human) (IG; IGIM)), 200t–201t
Cuvposa (glycopyrrolate), 879t, 886t
cyanocobalamin (vitamin B_{12}), 654t–656t
    administration, 660
    adverse effects, 660
    contraindications, 660
    nursing implications, 660
    patient teaching guidelines, 657b, 660
    pharmacokinetics, 659–660
    therapeutic effects, 660
    use, 660
Cyclen, 110t–111t
Cyclessa, 110t–111t
cyclic adenosine monophosphate (cAMP), 19–20
cyclobenzaprine (Amrix, Fexmid), 77
cyclobenzaprine hydrochloride (Amrix, Fexmid), 983t, 985t–986t, 989
Cyclogyl (cyclopentolate), 1078, 1078t–1079t
cyclooxygenase (COX), 286, 1107
cyclopentolate (Cyclogyl), 1078, 1078t–1079t

cyclophosphamide (Procytox), 235, 236t–245t, 245–246, 248b, 251b
cycloplegia, 880
cycloserine (Seromycin), 391–392
Cycloset (bromocriptine mesylate), 869t, 871t–872t, 874
cyclosporine (Gengraf, Neoral, SandIMMUNE), 211t, 212, 215–219, 217t, 225
    abnormal kidney function, 217
    action, 216
    adverse effects, 218
    contraindications, 218
    drug interactions, 218, 218b
    in hepatic impairment, 217
    nursing implications, 218–219
    pharmacokinetics, 216
    reproduction, pregnancy, and lactation, 217
    use, 216–218
cyclosporine emulsion (Cequa, Restasis, Verkazia; Restasis MultiDose), 1090t, 1094t–1095t, 1097
cyclothymia, 1010
Cyklokapron (tranexamic acid), 158, 158t
Cymbalta (duloxetine), 1009t, 1019
CYP (Cytochrome P450), 250
    definition of, 18
    polymorphisms of, 18
CYP3A4 inhibitors, 949
CYP2D6 functional deficiency, 165
cyproheptadine, 589–590, 590t–591t
cytarabine (Cytosar), 236t–245t, 246
cytochrome P450 (CYP), 250
    definition of, 18
    inhibitor, 412b, 438–441, 439t
    polymorphisms of, 18
CytoGam (CMV immune globulin, intravenous, human (CMV-IGIV)), 200t–201t
cytokines, 179, 209–210, 289b
    inhibitors, 226–227
    receptors, 179
cytomegalovirus (CMV) infection, 406b
    drugs for, 417–419
cytoprotectant drugs, 236t–238t, 264, 264t
Cytosar (cytarabine), 236t–245t, 246
Cytotec (misoprostol), 94–95, 94t, 692t, 701t, 702
cytotoxic antineoplastic drugs
    abnormal kidney function, 246
    administration, 250–251
    adverse effects, 247–249
    alkylating drugs, 235–238, 236t–238t
    antimetabolites, 236t–238t
    antitumor antibiotics, 236t–238t, 238–239
    cell cycle effects of, 232, 232f
    characteristics, 235b
    contraindications, 249–250
    with hepatic impairment, 246
    nursing implications, 250–251
    patient teaching guidelines, 251, 251b
    pharmacokinetics, 235
    plant alkaloids, 236t–238t, 239
    preventing interactions, 250
    route and dosage information for, 239, 239t–245t
    therapeutic effects, 251
    use of, 239–247
cytotoxic immunosuppressive agents, 210, 211t, 212–216, 213t
cytotoxic T cells, 210

D
dabigatran etexilate (Pradaxa), 140t–142t, 147, 148b
dabrafenib (Tafinlar), 236t–238t, 252t–257t, 258
dacarbazine, 236t–245t, 238, 248b
dactinomycin (Cosmegen), 236t–245t
Dalacin C Palmitate (clindamycin hydrochloride), 381t–382t
dalbavancin (Dalvance), 381t–382t, 383

dalteparin (Fragmin), 140, 140t–142t, 143, 156–157
Dalvance (dalbavancin), 381t–382t, 383
danazol, 119t–120t, 120, 122
Dantrium (dantrolene sodium), 983t, 985t–986t, 987
dantrolene, 983
dantrolene sodium (Dantrium, Revonto, Ryanodex), 983t, 985t–986t, 987
dapagliflozin (Farxiga), 562t, 564, 776t, 777
Dapagliflozin and saxagliptin (Qtern), 778
Dapagliflozin, saxagliptin, and metformin (Qternmet XR), 778
Daptacel (diphtheria, tetanus toxoids, and acellular pertussis (DTaP)), 195t–199t, 203
daptomycin (Cubicin), 381t–382t, 383–384
darbepoetin alfa (Aranesp), 180t–181t
daridorexant (Quviviq), 995t, 1003t, 1004
Darifenacin hydrobromide (APO-Darifenacin, Enablex, JAMP-Darifenacin), 887t
darifenacin hydrobromide (Enablex), 879t, 881t, 887t, 888
dasatinib (Sprycel), 236t–238t, 252t–257t, 258
daunorubicin (Cerubidine), 236t–245t, 238–239, 247, 248b
Daypro (oxaprozin), 290t, 298t–299t, 300
Daytrana (methylphenidate), 1047t, 1053t
Daytrana Methylin (methylphenidate), 1047t
DayVigo (lemborexant), 995t, 1003t, 1004
DDAVP (desmopressin acetate), 803–804, 804b
Decapeptyl (triptorelin), 236t–238t, 261t–263t, 264, 806t
decarboxylase inhibitor/dopamine precursor
  abnormal kidney function, 878
  administration, 878
  adverse effects, 878
  contraindications, 878
  drug interactions, 878
  in hepatic impairment patients, 878
  in lactation, 877
  mechanism of action, 877
  nursing implications, 878
  patient teaching guidelines, 878
  pharmacokinetics, 877
  in pregnancy, 877
  therapeutic effects, 878
  uses, 877–878
decitabine, 236t–245t
Declomycin (demeclocycline hydrochloride), 366t
decompensated shock, 541
decompensation, 551
defecation, 723
deferasirox (Exjade), 668
deferoxamine (Desferal), 668
dehydroepiandrosterone (DHEA), 123
delafloxacin (Baxdela), 353t, 358t, 360
delayed hypersensitivity, 588–589
Delsym (dextromethorphan), 574t, 578–580, 579t, 580b, 582, 583t
Delta-D (cholecalciferol), 816t
Deltasone (prednisone), 317, 318t, 320t–323t, 324–326, 328–329
delusions, 1030
Delyla, 110t–111t
Demadex (torsemide), 482t
demeclocycline hydrochloride (Declomycin), 365t–366t, 368
Demerol (meperidine), 894t, 896t–897t, 902
Demerol (meperidine hydrochloride), 77
Denavir (penciclovir), 417, 1115t
denosumab (Prolia, Xgeva), 823, 823t
Dentapaine (benzocaine), 912t, 916, 916t
11-deoxycortisol inhibitors, 834, 835t
  abnormal kidney function and hepatic impairment, 834
  administration of, 834
  adverse effects, 834–835

contraindications, 834
  in lactation, 834
  mechanism of action, 834
  nursing implications, 834–835
  patient teaching guidelines, 835, 836b
  pharmacokinetics, 834
  in pregnancy, 834
  preventing interactions, 834, 835b
  therapeutic effects, 834–835
  uses, 834
Depakote (valproate), 956t, 969t–972t, 974
Depakote ER (valproate), 956t, 969t–972t, 974
Depakote Sprinkles (valproate), 956t, 969t–972t
dependent edema, 630
Depo-Estradiol (estradiol cypionate), 103t
Depo-Estradiol (estradiol transdermal system), 103t
depolarizing neuromuscular blocking agent, 931
Depo-Medrol (methylprednisolone), 318t, 320t–323t
Depo-Medrol (methylprednisolone acetate), 320t–323t
Depo-Medrol (methylprednisolone sodium succinate), 616t
Depo-Provera (medroxyprogesterone acetate), 107t–108t
Depo-SubQ Provera 104 (medroxyprogesterone acetate), 107t–108t
depot medroxyprogesterone acetate SubQ, 107t–108t
Depo-Testosterone (testosterone cypionate), 120t
depression, 1008, 1008b
  clinical manifestations, 1008
  drug therapy, 1009–1010
  overview of, 1008–1010
  treatment of, 1009t
dermatitis, 1110
dermatologic drugs. See also specific drug
  creams, 42t–43t
dermatophyte infections, 1114
dermatophytes, 445
desensitization, 848
Desflurane (Suprane), 922t–923t, 924–925
desipramine (Norpramin), 1009t, 1012t
desirudin (Iprivask), 140t–142t, 147–148
desloratadine (Clarinex), 589–590, 590t, 596, 596t
desmopressin (Stimate, DDAVP, Apo-Desmopressin), 804t
desmopressin acetate (DDAVP, Stimate), 803–804, 804b
desoximetasone (Topicort Spray), 1112t
Desoxyn (methamphetamine), 1047t, 1050t
desvenlafaxine (Pristiq), 96b, 1009t, 1019
detection of antigens, 278
Detrol (tolterodine tartrate), 887t
Detrol LA (tolterodine tartrate), 879t, 881t, 887t
dexamethasone, 414, 714t, 716, 829–830
dexamethasone (Dextenza, Dexycu, Maxidex, Ozurdex), 1090t, 1094t–1095t, 1096
dexamethasone (TaperDex 12 Day; TaperDex 6 Day, TaperDex 7 Day, TopiDex, ZCort 7 Day, Apo-Dexamethasone, Dexamethasone Omega Unidose), 318t, 320t–323t, 324–325, 328–329
Dexamethasone Omega Unidose (dexamethasone), 318t, 320t–323t, 324–325, 328–329
dexchlorpheniramine (Polmon), 590t–591t, 593
Dexcom G6 Glucose Monitoring System, 755–758
Dexedrine (dextroamphetamine), 1047t, 1049, 1050t
Dexilant (dexlansoprazole), 692t, 699t, 700
dexlansoprazole (Dexilant), 692t, 699t, 700
Dexmedetomidine (Precedex), 922t, 932, 932t
dexmethylphenidate (Focalin, Focalin XR), 1047t, 1053t, 1054–1055
dexrazoxane, 236t–238t, 264t

dexrazoxane (Zinecard), 236t–238t, 264t
Dextenza (dexamethasone), 1090t, 1094t–1095t
dextroamphetamine (Dexedrine, ProCentra, Zenzedi, Xelstrym transdermal), 1047t, 1049, 1050t
dextroamphetamine and amphetamine (Adderall XR, Adderall, Mydayis), 1047t, 1050t, 1051
dextromethorphan (Delsym), 77, 574t, 578–580, 579t, 580b, 582, 583t
dextrose, 718
Dexycu (dexamethasone), 1090t, 1094t–1095t
D-Forte (ergocalciferol), 816t
Dhivy (Levodopa–carbidopa), 871t–872t
DiaBeta (glyburide), 754t, 763b, 764–765, 765t, 767b
diabetes insipidus, 798, 803–805
diabetes mellitus
  acute complications of, 752b
  adjuvant medications, 778–779, 778t
  alpha-glucosidase inhibitors, 767–769, 768t, 769b
  amylin analogs, 773, 773t, 774b
  assessment, 780b
  biguanides, 765–767, 766t, 767b
  clinical manifestations, 751–752, 752b
  complications of, 752b
  definition, 750
  dipeptidyl peptidase-4 inhibitors, 771–772, 772t, 772b
  drug therapy, 753, 754t, 755f
  evaluation, 780b
  glucagon-like peptide-1 receptor agonists (incretin mimetics), 774–776, 775t
  insulin (see insulin)
  meglitinides, 769–770, 770t, 771b
  nursing interventions, 780b
  nursing process, 780b
  obesity and, 676, 678
  outcomes of therapy, 780b
  overview of, 750–753
  sodium glucose cotransporter 2 inhibitors, 776–777, 776t, 777b
  sulfonylureas, 764–765, 765t
  thiazolidinediones, 769
  type 1, 750
  type 2 (see type 2 diabetes)
diabetic ketoacidosis (DKA), 751, 752b
Diacomit (stiripentol), 956t, 969t–972t, 983
diarrhea
  adjuvant medications
    antibacterial drugs, 741–743
    bile-binding drugs, 741–742
    bismuth salts, 741, 741t
    enzymatic replacement therapy, 741
    octreotide acetate, 741–742, 741t
    polycarbophil, 741t, 742
    selective 5-HT3 receptor antagonist, 738t, 741–743, 741t
  antibacterial drugs, 742–743
  antibiotic-associated colitis, 739
  assessment, 744b
  clinical considerations, 737
  clinical judgment, 555b
  clinical manifestations
  diphenoxylate with atropine for, 737–739, 738t, 740b
  drug therapy, 737, 738t, 740b
  evaluation, 744b
  functional disorders, 737
  human immunodeficiency virus/acquired immunodeficiency syndrome, 737
  hyperthyroidism, 737
  inflammatory bowel disorders, 737
  intestinal infections, 737
  intestinal neoplasms, 737
  irritable bowel syndrome, 737

lack of digestive enzymes, 737
laxative abuse, 738
nonpharmacologic therapy, 737
nursing interventions, 744b
nursing process, 744b
therapy, outcome of, 744b
Diastat (diazepam), 864t, 956t, 959
Diastat AcuDial (diazepam), 864t
Diastat Acudial (diazepam), 960t, 995, 995t
Diastat Pediatric (diazepam), 864t, 960t
Diazemuls (diazepam), 864t
diazepam, 87b, 96b, 960t, 983
 drug interactions, 961b
diazepam (Diastat Acudial, Diazepam Intensol, Valium, Valtoco), 995, 995t
diazepam (Valium, Diastat), 959
diazepam (Valium, Diastat Acudial, Diazepam, Diastat Pediatric, Diazepam Intensol), 960t
diazepam (Valium, Diastat, Acudial, Pediatric Diazepam Intensol), 956t
diazepam (Valium, Diastat AcuDial, Diastat Pediatric, Diazepam Intensol, Apo-Diazepam, Bio-Diazepam, Diastat, Valium), 864t
DiazePAM Intensol (diazepam), 864t
Diazepam Intensol (diazepam), 864t, 960t, 995, 995t
dibucaine, 1117
Diclegis (doxylamine succinate with pyridoxine ydrochloride), 708t, 711t, 712
diclofenac, 1090t, 1094t–1095t, 1096
diclofenac potassium (Cambia, Zorvolex, Apo-Diclo, Apo-Diclo SR Voltaren, Voltaren XR, Cambia, Zipsor), 290t, 302t–303t
dicloxacillin, 335t–337t, 339
dicyclomine hydrochloride (Bentyl), 885–886, 886t
Dicyclomine hydrochloride (Bentyl; JAMP Dicyclomine, Protylol, RIVA-Dicyclomine), 886t
didanosine, 432
dietary supplements
 administration of drug, 58–59, 59t–61t, 61b
 obesity treated with, 685–686, 685b
diethylpropion, 679, 679t, 681
Dificid (fidaxomicin), 378t
diflorasone diacetate (ApexiCon E, Psorcon), 1112t
Diflucan (fluconazole), 450, 451t–452t
diflunisal, 290t, 298t–299t, 300
digoxin (Lanoxin), 76–77, 562t, 564–565, 564b
dihydroergotamine mesylate (Trudhesa Migranal, Migranal), 942t, 943
dihydropyridines, 533
Dilantin (phenytoin), 956t, 964, 965t
Dilantin Infatabs (phenytoin), 965t
Dilaudid (hydromorphone), 894t, 896t–897t, 902, 932
diltiazem (Cardizem), 516–517, 516t, 517b, 524t, 532t, 533–534
diltiazem (Cardizem CD, Cartia XT), 482t, 491, 492t, 493
dimenhydrinate, 708t, 711t, 712
dimorphic fungi, 445
dinoprostone (Cervidil, Prepidil, Prostin E$_2$), 94, 94t
dinutuximab (Unituxin), 236t–238t, 252t–257t
Diopred (prednisolone), 320t–323t
Dioptics Atropine Solution (ophthalmic atropine), 882t
Diovan (valsartan), 482t, 490t, 491, 494, 495t–496t
diovan HCT, 495t–496t
dipeptidyl peptidase 4 (DPP-4) inhibitors, 772t
 administration, 772
 adverse effects, 771–772
 contraindications, 771–772
 mechanism of action, 771
 nursing implications, 772

 patient teaching guidelines, 772
 pharmacokinetics, 771
 therapeutic effects, 772
 uses, 771, 772t
Diphenhist (diphenhydramine), 590–593, 590t–591t, 592b
diphenhydramine (Diphenhist), 582, 583t, 590–593, 590t–591t, 592b
diphenhydramine hydrochloride, 77
diphenoxylate with atropine (Lomotil), 737–739, 738t, 740b
diphtheria, tetanus toxoids, and acellular pertussis (DTaP) (Daptacel, Infanrix; Adacel, Boostrix), 194b, 195t–199t, 203
Diprivan (propofol), 922t, 925, 926t
dipyridamole (Aggrenox), 151t–152t, 155
dipyridamole (Persantine), 140t, 151t–152t, 155–156
direct factor Xa inhibitors, 140t–142t
 abnormal kidney function, 149
 administration of, 149
 adverse effects, 149
 apixaban, 140t–142t, 148–149
 contraindications, 149
 drug interactions, 149b
 edoxaban, 140t–142t, 148–149
 in hepatic impairment patients, 149
 mechanism of action, 148
 nursing implications, 149
 patient teaching guidelines, 149
 pharmacokinetics, 148
 preventing interactions, 149
 reproduction, pregnancy, and lactation, 148
 therapeutic effects, 149
direct renin inhibitors, 494
direct thrombin inhibitors (DTIs), 141t–142t, 147
 abnormal kidney function and hepatic impairment, 147
 administration of, 147
 adverse effects, 147
 contraindications, 147
 drug interactions, 147, 148b
 mechanism of action, 147
 nursing implications, 147–148
 patient teaching guidelines, 144b, 146
 pharmacokinetics, 147
 preventing interactions, 147
 therapeutic effects, 148
direct-acting skeletal muscle relaxants, 987
 abnormal kidney function, 988
 adverse effects, 988
 contraindications, 988
 dose usage, 988
 hepatic impairment, 988
 mechanisms of action, 988
 nursing implications, 988
 patient teaching guidelines, 988b
 pharmacokinetics, 988
 preventing interactions, 988
 therapeutic effects, 988
directly observed therapy (DOT), 394
disease-modifying antirheumatic drugs, 221
disopyramide (Norpace), 508t, 510
disorganized thinking, 1030–1031
displacement, 22
disseminated intravascular coagulation (DIC), 140
distribution, 17–18
distributive shock, 540, 541t
disulfiram, 1061t–1063t, 1064
Ditropan XL (oxybutynin), 881t, 886, 887t
diuretics, 482t, 494, 561–563, 562t
 loop (see loop diuretics)
 osmotic, 21
 potassium-sparing (see potassium-sparing diuretics)

Diuril (chlorothiazide), 482t, 631t, 635–637, 636t, 637b
Divigel (estradiol transdermal system), 103t
DMARDs, 221
Doans Pills (magnesium salicylate), 290t, 292t, 294
dobutamine (Dobutrex), 543t, 547
Dobutrex (dobutamine), 543t, 547
Docefrez (docetaxel), 236t–245t, 249, 260–263
docetaxel (Docefrez), 236t–245t, 249, 260–263
docetaxel (Taxotere), 236t–245t, 249, 260–263
docosanol (Abreva), 416t, 417
docusate calcium, 724t
docusate sodium (Colace, Docusil), 724t, 726t
Docusil (docusate sodium), 724t, 726t
dofetilide (Tikosyn), 513t, 515
dolasetron (Anzemet), 708t, 713, 714t
dolutegravir, 432
Dom Minocycline (minocycline hydrochloride), 366t
DOM Selegiline (selegiline hydrochloride), 871t–872t
Dom-Azithromycin (azithromycin), 377, 378t, 380
DOMCandesartan (atacand HCT), 495t–496t
Dom-Cephalexin (cephalexin), 336t–337t
Dom-Clarithromycin (clarithromycin), 378t
DOM-Fluconazole, 451t–452t
DOM-Oxybutynin (oxybutynin), 887t
donepezil (Adlarity, Aricept, Aricept RDT), 855t, 858–859, 859t, 859b, 861
donepezil–memantine (Namzaric), 855t, 859t
dopamine, 543t, 546–547, 847–848
dopamine blocker, 1061t
dopamine receptor agonists, 869–875, 869t
 abnormal kidney function, 872
 administration, 873
 adverse effects, 872
 amantadine hydrochloride, 873–874
 apomorphine hydrochloride, 874
 bromocriptine mesylate, 874
 contraindications, 872–873
 drug interactions, 873, 873b
 in hepatic impairment patients, 872
 in lactation, 870
 mechanism of action, 869–870, 870f
 nursing implications, 873
 patient teaching guidelines, 873, 873b
 pharmacokinetics, 869
 pramipexole (Mirapex, Mirapex ER), 874
 in pregnancy, 870
 rasagiline (Azilect), 874
 ropinirole (Requip, Requip XL), 874
 rotigotine (Neupro), 874–875
 routes and dosage information, 871t–872t
 safinamide (Xadago), 875
 selegiline (Emsam, Zelapar), 875
 therapeutic effects, 873
 uses, 870–872
Doral (quazepam), 995t, 999
doripenem, 335t, 347t
dorzolamide (Cosopt, Cosopt PF), 1082t–1084t
dorzolamide (Trusopt), 1082t–1084t
dorzolamide hydrochloride (Trusopt), 1088
Dovonex (calcipotriene), 1116t–1117t
down-regulation, 848
doxazosin (Cardura), 119t, 128t, 129, 482t
Doxazosin XL (Cardura), 128t, 129
doxepin (Silenor), 96b, 1009t, 1012t
Doxil (doxorubicin liposomal), 236t–245t
doxorubicin (Adriamycin), 235, 236t–245t, 239, 245–247, 248b, 251b, 264t
doxorubicin liposomal (Doxil), 236t–238t
doxycycline (Vibramycin, Oracea, Monodox, Apprilon), 365t–366t, 367–368, 463, 464t
doxylamine, 583t
doxylamine succinate with pyridoxine ydrochloride (Diclegis, Bonjesta), 708t, 711t, 712

Dr. Gs Clear Gel (tolnaftate), 1115t
Drisdol (ergocalciferol), 816t
Drizalma Sprinkle (duloxetine), 1009t, 1019
dromotropic effect, 545–546
dronabinol (Marinol), 708t, 710b, 717t, 718
dronedarone (Multaq), 513t, 515
Droxia (hydroxyurea), 236t–245t, 238
Droxidopa, 946
drug(s). *See also specific drug*
    administration of, 8–9
    adverse effects of, 25–27, 26b
    American laws regarding, 5–8, 6t–7t
    Beers criteria, older adults medications, 11
    biotechnology of, 4
    classification of, 4
    clinical trials of, 8
    drug action
        age effects on, 22–23
        body weight effects on, 23
        ethnicity effects, 23–24
        genetics effect on, 23
        nonreceptor, 21
        pathologic conditions that affect, 24
        patient-related variables that affect, 22–25
        pharmacogenomic variations, 23–24
        psychological factors, 24–25
        receptor theory, 19–20
        sex (gender) effects on, 24
    Food and Drug Administration approval of, 8–9
    generic name, 4–5
    high-alert medications, 11
    information sources about, 12–13
    internet sites, 12–13
    marketing, 5
    names of, 4–5
    national patient safety goals, 10–11
    nonprescription, 5
    numerous handbooks, 12
    nurses initiative, 10
    overdose of, 27, 29t–31t
    over-the-counter, 5
    pregnancy categories, 11
    prescription, 5
    prototype, 4
    safety, 9–11
    sources of, 12–13
    testing procedure, 8
drug administration
    abbreviations commonly used in, 41t
    clinical judgment in practice, 34b
    drug actions after, 19
    ear and eye solutions, 42t–43t
    ear medications, 57
    gastrointestinal, 46b
    herbal and dietary supplements, 58–59, 59t–61t, 61b
    intramuscular injections
        advantages and disadvantages of, 45t–46t
        sites for, 56
    intravenous injections
        administration technique, 45t–46t, 46b
        advantages and disadvantages of, 45t–46t
        continuous infusion, 46b
        drug preparation for, 46b
        equipment for, 46b
        intermittent infusion, 46b
        needleless systems, 46b
        principles of, 46b
        sites for, 48–50, 50f
    legal responsibilities, 34
    medication errors, 34–40
    medication systems, 39
    nasogastric tube, 55
    needleless systems, 46b
    nose drops, 57
    nursing actions for, 50–57
    oral, 45
    parenteral
        ampules used in, 48
        definition of, 42t–43t, 45
        equipment for, 45, 47
        injection sites, 48–50, 49f
        patient teaching guidelines, 52b, 53b
        pharmacokinetics affected by, 16–19
        principles of, 33–34
        rectal suppositories, 42t–43t
        subcutaneous injections
            absorption after, 17
            advantages and disadvantages of, 45t–46t
            sites for, 48–50, 49f–50f
        using IV line already established, 56–57
        vaginal suppositories, 42t–43t
Drug Burden Index, 77
drug diversion, 894
drug dosages. *See also specific drug, dosage of*
    abbreviations commonly used in, 41t
    calculation of, 43–45
    definition of, 21
    forms of, 42t–43t
    loading, 21
    maintenance, 21
    measurement systems for, 43
    transdermal, 41–43
Drug Enforcement Administration, 7
drug interactions
    with drugs, 22
    effects of, 22
    with foods, 21
drug manufacturers, 35t–36t
drug receptors, 19–20
drug therapy, 210–211, 211t, 814, 853
    bipolar disorder, 1010
    depression, 1009–1010
    ear disorders, 1101–1102, 1101t
    epilepsy, 955, 956t
    eye disorders, 1077
    general anesthesia, 921–922
    otitis externa, 1101–1102
    psychotic disorders, 1031–1032
    spinal cord injury, 983
drug tolerance, 25
drug transport
    pathways and mechanisms, 16, 16b
    schematic diagram of, 17f
drug–diet interactions, 21–22
drug–drug interactions, 22
drug-induced parkinsonism, 1034
DSH Tar. Pentrax Gold, Psoriasin (coal tar), 1116t–1117t
Dsuvia (sufentanil), 932
D-Tabs (cholecalciferol), 816t
dual orexin receptor antagonists, 995t
dual receptor antagonists, 1003–1004
    adverse effects, 1003
    contraindications, 1003
    dose usage, 1003
    mechanisms of action, 1003
    nursing implications, 1003–1004
    patient teaching guidelines, 1004b
    pharmacokinetics, 1003
    preventing interactions, 1003
    therapeutic effects, 1004
dulaglutide (Trulicity), 754t, 775, 775t
Dulcolax (bisacodyl), 724t, 728–730, 729t, 730b
duloxetine (Cymbalta, Drizalma Sprinkle), 1009t, 1019
Duopa (Levodopa–carbidopa), 871t–872t
dupilumab (Dupixent), 1116t–1117t
Dupixent (dupilumab), 1116t–1117t
Duragesic (fentanyl), 896t–897t, 902, 902t, 932t
Duramorph (morphine sulfate), 894–903, 894t, 896t–897t
duration of action, 17

Durela (Tramadol), 896t–897t
Durham-Humphrey Amendment, 5–7, 6t–7t
Durysta (bimatoprost), 1082t–1084t
dutasteride (Avodart, ACT-Dutasteride, Apo-Dutasteride), 119t, 126, 126t
D-Vi-Sol (cholecalciferol), 816t
Dyazide, 495t–496t
Dynacin (minocycline hydrochloride), 365t
Dyrenium (triamterene), 482t, 631t, 638t, 639–640, 641t
dyslipidemia
    action site, 163–164, 165f
    assessment, 176b
    bile acid sequestrants (see bile acid sequestrants)
    cholesterol absorption inhibitor (see cholesterol absorption inhibitor)
    clinical manifestations, 162
    combination therapy, 174–175
    drugs administration, 163–164, 164t
    drugs categories, 163–164, 164t
    etiology, 162
    fibrates (see fibrates)
    HMG-CoA reductase inhibitors (see HMG-CoA reductase inhibitors)
    management, 162–164
    nursing interventions, 176b
    nursing process, 176b
    obesity and, 676, 676b, 683
    pathophysiology, 162
    screening, 162
    selection of drug, 163–164
    therapy outcomes, 176b
    treatment of, 164t
    types, 162, 162t
dyslipidemic drugs, 524t, 534
dysrhythmias
    antidysrhythmic drugs (see antidysrhythmic drugs)
    automaticity, 504
    class IA sodium channel blockers, 506, 507t–508t
    class IB sodium channel blockers, 507t–508t, 510
    class IC sodium channel blockers, 507t–508t, 510
    class II beta-adrenergic blockers, 507t, 511–513, 511t
    class III potassium channel blockers, 507t, 513–516, 513t
    class IV calcium channel blockers, 507t, 516–517
    clinical considerations, 504
    clinical manifestations, 504
    conductivity, 504
    drug therapy, 506, 507t
    ectopic, 504
    excitability, 511
    magnesium sulfate, 519
    nonpharmacologic management, 504–506
    overview of, 504–506
    prodysrhythmic effect, 506
    treatment of, 507t
    types of, 505b
dysthymia, 1010
dystonias, 1034

E

E. coli intestinal infections, 742
ear disorders, 1101–1102
    adjuvant medications, 1107
        nonnarcotic analgesic antipyretic, 1107
        propionic acid derivatives, 1107
        salicylates, 1107
    anti-infective, antiseptic, glucocorticoid, and acidifying agents, 1102–1104, 1102t
    assessment, 1108b
    clinical manifestations, 1101
    drug therapy, 1101–1102, 1101t
    evaluation, 1108b

fluoroquinolone, 1104–1105 (see also fluoroquinolone)
neomycin polymyxin B-hydrocortisone (see neomycin–polymyxin B–hydrocortisone)
nursing interventions, 1108b
nursing process, 1108b
outcomes of therapy, 1108b
penicillin, 1105–1106
ear solutions, 42t–43t
Ebixa (memantine), 855t, 859t
echinacea, 59t–61t
echinocandins
  abnormal kidney function, 455
  action, 454
  administration of, 455
  adverse effects, 455
  contraindications, 455
  drug interactions, 455t, 455b
  in hepatic impairment, 455
  lactation, 455
  nursing implications, 455–456
  patient teaching, 456
  pharmacokinetics, 454
  pregnancy, 455
  preventing interactions, 455, 455b
  reproduction, 455
  therapeutic effects, 455
  use, 454–455
eclampsia, 91
econazole (Ecoza, Zolpak), 447t, 1115t
Ecotrin (aspirin), 151t–152t
Ecoza (econazole), 447t, 1115t
ecstasy, 1059
ectopic, dysrhythmias, 504
eczema. See dermatitis
Edarbi (azilsartan), 482t
Edarbi (azilsartan medoxomil), 754t
Edecrin (ethacrynic acid), 631t–632t
edema, 288, 291, 298–299, 301, 630, 632t, 634, 636t
Edex powder (alprostadil), 119t
Edluar (zolpidem), 995t, 1002
edoxaban (Savaysa, Lixiana), 140t–142t, 148–149
Ed-Spaz (hyoscyamine sulfate), 882t
efavirenz (Sustiva), 433–435, 434t, 435b
Effexor XR (venlafaxine), 1009t
Effient (prasugrel), 150, 151t–152t, 152–154
Efgartigimod alfa (Vyvgart), 857, 861
Efudex (fluorouracil), 1116t–1117t
ejection fraction, 552
Eldepryl (selegiline hydrochloride), 871t–872t
electrolytes, 646. See also specific electrolyte
  definition, 646
  functions, 651t–653t
electronic infusion devices, 46b
Elepsia XR (levetiracetam), 969t–972t
Elestat (epinastine), 1090t
Elestrin (estradiol transdermal system), 103t
eletriptan (Relpax), 946
elevated blood lipids, 162
Elidel (pimecrolimus), 1116t–1117t
Eligard (leuprolide acetate), 236t–238t, 261t–263t, 263, 806t
elimination half-life, 19
Elinest, 110t–111t
Eliquis (apixaban), 141t–142t, 148–149
Elitek (rasburicase), 236t–245t, 238, 292t, 309t, 310
Elixophyllin (theophylline), 605t, 612–614, 613b
Ellence (epirubicin), 236t–245t
Elocon (mometasone), 318t, 320t–323t
elvitegravir, 432–433
embolus, 138
Emcyt (estramustine), 236t–245t
emedastine difumarate, 1090t
Emend (aprepitant), 708t, 715, 715t
emergence phase, in general anesthesia, 922
emergency resuscitation of adults, drug therapy
  atropine, 518
  calcium chloride, 518–519
  epinephrine, 518
  lidocaine, 518
  oxygen, 518
  sodium bicarbonate, 518
emetogenic drugs, 713
Emetrol (phosphorated carbohydrate solution), 708t, 717t, 718
Emo Cort (hydrocortisone), 320t–323t
emollients, 1117
empagliflozin (Jardiance), 562t, 564, 776t, 777
Emsam (selegiline), 871t–872t, 875, 1020t
Emsam (selegiline hydrochloride), 1009t
emtricitabine, 432–433
Enablex (darifenacin), 887t, 888
Enablex (darifenacin hydrobromide), 887t, 888
enalapril (Vasotec), 482t, 485t, 488, 495t–496t, 778, 778t
enalapril (Vasotec, ACT-Enalapril, APO-Enalapril), 482t
enalapril maleate (Epaned, Vasotec), 560–561, 562t
Enbrel (etanercept), 211t, 215, 227
Enbrel Mini (etanercept), 211t, 215, 227
Enbrel SureClick (etanercept), 211t, 215, 227
endogenous analgesia system, 895
Endometrin (progesterone), 107t–108t
endometriosis
  definition, 101
  drug therapy, 101
  prevalence, 101
  risk factors, 101
  symptoms, 101
endonuclease inhibitor, 412b, 422t, 424–425
endothelium, 479
end-stage shock, 541
enemas, 42t–43t
enfuvirtide (Fuzeon), 439–440, 439t
Engerix-B (hepatitis B vaccine), 193, 194b, 195t–199t, 202–203
enoxaparin (Lovenox, Lovenox HP, Lovenox with Preservative), 140, 140t–142t
Enpresse, 110t–111t
entacapone (Comtan, Stalevo), 869t, 876–877
Entamoeba histolytica, 377
enteral nutrition, 669
enteric-coated tablets, 41
Enterobacter species, 353
enterobiasis, 470t
Enterobius vermicularis, 469
Enterococci, 278b
Enterococcus faecalis, 275b, 383–386
Enterococcus faecium, 275b
enterohepatic recirculation, 18
Entocort (budesonide), 320t–323t
Entocort EC (budesonide), 318t, 320t–323t
Entresto (sacubitril/valsartan), 555–557, 556t, 556b, 557b
Entrophen (aspirin), 151t–152t
Enulose (lactulose), 724t, 732, 732t
enuresis, 1011
Envarsus (tacrolimus), 211t, 212, 215b, 216, 218–219
Envarsus XR (tacrolimus), 211t, 212, 215b, 216, 218–219
enzalutamide (Xtandi), 236t–238t, 260–263, 261t–263t
enzymatic replacement therapy, 741, 741t
enzyme inducers, 22
enzyme induction, 18
enzyme inhibition, 18
enzyme inhibitors for maintenance, 1064–1065
  adverse effects, 1065
  contraindications, 1065
  dose usage, 1064–1065
  mechanisms of action, 1064
  nursing implications, 1065
  patient teaching, 1065
  pharmacokinetics, 1064
  preventing interactions, 1065
  therapeutic effects, 1065
eosinophils, 289
Epaned (enalapril maleate), 560–561, 562t
epidural anesthesia, 911
epigastric pain, 299, 693, 697, 700
epilepsy, 954
  drug therapy, 955, 956t
  overview of, 954–955
epinastine, 1094t–1095t
epinastine (Elestat), 1090t
epinephrine (Adrenalin), 518, 541–542, 543t, 545–547, 605t, 607, 608t
epinephrine (Asthmanefrin Refill), 608t
EpiPen (epinephrine), 541–542, 543t, 545–547
epirubicin (Ellence, PMSEpirubicin), 236t–245t
Epitol (carbamazepine), 967t
eplerenone (Inspra), 631t, 638t, 640
epoetin alfa (Epogen, Procrit, Retacrit, Eprex), 180–181, 180t–181t, 183b, 236t–238t, 264t
epoetin beta (Mircera), 180t–181t, 183
Epogen (epoetin alfa), 180–181, 180t–181t, 183b, 236t–238t, 264t
epothilone B analogs, 236t–245t
Eprex (epoetin alfa), 180–181, 180t–181t, 183b, 236t–238t, 264t
Eprontia (topiramate), 969t–972t
eprosartan (Teveten), 482t
Eprosartan mesylate (Teveten), 754t
eptifibatide (Integrilin, eptifibatide injection), 151t–152t, 154, 156
Equalactin (polycarbophil), 738t, 741t, 742
Equetro (carbamazepine), 967t
eravacycline (Xerava), 365–366t, 368
Eraxis (anidulafungin), 447t, 455t, 456
Erbitux (cetuximab), 211t, 225, 236t–238t, 252t–257t, 257, 259f
erectile dysfunction
  phosphodiesterase type 5 inhibitors (see phosphodiesterase inhibitors)
erectile dysfunction (ED), 118
  adjuvant medications, 125–126, 126b
  assessment, 130b
  clinical considerations, 118
  clinical manifestations, 118
  evaluation, 130b
  nursing interventions, 130b
  nursing process, 130b
  outcomes of therapy, 130b
Erelzi (etanercept), 211t, 215, 227
Erfa-Amikacin (amikacin), 353–354, 353t, 355t, 357
ergocalciferol (Calciferol, Drisdol; D-Forte, SANDOZ D-Forte), 814, 816t
Ergomar (ergotamine tartrate), 938t, 942
ergot alkaloids, 942–943
  abnormal kidney function, 943
  adverse effects, 943
  age, 943
  contraindications, 943
  dihydroergotamine mesylate, 943
  dosage usage, 942–943
  hepatic impairment, 943
  mechanism of action, 942
  nursing implications, 943
  patient teaching guidelines, 943, 944b
  pharmacokinetics, 942
  preventing interactions, 943
  reproduction, pregnancy and lactation, 943
  therapeutic effects, 943
ergot derivatives, 946
ergotamine tartrate (Ergomar), 938t, 942
eribulin mesylate (Halaven), 236t–245t
Ermeza (levothyroxine), 791t

Errin (norethindrone), 107t–108t
ertapenem (Invanz), 335t, 347t, 348
Erwinaze (asparaginase), 236t–245t, 238, 246–247
Ery (erythromycin), 1113t
Erygel (erythromycin), 1113t
erythema, 248b, 1110
erythromycin, 377, 378t, 379b, 1090t
erythromycin (Ery, Erygel), 1091t, 1113t
erythromycin/benzoyl peroxide (Benzamycin), 1113t
erythropoiesis, 179
erythropoiesis-stimulating agents (ESA)
  administration of, 182
  adverse effects, 182
  contraindications, 182
  darbepoetin alfa, 182–183
  dosage information, 181t
  mechanism of action, 181
  nursing implications, 182
  pharmacokinetics, 181
  therapeutic effects, 182
erythropoietin, 179
Escherichia coli, 275b, 277, 353
escitalopram (Lexapro), 1009t, 1017, 1036
Esclim (estradiol transdermal system), 103t
Esketamine (Spravato), 927–928
eslicarbazepine (Aptiom), 956t, 967t, 968
esmolol (Brevibloc), 513, 524t
esomeprazole (Nexium), 692t, 699t, 700–701
esophageal candidiasis, 456
esophagitis, 690, 696
essential hypertension, 488
Estalis (estradiol/norethindrone), 112t
Estarylla, 110t–111t
estazolam, 995t
esterified estrogens (Menest, Estragyn), 103t
esters, 912t, 915–917
  adverse effects, 916
  chloroprocaine hydrochloride, 915
  contraindications, 916
  in lactation, 915
  mechanism of action, 915
  nursing implications, 916
  patient teaching guidelines, 916, 916b
  pharmacokinetics, 915
  in pregnancy, 915
  preventing interactions, 916
  therapeutic effects, 916
  uses, 915–916
estimated average requirement (EAR), 646b
Estrace (estradiol, micronized), 103t
estradiol, 947, 947t
  abnormal kidney function, 947
  adverse effects, 947
  age, 947
  contraindications, 947
  dosage usage, 947
  hepatic impairment, 947
  interactions, 948
  mechanism of action, 947
  nursing implications, 948
  patient teaching guidelines, 948
  pharmacokinetics, 947
  reproduction, pregnancy and lactation, 947
  therapeutic effects, 948
estradiol cypionate (Depo-Estradiol), 103t
estradiol, micronized (Estrace, Gynedol, Innofem, Estring, Vagifem; Estrace, Estring, Vagifem), 103t
estradiol transdermal system (Alora, Climara, Esclim, Menostar, Vivelle-Dot EstroGel, Elestrin, Divigel, Evamist; Climara, Depo-Estradiol, Estradot, Menostar, Oesclim, 103t
estradiol/drospirenone (Angeliq), 112t
estradiol/levonorgestrel (Climara Pro), 112t

estradiol/norethindrone (Activella, Amabelz;, CombiPatch, estalis), 112t
Estradiol/progesterone (Bijuva), 112t
Estradot (estradiol transdermal system), 103t
Estragyn (esterified estrogens), 103t
estramustine (Emcyt), 236t–245t
Estrasorb (estradiol transdermal system), 103t
Estring (estradiol, micronized), 103t
estrogen(s), 100–105, 947–948
  abnormal kidney function, 104
  administration of, 105
  adverse effects, 104–105
  contraindications, 104
  dosage information, 102, 103t
  drug interactions, 105, 105b
  effects of, 100
  in hepatic impairment patients, 104
  indications, 102
  mechanism of action, 102
  nursing implications, 104
  patient teaching guidelines, 105, 105b
  pharmacokinetics, 101–102
  physiology, 100
  reproduction, pregnancy, and lactation, 102
  therapeutic effects, 105
  uses, 102
estrogen replacement therapy, 102
estrogen–progestin combinations
  abnormal kidney function, 111
  administration of, 105
  adverse effects, 104
  contraindications, 104
  dosage information
    as contraceptives, 109, 110t–111t
    for noncontraceptive, 111, 112t
  drug interactions, 105, 105b
  in hepatic impairment patients, 111
  mechanism of actions, 109
  nursing implications, 104–105
  patient teaching guidelines, 105b
  pharmacokinetics, 109
  therapeutic effects, 113
  uses, 109–111
estropipate (Ogen, Ortho-Est), 103t
Estrostep Fe, 110t–111t
eszopiclone (Lunesta), 995t, 1001–1002
etanercept (Enbrel, Enbrel Mini, Enbrel SureClick, Brenzys, Erelzi), 211t, 215, 222t–224t, 227
ethacrynic acid (Edecrin), 631t–632t
ethambutol (Myambutol), 394b, 399t, 400
ethinyl estradiol–norethindrone (Ortho-Novum), 109, 112t
ethinyl estradiol/norethindrone acetate (femHRT), 112t
ethionamide (Trecator), 391
ethnicity, 23–24
ethosuximide (Zarontin), 956t, 969t–972t, 973
Ethyol (amifostine), 236t–238t, 264t
etodolac (Lodine, Taro-Etodolac), 290t, 302t–303t, 304
etomidate (Amidate), 835t, 836, 922t, 926t, 927
etonogestrel (Nexplanon), 106, 107t–108t
etoposide (Toposar, VePesid), 236t–245t, 239, 248b
Euflex (flutamide), 236t–238t, 261t–263t
Eulexin (flutamide), 236t–238t, 261t–263t
EURO-D (cholecalciferol), 816t
eutectic mixture of local anesthetics (EMLA), 912b
Euthyroid, 783
Euthyrox (levothyroxine), 791t
Evamist (estradiol transdermal system), 103t
everolimus (Afinitor Disperz, Zortress), 236t–238t, 252t–257t, 258
everolimus (Zortress, Afinitor, Afinitor Disperz), 211t, 217t, 219
Evidence-based practice (EBP), 58
Evista (raloxifene), 823t, 824

Evoclin (clindamycin), 1113t
evolocumab (Repatha, Repatha Pushtronex System, Repatha SureClick), 164t, 173–174, 173t
Evomela (melphalan), 236t–245t
excitability, dysrhythmias, 511
excretion, 18
Exelderm (sulconazole), 447t
Exelon (rivastigmine), 855t, 859, 859t
Exelon Patch (rivastigmine), 855t, 859, 859t
exemestane (Aromasin, ACT-Exemestane, APOExemestane, MEDexemestane), 236t–238t, 260, 261t–263t
exenatide (Byetta), 754t, 758b, 763b, 772b, 774–775, 775t, 777
exforge, 495t–496t
exogenous. See exogenous corticosteroids
exogenous corticosteroids
  abnormal kidney function and hepatic impairment, 326
  acute adrenocortical insufficiency, 325–326
  administration of, 327–328
  adverse effects, 327, 329
  allergic rhinitis, 323
  alternate-day therapy, 328
  arthritis, 323
  asthma, 323–324
  cancer, 324
  chronic obstructive pulmonary disease, 325
  contraindications, 327
  inflammatory bowel disease, 325
  inhibiting arachidonic acid metabolism, 317
  nursing implications, 327–331
  patient teaching guidelines, 329–331, 329b
  postoperative nausea and vomiting, 324–325
  preventing interactions, 327, 328b
  septic shock, 325
  spinal cord injury, 325
  strengthening/stabilizing biologic membranes, 317
  stress dosage therapy, 328
  therapeutic effects, 328–329
expectorants
  action, 580
  administration of, 581
  adverse effects, 580
  contraindications, 580
  drugs, 580
  guaifenesin, 580–581
  lactation, 580
  multi-ingredient nonprescription, 583t
  nursing implications, 581
  patient teaching guidelines, 577b, 581
  pharmacokinetics, 580
  pregnancy, 580
  reproduction, 580
  therapeutic effects, 581
  use, 580
Extavia (interferon beta-1b), 187t
extended-interval dosing, 356
extended-release capsules, 55
extended-spectrum drugs, 339
extensively drug-resistant tuberculosis (XDR-TB), 390
Extina (ketoconazole), 451t–452t, 453, 1115t
extraintestinal amebiasis, 463, 466, 467t
extrapyramidal effects, 1034
extrapyramidal reactions, 868–869, 885
extravasation, 248b
eye
  assessment, 1098b
  disorders, 1076–1077
    clinical manifestations, 1077
    drug therapy, 1077
    glaucoma, 1077
    ocular infections and inflammation, 1077, 1090–1097
    open-angle glaucoma, 1089

refractive errors, 1077
evaluation, 1098b
nursing interventions, 1098b
nursing process, 1098b
ointments, 42t–43t
outcomes of therapy, 1098b
structure and function, 1076
eye solutions, 42t–43t
eyeball, 1076
eyelid, 1076
ezetimibe (Zetia, Ezetrol), 21, 163–164, 164t, 171–173, 172t, 172b
Ezetrol (ezetimibe), 163–164, 164t, 171–173, 172t, 172b

F

Falmina, 110t–111t
famciclovir, 96b, 417
famotidine (Pepcid), 692t, 696t, 698
Fanapt (iloperidone), 1031t, 1039t–1040t, 1042
Fareston (toremifene), 236t–238t, 260, 261t–263t
Farxiga (dapagliflozin), 776t, 777
fasciculation, 931
Fasenra (benralizumab), 605t, 619t, 620
Faslodex (fulvestrant), 236t–238t, 260, 261t–263t
Fasturtec (rasburicase), 236t–245t, 238, 292t, 309t, 310
fat metabolism and insulin, 751
fatigue, 248b
fat-soluble vitamins, 645, 654–658
  vitamin A (retinol) (see vitamin A (retinol))
  vitamin E (see vitamin E)
  vitamin K (see vitamin K)
FDA (Food and Drug Administration), 68
  drug approval by, prescription and nonprescription, 8–9
  responsibilities of, 8–9
febuxostat (Uloric), 292t, 309–310, 309t
fecal impaction, 725
fedratinib (Inrebic), 211t, 220t, 221
felbamate (Felbatol), 956t, 969t–972t, 982
Felbatol (felbamate), 956t, 969t–972t, 982
Feldene (piroxicam), 290t, 301, 301t
felodipine (Plendil, Sandoz-Felodipine), 482t, 524t, 532t, 533
female reproductive health
  estrogen (see estrogen)
  overview of, 100–101
  progestins (see progestin(s))
Femara (letrozole), 84, 85t, 236t–238t, 260, 261t–263t
femHRT (ethinyl estradiol/norethindrone acetate), 112t
Femstat (butoconazole), 450
fenofibrate (Antara, Fenoglide, Fibricor, Lipofen, Tricor, Triglide, Trilipix, Lipidil EZ, Lipidil Supra), 164t, 170–171, 170t, 171b
Fenoglide (fenofibrate), 164t, 170–171, 170t, 171b
fenoldopam (Corlopam), 482t
fenoprofen (Fenortho, Nalfon), 290t, 298t–299t, 300
Fenortho (fenoprofen), 290t, 298t–299t, 300
Fensolvi (leuprolide acetate), 806t
fentanyl (Actiq, Abstral, Fentora, Matrix Patch, PMS-Fentanyl MTX), 894t, 896t–897t, 902
fentanyl (Sublimaze, Abstral, Fentora, Ionsys; Abstral, Duragesic, Fentora), 932t
fentanyl (Sublimaze, Actiq, Fentora, Lazanda, Subsys), 922t, 932
Fentora (fentanyl), 894t, 896t–897t, 902, 922t, 932, 932t
Feosol (ferrous sulfate), 662–666, 662t–664t
ferrous sulfate (Feosol), 662–666, 662t–664t
Fetroja (cefiderocol), 335t, 341, 342t–344t
fetus
  development of, 119
  drug effects, 86–87, 87f

Fetzima (levomilnacipran), 1009t, 1019
Fetzima Titration (levomilnacipran), 1009t, 1019
fever, 286, 288, 289b, 290t
feverfew, 59t–61t, 950
Fexmid (cyclobenzaprine), 77
Fexmid (cyclobenzaprine hydrochloride), 983t, 985t–986t, 989
fexofenadine (Allegra Allergy), 590t, 596–600, 596t, 597b
FiberCon (polycarbophil), 724t, 726t, 738t, 741t, 742
fibrates
  abnormal kidney function and hepatic impairment, 171
  administration of, 171
  adverse effects, 171
  contraindications, 171
  drugs interactions, 171, 171b
  gemfibrozil, 163–164, 164t, 170t, 171
  mechanism of action, 170
  nursing implications, 171
  pharmacokinetics, 170
  preventing interactions 171
  serum triglyceride, 170
  therapeutic effects, 171
Fibricor (fenofibrate), 164t, 170–171, 170t, 171b
fibrinolysin, 138
fidaxomicin (Dificid), 378t
field block anesthesia, 911
filgrastim (Granix, Neupogen, Nivestym, Releuko, Zarxio, Grastofil), 236t–238t, 248b, 264t
filgrastim (G-CSF) (Granix, Neupogen, Nivestym, Releuko, Zarxio, Nivestym, Grastofil), 180t, 184–186, 185t, 186b
Finacea (azelaic acid), 1113t
finasteride (Propecia, PMS-Finasteride), 126–128, 126t
finasteride (Proscar), 119t, 126–128, 126t
first messenger, 845–846
first-dose phenomenon, 499
first-generation antipsychotics, 1032–1036, 1033t
  abnormal kidney function, 1034
  adverse effects, 1034
  contraindications, 1034
  dose usage, 1032–1034
  drug interactions, 1035b
  drugs, 1033t
  hepatic impairment, 1034
  mechanisms of action, 1032
  nursing implications, 1034–1035
  patient teaching guidelines, 1035b
  pharmacokinetics, 1032
  preventing interactions, 1034
  therapeutic effects, 1035
first-generation H_1 receptor antagonists, 587–588, 587f
  abnormal kidney function, 592
  action, 590
  administration of, 592
  adverse effects, 592
  chlorpheniramine, 590t–591t, 593
  clemastine, 589–590, 590t–591t
  contraindications, 592
  cyproheptadine, 589–590, 590t–591t
  dexchlorpheniramine, 590t–591t, 593
  diphenhydramine, 587–588, 587f, 590–593, 591t, 592b
  dosage information, 590, 591t
  drug interactions, 592, 592b
  in hepatic impairment patients, 592
  hydroxyzine pamoate, 589–590, 590t–591t, 593
  lactation, 591
  nursing implications, 592–593
  patient teaching guidelines, 592–593, 593b
  pharmacokinetics, 590
  pregnancy, 591

promethazine, 590t–591t, 593
reproduction, 591
therapeutic effects, 592
uses, 590–592
first-generation nonphenothiazines, 1036–1038
  abnormal kidney function, 1037
  adverse effects, 1037
  contraindications, 1037
  dose usage, 1036–1037
  drug interactions, 1037b
  hepatic impairment, 1037
  mechanisms of action, 1036
  nursing implications, 1037–1038
  patient teaching guidelines, 1038b
  pharmacokinetics, 1036
  preventing interactions, 1037
  therapeutic effects, 1037
first-pass effect, 18
Firvanq (vancomycin), 381t–382t, 386
5-alpha reductase inhibitors, 119t
  abnormal kidney function, 126
  administration, 127
  adverse effects, 127
  contraindications, 127
  drug interactions, 127
  dutasteride, 128
  in hepatic impairment patients, 126
  mechanism of action, 126
  nursing implications, 127
  patient teaching guidelines, 127, 127b
  pharmacokinetics, 126
  reproduction, pregnancy, and lactation, 126
  therapeutic effects, 127
Flagyl (metronidazole), 381t–382t, 384, 464–465, 464t, 692t, 701t, 702
Flarex (fluorometholone), 1090t, 1094t–1095t
flatulence, 725
flavoxate hydrochloride, 879t, 881t, 887t
flecainide (Tambocor), 508t, 510
FloLipid (simvastatin), 164t, 166t, 167
Flomax (tamsulosin), 119t, 128, 128t
Flomax CR (tamsulosin), 119t, 128, 128t
Flonase (fluticasone), 605t
Flonase Allergy Relief OTC (fluticasone), 320t–323t
Florinef (fludrocortisone), 318t, 320t–323t, 830t, 832–833, 833b
Flovent (fluticasone aerosol), 605t
Flovent Diskus (fluticasone), 318t, 320t–323t, 616t
Flovent HFA (fluticasone), 318t, 320t–323t
Flovent Rota disk (fluticasone powder), 605t
floxuridine, 236t–245t
Fluad (influenza (IIV4)), 195t–199t
Fluad Pediatric (influenza (IIV4)), 195t–199t
Fluarix (influenza (IIV4)), 195t–199t
Flublok (influenza (IIV4)), 195t–199t
Flucelvax (influenza (IIV4)), 195t–199t
fluconazole (Diflucan), 450, 451t–452t
flucytosine (Ancobon), 456–457, 456t, 457b
fludrocortisone (Florinef), 318t, 320t–323t, 830t, 832–833, 833b
fluid volume excess
  assessment, 642b
  clinical considerations, 630
  clinical manifestations, 630
  combination products, 640–641, 641t
  drug therapy, 630–631, 630f
  evaluation, 642b
  loop diuretics (see loop diuretics)
  nephron, 630, 630f
  nursing interventions, 642b
  nursing process, 642b
  osmotic diuretics, 631t, 640, 640t
  overview, 630–631
  potassium-sparing diuretics (see potassium-sparing diuretics)
  thiazide diuretics (see thiazide diuretics)

fluid volume overload, 551
FluLaval (influenza (IIV4)), 195t–199t
FluLaval Tetra (influenza (IIV4)), 195t–199t
flumazenil (benzodiazepines), 1060–1061, 1061t–1063t
FluMist [LAIV4] live attenuated (influenza (IIV4)), 195t–199t
flunisolide, 318t, 320t–323t
flunisolide (Aerospan), 605t, 616t
fluocinonide (Vanos), 1112t
fluorometholone (Flarex, FML ForteFMLLiquifilm), 1090t, 1094t–1095t
Fluoroplex (fluorouracil), 1116t–1117t
fluoroquinolone, 1104–1105
　abnormal kidney function, 358
　administration of, 359, 1105
　adverse effects, 359–360, 1104
　assessment, 362b
　contraindications, 359, 1105
　dosage information, 358, 358t
　dose usage, 1104
　drug interactions, 359, 359b
　evaluation, 362b
　in hepatic impairment patients, 358
　herb and dietary interactions, 359, 359b
　mechanism of action, 357
　mechanisms of action, 1104
　nursing implications, 359–360, 1105
　nursing interventions, 362b
　nursing process, 362b
　patient teaching guidelines, 1105b
　pharmacokinetics, 354, 357, 1104
　preventing interactions, 1105
　therapeutic effects, 359–360, 1105
　uses, 358
fluorouracil (5-FU), 236t–245t, 238, 248b, 251b
fluorouracil (Carac, Efudex, Fluoroplex, Tolak), 1116t–1117t
fluoxetine (PROzac, Sarafem), 1009t, 1013
fluoxymesterone, 120
fluphenazine, 1031t, 1033t, 1035
flurandrenolide (Cordran, Nolix), 1112t
flurazepam, 995t
flurazepam hydrochloride, 77
flurbiprofen, 290t, 298t–299t, 300, 1094t–1095t
flurbiprofen (Ocufen), 1090t
flutamide (Eulexin, PMSFlutamide, Teva-Flutamide, NU-Flutamide, Euflex)), 236t–238t, 261t–263t
fluticasone (Arnuity Ellipta, Flovent Diskus, Flovent HFA, APOFluticasone HFa, Lovent Diskus, Flovent HFA, PMS-Fluticasone HFA), 318t, 320t–323t
fluticasone (Flonase), 605t, 617
fluticasone (Flonase Allergy Relief OTC; Apo-Fluticasone, RATIO-Flonase, TEVA-Fluticasone), 320t–323t
fluticasone (Xhance), 605t, 616t, 617, 621t
fluticasone aerosol (Flovent), 605t, 616t
fluticasone powder (Flovent Rota disk), 605t, 616t
fluticasone topical (Cutivate), 318t, 320t–323t
fluvastatin (Lescol, Lescol SL), 754t
fluvastatin (Lescol, Lescol XL), 164t, 166t, 167
Fluviral (influenza (IIV4)), 195t–199t
fluvoxamine (Luvox), 1009t
Fluzone (influenza (IIV4)), 195t–199t
Fluzone High Dose (influenza (IIV4)), 195t–199t
Fluzone High-Dose (influenza (IIV4)), 195t–199t
FML (fluorometholone), 1090t
FML ForteFMLLiquifilm (fluorometholone), 1094t–1095t
Focalin (dexmethylphenidate), 1047t, 1053t, 1054–1055
Focalin XR (dexmethylphenidate), 1047t, 1053t, 1054–1055
folic acid (folate), 654t–656t

administration, 660
adverse effects, 660
contraindications, 660
nursing implications, 660
patient teaching guidelines, 657b, 660
pharmacokinetics, 659–660
therapeutic effects, 660
use, 660
follicle-stimulating hormone (FSH), 798
folliculitis, 1110–1112
Follistim AQ (follitropin alfa), 799t
Follistim AQ (follitropin beta), 85, 85t, 799t
follitropin alfa (Gonal-F, Gonal-F RFF, Gonal-F Pen), 85, 85t
follitropin alfa/beta, 803
follitropin alfa/beta (Follistim AQ, Gonal-F, Gonal-F RFF Redi-Ject), 799t
follitropin alfa/beta (Gonal-t, Gonal-F RFF Redi-Ject; Gonal-F, Gonal-F Pen), 800t–801t
follitropin beta (Follistim AQ, Puregon), 85, 85t
Folotyn (pralatrexate), 236t–238t
fondaparinux (Arixtra), 140, 140t–142t
food allergies, 589
Food and Drug Administration (FDA), 68
　drug approval by, prescription and nonprescription, 8–9
　responsibilities of, 8–9
Food, Drug, and Cosmetic Act of 1938, 5–7, 6t–7t
Foradil (formoterol), 605t, 608t, 610, 621t
Forane (isoflurane), 922, 922t–923t
formoterol (Foradil), 605t, 608t, 610
formoterol (Performist, Foradil, Oxeze Turbuhaler), 608t
formoterol (Performist; Foradil, Oxeze Turbuhaler), 605t, 608t, 610, 621t
Fortaz (ceftazidime), 335t, 342t–344t
Forteo (teriparatide), 823t, 824
Fosamax (alendronate), 815t, 820–822, 820t–821t
fosinopril (APO-Fosinopril, CO Fosinopril), 482t
fosinopril (Monopril), 482t, 485t, 488, 495t–496t, 754t
fosphenytoin (Cerebyx), 956t, 965t, 966
Fragmin (dalteparin), 140, 140t–142t, 143, 156–157
FreeStyle Libre 2 System, 755–758
Fresenius Propoven (propofol), 922t, 925, 926t
Freya, 110t–111t
Frova (frovatriptan), 945t
frovatriptan (Frova), 945t, 946
fructose, 718
Fulphila (pegfilgrastim), 185–186, 185t
fulvestrant (Faslodex, TEVA-Fulvestrant)), 236t–238t, 260, 261t–263t
functionalized amino acids, 956t, 975
　abnormal kidney function, 976
　adverse effects, 976
　contraindications, 976
　dose usage, 976
　hepatic impairment, 976
　mechanisms of action, 975
　nursing implications, 976
　patient teaching guidelines, 976b
　pharmacokinetics, 975
　preventing interactions, 976
　therapeutic effects, 976
fungal infections. See also antifungal drugs
　assessment, 460b
　clinical manifestations, 445
　drug therapy, 445–446, 446f, 447t
　evaluation, 460b
　immunocompromised hosts, 445
　nursing interventions, 460b
　nursing process, 460b
　outcomes of therapy, 460b
fungi, 272–273, 445
Fungizone (amphotericin B deoxycholate), 446–449, 447t–448t, 449b

furosemide, 96b
furosemide (Lasix), 482t, 561, 562t, 631–635, 631t, 633b
furosemide (Lasix, APOFurosemide, Furosemide Special, MINT-Furosemide), 494, 496t–498t
fusion protein inhibitors, 211t, 222t–224t, 227–228, 412b, 439–440
Fuzeon (enfuvirtide), 439–440, 439t
Fycompa (perampanel), 956t, 969t–972t, 978

G

GABA agonist/glutamate antagonist, 1061t
GABA receptors, 998
GABA structural analogs, 956t
gabapentin (Neurontin, Gralise), 949, 956t, 961, 962t–963t
Gabitril (tiagabine), 962t–963t, 963–964
Gabitril (tiagabine hydrochloride), 956t
Gablofen (baclofen), 983t, 984, 985t–986t
galactagogues, 96
galantamine (Razadyne ER, Auro-Galantamine ER, Mylan-Galantamine ER), 855t, 859, 859t
galantamine hydrobromide (Razadyne ER), 859
gallstones, 676b
GamaSTAN S/D (immune globulin (human) (IG; IGIM)), 200t–201t
GamaSTAN S/D (immune globulin intravenous (IGIV)), 200t–201t, 203
gamma-aminobutyric acid, 949, 984
　abnormal kidney function, 985
　adverse effects, 985
　contraindications, 985
　dose usage, 985
　hepatic impairment, 985
　mechanisms of action, 985
　nursing implications, 985–987
　patient teaching guidelines, 987b
　pharmacokinetics, 984
　preventing interactions, 985
　therapeutic effects, 985
gamma-aminobutyric acid structural analogs, 961
　abnormal kidney function, 962
　adverse effects, 963
　contraindications, 963
　dose usage, 962
　hepatic impairment, 962
　mechanisms of action, 961
　nursing implications, 963
　patient teaching guidelines, 964b
　pharmacokinetics, 961
　preventing interactions, 963
　therapeutic effects, 963
Gammagard (immune globulin (human) (IG; IGIM)), 200t–201t
Gammagard (immune globulin intravenous (IGIV)), 200t–201t, 203
Gammagard S/D, Gamunex (immune globulin (human) (IG; IGIM)), 200t–201t
ganciclovir (Zirgan), 417–419, 418t, 1090t–1091t, 1092
Gardasil (human papillomavirus (HPV)), 194b, 195t–199t, 201
Gardasil 9 (human papillomavirus (HPV)), 194b, 195t–199t, 201
garlic, 59t–61t
gastric acid, 690–693
gastric juice, 695
gastric ulcers, 698–699, 699t, 702
gastritis, 692
gastroesophageal reflex disease (GERD), 90, 602, 692t
　adjuvant medications, 701–703, 701t
　assessment, 704b
　clinical considerations, 690
　clinical manifestations, 690

drug therapy, 690–691, 692t
evaluation, 704b
nursing interventions, 704b
nursing process, 704b
therapy, outcomes of, 704b
gastrointestinal anticholinergic drugs
administration, 886
adverse effects, 886
contraindications, 886
drug interactions, 886
in lactation, 886
mechanism of action, 885
nursing implications, 886
pharmacokinetics, 885
in pregnancy, 886
therapeutic effects, 886
uses, 885–886
gastrointestinal cation exchange, 668
gastrointestinal drugs, 675b
gastrointestinal (GI) effects, 785t–786t, 788, 831
gastrointestinal system, 316b
disorders, 24
drugs, 675b
gatifloxacin (Zymaxid), 1090t–1091t
gauge, 48
Gaviscon, 694t
Gazyva (obinutuzumab), 236t–238t, 252t–257t, 257
GD-Tranexamic Acid (tranexamic acid), 158t
Gelnique (oxybutynin), 887t
gelusil, 692t, 694t
gemcitabine (Infugem), 236t–245t, 246–247
gemfibrozil (Lopid), 163–164, 164t, 170t, 171
general anesthesia
adjuvant medications, 931–932, 932t
alpha-2 adrenergic agonist, 932
assessment, 933b
benzodiazepines, 931–932
clinical manifestations, 921
definition of, 921
drug therapy, 921–922
emergence phase, 922
evaluation, 933b
induction phase, 921–922
intravenous anesthetics (see intravenous anesthetics)
maintenance phase, 922
nursing interventions, 933b
nursing process, 933b
opioid analgesics, 932
outcomes of therapy, 933b
overview of, 921–922
general interventions, drug therapy, 52–57
generalized anxiety disorder, 993, 994b
generalized seizures, 955
genetics, 23
Gengraf (cyclosporine), 211t, 212, 215–219, 225
genital herpes, 406b
Genotropin (somatropin), 799, 799t–801t
Genotropin GoQuick (somatropin), 800t–801t
Genotropin MiniQuick (somatropin), 800t–801t
Gentak (gentamicin), 1090t
gentamicin, 1113t
gentamicin (Garamycin), 353–357, 353t, 355t, 356t
gentamicin (Gentak), 1090t
Geodon (ziprasidone), 1009t, 1024t, 1031t, 1039t–1040t, 1043
GERD (gastroesophageal reflex disease), 90, 602, 692t
adjuvant medications, 701–703, 701t
assessment, 704b
clinical considerations, 690
clinical manifestations, 690
drug therapy, 690–691, 692t
evaluation, 704b
nursing interventions, 704b
nursing process, 704b

therapy, outcomes of, 704b
gestational diabetes mellitus, 90
Gianvi, 110t–111t
giardiasis, 463, 464t, 465, 469
Gilotrif (afatinib), 236t–238t, 252t–257t
ginger, 59t–61t
Gingival hyperplasia, 964
ginkgo biloba, 59t–61t
glaucoma, 1077, 1082–1088, 1082t
Gleevec (imatinib), 236t–238t, 252, 252t–257t, 258–259
Gleostine (lomustine), 235, 236t–245t, 238
Gliadel (carmustine), 235, 236t–238t, 238–239
glimepiride (Amaryl), 754t, 763b, 765t, 767b, 777
glipizide (Glucotrol, Glucotrol XL), 754t, 763b, 765t
glitazone, 769, 777
Global Initiative for Asthma (GINA), 606
glomerular filtration rate (GFR), 79, 631
glucagon, 750
glucagon-like peptide-1 receptor agonists (incretin mimetics), 681b, 683–685, 683t, 774–776, 775t
administration, 774–775
adverse effects, 774–775
contraindication, 774
mechanism of action, 774
nursing implications, 774–775, 774b
patient teaching, 775
pharmacokinetics, 774
preventing interaction, 774
therapeutic effects, 775
uses, 774, 775t
glucan, 445–446, 446f, 456, 459
glucocorticoid agents, 1102–1104, 1102t
glucocorticoid receptor antagonists, 833–837, 835t
glucocorticoids, 314, 316b, 317, 318t, 319, 320t–323t. See also corticosteroids
thyroid eye disease medications, 790
glucomannan, 685b
gluconeogenesis, 774
Glucophage (metformin), 751, 754t, 760b, 765–767, 767b
Glucophage XR (metformin), 767b
glucosamine, 59t–61t
glucose, 668
glucose-6-phosphate dehydrogenase deficiency, 23
glucosuria, 751
Glucotrol (glipizide), 754t, 763b, 765t
Glumetza (metformin), 754t, 765, 766t
glyburide (DiaBeta), 754t, 763b, 764–765, 765t, 767b
glyburide (Glynase), 754t, 763b, 764–765, 765t, 767b, 777
Glycate (glycopyrrolate), 886t
glycerin (Pedia-Lax, Sani-Supp Pediatric), 724t, 729t
glycoprotein IIb/IIIa receptor antagonists, 154, 524t, 535
glycopyrrolate (Cuvposa, Robinul, Robinul-Forte), 879t, 886t
glycopyrrolate (Robinul, Cuvposa, Glycate; Cuvposa), 886t
glycylcyclines, 385–386
Glynase (glyburide), 754t, 763b, 764–765, 765t, 767b, 777
Glyset (miglitol), 754t, 758b, 763b, 767b, 768–769, 768t, 777
Gocovri (amantadine hydrochloride), 871t–872t
goiter, 784
golimumab (Simponi, Simponi Aria), 211t, 222t–224t
GoLYTELY (polyethylene glycol-electrolyte solution), 724t, 729t, 730
gonadotropin-releasing hormone (GnRH), 805, 807
gonadotropin-releasing hormone agonists, 236t–238t, 261t–263t, 263–264

Gonal-F (follitropin alfa), 85, 85t
Gonal-F (follitropin alfa/beta), 799t–801t
Gonal-F Pen (follitropin alfa), 85, 85t
Gonal-F Pen (follitropin alfa/beta), 800t–801t
Gonal-F RFF (follitropin alfa), 85, 85t
Gonal-F RFF Redi-Ject (follitropin alfa/beta), 799t–801t
Gonal-t (follitropin alfa/beta), 800t–801t
GoodSense Nasal Allergy Spray (triamcinolone acetonide), 318t, 320t–323t
GoodSense Oral Pain Relief (benzocaine), 912t, 916t
Gordofilm (salicylic acid), 1116t–1117t
goserelin (Zoladex), 236t–238t, 261t–263t, 263–264, 799t, 806t, 807
gout, 288–290, 290f
gouty attack, 288–290
gouty tophi projections, 290f
GP (glycoprotein) IIb/IIIa receptor antagonists, 524t, 535
graft rejection reaction, 209
graft versus host disease (GVHD), 209, 212, 216–217
Gralise (gabapentin), 962t–963t
gram-negative bacteria
Bacteroides, 275b, 277
Escherichia coli, 275b, 277
Klebsiella, 275b
Proteus, 275b
Pseudomonas, 275b
Salmonella, 275b
Serratia, 275b
Shigella, 275b
gram-positive bacteria
Enterococci, 275b
Staphylococci, 275b, 277
Streptococci, 275b, 277
Gram's stain, 273, 278, 281
granisetron (Sancuso, Sustol), 708t, 713, 714t
Granix (filgrastim), 184–186, 185t, 236t–238t, 248b, 264t
granulocyte colony-stimulating factors
administration of, 184
adverse effects, 184
contraindications, 184
dosage information, 184, 185t
filgrastim, 184–186, 185t, 186b
in hepatic function, 184
in kidney function, 184
mechanism of action, 184
nursing implications, 184–185
pegfilgrastim, 185–186, 185t
pharmacokinetics, 184
sargramostim, 185–186, 185t
therapeutic effects, 185
Grastofil (filgrastim), 184–186, 185t, 236t–238t, 248b, 264t
Graves' disease, 784
Graves orbitopathy. See Thyroid eye disease (TED)
gray syndrome, 382–383
griseofulvin, 457–459, 458t, 458b, 459b
group B streptococcus infection, 91
growth factor and tyrosine kinase inhibitors, 236t–238t, 248b
growth hormone (GH), 797
growth hormone deficiency, 797–798
growth hormone-releasing hormone (GHRH), 798
guaifenesin (Mucinex), 574t, 580–581, 580t
guanfacine (Intuniv), 1047t, 1055, 1056t
Guanylate cyclase-C (GC-C) agonists, 724t, 727b, 730–732, 731t
guar gum, 685b
guarana, 685b
guideline-directed medical therapy (GDMT), 554
Gynazole-1 (butoconazole), 447t
Gynedol (estradiol, micronized), 103t

H

Hadlima (adalimumab), 211t, 222t–224t, 227
Haemophilus influenzae, 377
haemophilus influenzae type b (Hib) (ActHIB, Hiberix, PedvaxHIB), 194, 194b, 195t–199t
Haemophilus influenzae type b (Hib) conjugate vaccine, 194b
hairy cell leukemia, 239t–245t
Halaven (eribulin mesylate), 236t–245t
Halcion (triazolam), 995t, 999
Haldol (haloperidol), 1031t, 1032, 1033t, 1061t–1063t
Haldol decanoate (haloperidol), 1033t
half-life, definition of, 19
hallucination, 1030
halobetasol propionate (Halobetasol Propionate, Lexette, Ultravate), 1112t
haloperidol (Haldol), 1031t, 1032, 1061t–1063t
haloperidol (Haldol, Haldol decanoate), 1033t
Halycil (propylthiouracil), 787t
hand–foot syndrome, 248b
Hashimoto's thyroiditis, 784
Havrix (hepatitis A vaccine), 194–203, 195t–199t
health care agencies, 35t–36t
health care-associated pneumonia, 278
heart
 automaticity of, 504
 conductivity of, 504
 electrophysiology of, 515
 excitability of, 511
heart disease, digoxin in, 76
heart failure
 adjuvant medications, 560–565
 administration, 554t
 assessment, 566b
 clinical conditions, 551
 clinical judgment, 555b
 clinical manifestations, 553
 drug therapy, 554
 evaluation, 566b
 nursing interventions, 566b
 nursing process, 566b
 pathophysiology, 552f
 phosphodiesterase inhibitor (*see* phosphodiesterase inhibitors)
 therapy, outcomes, 566b
 types, 552–553, 553t
heart failure with preserved ejection fraction (HFpEF), 552
heart failure with reduced ejection fraction (HFrEF), 552
heart valve disorders, 551
heartburn, 692–693, 696–697
heat stroke, 974
Helicobacter pylori, 690
 bismuth subsalicylate, 703
 combination therapy with antibiotics, 702–703
helminthiasis, 463, 469
helper T cells, 216
Hemabate (carboprost tromethamine), 94t, 95
Hemangeol (propranolol), 524t, 529, 530t, 531
Hemangeol (propranolol hydrochloride), 789t
hemangiol (propranolol), 511–512, 511t, 512b, 524t, 529, 530t, 531
hematologic effects, 788
hematologic malignancies, 233–234
hematopoiesis, 179
hematopoietic cytokines, 179
hematopoietic disorders
 adjuvant medications, 180, 180t, 188–189
 assessment, 190f
 clinical manifestations, 180
 erythrocyte hematopoietic drugs (*see* erythropoiesis-stimulating agents (ESA))
 evaluation, 190f

granulocyte colony-stimulating factors (*see* granulocyte colony-stimulating factors)
 immune function, 180
 immunostimulants, 180
 interferons (*see* interferon(s))
 interventions, 190f
 nursing process, 190f
 overview, 179–180, 179f
 patient teaching guidelines, 183b
 physiology, 179
 therapy outcomes, 190f
hemolytic–uremic syndrome, 246
hemostasis, 138, 139f
HepaGam B (hepatitis B immune globulin, human), 200t–201t
heparin(s), 139, 140t–142t
 abnormal kidney function, 142
 administration of, 143
 adverse effects, 143
 age, 140
 contraindications, 143
 drug interactions, 143b
 endogenous and exogenous, 139
 fondaparinux, 143–144
 LMWHs, 142–143, 157
 mechanism of action, 140
 nursing implications, 143
 patient teaching guidelines, 143, 144b
 patients with hepatic impairment, 142
 pharmacokinetics, 140
 preventing interactions, 143
 prototype, 140t
 reversal of, 157
 therapeutic effects, 143
Heparin-induced thrombocytopenia (HIT), 142
hepatic cytochrome P450 enzymes, 165
hepatic disorders, 24. *See also* liver
hepatic impairment
 cyclosporine use in, 217
 mycophenolate mofetil uses in, 213
hepatitis A
 description of, 194b
 vaccine (Havrix, Vaqta, Avaxim), 194–203, 194b, 195t–199t
hepatitis B virus (HBV), 193, 194b, 195t–199t, 202–203, 406b
 adefovir dipivoxil, 426
 entecavir, 426
 immune globulin, human (HBIG), 200t–201t
 lamivudine, 426t, 430t–431t
 nucleoside analogs, 412b, 425–426, 426t
 ribavirin, 426
 tenofovir disoproxil, 426
hepatitis C virus (HCV), 406b, 426–428, 426t
Heplisav-B (hepatitis B vaccine), 195t–199t, 203
Hepsera (adefovir dipivoxil), 408t–409t, 426, 426t
herbal drugs
 combination products, 574t, 582–585
 preparations, 582
 treating symptoms, 582, 583t
herbal preparations, for skin disorders, 1117, 1117b
herbal remedies and other preparations, 582, 582b
herbal supplements, 59t–61t, 950. *See also specific herb*
 anxiety and hypnosis, 996b
Herceptin (trastuzumab), 222t–224t, 226, 236t–238t, 252t–257t, 257–258
herpes simplex virus, 406b
 acyclovir, 415–417, 416t
 docosanol, 416t, 417
 drugs for, 415–417, 416t, 418t
 famciclovir, 417
 penciclovir, 417
 valacyclovir, 417
herpes virus infections, 406b
herpes zoster (Shingrix), 194b, 195t–199t, 406b

Hetlioz (tasimelteon), 995t, 1002
Hetlioz LQ (tasimelteon), 995t, 1002
Hexalen (altretamine), 236t–238t
Hiberix (haemophilus influenzae type b (Hib)), 194, 195t–199t
Hicon (sodium iodide ^{131}I), 787t, 789
high-alert medications, 11
high-density lipoprotein (HDL) cholesterol, 162, 164b
histamine, 289b, 590t, 594
histamine 1 receptor antagonists, 589–593, 590t–591t, 593b
histamine 2 receptor antagonists, 693–698, 694b, 696t
histamine and allergic response
 assessment, 599b
 clinical manifestations, 588–589, 588f
 drugs blocking, 589–590, 590t
 evaluation, 599b
 first-generation H$_1$ receptor antagonists, 587f, 590–593, 590t–591t, 592b
 histamine receptors, 594, 596
 hypersensitivity reactions, 589–590, 590t
 nursing interventions, 599b
 nursing process, 599b
 second-generation H1 receptor antagonists, 593b, 594–596, 595t
 therapy, outcomes of, 599b
 third-generation H1 receptor antagonists, 593b, 596–600, 596t
histone deacetylase inhibitor, 956t, 974
 abnormal kidney function, 975
 adverse effects, 975
 contraindications, 975
 dose usage, 974–975
 drug interactions, 975b
 hepatic impairment, 975
 mechanisms of action, 974
 nursing implications, 975
 patient teaching guidelines, 976b
 pharmacokinetics, 974
 preventing interactions, 975
 therapeutic effects, 975
histoplasmosis, 445, 447
histrelin (Vantas, Supprelin LA), 799t, 806t, 807
HIT (heparin-induced thrombocytopenia), 142
hives, 1115
Hizentra (immune globulin (human) (IG; IGIM)), 200t–201t
Hizentra (immune globulin intravenous (IGIV)), 200t–201t, 203
HMG-CoA reductase inhibitors, 754t, 779
 abnormal kidney function, 166
 action mechanism, 165
 administration of, 167
 adverse effects, 166–167
 cholesterol production, 164
 contraindications, 167
 drug interactions, 167, 167b
 fluvastatin, 164t, 166t, 167
 hepatic impairment patients, 166
 herb and dietary interactions, 167b
 lovastatin, 166t, 167
 nursing implications, 167
 pharmacokinetics, 164
 pitavastatin, 164t, 166t
 pravastatin, 166t, 167
 rosuvastatin, 166t
 simvastatin, 166t, 167
 therapeutic effects, 167
 treatment, 165
Hodgkin's disease, 233–234, 238, 239t–245t
Homatropaire (homatropine), 1078t
homatropine, 1079t
homatropine (Homatropaire), 1078t
Homatropine (homatropine bromide), 882t

Homatropine bromide, 881*t*
hookworm infections, 463
hormonal contraceptives
  estrogen-progestin combinations (*see* estrogen–progestin combinations)
  weight gain caused by, 675*b*
hormone(s)
  adrenal sex, 315
  anterior pituitary, 799–803
  corticotropin-releasing, 314
  hypothalamic, 799, 799*t*
  posterior pituitary, 799*t*, 803–805
  thyroid, 783, 783, c`, 784, 784, 784, 786, 786, 788, 789, 790, 791, 791–792, 792, 793*b*
hormone inhibitor drugs, 236*t*–238*t*, 260–264, 261*t*–263*t*, 261*f*
hormone replacement therapy (HRT)
  menopause, 101
hospital-acquired infections, 278
household system, 43
HP Acthar Gel (corticotropin), 799*t*, 802
H₁-receptor antagonists, 1090*t*, 1094*t*–1095*t*, 1095
Humalog (Insulin lispro), 753, 754*t*, 755, 756*t*–757*t*, 761, 763*b*
human chorionic gonadotropin (HCG) (Novarel, Pregnyl), 800*t*–801*t*
human chorionic gonadotropin (HCG) (Pregnyl), 85, 85*t*
human chorionic gonadotropin (HCG) (Pregnyl, Chorionic Gonadotropin), 799*t*, 800*t*, 803
human immunodeficiency virus (HIV), 79, 92, 406*b*, 428–438, 428*f*
  antiretroviral drugs, 428–438, 430*t*–431*t*, 433*b*, 434*t*
  combination medication for, 441
    action and use, 441
    administration of, 441
    adverse effects, 441
    contraindications, 441
    nursing implications, 441
    pharmacokinetics, 441
    preventing interactions, 441
    therapeutic effects, 441
  description, 406*b*
  drug therapy
    CCR5 antagonists, 439*t*, 440–441, 440*b*
    fusion protein inhibitors, 412*b*, 439–440
    integrase strand transfer inhibitors, 412*b*, 438–439, 439*t*
    non-nucleoside reverse transcriptase inhibitors, 412*b*, 433–435, 434*t*
    protease inhibitors, 435–438, 436*t*–437*t*
  immunizations in, 202
  infections, 445
  nucleoside reverse transcriptase inhibitors, 429–433, 430*t*–431*t*
    action, 429
    administration of, 432
    adverse effects, 429–432
    contraindications, 429–432
    nursing implications, 432
    pharmacokinetics, 429
    preventing interactions, 432
    therapeutic effects, 432
    use, 429
human papilloma virus (HPV) infection, 194*b*, 406*b*
human papillomavirus (HPV) (Gardasil 9; Gardasil, Cervarix), 194*b*, 195*t*–199*t*, 201
human papillomavirus (HPV) vaccine, 194*b*
Humatin (paromomycin), 355*t*
Humatrope (somatropin), 799, 800*t*–801*t*
Humira (adalimumab), 211*t*, 222*t*–224*t*, 227
Humira Pediatric Crohn's Start (adalimumab), 211*t*, 222*t*–224*t*, 227
Humira Pen (adalimumab), 211*t*, 222*t*–224*t*, 227

Humulin N (isophane insulin suspension), 754*t*, 756*t*–757*t*
Humulin R (insulin injection), 753, 754*t*, 756*t*–757*t*
Hurricaine (benzocaine), 912*t*
HurriCaine One (benzocaine), 912*t*, 916*t*
Hurricane Snap-n-Go (benzocaine), 912*t*, 916*t*
HurriPak Starter Kit (benzocaine), 912*t*, 916*t*
Hycamtin (topotecan), 236*t*–238*t*
hydantoins, 956*t*, 964
  abnormal kidney function, 964
  adverse effects, 964
  contraindications, 964–965
  dose usage, 964
  drug interactions, 965*b*
  hepatic impairment, 964
  mechanisms of action, 964
  nursing implications, 965–966
  patient teaching guidelines, 966*b*
  pharmacokinetics, 964
  preventing interactions, 965–966
  therapeutic effects, 965–966
Hyderm (hydrocortisone), 320*t*–323*t*
hydralazine, 23–24
hydralazine (Hydrazide, BiDil, APOHydrALAZINE, Apresoline), 482*t*
Hydra-zide (hydralazine), 482*t*
Hydrea (hydroxyurea), 236*t*–245*t*, 238
hydrochlorothiazide (HCTZ), 778–779, 778*t*
hydrochlorothiazide (HydroDiuril), 754*t*
hydrochlorothiazide (Microzide), 482*t*, 554*t*, 563
hydrochlorothiazide (Urozide), 631*t*, 635–637, 636*t*, 637*b*, 641*t*
hydrocodone, 578–580
  and acetaminophen products, 896*t*–897*t*
  ibuprofen, 896*t*–897*t*
hydrocodone (Hysingla), 893–894, 894*t*, 896*t*–897*t*, 902
hydrocodone (Hysingla ER), 896*t*–897*t*
hydrocodone bitartrate (Hysingla ER, pdp-Hydrocodone), 574*t*, 579*t*
hydrocortisone (A-Hydrocort, Cortef, Solu-Cortef; Cortef, Solu-Cortef), 320*t*–323*t*
hydrocortisone (Ala Cort, Ala Scalp, Anucort, Anusol, Colocort, Cortef, Cortenema, Cortifoam, Nutracort, Solu-Cortef, Barriere-HC, Emo Cort, Hyderm, Hydroval, NOVOHydrocort, Prevex HC, SANDOZ Hydrocortisone, Sama HC), 318*t*, 320*t*–323*t*
hydrocortisone (Alkindi Sprinkle, Cortef, Solu-CORTEF), 830–832, 830*t*, 832*b*
hydrocortisone acetate (Cortifoam), 320*t*–323*t*
hydrocortisone sodium phosphate, 605*t*
HydroDiuril (hydrochlorothiazide), 754*t*
Hydromorph Contin (hydromorphone), 894*t*, 896*t*–897*t*, 902
hydromorphone, 96*b*
hydromorphone (Dilaudid), 894*t*, 896*t*–897*t*, 902, 932
hydromorphone (Hydromorph Contin, Jurnista), 894*t*, 896*t*–897*t*, 902
Hydroval (hydrocortisone), 320*t*–323*t*
hydroxychloroquine (Plaquenil), 464*t*, 467*t*, 468
hydroxychloroquine (primaquine), 464*t*, 467*t*, 468
hydroxycitric acid, 685*b*
hydroxymethylglutaryl-coenzyme A (HMG-CoA), 163–164
5-Hydroxytryptamine 3 (5-HT3)
  abnormal kidney function, 713
  action, 713
  administration, 713
  adverse effects, 713
  contraindications, 713
  dolasetron, 708*t*, 713, 714*t*
  granisetron, 708*t*, 713, 714*t*
  in hepatic impairment patients, 713

nursing implications, 713
palonosetron, 708*t*, 713, 714*t*–715*t*, 716, 717*t*
patient teaching guidelines, 713
pharmacokinetics, 713
receptor antagonists, 714*t*
use, 713
hydroxyurea (Hydrea, Droxia, Siklos, Apo-Hydroxyurea, Mylan-Hydroxyurea, Hydrea)), 236*t*–245*t*, 238
hydroxyzine hydrochloride, 77
hydroxyzine pamoate (Vistaril), 589–590, 590*t*–591*t*, 593, 708*t*, 710, 711*t*, 712*b*
hyoscyamine sulfate (Anaspaz, Ed-Spaz, Hyosyne, Levsin), 882*t*
Hyosyne (hyoscyamine sulfate), 882*t*
Hyper HEP B S/D (hepatitis B immune globulin, human), 200*t*–201*t*
hyperaldosteronism, 316
hypercalcemia, 823–824
  calcitonin, 823
  denosumab, 823
  drugs, 823*t*
  emergency treatment of, 824
  phosphate salts, 823–824
  raloxifene, 824
  teriparatide, 824
hyperkalemia, 633*b*, 639–640, 666, 828–829
  agents, treatment, 668
hyperlipidemia. *See* dyslipidemia
hypermagnesemia, 692–693
hyperosmolar hyperglycemic nonketotic coma (HHNC), 752, 752*b*
hyperparathyroidism, 813
HyperRAB S/D (rabies immune globulin (HRIG)), 200*t*–201*t*
HyperRHO S/D Full Dose (Rh₀(D) immune globulin (human)), 200*t*–201*t*
hypersensitivity infusion reaction, 383
hypersensitivity (allergic) reactions, 587
  allergic contact dermatitis, 588, 588*f*
  allergic drug reactions, 589
  allergic rhinitis, 588, 588*f*
  drug therapy, 589–590, 590*t*
  food allergies, 589
  pseudoallergic drug reactions, 589
  type I, 587–588, 587*f*
  type II, 587*f*, 588
  type III, 587*f*, 588
  type IV, 587*f*, 588
hypersensitization, 848
hypertension
  adjuvant medications, 482*t*, 494–500, 496*t*–498*t*
  administration of, 482*t*
  in adolescents, 478
  angiotensin II receptor blockers (*see* angiotensin II receptor blockers)
  angiotensin-converting enzyme inhibitors (*see* angiotensin-converting enzyme inhibitors)
  antihypertensive–diuretic combination products, 494, 495*t*–496*t*
  assessment, 501*b*
  autoregulation, blood flow, 478
  benazepril (Lotensin), 482*t*, 485*t*, 488
  blood pressure regulation, 478
  cardiovascular disease, 76
  clinical manifestations, 479
  dietary management, 479–480
  drug interactions, 482*t*
  drug management, 480–484
  enalapril (Vasotec), 482*t*, 485*t*, 488, 495*t*–496*t*
  evaluation, 501*b*
  fosinopril (Monopril), 482*t*, 485*t*, 488, 495*t*–496*t*
  grades of, 478–479
  hypotension, 479
  lifestyle management, 480
  lisinopril (Zestril), 482*t*, 485*t*, 488, 495*t*–496*t*

hypertension (Continued)
  medications, 494–500, 496t–498t
  moexipril, 482t, 485t, 488
  nonpharmacologic treatment, 479–480
  nursing interventions, 501b
  nursing process, 501b
  obesity and, 676b, 680, 683
  outcomes of therapy, 501b
  overview of, 478–484
  perindopril (Coversyl), 482t, 485t, 488
  quinapril (Accupril), 482t, 485t, 488, 495t–496t
  ramipril (Altace), 482t, 485t, 488
  responses, 479
  therapy, 479–484
  trandolapril (Mavik), 482t, 485t, 488, 495t–496t
  types of, 478–479, 478b
hypertensive crisis, 872
hypertensive disorders in pregnancy, 91
hypertensive emergencies, 499
hypertensive urgencies, 478
HyperTET S/D (tetanus immune globulin), 200t–201t
hyperthyroidism, 551, 737
  adjuvant medication, 789
  antithyroid drug (see propylthiouracil (PTU))
  clinical considerations, 784
  clinical manifestations, 784
  drug therapy, 786
  propranolol, 789
  thyroid drugs (see thyroid drugs)
hyperuricemia, 248b, 288
hypnosis, 921
hypnotics, 993
hypocalcemia, 813, 813b, 815, 817–819
hypoglycemia, 753, 758–759, 758b, 762–765, 767b, 768–771, 774–775, 828–829
hypoglycemic drugs
  alpha-glucosidase inhibitors, 767–769, 768t, 769b
  biguanides, 765–767, 766t, 767b
  insulin (see insulin)
  meglitinides, 769–770, 770t, 771b
  sulfonylureas, 764–765, 765t
  thiazolidinediones, 769, 769t
hypoglycemic reaction, 758b, 761, 763b, 767b
hypogonadism, 118
hypokalemia, 633–634, 633b, 638, 640, 666
hypomagnesemia, 518
hypomania, 1010
hypoparathyroidism/hyperparathyroidism, 813
hypotension. See also shock
  acute, 540–541, 540f
  assessment, 548b
  clinical considerations, 540–541
  clinical manifestations, 541
  development of, 540f
  dobutamine, 543t, 547
  dopamine, 543t, 546–547
  drugs, 543t
  epinephrine, 545–547
  evaluation, 548b
  management, 541
  norepinephrine (see norepinephrine (Levophed))
  nursing interventions, 548b
  nursing process, 548b
  outcomes of therapy, 548b
  patient teaching guidelines, 545, 546b
  phenylephrine, 541–542, 547
  treatment of, 541
hypothalamic hormone drugs
  acromegaly, 807
    abnormal kidney function and hepatic impairment, 808
    administration of, 808
    adverse effects, 808
    contraindications, 808
    lactation, 808
    lanreotide, 808
    mechanism of action, 807
    nursing implications, 808
    octreotide acetate, 807–808, 809b
    pasireotide, 808–809
    patient teaching guidelines, 808, 809b
    pharmacokinetics, 807
    in pregnancy patients, 808
    preventing interactions, 808
    therapeutic effects, 808
    uses, 808
  central precocious puberty
    abnormal kidney function and hepatic impairment, 807
    administration of, 807
    adverse effects, 807
    contraindications, 807
    drugs, 806t
    goserelin, 807
    histrelin, 807
    in lactation, 807
    leuprolide acetate, 805
    mechanism of action, 805
    nafarelin, 807
    nursing implications, 807
    patient teaching guidelines, 807, 807b
    pharmacokinetics, 805
    in pregnancy patients, 807
    preventing interactions, 807
    therapeutic effects, 807
    triptorelin, 807
    uses, 806–807
hypothalamic hormones, 799, 799t
hypothalamic-pituitary-adrenal (HPA) axis, 828
hypothalamus, 261f, 288, 291, 295
hypothyroidism
  antithyroid drug (see propylthiouracil (PTU))
  clinical considerations, 784
  clinical manifestations, 784–786
  drug therapy, 786
  primary, 784
  signs and symptoms of, 788
  thyroid drugs (see thyroid drugs)
hypovolemic shock, 541t, 546–547, 546b
hypoxemia, 28
HypRho-D (Rh$_o$(D) immune globulin (human)), 200t–201t
Hysingla (hydrocodone), 893–894
Hysingla (hydrocodone bitartrate), 893–894, 894t, 896t–897t, 902
Hysingla ER (hydrocodone), 896t–897t
Hysingla ER (hydrocodone bitartrate), 574t, 579t
Hytrin (terazosin), 128t, 129
hyzaar (ACT Losartan/HCT, Hyzaar, ACT Losartan/HCT), 495t–496t
Hyzaar (hyzaar), 495t–496t

I

ibandronate (Boniva), 820t–821t
Ibavyr (ribavirin), 426t, 427–428
Ibrance (palbociclib), 236t–238t, 252t–257t
ibrexafungerp (Brexafemme), 458t, 459
ibritumomab, 87b
ibritumomab tiuxetan (Zevalin, Tiuxetan), 236t–238t, 252t–257t, 257–258
ibrutinib (Imbruvica), 236t–238t, 252t–257t, 258
ibudone (hydrocodone), 896t–897t
ibuprofen (hydrocodone), 896t–897t
ibuprofen (Motrin, Advil), 290t, 293, 295–300, 298t–299t, 300b, 1107
ibutilide (Corvert), 513t, 515
Iclusig (ponatinib), 236t–238t, 252t–257t, 259
Idamycin (idarubicin), 236t–245t, 247
idarubicin (Idamycin), 87b, 236t–245t, 247
idarucizumab (Praxbind), 140t, 148, 157–158, 158t
Ifex (ifosfamide), 236t–245t
ifosfamide, 87b
ifosfamide (Ifex), 236t–245t
IGIVnex (immune globulin (human) (IG; IGIM)), 200t–201t
Igm-mediated reaction, 588
iloperidone (Fanapt), 1031t, 1039t–1040t, 1042
imatinib (Gleevec, (Apo-Imatinib; ACT-Imatinib, Gleevec, Teva- Imatinib)), 236t–238t, 252, 252t–257t, 258–259
Imbruvica (ibrutinib), 236t–238t, 252t–257t, 258
Imdur (isosorbide mononitrate), 524t–525t, 528
imidazoline, 989
  adverse effects, 990
  contraindications, 990
  dose usage, 990
  mechanisms of action, 990
  nursing implications, 990
  patient teaching guidelines, 990b
  pharmacokinetics, 989
  preventing interactions, 990
  therapeutic effects, 990
iminostilbenes, 956t, 966, 967t
  abnormal kidney function, 966
  adverse effects, 966–967
  contraindications, 967
  dose usage, 966
  drug interactions, 967b
  hepatic impairment, 966
  mechanisms of action, 966
  nursing implications, 967–968
  patient teaching guidelines, 968b
  pharmacokinetics, 966
  preventing interactions, 967–968
  therapeutic effects, 968
imipenem-cilastatin (Primaxin), 335t, 347–350, 347t, 348b
imipenem-relebactam (Recarbrio), 335t–337t, 348
imipramine, 1009t, 1011, 1012t
imipramine (Tofranil), 950
Imitrex (sumatriptan), 944, 945t
immediate hypersensitivity, 587–588, 590–593. see also first-generation H_1 receptor antagonists
immune disorders, 210
immune globulin (human) (IG; IGIM) (Asceniv, Bivigam, Carimune NF, Gammagard, Hizentra, Privigen, GamaSTAN S/D, Hizentra, Privigen, Xembify; Cutaquig, Cuvitru, GamaSTAN S/D, Gammagard S/D, Gamunex, Hizentra, IGIVnex, Iveegam Immuno, Octagam, Panzyga), 200t–201t
immune globulin intravenous (IGIV), 200t–201t, 203
immune responses, 209
immune serums, 193, 200t–201t
immune system
  cytokines, 180
  glucocorticoids, 316b
  HIV infection, 406b
  hypersensitivity, 587
  latent tuberculosis infection, 389, 390b, 391t
immunity
  active, 193, 195t–199t
  passive, 193, 200t–201t
immunizations. See also vaccines
  in adolescents, 202
  adverse effects of, 203
  in cancer patients, 202
  changes in, 194b
  contraindications, 203
    administering the medication, 204, 204b
    adverse effects, assessing for, 203
    preventing interactions, 203–204
    therapeutic effects, assessing for, 204
  definition of, 193
  nursing process, 206b

patient teaching guidelines, 204, 205b
reproduction, pregnancy, and lactation, 202
routine childhood immunizations, vaccines used for, 202b
up-to-date with immunization recommendations, 205
immunocompetence, 179, 406b
immunodeficiency, 179
immunomodulators, 211, 227, 1116t–1117t
immunosuppressant drugs, 209–210, 212–216, 215b
　abnormal kidney function and hepatic impairment, 213
　activity of, 212f
　administration of, 211t
　adverse effects of, 214
　antibody preparations, 221–226
　antirejection agents, 216–219
　corticosteroids, 221
　cytokine inhibitors, 226–227
　definition of, 209
　drug interactions, 214, 214b
　monoclonal antibody, 224–226
　nursing process for, 229b
　reproduction, pregnancy, and lactation, 213
　self-administration of, 215b
　sites of action for, 212f
　therapeutic effects of, 214
immunosuppressant monoclonal antibodies, 605t, 619–620, 619t
immunosuppressants, 1090t, 1094t–1095t, 1097
　adverse effects, 1097
　contraindications, 1097
　dose usage, 1097
　mechanisms of action, 1097
　nursing implications, 1097
　patient teaching guidelines, 1097
　pharmacokinetics, 1097
　therapeutic effects, 1093
　thyroid eye disease medications, 790
immunosuppression, 324
　description of, 202, 209
　for organ transplantation, 209
Imodium (loperamide), 738t, 739
Imogam (rabies immune globulin (HRIG)), 200t–201t
Imogam Rabies HT (rabies immune globulin (HRIG)), 200t–201t
Imogam Rabies Pasteurized (rabies immune globulin (HRIG)), 200t–201t
Imovax Polio (poliomyelitis, inactivated (IPV)), 195t–199t
Imovax Rabies (rabies vaccine (HDCV CECV)), 195t–199t
impaired fasting glucose (IFG), 750
Impeklo (clobetasol propionate), 1112t
Imuran (azathioprine), 211t, 212, 216
inactivated poliomyelitis vaccine (IPV), 195t–199t
Inbrija, 874
incretin hormones, 771–772
indapamide (Lozide), 496t–498t, 631t, 636t, 637
Inderal (propranolol hydrochloride), 524t, 529, 530t, 531, 787t, 789, 789t
Inderal LA (propranolol hydrochloride), 482t, 511–512, 511t, 512b, 787t, 789
indirect-acting cholinergics
　abnormal kidney function, 854
　administration, 856
　adverse effects, 855–856
　contraindications, 856
　drug interactions, 856b
　in hepatic impairment patients, 854
　mechanism of action, 854
　muscarine, 855
　neostigmine, 854
　nursing implications, 856
　patient teaching guidelines, 856, 856b

pharmacokinetics, 854
pyridostigmine, 854
routes and dosage ranges, 854, 855t
therapeutic effects, 856
Indocin (indomethacin), 92–93, 93t, 290t, 297, 302–305, 302t–303t, 304b
indomethacin (Indocin, Tivorbex, Apo-Indomethacin, Sandoz-Indomethacin), 92–93, 93t, 290t, 297, 302–305, 302t–303t, 304b
induction phase, in general anesthesia, 921–922
Infanrix (diphtheria, tetanus toxoids, and acellular pertussis (DTaP)), 195t–199t
infants. See also pediatrics
　pharmacokinetics in, 18
infections, 248b
　ear (see ear disorders)
　fungal (see fungal infections)
　ocular, 1077
　parasitic infections (see parasitic infections)
infertility
　clomiphene citrate for, 84, 85t
　follitropins for, 85, 85t
　human chorionic gonadotropin for, 85, 85t
　letrozole, 84, 85t
　lupron for, 85, 85t
　menotropin for, 84, 85t
　routes and dosage ranges, 84, 85t
inflammation, 272, 288, 289b, 290t
inflammatory and immune responses, 316b
inflammatory bowel disorders, 325, 737
Inflectra (infliximab), 211t, 227
infliximab (Avsola, Remicade, Inflectra, Remsima, Renflexis), 211t, 222t–224t, 227
influenza A virus, 422–425, 422t
influenza B virus, 422–425, 422t
Influenza (IIV4) inactivated (Afluria; Fluad, Fluarix, Flublok, Flucelvax, FluLaval, Fluzone, Fluzone High-Dose, FluMist [LAIV4] live attenuated; Agriflu, Fluzone, Fluzone High Dose, Agriflu, Fluad, Fluad Pediatric, FluLaval Tetra, Fluviral, Quadrivalent Influvac), 195t–199t
influenza virus, 92
　influenza A virus, 422–425, 422t
　influenza B virus, 422–425, 422t
Infugem (gemcitabine), 236t–245t, 246–247
Infumorph (morphine sulfate), 894–903, 894t, 896t–897t
inhalation anesthetics, 922–925, 922t
　abnormal kidney function and hepatic impairment, 923
　administration of, 924
　adverse effects, 923–924
　contraindications, 924
　desflurane, 922t–923t, 924–925
　drugs, 923t
　isoflurane, 922
　in lactation, 923
　mechanism of action, 923
　nursing implications, 924
　patient teaching guidelines, 924, 925b
　pharmacokinetics, 922
　in pregnancy, 923
　preventing interactions, 924
　therapeutic effects, 924
　uses, 923
injections. See specific injection
Inlyta (axitinib), 236t–238t, 252t–257t
Innofem (estradiol, micronized), 103t
InnoPran (propranolol), 524t, 529, 530t, 531
InnoPran XL (propranolol hydrochloride), 787t, 789
inotropic effect, 545–546
inotropic medications, 506
Inrebic (fedratinib), 211t, 221
Inspra (eplerenone), 631t, 638t, 640

Instant Oral Pain Relief Max (benzocaine), 912t, 916t
Institute for Safe Medication Practices (ISMP), 10, 35
insulin, 48, 668
　abnormal kidney function, 759
　absorption of, 753–755
　administration, 768
　　continuous subcutaneous (sub-Q) insulin infusion pump, 761, 761f
　　food intake timing, 761
　　timing, 761
　adverse effects, 767
　choice of, 755
　contraindications, 759
　drug interactions, 760, 760b
　endogenous, 751, 753, 755, 759
　estimated average glucose (eAG), 762, 762t
　factors, increase insulin requirements, 758–759
　in hepatic impairment patients, 759
　human, 753
　intermediate-acting, 753, 754t, 756t–757t
　in lactation, 759
　long-acting, 753, 756t–757t
　mechanism of action, 755
　metabolism affected by, 751b
　nursing implications, 760–764
　patient teaching, 762–764, 763b, 764b
　perioperative therapy, 759, 760b
　pharmacokinetics, 755
　pork and bovine insulin, 753
　in pregnancy, 759
　preventing interactions, 760, 760b
　rapid-acting, 753
　regular, 753
　routes and dosages, 755, 756t–757t
　short-acting, 755, 756t–757t
　syringes for, 42t–43t
　therapeutic effects, 767
　type 2 diabetes (see type 2 diabetes)
　types of, 753–755
　uses, 755–759, 758b
insulin aspart (NovoLog), 753, 754t, 756t–757t, 763b, 764
insulin detemir (Levemir), 753, 754t, 755, 756t–757t, 764
insulin glargine (Lantus), 753, 754t, 755, 756t–757t, 761, 763b
insulin glulisine (Apidra), 753, 754t, 756t–757t
insulin lispro (Humalog), 753, 754t, 755, 756t–757t, 761, 763b
insulin lispro protamine, 756t–757t
insulin mixtures, 756t–757t
integrase strand transfer inhibitors (INSTIs), 412b, 438–439, 439t
Integrilin (eptifibatide), 140t, 151t–152t, 154, 156
integumentary effects, 785t–786t
Intensol (lorazepam), 960t
Intensol (prednisone), 317, 318t, 320t–323t, 324–326, 328–329
interference, 22
interferon(s), 180
　administration of, 187
　adverse effects, 186–187
　contraindications, 187
　dosage information, 186–188, 187t
　drug interactions, 187t
　in hepatic impairment patients, 186
　interferon alfa 3n, 187t, 188
　interferon beta 1a, 187t, 188
　interferon beta 1b, 187t
　mechanism of action, 186
　nursing implications, 187–188
　peginterferon alfa-2a, 187t, 188
　peginterferon alfa-2b, 187t
　pharmacokinetics, 186
　preventing interactions, 187, 188b
　therapeutic effects, 187

interferon alfa-2b (Intron-A), 186, 187t
interferon alfa-3n (Alferon N), 180t, 187t, 188
interferon beta-1a (Avonex, Rebif, Rebif Rebidose), 180t, 187t, 188
interferon beta-1b (Betaseron, Extavia), 180t, 187t
interferon gamma-1b (Actimmune), 180t, 187t, 188
interleukin-blocking agents, 211t, 227
interleukins, 180, 188
 -1, 188
 -2, 188
 -11, 188
 description of, 188–189
intermediate-acting insulins, 753, 754t, 756t–757t
intermittent infusion, 46b
International Society of Hypertension's current, evidence-based practice recommendations for the management and treatment of hypertension, 480, 483f
interventions, 52–57
intestinal amebiasis, 463–465
intestinal candidiasis, 453
intestinal infections, 737
intestinal neoplasms, 737
intima, 522
intramuscular injections
 advantages and disadvantages of, 45t–46t
 drug actions after, 17
 sites for, 56
intraocular pressure, 880
intraocular pressure (IOP), 1076
intravenous anesthetics, 922, 922t
intravenous general anesthetics, 925–928
 administration of, 927
 adverse effects, 927
 contraindications, 927
 drugs, 926t
 etomidate, 922t, 926t, 927
 in lactation, 927
 mechanism of action, 926
 methohexital sodium, 928
 nursing implications, 927
 patient teaching guidelines, 927
 pharmacokinetics, 926
 in pregnancy, 927
 preventing interactions, 927
 propofol, 925
 therapeutic effects, 927
 uses, 926–927
intravenous injections
 absorption after, 16–17
 administration technique, 45t–46t, 46b
 ampules used in, 48
 continuous infusion, 46b
 drug preparation for, 46b
 equipment for, 46b
 intermittent infusion, 46b
 needleless systems, 46b
 principles of, 46b
 sites for, 48–50, 50f
Intron A (interferon alfa-2b), 186, 187t
Intuniv (guanfacine), 1047t, 1055, 1056t
Invanz (ertapenem), 335t, 347t
invasive candidiasis, 454
Invega (paliperidone), 1031t, 1039t–1040t, 1042
Invega Sustenna (paliperidone), 1031t, 1039t–1040t
Invega Trinza (paliperidone), 1031t, 1039t–1040t
Invokana (canagliflozin), 776–777, 776t, 777b
i3odine Max (sodium iodide ¹³¹I), 787t
Iodotope (sodium iodide ¹³¹I), 787t
Ionsys (fentanyl), 932t
Iopidine (apraclonidine hydrochloride), 1082t–1084t
iOSAT (potassium iodide saturated solution of potassium iodide), 787t
ipilimumab (Yervoy), 211t, 222t–224t, 225–226, 236t–238t, 252t–257t, 257

iPLEDGE program, 1120b
IPOL (poliomyelitis, inactivated (IPV)), 195t–199t
ipratropium, 610–612, 611t, 692t
ipratropium bromide (Atrovent HFA), 879t, 881t–882t, 883
Ipratropium bromide (Atrovent HFA; Apo-Ipravent Solution, Apo-Ipravent Sterules, Atrovent HFA), 605t, 610–612, 611t, 882t
ipratropium/albuterol (Combivent Respimat Apo-Salvent-Ipravent Sterules, Combivent Respimat; Combivent UDV, ratio-Ipra Sal UDV, Teva-Combo Sterinebs), 610–612, 621t
Iprivask (desirudin), 141t–142t, 147–148
IPV (poliomyelitis vaccine, inactivated), 195t–199t
Irbesartan (Avapro), 754t
irbesartan (Avapro), 482t, 490–491, 490t, 495t–496t
Irbesartan-HCT (avalide), 495t–496t
irinotecan, 87b
irinotecan (Camptosar), 236t–245t, 246–247, 250
irinotecan (camptosar), 236t–238t
iris, 1076
iron deficiency
 ferrous sulfate (see ferrous sulfate)
iron dextran, 666
irreversible anticholinesterase toxicity, 863, 864t
irreversible shock, 541
irritable bowel syndrome (IBS), 737, 742–743
isavuconazole (Cresemba), 447t, 451t–452t, 454
Isentress (raltegravir), 438–439, 439t, 439b
isocarboxazid, 1021
isocarboxazid (Marplan), 1009t, 1020t
isoflurane (Forane), 922–924, 922t–923t
isoniazid (INH), 392–395
 abnormal kidney function, 393
 action, 393
 administration of, 395
 adverse effects, 394
 assessment, 395
 contraindications, 394
 dosage information, 393, 393t
 genetic variations that affect, 23
 in hepatic impairment patients, 393
 nursing implications, 394–395
 patient teaching guidelines, 395, 395b
 pharmacokinetics, 393
 preventing interactions, 394–395
 therapeutic effects, 395
 uses, 393–394
isophane insulin (NPH), 754t, 755
Isophane insulin suspension (NPH, Humulin N, Novolin N), 754t, 756t–757t
Isoptin SR (verapamil), 524t, 531–534, 532t
Isopto Atropine (atropine sulfate), 1077, 1078t–1079t
Isopto Atropine (ophthalmic atropine), 882t
Isopto Carpine (pilocarpine), 1082t
Isopto Homatropine (homatropine bromide), 882t
Isordil (isosorbide dinitrate), 524t, 526–528
isosorbide dinitrate (Isordil), 524t, 526–528
isosorbide mononitrate (Imdur), 524t–525t, 528
isotretinoin, 87b, 96b
isotretinoin (Absorica, Accutane, Amnesteem, Claravis, Myorisan), 1119
isotretinoin (Absorica, Accutane, Claravis, Amnesteem, Myorisan, Zenatane), 1118
isradipine, 482t, 524t
Istalol (timolol maleate), 1082t–1084t, 1085
itraconazole, 96b
itraconazole (Sporanox, Tolsura), 447t, 451t–452t, 453
IV calcium, 815
ivabradine (Corlanor), 559–560, 560t, 560b
Iveegam Immuno (immune globulin (human) (IG; IGIM)), 200t–201t
ivermectin (Stromectol), 464t, 469–470, 470t
Ivy-Rid (benzocaine), 912t, 916t

ixabepilone (Ixempra kit), 236t–245t
ixazomib (Ninlaro), 236t–238t, 252t–257t, 260
ixekizumab (Taltz), 211t, 222t–224t, 227
Ixempra kit (ixabepilone), 236t–245t

J

Jakafi (ruxolitinib), 211t, 219–221
JAMP Dicyclomine (dicyclomine hydrochloride), 886t
JAMP Methimazole (methimazole), 787t
JAMP-Colchicine (colchicine), 292t, 306–307, 307t, 308b
JAMP-Darifenacin (Darifenacin hydrobromide), 887t
JAMP-Letrozole (letrozole), 236t–238t, 260, 261t–263t
JAMP-Methotrexate (methotrexate), 211t, 212, 215b, 216, 226–227
JAMP-Quinine, 464t, 467t, 468
JAMP-Ropinirole (ropinirole hydrochloride), 871t–872t
Jamp-Sildenafil (sildenafil), 123, 124t
JAMP-Solifenacin (solifenacin succinate), 887t
JAMP-Terbinafine, 458t
JAMPVancomycin (vancomycin), 381t–382t
Jantoven (warfarin), 141t–142t
janus-kinase inhibitor, 211t, 219–221, 220t
Januvia (sitagliptin), 754t, 767b, 771–772, 772t
Jardiance (empagliflozin), 776t, 777
jaundice, 393
Jencycla (norethindrone), 107t–108t
Jevtana (cabazitaxel), 236t–245t
Johnson & Johnson (COVID-19), 194, 194b, 195t–199t, 201–203, 202b
Jolivette (norethindrone), 107t–108t
Jornay PM (methylphenidate), 1047t, 1053t
Junel Fe 1/20, 110t–111t
Jurnista (hydromorphone), 894t, 896t–897t, 902

K

Kadian (morphine sulfate), 894–903, 894t, 896t–897t
kanamycin, 390–391
Kanjinti (trastuzumab), 222t–224t, 226
Kariva, 110t–111t
Katerzia (amlodipine), 524t
kava, 996b
Keflex (cephalexin), 336t–337t
Kelnor 1/35, 110t–111t
Kelnor 1/50, 110t–111t
Kenalog (triamcinolone), 318t, 320t–323t
Kenalog-10 (triamcinolone), 320t–323t
Kenalog-40 (triamcinolone), 320t–323t
Kenalog 80 (triamcinolone), 318t, 320t–323t
Kengreal (cangrelor), 140t, 150, 151t–152t, 153
Kepivance (palifermin), 236t–238t, 264t
Keppra (levetiracetam), 956t, 969t–972t, 978
Keppra XR (levetiracetam), 969t–972t
keratitis, 1077
Kesimpta (ofatumumab), 236t–238t, 252t–257t, 257
Ketalar (ketamine), 922t, 926t, 927, 1009t, 1026
ketamine (Ketalar), 922t, 926t, 927, 1009t, 1026
ketoconazole (Apo-Ketoconazole, Teva-Ketoconazole), 834–835, 834t–835t, 835b, 836b
ketoconazole (Apo-Ketoconazole, Teva-Ketoconazole), 451t–452t, 453
ketoconazole (Extina, Nizoral), 447t, 451t–452t, 453
ketoconazole (Extina, Xolegel), 1115t
ketones, 751, 752b, 763b, 771
ketoprofen, 290t, 298t–299t, 300
ketorolac, 77, 290t, 302t–303t, 304–305
ketorolac (Acular, Acuvail), 1090t, 1094t–1095t
ketorolac tromethamine (ReadySharp Ketorolac), 938t
ketotifen (Alaway Children's Allergy, Claritin Eye, Zaditor), 1090t, 1096
ketotifen (Alaway, Claritin Eye, Zaditor), 1094t–1095t

Keytruda (pembrolizumab), 236t–238t, 252t–257t
kidney(s), 18
　transplantation, 213t
kidney disorders, 24. *See also* kidney(s)
kidney failure with replacement therapy (KFRT), 148, 771, 774
Kimyrsa (Oritavancin), 381t–382t
Kineret (anakinra), 211t, 227
Klebsiella pneumoniae, 275b
Klebsiella species, 353
Klonopin (clonazepam), 956t, 960t, 995t
Kristalose (lactulose), 724t, 732, 732t
Krystexxa (pegloticase), 292t, 309t, 310
Kupffer's cells, 138
Kurvelo, 110t–111t
Kussmaul respirations, 752b
Kynmobi (apomorphine hydrochloride), 871t–872t
Kynmobi Titration Kit (apomorphine hydrochloride), 871t–872t
Kyprolis (carfilzomib), 236t–238t, 252t–257t, 260

L

labetalol (Trandate, Normodyne), 482t
labor induction
　oxytocics, 94–95, 94t
　prostaglandins, 93–95, 94t
lacosamide (Vimpat), 956t, 969t–972t, 975
lacrimal system, 1076
lacrimation, 1076
lactation
　birth control, 96
　drug use during, 96, 96b
　induction, 95–96
lactulose (Constulose, Kristalose), 724t, 732, 732t
LaMICtal (lamotrigine), 956t, 969t–972t, 977
LaMICtal ODT (lamotrigine), 969t–972t
LaMICtal XR (lamotrigine), 969t–972t
Lamisil (terbinafine), 458t, 459, 1115t
lamivudine, 432
lamivudine (Dovato), 432
lamotrigine (LaMICtal), 956t, 977
lamotrigine (LaMICtal, LaMICtal ODT, LaMICtal XR, Subvenite), 969t–972t
lancet, 755–758
Lanoxin (digoxin), 76
lanreotide (Somatuline Depot, Somatuline Autogel), 799t, 806t, 808
lansoprazole, 692t, 699t
lansoprazole (Prevacid, Prevacid SoluTab), 692t, 699t, 700–701
Lantus (insulin glargine), 753, 754t, 755, 756t–757t, 761, 763b
lapatinib (Tykerb), 236t–238t, 248b, 252t–257t, 258
Larin 1/20, 110t–111t
Larotid (amoxicillin), 335t
larvae, 463
Lasix (furosemide), 482t, 496t–498t, 631–635, 631t, 633b
latanaprostene bunod, 1082t
latanoprost (Xalatan), 1083t–1084t, 1084
latanoprost (Xelpros), 1082t
latanoprostene bunod (Vyzulta), 1083t–1084t, 1084
latent tuberculosis infection, 391, 391t
Latisse (bimatoprost), 1082t–1084t
Latuda (lurasidone), 1031t, 1039t–1040t, 1042
laughing gas. *See* nitrous oxide
laxative(s). *See also* specific drug; specific drug
　action, 724
　administration of, 726
　adverse effects, 725
　bulk-forming, 724, 724t, 726t
　contraindications, 725
　definition of, 723–724
　diarrhea, 738
　and diuretic herbs, 685b
　dosage ranges, 726t

drug/herbal interactions, 726
lactation, 725
lubricant, 724t, 726–727, 726t
nursing implications, 726
patient teaching guidelines, 726, 727b
pharmacokinetics, 724
pregnancy, 725
reproduction, 725
surfactant, 727
therapeutic effects of, 726
uses, 724–725, 725t
Lazanda (fentanyl), 894t, 896t–897t, 902, 922t
Lederle Leucovorin (leucovorin), 236t–238t, 264t
Leena, 110t–111t
left-sided heart failure, 552
Lemborexant (DayVigo), 1003t
lemborexant (DayVigo), 995t, 1004
Lemtrada (alemtuzumab), 211t, 225, 236t–238t, 252t–257t
lens, 1076
lenvatinib (Lenvima), 236t–238t, 252t–257t, 258–259
Lenvima (lenvatinib), 236t–238t, 252t–257t, 258–259
Lescol (fluvastatin), 167, 164t, 166t, 754t
Lescol SL (fluvastatin), 754t
Lescol XL (fluvastatin), 164t, 166t, 167
Lessina-28, 110t–111t
letrozole (Femara, ACH-Letrozole, Apo-Letrozole, Bio- Letrozole, Femara, JAMP-Letrozole), 84, 85t, 236t–238t, 260, 261t–263t
leucovorin (Lederle Leucovorin), 236t–238t, 264t
leukemias, 233–234
Leukeran (chlorambucil), 236t–245t
Leukine (sargramostim), 185–186, 185t, 236t–238t, 248b, 264t
leukotriene(s), 289b, 615f, 617–619
leukotriene modifiers, 617–619
　abnormal kidney function, 618
　action, 617
　administration of, 618
　adverse effects, 618
　contraindications, 618
　drug, 618t
　drug interactions, 618b
　in hepatic impairment patients, 618
　nursing implications, 618–619
　patient teaching guidelines, 618–619
　pharmacokinetics, 617
　preventing interactions, 618
　therapeutic effects, 618
　use, 617–618
　zafirlukast, 605t, 618t, 619
　zileuton, 605t, 618t, 619
leuprolide (Eligard, Lupron Depot, Lupron), 85, 85t
leuprolide acetate (Camcevi, Eligard, Lupron Depot, Fensolvi, Lupron), 806t
leuprolide acetate (Eligard, Lupron Depot), 236t–238t, 261t–263t, 263
leuprolide acetate (Lupron), 806t
levalbuterol (Xopenex [MDI], Xopenex Concentrate, Xopenex HFA), 605t, 608t, 610
Levaquin (levofloxacin), 358t
levels of evidence, 58
Levemir (insulin detemir), 753, 754t, 755, 756t–757t, 764
levetiracetam (Elepsia XR, Keppra, Keppra XR, Roweepra, Roweepra XR, Spritam), 969t–972t
levetiracetam (Keppra), 956t, 978
Levitra (vardenafil), 119t, 124t, 125
levobunolol, 1082t–1084t
levocetirizine (Xyzal Allergy 24HR), 590t, 596–597, 596t
Levodopa, carbidopa, and entacapone (Stalevo), 869t, 877–878

Levodopa–carbidopa (Sinemet, Dhivy, Duopa, Rytary), 869–875, 871t–872t, 873b
levofloxacin, 1090t–1091t
levofloxacin (Levaquin), 353t, 358t, 360
levomilnacipran (Fetzima, Fetzima Titration), 1009t, 1019
levonorgestrel, 107t–108t
levonorgestrel-releasing intrauterine device, 107t–108t
Levophed (norepinephrine), 542, 543t. *See also* norepinephrine (Levophed)
　abnormal kidney function, 543
　action, 541–542, 542t
　administration of, 544
　adverse effects, 543–544
　contraindications, 544
　dobutamine, 543t, 547
　dopamine, 541–542, 543t, 546–547
　drug interactions, 544, 545b
　epinephrine, 541–542, 545–547
　lactation, 543
　nursing implications, 544–545
　patient teaching guidelines, 545, 546b
　pharmacokinetics, 542
　phenylephrine, 541–542, 547
　pregnancy, 543
　preventing interactions, 544, 545b
　reproduction, 543
　therapeutic effects, 544
　uses, 542–543
Levora, 110t–111t
Levothroid (levothyroxine), 790–792, 791t, 792b, 793b
levothyroxine (Levothroid), 790–792, 791t, 792b, 793b
levothyroxine (Ermeza, Euthyrox, Synthroid, Levoxyl, Tirosint, Levothroid), 791t
Levoxyl (levothyroxine), 791t
Levsin (hyoscyamine sulfate), 882t
Lexapro (escitalopram), 1009t, 1017, 1036
Lexette (halobetasol propionate), 1112t
LexiComp Online, 12
Leydig cells, 119
Librium (chlordiazepoxide), 1061, 1061t–1063t
lidocaine (Akten), 518, 1078t–1079t
lidocaine (Lidomark 1/5, Lidomark 2/5, Xylocaine, Xylocaine MPF), 912t
lidocaine (Xylocaine), 508t, 510, 518
lidocaine, epinephrine, and tetracaine (LET), 912b
ligands, 845
linaclotide (Linzess), 724t, 730–731, 731t
linagliptin (Tradjenta), 754t, 772, 772t
lincosamides, 383
lindane, 464t, 471t, 472
linezolid (Zyvox, Apo-Linezolid, Linezolid injection, Sandoz- Linezolid, Zyvoxam), 381t–382t, 384
Linezolid injection (linezolid), 381t–382t
Linzess (linaclotide), 724t, 730–731, 731t
Lioresal (baclofen), 983t, 984, 985t–986t
lipase inhibitors, 679t
　action, 682
　administration, 682
　in adolescents, 682
　adverse effects, 682
　contraindications, 682
　dosage information, 682, 682t
　drug interactions, 682
　lactation, 682
　nursing implications, 682–683
　patient teaching guidelines, 681b, 683
　pharmacokinetics, 681
　pregnancy, 682
　preventing interactions, 682
　reproduction, 682
　therapeutic effects, 683
　use, 682

lipid formulations (Abelcet, AmBisome), 446–447
lipid metabolism, 316b
lipid rescue therapy, 911
Lipidil EZ (fenofibrate), 164t, 170–171, 170t, 171b
Lipidil Supra (fenofibrate), 164t, 170–171, 170t, 171b
lipid-soluble drugs, 78
Lipitor (atorvastatin calcium), 164–167, 166t, 167b, 168b, 754t
lipodox 50 (Caelyx, Myocet), 236t–238t
Lipofen (fenofibrate), 164t, 170–171, 170t, 171b
lipopeptides, 383
lipoproteins, 162
liposomal amphotericin B (AmBisome), 446–447, 448t
liposomal lidocaine, 912b
Liquifilm (fluorometholone), 1090t
liraglutide (Saxenda, Victoza), 679t, 683–685, 683t, 754t, 775, 775t
liraglutide (Victoza), 754t, 775t
lisdexamfetamine (Vyvanse), 1047t, 1050t, 1051
Lisinopril (Prinivil, Zestril), 754t
lisinopril (Zestril), 482t, 485t, 488, 495t–496t
lithium, 96b
lithium carbonate (Lithobid), 1009t, 1023, 1024t
Lithobid (lithium carbonate), 1009t, 1023, 1024t
Lithotab (lithium carbonate). See lithium carbonate (Lithobid)
Livalo (pitavastatin), 164t, 166t
Livalo (pitavastatin calcium), 754t
liver, 17
  transplantation, 219
Lixiana (edoxaban), 140t–142t, 148–149
lixisenatide (Adlyxin), 754t, 775t
LMWHs (low-molecular-weight heparins), 142–143, 157
Lo Loestrin Fe, 110t–111t
loading dose, 21
local anesthetic systemic toxicity (LAST), 911–912
local anesthetics, 1081
  administration methods, 911
  adverse effects, 1081
  agents, 1117
  age-related considerations, 911
  amides (see amides)
  assessment, 918b
  dose usage, 1081
  drugs, 1078t–1079t
  drugs administered for, 912t
  epidural anesthesia, 911
  esters (see esters)
  evaluation, 918b
  interventions, 918b
  mechanisms of action, 1081
  nursing implications, 1081–1082
  nursing process, 918b
  outcomes of therapy, 918b
  overview of, 911–912
  pharmacokinetics, 1081
  spinal anesthesia, 911
  therapeutic effects, 1082
  topical anesthesia, 911
Lodalis (colesevelam), 164t, 169t, 170
Lodine (etodolac), 290t, 302t–303t, 304
lodoxamide (Alomide), 1090t, 1094t–1095t
Loestrin 1/20, 110t–111t
Loestrin Fe 1/20, 110t–111t
LolliCaine (benzocaine), 912t
Lolo, 110t–111t
Lomotil (diphenoxylate with atropine), 737–739, 738t, 740b
lomustine (Gleostine), 235, 236t–245t, 238
Lonapegsomatropin (Skytrofa), 802
long-acting injectable (LAI) antipsychotics, 1032
long-acting insulins, 753, 756t–757t
Loniten (minoxidil), 496t–498t

loop diuretics, 561, 562t
  abnormal kidney function, 632
  action, 631
  administration of, 633–634
  adverse effects, 633
  bumetanide, 631t–632t, 635
  contraindications, 633
  dosage information, 632t
  drug interactions, 633, 633b
  ethacrynic acid, 631t–632t
  furosemide, 631–635, 631t, 633b
  glomerular filtration rate, 631
  in hepatic impairment patients, 632
  herb, 633
  lactation, 632
  nursing implications, 633–634
  patient teaching guidelines, 634, 634b
  pharmacokinetics, 631
  pregnancy, 632
  prototype, 631t
  reproduction, 632
  therapeutic effects, 634
  torsemide, 631t–632t, 635
  use, 631–633
loperamide (Imodium), 738t, 739
Lopid (gemfibrozil), 163–164, 164t, 170t, 171
Lopressor (metoprolol), 524t, 530t, 531
lopressor HCT, 495t–496t
Loprox (ciclopirox), 447t
loratadine (Claritin), 595t, 596
lorazepam (Ativan, Lorazepam Intensol), 87b, 717, 956t, 960t, 995t, 999, 1061t–1063t
LORazepam (lorazepam), 956t
LORazepam Intensol (lorazepam), 956t
Lorazepam Intensol (lorazepam), 995t, 999
lorcaserin, 678–679
Loreev XR (lorazepam), 960t, 995t, 999
Lortab (hydrocodone), 896t–897t
Lorzone (chlorzoxazone), 985t–986t
losartan (Cozaar), 87b, 96b, 561, 562t
losartan (Cozaar, ACT Losartan), 778, 778t
LoSeasonique, 110t–111t
Lotemax (loteprednol), 1094t–1095t
Lotensin (benazepril), 482t, 485t, 488
Lotensin (Benazepril hydrochloride), 754t
loteprednol (Alrex), 1090t
loteprednol (Lotemax, Alrex), 1094t–1095t
lotrel, 495t–496t
Lotrimin (clotrimazole), 450
Lotrimin AF (clotrimazole), 1115t
Lotronex (alosetron), 738t, 741t, 742–743
lovastatin (Altoprev, Mevacor), 164t, 166t, 167, 754t
Lovenox (enoxaparin), 140, 141t–142t
Lovent Diskus (fluticasone), 318t, 320t–323t
low-calorie diet, 676b
low-density lipoprotein (LDL) cholesterol, 162, 164b
lower esophageal sphincter (LES), 690
low-molecular-weight heparins (LMWHs), 142–143, 157
  reversal of, 157
Low-Ogestrel, 110t–111t
loxapine, 1031t, 1033t, 1036
Lozide (indapamide), 631t, 636t, 637
lubiprostone (Amitiza), 724t, 732–733, 732t
lubricant laxative(s), 724t, 726–727, 726t
Lugol's solution (potassium iodide and iodine), 787t
Lugol's solution (strong iodine solution), 788–789
Lumify (brimonidine), 1082t–1084t, 1085
Lumigan (bimatoprost), 1082t–1084t
Lunesta (eszopiclone), 995t
Lupron (leuprolide), 85, 85t
Lupron (leuprolide acetate), 799t, 805, 806t
Lupron Depot (leuprolide acetate), 236t–238t, 261t–263t, 263, 806t
lurasidone (Latuda), 1031t, 1039t–1040t, 1042

luteinizing hormone (LH), 798
Lutera, 110t–111t
Luvox (fluvoxamine), 1009t
Luxiq (betamethasone, dipropionate), 1112t
lymphomas, 233–234
Lyrica (pregabalin), 956t, 962t–963t, 963
Lyrica CR (pregabalin), 956t, 962t–963t
Lysodren (mitotane), 835t, 836–837
Lysteda (tranexamic acid), 158t

M

Maalox suspension, 692t
Macrobid (nitrofurantoin), 365t, 372, 372t
Macrodantin (nitrofurantoin), 77, 365t, 372, 372t
macrolides
  abnormal kidney function, 377
  action, 377
  administration of, 379
  adverse effects, 377
  assessment, 387b
  contraindications, 378
  drugs, 378t
  evaluation, 387b
  in hepatic impairment patient, 377
  nursing implications, 378–379
  nursing interventions, 387b
  nursing process, 387b
  outcomes of therapy, 387b
  pharmacokinetics, 377
  preventing interactions, 378–379
  therapeutic effects, 379
  use, 377
mafenide acetate (Sulfamylon), 365t, 370t
magnesium, 950
magnesium citrate solution (Citroma, GoodSense Magnesium Citrate), 724t, 729t
magnesium hydroxide (Milk of Magnesia, Pedia-Lax, Phillips), 724t, 729t
magnesium oxide or hydroxide, 667
magnesium salicylate (Doans Pills), 290t, 292t, 294
magnesium sulfate, 91, 91t, 93, 93t, 518–519, 956t, 969t–972t, 977
maintenance anesthesia, 922
maintenance dose, 21
major depression, 1008b
malabsorption, 654
malaria, 463, 468–469
malaria prophylaxis, 468
Malarone (atovaquone/proguanil), 464t, 467t, 468
malathion (Ovide), 464t, 471t, 472
malignant hyperthermia, 923–924
malignant neoplasms
  development of, 234
  grading and staging of, 234
  types, 233–234
malignant otitis externa, 1101
mania, 1010
mannitol (Osmitrol), 631t, 640, 640t, 1082t–1084t
Mantoux skin test, 390b
MAO inhibitors, 946. See also monoamine oxidase (MAO) inhibitors
maraviroc (Selzentry), 440–441, 440b
Marcaine Preservative Free (bupivacaine), 912t
Marcaine Preservative free (bupivacaine), 915
Marcaine Spinal (bupivacaine), 912t, 915
marijuana (Cannabis), 718
Marinol (dronabinol), 708t, 717t, 718
marketing, 5
Marlissa, 110t–111t
Mar-Methimazole (methimazole), 787t
Marplan (isocarboxazid), 1009t, 1020t
Marvelon, 110t–111t
mast cell stabilizers, 620–621
maternal–placental–fetal circulation, 86
Matrix Patch (fentanyl), 894t, 896t–897t, 902
Matulane (procarbazine), 236t–245t, 246–247

Matzim LA (diltiazem), 524t, 532t, 533–534
Mavenclad (cladribine), 236t–245t
Mavik (trandolapril), 482t, 485t, 488, 495t–496t
Maxalt (rizatriptan), 945t
Maxidex (dexamethasone), 1090t, 1094t–1095t
Maxipime (cefepime), 335t, 342t–344t
maxzide, 495t–496t, 631t, 641t
measles, mumps, and rubella (MMR) (M–M–R II; M–M–R II, Priorix), 195t–199t, 202–203
measles, mumps, rubella, vaccine, 194b
mebendazole (Vermox), 464t, 469–470, 470t, 470b
meclizine (Antivert, Dramamine Less Drowsy, otion-Time), 708t, 711t, 712
meclofenamate sodium, 290t, 298t–299t, 300
MEDExemestane (exemestane), 236t–238t, 260, 261t–263t
media, 522
medication(s). *See also* drug(s); *specific drug*
 administration record, 55, 56f
 bar coding of, 39
 computerized ordering of, 35t–36t
 definition of, 33
 errors, 34–40
 history, 40, 51b
 orders, 39–41
 reconciliation of, 40
 systems, 39
Mediterranean fever, 307
Medrol (methylprednisolone sodium succinate), 320t–323t
medroxy progesterone acetate (Provera), 106–109, 107t–108t
mefenamic acid (Ponstan), 290t, 298t–299t, 300
mefloquine, 464t, 467t, 468–469
Mefoxin (cefoxitin), 340, 342t–344t
Megace ES (megestrol acetate), 107t–108t
Megace OS (megestrol acetate), 107t–108t
megaloblastic anemia, 660
megavitamins, 645
Megestrol (megestrol acetate), 107t–108t
megestrol acetate (Megace ES; Megace OS, Megestrol), 107t–108t
meglitinide, 777
meglitinides
 abnormal kidney function, 770
 administration, 770
 adverse effects, 770
 contraindications, 770
 drug interactions, 770, 771b
 in hepatic impairment patients, 770
 in lactation, 770
 mechanism of action, 770
 nursing implications, 770
 patient teaching guidelines, 770
 pharmacokinetics, 769
 in pregnancy patients, 770
 therapeutic effects, 770
 uses, 770, 770t
Mekinist (trametinib), 236t–238t, 252t–257t, 258
melatonin, 59t–61t, 996b
meloxicam (Anjeso, Apo-Meloxicam, Auro-Meloxicam), 290t, 300–301, 301t, 301b, 302b
melphalan (Evomela, Alkeran), 236t–245t
memantine (Namenda, Namenda XR, Namenda Titration Pack, Ebixa), 855t, 859t, 860
Menactra (meningococcal group ACWY vaccine (MenACWY-D)), 195t–199t
MenACWYCRM) (Menveo) (meingococcal group CWY vaccine (MenACWY-D), 195t–199t
MenACWY-TT (MenQuadfi) (meingococcal group CWY vaccine (MenACWY-D), 195t–199t
MenB-4C (Bexsero) (meningococcal group B vaccine (MenB-fHBP)), 195t–199t

MenB-fHBP (meningococcal group B vaccine (MenB-fHBP)), 195t–199t
Menest (esterified estrogens), 103t
meningococcal group ACWY vaccine (MenACWY-D) (Menactra), (MenACWYCRM) (Menveo), (MenACWY-TT) (MenQuadfi), 195t–199t
meningococcal group B vaccine (MenB-fHBP) (Trumenba, (MenB-4C) (Bexsero), 195t–199t
meningococcal vaccine, 194
menopause
 definition, 101
 drug therapy, 101
 symptoms, 101
 use of exogenous estrogens, 102
 vs. puberty, 100
Menopur (menotropin), 84, 85t, 799t–801t, 803
Menostar (estradiol transdermal system), 103t
menotropin (Menopur), 84, 85t, 799t–801t, 803
menotropins (Menopur), 803
menstrual cycle, 100
menstrual migraine headaches, 936
Mentax (butenafine), 1115t
meperidine (Demerol), 894t, 896t–897t, 902
meperidine hydrochloride (Demerol), 77
Mephyton (vitamin K), 140t, 158t
Mepivacaine (Carbocaine, Carbocaine Preservative Free, Polocaine, Polocaine Dental, Polocaine-MPF, Scandonest 3% Plain), 912t
Mepivacaine (Carbocaine, Polocaine), 915
mepolizumab (Nucala), 605t, 619t, 620
mercaptopurine (Purinethol, Purixan), 236t–245t, 238, 246–247
meropenem (Merrem), 335t, 347t, 348
meropenem-vaborbactam (Vabomere), 335t, 347t, 348
Merrem (meropenem), 335t, 347t
mesna (Mesnex), 236t–238t, 250, 264t
Mesnex (mesna), 236t–238t, 250, 264t
Mestinon (pyridostigmine), 854, 855t
metabolic effects, 785t–786t
metabolic syndrome, 162, 676b, 683
metabolism, 1009
 age effects on, 22–23
 definition of, 18
 drug–drug interaction effects on, 22
Metadol (methadone), 896t–897t
Metadol-D (methadone), 896t–897t
Metamucil (psyllium), 724t, 726, 726t
metaproterenol (Alupent), 605t, 608t, 610
metered dose inhalers, 42t–43t
metformin, 675b
metformin (Glucophage), 751, 754t, 760b, 765–767, 767b
methadone (Methadose), 894t, 896t–897t, 902, 1061t–1063t
Methadose (methadone), 894t, 896t–897t, 902, 1061t–1063t
methamphetamine (Desoxyn), 1047t, 1050t
Methergine (methylergonovine), 94t, 95
methicillin-resistant *Staphylococcus aureus* (MRSA), 278b, 385, 386, 396
methimazole (Tapazole, APO-Methimazole, JAMP Methimazole, Mar-Methimazole), 787t, 788
methocarbamol, 983t
methocarbamol (Robaxin), 77, 985t–986t, 987
methocarbamol (Robaxisal), 754t
Methohexital (Brevital Sodium), 922t, 926t
Methohexital sodium (Brevital), 928
methotrexate (MTX) (Otrexup, Rasuvo, RedTrex, Trexall, Xatmep), 87b, 211t, 212, 213t, 215b, 216, 226–227, 236t–245t, 238, 246–247, 248b, 251b
 administration, 216

autoimmune disorders and transplant therapy, 216
 excretion of, 216
 lower doses of, 216
 TNF-alpha-blocking agents, 226–227
methylcellulose (Citrucel), 724t, 726t
methyldopa, 77, 482t
methylergonovine (Methergine), 94t, 95
Methylin (methylphenidate), 1053t
methylphenidate (Adhansia XR, Aptensio, Concerta, Cotempla XR-ODT, Daytrana, Jornay PM, Concerta, Daytrana, Methylin, QuilliChew ER, Quillivant XR, Relexxiii, Ritalin, Ritalin LA), 1047t, 1053t
methylprednisolone (Depo-Medrol, Medrol, SOLU-Medrol, Uni-MED), 320t–323t, 716
methylprednisolone acetate (Depo-Medrol), 320t–323t
methylprednisolone sodium succinate, 605t, 616t
methylprednisolone sodium succinate (Solu-Medrol; Depo-Medrol, Medrol, Methylprednisolone acetate, Methylprednisolone sodium succinate, Solu-Medrol), 616t
methyltestosterone, 119t–120t, 122
metipranolol, 1082t–1084t
metoclopramide (Reglan), 95, 951t, 951t
Metoject (methotrexate), 211t, 212, 215b, 216, 226–227
metolazone (Zaroxolyn), 482t, 631t, 636t, 637
Metopirone (Metyrapone), 835t, 836
metoprolol (Lopressor, Toprol XL), 482t, 524t, 530t, 531
metoprolol succinate, 562t, 563–564
metric system, 43
MetroCream (metronidazole), 1113t
MetroLotion (metronidazole), 1113t
metronidazole (Flagyl), 381t–382t, 384, 464–465, 464t, 692t, 701t, 702
metronidazole (Flagyl; APO-MetroNIDAZOLE, Auro-MetroNIDAZOLE, PMSMetroNIDAZOLE), 381t–382t, 384
metronidazole (MetroCream, MetroLotion, Noritate, Nuvessa Rosadan, Vandazole), 1113t
Metyrapone (metopirone), 835t, 836
Mevacor (lovastatin), 754t
Miacalcin (calcitonin), 813–814, 823, 823t
micafungin (Mycamine), 447t, 455t, 456
Micardis (telmisartan), 482t, 490t, 491, 495t–496t
micardis HCT, 495t–496t
Micatin (miconazole), 1115t
miconazole (Micatin, Podactin), 1115t
miconazole (Oravig), 447t, 450
MICRhoGAM (Rh$_o$(D) immune globulin (human)), 200t–201t
Microgestin Fe 1/20, 110t–111t
microorganisms, 273–283
 antibiotic resistance pattern, 282
 antibiotic-resistant microorganisms, 278–280, 278b
 bacterial resistance, 280
 clinical manifestations, 278b, 280
 combination therapy, 283
 community-acquired vs. nosocomial infections, 278
 culture and sensitivity studies, 282
 drug therapy, 280–283
 empiric therapy, 282
 host defense mechanisms, 272, 277
 medication cost, 283
 normal flora, 277
 opportunistic pathogens, 277–278
 pathogen laboratory identification, 278
 penetrate infected tissues, 283
 toxicity and risk-to-benefit ratio, 283

Microzide (hydrochlorothiazide), 554t, 563
Midamor (amiloride), 482t, 496t–498t, 631t, 638t, 639–640
midazolam (Nayzilam), 922t, 931–932, 932t, 995t, 999
Middle East Respiratory Syndrome (MERS), 406b
miglitol, 777
miglitol (Glyset), 754t, 758b, 763b, 767b, 768–769, 768t, 777
migraine headaches, 936
  abortive therapy
    ergot alkaloids, 938t
    triptans, 944–947, 945t
  acetaminophen-aspirin-caffeine, 940–941, 940t, 941b
  adjuvant medications for, 951
  clinical manifestations, 936–937
  nonsteroidal anti-inflammatory agents, 938–940
  nursing process, 952b
  overview of, 936
  preventive therapy, 949–950
    angiotensin II receptor blockers, 950
    angiotensin-converting enzyme inhibitors, 950
    beta-adrenergic blocking agents, 949–950
    calcium channel blockers, 950
    carboxylic acid derivative, 949
    gamma-aminobutyric acid, 949
    herbal and vitamin supplements, 950
    sulfamate-substituted monosaccharide, 949
    tricyclic antidepressants, 950
  treatment of, 938t
Migranal, 942t
milk of magnesia (magnesium hydroxide), 724t, 729t
milliequivalents, 43
Millipred (prednisolone), 320t–323t
milnacipran (Savella, Savella Titration Pack), 1009t, 1019
milrinone, 557–559, 558t, 559b
mineral(s)
  adjuvants, 667
  excess
    deferasirox, 668
    deferoxamine, 668
    penicillamine, 667–668
    succimer, 668
  iron, 662–666, 665b
  potassium, 666–667
mineral electrolytes, 956t, 977
mineral oil (GoodSense Mineral Oil, Fleet Oil, Fleet Mineral Oil Enema), 724t, 726
mineralocorticoid(s), 314–315, 318t, 320t–323t, 830t
MinEstrin, 110t–111t
Minims Prednisolone (prednisolone), 320t–323t
minimum alveolar concentration (MAC), 924
minimum bactericidal concentration (MBC), 282
minimum effective concentration, 19
minimum inhibitory concentration (MIC), 282
Minipress (prazosin), 496t–498t
Minitran (nitroglycerin), 524–528, 524t–525t, 537b
Minocin (minocycline hydrochloride), 365t
minocycline hydrochloride (Minocin, Dynacin, Solodyn, Ximino, Dom Minocycline, Sandoz Minocycline), 365t–366t, 368
minoxidil (Loniten), 496t–498t, 499
MINT-Indomethacin (indomethacin), 92–93, 93t
MINT-Tolterodine (Tolterodine tartrate), 887t
miosis, 1076
Miralax (polyethylene glycol (PEG) solution), 724t, 729t, 730
Mirapex (pramipexole), 874
Mircera (epoetin beta), 180t–181t, 183
Mircette, 110t–111t
mirtazapine (Remeron), 1009t, 1021–1022, 1022t

miscellaneous antiepileptic drugs, 982
  abnormal kidney function, 982
  adverse effects, 982
  contraindications, 982
  dose usage, 982
  hepatic impairment, 982
  mechanisms of action, 982
  nursing implications, 982
  patient teaching guidelines, 983b
  pharmacokinetics, 982
  preventing interactions, 982
  therapeutic effects, 982
misoprostol (Cytotec), 94–95, 94t, 692t, 701t, 702
Mitigare (colchicine), 292t, 306–307, 307t, 308b
Mitigo (morphine sulfate), 894–903, 894t, 896t–897t
mitomycin (Mitosol), 236t–245t, 238–239
Mitosol (mitomycin), 236t–245t, 238–239
Mitotane (Lysodren), 835t, 836–837
mitoxantrone, 236t–245t
mitoxantrone (Novantrone), 236t–238t
Mivacurium, 922t, 931
MMR (measles, mumps, and rubella vaccine), 195t–199t, 202–203
modafinil (Provigil), 1047t, 1053t, 1054–1055
Moderna (COVID-19), 194, 194b, 195t–199t, 201–203, 202b
moexipril, 482t, 485t, 488
Moexipril hydrochloride (Univasc), 754t
moisturizers, 1117
molds, 445
mometasone (Asmanex Twisthaler), 605t, 616t, 617, 621t
mometasone (Asmanex, Asmanex HFA, Propel, Propel MiniSDS, Nasonex, Sinuva, Elocon; Asmanex Twisthaler, Apo-Mometasone, Mosaspray, Nasonex, SANDOZ Mometasone, Elocon PMS, TARO-Mometasone, TEVA-Mometasone), 318t, 320t–323t
mometasone/formoterol (Foradil), 621t
monitored anesthesia care, 926
monoamine oxidase (MAO) inhibitors, 384, 680, 685, 1009t. See also specific drug
  food interactions with, 21
  tyramine-containing foods and, 21
monoamine oxidase inhibitors (MOIs), 1019–1021
  abnormal kidney function, 1020
  adverse effects, 1016
  contraindications, 1020
  dose usage, 1019–1020
  drug interactions, 1020b
  hepatic impairment, 1020
  mechanisms of action, 1019
  nursing implications, 1020–1021
  patient teaching guidelines, 1021
  pharmacokinetics, 1019
  preventing interactions, 1020–1021
  therapeutic effects, 1021
monobactams
  abnormal kidney function and hepatic impairment, 349
  administeration, 350
  adverse effects, 349–350
  contraindications, 350
  mechanism of action, 349
  nursing implications, 350
  pharmacokinetics, 349
  route and dosage information, 349, 349t
  therapeutic effects, 350
monoclonal antibodies, 221–226, 222t–224t, 232, 236t–238t, 252, 252t–257t, 257–258
  for respiratory syncytial virus, 421
Monodox (doxycycline), 365t–366t, 367–368
Monopril (Fosinopril), 754t
Monopril (fosinopril), 482t, 485t, 488, 495t–496t

montelukast (Singulair), 617–619, 618t
mood disorders
  bipolar disorder (see bipolar disorder)
  depression (see depression)
mood-stabilizing agents, 675b, 1009t, 1023–1026
  abnormal kidney function, 1023
  adverse effects, 1023
  contraindications, 1023
  dose usage, 1023
  drug interactions, 1025b
  hepatic impairment, 1023
  mechanisms of action, 1023
  nursing implications, 1023
  patient teaching guidelines, 1025b
  pharmacokinetics, 1023
  preventing interactions, 1023
  therapeutic effects, 1024–1025
morphine (Mitigo, MorphaBond [ER]), 524t, 535, 893–894
morphine sulfate (Duramorph, Infumorph, Kadian, MS Contin, Mitigo), 894–903, 894t, 896t–897t
Mosaspray (mometasone), 320t–323t, 616t
M.O.S.-S.R (morphine sulfate), 896t–897t
Motegrity (prucalopride), 724t, 732t, 733
motion sickness, 718
Motrin (ibuprofen), 290t, 293, 295–300, 298t–299t, 300b, 1107
Motrin Sinus Headache Tablets, 583t
Movapo (apomorphine hydrochloride), 871t–872t
Moxatag (amoxicillin), 692t, 701t, 702
moxifloxacin (Auro-Moxifloxacin), 353t, 358t, 360
moxifloxacin (Vigamox), 1090t–1091t
MS Contin (morphine sulfate), 894–903, 894t, 896t–897t
MS Contin SRT (morphine sulfate), 896t–897t
Mucinex (guaifenesin), 574t, 580–581, 580t
mucolytics
  acetylcysteine, 581–582
  action, 581
  administration of, 582
  adverse reactions, 582
  contraindications, 582
  dosage ranges, 581, 581t
  lactation, 582
  nursing implications, 582
  patient teaching guidelines, 577b, 582
  pharmacokinetics, 581
  pregnancy, 582
  reproduction, 582
  therapeutic effects, 582
  use, 581–582
mucositis, 247, 248b
Multaq (dronedarone), 513t, 515
multidrug-resistant tuberculosis (MDR-TB), 279, 390–392, 400
multiple mineral–electrolyte preparations, 667
multiple myeloma, 233–234, 239t–245t
multivitamin, 646
mupirocin (Centany, Centany AT), 1113t
murine antibodies, 224
muscarine, 855
muscarinic receptors, 849, 879–880
muscle spasms, 954
  and spasticity, 984–990
    carbamate derivatives (see carbamate derivatives)
    centrally acting skeletal muscle relaxants, 987
    direct-acting skeletal muscle relaxants, 987
    gamma-aminobutyric acid derivatives, 984
    imidazoline derivatives, 989
    tricyclic antidepressant derivatives, 989
muscle spasms and spasticity
  carbamate derivatives (see carbamate derivatives)
  gamma-aminobutyric acid (see gamma-aminobutyric acid)

hydantoin derivatives (see hydantoins)
imidazoline derivatives (see imidazoline)
tricyclic antidepressant derivatives (see tricyclic antidepressant(s))
muscular effects, 785t–786t
musculoskeletal system, 316b
Muse (alprostadil), 119t
mutation, 233
Mvasi (bevacizumab), 211t, 225, 236t–238t, 252t–257t, 257–258
Mya, 110t–111t
Myambutol (ethambutol), 394b, 399t, 400
myasthenia crisis, 853
myasthenia gravis
 clinical manifestations, 853
 diagnosis, 853
 drug therapy for, 853, 854f
 immunosuppressive therapy for, 857
 indirect-acting cholinergics (see indirect-acting cholinergics)
 myasthenia crisis, 853
Mycamine (micafungin), 447t, 455t, 456
Mycobacterium avium complex (MAC) disease, 379, 389–392. See also tuberculosis
 treatment, drugs, 400–401
Mycobacterium tuberculosis, 389, 390b
Mycobutin (rifabutin), 397t, 398, 400
mycophenolate (CellCept), 857
mycophenolate mofetil (CellCept, Myfortic)
 action, 212
 adverse effects, 214
 contraindications, 214
 nursing implications, 214
 pharmacokinetics, 212
 reproduction, pregnancy, and lactation, 213
 uses, 213–214
  abnormal kidney function, 213
  in hepatic impairment, 213
mycophenolate mofetil IV (CellCept, CellCept Intravenous), 212–216
mycophenolate mofetil/mycophenolate sodium (CellCept, CellCept IV, Myfortic; ACH-Mycophenolate, APO-Mycophenolate), 213t
mycophenolate sodium PO (Myfortic), 211t
mycoses, 445
Mydayis (dextroamphetamine and amphetamine), 1047t, 1050t, 1051
Mydriacyl (tropicamide), 1078t–1079t
mydriasis, 880, 1076
myelosuppression, 247
Myfortic (mycophenolate mofetil/mycophenolate sodium), 213t
Myfortic (mycophenolate sodium PO), 211t
MYLAN Selegiline (selegiline hydrochloride), 871t–872t
Mylan-Almotriptan (almotriptan), 945t
Mylan-Amoxicillin (amoxicillin), 336t–337t
Mylan-Beclo AQ (beclomethasone), 320t–323t
Mylan-Budesonide AQ (budesonide), 320t–323t
Mylan-Buprenorphine/Naloxone (buprenorphine/naloxone), 904t
Mylan-Entacapone (Entacapone), 876t
Mylan-Galantamine ER (galantamine), 859t 855t, 859, 859t
Mylan-Hydroxyurea (hydroxyurea), 236t–245t, 238
Mylan-Leflunomide (leflunomide), 211t, 216
Mylan-Nabumetone (nabumetone), 290t, 298t–299t, 300, 302t–303t, 305
MYLAN-Oxybutynin (oxybutynin), 887t
Mylanta, 691–693, 692t, 694t
Mylanta Double Strength, 692t, 694t
Mylan-Tamoxifen (tamoxifen), 236t–238t, 260, 261t–263t
MYLAN-Tolterodine (Tolterodine tartrate), 887t
Myleran (busulfan), 236t–245t

myocardial infarction, 154
Myocet (lipodox 50), 236t–238t
Myorisan (isotretinoin), 1119
Myorisan (isotretinoin), 1118
Mysoline (primidone), 956t, 958–959, 958t
myxedema, 784, 792
 coma, 786, 791t

N
Nabi-HB (hepatitis B immune globulin, human), 200t–201t
nabilone (Cesamet), 708t, 717t, 718
nabumetone (Relafen, Relafen DS, Apo-Nabumetone, Mylan-Nabumetone, Teva-Nabumetone), 290t, 298t–299t, 300, 302t–303t, 305
N-acetyl-*p*-aminophenol (acetaminophen), 286, 288, 290, 290t, 294–297, 295t, 297b
nadolol (Corgard), 482t, 524t, 530t, 531
nafarelin (Synarel), 799t, 806t, 807
nafcillin, 335t–337t, 338–339
naftifine (Naftin), 1115t
Naftin (naftifine), 1115t
nalbuphine, 894t, 904t, 906
nalbuphine (Nubain), 894t, 904t, 906
Nalfon (fenoprofen), 290t, 298t–299t, 300
naloxone (Naloxone hydrochloride injection, Zimhi, Narcan), 894t, 898–899, 906, 907t
Naloxone (Narcan), 932
naloxone (Narcan), 1061t
naloxone (NarcanZimhi), 1062t–1063t
Naloxone hydrochloride injection (naloxone), 894t, 898–899, 906, 907t
naltrexone, 685, 1066
naltrexone (opioid narcotics), 1060–1061
naltrexone (Vivitrol), 894t, 907, 907t, 1061t–1063t
naltrexone–buprenorphine (Suboxone), 1061t
Namenda (memantine), 855t, 859t, 860
Namenda Titration Pack (memantine), 855t, 859t, 860
Namenda XR (memantine), 855t, 859t, 860
Namenda XR Titration Pack (memantine), 859t
Namzaric (donepezil-memantine), 855t, 859t, 861
Naprelan (naproxen sodium), 290t, 298t–299t
Naprosyn (naproxen sodium), 290t, 298t–299t
naproxen sodium (Aleve, Anaprox, Naprelan, Naprosyn), 938, 938t
naproxen sodium (Aleve, Anaprox, Naprelan, Naprosyn, Apo- Napro-Na), 290t, 298t–299t
naratriptan (Amerge), 945t, 946
Narcan (naloxone), 894t, 898–899, 906, 907t, 932, 1061t
NarcanZimhi (naloxone), 1062t–1063t
narcolepsy, 1047
 amphetamine-related drugs (see amphetamine-related drugs)
 amphetamines (see amphetamines)
 assessment, 1057b
 atomoxetine, 1055
 clinical manifestations, 1048
 drug therapy, 1048
 evaluation, 1057b
 guanfacine, 1055
 nursing interventions, 1057b
 nursing process, 1057b
 outcomes of therapy, 1057b
 overview of, 1047–1048
 sodium oxybate, 1055
 treatment of, 1047t
 xanthines (see xanthines)
narcotic antitussives, 579–580
narcotic codeine (Codeine Contin, Teva-Codeine), 574t, 578–580, 579t
Nardil (phenelzine), 1009t, 1020t
Naropin (ropivacaine), 912t

Nasacort Allergy (triamcinolone acetonide), 318t, 320t–323t
Nasacort AQ (triamcinolone acetonide), 320t–323t
nasal congestion
 antitussives (see nasal decongestants)
 assessment, 584b
 bronchial secretions, 574
 clinical manifestations, 574
 common cold, 574
 cough, 574
 drug therapy, 574–575, 574t
 drugs administration, 574t
 evaluation, 584b
 expectorants (see expectorants)
 herbal drugs (see herbal drugs)
 mucolytics (see mucolytics)
 multi-ingredient nonprescription, 583t
 nasal decongestants (see nasal decongestants)
 nonpharmacologic measures, 574
 nursing interventions, 584b
 nursing process, 584b
 outcomes of therapy, 584b
 rhinosinusitis, 574
nasal decongestants
 action, 575
 administration of, 576
 adverse effects, 576
 contraindications, 576
 dosage ranges, 575, 575t
 drug interactions, 576b
 lactation, 576
 nursing implications, 576
 oxymetazoline, 575t, 576–578
 patient teaching guidelines, 576, 577b
 pharmacokinetics, 575
 pregnancy, 576
 preventing interactions, 576
 reproduction, 576
 therapeutic effects, 576
 uses, 575–576, 575t
NasalCrom (cromolyn), 605t
nasogastric tube, 55
nasolacrimal occlusion, 1078
Nasonex (mometasone), 320t–323t, 616t
Natacyn (natamycin), 1090t–1091t, 1093
natamycin (Natacyn), 1090t–1091t, 1093
Natazia, 110t–111t
nateglinide (Starlix), 754t, 767b, 770, 770t
National Cholesterol Education Program (NCEP), 163
National Heart, Lung, and Blood Institute (NHLBI) Report, 678b
Natroba (spinosad), 464t, 471t, 472
nausea and vomiting, 248b, 707
 acupressure, 719
 acupuncture, 719
 antiemetic drug therapy, 707, 708t
 antihistamines, 710–712, 711t
 assessment, 720
 clinical manifestations, 707
 drug therapy, 707
 drugs administered for, 707, 708t
 evaluation, 720
 herbal supplements, 719
 5-hydroxytryptamine$_3$, 712–713, 714t
 miscellaneous antiemetics, 717–718, 717t
 nonpharmacological management, 719
 nursing interventions, 720
 nursing process, 720
 outcomes of therapy, 720
 overview, 707
 phenothiazines, 707–710, 709t, 709b
 substance P/neurokinin, 715–717, 715t, 716b
Navelbine (vinorelbine), 236t–238t
Nayzilam (midazolam), 922t, 931–932, 932t, 995t
Necon, 110t–111t

Necon 7/7/7, Dasetta 7/7/7, 110t–111t
Necon 0.5/35, Nortrel 0.5/35, 110t–111t
necrotizing otitis externa, 1101
needle-free lidocaine delivery, 912b
needleless systems, 46b
needles, 46b
nefazodone, 1009t, 1019
negative chronotropy, 530
negative feedback mechanism, 314, 315f
negative feedback system, 813
Neisseria gonorrhoeae, 341
nelarabine (Arranon, Atriance), 236t–245t
Nembutal (pentobarbital), 956t, 958–959, 958t
neoadjuvant chemotherapy, 232, 234
neomycin, 353t, 355t, 357, 1113t
neomycin–colistin–hydrocortisone– thonzonium (Coly-Mycin S Otic), 1102
neomycin–polymyxin B–hydrocortisone, 1102, 1102t
neonatal abstinence syndrome, 892b
neonates. *See also* infants
 pharmacokinetics, 69–70
neoplasms, 233–234
Neoral (cyclosporine), 211t, 212, 215–219, 225
neostigmine, 854
Neo-Synephrine (phenylephrine), 547, 574t–575t, 582, 583t
nephron, 630, 630f
nervous system, 316b
 central (*see* central nervous system)
 divisions of, 844f
Nesacaine (chloroprocaine hydrochloride), 912t, 915, 916t
Nesacaine-MPF (chloroprocaine hydrochloride), 912t, 915, 916t
Nesina (alogliptin), 754t, 772, 772t
netarsudil (Rhopressa), 1083t–1084t
netarsudil and latanoprost (Rocklatan), 1082t–1084t
netupitant/palonosetron (Akynzeo), 708t, 715t, 716
Neulasta (pegfilgrastim), 180t, 185–186, 185t
Neulasta Onpro (pegfilgrastim), 180t, 185–186, 185t
Neumega (oprelvekin), 188
Neupogen (filgrastim), 184–186, 185t, 236t–238t, 248b, 264t
Neupro (rotigotine transdermal), 869t
neuraminidase inhibitors, 412b, 422t, 423–424
neuraxial anesthesia, 911
neurogenic shock, 541
neurokinin 1 antagonist
 abnormal kidney function, 716
 action, 715
 administration, 716
 adverse effects, 716
 contraindications, 716
 in hepatic impairment patients, 716
 lactation, 716
 in mediating acute chemotherapy-induced nausea and vomiting, 715
 netupitant/palonosetron, 708t, 715t, 716
 nursing implications, 716
 patient teaching guidelines, 716
 pharmacokinetics, 715
 pregnancy, 716
 preventing interactions, 716, 716b
 reproduction, 716
 rolapitant, 708t, 715t, 717
 therapeutic effects, 716
 uses, 715–716, 715t
neuroleptic malignant syndrome, 1034
neuromuscular blocking agents, 922, 922t, 928–931, 929t
 abnormal kidney function, 929
 administration of, 930
 adverse effects, 929–930
 contraindications, 929
 depolarizing neuromuscular blocking agent, 931
 in hepatic impairment patients, 929
 in lactation, 929
 mechanism of action, 928
 nondepolarizing neuromuscular blocking agents, 930–931
 nursing implications, 929–930
 patient teaching guidelines, 930
 pharmacokinetics, 928
 in pregnancy, 929
 preventing interactions, 930
 uses, 928–929
 vecuronium, 928
Neurontin (gabapentin), 949, 956t, 961, 962t–963t
neuropathic pain, 898, 903
Neutra-Phos (phosphate salts), 823–824
Neutrogena Oil-Free Acne Wash (salicylic acid), 1116t–1117t
neutropenia, 180, 247
neutrophils, 180
nevirapine (Viramune), 408t–409t, 434t, 435
NexAVAR (sorafenib), 236t–238t, 248b, 252t–257t, 259
Nexium (esomeprazole), 692t, 699t, 700–701
Nexplanon (etonogestrel), 106, 107t–108t
Nexterone (amiodarone), 77, 513–515, 513t
niacin (Niacor, Slo-Niacin; Niaspan, Niaspan FCT, Niodan), 164t, 174, 174t
niacin (vitamin B$_3$), 654t–656t
 administration, 659
 adverse effects, 659
 contraindications, 659
 nursing implications, 659
 patient teaching guidelines for, 657b, 659
 pharmacokinetics and use, 659
 therapeutic effects, 659
Niacor (niacin), 164t, 174–175, 174t
Niaspan (niacin), 164t, 174–175, 174t
Niaspan FCT (niacin), 164t, 174–175, 174t
nicardipine (Cardene), 482t, 492t, 524t, 532t, 533
Nicoderm CQ (nicotine), 1061t–1063t
Nicorette mini (nicotine), 1061t–1063t
nicotine (Nicoderm CQ, Nicorette mini, Nicotrol NS), 1061t–1063t
nicotine receptor agonist, 1061t
nicotinic receptors, 849
nicotinic$_{CNS}$ receptors, 850
nicotinic$_m$ receptors, 850
nicotinic$_n$ receptors, 850
Nicotrol NS (nicotine), 1061t–1063t
nifedipine (Adalat), 524t, 531–533, 532t, 533b
nifedipine (Procardia, Procardia XL, Adalat CC, Afeditab CR; Adalat XL, Nifedipine ER), 93, 93t, 492t
Nifedipine ER (nifedipine), 93, 93t
Nikki, 110t–111t
Nilandron (nilutamide), 236t–238t, 261t–263t, 263
nilotinib (Tasigna), 236t–238t, 252t–257t, 258–259
nilutamide (Nilandron, Anandron), 236t–238t, 261t–263t, 263
Nimbex (cisatracurium), 922t, 929t
Ninlaro (ixazomib), 236t–238t, 252t–257t, 260
Niodan (niacin), 164t, 174–175, 174t
Nipent (pentostatin), 236t–238t
Nipride (sodium nitroprusside), 496t–498t
nirmatrelvir, 411t, 414–415
nisoldipine (Sular), 482t, 492t, 494
nitazoxanide (Alinia), 464t, 738t, 741t, 742
nitric oxide (NO), 289b
Nitro-Bid (nitroglycerin), 524–528, 524t–525t, 537b
Nitro-Dur (nitroglycerin), 524–528, 524t–525t, 537b
nitrofurantoin (Macrodantin), 77
nitrofurantoin (Macrodantin, Macrobid), 365t, 372, 372t
nitroglycerin (Nitro-Bid, Nitro-Dur, Nitrostat, Nitrolingual, Rectiv; Minitran), 524–528, 524t–525t, 537b
Nitrolingual (nitroglycerin), 524–528, 524t–525t, 537b
Nitropress (nitroprusside), 496t–498t
Nitropress (sodium nitroprusside), 482t, 496t–498t
nitroprusside (Nitropress), 496t–498t
Nitrostat (nitroglycerin), 524–528, 524t–525t, 537b
nitrous oxide, 922t–923t, 925
Nivestym (filgrastim), 184–186, 185t, 236t–238t, 248b, 264t
nivolumab (Opdivo), 211t, 222t–224t, 226, 236t–238t, 252t–257t, 258
nizatidine (Axid), 692t, 696t, 698
Nizoral (ketoconazole), 451t–452t, 453
NMDA receptor antagonist, 855t, 859t
N-methyl-D-aspartate receptor antagonist
 administration, 860
 adverse effects, 861
 contraindications, 860
 mechanism of action, 860
 nursing implications, 860–861
 patient teaching guidelines, 861
 pharmacokinetics, 860
 preventing interactions, 860
 therapeutic effects, 860
 use in, 860
Nolix (flurandrenolide), 1112t
Nolvadex-D (tamoxifen), 236t–238t, 260, 261t–263t
nonbenzodiazepine sedative hypnotics, 1001–1002
 eszopiclone, 1001–1002
 ramelteon, 1002
 tasimelteon, 1002
 zaleplon, 1002
 zolpidem, 1002
nondepolarizing neuromuscular blocking agents, 930–931
nondihydropyridines, 533–534
non-Hodgkin's lymphoma, 233–234, 239t–245t
nonnarcotic analgesic antipyretic, 290t, 294–297, 1107
nonnucleoside reverse transcriptase inhibitors (NNRTIs), 412b, 433–435, 434t
nonopioid medications, 922
nonprescription drugs, 5
non-ST-elevation myocardial infarction (NSTEMI), 523
nonsteroidal anti-inflammatory drugs (NSAIDs), 272–273, 286, 288, 290, 290t, 297, 305–306, 690
 abnormal kidney function, 939
 acetic acid derivatives, 290t, 302–305, 302t–303t
 adverse effects, 939
 contraindications, 939
 drug interactions, 939
 with hepatic impairment patients, 939
 ketorolac tromethamine, 939t, 940
 mechanism of action, 938–939
 naproxen sodium, 290t, 298t–299t
 nursing implications, 939–940
 oxicam derivatives, 290t, 300–301, 301t
 pharmacokinetics, 938
 propionic acid derivatives, 290t, 297–300, 298t–299t
 therapeutic effects, 939
Nora-BE (norethindrone), 107t–108t
noradrenergic neurotransmission system, 1060
noradrenergic sympathomimetic anorexiants, 679–681, 679t, 680b, 681b
Nordiflex (somatropin), 800t–801t
Norditropin (somatropin), 799t–801t
Norditropin FlexPro (somatropin), 800t–801t
Norditropin Simplex (somatropin), 800t–801t
norepinephrine, 845, 847
norepinephrine (Levophed), 542, 543t
 abnormal kidney function, 543
 action, 541–542, 542t
 administration of, 544

adverse effects, 543–544
contraindications, 544
dobutamine, 547
dopamine, 546–547
drug interactions, 544, 545b
epinephrine, 541–542, 545–547
lactation, 543
nursing implications, 544–545
patient teaching guidelines, 545, 546b
pharmacokinetics, 542
phenylephrine, 547
pregnancy, 543
preventing interactions, 544, 545b
reproduction, 543
therapeutic effects, 544
uses, 542–543
norethindrone (Errin, Jencycla, Ortho Micronor, Camila, Jolivette, Nor-Q-D, Nora-BE), 107t–108t
Noritate (metronidazole), 1113t
Norliqva (amlodipine), 524t
normal flora, 277
normal sinus rhythm, 506, 513–518
Normodyne (labetalol), 482t
normotensive blood pressure, 541
Norpace (disopyramide), 508t, 510
Norpramin (desipramine), 1009t, 1012t
Nor-Q-D (norethindrone), 107t–108t
Nortrel 1/35, 110t–111t
nortriptyline (Pamelor), 1009t, 1012t
Norvasc (amlodipine), 482t, 491–494, 492t, 524t, 532t, 533
nose drops, 57
Novamoxin (amoxicillin), 336t–337t, 692t, 701t, 702
Novantrone (mitoxantrone), 236t–238t
Novarel (human chorionic gonadotropin), 800t–801t
Novasen (aspirin), 140t, 151t–152t
Novo-Ampicillin (ampicillin), 335t–337t, 336–340, 338b
Novo-Cefaclor (cefaclor), 336t–337t
Novo-Cholamine (cholestyramine), 164t, 168–170, 169t
Novo-Clavamoxin (amoxicillin-clavulanate), 335t–337t, 338
Novo-Gesic (acetaminophen), 286, 288, 290, 290t, 294–297, 295t, 297b
NOVO-Hydrocort (hydrocortisone), 320t–323t
Novo-Hydroxyzin (hydroxyzine pamoate), 589–590, 590t–591t, 593
Novolin N (isophane insulin suspension), 754t, 756t–757t
Novolin R (insulin injection), 753, 754t, 756t–757t
NovoLog (insulin aspart), 753, 754t, 756t–757t, 763b, 764
Novo-Pen-VK (penicillin V), 336t–337t
Noxafil (posaconazole), 447t, 453–454
NPR-Amoxicillin (amoxicillin), 336t–337t
Nu-Amoxi (amoxicillin), 336t–337t
Nubain (nalbuphine), 894t, 904t, 906
Nucala (mepolizumab), 605t, 619t, 620
nucleoside reverse transcriptase inhibitors (NRTIs), 412b, 429–433, 430t–431t
NU-Flutamide (flutamide), 236t–238t, 261t–263t
Nulojix (belatacept), 211t, 227–228
NuLytely (polyethylene glycolelectrolyte solution), 724t, 729t, 730
numerous drug handbooks, 12
Nu-Pen-VK (penicillin V), 336t–337t
nurses initiative, 10
nursing diagnoses
description of, 51
for pain, 311b
Nurtec (rimegepant), 948–949, 948t
Nutracort (hydrocortisone), 318t, 320t–323t

Nutropin (somatropin), 799t–801t
Nutropin AQ NuSpin (somatropin), 800t–801t
Nutropin AQ pen (somatropin), 800t–801t
Nuvessa Rosadan (metronidazole), 1113t
Nuvigil (armodafinil), 1047t, 1053t, 1054–1055
Nuzyra (omadacycline), 365t–366t, 368
Nyamyc (nystatin), 1115t
nystatin (Bio-Statin), 447t–448t, 449
nystatin (Nyamyc, Nystop), 1115t
Nystop (nystatin), 1115t
Nyvepria (pegfilgrastim), 180t, 185–186, 185t

O

obesity
age considerations, 676
assessment, 687b
cancer and, 676b
cardiovascular disorders and, 676b
central, 676b
clinical manifestations, 678
description of, 674
diabetes mellitus and, 676b
drug therapy, 678–679
dyslipidemias, 676b
environmental factors, 674
evaluation, 687b
factors associated with, 674
gallstones and, 676b
genetic factors, 674
health risks of, 676b
herbal and dietary supplements for, 685–686, 685b
hypertension and, 676b, 680
medications, effects of, 675b
metabolic syndrome and, 676b
nursing interventions, 687b
nursing process, 687b
orlistat for, 21, 679t, 681–683, 682t
osteoarthritis and, 676b
phentermine hydrochloride for, 679t
physiologic factors, 674
psychosocial factors, 674
sleep apnea, 676b
therapy, outcomes of, 687b
obinutuzumab (Gazyva), 236t–238t, 252t–257t, 257
obsessive-compulsive disorder, 994b
obstructive shock, 540, 541t
Octagam (immune globulin (human) (IG; IGIM)), 200t–201t
Octaplex (prothrombin complex concentrate, human), 158t
octreotide acetate (Sandostatin, Sandostatin LAR Depot), 738t, 741–742, 741t, 799t, 806t, 807–808
abnormal kidney function and hepatic impairment, 808
administration of, 808
adverse effects, 808
contraindications, 808
in lactation, 808
lanreotide, 808
mechanism of action, 807
nursing implications, 808
octreotide acetate, 799t, 806t, 807–808
pasireotide, 808–809
pharmacokinetics, 807
in pregnancy, 808
preventing interactions, 808
therapeutic effects, 808
uses, 808
Ocufen (flurbiprofen), 1090t
Ocuflox (ofloxacin), 1090t–1091t
ocular infection and inflammation, 1077, 1090–1097
Ocusert Pilo-20 (pilocarpine ocular system), 1082t–1084t

Odrik (trandolapril), 485t
Oesclim (estradiol transdermal system), 103t
ofatumumab (Arzerra, Kesimpta), 236t–238t, 252t–257t, 257
ofloxacin (Apo-Oflox), 353t, 358t, 360
ofloxacin (Ocuflox), 1090t–1091t, 1102–1103
Ogen (estropipate), 103t
Ogestrel, 110t–111t
Ogivri (trastuzumab), 222t–224t, 226
olanzapine, 675b
olanzapine (Zyprexa), 708t, 715t, 717, 717t, 1039t–1040t, 1042
olanzapine (Zyprexa, Zyprexa Relprevv), 1031t
olanzapine (ZyPREXA, ZyPREXA Relprevv, ZyPREXA Zydis), 1009t, 1024t, 1025
olanzapine–fluoxetine (Symbyax), 1009t, 1024t
older adults
assessment, 81f
definition, 76
evaluation, 81f
evidence-based practice, 80b
infections, 79
medication adherence and aging, 80
nursing interventions, 81f
nursing process, 81b
patient-centered care, 77
pharmacodynamics, 76–77
adverse effects, prevention of, 77
Beers criteria, 76–77
cardiovascular disease, 76
digoxin, 76
Drug Burden Index, 77
physiologic changes, 76
pharmacokinetics
absorption, 78
distribution, 78
excretion, 79
metabolism, 78
therapy outcomes, 81f
Olestyr (cholestyramine), 164t, 168–170, 169t
oligohydrosis, 974
olmesartan, 950
olmesartan (Benicar), 482t, 490t, 491, 495t–496t
Olmesartan medoxomil (Benicar), 754t
Olmetec (benicar HCT), 495t–496t
olopatadine (Pataday, Pazeo), 1090t, 1094t–1095t
olopatadine (Patanase), 590t, 595–596, 595t
Olumiant (baricitinib), 211t, 221, 411t, 413–414
omadacycline (Nuzyra), 365t–366t, 368
omalizumab (Xolair), 226, 211t, 222t–224t, 619–620, 619t
omeprazole (Prilosec), 692t, 698–701, 699t
Omnitrope (somatropin), 800t–801t
ondansetron (Zofran), 708t, 712, 714t
Onfi (clobazam), 956t, 960t
Onglyza (saxagliptin), 754t, 772, 772t
Onzetra Xsail (sumatriptan), 944, 945t
Opdivo (nivolumab), 211t, 226, 236t–238t, 252t–257t, 258
open-angle glaucoma, 1089
Ophthalmic (ciprofloxacin), 1091t
ophthalmic atropine (Isopto Atropine; Dioptics Atropine Solution, Isopto Atropine), 882t
ophthalmic drugs. See also specific drug
adrenergic agonist (see adrenergic agonists)
alpha$_2$-adrenergic agonists (see alpha$_2$-adrenergic agonists)
antiallergic drugs, 1093
antibacterial drugs, 1090
anticholinergic drugs (see anticholinergic drugs)
antifungal drugs, 1093
anti-inflammatory drugs, 1096
antiviral drugs, 1092
assessment, 1098b
beta-adrenergic blocking drugs (see beta-adrenergic blocking drugs)

ophthalmic drugs. *See also specific drug (Continued)*
  carbonic anhydrase inhibitors (*see* carbonic anhydrase inhibitors)
  cholinergic drugs (*see* cholinergic drugs)
  clinical manifestations, 1077
  corticosteroids, 1096 (*see also* corticosteroids)
  evaluation, 1098b
  eye structure and function, 1076
  glaucoma, 1077, 1082–1088, 1082t
  H$_1$-receptor antagonists, 1095
  immunosuppressants, 1097
  inflammation, 1077
  local anesthetic drugs (*see* local anesthetics)
  nursing interventions, 1098b
  nursing process, 1098b
  ocular infections, 1077
  osmotic drugs, 1089
  outcomes of therapy, 1098b
  prostaglandin analogs (*see* prostaglandin analogs)
  refractive errors, 1077
  rho kinase inhibitor, 1087
  specific disorders, 1077
opiate-related antidiarrheal agents
  abnormal kidney function, 739
  action, 737
  administration, 739
  adverse effects, 739
  contraindications, 739
  diphenoxylate with atropine, 737–739, 738t, 740b
  drugs, 738t, 739, 740b
  in hepatic impairment, 739
  lactation, 738
  loperamide, 738t, 739
  nursing implications, 739
  paregoric, 738t, 739
  patient teaching guidelines, 739, 740b
  pharmacokinetics, 737
  pregnancy, 738
  preventing interactions, 739
  reproduction, 738
  therapeutic effects, 739
  uses, 738–739, 738t
opioid agonist–antagonist analgesic, 1061t
opioid agonists, 1066
  abnormal kidney function, 895, 905
  administration, 899, 905
  adverse effects, 898–899, 905
  analgesic, 1061t
  butorphanol, 903–905, 904t
  clinical manifestations, 893–894
  clinical uses of, 895–898, 904–905
  codeine, 901
  contraindications, 898, 905
  cytochrome P450 2D6981, 901
  dosage information, 904, 904t
  drug interactions, 898–899, 899b, 905
  fentanyl, 902
  in hepatic impairment patients, 895, 905
  hydrocodone, 902
  hydromorphone, 902
  in lactation, 895, 905
  mechanism of action, 895, 904
  meperidine, 902
  methadone, 902
  morphine sulfate, 894–903, 896t–897t
  nalbuphine, 894t, 904t, 906
  nursing implications, 898–900, 905
  oxycodone, 902–903
  oxymorphone, 903
  patient teaching guidelines, 899–900, 905
  pharmacokinetics, 895, 904
  in pregnancy, 895, 905
  therapeutic effects, 899, 905
  tramadol, 903
opioid analgesics, 39, 932

opioid antagonist, 1061t
  abnormal kidney function, 905–906
  administration, 905
  adverse effects, 905–907
  butorphanol, 903–905, 904t
  contraindications, 905, 907
  dosage information, 904, 904t
  drug interactions, 905
  in hepatic impairment patients, 905–906
  in lactation, 905–906
  mechanism of action, 904, 906
  nalbuphine, 894t, 904t, 906
  naloxone, 906–907, 907t
  naltrexone, 907
  nursing implications, 905, 907
  patient teaching guidelines, 905
  pharmacokinetics, 904, 906
  in pregnancy, 905–906
  therapeutic effects, 905, 907
  uses, 904–906
opioid medications, 922
opioid misuse, 892b
opioid narcotics (naltrexone), 1060–1061
opioid use disorder, opioid agonists and antagonists for, 1066
opioids with benzodiazepines and gabapentinoids, 77
opportunistic infections, 276–278, 280–281
opportunistic microorganisms, 277–278
oprelvekin (Neumega), 188
optic disk, 1076
Oracea (doxycycline), 365t–366t, 367–368
Oracort (triamcinolone), 318t, 320t–323t
Ora-film (benzocaine), 912t, 916t
oral candidiasis, 445
oral direct thrombin inhibitors, reversal of, 157–158
oral naltrexone (Vivitrol), 1065
oral solutions, 42t–43t
Oravig (miconazole), 447t
orbactiv (Oritavancin), 381t–382t, 384
Orencia (abatacept), 211t, 227
Orencia ClickJect (abatacept), 211t, 227
organ transplantation
  immunosuppression for, 202
  rejection reactions, 210
organic nitrates
  action, 524
  administration, 524t, 526
  adverse effects, 525
  contraindications, 526
  dosage ranges, 525t
  drug interactions, 526, 526b
  drugs administration, 524t
  lactation, 525
  nursing implications, 526
  patient teaching guidelines, 526, 527b
  pharmacokinetics, 524
  pregnancy, 525
  preventing interactions, 526
  reproduction, 525
  therapeutic effects, 526
  uses, 524–525, 524t
organogenesis, 87
organophosphate insecticides, 863
oritavancin (Orbactiv), 381t–382t, 384
orlistat (Xenical), 21
orlistat (Xenical, Alli), 679t, 681–683, 682t
orphenadrine citrate, 985t–986t, 989
Orsythia, 110t–111t
Ortho 1/35, 110t–111t
Ortho Micronor (norethindrone), 107t–108t
Ortho Tri-Cyclen, 110t–111t
Ortho Tri-Cyclen Lo Tri-Lo-Sprintec, 110t–111t
Ortho-Cyclen, 110t–111t
Ortho-Est (estropipate), 103t
Ortho-Novum (ethinyl estradiol-norethindrone), 109, 112t

Ortho-Novum 1/35, 110t–111t
orthophosphoric acid (Emetrol), 718
Os-Cal (calcium carbonate precipitated), 816t
oseltamivir (Tamiflu), 422t, 423–424
Osmitrol (mannitol), 631t, 640, 640t, 1082t–1084t
Osmolex ER (amantadine hydrochloride), 871t–872t
osmotic diuretics, 21, 631t, 640, 640t
osmotic drugs, 1082t–1084t, 1089
  adverse effects, 1089
  contraindications, 1089
  dose usage, 1089
  mechanisms of action, 1089
  nursing implications, 1089
  patient teaching guidelines, 1089
  pharmacokinetics, 1089
  therapeutic effects, 1089
osteoarthritis
  clinical manifestations, 288
  drug therapy, 290–291, 290t, 291f
  etiology, 288
  pathophysiology, 288
Osteocit (calcium citrate), 816t
osteoporosis, 813–814
  prevention and treatment of, 815t
otalgia, 1101
otic, 1101
Otiprio (ciprofloxacin), 1104t
otitis externa, 1101
  clinical manifestations, 1101
  drug therapy, 1101–1102
otitis media, 1101, 1101f
  clinical manifestations, 1101
  drug therapy, 1102
otorrhea, 1101
ototoxicity, 354
Otrexup (methotrexate), 211t, 212, 215b, 216, 226–227, 236t–245t, 238, 246–247, 248b, 251b
outpatient management of severe respiratory syndrome coronavirus 2 (SARS-CoV-2), 411t, 414
overdosage, 21, 29t–31t
overdose, 27, 29t–31t
over-the-counter medications, Food and Drug Administration approval of, 8–9
overweight management, 681, 681b, 685
Ovide (malathion), 464t, 471t, 472
Ovidrel (choriogonadotropin alpha), 799t–801t, 803
Ovidrel (recombinant chorionic gonadotropin alpha), 799t–801t
oxacillin, 335t–337t
oxaliplatin, 236t–245t, 251b
oxaprozin (Daypro), 290t, 298t–299t, 300
oxazepam, 995t
oxazolidinone, 384
oxcarbazepine (Oxtellar XR, Trileptal), 956t, 967t, 968
Oxeze Turbuhaler (formoterol), 605t, 608t, 610, 621t
oxicam derivatives, 290t, 300–301, 301t
  abnormal kidney function and hepatic impairment, 301
  administration of, 301
  adverse effects, 301
  contraindications, 301
  mechanism of action, 300
  nursing implications, 301
  pharmacokinetics, 300
  preventing interactions, 301, 301b
  therapeutic effects, 301
  use, 300–301
oxiconazole (Oxistat), 447t, 1115t
Oxistat (oxiconazole), 447t, 1115t
Oxtellar XR (oxcarbazepine), 956t, 967t
oxybutynin (Ditropan XL, Gelnique, Oxytrol), 881t, 886, 887t, 888b

Index **1163**

Oxybutynin (Ditropan XL, Gelnique, Oxytrol, Oxytrol for women; APO-Oxybutynin, Ditropan XL, DOM-Oxybutynin, Gelnique, MYLAN-Oxybutynin), 887t
Oxycodone (OxyContin, Xtampza ER, Oxy IR, OxyNEO, PMSOxycodone CR, Supeudol), 894t, 896t–897t, 902–903, 902t
oxycodone (Xtampza ER), 893–894
OxyContin, 903
oxygen, 518
oxymetazoline (Afrin), 574t–575t, 576–578
Oxymorphone, 896t–897t
oxymorphone, 896t–897t, 902t, 903
Oxymorphone Tramadol (Ultram, ConZip), 894t
OxyNEO (Oxycodone), 896t–897t
Oxytocic Agent (oxytocin), 804t
oxytocin (Pitocin), 94–95, 94t
oxytocin (Pitocin, Oxytocic Agent), 799t, 804t, 805
Oxytrol (oxybutynin), 881t, 886, 887t
Ozempic (semaglutide), 775–776, 775t
Ozobax (baclofen), 985t–986t
Ozurdex (dexamethasone), 1090t, 1094t–1095t, 1096

P

p53, 233
Pacerone (amiodarone), 77, 513–515, 513t
paclitaxel (conventional) (Apo-Paclitaxel), 236t–245t
paclitaxel (nanoparticle albumin bound) (Abraxane), 236t–245t
paclitaxel (nonparticle albumin bound) (Abraxane), 236t–238t
pacritinib (Vonjo), 211t, 220t, 221
Paget's disease, 813b, 820–821, 823
pain, 288, 289b, 290t
    acute, 901b
    assessment, 908b
    breakthrough, 897
    cancer, 898, 902
    chronic, 892, 894, 895, 898, 902–903
    classification of, 892
    clinical manifestations, 892–893
    definition of, 892
    description of, 892
    drug therapy, 893–894
    endogenous analgesia system for, 895
    evaluation, 908b
    intensity of, 892
    location of, 908
    management
        analgesics, 95
        anesthetics, 95
    neuropathic, 898, 903
    nursing interventions, 908b
    nursing process, 908b
    outcomes of therapy, 908b
    overview, 892–894
    perception of, 892
    somatic, 892
    treatment of
        opioid agonists (see opioid agonists)
        opioid antagonist (see opioid antagonist)
    visceral, 892
palbociclib (Ibrance), 236t–238t, 252t–257t
palifermin (Kepivance), 236t–238t, 264t
paliperidone (Invega, Invega Sustenna, Invega Trinza), 1031t, 1039t–1040t, 1042
palivizumab (Synagis), 420t, 421
palliation, 234
palliative chemotherapy, 247
palmar-plantar erythrodysesthesia, 248b
palonosetron (Aloxi), 708t, 714t–715t, 716, 717t

Pamelor (nortriptyline), 1009t, 1012t
pamidronate, 87b
pamidronate (Aredia, PMS-Pamidronate, Pamidronate Disodium Omega), 820t–821t, 822
Pamidronate Disodium Omega (pamidronate), 820t–821t
pancreatic juices, 690
Pancuronium, 922t, 929t, 930–931
panic disorder, 994b
panitumumab (Vectibix), 211t, 222t–224t, 225, 236t–238t, 252t–257t, 257–258
pantoprazole (Protonix, Protonix IV), 692t, 700–701
pantothenic acid (vitamin B$_5$), 647t–650t
Panzyga (immune globulin (human) (IG; IGIM)), 200t–201t
para-aminobenzoic acid (PABA, Paser), 369
para-aminosalicylic acid (Paser), 391
paracetamol (acetaminophen), 286, 288, 290, 290t, 294–297, 295t, 297t
Paracetamol (hydrocodone), 896t–897t
paranoia, 1030
Paraplatin (carboplatin), 236t–245t, 238, 250, 258
parasitic infections
    abnormal kidney function, 465
    action, 464–465
    amebicides, 463–465, 464t, 466b
    anthelmintics, 469–470, 470t, 470b
    antimalarials, 465–469, 467t, 468b
    assessment, 473b
    clinical manifestations, 463
    drug therapy, 463, 464t, 466b
    effects of, 463
    evaluation, 473b
    helminthiasis, 463, 469
    hepatic impairment, 465
    lactation, 464
    nursing interventions, 473b
    nursing process, 473b
    outcomes of therapy, 473b
    patient teaching guidelines, 466b
    pediculicides, 463, 464t, 471–472, 471t
    pregnancy, 464
    protozoa, 463
    reproduction, 464
    scabicides, 463, 464t, 471–472, 471t
    scabies, 463, 471–472, 471t
    use, 464–465
parasympathetic nervous system, 844, 853, 855
    body responses, 849
    cholinergic receptors, 849–850
    neurotransmitters, 849
parathyroid hormone (PTH), 813
paregoric, 738t, 739
parenteral nutrition, 669
parenteral solutions, 42t–43t
paricalcitol (Zemplar), 816t
parkinsonism, 868
Parkinson disease
    abnormal kidney function, 872
    administration, 873
    adverse effects, 873
    amantadine hydrochloride, 873–874
    assessment, 889b
    bromocriptine mesylate, 869t, 871t–872t, 874
    catechol-O-methyltrans-ferase inhibitors (see catechol-O-methyltransferase (COMT) inhibitors)
    clinical manifestations, 868–869
    contraindications, 872–873
    dopamine receptor agonists (see dopamine receptor agonists)
    drug interactions, 873, 873b
    drug therapy, 869
    evaluation, 889b

in hepatic impairment patients, 872
    manifestations, 868–869
    mechanism of action, 869–870
    nursing implications, 873
    nursing interventions, 889b
    nursing process, 889b
    outcomes of therapy, 889b
    patient teaching guidelines, 873, 873b
    pharmacokinetics, 869
    pramipexole, 874
    rasagiline, 871t–872t, 874
    ropinirole, 871t–872t, 874
    rotigotine, 871t–872t, 874–875
    selegiline, 871t–872t, 875
    therapeutic effects, 873
Parlodel (bromocriptine mesylate), 869t, 871t–872t, 874
Parnate (tranylcypromine), 1020t
paromomycin (Humatin), 353t, 355t, 357
paroxetine, 1017
paroxetine (Paxil), 1017
paroxetine (Paxil, Paxil CR, Brisdelle, Pexeva), 1009t
paroxysmal supraventricular tachycardia, 504
pasireotide (Signifor LAR), 806t
pasireotide (Signifor, Signifor LAR), 799t, 806t, 808–809, 833–834, 835t
Pataday (olopatadine), 1090t, 1094t–1095t
Patanase (olopatadine), 590t–595t, 595–596, 595t
Patanol (olopatadine), 1094t–1095t
patient-controlled analgesia (PCA), 897–898, 898b
patients, medication errors by, 34
Paxil (paroxetine), 1009t, 1017
Paxil CR (paroxetine), 1009t
Paxlovid (ritonavir), 411t, 414–415
Pazeo (olopatadine), 1090t, 1094t–1095t
pazopanib (Votrient), 236t–238t, 252t–257t, 258–259
P-Care K40 (triamcinolone), 318t, 320t–323t
P-Care K80 (triamcinolone), 318t, 320t–323t
PCSK9 inhibitors
    abnormal kidney function and hepatic impairment, 173
    administration of, 174
    adverse effects, 174
    contraindications, 173
    evolocumab, 164t, 173–174, 173t
    mechanism of action, 173
    nursing implications, 174
    patient teaching guidelines, 168b, 174
    pharmacokinetics, 173
    preventing interactions, 174
    therapeutic effects, 174
PDE5 inhibitors, 125
pdiatric type (DT), 195t–199t
PDP-Amantadine (amantadine hydrochloride), 871t–872t
pdp-Hydrocodone (hydrocodone bitartrate), 574t, 579t
peak expiratory flow rate (PEFR), 602
Pediapred (prednisolone), 320t–323t
Pediatric Diazepam Intensol (diazepam), 956t
pediatrics
    administration of in, 71–74
    age groups, 68, 68t
    drug safety in
        dose calculation, 68
        legislation and drug testing, 68
    infants, 71
    pharmacodynamics in, 68–69
    pharmacokinetics
        drug absorption, 69–70
        drug distribution, 70, 70f
        elimination, 70
        metabolism, 70
    school-aged children and adolescents, 71–74
    toddlers and preschoolers, 71

pediculicides, 463, 464t, 471–472, 471t
pediculosis, 463, 472
PedvaxHIB (haemophilus influenzae type b (Hib)), 194, 194b, 195t–199t
Pegasys (peginterferon alfa-2a), 180t, 187t, 188
pegfilgrastim (Neulasta, Neulasta Onpro, Fulphila, Nyvepria, Udenyca, Ziextenzo), 180t, 185–186, 185t
peginterferon alfa-2a (Pegasys), 180t, 187t, 188
peginterferon alfa-2b, 187t
pegloticase (Krystexxa), 292t, 309t, 310
pegvisomant (Somavert), 799t–801t, 803
pegylation, 188
pembrolizumab (Keytruda), 236t–238t, 252t–257t
pemetrexed (Alimta), 236t–245t
penciclovir (Denavir), 417, 1115t
penicillamine (Cuprimine), 667–668
penicillin(s), 335t–337t, 336–340, 339b, 1105–1106
　abnormal kidney function and hepatic impairment, 338
　administration of, 338, 1106
　adverse effects, 338–339, 1105
　aminopenicillins, 339
　antistaphylococcal penicillins, 339
　contraindications, 338, 1105–1106
　description of, 336
　dose usage, 1105
　drug interactions, 1106b
　mechanism of action, 336
　mechanisms of action, 1105
　nursing implications, 338–339, 1106
　patient teaching guidelines, 339, 339b, 1107b
　penicillin-beta-lactamase inhibitor combinations, 339–340
　pharmacokinetics, 336, 1105
　preventing interactions, 338, 338b, 1106
　route and dosage information, 336, 336t–337t
　therapeutic effects, 338–339, 1106
penicillin G benzathine (Pfizerpen; Crystapen; Bicillin LA), 335t–337t, 338
penicillin G procaine, 335t–337t
penicillin V (Apo-Pen VK, Novo-Pen-VK, Nu-Pen-VK, Penicillin VK), 335t–337t, 339
Penicillin VK (penicillin V), 335t
penicillinase-resistant (antistaphylococcal) penicillins, 336t–337t, 339
penicillin–beta-lactamase inhibitor combinations, 336t–337t, 339–340
penicillin-binding proteins (PBPs), 280
penicillin-resistant *Streptococcus pneumoniae*, 278b
Penlac (ciclopirox), 447t
pentazocine (Talwin), 894t, 903–904, 904t
pentobarbital (Nembutal), 956t, 958–959, 958t
pentostatin (Nipent), 236t–245t
Pepcid (famotidine), 692t, 696t, 698
pepsin, 690
peptic ulcer disease
　adjuvant medications, 701–703, 701t
　assessment, 704b
　clinical considerations, 690
　clinical manifestations, 690
　drug therapy, 690–691
　evaluation, 704b
　nursing interventions, 704b
　nursing process, 704b
　therapy, outcomes of, 704b
peptic ulcers, 829
Pepto-Bismol (bismuth subsalicylate), 703, 738t, 741, 741t
perampanel (Fycompa), 956t, 969t–972t, 978
Perforomist (formoterol), 605t, 608t, 610, 621t
perindopril (Coversyl), 482t, 485t, 488
Perindopril erbumine (Aceon, Coversyl), 754t
peripheral nerve block anesthesia, 911
peripheral nervous system (PNS), 844, 844f

peripherally inserted central catheters, 46b
Perjeta (pertuzumab), 236t–238t, 252t–257t, 257–258
permethrin, 466b, 471–472, 471t
perphenazine (PMS-Perphenazine), 708t–709t, 710, 1031t, 1033t, 1036
Persantine (dipyridamole), 151t–152t, 155–156
Perseris (risperidone), 1009t, 1024t, 1026, 1031t, 1039t–1040t, 1042
pertuzumab (Perjeta), 236t–238t, 252t–257t, 257–258
Pexeva (paroxetine), 1009t
Pfizer-BioNTech (COVID-19), 194, 194b, 195t–199t, 201–203, 202b
Pfizerpen (penicillin G benzathine), 336t–337t
phagocytosis, 273, 274f
pharmacists, 35t–36t
pharmacodynamics, 19–21
　older adults, 76–77
　　adverse effects, prevention of, 77
　　Beers criteria, 76–77
　　cardiovascular disease, 76
　　digoxin, 76
　　Drug Burden Index, 77
　　physiologic changes, 76
　pediatrics, 68–69
pharmacoeconomics, 5
pharmacogenomics, 5, 23–24
pharmacokinetics, 212
　absorption of, 16–17
　children, 22
　conventional antirejection agents, 216
　definition of, 16
　distribution, 17–18
　drug's bioavailability, 16–17
　elimination half-life, 19
　enzyme induction, 18
　enzyme inhibition, 18
　excretion, 18
　first-pass effect, 18
　infants, 18, 22
　lipase inhibitors, 681
　loop diuretics, 631
　metabolism, 18
　mycophenolate mofetil uses in, 212
　noradrenergic sympathomimetic anorexiants, 679
　older adults, 22–23
　　absorption, 78
　　distribution, 78
　　excretion, 79
　　metabolism, 78
　pathologic conditions that affect, 24
　patient-related variables that affect, 22–25
　pediatrics
　　drug absorption, 69–70
　　drug distribution, 70, 70f
　　elimination, 70
　　metabolism, 70
　polymorphisms, 18
　potassium-sparing diuretics, 638
　prodrugs, 18
　serum drug levels, 19
　serum half-life, 19
　sex differences, 24
　thiazide diuretics, 635
pharmacology, 5, 13
pharmacotherapy, 4
phenazopyridine hydrochloride (Pyridium), 365t, 372–373, 372t
phendimetrazine (Bontril PDM), 679t
phenelzine (Nardil), 1009t, 1020t
phenobarbital, 955, 956t, 958t
phenothiazine
　abnormal kidney function, 708
　action, 708

　administration, 709
　adverse effects, 709
　chlorpromazine, 710
　contraindications, 709
　dosage, 708, 709t
　first-generation (typical) antipsychotic drugs, 707–708
　in hepatic impairment patients, 708
　nursing implications, 709
　patient teaching guidelines, 709, 710b
　perphenazine, 710
　pharmacokinetics, 708
　preventing interactions, 709
　prochlorperazine, 710
　for schizophrenia/psychosis, 707–708
　therapeutic effects, 709
　uses, 708, 709t
phentermine, 679–681, 680b
phentermine hydrochloride (Adipex-P), 679t
phentermine–topiramate (Qsymia), 679t, 681
phenylephrine (Altafrin), 1078, 1079t
phenylephrine (Vazculep), 541–542, 543t, 547
phenylephrine (Vazculep, Neo-Synephrine), 574t–575t, 582, 583t
phenylephrine hydrochloride (Altafrin), 1078t
phenyltriazine derivatives, 956t, 977
　abnormal kidney function, 977
　adverse effects, 977
　contraindications, 977
　dose usage, 977
　drug interactions, 977b
　hepatic impairment, 977
　mechanisms of action, 977
　nursing implications, 977–978
　patient teaching guidelines, 978b
　pharmacokinetics, 977
　preventing interactions, 977
　therapeutic effects, 977
Phenytek (phenytoin), 965t
phenytoin (Dilantin), 956t, 964
phenytoin (Dilantin, Dilantin Infatabs, Phenytek, Phenytoin Infatabs), 965t
Phenytoin Infatabs (phenytoin), 965t
PHL-Amoxicillin (amoxicillin), 336t–337t
PhosLo (calcium acetate), 816t
phosphate salts (Neutra-Phos), 823–824
phosphene, 560
phosphodiesterase-3 enzyme inhibitor, 154
phosphodiesterase inhibitors (cardiotonic-inotropic agents), 557–559, 558t, 559b
phosphodiesterase type 5 inhibitors, 119t, 123–125
　administration, 124
　adverse effects, 124
　contraindications, 124
　drug interactions, 124, 124b
　mechanism of action, 124
　patient teaching guidelines, 125, 125b
　pharmacokinetics, 123
　route and dosage information, 124, 124t
　therapeutic effects, 125
phosphorated carbohydrate solution (Emetrol), 708t, 717t, 718
phosphorus, 813–814
physical dependence, 1059
physostigmine, 855t, 857
piggyback method, 57
Pilo-40 (pilocarpine ocular system), 1082t–1084t
pilocarpine, 1083t–1084t
pilocarpine (Isopto Carpine), 1082t
pilocarpine ocular system (Ocusert Pilo-20 or Pilo-40), 1082t–1084t
Pima (potassium iodide saturated solution of potassium iodide), 787t

pimecrolimus (Elidel), 1116t–1117t
pimozide, 1031t, 1033t, 1036
pindolol (APO-Pindol, Visken), 482t, 496t–498t
pinworm infections, 463, 469
pioglitazone (Actos), 754t, 767b, 769, 769t, 777
piperacillin, 335t–337t, 339
piperacillin/tazobactam (Zosyn; AJ-PIP/TAZ, piperacillin, and tazobactam for injection), 335t–337t, 340
piroxicam (Feldene, Apo-Piroxicam), 290t, 301, 301t
pitavastatin (Livalo, Zypitamag), 164t, 166t
Pitavastatin calcium (Livalo), 754t
Pitocin (oxytocin), 94–95, 94t, 799t, 804t, 805
pituitary and hypothalamic dysfunction
  acromegaly, 798
  anterior pituitary hormone, 799–803
  assessment, 810b
  clinical considerations, 797–798
  clinical manifestations, 797–798
  diabetes insipidus, 798
  drug therapy, 799
  evaluation, 810b
  growth hormone deficiency, 797–798
  hypothalamic hormones, 805–809
  nursing interventions, 810b
  nursing process, 810b
  outcomes of therapy, 810b
  overview of, 797–799
  posterior pituitary hormones, 803–805
  precocious puberty, 798
pituitary gland
  anterior, 783–784
  posterior, 797
pituitary hormones, 797f
placebo, 8
planning, 51–52
plant alkaloids, 236t–238t
Plaquenil (hydroxychloroquine), 464t, 467t, 468
plasma cholesterol, 162t
plasmin, 138
plasminogen, 138
Plasmodium spp., 463, 465–466
platelet-activating factor (PAF), 289b
Plavix (clopidogrel), 150, 151t–152t
plazomicin (Zemdri), 353t, 355t, 357
plecanatide (Trulance), 724t, 731–732, 731t
Plendil (felodipine), 492t, 524t, 532t, 533
PMS Cephalexin (cephalexin), 336t–337t
PMS Clarithromycin (clarithromycin), 377, 378t, 380
PMS Selegiline (selegiline hydrochloride), 871t–872t
PMS Vancomycin (vancomycin), 381t–382t
PMS-Benztropine (benztropine mesylate), 884t
PMSBortezomib (bortezomib), 236t–238t, 252t–257t, 259–260
PMS-Cholestyramine (cholestyramine), 164t, 168–170, 169t
PMS-Codeine (codeine), 896t–897t, 901
PMSColchicine (colchicine), 292t, 306–307, 307t, 308b
PMSEpirubicin (epirubicin), 236t–245t
PMS-Fentanyl MTX (fentanyl), 894t, 896t–897t
PMS-Finasteride (finasteride), 126–128, 126t
PMSFlutamide (flutamide), 236t–238t, 261t–263t
PMS-Fluticasone HFA (fluticasone), 318t, 320t–323t
PMS-Metronidazole, 464–465, 464t
PMS-MetroNIDAZOLE (metronidazole), 381t–382t
PMS-Oxycodone CR (Oxycodone), 894t, 896t–897t, 902–903, 902t
PMS-Pamidronate (pamidronate), 820t–821t
PMS-Prednisolone (prednisolone), 320t–323t
PMS-Ropinirole (ropinirole hydrochloride), 871t–872t

PMS-Sulfasalazine (sulfasalazine), 365t, 370t, 372
PMSTamoxifen (tamoxifen), 236t–238t, 260, 261t–263t
PMS-Tofacitinib (tofacitinib), 211t, 221
Pneumo 23 (pneumococcal 23 polysaccharide (PPSV 23)), 195t–199t
pneumococcal 23 polysaccharide (PPSV 23) (Pneumovax 23; Pneumo 23), 195t–199t
pneumococcal conjugate vaccine
  13-valent (PCV 13) (Prevnar 13), 195t–199t
  15-valent (PCV 15) (Vaxneuvance), 195t–199t
  20-valent (PCV 20) (Prevnar 20), 195t–199t
pneumococcal vaccine, 194b, 203
pneumococcal vaccine PPSV23 (Pneumovax), 194b
Pneumovax 23 (pneumococcal 23 polysaccharide (PPSV 23)), 195t–199t
PNS (peripheral nervous system), 844, 844f
Podactin (miconazole), 1115t
Podactin (tolnaftate), 1115t
Pod-Care 100K (triamcinolone), 318t, 320t–323t
podophyllotoxins, 236t–245t
polio vaccine, 203
poliomyelitis, inactivated (IPV) (IPOL, Imovax Polio), 195t–199t
Polmon (dexchlorpheniramine), 590t–591t, 593
Polocaine (mepivacaine), 912t, 915
Polocaine Dental (mepivacaine), 912t
Polocaine-MPF (mepivacaine), 912t
polycarbophil (FiberCon), 724t, 726t, 738t, 741t, 742
polyclonal antibodies, 222t–224t, 224, 226
polyenes
  abnormal kidney function, 448
  action, 447
  adverse effects, 449
  age, 447
  contraindications, 449
  drug administration, 448t, 449, 449b
  in hepatic impairment, 448
  lactation, 447
  nursing implications, 449
  patient teaching guidelines, 449, 449b
  pharmacokinetics, 446–447
  pregnancy, 447
  preventing interactions, 449, 449b
  reproduction, 447
  therapeutic effects, 449
  use, 447–448, 448t
polyethylene glycol (PEG) solution (GaviLAX, GlycoLax, HealthyLax, MiraLAX, PEGyLAX), 724t, 729t, 730
polyethylene glycol-electrolyte solution (PEG-ES) (Colyte, GaviLyte-N, GoLYTELY, NuLytely, TriLyte), 724t, 729t, 730
polymerase inhibitors, 412b, 426–427
polymorphisms, 18
polymyxin B, 1113t
polymyxin B (Polysporin), 1113t
polypharmacy, 76
Polysporin (bacitracin and polymyxin B), 1113t
polyuria, 798
ponatinib (Iclusig), 236t–238t, 252t–257t, 259
Ponstan (mefenamic acid), 290t, 298t–299t, 300
Portia, 110t–111t
Portia-28, 110t–111t
posaconazole (Noxafil), 447t, 453–454
postantibiotic effects, 356
postganglionic fibers, 499
postpartum depression, 1008b
posttraumatic stress disorder (PTSD), 993, 994b
potassium channel blockers, 506, 507t, 513–516
potassium imbalances
  prevention and management of, 633b
potassium iodide and iodine (Lugol solution), 787t
potassium iodide saturated solution of potassium iodide (iOSAT, ThyroSafe, ThyroShield, Pima, SSKI), 787t

potassium phosphate, 823–824, 823t
potassium-losing diuretics, 639–640
potassium-sparing diuretics
  abnormal kidney function, 638
  action, 638
  administration of, 639
  adverse effects, 639
  amiloride, 631t, 638t, 639–640
  contraindications, 639
  dosage information, 638t
  drug interactions, 639, 639b
  in hepatic impairment patients, 638
  herbs, 639
  lactation, 638
  nursing implications, 639
  nutritional needs, 89
  patient teaching guidelines, 634b, 639
  pharmacokinetics, 638
  physiologic and pharmacokinetic changes, 86t
  pregnancy, 638
  prototype, 637
  reproduction, 638
  spironolactone, 631t, 637–640, 638t, 639b, 641t
  tetanus–diphtheria–pertussis vaccine, 92
  therapeutic effects, 639
  triamterene, 631t, 638t, 639–640, 641t
  urinary tract infections, 92
  uses, 638–639
powders, 42t–43t
Pradaxa (dabigatran etexilate), 141t–142t, 147, 148b
Prader-Willi syndrome, 801
pralatrexate (Folotyn), 236t–238t
pralidoxime (Protopam), 863, 864t
Praluent (alirocumab), 164t, 173–174, 173t, 211t, 225
pramipexole (Mirapex, Mirapex ER), 874
pramlintide, 778
pramlintide acetate (Symlin), 773, 773t, 774b
pramoxine, 1117
Prandin (repaglinide), 754t, 767b, 769–770, 771b
prasugrel (Effient), 140t, 150, 151t–152t, 152–154
Pravachol (pravastatin), 164t, 166t, 167, 754t
Pravastatin (Pravachol), 754t
pravastatin (Pravachol), 164t, 166t, 167
Praxbind (idarucizumab), 148, 157–158, 158t
Praxis (aspirin), 140t, 151t–152t
prazosin (Minipress, APO-Prazo, Minipress), 482t, 496t–498t
Precedex (dexmedetomidine), 922t, 932, 932t
precocious puberty, 798
  central, 798
  gonadotropin-dependent, 798
  gonadotropin-independent, 798
  hypothalamic hormone drugs (see hypothalamic hormone drugs)
  incomplete, 798
Precose (acarbose), 754t, 758, 763, 767–769, 768t, 769b
Pred Forte (prednisolone), 318t, 320t–323t, 1090t, 1094t–1095t
Pred Mild (prednisolone), 318t, 320t–323t, 1094t–1095t
prednisolone (Millipred; Pediapred, PMS-Prednisolone), 320t–323t
prednisolone (Pred Forte), 1090t
prednisolone (Pred Forte, Pred Mild), 318t, 1094t–1095t
Prednisolone (Pred Forte, Pred Mild; Diopred, Minims Prednisolone, PMS-Prednisolone, Sod Phos Fort, Pred Forte, SANDOZ Prednisolone, TEVA-Prednisolone), 320t–323t
prednisone (Prednisone Intensol, Rayos, Apo-Prednisone, JAA-PredniSONE, Winpred), 317, 318t, 320t–323t, 324–326, 328–329, 616t

preeclampsia, 91
pregabalin (Lyrica), 963
pregabalin (Lyrica, Lyrica CR), 956t, 962t–963t
pregnancy
　anemia during, 90
　assessment, 97f
　constipation, 90
　drug(s), 11
　drug distribution during, 25
　drug therapy in
　　patient teaching guidelines, 88, 88b
　　principles of, 87–88, 88b
　evaluation, 97f
　gastroesophageal reflux disease, 90
　gestational diabetes mellitus, 90
　group B streptococcus, 91
　hypertension during, 93
　influenza, 92
　maternal-placental-fetal circulation, 86
　natural herbs, 89, 89b
　nausea and vomiting, 91
　nursing interventions, 97f
　nursing process, 97b
　outcomes of therapy, 97f
Pregnyl (human chorionic gonadotropin), 85, 85t, 799t, 800t, 803
preload, 524–525
Premarin (conjugated estrogens), 101–105, 103t
premature ventricular contractions, 505b
premenstrual dysphoric disorder (PMDD), 100
premenstrual syndrome
　characteristics, 100
　clinical manifestations, 100–101
　drug therapy, 101
　premenstrual dysphoric disorder, 100–101
Premphase (conjugated estrogens/medroxyprogesterone acetate), 112t
Premplus (conjugated estrogens/medroxyprogesterone acetate), 112t
Prempro (conjugated estrogen-medroxyprogesterone), 109, 112t
Prepidil (dinoprostone), 94, 94t
prescription medicine
　patient teaching guidelines, 53b
　self-administration of, 53b
preshock, 541
pressor effect, 546–547
presystemic metabolism, 18
preterm labor, 92
Prevacid (lansoprazole), 692t, 699t, 700–701
Prevalite (cholestyramine), 164t, 168–170, 169t, 738t, 741t, 742
Prevalite (cholestyramine), 738t
Preventive therapy, 937
Prevex HC (hydrocortisone), 320t–323t
Prevnar 13 (pneumococcal conjugate vaccine 13-valent (PCV 13)), 195t–199t
Prevnar 20 (pneumococcal conjugate vaccine 20-valent (PCV 20)), 195t–199t
Priftin (rifapentine), 391, 391t, 397t, 398
Prilosec (omeprazole), 692t, 698–701, 699t
primaquine, 464t, 467t, 468–469
primary adrenal insufficiency, 828
primary adrenocortical insufficiency, 828
primary hypothyroidism, 784
Primaxin (imipenem-cilastatin), 335t, 347t
primidone (Mysoline), 956t, 958–959, 958t
Prinivil (lisinopril), 482t, 754t
Priorix (M-M-R II (measles, mumps, and rubella (MMR)), 195t–199t, 202–203
Pristiq (desvenlafaxine), 1019
Privigen (immune globulin (human) (IG; IGIM)), 200t–201t
Privigen (immune globulin intravenous (IGIV)), 200t–201t, 203
ProAir RespiClick (albuterol), 605t, 606, 608t

Pro-Amox-250 (amoxicillin), 336t–337t
Pro-Amox-500 (amoxicillin), 336t–337t
PRO-Azithromycin (azithromycin), 378t
probenecid, 292t, 309t, 310
procainamide, 506–507, 507t–508t, 509, 509b
procarbazine (Matulane), 236t–245t, 246–247
Procardia (nifedipine), 93, 93t, 482t
Procardia XL (nifedipine), 482t
Pro-C-Dure 5 (triamcinolone), 318t, 320t–323t
Pro-C-Dure 6 (triamcinolone), 318t, 320t–323t
PRO-Cefadroxil (cefadroxil), 342t–344t
PRO-Cefuroxime (cefuroxime), 342t–344t
ProCentra (dextroamphetamine), 1047t, 1049, 1050t
prochlorperazine, 951
prochlorperazine (Compro), 708–709, 708t–709t, 709b, 951t
Procrit (epoetin alfa), 180–181, 180t–181t, 183b, 236t–238t, 264t
Procytox (cyclophosphamide), 235, 236t–245t, 245–246, 248b, 251b
prodrugs, 18
prodysrhythmic effects, 506
progesterone, 96
progesterone (Crinone, Endometrin, Prometrium), 100, 107t–108t
progestin(s), 100–101
　abnormal kidney function, 106
　administration of, 105
　adverse effects, 108
　contraindications, 108
　dosage information, 106, 107t–108t
　in hepatic impairment patients, 106
　mechanism of action, 106
　nursing implications, 104–105
　patient teaching guidelines, 105, 105b
　pharmacokinetics, 106
　physiology, 100
　preventing interactions, 105, 105b
　reproduction, pregnancy, and lactation, 106
　therapeutic effects, 105
　uses, 106
progestin-estrogen combinations
　in hepatic impairment patients, 111
　reproduction, pregnancy, and lactation, 111
progestin–estrogen combinations
　abnormal kidney function, 111
　administration of, 105
　adverse effects, 104
　contraindications, 104
　dosage information
　　as contraceptives, 109, 110t–111t
　　for noncontraceptive, 111, 112t
　drug interactions, 105, 105b
　in hepatic impairment patients, 111
　mechanism of actions, 109
　nursing implications, 104–105
　patient teaching guidelines, 105, 105b
　pharmacokinetics, 109
　therapeutic effects, 113
　uses, 109–111
Prograf (tacrolimus), 211t, 212, 215b, 216, 218–219
proguanil (Malarone), 464t, 467t, 468
Proleukin (aldesleukin), 188
Prolia (denosumab), 823, 823t
promethazine, 590t–591t, 593
Prometrium (progesterone), 107t–108t
propafenone (Rythmol), 508t, 510
proparacaine (Alcaine), 1078t–1079t
Propecia (finasteride), 119t, 126–128, 126t
Propel (mometasone), 320t–323t
Propel MiniSDS (mometasone), 320t–323t
propionibacterium acnes, 1110
propionic acid derivatives, 290t, 297–300, 298t–299t, 1107

　abnormal kidney function and hepatic impairment, 299
　administration of, 300
　adverse effects, 299–300
　contraindications, 299
　mechanism of action, 297
　nursing implications, 299–300
　patient teaching guidelines, 300, 300b
　pharmacokinetics, 297
　preventing interactions, 299, 300b
　reproduction, pregnancy, and lactation, 298
　therapeutic effects, 300
Propofol (Diprivan, Fresenius Propoven; Propofol-Lipuro; Diprivan, TEVAPropofol), 922t, 925
Propofol-Lipuro (propofol), 922t, 925, 926t
propranolol (Inderal LA, Hemangiol, InnoPran; Hemangiol), 482t, 496t–498t, 499, 511–512, 511t, 512t, 524t, 529, 530t, 531
propranolol hydrochloride (Inderal, Inderal LA, Innopran XL; Inderal, Inderal LA, Hemangeol, InnoPran XL), 787t, 789t
propylthiouracil, 87b
propylthiouracil (PTU)
　abnormal kidney function, 788
　administration of, 788
　adverse effects, 788
　contraindications, 788
　in hepatic impairment patients, 788
　iodine preparations, 788–789
　in lactation, 788
　mechanism of action, 786
　methimazole, 788
　nursing implications, 788
　patient teaching guidelines, 788, 789b
　pharmacokinetics, 786
　in pregnancy patients, 788
　preventing interactions, 788
　strong iodine solution, 788–789
　therapeutic effects, 788
　uses, 786–788
propylthiouracil (PTU) (Halycil), 787t
Proscar (finasteride), 119t, 126–128, 126t
prostaglandin analogs, 702, 1082, 1082t–1084t
　adverse effects, 1082
　contraindications, 1082
　dose usage, 1082
　mechanisms of action, 1082
　nursing implications, 1084
　patient teaching guidelines, 1084
　pharmacokinetics, 1082
　therapeutic effects, 1084
prostaglandins, 93–94, 94t, 119t, 286, 287t
Prostin E$_2$ (dinoprostone), 94, 94t
protamine sulfate, 140t, 143, 157, 158t
protease inhibitors (PIs), 435–438, 436t–437t
proteasome inhibitor, 236t–238t, 252t–257t, 259–260
protein binding, 17
protein metabolism, 316b, 751
Proteus spp., 275b, 277
prothrombin complex concentrate, human (Beriplex P/N, Octaplex), 158t
proton pump inhibitors
　abnormal kidney function, 700
　action, 698
　administration, 700
　adverse effects, 33, 700
　contraindications, 700
　drug interactions, 700
　in hepatic impairment patients, 700
　lactation, 700
　nursing implications, 700
　patient teaching guidelines, 694b, 700
　pharmacokinetics, 698
　pregnancy, 700
　reproduction, 700

routes and dosage ranges, 699*t*
therapeutic effects, 700
use, 698–700
Protonix (pantoprazole), 692*t*, 700–701
protooncogenes, 233
Protopam (pralidoxime), 863, 864*t*
Protopic (tacrolimus), 1116*t*–1117*t*
prototype drugs, 4, 854
protriptyline hydrochloride, 1009*t*, 1012*t*
Protylol (dicyclomine hydrochloride), 886*t*
Proventil HFA (albuterol), 605*t*, 606, 608*t*
Provera (medroxyprogesterone acetate), 106–109, 107*t*–108*t*
Provigil (modafinil), 1047*t*, 1053*t*, 1054–1055
PROzac (fluoxetine), 1009*t*, 1013
prucalopride (Motegrity), 724*t*, 732*t*, 733
pruritus, 1110
pseudoallergic drug reactions, 589
pseudoephedrine (Semprex-D), 590*t*, 595–596, 595*t*
pseudoephedrine (Sudafed), 575–578, 575*t*
Pseudomonas, 275*b*
Pseudomonas aeruginosa, 275*b*, 354, 1101
Pseudomonas and *Proteus* species, 353
Psorcon (diflorasone diacetate), 1112*t*
psoriasis, 209–210, 216–217, 227, 1110
psoriatic arthritis, 210, 216, 219, 220*t*
psychoactive substance use, 1067
psychological considerations, 24–25
psychological dependence, 1059
psychosis, 1030
psychotic disorders
  antipsychotics (*see* antipsychotic drugs)
  assessment, 1044*b*
  clinical considerations, 1030
  clinical manifestations, 1030–1031
  drug therapy, 1031–1032
  evaluation, 1044*b*
  first-generation antipsychotics, 1032–1036
  first-generation nonphenothiazines, 1036–1038
  nursing interventions, 1044*b*
  nursing process, 1044*b*
  outcomes of therapy, 1044*b*
  overview, 1030–1032
  phenothiazine antipsychotics (*see* phenothiazine)
  recommendations for, 1031*b*
  second-generation "atypical" antipsychotics, 1038–1043
  treatment of, 1031*t*
psyllium preparations (Metamucil), 724*t*, 726, 726*t*
Pulmicort (budesonide), 320*t*–323*t*
Pulmicort Flexhaler (budesonide), 320*t*–323*t*
Pulmicort Nebuamp (budesonide), 320*t*–323*t*
Pulmicort Turbuhaler (budesonide), 320*t*–323*t*, 605*t*, 616*t*
pupil, 1076
Puregon (follitropin beta), 85, 85*t*
purine antagonist, 236*t*–238*t*, 238
Purinethol (mercaptopurine), 236*t*–245*t*, 238, 246–247
Purixan (mercaptopurine), 236*t*–245*t*, 238, 246–247
pyrazinamide, 391, 394*b*, 399–400, 399*t*
Pyridium (phenazopyridine hydrochloride), 365*t*, 372–373, 372*t*
pyridostigmine (Mestinon, Reginol, Mestinon-SR), 854–856, 864*t*
pyridoxine (vitamin B6), 654*t*–656*t*
  administration, 659
  adverse effects, 659
  contraindications, 659
  nursing implications, 659
  patient teaching guidelines for, 657*b*, 659
  pharmacokinetics and use, 659
  therapeutic effects, 659
pyrimidine, 236*t*–245*t*, 238
pyrimidine analog
  abnormal kidney function, 456
  action, 456
  administration of, 457
  adverse effects, 457
  contraindications, 457
  hemodialysis, 457
  in hepatic impairment, 456
  lactation, 456
  nursing implications, 457
  patient teaching guidelines, 457, 457*b*
  pharmacokinetics, 456
  pregnancy, 456
  preventing interactions, 457, 457*b*
  reproduction, 456
  therapeutic effects, 457
  use, 456–457
pyrogens, 288, 291
pyrosis, 690
pyrrolidine derivatives, 956*t*, 978
  abnormal kidney function, 978
  adverse effects, 978
  contraindications, 978
  dose usage, 978
  hepatic impairment, 978
  mechanisms of action, 978
  nursing implications, 978
  patient teaching guidelines, 979*b*
  pharmacokinetics, 978
  preventing interactions, 978
  therapeutic effects, 978

Q

Qsymia (phentermine–topiramate), 679*t*, 681
Qtern (dapagliflozin and saxagliptin), 778
Qternmet XR (dapagliflozin, saxagliptin, and metformin), 778
Quadrivalent Influvac (influenza (IIV4)), 195*t*–199*t*
Qualaquin (quinine), 464*t*, 467*t*, 468
Quality and Safety Education for Nurses (QSEN)
  QNASL (beclomethasone), 320*t*–323*t*, 616*t*
  QNASL Children's (beclomethasone), 320*t*–323*t*, 616*t*
Quasense, 110*t*–111*t*
quazepam (Doral), 995*t*, 999
Qudexy XR (topiramate), 969*t*–972*t*
Quelicin (succinylcholine), 922*t*, 929*t*, 931
Quelicin chloride (succinylcholine), 929*t*
Questran (cholestyramine), 164*t*, 168–170, 169*t*
quetiapine (Seroquel), 1009*t*
quetiapine (Seroquel, Seroquel XR), 1024*t*, 1025–1026, 1031*t*, 1039*t*–1040*t*, 1042
QuilliChew ER (methylphenidate), 1047*t*, 1053*t*
Quillivant XR (methylphenidate), 1047*t*, 1053*t*
quinapril (Accupril), 482*t*, 485*t*, 488, 495*t*–496*t*
Quinapril hydrochloride (Accupril), 754*t*
Quinate (quinidine), 508*t*, 510
quinidine, 77
quinidine (Apo-Quinidine, Quinate, Novo-Quinidin), 508*t*, 510
quinine (Qualaquin; APO-Quinine, JAMP-Quinine), 464*t*, 467*t*, 468
quinupristin–dalfopristin (Synercid), 381*t*–382*t*, 384–385
Qulipta (atogepant), 948*t*, 949
Quviviq (daridorexant), 995*t*, 1003*t*, 1004
QVAR (beclomethasone), 318*t*, 320*t*–323*t*, 605*t*, 616*t*
Qvar RediHaler (beclomethasone), 318*t*, 320*t*–323*t*, 605, 614, 616*t*
Qvar RediHaler Beconase AQ (beclomethasone), 605*t*, 614–615, 616*t*

R

RabAvert (rabies vaccine (HDCV CECV)), 195*t*–199*t*
rabeprazole (AcipHex, AcipHex Sprinkle), 96*b*, 692*t*, 699*t*, 700
rabies immune globulin (HRIG) (HyperRAB S/D, Imogam Rabies HT; HyperRAB S/D, Imogam Rabies Pasteurized), 200*t*–201*t*
rabies vaccine (HDCV CECV) (Imovax Rabies, RabAvert), 195*t*–199*t*
radioactive iodine, 786–789
raloxifene (Evista, ACT Raloxifene, APORaloxifene, Evista), 823*t*, 824
raltegravir (Isentress), 438–439, 439*t*, 439*b*
ramelteon, 96*b*, 1002
ramelteon (Rozerem), 995*t*
Ramipril (Altace), 754*t*
ramipril (Altace), 482*t*, 485*t*, 488
Ranexa (ranolazine), 524*t*, 534, 534*t*
ranolazine (Ranexa), 524*t*, 534, 534*t*
RANRosuvastatin (rosuvastatin), 164*t*, 166*t*
Rapaflo (silodosin), 119*t*, 128*t*, 129
Rapamune (sirolimus), 211*t*, 215*b*, 219
rapid sequence induction, 931
rasagiline (Azilect), 869*t*, 871*t*–872*t*, 874
rasburicase (Elitek, Fasturtec), 236*t*–245*t*, 238, 292*t*, 309*t*, 310
Rasilez (aliskiren), 496*t*–498*t*
Rasuvo (methotrexate), 211*t*, 212, 215*b*, 216, 226–227, 236*t*–245*t*, 238, 246–247, 248*b*, 251*b*
RATIO- Flonase (fluticasone), 320*t*–323*t*
ratio-Aclavulanate (amoxicillin-clavulanate), 335*t*–337*t*, 338
Ratio-Codeine (codeine), 896*t*–897*t*, 901
ratio-Ipra Sal UDV (ipratropium/albuterol), 621
Rayos (prednisone), 317, 318*t*, 320*t*–323*t*, 324–326, 328–329
Razadyne ER (galantamine, galantamine hydrobromide) 855*t*, 859, 859*t*
Reactine (cetirizine), 590*t*, 594–597, 595*t*
Rebif (interferon beta-1a), 187*t*, 188
Rebif Rebidose (interferon beta-1a), 187*t*
Recarbrio (imipenem-relebactam), 335*t*–337*t*, 348
receptor(s)
  alpha$_2$, 848
  alpha$_1$ receptors, 848
  beta$_1$, beta$_2$, and beta$_3$, 848
  dopaminergic
    D$_1$ and D$_5$, 848
    D$_2$, D$_3$, and D$_4$, 848
  muscarinic, 849, 879–880
  nicotinic$_{CNS}$, 850
  nicotinic$_m$, 850
  nicotinic$_n$, 850
  protein, 20
  serotonin, 708*t*, 712–713, 714*t*
receptor theory of drug action, 19–20
Reclast (zoledronic acid), 820*t*–821*t*
recombinant hCG choriogonadotropin alpha (Ovidrel), 799*t*–801*t*, 803
Recombivax HB (hepatitis B vaccine), 193, 194*b*, 195*t*–199*t*, 202–203
recommended dietary allowance, 645, 646*b*
rectal suppositories, 42*t*–43*t*
Rectiv (nitroglycerin), 524–528, 524*t*–525*t*, 537*b*
RediTrex (methotrexate), 211*t*, 212, 215*b*, 216, 226–227, 236*t*–245*t*, 238, 246–247, 248*b*, 251*b*
refraction, 1076
refractive errors, 1077
Reginol, Mestinon-SR (pyridostigmine), 854, 855*t*
Reglan (metoclopramide), 95, 951*t*
Regonol (pyridostigmine), 854, 855*t*
regorafenib (Stivarga), 236*t*–238*t*, 252*t*–257*t*, 259
Regranex (becaplermin), 1116*t*–1117*t*
regular insulin (Humulin R, Novolin R), 753, 755, 756*t*–757*t*, 759
rejection reactions
  antirejection agents, 216–219
  description of, 210

Relafen (nabumetone), 290t, 298t–299t, 300, 302t–303t, 305
Relafen DS (nabumetone), 290t, 298t–299t, 300, 302t–303t, 305
Releuko (filgrastim), 184–186, 185t, 236t–238t, 248b, 264t
Relexxiii (methylphenidate), 1047t, 1053t
remdesivir, 411–412, 411t
Remeron (mirtazapine), 1009t, 1021–1022, 1022t
Remicade (infliximab), 211t, 227
remifentanil (Ultiva), 932
Remimazolam (Byfavo), 932
remission, 234
Remsima (infliximab), 211t, 227
Renflexis (infliximab), 211t, 227
renin–angiotensin system, 555
ReoPro (abciximab), 151t–152t
Repaglinide, 770
repaglinide (Prandin), 754t, 767b, 769–770, 771b
Repatha (evolocumab), 164t, 173–174, 173t
Repatha Pushtronex System (evolocumab), 164t, 173–174, 173t
Repatha SureClick (evolocumab), 164t, 173–174, 173t
Reprexain (hydrocodone), 896t–897t
reproductive effects, 785t–786t
reproductive health problems in males
 androgen deficiency, 118
  abuse of, 122–123
  assessment, 130b
  clinical considerations, 118
  clinical manifestations, 118
  evaluation, 130b
  nursing interventions, 130b
  nursing process, 130b
  outcomes of therapy, 130b
 benign prostatic hypertrophy
  assessment, 130b
  clinical considerations, 118
  clinical manifestations, 118
  evaluation, 130b
  nursing interventions, 130b
  nursing process, 130b
  therapy, outcomes of, 130b
 clinical judgment in practice, 119b
 erectile dysfunction
  adjuvant medications, 125–126, 126b
  assessment, 130b
  clinical considerations, 118
  clinical manifestations, 118
  evaluation, 130b
  nursing interventions, 130b
  nursing process, 130b
  outcomes of therapy, 130b
Requip (ropinirole), 874
Requip XL (ropinirole), 874
rescue inhalant medications, 606
research, 23
residual neuromuscular blockade, 930
resistant organisms, 278b
reslizumab (Cinqair), 605, 619t, 620
respiratory disorders
 asthma, 602–606
 common cold, 574
 nasal congestion associated with, 574–575
 rhinosinusitis, 574
 sinusitis, 574
respiratory syncytial virus (RSV), 406b, 419–421
 monoclonal antibody, 421
respiratory system, 316b
Restasis (cyclosporine emulsion), 1090t, 1094t–1095t, 1097
Restasis MultiDose (cyclosporine emulsion), 1090t, 1094t–1095t, 1097
Restoril (temazepam), 995t
Retacrit (epoetin alfa), 180–181, 180t–181t, 183b, 236t–238t, 264t

retapamulin (Altabax), 1113t
retina, 1076
retinitis, 406b
retinoids, 1118–1121, 1119t
 abnormal kidney function, 1119
 administration of, 1120
 adverse effects, 1119
 contraindications, 1120
 dose usage, 1119
 drug interactions, 1120b
 hepatic impairment, 1119
 iPLEDGE program, 1120b
 mechanisms of action, 1119
 nursing implications, 1120–1121
 patient teaching guidelines, 1121b
 pharmacokinetics, 1119
 preventing interactions, 1120
 therapeutic effects, 1120
retinol (vitamin A), 654t–656t
 administration, 656
 adverse effects, 656
 contraindications, 656
 drug interaction, 654t–656t
 nursing implications, 656
 patient teaching guidelines, 656, 657b
 pharmacokinetics and use, 654–656
 therapeutic effects, 656
Retrovir (zidovudine), 412b, 429–433, 432t
Revatio (sildenafil), 119t, 123, 124t
reversible indirect-acting cholinergics
 administration, 858–859
 adverse effects, 858–859
 contraindications, 858
 donepezil, 858
 drug interactions, 858, 859b
 galantamine hydrobromide, 859
 mechanism of action, 858
 nursing implications, 858–859
 patient teaching guidelines, 859, 860b
 pharmacokinetics, 858
 preventing interactions, 858, 859b
 in reanl and hepatic impairment patients, 858
 rivastigmine, 859, 859t
 routes and dosage ranges, 859t
 therapeutic effects, 859
 uses, 858
ReVia (naltrexone), 894t, 905–907, 907t
Revonto (dantrolene sodium), 983t, 985t–986t, 987
Reye syndrome, 292
rheumatoid arthritis, 210, 216–217, 219, 220t, 226–227
rhinitis, 574
Rhinocort Allergy (budesonide), 318t, 320t–323t
Rhinocort Aqua (budesonide), 320t–323t
Rhinocort Turbuhaler (budesonide), 320t–323t
rhinosinusitis, 574
rho kinase inhibitor, 1083t–1084t, 1087
 adverse effects, 1087
 contraindications, 1087
 dose usage, 1087
 mechanisms of action, 1087
 nursing implications, 1087
 patient teaching guidelines, 1087
 pharmacokinetics, 1086
 preventing interactions, 1087
 therapeutic effects, 1087
RhoGAM (Rh$_o$(D) immune globulin (human)), 200t–201t
Rh$_o$(D) immune globulin (human) (HyperRHO S/D Full Dose, MICRhoGAM, RhoGAM, WinRho SDF; HyperRHO S/D Full Dose, HypRho-D, WinRho SDF), 200t–201t
Rhopressa (netarsudil), 1083t–1084t
Riabni (rituximab), 236t–238t, 252t–257t, 257
ribavirin, 87b
ribavirin (Ibavyr), 426t, 427–428

ribavirin (Virazole), 419–421, 420t
riboflavin (vitamin B$_2$), 654t–656t, 950
rifabutin (Mycobutin), 397t, 398, 400
Rifadin (rifampin), 389, 394b, 396–398, 397t
rifampin (Rifadin), 389, 394b, 396–398, 397t
rifamycins, 396–398, 398b
 abnormal kidney function, 396
 action, 396
 administration of, 397
 adverse effects, 396
 contraindications, 396
 dosage information, 396, 397t
 in hepatic impairment patient, 396
 nursing implications, 396–398
 patient teaching guidelines, 396, 398, 398b
 pharmacokinetics, 396
 preventing interactions, 396–397
 therapeutic effects, 397
 uses, 396
rifapentine (Priftin), 391, 391t, 397t, 398
Rifater, 400
rifaximin (Xifaxan), 738t, 741t, 742
rifaximin (Xifaxan; Zaxine), 381t–382t, 385
right-sided heart failure, 552–553
rimantadine, 423
rimegepant (Nurtec), 948–949, 948t
rimexolone, 1090t
Rinvoq (upadacitinib), 211t, 221
Riomet (metformin), 754t, 765, 766t
risedronate (Actonel, Actonel DR), 820t–821t
risk evaluation and mitigation strategy (REMS), 893–894
risk-to-benefit ratio, 76
RisperDAL (risperidone), 1009t, 1024t, 1026
Risperdal (risperidone), 1031t, 1039t–1040t, 1042
Risperdal Consta (risperidone), 1009t, 1024t, 1026, 1031t, 1039t–1040t
risperidone (Perseris, RisperDAL, RisperDAL Consta), 1009t, 1024t, 1026
risperidone (Risperdal Consta), 1039t–1040t
risperidone (Risperdal, Perseris), 1039t–1040t, 1042
risperidone (Risperdal, Perseris, Risperdal Consta), 1031t
Ritalin (methylphenidate), 1047t, 1053t
Ritalin LA (methylphenidate), 1047t, 1053t
ritonavir (Paxlovid), 411t, 414–415
Rituxan (rituximab), 211t, 226, 236t–238t, 252t–257t, 257
rituximab, 411t, 412–413
rituximab (Riabni, Rituxan, Ruxience, Truxima), 236t–238t, 252t–257t, 257
rituximab (Rituxan, Truxima), 211t, 222t–224t, 226
Riva Clindamycin (clindamycin hydrochloride), 381t–382t
RIVA-Dicyclomine (dicyclomine hydrochloride), 886t
Rivanase AQ (beclomethasone), 320t–323t
RIVAO-lmesartan (benicar HCT), 495t–496t
Riva-Rosuvastatin (rosuvastatin), 164t, 166t
Rivaroxaban, 77
rivaroxaban (Xarelto), 140t–142t, 148
Rivastigmine (Exelon, Rivastigmine Patch 5, or 15, SANDOZ Rivastigmine), 859, 859t
Rivastigmine Patch 5, or 15 (rivastigmine), 859, 855t, 859t
rizatriptan (Maxalt, Maxalt-MLT, Maxalt, Maxalt RPD), 945t, 946
RNA viruses, 419, 422
Robaxin (methocarbamol), 77, 985t–986t, 987
Robaxisal (acetylsalicylic acid/methocarbamol), 754t
Robinul (glycopyrrolate), 878–879, 879t, 881t, 885, 886t
Robitussin Severe Multisymptom Cough Cold & Flu, 583t

Rocaltrol (calcitriol), 816t
Rocklatan (netarsudil and latanoprost), 1082t–1084t
Rocuronium, 922t, 929t, 930–931
rolapitant (Varubi), 708t, 715t, 717
Rome III criteria for functional constipation, 723
ropinirole (Requip, Requip XL), 871t–872t, 874
ropivacaine (Naropin), 912t
rosacea, 1110–1112
rosiglitazone maleate (Avandia), 754t, 767b, 769, 769t, 772t
Rosuvastatin (Crestor), 754t
rosuvastatin (Crestor; RANRosuvastatin, Riva-Rosuvastatin, Sandoz-Rosuvastatin, Teva-Rosuvastatin), 164t, 166t
Rotarix (rotavirus (RV)), 194, 194b, 195t–199t
RotaTeq (rotavirus (RV)), 194, 194b, 195t–199t
rotavirus (RV) (RotaTeq; Rotarix), 194, 194b, 195t–199t
   vaccine, 194b
rotigotine, 871t–872t, 874–875
rotigotine transdermal (Neupro), 869t
roundworm infections, 463, 470
Roweepra (levetiracetam), 969t–972t
Roweepra XR (levetiracetam), 969t–972t
Rozerem (ramelteon), 995t
rufinamide (Banzel), 956t, 969t–972t, 981
Ruxience (rituximab), 236t–238t, 252t–257t, 257
ruxolitinib (Jakafi), 211t, 219–221, 220t
   action, 220
   adverse effects, 221
   contraindications, 221
   nursing implications, 221
   pharmacokinetics, 220
   use, 220
Ryanodex (dantrolene sodium), 983t, 985t–986t, 987
Rybelsus, 684
Rytary (Levodopa–carbidopa), 871t–872t
Rythmodan (disopyramide), 508t, 510
Rythmol (propafenone), 508t, 510

S

Sabril (vigabatrin), 956t, 962t–963t, 964
sacubitril/valsartan, 555–557, 556t, 556b, 557b
Safinamide (Xadago), 871t–872t
Safyral, 110t–111t
Saizen (somatropin), 800t–801t
Salazopyrin (sulfasalazine), 365t, 370t, 372
salicylates, 290t, 291–294, 292t, 1107
   abnormal kidney function and hepatic impairment, 292
   administration of, 293
   adverse effects, 293
   contraindications, 293
   drug interactions, 293, 293b
   intoxication, 294
   mechanism of action, 291
   overdose treatment, 294
   patient teaching guidelines, 294, 294b
   pharmacokinetics, 291
   therapeutic effects, 293
   toxicity, 294
   use, 291–293
salicylic acid (AcNesic, Bensal HP, Gordofilm, Clear Away One Step Wart Remover, Neutrogena Oil-Free Acne Wash), 1116t–1117t
salicylism, 293
saline cathartics, 724t, 728, 729t, 730
salmeterol (Serevent), 605t, 608t, 610
Salmonella, 275b
Salmonella infections, 742
salsalate, 290t, 292t, 294
Sama HC (hydrocortisone), 320t–323t
Sanctura XR (trospium chloride), 887t
Sancuso (granisetron), 708t, 714t
SandIMMUNE (cyclosporine), 211t, 212, 215–219, 225
Sandostatin (octreotide acetate), 738t, 741–742, 741t, 799t, 806t, 807–808
Sandostatin LAR (octreotide acetate), 799t, 806t, 807–808
Sandoz Almotriptan (almotriptan), 945t
Sandoz Colchicine (colchicine), 292t, 306–307, 307t, 308b
SANDOZ D-Forte (ergocalciferol), 816t
SANDOZ Hydrocortisone (hydrocortisone), 320t–323t
Sandoz Minocycline (minocycline hydrochloride), 366t
SANDOZ Mometasone (mometasone), 320t–323t
SANDOZ Prednisolone (prednisolone), 320t–323t
SANDOZ Rivastigmine (rivastigmine), 855t, 859, 859t
Sandoz Silodosin (silodosin), 128t, 129
Sandoz Tacrolimus (tacrolimus), 211t, 212, 215b, 216, 218–219
SANDOZ Trandolapril (trandolapril), 485t
Sandoz-Alfuzosin (alfuzosin), 128t, 129
Sandoz-Indomethacin (indomethacin), 290t, 297, 302–305, 302t–303t, 304b
Sandoz-Linezolid (linezolid), 381t–382t
Sandoz-Rosuvastatin (rosuvastatin), 164t, 166t
Sandoz-Tamsulosin (tamsulosin), 119t, 128, 128t
Saphris (asenapine), 1031t, 1039t–1040t, 1042
saquinavir mesylate, 435–438, 436t–437t
Saracoll (bupivacaine), 912t, 915
Sarafem (fluoxetine), 1013
sarecycline (Seysara), 365t–366t, 368
sargramostim (Leukine), 185–186, 185t, 236t–238t, 248b, 264t
sarilumab, 411t, 412–413
SARS-CoV$_2$, 79
saturated solution of potassium iodide (SSKI), 787t, 788–789
Savaysa (edoxaban), 140t–142t, 148–149
Savella (milnacipran), 1009t, 1019
Savella Titration Pack (milnacipran), 1009t, 1019
saw palmetto, 59t–61t
saxagliptin (Onglyza), 754t, 772, 772t
Saxenda (liraglutide), 679t, 683–685, 683t, 754t, 775, 775t
scabicides, 463, 464t, 471–472, 471t
scabies, 463, 471–472, 471t
schizophrenia, 1030–1031
Schlemm's canal, 1076f
sclera, 1076
scopolamine (Transderm Scop), 708t, 717t, 718, 879t, 882t, 883
Scopolamine (Transderm Scop; Buscopan), 882t
Scopolamine hydrobromide, 881t
seasonal affective disorder (SAD), 1008b, 1021
Seasonale, 110t–111t
Seasonique, 110t–111t
second messenger, 845–846
secondary adrenal cortical insufficiency, 828–829
secondary adrenal insufficiency, 828
second-generation "atypical" antipsychotics, 1038–1043
   abnormal kidney function, 1041
   adverse effects, 1040
   contraindications, 1040–1041
   dose usage, 1038–1040
   drug interactions, 1041b
   hepatic impairment, 1040
   mechanisms of action, 1038
   nursing implications, 1041
   patient teaching guidelines, 1041b
   pharmacokinetics, 1038
   preventing interactions, 1041
   therapeutic effects, 1037
second-generation H_1 receptor antagonists
   abnormal kidney function, 594
   acrivastine, 590t, 595–596, 595t
   action, 594
   administration of, 595
   adverse effects, 595
   azelastin, 590t, 595–596, 595t
   cetirizine, 590t, 594–597, 595t
   contraindications, 595
   dosage information, 594, 595t
   drug interactions, 595
   in hepatic impairment patients, 594
   lactation, 594
   loratadine, 595t, 596
   nursing implications, 595
   olopatadine, 590t, 595–596, 595t
   patient teaching guidelines, 593b, 595
   pharmacokinetics, 594
   pregnancy, 594
   reproduction, 594
   therapeutic effects, 595
   uses, 594–595
Sectral (acebutolol), 511t, 512
Secuado (asenapine), 1031t, 1039t–1040t
sedative–hypnotics, 995t
sedatives, 993
seizure, 954
   clinical considerations and manifestations, 954–955
   overview of, 954–955
seizure disorders
   AMPA glutamate receptor antagonist, 978
   barbiturates, 955
   benzodiazepines, 959
   histone deacetylase inhibitor, 974
   hydantoins, 964
   magnesium sulfate, 977
   nursing process, 990b
   tetrazole alkyl carbamate derivative, 980
Select 1/35, 110t–111t
selective COX-2 inhibitor, 290t, 305–306
   abnormal kidney function and hepatic impairment, 305
   administration of, 306
   adverse effects, 306
   contraindications, 306
   description, 305
   mechanism of action, 305
   nursing implications, 306
   patient teaching guidelines, 306, 306b
   pharmacokinetics, 305
   preventing interactions, 306
   therapeutic effects, 306
selective estrogen receptor modulator bazedoxifene (Duavee), 101
selective norepinephrine reuptake inhibitors, 1047t, 1056t
selective serotonin reuptake inhibitors (SSRIs), 1009t, 1013–1017
   abnormal kidney function, 1016
   adverse effects, 1016
   contraindications, 1016
   dose usage, 1015–1016
   hepatic impairment, 1016
   mechanisms of action, 1015
   nursing implications, 1016–1017
   pharmacokinetics, 1013–1015
   PMS and PMDD, 101
   preventing interactions, 1016
   sex and, 24
   therapeutic effects, 1017
selegiline, 1021
selegiline (Eldepryl, Emsam, Zelapar), 871t–872t, 875, 1020t
selegiline hydrochloride (Emsam, Zelapar), 1009t
selenium sulfide (Anti-Dandruff), 1116t–1117t

self-antigens, 209
Selzentry (maraviroc), 440–441, 440b
semaglutide (Ozempic), 679t, 684, 775–776, 775t
Semprex-D (acrivastine), 590t, 595–596, 595t
Semprex-D (pseudoephedrine), 590t, 595–596, 595t
senna preparations (Senokot), 724t, 729t
Senokot (senna preparations), 724t, 729t
Sensorcaine (bupivacaine), 912t, 915
septic shock, 276, 325, 542, 546b
Septra (trimethoprim-sulfamethoxazole), 365t, 367, 369, 371
serdexmethylphenidate and dexmethylphenidate (Azstarys), 1053t, 1054–1055
serdexmethylphenidate-dexmethylphenidate (Azstarys), 1047t
Serevent (salmeterol), 605t, 608t, 610
Serevent Diskhaler Disk (salmeterol), 608t
Serevent Diskus (salmeterol), 608t
Sernivo (betamethasone, dipropionate), 1112t
serology, 278
Seromycin (cycloserine), 391–392
Serophene (clomiphene citrate), 84, 85t
Seroquel (quetiapine), 1009t, 1024t, 1025–1026, 1031t, 1039t–1040t, 1042
Seroquel XR (quetiapine), 1024t, 1031t, 1039t–1040t, 1042
Serostim (somatropin), 799t–801t
serotonergic agents, 946
serotonin receptor antagonists, 708t, 712–713, 714t
serotonin syndrome, 946
serotonin-norepinephrine reuptake inhibitors (SNRIs), 77, 1009t, 1017–1019
  abnormal kidney function, 1018
  adverse effects, 1018–1019
  contraindications, 1019
  dose usage, 1017–1018
  hepatic impairment, 1018
  mechanisms of action, 1017
  nursing implications, 1019
  patient teaching guidelines, 1019
  pharmacokinetics, 1017
  PMS and PMDD, 101
  preventing interactions, 1019
  therapeutic effects, 1019
Serratia species, 275b, 353
  S. marcescens, 275b
sertraline (Zoloft), 1009t, 1017, 1036
serum creatinine, 360
serum drug levels, 19
serum half-life, 19
serum sickness, 588–589
severe acute respiratory syndrome (SARS), 406b
severe respiratory syndrome coronavirus 2 (SARS-CoV-2)
  acute, 410–411, 411t
  outpatient management, 411t, 414
sevoflurane (SoJourn, Ultane), 922t–923t, 925
sex (gender), 24
sex hormones, 260
Seysara (sarecycline), 365t–366t, 368
Shigella, 275b
Shingrix (herpes zoster), 194b, 195t–199t
shock
  acute, 540–541, 540f
  adrenergic receptors (see adrenergic drugs)
  anaphylactic, 541, 546, 546b
  assessment, 548b
  cardiogenic, 540, 541t, 542, 546b
  clinical considerations, 540–541
  clinical manifestations, 541
  compensated, 541
  decompensated, 541
  development of, 540, 540f
  distributive, 540, 541t
  drugs, 543t
  evaluation, 548b

hemodynamic profiles, 541t
hypovolemic, 319, 541t, 546–547, 546b
irreversible, 541
management, 541
nursing interventions, 548b
nursing process, 548b
obstructive, 540, 541t
outcomes of therapy, 548b
patient teaching guidelines, 545, 546b
septic, 319, 325
stages of, 541
treatment, 541
types, 540
Shopko Athletes Foot (clotrimazole), 1115t
short-acting insulins, 755, 756t–757t
sibutramine, 678–679
signal transduction, 845
  for adrenergic beta receptor, 846f
Signifor (pasireotide), 799t, 808–809, 833–834, 835t
Signifor LAR (pasireotide), 799t, 806t, 808–809, 833–834, 835t
Siklos (hydroxyurea), 236t–245t, 238
sildenafil (Viagra, Revatio, AG-Sildenafil, Jamp-Sildenafil), 119t, 123–125, 124t
Silenor (doxepin), 1009t, 1012t
silodosin (Rapaflo), 119t
silodosin (Rapaflo, Sandoz Silodosin), 128t, 129
Silvadene (silver sulfadiazine), 365t, 370t, 372, 1113t
silver sulfadiazine (Silvadene), 365t, 370t, 372, 1113t
Simbrinza (brinzolamide and brimonidine), 1082t–1084t
Simponi (golimumab), 211t
Simponi Aria (golimumab), 211t
Simulect (basiliximab), 211t, 224–225
simvastatin, 96b
simvastatin (Zocor, FloLipid), 164t, 166t, 167, 754t, 778t, 779
Sinemet (Levodopa-carbidopa), 871t–872t
Singulair (montelukast), 617–619, 618t
sinoatrial node modulators, 559–560, 560t, 560b
sinus bradycardia, 505b
sinus rhythm, 504
sinus tachycardia, 505b
sinusitis, 574
Sinutab Sinus Allergy Maximum Strength Caplets, 583t
Sinuva (mometasone), 318t, 320t–323t
sirolimus (Rapamune), 211t, 215b, 217t, 219
sitagliptin, 777
sitagliptin phosphate (Januvia), 754t, 767b, 771–772, 772t
Sitavig (acyclovir), 1115t
Sivextro (tedizolid phosphate), 381t–382t, 385
skin disorders, 1110–1117
  acne vulgaris, 1117–1118
  assessment, 1122b
  corticosteroid drug therapy, 1110
  drug therapy
    antibacterial, 1110–1117
    antifungal, 1114
    antihistamines, 1115
    antiviral, 1114
    emollients and moisturizers, 1117
    enzymes, 1114
    immunosuppressant, 1114–1115
    local anesthetic agents, 1117
    retinoids, 1119–1121, 1119t
  evaluation, 1122b
  herbal preparations for, 1117, 1117b
  nursing interventions, 1122b
  nursing process, 1122b
  outcomes of therapy, 1122b
  patient teaching guidelines for, 1111b
skin, drug administration to, 45t–46t, 57

Skytrofa (Lonapegsomatropin), 802
sleep and insomnia
  assessment, 1005b
  benzodiazepines (see benzodiazepines)
  dual receptor antagonists, 1003–1004
  evaluation, 1005b
  nursing interventions, 1005b
  outcomes of therapy, 1005b
  sedative hypnotics (see nonbenzodiazepine sedative hypnotics)
sleep apnea, 676b, 678
Slo-Niacin (niacin), 164t, 174–175, 174t
smoking, 523
  deterrent, 1061t
Soaanz (torsemide), 631t–632t, 635
social anxiety disorder (SAD), 994b
Sod Phos Fort (prednisolone), 320t–323t
sodium bicarbonate, 518, 668
sodium glucose cotransporter 2 (SGLT2) inhibitors
  abnormal kidney function, 776
  administration, 777
  adverse effects, 776–777
  contraindications, 777
  in hepatic impairment patients, 776
  in lactation, 776
  mechanism of action, 776
  nursing implications, 777, 777b
  patient teaching guidelines, 777, 777b
  pharmacokinetics, 776
  therapeutic effects, 777
  use, 776, 776t
sodium iodide ^{131}I (Iodotope, i3odine Max, Hicon), 787t, 789
sodium nitroprusside (Nitropress, Nipride), 482t, 496t–498t
sodium oxybate (Xyrem), 1047t, 1055, 1056t
sodium phosphate (betamethasone), 320t–323t, 823–824, 823t
sodium succinate, 605t
sodium-glucose cotransporter 2 inhibitors (SGLT2i), 562t, 564
sofosbuvir (Sovaldi), 426–427, 426t
SoJourn (Sevoflurane), 922t
solid neoplasms, 234
solid organ transplantation, rejection reactions with, 210
solifenacin succinate (Vesicare), 879t, 881t, 887t, 888
Solifenacin succinate (Vesicare; ACT-Solifenacin, APO-Solifenacin, JAMP-Solifenacin, Vesicare), 887t
Solodyn (minocycline hydrochloride), 365t
Soltamox (tamoxifen), 236t–238t, 260, 261t–263t
Solu-CORTEF (hydrocortisone), 830–832, 830t, 832b
Solu-Cortef (hydrocortisone), 318t, 320t–323t
Solu-Medrol (methylprednisolone sodium succinate), 320t–323t, 616t
Soluspan (betamethasone), 318t, 320t–323t
Soma (carisoprodol), 983t, 984, 985t–986t
somatic nervous system, 844f
  organization of, 845f
somatic pain, 892
somatropin (Genotropin, Genotropin MiniQuick, Humatrope, Norditropin FlexPro, Nutropin AQ NuSpin 10, Serostim, Omnitrope, Genotropin GoQuick, Norditropin, Nordiflex, Norditropin Simplex, Nutropin AQ NuSpin, Nutropin AQ pen, Saizen, Serostim), 799, 800t–801t
Somatuline Autogel (lanreotide), 806t
Somatuline Depot (lanreotide), 799t, 806t, 808
Somavert (pegvisomant), 799t–801t, 803
sorafenib (NexAVAR), 236t–238t, 248b, 252t–257t, 259
sorbitol, 723, 724t, 732t, 733

Sorilux (calcipotriene), 1116t–1117t
Sorine (sotalol), 511t, 513, 513t, 515
sotalol (Betapace, Sorine, Sotylize), 511t, 513, 513t, 515
Sotylize (sotalol), 511t, 513, 513t, 515
Sovaldi (sofosbuvir), 426–427, 426t
spasticity, 954
Spectazole (econazole), 447t
spinal anesthesia, 911, 917
spinal cord injury, 325
    clinical manifestations, 983
    drug therapy, 983
    overview of, 983
    skeletal muscle, classes of, 983, 983t
spinosad (Natroba), 464t, 471t, 472
Spiriva (tiotropium), 605t, 611–612, 611t
Spiriva HandiHaler (tiotropium bromide), 881t–882t, 883
Spiriva Respimat (tiotropium bromide), 882t, 883
spironolactone (Aldactone), 482t, 496t–498t, 554t, 563, 631t, 637–640, 638t, 639b, 641t
Sporanox (itraconazole), 447t, 451t–452t, 453
Sporotrichosis, 445, 447
Spravato (esketamine), 927–928
Sprintec, 110t–111t
Spritam (levetiracetam), 969t–972t
Sprycel (dasatinib), 236t–238t, 252t–257t, 258
Sronyx, 110t–111t
SSKI (potassium iodide saturated solution of potassium iodide), 787t, 788–789
SSRIs. *See* selective serotonin reuptake inhibitors (SSRIs)
St. John's Wort, 59t–61t
    antidepressant, 1022b
Stable angina, 522–523, 522f
Stalevo (entacapone), 869t, 877–878, 877t
Stalevo (levodopa), 869t, 877–878
staphylococcal species nonaureus (SSNA), 386
Staphylococci, 275b, 277
Staphylococcus aureus, 275, 278
    description of, 275
    methicillin-resistant, 278b, 385, 386, 396
    Staphylococcus epidermidis, 386
Staphylococcus pneumoniae, 386
Staphylococcus species, non-aureus (SSNA), 275
Starlix (nateglinide), 754t, 767b, 770, 770t
Statex (morphine sulfate), 896b–897t
statins, 164–167, 166t
status asthmaticus, 606
status epilepticus, 955
Staxyn (vardenafil), 124t
steady-state concentration, 19
Stelara (ustekinumab), 211t, 227
stem cells, 179, 184
    transplantation, 210
Stendra (avanafil), 119t, 124t, 125
steroids, 314
Stevens–Johnson syndrome, 957, 974
Stimate (DDAVP), 799t, 803–804, 804t, 804b
Stimate (desmopressin), 799t, 803–804, 804t, 804b
stimulant abuse
    central nervous system, 1067
stimulant cathartics, 724t, 728, 729t, 730
stimulants, 1048–1049. *See also* central nervous
stiripentol (Diacomit), 956t, 969t–972t, 983
Stivarga (regorafenib), 236t–238t, 252t–257t, 259
stomatitis, 248b
stool softeners, 724, 727
Strattera (atomoxetine), 1047t, 1055, 1056t
Streptococci, 275b, 277
Streptococcus pneumoniae penicillin-resistant, 278b
Streptococcus pyogenes, 275
streptogramins, 384–385
streptomycin, 353t, 355t, 357, 391, 400
streptozocin (Zanosar), 236t–245t
stress dosage therapy, 328

stress response, 314
stress ulcers, 692, 696
Stromectol (ivermectin), 464t, 469–470, 470t
strong iodine solution (Lugol's solution), 788–789
Strongyloides stercoralis, 470
strongyloidiasis, 470
subclinical hyperthyroidism, 784
subcutaneous injections
    absorption after, 17
    advantages and disadvantages of, 45t–46t
    sites for, 48–50, 49f–50f
Sublimaze (fentanyl), 922t, 932, 932t
Sublocade (buprenorphine), 896t–897t, 904t, 1061t–1063t, 1066
Suboxone (buprenorphine/naloxone), 904t, 1062t–1063t
Suboxone (naltrexone-buprenorphine), 1061t
substance dependence, 1059
substance misuse and dependence, 1061t
    assessment, 1068b
    central nervous system depressant, 1061
    central nervous system stimulant abuse, 1067
    characteristics, 1059b
    clinical considerations, 1060
    clinical manifestations, 1060
    drug therapy, 1060–1061
        benzodiazepines (*see* benzodiazepines)
    enzyme inhibitors for maintenance, 1064–1065
    evolution, 1068b
    nursing interventions, 1068b
    nursing process, 1068b
    opioid use disorder, 1066
    outcomes of theraphy, 1068b
    overview of, 1059–1061
    physical dependence, 1059
    psychoactive substance use, 1067
    psychological dependence, 1059
    therapy, 1060–1061
        general approach, 1060
    tolerance, 1059–1060
substance P
    abnormal kidney function, 716
    action, 715
    administration, 716
    adverse effects, 716
    contraindications, 716
    in hepatic impairment patients, 716
    lactation, 716
    in mediating acute chemotherapy-induced nausea and vomiting, 715
    netupitant/palonosetron, 708t, 715t, 716
    nursing implications, 716
    patient teaching guidelines, 716
    pharmacokinetics, 715
    pregnancy, 716
    preventing interactions, 716, 716b
    reproduction, 716
    rolapitant, 708t, 715t, 717
    therapeutic effects, 716
    uses, 715–716, 715t
substantia nigra, 868
Subsys (fentanyl), 894t, 896t–897t, 902, 922t, 932
Subutex (buprenorphine), 894t, 896t–897t
Subvenite (lamotrigine), 969t–972t
succimer (or dimercaptosuccinic acid), 668
succinimide, 956t
succinimides, 973
    adverse effects, 973
    contraindications, 973
    dose usage, 973
    mechanisms of action, 973
    nursing implications, 973
    patient teaching guidelines, 973b
    pharmacokinetics, 973
    preventing interactions, 973
    therapeutic effects, 973

Succinylcholine (Anectine, Quelicin, Quelicin Chloride), 922t, 929t, 931
sucralfate (Carafate), 692t, 701t, 702
Sudafed (pseudoephedrine), 575–578, 575t
sufentanil (Dsuvia), 932
Sugammadex (Bridion), 930
Sular (nisoldipine), 482t, 492t, 494
sulconazole (Exelderm), 447t
sulfacetam, 1090t
sulfacetamide, 1091t
sulfadiazine, 365t, 370t, 371–372
sulfamate-substituted monosaccharide, 949
sulfamate-substituted monosaccharides, 956t, 979
    adverse effects, 980
    contraindications, 980
    dose usage, 980
    drug interactions, 980b
    mechanisms of action, 980
    nursing implications, 980
    patient teaching guidelines, 980b
    pharmacokinetics, 979–980
    preventing interactions, 980
    therapeutic effects, 980
sulfamethoxazole, 96b
Sulfamylon (mafenide acetate), 365t, 370t
sulfasalazine (Azulfidine, PMS-Sulfasalazine, Salazopyrin), 365t, 370t, 372
sulfonamide, 956t, 973
    abnormal kidney function, 974
    adverse effects, 974
    contraindications, 974
    dose usage, 974
    hepatic impairment, 974
    mechanisms of action, 974
    nursing implications, 974
    patient teaching, 974
    pharmacokinetics, 974
    preventing interactions, 974
    therapeutic effects, 974
sulfonamides, 365, 365t, 368–372, 370t
sulfonylurea, 777
sulfonylureas, 764–765, 765t
sulindac (Apo-Sulin, Teva-Sulindac), 290t, 302t–303t, 305
sulphonamides
    abnormal kidney function, 370
    administration of, 371
    adverse effects, 370–371
    assessment, 374
    contraindications, 370
    evaluation, 374
    in hepatic impairment patients, 370
    nursing implications, 371
    nursing interventions, 374
    nursing process, 374b
    outcomes of therapy, 374
    para-aminobenzoic acid, 369
    patient teaching guidelines, 371, 371b
    pharmacokinetics, 369
    preventing interactions, 371, 371b
    therapeutic effects, 371
    use of, 369–370
sumatriptan (Imitrex, Onzetra Xsail), 944, 945t
sumatriptan and naproxen (Treximet, Suvexx), 945t
sumatriptan–naproxen sodium (Treximet), 946
sunitinib (Sutent), 236t–238t, 248b, 252t–257t, 259
superficial mycoses
    miscellaneous antifungal agents, 457–459, 458t, 458b, 459b
Superinfections, 338
Supeudol (Oxycodone), 894t, 896t–897t, 902–903, 902t
suppositories
    rectal, 42t–43t
    vaginal, 42t–43t
Supprelin LA (histrelin), 799t, 806

Suprane (desflurane), 922t–923t, 924–925
Suprax (cefixime), 342t–344t
surfactant laxative(s), 724, 727
susceptibility, 282
susceptible organisms, 282
suspensions, 42t–43t
Sustol (granisetron), 708t, 714t
Sutent (sunitinib), 236t–238t, 248b, 252t–257t, 259
Suvexx (sumatriptan and naproxen), 945t
suvorexant (Belsomra), 995t, 1003t
Syeda, 110t–111t
Symbicort (budesonide/formoterol), 621
Symbyax (olanzapine-fluoxetine), 1009t, 1024t
Symlin (pramlintide acetate), 773, 773t, 774b
sympathetic nervous system (SNS), 844–848
    adrenergic receptors, 847–848
    alpha and beta receptors, 847b
    blood pressure regulation by, 478
    neurotransmitters, 847
sympatholytic drugs, 499
sympatholytics, 1047t, 1056t
Sympazan (clobazam), 956t, 960t
Synacthen Depot (cosyntropin), 800t–801t
Synagis (palivizumab), 420t, 421
Synarel (nafarelin), 799t, 806t, 807
Syndros (dronabinol), 708t, 717t, 718
Synercid (quinupristin-dalfopristin), 381t–382t, 384–385
synergism, 22
synthetic conjugated (conjugated estrogens), 101–105, 103t
synthetic vitamins, 657b
Synthroid (levothyroxine), 787t, 790–792, 791t, 792b, 793b
syringes, 48
systemic lupus erythematosus, 589

T
T cells, 209–211, 216, 226–227
    blockage, 227
T Tri-Sprintec, 110t–111t
tablets, 42t–43t
Tabloid (thioguanine), 236t–245t
tachydysrhythmias, 504, 506
tacrolimus (Prograf, Astagraf XL, Envarsus XR, Prograf; Advagraf, Envarsus, Prograf, Sandoz Tacrolimus), 211t, 212, 215b, 216, 217t, 218–219
tacrolimus (Protopic), 1116t–1117t
tadalafil (Cialis, Adcirca), 119t, 124t, 125
Tafinlar (dabrafenib), 236t–238t, 252t–257t, 258
tafluprost (Zioptan), 1082t–1084t, 1084
Tagamet (cimetidine), 692t, 693, 695–698, 696t
Taltz (ixekizumab), 211t, 227
Talwin (pentazocine), 894t, 903–904, 904t
Tambocor (flecainide), 508t, 510
Tamiflu (oseltamivir), 422t, 423–424
tamoxifen (Soltamox, Apo-Tamox, Mylan-Tamoxifen, Nolvadex-D, Teva-Tamoxifen, PMSTamoxifen)), 236t–238t, 260, 261t–263t
tamsulosin (Flomax, APO-Tamsulosin CR, Flomax CR, Sandoz-Tamsulosin), 119t, 128, 128t
Tanzeum (albiglutide), 754t
Tapazole (methimazole), 787t, 788
TaperDex 6 Day (dexamethasone), 318t, 320t–323t, 324–325, 328–329
TaperDex 7 Day (dexamethasone), 318t, 320t–323t, 324–325, 328–329
TaperDex 12 Day (dexamethasone), 318t, 320t–323t, 324–325, 328–329
tapeworms, 463
tardive dyskinesia, 1034
Tarka (verapamil), 482t, 495t–496t
Taro-Etodolac (etodolac), 290t, 302t–303t, 304
TARO-Mometasone (mometasone), 320t–323t

TARO-Tofacitinib (tofacitinib), 211t, 221
Taro-Warfarin (warfarin), 141t–142t
TARO-Zoledronic Acid (zoledronic acid), 820t–821t
Tasigna (nilotinib), 236t–238t, 252t–257t, 258–259
tasimelteon (Hetlioz, Hetlioz LQ), 995t, 1002
Tasmar (tolcapone), 869t, 876t
taxanes, 236t–245t, 239, 249–250
Taxotere (docetaxel), 236t–245t, 249, 260–263
tazarotene, 1119t, 1121
Tazicef (ceftazidime), 342t–344t
tazobactam for injection (Piperacillin/tazobactam), 336t–337t
Td Absorbed (tetanus and diphtheria toxoids (adult type) (Td)), 195t–199t
Tdap vaccine booster, 194b
TDVax (tetanus and diphtheria toxoids (adult type) (Td)), 195t–199t
tears, 1076
tedizolid (Sivextro), 381t–382t, 385
tedizolid phosphate (Sivextro), 381t–382t, 385
Teflaro (ceftaroline), 335t, 341, 342t–344t
tegaserod (Zelnorm), 724t, 732t, 733
Tegretol (carbamazepine), 956t, 966, 967t
TEGretol-SR (carbamazepine), 956t, 967t
Tekturna (aliskiren), 482t, 494, 496t–498t
telavancin (Vibativ), 381t–382t, 385
telmisartan (Micardis), 482t, 490t, 491, 495t–496t
temazepam (Restoril), 87b, 995t
temsirolimus (Torisel), 236t–238t, 252t–257t, 258
tenecteplase (TNKase), 140t, 155t, 157
teniposide (Vumon), 236t–238t
Tenivac (tetanus and diphtheria toxoids (adult type) (Td)), 195t–199t
tenofovir disoproxil fumarate (Stribild), 432–433
tenoretic, 495t–496t
Tenormin (atenolol), 482t, 524t, 529–531, 530t, 531b
tension headaches
    clinical manifestations, 937
    treatment of, 938
tension-type headache, 936
Tepadina (thiotepa), 236t–245t
Teprotumumab, 790
teratogenic drugs, 87, 87b, 87f
Terazol 3 (terconazole), 447t
Terazol 7 (terconazole), 447t
terazosin (APO-Terazosin, PMS-Terazosin, Hytrin), 128t, 129, 482t, 496t–498t
terbinafine, 96b
terbinafine (Lamisil), 458t, 459, 1115t
terbutaline, 605t, 608t, 610, 850
terbutaline sulfate, 93, 93t
terconazole (Terazol), 447t
teriparatide (Forteo), 823t, 824
Tessalon (benzonatate), 574t, 579, 579t
Testim (testosterone cypionate), 120t
Testim (testosterone enanthate), 120t
testosterone, 120, 120t
    administration, 121
    adverse effects, 121
    body effects, 119b
    contraindications, 121
    danazol, 119t–120t, 122
    drug interactions, 121, 121b
    mechanism of action, 120
    methyltestosterone, 120t
    nursing implications, 121
    patient teaching guidelines, 121
    pharmacokinetics, 120
    route and dosage information, 120, 120t
    therapeutic effects, 121
testosterone cypionate (Depo-Testosterone, Andriol, Androderm, Axiron, Testim), 120t

testosterone enanthate (Xyosted; Andriol, Androderm, Axiron, Testim), 120t
testosterone gel (AndroGel 1%), 120t
testosterone pellets, 120t
testosterone transdermal systems (Androderm, Andriol, Androderm, AndroGel, Axiron), 120t
tetanus and diphtheria toxoids (adult type) (Td) (TDVax, Tenivac; Td Absorbed), 195t–199t
tetanus immune globulin (HyperTET S/D), 200t–201t
tetanus, reduced diphtheria, acellular pertussis (Tdap) (Adacel, Boostrix), 195t–199t
tetanus toxoid, 195t–199t
tetanus–diphtheria–pertussis (Tdap) vaccine, 92
tetany, 814, 817
Tetcaine (tetracaine), 1078t–1079t
Tetracaine (Altacaine, Ametop), 912t, 917
tetracaine (Altacaine, Tetcaine, TetraVisc), 1078t–1079t
tetracycline (Achromycin V), 87b, 365t, 692t, 693, 697, 701t, 702
    abnormal kidney function and hepatic impairment, 367
    administration of, 367
    adverse effects, 367–368
    assessment, 374
    contraindications, 367
    dairy products interaction with, 21–22
    drug interactions, 367, 367b
    evaluation, 374
    nursing implications, 367–368
    nursing interventions, 374
    nursing process, 374b
    outcomes of therapy, 374
    patient teaching guidelines, 368, 368b
    pharmacokinetics, 367
    therapeutic effects, 367
TetraVisc (tetracaine), 1078t–1079t
tetrazole alkyl carbamate derivative, 956t, 980
    adverse effects, 981
    contraindications, 981
    dose usage, 981
    mechanisms of action, 981
    nursing implications, 981
    patient teaching guidelines, 981b
    pharmacokinetics, 981
    preventing interactions, 981
    therapeutic effects, 981
TEVA Azathioprine (azathioprine), 211t, 212, 216
Teva- Rosuvastatin (rosuvastatin), 164t, 166t
TEVA Selegiline (selegiline hydrochloride), 871t–872t
TEVA-Budesonide (budesonide), 320t–323t
Teva-Cefadroxil (cefadroxil), 342t–344t
Teva-Cephalexin (cephalexin), 336t–337t
TEVA-Chlorpromazine (chlorpromazine hydrochloride), 951t
Teva-Clindamycin (clindamycin hydrochloride), 381t–382t
Teva-Codeine (narcotic codeine), 574t, 578–580, 579t
Teva-Combo Sterinebs (ipratropium/albuterol), 621
Teva-Doxazosin (Cardura), 128t, 129
Teva-Flutamide (flutamide), 236t–238t, 261t–263t
TEVA-Fluticasone (fluticasone), 320t–323t
TEVA-Fulvestrant (fulvestrant), 236t–238t, 260, 261t–263t
Teva-Imatinib (imatinib), 236t–238t, 252, 252t–257t, 258–259
Teva-Ketoconazole, 451t–452t, 453
Teva-Ketoconazole (ketoconazole), 835t
TEVA-Levocarbidopa (Levodopa–carbidopa), 871t–872t
TEVA-Mometasone (mometasone), 320t–323t
Teva-Morphine SR (morphine sulfate), 896t–897t

Teva-Nabumetone (nabumetone), 290t, 298t–299t, 300, 302t–303t, 305
TEVA-Prednisolone (prednisolone), 320t–323t
TEVA-PredniSONE (prednisone), 317, 318t, 320t–323t, 324–326, 328–329
TEVAPropofol (propofol), 926t
TEVA-Rasagiline (rasagiline), 871t–872t
Teva-Sulindac (sulindac), 290t, 302t–303t, 305
Teva-Tamoxifen (tamoxifen), 236t–238t, 260, 261t–263t
Teveten (eprosartan mesylate), 754t
Thalitone (chlorothiazide), 631t, 635–637, 636t, 637b
Theo-24 (short-acting theophylline, theophylline), 605t, 612, 612t
Theochron, 605t, 612, 612t
Theochron (long-acting theophylline, theophylline), 679t
Theolair (short-acting theophylline), 612t
theophylline, 22
theophylline (Elixophyllin, Theo-24, Theochron, minophylline, Theochron), 605t, 612–614, 613b
Theraflu Flu, Nighttime Severe Cold & Cough Hot Liquid Powder, 583t
therapeutic effects. *See specific drug, therapeutic effects of*
therapeutic index, 353–354, 564–565
thiamine (vitamin B$_1$), 654t–656t
  administration, 659
  adverse effects, 659
  contraindications, 659
  nursing implications, 659
  patient teaching guidelines for, 657b, 659
  pharmacokinetics and use, 659
  therapeutic effects, 659
thiazide diuretics, 554t, 563
  abnormal kidney function, 635
  action, 635
  administration of, 636
  adverse effects, 635
  chlorothiazide, 631t, 636t, 637
  chlorthalidone, 631t, 636t, 637
  contraindications, 636
  dosage information, 636t
  drug interactions, 636, 637b
  in hepatic impairment patients, 635
  herbs, 636
  hydrochlorothiazide, 631t, 635–637, 636t
  indapamide, 631t, 636t, 637
  lactation, 635
  metolazone, 631t, 636t, 637
  nursing implications, 636–637
  patient teaching guidelines, 634b, 637
  pharmacokinetics, 635
  pregnancy, 635
  prototype, 631t
  reproduction, 635
  therapeutic effects, 636
  use, 635
thiazide-like diuretics, 754t, 778–779
thiazolidinediones, 754t, 769–771, 769t, 774, 777–778
thioguanine (Tabloid), 236t–245t
thioridazine, 1031t, 1033t, 1036
thiotepa (Tepadina), 236t–245t
thiothixene, 1031t, 1033t, 1038
third-generation H$_1$ receptor antagonists
  abnormal kidney function, 597
  action, 596
  administration of, 597
  adverse effects, 597
  contraindications, 597
  desloratadine, 590t, 596–597, 596t
  dosage ranges, 596, 596t
  drug interactions, 597, 597b

fexofenadine, 590t, 596–600, 596t, 597b
  in hepatic impairment patients, 597
  herbs and foods, 597
  lactation, 596
  levocetirizine, 590t, 596–597, 596t
  nursing implications, 597
  patient teaching guidelines, 593b, 597
  pharmacokinetics, 596
  pregnancy, 596
  reproduction, 596
  therapeutic effects, 597
  uses, 596–597
thorazine (chlorpromazine), 708t–709t, 710
threadworm infections, 463
throat lozenges, 42t–43t
thrombocytopenia, 247
thrombogenesis, 138
thrombolysis, 138
thrombolytic drugs, 155–157, 535–536
  abnormal kidney function and hepatic impairment, 155
  administration of, 156
  adverse effects, 156
  alteplase, 140t, 155–157, 155t
  contraindications, 156
  drug interactions, 156, 156b
  mechanism of action, 155
  nursing implications, 156
  pharmacokinetics, 155
  preventing interactions, 156–157
  reversal of, 158
  tenecteplase, 140t, 155t, 157
  therapeutic effects, 143
thrombosis, 138
thromboxane A$_2$ inhibitors, 154
thrombus, 138
thymoglobulin (antithymocyte globulin (ATG)), 222t–224t, 224, 226
thyrogen (thyrotropin alfa), 799t–801t, 803
thyroid disorders, 24
  body systems, 785t–786t
  hyperthyroidism (*see* hyperthyroidism)
  hypothyroidism (*see* hypothyroidism)
  nursing process, 794b
thyroid drugs, 787t, 790–793
  abnormal kidney function, 791
  administration of, 792
  adverse effects, 791–792
  contraindications, 791–792
  drugs, 791t
  in hepatic impairment patients, 791
  in lactation, 791
  mechanism of action, 790
  nursing implications, 792–793
  patient teaching guidelines, 792–793, 793b
  pharmacokinetics, 790
  in pregnancy patients, 791
  preventing interactions, 792, 792b
  therapeutic effects, 792
  uses, 790–791
thyroid eye disease (TED), 790
  clinical presentation, 790
  medication, 790
  treatment for, 790
thyroid gland
  physiology, 783–784, 783f
  thyroxine, 783
thyroid replacement therapy, 786
thyroid storm, 784
thyroiditis, 784
thyroid-releasing hormone (TRH), 783, 783f
thyroid-stimulating hormone (TSH), 807
ThyroSafe (potassium iodide saturated solution of potassium iodide), 787t
ThyroShield (potassium iodide saturated solution of potassium iodide), 787t

thyrotropin alfa (Thyrogen), 799t–801t, 803
thyroxine, 783
tiagabine (Gabitril), 962t–963t, 963–964
tiagabine hydrochloride (Gabitril), 956t
Tiazac (diltiazem), 516–517, 516t, 517b, 524t, 532t, 533–534
ticagrelor (Brilinta), 140t, 151t–152t, 152–153
ticarcillin, 339
tigecycline (Tygacil), 87b, 96b, 365t–366t, 368, 381t–382t, 385–386
Tikosyn (dofetilide), 513t, 515
timolol (Blocadren), 482t, 496t–498t, 499
timolol (Combigan), 1082t
timolol (Cosopt, Cosopt PF), 1082t
timolol maleate (Betamol, Istalol, Timolol Maleate Ocudose, Timoptic, Timoptic Maleate-EX, Timoptic-XE), 1085
timolol maleate (Betamol, Istalol, Timoptic, Timoptic Ocudose, Timoptic-XE), 1082t–1084t
Timolol Maleate Ocudose (timolol maleate), 1083t–1084t, 1085
Timoptic (timolol maleate), 1082t–1084t, 1085
Timoptic Maleate-EX (timolol maleate), 1085
tinidazole, 464–465, 464t
tioconazole (Vagistat-1), 447t
tiotropium (Spiriva), 605t, 611–612, 611t
tiotropium bromide (Spiriva HandiHaler, Spiriva Respimat), 879t, 881t–882t, 883
tirofiban (Aggrastat), 151t–152t, 154, 156
Tirosint (levothyroxine), 791t
Titralac, 692t, 693, 694t
Tiuxetan (ibritumomab tiuxetan), 236t–238t, 252t–257t, 257–258
Tivorbex (indomethacin), 92–93, 93t, 290t, 297, 302–305, 302t–303t, 304b
TMP-SMZ (trimethoprim-sulfamethoxazole), 365t, 367, 369
TNKase (tenecteplase), 155t, 157
tobramycin, 353–354, 353t, 355t, 357
tocilizumab (Actemra, Actemra ACTPen), 211t, 222t–224t, 227, 411t, 412–413, 790
tocolytics, 92–93
  magnesium sulfate, 93, 93t
  nifedipine, 93, 93t
  nonsteroidal anti-inflammatory drugs, 92–93
  route and dosage information for, 92, 93t
  terbutaline sulfate, 93, 93t
tofacitinib (Xeljanz, Xeljanz XR; AURO Tofacitinib, PMS-Tofacitinib, TARO-Tofacitinib), 211t, 220t, 221
Tolazamide, 754t, 765t
Tolbutamide, 754t, 765t
tolcapone (Tasmar), 869t, 876t
tolerable upper intake level, 645
tolerance, 25, 893
tolmetin sodium, 290t
Tolsura (itraconazole), 447t, 451t–452t, 453
tolterodine tartrate (Detrol, Detrol LA; Detrol, Detrol LA, APOTolterodine, MINT-Tolterodine, MYLAN-Tolterodine), 879t, 881t, 887t, 888
Topex Topical Anesthetic (benzocaine), 916
tophi, 288–290, 290f
topical anesthesia, 911
  in children, 912b
TopiDex (dexamethasone), 318t, 320t–323t, 324–325, 328–329
topiramate, 96b
Toposar (etoposide), 236t–245t, 239, 248b
topotecan (Hycamtin, TEVATopotecan), 236t–245t, 247
Toprol XL (metoprolol), 524t, 530t, 531
toremifene (Fareston), 236t–238t, 260, 261t–263t
Torisel (temsirolimus), 236t–238t, 252t–257t, 258
torsemide (demadex), 482t

Index

torsemide (Soaanz), 631t–632t, 635
tositumomab (Bexxar), 236t–238t, 252t–257t, 258
total body water, 68–69, 70f
total intravenous anesthesia (TIVA), 924
total serum cholesterol, 162t
toxicity
    acetaminophen, 297
    aminoglycosides, 353–354, 356
    anticholinesterase agents, 863, 864t
    antimicrobial drugs, 283
    concentration, 19
    doses, 19, 19f
    irreversible anticholinesterase, 863, 864t
    isoniazid, 393
    opioids, 899b
    quinupristin–dalfopristin, 385
    salicylates, 294
toxoids, 195t–199t
    definition of, 193
    indications for, 194
    types of, 195t–199t
trade name, 4–5
Tradjenta (linagliptin), 754t, 772, 772t
tramadol (Ultram), 894t, 896t–897t, 902t, 903
trametinib (Mekinist), 236t–238t, 252t–257t, 258
Trandate (labetalol), 482t, 496t–498t
trandolapril (Mavik, Gopten), 482t, 485t, 488, 495t–496t, 754t
tranexamic acid (Cyklokapron, Lysteda, GD-Tranexamic Acid, Tranexamic Acid Injection BP), 140t, 158, 158t
tranexamic acid (TXA; Cyklokapron, Lysteda), 95
Tranexamic Acid Injection BP (tranexamic acid), 158t
Transderm Scop (scopolamine), 708t, 717t, 718, 879t, 882t, 883
transdermal formulations, 41–43
transient ischemic attacks (TIA), 154
transplantation
    antirejection agents, 217
    bone marrow, 209–210, 216, 226
    immunosuppressants use in, 209
    solid organ, 210
    stem cell, 210
    tissue and organ, 209
trastuzumab (Herceptin, Kanjinti, Ogivri), 211t, 222t–224t, 226, 236t–238t, 252t–257t, 257–258
traveler's diarrhea, 742
Treanda (bendamustine), 236t–245t
Trecator (ethionamide), 391
Trelstar (triptorelin), 236t–238t, 261t–263t, 264, 806t
Trelstar Mixject (triptorelin), 236t–238t, 261t–263t, 264, 799t, 806t, 807
Trexall (methotrexate), 236t–245t, 238, 246–247, 248b, 251b
Triaderm (triamcinolone), 320t–323t
triamcinolone (Kenalog, Kenalog 80, P-Care K40, P-Care K80, Pod-Care 100K, Pro-C-Dure 5, Pro-C-Dure 6, Zilretta), 318t
triamcinolone (Kenalog, Kenalog 80, P-Care K40, P-Care K80, Pod-Care 100K, Pro-C-Dure 5, Pro-C-Dure 6, Zilretta; Kenalog-10, Kenalog-40), 318t, 320t–323t
triamcinolone (Trianex, Triderm; Aristocort, Aristocort R, Oracort, Triaderm), 320t–323t
triamcinolone (topical) (Trianex, Triderm), 318t
triamcinolone acetonide (GoodSense Nasal Allergy Spray, Nasacort Allergy; Nasacort Allergy (all over thecounter; Apo-Triamcinolone AQ, Nasacort AQ), 318t, 320t–323t, 617
triamterene (Dyrenium), 482t, 496t–498t, 631t, 638t, 639–640, 641t
Trianex (triamcinolone), 320t–323t

triazene, 235, 236t–245t, 238
triazolam, 87b, 96b
trichomoniasis, 463–465, 464t
triclabendazole, 464t
Tricor (fenofibrate), 164t, 170–171, 170t, 171b
Tri-Cyclen, 110t–111t
Tri-Cyclen Lo, 110t–111t
tricyclic antidepressant(s), 950, 989, 1011–1013. See also specific drug
    derivatives, 989
Triderm (triamcinolone), 318t, 320t–323t
Tridural (Tramadol), 896t–897t
trifluridine, 417
triggers, 605
Triglide (fenofibrate), 164t, 170–171, 170t, 171b
triglyceride levels, 162t
trihexyphenidyl, 879t, 881t, 884
triiodothyronine, 783
Tri-Legest Fe, 110t–111t
Trilipix (fenofibrate), 164t, 170–171, 170t, 171b
trimethoprim, 365t, 370–371, 372t, 373
trimethoprim-sulfamethoxazole (TMP-SMZ, Bactrim, Septra, Apo-Sulfatrim), 77
trimethoprim–sulfamethoxazole (TMP-SMZ, Bactrim, Septra, Apo-Sulfatrim), 365t, 367, 369
Tri-Norinyl, 110t–111t
Triptodur (Triptorelin), 806t
triptorelin (Trelstar Mixject, Trelstar, Decapeptyl), 799t, 806t, 807
triptorelin (Trelstar, Trelstar Mixject, Decapeptyl), 236t–238t, 261t–263t, 264
Trivora-28, 110t–111t
trophozoites, 465
Trosec (trospium chloride), 887t
trospium chloride (Sanctura XR, Trosec), 879t, 881t, 887t, 888
Trousseau's sign, 817
Trulance (plecanatide), 724t, 731–732, 731t
Trulicity (dulaglutide), 754t, 775, 775t
Trumenba (meningococcal group B vaccine (MenB-fHBP)), 195t–199t
Truxima (rituximab), 211t, 226, 236t–238t, 252t–257t, 257
tuberculin, 48
tuberculosis
    active, 389
    adjuvant first-line antitubercular drugs, 399–400
    anti-TB drugs in pregnancy, 393, 394b, 396
    antitubercular drugs
        adjuvant first-line, 399–400, 399t
        special strategies to increase adherence to, 401
    assessment, 402b
    clinical considerations, 389–391
    clinical manifestations, 389–391
    drug therapy, 391–392, 391t–392t
    evaluation, 402b
    first-line drug combinations, 391
    guidelines, 390b
    isoniazid, 392–395, 393t, 394b, 395b
    latent tuberculosis infection, 391, 391t
    multidrug-resistant tuberculosis, 390–392, 400
    nursing interventions, 402b
    nursing process, 402b
    primary infection, 389
    rifamycins, 396–398, 397t, 398b
    second-line anti-TB drugs, 389–391, 400
    tests for, 390, 390b
    transmission, 389
tubular secretion, 79
tumor lysis syndrome, 247–249
tumor necrosis factor (TNF)-alpha, 210
    blocking agents, 222t–224t, 226–227
    description of, 226–227

tumor necrosis factor alpha–blocking agents, 211t, 226–227
tumor suppressor genes, 233
tums (calcium carbonate precipitated), 692t, 693, 694t
Turner syndrome, 801
two serogroup B meningococcal (MenB) vaccines, 194
two-ratio method, 44–45
twynsta, 495t–496t
Tygacil (tigecycline), 365t–366t, 368, 381t–382t, 385–386
Tykerb (lapatinib), 236t–238t, 248b, 252t–257t, 258
Tylenol (acetaminophen), 286, 288, 290, 290t, 294–297, 295t, 297b, 581–583, 583t
type 1 diabetes
    amylin analogs, 773, 773t
    insulin (see insulin)
    nursing process, 780b
type 2 diabetes
    amylin analogs, 773, 773t
    combination drug therapy for, 777–778
    dipeptidyl peptidase-4 inhibitors, 771–772
    enalapril maleate, 778
    glucagon-like peptide-1 receptor agonists (incretin mimetics), 774–776
    insulin (see insulin)
    nursing process, 780b
    risk factor, 751
    thiazolidinediones, 769

U

Uceris (budesonide), 318t
Udenyca (pegfilgrastim), 180t, 185–186, 185t
ulcerative colitis, 328
Uloric (febuxostat), 292t, 309–310, 309t
Ultane (Sevoflurane), 922t–923t, 925
Ultiva (remifentanil), 932
Ultram (Oxymorphone Tramadol), 894t, 896t–897t, 902t, 903
Unasyn (ampicillin-sulbactam), 335t–337t
Unclassified antidysrhythmic drugs, 507t, 517–518
Uni-MED (methylprednisolone), 320t–323t
Uniphyl (short-acting theophylline), 612t
units, 33
Unituxin (dinutuximab), 236t–238t, 252t–257t
Univasc (moexipril hydrochloride), 754t
upadacitinib (Rinvoq), 211t, 220t, 221
up-regulation, 848
Urecholine (bethanechol), 855t, 862–863
uricosuric agents, 290, 292t, 308–310, 309t
    abnormal kidney function and hepatic impairment, 308
    administration of, 308
    adverse effects, 308
    contraindications, 308
    mechanism of action, 308
    nursing implications, 308–309
    patient teaching guidelines, 309, 309b
    pharmacokinetics, 308
    preventing interactions, 308
    therapeutic effects, 308
urinary antiseptics, 365t
    nitrofurantoin, 372, 372t
    nursing process, 374b
    phenazopyridine, 372–373, 372t
    trimethoprim, 372t, 373
urinary tract infections (UTI), 79, 92
    drug therapy for
        nitrofurantoin, 372, 372t
        nursing process, 374b
        phenazopyridine, 372–373, 372t
        trimethoprim, 372t, 373
    during pregnancy, 92
Uroxatral (alfuzosin), 119t, 128t, 129
Urozide (hydrochlorothiazide), 631t, 635–637, 636t, 637b, 641t

ustekinumab (Stelara), 211t, 222t–224t, 227
uterine motility, drugs altering
　magnesium sulfate, 93, 93t
　nifedipine, 93, 93t
　nonsteroidal anti-inflammatory drugs, 92–93
　route and dosage information for, 92, 93t
　terbutaline sulfate, 93, 93t
uterotonics, 95

V

Vabomere (meropenem-vaborbactam), 335t, 347t
vaccines. *See also* immunizations
　definition, 193
　indications for, 195t–199t
　types of, 195t–199t
Vagifem (estradiol, micronized), 103t
vaginal candidiasis, 449, 453
vaginal creams, 42t–43t
vaginal suppositories, 42t–43t
vaginal trichomoniasis, 464
Vagistat-1 (tioconazole), 447t
valacyclovir (Valtrex), 417
valerian, 59t–61t
Valium (diazepam), 864t
valproate, 87b
valrubicin (Valstar), 236t–245t
valsartan (Diovan), 482t, 490t, 491, 494, 495t–496t
valsartan-HCT, 495t–496t
Valstar (valrubicin), 236t–245t
Vancocin (vancomycin), 381t–382t, 386
Vancocin HCl (vancomycin), 381t–382t
vancomycin (Firvanq, Vancocin, Vancocin HCl; JAMPVancomycin, PMS Vancomycin, Vancocin), 381t–382t, 386
Vancomycin-resistant enterococci (VRE), 278b, 381–382, 386
vancomycin-resistant *Enterococcus faecium* (VREF), 384
Vantas (histrelin), 799t, 806t, 807
Vaqta (hepatitis A vaccine), 194–203, 195t–199t
vardenafil (Levitra), 119t, 125
vardenafil (Levitra, Staxyn), 124t
varicella (VAR) (Varivax; Varilrix, Varivax III), 195t–199t
varicella vaccine, 203
varicella-zoster immune globulin (human) (VZIG) (VariZIG), 200t–201t
varicella-zoster virus, 415–417, 416t
Varilrix (varicella (VAR)), 195t–199t
Varivax (varicella (VAR)), 195t–199t
Varivax III (varicella (VAR)), 195t–199t
VariZIG (varicella-zoster immune globulin (human) (VZIG)), 200t–201t
Varubi (rolapitant), 708t, 715t, 717
Vascular stage of acute inflammation, 272, 273f
vaseretic, 495t–496t
vasoconstrictors, 484
vasodilators, 499–500
vasopressin (Vasostrict), 799t, 804t, 805
Vasostrict (vasopressin), 799t, 804t, 805
Vasotec (enalapril), 482t, 485t, 488, 495t–496t
Vasotec (enalapril maleate), 560–561, 562t, 778, 778t
Vaxneuvance (pneumococcal conjugate vaccine 15-valent (PCV 15)), 195t–199t
Vazculep (phenylephrine), 541–542, 543t, 547, 574t–575t, 582, 583t
Vectibix (panitumumab), 211t, 225, 236t–238t, 252t–257t, 257–258
Vecuronium, 922t, 929t
Velcade (bortezomib), 236t–238t, 252t–257t, 259–260
Velivet, 110t–111t
venipuncture, 45–46t, 46b, 56
venous thrombosis, 138
Ventolin (albuterol, Proventil, AccuNeb), 605t

Ventolin Discus (albuterol), 608t
Ventolin HFA (albuterol), 605t, 606, 608t
Ventolin I.V. infusion (albuterol), 605t, 608t
Ventolin Nebules P.F., 608t
ventricular fibrillation, 505b
ventricular remodeling, 563
ventricular tachycardia, 505b
VePesid (etoposide), 236t–245t, 239, 248b
verapamil (Calan SR, Verelan; Covera-HS, Verapamil Hydrochloride, Isoptin SR), 482t, 491, 492t, 493–494, 524t, 531–534, 532t
verapamil (Calan, Calan SR, Verelan), 512b, 516–517, 516t
Verelan (verapamil), 482t, 491, 492t, 493–494, 512b, 516–517, 516t, 524t, 531–534, 532t
Vermox (mebendazole), 464t, 469–470, 470t, 470b
Vesicare (solifenacin succinate), 887t
Vfend (voriconazole), 447t, 453–454
Viagra (sildenafil), 119t, 123, 124t
vials, 48
Vibativ (telavancin), 381t–382t, 385
Vibramycin (doxycycline), 365t–366t, 367–368
Vicks NyQuil Severe Cough, Cold & Flu LiquiCaps, 583t
Vicodin HP (hydrocodone), 896t–897t
vicoprofen (hydrocodone), 896t–897t
Victoza (liraglutide), 679t, 683–685, 683t, 754t, 775t
Vidaza (azacitidine), 236t–245t
vinblastine, 236t–245t, 239, 247, 248b
vinca alkaloids, 236t–245t, 239, 248b, 250
Vincasar PFS (vincristine sulfate), 236t–245t, 239
vincristine sulfate (Vincasar PFS), 236t–245t, 239
vinorelbine (Navelbine), 236t–245t, 239
viral hepatitis, 406b
viral infection(s), 406b
　administration, 408t–409t
　assessment, 442b
　clinical manifestations, 405
　drug therapy, 405
　evaluation, 442b
　nursing interventions, 442b
　nursing process, 442b
　outcomes of therapy, 442b
viral load, 406b
Viramune (nevirapine), 408t–409t, 434t, 435
Virazole (ribavirin), 408t–409t, 419–421, 420t
Viread (tenofovir disoproxil fumarate), 408t–409t, 426, 426t, 430t–431t, 432–433
viruses, 272–273
visceral pain, 892
Vistaril (hydroxyzine pamoate), 589–590, 590t–591t, 593, 708t, 710, 711t
vitamin(s)
　abnormal kidney function and hepatic impairment, 654
　deficiencies, 654t–656t
　fat-soluble, 645, 647t–650t, 654–658
　recommended daily intakes, 645, 646b
　upper intake levels, 645, 646b
　water-soluble, 645, 654t–656t, 658–661
vitamin A (retinol), 654t–656t
　administration, 656
　adverse effects, 656
　contraindications, 656
　drug interaction, 654t–656t
　nursing implications, 656
　patient teaching guidelines, 656, 657b
　pharmacokinetics and use, 654–656
　therapeutic effects, 656
vitamin B1 (thiamine), 654t–656t
　administration, 659
　adverse effects, 659
　contraindications, 659
　nursing implications, 659
　patient teaching guidelines for, 657b, 659

pharmacokinetics and use, 659
　therapeutic effects, 659
vitamin B2 (riboflavin), 654t–656t
vitamin B3 (niacin), 654t–656t
　administration, 659
　adverse effects, 659
　contraindications, 659
　nursing implications, 659
　patient teaching guidelines for, 657b, 659
　pharmacokinetics and use, 659
　therapeutic effects, 659
vitamin B5 (pantothenic acid), 647t–650t
vitamin B6 (pyridoxine), 654t–656t
　administration, 659
　adverse effects, 659
　contraindications, 659
　nursing implications, 659
　patient teaching guidelines for, 657b, 659
　pharmacokinetics and use, 659
　therapeutic effects, 659
vitamin B12 (cyanocobalamin), 654t–656t
　administration, 660
　adverse effects, 660
　contraindications, 660
　nursing implications, 660
　patient teaching guidelines, 657b, 660
　pharmacokinetics, 659–660
　therapeutic effects, 660
　use, 660
vitamin C (ascorbic acid), 654t–656t
　administration, 661
　adverse effects, 661
　contraindications, 661
　nursing implications, 661
　patient teaching guidelines, 657b, 661
　pharmacokinetics, 660
　therapeutic effects, 661
　use, 660–661
vitamin D2, 816t
vitamin D3, 816t
vitamin D (calciferol), 818–820
vitamin E, 654t–656t
　administration, 658
　adverse effects, 658
　contraindications, 658
　nursing implications, 658
　patient teaching guidelines, 657b, 658
　pharmacokinetics and use, 656
　preventing interactions, 658
　therapeutic effects, 658
vitamin K (Mephyton), 140t, 158t
vitamin K (phytonadione)
　administration, 658
　adverse effects and contraindications, 658
　antagonists
　　reversal of, 157
　　warfarin (*see* Apo-Warfarin, Coumadin, Taro-Warfarin); warfarin (Coumadin, Jantoven)
　nursing implications, 658
　patient teaching guidelines, 657b, 658
　pharmacokinetics and use, 658
　preventing interactions, 658
　routes and dosage ranges, 654t–656t
　therapeutic effects, 658
Vivelle-Dot EstroGel (estradiol transdermal system), 103t
vivitrol (naltrexone), 894t, 907, 907t
Voltaren XR (diclofenac potassium), 290t, 302t–303t
vomiting center, 717, 720f
Vonjo (pacritinib), 211t, 221
vorapaxar (Zontivity), 140t, 148–149, 151t–152t
voriconazole (Vfend), 447t, 453–454
Votrient (pazopanib), 236t–238t, 252t–257t, 258–259

VPI-Amikacin (amikacin), 353–354, 353t, 355t, 357
vulvovaginal candidiasis, 445
Vumon (teniposide), 236t–238t
Vyvgart (Efgartigimod alfa), 857

W

warfarin (Coumadin, Jantoven; Apo-Warfarin, Coumadin, Taro-Warfarin), 87b, 140t–142t, 144
   administration, 145
   adverse effects, 145
   contraindications, 145
   dosage information, 141t–142t, 144
   drug interactions, 145, 146b
   mechanism of action, 144–145
   nursing implications, 145–146
   patient teaching guidelines, 144b, 146
   patients with hepatic impairment, 145
   pharmacokinetics, 144
   preventing interactions, 146b
   reproduction, pregnancy, and lactation, 145
   therapeutic effects, 145
water-soluble vitamins, 645, 658–661
   vitamin B_{12} and folic acid, 659–660
   vitamin B complex, 658–659
   vitamin C, 660–661
wearing off, 874
weight loss
   orlistat for, 21, 679t, 681–683, 682t
   patient teaching guidelines, 681b
   phentermine hydrochloride for, 679t
   sibutramine for, 678–679
weight management
   amphetamines, 685
   bupropion, 685
   bupropion–naltrexone, 685, 685t
   drug administration, 679t
   herbal and dietary supplements, 685–686, 685b
   metformin for, 675b
   monoamine oxidase inhibitors, 680, 685
   naltrexone, 685
   sibutramine for, 678–679
Welchol (colesevelam), 164t, 169t, 170
whipworm infections, 469
Winpred (prednisone), 317, 318t, 320t–323t, 324–326, 328–329
WinRho SDF ($Rh_o(D)$ immune globulin (human)), 200t–201t
work-exacerbated asthma (WEA), 602

X

Xadago (safinamide), 871t–872t
Xanax (alprazolam), 101
xanthines, 612–614
   abnormal kidney function, 613
   action, 612
   administration of, 613
   adverse effects, 613
   contraindications, 613
   dosage ranges, 612t
   drug interactions, 613b
   drugs, 612t
   in hepatic impairment patients, 613
   nursing implications, 613–614
   patient teaching guidelines, 614
   pharmacokinetics, 612
   preventing interactions, 613
   therapeutic effects, 613
   use, 612–613
Xarelto (rivaroxaban), 141t–142t, 148
Xatmep (methotrexate), 211t, 212, 215b, 216, 226–227, 236t–245t, 238, 246–247, 248b, 251b
Xatral (alfuzosin), 119t, 128t, 129
Xeljanz (tofacitinib), 211t, 221
Xeljanz XR (tofacitinib), 211t, 221
Xeloda (capecitabine), 236t–245t
Xembify (immune globulin (human) (IG; IGIM)), 200t–201t
Xenical (orlistat), 21, 679t, 681–683, 682t
Xerava (eravacycline), 365t–366t, 368
Xgeva (denosumab), 823, 823t
Xhance (fluticasone), 616t
Xifaxan (rifaximin), 381t–382t, 385, 738t, 741t, 742
Ximino (minocycline hydrochloride), 365
Xofluza (baloxavir marboxil), 412b, 422t, 424–425
Xolair (omalizumab), 211t, 226, 605t, 619–620, 619t
Xopenex (levalbuterol), 605t, 608t, 610
Xopenex Concentrate (levalbuterol), 605t, 608t, 610
Xopenex HFA (levalbuterol), 605t, 608t
Xtampza ER (Oxycodone), 894t, 896t–897t, 902–903, 902t
Xtandi (enzalutamide), 236t–238t, 260–263, 261t–263t
Xylocaine (lidocaine), 508t, 510, 518
Xylocard (lidocaine), 508t, 510, 518
Xylon (hydrocodone), 896t–897t
Xyosted (testosterone enanthate), 120t
Xyzal Allergy 24HR (levocetirizine), 590t, 596–597, 596t

Y

Yasmin, 110t–111t
Yaz, 110t–111t
Yaz Plus, 110t–111t
yeasts, 445
Yervoy (ipilimumab), 211t, 225–226, 236t–238t, 252t–257t, 257
Yonsa (abiraterone), 236t–238t, 260–263, 261t–263t

Z

zafirlukast (Accolate), 619, 605t, 618t
Zamine, 110t–111t
Zanosar (streptozocin), 236t–245t
Zarah, 110t–111t
Zaroxolyn (metolazone), 482t, 631t, 636t, 637
Zarxio (filgrastim), 184–186, 185t, 236t–238t, 248b, 264t
Zaxine (rifaximin), 381t–382t
ZCort 7 Day (dexamethasone), 318t, 320t–323t, 324–325, 328–329
Zelapar (selegiline), 869t, 875
Zelnorm (tegaserod), 724t, 732t, 733
Zemdri (plazomicin), 353t, 355t, 357
Zemplar (paricalcitol), 816t
Zenhale (mometasone/formoterol), 605t, 616t, 617, 621t
Zerbaxa (ceftolozane-tazobactam), 335t, 342t–344t, 346
zestoretic, 495t–496t
Zestril (lisinopril), 482t, 485t, 488, 495t–496t, 754t
Zetia (ezetimibe), 21, 163–164, 164t, 171–173, 172t, 172b
Zevalin (ibritumomab tiuxetan), 236t–238t, 252t–257t, 257–258
ziac, 495t–496t
zidovudine (Retrovir), 412b, 429–433, 432b
Ziextenzo (pegfilgrastim), 180t, 185–186, 185t
Zilactin Baby (benzocaine), 912t, 916t
zileuton (Zyflo, Zyflo CR), 619, 605t, 618t
Zilretta (triamcinolone), 318t, 320t–323t
Zimhi (naloxone), 894t, 906, 907t
Zinacef (cefuroxime), 342t–344t
zinc sulfate and zinc gluconate, 667
Zinecard (dexrazoxane), 236t–238t, 264t
Zipsor (diclofenac potassium), 290t, 302t–303t
Zirabev (bevacizumab), 211t, 225, 236t–238t, 252t–257t, 257–258
Zithromax (azithromycin), 378t
Zithromax Tri-Pak (azithromycin), 378t
Zocor (simvastatin), 164t, 166t, 167, 754t, 778t, 779
Zofran (ondansetron), 708t, 712, 714t
Zoladex (goserelin), 236t–238t, 261t–263t, 263–264, 799t, 806t, 807
zoledronic acid, 87b
zoledronic acid (Reclast, Zometa; Aclasta, TAROZoledronic Acid), 820t–821t
Zollinger-Ellison syndrome, 696, 696t, 698–699
zonisamide, 96b
Zontivity (vorapaxar), 148–149, 151t–152t
Zortress (everolimus), 211t, 219, 236t–238t, 252t–257t, 258
Zorvolex (diclofenac potassium), 290t, 302t–303t
Zosyn (piperacillin/tazobactam), 335t–337t
Zovia 1/35E, 110t–111t
Zovirax (acyclovir), 415–417, 416t
Zubsolv (buprenorphine/naloxone), 904t
Zyflo (zileuton), 605t, 618t, 619
Zyflo CR (zileuton), 605t, 618t, 619
Zykadia (ceritinib), 236t–238t, 252t–257t, 258
Zyloprim (allopurinol), 292t, 308–310, 309t, 309b
Zypitamag (pitavastatin), 164t, 166t
Zyrtec Allergy (cetirizine), 590t, 594–597, 595t
Zytiga (abiraterone), 236t–238t, 260–263, 261t–263t
Zytram XL (Tramadol), 896t–897t
Zyvox (linezolid), 381t–382t, 384
Zyvoxam (linezolid), 381t–382t